DUNHAM PUBLIC LIBRARY
WHITESBORO, NY 13492

CASTLE CONNOLLY
TOP DOCTORS
New York Metro Area
10th Edition

America's Trusted Source For
Identifying Top Doctors

S0-DTC-709

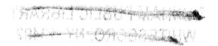

All Rights Reserved

Copyright © 2006, by Castle Connolly Medical Ltd.

The selection of medical providers for inclusion in this book was based in part on opinions solicited from physicians, nurses, and other healthcare professionals. The author and publishers cannot assure the accuracy of information provided to them by third parties, since such opinions are necessarily subjective and may be incomplete. The omission from this book of particular healthcare providers does not mean that such providers are not competent or reputable.

The purpose of this book is educational and informational. It is not intended to replace the advice of your physician or to assist the layman in diagnosing or treating illness, disease, or injury. Following the advice or recommendations set forth in this book is entirely at the reader's own risk. The author and publishers cannot ensure accuracy of, or assume responsibility for, the information in the book as such information is affected by constant change. Liability to any person or organization for any loss or damage caused by errors or omissions in this book is hereby disclaimed. Whenever possible, readers should consult their own primary care physician when selecting healthcare providers, including any selection based upon information contained in this book. In order to protect patient privacy, the names of patients cited in anecdotes throughout the book have been omitted.

Reproduction in whole or part, or storage in any data retrieval system and reproduction therefrom, is strictly prohibited and violates federal copyright and trademark laws. The contents of this book are intended for the personal use of the buyer. Use for any commercial purpose is strictly prohibited and will be pursued vigorously.

The confidence of our readers in our editorial integrity is crucial to the success of the Castle Connolly Guides. Any use of the Castle Connolly name, or of any list or listing (or portion of either) from any Castle Connolly Guide, for advertising or for any commercial purpose, without prior written consent, is strictly prohibited and may result in legal action.

For more information, please contact:

Castle Connolly Medical Ltd., 42 West 24th St, New York, New York 10010
212-367-8400x10
E-mail: info@castleconnolly.com
Web site: http://www.castleconnolly.com.

Library of Congress Control Number: 2006925013
ISBN   1-883769-20-5;   978-1-883769-20-8   (paperback)
ISBN   1-883769-21-3;   978-1-883769-21-5   (hardcover)
Printed in the United States of America

Table of Contents

DUNHAM PUBLIC LIBRAR
WHITESBORO, NY 13492

Table of Contents

Table of Contents

Table of Contents

Table of Contents

Table of Contents

Hippocratic Oath

I swear by Apollo the physician, and Asklepios, and health, and All-Heal and all the gods and goddesses, that, according to my ability and judgement, I will keep this Oath and this stipulation — to reckon him who taught me this Art equally dear to me as my parents, to share my substance with him, and relieve his necessities if required; to look upon his offspring in the same footing as my own brothers, and to teach them this Art, if they should wish to learn it, without fee or stipulation; and that by precept, lecture and every other mode of instruction, I will impart a knowledge of the Art to my own sons, and those of my teachers, and to disciples bound by a stipulation and oath according to the law of medicine, but to none others.

I will follow that system of regimen which, according to my ability and judgement, I consider for the benefit of my patients, and abstain from whatever is deleterious and mischievous. I will give no deadly medicine to anyone if asked nor suggest any such counsel; and in like manner I will not give to a woman a pessary to produce abortion. With purity and wholeness I will pass my life and practice my Art.

I will not cut persons labouring under the stone, but will leave this to be done by men who are practitioners of this work. Into whatever houses I enter, I will go into them for the benefit of the sick, and will abstain from every voluntary act of mischief and corruption; and, further, from the seduction of females or males, of freemen and slaves. Whatever, in connection with my professional practice, or not in connection with it, I see or hear, in the life of men, which ought not to be spoken of abroad, I will not divulge, as reckoning that all such should be kept secret. While I continue to keep this Oath unviolated, may it be granted to me to enjoy life and the practice of the art, respected by all men, in all times! But should I trespass and violate this Oath, may the reverse be my lot!

from *Dorland's Illustrated Medical Dictionary.* 27th ed. (Philadelphia) W.B. Saunders Co., 1988. Hippocratic Oath. [Hippocrates. Greek physician, 460-377 B.C.]

About the Publishers

John K. Castle has spent much of the last three decades involved with healthcare institutions and issues. Mr. Castle served as Chairman of the Board of New York Medical College for eleven years, an institution where he served on the Board of Trustees for twenty-two years.

Mr. Castle has been extensively involved in other healthcare and voluntary activities as well. He served for five years as a public commissioner on the Joint Commission on Accreditation of Healthcare Organizations (JCAHO), the body which accredits most public and private hospitals throughout the United States. Mr. Castle has also served as a trustee of five different hospitals in the metropolitan New York region, including NewYork-Presbyterian Hospital, where he continues to serve.

Mr. Castle is also the Chairman of the Columbia Presbyterian Science Advisory Council and a Director of the Whitehead Institute for Biomedical Research. He is a Fellow of New York Academy of Medicine and has served as a Trustee of the Academy. He is Chairman of the United Hospital Fund of New York's Capital Campaign. He continues as Director Emeritus of the United Hospital Fund. He is a Life Member of the MIT Corporation, the governing body of the Massachusetts Institute of Technology.

Mr. Castle is the Chairman of Castle Connolly Medical Ltd. and affiliated companies which publish and co-publish *Castle Connolly America's Top Doctors™ 6th Edition*; *Castle Connolly **Top Doctors: New York Metro Area 10th Edition*** and other books to help people find the best healthcare. Castle Connolly Healthcare Navigation LTD is a company that assists individuals and families obtain the best healthcare from the U.S.'s excellent, but often confusing, healthcare system.

John J. Connolly, Ed.D. is the President & CEO of Castle Connolly Medical Ltd., and is the nation's foremost authority on identifying top physicians. Dr. Connolly's experience in healthcare is extensive.

For more than a decade he served as President of New York Medical College, the nation's second largest private medical college. He is a Fellow of the New York Academy of Medicine, a Fellow of the New York Academy of Sciences, a Director of the New York Business Group on Health, a member of the President's Council of the United Hospital Fund, and a member of the Board of Advisors of Funding First, a Lasker Foundation initiative. Dr. Connolly has served as a trustee of two hospitals and as Chairman of the Board of one. He is extensively involved in healthcare and community activities and has served on a number of voluntary and corporate boards including the Board of the American Lyme Disease Foundation, of which he is a founder and past chairman, and the Board of Advisors of the Whitehead Institute for Biomedical Research. He is also a Director and Chairman of the Professional Examination Service. He holds a Bachelor of Science degree from Worcester State College, a Master's degree from the University of Connecticut, and a Doctor of Education degree in College and University Administration from Teacher's College, Columbia University.

Dr. Connolly has appeared on or been interviewed by over 100 television and radio stations nationwide including *The Today Show* (NBC-TV), *Good Morning America* (ABC-TV), *20/20* (ABC-TV), *48 Hours* (CBS-TV), *Fox Cable News* (national), *Morning News* (CNN) and *Weekend Today in New York* (WNBC-TV). *The New York Times*, the *Chicago Tribune*, the *Daily News* (New York), the *Boston Herald* and other newspapers, as well as many national and regional magazines, have featured Castle Connolly Guides and/or Dr. Connolly in stories. He is the author and/or editor of eight books, all written to help families and individuals find the best healthcare.

Medical Advisory Board

Castle Connolly Medical Ltd. is pleased to have associated with a distinguished group of medical leaders who offer invaluable advice and wisdom in our efforts to assist consumers in making good healthcare choices. We thank each member of the Medical Advisory Board for their valuable contributions.

Charles Bechert, M.D.
> The Sight Foundation

Roger Bulger, M.D.
> National Institutes of Health

Harry J. Buncke, M.D.
> California Pacific Medical Center

Joseph Cimino, M.D.
> Professor and Chairman, Community and Preventative Medicine,
> New York Medical College

Menard M. Gertler, M.D., D.Sc.
> Clinical Professor of Medicine
> Cornell University Medical School

Leo Henikoff, M.D.
> President and CEO (retired)
> Rush Presbyterian-St. Luke's Medical Center

Yutaka Kikkawa, M.D.
> Professor and Chairman Emeritus
> Department of Pathology, University of California,
> Irvine College of Health Sciences

David Paige, M.D.
> Professor
> Bloomberg School of Public Health,
> Johns Hopkins University

Ronald Pion, M.D.
> Chairman and CEO
> Medical Telecommunications Associates

Richard L. Reece, M.D.
> Editor
> *Physician Practice Options*

Leon G. Smith, M.D.
> Chairman of Medicine
> St. Michael's Medical Center, NJ

Helen Smits, M.D.
> Former Deputy Director
> Healthcare Financing Administration (HCFA)

Ralph Snyderman, M.D.
> Chairman Emeritus
> Duke University Health System

Foreword

Dear Reader:

Choosing a doctor is one of the most important choices in your life. However, most of us put little effort into this selection. We simply pick a name from a list or get a recommendation from a friend.

Most of us have very little information about our doctors, and/or don't know where to get it. Now with the publication of this Castle Connolly Guide—*Top Doctors: New York Metro Area*, you can learn about doctors' medical school education, residency training, fellowships, board certifications, hospital appointments and much more. The Guide also describes in simple terms what information you should ascertain about each doctor and how to evaluate it. This information gathering is essential for anyone who wants to find a good doctor to truly meet his or her healthcare needs.

As an administrator and nurse who deals with the problems of health on a daily basis, I know well the importance of getting the best healthcare. Our center assists medical malpractice victims. The human tragedy we often encounter is heartbreaking.

In many cases, had the patient taken a few minutes to make a modest effort to learn more about his or her doctor's background, a serious incident may have been avoided.

That is why *Top Doctors: New York Metro Area* is so important to consumers. In this new and rapidly changing healthcare environment, patients must be well informed. Many do not trust the healthcare system. They are not confident their HMO, their hospital, or even their doctor, is motivated to protect them and to ensure that they get excellent care.

The Castle Connolly Guide is a comprehensive guide chock full of valuable information. It is completely consumer-friendly, giving readers all they need to know to make intelligent, informed choices.

Use it well and in good health!

Sincerely,

Sandra Gainer, R.N.
Associate Director
National Center for Patient Rights

Introduction

A savvy consumer, searching for a car, restaurant, house or even a spouse, can easily find a guidebook to help. Yet, when it comes to choosing healthcare providers, the bookshelves are nearly bare.

Top Doctors has been written to fill that void. It will guide you in making critical —even lifesaving—choices.

This Guide Has Two Goals:

- To provide you with a base of information and a framework of understanding so that you can participate in the important healthcare choices that will maximize your own health, your family's health and the quality of your life.

- To provide detailed information on more than 6,000 well-trained, highly competent physicians from which you may confidently choose your personal best doctors for your own healthcare needs and those of your family.

Medicine is often described as a combination of art and science. This description holds true for the process of selecting the best medical care. This book describes the "science" of making that selection. It is not magical or even difficult. It is simply a matter of knowing what information you should have and where to find it.

The "art" is what you will bring to the selection process. It is based upon your feelings, your needs and the chemistry that develops between you and those who provide your healthcare. Castle Connolly *Top Doctors: New York Metro Area* will help you prepare for that interaction and will guide you in getting the most from it.

Most importantly, Castle Connolly *Top Doctors: New York Metro Area* will tell you how to combine the art and science so that you can make the best choices.

How to Use This Guide

This book has been written as a basic, "how to" guide for selecting the best healthcare. Section One provides important information on how to choose the best doctors. Doctors are the most important providers of healthcare and whether you are part of an HMO or covered by traditional medical insurance, you want the very best doctors to attend to your healthcare needs. Section Three contains listings of doctors as well as information on hospitals invited to participate in the Guide's *Partnership for Excellence* program. Section Four includes information on "Centers of Excellence"—special programs and services—offered by a number of the hospitals participating in the *Partnership for Excellence* program. Section Five contains seven appendices with important and interesting information.

Introduction

There Are Two Effective Ways to Use This Guide:

- Start at the beginning. This method will give you a broad understanding of the healthcare field and a clearer perspective of where you, the patient, fit in it. This method will arm you with necessary information for making informed choices and will help you find the best doctors.

- Study the doctor listings. While at least a brief reading of some or all of the introductory chapters is recommended so that, in the end, you will make well-informed choices, it is understandable that you may wish to go straight to the physician listings. The organization of these listings is outlined on pages 71 to 84. You will find guidelines for effectively using the listings on these pages.

Each chapter begins with explanations of terms that may be new to you. Reviewing these terms will help you read the section more easily.

In preparing this book, we've left little to chance or question. We hope to inspire you to assume a curious and insistent attitude as you make the healthcare choices that will take you and your family through life.

Section One

The Doctor of Choice

Chapter 1

Primary Care Physicians

Key Terms: Chapter 1

LUPUS ERYTHEMATOSUS

An autoimmune disorder, also referred to as SLE, or simply "lupus." It can cause inflammation and possible damage to a number of vital organs and is commonly marked by joint pain, facial and other rashes, abnormally high antibody levels, and diminished red blood cell levels.

LYME DISEASE

An infectious disease, transmitted through the bite of a deer tick, which may or may not produce a distinctive bull's-eye rash at the site of the tick bite. First identified in Lyme, Connecticut, the infection may also produce other symptoms, including flu-like aches, arthritic joint pain, and, in complicated cases, cardiac abnormalities.

MANAGED CARE

The process of integrating the finance and delivery of healthcare to control costs and improve quality. A managed care plan typically involves a group of practitioners who "manage" care for a specified population.

OSTEOPATH

A healthcare professional who has earned a degree in osteopathic medicine, a D.O. Osteopathic Medicine emphasizes massage and bone manipulation while traditional Western Allopathic Medicine emphasizes treatment with drugs and surgery.

PREVENTIVE MEDICINE/CARE

Health services that are aimed at maintaining good health and preventing illness. These services include routine physical examinations, immunizations, certain screening tests such as mammograms or Pap tests, as well as the practice of good health habits.

PRIMARY CARE PHYSICIAN

The first doctor consulted for any health problem, a primary care physician is a specialist who offers basic, including preventive, medical care. It is important to maintain an ongoing relationship with your primary care physician.

SPECIALIST

A physician who practices in one or more of the 25 specialties defined by the American Board of Medical Specialties (ABMS). The term is also used to denote a physician's area of practice, such as pediatrics, geriatrics, surgery, etc.

SUBSPECIALIST

A specialist who obtains further training and certification in one or more of the 70 subspecialties approved by the American Board of Medical Specialties.

Quick Tips

1. The time to establish a relationship with a doctor is *while you are healthy*. The Top Doctor to establish your relationship with is the one who is most likely to keep you healthy: a primary care doctor.

2. Primary means first, so a primary care doctor is the first one you see for most health problems.

3. It is difficult for any doctor, however skilled, to make judgments based on only one visit or a single test.

4. Your primary care doctor can educate you about the hows and whys of health maintenance and disease prevention and follow up to help you stay faithful to the course the two of you have agreed upon.

Quick Take

…Primary care physician. That's a hot term in healthcare today. Who is this physician? And how do you find one?…

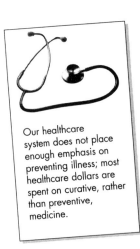

Our healthcare system does not place enough emphasis on preventing illness; most healthcare dollars are spent on curative, rather than preventive, medicine.

Chapter 1
Primary Care Physicians

When it comes to choosing a doctor, too many people let the decision slide until they are sick or hurt and need medical attention fast. That's unfortunate if an illness that could have been managed successfully develops to a stage where it becomes difficult to control or cure. It's even more unfortunate if the illness could have been prevented in the first place.

The time to establish a relationship with a doctor is *while you are healthy*, and the best one to establish your relationship with is the one who is most likely to keep you healthy: a primary care doctor.

Primary means "first", so a primary care doctor is the first one you see for any health problem. Primary also means "basic", so a primary care doctor offers the kind of fundamental care that can keep you healthy.

Yes, You Do Need a Doctor When You're Healthy

Here are four good reasons why you should start your search for a primary care doctor now:

Reason One

A primary care doctor can put your current medical condition into context consisting of your medical history, current condition as compared with past medical status, and changes in your body and environment over time. It is difficult for any doctor, however skilled, to make informed medical judgments based on only one visit or a single test. Conditions well out of normal range are easy to pick up, but extreme variations do not always occur, and a serious illness may develop slowly with only a gradual increase in symptoms. The operative word is continuity: ideally, your medical care should not be interrupted by changes in providers.

Reason Two

A primary care doctor is better able to treat you as a whole person. Medicine has become very specialized and procedure-oriented, but the human body is not a loose collection of unrelated parts. It is a "whole" with strong interrelationships among all biological systems. Some of the poorest medical care results from people jumping from subspecialist to subspecialist. Despite talent, skill and training, no specialist knows the patient well enough, or for long enough, to be able to take the whole person into consideration and track the normal patterns of evolution and change. We end up with a specialist for every organ and system instead of a doctor who will care for the whole person.

Reason Three

A primary care doctor can establish preventive programs. Our healthcare system does not place enough emphasis on preventing illness; most healthcare dollars are spent on curative, rather than preventive, medicine. However, the status quo is slowly changing, and it is within primary care that the change is most evident. Your primary care doctor can educate you about the hows and whys of health maintenance and disease prevention and can follow up to help you stay faithful to the course the two of you have agreed upon. Only an ongoing relationship makes this possible.

Reason Four

A primary care doctor can save you money. Managed care advocates, among others, have long deplored the waste inherent in a system in which patients can simply call any specialist any time they have an ache or pain or are not feeling well. Primary care doctors can monitor referrals to specialists, following the patient closely to put together a variety of observations, opinions, and test results in order to treat each person on an individual basis. This improves the quality of care and also controls costs.

A businessman in his late fifties, a long-time competitive runner, had surgery in one of New York's top hospitals to repair a badly torn Achilles tendon. At his first follow-up visit to the orthopaedic surgeon, he was assured that "everything was healing perfectly," that he had nothing to be concerned about, and that he would soon be up and running again. Shortly thereafter, just before a summer camping trip, he decided to have his yearly physical examination. The primary care doctor examined the site of the surgery, probing up and down the whole length of the leg. Explaining that he was concerned about certain swelling and discoloration, the doctor arranged for a further examination with ultrasound imaging. This sophisticated test showed that a blood clot had formed in the upper part of the leg, which could have caused severe disability and even death had it gotten into the bloodstream and traveled to the heart or brain. It was the primary care doctor, who knew the patient well, who discovered the potentially fatal condition while carefully conducting a full physical exam.

Patients who visit specialists without some guidance from a primary care doctor may choose the wrong specialist based on a general observation and self-diagnosis about the problem or illness they're experiencing. While in some cases the problem may be obvious (for example, an eye injury), in others it may be more subtle. Diseases such as lupus erythematosus and Lyme disease, for example, often have myriad symptoms that are easily misinterpreted by laypersons; in fact, they are often difficult even for doctors to diagnose accurately. While certain problems may require the collaboration of several specialists, it is important to have a primary care doctor navigating the course.

Finally, it is estimated that almost half of all emergency room visits in some areas are for non-emergencies; it's the most expensive place to receive primary care. When people have primary care doctors, they tend to turn to them rather than to hospital emergency departments.

If you are enrolled in any kind of managed care program, health maintenance organization (HMO) or other, you will almost always be required to select a primary care doctor from its roster. Managed care executives recognize the necessity of a primary care doctor, not only for delivering quality healthcare, but also for controlling costs.

1. How to Find a Doctor

Unless you already have a primary care doctor you are satisfied with, you will have to find one. How? Here are five possible avenues to *begin* the process of finding the doctor that best suits your needs; each has limits, however.

2. Doctor Referrals

If you are moving and are leaving a trusted doctor behind, get a recommendation or two before you go. Furthermore, ask in what context and how well your doctor knows the new doctor—they may not have met since medical school.

3. Friends and Relatives

Always keep in mind that such recommendations are based largely on what may be "simpatico," or a personal affinity. Ask *why* your friend likes the doctor. It might be because the fees are low or the doctor makes house calls or is warm and sociable—all valid considerations, but certainly not principal determinants. So be wary of the generalized recommendation that "Dr. Jones is just wonderful." When considering recommendations, use the old navigational technique of triangulation: focus on doctors whose names are mentioned by three or more people.

4. Hospital Referral Services

Hospital telephone referral lines are not designed to distinguish among hundreds of doctors who may be more or less well regarded by other doctors, or who may be better suited to a particular caller when factors other than location, insurance coverage and office hours are taken into consideration. It would be impolitic for hospital referral services to rate their doctors. Their recommendations are based on specialty and geographic proximity, usually by way of a computer that rotates through the lists to "recommend" the next three names in line, and all members of the medical staff are eligible to participate.

Quick Tips

5. Any doctor with a license can practice in any specialty he/she chooses. Board certification is your assurance that the doctor has appropriate training in the specialty.

6. When considering recommendations, use the old navigational technique of triangulation: focus on doctors whose names are mentioned by three or more people.

7. Hospital telephone referral lines are not designed to distinguish among hundreds of doctors who may be more or less well regarded by other doctors, or who may be better suited to a particular caller when factors other than location, insurance coverage and office hours are taken into consideration.

8. Many local medical societies publish directories, some of which are intended primarily for doctor-to-doctor referrals, while others are distributed to the public. They provide information but do not address quality.

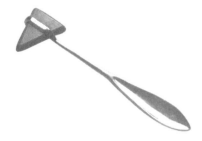

One woman—a long-time city resident who moved to the suburbs to be near her children—found out the hard way about advice when she selected a doctor on the basis of her neighbor's glowing praise. During the initial visit, the patient's numerous questions about her chronic arthritis condition went unanswered while the doctor merely patted her on the shoulder and assured her that he would "take care of everything." While this paternalistic attitude might have suited the neighbor's needs, it fell far short for this senior patient, who was used to a good give-and-take with her former internist. She resumed her search for a doctor—this time with the assistance of the Castle Connolly Guide, a more reliable source than a friend's recommendation.

5. Medical Society Directories

Many local medical societies publish directories, some of which are intended primarily for doctor-to-doctor referrals, while others are distributed to the public. These directories usually provide names, addresses, phone numbers and specialties and can be useful sources. However, they do not distinguish among doctors in any way. All members of the medical society, usually a countywide organization, are eligible for inclusion. This also applies to the referral lines offered by many medical societies.

Advertising

Responding to advertising is the least effective way to find a doctor. While more and more health professionals now advertise, a practice which is no longer considered unethical, some stigma still remains. Advertising could lead you to a doctor who receives few or no referrals from colleagues and whose orientation to the profession is more entrepreneurial than medical. Most referral lines not sponsored by hospitals charge a fee to doctors who want to be listed. This is simply another form of advertising.

Many Ways to Say Doctor

In this guide, the term "doctor" is used to describe only medical doctors who have received a Doctor of Medicine degree (MD) and osteopaths who have received a Doctor of Osteopathic Medicine degree (DO). Doctors who have been trained in the British system may hold a degree of Bachelor of Medicine (MB), Bachelor of Surgery (BS), or Bachelor of Chirurgia (BCh), which is based on the ancient Greek term that refers to surgery.

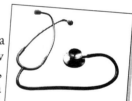

A recent poll of consumers sponsored by the American Medical Association (AMA) concluded that approximately 70 percent of those who responded agreed with the statement that "people are beginning to lose faith in their doctors," and that 69 percent of respondents agreed that doctors "are too interested in making money."

The more formal term for any of these practitioners is "physician." However, most people use the more popular term "doctor," which is the one generally used in this book. Our discussions do not include other kinds of doctors such as dentists, podiatrists, psychologists or chiropractors, who also deliver healthcare.

Primary Care: The Fundamental Four

There is not complete agreement in medicine on which specialties are practiced by the group of doctors known as primary care specialists. For the purposes of this book, we have included the following specialties: Internal Medicine, Pediatrics, Family Practice, and Obstetrics and Gynecology. Most adults choose general internists as their primary care doctors and select pediatricians for their children. There is also another type of specialist, the family practitioner, who cares for both children and adults. In addition to such generalists, many women also select obstetrician/gynecologists as primary care providers.

- A **general internist**, specializing in internal medicine, is trained to treat all internal organs and systems of the body. Many internists also are board certified in a subspecialty such as cardiology, gastroenterology or geriatric medicine. Therefore, if you have a history of heart disease, you may wish to select an internist who has additional training in cardiology, but who primarily practices general internal medicine. On the other hand, your primary care doctor may refer you to a cardiologist when necessary, and both may treat you over a period of years. In fact, it is not unusual for a patient with a serious or complex illness to be followed by two or three doctors, with the primary care doctor "quarterbacking" the team.

- A **family practitioner** is very broadly trained. Such doctors come closest to the general practitioner of the past. They are qualified to treat all family members, including children.

- A **pediatrician** is the doctor you would choose for the care of your children. As with doctors in internal medicine, pediatricians often have a subspecialty such as cardiology, rheumatology or endocrinology.

- **Obstetricians** and **Gynecologists** are the subject of significant debate in terms of their appropriateness as primary care doctors. The American Board of Obstetrics and Gynecology states that these doctors are specialists and are not generally trained for primary care. However, the reality is that many, particularly those who solely practice gynecology, often serve as a woman's primary care doctor. Gynecologists are divided on the issue. One recent study showed that 95 percent of visits to ob/gyns are self-referred and that about 60 percent of visits to these specialists are for diagnostic services and preventive services. Another study, by the American College of Obstetricians and Gynecologists, showed that 54 percent of women who see a gynecologist use these doctors for primary care. Reflecting the reality of current medical practice, we have included these specialists in the primary care category.

Chapter 2

What Makes a "Top Doctor?"

Key Terms: Chapter 2

ACADEMIC MEDICAL CENTER

A large medical complex that centers around a teaching hospital in which residency and fellowship programs are offered, where the medical school faculty practices full time, and where major clinical research activities occur.

BOARD CERTIFIED

Term signifying that a doctor is qualified for specialization by one of the American Board of Medical Specialties (ABMS) boards. Qualification includes completing an approved residency and passing a rigid exam.

BOARD ELIGIBLE

Term signifying that a doctor has completed an approved residency but has not yet taken the exam given by one of the ABMS recognized boards. The term conveys no official status in the eyes of the ABMS.

CLINICAL

Medical care that involves direct contact with patients.

CREDENTIALING

A process of screening conducted by hospitals by means of which they review the training and licenses of doctors applying to practice on their medical staffs.

INDEMNITY

A form of health insurance coverage that pays for healthcare but permits the patients to select their provider. Until 1990, indemnity insurance covered most insured people in the United States.

LICENSURE

Official credentials by individual states that permit a doctor to practice medicine in that state. In some states, doctors may be licensed with no more than one year of post-graduate training.

RESIDENCY

A training period spent in a hospital by a graduate of a medical school before going into practice. Residents have earned a medical degree and, therefore, are doctors but must complete an approved residency and pass an exam to become board certified.

TERTIARY CARE

Medical services provided by a hospital or medical center that include complex treatments and procedures such as open heart surgery, organ transplants, and burn care.

Quick Tips

9. Responding to advertising is the least effective way to find a doctor.

10. Many women select obstetrician/gynecologists as primary care providers.

11. To check on a doctor's (MD) Board certification call the American Board of Medical Specialties Information Line established for that purpose 866-275-2267 or check their website at www.abms.org.

12. Since most people will obtain all, or certainly most, of their medical care near where they live or work, it is important for you to identify which doctors are among the best in your own community.

13. If in doubt about a doctor's training, ask the doctor if the residency completed was in the specialty of his/her practice. If not, ask why not.

14. Board certification and recertification are the best ways to measure competence and training.

15. The easiest way you can assess the quality of a doctor's residency program is to see if it took place in a large medical center with a name you recognize.

16. If a doctor does not have admitting privileges or is not on the attending staff of a hospital, you may wish to consider choosing another doctor.

17. There are many excellent, well-trained doctors at community hospitals and they should be as carefully evaluated and considered in your search as a doctor at a teaching hospital.

Quick Take

…You should consider four broad criteria when selecting a primary care doctor: professional preparation, professional reputation, office and practice arrangements and professional or bedside manner…

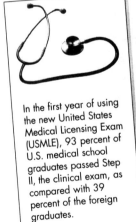

In the first year of using the new United States Medical Licensing Exam (USMLE), 93 percent of U.S. medical school graduates passed Step II, the clinical exam, as compared with 39 percent of the foreign graduates.

Chapter 2
What Makes a "Top Doctor?"

While the overwhelming majority of doctors are competent practitioners, some are less well trained or, for various other reasons, lack a desired level of professional skill or personal characteristics. They have met certain minimum standards, passed the necessary exams and are licensed, but you would still be better off to avoid them. At the same time, among the many good doctors you could choose from, there will be some who are better for you and your family for a variety of reasons.

Identifying the "top" doctors in a particular specialty is a challenge. There may be some who are generally acknowledged as leaders in a particular field, but that level of national reputation is typically built on appointments to important academic positions, innovative research, or the development of cutting-edge clinical techniques and treatments. Unless you are in need of those techniques and treatments, those doctors may not be the best for you. Since most people will obtain all, or certainly most, of their medical care near where they live, it is important for you to identify which doctors are among the best in your own community.

There are four basic criteria for selecting your own best doctor: professional preparation, professional reputation, office and practice arrangements and personal or bedside manner. The first three of these assessments can be made prior to your first visit, which is when you can make your fourth evaluation.

Professional Preparation—Education

Your review of your prospective doctor's education and training should begin with medical school. While you may feel that the institution where someone earned a bachelor's degree could be an indication of the quality of the doctor, most people in the medical field do not believe it plays a major role. A degree from a highly selective undergraduate college or university will help an aspiring doctor gain admission to a medical school, but once there, all students are peers. However, the information on undergraduate colleges, if important to you, is available in the American Board of Medical Specialties (ABMS) *Compendium of Certified Medical Specialists* and other medical directories.

American medical schools are highly standardized, at least in terms of minimum quality. All U.S. medical schools that grant medical degrees (MDs) and osteopathic degrees (DOs) are accredited by a group known as the LCME (Liaison Committee for Medical Education). Most are also accredited by the appropriate state agency, if one exists, and by regional accrediting agencies that accredit colleges and universities of all kinds.

Furthermore, U.S. medical schools have universally high standards for admission, including success at the undergraduate level and on the Medical College Admissions Tests (MCATs). Although frequently criticized for being slow to change and for training too many specialists, the system of medical education in the United States has insured high quality in medical practice. One recent positive change is a strong effort in most medical schools to diversify the composition of the student body. While these schools have been less successful in enrolling racial minorities, the number of women in U.S. medical schools has increased to the point where they now make up about 50 percent of most classes. In certain specialties preferred by women medical graduates (pediatrics, for example), it is possible that, in coming years, the majority of specialists will be female.

Most doctors practicing in the United States are graduates of U.S. medical schools. There are two other groups of doctors in practice who make up a relatively small proportion of the total doctor population. They are: (1) foreign nationals who graduated from foreign schools; and (2) U.S. nationals who graduated from foreign schools (Canadian medical schools are not considered foreign).

Foreign Medical Graduates

Foreign medical schools vary greatly in quality. Even some of the oldest and finest European schools have become virtually "open door," with huge numbers of unscreened students making teaching and learning difficult. Others are excellent and provided the model for our own system of medical education.

The fact that someone graduated from a foreign school does not mean that he or she is a poor doctor. Foreign schools, like U.S. schools, produce good doctors and poor doctors. Foreign medical graduates must pass the same exam taken by U.S. graduates for licensure, but the failure rate for foreign graduates is significantly higher. In the first year of using the new United States Medical Licensing Exam (USMLE), 93 percent of U.S. medical school graduates passed Step II, the clinical exam, as compared with 39 percent of foreign graduates. It is clear that the quality of foreign schools, if not individual doctors, is not the same as U.S. medical schools, at least as measured by our standards. Nonetheless, many communities and patients have been well served by foreign medical graduates practicing in this country—often in areas where it has been difficult to attract graduates of American schools.

Residency

Most doctors practicing today have at least three years of postgraduate training (following the MD or DO) in an approved residency program. This is not only an important step in the process of becoming a competent doctor, but it is also a requirement for board (specialty) certification. Most people assume that a prospective doctor needs to complete a three-year residency program to obtain a medical license. This is not true in some states. New York State, for example, requires only one postgraduate year. However, since all approved residencies last at least three years and some, such as those in neurosurgery, general surgery, orthopaedic surgery and urology may extend for five or more years, it is important to know the details of a doctor's training. Licensure alone is not enough of a basis on which to make a good choice.

Without undertaking extensive and detailed research on every residency program, the best assessment you can make of a doctor's residency program is to see if it took place in a large medical center whose name you recognize. The more prestigious institutions tend to attract the best medical students, sometimes regardless of the quality of the individual residency program. If in doubt about a doctor's training, ask the doctor if the residency completed was in the specialty of his/her practice. If not, ask why.

It is also important to be certain that a doctor completed a residency that has been approved by the appropriate governing board of the specialty such as the American Board of Surgery, the American Board of Radiology or the American Osteopathic Board of Pediatrics. These board groups are listed in Appendix A. If you are really concerned about a doctor's training, you should first call the hospital that offered the residency and ask if the residency was approved by the appropriate specialty group. If still in doubt, review the publication *Directory of Graduate Medical Education Programs*, often called the "green book," found in medical school or hospital libraries, which lists all approved residencies.

Board Certification

With an MD or DO degree and a license, an individual may practice any kind of medicine—with or without additional special training. For example, doctors with a license but no special training may call themselves cardiologists or pediatricians. This is why board certification is such an important factor. Twenty-five specialties are recognized by the American Board of Medical Specialties (ABMS). (Visit www.abms.org or call 866-275-2267 for more information.) Eighteen boards certify in 106 specialties under the aegis of the American Osteopathic Association (AOA). (Visit www.osteopathic.org or call 800-621-1773 for more information.) Doctors who have qualified for such specialization are called board certified; they have completed an

> All U.S. medical schools that grant medical degrees (MDs) and osteopathic degrees (DOs) are accredited by a group known as the LCME (Liaison Committee for Medical Education).

approved residency and passed the board's exam. (See Appendix A for an approved ABMS and AOA list; see pages 80-84 for a description of each specialty and subspecialty.) While many doctors who are not board certified do call themselves specialists, board certification is the best standard by which to measure competence and training.

You can be confident that doctors who are board certified have at a minimum the proper training in their specialty and have demonstrated their proficiency through supervision and testing. While there are many non-board certified doctors who are highly competent, it is more difficult to assess the level of their training. Board certification alone does not guarantee competence, but it is a standard that reflects successful completion of an appropriate training program.

Recertification

A relatively new focus of the specialty boards is the area of recertification. Until recently, board certification lasted for an unlimited time period. Now, almost all the boards have put time limits on the certification period. For example, in internal medicine, it is ten years; in family practice, seven years. In osteopathic medicine, some of the boards need to set a recertification period within 10 years. Many have done so already. These more stringent standards reflect an increasing emphasis, by both the medical boards and state agencies responsible for licensing doctors, on recertification.

Since the policies of the boards vary widely, it is good procedure to ask a doctor if certification was awarded and when. If the date was seven to ten years ago, ask if he/she has been recertified. **Note: The most recent date of board certification or recertification is indicated in each physician's listing in this guide.**

Unfortunately, many boards permit "grandfathering," whereby already certified doctors do not have to be recertified, and recertification demands apply only to newly certified doctors. Appendix A contains a list of the names and addresses of the boards and the certification period for each board specialty. Even if recertification is not required, it is good professional practice for doctors to undertake the process. It assures you, the patient, that they are attempting to stay current.

Many states have a continuing medical education (CME) requirement for doctors. These states typically require a minimum number of CME credits for a doctor to maintain a medical license. Seven states require 150 CME credits over a three-year period. Osteopathic doctors are required to take 120 hours of CME credits within three years to maintain certification.

Board Eligibility

Many doctors who have been recently trained are waiting to take the boards. They are sometimes described as "board eligible," a common term that the ABMS advocates abandoning because of its ambiguity. Board eligible means that the doctor has completed an approved residency and is qualified to sit for the related board's exam.

Each member board of the ABMS has its own policy regarding the use and recognition of the board eligible term. Therefore, the description "board eligible" should not be viewed as a genuine qualification, especially if a doctor has been out of medical school long enough to have taken the certification exam. To the boards, a doctor is either board certified or not. Furthermore, most of the specialty boards permit unlimited attempts to pass the exam and, in some cases, doctors who have failed the exam twice or even ten times continue to call themselves board eligible. In osteopathic medicine, the board eligible status is recognized only for the first six years after completion of a residency.

Self-Designated Medical Specialties

In addition to the ABMS and AOA-approved list of specialties and subspecialties, there is a wide variety of other doctors, and groups of doctors, who may call themselves "specialists." There are, at present, at least 100 such groups called self-designated medical specialties. They range from doctors who are working to create a recognized body of knowledge and subspecialty training to less formal groups interested in a particular approach to the practice of medicine. These groups may or may not have standards for membership. There is no way of determining the true extent of their members' training, and they are not recognized by the ABMS* or the AOA. While you should be cautious of doctors who claim they are specialists in these areas, many do have advanced training and the groups at least offer a listing of people interested in a particular approach to medical care. Rely on board certification to assure yourself of basic competence and use membership in one of these groups to indicate strong interest and possible additional training in a particular aspect of medicine. A list of these self-designated medical specialties may be found in Appendix B.

Fellowships

The purpose of a fellowship is to provide advanced training in the clinical techniques and research of a particular subspecialty. In the U.S. there are a variety of fellowship programs available to doctors, and they fall into two broad categories: approved and unapproved. Approved fellowships are those approved by the appropriate medical specialty board (e.g., the American Board of Radiology) and that lead to a subspecialty certificate. Fellowship programs that are not approved are often in the same areas of training as those that are, but they do not lead to a subspecialty certificate. Unfortunately, all too often, unapproved fellowships exist only to provide relatively inexpensive labor for the research and/or patient care activities of a clinical department in a medical school or hospital. In such cases, the learning that takes place is secondary and may be a good deal less than in an approved fellowship. On the other hand, any fellowship is better than none at all, and some unapproved fellowships have that status for a valid reason, which should not reflect negatively on the program. For example, the fellowship may have been recently created with approval being sought. To check that a fellowship is an approved one, call the hospital where the training took place or the medical board for that specialty.

Professional Reputation

There are doctors who meet every professional standard on paper, but who are simply not good doctors. In all probability the medical community has ascertained that and, while the individual may still practice medicine, his or her reputation will reflect that collective assessment. There are also doctors who are outstanding leaders in their fields because of research or professional activities, but who are not particularly strong or perhaps even active in patient care. It is important to distinguish that kind of professional reputation from a reputation as a competent, caring doctor in delivering patient care. In a consumer survey conducted by Towers Perrin, the management consulting firm, the chief criterion by which the respondents selected doctors was reputation. This was the most important factor for those enrolled in either managed care or indemnity plans.

---

* Subspecialties, not yet recognized by the ABMS—Pediatric Neurosurgery, Facial Plastic & Reconstructive Surgery, have been included because the training and certification process is rigorous and meaningful.

Hospital Appointment

Most doctors are on the medical staff of one or more hospitals and are known as "attendings." If a doctor does not have admitting privileges or is not on the attending staff of a hospital, you may wish to consider choosing another doctor. It can be very difficult to ascertain whether the lack of hospital appointment is for a good reason or not. For example, it is understandable that some doctors who are raising families or heading toward retirement choose not to meet the demands (meetings, committees, etc.) of being an attending. However, if you need care in a hospital, the lack of such an appointment means that another doctor will have to oversee that care. In some specialties such as dermatology and psychiatry, doctors may conduct their entire practices in the office, and a hospital appointment is not as essential, or as good a criterion for assessment, as in other specialties.

While mistakes are made, most hospitals are quite careful about admissions to their medical staffs. The best hospitals are highly selective, so a degree of screening (or "credentialing") has been done for you. In other words, the best doctors practice at the best hospitals. Since caring for a patient in the hospital also is often a team effort involving a number of specialists, the reputation of the hospital where the doctor admits patients carries special weight. Hospital medical staffs also review their colleagues' credentials before authorizing them to perform specific procedures. In addition, they typically reappoint their medical staffs—and review them—every two or three years. In effect, this is an additional screening to protect patients. It is especially true of hospitals that have what are known as "closed staffs," where it is impossible to obtain admitting privileges unless there is a vacancy that the administration and medical staff deem necessary to fill. If you are having some type of surgical procedure and are concerned about the doctor's skill or experience with it, it may be worthwhile to call the Medical Affairs office at the doctor's hospital to see if he or she is authorized to perform that procedure in the hospital.

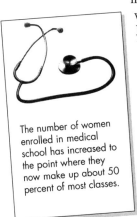

The number of women enrolled in medical school has increased to the point where they now make up about 50 percent of most classes.

The reasons for a hospital's selectivity are easy to understand: every hospital wants to have the best reputation possible in order to attract patients, and no hospital, excellent or not, wishes to expose itself to liability. Obviously, the quality of the medical staff is immensely important in creating that reputation. Unfortunately, some hospitals are less diligent when a major group practice of doctors, all of whom have previously been affiliated with the institution, adds new members. In such cases, the hospital may almost automatically grant privileges without conducting the same intensive review given to individual doctors who are not members of a group practice. Also, some hospitals are less selective in granting privileges when beds are empty than when beds are full, since additional attendings provide additional patients.

A last and very important reason why a hospital appointment is an essential requirement in your choice of a doctor is that many states permit doctors to practice *without* malpractice insurance. If you are injured as a result of the doctor's poor care, you could be without recourse. However, few *hospitals* permit doctors to practice in them unless they carry malpractice insurance. This not only protects the hospital, but the patient as well.

Many people believe that they should choose a doctor with an appointment at a major medical center as opposed to a community hospital. This assumption is incorrect on two counts. For one thing, there are many excellent, well-trained doctors at community hospitals and they should be as carefully evaluated and considered in your search as a doctor at a large institution. What's more, the term "medical center" has less significance today than it did years ago when the term was used to describe only the major university hospitals of medical schools. A true medical center is a teaching hospital that offers multiple residency programs and at which the medical school faculty practices full-time, with fellowship programs and major clinical research activities an integral part of the teaching of medical students. These large centers also are involved in tertiary care, offering services such as organ transplants, burn care and cardiovascular surgery.

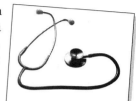

In a consumer survey conducted by Towers Perrin, the management consulting firm, the chief criterion by which the respondents selected doctors was reputation. This was the most important factor for those enrolled in either managed care or indemnity plans.

Today many community hospitals have added the term "medical center" to their name. They do this for two purposes: to indicate that they, too, offer advanced and sophisticated medical programs, and to compete for patients with the academic medical centers. With academic medical centers turning out many well-trained specialists and subspecialists who establish practices in nearby communities and then want to continue the highly specialized techniques they have learned, many community hospitals have initiated tertiary care programs of their own, further blurring the distinction between medical centers and hospitals.

In any case, most of our healthcare today is delivered *outside* of the hospital in ambulatory outpatient settings. Those who are hospitalized for acute illness (e.g., surgery, serious infection) will find that community hospitals and their staffs are well-suited to the task.

When extremely difficult and complex problems develop, or when tertiary care is needed, many communities have excellent academic medical centers. Of course, they offer primary care as well, especially to those who live nearby. This illustrates the point, once again, that medical care is a local issue.

Medical School Faculty Appointment

Many doctors have appointments on the faculties of medical schools. There is a range of categories from "straight" appointments—meaning full-time appointment as professor, associate professor, assistant professor or instructor—to clinical ranks that may reflect lesser degrees of involvement in teaching or research. If someone carries what is known as a straight academic rank (i.e., professor of surgery, without "clinical" in the title), this usually means that the individual is engaged full-time in medical school research and/or teaching activities. The title "professor of clinical surgery" usually describes a doctor who has a full-time appointment in a medical school, but who puts a greater emphasis on clinical practice (patient care) than on research or teaching. The title "clinical professor of surgery" usually specifies a part-time or adjunct appointment and less direct involvement in medical school activities.

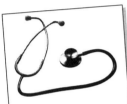

The newest approaches and techniques in medicine, for the most part, are explored and developed by medical school faculties in their laboratories and clinical practice settings.

Doctors who are full-time academicians may be in the forefront of new techniques and research, but they are not necessarily better doctors. Nonetheless, you can be assured that they have the support of other faculty, residents and medical students.

When you are seeking a subspecialist, a doctor's relationship to a medical school becomes more meaningful since medical school faculties tend to be made up of subspecialists. You are less likely to find large numbers of general or primary care practitioners engaged full-time on a medical school faculty. The newest approaches and techniques in medicine, for the most part, are explored and developed by medical school faculties in their laboratories and clinical practice settings. This is where they practice their subspecialties, as well as teach and perform research. Such leading specialists are not necessarily better doctors than community doctors—they are trained to provide a *different* kind of medical care. The best care is provided by a combination of primary care doctors and other specialists and subspecialists.

Medical Society Membership

Most medical society memberships sound very prestigious and some are; however, there are many societies that are not selective and which virtually any doctor can join. In addition, membership in many of the more prestigious societies is based on research and publication, or on leadership in the field, and may have little to do with direct patient care. While it is clearly an honor to be invited to join these groups, membership may be less than helpful in discerning whether a doctor can meet your needs.

Board certified doctors are referred to as Diplomates of the Board. Some of the colleges of medical specialties (e.g., the American College of Radiology and the American College of Surgeons) have multiple levels of recognition. The first is basic membership and the second, more prestigious and difficult to obtain, is status as a Fellow.

Fellowship status in the colleges is meaningful and is based on experience, professional achievement and recognition by one's peers, including extensive experience in patient care. It should be viewed as a significant professional qualification.

Experience

Experience is difficult to assess. Obviously, in most cases, an older doctor has more experience; on the other hand, a younger doctor has been more recently immersed in residency, the challenge of medical school, or even a fellowship, and may be the most up-to-date. If a doctor is board certified, you may assume that assures at least a minimal amount of experience, but it could be as little as a year. In this guide the board certification date may reflect a doctor's most recent recertification, so check the date of graduation from medical school or completion of residency if you want to know precisely how long a doctor has been in practice.

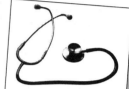

There is a good deal of evidence that there is a positive relationship between quantity of experience and quality of care. That is, the more often a doctor performs a procedure, the better he/she becomes at it. That is why it is important to ask a doctor about his or her experience with the procedure that you need. Does the doctor see and treat similar cases every day, every week or only rarely? Of course, with some rare conditions, rarely is the only possible answer, but it is relative frequency that is critical. Major metropolitan areas, especially New York and San Francisco, became leaders in the treatment of AIDS because of the large number of patients seen in those metropolitan areas. Doctors in the suburbs of New York City (especially in New York's Westchester, Nassau and Suffolk counties) and in Fairfield County, Connecticut became leaders in the research and treatment of Lyme disease because that region is the epicenter of the disease.

Many states typically require a minimum number of continuing medical education (CME) credits for a doctor to maintain a medical license. Seven states require 150 CME credits over a three-year period. Osteopathic doctors are required to take 150 hours of CME credits within three years to maintain certification.

In some states, data is available on volume or numbers of certain procedures performed at hospitals. For this information in New York you can call the Center for Medical Consumers, a non-profit advocacy organization, or visit its website at www.medicalconsumers.org. For volume and outcome information in other states, visit the website of Health Care Choices at www.healthcarechoices.org. There is a good deal of controversy, however, on the validity and usefulness of such data. Opponents cite the fact that some of the data is produced from Medicare patient records only and, thus, is based solely on an elderly population that does not represent the total activity of a hospital or doctor. Proponents of the use of such volume data agree that it is not perfect, but suggest that it can be one useful criterion in selecting the best places to receive care for these specific problems. Recognizing the limitations of such data, the healthcare consumer may, nonetheless, find it of interest and use.

Office and Practice Arrangements

Although clearly not as important as training or reputation, office and practice arrangements are usually of great significance to patients. Practice arrangements include office hours, office location, billing procedures and office testing among the many factors that result in how well the office is run.

Many years ago most doctors practiced independently in private offices. They were called "solo practitioners" and usually had agreements with other doctors to respond to their patients' calls when they were unavailable. In recent decades, most doctors have entered group practices; indeed, this is becoming the most common way for young doctors to begin to practice. Two or more doctors in the same specialty, or in different specialties (a multi-specialty group), share offices and staff to lower their costs of operations. They also cover for each other on rotation for weekends, evenings and vacations. As a patient you may prefer one of the following: a solo practitioner who is covered occasionally; a group where you usually, but not always, see the same doctor; or a multi-specialty group where, if a consultation or referral is necessary, the specialist is at the same location. The choice is really one of personal preference.

There are other factors relating to practice arrangements that may or may not be important to an individual when choosing a doctor. One is the location of the office. A consumer poll conducted for the Robert Wood Johnson Foundation identified office location as one of the two most important factors in the selection of a doctor (the other was a recommendation by a relative or friend). Actually, the site of the office can be very important in choosing a doctor you may visit on a regular basis. If the location is inconvenient, you may be discouraged from making needed visits.

Another important factor concerns the use of nurse practitioners and physician's assistants in the office. Licensed nurse practitioners are advanced practice nurses in primary care. They have additional training beyond the basic requirements for nursing licensure, usually a master's degree or special certificate. They perform a broad range of nursing functions as well as functions that, historically, have been performed by doctors, including assessing and diagnosing, conducting physical examinations, ordering diagnostic tests, implementing treatment plans and monitoring patient status. Physician's assistants are licensed to provide medical care in many states. However, unlike nurses, they may practice only under a doctor's direction and supervision. According to an article in the professional journal *Family Practice Management*, these "midlevel providers," as they are called, "can handle 80 to 90 percent of the problems that occasion office visits." These providers have become more of a presence in healthcare in recent years, especially in medical groups and HMOs. If you don't think you will be satisfied having your office visit and examination conducted by anyone but the doctor, you should determine up front how many midlevel providers are on staff and how extensive their responsibilities are.

Quick Tips

18. Doctors who are full-time academicians may be in the forefront of new techniques and research, but they are not necessarily better doctors.

19. The best care is provided by a combination of primary care doctors and other specialists and subspecialists.

20. Do not hesitate to ask how frequently your doctor has performed a procedure and with what degree of success. Practice may not lead to perfection, but it improves skills and enhances the probability of success.

21. Check the date of graduation from medical school or completion of residency if you want to know precisely how long a doctor has been in practice.

22. If you don't think you will be satisfied having your office visit and examination conducted by anyone but the doctor, you should determine up front how many midlevel providers are on staff and how extensive their responsibilities are.

23. The site of the office can be very important in choosing a doctor you may visit on a regular basis. If the location is inconvenient, you may be discouraged from making needed visits.

24. You should discuss any chronic problem when first establishing a relationship with a doctor. In fact, you may want to find a doctor with special interest or training in that problem.

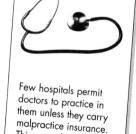

Few hospitals permit doctors to practice in them unless they carry malpractice insurance. This not only protects the hospital, but the patient as well.

Chapter Two

Narrowing the Choice

Here are 10 additional questions that will guide you in assessing if the practice patterns or arrangements of a doctor meet your needs. If there are other items not listed that are important to you, add them to the list before you make your initial appointment. You should try to obtain as much of the information as possible from the staff.

- *Are you currently accepting new patients and, if so, is a referral required?*

- *On average, how long does a patient have to wait for an appointment?*

- *Are you open on weekends? In the evening?*

- *If lab work and X-rays are performed in the office, what are the qualifications of the people doing the tests?*

- *Are full payment, deductibles or co-payments required at the time of the appointment?*

- *Do you accept my insurance plan? Medicare? Medicaid? Workers' compensation? No-fault insurance?*

- *Do you accept credit cards and, if so, which do you accept?*

- *Do you accept patient phone calls?*

- *Will you care for patients in their homes?*

- *Is your office handicapped-accessible?*

If you have a chronic illness or disease, there may be certain additional aspects of a doctor's practice that could be particularly important to you. You should discuss any chronic problems when first establishing a relationship with a doctor. In fact, you may want to find a doctor with special interest or training in that problem.

House calls also continue to be important to some people. Yes, some doctors still do make house calls! In fact, a recent *American Medical News* article suggested that 43 percent of internal medicine specialists and 65 percent of family practice specialists made one or more house calls a year. However, it is important to point out that the number of doctors making house calls has declined because of technology, liability risks and time pressures. Important diagnostic equipment often cannot be carried around in a doctor's little black bag and is only available in the office or hospital. Also, the time required to visit one patient at home markedly reduces the time available to see other patients.

Personal or Bedside Manner

To many patients, once they have determined that a doctor is competent, the doctor's professional manner—also known as bedside manner—is the most important part of their choice. The Towers Perrin report cited earlier indicated that after reputation, skill in communicating was the most important factor sought in doctors. Patients prefer sensitive and caring doctors who listen carefully and demonstrate their concern. Studies show that such doctors are sued less often than others!

What characteristics make up a doctor's personal manner? The four described below may, when considered together, give you a clear idea of whether a particular doctor will be your personal "top" doctor.

- **Listening**. Professional manner includes the doctor's willingness to listen to patients, be supportive and understanding, explain procedures and exhibit concern and respect. These skills are expressed at the bedside, in the office, or in any setting where there is doctor-patient contact. Listening is also a valuable diagnostic tool. Unfortunately, these skills often have not been taught well in medical schools and the lack of them forms the primary basis for complaints from patients. However, there is growing emphasis on these vital interpersonal and communications skills in medical schools today and with good reason. They are critically important to most patients.

- **Cultural Sensitivity**. Some patients may prefer doctors who speak their language or are familiar with their cultural background. The term "culturally competent physician" is a relatively new one describing doctors who have the needed skills and attitudes to effectively treat patients from minority cultures.

- **Ethical, Religious** and **Philosophical Views**. Religion, or at least views on issues such as abortion, utilization of life-sustaining measures, natural childbirth, breast-feeding and other such matters can also be important. It is perfectly appropriate to ask doctors their views on sensitive issues.

- **Decision-Making Procedures**. Years ago patients took the words of the doctor as law, not to be questioned or perhaps even discussed. That is not the case today. Consumers are better informed about health issues and may want to be actively involved in the decision-making affecting their health. Some patients do not feel this way and are comfortable accepting a doctor's diagnosis or course of treatment without question. Some doctors—in diminishing numbers, thankfully—feel uncomfortable with patients who want everything explained to them or want to be involved in decision-making. Consider how you feel about this issue and discuss it with your doctor to be certain you are on compatible wavelengths.

Of course, what ultimately makes a "top" doctor are the results, the "outcomes," of care. Unfortunately, there is relatively little information available to consumers on the outcomes of physicians and hospitals. Some states, New York for example, have produced studies on outcomes for cardiac surgery. Also, some HMOs are talking about producing report cards for doctors. Generally, however, consumers will have difficulty finding outcome studies for individual doctors.

On the other hand, there is a growing movement to track and publish outcomes data on hospitals. The federal government has taken the lead by releasing outcomes data by hospitals for selected procedures. Visit www.hospitalcompare.hhs.gov.

Chapter 3

You and Your Doctor:
A Team

Key Terms: Chapter 3

AMERICAN MEDICAL ASSOCIATION

A membership organization of physicians and their professional associations dedicated to promoting the art and science of medicine and the betterment of public health through establishing and promoting ethical, educational, and clinical standards for the medical profession. It represents the interests of physicians on the national level.

BASELINE TESTS

A series of basic, routine medical tests—such as electrocardiogram, complete blood count, blood pressure measurement, weight measurement, and chest X-ray—that are usually completed by a physician upon a patient's initial visit in order to provide a standard for comparison during subsequent health examinations.

GENERIC DRUGS

Prescription medications that have been marketed by one company under a proprietary or brand name and which may be sold, after the original exclusive 17-year patent expires, under a generic name or the name assigned to it during an early stage of development. Most generic drugs are less expensive than proprietary versions and are just as effective except in cases when, because of different manufacturing processes, they are not bioequivalent or handled by the body in an identical manner.

THIRD PARTY PAYER

An organization such as indemnity insurance company or managed care organization that provides individual and group health insurance, or a governmental department that assumes responsibility for the payment of an individual's healthcare, either directly to the healthcare provider or by means of reimbursement to the individual (Medicare and Medicaid are such government programs).

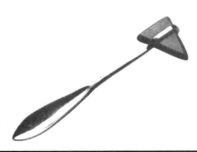

Quick Tips

25. Always obtain copies of all medical records and tests for your files.

26. When selecting a doctor, especially a primary care doctor, it is appropriate to request an interview to get acquainted.

27. Good doctors listen, good patients talk.

28. Always bring a pad and pencil with you to medical appointments. When the doctor gives you instructions, take notes.

29. The *Physician's Desk Reference*, commonly known as the PDR, is available in most libraries and is an excellent resource for learning more about medications. (The PDR web page is at http://www.pdr.net)

30. Do not hesitate to ask your pharmacist about side effects, generic substitutions and other questions related to your medications.

Quick Take

...The best doctor-patient relationship is based on a two-way dialogue. Be open and honest and seek a doctor who is the same...

Chapter 3
You and Your Doctor: A Team

Trust and respect between doctors and patients have reached a low point in modern American society. A recent poll of consumers sponsored by the American Medical Association (AMA) concluded that approximately 70 percent of those who responded agreed with the statement that "people are beginning to lose faith in their doctors." (Despite concerns about doctors in general, much research has shown that patients tend to rate their own doctors well.)

Trust between doctors and patients has declined for many reasons, including unrealistic expectations on the part of some patients and the patronizing attitudes of some doctors, which clash with the higher education level and medical sophistication of many patients. This has been further complicated by changing financial arrangements, particularly those involving the government and third-party payers, and the perception that some doctors seem to be motivated not by the values of the Hippocratic Oath (See page xiii), but by those of the marketplace. The AMA poll cited earlier found that 69 percent of respondents agreed that doctors "are too interested in making money." Perhaps a significant factor in creating this atmosphere is that in many cases the relationship between doctor and patient now has another dimension, the managed care organization. Another significant contributor is the huge amount of paperwork required from doctors. Generated by quality-assurance efforts, regulation, complex billing and managed care procedures, this burden reduces the time doctors are able to spend with patients.

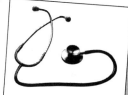

According to an article in the professional journal *Family Practice Management*, these "midlevel providers," as they are called, "can handle 80 to 90 percent of the problems that occasion office visits."

Given the formidable obstacles, it might seem impossible to find a primary care doctor who is well suited to your needs. If you have carefully read the preceding chapters, your work is half done. What remains is to find that special individual who fits the criteria.

The Initial Interview

When selecting a doctor, especially a primary care doctor, it is appropriate to request an exploratory interview. Frequently, doctors will engage in such brief interviews at no charge or at a reduced fee or by telephone. It is preferable to find out about a doctor's credentials, office hours and billing procedures from the staff beforehand so you don't waste time asking about basic facts. This leaves time to ask the doctor questions that will allow you to determine what kind of relationship could develop. It is interesting that many parents will insist on interviewing a pediatrician for their child but wouldn't think of interviewing a physician for themselves.

Ask the Right Questions

The most important aspect of this session is to see if you can develop a positive doctor-patient relationship. Are you comfortable with the doctor's manner, style and general personality? Do you feel a strong sense of trust in the doctor? Here are five questions to ask the doctor plus two questions to ask yourself that may lead you closer to a selection.

- *What is your experience in treating _____ (if you are seeking care for a particular illness or condition)?*

- *Are you open to treatments and therapies that do not rely heavily on medication?*

- *What preventive programs do you suggest for someone of my age, sex and health status?*

- *How do you feel about involving patients in decision-making?*

- *What are your views on_____(ethical and moral issues of importance to you as a patient)?*

Even when the doctor is responding to your questions, you should ask yourself:

- *Is the doctor paying attention to me and really considering my questions or do the impersonal, "stock" answers indicate that the doctor's thoughts are elsewhere?*

- *Does this doctor speak about good health and prevention with the personal knowledge of someone who seems to practice it?*

If your prospective doctor seems to measure up to your standards, get the relationship off to a good start by making an appointment for a complete check-up. During this appointment, you will have an opportunity to share your medical and family history, and baseline tests will be performed to serve as a standard in the years ahead.

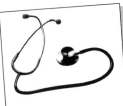

Analysis of doctor-patient conversations has revealed that many patients wait until the end of a conversation, even until they are saying goodbye, to tell their doctors what is really bothering them.

Talking with Your Doctor

After you have selected your doctor, your first appointment should include an extensive medical history. Your doctor should spend time with you, ask questions and listen to your responses carefully.

Medical students are often told, "Listen to your patients. They'll tell you what's wrong with them." This conveys an important lesson not only for doctors, but for patients: *Good doctors listen, good patients talk.*

One woman, imbued with her new "take charge" role in her healthcare, carried the interviewing process to the limit when she visited more than 20 doctors for exploratory interviews in the course of a single year. Each time there was some little problem: the doctor was behind schedule, the doctor was very brusque, the doctor discussed everything in complicated medical language, even one instance when she concluded that the doctor was just too young. Not only was she imposing on the professionalism of the doctors who conducted the interviews with her, but she was actually neglecting her healthcare; during that year, she never had a single medical examination. If a serious health problem had been in the developing stages, a year would have been too long to go without medical treatment.

Analysis of doctor-patient conversations has revealed that many patients wait until the end of a conversation, even until they are saying goodbye, to tell their doctors what is really bothering them. This is just a small example of the dynamics of doctor-patient relationships. It is also a good example of a waste of valuable time—the doctor's and the patient's. One reason doctors need to be trained to be good listeners is that they frequently must ascertain what is troubling the patient not by what is said directly, but by what is said indirectly, not at all or through body language and other signs. However, it is always easier, less time-consuming and certainly more effective if a patient can describe problems completely and accurately.

Before you even see a doctor, you should prepare thoroughly. You should have a complete record of your medical history, including a record of X-rays and any other diagnostic tests, as well as blood workups. You need information about childhood diseases, chronic conditions, hospitalizations, past and present medications, doses and drug reactions, if any, and, if possible, something about the health history of your parents and even their siblings. Except for the last item, these are available to patients from their previous doctors or hospitals. That is why it is useful to obtain copies of all medical records and tests for your own files. Not only will this save you time and effort, but may avoid additional testing and expense. Your doctor will also ask many seemingly personal questions about your work, education, sex life and even drug and alcohol use. These are all part of a complete medical history and will help your doctor better understand you and your state of health.

A consumer poll conducted for the Robert Wood Johnson Foundation identified office location as one of the two most important factors in the selection of a doctor.

If you have a particular problem or concern, describe all your symptoms. Try not to minimize or exaggerate and, most of all, don't deny.

An executive of a large computer software firm assured his doctor that he was "feeling fit," choosing not to mention the sometimes severe pain in his scrotum. Six months later the pain had worsened to the degree that it demanded attention. Unfortunately, the diagnosis was advanced testicular cancer.

If you have questions to ask your doctor, make a list. Always bring a pad and pencil with you to medical appointments. When the doctor gives you instructions, take notes or ask the doctor to write them down for you. If a prescription is written, ask about doses, side effects, efficacy and alternative medications as well as generic substitutes. The *Physician's Desk Reference*, commonly known as the PDR, is available in most libraries and is an excellent resource for learning more about medications. There is also a PDR web page on the Internet at http://www.pdr.net. You can also get a great deal of information on medications from another health professional, your pharmacist. Do not hesitate to ask your pharmacist about side effects, generic substitutions and other questions related to your medications. However, if the information you receive conflicts with that given by your doctor, consult with the doctor and follow his or her directions.

A Matter of Time

Patients want and expect doctors who listen, express concern, explain conditions and procedures in a clear and understandable manner, discuss medications and their effects and side effects thoroughly, return calls, are available when needed and, perhaps most importantly, spend sufficient time with them. With increasing demands on their time, many doctors are left with an uneasy feeling of "running to stay in place." The end result may be a tendency, unintended for the most part, to rush through a patient visit. This situation contributes to the erosion of the doctor-patient relationship.

Also contributing to this problem is pervasive lateness on the part of doctors. Patients frequently complain that they spend hours in a doctor's waiting room, long past the appointed hour (research has shown the average wait is 20 minutes). Unfortunately, the duration of a patient visit is not always predictable and unexpected delays may occur if the diagnosis is complicated or if a patient needs to discuss what is on his or her mind. The doctor who spends extra time with another patient is probably the doctor you want for yourself. If the lateness is excessive, persistent and without apparent good reason, discuss it with your doctor and, if it is interfering with your relationship, consider changing doctors. After a delay of two hours in his doctor's office, one patient, a self-employed marketing consultant, made sure that it would never happen again. Did he have a showdown with the doctor? Did he decide never to return? Not at all. He simply made it a point to call the doctor's office two hours before his scheduled appointment to see how the schedule was running. He then adjusted his own schedule to coincide with the doctor's.

Chapter 4

Strengthening Your Team

Key Terms: Chapter 4

ALTERNATIVE THERAPY

Non-traditional forms of healthcare—including acupuncture, homeopathy, naturopathy, massage, reflexology, biofeedback, hypnotherapy, herbology, therapeutic touch, and prayer—that are often based on ancient healing methods and have not been tested in a conventional scientific manner.

CLINICAL TRIAL

An experimental trial of a new drug or therapy in a selected group of human volunteers who suffer from the condition for which the experimental drug or treatment is to be used.

DOUBLE BLIND STUDY

One form of a clinical trial in which two groups of volunteers—one group receiving the real drug or treatment and the other receiving a placebo or dummy—are followed for a specific period of time by researchers who do not know themselves who is receiving which therapy.

PROTOCOL

A rigid set of rules set up for a clinical trial by the Food and Drug Administration (FDA) which must be followed strictly by all researchers and volunteers participating in the trial.

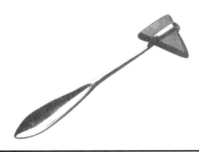

Quick Tips

31. The more complex and difficult the problem, the more important reputation is. In fact, you might well narrow your focus to doctors on the staffs of certain medical centers noted for excellence with specific problems.

32. Doctors typically refer patients to doctors on the staffs of the same hospitals where they practice.

33. If the lateness of your doctor is excessive, persistent and without apparent good reason, discuss it with him/her.

34. If you are not comfortable with your primary care doctor's referral, ask for a number of options. If necessary, you may consider going "out of network" even if you have to pay some or all of the fee.

Quick Take

...The old adage, two heads are better than one, often applies in healthcare, too. Expanded options include referrals, second opinions, alternative therapies and clinical trials...

Chapter 4
Strengthening Your Team

When You Need a Specialist

For the most part, selecting a specialist is similar to choosing a primary care doctor. There is one major difference, however; typically you will be referred to a specialist by your primary care doctor. Suggesting a consultation does not show a weakness on the part of the doctor. On the contrary, the real weakness lies in a doctor's reluctance to suggest consultations when advisable. Your primary care doctor will receive a written report from any consultation or referral. You should request a copy as well.

Ask your doctor why this particular specialist is being recommended. Find out about the specialist's training and experience. If your doctor has sent many patients to the same doctor for the same treatment, you should find out how successful the treatment was and if the patients were satisfied. You might also ask if the specialist would be the one selected for your doctor's own personal care. You should feel comfortable about seeing the specialist and, if you are not, ask for another recommendation or find a different one on your own.

Frequently, patients do seek out specialists on their own. If you are attempting to find a specialist or subspecialist without the guidance of your primary care doctor, use the various selection procedures described in Chapters 1, 2 and 3. When selecting a physician on your own, even greater emphasis should be placed on board certification in the relevant specialty. If you are trying to find someone to treat a very specific problem, make certain that the individual is well trained in that area. You may check to see if a doctor is board certified by calling the American Board of Medical Specialties at 866-275-2267 or visiting their website at www.abms.org.

You will also want to know if the specialist you select is well respected. The more complex and difficult the problem, the more important reputation is. In fact, you might narrow your focus to doctors on the staffs of certain medical centers noted for excellence in your specific problem. There are a number of books and magazine articles such as the annual *U.S. News & World Report* issue on America's best hospitals, that offer views on the best medical centers for specific problems.

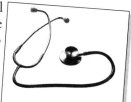

Our healthcare system does not place enough emphasis on preventing illness; most healthcare dollars are spent on curative, rather than preventive, medicine.

Last, make certain your doctor and the specialist communicate easily about your case. If you should have a problem with a specialist, or if you are not pleased with the care given, let your primary care doctor know about it right away.

Easy access to specialists and subspecialists, especially in large metropolitan areas, presents certain problems in coordination of care that a patient should be aware of. This difficulty is probably epitomized by one woman who was treated by a dermatologist, an ophthalmologist, a rheumatologist, a psychiatrist and an allergist, all of whom had office space in her very large apartment complex on Manhattan's Upper West Side, thus eliminating her need to even to put on her coat. Fortunately, all were quite competent and had all the necessary qualifications. Unfortunately, each was affiliated with a different medical center, which made coordinating her care with her primary care doctor very complex.

Doctors typically refer patients to doctors on the staffs of the same hospitals at which they practice. There are good and poor reasons for this, as explained below.

Why Doctors Usually Refer to Doctors in the Same Hospitals
Good Reasons:

- They know the doctors better.

- They continue to be involved in the case.

- Coordination of multiple specialists may be easier.

Poor Reasons:

- It is easier.

- They will get referrals back.

- It reduces the chance of losing the patient to another doctor.

- It may help build social or professional relationships.

- The hospital may pressure doctors to refer within the institution.

In today's managed care environment, doctor referrals usually are restricted to other doctors in the managed care organization's network. Sometimes the referring doctor may not even be familiar with the other doctor's qualifications. If you are not comfortable with your primary care doctor's referral, ask for a number of options. If necessary, you may consider going "out of network" even if you have to pay some or all of the fee.

Second Opinions

Second opinions are a valuable medical tool, infrequently used in many instances, overused in others. Clearly, you do not want to get another doctor's opinion on every ailment or problem, but there are definitely times you should seek out a second opinion:

- Before major surgery.

- When the diagnosis is serious or life-threatening.

- If a rare disease is diagnosed.

- If the diagnosis is uncertain.

- If you think the number of tests or procedures recommended is excessive.

- If a test result has serious implications—a positive Pap smear for example—have the test re-done immediately before taking further action.

- If the treatment suggested is risky or expensive.

- If you are uncomfortable with the diagnosis and treatment recommended.

- If a course of treatment is not working.

- If you question your doctor's competence.

- If your insurance company requires it.

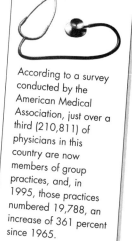

Most doctors will be supportive if you request a second opinion, and many will even recommend it. In many cases, insurance companies will pay for second opinions, but check ahead of time to make sure your insurance plan does cover them. In an HMO, you may have to be more assertive because one way that HMOs control costs is by limiting second opinions. This is especially true if you want an opinion outside the plan's network.

According to a survey conducted by the American Medical Association, just over a third (210,811) of physicians in this country are now members of group practices, and, in 1995, those practices numbered 19,788, an increase of 361 percent since 1965.

Often, the opinion of a second doctor will affirm the opinion of the first, but the reassurance may be worth the time and extra cost. On the other hand, if the second opinion differs from the first, you have two remaining alternatives: seek the opinion of a third doctor, or educate yourself as much as possible by talking with both doctors and reading up on the problem (trusting your instincts about which diagnosis is correct). If the diagnosis is the same but the recommended treatments differ, remember that doctors may have different solutions to the same problem—and any one or more could be efficient. For example, an orthopaedic surgeon may recommend surgery to correct a knee injury while a physiatrist (a doctor certified in physical medicine and rehabilitation) may recommend rehabilitation. One might work better than the other or they could both work equally well. The choice may be based on your preference. Remember, however, that surgical solutions can rarely be reversed. It usually is best to try a non-surgical solution first, if possible.

Complementary Medicine: Exploring Your Options

A recent study conducted by the University of Florida estimated that 86 percent of households in the U.S. use some type of complementary therapies (a term that implies that these therapies are used along with conventional medical treatment rather than in place of them). Total out-of-pocket expenditures for complementary/alternative medicine approach $30 billion annually, estimates David Eisenberg, MD and colleagues at the Harvard/Beth Israel Center for the Study of Alternative Medicine Research. They further point out that total visits to complementary/alternative providers numbered 629 million in 1997 as compared to 386 million visits to primary care physicians.

One of the reasons conventional medical therapies are conventional is that most have been proven to be effective in a rigorous scientific manner, while many complementary /alternative therapies have not been tested under accepted scientific conditions. You should always consider the possibility that some alternative therapies, since they are unproven, may do more harm than good. The alternative approaches in use today range from legitimate searches for new therapies to outright quackery and fraud. Without the guidance of the scientific and medical community, it is sometimes impossible for doctors, let alone consumers, to tell the difference.

Nonetheless, doctors are becoming more open to the use of complementary/alternative approaches. One study reported that about 30 percent of doctors questioned in the Los Angeles area said that they were open to complementary/ alternative practices in one form or another and that acceptance is growing. Medical scientists are also indicating a new interest in studying approaches to health that may complement the strengths of Western medicine. Some of the therapies being explored include mind-body medicine, hypnotherapy, biofeedback, chiropractic, vital energy, metabolic therapy, naturopathy, homeopathy, therapeutic touch, acupuncture, prayer, and the use of herbs.

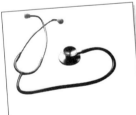

Total out-of-pocket expenditures for alternative and complementary medicine approach $30 billion annually, estimated David Eisenberg MD and colleagues at the Harvard/Beth Israel Center for the study of Alternative Medicine Research.

Alternative healthcare often complements rather than replaces Western Medicine. As such, the terms "complementary" or "integrative," which accurately describe the relationship between Western and alternative healthcare, are used with increased frequency as this type of approach towards medicine becomes more commonplace.

In a *New England Journal of Medicine* study, 72 percent of the respondents who used unconventional therapies did not inform their medical doctor that they had done so.

That is unfortunate, because such treatments could be greatly enhanced with the support and advice of a primary care doctor. More worrisome is the great danger that some people may use alternative treatments in lieu of, rather than as a supplement to, more conventional and proven medical therapies. A classic and tragic example of this was the surge of patients who traveled to Mexico to seek a "magic bullet" cure for cancer promised by the drug Laetrile (made from apricot pits). There was no magic; indeed, patients lost money, hope and, in some cases, the opportunity for timely use of proven treatment. If you do explore alternative therapies, be certain to let your doctor know about it. Some may be harmful, especially if you are undergoing another treatment under your doctor's direction.

To learn more about complementary/alternative medicine, contact the National Center for Complementary and Alternative Medicine Clearinghouse to locate a source of reliable information on the practice you are considering (see Appendix D).

How to Use Complementary/Alternative Medicine Wisely and Well

- Try to learn everything you can about the particular therapy you are interested in. Your local library and the Internet both have substantial materials on complementary/alternative medicine.

- Discuss your plans with your doctor. You might gain some insight into the therapy in terms of its possible risks. Furthermore, if you are currently under medical treatment, you should make certain that the two approaches will not conflict in some way.

- If you start an alternative therapy and it does not appear to be providing relief, or worse, seems to be worsening the condition, contact your doctor immediately.

In the *New England Journal of Medicine* study, 72 percent of the respondents who used unconventional therapies did not inform their medical doctor that they had done so.

Clinical Trials: Should You Participate?

Each year, more than half a million Americans, some of them sick, but even more of them healthy, volunteer to take part in experimental trials of new drugs and therapies. Before drugs, vaccines, biological agents and medical devices are made available for general use by doctors and their patients, they must go through extensive testing on animals and humans called "clinical trials." There is probably at least one clinical trial in process at some medical center for almost every serious disease.

On the plus side, a clinical trial offers the opportunity for prompt use of a drug or other treatment that seems promising, and comes with the bonus of regular and thorough medical examinations at no cost to you (some trials even make allowances for participants' travel and other expenses). Moreover, patients are encouraged to discuss all of their experiences regarding the trial. You will probably learn more about your condition and feel more in control, which can have a very positive effect. On the downside, you may be giving up standard treatment for something that may or may not be better. There is even the possibility that you will not get a drug at all, because most trials are conducted by the double-blind method, in which half of the participants get the drug and half get a placebo, or "dummy" medicine. Even the doctors conducting the trials do not know who is getting which.

What to Know Before You Get Involved

If you are considering participating in a clinical trial, you will want to know:

- Who is the sponsor? Look for a federal government, major health organization, drug company or university-sponsored trial.

- Do any impartial authorities monitor the trial? Every hospital conducting research has an institutional review board (IRB) consisting of medical professionals and community leaders who approve that hospital's participation. There are also data and safety monitoring boards that oversee trials.

- What is the financial relationship, if any, between the doctor, hospital and the company or agency sponsoring the trial?

- Will there be pain or discomfort? Will diagnostic tests be involved? Get detailed answers to these concerns before you sign any form.

- How often will I be examined? This depends on the guidelines of the trial (called the protocol). You should make every effort to keep your appointments.

- Does my own doctor get a record of my participation in the trial? Routine health information is sent to your doctor, but details relevant to a "blinded" trial are not disclosed until the trial is over.

- Is the drug in this trial approved for treatment of any other disorder? If the answer is yes, you then know that the drug has a prior safety record.

- After the study has ended, if I have responded well to the drug, will I be able to continue using it, even before it is approved?

- Can I drop out?

If you are interested in participating in a clinical trial, make your desire known to your doctor, who can track down openings in trials being conducted by medical centers, private foundations, drug companies, physician groups and the federal government. You can also access information on clinical trials by visiting the CenterWatch Clinical Trials Listing Service at www.centerwatch.com or the website of the National Cancer Institute at www.cancer.gov/clinical_trials/.

Chapter 5

Changing Your Doctor

Key Terms: Chapter 5

NATIONAL PRACTITIONER DATA BANK

A computerized listing, created in 1986 by an Act of Congress, to track health professionals who are disciplined for unprofessional behavior and to deter them from simply moving their practices from one state to another.

PUBLIC CITIZENS' HEALTH RESEARCH GROUP

A Washington, D.C. based consumer advocacy group that has been publicly critical of many medical practices that the group considers detrimental to public healthcare.

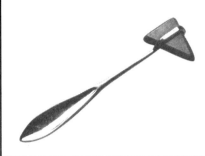

Quick Tips

35. In many cases, insurance companies will pay for second opinions, but check ahead of time to make sure your insurance plan does cover them.

36. One way HMOs control costs is by limiting second opinions.

37. Doctors may have different solutions to the same problem—and any one or more could work.

38. Surgical solutions can rarely be reversed. It usually is best to try a non-surgical solution first, if possible.

39. You should always consider the possibility that alternative therapies, simply because they are unproven, may do more harm than good.

40. If you do explore alternative therapies, be certain to let your doctor know about it. Some may be harmful, especially if you are undergoing another treatment under your doctor's direction.

41. Before you decide to part company with your doctor, ask yourself if you've been a responsible patient.

42. A doctor-patient relationship is like a marriage—both sides have to work to make it successful.

43. Expressing your dissatisfaction may open the communication lines between you and your doctor. You might even end up in a better relationship with your present doctor.

44. Unless the situation is intolerable or the doctor is impaired, stay with your current doctor until you have found another one that you like.

45. When changing doctors you may have to sign a release with your new doctor approving the transfer of all your medical records to the new office. These records cannot be withheld for any reason, even if you have not yet paid your last bill.

Quick Take

... There's a big difference between doctor-hopping and changing doctors for a good reason. Most failed doctor-patient relationships can be attributed to some common complaints but sometimes it is a matter of self-defense...

Chapter 5
Changing Your Doctor

Obviously, at times there are good reasons for changing doctors. Some are very simple and straightforward, such as a doctor's retirement, illness or death, your own relocation or a change in your health plan. About 40 percent of people enrolling in managed care plans have to change their doctor to one who is affiliated with the plan.

The onset of a chronic condition may also prompt a change to a different medical specialist, such as a rheumatologist or cardiologist, if a condition needs to be managed by a specialist other than a primary care doctor.

If you have continuing symptoms that your doctor has been unable to diagnose or if, after a diagnosis, your problems continue to linger without improvement, you should at least consider getting a second opinion and, depending on that opinion, possibly changing doctors. Doctors often have different approaches to the same problem. A different doctor may offer a different perspective and, perhaps, a solution.

You might also change doctors in order to find one who includes complementary/alternative medicine in the treatment or to find one who can help you enroll in a clinical trial.

People who have hostile feelings toward organized medicine tend to change doctors frequently; their complaints then become a self-fulfilling prophecy. They don't get continuous, quality care because it's impossible for anyone to deliver it. On the other hand, negative feelings may be prompted by unfortunate encounters with incompetent doctors or by the patronizing or otherwise inappropriate attitudes expressed by some doctors toward patients. Patients on the receiving end of such a relationship should continue their search for a doctor who better meets their needs.

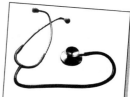

Eight Reasons to Say Goodbye

Here are the eight most common complaints about "doctors I don't go to anymore."

Poor Bedside Manner

Good medical care is more than diagnosis and treatment; it's also an attitude on the part of the doctor that sparks a sense of trust in the patient. Being under the care of a doctor who is impersonal, abrupt, bored, arrogant, condescending or sarcastic may, in the end, be counterproductive.

The National Practitioner Data Bank contains the names of more than 170,000 health practitioners who have either a licensing action or malpractice judgment or settlement against them. You can write directly to the National Practitioner Data Bank if you wish more information.

The doctor's aloofness could have a more serious explanation: substance abuse or psychological impairment, which, according to a recent American Medical Association report, affect 30,000 to 40,000 physicians. Mood swings and detachment are signs to watch for.

Too Vague and Evasive

A doctor who dismisses problems with "it's nothing to worry about" or "let me take care of it" or who uses medical jargon isn't interested in having you as a partner in your healthcare. The effect of this evasiveness can be anger, fear and confusion, leading to failure to follow directions and failure of treatment.

Never on Schedule

Medical emergencies can make appointment scheduling an inexact science, but when snafus become chronic, it's a sign of trouble. An explanation can ease the frustration, but make-up time should not be at your expense.

Couldn't Diagnose the Problem

Some conditions can't be diagnosed on-the-spot. Others aren't attributable to one specific cause. That doesn't excuse an incomplete workup, however, which may leave you with a condition that could have been treated earlier.

Ordered Too Many Tests

Sophisticated technology is available and doctors tend to use it, although some testing may not be necessary. The number of tests performed for diagnosis seems to be reduced in patient-doctor relationships where communication is strong.

Discouraged Second Opinions

A doctor who dissuades you from talking to another doctor may perceive it as questioning his or her professional abilities.

Didn't Protect My Medical Privacy

No patient should have to discuss the reason for a visit, payment or payment problems within earshot of other patients or staff.

Under certain conditions, medical records can be requested by and turned over to insurance companies, lawyers, employers and certain others without your consent, but you can certainly see them, too, to make sure they contain the proper information. In all 50 states and the District of Columbia, federal law grants patients access to their medical records.

Unpleasant Office Staff

Repeated incidents such as rudeness over the telephone, a brusque physician's assistant or being kept waiting in an examining room for a long time before the doctor shows up are all annoying indications that a staff could do better.

The staff takes its cues from the chief. A doctor who doesn't demand the highest level of performance from a staff may be sending a message about his or her own laxity in diagnosis and treatment.

Should You Switch?

If these conditions exist in your doctor-patient relationship, it may be time to consider finding a new doctor. But before you decide to part company with your doctor, ask yourself if you've been a responsible patient. Often problems arise when patients don't reveal their full medical history or if they forget to alert their doctor about other drugs they are taking. A doctor-patient relationship is like a marriage—both sides have to work to make it successful.

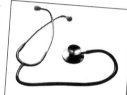

If you're sure the problem isn't on your side, however, confront your doctor with your grievances. Or if it's easier for you, you may want to write them in a letter. Expressing your dissatisfaction may open the communication lines between you and your doctor. You might even end up in a better relationship with your present doctor. Sometimes doctors aren't aware that they are in the midst of a deteriorating relationship until a patient wants to leave.

In all 50 states and the District of Columbia, federal law grants patients access to their medical records.

But if you are still unhappy with your doctor and you've decided a change is necessary, you can make a clean break by simply going to another doctor. Keep in mind, however, that your most important concern should be continuity of care. So, unless the situation is intolerable or the doctor is impaired, stay with your current doctor until you have found another one that you like.

Generally, medical records are kept by your doctor until you have found a new one. You will then have to sign a release with your new doctor approving the transfer of all your medical records to the new office. These records cannot be withheld for any reason, even if you have not yet paid your last bill.

Finally, don't feel embarrassed or guilty if you decide to change doctors. Remember, good quality medical care is your right!

Self Defense: Avoiding Questionable Doctors

In addition to finding good doctors, you also want to be able to identify and avoid doctors who have a history of professional problems. One way to do this is to make certain a doctor has not been disciplined by your state or, in fact, any state. You can call the appropriate state agency (listed in Appendix E) or check the websites of those state agencies that make this information available. These sites list the names of doctors who have been disciplined by their state or by the federal government. The disciplinary actions were taken for a variety of reasons, including overprescribing or misprescribing medications, criminal convictions, alcohol or drug abuse and patient sexual abuse.

You also may visit the 'Vital Healthcare Info' section of the Castle Connolly Medical Ltd. website (www.CastleConnolly.com) for links to those states with discipline information on their sites. You may also visit www.docboard.org, a website that lists disciplined doctors, or link to the American Medical Association (AMA) at www.ama-assn.org and American Board of Medical Specialities (ABMS) at www.abms.org. For the websites for biographical information about doctors, including board certification, see Appendix D.

The Public Citizens' Health Research Group, which publishes a report on the number of physicians disciplined in each state, believes that many states are not aggressive enough in monitoring doctors. They have been leading the call for public access to the National Practitioner Data Bank. The Data Bank was created in 1986 by an Act of Congress to track professionals who are disciplined for unprofessional behavior and to deter them from simply moving their practices from one state to another. The Data Bank became operational in 1990 and contains a record of adverse actions such as license removal, loss of clinical privileges and professional society membership actions taken against doctors and other licensed health professionals such as dentists. It contains the names of more than 170,000 health practitioners who have either a licensing action or malpractice judgment or settlement against them. There is strong pressure from some medical groups either to do away with the Data Bank or to place even stricter controls on access to it. They support their position with examples of errors in the handling of sensitive information. It is unlikely that Congress would permit the elimination of the Data Bank, however. In fact, it is possible that at some time in the future, access may be made more available to the public. However, at the present time there is no public access to this information.

A data service used by lawyers to check on a doctor's or hospital's malpractice history is LEXIS/NEXIS, the computerized legal information service. Some libraries will do a LEXIS/NEXIS search for a fee, usually more than $75.00. Public access to the listing of malpractice payments is one issue on which doctors are very sensitive, and rightfully so. Many malpractice payments are made by insurance companies over the objections of doctors because the insurers feel it's cheaper to settle than to fight. Yet, doctors who feel they are blameless contend that these settlements reflect negatively on them. Also, since so many specialists, such as those in obstetrics and gynecology, are subject to more frequent lawsuits because of the nature of their practices, doctors are concerned about how patients will interpret a malpractice settlement. A few states, for example Massachussetts, make this information available on the State Health Department website. Check to see if it is available in your state. (See Vital Healthcare Information on the Castle Connolly Medical Ltd website (www.CastleConnolly.com.)

People who believe they have a problem with a doctor, whether in regard to fees, treatment or ethics, may contact the appropriate local medical society in the county in which the doctor practices or the state medical society. State health departments are also resources consumers may turn to for assistance or information on disciplinary actions taken against doctors. The health department, typically, will only divulge that an action has been taken but will not give you any specific information about it (See Appendix E for phone numbers and addresses).

Changing your doctor should not be considered a setback in your search for the best doctor to meet your needs. As you may have come to understand throughout preceding chapters in this book, the personal and treatment styles doctors bring to their practices vary greatly. What is important for you, as a patient, to realize is that these subtle and immeasurable characteristics can be as important as clinical skills. There is, in fact, substantial empirical and anecdotal evidence demonstrating that confidence in the healer and the healing process plays a major role in many cures. Your main objective is to find the therapy—in combination with the professional who is providing the therapy—that works best for you.

In one case involving a woman in her mid-thirties, the doctor-patient relationship was severed over what was basically a conflict in personalities: the woman wished to have more control over her healthcare, and the doctor was reluctant to give it. The impasse was reached before the two could attempt any kind of a compromise, and the woman went off in search of a doctor who would better suit her personal needs. A year later, after a fruitless search for a doctor whose medical expertise she respected, she returned to her original doctor.

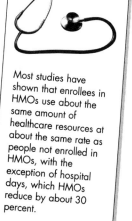

Most studies have shown that enrollees in HMOs use about the same amount of healthcare resources at about the same rate as people not enrolled in HMOs, with the exception of hospital days, which HMOs reduce by about 30 percent.

Chapter 6

Choosing a Doctor in an HMO

Key Terms: Chapter 6

CAPITATION
A method of payment to physicians and other healthcare providers whereby a fixed amount of money is allotted for each patient served.

EPO
An Exclusive Provider Organization is similar to a PPO except the patients must use only providers in the EPO.

GROUP MODEL HMO
A model of an HMO in which the HMO contracts with large multi-specialty groups of doctors to provide care, usually from a number of central locations.

HEALTH MAINTENANCE ORGANIZATION (HMO)
One type of managed care organization that provides for a wide range of comprehensive healthcare services for its members in return for a fixed, predetermined fee. The care is provided by a network or group of physicians affiliated with the organization and possibly other healthcare professionals.

IPA
An Independent Practice Association is one model of health maintenance organization (HMO) in which the organization contracts with individual doctors, or groups of doctors, to provide care for the enrolled patients in the doctors' own offices.

PHO
A Physician Hospital Organization is an organization of a hospital and its physicians that may contract with managed care organizations (MCO) or may become licensed as an MCO itself.

PPO
A Preferred Provider Organization is a managed care model that offers healthcare provided by a group of doctors and/or hospitals that have negotiated discounted rates, either capitated or fee-for-service, for enrollees while continuing to provide care for other patients. Patients typically pay less if they use the PPO provider.

PSO
A Provider Service Organization, sometimes called a provider service network (PSN), is a group of doctors that are organized to provide care to a large number of patients, typically under contract to managed care organizations.

STAFF MODEL HMO
A managed care model where the HMO employs the doctors, usually on salary. Care is provided out of a number of centralized locations.

Quick Tips

46. A data service used by lawyers to check on a doctor's or hospital's malpractice history is LEXIS/NEXIS, the computerized legal information service. LEXIS will do a search and issue a report on any malpractice awards or settlements ordered by a court.

47. State health departments are also places consumers may turn to for assistance or information on disciplinary actions taken against doctors.

48. There is substantial empirical and anecdotal evidence demonstrating that confidence in the healer and the healing process plays a major role in many cures.

49. People who believe they have a problem with a doctor, whether in regard to fees, treatment, or ethics, may contact the appropriate local medical society in the county in which the doctor practices, or the state medical society.

50. The main factor to focus on in assessing an HMO is its resources, primarily doctors and hospitals.

51. HMOs may list hundreds of doctors but not all of them are necessarily accessible to all members.

52. When you need a specialist, it is your primary care doctor who will refer you, as in traditional indemnity plans. But, unlike indemnity plans in which you can find a specialist on your own if you choose, in managed care plans you typically must be referred to see a specialist.

Quick Take

...The rules are different but they are not difficult to play by. The first step is to sort out the alphabet soup of models. The model of HMO usually determines how your care will be delivered and often your satisfaction with it...

Chapter 6
Choosing a Doctor in an HMO

At one time only doctors looking for new patients joined HMOs. Today, there is a new reality. Almost *all* doctors—more than 80 percent—participate in some kind of managed care arrangement. So it is likely that you will find the best for your own care if you know how to work the system.

When managed care achieves a significant market penetration and begins to control the flow of large numbers of patients, more doctors sign on. Also, many hospitals encourage their doctors to sign on with as many different plans as possible in order to ensure that the hospital does not lose any potential patients. Managed care now enrolls more than one out of every three people in the country, and more than 80 percent of workers who get health insurance through their employer are in some form of managed care. Today, more people are enrolled in PPOs (Preferred Provider Organization), which tend to be more flexible in choices of physicians, than are enrolled in HMOs. However, we will use HMO as "shorthand" for both.

The main factor to focus on in assessing an HMO or a PPO is its resources, primarily doctors and hospitals. First, is there an ample selection of primary care doctors near where you live and work? Second, are the doctors well qualified? This can be answered by following the approach outlined in this book for finding the best doctors. When choosing doctors, it is usually a good idea to call their offices to confirm they are still affiliated with the particular plan. Doctors frequently change affiliations with managed care plans. Also, it is a good idea to check on the procedure for using the doctor listed.

HMOs may list hundreds of doctors but not all of them are necessarily accessible to all members. A large HMO, for example, may restrict the number of specialists that primary care doctors can refer to for various reasons, including location, hospital capacity, and general resource allocation. So although you may see the name of an ophthalmologist, gynecologist, or other specialist you want to use, and indeed that doctor may be affiliated with the HMO, it does not necessarily follow that your primary care doctor is free to refer you to them. Those specialists may see HMO patients only on a certain basis—for specific procedures, for example, or in a certain geographic region—and then possibly only after a rigorous screening process. These possibilities illustrate the varying styles of operation you will find in managed care plans.

Doctors in HMOs are bound by the same professional ethics that guide all doctors. However, there is a major difference; in an HMO, the plan is responsible for providing you with care as well as with a doctor. If your doctor leaves the plan, you don't follow him or her. The plan provides a new doctor for you.

Selecting Doctors in an HMO

Selecting a doctor in an HMO can be a greater challenge than selecting one when you have indemnity insurance that leaves you free to select a doctor without the restrictions of the plan. Obviously, in an HMO arrangement you need to select a doctor who belongs to that plan. Studies have shown that about 40 percent of enrollees in managed care plans have to choose a new doctor when they join. However, even in a plan of small size, you will usually have the option of choosing among a number of primary care doctors as well as other specialists and subspecialists. In doing so, utilize the same criteria you would apply to selecting a doctor in a fee-for-service practice.

The first doctor you select in an HMO plan is your primary care doctor. Typically, you will be sent a list with little information other than the doctor's name, specialty, and address. *Find out more about those doctors you may be considering.* Use the process described earlier in this book. If you make a selection and are not satisfied, request a change. Ask about the procedure for changing doctors before you join the plan.

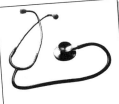

Typically a member will pay an additional 20 - 30 percent more of the total cost to go "out-of-network."

When you need a specialist, it is your primary care doctor who will refer you, as in traditional indemnity plans. But, unlike indemnity plans in which you can find a specialist on your own if you choose, in managed care plans you must be referred to see a specialist. Again, your choices will be limited in selecting specialists, but be assertive. Ask for a choice of doctors and ask why your primary care doctor recommends a particular specialist. One disadvantage to the IPA model and the network referral process is that primary care doctors can end up making referrals to specialists and/or subspecialists they do not know. This may result in poor communication between the primary care doctor and the specialist, which is not in the patient's best interest. If you are not satisfied with the choices offered, ask to go outside the plan. Choice of providers outside a plan is built into certain managed care plans (PPOs or POS, Point of Service) and is permitted in many others under certain conditions.

However, if you do not have a choice, or if the choices are not ones with which you agree, consider going outside the HMO. Although you are likely to have to pay more, it may be worth it if you get a correct diagnosis and appropriate treatment for your problem. In some cases, the HMO will agree to pay at least a consultation fee if you feel strongly that you need to discuss your problem with another doctor outside the HMO network. After the consultation, if you still feel the need for a different doctor, at least your choice will be based on more complete information.

One of the most popular plans offered by HMOs permits going outside of the network of doctors and hospitals—but at an added cost. The point of service, or POS plan, one of the fastest growing offerings of many HMOs, permits the HMO member to use doctors, hospitals, and other services that are not part of the HMO network. Typically, the member will pay an additional fee for this choice—for example, 20 percent or 30 percent of the cost—whereas if the member stays "in-network" the HMO will pay all or close to all of the cost.

When leaving the network of a POS, however, patients should find out exactly how much it will cost to do so. Some HMOs will pay a percentage of "usual and customary fees" while others will pay a percentage of their own fee schedule, which is usually lower.

HMO Models

Although a large alphabet soup of HMO models has appeared since the big move toward managed care began in the late 1980s, and we now have PPOs, PSOs, and EPOs, two models are most important to the healthcare consumer. One is the staff or group model where patients visit their doctors in a single, or perhaps in a few, locations and where all the doctors and most, if not all, diagnostic and treatment facilities are located. The second is the independent practice association or IPA model where doctors see patients in their private offices. Organizations such as PPOs, EPOs and PSOs tend to be organized on the IPA model.

Whether a group/staff model or an IPA, all HMOs require a primary care physician and all have certain protocols, usually involving referral by the primary care physician, to access a specialist.

Doctor Compensation

There is virtually no difference in the types of doctors who practice in the two HMO models and each should be evaluated in terms of benefits to the individual patient. There is, however, a separate matter of how doctors in HMOs are compensated, and this issue has become a major concern to both patients and doctors.

HMOs compensate doctors in a number of ways. Doctors who are employed by staff model HMOs are usually on salary, perhaps with a quality bonus based on patient satisfaction. In group model HMOs the physician group has a contract with the HMO and the doctors are employed by the group, usually on salary and, again, often with a quality bonus.

In the IPA model HMOs, or in PPOs, EPOs, PSOs and other types of managed care organizations, the doctors are usually paid in one of two ways. In the past, the predominant payment method was a negotiated fee schedule, typically designed at some discount to the doctor's normal fee. Doctors simply traded the promise of higher volume for a reduced fee. Today, a major method of payment in an IPA is capitation. While this is fast becoming the most common method of payment in IPAs it is also the one generating the most controversy.

Under a capitated or capitation system doctors are paid a set amount per month or per year to provide care to a patient during that time period. So, for example, a primary care physician may be paid $25 per member per month.

HMOs have moved toward capitation as a method of payment because they found that discounted fee-for-service payment methods did not reduce costs as much as had been hoped, if at all. To make up for discounted fees of 20 percent, for instance, some doctors simply scheduled 20 percent more patient visits so that their incomes would not decrease. Doctors openly comment that discounted fees translate to discounted time with patients!

Capitation has helped to control costs. However, it also has introduced a number of important ethical issues for doctors, other healthcare providers, and for patients. Many are troubled by the notion that a doctor could be placed in a situation that appears to promise rewards for *not* providing care. It is generally recognized that under a fee-for-service system doctors have an incentive to provide more care, even if it is not necessary, because they are paid by the amount of care they deliver. But the reverse is not accepted in such a benign fashion: the concept of a doctor being rewarded to provide *less* care is of major concern to many people, including many doctors.

Another technique involved in payment systems utilized by managed care companies is called "withholds" or "set-asides." This method is also used to motivate doctors to control costs and, as in capitation, raises similar ethical concerns. Under this method, for example, a group of pediatricians is contracted to care for 1,000 children. That contract is based on a budget of $15,000 a month. A certain amount of that budget, say 20 percent, is reserved for referrals to subspecialists and another 20 percent is set aside or withheld. If the group of doctors uses fewer subspecialist referrals than budgeted they receive the 20 percent that was set aside. If they use more subspecialist referrals than were budgeted the extra amount comes out of the set-aside. The more set-aside that is used for referrals, the less doctors will be able to receive from it.

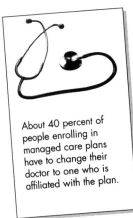

About 40 percent of people enrolling in managed care plans have to change their doctor to one who is affiliated with the plan.

A great deal of controversy has ensued over these payment mechanisms. Some states, in fact, are legislating to prohibit or restrict these practices. Individual "horror stories" of patients who have been denied appropriate care, such as not being referred to a subspecialist in a timely manner, have been used to demonstrate the issue in human terms.

Some studies demonstrate that when physician-run health plans are paid by capitation and are in control they reduce costs more substantially than other plans. Some doctors strongly support capitation. They believe it makes them, rather than managers, responsible for allocating resources and making medical decisions.

And, despite the outcry, most of the studies of HMO patients versus non-HMO patients demonstrate no differences in their health status.

In fact, there is a substantial body of research suggesting that HMO members receive more in the way of preventive services than do non-HMO populations.

If method of payment is an issue of concern to you, it may be wise to ask your doctor about the method of compensation in the HMO in which you are enrolled. If you believe the method would work against you as a patient, you should discuss it with your doctor and ask if and how it influences the manner of care for patients. If you are not satisfied by the answer, you may want to change doctors or, better yet, change HMOs, if possible.

While the wisest course of action is to ask about this issue before joining an HMO, rather than after you have become a member, most HMO members have not done this. If you believe you are not receiving appropriate care because of an HMO policy, you can contact your state health insurance department (see Appendix E).

In response to patient and physician concerns about payment policies, groups of doctors in various parts of the country have formed organizations to receive and investigate complaints against HMOs. You can contact them with any grievances you have about your HMO (see Physicians Who Care, Appendix D).

How Doctors and Patients Feel About Managed Care

People enrolled in HMOs tend to like them. However, most doctors do not like managed care—and understandably so! Managed care organizations negotiate deep discounts in fees for doctors. There is no reason doctors should prefer this process, but when managed care controls so many patients there is little choice but to join managed care and negotiate.

Managed care organizations also require doctors to do a substantial amount of paperwork and to follow policies and procedures that control costs and monitor quality. All of this creates a level of business management most doctors resent.

At least a portion of these negative attitudes toward managed care can be ascribed to differences in the organization of medical practices in different parts of the country.

The Northeast, South, and Southwest regions have been the slowest to accept managed care because doctors generally resisted it more strongly than those in other parts of the country. Doctors in large group practices, which are more common in the far west and midwest than in the east, adapted to managed care more readily. In the northeast, where doctors practice solo or in small groups, the change has been greater and the adjustment more difficult.

Most doctors have adapted and learned to practice successfully in this new medical environment. According to a survey conducted by the American Medical Association, just over a third (210,811) of physicians in this country are now members of group practices. In 1995 group practices numbered 19,788, an increase of 361 percent since 1965. From 1991 to 1995, the number of groups increased by 16.4 percent and the number of group physicians by 14.3 percent.

The survey shows that, in an environment that is organizationally complex, medical groups have changed how they are organized legally, with partnerships declining to 13.8 percent and professional corporations increasing to 77.9 percent. In the latter group, control of decision making remains largely in physician hands. This ability to retain decision making power has dramatically altered physicians' attitudes towards managed care.

The view of patients and the public, however, is decidedly more positive about managed care.

A study sponsored by the Medstat Group, J.D. Power and Associates and the New England Medical Center reported that in 20 markets across the United States, HMOs received more top scores than PPOs and fee-for-service plans.

The study asked plan members to assess their health plans on choice of providers, physician care, premiums and deductibles and access to care. HMOs topped fee-for-service and point-of-service plans in more than half the markets.

One of the findings uncovered in a Louis Harris Associates poll of consumers was that the majority surveyed, 59 percent, believed the trend toward managed care was a good thing as compared to 28 percent who viewed it as a bad thing. Also, 48 percent as compared to 39 percent believed managed care would improve quality, and 59 percent versus 30 percent believed it would help contain the costs of care. Of note was that the response of those people in communities with a high penetration by managed care tended to be the most positive!

There are many studies that have examined the quality of care and the satisfaction of patients in managed care settings. Most show that members of HMOs and other managed care organizations are at least as satisfied or more satisfied with their care than people covered by indemnity insurance. Some studies have shown indemnity-covered people are more satisfied, particularly when it relates to choice of doctors. In fact, the issue of greatest concern to HMO enrollees is usually access, particularly to specialists. Advocates of either view can point to studies to support managed care or to criticize it. The key may lie in the studies that have demonstrated that when individuals have a choice, and select a managed care plan, they tend to be more satisfied than those who have no choice.

In terms of quality the conclusion is similar. While critics may contend that the care delivered by managed care organizations is not adequate, and a study of Medicaid patients is frequently cited to support this view, the overwhelming majority of studies demonstrate no difference in health status and quality of care between those people covered by managed care plans and those covered by indemnity insurance.

The variability in the results of all of the studies on quality and satisfaction in managed care reinforces the important premise that, as there are good doctors and poor doctors, there are good HMOs and poor HMOs. It is important for consumers to know how to discern the difference and to put some effort, however modest, into finding the best.

Points to Remember

- To summarize, there is basically no difference in quality between doctors in HMOs and those in private practice. You can find excellent doctors if you're a member of an HMO and you can find poor ones, just as you can find excellent and poor doctors if you carry indemnity insurance. The key is making sure that you find the best available for your own needs and the needs of your family.

Some simple guidelines to remember:

- Review the credentials and training of *any* doctor who cares for you.

- Make certain a doctor you select is taking new patients and the waiting period for an appointment is not unreasonable.

- Be sure the HMO has a sufficient number of specialists and subspecialists you may need to see and that they are of high quality. For example, if you have diabetes, you will want to make sure that the HMO has endocrinologists on staff or as part of its network. If you have coronary heart disease, you will want to make sure that the HMO has first rate cardiologists and an arrangement with an outstanding center where the doctors perform invasive and non-invasive diagnostic techniques and which has a good record for open heart surgery.

- Determine beforehand the HMO's policy for patient referral to subspecialists, especially whether you will have a choice and how it may be exercised.

- Inquire about the rules for changing doctors in the HMO if you are not satisfied with your initial choice. You will want to know not only the procedure but how often such change is allowed.

- Ask about your options to go out of network and what your additional percentage of payment will be if you exercise this option. In determining what percentage the HMO pays, try to find out whether their payment is based on the HMO fee scale or "usual and customary" fees.

- Ask your doctor about the HMO's compensation system. You want to be sure that the system for paying your doctor will not have a negative influence on your care.

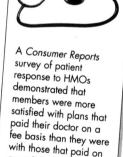

A Consumer Reports survey of patient response to HMOs demonstrated that members were more satisfied with plans that paid their doctor on a fee basis than they were with those that paid on a capitated, or per person, basis.

Quick Tips

53. When leaving the network in a POS plan, patients should find out exactly how much it will cost to do so.

54. When choosing doctors, it is usually a good idea to call their offices to confirm that they are still affiliated with the particular plan.

55. When choosing a doctor in an HMO, use the same criteria you would apply to selecting a doctor in a fee-for-service practice.

56. Typically, you will be sent a list with little information other than the doctor's name, specialty, and address. Find out more about those doctors you may be considering.

57. In some cases, an HMO will agree to pay at least a consultation fee if you feel strongly that you need to discuss your problem with another doctor outside the HMO network.

58. If method of HMO payment to physicians is an issue of concern to you, it may be wise to ask your doctor about the method of compensation in the HMO in which you are enrolled.

59. If you believe you are not receiving appropriate care because of an HMO policy you can contact your state health or insurance department.

60. People in communities with a high penetration by managed care tended to be the most positive about it.

61. The issue of greatest concern to HMO enrollees is usually access, particularly to specialists.

62. The variability in the results of all of the studies on quality and satisfaction in managed care reinforces the important premise that as there are good doctors and poor doctors, there are good HMOs and poor HMOs.

Section Two

How to Use the Directory of Doctors

Includes
Partnership for Excellence
Program

How to Use the Directory of Doctors

Castle Connolly Medical Ltd. provides healthcare consumers with an invaluable source of information to identify leading physicians in their own community. This tenth edition of the Castle Connolly Guide, *Top Doctors: New York Metro Area*, contains vital information on more than 6,000 of the finest doctors in the region. Our guides are the result of a methodical process requiring a complete credential, licensing and disciplinary review of all doctors nominated for inclusion in the guide.

Why This Book Is Your Best Guide

Top Doctors is unique in a number of ways. The first edition of the Guide, published in 1994, was the first selective directory of doctors who practice in the New York metropolitan region. Castle Connolly recognizes that most healthcare is provided locally and people generally obtain their healthcare where they live or work. Therefore, by identifying excellent, caring physicians in every community and in every hospital, we apprise consumers of the best healthcare available to them within their own communities. Healthcare consumers in the New York metropolitan region are very fortunate in the abundance of doctors—approximately 55,000—who practice in the area. On the other hand, making a selection of one out of such a multitude can be a daunting task; it's hard even to know where to start. With *Top Doctors: New York Metro Area* in hand, you are already well on your way to finding the very best doctor for your individual needs and the needs of your family members.

With the profusion of outstanding academic medical centers, tertiary care teaching hospitals and fine regional hospitals in the New York metropolitan area, virtually any medical procedure or treatment can be found close to home. By virtue of this fact, it would be a simple matter to compile a book identifying the outstanding leaders in medical research and academic medicine in the region. Although many of these doctors are included in the listings, their names are to be found among the many excellent and caring doctors who deliver outstanding patient care in every community in the area. The goal—first and foremost—is to help you find the best doctors to meet your healthcare needs where you live and work. Again, a good reason why the Castle Connolly Guide is exceptional.

Further, the Castle Connolly Guide is different from most other listings of doctors in its selection process. Our selection is predicated on an extensive nomination procedure and a set of exacting standards which each nominated doctor was required to meet. To you, this means that the basis for inclusion of every one of the doctors in the listings was twofold: respect of their peers and medical excellence. Doctors do not pay to be listed. Our goal is to serve consumers, not doctors, hospitals or health plans.

How Castle Connolly Selects the Top Doctors

The basis of the Castle Connolly selection process is peer nomination. In some ways, this resembles an enhancement of the process in which a personal physician provides a patient with a referral to another physician for a particular problem. However, if the recommendation of one doctor is good, the recommendation of many doctors is even better. So, we ask thousands of randomly selected physicians in the New York metropolitan area for their nominations.

How do we accomplish this enormous task? Over the years, the Castle Connolly physician-directed research team developed its extensive database of physicians through periodic mail, telephone and email surveys in the following counties:

New York State: New York (Manhattan), Bronx, Kings (Brooklyn), Queens, Richmond, Nassau, Suffolk, Rockland, Westchester

New Jersey: Bergen, Essex, Hudson, Mercer, Middlesex, Monmouth, Morris, Passaic, Somerset, Union

Connecticut: Fairfield, New Haven

This cumulative database is systematically maintained and continuously updated. Surveyed physicians nominate top doctors in both their own and related specialties—especially those to whom they would refer their patients and their own family members. The database is also updated through further mail and telephone surveys. Each year we build on our prior research and supplement our database by inviting leading physicians at major medical centers in the metropolitan area, the thousands of top doctors included in earlier editions of our guide, and local leaders in the various medical specialties to offer their nominations for *Top Doctors: New York Metro Area.*

In addition to nominations obtained directly from practicing physicians, Castle Connolly solicits nominations from each area hospital's:

- President or Chief Executive Officer
- Vice President of Medical Affairs or the equivalent position
- Chief of Service in:
  - Anesthesiology
  - Medicine
  - Neurology
  - Obstetrics/Gynecology
  - Pathology
  - Pediatrics
  - Radiology
  - Surgery

Considerations for Inclusion Among the Top Doctors

Castle Connolly considers the following among the varied criteria used to determine physician eligibility for inclusion in our guides.

Professional Qualifications

- Education
- Residency
- Board certification
- Fellowships

- Professional reputation
- Hospital appointment
- Medical school faculty appointment
- Experience
- Disciplinary history

Personal Characteristics/Qualities

Not only do we seek nominations of physicians who excel in academic medicine and research, but most importantly, those who exhibit excellence in patient care. We ask physicians in our survey to consider not only the training and clinical skills of the physicians they nominate, but also interpersonal skills such as the following:

- Listening and communicating effectively
- Demonstrating empathy
- Educating and informing
- Instilling trust and confidence

Verification/Credential Review

The Castle Connolly research staff reviews and refines the pool of nominated physicians in a region, validates nominations, and verifies credentials. This results in the development of a preliminary list of physicians. Each provisionally selected physician is then required to complete a comprehensive professional biographical form including their special practice interests (see the "SPECIAL EXPERTISE INDEX"). The information contained in the biographical form becomes an integral part of each selected physician's listing in the guide.

The last phase of the process refines the list of provisionally selected doctors by cross-referencing their names against a variety of databases providing confirmation of:

- Board certification and recertification
- Licensing
- Disciplinary history

In some regions, a small number of peer-nominated physicians who are not board-certified may be included in a guide. These are doctors recognized by their colleagues as having exceptional demonstrated clinical practice experience.

Physicians ultimately selected for inclusion in *Top Doctors: New York Metro Area* receive formal notification of their nomination for listing upon completion of the final confirmation of their professional credentials.

How You Can Select the Top Doctors

How can you begin to make a choice from such a compilation of names? There is, in fact, a basic step-by-step process which varies somewhat depending on your individual needs as you approach the list. Here are the possibilities:

One: If You Are Looking for a Doctor in a Particular County

The key: Physicians listed in the following pages are organized under the county in which their office is located so that you can go directly to the section listing doctors in your county of residence.

Key fact: Like most healthcare consumers, you probably receive your healthcare locally. If you think about it, you usually have been treated by doctors close to where you live and in community hospitals. If necessary, you may be referred to regional specialists and nearby medical centers.

Two: If You Are Looking for a Primary Care Physician— a Generalist

The key: The doctors who practice predominantly primary care, in the specialties of internal medicine, family practice, pediatrics, and obstetrics/gynecology, are designated by the notation **PCP** in the listing.

Key fact: Every board certified physician is a specialist. The term "having boards" signifies that a physician has completed an approved residency in a given specialty and has passed a rigorous examination given by that particular board. Therefore, doctors who practice primary care—internists, family practitioners, pediatricians, and ob/gyns—are specialists in their respective fields, as are urologists, otolaryngologists, and radiologists. These specialists are considered primary care physicians.

Three: If You Are Looking for a Physician in a Particular Specialty

The key: Each entry contains the specialty practiced by the doctor and, in most cases, the most recent year of board certification.

Key fact: Many physicians specialize in fields of medicine that are not primary care. These specialists have completed an approved residency in a given specialty and have passed a rigorous exam given by that specialty board. For example, some physicians are board certified in psychiatry, surgery, allergy and immunology, or dermatology.

Many doctors choose to specialize further. They choose an additional training program called a fellowship and upon completion of the program, they are required to take another exam in order to be certified as a subspecialist. An example of such subspecialization is an internist (initially board certified in internal medicine) who subspecialize in nephrology or cardiology. This doctor would be termed "double boarded" and would very likely practice nephrology or cardiology rather than internal medicine as a primary care physician.

Four: If You Are Looking for a Doctor with Expertise in a Particular Disease or Technique

The key: Particular skills and interests of the doctors are found under the heading "SPECIAL EXPERTISE INDEX."

Key fact: A physician may have a special expertise interest in a particular field of medicine without actually being board certified in that area. Special expertise interests should not be confused with a board certified medical specialty. For example, cosmetic surgery is not an American Board of Medical Specialties recognized specialty, but it may constitute a major practice activity for many plastic surgeons. Certain doctors may develop a reputation as "specialists" in AIDS, diabetes or arthroscopic surgery. None of these are recognized medical specialties, yet they are indications of a doctor's expertise in a disease or medical or surgical procedure which may be helpful if you have the disease or need the procedure.

Many doctors who have a strong interest in, or consider themselves "specializing in," a particular health problem or medical technique form special interest groups referred to as "self-designated medical specialties." These groups are often confused with recognized medical specialties, which they are not. Some of the groups would like to be recognized by the ABMS and may even work toward that goal. For example, adolescent medicine was a special interest and self-designated specialty that is now an ABMS recognized subspecialty.

Choosing a doctor with a special practice interest is an additional step to be considered after you have already narrowed your choices to particular specialists and/or subspecialists. The "SPECIAL EXPERTISE INDEX" lists the doctors' special area or areas of expertise and can be particularly useful in identifying physicians who embrace alternative or complementary practices. Self-designated medical specialties are listed in Appendix B.

Five: If You Are Looking for a Doctor by Name

The key: The "ALPHABETICAL LISTING OF DOCTORS" indicates the page on which information on the doctor's credentials can be found. The listing is arranged in last name, first name order.

Key fact: Most people start their search for a doctor through recommendation by family and friends. As a savvy healthcare consumer you realize that such recommendations are often based on personal "chemistry" and may be made by someone who actually knows very little about doctors or healthcare. Therefore, you will want to check the credentials of any recommended doctor and follow the additional recommendations we have outlined in Sections One and Two.

Six: If You Want Detailed Information on a Particular Doctor

The key: Each doctor's listing includes a substantial amount of information about the doctor.

Key fact: Wise choices in healthcare are made by consumers who have gathered as much information as possible about a particular doctor. If a professional information form was not returned by a doctor in time for inclusion in the book, our research staff verified certain major points of information (name, address, telephone, hospital affiliation, and specialty) from public sources and we have included this limited information. Even if a doctor's full credentials are included in this book, it is possible that, since the time of publication, the doctor has moved his or her office(s), changed telephone number(s), joined new medical groups, resigned from or joined hospital staffs, and, especially, changed relationships with HMOs and PPOs. Nonetheless, you can, in most cases, track down the doctor by using the following sources:

- Doctor's office—call the office number listed in the directory and ask for a new number.
- Hospitals—call the hospital listed in the directory and ask for help in locating a particular doctor.
- State Health Department—all state health department numbers are listed in Appendix E.
- American Board of Medical Specialties—a complete listing of ABMS Specialty Boards is found in Appendix A.
- American Osteopathic Association—a complete listing of AOA Specialty Boards is found in Appendix A.

Conclusion

You are now ready to work with our directory of more than 6,000 of the finest doctors in the New York metropolitan area. Although you may be well-informed as a result of reading Sections One and Two of this book, it is possible that choosing the doctor will seem to be a complex endeavor. The tendency might be to try to get the job done as quickly as possible by picking a doctor based solely on the convenience of the office's location. To do so would be a big mistake. You want the best healthcare. You deserve it. A little effort will help you get the best.

There are many excellent doctors in the region not listed in this book. You can identify them by using the process we have described in Sections One and Two or, if a doctor in this book is unable to meet your needs, ask about other physicians that doctor regards highly.

We believe that this book will educate and enlighten you throughout its pages and that it will prove its value in the end—when you decide on the doctor with whom you plan to have a lasting relationship.

Obtaining Additional Doctor Information

You may wish to call a doctor's office to make an appointment or to help determine if the doctor is the one you want to care for you. Here are some questions you may want to ask:

1. Is a referral required?
2. Are you accepting new patients?
3. Which health plans/insurance do you accept?
4. Do you accept Medicare? Medicaid? Workers' compensation? No-fault insurance?
5. Are payments of deductible and co-payments required at the time of appointment?
6. Do you accept credit cards?
7. Do you see patients in the evening? On weekends?
8. Is the office handicapped-accessible?
9. Do you accept phone calls from patients?
10. If you are not comfortable addressing the doctor in English, ask if your native language is spoken by the doctor or by someone else in the office.

Smith, John MD [IM] PCP - *Spec Exp:* *Ulcers; Crohn's Disease;*
Name [specialty] &   Special Expertise(s)
Primary Care Physician symbol

Hospital: NYU Med Ctr (page 130); **Address:** 100 Tenth St, FL 5 - Ste 3A, MC-1234, New York, NY 10010;
admitting hospital(s) &   Office address   Mail code   City, state zip
Hospital Information page(s)

Phone: (904) 296-0000; **Board Cert:** IM 1970, GE 1974; **Med School:** U Fla Coll Med 1966;
Office phone   *Board certification(s) & date(s)   Medical school & year of degree

Resid: IM, NYU Med Ctr 1969; **Fellow:** GE, Lenox Hill Hosp 1972;
Residency(ies) & location(s)   Fellowship(s) & location(s)

Fac Appt: Assoc Clin Prof Med, NYU Sch Med
Faculty appointment & location

* Indicates the most recent date of board certification or recertification.

In our listings of the professional information on doctors, we have abbreviated hospitals and medical schools. The abbreviations are designed to be self-explanatory, but if you need assistance, refer to Appendix C: Hospital Listings.

Note on Special Expertise(s)

These are not medical specialties as described on pages 79-84, but the areas of expertise or practice interests indicated by the doctor.

The information reported in each doctor's listing is, for the most part, provided by the doctor or his/her office staff. Castle Connolly attempts to verify the data through other sources but cannot guarantee that in all cases all data have been so verified or are accurate. All such information is subject to change from time to time due to changes in physician practices. Many doctors participate in several health plans and/or switch plans frequently. Therefore, you should verify with the doctor's office whether your health plan is currently accepted.

Medical Specialties and Subspecialties

In the pages that follow, each list of doctors in a medical specialty or subspecialty is preceded by a brief description of that specialty (or subspecialty) and the training required for board certification.

Critical Care Medicine has been excluded because in emergency situations there is neither time nor opportunity for choice. A number of other specialities not relevant to most patients (e.g., Forensic Psychiatry) have not been included as well.

The following descriptions of medical specialties and subspecialties were provided by the American Board of Medical Specialties (ABMS), an organization comprised of the 24 medical specialty boards that provide certification in 25 medical specialties. A complete listing of all specialists certified by the ABMS can be found in *The Official ABMS Directory of Board Certified Medical Specialists*, is published by *Marquis Who's Who*. It is available (either in a multi-volume directory or on CD-ROM) in most public libraries, hospital libraries, university libraries and medical libraries. The ABMS also operates a toll-free phone line at 1-866-275-2267 and a website at www.abms.org to verify the certification status of individual doctors.

The following important policy statement, approved by the ABMS Assembly on March 19, 1987, remains valid.

The Purpose of Certification

The intent of the certification process, as defined by the member boards of the American Board of Medical Specialties, is to provide assurance to the public that a certified medical specialist has successfully completed an approved educational program and an evaluation, including an examination process designed to assess the knowledge, experience and skills requisite to the provision of high quality patient care in that specialty.

Medical Specialties and Subspecialties

Medical Specialty and Subspecialty Descriptions and Abbreviations

The following medical specialties and subspecialties are indicated in the doctors' listings by their abbreviations. Specialties are indicated in bold, subspecialties in italics, and the four primary care specialties in bold capitals. To review the official American Board of Medical Specialties (ABMS) organization of specialties, refer to Appendix A.

Addiction Psychiatry   *AdP*

Deals with habitual psychological and physiological dependence on a substance or practice which is beyond voluntary control.

Adolescent Medicine   *AM*

Involves the primary care treatment of adolescents and young adults.

Allergy & Immunology   **A&I**

Diagnosis and treatment of allergies, asthma, and skin problems such as hives and contact dermatitis.

Anesthesiology   **Anes**

Provides pain relief in maintenance or restoration of a stable condition during and following an operation. Anesthesiologists also diagnose and treat acute and long standing pain problems.

Cardiac Electrophysiology (Clinical)   *CE*

Involves complicated technical procedures to evaluate heart rhythms and determine appropriate treatment for them.

Cardiovascular Disease   *Cv*

Involves the diagnosis and treatment of disorders of the heart, lungs, and blood vessels.

Child & Adolescent Psychiatry   *ChAP*

Deals with the diagnosis and treatment of mental diseases in children and adolescents.

Child Neurology   *ChiN*

Diagnosis and medical treatment of disorders of the brain, spinal cord, and nervous system in children.

Clinical Genetics   **CG**

Deals with identifying the genetic causes of inherited diseases and ailments and preventing, when possible, their occurrence.

Colon and Rectal Surgery   **CRS**

Surgical treatment of diseases of the intestinal tract, colon and rectum, anal canal, and perianal area.

Critical Care Medicine   *CCM*

Involves diagnosing and taking immediate action to prevent death or further injury of a patient. Examples of critical injuries include shock, heart attack, drug overdose, and massive bleeding.

Dermatology   **D**

Diagnosis and treatment of benign and malignant disorders of the skin, mouth, external genitalia, hair and nails, as well as a number of sexually transmitted diseases.

Diagnostic Radiology   *DR*

Involves the study of all modalities of radiant energy in medical diagnoses and therapeutic procedures utilizing radiologic guidance.

Endocrinology, Diabetes & Metabolism   *EDM*

Involves the study and treatment of patients suffering from hormonal and chemical disorders.

FAMILY MEDICINE   **FP**

Deals with and oversees the total healthcare of individual patients and their family members. Family practitioners are more common in rural areas and may perform procedures more commonly performed by specialists (e.g., minor surgery).

Forensic Psychiatry   *FPsy*

Concerns the evaluation of certain diagnostic groups of patients that include those with sexual disorders, antisocial personality disorders, paranoid disorders, and addictive disorders.

Gastroenterology   *Ge*

The study, diagnosis and treatment of diseases of the digestive organs including the stomach, bowels, liver, and gallbladder.

Geriatric Medicine   *Ger*

Deals with diseases of the elderly and the problems associated with aging.

Geriatric Psychiatry   *GerPsy*

Involves the diagnosis, prevention, and treatment of mental illness in the elderly.

Gynecologic Oncology   *GO*

Deals with cancers of the female genital tract and reproductive systems.

Hand Surgery   *HS*

Involves the treatment of injury to the hand through surgical techniques.

Hematology   *Hem*

Involves the diagnosis and treatment of diseases and disorders of the blood, bone marrow, spleen, and lymph glands.

Infectious Disease   *Inf*

The study and treatment of diseases caused by a bacterium, virus, fungus, or animal parasite.

INTERNAL MEDICINE   **IM**

Diagnosis and nonsurgical treatment of diseases, especially those of adults. Internists may act as primary care specialists, highly trained family doctors, or they may subspecialize in specialties such as cardiology or nephrology.

Maternal & Fetal Medicine   *MF*

Involves the care of women with high-risk pregnancies and their unborn fetuses.

Medical Oncology   *Onc*

Refers to the study and treatment of tumors and other cancers.

Neonatal-Perinatal Medicine   *NP*

Involves the diagnosis and treatments of infants prior to, during, and one month beyond birth.

Medical Specialties and Subspecialties

Nephrology   *Nep*

Concerned with disorders of the kidneys, high blood pressure, fluid and mineral balance, dialysis of body wastes when the kidneys do not function, and consultation with surgeons about kidney transplantation.

Neurological Surgery   **NS**

Involves surgery of the brain, spinal cord, and nervous system.

Neurology   **N**

Diagnosis and medical treatment of disorders of the brain, spinal cord, and nervous system.

Neuroradiology   *NRad*

Involves the utilization of imaging procedures during diagnosis as they relate to the brain, spine and spinal cord, head, neck, and organs of special sense in adults and children.

Nuclear Medicine   **NuM**

Evaluation of the functions of all the organs in the body and treatment of thyroid disease, benign and malignant tumors, and radiation exposure through the use of radioactive substances.

Nuclear Radiology   *NR*

Involves the use of radioactive substances to diagnose and treat certain functions and diseases of the body.

OBSTETRICS & GYNECOLOGY   **ObG**

Deals with the medical aspects of and intervention in pregnancy and labor and the overall health of the female reproductive system.

Occupational Medicine   *OM*

Concentrates on the effect of the work environment on the health of employees.

Ophthalmology   **Oph**

Diagnosis and treatment of diseases of and injuries to the eye.

Orthopaedic Surgery   **OrS**

Involves operations to correct injuries which interfere with the form and function of the extremities, spine, and associated structures.

Otolaryngology   **Oto**

Explores and treats diseases in the interrelated areas of the ears, nose and throat.

Otology/Neurotology   *ON*

Concentrates on the management, prevention, cure and care of patients with diseases of the ear and temporal bone, including disorders of hearing and balance.

Pain Medicine   *PM*

Involves providing a high level of care for patients experiencing problems with acute or chronic pain in both hospital and ambulatory settings.

Pediatric Cardiology   *PCd*

Involves the diagnosis and treatment of heart disease in children.

Pediatric Critical Care Medicine   *PCCM*

Involves the care of children who are victims of life threatening disorders such as severe accidents, shock, and diabetes acidosis.

Pediatric Dermatology   *PD*

Diagnosis and treatment of benign and malignant disorders of the skin, mouth, external genitalia, hair and nails in children.

Pediatric Endocrinology   *PEn*

Involves the study and treatment of children with hormonal and chemical disorders.

Pediatric Gastroenterology   *PGe*

The study, diagnosis, and treatment of diseases of the digestive tract in children.

Pediatric Hematology-Oncology   *PHO*

The study and treatment of cancers of the blood and blood-forming parts of the body in children.

Pediatric Infectious Disease   *PInf*

The study and treatment of diseases caused by a virus, bacterium, fungus, or animal parasite in children.

Pediatric Nephrology   *PNep*

Deals with the diagnosis and treatment of disorders of the kidneys in children.

Pediatric Otolaryngology   *POto*

Involves the diagnosis and treatment of disorders of the ear, nose, and throat which affect children.

Pediatric Pulmonology   *PPul*

Involves the diagnosis and treatment of diseases of the chest, lungs, and chest tissue in children.

Pediatric Radiology   *PR*

Involves diagnostic imaging as it pertains to the newborn, infant, child, and adolescent.

Pediatric Rheumatology   *PRhu*

Involves the treatment of diseases of the joints and connective tissues in children.

Pediatric Surgery   *PS*

Treatment of disease, injury, or deformity in children through surgical techniques.

PEDIATRICS   **Ped**

Diagnosis and treatment of diseases of childhood and monitoring of the growth, development, and well-being of preadolescent.

Physical Medicine & Rehabilitation   **PMR**

The use of physical therapy and physical agents such as water, heat, light electricity, and mechanical manipulations in the diagnosis, treatment, and prevention of disease and body disorders.

Plastic Surgery   **PlS**

Involves reconstructive and cosmetic surgery of the face and other body parts.

Preventive Medicine   **PrM**

A specialty focusing on the prevention of illness and on the health of groups rather than individuals.

Psychiatry   **Psyc**

Examination, treatment, and prevention of mental illness through the use of psychoanalysis and/or drugs.

Medical Specialties and Subspecialties

Public Health & General Preventive Medicine   *PHGPM*
Involves the investigation of the causes of epidemic disease and the prevention of a wide variety of acute and chronic illness.

Pulmonary Disease   *Pul*
Involves the diagnosis and treatment of diseases of the chest, lungs, and airways.

Radiation Oncology   *RadRo*
Involves the use of radiant energy and isotopes in the study and treatment of disease, especially malignant cancer.

Reproductive Endocrinology   *RE*
Deals with the endocrine system (including the pituitary, thyroid, parathyroid, adrenal glands, placenta, ovaries, and testes) and how its failure relates to infertility.

Rheumatology   *Rhu*
Involves the treatment of diseases of the joints, muscles, bones and associated structures.

Sleep Medicine   *Sleep Med*
Involves the investigation and treatment of patients with sleep disorders.

Spinal Cord Injury Medicine   *SpCdInj*
Involves the prevention, diagnosis, treatment and management of traumatic spinal cord injuries.

Sports Medicine   *SM*
Refers to the practice of an orthopedist or other physician who specializes in injuries to the bone or other soft tissues (muscles, tendons, ligaments) caused by participation in athletic activity.

Surgery   **S**
Treatment of disease, injury, and deformity by surgical procedures.

Surgery of the Hand   *SHd*
Involves providing appropriate care for all structures in the upper extremity directly affecting the hand and wrist function.

Surgical Critical Care   *SCC*
Involves specialized care in the management of the critically ill patient, particularly the trauma victim and postoperative patient in the emergency department, intensive care unit, trauma unit, burn unit, and other similar settings.

Thoracic Surgery (includes open heart surgery)   **TS**
Involves surgery on the heart, lungs, and chest area.

Urology   **U**
Diagnosis and treatment of diseases of the genitals in men and disorders of the urinary tract and bladder in both men and women.

Vascular & Interventional Radiology   *VIR*
Involves diagnosing and treating diseases by percutaneous methods guided by various radiologic imaging modalities.

Vascular Surgery   *VascS*
Involves the operative treatment of disorders of the blood vessels excluding those to the heart, lungs, or brain.

Partnership for Excellence

Partnership for Excellence
The Hospital Information Program

There are more than 200 acute care and specialty hospitals in the New York metropolitan area, many of which have extraordinary capabilities for superior patient care. Castle Connolly Medical Ltd. has received many requests from book buyers to provide information about hospitals. In response, we have invited a select group of outstanding hospitals to profile their services in this guide through the medium of paid advertorials. This program, called the Hospital Information Program, is totally separate from the physician selection process, which is based upon a completely independent review system. Hospitals that sponsored pages in the Hospital Information Program are organized into three groups: Major Medical Centers, Specialty Hospitals and Regional Medical Centers.

Major Medical Centers begin on the next page and are followed by the Specialty Hospital pages. This section is followed by the listings of doctors. Regional Medical Centers and Hospitals are found at the end of each county section–within the doctor listings. The information gives you an overview of programs and services offered by these hospitals, as well as vital information related to their accreditation and sponsorship. Each hospital profile also contains a physician referral number, should you wish to ask the hospitals for recommendations of physicians not listed in the Castle Connolly Guide.

The "Centers of Excellence" section was also developed in response to requests from our readers who want to know which hospitals have special programs or services focusing on a particular illness or health need. The "Centers of Excellence" described here are also offered by hospitals participating in the *Partnership for Excellence* section of this guide. They reflect the depth of commitment of these hospitals, which provides the staff, resources and financial support necessary to develop these special programs. We believe you will find this information helpful in your search for the best healthcare —from both physicians and hospitals—for you and your family.

We are pleased to have these distinguished institutions as partners in our effort to help you meet your healthcare needs.

The following pages contain vital information on eight of the region's Major Medical Centers. A Major Medical Center is an acute care hospital with tertiary care services, residency programs, a major affiliation with a medical school and clinical research programs. A major medical center draws its patients from a broad geographic region, even nationally and internationally and, in many instances, is the center of a network or consortium of hospitals.

The New York metropolitan region is nationally and internationally known for its major medical centers and their excellent programs and services. Some of the nation's leading academic centers are in this region and, in addition to superior patient care and cutting edge patient research, they produce thousands of talented, well trained physicians and other health professionals each year. Castle Connolly Medical Ltd. has invited a number of major medical centers in the region to sponsor the profiles and information that follows.

Major Medical Centers

Atlantic Health System

Continuum Health Partners

Hackensack University Medical Center

Lenox Hill Hospital

Maimonides Medical Center

Mount Sinai Medical Center

NewYork-Presbyterian Hospital

NYU Medical Center

ATLANTIC HEALTH

Morristown Memorial Hospital • Overlook Hospital

THE PASSION TO LEAD

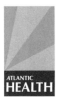

Goryeb Children's Hospital • Atlantic Neuroscience Institute
Carol G. Simon Cancer Center/The Cancer Center at Overlook Hospital
Gagnon Heart Hospital • Atlantic Rehabilitation Institute

P.O. Box 1905, Morristown, NJ 07962 • 1-800-247-9580 • atlantichealth.org

Sponsorship:	**Voluntary Not–for–Profit**
Beds:	**1133**
Accreditation:	**Joint Commission on Accreditation of Healthcare Organizations (JCAHO)**

Atlantic Health is on the forefront of medicine, setting standards for quality health care in New Jersey and beyond.

Our nationally recognized physicians, experienced nurses and skilled staff provide outstanding and compassionate care. Renowned for its breadth of cardiac services, Morristown Memorial Hospital performs the second most heart surgeries in the New York metropolitan area. Overlook Hospital, the regional leader in comprehensive stroke care and neurosciences, was the first hospital in the Northeast to utilize revolutionary CyberKnife technology.

In all our specialties, such as pediatrics, orthopedics, cancer care, rehabilitation medicine, women's health, cardiovascular care and neuroscience, Atlantic Health physicians are leaders in their fields, always searching for the most effective diagnosis and treatment options for each patient. Our world-class facilities feature state-of-the-art equipment in a comfortable, family-friendly environment that puts patients first.

◢ MORRISTOWN MEMORIAL HOSPITAL – 100 Madison Avenue, Morristown, NJ 07962

Morristown Memorial Hospital has been serving the Morris County community for more than 100 years, setting high standards for patient care in state-of-the-art facilities with a full range of medical specialties and services.

Named a Level I Regional Trauma Center by the American College of Surgeons and a Level II Trauma Center by the state, Morristown Memorial offers superlative care with our highly trained trauma teams. Our cardiac surgery program is the largest in the state. Our Level III Regional Perinatal Center provides specialized care to sick or premature infants, and the Goryeb Children's Hospital has more than 100 pediatric specialists caring for patients in a child-centered facility. Our mission at the Carol G. Simon Cancer Center, where we treat all types of cancer with the most advanced methods, is to provide comprehensive, compassionate and individualized service.

Our quality of care has earned us national recognition. Recently, Morristown Memorial was re-designated a **Magnet Hospital for Excellence in Nursing Service**, the highest level of recognition by American Nurses Credentialing Center for facilities that provide acute care services. Less than three percent of US hospitals receive the prestigious Magnet designation.

We are a winner of the **National Research Corporation's 2006 Consumer Choice Award** and *Advanced Newsmagazines* named our **Sleep Disorder Center "Best Sleep Facility in the US."** TeenHealthFX.com, our online resource for adolescents and young adults, has won numerous awards including "Best Overall Site" for the 2005 Medicine on the Net Awards.

Morristown Memorial is accredited by the Joint Commission on Accreditation of Healthcare Organizations (JCAHO). We are an affiliate of the University of Medicine and Dentistry of New Jersey-New Jersey Medical School and a partner with the Cancer Institute of New Jersey.

◢ OVERLOOK HOSPITAL - 99 Beauvoir Avenue, Summit, NJ 07902

Overlook is at the forefront of leading medical technology. We have the state's first combined PET/CT scanner and stereotactic radiosurgery cancer treatment program; our new Neuroscience Institute offers a brain tumor center, stroke center and epilepsy program, as well as neurointerventional radiology; and we are the first center in the NYC area to offer the revolutionary **CyberKnife**. Nationally recognized for our Emergency Department, we are one of five New Jersey hospitals approved to provide emergency angioplasty in a community hospital setting.

Sponsored Page

We are proud that our accomplishments in expert medical care have been recognized in prestigious awards. Recently, our **"Women's Heart Awareness" program won the 2006 Circle of Excellence Community Service Award from the American Association of Critical Care Nurses.** In 2005, we were **New Jersey Hospital Association's (NJHA) honorable mention winner for our "Closing the Healthcare Loop"** program. In addition, the Intensive Care Unit at Overlook won the **American Association of Critical Care Nurses' 2005 Beacon Award for Critical Care Excellence**, an award designated to recognize the nation's top hospital critical care units. Overlook Hospital was the first New Jersey hospital to obtain this national award.

Overlook Hospital is a clinical affiliate of the University of Medicine and Dentistry of New Jersey-New Jersey Medical School. We are also a partner with The Cancer Institute of New Jersey. Overlook is accredited by the Joint Commission for Accreditation of Health Care Organizations (JCAHO).

◢ GORYEB CHILDREN'S HOSPITAL

Your child will benefit from the expertise of nationally-recognized, board certified pediatric specialists who are actively involved in clinical research, enabling them to offer your child the newest medications, treatments and technologies. Experts at the Goryeb Children's Hospital at Morristown Memorial Hospital and the Goryeb Inpatient Pediatric Unit at Overlook Hospital are dedicated to helping you with your child's health. We partner with you and your child's physicians to manage emergencies, chronic conditions and serious illnesses. Both facilities feature a family-focused, child-friendly environment. In addition, the Morristown campus includes a pediatric intensive care unit and more.

◢ ATLANTIC NEUROSCIENCE INSTITUTE

The Atlantic Neuroscience Institute, the premier provider of neuroscience services in the New Jersey region, delivers quality health care that is compassionate, multidisciplinary and broadly accessible. We apply the most advanced new treatments and diagnostic tools, leading the way in the application of evidence-based medicine and technological innovation. We collaborate with other Atlantic Health professionals to provide superior, comprehensive, multidisciplinary care to all of our patients.

Based at Overlook Hospital, the Atlantic Neuroscience Institute utilizes the expertise of adult and pediatric neurologists and neurosurgeons, neuroradiologists, and specialists in related fields. Our Institute, including our state-of-the-art Neuroscience Inpatient Unit and Intensive Care Unit, is staffed by some of the most dedicated, highly rated neuroscience physicians and nurses. Among the many cutting edge technologies we use are neuro-imaging, image-guided neurosurgery and CyberKnife radiosurgery to provide optimal diagnostic and treatment services.

◢ CAROL G. SIMON CANCER CENTER/THE CANCER CENTER AT OVERLOOK HOSPITAL

The Carol G. Simon Cancer Center and the Cancer Center at Overlook Hospital offer the most advanced methods to diagnose, treat, and manage all types of cancers. Our mission is to provide comprehensive, compassionate, and individualized care to our patients. We combine the latest medical technologies, such as minimally invasive surgeries, image-guided radiation, and cytogenetics, with complementary medicine, including relaxation, guided imagery, meditation, yoga, and massage. Our highly trained physicians and oncology professionals work together in a collaborative setting that promotes a coordinated, multidisciplinary approach to cancer care.

◢ GAGNON HEART HOSPITAL

We are a national leader in the research and treatment of cardiac disease, and more heart surgery is performed at Morristown Memorial than at any other NJ hospital. In fact, Morristown Memorial is second in the New York Metro region in the number of heart surgeries performed. The Gagnon Heart Hospital's new flagship facility, opening at Morristown Memorial in 2008, will feature private patient rooms, new operating and procedure rooms and convenient access to all facets of cardiac care. Our Cardiac Care Units provide a full range of diagnostic testing procedures, including the 64-image Cardiac CT Angiography - the latest technology in non-invasive cardiac imaging - and our cardiac specialists develop comprehensive treatment and recovery plans for each patient. During the recovery process, you have the benefit of cardiac rehabilitation experts who help you to gain physical and emotional strength, and to plan heart-healthy routines when you return home.

PHYSICIAN REFERRAL **For a physician referral or for more information please contact Atlantic Health at: 1-800-427-9580 or atlantichealth.org**

Sponsored Page

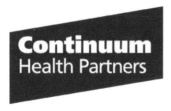

Continuum Health Partners

Phone (800) 420-4004
www.chpnyc.org

Sponsorship: Voluntary Not-for-Profit
Beds: 2,995 certified beds
Accreditation: Joint Commission of Accreditation of Healthcare Organizations (JCAHO). Accreditation
                 Council for Graduate Medical Education, Medical Society of New York, in cooperation with
                 the Accreditation Council for Continuing Medical Education

A STRONG PARTNERSHIP WITH A PROUD HERITAGE

Continuum Health Partners, Inc. is a partnership of five venerable health care providers, Beth Israel Medical Center, St. Luke's Hospital, Roosevelt Hospital, Long Island College Hospital, and the New York Eye and Ear Infirmary. Each of the five partner institutions was established more than a century ago by individuals committed to improving health and health care in their communities. Today, the system represents more than 4,800 physicians and dentists and is superbly equipped to respond to the health care needs of the populations we serve. Continuum providers also see patients in group and private practice settings and in ambulatory centers.

LOCATIONS

Continuum Health Partners has campuses throughout Manhattan and Brooklyn. Beth Israel Medical Center has two divisions: the Milton and Caroll Petrie Division on the East Side, and the Kings Highway Division in Brooklyn. The Phillips Ambulatory Care Center, a state-of-the art outpatient center, is located at Union Square. St. Luke's Hospital is in Morningside Heights and Roosevelt Hospital is in the Columbus Circle and Lincoln Center neighborhoods on the West Side. Long Island College Hospital is located in the Brooklyn Heights/Cobble Hill section of Brooklyn. The New York Eye and Ear Infirmary is located on Second Avenue and 14th Street.

ACADEMIC AFFILIATIONS

Beth Israel Medical Center is the University Hospital and Manhattan Campus for the Albert Einstein College of Medicine. St. Luke's-Roosevelt Hospital Center is the University Hospital for Columbia University College of Physicians and Surgeons. Long Island College Hospital is the primary teaching affiliate of the SUNY-Health Science Center in Brooklyn. The New York Eye and Ear Infirmary is the primary teaching center of the New York Medical College and affiliated teaching hospitals in the areas of ophthalmology and otolaryngology.

Physician Referral For a referral to a doctor in your neighborhood, call (800) 420-4004. Continuum's Referral Service can help you find a primary care physician or specialist affiliated with Beth Israel, St. Luke's, Roosevelt, Long Island College Hospital, or the New York Eye and Ear Infirmary. **Visit our Website at www.chpnyc.org**

535

CENTERS OF EXCELLENCE AT CONTINUUM HEALTH PARTNERS

Cancer

The Continuum Cancer Centers of New York offer early detection, diagnosis, and treatment of a wide range of cancers. Our nationally recognized physicians offer innovative and highly successful programs coupled with superb support services for patients and caregivers. Our cancer services are state of the art, supported by sophisticated programs in medical oncology, surgical oncology, and radiation oncology.

Cardiology

The cardiology, cardiac surgery, and cardiac rehabilitation team at the Continuum Heart Institute offers a full range of diagnostic and treatment services. Our Heart Institute is one of only a handful of programs to offer minimally invasive coronary bypass surgery using The DaVinci Surgical System™, the most advanced piece of cardiovascular technology. Our cardiac surgical mortality rates are among the lowest in New York State.

Neurology, Neurosurgery & Interventional Neuroradiology

Continuum is home to many world leaders in neurology, neurosurgery and interventional neuroradiology. Our physicians are recognized authorities who establish innovative care protocols, chart new venues in therapy and develop the technologies that set the standards in the neuroscience fields.

Musculoskeletal

Continuum Health Partners physicians are leading providers of general orthopedic, sports medicine, spine and rheumatologic care. With services offered at Beth Israel Medical Center, Roosevelt Hospital, St. Luke's Hospital and Long Island College Hospital, our orthopedic specialists offer state-of-the-art care to patients throughout the New York metropolitan region. Many of our orthopedic surgeons are leaders in their field and are fellowship trained in their area of sub-specialty.

Ear, Nose and Throat

Continuum offers eye, ear, nose and throat services throughout our system. The New York Eye and Ear Infirmary is the largest provider of eye care in America and operates one of the nation's most extensive ear, nose and throat clinics. New York Eye and Ear Infirmary is also a recognized leader in plastic and reconstructive surgery.

HIV/AIDS Services

We are one of the largest providers of HIV/AIDS care in New York City, with comprehensive-care clinics and facilities in multiple locations. Our facilities offer a complete range of health care services for individuals with HIV: diagnostic procedures, the latest treatments, and support services for individuals of all ages and their families.

Pain Management

Our Department of Pain Medicine and Palliative Care began in 1997 and is the first combined department in these fields in the United States. The department provides services by a multidisciplinary team of specialists who work with patients to assess and treat pain and its symptoms. Among the department's programs are Continuum Hospice Care for end-of-life care, the Family Caregiver Program, and Net of Care.

Substance Abuse

The Continuum hospitals offer extensive chemical dependency treatment services through The Addiction Institute of New York, the Stuyvesant Square Chemical Dependency Treatment Program, and the Department of Psychiatry. Our services include inpatient detoxification and outpatient programs, services for the mentally ill, family services, and after-care programs.

HACKENSACK UNIVERSITY MEDICAL CENTER

30 Prospect Avenue
Hackensack, New Jersey 07601
phone 201-996-3760
fax 201-996-3452

www.humc.com

Sponsorship	A not-for-profit, teaching and research hospital affiliated with the University of Medicine and Dentistry of New Jersey – New Jersey Medical School.
Beds	A 781-bed, Level II Trauma Center, providing tertiary and regional services for the New York/New Jersey metropolitan area.
Accreditation	Joint Commission on the Accreditation of Healthcare Organizations (JCAHO).
	Record Number of Gold Seals of Approval™ For Healthcare Quality from JCAHO in these areas: The Stroke Center, Heart Failure, Acute Myocardial Infarction (AMI), Asthma, Coronary Artery Disease, Joint Replacement, Pneumonia, and Chronic Kidney Disease.

Hackensack University Medical Center's standing as one of New Jersey's and the nation's healthcare leaders is driven by a commitment to quality. Founded in 1888, HUMC is a nationally recognized organization offering patients the most comprehensive services, state-of-the-art technologies and facilities, cutting-edge research with an annual budget of more than $1 billion. A leader in providing the highest quality care, Hackensack University Medical Center offers one of the region's most modern campuses, which is continually updated and expanded to incorporate emerging clinical approaches, medicine, and technologies.

MEDICAL AND DENTAL STAFF
Since Hackensack University Medical Center is one of the region's most comprehensive and progressive medical centers, it easily attracts many of the area's leading physicians. These doctors, many of whom are on the cutting edge in their fields and have received their training at our nation's most prominent institutions, have selected Hackensack University Medical Center as their place to practice their best medicine.

NURSING EXCELLENCE
Our medical staff is joined by a team of extraordinary nurses. As a Magnet Hospital, Hackensack University Medical Center attracts and retains nurses who are tops in their fields.

Hackensack University Medical Center is in its eleventh year as a Magnet Hospital. In 1995, it became the first hospital in the country – after the pilot program – to receive the Magnet Award for Nursing Excellence. This honor is the highest recognition that can be bestowed by The American Nurses Credentialing Center. The medical center received redesignation as a Magnet Hospital in 1999 and again in 2003.

NATIONAL RECOGNITIONS HIGHLIGHT SUPERIOR PATIENT CARE
Throughout its history, Hackensack University Medical Center has been recognized by many of the nation's most prestigious organizations for its high level of clinical and organizational excellence. Not only do these recognitions set us apart from our competitors, more importantly they provide consumers with valuable objective data on which to make informed decisions about their healthcare. More than a plaque on the wall, our vast recognitions, rankings, and ratings highlight medical excellence at Hackensack University Medical Center – the hallmark of our success.

Third in the Nation for Hospital Safety – Hackensack University Medical Center has been ranked number three in the U.S. for hospital safety and quality in *Consumers Digest*. The article, entitled "Hospital Safety: Where to Get the Best Care," includes a list of America's 50 exceptional hospitals. Hackensack University Medical Center came in third, following Massachusetts General Hospital (No.1) and Brigham and Women's Hospital (No.2).

 Sponsored Page

Region 2 Quality Award/U.S. Environmental Protection Agency – The regional office of the U.S. Environmental Protection Agency recognized Hackensack University Medical Center and The Deirdre Imus Environmental Center for Pediatric Oncology® for its contributions to environmental health.

HealthGrades® Distinguished Hospital Award for Clinical Excellence™ – Every year since 2003, Hackensack University Medical Center has received the HealthGrades Distinguished Hospital Award for Clinical Excellence™. The award places Hackensack University Medical Center in the top five percent in the U.S. for clinical quality performance for the third consecutive year.

2006 HealthGrades Specialty Excellence Awards

- Cardiac Care Excellence Award™
- Gastrointestinal Care Excellence Award™
- Orthopaedic Care Excellence Award™
- General Surgery Excellence Award™

J.D. Power and Associates Distinguished Hospital Program℠ for Inpatient and Outpatient Services

Consumer's Choice Award Winner – Bergen-Passaic's Most Preferred Hospital for Overall Quality and Image for ten consecutive years. The award is based on a survey of more than 140,000 households nationwide by The National Research Corporation of Lincoln, Nebraska.

One of the nation's "100 Most Wired Hospitals and Health Systems" – Eight years in a row ranking from *Hospitals & Health Networks,* a publication of The American Hospital Association.

WORLD-CLASS CARDIAC CARE

Hackensack University Medical Center is one of America's most comprehensive cardiac care hospitals. The Heart Center provides a full-range of state-of-the-art invasive and non-invasive diagnostic and treatment services including electrophysiology studies, a state-designated cardiac catheterization center, and one of the largest cardiac surgery programs in the state.

Our national rankings include:

- One of "America's Best Hospitals" for heart and heart surgery by *U.S. News & World Report*® 2006. The medical center was the only acute care hospital in New Jersey to receive a national ranking.

- HealthGrades® Five-Star Rating for Women's Health Services. In its study, *Women's Health Outcomes in U.S. Hospitals,* HealthGrades ranked Hackensack University Medical Center in the top 10 percent in the nation for women's health services. This ranking includes cardiac and stroke outcomes for women, as well as maternity care.

NEW JERSEY'S LARGEST AND MOST COMPREHENSIVE CANCER CENTER

The Cancer Center at Hackensack University Medical Center is New Jersey's largest and most comprehensive and is among the nation's top 10 in patient volume.

ONE OF THE NATION'S RENOWNED PEDIATRIC PROGRAMS

Hackensack University Medical Center is a state-designated New Jersey Children's Hospital. It is also a full-voting member in the National Association of Children's Hospitals and Related Institutions, the non-profit association that speaks on behalf of children's health needs and their caregivers.

THE JOSEPH M. SANZARI CHILDREN'S HOSPITAL

The Joseph M. Sanzari Children's Hospital has been selected twice as one of the top 25 Children's Hospitals in the country and the top ranked Children's Hospital in New Jersey by *Child* Magazine. The Joseph M. Sanzari Children's Hospital is located in The Sarkis and Siran Gabrellian Women's and Children's Pavilion, a 300,000-square-foot pavilion that also houses The Donna A. Sanzari Women's Hospital and The Mark Messier Skyway for Tomorrows Children. This new facility is one of the country's first environmentally responsible and sustainable healthcare facilities and is ranked as one of the Top 10 Green Hospitals by *The Green Guide.*

PHYSICIAN REFERRAL

Hackensack University Medical Center's Physician Referral Service representatives offer information on the nearly 1,400 medical and dental staff members representing more than 50 specialties. Call 201-996-2020.

Lenox Hill Hospital

100 East 77th Street, New York, NY 10021

Tel: 212-434-2000

www.lenoxhillhospital.org

Beds: 652

Sponsorship: Voluntary Not-for-Profit

Accreditation: Joint Commission on Accreditation of Healthcare Organizations, College of American Pathologists, American Association of Blood Banks, Accreditation Council for Graduate Medical Education, Accreditation Council for Continuing Medical Education, Commission on Accreditation of Allied Health Education Programs

GENERAL PROFILE

Lenox Hill Hospital, located on Manhattan's Upper East Side, is a 652-bed, fully accredited, acute care hospital. Founded in 1857, the Hospital has earned a national reputation for providing the highest quality care, training new physicians, and contributing to progress in research. The Hospital, recognized nationally as a leader in cardiac care, orthopedics and maternal/child health, offers a wide range of services in radiology, and medical and surgical specialties.

Manhattan Eye, Ear & Throat Hospital, a world-renowned specialty hospital serving the community since 1869, is a subsidiary of Lenox Hill Hospital.

MEDICAL STAFF AND TEACHING PROGRAMS

Lenox Hill Hospital has nearly 1,400 physicians on staff, with outstanding national and international reputations in their fields. The Hospital offers 20 residency and fellowship programs.

CENTERS OF EXCELLENCE

LENOX HILL HEART AND VASCULAR INSTITUTE OF NEW YORK

Since 1938, when Lenox Hill Hospital cardiologists performed the first angiogram in the country, the Hospital has been recognized as a leader in cardiovascular care. This has been followed by other groundbreaking procedures, including the first coronary angioplasty in the nation performed in 1978; the implantation of the first coronary stent in NYC in 1991; the first minimally invasive direct coronary artery bypass surgery in the U.S. in 1994; and the implantation of the first FDA-approved drug coated stent in the nation in 2003.

94

The Institute continues today as a leader in the field, developing groundbreaking techniques to minimize heart damage and speed recovery. These include the largest carotid stent program in the nation (2004) and the largest minimally invasive heart assist program in the tri-state area (2005). Today, Lenox Hill Heart and Vascular Institute physicians and surgeons continue to offer a comprehensive approach to total cardiac and vascular care, providing patients with diagnoses of simple and highly complex conditions.

ORTHOPEDIC SURGERY AND SPORTS MEDICINE

Lenox Hill Hospital is recognized internationally as a leader in orthopedic surgery and sports medicine, and provides treatment for a broad range of musculoskeletal conditions. The Hospital's Nicholas Institute of Sports Medicine and Athletic Trauma was the first hospital-based center in the U.S. dedicated to the advancement of research in sports medicine. Its expert staff provides treatment and rehabilitation to injured athletes, including players on the NY Jets and Islanders. The Hospital's orthopedic surgeons are leaders in total and partial joint replacement surgery, and in surgery of the spine, foot, ankle and hand.

MATERNAL/CHILD HEALTH

Lenox Hill Hospital is renowned for its exceptional obstetrical services, from prenatal to postpartum care. The Hospital's obstetricians and gynecologists manage routine and high-risk concerns and offer specialized expertise in breast disease, reproductive endocrinology, bladder disorders, infertility, and gynecologic oncology. Expectant mothers with high-risk pregnancies benefit from the expertise of a highly skilled team of specialists at the Hospital's Center for Maternal-Fetal Medicine. Services include a full range of prenatal testing, as well as ongoing monitoring of both mother and fetus. Premature infants and those born with special needs receive specialized attention in the Hospital's Neonatal Critical Care Unit.

To find a doctor who's right for you, call our 24-hour physician referral service toll free at 1-888-RIGHT MD (1-888-744-4863).

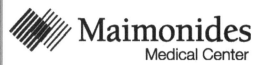

MAIMONIDES MEDICAL CENTER

4802 Tenth Avenue
Brooklyn, New York 11219
Phone: (718) 283-6000
Physician Referral: 1-888 MMC DOCS
http://www.maimonidesmed.org

Sponsorship:	Voluntary, Not-for-Profit
Beds:	705 acute, 70 psychiatric
Accreditation:	Joint Commission on Accreditation of Healthcare Organizations (JCAHO)
	American College of Surgeons
	American Council of Graduate Medical Education (ACGME)

The nation's third largest independent teaching hospital, Maimonides Medical Center is a conductor of clinical trials for new treatments and therapies. Cited for overall clinical excellence by numerous healthcare report cards and evaluation services, Maimonides is a celebrated leader in the use of information technology to enhance patient care.

Significant Accomplishments

• Maimonides is one of a select few hospitals in the US to meet the criteria for excellence in healthcare established by the Leapfrog Group, a coalition of some of the nation's largest employers.

• Excellence in cardiac care is historic: the first successful human heart transplant in the US was performed at Maimonides in 1967, and our current interventional cardiology program provides the best patient outcomes in the state of New York.

• Physicians at Maimonides are among the eight percent nationwide who use computers to enter patient orders, thereby reducing the risk of errors, increasing efficiency, and speeding the healing process.

• Maimonides has appeared on the American Hospital Association's "Most Wired" and "Most Wireless" lists more often than any other healthcare institution in the metropolitan area.

• More babies were born at Maimonides in 2005 than at any other facility in the state of New York – due in no small part to its designation as a Regional Perinatal Center with Obstetric and Pediatric services that are unrivaled in this area.

Centers of Excellence

Cancer Center

• Maimonides Cancer Center offers a fully integrated approach to cancer care that includes prevention, screening, diagnostics, treatment, palliative care and clinical research – all in one location. Staffed by leading oncologists, radiologists, nurses, social workers and treatment specialists, the Center provides compassionate, patient-centered, state-of-the-art care. The Radiologic Oncology division provides the most advanced imaging and treatment technology.

Sponsored Page

Cardiac Institute

• Renowned for its Catheterization Lab and pioneering new surgical procedures, the Institute includes an electrophysiology (EP) lab, two ICUs, Chest Pain Observation Unit, Advanced Cardiac Care Unit, and Congestive Heart Failure Program. The first successful heart transplant in America was performed at Maimonides in 1967. Today, its Cath Lab provides the best patient outcomes in the state of New York.

Stroke Center

• The Stroke Center at Maimonides is ranked among the best in the nation – and one of the top two Centers in New York state. It is currently the site of two clinical trials for new stroke medications. The Center is one of the few that provides interventional neuroradiology techniques to remove stroke-causing blood clots from the brain – without surgery – significantly reducing the debilitating effects of stroke.

Infants and Children's Hospital

• Accredited by the National Association of Children's Hospitals and Related Institutions (NACHRI), Maimonides Infants and Children's Hospital includes comprehensive Inpatient Services and over 30 pediatric subspecialties. With a Child Life program fully integrated with family-centered care, the Maimonides Infants and Children's Hospital also provides a Pediatric ICU, Neonatal ICU, Outpatient Pavilion, and Pediatric ER.

Vascular Institute

• The Vascular Institute at Maimonides provides comprehensive diagnostic, clinical and vascular surgical services for patients with circulatory complications related to hypertension, diabetes, arteriosclerosis and other diseases. One of only five centers in New York certified to train vascular surgeons, the Institute includes a Diagnostic Lab, Vein Center, Vascular Surgery Center and Wound Center with Hyperbaric Unit.

Stella & Joseph Payson Birthing Center

• Maimonides is ranked among the best in the nation for maternity care by HealthGrades, the leading source for independent healthcare quality information. More babies were delivered at Maimonides in 2005 than at any other hospital in New York State. The Payson Birthing Center offers a home-like setting with doulas and midwives, combined with advanced technology, including a perinatal testing center with 3-D ultrasound and 24/7 neonatology.

Geriatrics Program

• Maimonides serves one of the oldest populations in New York City, with one in ten of our patients over the age of 85. The Geriatrics Program is fully equipped to meet the special needs of these seniors, including the assessment of memory loss and expertise in geriatric syndromes such as incontinence, falls and frailty. The Program encompasses inpatient and outpatient services, features the Acute Care for Elderly (ACE) Unit, and provides home-visiting services.

THE MOUNT SINAI MEDICAL CENTER

One Gustave L. Levy Place (Fifth Avenue and 98th Street)
New York, NY 10029
Physician Referral: 1-800-MD-SINAI
www.mountsinai.org

Sponsorship	Voluntary Not-for-Profit
Beds	1,171
Accreditation	Joint Commission on Accreditation of Healthcare Organizations (JACHO), Commission for Accreditation of Rehabilitation Facilities (CARF), Magnet Award for Nursing Excellence

The Mount Sinai Medical Center, located on the Upper East Side in New York City, consists of The Mount Sinai Hospital, a tertiary and quaternary care facility known for excellence in patient care, and Mount Sinai School of Medicine, a leader in medical research and in the education of tomorrow's physicians by internationally known faculty. Founded in 1852, The Mount Sinai Hospital is one of the oldest voluntary teaching hospitals in the country. The patients of Mount Sinai receive attentive care from the Medical Center's award winning nursing staff and benefit as teams of physicians and scientists work together to rapidly translate laboratory research into new patient treatments. Many of the groundbreaking approaches that result from these collaborations are initially available at only a handful of facilities in the country—some, only at Mount Sinai. These advances make Mount Sinai the first choice for patients with complex medical and surgical needs.

SPECIAL PROGRAMS

Recognized for excellence in numerous specialties, The Mount Sinai Medical Center and its medical staff have been consistently ranked among the best in New York City and the country by such respected publications as *U.S. News & World Report* and *New York* magazine.

Mount Sinai Heart, under the direction of Valentin Fuster, MD, PhD, combines all of Mount Sinai's world-class resources with innovative thinking, creative programs, and an unwavering commitment to the prevention and treatment of cardiovascular disease. Capitalizing upon the talent and expertise of internationally renowned Mount Sinai physicians David Adams, MD; Michael Marin, MD; Samin Sharma, MD, and a host of other highly regarded cardiac surgeons, interventionalists, and cardiologists, Mount Sinai Heart provides an integrated approach to clinical care utilizing basic and clinical research. With the rapid translation of innovative research concepts into improved preventive, diagnostic, and therapeutic care, patients receive multidisciplinary treatment of unprecedented quality.

Mount Sinai's **Neurology and Neurosurgery** specialists are experts in skull-base surgery and neuroendoscopy for adults and children with primary brain tumors, cerebrovascular, pituitary and acoustic conditions as well as epilepsy, disorders in neuromuscular transmission, peripheral nerve problems, and spinal reconstruction. Computerized stereotactic techniques allow three-dimensional localization of specific sites within the nervous system. Functional neurosurgery precisely targets abnormalities in the brain and spinal cord in combination with minimally invasive surgical approaches. Outpatient radiosurgery uses computer-assisted radiation to treat lesions without opening the skull.

Sponsored Page

Mount Sinai's **Gastrointestinal and Surgical Specialties** has a rich history of excellence and offers superior care in the diagnosis and treatment of all diseases of the digestive system. In 1932, Crohn's disease was first identified at Mount Sinai. Since then, Mount Sinai physicians have pioneered countless techniques to help patients with Crohn's disease and other digestive disorders lead better lives. Recognized for expertise and skill, Mount Sinai is ranked #7 in the United States for treatment of digestive disorders by *U.S. News & World Report.*

The **Multidisciplinary Head and Neck Cancer Center**, under the leadership of Eric Genden, MD, FACS, provides each patient with a team of nationally recognized physicians and surgeons who work together to provide state-of-the-art curative management of tumors of the oral cavity, larynx, skull-base, and thyroid gland.

Recognized as a national leader in organ transplantation, The **Recanati/Miller Transplantation Institute** is one the few institutes in the country to provide combined organ transplantation. Renowned for its long-term experience in the field, The Mount Sinai Hospital was the site of the first liver transplant in New York State.

Complete care for people with disabilities is delivered through **Rehabilitation Medicine** at Mount Sinai. A wide range of comprehensive patient care services are available for individuals with spinal cord injuries, brain injuries, and a variety of neuromuscular, musculoskeletal, and chronic conditions. Mount Sinai's Rehabilitation Medicine program is CARF-accredited for treatment of both inpatient spinal cord and brain injury and is home to a comprehensive outpatient physical and occupational therapy facility.

Mount Sinai's Department of **Orthopaedics** is dedicated to the preservation, restoration, and development of the musculoskeletal system. Experts in surgery of the foot and ankle, knee, hip, hand, elbow, shoulder, and spine; total joint replacement (knee, hip, foot and ankle, and shoulder); microvascular surgery; cancer surgery; and minimally invasive surgery, provide personalized treatments using the latest technological innovations, including 3-D imaging technology.

Minimally Invasive Surgery at Mount Sinai continues to be at the forefront of providing advanced procedures using state-of-the-art instruments. We also provide specialized and unique expertise in the use of minimally invasive procedures as well as to traditional surgery options.

Geriatrics and Adult Development specialists at Mount Sinai work hard to improve life and longevity for New York's elderly. Ranked third in the nation for the second straight year by *U.S. News & World Report* in its "Best Graduate Schools" issue, Mount Sinai is a pioneer in geriatric medicine and continues to break new ground, offering comprehensive care, disease prevention, and the promotion of healthy and productive aging. Medical staff and social workers address patients' needs as a team through comprehensive patient-centered care.

To find a Mount Sinai physician, surgeon, or specialist, please call
1-800-MD-SINAI or visit www.mountsinai.org
Both services are available 24 hours a day / 7 days a week

⌐ NewYork-Presbyterian
⌐ The University Hospital of Columbia and Cornell

Affiliated with Columbia University College of Physicians and Surgeons and Weill Medical College of Cornell University

NewYork-Presbyterian Hospital
Weill Cornell Medical Center
525 East 68th Street
New York, NY 10021

NewYork-Presbyterian Hospital
Columbia University Medical Center
622 West 168th Street
New York, NY 10032

Sponsorship:	Voluntary Not-for-Profit
Beds:	2,369
Accreditation:	Joint Commission on Accreditation of Healthcare Organizations (JCAHO), Commission on Accreditation of Rehabilitation Facilities (CARF) and College of American Pathologists (CAP)

The *U.S. News & World Report* has ranked NewYork-Presbyterian Hospital higher in more specialties than any other hospital in the New York area. NewYork-Presbyterian Hospital was named to the *Honor Roll of America's Best Hospitals.*

OVERVIEW:

NewYork-Presbyterian Hospital is the largest hospital in New York and one of the most comprehensive healthcare institutions in the nation with 5,500 physicians, approximately 105,000 discharges and nearly 1 million outpatient visits annually, and with its affiliated medical schools, more than $400 million in research support. NewYork-Presbyterian is dedicated to providing top-quality care with sensitivity, warmth and compassion. The Hospital's world-class medical staff provides state-of-the-art diagnosis and treatment in all areas of medicine — including preventive and primary care—and in all specialties and subspecialties. The Hospital also offers inpatient and outpatient services at The Allen Pavilion in northern Manhattan, and at the Westchester Division, one of the nation's top ranked and the region's largest psychiatric facility.

AMONG ITS RENOWNED CENTERS OF EXCELLENCE ARE:

Morgan Stanley Children's Hospital and the Komansky Center for Children's Health— One of the largest, most comprehensive children's hospitals in the world providing highly sophisticated pediatric medical, surgical and intensive care, including a pediatric cardiovascular center, in a compassionate environment.

NewYork-Presbyterian Cancer Centers — Coordinated, multidisciplinary care and the latest therapeutic options and clinical trials. The Herbert Irving Comprehensive Cancer Center, located at Columbia Presbyterian, is one of only two cancer centers in the metropolitan area to have received the designation "comprehensive" from the National Cancer Institute.

NewYork-Presbyterian Heart — Expert diagnostic capabilities and medical and surgical innovations for simple to complex heart conditions. The Hospital's cardiac surgical mortality rates are among the lowest in the nation.

NewYork-Presbyterian Neuroscience Centers — Latest research, diagnosis and treatment capabilities in Alzheimer's disease, Multiple Sclerosis, Parkinson's disease, aneurysms, epilepsy, brain tumors, stokes and other neurological disorders.

NewYork-Presbyterian Psychiatry — World-renowned center of excellence in psychiatric treatment, research and education.

NewYork-Presbyterian Transplant Institute — Adult and pediatric heart, liver and kidney, and adult lung and pancreas transplantation and cutting-edge research.

Sponsored Page

NewYork-Presbyterian Vascular Care Center — Comprehensive and integrated preventive, diagnostic and treatment program for diverse problems related to arteries and veins throughout the body.

NewYork-Presbyterian Digestive Disease Services — Expert capabilities in the broad range of conditions that affect the organs as well as other components of the digestive system.

William Randolph Hearst Burn Center — Largest and busiest burn center in the nation which also conducts research to improve survival and enhance quality of life for burn victims.

In addition, the Hospital offers extraordinary expertise, comprehensive programs and specialized resources in the fields of:

AIDS — The Center for Special Studies at NewYork Weill Cornell and the AIDS Care Program at Columbia Presbyterian provide continuous, comprehensive care for men, women and children with HIV/AIDS. Both sites are designated AIDS centers by New York State and by the National Institutes of Health.

Gene Therapy — Research by Hospital physicians and scientists have made possible advances in the treatment of cardiac ischemia, atherosclerosis, breast cancer and cystic fibrosis.

Reproductive Medicine and Infertility — National leader in the field, the Hospital's prestigious IVF programs enjoy outstanding success rates.

Trauma Center — Level 1 designations as an Adult Trauma Unit and a Pediatric Trauma Unit ensure the Hospital upholds the highest standards of 24-hour preparedness and treatment.

Women's Health Care — One of the first hospitals dedicated to women's health, NewYork-Presbyterian has established comprehensive programs which provide healthcare to women through all stages of their lives.

ACADEMIC AFFILIATIONS:

NewYork-Presbyterian is the only hospital in the world affiliated with two Ivy League medical schools; The Joan and Sanford I Weill Medical College of Cornell University and the Columbia University College of Physicians and Surgeons.

NEWYORK-PRESBYTERIAN HEALTHCARE SYSTEM:

NewYork-Presbyterian Hospital is at the center of a premier healthcare system, which provides a comprehensive network of healthcare providers throughout the New York metropolitan area, including northern New Jersey, Westchester, the Hudson Valley and Fairfield, Connecticut. The full-service system includes 31 acute-care and community hospitals, 3 specialty institutions, 15 long-term facilities, 10 certified home-health agencies, and over 100 ambulatory-care centers.

Physician Referral: To find a NewYork-Presbyterian Hospital affiliated physician to meet your needs, call toll free **1-877-NYP-WELL** (1-877-697-9355) or visit our website at www.nyp.org.

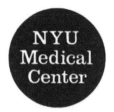

NYU Medical Center
550 First Avenue (31st Street)
New York, NY 10016
Physician Referral:
(888) 7-NYU-MED (888-769-8633)
www.nyumc.org

Sponsorship: Private, Not-for-Profit
Beds: 1069
Accreditation: Joint Commission on Accreditation of Healthcare Organizations (JACHO), Commission for Accreditation of Rehabilitation Facilities (CARF) and Magnet Status

A LEADER IN PATIENT CARE

NYU Medical Center is one of the nation's leading academic medical centers, combining excellence in patient care, research and medical education. A not-for-profit institution, NYU medical Center includes Tisch Hospital, a voluntary 705-bed tertiary care facility serving more than 35,000 inpatients annually, and the Rusk Institute of Rehabilitation Medicine which has 174 beds and serves 2,400 inpatients and more than 41,300 outpatients annually and the NYU Hospital for Joint Disease, which has 190 beds and is one of the nation's premier hospitals for treating orthopaedic and rheumatological disorders.

A DISTINGUISHED FACULTY
NYU School of Medicine has approximately 3,840 faculty members who are attending physicians at Tisch Hospital, Rusk Institute, the Hospital for Joint Diseases, NYU Downtown Hospital, Bellevue Hospital Center, one of the largest and oldest municipal hospitals in North America and an affiliate of NYU Medical Center and the Harborview Veterans Administration system. Many faculty members have distinguished national and international reputations.

A LEADER IN EDUCATION
NYU School of Medicine enrolls more than 678 students and has over 960 resident physicians who are graduates of the nation's finest medical schools. NYU School of Medicine offers a rich research and educational experience, providing residency training programs in virtually every medical specialty. The rich environment of research and training is translated into leading-edge care at our hospitals.

SPECIAL PROGRAMS AT TISCH HOSPITAL

Cancer
The NYU Cancer Institute, home to The Rita J. & Stanley H. Kaplan Comprehensive Cancer Center, an NCI-designated facility, provides state-of-the-art cancer therapy, supportive care, screening and early detection services, and educational programs on prevention.

Cardiac Surgery
NYU Medical Center's cardiovascular surgeons are leaders in the development of minimally invasive techniques for heart valve and bypass surgery, which are significantly less painful and require a much shorter recovery period. More minimally invasive cardiac surgeries have been performed at Tisch than at any other hospital in the world.

Cardiology
A complete range of services is available, including non-invasive cardiology services, cardiac stress testing, and the full range of diagnostic and interventional procedures in cardiac catheterization and electrophysiology. The Pediatric Cardiology Program provides comprehensive care to children who have congenital or acquired heart diseases. The Joan and Joel Smilow Cardiac Prevention and Rehabilitation Center provides an array of services for people at risk for heart disease and those recovering from cardiac surgery.

Sponsored Page

Epilepsy	The Comprehensive Epilepsy Center for treatment of adults and children is the largest facility of its kind on the east coast. The Center's unique team approach includes evaluations conducted jointly by epileptologists, neuropsychologists and neurosurgeons, as well as diagnostic studies and therapies for seizure control.
Gamma Knife	The Gamma Knife Unit is used to remove certain types of tumors, aneurysms, and arteriovenous malformations too deep within the brain to reach with a scalpel. This alternative to traditional surgery is bloodless, usually allowing patients to return home the next day.
Obstetrics	NYU Medical Center offers unparalleled diagnostic techniques and surgical & Gynecology innovations to treat women of all ages, with world-class expertise in infertility treatment and management of high-risk pregnancies.
Pain Management	The Pain Management Center team works closely with a broad range of specialists to provide highly individualized care for each patient. Acute cancer and chronic pain management services are among the Center's specialties.
Pregnancy (High-Risk)	NYU Medical Center provides a host of services for high-risk pregnancies. The Program for IVF, Reproductive Surgery, and Infertility is at the leading edge of assisting couples who have trouble conceiving. The Maternal-Fetal Medicine Program helps women with special risks, such as multiple births, hypertension, diabetes, and heart problems. The Recurrent Pregnancy Loss Program treats women who have a history of miscarriage.
Reconstructive Plastic Surgery	The Institute of Reconstructive Plastic Surgery is the largest facility of its kind in the world, performing 1,500 operations a year and treating problems ranging from severe deformities stemming from congenital birth defects, to injuries and burns. Its staff has pioneered techniques in craniofacial surgery, microsurgery, hand surgery, breast reconstruction, and aesthetic surgery.
Skin Diseases	The Charles C. Harris Skin and Cancer Unit is an internationally-acclaimed center for the treatment of serious and rare skin diseases. It also provides regular outpatient services in specialty clinics for a wide range of common skin problems.
Surgery	Leading the nation in advancement of minimally invasive procedures and surgical techniques.
Transplant	The Mary Lea Johnson Richards Organ Transplant Center is one of the nation's leading centers for liver, kidney, and pancreas transplants including a living donor program. Its clinical team is one of the most experienced in the world, with some of the best patient and graft survival statistics in the nation.
Urology	NYU Medical Center's urologists are leaders in treating prostate disorders, including prostate cancer, as well as many other male and female urological problems. They helped pioneer minimally invasive surgical techniques to preserve a man's sexual function after surgery, and they were leaders in clinical trials of Viagra.

REHABILITATION MEDICINE

Founded by Dr. Howard A. Rusk in 1948, the Rusk Institute of Rehabilitation Medicine is the world's first and one of the largest university centers for the treatment of adults and children with disabilities. The Rusk Institute has been ranked the #1 rehabilitation medicine center in the New York area by the *U.S.News & World Report*'s annual "Best Hospitals" survey for the last fourteen years.

Physician Referral (888) 7-NYU-MED (888-769-8633)
NYU Medical Center provides a free telephone referral service from
9 a.m. to 5 p.m. weekdays. The service provides access to nearly 1,400 NYU physicians.

796

Directory of Doctors

The New York metropolitan region is unique in its concentration of excellent Specialty Hospitals. Specialty Hospitals include those with a specific patient and disease focus such as cardiac care, psychiatric care and care of diseases and problems of eyes and ears. Many of these hospitals are nationally and internationally known for their outstanding care in these specialty areas and draw patients from the region and beyond who seek their excellent specialized care.

Castle Connolly Medical Ltd. has invited the following outstanding Specialty Hospitals to present important facts and information on their hospitals by sponsoring the profiles that follow.

Specialty Hospitals

Burke Rehabilitation Hospital

Calvary Hospital

NYU-Hospital for Joint Diseases

Hospital for Special Surgery

Memorial Sloan-Kettering Cancer Center

New York Eye & Ear Infirmary

Rusk Institute of Rehabilitation Medicine

St. Francis Hospital - The Heart Center

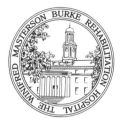

THE BURKE REHABILITATION HOSPITAL

785 Mamaroneck Avenue
White Plains, NY 10605
914-597-2500   1-888-99-BURKE
Admission Hotline 914-946-0865
www.burke.org

Sponsorship: **Private, not-for-profit**
Beds: **150**
Accreditation: **The Joint Commission on Accreditation of Healthcare Organizations (JCAHO) and The Commission on Accreditation of Rehabilitation Facilities (CARF)**
Academic Affiliation: Weill Medical College of Cornell University and the New York- Presbyterian Healthcare System.

The Burke Rehabilitation Hospital, founded in April 1915, is the only provider of dedicated rehabilitation services in Westchester County, New York. Our mission is helping people regain a maximum level of mobility and independence following a disabling illness or injury; to engage in research to improve medical care and to offer health care services appropriate to the needs of our community.

BURKE REHABILITATION HOSPITAL: Burke's beautiful, 60-acre main campus is home to the 150-bed inpatient hospital, which serves patients 16 years and older. Each of the five 30-bed units is focused on a specific disease or related conditions. Burke specializes in treating physical disabilities including stroke, brain injuries, spinal cord injuries, Parkinson's disease and other neurological disorders, cardiac disease, chronic pulmonary disease, arthritis, orthopedics and amputation. We utilize a multidisciplinary team approach to patient care. Under the direction of full-time board-certified physicians, each rehabilitation team may include internists, neurologists, pulmonologists, or rheumatologists; physical, occupational, speech or recreation therapists; audiologists; nurses; social workers; dieticians and respiratory therapists. Burke's brain injury, spinal cord injury and general medical rehabilitation programs are CARF-accredited.

OUTPATIENT SERVICES: The acute, intensive inpatient experience at Burke is complemented by an individually tailored outpatient program. Former inpatients can continue their progress while community residents have access to rehabilitative services on Burke's main campus and at our Rehabilitation & Sports Medicine Clinics in Purchase, White Plains and in the Bronx.

AT THE **BURKE MEDICAL RESEARCH INSTITUTE**, located on our main campus, a world-class group of scientists are currently conducting research in neurodegenerative and inflammatory diseases; stroke prevention and recovery; mechanisms in Parkinson's disease and spinal cord injury and recovery. The Institute is affiliated with the Weill Medical College of Cornell University. We are using discoveries made in the laboratory to improve patient care.

Whether our doctors, nurses, and therapists are providing state-of-the-art treatment, or our research scientists are exploring the frontiers of neurological and pulmonary medicine, they share a central commitment—to ensure that every patient at Burke makes the fullest possible recovery from their illness or injury.

"When they said rehab, I said Burke."
1-888-99BURKE Admission Hotline 914-946-0865

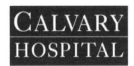

The Model for the Relief
of Cancer Pain and Symptoms
for Over a Century

1740 Eastchester Road
Bronx, NY 10461
Tel: (718) 518-2300
Fax: (718) 518-2670

150 55th Street
Brooklyn, NY 1122(
Tel: (718) 518-2300
Fax: (718) 518-2670

www.calvaryhospital.org

Beds	225: 200 in Bronx; 25 at Brooklyn satellite, Lutheran Medical Center
Accreditation	Joint Commission on Accreditation of Healthcare Organizations (JCAHO), College of American Pathologists (CAP), JCAHO for Home Care and Hospice

Setting the Standard for Palliative Care

Founded in 1899. Voluntary, not-for-profit Archdiocesan hospital specializing in palliative care for adults with advanced cancer. We serve patients and families of all faith traditions in a restraint-free setting, with 24/7 visiting hours. Extensive bereavement support for family and friends.

Palliative Care Institute

Calvary's research and education arm, offering a curriculum for medical students, residents, and postdoctoral fellows. Health lectures for the community. The INSIDE CALVARY 3-day curriculum for healthcare professionals provides direct observation of palliative care.

Acute Inpatient Care

1-page form expedites admission process. Adults with advanced cancer are assigned a primary physician and a care team: nurse, social worker, dietitian, case manager. Goal is to maximize physical, spiritual, and emotional comfort. Pastoral care and bereavement support are integral to care. Calvary consistently ranks in the top 1% of its peers for patient satisfaction.

Outpatient and Wound Care

Outpatient clinic for cancer patients undergoing active treatment or who do not require acute inpatient care. Center for Curative and Palliative Wound Care treats complex wounds related to cancer, diabetes, vascular disease, and other illnesses.

CALVARY@HOME: Home Care, Hospice, Nursing Home Hospice

Certified Home Health Agency

Provides full range of home care services, not limited to patients with advanced cancer, in Bronx, Queens, northern Manhattan and southern Westchester. Care is coordinated by patient's community physician or Calvary doctor. Nurse is available 24/7 for telephone consults.

Hospice

For people with all terminal diagnoses who are primarily cared for at home. Emphasis on quality of life, control of pain and symptoms, and support for family. Serves patients in Bronx, Brooklyn, Manhattan, Queens, Westchester, Nassau, and Rockland. Care may be coordinated by community physician or Calvary doctor. Nurse is available 24/7 by telephone. Bereavement support. Short-term hospitalization is available for acute symptom mangement.

Nursing Home Hospice

For nursing home residents suffering from all end-stage illnesses. Goal is to promote quality of life.

Satellite Program

Calvary plans to develop new satellites, to serve increasing numbers of people in our area.

Family Care

Focuses on the impact of cancer on the family.

Extensive bereavement support for adults, teens, and children, including bereavement camp for children and teens who participate in our support groups.

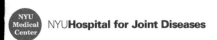 NYU**Hospital for Joint Diseases**

301 East 17th Street (at Second Avenue)
New York, NY 10003
212-598-6000   FAX: 212-260-1203
Website: www.nyuhjd.org

Sponsorship:	NYU Medical Center
Beds:	190
Accreditation:	Joint Commission on Accreditation of Healthcare Organizations (JCAHO), Commission of Accreditation for Rehabilitation Facilities (CARF)

PROFILE
NYU Hospital for Joint Diseases is one of the nation's leading orthopaedic, rheumatologic, rehabilitation and neurologic specialty sites dedicated to the prevention and treatment of neuromusculoskeletal diseases. NYUHJD is a voluntary, not-for-profit teaching institution and is part of NYU Medical Center.

MEDICAL STAFF
NYU Hospital for Joint Diseases has over 500 board certified members of the attending medical staff specializing in orthopaedics, rheumatology, rehabilitation medicine and neurology.

TEACHING PROGRAMS
NYUHJD sponsors a fully accredited five-year orthopaedic surgery residency program with twelve residents each year. In addition, seven different fellowships are offered in the subspecialty areas of orthopaedics including hand, foot and ankle, spine, sports medicine, shoulder, and total joint replacement..

SPECIAL PROGRAMS
Orthopaedic Surgery: Joint Replacement Center, The Spine Center, Arthroscopic Surgery, Pediatric Orthopaedics, Bone Tumor Service, Foot and Ankle Surgery, Hand Surgery, Limb Lengthening and Bone Growth, Occupational and Industrial Orthopaedic Care, Sports Medicine, Shoulder Institute, Center for Neuromuscular and Developmental Disorders, Diabetes Foot and Ankle Center, The Harkness Center for Dance Injuries, and an Immediate Orthopaedic Care Center.

Department of Rheumatology and Medicine: Center for Arthritis & Autoimmunity and the Peter D. Seligman Center for Advanced Therapeutics. Rheumatoid Arthritis, Osteoarthritis, Psoriatic Arthritis, Lupus, Osteoporosis, Fibromyalgia, Scleroderma, Sjogren's Syndrome.

Rehabilitation Medicine: The Rusk Institute of Rehabilitation Medicine at 17th Street offers comprehensive inpatient (orthopaedic and neurological rehabilitation, pain management) and outpatient rehabilitation services at NYUHJD and other locations.

Additional Programs: Orthopaedic Neurology, Initiative for Women with Disabilities, Multiple Sclerosis, Neuroimmunology, Neurosurgery, Comprehensive Pain Treatment Center, Clinical Neurophysiology, Movement Disorders, and Neurorehabilitation.

OTHER SERVICES
Managed Care Plans: NYU Hospital for Joint Diseases participates in over 45 managed care plans covering 72 different products (i.e., HMO, POS, PPO, Medicare, Medicaid, etc.).

Physician Referral	NYUHJD offers a free telephone physician referral service, Monday-Friday, 8:30 am to 6:00 pm. The physician referral service can be reached at 1-888-HJD-DOCS (1-888-453-3627).

690

HOSPITAL
FOR
SPECIAL
SURGERY

HOSPITAL FOR SPECIAL SURGERY

535 East 70th Street • New York, NY 10021
Physician Referral: 800-854-0071

hss.edu

Sponsorship: Private, Non-Profit
Beds: 138
Accreditation: Joint Commission on Accreditation of Healthcare Organizations (JCAHO)

FIRST IN ITS FIELD
Founded in 1863, Hospital for Special Surgery is the nation's leading specialty hospital for orthopaedics and rheumatology.

FIRST IN JOINT REPLACEMENTS
HSS pioneered designs and surgical techniques for the first modern total knee replacement in the 1970's. Today, HSS performs more joint replacements than any other hospital in America.

PIONEERING MINIMALLY INVASIVE SURGERY
HSS surgeons developed smaller instruments and surgical techniques allowing minimally invasive total hip replacement and minimally invasive total knee replacement. HSS anesthesiologists, world leaders in regional anesthesia, developed special pain blocks required for minimally invasive surgery. HSS surgeons are innovators in hand, elbow, shoulder, and spine surgery techniques. They are leading experts in arthroplasty. Over 75% of all knee procedures performed at HSS are minimally invasive.

AMERICA'S LARGEST GROUP OF RHEUMATOLOGISTS
HSS Rheumatologists are international authorities and pioneering researchers in all rheumatological and autoimmune conditions and treatments, including lupus, rheumatoid arthritis, juvenile rheumatoid arthritis, and osteoarthritis. The Godsen-Robinson Early Arthritis Center provides treatment plans and education for patients and primary care physicians about the importance of early intervention in osteoarthritis and rheumatoid arthritis.

WORLD'S LARGEST, MOST EXPERIENCED GROUP OF MUSCULOSKELETAL RADIOLOGISTS
HSS is the largest academic center in the world dedicated to musculoskeletal imaging. HSS Radiologists developed the revolutionary MRI pulse-sequencing techniques that reveal early degenerative changes in cartilage and other soft tissue. No other academic institution has five high field MR Units dedicated exclusively to musculoskeletal imaging.

**Top Ranked in Orthopaedics
& Rheumatology in the Northeast
by** *U.S. News & World Reports*
for 16 Years in a Row

**Winner of Nursing's Highest Honor:
Magnet Status for Nursing Excellence**

**Winner of New York State's
First Patient Safety Award**

**Over 200 Attending Physicians and
74 Noted Research Scientists–
All are Faculty Members of
Weill Medical College of
Cornell University Faculty**

**Team Physicians for NY Mets,
NY Giants, Association of Tennis
Professionals, St. John's University and
other Professional and College Teams**

Sponsored Page

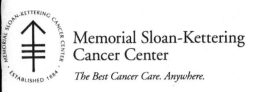

Memorial Sloan-Kettering Cancer Center

The Best Cancer Care. Anywhere.

1275 York Avenue
New York, NY 10021
Phone: (212) 639-2000
Physician Referral: (800) 525-2225
www.mskcc.org

Beds: 432
Sponsorship/Network Affiliation: Private, Non-Profit
Physician Referral: (800) 525-2225

THE MSKCC ADVANTAGE: CANCER IS OUR ONLY FOCUS

At Memorial Sloan-Kettering Cancer Center, our only focus is cancer as it has been for more than a century. Internationally recognized as one of the world's premier facilities for cancer care, Memorial Sloan-Kettering was ranked #1 in the United States for cancer care 2006 by *US News & World Report*. We are proud of our designation as a National Cancer Institute (NCI) Comprehensive Cancer Center.

A TEAM APPROACH TO CANCER CARE

Multidisciplinary teams of physicians, defined by cancer type (lung, breast, etc.), work together to guide each patient through diagnosis, treatment and recovery. The combined expertise of many doctors—surgeons, medical oncologists, radiologists, radiation oncologists and pathologists—ensures that patients who need several different therapies to treat their cancer will receive the best combination for them.

GREATER PRECISION IN DIAGNOSIS

At Memorial Sloan-Kettering, we offer the most advanced imaging technologies, such as combined PET/CT imaging, to accurately diagnose and stage cancers. Our highly specialized pathologists are increasingly able to identify the molecular differences among tumors, providing even greater precision in diagnosis. This allows our physicians to determine the optimal therapy that is available to treat each individual's specific cancer.

UNPARALLELED SURGICAL EXPERTISE

Recent studies have shown that, for many cancers, patients have fewer complications and better outcomes if they have surgery at a hospital that performs high volumes of these operations and if the surgery is performed by a surgeon who is very experienced in the procedure. Because of their sole focus on cancer, our surgeons are among the most skilled and experienced cancer surgeons in the world. Over the years, they have pioneered scores of surgical innovations, including the use of minimally invasive techniques for many cancers, as well as procedures to spare or reconstruct organs and preserve function. They are renowned for not only saving lives, but saving the quality of life.

ADVANCES IN CHEMOTHERAPY

Our medical oncologists are leaders in developing new chemotherapy drugs that are safer and more effective than standard therapies. They can also help patients manage the side effects of chemotherapy, such as nausea and fatigue. Increasingly, our medical oncologists employ sophisticated technologies, such as immunotherapies or vaccines, often in combination with chemotherapy, to more effectively treat cancer.

LEADERS IN RADIATION THERAPY

Memorial Sloan-Kettering's radiation oncologists pioneered intensity-modulated radiation therapy, which allows higher, more effective doses of radiation to be delivered to tumors while minimizing exposure to surrounding healthy tissues and organs. They are experts in the use of brachytherapy, where tiny radioactive seeds are implanted to provide high doses of radiation directly to the tumor. Our doctors have also developed the use of radiation therapy with chemotherapy, which makes tumor cells more sensitive to the effects of radiation, enhancing the success of therapy.

RESEARCH EXPANDS TREATMENT OPTIONS

Our doctors and research scientists work closely together to improve the standard of care through the integration of clinical trials into clinical practice. This close collaboration means that new drugs and therapies developed in the laboratory can be moved quickly to the bedside, offering patients improved treatment options and better chances for cure. There are approximately 400 active clinical trials being conducted here at Memorial Sloan-Kettering.

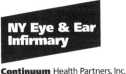

THE NEW YORK EYE AND EAR INFIRMARY

310 East 14th Street
New York, New York 10003
Tel. 212.979.4000   Fax. 212.228.0664
http://www.nyee.edu

BEDS:	34; Operating Rooms: 17; Surgical Cases: 20,000+ a year
Sponsorship:	Voluntary Not-for-Profit
Accreditation:	Joint Commission on the Accreditation of Healthcare Organizations
	College of American Pathologists

GENERAL OVERVIEW

The New York Eye and Ear Infirmary is one of the world's leading facilities for the diagnosis and treatment of diseases of the eyes, ears, nose, throat and related conditions. Founded in 1820, it is the oldest continuously operating specialty hospital in the nation, as well as one of the busiest.

ACADEMIC AND CLINICAL AFFILIATIONS

A voluntary, not-for-profit institution, the Infirmary is a member of Continuum Health Partners, Inc. and an affiliated teaching hospital of New York Medical College. There are highly regarded residency programs in ophthalmology and otolaryngology, plus some two dozen post-graduate fellowship positions.

THE MEDICAL STAFF

The Medical Staff includes more than 500 board-certified attending physicians and surgeons throughout the metropolitan area. Many are renowned for their breakthrough research introducing widely practiced techniques.

SPECIALTIES

Ophthalmology: Within this area are subspecialties of cataract, glaucoma, retina, cornea and refractive surgery, ocular plastic surgery, pediatric ophthalmology and strabismus, neuro-ophthalmology and ocular tumor. Laser, photography, fluorescein angiography and electrophysiological testing are among the most advanced services available anywhere.

Otolaryngology: The department is in the forefront of treatment modalities using highly sophisticated endoscopic and laser equipment. Subspecialties include rhinology, laryngology, head & neck surgery, otology/neurotology, pediatric otolaryngology, audiology, speech therapy and hearing aid dispensing.

Plastic & Reconstructive Surgery: Microsurgical capabilities and premium patient accommodations provide an optimum environment for facial plasty, liposuction and repair of defects from disease or trauma.

RELATED SERVICES

New York Eye Trauma Center: An advanced program for emergency treatment of eye injuries, it also is the Eye Injury Registry of New York State and leading collector of data which will help develop preventative strategies.

Ambulatory Surgery: A comprehensive Ambulatory Surgery Center is designed to expedite admission testing, pre-op preparation and post-op recovery in an efficient and comfortable setting.

Pediatric Specialty Care: Services of eye and ear, nose and throat specialists are coordinated with other professional and support staff especially sensitive to the youngest patients.

RESEARCH AND EDUCATION

The New York Eye and Ear Infirmary is a national and international leader in research in its specialties, achieving many "firsts" in successful surgical procedures and medical treatments. Laboratories include Cell Culture, Ocular Imaging, and Microsurgical Education. Over a hundred studies and clinical trials are currently being conducted.

Physician Referral: Call 1.800.449.HOPE (4673)

Sponsored Page

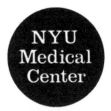

RUSK INSTITUTE OF REHABILITATION MEDICINE
At NYU Medical Center

400 East 34th Street (between 1st Avenue and FDR Drive)
New York, NY 10016
Physician Referral (888) 7-NYU-MED
(888-769-8633)
www.msnyuhealth.org/ri/rusk

Sponsorship:	Private, Not-for-Profit
Beds:	174
Accreditation:	Joint Commission on Accreditation of Healthcare Organizations (JCAHO), Commission for Accreditation of Rehabilitation Facilities (CARF)

LEADING THE WAY IN REHABILITATION MEDICINE

Yesterday, Today and Tomorrow

The Rusk Institute of Rehabilitation Medicine, an integral component of NYU Medical Center, is the world's first facility devoted entirely to rehabilitation medicine. Founded in 1948 by Dr. Howard A. Rusk, it is the largest university-affiliated center for the treatment of adults and children with disabilities, as well as for research and training in rehabilitation medicine.

The relationship between Rusk Institute and other clinical and research units within the Medical Center – including Tisch Hospital, a 726-bed acute-care facility – contributes to an environment which provides the optimal rehabilitation setting for patients. Should the need arise, patients at Rusk Institute have immediate access to Tisch Hospital's superb tertiary-care facilities, with its full range of medical and surgical services and equipment.

Rusk Institute treats neurological, orthopedic and a wide variety of physical disabilities in children and adults on an inpatient and outpatient basis. Rusk Institute has continuously succeeded both in improving the lives of the physically challenged and in delivering on its commitment to quality patient care.

SPECIAL PROGRAMS AT RUSK:

Amputee Program	Aphasia Rehabilitation
Arthritis Program	Back Pain Program
Barrier-Free Design Unit	Biofeedback for Motor Disorders
Brain Injury Program	Cancer Rehabilitation
Cardiac Rehabilitation	Cerebral Palsy
Chronic Pain Treatment	Cognitive Remediation
Dysphagia/Swallowing Program	Hand Therapy
Hip and Lower Extremity Fractures	Horticultural Therapy
Jerry Lewis Muscular Dystrophy Clinic	Job Placement Services
Joint replacements	Lymphedema Program
Mild Trauatic Brain Injury Program	Music/Art Therapy
Multiple Sclerosis Program	Neuromuscular Diseases
Pain (acute and chronic) Management	Parkinson' Disease Program
Patient/Family Support Groups	Pediatric Communications Skills Program
Pediatric Rehabilitation	Pre-School and Early Intervention
Pulmonary Rehabilitation	Rehabilitation Services for Women
Rhizotomy Program	Scoliosis Program
Spasticity Management	Spina Bifida Program
Spinal Cord Injury Program	Splinting Program for Neurological Patients
Sports Injuries Rehabilitation	Stroke Rehabilitation
Swallowing Disorders (Dysphagia) Program	Vestibular (Balance) Disorders Program

The Rusk Institute has trained more Rehabilitation specialists than any other center in the world and has been ranked the #1 rehabilitation hospital in New York by *U.S. News & World Reports* for seventeen consecutive years.

688

St. Francis Hospital, The Heart Center®

100 Port Washington Blvd.
Roslyn, New York 11576
www.stfrancisheartcenter.com
(516) 562-6000

Sponsorship:	Voluntary not-for-profit
Beds:	279
Accreditation:	Awarded accreditation from the Joint Commission on Accreditation of Healthcare Organizations
Affiliation:	A member of Catholic Health Services of Long Island

St. Francis Hospital, The Heart Center® is New York State's only specialty designated cardiac center, offering one of the leading cardiac care programs in the nation. Founded in 1922 by the Franciscan Missionaries of Mary, the Hospital is recognized as an innovator in the delivery of specialized cardiovascular services in an environment where excellence and compassion are emphasized. St. Francis also offers a superb program in non-cardiac surgery, including some of the most advanced technology and minimally invasive techniques available for vascular, prostate, ear-nose-throat (ENT), and orthopedic surgery.

Cardiac Diagnostics and Treatment
St. Francis Hospital performs more cardiac procedures than any other hospital in the Northeast and has been consistently recognized for its outstanding quality of care. In recent years, the Hospital has been named one of America's best heart centers by *U.S.News & World Report* and by *Modern Maturity*, the magazine of AARP.

Cardiac surgery: In 2005, 1,642 open heart surgeries were performed at St. Francis Hospital. It was the only hospital in the New York metropolitan area with risk-adjusted mortality rates significantly below the statewide average for heart valve and valve/coronary artery bypass surgery, the most challenging forms of common cardiac surgery. St. Francis is also a leading center for off-pump bypass surgery and some of the most advanced minimally invasive techniques.

Cardiac catheterization: In 2005, St. Francis interventional cardiologists performed 10,536 cardiac catheterizations and 4,262 percutaneous coronary interventions (angioplasty and insertion of stents). In the last year reported by the Department of Health, St. Francis had the highest caseload in New York State. The Hospital is also recognized as one of the East Coast's highest volume centers for catheter-based techniques to close atrial septal defects (ASDs) and patent foramen ovale (PFO).

Arrhythmia and Pacemaker Center: St. Francis has a leading national program for pacemaker implantation and the diagnosis and treatment of cardiac rhythm abnormalities. The Center has unparalleled expertise in radiofrequency cardiac ablation, including treatment of atrial fibrillation.

Research and Technology
At the St. Francis Cardiac Research Institute, a team of world-renowned researchers is working with the latest non-invasive imaging technology, including the new 64-slice CT scanner, 3-dimensional echocardiography system, and the area's first dedicated cardiac magnetic resonance (MRI) unit. This multi-modality approach to investigating the heart's function and disease processes is aimed at improving methods of diagnosing heart disease.

Prevention and Education
St. Francis Hospital's satellite campus, The DeMatteis Center for Cardiac Research and Education, in Old Brookville, New York, is one of the few freestanding campuses in the U.S. dedicated to the prevention of heart disease. It is the site of community health lectures, as well as the largest medically staffed cardiac fitness and rehabilitation program on Long Island.

Physician referral: 1-888-HEARTNY

644

Sponsored Page

New York State Metropolitan Regional Medical Centers and Hospitals

The New York metropolitan region is fortunate to have a large number of truly excellent Regional Medical Centers and Hospitals. Many of these institutions offer sophisticated services that in years past were offered only at academic medical centers. However, with advancements in medical technology, Regional Medical Centers and Hospitals have access to the equipment, and by virtue of the medical schools and teaching hospitals in the region, the well-trained physicians and staff, to offer these programs.

Regional Medical Centers and Hospitals range in size from the small (100 beds) to the very large (800 beds) but they share a common theme: a primary focus on patient care.

We have invited a select number of excellent Regional Medical Centers and Hospitals to provide readers of the Castle Connolly Guide with information on their institutions and services by sponsoring profiles, which are included at the end of individual county sections in the physician listings that follow.

Regional Medical Centers and Hospitals

Cabrini Medical Center

Saint Vincent Catholic Medical Centers

New York Medthodists Hospital

Sound Shore Medical Center

The Mount Vernon Hospital

Westchester Medical Center

White Plains Hospital Center

Englewood Hospital & Medical Center

Holy Name Hospital

The Valley Hospital

Robert Wood Johnson University Hospital

Yale-New Haven Hospital

Section Three

Physician Listings

The State of New York

New York (Manhattan)

ADDICTION PSYCHIATRY

Frances, Richard J MD (AdP) - **Spec Exp:** Alcohol Abuse; Substance Abuse; Forensic Psychiatry; **Hospital:** Silver Hill Hosp, NYU Med Ctr (page 102); **Address:** 510 E 86th St, Ste 1D, New York, NY 10028; **Phone:** 212-861-0570; **Board Cert:** Psychiatry 1976; Addiction Psychiatry 2002; **Med School:** NYU Sch Med 1971; **Resid:** Psychiatry, Bronx Meml Hosp 1974; **Fellow:** Psychoanalysis, NY Psychanal Inst 1978; **Fac Appt:** Clin Prof Psyc, NYU Sch Med

Galanter, Marc MD (AdP) - **Spec Exp:** Alcohol Abuse; Drug Abuse; **Hospital:** NYU Med Ctr (page 102); **Address:** 285 Central Park West, New York, NY 10024-3006; **Phone:** 212-877-4093; **Board Cert:** Psychiatry 1974; Addiction Psychiatry 2002; **Med School:** Albert Einstein Coll Med 1967; **Resid:** Psychiatry, Bronx Muni Hosp-Einstein 1971; **Fac Appt:** Prof Psyc, NYU Sch Med

Kleber, Herbert MD (AdP) - **Spec Exp:** Opiate Addiction; Cocaine Addiction; Marijuana Abuse; Drug Abuse; **Hospital:** NY-Presby Hosp (page 100), NY State Psychiatric Inst (page 100); **Address:** 1051 Riverside Dr, New York, NY 10032-1007; **Phone:** 212-543-5570; **Med School:** Jefferson Med Coll 1960; **Resid:** Psychiatry, Yale-New Haven Hosp 1964; **Fac Appt:** Prof Psyc, Columbia P&S

Levin, Frances R MD (AdP) - **Spec Exp:** Addiction/Substance Abuse; Dual Diagnosis; Substance Abuse in ADHD Patients; **Hospital:** NY State Psychiatric Inst (page 100), NY-Presby Hosp (page 100); **Address:** NYSPI, Dept Psychiatry, 1051 Riverside Drive, Unit 66, New York, NY 10032; **Phone:** 212-923-3031; **Board Cert:** Psychiatry 1990; Addiction Psychiatry 1993; **Med School:** Cornell Univ-Weill Med Coll 1985; **Resid:** Psychiatry, Payne Whitney Clin 1989; **Fellow:** Substance Abuse, Univ Maryland/NIDA 1990; **Fac Appt:** Assoc Prof Psyc, Columbia P&S

Paul, Edward MD (AdP) - **Spec Exp:** Opiate Addiction; Alcohol Abuse; Nicotine Dependence; **Hospital:** NYU Med Ctr (page 102); **Address:** 155 E 31st St, Ste 25J, New York, NY 10016; **Phone:** 212-447-5712; **Board Cert:** Psychiatry 1987; Addiction Psychiatry 2003; **Med School:** Columbia P&S 1982; **Resid:** Psychiatry, Payne Whitney Clinic 1987; Psychoanalysis, NYU Med Ctr 1993; **Fellow:** Substance Abuse, New York Hosp 1987; **Fac Appt:** Asst Clin Prof Psyc, NYU Sch Med

Rosenberg, Kenneth P MD (AdP) - **Spec Exp:** Addiction/Substance Abuse; Sexual Dysfunction; Physicians' Health-Psychiatric; **Hospital:** NY-Presby Hosp (page 100); **Address:** 110 E 71st St, New York, NY 10021; **Phone:** 212-861-8807; **Board Cert:** Psychiatry 1992; Addiction Psychiatry 1998; **Med School:** Albert Einstein Coll Med 1983; **Resid:** Psychiatry, NY Hosp-Cornell Med Ctr 1988; **Fellow:** Substance Abuse, NY Hosp-Cornell Med Ctr 1991; Public Health, NY Hosp-Cornell Med Ctr 1992; **Fac Appt:** Assoc Clin Prof Psyc, Cornell Univ-Weill Med Coll

Weiss, Carol J MD (AdP) - **Spec Exp:** Drug Abuse; Alcohol Abuse; **Hospital:** NY-Presby Hosp (page 100); **Address:** 1044 Madison Ave, New York, NY 10022; **Phone:** 212-988-1209; **Board Cert:** Psychiatry 1989; Addiction Psychiatry 1993; **Med School:** Johns Hopkins Univ 1983; **Resid:** Psychiatry, New York Hosp 1987; **Fellow:** Addiction Psychiatry, New York Hosp 1989; **Fac Appt:** Asst Clin Prof Psyc, Cornell Univ-Weill Med Coll

ADOLESCENT MEDICINE

Diaz, Angela MD (AM) - **Spec Exp:** Adolescent Gynecology; Adolescent Medicine; Abuse/Neglect; **Hospital:** Mount Sinai Med Ctr (page 98); **Address:** 320 E 94th St Fl 2, New York, NY 10128-5604; **Phone:** 212-423-2900; **Board Cert:** Pediatrics 1987; Adolescent Medicine 2004; **Med School:** Columbia P&S 1981; **Resid:** Pediatrics, Mt Sinai Med Ctr 1984; **Fellow:** Adolescent Medicine, Mt Sinai Med Ctr 1985; **Fac Appt:** Prof Ped, Mount Sinai Sch Med

Levin Carmine, Linda MD (AM) `PCP` - **Spec Exp:** AIDS/HIV in Adolescents; **Hospital:** Mount Sinai Med Ctr (page 98); **Address:** 312 E 94th St, New York, NY 10128-5604; **Phone:** 212-423-2887; **Board Cert:** Pediatrics 1987; Adolescent Medicine 2002; **Med School:** NYU Sch Med 1982; **Resid:** Pediatrics, Montefiore Hosp Med Ctr 1985; **Fellow:** Adolescent Medicine, Montefiore Hosp Med Ctr 1986; **Fac Appt:** Assoc Clin Prof Ped, Mount Sinai Sch Med

Lopez, Ralph MD (AM) - **Spec Exp:** Growth/Development Disorders; Eating Disorders; Learning Disorders; **Hospital:** NY-Presby Hosp (page 100), Lenox Hill Hosp (page 94); **Address:** 418 E 71st St, New York, NY 10021-4894; **Phone:** 212-772-8989; **Board Cert:** Pediatrics 1972; **Med School:** NYU Sch Med 1967; **Resid:** Pediatrics, Bellevue Hosp 1969; Pediatrics, Chldns Hosp 1970; **Fellow:** Adolescent Medicine, Chldns Hosp 1971, **Fac Appt:** Assoc Clin Prof Ped, Cornell Univ-Weill Med Coll

Marks, Andrea MD (AM) - **Spec Exp:** Eating Disorders; Adolescent Gynecology; Psychosomatic Disorders; Parenting Issues; **Hospital:** Mount Sinai Med Ctr (page 98); **Address:** 14 E 90th St, New York, NY 10128-0671; **Phone:** 212-987-1414; **Board Cert:** Pediatrics 1977; Adolescent Medicine 2002; **Med School:** Univ Pennsylvania 1972; **Resid:** Pediatrics, Chldns Hosp 1974; **Fellow:** Adolescent Medicine, Chldns Hosp 1975; **Fac Appt:** Assoc Clin Prof Ped, Mount Sinai Sch Med

Pegler, Cynthia MD (AM) `PCP` - **Spec Exp:** Adolescent Gynecology; Eating Disorders; **Hospital:** Lenox Hill Hosp (page 94); **Address:** 992 5th Ave, New York, NY 10028; **Phone:** 212-517-5313; **Board Cert:** Pediatrics 1998; Adolescent Medicine 2002; **Med School:** Albany Med Coll 1984; **Resid:** Pediatrics, N Shore Univ Hosp 1987; **Fellow:** Adolescent Medicine, N Shore Univ Hosp 1990

ALLERGY & IMMUNOLOGY

Buchbinder, Ellen MD (A&I) - **Spec Exp:** Asthma; Allergy; Rhinitis; **Hospital:** Mount Sinai Med Ctr (page 98); **Address:** 111B E 88th St, New York, NY 10128; **Phone:** 212-410-3246; **Board Cert:** Internal Medicine 1981; Allergy & Immunology 1983; **Med School:** Tulane Univ 1978; **Resid:** Internal Medicine, New England Deaconess Hosp 1981; **Fellow:** Allergy & Immunology, Mass Genl Hosp 1983; **Fac Appt:** Asst Clin Prof Med, Mount Sinai Sch Med

Chandler, Michael MD (A&I) - **Spec Exp:** Asthma; Sinus Disorders; **Hospital:** Lenox Hill Hosp (page 94), Mount Sinai Med Ctr (page 98); **Address:** 115 E 61st St, New York, NY 10021-8183; **Phone:** 212-486-6715; **Board Cert:** Internal Medicine 1984; Allergy & Immunology 1987; **Med School:** Wayne State Univ 1981; **Resid:** Internal Medicine, Northwestern Meml Hosp 1984; **Fellow:** Allergy & Immunology, Northwestern Meml Hosp 1986; **Fac Appt:** Asst Clin Prof Med, Mount Sinai Sch Med

Corn, Beth E MD (A&I) - **Spec Exp:** Asthma; **Hospital:** Mount Sinai Med Ctr (page 98); **Address:** 5 E 98th St Fl 10, New York, NY 10029; **Phone:** 212-241-0764; **Board Cert:** Internal Medicine 1995; Allergy & Immunology 1997; **Med School:** Albert Einstein Coll Med 1989; **Resid:** Internal Medicine, St Lukes-Roosevelt Hosp 1992; **Fellow:** Clinical Immunology, Mt Sinai Med Ctr 1994; **Fac Appt:** Asst Prof Med, Mount Sinai Sch Med

Cunningham-Rundles, Charlotte MD/PhD (A&I) - **Spec Exp:** Immunotherapy; Immunodeficiency Disorders; **Hospital:** Mount Sinai Med Ctr (page 98); **Address:** 1425 Madison Ave, rm 11-20, New York, NY 10029; **Phone:** 212-659-9268; **Board Cert:** Internal Medicine 1972; **Med School:** Columbia P&S 1969; **Resid:** Internal Medicine, Bellevue Hosp Ctr 1972; **Fellow:** Allergy & Immunology, NYU Med Ctr 1974; **Fac Appt:** Prof Med, Mount Sinai Sch Med

Feldman, B Robert MD (A&I) - **Spec Exp:** Asthma; Allergic Rhinitis; Food Allergy; **Hospital:** NY-Presby Hosp (page 100); **Address:** Morgan Stanley Chlds Hosp NY-Presby, 3959 Broadway, New York, NY 10032; **Phone:** 212-305-2300; **Board Cert:** Pediatrics 1965; Allergy & Immunology 1972; **Med School:** Univ Hlth Sci/Chicago Med Sch 1959; **Resid:** Pediatrics, Michael Reese Hosp 1962; Allergy & Immunology, Michael Reese Hosp 1963; **Fellow:** Allergy & Immunology, Columbia-Presby Med Ctr 1964; **Fac Appt:** Clin Prof Ped, Columbia P&S

Frenkel, Renata MD (A&I) - **Spec Exp:** Asthma; Allergy; Sinus Disorders; **Hospital:** St Luke's - Roosevelt Hosp Ctr - Roosevelt Div (page 90), Lenox Hill Hosp (page 94); **Address:** 30 W 60th St, Ste 1U, New York, NY 10023-7906; **Phone:** 212-265-1990; **Board Cert:** Allergy & Immunology 1979; **Med School:** Austria 1968; **Resid:** Allergy & Immunology, Roosevelt Hosp 1975; **Fac Appt:** , Columbia P&S

Grubman, Samuel MD (A&I) - **Spec Exp:** Allergy; Asthma; Food Allergy; **Hospital:** St Vincent Cath Med Ctrs - Manhattan (page 375); **Address:** 222 W 14th St, New York, NY 10011; **Phone:** 212-604-1880; **Board Cert:** Allergy & Immunology 1999; Pediatrics 1987; **Med School:** Mount Sinai Sch Med 1983; **Resid:** Pediatrics, NYU Med Ctr 1986; **Fellow:** Allergy & Immunology, Montefiore Med Ctr 1988; **Fac Appt:** Assoc Clin Prof Ped, NY Med Coll

Kadar, Avraham MD (A&I) - **Spec Exp:** Asthma & Allergy; Immune Deficiency; Autoimmune Disease; **Hospital:** Beth Israel Med Ctr - Petrie Division (page 90), Northern Westchester Hosp; **Address:** 530 Park Ave Fl 1, New York, NY 10021; **Phone:** 212-755-3456; **Board Cert:** Pediatrics 1988; Clinical & Laboratory Immunology 1990; **Med School:** Israel 1983; **Resid:** Pediatrics, Albert Einstein 1986; **Fellow:** Allergy & Immunology, Nat Inst Health 1989; **Fac Appt:** Asst Clin Prof A&I, Albert Einstein Coll Med

Mazza, David S MD (A&I) - **Spec Exp:** Asthma; Sinus Disorders; Eczema; **Hospital:** St Luke's - Roosevelt Hosp Ctr - Roosevelt Div (page 90), St Vincent Cath Med Ctrs - Manhattan (page 375); **Address:** 7 Lexington Ave, Ste 3, New York, NY 10010-5517; **Phone:** 212-677-7170; **Board Cert:** Pediatrics 1983; Allergy & Immunology 1999; **Med School:** Univ VT Coll Med 1977; **Resid:** Pediatrics, NYU-Bellevue Hosp 1980; **Fellow:** Pediatrics, Bellevue Hosp 1982; Allergy & Immunology, St Luke's-Roosevelt Hosp Ctr 1989; **Fac Appt:** Assoc Prof Ped, Columbia P&S

Rubin, James MD (A&I) - **Spec Exp:** Asthma; Rhinitis; Sinus Disorders; **Hospital:** Beth Israel Med Ctr - Petrie Division (page 90); **Address:** 35 E 35th St, Ste 202, New York, NY 10016-3823; **Phone:** 212-685-4225; **Board Cert:** Internal Medicine 1968; Allergy & Immunology 1971; **Med School:** NY Med Coll 1960; **Resid:** Internal Medicine, Beth Israel Hosp 1964; **Fellow:** Allergy & Immunology, Jewish Hosp 1965; **Fac Appt:** Assoc Clin Prof Med, Albert Einstein Coll Med

New York (Manhattan)

Shepherd, Gillian M MD (A&I) - **Spec Exp:** Food & Drug Allergy; Rhinosinusitis & Asthma; Urticaria; Insect Allergies; **Hospital:** NY-Presby Hosp (page 100), Meml Sloan Kettering Cancer Ctr (page 109); **Address:** 235 E 67th St, Ste 203, New York, NY 10021-6040; **Phone:** 212-288-9300; **Board Cert:** Internal Medicine 1979; Allergy & Immunology 1981; **Med School:** NY Med Coll 1976; **Resid:** Internal Medicine, Lenox Hill Hosp 1979; **Fellow:** Allergy & Immunology, New York Hosp-Cornell 1981; **Fac Appt:** Assoc Clin Prof Med, Cornell Univ-Weill Med Coll

Siegal, Frederick P MD (A&I) - **Spec Exp:** AIDS/HIV; Immune Deficiency; **Hospital:** St Vincent Cath Med Ctrs - Manhattan (page 375); **Address:** 222 W 14th St Fl Ground, New York, NY 10011; **Phone:** 212-604-2941; **Board Cert:** Internal Medicine 1971; Allergy & Immunology 1973; **Med School:** Columbia P&S 1965; **Resid:** Internal Medicine, Mt Sinai Hosp 1970; **Fellow:** Immunology, Rockefeller Univ 1973

Slankard, Marjorie MD (A&I) - **Spec Exp:** Rhinitis; Asthma; Sinusitis; Food Allergy; **Hospital:** NY-Presby Hosp (page 100), Valley Hosp (page 762); **Address:** 16 E 60th St, Ste 321, New York, NY 10022; **Phone:** 212-326-8410; **Board Cert:** Internal Medicine 1974; Allergy & Immunology 1977; **Med School:** Univ MO-Columbia Sch Med 1971; **Resid:** Internal Medicine, New York Hosp 1974; Internal Medicine, Rockefeller Univ Hosp 1974; **Fellow:** Immunology, New York Hosp-Cornell 1976; Immunology, Mount Sinai Med Ctr 1980; **Fac Appt:** Clin Prof Med, Columbia P&S

Tolston, Evelyn MD (A&I) - **Spec Exp:** Rhinitis; Asthma; Allergy; **Hospital:** Cabrini Med Ctr (page 374); **Address:** 161 Madison Ave, Ste 3A, New York, NY 10016; **Phone:** 646-424-0400; **Board Cert:** Internal Medicine 1994; Allergy & Immunology 1995; **Med School:** Ukraine 1982; **Resid:** Internal Medicine, Cabrini Med Ctr 1993; Allergy & Immunology, Albert Einstein Coll Med 1995

Young, Stuart H. MD (A&I) - **Spec Exp:** Asthma; Nasal & Sinus Disorders; Urticaria; **Hospital:** Mount Sinai Med Ctr (page 98); **Address:** 121 E 60th St, Ste 1D, New York, NY 10022-1102; **Phone:** 212-826-0815; **Board Cert:** Pediatrics 1968; Allergy & Immunology 1972; **Med School:** SUNY Downstate 1963; **Resid:** Pediatrics, Kings Co Hosp 1966; **Fellow:** Allergy & Immunology, Natl Jewish Hosp 1970; **Fac Appt:** Assoc Clin Prof Med, Mount Sinai Sch Med

CARDIAC ELECTROPHYSIOLOGY

Chinitz, Larry MD (CE) - **Spec Exp:** Arrhythmias; Pacemakers; Defibrillators; **Hospital:** NYU Med Ctr (page 102); **Address:** 403 E 34th St Fl 2, New York, NY 10016-6402; **Phone:** 212-263-7149; **Board Cert:** Internal Medicine 1982; Cardiovascular Disease 1985; Cardiac Electrophysiology 1998; **Med School:** NYU Sch Med 1979; **Resid:** Internal Medicine, Bellevue Hosp 1983; **Fellow:** Cardiovascular Disease, NYU Med Ctr/Bellevue 1985; Cardiac Electrophysiology, Montefiore/NYU 1985; **Fac Appt:** Assoc Prof Med, NYU Sch Med

Evans, Steven J MD (CE) - **Spec Exp:** Arrhythmias; Electrophysiologic Testing; Defibrillators; Pacemakers; **Hospital:** Beth Israel Med Ctr - Petrie Division (page 90); **Address:** Beth Israel Med Ctr, 5 Baird Hall, 1st Ave @ 16th St, New York, NY 10003; **Phone:** 212-844-1261; **Board Cert:** Internal Medicine 1987; Cardiovascular Disease 1989; Cardiac Electrophysiology 2002; **Med School:** NYU Sch Med 1984; **Resid:** Internal Medicine, Manhattan VA Med Ctr 1987; **Fellow:** Cardiovascular Disease, Cedars-Sinai Med Ctr 1990; **Fac Appt:** Asst Prof Med, Albert Einstein Coll Med

Garan, Hasan MD (CE) - **Spec Exp:** Arrhythmias; Cardiac Catheterization; Pacemakers/Defibrillators; **Hospital:** NY-Presby Hosp (page 100); **Address:** 161 Fort Washington Ave, rm 546, New York, NY 10032; **Phone:** 212-305-8559; **Board Cert:** Internal Medicine 1977; Cardiovascular Disease 1979; Cardiac Electrophysiology 1996; **Med School:** Harvard Med Sch 1974; **Resid:** Internal Medicine, Hosp Univ Penn 1976; **Fellow:** Cardiovascular Disease, Mass Genl Hosp 1978; Cardiac Electrophysiology, Mass Genl Hosp 1979; **Fac Appt:** Prof Med, Columbia P&S

Gomes, J Anthony MD (CE) - **Spec Exp:** Arrhythmias; Heart Attack; Atrial Fibrillation; Pacemakers; **Hospital:** Mount Sinai Med Ctr (page 98); **Address:** Mount Sinai Medical Ctr, One Gustave L Levy Pl, Box 1054, New York, NY 10029-6500; **Phone:** 212-241-7272; **Board Cert:** Internal Medicine 1974; Cardiovascular Disease 1975; Cardiac Electrophysiology 1994; **Med School:** India 1970; **Resid:** Internal Medicine, Mt Sinai Med Ctr 1973; **Fellow:** Cardiovascular Disease, Mt Sinai Med Ctr 1975; **Fac Appt:** Prof Med, Mount Sinai Sch Med

Lerman, Bruce MD (CE) - **Spec Exp:** Catheter Ablation; Defibrillators; Arrhythmias; **Hospital:** NY-Presby Hosp (page 100); **Address:** NY Weill Cornell Med Ctr, 520 E 70th St, Starr 4, New York, NY 10021-9800; **Phone:** 212-746-2169; **Board Cert:** Internal Medicine 1980; Cardiovascular Disease 1985; Cardiac Electrophysiology 2002; **Med School:** Loyola Univ-Stritch Sch Med 1977; **Resid:** Internal Medicine, Northwestern Univ Hosp 1980; Internal Medicine, Univ Michigan Med Ctr 1981; **Fellow:** Cardiovascular Disease, Hosp Univ Penn 1982; Cardiovascular Disease, Johns Hopkins Hosp 1983; **Fac Appt:** Prof Med, Cornell Univ-Weill Med Coll

Matos, Jeffrey MD (CE) - **Spec Exp:** Arrhythmias; Pacemakers; Defibrillators; **Hospital:** Lenox Hill Hosp (page 94); **Address:** 1421 Third Ave Fl 5, New York, NY 10028; **Phone:** 212-772-6384; **Board Cert:** Internal Medicine 1980; Cardiovascular Disease 1983; Cardiac Electrophysiology 1994; **Med School:** Harvard Med Sch 1975; **Resid:** Internal Medicine, Beth Israel Hosp 1978; **Fellow:** Cardiovascular Disease, Peter Bent Brigham Hosp 1980; **Fac Appt:** Assoc Clin Prof Med, NYU Sch Med

Slater, William MD (CE) - **Spec Exp:** Arrhythmias; Pacemakers; Defibrillators; **Hospital:** NYU Med Ctr (page 102); **Address:** NYU Medical Ctr, Div Cardiology, 530 First Ave, Ste 7B, New York, NY 10016; **Phone:** 212-263-7463; **Board Cert:** Internal Medicine 1981; Cardiovascular Disease 1985; Cardiac Electrophysiology 2002; **Med School:** Harvard Med Sch 1978; **Resid:** Internal Medicine, NYU-Bellevue Med Ctr 1981; **Fellow:** Cardiovascular Disease, Mt Sinai Hosp 1984; Cardiovascular Disease, Mass Genl Med Ctr 1986; **Fac Appt:** Assoc Prof Med, NYU Sch Med

Steinberg, Jonathan S MD (CE) - **Spec Exp:** Atrial Fibrillation; Catheter Ablation; Defibrillators; Arrhythmias; **Hospital:** St Luke's - Roosevelt Hosp Ctr - Roosevelt Div (page 90), Valley Hosp (page 762); **Address:** St Luke's-Roosevelt Hospital S&R Bldg, 1111 W 114th St Fl 3 - rm 8-325, New York, NY 10025; **Phone:** 212-523-4007; **Board Cert:** Internal Medicine 1983; Cardiovascular Disease 1987; Cardiac Electrophysiology 2002; **Med School:** Mount Sinai Sch Med 1980; **Resid:** Internal Medicine, NYU Med Ctr/Manhattan VA Hosp 1984; **Fellow:** Cardiovascular Disease, Geo Wash Univ Med Ctr 1986; Cardiac Electrophysiology, Columbia Presby Med Ctr 1988; **Fac Appt:** Prof Med, Columbia P&S

CARDIOVASCULAR DISEASE

Askanas, Alexander MD (Cv) - **Spec Exp:** Arrhythmias; Angina; Congestive Heart Failure; **Hospital:** Beth Israel Med Ctr - Petrie Division (page 90); **Address:** 1085 Park Ave, New York, NY 10128-1168; **Phone:** 212-369-3080; **Board Cert:** Internal Medicine 1972; Cardiovascular Disease 1974; **Med School:** Poland 1960; **Resid:** Internal Medicine, VA Med Ctr 1971; **Fellow:** Cardiovascular Disease, VA Med Ctr 1972; **Fac Appt:** Asst Prof Med, Mount Sinai Sch Med

Berdoff, Russell MD (Cv) - **Spec Exp:** Coronary Artery Disease; Heart Valve Disease; **Hospital:** Beth Israel Med Ctr - Petrie Division (page 90); **Address:** 67 Irving Pl, Fl 7, New York, NY 10003-2202; **Phone:** 212-979-9224; **Board Cert:** Internal Medicine 1978; Cardiovascular Disease 1981; **Med School:** NY Med Coll 1975; **Resid:** Internal Medicine, DC Genl Hosp 1978; **Fellow:** Cardiovascular Disease, Johns Hopkins Hosp 1980; **Fac Appt:** Assoc Clin Prof Med, Albert Einstein Coll Med

Berger, Marvin MD (Cv) - **Spec Exp:** Echocardiography; **Hospital:** Beth Israel Med Ctr - Petrie Division (page 90); **Address:** 1 St Ave & 16th St, New York, NY 10003; **Phone:** 212-420-2068; **Board Cert:** Internal Medicine 1969; Cardiovascular Disease 1977; **Med School:** Univ Hlth Sci/Chicago Med Sch 1961; **Resid:** Internal Medicine, Beth Israel Hosp 1964; **Fellow:** Cardiovascular Disease, Mount Sinai Hosp 1965; **Fac Appt:** Clin Prof Med, Albert Einstein Coll Med

Bergmann, Steven MD (Cv) - **Spec Exp:** Nuclear Cardiology; Cardiac Imaging; **Hospital:** Beth Israel Med Ctr - Petrie Division (page 90), NY-Presby Hosp (page 100); **Address:** Beth Israel Med Ctr, Heart Institute, 1st Ave at 16th St, Baird Hall, 5th fl, New York, NY 10003; **Phone:** 212-420-4681; **Board Cert:** Internal Medicine 1998; **Med School:** Washington Univ, St Louis 1985; **Resid:** Internal Medicine, Barnes-Jewish Hosp 1988; **Fellow:** Cardiovascular Disease, Barnes-Jewish Hosp 1990; Cardiovascular Disease, Beth Israel Med Ctr 2003; **Fac Appt:** Prof Med, Albert Einstein Coll Med

Blake, James MD (Cv) - **Spec Exp:** Congestive Heart Failure; Nuclear Cardiology; Echocardiography; **Hospital:** NY-Presby Hosp (page 100), Hosp For Special Surgery (page 108); **Address:** 328 E 61st St, New York, NY 10021; **Phone:** 212-755-8700; **Board Cert:** Internal Medicine 1984; Cardiovascular Disease 1987; **Med School:** Albert Einstein Coll Med 1981; **Resid:** Internal Medicine, New York Hosp 1984; **Fellow:** Cardiovascular Disease, New York Hosp 1987; **Fac Appt:** Assoc Clin Prof Med, Cornell Univ-Weill Med Coll

Blumenthal, David S MD (Cv) - **Spec Exp:** Heart Valve Disease; Preventive Cardiology; Coronary Artery Disease; **Hospital:** NY-Presby Hosp (page 100); **Address:** 407 E 70th St, Fl 1, New York, NY 10021-5302; **Phone:** 212-861-3222; **Board Cert:** Internal Medicine 1978; Cardiovascular Disease 1981; **Med School:** Cornell Univ-Weill Med Coll 1975; **Resid:** Internal Medicine, New York Hosp 1978; Internal Medicine, New York Hosp 1981; **Fellow:** Cardiovascular Disease, Johns Hopkins Hosp 1980; **Fac Appt:** Clin Prof Med, Cornell Univ-Weill Med Coll

Borer, Jeffrey MD (Cv) - **Spec Exp:** Heart Valve Disease; Heart Failure; Nuclear Cardiology; **Hospital:** NY-Presby Hosp (page 100); **Address:** NY Presby Hosp, H Gilman Inst Heart Disease, 525 E 68th St, Box 118, New York, NY 10021-4870; **Phone:** 212-746-4646; **Board Cert:** Internal Medicine 1973; Cardiovascular Disease 1975; **Med School:** Cornell Univ-Weill Med Coll 1969; **Resid:** Internal Medicine, Mass Genl Hosp 1971; **Fellow:** Cardiovascular Disease, Natl Heart, Lung & Blood Inst 1974; Cardiovascular Disease, Guy's Hosp 1975; **Fac Appt:** Prof Med, Cornell Univ-Weill Med Coll

Braff, Robert MD (Cv) - **Spec Exp:** Angiography-Coronary; Echocardiography; **Hospital:** St Vincent Cath Med Ctrs - Manhattan (page 375); **Address:** 36 7th Ave, Ste 402, New York, NY 10011-6609; **Phone:** 212-242-3337; **Board Cert:** Internal Medicine 1976; Cardiovascular Disease 1981; **Med School:** SUNY Hlth Sci Ctr 1973; **Resid:** Internal Medicine, St Vincents Hosp 1976; **Fellow:** Cardiovascular Disease, Georgetown Univ Hosp 1978; **Fac Appt:** Asst Clin Prof Med, NY Med Coll

Cemaletin, Nevber MD (Cv) - **Hospital:** Lenox Hill Hosp (page 94), Manhattan Eye, Ear & Throat Hosp; **Address:** 110 E 59th St, Ste 9B, New York, NY 10022; **Phone:** 212-583-2899; **Board Cert:** Internal Medicine 1988; Cardiovascular Disease 1989; **Med School:** NY Med Coll 1984; **Resid:** Internal Medicine, Lenox Hill Hosp 1987; **Fellow:** Cardiovascular Disease, Lenox Hill Hosp 1989

Cohen, Howard A MD (Cv) - **Spec Exp:** Interventional Cardiology; **Hospital:** Lenox Hill Hosp (page 94); **Address:** Lenox Hill Hosp, Interventional Cardiology, 130 E 77th St Fl 9, New York, NY 10021; **Phone:** 212-434-2606; **Board Cert:** Internal Medicine 1974; Cardiovascular Disease 1977; **Med School:** NYU Sch Med 1970; **Resid:** Internal Medicine, Bellevue Hosp Ctr 1974; **Fellow:** Cardiovascular Disease, Johns Hopkins Hosp 1976

Cole, William J MD (Cv) - **Spec Exp:** Coronary Heart Disease; Hypertension; Cholesterol/Lipid Disorders; **Hospital:** NYU Med Ctr (page 102), NY Downtown Hosp; **Address:** 530 First Ave, Ste 3-D, New York, NY 10016; **Phone:** 212-263-7071; **Board Cert:** Internal Medicine 1983; Cardiovascular Disease 1987; **Med School:** NYU Sch Med 1980; **Resid:** Cardiovascular Disease, NYU Med Ctr 1984; **Fac Appt:** Asst Clin Prof Med, NYU Sch Med

Coppola, John T MD (Cv) - **Spec Exp:** Cardiac Catheterization; Angioplasty; **Hospital:** St Vincent Cath Med Ctrs - Manhattan (page 375); **Address:** 275 7th Ave Fl 3, New York, NY 10001; **Phone:** 646-660-9999; **Board Cert:** Internal Medicine 1981; Cardiovascular Disease 1983; Interventional Cardiology 1999; **Med School:** NY Med Coll 1978; **Resid:** Internal Medicine, St Vincent Catholic Med Ctr 1981; **Fellow:** Cardiovascular Disease, St Vincent Catholic Med Ctr 1983

Devereux, Richard B MD (Cv) - **Spec Exp:** Hypertension; Marfan's Syndrome; Heart Valve Disease; **Hospital:** NY-Presby Hosp (page 100); **Address:** 525 E 68th St, rm K-415, New York, NY 10021-4870; **Phone:** 212-746-4655; **Board Cert:** Internal Medicine 1974; Cardiovascular Disease 1977; **Med School:** Univ Pennsylvania 1971; **Resid:** Internal Medicine, New York Hosp 1974; **Fellow:** Cardiovascular Disease, Hosp Univ Penn 1976; **Fac Appt:** Prof Med, Cornell Univ-Weill Med Coll

Drusin, Ronald MD (Cv) - **Spec Exp:** Heart Failure; Coronary Artery Disease; Heart Valve Disease; **Hospital:** NY-Presby Hosp (page 100); **Address:** 161 Fort Washington Ave, rm 338, New York, NY 10032; **Phone:** 212-305-5371; **Board Cert:** Internal Medicine 1973; Cardiovascular Disease 1975; **Med School:** Columbia P&S 1966; **Resid:** Internal Medicine, Presbyterian Hosp 1969; **Fellow:** Cardiovascular Disease, Columbia-Presby Hosp 1973; **Fac Appt:** Clin Prof Med, Columbia P&S

Friedman, Howard S MD (Cv) - **Spec Exp:** Atrial Fibrillation; Coronary Artery Disease; Hypertension; **Hospital:** NYU Med Ctr (page 102); **Address:** 650 First Ave, Fl 3, New York, NY 10016-3240; **Phone:** 212-889-9393; **Board Cert:** Internal Medicine 1971; Cardiovascular Disease 1974; Critical Care Medicine 2001; Geriatric Medicine 2004; **Med School:** SUNY Buffalo 1966; **Resid:** Internal Medicine, Mt Sinai Med Ctr 1969; Cardiovascular Disease, Mt Sinai Med Ctr 1973; **Fac Appt:** Clin Prof Med, NYU Sch Med

Friedman, Sanford MD (Cv) - **Spec Exp:** Preventive Cardiology; **Hospital:** Mount Sinai Med Ctr (page 98); **Address:** 941 Park Ave, New York, NY 10028; **Phone:** 212-988-3772; **Board Cert:** Internal Medicine 1980; Cardiovascular Disease 1977; **Med School:** Tufts Univ 1971; **Resid:** Internal Medicine, Mt Sinai Med Ctr 1974; **Fellow:** Cardiovascular Disease, Mt Sinai Med Ctr 1976; **Fac Appt:** Assoc Clin Prof Med, Mount Sinai Sch Med

Fuchs, Richard MD (Cv) - **Spec Exp:** Coronary Artery Disease; Heart Valve Disease; **Hospital:** NY-Presby Hosp (page 100); **Address:** 310 E 72nd St, Fl 2, New York, NY 10021; **Phone:** 212-717-2254; **Board Cert:** Internal Medicine 1979; Cardiovascular Disease 1981; **Med School:** Harvard Med Sch 1976; **Resid:** Internal Medicine, New York Hosp 1979; **Fellow:** Cardiovascular Disease, Johns Hopkins Hosp 1982; **Fac Appt:** Assoc Prof Med, Cornell Univ-Weill Med Coll

Fuster, Valentin MD/PhD (Cv) - **Spec Exp:** Coronary Artery Disease; Heart Valve Disease; Congenital Heart Disease; **Hospital:** Mount Sinai Med Ctr (page 98); **Address:** One Gustave Levy Pl, Box 1030, New York, NY 10029-6500; **Phone:** 212-241-7911; **Board Cert:** Internal Medicine 1976; Cardiovascular Disease 1977; **Med School:** Spain 1967; **Resid:** Internal Medicine, Mayo Clinic 1972; Cardiovascular Disease, Mayo Clinic 1974; **Fellow:** Cardiovascular Disease, Univ Edinburgh 1971; **Fac Appt:** Prof Med, Mount Sinai Sch Med

Garfein, Oscar MD (Cv) - **Spec Exp:** Coronary Artery Disease; Congestive Heart Failure; Physicians' Health-Cardiac; **Hospital:** St Luke's - Roosevelt Hosp Ctr - Roosevelt Div (page 90), NY-Presby Hosp (page 100); **Address:** 425 W 59th St, Ste 9A, New York, NY 10019-1104; **Phone:** 917-584-1171; **Board Cert:** Internal Medicine 1971; Cardiovascular Disease 1975; **Med School:** Columbia P&S 1965; **Resid:** Internal Medicine, Columbia-Presby Hosp 1967; Internal Medicine, Mass Genl Hosp 1970; **Fellow:** Cardiovascular Disease, Beth Israel Hosp 1971; Cardiovascular Disease, St Luke's Hosp 1972; **Fac Appt:** Assoc Clin Prof Med, Columbia P&S

Giardina, Elsa-Grace MD (Cv) - **Spec Exp:** Heart Disease in Women; Arrhythmias; Preventive Cardiology; **Hospital:** NY-Presby Hosp (page 100); **Address:** 16 E 60th St, Ste 321, New York, NY 10022-1002; **Phone:** 212-326-8540; **Board Cert:** Internal Medicine 1971; Cardiovascular Disease 1983; **Med School:** NY Med Coll 1965; **Resid:** Internal Medicine, St Luke's-Roosevelt Hosp 1969; **Fellow:** Cardiovascular Disease, Columbia-Presby Hosp 1971; **Fac Appt:** Prof Med, Columbia P&S

Gliklich, Jerry MD (Cv) - **Spec Exp:** Heart Valve Disease; Arrhythmias; **Hospital:** NY-Presby Hosp (page 100); **Address:** 161 Fort Washington Ave, Ste 535, New York, NY 10032-3713; **Phone:** 212-305-5588; **Board Cert:** Internal Medicine 1978; Cardiovascular Disease 1981; **Med School:** Columbia P&S 1975; **Resid:** Internal Medicine, New York Hosp 1978; **Fellow:** Cardiovascular Disease, Columbia-Presby Hosp 1981; **Fac Appt:** Clin Prof Med, Columbia P&S

Goldberg, Harvey MD (Cv) - **Spec Exp:** Angina; Preventive Cardiology; **Hospital:** NY-Presby Hosp (page 100), Lenox Hill Hosp (page 94); **Address:** 425 E 61st St Fl 6, New York, NY 10021-8722; **Phone:** 212-752-2000; **Board Cert:** Internal Medicine 1979; Cardiovascular Disease 1981; **Med School:** Cornell Univ-Weill Med Coll 1976; **Resid:** Internal Medicine, New York Hosp 1979; **Fellow:** Cardiovascular Disease, New York Hosp 1981; **Fac Appt:** Assoc Clin Prof Med, Cornell Univ-Weill Med Coll

Goldberg, Nieca MD (Cv) - **Spec Exp:** Heart Disease in Women; Preventive Cardiology; Echocardiography; **Hospital:** Lenox Hill Hosp (page 94); **Address:** 177 E 87th St, New York, NY 10028; **Phone:** 212-289-2045; **Board Cert:** Internal Medicine 1987; Cardiovascular Disease 1995; **Med School:** SUNY Downstate 1984; **Resid:** Internal Medicine, St Lukes Roosevelt Hosp Ctr 1987; **Fellow:** Cardiovascular Disease, SUNY Hlth Sci Ctr 1990; **Fac Appt:** Asst Clin Prof Med, NYU Sch Med

Goldman, Martin E MD (Cv) - **Spec Exp:** Echocardiography; Heart Valve Disease; **Hospital:** Mount Sinai Med Ctr (page 98); **Address:** 1 Gustave Levy Pl, Box 1030, New York, NY 10029-6504; **Phone:** 212-241-3078; **Board Cert:** Internal Medicine 1979; Cardiovascular Disease 1981; **Med School:** Albert Einstein Coll Med 1976; **Resid:** Internal Medicine, Peter Bent Brigham Hosp 1978; **Fellow:** Cardiovascular Disease, Mount Sinai Hosp 1980; **Fac Appt:** Prof Med, NYU Sch Med

Grossman, Will MD (Cv) - **Spec Exp:** Coronary Artery Disease; Heart Valve Disease; Congestive Heart Failure; **Hospital:** Beth Israel Med Ctr - Petrie Division (page 90); **Address:** 30 E 72nd St, FL 1, New York, NY 10021-4265; **Phone:** 212-535-5110; **Board Cert:** Internal Medicine 1972; Cardiovascular Disease 1977; **Med School:** NYU Sch Med 1957; **Resid:** Internal Medicine, Cincinnati Genl Hosp 1959; Internal Medicine, Henry Ford Hosp 1963; **Fellow:** Cardiovascular Disease, New Jersey Coll Med 1964; **Fac Appt:** Asst Prof Med, Albert Einstein Coll Med

Halperin, Jonathan L MD (Cv) - **Spec Exp:** Peripheral Vascular Disease; Atrial Fibrillation; **Hospital:** Mount Sinai Med Ctr (page 98); **Address:** Fifth Ave at 100th St, New York, NY 10029; **Phone:** 212-241-7243; **Board Cert:** Internal Medicine 1980; Cardiovascular Disease 1981; **Med School:** Boston Univ 1975; **Resid:** Internal Medicine, Mass Genl Hosp 1977; **Fellow:** Vascular Medicine, Boston Univ Med Ctr 1978; Cardiovascular Disease, Boston Univ Med Ctr 1980; **Fac Appt:** Prof Med, Mount Sinai Sch Med

Hayes, Joseph MD (Cv) - **Spec Exp:** Atrial Fibrillation; Heart Failure; Coronary Artery Disease; **Hospital:** NY-Presby Hosp (page 100); **Address:** 505 E 70th St, New York, NY 10021; **Phone:** 212-746-2670; **Board Cert:** Internal Medicine 1972; Cardiovascular Disease 1975; **Med School:** Georgetown Univ 1963; **Resid:** Internal Medicine, NY Hosp-Cornell Med Ctr 1966; **Fellow:** Cardiovascular Disease, NY Hosp-Cornell Med Ctr 1968; **Fac Appt:** Prof Med, Cornell Univ-Weill Med Coll

Hecht, Alan MD (Cv) - **Spec Exp:** Heart Valve Disease; Coronary Artery Disease; Arrhythmias; **Hospital:** Mount Sinai Med Ctr (page 98); **Address:** 1075 Park Ave, New York, NY 10128; **Phone:** 212-876-0845; **Board Cert:** Internal Medicine 1984; Cardiovascular Disease 1987; **Med School:** Northwestern Univ 1981; **Resid:** Internal Medicine, Mount Sinai Hosp 1984; **Fellow:** Cardiovascular Disease, Mount Sinai Hosp 1986; **Fac Appt:** Assoc Clin Prof Med, Mount Sinai Sch Med

Hochman, Judith S MD (Cv) - **Spec Exp:** Coronary Artery Disease; **Hospital:** NYU Med Ctr (page 102); **Address:** NYU Medical Ctr, 550 First Ave, rm 8CC1173, New York, NY 10016; **Phone:** 212-263-6927; **Board Cert:** Internal Medicine 1980; Cardiovascular Disease 1983; **Med School:** Harvard Med Sch 1977; **Resid:** Internal Medicine, Peter Bent Brigham Hosp 1979; Internal Medicine, U Mass Med Ctr 1980; **Fellow:** Cardiovascular Disease, Johns Hopkins Hosp 1982; **Fac Appt:** Prof Med, NYU Sch Med

Inra, Lawrence A MD (Cv) - **Spec Exp:** Coronary Artery Disease; Heart Valve Disease; Cholesterol/Lipid Disorders; Preventive Cardiology; **Hospital:** NY-Presby Hosp (page 100), Hosp For Special Surgery (page 108); **Address:** 407 E 70th St, New York, NY 10021; **Phone:** 212-249-1011; **Board Cert:** Internal Medicine 1979; Cardiovascular Disease 1981; **Med School:** Johns Hopkins Univ 1976; **Resid:** Internal Medicine, New York Hosp 1979; **Fellow:** Cardiovascular Disease, Mount Sinai Hosp 1981; **Fac Appt:** Asst Clin Prof Med, Cornell Univ-Weill Med Coll

Kahn, Martin MD (Cv) - **Spec Exp:** Coronary Artery Disease; **Hospital:** NYU Med Ctr (page 102); **Address:** 530 First Ave, Ste 4-H, New York, NY 10016; **Phone:** 212-263-7228; **Board Cert:** Internal Medicine 1977; Cardiovascular Disease 1975; **Med School:** NYU Sch Med 1963; **Resid:** Internal Medicine, Bellevue Hosp 1965; Internal Medicine, Bellevue Hosp 1970; **Fellow:** Cardiovascular Disease, Bellevue Hosp 1972; **Fac Appt:** Prof Med, NYU Sch Med

Kamen, Mazen MD (Cv) - **Spec Exp:** Heart Valve Disease; Cholesterol/Lipid Disorders; Hypertension; **Hospital:** NY-Presby Hosp (page 100); **Address:** 1021 Park Ave, New York, NY 10028; **Phone:** 212-427-5800; **Board Cert:** Internal Medicine 1990; Cardiovascular Disease 1995; **Med School:** NYU Sch Med 1983; **Resid:** Internal Medicine, NYU Med Ctr 1986; **Fellow:** Cardiovascular Disease, NY Cornell Med Ctr 1990; **Fac Appt:** Asst Prof Med, Cornell Univ-Weill Med Coll

Katz, Edward MD (Cv) - **Spec Exp:** Echocardiography; Cholesterol/Lipid Disorders; Coronary Artery Disease; **Hospital:** Hosp For Joint Diseases (page 107), NYU Med Ctr (page 102); **Address:** 305 2nd Ave, Ste 16, New York, NY 10003; **Phone:** 212-598-6516; **Board Cert:** Cardiovascular Disease 1991; Internal Medicine 1988; **Med School:** NYU Sch Med 1985; **Resid:** Internal Medicine, NYU Med Ctr 1988; **Fellow:** Cardiovascular Disease, NYU Med Ctr 1991; **Fac Appt:** Asst Clin Prof Med, NYU Sch Med

Kligfield, Paul MD (Cv) - **Hospital:** NY-Presby Hosp (page 100); **Address:** Dept Cardiology, 520 E 70th St, New York, NY 10021; **Phone:** 212-746-4686; **Board Cert:** Internal Medicine 1973; Cardiovascular Disease 1975; **Med School:** Harvard Med Sch 1970; **Resid:** Internal Medicine, Beth Israel Hosp 1972; Cardiovascular Disease, St George's Hosp 1973; **Fellow:** Cardiovascular Disease, New York Hosp 1975; **Fac Appt:** Prof Med, Cornell Univ-Weill Med Coll

Kronzon, Itzhak MD (Cv) - **Spec Exp:** Heart Valve Disease; Echocardiography; Pericardial Diseases; **Hospital:** NYU Med Ctr (page 102); **Address:** NYU Med Ctr, 560 1st Ave, rm HW228, New York, NY 10016; **Phone:** 212-263-5665; **Board Cert:** Internal Medicine 1979; Cardiovascular Disease 1981; **Med School:** Israel 1964; **Resid:** Internal Medicine, Jerusalem 1969; **Fellow:** Cardiovascular Disease, Montefiore Med Ctr 1973; Cardiovascular Disease, NYU Med Ctr 1974; **Fac Appt:** Prof Med, NYU Sch Med

Kutnick, Richard MD (Cv) - **Spec Exp:** Echocardiography; **Hospital:** Lenox Hill Hosp (page 94); **Address:** 898 Park Ave, New York, NY 10021-2897; **Phone:** 212-879-2628; **Board Cert:** Internal Medicine 1979; Cardiovascular Disease 1981; **Med School:** Tufts Univ 1976; **Resid:** Internal Medicine, Lenox Hill Hosp 1979; **Fellow:** Cardiovascular Disease, Lenox Hill Hosp 1981; **Fac Appt:** Asst Prof Med, NYU Sch Med

Lazar, Eliot J MD (Cv) - **Spec Exp:** Hypertension; Coronary Artery Disease; **Hospital:** NY-Presby Hosp (page 100); **Address:** Box 569 NYPH, 525 E 68th St, New York, NY 10021; **Phone:** 212-746-4241; **Board Cert:** Internal Medicine 1984; Cardiovascular Disease 1987; Critical Care Medicine 2000; Geriatric Medicine 1996; **Med School:** SUNY Upstate Med Univ 1981; **Resid:** Internal Medicine, Bronx Muni Hosp 1984; **Fellow:** Cardiovascular Disease, Mount Sinai Hosp 1987; **Fac Appt:** Assoc Clin Prof Med, Cornell Univ-Weill Med Coll

Lewis, Benjamin H MD (Cv) - **Spec Exp:** Cardiac Stress Testing; Heart Disease & Gender; **Hospital:** NY-Presby Hosp (page 100), Lenox Hill Hosp (page 94); **Address:** 16 E 60th St Fl 3, New York, NY 10022-1002; **Phone:** 212-326-8425; **Board Cert:** Internal Medicine 1980; Cardiovascular Disease 1983; **Med School:** UCSF 1977; **Resid:** Internal Medicine, Hosp Univ Penn 1978; Internal Medicine, Columbia-Presby Hosp 1980; **Fellow:** Cardiovascular Disease, Brigham Womens Hosp 1982; **Fac Appt:** Asst Prof Med, Columbia P&S

Matta, Raymond J MD (Cv) - **Hospital:** Mount Sinai Med Ctr (page 98); **Address:** 1120 Park Ave, New York, NY 10128-1242; **Phone:** 212-410-5800; **Board Cert:** Internal Medicine 1973; Cardiovascular Disease 1975; **Med School:** Univ Pittsburgh 1969; **Resid:** Internal Medicine, Mass Genl Hosp 1971; **Fellow:** Cardiovascular Disease, Peter Bent Brigham Hosp 1975; **Fac Appt:** Assoc Clin Prof Med, Mount Sinai Sch Med

Mattes, Leonard MD (Cv) - **Hospital:** Mount Sinai Med Ctr (page 98); **Address:** 1199 Park Ave, Ste 1F, New York, NY 10128-1713; **Phone:** 212-876-7045; **Board Cert:** Internal Medicine 1972; Cardiovascular Disease 1975; **Med School:** Tulane Univ 1962; **Resid:** Internal Medicine, Mount Sinai 1967; Cardiovascular Disease, Mount Sinai 1969; **Fellow:** Cardiovascular Disease, Mount Sinai 1968; **Fac Appt:** Asst Clin Prof Med, Mount Sinai Sch Med

Meller, Jose MD (Cv) - **Spec Exp:** Cardiac Catheterization; Hypertension; Angioplasty; **Hospital:** Mount Sinai Med Ctr (page 98); **Address:** 941 Park Ave, New York, NY 10028; **Phone:** 212-988-3772; **Board Cert:** Internal Medicine 1973; Cardiovascular Disease 1975; **Med School:** Chile 1969; **Resid:** Internal Medicine, Elmhurst Hosp 1971; Internal Medicine, Mt Sinai Med Ctr 1972; **Fellow:** Cardiovascular Disease, Mt Sinai Med Ctr 1974; **Fac Appt:** Prof Med, Mount Sinai Sch Med

Mosca, Lori J MD/PhD (Cv) - **Spec Exp:** Preventive Cardiology; **Hospital:** NY-Presby Hosp (page 100); **Address:** NY Presby Med Ctr, Div Preventive Cardiology, 622 W 168th St, PH10-203D, New York, NY 10032; **Phone:** 212-305-4866; **Board Cert:** Internal Medicine 1989; **Med School:** SUNY Upstate Med Univ 1984; **Resid:** Internal Medicine, SUNYHealth Sci Ctr 1987; **Fellow:** Cardiovascular Disease, Columbia Presby Med Ctr 1991; Epidemiology, Columbia Presby Med Ctr 1992; **Fac Appt:** Assoc Prof Med, Columbia P&S

Mueller, Richard L MD (Cv) - **Spec Exp:** Echocardiography; Cholesterol/Lipid Disorders; Hypertension; **Hospital:** NY-Presby Hosp (page 100), St Luke's - Roosevelt Hosp Ctr - Roosevelt Div (page 90); **Address:** 401 E 55th St, New York, NY 10022-1236; **Phone:** 212-593-9800; **Board Cert:** Internal Medicine 2000; Cardiovascular Disease 2000; **Med School:** UCSF 1987; **Resid:** Internal Medicine, N Shore Univ Hosp 1991; Internal Medicine, Meml Sloan Kettering Cancer Ctr 1990; **Fellow:** Cardiovascular Disease, New York Hosp 1994

Poon, Michael MD (Cv) - **Spec Exp:** Coronary Artery Disease; Pulmonary Hypertension; Coronary Imaging CT-MR; Cardiac Imaging; **Hospital:** Cabrini Med Ctr (page 374), Mount Sinai Med Ctr (page 98); **Address:** Cabrini Medical Ctr Bldg B, 227 E 19th St, rm 549, New York, NY 10003; **Phone:** 212-995-6865; **Board Cert:** Cardiovascular Disease 1997; **Med School:** Mount Sinai Sch Med 1987; **Resid:** Internal Medicine, Mount Sinai Med Ctr 1991; **Fellow:** Cardiovascular Disease, Mount Sinai Med Ctr 1993; **Fac Appt:** Assoc Prof Med, Mount Sinai Sch Med

Porder, Joseph B MD (Cv) - **Spec Exp:** Preventive Cardiology; Nutrition; Echocardiography; **Hospital:** Mount Sinai Med Ctr (page 98); **Address:** 1160 5th Ave, Ste 102, New York, NY 10029; **Phone:** 212-860-5500; **Board Cert:** Internal Medicine 1985; Cardiovascular Disease 1987; **Med School:** Columbia P&S 1982; **Resid:** Internal Medicine, Mt Sinai Hosp 1985; **Fellow:** Cardiovascular Disease, Mt Sinai Hosp 1987

Post, Martin MD (Cv) - **Spec Exp:** Coronary Artery Disease; Cholesterol/Lipid Disorders; **Hospital:** NY-Presby Hosp (page 100); **Address:** 425 E 61st St, New York, NY 10021; **Phone:** 212-752-2000; **Board Cert:** Internal Medicine 1974; Cardiovascular Disease 1974; **Med School:** SUNY Upstate Med Univ 1967; **Resid:** Internal Medicine, Ohio State Univ Hosp 1970; **Fellow:** Cardiovascular Disease, New York Hosp 1972; **Fac Appt:** Asst Prof Med, Cornell Univ-Weill Med Coll

Reichstein, Robert P MD (Cv) - **Spec Exp:** Preventive Cardiology; Cholesterol/Lipid Disorders; Cardiac Imaging; **Hospital:** Mount Sinai Med Ctr (page 98); **Address:** 1185 Park Ave, Ste 1L, New York, NY 10128; **Phone:** 212-996-2900; **Board Cert:** Internal Medicine 1980; Cardiovascular Disease 1983; **Med School:** Univ Hlth Sci/Chicago Med Sch 1977; **Resid:** Internal Medicine, Mount Sinai Hosp 1981; **Fellow:** Cardiovascular Disease, Mount Sinai Hosp 1984; **Fac Appt:** Asst Clin Prof Med, Mount Sinai Sch Med

Reiffel, James MD (Cv) - **Spec Exp:** Arrhythmias; **Hospital:** NY-Presby Hosp (page 100); **Address:** 161 Fort Washington Ave, New York, NY 10032-3713; **Phone:** 212-305-5206; **Board Cert:** Internal Medicine 1972; Cardiovascular Disease 1975; Cardiac Electrophysiology 1992; **Med School:** Columbia P&S 1969; **Resid:** Internal Medicine, Columbia-Presby Med Ctr 1972; **Fellow:** Cardiovascular Disease, Columbia-Presby Med Ctr 1974; **Fac Appt:** Prof Med, Columbia P&S

Reison, Dennis MD (Cv) - **Spec Exp:** Interventional Cardiology; **Hospital:** NY-Presby Hosp (page 100), Valley Hosp (page 762); **Address:** New York Physicians, 635 Madison Ave, New York, NY 10022-1002; **Phone:** 212-857-4501; **Board Cert:** Internal Medicine 1978; Cardiovascular Disease 1981; Interventional Cardiology 1999; **Med School:** Stanford Univ 1975; **Resid:** Internal Medicine, Columbia Presby Med Ctr 1978; **Fellow:** Cardiovascular Disease, Mt Sinai Hosp 1979; Cardiovascular Disease, Columbia Univ 1981; **Fac Appt:** Asst Clin Prof Med, Columbia P&S

Rentrop, K Peter MD (Cv) - **Hospital:** St Vincent Cath Med Ctrs - Manhattan (page 375), St Luke's - Roosevelt Hosp Ctr - Roosevelt Div (page 90); **Address:** 928 Broadway, New York, NY 10010; **Phone:** 212-475-8066; **Board Cert:** Internal Medicine 1973; **Med School:** Germany 1966; **Resid:** Internal Medicine, Detroit Med Ctr 1970; Internal Medicine, Cleveland Clinic 1971; **Fellow:** Cardiovascular Disease, Cleveland Clinic 1973; **Fac Appt:** Prof Med, NY Med Coll

Romanello, Paul P MD (Cv) - **Spec Exp:** Cholesterol/Lipid Disorders; Coronary Artery Disease; Hypertension; **Hospital:** Lenox Hill Hosp (page 94); **Address:** 158 E 84th St, New York, NY 10028; **Phone:** 212-535-6340; **Board Cert:** Internal Medicine 1987; Cardiovascular Disease 1989; **Med School:** SUNY Upstate Med Univ 1983; **Resid:** Internal Medicine, Lenox Hill Hosp 1987; **Fellow:** Cardiovascular Disease, Lenox Hill Hosp 1989

Rosenfeld, Isadore MD (Cv) - **Spec Exp:** Cardiac Stress Testing; Hypertension; Coronary Artery Disease; **Hospital:** NY-Presby Hosp (page 100); **Address:** 125 E 72nd St, New York, NY 10021-4250; **Phone:** 212-628-6100; **Med School:** McGill Univ 1951; **Resid:** Internal Medicine, Royal Victoria Hosp 1953; Internal Medicine, Johns Hopkins Med Ctr 1954; **Fellow:** Cardiovascular Disease, Jewish Genl Hosp 1955; Cardiovascular Disease, Mount Sinai Hosp 1956; **Fac Appt:** Prof Med, Cornell Univ-Weill Med Coll

Rozanski, Alan MD (Cv) - **Spec Exp:** Nuclear Cardiology; Stress Management; **Hospital:** St Luke's - Roosevelt Hosp Ctr - Roosevelt Div (page 90); **Address:** 1111 Amsterdam Ave, New York, NY 10025; **Phone:** 212-523-4011; **Board Cert:** Internal Medicine 1978; Cardiovascular Disease 1983; **Med School:** Tufts Univ 1975; **Resid:** Internal Medicine, Mount Sinai 1977; **Fellow:** Cardiovascular Disease, Mount Sinai 1980; Nuclear Medicine, Cedars-Sinai Med Ctr 1982; **Fac Appt:** Prof Med, Columbia P&S

Scheidt, Stephen MD (Cv) - **Spec Exp:** Coronary Artery Disease; Heart Valve Disease; **Hospital:** NY-Presby Hosp (page 100); **Address:** 520 E 70th St, New York, NY 10021-9800; **Phone:** 212-746-2148; **Board Cert:** Internal Medicine 1974; Cardiovascular Disease 1974; **Med School:** Columbia P&S 1965; **Resid:** Internal Medicine, Bellevue Hosp- Columbia Div 1968; **Fellow:** Cardiovascular Disease, New York Hosp 1970; **Fac Appt:** Prof Med, Cornell Univ-Weill Med Coll

Schiffer, Mark B MD (Cv) - **Spec Exp:** Preventive Cardiology; Coronary Artery Disease; Cholesterol/Lipid Disorders; **Hospital:** Lenox Hill Hosp (page 94); **Address:** 158 E 84th St Fl 5, New York, NY 10028-1802; **Phone:** 212-535-6340; **Board Cert:** Internal Medicine 1980; Cardiovascular Disease 1983; **Med School:** Northwestern Univ 1977; **Resid:** Internal Medicine, Lenox Hill Hosp 1981; **Fellow:** Cardiovascular Disease, Lenox Hill Hosp 1983; **Fac Appt:** Assoc Clin Prof Med, NYU Sch Med

Schulman, Ira MD (Cv) - **Spec Exp:** Angina; Heart Failure; **Hospital:** NY Downtown Hosp, NYU Med Ctr (page 102); **Address:** 170 William St, Ste 818, New York, NY 10038; **Phone:** 212-233-5308; **Board Cert:** Internal Medicine 1977; Cardiovascular Disease 1979; **Med School:** NYU Sch Med 1974; **Resid:** Internal Medicine, Bellevue Hosp 1977; **Fellow:** Cardiovascular Disease, Montefiore Med Ctr 1979; **Fac Appt:** Asst Prof Med, Cornell Univ-Weill Med Coll

Schwartz, Allan MD (Cv) - **Spec Exp:** Interventional Cardiology; Cardiac Catheterization; Mitral Valve Disease; **Hospital:** NY-Presby Hosp (page 100); **Address:** 161 Ft Washington Ave, Ste 551, New York, NY 10032-3713; **Phone:** 212-305-5367; **Board Cert:** Internal Medicine 1977; Cardiovascular Disease 1979; **Med School:** Columbia P&S 1974; **Resid:** Internal Medicine, Columbia-Presby Med Ctr 1976; **Fellow:** Cardiovascular Disease, Mass Genl Hosp 1978; **Fac Appt:** Clin Prof Med, Columbia P&S

Schwartz, William MD (Cv) - **Spec Exp:** Coronary Artery Disease; Cardiac Catheterization; **Hospital:** Lenox Hill Hosp (page 94), Mount Sinai Med Ctr (page 98); **Address:** 150 E 77th St, Ste 1E, New York, NY 10021; **Phone:** 212-439-6000; **Board Cert:** Internal Medicine 1978; Cardiovascular Disease 1981; **Med School:** Albert Einstein Coll Med 1975; **Resid:** Internal Medicine, Bronx Municipal Hosp 1978; **Fellow:** Cardiovascular Disease, Bronx Municipal Hosp 1979

Seinfeld, David MD (Cv) - **Hospital:** Lenox Hill Hosp (page 94), Montefiore Med Ctr; **Address:** 35 E 75th St, New York, NY 10021-2761; **Phone:** 212-288-1538; **Board Cert:** Internal Medicine 1976; Cardiovascular Disease 1979; **Med School:** Albert Einstein Coll Med 1973; **Resid:** Internal Medicine, Montefiore Hosp Med Ctr 1976; **Fellow:** Cardiovascular Disease, Montefiore Hosp Med Ctr 1978; **Fac Appt:** Assoc Clin Prof Med, Albert Einstein Coll Med

Sherman, Warren MD (Cv) - **Spec Exp:** Angioplasty; Interventional Cardiology; **Hospital:** NY-Presby Hosp (page 100); **Address:** 161 Fort Washington Ave, Irving 5, New York, NY 10032; **Phone:** 212-342-0886; **Board Cert:** Internal Medicine 1980; Cardiovascular Disease 1983; Interventional Cardiology 2000; **Med School:** SUNY Upstate Med Univ 1977; **Resid:** Internal Medicine, Rochester Genl Hosp 1980; **Fellow:** Cardiovascular Disease, Oregon Hlth Sci Univ 1982; **Fac Appt:** Assoc Clin Prof Med, Columbia P&S

Shimony, Rony MD (Cv) - **Spec Exp:** Coronary Artery Disease; Arrhythmias & Pacemakers; Atrial Fibrillation; **Hospital:** Lenox Hill Hosp (page 94), NY-Presby Hosp (page 100); **Address:** 425 E 61 St Fl 4, New York, NY 10021-7216; **Phone:** 212-752-2700; **Board Cert:** Internal Medicine 1987; Cardiovascular Disease 1989; **Med School:** SUNY Buffalo 1984; **Resid:** Internal Medicine, Lenox Hill Hosp 1987; **Fellow:** Cardiovascular Disease, Lenox Hill Hosp 1989; Cardiac Electrophysiology, Lenox Hill Hosp 1992

Siegal, Michael S MD (Cv) - **Spec Exp:** Coronary Artery Disease; **Hospital:** St Luke's - Roosevelt Hosp Ctr - Roosevelt Div (page 90); **Address:** 115 E 57th St Fl 15, New York, NY 10022; **Phone:** 212-319-1700; **Board Cert:** Internal Medicine 1980; Cardiovascular Disease 1983; **Med School:** Columbia P&S 1970; **Resid:** Internal Medicine, Bellevue/NYU Med Ctr 1980; **Fellow:** Cardiovascular Disease, Mt Sinai Hosp 1982

Siegel, Stephen MD (Cv) - **Spec Exp:** Sports Cardiology; Preventive Cardiology; Cholesterol/Lipid Disorders; Hypertension; **Hospital:** NYU Med Ctr (page 102), NY Downtown Hosp; **Address:** 245 E 35th St, New York, NY 10016; **Phone:** 212-684-1108; **Board Cert:** Internal Medicine 1981; Cardiovascular Disease 1983; **Med School:** Med Coll VA 1978; **Resid:** Internal Medicine, NYU Med Ctr 1981; Internal Medicine, Bellevue Hosp Ctr 1981; **Fellow:** Cardiovascular Disease, NYU Med Ctr 1983; Cardiovascular Disease, Bellevue Hosp Ctr 1983; **Fac Appt:** Asst Clin Prof Med, NYU Sch Med

Sklaroff, Herschel MD (Cv) - **Spec Exp:** Angina; Syncope; Hypertension; **Hospital:** Mount Sinai Med Ctr (page 98); **Address:** 1175 Park Ave, New York, NY 10128; **Phone:** 212-289-6500 x2; **Board Cert:** Internal Medicine 1969; Cardiovascular Disease 1977; **Med School:** Univ Pennsylvania 1961; **Resid:** Internal Medicine, Mt Sinai Hosp 1965; Cardiovascular Disease, Mt Sinai Hosp 1966; **Fac Appt:** Clin Prof Med, Mount Sinai Sch Med

Squire, Anthony MD (Cv) - **Spec Exp:** Echocardiography; Coronary Artery Disease; Cardiac Stress Testing; **Hospital:** Mount Sinai Med Ctr (page 98); **Address:** 1120 Park Ave, Ste 1C, New York, NY 10128-1242; **Phone:** 212-410-4800; **Board Cert:** Internal Medicine 1981; Cardiovascular Disease 1983; **Med School:** Mount Sinai Sch Med 1978; **Resid:** Internal Medicine, Mount Sinai Hosp 1981; **Fellow:** Cardiovascular Disease, Mount Sinai Hosp 1983; **Fac Appt:** Assoc Clin Prof Med, Mount Sinai Sch Med

Stein, Richard A MD (Cv) - **Spec Exp:** Preventive Cardiology; Coronary Artery Disease; Cardiac Rehabilitation; **Hospital:** Beth Israel Med Ctr - Petrie Division (page 90), Lenox Hill Hosp (page 94); **Address:** Beth Israel Hosp, Heart Inst, 5 Baird Hall, 1st Ave & 16th St, New York, NY 10003; **Phone:** 212-420-4126; **Board Cert:** Internal Medicine 1973; Cardiovascular Disease 1975; Sports Medicine 1997; **Med School:** NYU Sch Med 1967; **Resid:** Internal Medicine, Univ Hosp 1969; **Fellow:** Cardiovascular Disease, Univ Hosp 1974; **Fac Appt:** Clin Prof Med, Albert Einstein Coll Med

Steingart, Richard MD (Cv) - **Spec Exp:** Heart Failure; Nuclear Cardiology; Heart Disease in Cancer Patients; **Hospital:** Meml Sloan Kettering Cancer Ctr (page 109); **Address:** Meml Sloan-Kettering Cancer Ctr, Cardiology, 1275 York Ave, New York, NY 10021; **Phone:** 212-639-8488; **Board Cert:** Internal Medicine 1977; Cardiovascular Disease 1979; **Med School:** Mount Sinai Sch Med 1974; **Resid:** Internal Medicine, Yale-New Haven Hosp 1977; **Fellow:** Cardiovascular Disease, Mt Sinai Med Ctr 1979; **Fac Appt:** Prof Med, Cornell Univ-Weill Med Coll

Tenenbaum, Joseph MD (Cv) - **Spec Exp:** Heart Valve Disease; Coronary Artery Disease; Atrial Fibrillation; **Hospital:** NY-Presby Hosp (page 100); **Address:** 161 Ft Washington Ave Bldg IP - Ste 535, New York, NY 10032-3713; **Phone:** 212-305-5288; **Board Cert:** Internal Medicine 1977; Cardiovascular Disease 1979; **Med School:** Harvard Med Sch 1974; **Resid:** Internal Medicine, Columbia-Presby Med Ctr 1977; **Fellow:** Cardiovascular Disease, Mt Sinai Hosp 1979; **Fac Appt:** Clin Prof Med, Columbia P&S

Tyberg, Theodore MD (Cv) - **Spec Exp:** Coronary Artery Disease; Cholesterol/Lipid Disorders; **Hospital:** NY-Presby Hosp (page 100); **Address:** 425 E 61st St, Fl 6, New York, NY 10021-4032; **Phone:** 212-752-2000; **Board Cert:** Internal Medicine 1978; Cardiovascular Disease 1981; **Med School:** Rush Med Coll 1975; **Resid:** Internal Medicine, New York Hosp 1978; **Fellow:** Cardiovascular Disease, Yale-New Haven Hosp 1980; **Fac Appt:** Assoc Clin Prof Med, Cornell Univ-Weill Med Coll

Unger, Allen MD (Cv) - **Spec Exp:** Cholesterol/Lipid Disorders; Hypertension; **Hospital:** Mount Sinai Med Ctr (page 98); **Address:** 12 E 86th St, New York, NY 10028-0506; **Phone:** 212-734-6000; **Board Cert:** Internal Medicine 1968; Cardiovascular Disease 1977; **Med School:** SUNY Upstate Med Univ 1960; **Resid:** Internal Medicine, Mount Sinai Hosp 1967; **Fellow:** Cardiovascular Disease, Mount Sinai Hosp 1966; **Fac Appt:** Asst Clin Prof Med, Mount Sinai Sch Med

Varriale, Philip MD (Cv) - **Spec Exp:** Coronary Artery Disease; Arrhythmias & Pacemakers; Congestive Heart Failure; **Hospital:** Cabrini Med Ctr (page 374), St Vincent Cath Med Ctrs - Manhattan (page 375); **Address:** 222 E 19th St, Ste 2D, New York, NY 10003-2666; **Phone:** 212-777-3219; **Board Cert:** Internal Medicine 1966; Cardiovascular Disease 1970; **Med School:** SUNY Hlth Sci Ctr 1959; **Resid:** Internal Medicine, VA Med Ctr 1962; Internal Medicine, St Vincent's Hosp & Med Ctr 1963; **Fellow:** Cardiovascular Disease, St Vincent's Hosp & Med Ctr 1964; **Fac Appt:** Assoc Clin Prof Med, Mount Sinai Sch Med

Weisenseel, Arthur Charles MD (Cv) - **Spec Exp:** Coronary Artery Disease; Cholesterol/Lipid Disorders; Congestive Heart Failure; **Hospital:** Mount Sinai Med Ctr (page 98); **Address:** 12 E 86th St, New York, NY 10028-0506; **Phone:** 212-734-6000; **Board Cert:** Internal Medicine 1969; Cardiovascular Disease 1973; **Med School:** Georgetown Univ 1963; **Resid:** Internal Medicine, Mount Sinai 1966; **Fellow:** Cardiovascular Disease, Mount Sinai 1967; **Fac Appt:** Asst Clin Prof Med, Mount Sinai Sch Med

Woldenberg, David MD (Cv) - **Spec Exp:** Geriatric Cardiology; **Hospital:** Lenox Hill Hosp (page 94), Mount Sinai Med Ctr (page 98); **Address:** 121 E 60 St, Ste 9B, New York, NY 10022; **Phone:** 212-230-1144; **Board Cert:** Internal Medicine 1980; Cardiovascular Disease 1981; **Med School:** Univ Hlth Sci/Chicago Med Sch 1958; **Resid:** Internal Medicine, Beth Israel Med Ctr 1961; **Fellow:** Cardiovascular Disease, Mt Sinai Hosp 1962; **Fac Appt:** Asst Clin Prof Med, Mount Sinai Sch Med

Wolk, Michael MD (Cv) - **Spec Exp:** Coronary Artery Disease; Heart Failure; Hypertension; **Hospital:** NY-Presby Hosp (page 100); **Address:** 425 E 61st St Fl 6, New York, NY 10021; **Phone:** 212-752-2000; **Board Cert:** Internal Medicine 1971; Cardiovascular Disease 1973; **Med School:** Columbia P&S 1964; **Resid:** Internal Medicine, Univ Hosp 1967; **Fellow:** Cardiovascular Disease, New England Med Ctr 1969; Cardiovascular Disease, New York Hosp-Cornell 1970; **Fac Appt:** Clin Prof Med, Cornell Univ-Weill Med Coll

Zaremski, Benjamin MD (Cv) - **Hospital:** Beth Israel Med Ctr - Petrie Division (page 90), Lenox Hill Hosp (page 94); **Address:** 510 E 80th St, New York, NY 10021; **Phone:** 212-517-0022; **Board Cert:** Internal Medicine 1986; **Med School:** Dominican Republic 1981; **Resid:** Internal Medicine, Metropolitan Hosp 1984; **Fellow:** Cardiovascular Disease, St Francis Hosp/Metropolitan Hosp 1986

CHILD & ADOLESCENT PSYCHIATRY

Abright, Arthur Reese MD (ChAP) - **Spec Exp:** Bipolar/Mood Disorders; ADD/ADHD; Post Traumatic Stress Disorder; Autism; **Hospital:** St Vincent Cath Med Ctrs - Manhattan (page 375); **Address:** 144 W 12th St, New York, NY 10011-8202; **Phone:** 212-604-8213; **Board Cert:** Psychiatry 1978; Child & Adolescent Psychiatry 1981; **Med School:** Univ Tex SW, Dallas 1973; **Resid:** Psychiatry, St Vincent's Hosp 1974; Psychiatry, NY Hosp-Cornell Med Ctr 1977; **Fellow:** Child & Adolescent Psychiatry, NY Hosp-Cornell Med Ctr 1979; **Fac Appt:** Clin Prof Psyc, NY Med Coll

Bird, Hector MD (ChAP) - **Spec Exp:** ADD/ADHD; Anxiety & Depression; Personality Disorders; **Hospital:** NY-Presby Hosp (page 100); **Address:** 145 Central Park West, Ste 1CC, New York, NY 10023-2004; **Phone:** 212-874-5311; **Board Cert:** Psychiatry 1975; Child & Adolescent Psychiatry 1977; **Med School:** Yale Univ 1965; **Resid:** Psychiatry, NY State Psych Inst 1971; Child & Adolescent Psychiatry, NY State Psych Inst 1972; **Fellow:** Psychoanalysis, WA White Institute 1977; **Fac Appt:** Prof Psyc, Columbia P&S

Burkes, Lynn MD (ChAP) - **Spec Exp:** Diagnostic Problems; ADD/ADHD; Divorce/Family Issues; **Hospital:** NYU Med Ctr (page 102); **Address:** 185 West End Ave, New York, NY 10023-5539; **Phone:** 212-362-5920; **Board Cert:** Psychiatry 1977; Child & Adolescent Psychiatry 1978; **Med School:** Med Coll PA Hahnemann 1970; **Resid:** Psychiatry, Albert Einstein 1973; **Fellow:** Psychiatry, Bellevue Hosp 1975; **Fac Appt:** Assoc Clin Prof Psyc, NYU Sch Med

Coffey, Barbara J MD (ChAP) - **Spec Exp:** Tourette's Syndrome; ADD/ADHD; Obsessive-Compulsive Disorder; **Hospital:** NYU Med Ctr (page 102), McLean Hosp; **Address:** NYU Child Study Ctr, 577 1st Ave, New York, NY 10016; **Phone:** 212-263-3926; **Board Cert:** Psychiatry 1981; Child & Adolescent Psychiatry 1986; **Med School:** Tufts Univ 1975; **Resid:** Psychiatry, Boston Univ 1978; Child & Adolescent Psychiatry, Tufts Univ 1980; **Fac Appt:** Assoc Prof Psyc, NYU Sch Med

Fox, Sarah J MD (ChAP) - **Spec Exp:** Anxiety & Mood Disorders; Eating Disorders; Psychoanalysis; **Hospital:** NY-Presby Hosp (page 100); **Address:** 210 W 89th St, Ste 1E, New York, NY 10024-1803; **Phone:** 212-874-4558; **Board Cert:** Psychiatry 1991; Child & Adolescent Psychiatry 1994; **Med School:** Tufts Univ 1982; **Resid:** Pediatrics, Jacobi Med Ctr 1983; Psychiatry, Albert Einstein 1985; **Fellow:** Child & Adolescent Psychiatry, Columbia-Presby Med Ctr 1987

Hertzig, Margaret MD (ChAP) - **Spec Exp:** Developmental Disorders; ADD/ADHD; **Hospital:** NY-Presby Hosp (page 100); **Address:** 525 E 68th St, Box 140, New York, NY 10021; **Phone:** 212-746-5712; **Board Cert:** Psychiatry 1968; Child & Adolescent Psychiatry 1975; **Med School:** NYU Sch Med 1960; **Resid:** Pediatrics, Jewish Hosp 1962; Psychiatry, Bellevue Psych Hosp 1964; **Fellow:** Psychiatric Research, NYU Sch Med 1966; **Fac Appt:** Prof Psyc, Cornell Univ-Weill Med Coll

Hirsch, Glenn S MD (ChAP) - **Spec Exp:** Anxiety & Mood Disorders; Tourette's Syndrome; Bipolar/Mood Disorders; ADD/ADHD; **Hospital:** NYU Med Ctr (page 102), Bellevue Hosp Ctr; **Address:** NYU Child Study Center, 577 First Ave, New York, NY 10016; **Phone:** 212-263-8704; **Board Cert:** Psychiatry 1984; Child & Adolescent Psychiatry 1985; **Med School:** Albert Einstein Coll Med 1979; **Resid:** Psychiatry, New York Hosp-Cornell 1982; **Fellow:** Child & Adolescent Psychiatry, Columbia-Presby Med Ctr 1984; **Fac Appt:** Asst Prof Psyc, NYU Sch Med

Kestenbaum, Clarice J MD (ChAP) - **Spec Exp:** Anxiety Disorders; Psychodynamic Psychotherapy; **Hospital:** NY-Presby Hosp (page 100), NY-Presby Hosp (page 100); **Address:** 1051 Riverside Drive, Box 74, New York, NY 10032; **Phone:** 212-873-1020; **Board Cert:** Psychiatry 1971; Child & Adolescent Psychiatry 1975; **Med School:** UCLA 1960; **Resid:** Psychiatry, Columbia Presby Med Ctr 1963; Child & Adolescent Psychiatry, Columbia Presby Med Ctr 1965; **Fac Appt:** Clin Prof Psyc, Columbia P&S

Koplewicz, Harold MD (ChAP) - **Spec Exp:** Anxiety Disorders; Psychopharmacology; **Hospital:** NYU Med Ctr (page 102), Bellevue Hosp Ctr; **Address:** NYU Child Study Center, 577 First Ave, Ste 221A, New York, NY 10016; **Phone:** 212-263-6205; **Board Cert:** Psychiatry 1983; Child & Adolescent Psychiatry 1984; **Med School:** Albert Einstein Coll Med 1978; **Resid:** Psychiatry, New York Hosp-Westchester Div 1981; Child & Adolescent Psychiatry, NY State Psyc Inst 1983; **Fellow:** Psychiatric Research, NY State Psyc Inst 1985; **Fac Appt:** Prof Psyc, NYU Sch Med

Kron, Leo MD (ChAP) - **Spec Exp:** Psychopharmacology; Psychotherapy; **Hospital:** St Luke's - Roosevelt Hosp Ctr - Roosevelt Div (page 90); **Address:** 30 E 76th St, Ste 3A, New York, NY 10021; **Phone:** 212-861-7001; **Board Cert:** Child & Adolescent Psychiatry 1986; Psychiatry 1976; **Med School:** Univ British Columbia Fac Med 1961; **Resid:** Psychiatry, Montefiore Hosp Med Ctr 1976; **Fellow:** Child & Adolescent Psychiatry, St Luke's-Roosevelt Hosp Ctr 1978; **Fac Appt:** Asst Clin Prof Psyc, Columbia P&S

Moreau, Donna MD (ChAP) - **Spec Exp:** Psychotherapy & Psychopharmacology; Anxiety & Mood Disorders; Psychiatry-Adult; **Hospital:** NY-Presby Hosp (page 100); **Address:** 110 East End Ave, New York, NY 10028-7412; **Phone:** 212-772-9205; **Board Cert:** Psychiatry 1985; Child & Adolescent Psychiatry 1991; **Med School:** SUNY Hlth Sci Ctr 1976; **Resid:** Psychiatry, NY Hosp 1984; **Fellow:** Child & Adolescent Psychiatry, NY Hosp 1986; **Fac Appt:** Assoc Clin Prof Psyc, Columbia P&S

Newcorn, Jeffrey H MD (ChAP) - **Spec Exp:** Psychopharmacology; ADD/ADHD; **Hospital:** Mount Sinai Med Ctr (page 98); **Address:** Mount Sinai Hosp, Dept Psychiatry, One Gustave Levy Pl, Box 1230, New York, NY 10029; **Phone:** 212-659-8705; **Board Cert:** Psychiatry 1982; Child & Adolescent Psychiatry 1984; **Med School:** Univ Rochester 1977; **Resid:** Psychiatry, Tufts-New England Med Ctr 1980; **Fellow:** Child & Adolescent Psychiatry, Tufts-New England Med Ctr 1982; **Fac Appt:** Assoc Prof Psyc, Mount Sinai Sch Med

Perry, Richard MD (ChAP) - **Spec Exp:** Pervasive Development Disorders; Behavioral Disorders; Psychopharmacology; **Address:** 55 W 74th St, New York, NY 10023-2429; **Phone:** 212-595-0116; **Board Cert:** Psychiatry 1976; Child & Adolescent Psychiatry 1985; **Med School:** Belgium 1970; **Resid:** Psychiatry, Bellevue Hosp 1972; **Fellow:** Child & Adolescent Psychiatry, Bellevue Hosp 1974; **Fac Appt:** Clin Prof Psyc, NYU Sch Med

Rosenfeld, Alvin MD (ChAP) - **Spec Exp:** Family Therapy; Psychotherapy; Sexual Development Problems; **Hospital:** Mass Genl Hosp; **Address:** 4 E 89th St, Ste 1F, New York, NY 10128-0656; **Phone:** 212-348-5900; **Board Cert:** Psychiatry 1976; Child & Adolescent Psychiatry 1978; **Med School:** Harvard Med Sch 1970; **Resid:** Psychiatry, Mass Mental Hlth Ctr/Harvard Med Sch 1973; **Fellow:** Child & Adolescent Psychiatry, Beth Israel Med Ctr/Harvard Med Sch 1975

Shaffer, David MD (ChAP) - **Spec Exp:** Anxiety Disorders; Suicide; **Hospital:** NY-Presby Hosp (page 100); **Address:** 1051 Riverside, Unit 78, New York, NY 10032-1007; **Phone:** 212-543-5948; **Med School:** England 1961; **Resid:** Psychiatry, Univ Coll Hosp & Hosp For Sick Chldn 1966; **Fellow:** Child Psychiatry, Yale-New Hosp 1967; **Fac Appt:** Prof Psyc, Columbia P&S

Spencer, E Kay MD (ChAP) - **Hospital:** NYU Med Ctr (page 102); **Address:** 22 E 36th St, Ste 2D, New York, NY 10016; **Phone:** 212-684-3810; **Board Cert:** Psychiatry 1990; Child & Adolescent Psychiatry 1992; **Med School:** Geo Wash Univ 1979; **Resid:** Pediatrics, Univ Maryland Hosp 1982; Psychiatry, NYU Med Ctr 1986; **Fellow:** Behavioral Pediatrics, Univ Maryland Hosp 1984; Child & Adolescent Psychiatry, NYU Med Ctr 1988; **Fac Appt:** Asst Prof Psyc, NYU Sch Med

Turecki, Stanley K MD (ChAP) - **Spec Exp:** Temperamentally Difficult Child; ADD/ADHD; Parenting Issues; **Hospital:** Lenox Hill Hosp (page 94), Beth Israel Med Ctr - Petrie Division (page 90); **Address:** 136 E 64th St, Ste 1B, New York, NY 10021-2137; **Phone:** 212-355-2535; **Board Cert:** Psychiatry 1978; Child & Adolescent Psychiatry 1981; **Med School:** South Africa 1961; **Resid:** Psychiatry, Tara Hospital 1969; Child & Adolescent Psychiatry, Mt Sinai Hosp 1971

CHILD NEUROLOGY

Allen, Jeffrey MD (ChiN) - **Spec Exp:** Neuro-Oncology; Brain Tumors; **Hospital:** NYU Med Ctr (page 102), St Luke's - Roosevelt Hosp Ctr - Roosevelt Div (page 90); **Address:** 317 E 34 St Fl 8, New York, NY 10016; **Phone:** 212-263-6725; **Board Cert:** Child Neurology 1977; **Med School:** Harvard Med Sch 1969; **Resid:** Pediatrics, Montreal Chldns Hosp 1973; Pediatric Neurology, Montreal Neur Inst/McGill 1976; **Fac Appt:** Prof Ped, NYU Sch Med

Aron, Alan MD (ChiN) - **Spec Exp:** Neurofibromatosis; Movement Disorders; Developmental Delay; **Hospital:** Mount Sinai Med Ctr (page 98); **Address:** Mt Sinai Hosp, Child Neurology, 5 E 98th St, Box 1206, New York, NY 10029; **Phone:** 212-831-4393; **Board Cert:** Pediatrics 1963; Neurology 1967; Child Neurology 1969; **Med School:** Columbia P&S 1958; **Resid:** Pediatrics, Babies Hosp-Columbia-Presby Hosp 1961; **Fellow:** Pediatric Neurology, Babies Hosp-Columbia Presby Hosp 1964; **Fac Appt:** Prof N, Mount Sinai Sch Med

Chutorian, Abraham MD (ChiN) - **Spec Exp:** Autoimmune Disease; Movement Disorders; Headache; Migraine; **Hospital:** NY-Presby Hosp (page 100), Hosp For Special Surgery (page 108); **Address:** 654 Madison Ave, New York, NY 10021; **Phone:** 212-750-2800; **Board Cert:** Pediatrics 1962; Neurology 1964; Child Neurology 1968; **Med School:** Univ Manitoba 1957; **Resid:** Pediatrics, Chldns Hosp 1960; **Fellow:** Neurology, Columbia-Presby Med Ctr 1963; **Fac Appt:** Prof N, Cornell Univ-Weill Med Coll

De Vivo, Darryl C MD (ChiN) - **Spec Exp:** Metabolic Disorders; Neuromuscular Disorders; Spinal Muscular Atrophy (SMA); **Hospital:** NY-Presby Hosp (page 100); **Address:** 710 W 168th St, rm 201, Neurological Inst, New York, NY 10032; **Phone:** 212-305-5244; **Board Cert:** Child Neurology 1972; **Med School:** Univ VA Sch Med 1964; **Resid:** Pediatrics, Mass Genl Hosp 1966; Neurology, Mass Genl Hosp 1967; **Fellow:** Neurology, Natl Inst Hlth 1969; Child Neurology, Children's Hosp-Wash Univ 1970; **Fac Appt:** Prof N, Columbia P&S

Fish, Irving MD (ChiN) - **Spec Exp:** Headache; **Hospital:** NYU Med Ctr (page 102), Bellevue Hosp Ctr; **Address:** NYU Dept Neurology-Bellevue Hosp Ctr, 462 First Ave, rm NBV-7W11, New York, NY 10016; **Phone:** 212-263-6464; **Med School:** Canada 1964; **Resid:** Pediatrics, Chldns Hosp 1965; Child Neurology, NY Hosp-Cornell Med Ctr 1968; **Fac Appt:** Assoc Prof N, NYU Sch Med

Gold, Arnold MD (ChiN) - **Spec Exp:** Learning Disorders; Autism; Epilepsy; **Hospital:** NY-Presby Hosp (page 100); **Address:** 710 W 168th St, New York, NY 10032-2603; **Phone:** 212-305-5483; **Board Cert:** Neurology 1962; Pediatrics 1960; **Med School:** Switzerland 1954; **Resid:** Pediatrics, Charity Hosp 1955; Pediatrics, Chldns Hosp 1958; **Fellow:** Child Neurology, Columbia-Presby 1961; **Fac Appt:** Clin Prof N, Columbia P&S

Kaufman, David M MD (ChiN) - **Spec Exp:** Epilepsy/Seizure Disorders; Headache; Learning Disorders; **Hospital:** Mount Sinai Med Ctr (page 98), Lenox Hill Hosp (page 94); **Address:** 3 E 83rd St, New York, NY 10028-0459; **Phone:** 212-737-4911; **Board Cert:** Pediatrics 1980; **Med School:** Boston Univ 1975; **Resid:** Pediatrics, NY Hosp-Cornell Med Ctr 1977; Neurology, Mount Sinai Hosp 1978; **Fellow:** Child Neurology, Mount Sinai Hosp 1980; **Fac Appt:** Asst Clin Prof N, Mount Sinai Sch Med

Miles, Daniel K MD (ChiN) - **Spec Exp:** Pediatric Neurology; Tuberous Sclerosis; Epilepsy-Pediatric; **Hospital:** NYU Med Ctr (page 102); **Address:** NYU Comprehensive Epilepsy Ctr, 403 E 34th St Fl 4, New York, NY 10016; **Phone:** 212-263-8318; **Board Cert:** Child Neurology 1994; Clinical Neurophysiology 1996; **Med School:** UMDNJ-NJ Med Sch, Newark 1983; **Resid:** Pediatrics, St Christopher's Hosp 1986; Pediatric Neurology, Chlds Meml Hosp 1989; **Fellow:** Epilepsy, Boston Chlds Hosp 1990

Molofsky, Walter MD (ChiN) - **Spec Exp:** Headache; ADD/ADHD; Seizure Disorders; **Hospital:** Beth Israel Med Ctr - Petrie Division (page 90), St Luke's - Roosevelt Hosp Ctr - Roosevelt Div (page 90); **Address:** Beth Israel Med Ctr, 10 Union Square E, New York, NY 10128-7603; **Phone:** 212-844-6910; **Board Cert:** Pediatrics 1982; Child Neurology 1986; **Med School:** NYU Sch Med 1976; **Resid:** Pediatrics, Columbia-Presby Med Ctr 1978; **Fellow:** Child Neurology, Columbia-Presby Med Ctr 1981; **Fac Appt:** Assoc Prof N, Albert Einstein Coll Med

Nass, Ruth MD (ChiN) - **Spec Exp:** Learning Disorders; ADD/ADHD; Asperger's Syndrome; **Hospital:** NYU Med Ctr (page 102); **Address:** 400 E 34th St, Ste RR311, New York, NY 10016-4901; **Phone:** 212-263-7753; **Board Cert:** Pediatrics 1980; Child Neurology 1981; **Med School:** Albert Einstein Coll Med 1975; **Resid:** Pediatrics, NY Hosp 1977; Child Neurology, Columbia-Presby 1978; **Fellow:** Neurology, NY Hosp 1982; **Fac Appt:** Clin Prof N, NYU Sch Med

Patterson, Marc MD (ChiN) - **Spec Exp:** Neurogenetics; Developmental Delay; Metabolic Disorders; **Hospital:** NY-Presby Hosp (page 100); **Address:** Division of Ped Neurology, 180 Fort Washington Ave Bldg HP Fl 5 - Ste 542, MC 540, New York, NY 10032-3710; **Phone:** 212-305-6038; **Board Cert:** Child Neurology 2004; Neurodevelopmental Disabilities 2001; **Med School:** Australia 1981; **Resid:** Neurology, Univ Queenland 1988; Child Neurology, Mayo Clinic 1990; **Fellow:** Metabolic Neurology, Natl Inst Health 1992; Pediatrics, Mayo Cilnic 1993; **Fac Appt:** Prof N, Columbia P&S

Wolf, Steven M MD (ChiN) - **Spec Exp:** Epilepsy; Headache; Migraine; **Hospital:** Beth Israel Med Ctr - Petrie Division (page 90), St Luke's - Roosevelt Hosp Ctr - Roosevelt Div (page 90); **Address:** Beth Israel Med Ctr, Dept Ped Neurology, 10 Union Square East, Ste 5J, New York, NY 10003; **Phone:** 212-870-8506; **Board Cert:** Child Neurology 1996; Clinical Neurophysiology 1997; **Med School:** Albany Med Coll 1989; **Resid:** Pediatrics, Montefiore Med Ctr 1991; Child Neurology, Montefiore Med Ctr 1994; **Fellow:** Epilepsy, Montefiore Med Ctr 1995; **Fac Appt:** Asst Prof N, Albert Einstein Coll Med

CLINICAL GENETICS

Anyane-Yeboa, Kwame MD (CG) - **Spec Exp:** Dysmorphology; Prenatal Diagnosis; **Hospital:** NY-Presby Hosp (page 100); **Address:** Morgan Stanley Children's Hospital of NY, 3959 Broadway Fl 6N - rm 601A, New York, NY 10032; **Phone:** 212-305-6731; **Board Cert:** Pediatrics 1979; Clinical Genetics 1982; **Med School:** Ghana 1972; **Resid:** Pediatrics, Harlem Hosp 1977; **Fellow:** Clinical Genetics, Babies Hosp-Columbia Presby 1980; **Fac Appt:** Assoc Prof Ped, Columbia P&S

Davis, Jessica G MD (CG) - **Spec Exp:** Marfan's Syndrome; Mental Retardation; Neurofibromatosis; Ehlers-Danlos Syndrome; **Hospital:** NY-Presby Hosp (page 100), Hosp For Special Surgery (page 108); **Address:** 525 E 68th St, Box 128, New York, NY 10021-4870; **Phone:** 212-746-1496; **Board Cert:** Clinical Genetics 1984; **Med School:** Columbia P&S 1959; **Resid:** Pediatrics, St Luke's Hosp 1962; Clinical Genetics, Albert Einstein Coll Med 1965; **Fellow:** Cytogenetics, Albert Einstein Coll Med 1966; Pediatrics, Albert Einstein Col Med 1968; **Fac Appt:** Assoc Clin Prof Ped, Cornell Univ-Weill Med Coll

Desnick, Robert J MD/PhD (CG) - **Spec Exp:** Inherited Metabolic Disorders; Fabry's Disease; Gaucher Disease; Porphyria; **Hospital:** Mount Sinai Med Ctr (page 98), Elmhurst Hosp Ctr; **Address:** Mt Sinai Sch Med, Box 1498, Fifth Ave @ 100th St, New York, NY 10029; **Phone:** 212-241-6947; **Board Cert:** Clinical Genetics 1982; Clinical Molecular Genetics 1999; Clinical Biochemical Genetics 1982; **Med School:** Univ Minn 1971; **Resid:** Pediatrics, Univ Minn Hosps 1973; **Fac Appt:** Prof CG, Mount Sinai Sch Med

Gilbert, Fred MD (CG) - **Spec Exp:** Cancer Genetics; Prenatal Diagnosis; **Hospital:** NY-Presby Hosp (page 100); **Address:** 525 E 68th St, Box 53, New York, NY 10021; **Phone:** 212-746-1496; **Board Cert:** Clinical Genetics 1982; Clinical Cytogenetics 1982; Clinical Molecular Genetics 2004; **Med School:** Albert Einstein Coll Med 1966; **Resid:** Internal Medicine, Barnes Hosp 1968; Internal Medicine, Natl Inst Hlth 1971; **Fellow:** Clinical Genetics, Yale-New Haven Hosp 1974; **Fac Appt:** Assoc Prof Ped, Cornell Univ-Weill Med Coll

Hirschhorn, Kurt MD (CG) - **Spec Exp:** Inherited Diseases; Congenital Anomalies; Prenatal Diagnosis; **Hospital:** Mount Sinai Med Ctr (page 98); **Address:** Human Genetics, Pediatrics and Medicine, Mt Sinai Hosp, New York, NY 10029-6574; **Phone:** 212-241-4305; **Board Cert:** Internal Medicine 1963; Clinical Genetics 1984; Clinical Cytogenetics 1984; Clinical Biochemical Genetics 1984; **Med School:** NYU Sch Med 1954; **Resid:** Internal Medicine, Bellevue Hosp 1956; **Fellow:** Metabolic Diseases, NYU Sch Med 1957; Clinical Genetics, State Inst Human Genetics 1958; **Fac Appt:** Prof Ped, Mount Sinai Sch Med

Ostrer, Harry MD (CG) - **Spec Exp:** Genetic Disorders; Hereditary Cancer; **Hospital:** NYU Med Ctr (page 102); **Address:** NYU Medical Ctr, 550 1st Ave, rm MSB136, New York, NY 10016; **Phone:** 212-263-5746; **Board Cert:** Clinical Genetics 1984; Pediatrics 1985; Clinical Cytogenetics 1990; Clinical Molecular Genetics 2004; **Med School:** Columbia P&S 1976; **Resid:** Pediatrics, Johns Hopkins Hosp 1978; Clinical Genetics, Natl Inst Health 1981; **Fellow:** Molecular Genetics, Johns Hopkins Hosp 1983; **Fac Appt:** Prof Ped, NYU Sch Med

Willner, Judith P MD (CG) - **Spec Exp:** Prenatal Diagnosis; Dysmorphology; Metabolic Genetic Disorders; **Hospital:** Mount Sinai Med Ctr (page 98), Englewood Hosp & Med Ctr (page 760); **Address:** Mount Sinai Med Ctr, Dept Clinical Genetics, 1 Gustave Levy Pl, Box 1497, New York, NY 10029-6500; **Phone:** 212-241-6947; **Board Cert:** Pediatrics 1977; Clinical Genetics 1982; **Med School:** NYU Sch Med 1971; **Resid:** Pediatrics, Chldns Hosp Natl Med Ctr 1973; **Fellow:** Clinical Genetics, Mount Sinai Hosp 1977; **Fac Appt:** Prof CG, Mount Sinai Sch Med

COLON & RECTAL SURGERY

Brandeis, Steven MD (CRS) - **Spec Exp:** Laparoscopic Surgery; Colon & Rectal Cancer; Hemorrhoids; **Hospital:** NY Downtown Hosp, NYU Med Ctr (page 102); **Address:** 251 E 33rd St, FL 2, New York, NY 10016; **Phone:** 212-696-5411; **Board Cert:** Surgery 1981; Colon & Rectal Surgery 2001; **Med School:** NYU Sch Med 1975; **Resid:** Surgery, NYU Med Ctr-Bellevue Hosp 1980; **Fellow:** Colon & Rectal Surgery, RWJ Univ Hosp 1981

Gingold, Bruce S MD (CRS) - **Spec Exp:** Colostomy Avoidance; Inflammatory Bowel Disease/Crohn's; Colonoscopy; **Hospital:** St Vincent Cath Med Ctrs - Manhattan (page 375), Beth Israel Med Ctr - Petrie Division (page 90); **Address:** 36 7th Ave, Ste 522, New York, NY 10011-6600; **Phone:** 212-675-2997; **Board Cert:** Colon & Rectal Surgery 1976; Surgery 1977; **Med School:** Jefferson Med Coll 1970; **Resid:** Surgery, St Vincent's Hosp & Med Ctr 1975; **Fellow:** Colon & Rectal Surgery, Cleveland Clinic 1976; **Fac Appt:** Assoc Clin Prof S, NY Med Coll

Gorfine, Stephen MD (CRS) - **Spec Exp:** Anal Disorders & Reconstruction; Hemorrhoids; Rectal Cancer; **Hospital:** Mount Sinai Med Ctr (page 98), Lenox Hill Hosp (page 94); **Address:** 25 E 69th St, New York, NY 10021-4925; **Phone:** 212-517-8600; **Board Cert:** Internal Medicine 1981; Surgery 1996; Colon & Rectal Surgery 1988; **Med School:** Univ Mass Sch Med 1978; **Resid:** Internal Medicine, Mount Sinai Hosp 1981; Surgery, Mount Sinai Hosp 1985; **Fellow:** Colon & Rectal Surgery, Ferguson Hosp 1987; **Fac Appt:** Clin Prof S, Mount Sinai Sch Med

Gottesman, Lester MD (CRS) - **Spec Exp:** Anorectal Disorders; Incontinence-Fecal; **Hospital:** St Luke's - Roosevelt Hosp Ctr - Roosevelt Div (page 90); **Address:** 425 W 59th St, Ste 9A, New York, NY 10019-1104; **Phone:** 212-523-8417; **Board Cert:** Surgery 1993; Colon & Rectal Surgery 1988; **Med School:** Univ Pittsburgh 1978; **Resid:** Surgery, St Luke's-Roosevelt Hosp Ctr 1983; **Fellow:** Surgery, Meml Sloan Kettering Cancer Ctr 1985; Colon & Rectal Surgery, Ferguson Clinic 1987; **Fac Appt:** Assoc Prof S, Columbia P&S

Guillem, Jose MD (CRS) - **Spec Exp:** Colon & Rectal Cancer; Rectal Cancer/Sphincter Preservation; Minimally Invasive Surgery; Colon & Rectal Cancer-Familial Polyposis; **Hospital:** Meml Sloan Kettering Cancer Ctr (page 109); **Address:** Meml Sloan Kettering Cancer Ctr, 1275 York Ave, rm C1077, New York, NY 10021; **Phone:** 212-639-8278; **Board Cert:** Colon & Rectal Surgery 2004; Surgery 2004; **Med School:** Yale Univ 1983; **Resid:** Surgery, Columbia-Presby Med Ctr 1990; **Fellow:** Colon & Rectal Surgery, Lahey Clinic 1991; **Fac Appt:** Prof CRS, Cornell Univ-Weill Med Coll

Milsom, Jeffrey W MD (CRS) - **Spec Exp:** Inflammatory Bowel Disease; Laparoscopic Surgery; Colon & Rectal Cancer; Crohn's Disease; **Hospital:** NY-Presby Hosp (page 100); **Address:** NY Cornell Med Ctr, Div Colorectal Surgery, 525 E 68th St, Box 172, New York, NY 10021; **Phone:** 212-746-6030; **Board Cert:** Surgery 1992; Colon & Rectal Surgery 1986; **Med School:** Univ Pittsburgh 1979; **Resid:** Surgery, Roosevelt Hosp 1981; Surgery, Univ Virginia Med Ctr 1984; **Fellow:** Colon & Rectal Surgery, Ferguson Hosp 1985; **Fac Appt:** Prof S, Columbia P&S

Sonoda, Toyooki MD (CRS) - **Spec Exp:** Inflammatory Bowel Disease; Laparoscopic Surgery; Colon & Rectal Cancer & Surgery; Crohn's Disease; **Hospital:** NY-Presby Hosp (page 100); **Address:** NY Presbyterian-Cornell Medical Ctr, 525 E 68th St, Box 172, New York, NY 10021; **Phone:** 212-746-6030; **Board Cert:** Surgery 1999; Colon & Rectal Surgery 2001; **Med School:** Yale Univ 1993; **Resid:** Surgery, UCSF Med Ctr; Colon & Rectal Surgery, Cleveland Clinic; **Fellow:** Laparoscopic Surgery, Mt Sinai Med Ctr; **Fac Appt:** Asst Prof S, Cornell Univ-Weill Med Coll

Steinhagen, Randolph MD (CRS) - **Spec Exp:** Colostomy Avoidance; Colon & Rectal Cancer; Inflammatory Bowel Disease/Crohn's; **Hospital:** Mount Sinai Med Ctr (page 98); **Address:** Div Colon & Rectal Surgery, 5 E 98th St Fl 14, Box 1259, New York, NY 10029-6501; **Phone:** 212-241-3547; **Board Cert:** Surgery 2002; Colon & Rectal Surgery 1985; **Med School:** Wayne State Univ 1977; **Resid:** Surgery, Mount Sinai Hosp 1982; **Fellow:** Colon & Rectal Surgery, Cleveland Clinic 1983; **Fac Appt:** Assoc Prof S, Mount Sinai Sch Med

New York (Manhattan)

Weinstein, Michael A MD (CRS) - **Hospital:** Lenox Hill Hosp (page 94); **Address:** 475 E 72nd St, Ste 102, New York, NY 10021; **Phone:** 212-249-9010; **Board Cert:** Surgery 1974; Colon & Rectal Surgery 1976; **Med School:** SUNY Hlth Sci Ctr 1968; **Resid:** Surgery, Albert Einstein 1970; Surgery, Beth Israel Med Ctr 1973; **Fellow:** Colon & Rectal Surgery, Muhlenberg Med Ctr 1976

Whelan, Richard L MD (CRS) - **Spec Exp:** Laparoscopic Surgery; Colon & Rectal Cancer; **Hospital:** NY-Presby Hosp (page 100); **Address:** 161 Ft Washington Ave, rm 820, New York, NY 10032; **Phone:** 212-342-1155; **Board Cert:** Surgery 1997; Colon & Rectal Surgery 1989; **Med School:** Columbia P&S 1982; **Resid:** Surgery, Columbia Presby Hosp 1987; **Fellow:** Colon & Rectal Surgery, Univ Minn Med Ctr 1988; **Fac Appt:** Assoc Clin Prof S, Columbia P&S

Wong, W Douglas MD (CRS) - **Spec Exp:** Rectal Cancer/Sphincter Preservation; Colon & Rectal Cancer; Anal Disorders & Reconstruction; **Hospital:** Meml Sloan Kettering Cancer Ctr (page 109); **Address:** Meml Sloan Kettering Cancer Ctr, 1275 York Ave, rm C-1067, New York, NY 10021-6094; **Phone:** 212-639-5117; **Board Cert:** Surgery 1997; Colon & Rectal Surgery 2004; **Med School:** Canada 1972; **Resid:** Surgery, Univ Manitoba Hosp 1977; **Fellow:** Colon & Rectal Surgery, Univ Minn Med Ctr 1984; **Fac Appt:** Prof S, Cornell Univ-Weill Med Coll

CRITICAL CARE MEDICINE

Bahr, Gerald MD (CCM) - **Spec Exp:** Ethics; **Hospital:** Lenox Hill Hosp (page 94); **Address:** Lenox Hill Hosp - Medicine, 110 E 59th St, Ste 9A, New York, NY 10022-1304; **Phone:** 212-583-2878; **Board Cert:** Internal Medicine 1976; Critical Care Medicine 1998; **Med School:** NY Med Coll 1972; **Resid:** Internal Medicine, Lenox Hill Hosp 1976; **Fellow:** Internal Medicine, Lenox Hill Hosp 1976; **Fac Appt:** Assoc Clin Prof Med, NYU Sch Med

Benjamin, Ernest MD (CCM) - **Spec Exp:** Respiratory Distress Syndrome; **Hospital:** Mount Sinai Med Ctr (page 98); **Address:** Mount Sinai Hosp, SICU Box 1264, 1 Gustave Levy Pl, New York, NY 10029; **Phone:** 212-241-8867; **Board Cert:** Anesthesiology 1988; Critical Care Medicine 1989; **Med School:** France 1971; **Resid:** Anesthesiology, Univ Claude Bernard 1978; Internal Medicine, North Genl Hosp 1982; **Fellow:** Anesthesiology, Mount Sinai 1980; Anesthesiology, Mount Sinai 1983; **Fac Appt:** Prof S, Mount Sinai Sch Med

Halpern, Neil MD (CCM) - **Spec Exp:** Hypertension-Postoperative; **Hospital:** Meml Sloan Kettering Cancer Ctr (page 109); **Address:** Memorial Sloan Kettering Cancer Ctr, 1275 York Ave, rm M210, New York, NY 10021; **Phone:** 212-639-6731; **Board Cert:** Internal Medicine 1984; Critical Care Medicine 1998; **Med School:** Mount Sinai Sch Med 1981; **Resid:** Internal Medicine, Mount Sinai Hosp 1984; **Fellow:** Critical Care Medicine, Univ Pittsburgh 1985; **Fac Appt:** Clin Prof Med, Cornell Univ-Weill Med Coll

Nierman, David MD (CCM) - **Spec Exp:** Critical Illness-Prolonged; Respiratory Failure; Sepsis; Critical Care; **Hospital:** Mount Sinai Med Ctr (page 98); **Address:** Mt Sinai Med Ctr, One Gustave L Levy Pl, Box 1232, New York, NY 10029-6574; **Phone:** 212-241-1386; **Board Cert:** Internal Medicine 1984; Pulmonary Disease 1988; Critical Care Medicine 2002; **Med School:** Israel 1981; **Resid:** Internal Medicine, LI Jewish-Hillside Med Ctr 1984; Emergency Medicine, LI Jewish-Hillside Med Ctr 1986; **Fellow:** Pulmonary Disease, St Lukes-Roosevelt Med Ctr 1988; **Fac Appt:** Assoc Prof Med, Mount Sinai Sch Med

Wagner, Ira J MD (CCM) - **Spec Exp:** Respiratory Failure; Ethics; **Hospital:** St Vincent Cath Med Ctrs - Manhattan (page 375); **Address:** St Vincent's Hospital, 153 W 11th St, Coleman Bldg, 1050E, New York, NY 10011-8305; **Phone:** 212-604-8336; **Board Cert:** Internal Medicine 1980; Critical Care Medicine 1998; **Med School:** SUNY Downstate 1976; **Resid:** Internal Medicine, St Vincent's Hosp 1979; **Fellow:** Critical Care Medicine, Univ Pittsburgh 1980; **Fac Appt:** Assoc Clin Prof Med, NY Med Coll

DERMATOLOGY

Ackerman, A Bernard MD (D) - **Spec Exp:** Dermatopathology; Melanoma Consultation; Inflammatory Diseases of Skin; **Hospital:** St Luke's - Roosevelt Hosp Ctr - Roosevelt Div (page 90), NY-Presby Hosp (page 100); **Address:** 145 E 32nd St Fl 10, New York, NY 10016; **Phone:** 212-889-6225; **Board Cert:** Dermatology 1970; Dermatopathology 1974; **Med School:** Columbia P&S 1962; **Resid:** Dermatology, Columbia Presby Hosp 1964; Dermatology, Univ Penn Hosp 1967; **Fellow:** Dermatopathology, Mass Genl Hosp 1969

Albom, Michael MD (D) - **Spec Exp:** Mohs' Surgery; Cosmetic Dermatology; Botox Therapy; **Hospital:** NYU Med Ctr (page 102), Manhattan Eye, Ear & Throat Hosp; **Address:** 33 E 70th St, New York, NY 10021; **Phone:** 212-517-2121; **Board Cert:** Dermatology 1976; **Med School:** Boston Univ 1970; **Resid:** Dermatology, Boston Univ Med Ctr 1974; **Fellow:** Mohs Surgery, NYU Med Ctr 1975; **Fac Appt:** Clin Prof D, NYU Sch Med

Aranoff, Shera MD (D) - **Spec Exp:** Acne; Skin Cancer; Cosmetic Dermatology; Psoriasis/Eczema; **Hospital:** Lenox Hill Hosp (page 94); **Address:** 975 Park Ave, Ste 1-A, New York, NY 10028; **Phone:** 212-772-9305; **Board Cert:** Dermatology 1980; **Med School:** NY Med Coll 1973; **Resid:** Dermatology, Westchester Co Med Ctr 1980

Auerbach, Robert MD (D) - **Spec Exp:** Skin Tumors; Psoriasis; Aging Skin; **Hospital:** NYU Med Ctr (page 102), Bellevue Hosp Ctr; **Address:** 116 E 68th St, New York, NY 10021; **Phone:** 212-396-2515; **Board Cert:** Dermatology 1964; **Med School:** NYU Sch Med 1958; **Resid:** Dermatology, Univ Chicago Clins 1961; **Fellow:** Dermatology, Natl Cancer Inst - NIH 1963; **Fac Appt:** Clin Prof D, NYU Sch Med

Avram, Marc R MD (D) - **Spec Exp:** Hair Restoration/Transplant; Laser Surgery; **Hospital:** NY-Presby Hosp (page 100), Long Island Coll Hosp (page 90); **Address:** 905 5th Ave, New York, NY 10021-2650; **Phone:** 212-734-4007; **Board Cert:** Dermatology 1994; **Med School:** SUNY Downstate 1989; **Resid:** Dermatology, Mass Genl Hosp 1994; **Fac Appt:** Asst Prof D, Cornell Univ-Weill Med Coll

Bernstein, Robert M MD (D) - **Spec Exp:** Hair Restoration/Transplant; **Hospital:** NY-Presby Hosp (page 100), Englewood Hosp & Med Ctr (page 760); **Address:** 125 E 63rd St, New York, NY 10021; **Phone:** 212-826-2400; **Board Cert:** Dermatology 1982; **Med School:** UMDNJ-NJ Med Sch, Newark 1978; **Resid:** Dermatology, Albert Einstein Med Ctr 1982; **Fac Appt:** Assoc Clin Prof D, Columbia P&S

Berson, Diane S MD (D) - **Spec Exp:** Aging Skin; Acne; Skin Cancer; **Hospital:** NY-Presby Hosp (page 100); **Address:** 211 E 53rd St, Ste 3, New York, NY 10022; **Phone:** 212-355-3511; **Board Cert:** Dermatology 1988; **Med School:** NYU Sch Med 1984; **Resid:** Dermatology, SUNY Downstate Med Ctr 1988; **Fac Appt:** Assoc Prof D, Cornell Univ-Weill Med Coll

Bickers, David MD (D) - **Spec Exp:** Skin Cancer; Phototherapy; Psoriasis; **Hospital:** NY-Presby Hosp (page 100); **Address:** 16 E 60th St, Ste 300, New York, NY 10022-1002; **Phone:** 212-326-8465; **Board Cert:** Dermatology 1974; **Med School:** Univ VA Sch Med 1967; **Resid:** Dermatology, NYU Med Ctr 1973; **Fellow:** Pharmacology, Rockefeller Univ Hosp 1974; **Fac Appt:** Prof D, Columbia P&S

Brademas, Mary Ellen MD (D) - **Spec Exp:** Skin Diseases; Cosmetic Dermatology; Nail Diseases; **Hospital:** NYU Med Ctr (page 102); **Address:** 11 5th Ave, New York, NY 10003; **Phone:** 212-477-1515; **Board Cert:** Dermatology 1983; **Med School:** Georgetown Univ 1979; **Resid:** Dermatology, Johns Hopkins Hosp 1981; Dermatology, NYU Med Ctr 1983; **Fac Appt:** Assoc Clin Prof D, NYU Sch Med

Buchness, Mary Ruth MD (D) - **Spec Exp:** Skin Infections; Skin Cancer; Cosmetic Dermatology; **Hospital:** St Vincent Cath Med Ctrs - Manhattan (page 375); **Address:** 36 7th Ave, Ste 423, New York, NY 10011; **Phone:** 212-242-5815; **Board Cert:** Dermatology 1986; **Med School:** Columbia P&S 1982; **Resid:** Dermatology, Columbia Univ 1986; **Fac Appt:** Assoc Prof Med, NY Med Coll

Burke, Karen MD/PhD (D) - **Spec Exp:** Skin Cancer; Acne; Aging Skin; **Hospital:** Cabrini Med Ctr (page 374), Mount Sinai Med Ctr (page 98); **Address:** 429 E 52nd St, New York, NY 10022; **Phone:** 212-754-1100; **Board Cert:** Dermatology 1985; **Med School:** NYU Sch Med 1978; **Resid:** Dermatology, NYU Med Ctr 1983

Bystryn, Jean-Claude MD (D) - **Spec Exp:** Melanoma; Blistering Diseases; Skin Cancer; Hair Loss; **Hospital:** NYU Med Ctr (page 102); **Address:** 530 1st Ave, Ste 7F, New York, NY 10016; **Phone:** 212-889-3846; **Board Cert:** Dermatology 1970; Clinical & Laboratory Dematologic Immunology 1985; **Med School:** NYU Sch Med 1962; **Resid:** Internal Medicine, Montefiore Hosp 1964; Dermatology, NYU Med Ctr 1969; **Fellow:** Immunology, New York Univ 1972; **Fac Appt:** Prof D, NYU Sch Med

Cipollaro, Vincent MD (D) - **Spec Exp:** Skin Cancer; **Hospital:** NY-Presby Hosp (page 100); **Address:** 121 E 60th St, Ste 10-D, New York, NY 10022; **Phone:** 212-588-1963; **Board Cert:** Dermatology 1965; **Med School:** Italy 1958; **Resid:** Dermatology, VA Med Ctr 1962; Dermatology, New York Hosp 1963; **Fac Appt:** Assoc Prof D, Cornell Univ-Weill Med Coll

Clark, Sheryl MD (D) - **Spec Exp:** Melanoma & Skin Cancer; Cosmetic Dermatology; Skin Laser Surgery; **Hospital:** NY-Presby Hosp (page 100); **Address:** 109 E 61st St, New York, NY 10021-8101; **Phone:** 212-750-2905; **Board Cert:** Dermatology 1988; **Med School:** Case West Res Univ 1982; **Resid:** Internal Medicine, Mount Sinai-Univ Hosp 1983; Dermatology, Barnes Hosp-Wash Univ 1988; **Fellow:** Dermatology, Barnes Hosp-Wash Univ 1985; **Fac Appt:** Asst Prof D, Cornell Univ-Weill Med Coll

Davis, Joyce MD (D) - **Spec Exp:** Acne; Hair Loss; Cosmetic Dermatology; **Hospital:** Beth Israel Med Ctr - Petrie Division (page 90), Mount Sinai Med Ctr (page 98); **Address:** 69 Fifth Avenue at 15th St, New York, NY 10003; **Phone:** 212-242-3066; **Board Cert:** Dermatology 1983; **Med School:** Albert Einstein Coll Med 1979; **Resid:** Internal Medicine, Beth Israel Med Ctr 1980; Dermatology, Mount Sinai Med Ctr 1983

Deleo, Vincent A MD (D) - **Spec Exp:** Photosensitive Skin Diseases; Contact Dermatitis; Occupational Dermatology; **Hospital:** St Luke's - Roosevelt Hosp Ctr - Roosevelt Div (page 90), Beth Israel Med Ctr - Petrie Division (page 90); **Address:** 425 W 59th St, Ste 5C, New York, NY 10019-1104; **Phone:** 212-523-6003; **Board Cert:** Dermatology 1976; **Med School:** Louisiana State Univ 1969; **Resid:** Dermatology, Columbia Univ-USPHS 1976; **Fac Appt:** Assoc Prof D, Columbia P&S

Demar, Leon MD (D) - **Spec Exp:** Skin Cancer; Pediatric Dermatology; Acne; **Hospital:** Lenox Hill Hosp (page 94), NY-Presby Hosp (page 100); **Address:** 985 5th Ave, New York, NY 10021-0142; **Phone:** 212-988-9010; **Board Cert:** Dermatology 1977; **Med School:** NYU Sch Med 1973; **Resid:** Dermatology, Stanford Med Ctr 1975; Dermatology, Columbia-Presby Med Ctr 1977; **Fac Appt:** Assoc Clin Prof D, Columbia P&S

Felderman, Leonora MD (D) - **Spec Exp:** Cosmetic Dermatology; **Hospital:** Lenox Hill Hosp (page 94); **Address:** 1317 3rd Ave Fl 8, New York, NY 10021-2995; **Phone:** 212-734-0091; **Board Cert:** Dermatology 1985; **Med School:** NY Med Coll 1981; **Resid:** Dermatology, Montefiore Med Ctr 1985

Franks Jr, Andrew G MD (D) - **Spec Exp:** Lupus/SLE; Raynaud's Disease; Scleroderma; **Hospital:** NYU Med Ctr (page 102), Lenox Hill Hosp (page 94); **Address:** 60 Gramercy Park N, Ste 1N, New York, NY 10010-5429; **Phone:** 212-475-2312; **Board Cert:** Internal Medicine 1975; Dermatology 1977; Rheumatology 1978; **Med School:** NYU Sch Med 1971; **Resid:** Internal Medicine, Beth Israel Med Ctr 1974; Dermatology, Columbia-Presby Med Ctr 1975; **Fellow:** Rheumatology, Columbia-Presby Med Ctr 1977; **Fac Appt:** Prof D, NYU Sch Med

Friedman-Kien, Alvin MD (D) - **Spec Exp:** AIDS/HIV; Herpes Simplex; Warts; **Hospital:** NYU Med Ctr (page 102); **Address:** 530 1st Ave, Ste 7C, New York, NY 10016-6402; **Phone:** 212-263-7380; **Board Cert:** Dermatology 1965; **Med School:** Yale Univ 1960; **Resid:** Dermatology, Mass Genl Hosp 1962; Dermatology, Natl Inst Health 1964; **Fellow:** Dermatology, NYU Med Ctr 1965; **Fac Appt:** Prof D, NY Med Coll

Garzon, Maria C MD (D) - **Spec Exp:** Pediatric Dermatology; Vascular Anomalies; Mycosis Fungoides; **Hospital:** NY-Presby Hosp (page 100); **Address:** Columbia Univ, Dept Dermatology, 161 Ft Washington Ave Fl 12, New York, NY 10032; **Phone:** 212-305-5293; **Board Cert:** Dermatology 1995; Pediatrics 1999; Pediatric Dermatology ; **Med School:** Columbia P&S 1988; **Resid:** Pediatrics, Columbia Presby-Babies Hosp 1991; **Fellow:** Dermatology, Columbia Univ 1995; **Fac Appt:** Assoc Clin Prof D, Columbia P&S

Gendler, Ellen C MD (D) - **Spec Exp:** Cosmetic Dermatology; Contact Dermatitis; Botox Therapy; **Hospital:** NYU Med Ctr (page 102); **Address:** 1035 Fifth Ave, New York, NY 10028; **Phone:** 212-288-8222; **Board Cert:** Dermatology 1985; **Med School:** Columbia P&S 1981; **Resid:** Dermatology, NYU Med Ctr 1985; **Fac Appt:** Assoc Clin Prof D, NYU Sch Med

Geronemus, Roy MD (D) - **Spec Exp:** Skin Laser Surgery; Cosmetic Dermatology; Mohs' Surgery; Skin Cancer; **Hospital:** NYU Med Ctr (page 102), New York Eye & Ear Infirm (page 110); **Address:** 317 E 34 St, Ste 11N, New York, NY 10016-4974; **Phone:** 212-686-7306; **Board Cert:** Dermatology 1983; **Med School:** Univ Miami Sch Med 1979; **Resid:** Dermatology, NYU-Skin Cancer Unit 1983; **Fellow:** Mohs Surgery, NYU-Skin Cancer Unit 1984; **Fac Appt:** Clin Prof D, NYU Sch Med

Gordon, Marsha MD (D) - **Spec Exp:** Cosmetic Dermatology; Botox Therapy; Acne; **Hospital:** Mount Sinai Med Ctr (page 98); **Address:** 5 E 98th St Fl 5, New York, NY 10029-6501; **Phone:** 212-241-9728; **Board Cert:** Dermatology 1988; **Med School:** Univ Pennsylvania 1984; **Resid:** Dermatology, Mount Sinai Hosp 1988; **Fac Appt:** Clin Prof D, Mount Sinai Sch Med

Granstein, Richard MD (D) - **Spec Exp:** Autoimmune Disease; Skin Cancer; Psoriasis; **Hospital:** NY-Presby Hosp (page 100); **Address:** 520 E 70th St Fl 3 - Ste 326, New York, NY 10021; **Phone:** 212-746-2007; **Board Cert:** Dermatology 1983; Clinical & Laboratory Dematologic Immunology 1985; **Med School:** UCLA 1978; **Resid:** Dermatology, Mass Genl Hosp 1981; **Fellow:** Research, Natl Cancer Inst-Frederick Cancer Rsch Facl 1982; Dermatology, Mass Genl Hosp 1983; **Fac Appt:** Prof D, Cornell Univ-Weill Med Coll

Greenberg, Robert MD (D) - **Spec Exp:** Skin Laser Surgery; Cosmetic Dermatology; Botox Therapy; **Hospital:** NYU Med Ctr (page 102); **Address:** 117 E 72nd St, New York, NY 10021-4249; **Phone:** 212-861-2580; **Board Cert:** Dermatology 1977; **Med School:** Univ Mich Med Sch 1970; **Resid:** Dermatology, Univ of Miami Hosps 1975; Dermatology, New York Univ 1977; **Fellow:** Dermatology, Univ Miami Hosp 1974; **Fac Appt:** Asst Clin Prof D, NYU Sch Med

Greenspan, Alan H MD (D) - **Spec Exp:** Skin Cancer; Dermatologic Surgery; **Hospital:** NYU Med Ctr (page 102), NY Downtown Hosp; **Address:** 39 Broadway, Ste 1911, New York, NY 10006; **Phone:** 212-509-5200; **Board Cert:** Dermatology 1984; **Med School:** Northwestern Univ 1979; **Resid:** Internal Medicine, Northwestern Univ 1981; Dermatology, NYU Med Ctr 1984; **Fac Appt:** Asst Clin Prof D, NYU Sch Med

Gross, Dennis MD (D) - **Hospital:** NYU Med Ctr (page 102); **Address:** 105 E 37th St, Ground Fl, New York, NY 10016; **Phone:** 212-725-4555; **Board Cert:** Dermatology 1990; **Med School:** SUNY Stony Brook 1986; **Resid:** Dermatology, NYU Med Ctr 1990; **Fac Appt:** Asst Clin Prof D, NYU Sch Med

Grossman, Melanie MD (D) - **Spec Exp:** Skin Laser Surgery; Tattoo Removal; Cosmetic Dermatology; Botox Therapy; **Hospital:** NY-Presby Hosp (page 100), NY-Presby Hosp (page 100); **Address:** 161 Madison Ave, Ste 4NW, New York, NY 10016-5405; **Phone:** 212-725-8600; **Board Cert:** Dermatology 1999; **Med School:** NYU Sch Med 1988; **Resid:** Internal Medicine, Yale-New Haven Hosp 1989; Dermatology, Columbia/Presby Hosp 1992; **Fellow:** Laser Surgery, Mass Genl Hosp/Harvard 1995; **Fac Appt:** Asst Clin Prof D, Columbia P&S

Halpern, Allan C MD (D) - **Spec Exp:** Skin Cancer; Melanoma; Melanoma Early Detection/Prevention; **Hospital:** Meml Sloan Kettering Cancer Ctr (page 109); **Address:** 160 E 53rd St, New York, NY 10022; **Phone:** 212-610-0766; **Board Cert:** Internal Medicine 1984; Dermatology 1988; **Med School:** Albert Einstein Coll Med 1981; **Resid:** Dermatology, Hosp Univ Penn 1988; **Fellow:** Epidemiology, Hosp Univ Penn 1989; **Fac Appt:** Assoc Prof Med, Cornell Univ-Weill Med Coll

Hatcher, Virgil MD (D) - **Spec Exp:** Cosmetic Dermatology; Psoriasis; Viral Infections; **Hospital:** NYU Med Ctr (page 102); **Address:** 420 W 23rd St, Ste A-GF, New York, NY 10011-2172; **Phone:** 212-675-4244; **Board Cert:** Dermatology 1982; **Med School:** UCSF 1978; **Resid:** Dermatology, NYU Med Ctr 1982; **Fellow:** Virology, NYU Med Ctr 1983; **Fac Appt:** Asst Clin Prof D, NYU Sch Med

Hochman, Herbert MD (D) - **Spec Exp:** Cosmetic Dermatology; Laser Surgery; Botox Therapy; **Hospital:** Lenox Hill Hosp (page 94); **Address:** 1020 Park Ave, New York, NY 10028-0913; **Phone:** 212-861-1656; **Board Cert:** Dermatology 1977; **Med School:** Tulane Univ 1970; **Resid:** Dermatology, Montefiore Hosp-Albert Einstein 1976

Jacobs, Michael MD (D) - **Spec Exp:** Skin Cancer; Melanoma; Lupus/SLE; **Hospital:** NY-Presby Hosp (page 100), Hosp For Special Surgery (page 108); **Address:** 407 E 70th St Fl 2, New York, NY 10021-5302; **Phone:** 212-772-7190; **Board Cert:** Dermatology 1981; **Med School:** Cornell Univ-Weill Med Coll 1977; **Resid:** Dermatology, New York Hosp-Cornell 1981; **Fac Appt:** Assoc Clin Prof D, Cornell Univ-Weill Med Coll

Katz, Bruce MD (D) - **Spec Exp:** Skin Laser Surgery; Liposuction; Cosmetic Dermatology; **Hospital:** Mount Sinai Med Ctr (page 98); **Address:** 60 E 56th St Fl 2, New York, NY 10022-3350; **Phone:** 212-688-5882; **Board Cert:** Dermatology 1983; **Med School:** McGill Univ 1977; **Resid:** Internal Medicine, Columbia Presby Med Ctr 1979; Dermatology, Columbia Presby Med Ctr 1982; **Fac Appt:** Clin Prof D, Mount Sinai Sch Med

Kauvar, Arielle MD (D) - **Spec Exp:** Laser Surgery; Mohs' Surgery; Cosmetic Dermatology; **Hospital:** NYU Med Ctr (page 102), New York Eye & Ear Infirm (page 110); **Address:** 994 Fifth Ave, New York, NY 10028; **Phone:** 212-249-9440; **Board Cert:** Dermatology 2001; **Med School:** Harvard Med Sch 1989; **Resid:** Dermatology, NYU Med Ctr 1993; **Fellow:** Mohs Surgery, Laser & Skin Surgery Ctr 1994; **Fac Appt:** Assoc Clin Prof D, NYU Sch Med

Kenet, Barney J MD (D) - **Spec Exp:** Dermatologic Surgery; Cosmetic Dermatology; Liposuction; **Hospital:** NY-Presby Hosp (page 100); **Address:** 25 E 86th St, New York, NY 10028; **Phone:** 212-535-9753; **Board Cert:** Dermatology 2001; **Med School:** Brown Univ 1988; **Resid:** Dermatology, New York Hosp 1992

Kline, Mitchell MD (D) - **Spec Exp:** Melanoma & Skin Cancer; Aging Skin; Botox Therapy; **Hospital:** NY-Presby Hosp (page 100); **Address:** 700 Park Ave, New York, NY 10021; **Phone:** 212-517-6555; **Board Cert:** Dermatology 1990; **Med School:** Univ Pennsylvania 1985; **Resid:** Internal Medicine, Graduate Hosp 1987; Dermatology, New York Hosp 1990

Kriegel, David MD (D) - **Spec Exp:** Mohs' Surgery; Cosmetic Dermatology; Skin Laser Surgery; **Hospital:** Mount Sinai Med Ctr (page 98); **Address:** 315 W 57th St, Ste LL3, New York, NY 10019; **Phone:** 212-489-6669; **Board Cert:** Dermatology 1993; **Med School:** Boston Univ 1987; **Resid:** Dermatology, New England Med Ctr 1991; **Fellow:** Mohs Surgery, Stony Brook Univ Hosp 1993; **Fac Appt:** Assoc Prof D, Mount Sinai Sch Med

Kurtin, Stephen MD (D) - **Spec Exp:** Skin Cancer; Cosmetic Dermatology; Botox Therapy; **Hospital:** Mount Sinai Med Ctr (page 98); **Address:** 111 E 71st St, New York, NY 10021; **Phone:** 212-772-1717; **Board Cert:** Dermatology 1970; **Med School:** Columbia P&S 1965; **Resid:** Dermatology, Bellevue Hosp Ctr-NYU 1969; **Fac Appt:** Assoc Clin Prof D, Mount Sinai Sch Med

Lebwohl, Mark MD (D) - **Spec Exp:** Skin Cancer; Psoriasis; **Hospital:** Mount Sinai Med Ctr (page 98); **Address:** 5 E 98th St Fl 5, New York, NY 10029-6501; **Phone:** 212-241-9728; **Board Cert:** Internal Medicine 1981; Dermatology 1983; **Med School:** Harvard Med Sch 1978; **Resid:** Internal Medicine, Mount Sinai Hosp 1981; **Fellow:** Dermatology, Mount Sinai Hosp 1983; **Fac Appt:** Prof D, Mount Sinai Sch Med

Lombardo, Peter C MD (D) - **Spec Exp:** Skin Laser Surgery; Skin Cancer; Cosmetic Dermatology; **Hospital:** St Luke's - Roosevelt Hosp Ctr - Roosevelt Div (page 90), NY-Presby Hosp (page 100); **Address:** 445 E 58th St, New York, NY 10022; **Phone:** 212-838-0270; **Board Cert:** Dermatology 1999; **Med School:** Albany Med Coll 1959; **Resid:** Dermatology, Columbia-Presby 1965; Internal Medicine, St Luke's-Roosevelt Hosp Ctr 1966; **Fac Appt:** Assoc Clin Prof D, Columbia P&S

Myskowski, Patricia L MD (D) - **Spec Exp:** AIDS-Kaposi's Sarcoma; Cutaneous Lymphoma; Skin Cancer; **Hospital:** Meml Sloan Kettering Cancer Ctr (page 109); **Address:** Memorial Sloan Kettering Cancer Ctr, OPD, 160 E 53rd St Fl 10, New York, NY 10021; **Phone:** 212-639-5807; **Board Cert:** Dermatology 1980; Clinical & Laboratory Dematologic Immunology 1985; **Med School:** Brown Univ 1975; **Resid:** Internal Medicine, Bronx VA Hosp; Dermatology, NY Hosp-Cornell Med Ctr 1980; **Fellow:** Dermatology, Meml Sloan Kettering Cancer Ctr 1981; **Fac Appt:** Assoc Prof D, Cornell Univ-Weill Med Coll

Orbuch, Philip MD (D) - **Spec Exp:** Pediatric Dermatology; Skin Cancer; **Hospital:** NYU Med Ctr (page 102), Bellevue Hosp Ctr; **Address:** 345 E 37th St, Ste 307, New York, NY 10016; **Phone:** 212-532-5355; **Board Cert:** Dermatology 1986; **Med School:** Israel 1981; **Resid:** Dermatology, New York Univ Med Ctr 1985; **Fellow:** Dermatology, New York Univ Med Ctr 1986; **Fac Appt:** Assoc Clin Prof D, NYU Sch Med

Orentreich, David MD (D) - **Spec Exp:** Dermatologic Surgery; Liposuction; Hair Restoration/Transplant; **Hospital:** Mount Sinai Med Ctr (page 98); **Address:** 909 5th Ave, New York, NY 10021; **Phone:** 212-794-0800; **Board Cert:** Dermatology 1984; **Med School:** Columbia P&S 1980; **Resid:** Dermatology, Mt Sinai Hosp 1981; **Fac Appt:** Asst Clin Prof D, Mount Sinai Sch Med

Orlow, Seth MD/PhD (D) - **Spec Exp:** Pediatric Dermatology; Hemangiomas/Birthmarks; Psoriasis/Eczema; **Hospital:** NYU Med Ctr (page 102), Lenox Hill Hosp (page 94); **Address:** 530 1st Ave, Ste 7R, New York, NY 10016-6402; **Phone:** 212-263-5889; **Board Cert:** Dermatology 1990; **Med School:** Albert Einstein Coll Med 1986; **Resid:** Pediatrics, Mt Sinai Hosp 1987; Dermatology, Yale-New Haven Hosp 1989; **Fellow:** Dermatology, Yale-New Haven Hosp 1990; **Fac Appt:** Prof D, NYU Sch Med

Podwal, Mark MD (D) - **Spec Exp:** Skin Cancer; Rashes; **Hospital:** NYU Med Ctr (page 102); **Address:** 55 E 73rd St, New York, NY 10021; **Phone:** 212-288-7488; **Board Cert:** Dermatology 1975; **Med School:** NYU Sch Med 1970; **Resid:** Dermatology, Bellevue Hosp 1974; **Fac Appt:** Assoc Clin Prof D, NYU Sch Med

Polis, Laurie MD (D) - **Spec Exp:** Cosmetic Dermatology; Skin Laser Surgery; Botox Therapy; **Hospital:** Beth Israel Med Ctr - Petrie Division (page 90), Mount Sinai Med Ctr (page 98); **Address:** 62 Crosby St, New York, NY 10012; **Phone:** 212-431-1600 x227; **Board Cert:** Dermatology 1989; **Med School:** Mount Sinai Sch Med 1983; **Resid:** Dermatology, Montefiore Med Ctr 1989; **Fac Appt:** Asst Prof D, Albert Einstein Coll Med

Prioleau, Philip G MD (D) - **Spec Exp:** Melanoma; Skin Cancer; Mohs' Surgery; **Hospital:** NY-Presby Hosp (page 100); **Address:** 1035 Fifth Ave, Ste C, New York, NY 10028; **Phone:** 212-794-3548; **Board Cert:** Surgery 1973; Anatomic Pathology 1979; Dermatopathology 1980; Dermatology 1983; **Med School:** Med Univ SC 1967; **Resid:** Surgery, Univ Va Hosp 1972; Plastic Surgery, Duke Univ Hosp 1975; **Fellow:** Pathology, Barnes Hosp 1980; Dermatopathology, NYU Med Ctr 1981; **Fac Appt:** Assoc Prof D, Cornell Univ-Weill Med Coll

Prystowsky, Janet MD (D) - **Spec Exp:** Mohs' Surgery; Cosmetic Dermatology; Skin Cancer; **Hospital:** St Luke's - Roosevelt Hosp Ctr - Roosevelt Div (page 90), Montefiore Med Ctr; **Address:** 225 E 64th St, New York, NY 10021; **Phone:** 212-230-1212; **Board Cert:** Dermatology 1987; **Med School:** Univ Chicago-Pritzker Sch Med 1983; **Resid:** Internal Medicine, Univ Chicago 1984; Dermatology, Hosp Univ Penn 1987; **Fellow:** Mohs Surgery, SUNY Stony Brook

Ramsay, David L MD (D) - **Spec Exp:** Cutaneous Lymphoma; Skin Cancer; **Hospital:** NYU Med Ctr (page 102); **Address:** 530 1st Ave, Ste 7G, New York, NY 10016; **Phone:** 212-683-6283; **Board Cert:** Dermatology 1974; **Med School:** Indiana Univ 1969; **Resid:** Dermatology, New York Univ Med Ctr 1973; **Fellow:** Nat Inst Health 1973; **Fac Appt:** Clin Prof D, NYU Sch Med

Ratner, Desiree MD (D) - **Spec Exp:** Mohs' Surgery; Skin Cancer; Dermatologic Surgery; **Hospital:** NY-Presby Hosp (page 100); **Address:** 161 Fort Washington Ave Fl 12, Columbia Presbyterian Medical Ctr, New York, NY 10032; **Phone:** 212-305-3625; **Board Cert:** Dermatology 2003; **Med School:** Johns Hopkins Univ 1989; **Resid:** Dermatology, Univ Michigan Med Ctr 1993; **Fellow:** Mohs Surgery, New England Med Ctr 1994; Mohs Surgery, Lahey Clinic 1995; **Fac Appt:** Assoc Clin Prof D, Columbia P&S

Rigel, Darrell S MD (D) - **Spec Exp:** Melanoma; Skin Cancer; Cosmetic Dermatology; **Hospital:** NYU Med Ctr (page 102), Mount Sinai Med Ctr (page 98); **Address:** 35 E 35th Street, Ste 208, New York, NY 10016-3823; **Phone:** 212-684-5964; **Board Cert:** Dermatology 1983; **Med School:** Geo Wash Univ 1978; **Resid:** Dermatology, NYU Med Ctr 1982; **Fellow:** Dermatologic Surgery, NYU Med Ctr 1983; **Fac Appt:** Clin Prof D, NYU Sch Med

Robins, Perry MD (D) - **Spec Exp:** Mohs' Surgery; Skin Cancer; Melanoma; **Hospital:** NYU Med Ctr (page 102), Bellevue Hosp Ctr; **Address:** 530 First Ave, Ste 7H, New York, NY 10016; **Phone:** 212-263-7222; **Med School:** Germany 1961; **Resid:** Dermatology, VA Med Ctr 1964; **Fellow:** Dermatology, NYU Med Ctr 1967; **Fac Appt:** Prof D, NYU Sch Med

Romano, John MD (D) - **Spec Exp:** Aging Skin; Cosmetic Dermatology; Skin Cancer; **Hospital:** St Vincent Cath Med Ctrs - Manhattan (page 375), NY-Presby Hosp (page 100); **Address:** 36 7th Ave, Ste 423, New York, NY 10011; **Phone:** 212-242-5815; **Board Cert:** Dermatology 1980; **Med School:** Cornell Univ-Weill Med Coll 1973; **Resid:** Internal Medicine, St. Vincents Hosp 1976; Dermatology, New York Hosp 1978; **Fellow:** Dermatology, New York Hosp 1978; **Fac Appt:** Asst Clin Prof D, Cornell Univ-Weill Med Coll

Sadick, Neil MD (D) - **Spec Exp:** Cosmetic Dermatology; Laser Surgery; Hair Restoration/Transplant; Varicose Veins; **Hospital:** NY-Presby Hosp (page 100), N Shore Univ Hosp at Manhasset; **Address:** 772 Park Ave, New York, NY 10021; **Phone:** 212-772-7242; **Board Cert:** Internal Medicine 1980; Dermatology 1983; **Med School:** SUNY Downstate 1977; **Resid:** Internal Medicine, N Shore Univ Hosp 1980; Internal Medicine, Meml Sloan Kettering Cancer Ctr 1980; **Fellow:** Dermatology, New York Hosp 1982; Dermatology, Meml Sloan-Kettering Cancer Ctr 1982; **Fac Appt:** Clin Prof D, Cornell Univ-Weill Med Coll

Safai, Bijan MD (D) - **Spec Exp:** Dermatologic Surgery; Skin Cancer; Skin Laser Surgery; **Hospital:** Metropolitan Hosp Ctr - NY, Westchester Med Ctr (page 713); **Address:** 625 Park Ave, New York, NY 10021; **Phone:** 212-988-8918; **Board Cert:** Dermatology 1974; **Med School:** Iran 1965; **Resid:** Internal Medicine, VA Med Ctr 1970; Dermatology, NYU Med Ctr 1973; **Fellow:** Immunology, Mem Sloan-Kettering Cancer Ctr 1974; **Fac Appt:** Prof D, NY Med Coll

Sanchez, Miguel R MD (D) - **Spec Exp:** Genital Warts; Sexually Transmitted Diseases; Ethnic Dermatology; **Hospital:** NYU Med Ctr (page 102), Bellevue Hosp Ctr; **Address:** NYU Med Ctr, Dept Dermatology, 550 1st Ave, New York, NY 10016; **Phone:** 212-263-6484; **Board Cert:** Dermatology 1986; **Med School:** Albert Einstein Coll Med 1974; **Resid:** Family Medicine, Montefiore Hosp 1978; Dermatology, NYU Med Ctr 1983; **Fac Appt:** Assoc Prof D, NYU Sch Med

Schultz, Neal MD (D) - **Spec Exp:** Cosmetic Dermatology; Skin Cancer & Moles; Skin Laser Surgery; Tattoo Removal; **Hospital:** Mount Sinai Med Ctr (page 98), Lenox Hill Hosp (page 94); **Address:** 1130 Park Ave, New York, NY 10128; **Phone:** 212-369-9600; **Board Cert:** Dermatology 1978; **Med School:** Columbia P&S 1973; **Resid:** Internal Medicine, Mount Sinai Hosp 1975; Dermatology, Mount Sinai Hosp 1978

Shelton, Ronald M MD (D) - **Spec Exp:** Liposuction; Mohs' Surgery; Skin Laser Surgery; **Hospital:** Mount Sinai Med Ctr (page 98); **Address:** 260 E 66 St, New York, NY 10021; **Phone:** 212-593-1818; **Board Cert:** Dermatology 1990; **Med School:** SUNY Hlth Sci Ctr 1984; **Resid:** Surgery, LI Jewish Med Ctr 1985; Dermatology, Brooke Army Med Ctr 1990; **Fellow:** Mohs Surgery, UCSF Med Ctr 1993; **Fac Appt:** Asst Prof D, Mount Sinai Sch Med

Shupack, Jerome L MD (D) - **Spec Exp:** Rare Skin Disorders; Psoriasis; **Hospital:** NYU Med Ctr (page 102); **Address:** 530 1st Ave, New York, NY 10016-6402; **Phone:** 212-263-7344; **Board Cert:** Dermatology 1970; **Med School:** Columbia P&S 1963; **Resid:** Internal Medicine, Mt Sinai Hosp 1965; Dermatology, NYU Med Ctr 1970; **Fac Appt:** Prof D, NYU Sch Med

Sibulkin, David MD (D) - **Hospital:** St Luke's - Roosevelt Hosp Ctr - Roosevelt Div (page 90), NY-Presby Hosp (page 100); **Address:** 1886 Broadway Fl 2, New York, NY 10023; **Phone:** 212-753-1470; **Board Cert:** Dermatology 1973; **Med School:** NYU Sch Med 1966; **Resid:** Dermatology, Bellevue Hosp 1972; **Fac Appt:** Assoc Clin Prof D, Columbia P&S

Silvers, David MD (D) - **Spec Exp:** Dermatopathology; **Hospital:** NY-Presby Hosp (page 100); **Address:** Vanderbilt Clinic 15, rm 207, 630 W 168th St, New York, NY 10032-3702; **Phone:** 212-305-2155; **Board Cert:** Dermatology 1973; Dermatopathology 1974; **Med School:** Duke Univ 1968; **Resid:** Dermatology, NYU Med Ctr 1971; **Fellow:** Dermatopathology, Armed Forces Inst Path 1973; **Fac Appt:** Clin Prof D, Columbia P&S

Sobel, Howard MD (D) - **Spec Exp:** Cosmetic Dermatology; Botox Therapy; Liposuction; Laser Surgery; **Hospital:** Lenox Hill Hosp (page 94), Beth Israel Med Ctr - Petrie Division (page 90); **Address:** 960A Park Ave, New York, NY 10028-0325; **Phone:** 212-288-0060; **Med School:** Albert Einstein Coll Med 1975; **Resid:** Dermatology, Emory Univ Hosp 1979

Soter, Nicholas A MD (D) - **Spec Exp:** Urticaria; Psoriasis; Vasculitis; **Hospital:** NYU Med Ctr (page 102); **Address:** 530 1st Ave, Ste 7R, New York, NY 10016; **Phone:** 212-263-5889; **Board Cert:** Dermatology 1970; **Med School:** Univ Tex SW, Dallas 1965; **Resid:** Dermatology, Baylor Med Ctr 1968; Dermatology, Mass Genl Hosp 1969; **Fellow:** Immunology, Harvard 1973; **Fac Appt:** Prof D, NYU Sch Med

Tanenbaum, Diane MD (D) - **Spec Exp:** Skin Cancer; **Hospital:** Lenox Hill Hosp (page 94); **Address:** 16 E 79th St, Ste 22, New York, NY 10021-0150; **Phone:** 212-249-6122; **Board Cert:** Dermatology 1971; **Med School:** SUNY Downstate 1964; **Resid:** Dermatology, NYU Med Ctr 1970; **Fac Appt:** Assoc Clin Prof D, NYU Sch Med

Tesser, Mark MD (D) - **Spec Exp:** Cosmetic Dermatology; Botox Therapy; **Hospital:** Mount Sinai Med Ctr (page 98); **Address:** 1107 Park Ave, New York, NY 10128; **Phone:** 212-996-9600; **Board Cert:** Internal Medicine 1977; Dermatology 1980; **Med School:** Albert Einstein Coll Med 1974; **Resid:** Internal Medicine, Mount Sinai 1977; Dermatology, Mount Sinai 1979

Vogel, Louis MD (D) - **Spec Exp:** Cosmetic Dermatology; Botox Therapy; Hair Removal-Laser; **Hospital:** NYU Med Ctr (page 102); **Address:** 16 Park Ave, Ste 1D, New York, NY 10016-4329; **Phone:** 212-447-5443; **Board Cert:** Internal Medicine 1980; Dermatology 1983; **Med School:** Boston Univ 1977; **Resid:** Internal Medicine, NYU Med Ctr 1980; Dermatology, NYU Med Ctr 1982; **Fac Appt:** Asst Clin Prof D, NYU Sch Med

Walther, Robert MD (D) - **Spec Exp:** Acne; Skin Cancer; Psoriasis; **Hospital:** NY-Presby Hosp (page 100); **Address:** 16 E 60th St, Ste 300, New York, NY 10022; **Phone:** 212-326-8465; **Board Cert:** Dermatology 1999; Internal Medicine 1977; **Med School:** Univ NC Sch Med 1973; **Resid:** Internal Medicine, Univ Miami Hosps 1975; Dermatology, Columbia-Presby Hosp 1978; **Fellow:** Dermatology, Rockefeller Univ Hosp; **Fac Appt:** Clin Prof D, Columbia P&S

Warner, Robert MD (D) - **Spec Exp:** Laser Surgery; Hair Removal-Laser; Cosmetic Dermatology; **Hospital:** Mount Sinai Med Ctr (page 98); **Address:** 580 Park Ave, New York, NY 10021-7313; **Phone:** 212-752-3692; **Board Cert:** Dermatology 1981; **Med School:** SUNY Hlth Sci Ctr 1977; **Resid:** Internal Medicine, Kings County Hosp 1978; Dermatology, Mount Sinai 1981; **Fac Appt:** Asst Clin Prof D, Mount Sinai Sch Med

Wexler, Patricia MD (D) - **Spec Exp:** Skin Laser Surgery; Liposuction & Fat Transplantation; Botox Therapy; Acne; **Hospital:** Mount Sinai Med Ctr (page 98); **Address:** 145 E 32nd St Fl 7, New York, NY 10016; **Phone:** 212-684-2626; **Board Cert:** Internal Medicine 1983; Dermatology 1986; **Med School:** Belgium 1979; **Resid:** Internal Medicine, Beth Israel Med Ctr 1982; Dermatology, Mt Sinai Hosp 1986; **Fellow:** Infectious Disease, Beth Israel Med Ctr 1983; **Fac Appt:** Assoc Clin Prof D, Mount Sinai Sch Med

DIAGNOSTIC RADIOLOGY

Abramson, Sara MD (DR) - **Spec Exp:** Pediatric Radiology; **Hospital:** Meml Sloan Kettering Cancer Ctr (page 109); **Address:** 1275 York Ave, New York, NY 10021-6007; **Phone:** 212-639-2184; **Board Cert:** Diagnostic Radiology 1976; Pediatric Radiology 1994; **Med School:** Mount Sinai Sch Med 1971; **Resid:** Pediatrics, Mt Sinai Hosp 1973; Radiology, Chldns Mercy Hosp 1976; **Fellow:** Pediatric Radiology, Chldns Hosp 1981; **Fac Appt:** Prof Rad, Cornell Univ-Weill Med Coll

Adler, Ronald S MD/PhD (DR) - **Spec Exp:** Musculoskeletal Imaging; Ultrasound; Power Doppler Imaging; **Hospital:** Hosp For Special Surgery (page 108), NY-Presby Hosp (page 100); **Address:** 535 E 70th St, Hospital for Special Surgery, New York, NY 10021; **Phone:** 212-606-1635; **Board Cert:** Diagnostic Radiology 1988; **Med School:** Wayne State Univ 1984; **Resid:** Radiology, Univ Mich Med Ctr 1988; **Fellow:** Ultrasound/CT/MRI, Univ Mich Med Ctr 1989; **Fac Appt:** Prof Rad, Cornell Univ-Weill Med Coll

Alderson, Philip MD (DR) - **Spec Exp:** Pulmonary Embolism; Lung Cancer; **Hospital:** NY-Presby Hosp (page 100); **Address:** Columbia Univ Radiology, 630 W 168th St, Harkness 3-320, New York, NY 10032; **Phone:** 212-305-8994; **Board Cert:** Diagnostic Radiology 1976; Nuclear Medicine 1974; Nuclear Radiology 1981; **Med School:** Washington Univ, St Louis 1970; **Resid:** Radiology, Barnes Hosp 1974; **Fellow:** Nuclear Medicine, Barnes Hosp 1975; **Fac Appt:** Prof Rad, Columbia P&S

Amodio, John MD (DR) - **Spec Exp:** Pediatric Radiology; **Hospital:** NYU Med Ctr (page 102); **Address:** NYU Med Ctr-Tisch Hosp, Div Ped Radiology, 550 1st Ave, New York, NY 10016; **Phone:** 212-263-5362; **Board Cert:** Diagnostic Radiology 1984; Pediatric Radiology 2005; **Med School:** NY Med Coll 1980; **Resid:** Diagnostic Radiology, Montefiore Hosp Med Ctr 1984; **Fellow:** Pediatric Radiology, Columbia-Presby Med Ctr 1985

Austin, John H M MD (DR) - **Spec Exp:** Lung Cancer; **Hospital:** NY-Presby Hosp (page 100); **Address:** Columbia Presby Hosp, Dept Radiology, 622 W 168th St, MHB 3-202C, New York, NY 10032-3784; **Phone:** 212-305-2986; **Board Cert:** Diagnostic Radiology 1970; **Med School:** Yale Univ 1965; **Resid:** Radiology, UCSF Med Ctr 1968; **Fellow:** Radiology, UCSF Med Ctr 1970; **Fac Appt:** Prof Rad, Columbia P&S

Baer, Jeanne MD (DR) - **Spec Exp:** Abdominal Imaging; **Hospital:** St Luke's - Roosevelt Hosp Ctr - St Luke's Hosp (page 90); **Address:** St Luke's Hosp, Dept Radiology, 1111 Amsterdam Ave, New York, NY 10025-1716; **Phone:** 212-523-4272; **Board Cert:** Radiology 1971; **Med School:** Columbia P&S 1964; **Resid:** Internal Medicine, Geo Wash Univ Med Ctr 1967; **Fellow:** Radiology, St Luke's-Roosevelt Hosp Ctr 1970; **Fac Appt:** Assoc Clin Prof Rad, Columbia P&S

Barone, Clement MD (DR) - **Spec Exp:** Women's Imaging; Mammography; Bone Densitometry; **Address:** 1440 York Ave, Ste P-1, New York, NY 10021-2577; **Phone:** 212-988-1303; **Board Cert:** Diagnostic Radiology 1974; **Med School:** NY Med Coll 1968; **Resid:** Diagnostic Radiology, Mt Sinai Hosp 1970; Diagnostic Radiology, Mt Sinai Hosp 1974; **Fac Appt:** Asst Clin Prof Rad, Mount Sinai Sch Med

Berson, Barry MD (DR) - **Spec Exp:** Mammography; Breast Imaging; Bone Densitometry; **Hospital:** Mount Sinai Med Ctr (page 98); **Address:** 165 E 84th St, New York, NY 10028-0302; **Phone:** 212-535-9770; **Board Cert:** Diagnostic Radiology 1990; Neuroradiology 1992; **Med School:** Mount Sinai Sch Med 1984; **Resid:** Radiology, Mount Sinai Hosp 1990; **Fellow:** Neuroradiology, NYU Med Ctr 1992; **Fac Appt:** Asst Clin Prof Rad, Mount Sinai Sch Med

Brill, Paula MD (DR) - **Spec Exp:** Pediatric Radiology; Bone Disorders; **Hospital:** NY-Presby Hosp (page 100), NY-Presby Hosp (page 100); **Address:** 525 E 68th St, New York, NY 10021-4873; **Phone:** 212-746-2554; **Board Cert:** Pediatrics 1970; Diagnostic Radiology 1971; Pediatric Radiology 2005; **Med School:** Cornell Univ-Weill Med Coll 1962; **Resid:** Pediatrics, New York Hosp 1968; Radiology, New York Hosp 1971; **Fellow:** Radiology, Cornell Univ 1971; **Fac Appt:** Prof Rad, Cornell Univ-Weill Med Coll

Cohen, Burton A MD (DR) - **Spec Exp:** CT Scan; MRI; Ovarian Cancer; **Hospital:** Mount Sinai Med Ctr (page 98); **Address:** 165 E 84th St, New York, NY 10028; **Phone:** 212-535-9770; **Board Cert:** Diagnostic Radiology 1979; **Med School:** NY Med Coll 1975; **Resid:** Diagnostic Radiology, Mount Sinai Hosp 1979; **Fac Appt:** Assoc Clin Prof Rad, Mount Sinai Sch Med

Dershaw, D David MD (DR) - **Spec Exp:** Breast Imaging; Breast Cancer; **Hospital:** Meml Sloan Kettering Cancer Ctr (page 109); **Address:** 1275 York Ave, New York, NY 10021-6007; **Phone:** 212-639-7295; **Board Cert:** Diagnostic Radiology 1978; **Med School:** Jefferson Med Coll 1974; **Resid:** Diagnostic Radiology, New York Hosp 1978; **Fellow:** Ultrasound, Thomas Jefferson Univ Hosp 1979; **Fac Appt:** Prof Rad, Cornell Univ-Weill Med Coll

Edelstein, Barbara A MD (DR) - **Spec Exp:** Breast Cancer; Women's Imaging; **Address:** 1045 Park Ave, New York, NY 10028; **Phone:** 212-860-7700; **Board Cert:** Diagnostic Radiology 1983; **Med School:** NY Med Coll 1977; **Resid:** Diagnostic Radiology, Montefiore Hosp 1982

Feldman, Frieda MD (DR) - **Spec Exp:** Musculoskeletal Imaging; **Hospital:** NY-Presby Hosp (page 100); **Address:** Columbia Presby Med Ctr, Harkness Pavilion 3, 622 W 168th St, rm 326, New York, NY 10032; **Phone:** 212-305-2986; **Board Cert:** Radiology 1962; **Med School:** NYU Sch Med 1957; **Resid:** Diagnostic Radiology, Bellevue Hosp 1961; **Fellow:** Diagnostic Radiology, Columbia-Presby Hosp 1962; **Fac Appt:** Prof Rad, Columbia P&S

Fried, Karen O MD (DR) - **Spec Exp:** Ultrasound; Thyroid Ultrasound; Vascular Ultrasound; **Address:** Lenox Hill Radiology, 61 E 77th St, New York, NY 10021; **Phone:** 212-772-3111; **Board Cert:** Diagnostic Radiology 1990; **Med School:** Albany Med Coll 1985; **Resid:** Diagnostic Radiology, LIJ Med Ctr 1990; **Fellow:** Cross Sectional Imaging, LIJ Med Ctr 1991

Genieser, Nancy B MD (DR) - **Spec Exp:** Neonatal Radiology; Pediatric Radiology; Child Abuse Imaging; **Hospital:** NYU Med Ctr (page 102), Bellevue Hosp Ctr; **Address:** 462 1st Ave, NBV 3W33, New York, NY 10016; **Phone:** 212-263-6373; **Board Cert:** Pediatric Radiology 1995; Radiology 1967; **Med School:** Med Coll PA Hahnemann 1962; **Resid:** Radiology, NYU Med Ctr 1966; **Fac Appt:** Prof Rad, NYU Sch Med

Gross, Joshua MD (DR) - **Spec Exp:** Breast Imaging; Breast Cancer; **Hospital:** Beth Israel Med Ctr - Petrie Division (page 90); **Address:** 10 Union Square E, Breast Imaging Dept, Ste 4L, New York, NY 10003; **Phone:** 212-844-8776; **Board Cert:** Diagnostic Radiology 1984; **Med School:** Albert Einstein Coll Med 1980; **Resid:** Diagnostic Radiology, Einstein/Jacobi Hosp 1984

Hann, Lucy MD (DR) - **Spec Exp:** Liver & Biliary Cancer Ultrasound; Ovarian Cancer Ultrasound Diagnosis; Thyroid Ultrasound; **Hospital:** Meml Sloan Kettering Cancer Ctr (page 109); **Address:** Memorial Sloan-Kettering Cancer Ctr, 1275 York Ave, rm C278, New York, NY 10021; **Phone:** 212-639-2179; **Board Cert:** Diagnostic Radiology 1977; **Med School:** Harvard Med Sch 1971; **Resid:** Diagnostic Radiology, Hosp Univ Penn 1974; Diagnostic Radiology, Mass General Hosp 1977; **Fellow:** Body Imaging, Mass General Hosp 1978; **Fac Appt:** Prof Rad, Cornell Univ-Weill Med Coll

Henschke, Claudia L MD/PhD (DR) - **Spec Exp:** Lung Cancer; Lung Disease Imaging; **Hospital:** NY-Presby Hosp (page 100); **Address:** NY Weill Medical College, Dept Radiology, 525 E 68th St, Box 586, New York, NY 10021; **Phone:** 212-746-1325; **Board Cert:** Diagnostic Radiology 1981; **Med School:** Howard Univ 1977; **Resid:** Diagnostic Radiology, Brigham & Womens Hosp 1983; **Fac Appt:** Prof Rad, Cornell Univ-Weill Med Coll

Hricak, Hedvig MD/PhD (DR) - **Spec Exp:** Prostate Cancer-MR Spectroscopy (MRSI); Breast Imaging; Breast Cancer; **Hospital:** Meml Sloan Kettering Cancer Ctr (page 109); **Address:** Meml Sloan Kettering Cancer Ctr, Dept Radiology, 1275 York Ave, New York, NY 10021; **Phone:** 212-639-7284; **Board Cert:** Diagnostic Radiology 1978; **Med School:** Yugoslavia 1970; **Resid:** Diagnostic Radiology, St Joseph Mercy Hosp 1977; **Fellow:** Ultrasound/CT, Henry Ford Hosp 1978; **Fac Appt:** Prof Rad, Cornell Univ-Weill Med Coll

Jacobs, Morton MD (DR) - **Hospital:** NY-Presby Hosp (page 100); **Address:** 203 E 60th St, New York, NY 10022; **Phone:** 212-486-5529; **Board Cert:** Diagnostic Radiology 1976; Neuroradiology 1996; **Med School:** Univ Chicago-Pritzker Sch Med 1972; **Resid:** Diagnostic Radiology, New York Hosp 1976; **Fellow:** Neuroradiology, New York Hosp 1979; **Fac Appt:** Asst Clin Prof Rad, Cornell Univ-Weill Med Coll

Kazam, Elias MD (DR) - **Spec Exp:** CT Scan; Ultrasound; MRI; **Hospital:** NY-Presby Hosp (page 100); **Address:** 400 E 66th St, New York, NY 10021-9314; **Phone:** 212-838-4243; **Board Cert:** Diagnostic Radiology 1974; Nuclear Medicine 1976; **Med School:** Albert Einstein Coll Med 1966; **Resid:** Radiology, Peter Bent Brigham Hosp 1972; Radiology, New York Hosp 1973; **Fellow:** Natl Cancer Inst-NIH 1969; **Fac Appt:** Prof Emeritus Rad, Cornell Univ-Weill Med Coll

Klug, Jonathan MD (DR) - **Spec Exp:** Musculoskeletal Imaging; **Hospital:** NYU Med Ctr (page 102); **Address:** NYU Medical Ctr, Dept Radiology, 540 First Ave Fl 2, New York, NY 10016; **Phone:** 212-263-5941; **Board Cert:** Diagnostic Radiology 1994; **Med School:** NYU Sch Med 1988; **Resid:** Diagnostic Radiology, NYU Medical Ctr 1994; **Fellow:** Skeletal Radiology, NYU Medical Ctr 1995; **Fac Appt:** Asst Prof Rad, NYU Sch Med

Knopp, Edmond A. MD (DR) - **Spec Exp:** MRI; Neuroradiology; Endocrine Radiology; CT Scan; **Hospital:** NYU Med Ctr (page 102); **Address:** NYU Med Ctr, Neuro MRI Dept, 530 First Ave, New York, NY 10016; **Phone:** 212-263-8723; **Board Cert:** Diagnostic Radiology 1992; Neuroradiology 1995; **Med School:** SUNY Downstate 1986; **Resid:** Surgery, Maimonides MC 1988; Radiology, St Lukes\Roosevelt Hosp 1991; **Fellow:** Neuroradiology, NYU Med Ctr 1994; **Fac Appt:** Assoc Prof Rad, NYU Sch Med

Lefkovitz, Zvi MD (DR) - **Spec Exp:** Chest Radiology; Bone Imaging; **Hospital:** Mount Sinai Med Ctr (page 98), Queens Hosp Ctr - Jamaica; **Address:** 1 Gustave L Levy Pl, Dept Rad, Box 1234, New York, NY 10029-6500; **Phone:** 212-241-8730; **Board Cert:** Diagnostic Radiology 1986; **Med School:** Univ Hlth Sci/Chicago Med Sch 1982; **Resid:** Diagnostic Radiology, Maimonides Med Ctr 1986; **Fellow:** Interventional Radiology, Univ Hosp 1987; **Fac Appt:** Assoc Prof Rad, Mount Sinai Sch Med

Levy, Miriam MD (DR) - **Spec Exp:** Breast Imaging; Mammography; Women's Imaging; **Address:** 635 Madison Ave Fl 16, New York, NY 10022; **Phone:** 212-794-2500; **Board Cert:** Diagnostic Radiology 1983; **Med School:** Albert Einstein Coll Med 1979; **Resid:** Diagnostic Radiology, Geo Wash Univ Hosp 1982; Diagnostic Radiology, St Vincent's Hosp & Med Ctr 1983; **Fellow:** Ultrasound/CT/MRI, New York Hosp 1984; **Fac Appt:** Asst Clin Prof Path, Mount Sinai Sch Med

Maklansky, Daniel MD (DR) - **Spec Exp:** Gastrointestinal Imaging; **Hospital:** Mount Sinai Med Ctr (page 98); **Address:** 165 E 84th St, New York, NY 10028; **Phone:** 212-289-5611; **Board Cert:** Radiology 1962; **Med School:** SUNY Downstate 1956; **Resid:** Radiology, Mt Sinai Hosp 1962; **Fac Appt:** Assoc Clin Prof Rad, Mount Sinai Sch Med

Megibow, Alec J MD (DR) - **Spec Exp:** Abdominal Imaging; Gastrointestinal Imaging; CT Scan-Body; **Hospital:** NYU Med Ctr (page 102); **Address:** 550 1st Ave, HHC 232, New York, NY 10016; **Phone:** 212-263-5222; **Board Cert:** Diagnostic Radiology 1978; **Med School:** SUNY Upstate Med Univ 1974; **Resid:** Diagnostic Radiology, Bellevue Hosp 1978; **Fellow:** NYU Med Ctr 1978; **Fac Appt:** Prof Rad, NYU Sch Med

Mitnick, Julie MD (DR) - **Spec Exp:** Mammography; Breast Cancer; **Hospital:** NYU Med Ctr (page 102); **Address:** 650 1st Ave Fl 2, New York, NY 10016; **Phone:** 212-686-4440; **Board Cert:** Diagnostic Radiology 1977; **Med School:** NYU Sch Med 1973; **Resid:** Diagnostic Radiology, NYU Med Ctr 1977; **Fellow:** Pediatric Radiology, NYU Med Ctr 1978; **Fac Appt:** Assoc Clin Prof Rad, NYU Sch Med

Mitty, Harold MD (DR) - **Spec Exp:** Kidney Imaging; Bladder Imaging; **Hospital:** Mount Sinai Med Ctr (page 98); **Address:** Mount Sinai Med Ctr, 1 Gustave Levy Pl, Box 1234, New York, NY 10029-6504; **Phone:** 212-241-7409; **Board Cert:** Radiology 1966; **Med School:** SUNY Downstate 1958; **Resid:** Radiology, Mount Sinai Med Ctr 1965; **Fac Appt:** Prof Rad, Mount Sinai Sch Med

Naidich, David P MD (DR) - **Spec Exp:** Chest Radiology; Chronic Lung Disease; **Hospital:** NYU Med Ctr (page 102), Bellevue Hosp Ctr; **Address:** NYU Medical Center, Dept Radiology, 560 1st Ave, rm 236, New York, NY 10016; **Phone:** 212-263-5229; **Board Cert:** Diagnostic Radiology 1980; **Med School:** NYU Sch Med 1975; **Resid:** Diagnostic Radiology, Johns Hopkins Hosp 1979; **Fellow:** Cross Sectional Imaging, Johns Hopkins Hosp 1980; **Fac Appt:** Prof Rad, NYU Sch Med

Newhouse, Jeffrey MD (DR) - **Spec Exp:** Abdominal Radiology; Pelvic Imaging; **Hospital:** NY-Presby Hosp (page 100); **Address:** 177 Fort Washington Ave, Millstein Bldg, 3rd Fl-Radiology, New York, NY 10032; **Phone:** 212-305-7898; **Board Cert:** Diagnostic Radiology 1972; **Med School:** Harvard Med Sch 1967; **Resid:** Radiology, Mass Genl Hosp 1972; **Fac Appt:** Prof Rad, Columbia P&S

Novick, Mark D MD (DR) - **Spec Exp:** Breast Imaging; Mammography; MRI; **Address:** Manhattan East Breast Imaging, 130 W 79th St, New York, NY 10024; **Phone:** 212-362-5300; **Board Cert:** Diagnostic Radiology 1983; **Med School:** Univ Tenn Coll Med, Memphis 1978; **Resid:** Radiology, Univ Tenn Med Ctr 1982; **Fellow:** Magnetic Resonance Imaging, UCSF Med Ctr

Ostrovsky, Paul MD (DR) - **Spec Exp:** Obstetric Ultrasound; Breast Imaging; **Hospital:** Mount Sinai Med Ctr (page 98); **Address:** 121A E 83rd St, New York, NY 10028; **Phone:** 212-879-6200 x108; **Board Cert:** Diagnostic Radiology 1982; **Med School:** NY Med Coll 1978; **Resid:** Radiology, Mount Sinai Hosp 1982

Panicek, David MD (DR) - **Spec Exp:** Bone Cancer; Soft Tissue Tumors; **Hospital:** Meml Sloan Kettering Cancer Ctr (page 109); **Address:** Memorial Hosp - Dept Radiology, 1275 York Ave, rm C276G, New York, NY 10021; **Phone:** 212-639-5825; **Board Cert:** Diagnostic Radiology 1984; **Med School:** Cornell Univ-Weill Med Coll 1980; **Resid:** Radiology, New York Hosp-Cornell 1984; **Fac Appt:** Prof Rad, Cornell Univ-Weill Med Coll

Pavlov, Helene MD (DR) - **Spec Exp:** Sports Medicine Radiology; **Hospital:** Hosp For Special Surgery (page 108); **Address:** Hosp for Special Surg, 535 E 70th St, New York, NY 10021-4892; **Phone:** 212-606-1132; **Board Cert:** Radiology 1976; **Med School:** Temple Univ 1976; **Resid:** Radiology, Germantown Hosp 1976; **Fellow:** Musculoskeletal Imaging, Hosp For Special Surg 1977; **Fac Appt:** Prof Rad, Cornell Univ-Weill Med Coll

Potter, Hollis J MD (DR) - **Spec Exp:** Musculoskeletal Imaging; Cartilage Damage; Arthroplasty Imaging; **Hospital:** Hosp For Special Surgery (page 108); **Address:** Hospital for Special Surgery, MRI-basement, 535 E 70th St, New York, NY 10021-4892; **Phone:** 212-606-1023; **Board Cert:** Diagnostic Radiology 1990; **Med School:** NY Med Coll 1985; **Resid:** Radiology, North Shore Univ Hosp 1990; **Fellow:** Radiology, Hosp Special Surgery 1991; **Fac Appt:** Prof Rad, Cornell Univ-Weill Med Coll

Rosenblatt, Ruth MD (DR) - **Spec Exp:** Breast Cancer; **Hospital:** NY-Presby Hosp (page 100); **Address:** 425 E 61st St Fl 9, New York, NY 10021; **Phone:** 212-821-0600; **Board Cert:** Radiology 1969; **Med School:** Med Coll PA Hahnemann 1964; **Resid:** Radiology, Montefiore Hosp Med Ctr 1968; **Fac Appt:** Clin Prof Rad, Cornell Univ-Weill Med Coll

Rosenfeld, Stanley MD (DR) - **Spec Exp:** Mammography; Ultrasound; **Hospital:** Mount Sinai Med Ctr (page 98); **Address:** 945 5th Ave, New York, NY 10021-2661; **Phone:** 212-744-5538; **Board Cert:** Diagnostic Radiology 1978; **Med School:** Albert Einstein Coll Med 1974; **Resid:** Radiology, Montefiore Hosp Med Ctr 1978

Som, Peter MD (DR) - **Spec Exp:** Head & Neck Imaging; **Hospital:** Mount Sinai Med Ctr (page 98); **Address:** Mount Sinai Med Ctr, Dept Radiology, 1 Gustave Levy Pl, New York, NY 10029-6504; **Phone:** 212-241-7420; **Board Cert:** Radiology 1972; **Med School:** NYU Sch Med 1967; **Resid:** Radiology, Mount Sinai Hosp 1971; **Fac Appt:** Prof Rad, Mount Sinai Sch Med

Sonnenblick, Emily MD (DR) - **Spec Exp:** Women's Imaging; **Hospital:** Mount Sinai Med Ctr (page 98); **Address:** 945 Fifth Ave, New York, NY 10021-2655; **Phone:** 212-744-5538; **Board Cert:** Diagnostic Radiology 1987; **Med School:** Cornell Univ-Weill Med Coll 1982; **Resid:** Radiology, Hosp Univ Penn 1984; Radiology, Columbia-Presby Hosp 1986; **Fellow:** Ultrasound, Mt Sinai Hosp 1987

Winchester, Patricia MD (DR) - **Spec Exp:** Pediatric Radiology; **Hospital:** NY-Presby Hosp (page 100); **Address:** Cornell Univ Med Ctr, Dept Radiology, 525 E 68th St, New York, NY 10021-4873; **Phone:** 212-746-2555; **Board Cert:** Pediatrics 1969; Diagnostic Radiology 1967; Pediatric Radiology 1995; **Med School:** Duke Univ 1959; **Resid:** Pediatrics, New York Hosp 1962; Radiology, New York Hosp 1968; **Fac Appt:** Prof Rad, Cornell Univ-Weill Med Coll

Wolff, Steven D MD/PhD (DR) - **Spec Exp:** Cardiovascular Imaging; **Hospital:** Lenox Hill Hosp (page 94); **Address:** 62 E 88th St, New York, NY 10128; **Phone:** 212-369-9200; **Board Cert:** Diagnostic Radiology 1994; **Med School:** Duke Univ 1989; **Resid:** Radiology, Johns Hopkins Hosp 1994

ENDOCRINOLOGY, DIABETES & METABOLISM

Barandes, Martin MD (EDM) - **Spec Exp:** Thyroid Disorders; Nuclear Medicine; Nuclear Cardiology; **Hospital:** St Vincent Cath Med Ctrs - Manhattan (page 375), Manhattan Eye, Ear & Throat Hosp; **Address:** 155 E 76th St, New York, NY 10021-2810; **Phone:** 212-249-0622; **Board Cert:** Internal Medicine 1975; Endocrinology 1975; Nuclear Medicine 1972; **Med School:** Albany Med Coll 1963; **Resid:** Internal Medicine, Roosevelt Hosp 1966; Internal Medicine, Meml Sloan Kettering Cancer Ctr 1967; **Fellow:** Endocrinology, New York Hosp 1971

Becker, Carolyn MD (EDM) - **Spec Exp:** Osteoporosis; Parathyroid Disorders; Bone Disorders-Metabolic; **Hospital:** NY-Presby Hosp (page 100); **Address:** 180 Ft Washington Ave, Harkness Pavilion - FL 9, Rm 904, New York, NY 10032-3710; **Phone:** 212-305-0066; **Board Cert:** Internal Medicine 1985; Endocrinology, Diabetes & Metabolism 1989; **Med School:** Harvard Med Sch 1982; **Resid:** Internal Medicine, Michael Reese Hosp 1985; **Fellow:** Endocrinology, Diabetes & Metabolism, Mass Genl Hosp 1988; **Fac Appt:** Assoc Clin Prof Med, Columbia P&S

Bergman, Donald MD (EDM) - **Spec Exp:** Osteoporosis; Thyroid Disorders; Calcium Disorders; **Hospital:** Mount Sinai Med Ctr (page 98); **Address:** 1199 Park Ave, Ste 1F, New York, NY 10128; **Phone:** 212-876-7333; **Board Cert:** Internal Medicine 1975; Endocrinology, Diabetes & Metabolism 1977; **Med School:** Jefferson Med Coll 1971; **Resid:** Obstetrics & Gynecology, Mount Sinai Hosp 1972; Internal Medicine, Mount Sinai Hosp 1975; **Fellow:** Endocrinology, Diabetes & Metabolism, Mount Sinai Hosp 1977; **Fac Appt:** Clin Prof Med, Mount Sinai Sch Med

Bilezikian, John P MD (EDM) - **Spec Exp:** Osteoporosis; Bone Disorders-Metabolic; Parathyroid Disease; **Hospital:** NY-Presby Hosp (page 100); **Address:** New York Presby Hosp - Metabolic Bone Diseases Prog, 180 Fort Washington Ave, Harkness Pav Fl 9 - Ste 920, New York, NY 10032; **Phone:** 212-305-2663; **Board Cert:** Internal Medicine 1975; Endocrinology, Diabetes & Metabolism 1977; **Med School:** Columbia P&S 1969; **Resid:** Internal Medicine, Columbia-Presby Hosp 1975; **Fellow:** Endocrinology, Diabetes & Metabolism, Natl Inst Health 1977; **Fac Appt:** Prof Med, Columbia P&S

Bloomgarden, Zachary MD (EDM) - **Spec Exp:** Diabetes; Diabetic Kidney Disease; Cholesterol/Lipid Disorders; **Hospital:** Mount Sinai Med Ctr (page 98); **Address:** 35 E 85th St, New York, NY 10028-0954; **Phone:** 212-879-5933; **Board Cert:** Internal Medicine 1977; Endocrinology, Diabetes & Metabolism 1979; **Med School:** Albert Einstein Coll Med 1974; **Resid:** Internal Medicine, Montefiore Hosp Med Ctr 1977; **Fellow:** Endocrinology, Diabetes & Metabolism, Vanderbilt Univ Med Ctr 1979; **Fac Appt:** Assoc Clin Prof Med, Mount Sinai Sch Med

Blum, Conrad MD (EDM) - **Spec Exp:** Cholesterol/Lipid Disorders; Thyroid Disorders; Diabetes; **Hospital:** NY-Presby Hosp (page 100); **Address:** 16 E 60th St, Ste 320, New York, NY 10022-1002; **Phone:** 212-326-8421; **Board Cert:** Internal Medicine 1976; Endocrinology, Diabetes & Metabolism 1977; **Med School:** Northwestern Univ 1971; **Resid:** Internal Medicine, Brigham Hosp 1976; **Fellow:** Endocrinology, Diabetes & Metabolism, Northwestern Univ Med Sch 1977; **Fac Appt:** Clin Prof Med, Columbia P&S

Blum, Manfred MD (EDM) - **Spec Exp:** Thyroid Disorders; Parathyroid Disorders; **Hospital:** NYU Med Ctr (page 102); **Address:** 530 1st Ave, Ste 4E, New York, NY 10016; **Phone:** 212-263-7444; **Board Cert:** Internal Medicine 1974; Endocrinology 1975; **Med School:** NYU Sch Med 1957; **Resid:** Internal Medicine, Montefiore Hosp 1959; Internal Medicine, Bellevue Hosp 1960; **Fellow:** Endocrinology, Harvard-Beth Israel Hosp 1961; **Fac Appt:** Clin Prof Med, NYU Sch Med

Bockman, Richard MD/PhD (EDM) - **Spec Exp:** Bone Disorders-Metabolic; Osteoporosis; Thyroid Disorders; **Hospital:** Hosp For Special Surgery (page 108), NY-Presby Hosp (page 100); **Address:** 519 E 72nd St, New York, NY 10021-4028; **Phone:** 212-606-1458; **Board Cert:** Internal Medicine 1975; **Med School:** Yale Univ 1968; **Resid:** Internal Medicine, NYU Med Ctr 1975; **Fellow:** Internal Medicine, Weill Med Coll-Cornell 1973; **Fac Appt:** Prof Med, Cornell Univ-Weill Med Coll

Bukberg, Phillip MD (EDM) - **Spec Exp:** Diabetes; Cholesterol/Lipid Disorders; **Hospital:** St Vincent Cath Med Ctrs - Manhattan (page 375); **Address:** 36 7th Ave, Ste 517, New York, NY 10011-6688; **Phone:** 212-807-8129; **Board Cert:** Internal Medicine 1977; Endocrinology, Diabetes & Metabolism 1979; **Med School:** SUNY Downstate 1973; **Resid:** Internal Medicine, St Vincent's Hosp & Med Ctr 1977; **Fellow:** Endocrinology, Meml Sloan Kettering Cancer Ctr 1979; Endocrinology, Mount Sinai Hosp 1982

Burroughs, Valentine MD (EDM) - **Spec Exp:** Diabetes; Thyroid Disorders; Hypertension; **Hospital:** N Genl Hosp, Mount Sinai Med Ctr (page 98); **Address:** 1789 Madison Ave, New York, NY 10035; **Phone:** 212-360-5090; **Board Cert:** Internal Medicine 1978; Endocrinology 1981; **Med School:** Univ Mich Med Sch 1975; **Resid:** Internal Medicine, Columbia-Presby Med Ctr 1979; **Fellow:** Endocrinology, NYU Med Ctr 1981; **Fac Appt:** Asst Clin Prof Med, Columbia P&S

Davies, Terry MD (EDM) - **Spec Exp:** Thyroid Disorders; Graves' Disease; Hashimoto's Disease; **Hospital:** Mount Sinai Med Ctr (page 98); **Address:** 1 Gustave Levy Pl, Box 1055, New York, NY 10029-6500; **Phone:** 212-241-7975; **Med School:** England 1971; **Resid:** Internal Medicine, Univ Newcastle 1975; **Fellow:** Endocrinology, Diabetes & Metabolism, Univ Newcastle 1977; Endocrinology, Diabetes & Metabolism, Natl Inst Hlth 1979; **Fac Appt:** Prof Med, Mount Sinai Sch Med

Felig, Philip MD (EDM) - **Spec Exp:** Diabetes; Thyroid Disorders; Osteoporosis; **Hospital:** Lenox Hill Hosp (page 94), Beth Israel Med Ctr - Petrie Division (page 90); **Address:** 1056 5th Ave, New York, NY 10028-0112; **Phone:** 212-534-5900; **Board Cert:** Internal Medicine 1968; **Med School:** Yale Univ 1961; **Resid:** Internal Medicine, Yale-New Haven Hosp 1967; **Fellow:** Endocrinology, Diabetes & Metabolism, Peter Bent Brigham Hosp-Harvard 1969

Goland, Robin MD (EDM) - **Spec Exp:** Diabetes; **Hospital:** NY-Presby Hosp (page 100); **Address:** 1150 St Nicholas Ave Fl 2, New York, NY 10032; **Phone:** 212-851-5494; **Board Cert:** Internal Medicine 1983; Endocrinology 1989; **Med School:** Columbia P&S 1980; **Resid:** Internal Medicine, Columbia-Presby Med Ctr 1984; **Fellow:** Endocrinology, Diabetes & Metabolism, Columbia-Presby Med Ctr 1987; **Fac Appt:** Assoc Prof Med, Columbia P&S

Greene, Loren Wissner MD (EDM) - **Spec Exp:** Diabetes; Thyroid Disorders; Osteoporosis; **Hospital:** NYU Med Ctr (page 102), NY Downtown Hosp; **Address:** 530 1st Ave, Ste 4B, New York, NY 10016-6402; **Phone:** 212-263-7449; **Board Cert:** Internal Medicine 1978; Endocrinology, Diabetes & Metabolism 1981; **Med School:** NYU Sch Med 1975; **Resid:** Internal Medicine, Bellevue Hosp Ctr-NYU 1978; **Fellow:** Endocrinology, Diabetes & Metabolism, Bellevue Hosp Ctr-NYU 1980; **Fac Appt:** Assoc Clin Prof Med, NYU Sch Med

Hembree, Wylie MD (EDM) - **Spec Exp:** Reproductive Endocrinology-Male; Andrology; **Hospital:** NY-Presby Hosp (page 100); **Address:** 101 Central Park West, Ste 1-B, New York, NY 10023; **Phone:** 212-721-3622; **Board Cert:** Internal Medicine 1972; Endocrinology 1973; **Med School:** Washington Univ, St Louis 1964; **Resid:** Internal Medicine, Boston City Hosp 1966; Internal Medicine, Columbia-Presby Hosp 1971; **Fellow:** Endocrinology, NIH Endo Br/Natl Cancer Inst 1968; **Fac Appt:** Assoc Clin Prof Med, Columbia P&S

Imperato-McGinley, Julianne MD (EDM) - **Spec Exp:** Sexual Differentiation Disorders; **Hospital:** NY-Presby Hosp (page 100); **Address:** 525 E 68th St, rm F-2006, Box 149, New York, NY 10021; **Phone:** 212-746-6276; **Med School:** SUNY Downstate 1965; **Resid:** Internal Medicine, Lenox Hill Hosp 1969; **Fellow:** Endocrinology, Diabetes & Metabolism, NY Weill Cornell Med Ctr 1970

Jacobs, David R MD (EDM) - **Spec Exp:** Thyroid Disorders; Osteoporosis; **Hospital:** Lenox Hill Hosp (page 94), Mount Sinai Med Ctr (page 98); **Address:** 240 E 82nd St, New York, NY 10028; **Phone:** 212-628-0300; **Board Cert:** Internal Medicine 1963; Endocrinology, Diabetes & Metabolism 1972; **Med School:** Case West Res Univ 1956; **Resid:** Internal Medicine, Mount Sinai Hosp 1959; **Fellow:** Endocrinology, Mount Sinai Hosp 1960; **Fac Appt:** Clin Prof Med, NYU Sch Med

Jacobs, Thomas MD (EDM) - **Spec Exp:** Adrenal Disorders; Pituitary Disorders; Calcium Disorders; **Hospital:** NY-Presby Hosp (page 100); **Address:** 161 Fort Washington Ave, rm 210, New York, NY 10032-3713; **Phone:** 212-305-5578; **Board Cert:** Internal Medicine 1973; Endocrinology, Diabetes & Metabolism 1975; **Med School:** Johns Hopkins Univ 1968; **Resid:** Internal Medicine, Columbia Presby Hosp 1973; **Fellow:** Endocrinology, Diabetes & Metabolism, Univ Wash Med Ctr 1975; **Fac Appt:** Clin Prof Med, Columbia P&S

Kleinberg, David MD (EDM) - **Spec Exp:** Neuroendocrinology; Pituitary Disorders; **Hospital:** NYU Med Ctr (page 102); **Address:** 530 1st Ave, Ste 4C, New York, NY 10016; **Phone:** 212-263-6772; **Board Cert:** Internal Medicine 1972; Endocrinology 1975; **Med School:** Univ Miami Sch Med 1966; **Resid:** Internal Medicine, Maimonides Med Ctr 1968; Internal Medicine, Columbia-Presby Med Ctr 1971; **Fellow:** Endocrinology, Diabetes & Metabolism, Columbia-Presby Med Ctr 1970; **Fac Appt:** Prof Med, NYU Sch Med

Klyde, Barry J MD (EDM) - **Spec Exp:** Thyroid Disorders; Sexual Dysfunction; **Hospital:** NY-Presby Hosp (page 100), NY Hosp Queens; **Address:** 520 E 72nd St, Ste LO, New York, NY 10021-4881; **Phone:** 212-772-3333; **Board Cert:** Internal Medicine 1977; Endocrinology, Diabetes & Metabolism 1981; **Med School:** Stanford Univ 1974; **Resid:** Internal Medicine, New York Hosp 1977; **Fellow:** Endocrinology, Diabetes & Metabolism, New York Hosp 1979; **Fac Appt:** Asst Prof Med, Cornell Univ-Weill Med Coll

Mahler, Richard J MD (EDM) - **Spec Exp:** Thyroid Disorders; Diabetes; **Hospital:** NY-Presby Hosp (page 100); **Address:** 220 E 69th St, New York, NY 10021-5737; **Phone:** 212-879-4073; **Board Cert:** Internal Medicine 1987; **Med School:** NY Med Coll 1959; **Resid:** Internal Medicine, NY Med-Metro Med 1962; Endocrinology, Diabetes & Metabolism, NY Med Coll 1963; **Fellow:** Endocrinology, Diabetes & Metabolism, Univ Durham/Univ New Castle 1964; **Fac Appt:** Assoc Clin Prof Med, Cornell Univ-Weill Med Coll

McConnell, Robert John MD (EDM) - **Spec Exp:** Thyroid Disorders; Thyroid Ultrasound; **Hospital:** NY-Presby Hosp (page 100); **Address:** 161 Fort Washington Ave, Ste 210, New York, NY 10032-3713; **Phone:** 212-305-5579; **Board Cert:** Internal Medicine 1978; Endocrinology, Diabetes & Metabolism 1981; **Med School:** Columbia P&S 1973; **Resid:** Internal Medicine, Barnes Hosp 1975; **Fellow:** Endocrinology, Diabetes & Metabolism, Columbia-Presby Hosp 1978; **Fac Appt:** Prof Med, Columbia P&S

Mechanick, Jeffrey I MD (EDM) - **Spec Exp:** Nutrition; Thyroid Disorders; Thyroid Cancer; **Hospital:** Mount Sinai Med Ctr (page 98); **Address:** 1192 Park Ave, New York, NY 10128; **Phone:** 212-831-2100; **Board Cert:** Internal Medicine 1988; Endocrinology, Diabetes & Metabolism 1993; **Med School:** Mount Sinai Sch Med 1985; **Resid:** Internal Medicine, Baylor Coll Med 1988; **Fellow:** Endocrinology, Diabetes & Metabolism, Mount Sinai Hosp 1990; **Fac Appt:** Assoc Clin Prof Med, Mount Sinai Sch Med

Nydick, Martin MD (EDM) - **Spec Exp:** Metabolic Bone Disease; Osteoporosis; **Hospital:** NY-Presby Hosp (page 100), Hosp For Special Surgery (page 108); **Address:** 475 E 72nd St, Ste L2, New York, NY 10021-4458; **Phone:** 212-249-1260; **Board Cert:** Internal Medicine 1974; Endocrinology 1977; **Med School:** Columbia P&S 1957; **Resid:** Internal Medicine, Bellevue Hosp 1960; **Fellow:** Endocrinology, NCI-Natl Inst Hlth 1962; Endocrinology, Diabetes & Metabolism, Univ Wash Med Ctr 1964; **Fac Appt:** Assoc Clin Prof Med, Cornell Univ-Weill Med Coll

Park, Constance MD/PhD (EDM) - **Spec Exp:** Thyroid Disorders; Osteoporosis; Menopause Problems; **Hospital:** NY-Presby Hosp (page 100); **Address:** 903 Park Ave, New York, NY 10021; **Phone:** 212-639-9850; **Board Cert:** Internal Medicine 1980; Endocrinology, Diabetes & Metabolism 1997; **Med School:** Albert Einstein Coll Med 1974; **Resid:** Internal Medicine, Bellevue Hosp 1976; **Fellow:** Endocrinology, Diabetes & Metabolism, Albert Einstein 1978; **Fac Appt:** Assoc Clin Prof Med, Columbia P&S

Poretsky, Leonid MD (EDM) - **Spec Exp:** Diabetes; Thyroid Disorders; **Hospital:** Beth Israel Med Ctr - Petrie Division (page 90); **Address:** 317 E 17th St Fl 7, New York, NY 10003; **Phone:** 212-420-2226; **Board Cert:** Internal Medicine 1983; Endocrinology, Diabetes & Metabolism 1995; **Med School:** Russia 1977; **Resid:** Internal Medicine, Coney Island Hosp 1983; **Fellow:** Endocrinology, Beth Israel Hosp 1985

Seplowitz, Alan MD (EDM) - **Spec Exp:** Thyroid Disorders; Cholesterol/Lipid Disorders; **Hospital:** NY-Presby Hosp (page 100); **Address:** 161 Fort Washington Ave, New York, NY 10032-3713; **Phone:** 212-305-5503; **Board Cert:** Internal Medicine 1975; Endocrinology 1977; **Med School:** Columbia P&S 1972; **Resid:** Internal Medicine, Columbia-Presby Med Ctr 1974; **Fellow:** Endocrinology, Diabetes & Metabolism, Columbia-Presby Med Ctr 1978; **Fac Appt:** Assoc Clin Prof Med, Columbia P&S

Shane, Elizabeth MD (EDM) - **Spec Exp:** Bone Disorders-Metabolic; Osteoporosis; Parathyroid Disorders; **Hospital:** NY-Presby Hosp (page 100); **Address:** 180 Ft Washington Ave, New York, NY 10032; **Phone:** 212-305-2663; **Board Cert:** Internal Medicine 1978; Endocrinology 1981; **Med School:** Univ Toronto 1975; **Resid:** Internal Medicine, Toronto Genl Hosp 1976; Internal Medicine, Columbia-Presby Hosp 1978; **Fellow:** Endocrinology, Columbia-Presby Hosp 1981; **Fac Appt:** Clin Prof Med, Columbia P&S

Sheehan, Peter MD (EDM) - **Spec Exp:** Diabetic Leg/Foot; Diabetes; **Hospital:** Cabrini Med Ctr (page 374); **Address:** Cabrini Medical Ctr, Diabetic Ctr, Bldg D, 227 E 19th St Fl 5, New York, NY 10003; **Phone:** 212-995-7120; **Board Cert:** Internal Medicine 1984; Endocrinology, Diabetes & Metabolism 1987; **Med School:** SUNY Downstate 1981; **Resid:** Internal Medicine, Staten Island Hosp 1984; **Fellow:** Endocrinology, Yale-New Haven Hosp 1986; **Fac Appt:** Assoc Clin Prof Med, NYU Sch Med

Silverberg, Shonni J MD (EDM) - **Spec Exp:** Osteoporosis; Parathyroid Disorders; Calcium Disorders; **Hospital:** NY-Presby Hosp (page 100); **Address:** 180 Fort Washington Ave, rm 920, New York, NY 10032-3702; **Phone:** 212-305-2663; **Board Cert:** Internal Medicine 1983; Endocrinology, Diabetes & Metabolism 1985; **Med School:** Cornell Univ-Weill Med Coll 1980; **Resid:** Internal Medicine, New York Hosp 1983; **Fellow:** Endocrinology, Diabetes & Metabolism, Columbia-Presby Med Ctr 1986; **Fac Appt:** Prof Med, Columbia P&S

New York (Manhattan)

Siris, Ethel MD (EDM) - **Spec Exp:** Osteoporosis; Paget's Disease of Bone; Bone Disorders-Metabolic; **Hospital:** NY-Presby Hosp (page 100); **Address:** 180 Ft Washington Ave, Harkness Bldg - rm 9-964, New York, NY 10032-3710; **Phone:** 212-305-9531; **Board Cert:** Internal Medicine 1974; Endocrinology, Diabetes & Metabolism 1977; **Med School:** Columbia P&S 1971; **Resid:** Internal Medicine, Columbia-Presby Med Ctr 1974; **Fellow:** Endocrinology, Diabetes & Metabolism, Natl Inst Hlth 1976; Endocrinology, Diabetes & Metabolism, Columbia-Presby Med Ctr 1977; **Fac Appt:** Prof Med, Columbia P&S

Szabo, Andrew John MD (EDM) - **Spec Exp:** Diabetes; Thyroid Disorders; **Hospital:** Lenox Hill Hosp (page 94), NY-Presby Hosp (page 100); **Address:** 860 Fifth Ave, New York, NY 10022-1304; **Phone:** 212-583-2816; **Board Cert:** Internal Medicine 1987; Endocrinology, Diabetes & Metabolism 1989; **Med School:** McGill Univ 1959; **Resid:** Internal Medicine, Montreal General Hosp 1962; Internal Medicine, Queen Mary Veteran's Hosp 1962; **Fellow:** Endocrinology, Diabetes & Metabolism, Montreal General Hosp 1964; Endocrinology, Diabetes & Metabolism, New England Med Ctr-Deaconess Hosp 1965; **Fac Appt:** Assoc Clin Prof Med, Cornell Univ-Weill Med Coll

Wardlaw, Sharon MD (EDM) - **Spec Exp:** Pituitary Disorders; Neuroendocrinology; **Hospital:** NY-Presby Hosp (page 100); **Address:** 650 W 168th St, Ste BB 9-904, New York, NY 10032-3702; **Phone:** 212-305-2254; **Board Cert:** Internal Medicine 1978; Endocrinology, Diabetes & Metabolism 1979; **Med School:** Cornell Univ-Weill Med Coll 1975; **Resid:** Internal Medicine, Case Western Univ Hosp 1977; **Fellow:** Endocrinology, Diabetes & Metabolism, Columbia-Presby 1980; **Fac Appt:** Prof Med, Columbia P&S

Young, Iven MD (EDM) - **Spec Exp:** Thyroid Disorders; Osteoporosis; Pituitary Disorders; **Hospital:** St Vincent Cath Med Ctrs - Manhattan (page 375), NYU Med Ctr (page 102); **Address:** 130 W 12th St, Ste 7D, New York, NY 10011-8250; **Phone:** 212-675-9332; **Board Cert:** Internal Medicine 1966; Endocrinology, Diabetes & Metabolism 1973; **Med School:** NYU Sch Med 1959; **Resid:** Internal Medicine, VA Med Ctr 1963; **Fellow:** Endocrinology, NYU Med Ctr 1966; **Fac Appt:** Assoc Clin Prof Med, NY Med Coll

FAMILY MEDICINE

Calman, Neil MD (FMed) **PCP** - **Hospital:** Beth Israel Med Ctr - Petrie Division (page 90), Bronx Lebanon Hosp Ctr; **Address:** 16 E 16th St Fl 4, New York, NY 10003-3105; **Phone:** 212-924-7744; **Board Cert:** Family Medicine 2003; **Med School:** Rush Med Coll 1975; **Resid:** Family Medicine, Montefiore Hosp Med Ctr 1978; **Fac Appt:** Prof FMed, Albert Einstein Coll Med

Clements, Jerry MD (FMed) **PCP** - **Spec Exp:** Pediatrics; Travel Medicine; **Hospital:** Beth Israel Med Ctr - Petrie Division (page 90), St Vincent Cath Med Ctrs - Manhattan (page 375); **Address:** 25 5th Ave, Ste 1A, New York, NY 10003-4308; **Phone:** 212-477-1750; **Board Cert:** Family Medicine 1999; **Med School:** West Indies 1983; **Resid:** Family Medicine, St Joseph's Hosp 1986

Leeds, Gary MD (FMed) **PCP** - **Spec Exp:** Asthma & Allergy; Hypertension; Cholesterol/Lipid Disorders; **Hospital:** Beth Israel Med Ctr - Petrie Division (page 90), Cabrini Med Ctr (page 374); **Address:** 22 W 15th St, New York, NY 10011-6842; **Phone:** 212-206-7717; **Board Cert:** Family Medicine 2002; **Med School:** Brown Univ 1978; **Resid:** Family Medicine, Georgetown Univ Hosp 1981

Levy, Albert MD (FMed) **PCP** - **Spec Exp:** Hypertension; Diabetes; Sexual Dysfunction; **Hospital:** Mount Sinai Med Ctr (page 98), Lenox Hill Hosp (page 94); **Address:** 911 Park Ave, New York, NY 10021-0337; **Phone:** 212-288-7193; **Board Cert:** Family Medicine 2000; Geriatric Medicine 1996; **Med School:** Brazil 1973; **Resid:** Family Medicine, Kings County Hosp 1980; **Fac Appt:** Asst Clin Prof Med, Mount Sinai Sch Med

Lyon, Valerie MD (FMed) `PCP` - **Spec Exp:** Preventive Medicine; **Hospital:** Lenox Hill Hosp (page 94); **Address:** 59 E 54th St Fl 2, New York, NY 10022; **Phone:** 212-750-8330; **Board Cert:** Family Medicine 1999; **Med School:** Temple Univ 1986; **Resid:** Family Medicine, South Nassau Comm Hosp 1989

Schiller, Robert MD (FMed) `PCP` - **Spec Exp:** Complementary Medicine; Pediatrics; **Hospital:** Beth Israel Med Ctr - Petrie Division (page 90), Long Island Coll Hosp (page 90); **Address:** 16 E 16th St, New York, NY 10003-3105; **Phone:** 212-924-7744 x277; **Board Cert:** Family Medicine 1999; **Med School:** NYU Sch Med 1982; **Resid:** Family Medicine, Montefiore Med Ctr 1985; **Fac Appt:** Asst Prof FMed, Albert Einstein Coll Med

Tamarin, Steven MD (FMed) `PCP` - **Spec Exp:** Diagnostic Problems; Preventive Medicine; **Hospital:** St Luke's - Roosevelt Hosp Ctr - Roosevelt Div (page 90); **Address:** 441 West End Ave, Ste 1J, New York, NY 10024; **Phone:** 212-496-2291; **Board Cert:** Family Medicine 2002; **Med School:** Mexico 1975; **Resid:** Family Medicine, SUNY Downstate Med Ctr 1980

GASTROENTEROLOGY

Abreu, Maria T MD (Ge) - **Spec Exp:** Inflammatory Bowel Disease/Crohn's; Ulcerative Colitis; **Hospital:** Mount Sinai Med Ctr (page 98); **Address:** 5 East 98th Street, Box 1625, New York, NY 10029; **Phone:** 212-241-4299; **Board Cert:** Gastroenterology 2005; **Med School:** Univ Miami Sch Med 1990; **Resid:** Internal Medicine, Brigham & Women's Hosp 1992; **Fellow:** Gastroenterology, UCLA Med Ctr 1995; **Fac Appt:** Assoc Prof Med, Mount Sinai Sch Med

Ackert, John MD (Ge) - **Spec Exp:** Colonoscopy; **Hospital:** NYU Med Ctr (page 102); **Address:** 232 E 30th St, New York, NY 10016; **Phone:** 212-889-5544; **Board Cert:** Internal Medicine 1975; Gastroenterology 1977; **Med School:** NYU Sch Med 1972; **Resid:** Internal Medicine, NYU Med Ctr 1975; **Fellow:** Gastroenterology, NYU Med Ctr 1977; **Fac Appt:** Asst Prof Med, NYU Sch Med

Adler, Howard MD (Ge) - **Spec Exp:** Colon Cancer; Colonoscopy; Endoscopy; **Hospital:** Lenox Hill Hosp (page 94); **Address:** 35 Sutton Pl, New York, NY 10022-2464; **Phone:** 212-421-3696; **Board Cert:** Internal Medicine 1967; Gastroenterology 1977; **Med School:** Albert Einstein Coll Med 1960; **Resid:** Internal Medicine, Herbert C Moffitt Hosp 1962; Internal Medicine, Bronx Municipal Hosp 1965; **Fellow:** Gastroenterology, Cornell U-Bellevue Hosp 1967; **Fac Appt:** Assoc Clin Prof Med, Albert Einstein Coll Med

Agus, Saul G MD (Ge) - **Spec Exp:** Endoscopy; **Hospital:** Mount Sinai Med Ctr (page 98); **Address:** 1080 5th Ave, New York, NY 10128; **Phone:** 212-860-0841; **Board Cert:** Internal Medicine 1973; Gastroenterology 1975; **Med School:** NYU Sch Med 1968; **Resid:** Internal Medicine, Mass Genl Hosp 1970; **Fellow:** Gastroenterology, Mt Sinai Med Ctr 1974; **Fac Appt:** Asst Clin Prof Med, Mount Sinai Sch Med

Aisenberg, James MD (Ge) - **Spec Exp:** Colon Cancer Screening; Inflammatory Bowel Disease; Gastroesophageal Reflux Disease (GERD); **Hospital:** Mount Sinai Med Ctr (page 98); **Address:** 311 E 79th St, Ste 2-A, New York, NY 10021; **Phone:** 212-996-6633; **Board Cert:** Internal Medicine 2000; Gastroenterology 2000; **Med School:** Harvard Med Sch 1987; **Resid:** Internal Medicine, Columbia-Presby Med Ctr 1990; **Fellow:** Gastroenterology, Mount Sinai Hosp 1993; **Fac Appt:** Asst Clin Prof Med, Mount Sinai Sch Med

Attia, Albert MD (Ge) - **Spec Exp:** Inflammatory Bowel Disease/Crohn's; Irritable Bowel Syndrome; Gastroesophageal Reflux Disease (GERD); **Hospital:** St Luke's - Roosevelt Hosp Ctr - Roosevelt Div (page 90); **Address:** 350 W 58th St, New York, NY 10019-1804; **Phone:** 212-307-7210; **Board Cert:** Internal Medicine 1970; Gastroenterology 1972; **Med School:** Cornell Univ-Weill Med Coll 1958; **Resid:** Internal Medicine, St Luke's-Roosevelt Hosp Ctr 1961; **Fellow:** Gastroenterology, Seton Hall Univ Hosp 1963; **Fac Appt:** Clin Prof Med, Columbia P&S

Basuk, Paul M MD (Ge) - **Spec Exp:** Gallbladder Disease; Pancreatic Disease; Esophageal Disorders; **Hospital:** NY-Presby Hosp (page 100); **Address:** 310 E 72nd St, New York, NY 10021-4726; **Phone:** 212-861-9715; **Board Cert:** Internal Medicine 1983; Gastroenterology 1987; **Med School:** Northwestern Univ 1980; **Resid:** Internal Medicine, UCSF Med Ctr 1983; **Fellow:** Gastroenterology, UCSF Med Ctr 1987; **Fac Appt:** Asst Prof Med, Cornell Univ-Weill Med Coll

Bednarek, Karl MD (Ge) - **Spec Exp:** Liver Disease; **Hospital:** Beth Israel Med Ctr - Petrie Division (page 90), Hosp For Joint Diseases (page 107); **Address:** 10 Union Square E, Ste 2G, New York, NY 10003; **Phone:** 212-844-6335; **Board Cert:** Internal Medicine 1985; Gastroenterology 1993; **Med School:** Mount Sinai Sch Med 1982; **Resid:** Internal Medicine, Beth Israel Med Ctr 1986; **Fellow:** Gastroenterology, Beth Israel Med Ctr 1988

Ben-Zvi, Jeffrey MD (Ge) - **Spec Exp:** Inflammatory Bowel Disease/Crohn's; Gastroesophageal Reflux Disease (GERD); Pancreatic/Biliary Endoscopy (ERCP); **Hospital:** Lenox Hill Hosp (page 94), NY-Presby Hosp (page 100); **Address:** 911 Park Avenue, New York, NY 10021-0337; **Phone:** 212-772-8730; **Board Cert:** Internal Medicine 2004; Gastroenterology 2004; Geriatric Medicine 2004; **Med School:** Columbia P&S 1983; **Resid:** Internal Medicine, St Luke's-Roosevelt Hosp Ctr 1986; **Fellow:** Gastroenterology, St Luke's-Roosevelt Hosp Ctr 1988; **Fac Appt:** Asst Clin Prof Med, Columbia P&S

Berenson, Murray J MD (Ge) - **Hospital:** St Vincent Cath Med Ctrs - Manhattan (page 375); **Address:** 115 E 61st St Fl 14, New York, NY 10021-8101; **Phone:** 212-421-8340; **Board Cert:** Internal Medicine 1969; Gastroenterology 1979; **Med School:** NYU Sch Med 1961; **Resid:** Internal Medicine, St Vincents Hosp 1963; **Fellow:** Gastroenterology, Hosp Univ Penn 1963

Bernstein, Brett B MD (Ge) - **Spec Exp:** Gastroesophageal Reflux Disease (GERD); Capsule Endoscopy; **Hospital:** Beth Israel Med Ctr - Petrie Division (page 90); **Address:** 10 Union Square East, Ste 2G, New York, NY 10003; **Phone:** 212-844-6330; **Board Cert:** Internal Medicine 2001; Gastroenterology 1995; **Med School:** Mount Sinai Sch Med 1988; **Resid:** Internal Medicine, Beth Israel Med Ctr 1991; **Fellow:** Gastroenterology, Beth Israel Med Ctr 1994; **Fac Appt:** Asst Prof Med, Albert Einstein Coll Med

Bodenheimer, Jr, Henry C MD (Ge) - **Spec Exp:** Hepatitis; Transplant Medicine-Liver; Liver & Biliary Disease; **Hospital:** Beth Israel Med Ctr - Petrie Division (page 90); **Address:** Beth Israel Med Ctr, Div Digestive Diseases, 1st Ave @ 16th St, New York, NY 10003; **Phone:** 212-420-4015; **Board Cert:** Internal Medicine 1978; Gastroenterology 1981; **Med School:** Tufts Univ 1975; **Resid:** Internal Medicine, Mount Sinai Hosp 1978; **Fellow:** Gastroenterology, Mount Sinai Hosp 1979; Gastroenterology, Rhode Island Hosp 1981; **Fac Appt:** Prof Med, Albert Einstein Coll Med

Brenner, David A MD (Ge) - **Spec Exp:** Porphyria; Hepatitis; **Hospital:** NY-Presby Hosp (page 100); **Address:** Columbia Univ, Dept Med, 622 W 168th St, PH8 East Rm 105, New York, NY 10032; **Phone:** 212-305-5838; **Board Cert:** Internal Medicine 1982; Gastroenterology 1987; **Med School:** Yale Univ 1979; **Resid:** Internal Medicine, Yale-New Haven Med Ctr 1982; **Fellow:** Research, Natl Inst Hlth 1985; Gastroenterology, UCSD Med Ctr 1986; **Fac Appt:** Prof Med, Columbia P&S

Cantor, Michael C MD (Ge) - **Spec Exp:** Colon Cancer; Hepatitis; Liver Disease; **Hospital:** NY-Presby Hosp (page 100); **Address:** 310 E 72nd St, New York, NY 10021-4703; **Phone:** 212-472-3333; **Board Cert:** Internal Medicine 1985; Gastroenterology 1989; **Med School:** Columbia P&S 1982; **Resid:** Internal Medicine, New York Hosp 1985; **Fellow:** Gastroenterology, New York Hosp 1988; **Fac Appt:** Asst Clin Prof Med, Cornell Univ-Weill Med Coll

Chapman, Mark MD (Ge) - **Spec Exp:** Inflammatory Bowel Disease/Crohn's; Peptic Ulcer Disease; Motility Disorders; **Hospital:** Mount Sinai Med Ctr (page 98); **Address:** 12 E 86th St, New York, NY 10028-0506; **Phone:** 212-861-2000; **Board Cert:** Internal Medicine 1968; Gastroenterology 1970; **Med School:** SUNY Downstate 1961; **Resid:** Internal Medicine, Mt Sinai Hosp 1962; Internal Medicine, Montefiore Med Ctr 1963; **Fellow:** Internal Medicine, Mt Sinai Hosp 1964; Gastroenterology, Mt Sinai Hosp 1966; **Fac Appt:** Assoc Clin Prof Med, Mount Sinai Sch Med

Clain, David MD (Ge) - **Spec Exp:** Liver Disease; Hepatitis; Pancreatic/Biliary Endoscopy (ERCP); Colonoscopy; **Hospital:** Beth Israel Med Ctr - Petrie Division (page 90); **Address:** Phillips Ambulatory Care Ctr, Ste 2G, 10 Union Square E, New York, NY 10003; **Phone:** 212-420-4521; **Board Cert:** Internal Medicine 1980; Gastroenterology 1981; **Med School:** South Africa 1959; **Resid:** Internal Medicine, Birmingham General 1964; Internal Medicine, Charing Cross 1965; **Fellow:** Gastroenterology, Royal Free Hosp 1966; **Fac Appt:** Prof Med, Albert Einstein Coll Med

Cohen, Jonathan MD (Ge) - **Spec Exp:** Pancreatic/Biliary Endoscopy (ERCP); Pancreatic Disease; Liver Disease; Colonoscopy; **Hospital:** NYU Med Ctr (page 102); **Address:** 232 E 30th St, New York, NY 10016-8202; **Phone:** 212-889-5544; **Board Cert:** Internal Medicine 1993; Gastroenterology 1995; **Med School:** Harvard Med Sch 1990; **Resid:** Internal Medicine, Beth Israel Hosp 1993; **Fellow:** Gastroenterology, UCLA Med Ctr 1995; Endoscopy, Wellesley Hosp 1995; **Fac Appt:** Assoc Clin Prof Med, NYU Sch Med

Cohen, Lawrence B MD (Ge) - **Spec Exp:** Gastroesophageal Reflux Disease (GERD); Esophageal Disorders; Colon & Rectal Cancer; **Hospital:** Mount Sinai Med Ctr (page 98); **Address:** 311 E 79th St, Ste A, New York, NY 10021; **Phone:** 212-996-6633; **Board Cert:** Internal Medicine 1981; Gastroenterology 1983; **Med School:** Hahnemann Univ 1978; **Resid:** Internal Medicine, Mount Sinai Hosp 1981; **Fellow:** Gastroenterology, Mount Sinai Hosp 1983; **Fac Appt:** Assoc Clin Prof Med, Mount Sinai Sch Med

Cohen, Seth A MD (Ge) - **Spec Exp:** Pancreatic/Biliary Endoscopy (ERCP); Colonoscopy; Endoscopy; **Hospital:** Beth Israel Med Ctr - Petrie Division (page 90), Mount Sinai Med Ctr (page 98); **Address:** 60 East End Ave, New York, NY 10028-0305; **Phone:** 212-734-8874; **Board Cert:** Internal Medicine 1989; Gastroenterology 2004; **Med School:** Columbia P&S 1986; **Resid:** Internal Medicine, Mount Sinai Med Ctr 1989; Gastroenterology, St Luke's-Roosevelt Hosp Ctr 1991; **Fellow:** Gastroenterology, Beth Israel Hosp 1992

Connor, Bradley A MD (Ge) - **Spec Exp:** Travel Medicine; Parasitic Infections; **Hospital:** NY-Presby Hosp (page 100); **Address:** 50 E 69th St, New York, NY 10021; **Phone:** 212-988-2800; **Board Cert:** Internal Medicine 1982; Gastroenterology 1985; **Med School:** Univ Tex SW, Dallas 1978; **Resid:** Internal Medicine, Univ Tex Hlth Sci Ctr-Bexar Co/A Murphy VA Hosps 1981; **Fellow:** Gastroenterology, NY Hosp 1984; **Fac Appt:** Assoc Clin Prof Med, Cornell Univ-Weill Med Coll

Cooper, Robert B MD (Ge) - **Hospital:** NY-Presby Hosp (page 100); **Address:** 635 Madison Ave Fl 17, New York, NY 10022; **Phone:** 212-717-4967; **Board Cert:** Internal Medicine 1984; Gastroenterology 1989; **Med School:** Cornell Univ-Weill Med Coll 1981; **Resid:** Internal Medicine, New York Hosp 1984; **Fellow:** Gastroenterology, New York Hosp 1987

Dieterich, Douglas MD (Ge) - **Spec Exp:** Hepatitis; AIDS/HIV; Liver Disease; Endoscopy; **Hospital:** Mount Sinai Med Ctr (page 98), NYU Med Ctr (page 102); **Address:** 5 E 98th St Fl 11, New York, NY 10029; **Phone:** 212-241-7270; **Board Cert:** Internal Medicine 1981; Gastroenterology 1987; **Med School:** NYU Sch Med 1978; **Resid:** Internal Medicine, Bellevue Hosp Ctr-NYU 1981; **Fellow:** Gastroenterology, Bellevue Hosp Ctr-NYU 1983; **Fac Appt:** Prof Med, Mount Sinai Sch Med

Field, Steven P MD (Ge) - **Spec Exp:** Inflammatory Bowel Disease/Crohn's; Irritable Bowel Syndrome; **Hospital:** NYU Med Ctr (page 102); **Address:** 245 E 35th St, New York, NY 10016; **Phone:** 212-686-9477; **Board Cert:** Internal Medicine 1980; Gastroenterology 1983; **Med School:** NYU Sch Med 1977; **Resid:** Internal Medicine, Bellevue Hosp 1981; **Fellow:** Gastroenterology, Mt Sinai Hosp 1983; **Fac Appt:** Asst Clin Prof Med, NYU Sch Med

Fochios, Steven MD (Ge) - **Spec Exp:** Endoscopy; **Hospital:** Lenox Hill Hosp (page 94), Manhattan Eye, Ear & Throat Hosp; **Address:** 117 E 65th St, New York, NY 10021; **Phone:** 212-861-4278; **Board Cert:** Internal Medicine 1980; Gastroenterology 1985; **Med School:** Geo Wash Univ 1976; **Resid:** Internal Medicine, Lenox Hill Hosp 1979; **Fellow:** Gastroenterology, Lenox Hill Hosp 1981

Foong, Anthony MD (Ge) - **Spec Exp:** Endoscopy; Colonoscopy; Gastrointestinal Disorders; **Hospital:** St Vincent Cath Med Ctrs - Manhattan (page 375), Cabrini Med Ctr (page 374); **Address:** 210 Canal St, Ste 601, New York, NY 10013; **Phone:** 212-693-2100; **Board Cert:** Internal Medicine 1984; Gastroenterology 1987; **Med School:** Tufts Univ 1981; **Resid:** Internal Medicine, Univ Md Hosp 1984; **Fellow:** Gastroenterology, St Luke's-Roosevelt Hosp Ctr 1986

Frank, Michael MD (Ge) - **Spec Exp:** Inflammatory Bowel Disease/Crohn's; Colonoscopy; Endoscopy; **Hospital:** Lenox Hill Hosp (page 94), Montefiore Med Ctr - Weiler-Einstein Div; **Address:** 9 E 63rd St, New York, NY 10021-7236; **Phone:** 212-593-7170; **Board Cert:** Internal Medicine 1977; Gastroenterology 1979; **Med School:** Albert Einstein Coll Med 1974; **Resid:** Internal Medicine, Bronx Municipal Hosp Ctr 1977; **Fellow:** Gastroenterology, Montefiore Hosp Med Ctr 1979; **Fac Appt:** Assoc Clin Prof Med, Albert Einstein Coll Med

Freiman, Hal MD (Ge) - **Spec Exp:** Gastroesophageal Reflux Disease (GERD); Colon Cancer Screening; Biliary Disease; **Hospital:** St Vincent Cath Med Ctrs - Manhattan (page 375); **Address:** 59 W 12th St, Ste 1D, New York, NY 10011-8520; **Phone:** 212-206-0074; **Board Cert:** Internal Medicine 1981; Gastroenterology 1983; **Med School:** Albany Med Coll 1978; **Resid:** Internal Medicine, St Vincent's Hosp 1981; **Fellow:** Gastroenterology, Westchester Co Med Ctr 1983; **Fac Appt:** Asst Clin Prof Med, NY Med Coll

Friedlander, Charles MD (Ge) - **Spec Exp:** Colonoscopy; Irritable Bowel Syndrome; **Hospital:** NYU Med Ctr (page 102); **Address:** 232 E 30th St, New York, NY 10016-8202; **Phone:** 212-889-5544; **Board Cert:** Internal Medicine 1974; Gastroenterology 1977; **Med School:** SUNY Downstate 1968; **Resid:** Internal Medicine, Bellevue Hosp 1971; **Fellow:** Gastroenterology, NYU Med Ctr 1976; **Fac Appt:** Assoc Prof Med, NYU Sch Med

Friedman, Gerald MD/PhD (Ge) - **Spec Exp:** Irritable Bowel Syndrome; Inflammatory Bowel Disease/Crohn's; Nutrition; **Hospital:** Mount Sinai Med Ctr (page 98); **Address:** 1751 York Ave, New York, NY 10128; **Phone:** 212-860-6660; **Board Cert:** Internal Medicine 1965; Gastroenterology 1971; **Med School:** SUNY Buffalo 1957; **Resid:** Internal Medicine, Montefiore Hosp Med Ctr 1959; Internal Medicine, Mount Sinai Hosp 1960; **Fellow:** Gastroenterology, Mount Sinai Hosp 1962; **Fac Appt:** Clin Prof Med, Mount Sinai Sch Med

Friedman, Scott L MD (Ge) - **Spec Exp:** Liver Disease; **Hospital:** Mount Sinai Med Ctr (page 98); **Address:** Mt Sinai Medical Ctr, Div Gastroenterology, One Gustave L Levy Pl, New York, NY 10029; **Phone:** 212-659-9501; **Board Cert:** Internal Medicine 1982; Gastroenterology 1985; **Med School:** Mount Sinai Sch Med 1979; **Resid:** Internal Medicine, Beth Israel Hosp 1982; **Fellow:** Gastroenterology, UCSF Med Ctr 1985; **Fac Appt:** Prof Med, Mount Sinai Sch Med

Gerson, Charles MD (Ge) - **Spec Exp:** Irritable Bowel Syndrome; Diarrheal Diseases; **Hospital:** Mount Sinai Med Ctr (page 98); **Address:** 80 Central Park West, Ste B, New York, NY 10023-5204; **Phone:** 212-496-6161; **Board Cert:** Internal Medicine 1970; Gastroenterology 1972; **Med School:** SUNY Downstate 1962; **Resid:** Internal Medicine, Bellevue Hosp 1964; Internal Medicine, Mount Sinai Hosp 1965; **Fellow:** Gastroenterology, Bellevue Hosp 1968; Gastroenterology, Mount Sinai Hosp 1969; **Fac Appt:** Clin Prof Med, Mount Sinai Sch Med

Goldberg, Myron D MD (Ge) - **Spec Exp:** Inflammatory Bowel Disease/Crohn's; Endoscopy; Colonoscopy; **Hospital:** Lenox Hill Hosp (page 94); **Address:** 110 E 59th St, Ste 10D, New York, NY 10022-1304; **Phone:** 212-583-2900; **Board Cert:** Internal Medicine 1977; Gastroenterology 1979; **Med School:** Albert Einstein Coll Med 1971; **Resid:** Internal Medicine, Montefiore Hosp Med Ctr 1973; Internal Medicine, Lenox Hill Hosp 1974; **Fellow:** Gastroenterology, Columbia-Presby 1977; Gastroenterology, Lenox Hill Hosp 1978; **Fac Appt:** Asst Clin Prof Med, NYU Sch Med

Goldin, Howard MD (Ge) - **Spec Exp:** Inflammatory Bowel Disease/Crohn's; Endoscopy; Liver Disease; **Hospital:** NY-Presby Hosp (page 100), Rockefeller Univ; **Address:** 646 Park Ave, New York, NY 10021-6105; **Phone:** 212-249-0404; **Board Cert:** Internal Medicine 1968; Gastroenterology 1973; **Med School:** Cornell Univ-Weill Med Coll 1961; **Resid:** Internal Medicine, New York Hosp 1964; **Fellow:** Gastroenterology, New York Hosp 1966; **Fac Appt:** Clin Prof Med, Cornell Univ-Weill Med Coll

Green, Peter MD (Ge) - **Spec Exp:** Celiac Disease; Endoscopy; Colonoscopy; Malabsorption; **Hospital:** NY-Presby Hosp (page 100); **Address:** Celiac Disease Ctr, Harkness Bldg, 180 Fort Washington Ave, rm 956, New York, NY 10032-3713; **Phone:** 212-305-5590; **Med School:** Australia 1970; **Resid:** Internal Medicine, North Shore Med Ctr 1974; **Fellow:** Gastroenterology, North Shore Med Ctr 1976; Gastroenterology, Beth Israel Hosp 1977; **Fac Appt:** Clin Prof Med, Columbia P&S

Hammerman, Hillel MD (Ge) - **Spec Exp:** Swallowing Disorders; Liver Disease; **Hospital:** Lenox Hill Hosp (page 94); **Address:** 210 E 73rd St, New York, NY 10021; **Phone:** 212-288-1030; **Board Cert:** Internal Medicine 1981; Gastroenterology 1983; **Med School:** Cornell Univ-Weill Med Coll 1978; **Resid:** Internal Medicine, Baltimore City Hosps 1981; **Fellow:** Gastroenterology, Lahey Clinic 1983

Harary, Albert MD (Ge) - **Spec Exp:** Endoscopy & Colonoscopy; Gastroesophageal Reflux Disease (GERD); Swallowing Disorders; **Hospital:** Lenox Hill Hosp (page 94); **Address:** 654 Madison Ave, Fl 6, New York, NY 10021-8404; **Phone:** 212-702-0123; **Board Cert:** Internal Medicine 1982; Gastroenterology 1985; **Med School:** Columbia P&S 1979; **Resid:** Internal Medicine, Univ Miami Affil Hosp 1982; **Fellow:** Gastroenterology, Univ Miami Affil Hosp 1984; **Fac Appt:** Asst Clin Prof Med, NYU Sch Med

Horowitz, Lawrence MD (Ge) - **Spec Exp:** Esophageal Disorders; Irritable Bowel Syndrome; Ulcerative Colitis; **Hospital:** NYU Med Ctr (page 102); **Address:** 530 1st Ave, New York, NY 10016-6402; **Phone:** 212-263-7236; **Board Cert:** Internal Medicine 1962; Gastroenterology 1966; **Med School:** SUNY Downstate 1955; **Resid:** Internal Medicine, Albert Einstein 1968; Gastroenterology, VA Med Ctr 1969; **Fac Appt:** Clin Prof Med, NYU Sch Med

Itzkowitz, Steven H MD (Ge) - **Spec Exp:** Colon & Rectal Cancer; Colon & Rectal Cancer Detection; Inflammatory Bowel Disease; **Hospital:** Mount Sinai Med Ctr (page 98); **Address:** 5 E 98th St, Box 1625, New York, NY 10029; **Phone:** 212-241-4299; **Board Cert:** Internal Medicine 1982; Gastroenterology 1985; **Med School:** Mount Sinai Sch Med 1979; **Resid:** Internal Medicine, Bellevue Hosp/ NYU Med Ctr 1982; **Fellow:** Gastroenterology, UCSF Med Ctr 1984; **Fac Appt:** Prof Med, Mount Sinai Sch Med

Jacobson, Ira MD (Ge) - **Spec Exp:** Liver Disease; Pancreatic/Biliary Endoscopy (ERCP); Colonoscopy; Hepatitis; **Hospital:** NY-Presby Hosp (page 100); **Address:** 450 E 69th St, New York, NY 10021-5016; **Phone:** 212-746-2115; **Board Cert:** Internal Medicine 1982; Gastroenterology 1985; **Med School:** Columbia P&S 1979; **Resid:** Internal Medicine, UCSF Med Ctr 1982; **Fellow:** Gastroenterology, Mass Genl Hosp 1984; **Fac Appt:** Prof Med, Cornell Univ-Weill Med Coll

Januzzi, James MD (Ge) - **Hospital:** St Vincent Cath Med Ctrs - Manhattan (page 375); **Address:** 29 Washington Square W, New York, NY 10011; **Phone:** 212-982-5551; **Board Cert:** Internal Medicine 1972; Gastroenterology 1977; **Med School:** NY Med Coll 1966; **Resid:** Internal Medicine, St Vincents Hosp 1972; **Fac Appt:** Asst Clin Prof Med, NY Med Coll

Kairam, Indira MD (Ge) - **Spec Exp:** Colon Cancer; Peptic Ulcer Disease; Hepatitis C; **Hospital:** St. Vincent's Midtown, Roosevelt Care Ctr - Edison; **Address:** 945 West End Ave, Ste 1D, New York, NY 10025-3573; **Phone:** 212-865-7355; **Board Cert:** Internal Medicine 1978; **Med School:** India 1973; **Resid:** Internal Medicine, St Clare's Hosp 1978; **Fellow:** Gastroenterology, Lahey Clinic 1980; **Fac Appt:** Asst Prof Med, NY Med Coll

Kimball, Annetta MD (Ge) - **Spec Exp:** Hepatitis; Inflammatory Bowel Disease/Crohn's; **Hospital:** St Luke's - Roosevelt Hosp Ctr - Roosevelt Div (page 90); **Address:** 315 W 57th St, Ste 301, New York, NY 10019; **Phone:** 212-371-8900; **Board Cert:** Internal Medicine 1972; Gastroenterology 1973; **Med School:** Boston Univ 1968; **Resid:** Internal Medicine, Roosevelt Hosp 1970; Internal Medicine, Mount Sinai Hosp 1971; **Fellow:** Gastroenterology, Mount Sinai Hosp 1973; **Fac Appt:** Assoc Clin Prof Med, Columbia P&S

Klion, Franklin MD (Ge) - **Spec Exp:** Liver Disease; Hepatitis; **Hospital:** Mount Sinai Med Ctr (page 98); **Address:** 1060 5th Ave, New York, NY 10128-0104; **Phone:** 212-369-1541; **Board Cert:** Internal Medicine 1965; Gastroenterology 1968; **Med School:** NY Med Coll 1958; **Resid:** Internal Medicine, Kingsbridge VA Hosp 1960; Internal Medicine, Mount Sinai Hosp 1963; **Fellow:** Gastroenterology, Mount Sinai Hosp 1964; Hepatology, Mount Sinai Hosp 1965; **Fac Appt:** Clin Prof Med, Mount Sinai Sch Med

Knapp, Albert B MD (Ge) - **Spec Exp:** Colonoscopy/Polypectomy; Endoscopy; Liver Disease; **Hospital:** NYU Med Ctr (page 102), Lenox Hill Hosp (page 94); **Address:** 21 E 79th St, New York, NY 10021-0125; **Phone:** 212-737-3446; **Board Cert:** Internal Medicine 1982; Gastroenterology 1987; **Med School:** Columbia P&S 1979; **Resid:** Internal Medicine, Albert Einstein Med Ctr 1982; **Fellow:** Gastroenterology, Brigham & Women's Hosp/Harvard 1985; **Fac Appt:** Assoc Prof Med, NYU Sch Med

Korelitz, Burton I MD (Ge) - **Spec Exp:** Inflammatory Bowel Disease; Ulcerative Colitis; Crohn's Disease; **Hospital:** Lenox Hill Hosp (page 94); **Address:** 115 E 57th St, Ste 510, New York, NY 10022; **Phone:** 212-988-3800; **Board Cert:** Internal Medicine 1958; Gastroenterology 1961; **Med School:** Boston Univ 1951; **Resid:** Internal Medicine, VA Hosp 1953; Gastroenterology, Beth Israel Hosp 1954; **Fellow:** Gastroenterology, Mt Sinai Hosp 1956; **Fac Appt:** Clin Prof Med, NYU Sch Med

Kornbluth, Arthur Asher MD (Ge) - **Spec Exp:** Inflammatory Bowel Disease; Diarrheal Diseases; Colonoscopy; **Hospital:** Mount Sinai Med Ctr (page 98); **Address:** 1751 York Ave, New York, NY 10128-6812; **Phone:** 212-369-2490; **Board Cert:** Internal Medicine 1989; Gastroenterology 2002; **Med School:** SUNY Hlth Sci Ctr 1984; **Resid:** Internal Medicine, Albert Einstein 1988; **Fellow:** Gastroenterology, Mount Sinai Hosp 1990; **Fac Appt:** Assoc Clin Prof Med, Mount Sinai Sch Med

Kotler, Donald P MD (Ge) - **Spec Exp:** Esophageal Disorders; Nutrition & AIDS; **Hospital:** St Luke's - Roosevelt Hosp Ctr - St Luke's Hosp (page 90); **Address:** 1111 Amsterdam Ave, S&R 12, New York, NY 10025; **Phone:** 212-523-3670; **Board Cert:** Internal Medicine 1976; Gastroenterology 1979; **Med School:** Albert Einstein Coll Med 1973; **Resid:** Internal Medicine, Jacobi Med Ctr 1976; **Fellow:** Gastroenterology, Hosp Univ Penn 1978; **Fac Appt:** Assoc Prof Med, Columbia P&S

Krumholz, Michael MD (Ge) - **Spec Exp:** Colonoscopy; Colon Cancer Screening; Peptic Ulcer Disease; **Hospital:** Lenox Hill Hosp (page 94); **Address:** 111 E 80th St, Ste 1C, New York, NY 10021-0350; **Phone:** 212-734-5533; **Board Cert:** Internal Medicine 1983; Gastroenterology 1987; **Med School:** Mount Sinai Sch Med 1980; **Resid:** Internal Medicine, Beth Israel Hosp 1984; **Fellow:** Gastroenterology, Lenox Hill Hosp 1986; **Fac Appt:** Med, NYU Sch Med

Kummer, Bart MD (Ge) - **Spec Exp:** Colonoscopy; Endoscopy; **Hospital:** NY Downtown Hosp, NYU Med Ctr (page 102); **Address:** 19 Beekman St Fl 6, New York, NY 10038-1522; **Phone:** 212-406-7050; **Board Cert:** Internal Medicine 1982; Gastroenterology 1985; **Med School:** Cornell Univ-Weill Med Coll 1979; **Resid:** Internal Medicine, Harlem Hosp 1982; **Fellow:** Gastroenterology, St Luke's-Roosevelt Hosp Ctr 1985; **Fac Appt:** Asst Prof Med, NYU Sch Med

Kurtz, Robert C MD (Ge) - **Spec Exp:** Gastrointestinal Cancer; Colon & Rectal Cancer Detection; Endoscopy; Nutrition; **Hospital:** Meml Sloan Kettering Cancer Ctr (page 109); **Address:** Meml Sloan Kettering Cancer Ctr, 1275 York Ave, rm H510, New York, NY 10021-6007; **Phone:** 212-639-7620; **Board Cert:** Internal Medicine 1971; Gastroenterology 1977; **Med School:** Jefferson Med Coll 1968; **Resid:** Internal Medicine, NY Hosp/Meml Sloan Kettering Cancer Ctr 1971; **Fellow:** Gastroenterology, Meml Sloan Kettering Cancer Ctr 1973; **Fac Appt:** Prof Med, Cornell Univ-Weill Med Coll

Lambroza, Arnon MD (Ge) - **Spec Exp:** Swallowing Disorders; Gastroesophageal Reflux Disease (GERD); Barrett's Esophagus; **Hospital:** NY-Presby Hosp (page 100), Lenox Hill Hosp (page 94); **Address:** 950 Park Ave, New York, NY 10028-0320; **Phone:** 212-517-7570; **Board Cert:** Internal Medicine 1987; Gastroenterology 2001; **Med School:** Albert Einstein Coll Med 1984; **Resid:** Internal Medicine, Hosp Univ Penn 1987; **Fellow:** Gastroenterology, New York Hosp 1990; **Fac Appt:** Assoc Clin Prof Med, Cornell Univ-Weill Med Coll

Lax, James MD (Ge) - **Spec Exp:** Liver Disease; Gastroesophageal Reflux Disease (GERD); Barrett's Esophagus; **Hospital:** St Luke's - Roosevelt Hosp Ctr - Roosevelt Div (page 90), Lenox Hill Hosp (page 94); **Address:** 160 E 72nd St, New York, NY 10021-4364; **Phone:** 212-988-5740; **Board Cert:** Internal Medicine 1984; Gastroenterology 1987; **Med School:** NYU Sch Med 1981; **Resid:** Internal Medicine, St Luke's-Roosevelt Hosp Ctr 1984; **Fellow:** Gastroenterology, St Luke's-Roosevelt Hosp Ctr 1986; **Fac Appt:** Asst Clin Prof Med, Columbia P&S

Lebwohl, Oscar MD (Ge) - **Spec Exp:** Endoscopy; Inflammatory Bowel Disease/Chrohn's; Ulcerative Colitis; **Hospital:** NY-Presby Hosp (page 100); **Address:** 161 Fort Washington Ave, New York, NY 10032-3713; **Phone:** 212-305-5363; **Board Cert:** Internal Medicine 1975; Gastroenterology 1977; **Med School:** Harvard Med Sch 1972; **Resid:** Internal Medicine, Mt Sinai Med Ctr 1975; **Fellow:** Gastroenterology, Columbia-Presby Med Ctr 1976; Hepatology, Mt Sinai Med Ctr 1977; **Fac Appt:** Clin Prof Med, Columbia P&S

Lewis, Blair MD (Ge) - **Spec Exp:** Endoscopy; Capsule Endoscopy; **Hospital:** Mount Sinai Med Ctr (page 98); **Address:** 1067 5th Ave, New York, NY 10128-0101; **Phone:** 212-369-6600; **Board Cert:** Internal Medicine 1985; Gastroenterology 1987; **Med School:** Albert Einstein Coll Med 1982; **Resid:** Internal Medicine, Montefiore Hosp Med Ctr 1985; **Fellow:** Gastroenterology, Mount Sinai Med Ctr 1987; **Fac Appt:** Asst Clin Prof Med, Mount Sinai Sch Med

Lightdale, Charles MD (Ge) - **Spec Exp:** Barrett's Esophagus; Gastrointestinal Cancer; Endoscopic Ultrasound; **Hospital:** NY-Presby Hosp (page 100); **Address:** Columbia-Presby Med Ctr, Irving Pavilion, 161 Fort Washington Ave, rm 812, New York, NY 10032-3713; **Phone:** 212-305-3423; **Board Cert:** Internal Medicine 1972; Gastroenterology 1973; **Med School:** Columbia P&S 1966; **Resid:** Internal Medicine, Yale-New Haven Hosp 1968; Internal Medicine, New York Hosp 1969; **Fellow:** Gastroenterology, New York Hosp-Cornell 1973; **Fac Appt:** Prof Med, Columbia P&S

Lucak, Basil K MD (Ge) - **Spec Exp:** Gastroesophageal Reflux Disease (GERD); Peptic Acid Disorders; Cancer Screening; **Hospital:** NYU Med Ctr (page 102), VA Med Ctr - Manhattan; **Address:** 530 1st Ave, Ste 9N, New York, NY 10016; **Phone:** 212-263-3095; **Board Cert:** Internal Medicine 1977; Gastroenterology 1981; **Med School:** NYU Sch Med 1974; **Resid:** Internal Medicine, New York Hosp 1976; Internal Medicine, VA Med Ctr 1977; **Fellow:** Gastroenterology, Bellevue Hosp 1979; **Fac Appt:** Asst Clin Prof Med, NYU Sch Med

Lustbader, Ian J MD (Ge) - **Spec Exp:** Hepatitis C; Colonoscopy; Ulcerative Colitis/Crohn's; **Hospital:** NYU Med Ctr (page 102); **Address:** 245 E 35th St, New York, NY 10016-4283; **Phone:** 212-685-5252; **Board Cert:** Internal Medicine 1985; Gastroenterology 1987; **Med School:** Columbia P&S 1982; **Resid:** Internal Medicine, St Luke's-Roosevelt Hosp Ctr 1985; **Fellow:** Gastroenterology, Bellevue Hosp 1987; **Fac Appt:** Asst Clin Prof Med, NYU Sch Med

Magun, Arthur MD (Ge) - **Spec Exp:** Hepatitis; Ulcerative Colitis/Crohn's; Endoscopy; Liver Disease; **Hospital:** NY-Presby Hosp (page 100); **Address:** 161 Fort Washington Ave, rm 338, New York, NY 10032-3713; **Phone:** 212-305-5287; **Board Cert:** Internal Medicine 1980; Gastroenterology 1983; **Med School:** Mount Sinai Sch Med 1977; **Resid:** Internal Medicine, Columbia-Presby Med Ctr 1980; **Fellow:** Gastroenterology, Columbia-Presby Med Ctr 1983; **Fac Appt:** Clin Prof Med, Columbia P&S

Markowitz, David MD (Ge) - **Spec Exp:** Gastroesophageal Reflux Disease (GERD); Esophageal Disorders; Endoscopy; **Hospital:** NY-Presby Hosp (page 100); **Address:** 161 Ft Washington Ave, rm 3-301, New York, NY 10032; **Phone:** 212-305-1024; **Board Cert:** Internal Medicine 1988; Gastroenterology 2001; **Med School:** Columbia P&S 1985; **Resid:** Internal Medicine, Columbia-Presby Hosp 1988; **Fellow:** Gastroenterology, Columbia-Presby Hosp 1991; **Fac Appt:** Asst Clin Prof Med, Columbia P&S

Marsh Jr, Franklin MD (Ge) - **Spec Exp:** Colon Cancer; Liver Disease; Motility Disorders; **Hospital:** NY-Presby Hosp (page 100), N Genl Hosp; **Address:** 342 E 67th St, New York, NY 10021-6238; **Phone:** 212-288-8820; **Board Cert:** Internal Medicine 1981; Gastroenterology 1985; **Med School:** SUNY Buffalo 1978; **Resid:** Internal Medicine, Harlem Hosp 1982; **Fellow:** Gastroenterology, New York Hosp 1995; **Fac Appt:** Asst Clin Prof Med, Cornell Univ-Weill Med Coll

Martin, Paul MD (Ge) - **Spec Exp:** Liver Disease; Hepatitis; Transplant Medicine-Liver; **Hospital:** Mount Sinai Med Ctr (page 98); **Address:** 5 E 98th St Fl 11, New York, NY 10029; **Phone:** 212-241-0034; **Board Cert:** Internal Medicine 1984; Gastroenterology 1987; **Med School:** Ireland 1978; **Resid:** Internal Medicine, St Vincent's Hosp 1982; Internal Medicine, Univ Alberta 1984; **Fellow:** Gastroenterology, Queen Univ 1986; Hepatology, Natl Inst Hlth 1989; **Fac Appt:** Prof Med, Mount Sinai Sch Med

Mayer, Lloyd MD (Ge) - **Spec Exp:** Inflammatory Bowel Disease/Crohn's; Ulcerative Colitis; **Hospital:** Mount Sinai Med Ctr (page 98); **Address:** 1425 Madison Ave Fl 11 - rm 1120, Box 1089, New York, NY 10029; **Phone:** 212-659-9266; **Board Cert:** Internal Medicine 1979; Gastroenterology 1981; **Med School:** Mount Sinai Sch Med 1976; **Resid:** Internal Medicine, Bellevue Hosp 1979; **Fellow:** Gastroenterology, Mount Sinai Hosp 1981; **Fac Appt:** Prof Med, Mount Sinai Sch Med

Milano, Andrew MD (Ge) - **Spec Exp:** Endoscopy; Inflammatory Bowel Disease/Crohn's; Esophageal Disorders; **Hospital:** NYU Med Ctr (page 102); **Address:** 530 1st Ave, Ste 4K, New York, NY 10016-6402; **Phone:** 212-263-7483; **Board Cert:** Internal Medicine 1977; Gastroenterology 1972; **Med School:** NYU Sch Med 1964; **Resid:** Internal Medicine, NYU-Bellevue Hosp 1967; **Fellow:** Gastroenterology, NYU-Bellevue Hosp 1968; **Fac Appt:** Clin Prof Med, NYU Sch Med

Miskovitz, Paul MD (Ge) - **Spec Exp:** Endoscopy; Liver Disease; **Hospital:** NY-Presby Hosp (page 100); **Address:** 50 E 70th St, New York, NY 10021-4928; **Phone:** 212-717-4966; **Board Cert:** Internal Medicine 1978; Gastroenterology 1981; **Med School:** Cornell Univ-Weill Med Coll 1975; **Resid:** Internal Medicine, NY Hosp 1978; **Fellow:** Gastroenterology, NY Hosp 1980; **Fac Appt:** Clin Prof Med, Cornell Univ-Weill Med Coll

Nagler, Jerry MD (Ge) - **Spec Exp:** Inflammatory Bowel Disease; Irritable Bowel Syndrome; **Hospital:** NY-Presby Hosp (page 100); **Address:** 407 E 70th St, FL 5, New York, NY 10021-5302; **Phone:** 212-628-7777; **Board Cert:** Internal Medicine 1976; Gastroenterology 1983; **Med School:** Yale Univ 1973; **Resid:** Internal Medicine, Columbia-Presby Hosp 1976; **Fellow:** Gastroenterology, New York Hosp 1978; **Fac Appt:** Asst Clin Prof Med, Cornell Univ-Weill Med Coll

New York (Manhattan)

Ottaviano, Lawrence MD (Ge) - **Spec Exp:** Peptic Ulcer Disease; Colitis; **Hospital:** Cabrini Med Ctr (page 374), St Vincent Cath Med Ctrs - Manhattan (page 375); **Address:** 60 Gramercy Park North, Ste 1B, New York, NY 10010; **Phone:** 212-254-1220; **Board Cert:** Internal Medicine 1988; Gastroenterology 1993; **Med School:** West Indies 1984; **Resid:** Internal Medicine, Cabrini Med Ctr 1987; **Fellow:** Gastroenterology, Cabrini Med Ctr 1989; **Fac Appt:** Asst Clin Prof Med, NY Med Coll

Pochapin, Mark B MD (Ge) - **Spec Exp:** Pancreatic Cancer; Endoscopic Ultrasound; Colon & Rectal Cancer Prevention; Diarrheal Diseases; **Hospital:** NY-Presby Hosp (page 100); **Address:** The Jay Monahan Ctr for GI Hlth, 1315 York Ave, New York, NY 10022; **Phone:** 212-746-4014; **Board Cert:** Internal Medicine 1991; Gastroenterology 1993; **Med School:** Cornell Univ-Weill Med Coll 1988; **Resid:** Internal Medicine, New York Hosp-Cornell Med Ctr 1991; **Fellow:** Gastroenterology, Montefiore Med Ctr/Albert Einstein 1993; **Fac Appt:** Assoc Clin Prof Med, Cornell Univ-Weill Med Coll

Present, Daniel MD (Ge) - **Spec Exp:** Inflammatory Bowel Disease/Crohn's; Ulcerative Colitis; Crohn's Disease; **Hospital:** Mount Sinai Med Ctr (page 98); **Address:** 12 E 86th St, New York, NY 10028-0506; **Phone:** 212-861-2000; **Board Cert:** Internal Medicine 1966; Gastroenterology 1970; **Med School:** SUNY Downstate 1959; **Resid:** Internal Medicine, Mount Sinai Hosp 1964; **Fellow:** Gastroenterology, Mount Sinai Hosp 1966; **Fac Appt:** Clin Prof Med, Mount Sinai Sch Med

Robilotti, James MD (Ge) - **Spec Exp:** Irritable Bowel Syndrome; Peptic Ulcer; Gastroesophageal Reflux Disease (GERD); Endoscopy; **Hospital:** St Vincent Cath Med Ctrs - Manhattan (page 375); **Address:** 29 Washington Sq West, New York, NY 10011-9180; **Phone:** 212-475-4030; **Board Cert:** Internal Medicine 1972; Gastroenterology 1981; **Med School:** UMDNJ-NJ Med Sch, Newark 1965; **Resid:** Internal Medicine, St Vincent's Hosp & Med Ctr 1967; **Fellow:** Gastroenterology, St Vincent's Hosp & Med Ctr 1970; **Fac Appt:** Assoc Clin Prof Med, NY Med Coll

Romeu, Jose MD (Ge) - **Spec Exp:** Colonoscopy/Polypectomy; Gastroscopy; Gastrointestinal Cancer; **Hospital:** Mount Sinai Med Ctr (page 98), Lenox Hill Hosp (page 94); **Address:** 1107 5th Ave, New York, NY 10128-0145; **Phone:** 212-534-6747; **Board Cert:** Internal Medicine 1973; Gastroenterology 1975; **Med School:** NYU Sch Med 1970; **Resid:** Internal Medicine, Mount Sinai Hosp 1973; **Fellow:** Gastroenterology, Mount Sinai Hosp 1976; **Fac Appt:** Asst Prof Med, Mount Sinai Sch Med

Rubin, Moshe MD (Ge) - **Spec Exp:** Endoscopy; Capsule Endoscopy; Colonoscopy; **Hospital:** NY-Presby Hosp (page 100); **Address:** 16 E 60th St, Ste 321, New York, NY 10022-4813; **Phone:** 212-326-5530; **Board Cert:** Internal Medicine 1986; Gastroenterology 1988; **Med School:** Yale Univ 1983; **Resid:** Internal Medicine, NY Hosp 1986; **Fellow:** Gastroenterology, Columbia-Presby 1988; **Fac Appt:** Assoc Clin Prof Med, Columbia P&S

Rubin, Peter MD (Ge) - **Spec Exp:** Endoscopy; Inflammatory Bowel Disease; **Hospital:** Mount Sinai Med Ctr (page 98); **Address:** 920 Park Ave, New York, NY 10028; **Phone:** 212-535-3400; **Board Cert:** Internal Medicine 1973; Gastroenterology 1975; **Med School:** Univ Rochester 1970; **Resid:** Internal Medicine, Mount Sinai Hosp 1973; **Fellow:** Gastroenterology, Mount Sinai Hosp 1975; **Fac Appt:** Assoc Clin Prof Med, Mount Sinai Sch Med

Ruoff, Michael MD (Ge) - **Spec Exp:** Esophageal Disorders; Malabsorption; **Hospital:** NYU Med Ctr (page 102); **Address:** 232 E 30 St, New York, NY 10016; **Phone:** 212-889-5544; **Board Cert:** Internal Medicine 1980; Gastroenterology 1972; **Med School:** NYU Sch Med 1963; **Resid:** Internal Medicine, Bellevue Hosp 1966; **Fellow:** Gastroenterology, NYU Med Ctr 1967; **Fac Appt:** Clin Prof Med, NYU Sch Med

Sachar, David MD (Ge) - **Spec Exp:** Crohn's Disease; Ulcerative Colitis; Inflammatory Bowel Disease; **Hospital:** Mount Sinai Med Ctr (page 98); **Address:** 5 E 98th St Fl 11, New York, NY 10029-6574; **Phone:** 212-241-4299; **Board Cert:** Internal Medicine 1969; Gastroenterology 1972; **Med School:** Harvard Med Sch 1963; **Resid:** Internal Medicine, Beth Israel Hosp 1965; Internal Medicine, Beth Israel Hosp 1968; **Fellow:** Gastroenterology, Mount Sinai Hosp 1970; **Fac Appt:** Clin Prof Med, Mount Sinai Sch Med

Salik, James MD (Ge) - **Spec Exp:** Colonoscopy; Liver Disease; Inflammatory Bowel Disease; **Hospital:** NYU Med Ctr (page 102); **Address:** 232 E 30th St, New York, NY 10016-8202; **Phone:** 212-889-5544; **Board Cert:** Internal Medicine 1983; Gastroenterology 1985; **Med School:** NYU Sch Med 1980; **Resid:** Internal Medicine, Bellevue Hosp 1983; **Fellow:** Gastroenterology, Bellevue Hosp 1985; **Fac Appt:** Asst Prof Med, NYU Sch Med

Scherl, Ellen MD (Ge) - **Spec Exp:** Inflammatory Bowel Disease; **Hospital:** NY-Presby Hosp (page 100), Beth Israel Med Ctr - Petrie Division (page 90); **Address:** 1315 York Ave, Mezzanine Level, New York, NY 10021; **Phone:** 212-746-5077; **Board Cert:** Internal Medicine 1983; Gastroenterology 1997; **Med School:** NY Med Coll 1977; **Resid:** Internal Medicine, Beth Israel Med Ctr 1981; **Fellow:** Gastroenterology, MT Sinai Med Ctr 1983; **Fac Appt:** Asst Prof Med, Cornell Univ-Weill Med Coll

Schmerin, Michael MD (Ge) - **Spec Exp:** Colonoscopy; Gastroscopy; Gastroesophageal Reflux Disease (GERD); **Hospital:** NY-Presby Hosp (page 100), Lenox Hill Hosp (page 94); **Address:** 1060 Park Ave, Ste 1G, New York, NY 10128-1095; **Phone:** 212-348-3166; **Board Cert:** Internal Medicine 1976; Gastroenterology 1977; **Med School:** Jefferson Med Coll 1973; **Resid:** Internal Medicine, New York Hosp-Cornell 1975; **Fellow:** Gastroenterology, New York Hosp-Cornell 1977

Schneider, Lewis MD (Ge) - **Spec Exp:** Colon Cancer; Colonoscopy/Polypectomy; Ulcerative Colitis; **Hospital:** NY-Presby Hosp (page 100); **Address:** 16 E 60th St, rm 322, New York, NY 10022; **Phone:** 212-326-8426; **Board Cert:** Internal Medicine 1981; **Med School:** SUNY Downstate 1978; **Resid:** Internal Medicine, Columbia-Presby Hosp 1981; **Fellow:** Gastroenterology, Columbia-Presby Hosp 1983

Shike, Moshe MD (Ge) - **Spec Exp:** Gastrointestinal Cancer; Nutrition & Cancer Prevention; Endoscopy; **Hospital:** Meml Sloan Kettering Cancer Ctr (page 109); **Address:** 1275 York Ave, rm S-536, New York, NY 10021; **Phone:** 212-639-7230; **Board Cert:** Internal Medicine 1977; Gastroenterology 1981; **Med School:** Israel 1975; **Resid:** Internal Medicine, Mt Auburn Hosp 1977; **Fellow:** Gastroenterology, Toronto Genl Hosp 1981; **Fac Appt:** Prof Med, Cornell Univ-Weill Med Coll

Shinya, Hiromi MD (Ge) - **Spec Exp:** Colonoscopy; Gastroscopy; Nutrition; **Hospital:** Beth Israel Med Ctr - Petrie Division (page 90); **Address:** 305 E 55th St, Ste 102, New York, NY 10022-4148; **Phone:** 212-751-9714; **Med School:** Japan 1961; **Resid:** Surgery, Beth Israel Med Ctr 1968; **Fellow:** Surgery, Beth Israel Med Ctr 1970; **Fac Appt:** Clin Prof S, Albert Einstein Coll Med

Siegel, Jerome H MD (Ge) - **Spec Exp:** Pancreatic/Biliary Endoscopy (ERCP); Colonoscopy; Colon Cancer Screening; **Hospital:** Beth Israel Med Ctr - Petrie Division (page 90), Hackensack Univ Med Ctr (page 92); **Address:** 60 E End Ave, New York, NY 10028-7907; **Phone:** 212-734-8874; **Board Cert:** Internal Medicine 1978; Gastroenterology 1979; **Med School:** Med Coll GA 1960; **Resid:** Internal Medicine, NY VA Med Ctr 1965; Gastroenterology, NY VA Med Ctr 1966; **Fellow:** Gastroenterology, Royal Free Hosp 1975; **Fac Appt:** Clin Prof Med, Albert Einstein Coll Med

Stein, Jeffrey A MD (Ge) - **Spec Exp:** Gallbladder Disease; Pancreatic Disease; **Hospital:** NY-Presby Hosp (page 100); **Address:** 161 Ft Washington Ave, rm 328, New York, NY 10032; **Phone:** 212-305-5444; **Board Cert:** Internal Medicine 1971; Gastroenterology 1973; **Med School:** Harvard Med Sch 1965; **Resid:** Internal Medicine, Presbyterian Hosp 1970; **Fellow:** Gastroenterology, Presbyterian Hosp 1971; **Fac Appt:** Clin Prof Med, Columbia P&S

Stevens, Peter D MD (Ge) - **Spec Exp:** Endoscopy; Pancreatic Disease; Pancreatic/Biliary Endoscopy (ERCP); **Hospital:** NY-Presby Hosp (page 100); **Address:** NY Presby-Columbia Presbyterian Med Ctr, 161 Fort Washington St, Ste 301, New York, NY 10032; **Phone:** 212-305-1909; **Board Cert:** Gastroenterology 2003; **Med School:** Columbia P&S 1987; **Resid:** Internal Medicine, Columbia Presby Med Ctr 1991; **Fellow:** Gastroenterology, Columbia Presby Med Ctr 1993; Endoscopy, Columbia Presby Med Ctr 1994; **Fac Appt:** Asst Clin Prof Med, Columbia P&S

Tobias, Hillel MD (Ge) - **Spec Exp:** Liver Disease; Hepatitis B & C; Liver & Biliary Disease; **Hospital:** NYU Med Ctr (page 102); **Address:** 232 E 30th St, New York, NY 10016-8202; **Phone:** 212-889-5544; **Board Cert:** Internal Medicine 1967; Gastroenterology 1979; **Med School:** Washington Univ, St Louis 1960; **Resid:** Internal Medicine, Bellevue Hosp 1963; **Fellow:** Hepatology, Royal Free Hosp 1965; Hepatology, Mount Sinai Hosp 1967; **Fac Appt:** Prof Med, NYU Sch Med

Ullman, Thomas A MD (Ge) - **Spec Exp:** Irritable Bowel Syndrome; Ulcerative Colitis; Inflammatory Bowel Disease/Crohn's; **Hospital:** Mount Sinai Med Ctr (page 98); **Address:** 5 E 98th St Fl 11, New York, NY 10029; **Phone:** 212-241-4299; **Board Cert:** Internal Medicine 1995; Gastroenterology 1999; **Med School:** Cornell Univ-Weill Med Coll 1992; **Resid:** Internal Medicine, NY Hosp 1995; **Fellow:** Gastroenterology, Yale-New Haven Hosp 1999; **Fac Appt:** Asst Prof Med, Mount Sinai Sch Med

Walfish, Jacob MD (Ge) - **Spec Exp:** Irritable Bowel Syndrome; Diagnostic Problems; **Hospital:** Mount Sinai Med Ctr (page 98); **Address:** 1150 Park Ave, New York, NY 10128; **Phone:** 212-831-5000; **Board Cert:** Internal Medicine 1977; Gastroenterology 1979; **Med School:** Harvard Med Sch 1974; **Resid:** Internal Medicine, Mount Sinai Hosp 1977; **Fellow:** Gastroenterology, Mount Sinai Hosp 1979

Waye, Jerome MD (Ge) - **Spec Exp:** Endoscopy; Colon Cancer; Colonoscopy; **Hospital:** Mount Sinai Med Ctr (page 98), Lenox Hill Hosp (page 94); **Address:** 650 Park Ave, New York, NY 10021-6115; **Phone:** 212-439-7779; **Board Cert:** Internal Medicine 1965; Gastroenterology 1970; **Med School:** Boston Univ 1958; **Resid:** Internal Medicine, Mount Sinai Hosp 1961; **Fellow:** Gastroenterology, Mount Sinai Hosp 1962; **Fac Appt:** Clin Prof Med, Mount Sinai Sch Med

Weiss, Robert A MD (Ge) - **Spec Exp:** Colon Cancer; Gastroesophageal Reflux Disease (GERD); Endoscopy; **Hospital:** Beth Israel Med Ctr - Petrie Division (page 90); **Address:** 2 W 86th St, Ste 4, New York, NY 10024-3625; **Phone:** 212-769-1700; **Board Cert:** Internal Medicine 1987; Gastroenterology 1989; **Med School:** Mount Sinai Sch Med 1983; **Resid:** Internal Medicine, Beth Israel Med Ctr 1986; **Fellow:** Gastroenterology, Elmhurst Hosp Ctr-Mt Sinai 1988; **Fac Appt:** Asst Clin Prof Med, Albert Einstein Coll Med

Winawer, Sidney J MD (Ge) - **Spec Exp:** Colonoscopy; Colon Cancer; Cancer Prevention; **Hospital:** Meml Sloan Kettering Cancer Ctr (page 109); **Address:** 1275 York Ave, Box 90, New York, NY 10021-6094; **Phone:** 212-639-7678; **Board Cert:** Internal Medicine 1965; Gastroenterology 1973; **Med School:** SUNY Downstate 1956; **Resid:** Internal Medicine, VA Hosp 1961; Internal Medicine, Maimonides Hosp 1962; **Fellow:** Gastroenterology, Boston City Hosp 1964; **Fac Appt:** Prof Med, Cornell Univ-Weill Med Coll

GERIATRIC MEDICINE

Adelman, Ronald MD (Ger) - **Hospital:** NY-Presby Hosp (page 100); **Address:** 1484 1st Ave, New York, NY 10021; **Phone:** 212-746-7000; **Board Cert:** Internal Medicine 1982; Geriatric Medicine 1998; **Med School:** Albert Einstein Coll Med 1978; **Resid:** Internal Medicine, Montefiore Hosp Med Ctr 1981

Bloom, Patricia A MD (Ger) - **Spec Exp:** Dementia; Geriatric Functional Assessment; Osteoporosis; **Hospital:** Mount Sinai Med Ctr (page 98); **Address:** 1470 Madison Ave, New York, NY 10029-6542; **Phone:** 212-659-8552; **Board Cert:** Internal Medicine 1978; Geriatric Medicine 1998; **Med School:** Univ Minn 1975; **Resid:** Internal Medicine, Montefiore Hosp 1978; **Fac Appt:** Assoc Prof Med, Mount Sinai Sch Med

Finkelstein, Martin S MD (Ger) - **Hospital:** NYU Med Ctr (page 102); **Address:** 530 1st Ave, Ste 4J, New York, NY 10016-6402; **Phone:** 212-263-7043; **Board Cert:** Internal Medicine 1970; Geriatric Medicine 1988; **Med School:** NYU Sch Med 1964; **Resid:** Internal Medicine, Bellevue Hosp 1966; Internal Medicine, Stanford Univ Med Ctr 1967; **Fellow:** Infectious Disease, Stanford Univ Med Ctr 1968; **Fac Appt:** Assoc Clin Prof Med, NYU Sch Med

Fogel, Joyce MD (Ger) **PCP** - **Spec Exp:** Memory Disorders; Geriatric Functional Assessment; **Hospital:** St Vincent Cath Med Ctrs - Manhattan (page 375); **Address:** 275 8th Ave, New York, NY 10011-8305; **Phone:** 212-463-0101; **Board Cert:** Internal Medicine 1986; Geriatric Medicine 2000; **Med School:** SUNY Downstate 1982; **Resid:** Internal Medicine, Kings Co Hosp 1986; **Fellow:** Geriatric Medicine, Bellevue/NYU Med Ctr 1989; **Fac Appt:** Assoc Clin Prof Med, NY Med Coll

Freedman, Michael L MD (Ger) - **Spec Exp:** Alzheimer's Disease; Anemia; Nutrition; **Hospital:** NYU Med Ctr (page 102), Bellevue Hosp Ctr; **Address:** 530 First Ave, Ste 4J, New York, NY 10016-6402; **Phone:** 212-263-7043; **Board Cert:** Internal Medicine 1971; Hematology 1974; Geriatric Medicine 1998; **Med School:** Tufts Univ 1963; **Resid:** Internal Medicine, Bellevue Hosp 1965; Internal Medicine, Bellevue Hosp 1969; **Fellow:** Hematology, Natl Inst Hlth-NCI 1968; **Fac Appt:** Prof Med, NYU Sch Med

Kellogg, F Russell MD (Ger) **PCP** - **Spec Exp:** Hypertension; **Hospital:** St Vincent Cath Med Ctrs - Manhattan (page 375); **Address:** 222 W 14th St, Ground Fl, New York, NY 10011; **Phone:** 212-604-1800; **Board Cert:** Internal Medicine 1998; Geriatric Medicine 1997; **Med School:** NY Med Coll 1974; **Resid:** Internal Medicine, St Vincent's Hosp 1977; **Fac Appt:** Asst Prof Med, NY Med Coll

Lachs, Mark MD (Ger) - **Spec Exp:** Abuse/Neglect; **Hospital:** NY-Presby Hosp (page 100); **Address:** Irving Sherwood Wright Center on Aging, 1484 First Ave, New York, NY 10021; **Phone:** 212-746-7000; **Board Cert:** Internal Medicine 1988; Geriatric Medicine 1992; **Med School:** NYU Sch Med 1985; **Resid:** Internal Medicine, Hosp Univ Penn 1988; **Fellow:** Geriatric Medicine, Yale Univ 1990; **Fac Appt:** Assoc Prof Med, Cornell Univ-Weill Med Coll

Leipzig, Rosanne MD (Ger) **PCP** - **Spec Exp:** Medications in the Elderly; **Hospital:** Mount Sinai Med Ctr (page 98); **Address:** 1 Gustave L. Levy Pl, Box 1070, New York, NY 10029-6500; **Phone:** 212-241-4274; **Board Cert:** Internal Medicine 1982; Geriatric Medicine 1998; **Med School:** Univ Mich Med Sch 1978; **Resid:** Internal Medicine, Strong Meml Hosp 1982; **Fellow:** Clinical Pharmacology, New York Hosp 1985; **Fac Appt:** Prof Med, Mount Sinai Sch Med

Libow, Leslie MD (Ger) - **Spec Exp:** Diagnostic Problems; **Hospital:** Mount Sinai Med Ctr (page 98); **Address:** 1 Gustave Levy Pl, Box 1070, New York, NY 10029; **Phone:** 212-659-8552; **Board Cert:** Internal Medicine 1977; Geriatric Medicine 1988; **Med School:** Univ Hlth Sci/Chicago Med Sch 1958; **Resid:** Internal Medicine, Bronx VA Hosp 1960; Internal Medicine, Mt Sinai Hosp 1964; **Fac Appt:** Prof Med, Mount Sinai Sch Med

Meier, Diane MD (Ger) - **Spec Exp:** Palliative Care; **Hospital:** Mount Sinai Med Ctr (page 98); **Address:** Mt Sinai School Medicine, Box 1070, New York, NY 10029-6501; **Phone:** 212-241-1446; **Board Cert:** Internal Medicine 1981; Geriatric Medicine 1999; **Med School:** Northwestern Univ 1977; **Resid:** Internal Medicine, Oregon Hlth Sci Univ 1981; **Fellow:** Geriatric Medicine, VA Med Ctr 1983; **Fac Appt:** Prof Med, Mount Sinai Sch Med

Nichols, Jeffrey MD (Ger) - **Spec Exp:** Dementia; Long Term Care; Home Care; **Hospital:** Cabrini Med Ctr (page 374); **Address:** 220 E 19th St, New York, NY 10019; **Phone:** 212-358-6255; **Board Cert:** Internal Medicine 1979; Geriatric Medicine 1998; **Med School:** Cornell Univ-Weill Med Coll 1976; **Resid:** Internal Medicine, St Vincent's Hosp & Med Ctr 1979; **Fac Appt:** Assoc Clin Prof Med, Mount Sinai Sch Med

Perskin, Michael MD (Ger) **PCP** - **Spec Exp:** Alzheimer's Disease; Dementia; Cholesterol/Lipid Disorders; Hypertension; **Hospital:** NYU Med Ctr (page 102), Hosp For Joint Diseases (page 107); **Address:** 235 E 38th St, New York, NY 10016-2709; **Phone:** 212-679-1410; **Board Cert:** Internal Medicine 1989; Geriatric Medicine 2000; **Med School:** Brown Univ 1986; **Resid:** Internal Medicine, St Luke's-Roosevelt Hosp Ctr 1989; **Fellow:** Geriatric Medicine, NYU Med Ctr 1991; **Fac Appt:** Asst Clin Prof Med, NYU Sch Med

Sherman, Fredrick T MD (Ger) **PCP** - **Spec Exp:** Alzheimer's Disease; Frail Elderly; Falls in the Elderly; **Hospital:** Mount Sinai Med Ctr (page 98); **Address:** Brookdale Dept Geriatrics-Mt Sinai Med Ctr, 1 Gustave Levy Pl, Box 1070, New York, NY 10029; **Phone:** 212-659-8552; **Board Cert:** Internal Medicine 1975; Geriatric Medicine 1998; **Med School:** Temple Univ 1972; **Resid:** Internal Medicine, Hosp Univ Penn 1975; **Fac Appt:** Prof Med, Mount Sinai Sch Med

Siegler, Eugenia MD (Ger) **PCP** - **Spec Exp:** Dementia; **Hospital:** NY-Presby Hosp (page 100); **Address:** Irving Sherwood Wright Ctr on Aging, 1484 First Ave, New York, NY 10021; **Phone:** 212-746-7000; **Board Cert:** Internal Medicine 1986; Geriatric Medicine 1998; **Med School:** Johns Hopkins Univ 1983; **Resid:** Internal Medicine, Bellevue Hosp 1987; **Fellow:** Geriatric Medicine, Hosp Univ Penn 1989; **Fac Appt:** Assoc Prof Med, Cornell Univ-Weill Med Coll

GERIATRIC PSYCHIATRY

Reisberg, Barry MD (GerPsy) - **Spec Exp:** Alzheimer's Disease; Dementia; Depression; **Hospital:** NYU Med Ctr (page 102); **Address:** Aging & Dementia Rsch Ctr - NYU, 550 First Ave, THN 316, New York, NY 10016; **Phone:** 212-263-8550; **Board Cert:** Psychiatry 1976; Geriatric Psychiatry 2000; **Med School:** NY Med Coll 1972; **Resid:** Psychiatry, Metropolitan Hosp 1975; **Fellow:** Psychiatric Research, Univ London 1975; **Fac Appt:** Prof Psyc, NYU Sch Med

Serby, Michael J MD (GerPsy) - **Spec Exp:** Alzheimer's Disease; Depression; Parkinson's Disease; **Hospital:** Beth Israel Med Ctr - Petrie Division (page 90); **Address:** Beth Israel Med Ctr, Dept Psychiatry, 1st Ave at 16th St, New York, NY 10003; **Phone:** 212-420-2421; **Board Cert:** Psychiatry 1979; Geriatric Psychiatry 2000; **Med School:** Emory Univ 1969; **Resid:** Psychiatry, Bellevue Hosp-NYU 1976; **Fac Appt:** Clin Prof Psyc, Albert Einstein Coll Med

GYNECOLOGIC ONCOLOGY

Abu-Rustum, Nadeem R MD (GO) - **Spec Exp:** Ovarian Cancer; Uterine Cancer; Cervical Cancer; Vulvar Disease/Cancer; **Hospital:** Meml Sloan Kettering Cancer Ctr (page 109); **Address:** Meml Sloan Kettering Cancer Ctr, 1275 York Ave, rm C1096, New York, NY 10021; **Phone:** 212-639-7051; **Board Cert:** Obstetrics & Gynecology 1998; Gynecologic Oncology 2000; **Med School:** Lebanon 1990; **Resid:** Obstetrics & Gynecology, Greater Baltimore Med Ctr 1994; **Fellow:** Gynecologic Oncology, Meml Sloan Kettering Cancer Ctr 1997; **Fac Appt:** Asst Prof ObG, Cornell Univ-Weill Med Coll

Barakat, Richard MD (GO) - **Spec Exp:** Laparoscopic Surgery; Ovarian Cancer; Uterine Cancer; **Hospital:** Meml Sloan Kettering Cancer Ctr (page 109); **Address:** Memorial Sloan Kettering Cancer Ctr, 1275 York Ave, rm C1091, New York, NY 10021; **Phone:** 212-639-2453; **Board Cert:** Obstetrics & Gynecology 1992; Gynecologic Oncology 1994; **Med School:** SUNY Hlth Sci Ctr 1985; **Resid:** Obstetrics & Gynecology, Bellevue Hosp 1989; **Fellow:** Gynecologic Oncology, Meml Sloan Kettering Cancer Ctr 1991; **Fac Appt:** Assoc Prof ObG, Cornell Univ-Weill Med Coll

Brown, Carol MD (GO) - **Spec Exp:** Gynecologic Cancer; DES-Exposed Females; Fertility Preservation in Cancer; **Hospital:** Meml Sloan Kettering Cancer Ctr (page 109); **Address:** Meml Sloan Kettering Cancer Ctr, 1275 York Ave, rm C1086, New York, NY 10021; **Phone:** 212-639-7659; **Board Cert:** Obstetrics & Gynecology 2005; Gynecologic Oncology 2005; **Med School:** Columbia P&S 1986; **Resid:** Obstetrics & Gynecology, Hosp Univ Penn 1990; **Fellow:** Gynecologic Oncology, Meml Sloan Kettering Cancer Ctr 1992; Research, Meml Sloan Kettering Cancer Ctr 1994; **Fac Appt:** Asst Prof ObG, Cornell Univ-Weill Med Coll

Calanog, Anthony MD (GO) - **Spec Exp:** Ovarian Cancer; Cervical Cancer; Uterine Cancer; **Hospital:** Lenox Hill Hosp (page 94); **Address:** 907 Fifth Ave, New York, NY 10021-4156; **Phone:** 212-838-0886; **Board Cert:** Obstetrics & Gynecology 1972; Gynecologic Oncology 1975; **Med School:** Philippines 1962; **Resid:** Obstetrics & Gynecology, St Thomas Hosp 1964; Obstetrics & Gynecology, NY Med Coll 1967; **Fellow:** Gynecologic Oncology, NY Med Coll 1972; **Fac Appt:** Clin Prof ObG, NYU Sch Med

Caputo, Thomas A MD (GO) - **Spec Exp:** Cervical Cancer; Ovarian Cancer; Uterine Cancer; **Hospital:** NY-Presby Hosp (page 100); **Address:** 525 E 68th St, Ste J130, New York, NY 10021; **Phone:** 212-746-3179; **Board Cert:** Obstetrics & Gynecology 1993; Gynecologic Oncology 1977; **Med School:** UMDNJ-NJ Med Sch, Newark 1965; **Resid:** Obstetrics & Gynecology, Martland Hosp 1969; **Fellow:** Gynecologic Oncology, Emory Univ Hosp 1974; **Fac Appt:** Clin Prof ObG, Cornell Univ-Weill Med Coll

Chuang, Linus MD (GO) - **Spec Exp:** Laparoscopic Surgery; Ovarian Cancer; Gynecologic Cancer; Minimally Invasive Surgery; **Hospital:** Mount Sinai Med Ctr (page 98), Westchester Med Ctr (page 713); **Address:** 5 E 98th St Fl 2, Box 1173, New York, NY 10029; **Phone:** 212-241-1111; **Board Cert:** Obstetrics & Gynecology 2003; Gynecologic Oncology 2003; **Med School:** Taiwan 1981; **Resid:** Obstetrics & Gynecology, Flushing Hosp 1990; **Fellow:** Gynecologic Oncology, MD Anderson Cancer Ctr 1994; **Fac Appt:** Asst Prof ObG, Mount Sinai Sch Med

Cohen, Carmel MD (GO) - **Spec Exp:** Ovarian Cancer; Cervical Cancer; Pelvic Tumors; **Hospital:** NY-Presby Hosp (page 100); **Address:** Columbia Presby Med Ctr, Div Gyn Oncol, 161 Ft Washington Ave Fl 8th - rm 837, New York, NY 10032; **Phone:** 212-305-3410; **Board Cert:** Obstetrics & Gynecology 2004; Gynecologic Oncology 2004; **Med School:** Tulane Univ 1958; **Resid:** Obstetrics & Gynecology, Mount Sinai Hosp 1964; **Fellow:** Gynecologic Oncology, Mount Sinai Hosp 1965; **Fac Appt:** Prof ObG, Columbia P&S

Curtin, John P MD (GO) - **Spec Exp:** Uterine Cancer; Ovarian Cancer; Laparoscopic Surgery; **Hospital:** NYU Med Ctr (page 102); **Address:** NYU Clinical Cancer Ctr, 160 S 34th St Fl 4, New York, NY 10016-6402; **Phone:** 212-731-5345; **Board Cert:** Obstetrics & Gynecology 1996; Gynecologic Oncology 1996; **Med School:** Creighton Univ 1979; **Resid:** Obstetrics & Gynecology, Univ Minn Med Ctr 1984; **Fellow:** Gynecologic Oncology, Meml Sloan-Kettering Cancer Ctr 1988; **Fac Appt:** Prof ObG, NYU Sch Med

Dottino, Peter R MD (GO) - **Spec Exp:** Laparoscopic Surgery; **Hospital:** Mount Sinai Med Ctr (page 98), Hackensack Univ Med Ctr (page 92); **Address:** 800 5th Ave Bldg 405, New York, NY 10021-7215; **Phone:** 212-888-8439; **Board Cert:** Obstetrics & Gynecology 1996; Gynecologic Oncology 1996; **Med School:** Georgetown Univ 1979; **Resid:** Obstetrics & Gynecology, SUNY Downstate Med Ctr 1983; **Fellow:** Gynecologic Oncology, Mount Sinai Hosp 1985

Fishman, David A MD (GO) - **Spec Exp:** Ovarian Cancer; Ovarian Cancer-Early Detection; Gynecologic Cancer; **Hospital:** NYU Med Ctr (page 102); **Address:** NYU Clinical Cancer Ctr, 160 E 34 St Fl 4, New York, NY 10016; **Phone:** 212-731-5345; **Board Cert:** Obstetrics & Gynecology 1995; Gynecologic Oncology 1998; **Med School:** Texas Tech Univ 1988; **Resid:** Obstetrics & Gynecology, Yale-New Haven Hosp 1992; **Fellow:** Gynecologic Oncology, Yale-New Haven Hosp 1994; **Fac Appt:** Prof ObG, NYU Sch Med

Herzog, Thomas J MD (GO) - **Spec Exp:** Cervical Cancer; Laparoscopic Surgery; **Hospital:** NY-Presby Hosp (page 100); **Address:** Herbert Irving Pavilian, 161 Fort Washington Ave, 8-837, New York, NY 10032; **Phone:** 212-305-3410; **Board Cert:** Obstetrics & Gynecology 2005; Gynecologic Oncology 2005; **Med School:** Univ Cincinnati 1986; **Resid:** Obstetrics & Gynecology, Good Samaritan Hosp 1990; **Fellow:** Gynecologic Oncology, Wash Univ Sch Med 1993; **Fac Appt:** Assoc Prof ObG, Washington Univ, St Louis

Koulos, John MD (GO) - **Spec Exp:** Cervical Cancer; Uterine Cancer; Ovarian Cancer; **Hospital:** Beth Israel Med Ctr - Petrie Division (page 90); **Address:** Beth Israel Hosp Cancer Ctr, 10 Union Square E, Ste 4C, New York, NY 10003; **Phone:** 212-844-5729; **Board Cert:** Obstetrics & Gynecology 2005; Gynecologic Oncology 2005; **Med School:** Northwestern Univ 1978; **Resid:** Obstetrics & Gynecology, Northwestern Univ Med Sch 1982; **Fellow:** Gynecologic Oncology, Meml Sloan Kettering Cancer Ctr 1984; **Fac Appt:** Assoc Prof ObG, NY Med Coll

Rahaman, Jamal MD (GO) - **Spec Exp:** Minimally Invasive Surgery; Gynecologic Cancer; Pelvic Reconstruction; **Hospital:** Mount Sinai Med Ctr (page 98); **Address:** Mt Sinai Med Ctr, Div Gynecologic Oncology, 5 E 98th St Fl 2, Box 1173, New York, NY 10029; **Phone:** 212-427-9898; **Board Cert:** Obstetrics & Gynecology 1996; Gynecologic Oncology 2000; **Med School:** West Indies 1984; **Resid:** Obstetrics & Gynecology, Lincoln Med Ctr 1991; Obstetrics & Gynecology, Mount Sinai Med Ctr 1993; **Fellow:** Cardiovascular Surgery, Texas Heart Inst 1990; Gynecologic Oncology, Mount Sinai Med Ctr 1995; **Fac Appt:** Asst Prof ObG, Mount Sinai Sch Med

Wallach, Robert C MD (GO) - **Spec Exp:** Vulvar & Vaginal Cancer; Ovarian Cancer; Cervical Cancer; Uterine Cancer; **Hospital:** NYU Med Ctr (page 102); **Address:** NYU Clinical Cancer Ctr, 160 E 34th St, New York, NY 10016; **Phone:** 212-735-5345; **Board Cert:** Obstetrics & Gynecology 1967; Gynecologic Oncology 1974; **Med School:** Yale Univ 1960; **Resid:** Obstetrics & Gynecology, Beth Israel Med Ctr 1965; **Fellow:** Gynecologic Oncology, SUNY Downstate Med Ctr 1966; **Fac Appt:** Prof ObG, NYU Sch Med

HAND SURGERY

Athanasian, Edward MD (HS) - **Spec Exp:** Bone & Soft Tissue Tumors; Hand & Upper Extremity Tumors; Hand & Upper Extremity Fractures; **Hospital:** Hosp For Special Surgery (page 108), Meml Sloan Kettering Cancer Ctr (page 109); **Address:** Hospital for Special Surgery, 535 E 70th St, New York, NY 10021; **Phone:** 212-606-1962; **Board Cert:** Orthopaedic Surgery 1997; Hand Surgery 1999; **Med School:** Columbia P&S 1988; **Resid:** Surgery, Beth Israel Hosp 1989; Orthopaedic Surgery, Hosp Special Surgery 1993; **Fellow:** Hand Surgery, Mayo Clinic 1994; Orthopaedic Oncology, Meml Sloan Kettering Cancer Ctr 1995; **Fac Appt:** Asst Prof OrS, Cornell Univ-Weill Med Coll

Barron, O Alton MD (HS) - **Spec Exp:** Shoulder Arthroscopic Surgery; Elbow Surgery; Nerve & Tendon Reconstruction; Shoulder Reconstruction; **Hospital:** St Luke's - Roosevelt Hosp Ctr - Roosevelt Div (page 90); **Address:** CV Starr Hand Surgery Ctr, 1000 10th Ave, Fl 3, New York, NY 10019; **Phone:** 212-523-7590; **Board Cert:** Orthopaedic Surgery 1998; Hand Surgery 2000; **Med School:** Tulane Univ 1989; **Resid:** Surgery, Tulane Univ Affil Hosps 1994; **Fellow:** Shoulder Surgery, Columbia Presby Hosp 1995; Hand Surgery, St Lukes Roosevelt Hosp; **Fac Appt:** Asst Clin Prof S, Columbia P&S

Beasley, Robert MD (HS) - **Spec Exp:** Hand Reconstruction; Hand Paralytic Disorders; Arthritis; **Hospital:** NYU Med Ctr (page 102), Bellevue Hosp Ctr; **Address:** 345 E 37th St, Ste 201, New York, NY 10016-3256; **Phone:** 212-986-9494; **Board Cert:** Plastic Surgery 1968; **Med School:** Univ Tenn Coll Med, Memphis 1953; **Resid:** Hand Surgery, Roosevelt Hosp 1961; Plastic Surgery, Columbia-Presby Med Ctr 1963; **Fac Appt:** Prof S, NYU Sch Med

Botwinick, Nelson MD (HS) - **Spec Exp:** Trauma; Carpal Tunnel Syndrome; Arthritis Hand Surgery; **Hospital:** NY Downtown Hosp; **Address:** 19 Beekman St, New York, NY 10038-1522; **Phone:** 212-513-7711; **Board Cert:** Orthopaedic Surgery 1999; Hand Surgery 2004; **Med School:** NYU Sch Med 1980; **Resid:** Orthopaedic Surgery, NYU Med Ctr 1985; **Fellow:** Orthopaedic Surgery, NYU Med Ctr 1986; **Fac Appt:** Assoc Clin Prof OrS, NYU Sch Med

Carlson, Michelle Gerwin MD (HS) - **Spec Exp:** Sports Injuries; Hand & Upper Extremity Surgery; Pediatric Hand/Arm Surgery; Hand Surgery in Women; **Hospital:** Hosp For Special Surgery (page 108), NY-Presby Hosp (page 100); **Address:** 523 E 72nd St Fl 4 - rm 439, New York, NY 10021; **Phone:** 212-606-1546; **Board Cert:** Orthopaedic Surgery 1995; Hand Surgery 1996; **Med School:** Cornell Univ-Weill Med Coll 1989; **Resid:** Surgery, Hosp Special Surg 1994; **Fellow:** Hand Surgery, Hosp Special Surg 1996; **Fac Appt:** Asst Prof OrS, Cornell Univ-Weill Med Coll

Choi, Mihye MD (HS) - **Spec Exp:** Hand Reconstruction; Peripheral Nerve Surgery; **Hospital:** NYU Med Ctr (page 102); **Address:** 530 1st Ave, Ste 8Y, New York, NY 10016; **Phone:** 212-263-6004; **Board Cert:** Plastic Surgery 1998; Hand Surgery 2000; **Med School:** Univ Rochester 1987; **Resid:** Surgery, Beth Israel Hosp 1990; Plastic Surgery, Mount Sinai Med Ctr 1995; **Fellow:** Hand Surgery, NYU Med Ctr 1996; **Fac Appt:** Assoc Prof S, NYU Sch Med

Friedman, David Wayne MD (HS) - **Spec Exp:** Hand Reconstruction; **Hospital:** NYU Med Ctr (page 102); **Address:** 345 E 37th St, Ste 201, New York, NY 10016; **Phone:** 212-986-9494; **Board Cert:** Surgery 1995; Plastic Surgery 1999; Hand Surgery 2000; **Med School:** Univ Tex SW, Dallas 1988; **Resid:** Surgery, UMDNJ Med Ctr 1994; Plastic Surgery, NYU Med Ctr 1996; **Fellow:** Hand Surgery, NYU Med Ctr 1997; **Fac Appt:** Assoc Prof S, NYU Sch Med

Glickel, Steven MD (HS) - **Spec Exp:** Hand & Wrist Surgery; Elbow Surgery; Peripheral Nerve Surgery; **Hospital:** St Luke's - Roosevelt Hosp Ctr - Roosevelt Div (page 90); **Address:** 1000 10th Ave Fl 3, New York, NY 10019; **Phone:** 212-523-7590; **Board Cert:** Orthopaedic Surgery 1985; Hand Surgery 1998; **Med School:** Harvard Med Sch 1976; **Resid:** Surgery, Columbia Presby Hosp 1978; Orthopaedic Surgery, Harvard Comb Ortho 1981; **Fellow:** Hand Surgery, St Luke's-Roosevelt Hosp Ctr 1983; Research, Columbia Presby Hosp 1982; **Fac Appt:** Assoc Clin Prof OrS, Columbia P&S

Grad, Joel MD (HS) - **Spec Exp:** Carpal Tunnel Syndrome; Tendon Surgery; **Hospital:** St Vincent Cath Med Ctrs - Manhattan (page 375), NY-Presby Hosp (page 100); **Address:** 95 University Place, New York, NY 10003; **Phone:** 212-604-1362; **Board Cert:** Orthopaedic Surgery 1984; **Med School:** SUNY Downstate 1976; **Resid:** Surgery, St Vincents Hosp 1978; Orthopaedic Surgery, NYU Med Ctr 1981; **Fellow:** Hand Surgery, Hand Surg Assoc 1982; **Fac Appt:** Asst Prof OrS, NYU Sch Med

King, William MD (HS) - **Spec Exp:** Carpal Tunnel Syndrome; Hand Reconstruction; Microvascular Surgery; **Hospital:** Hosp For Joint Diseases (page 107), Beth Israel Med Ctr - Petrie Division (page 90); **Address:** 159 E 74th St Fl 2, New York, NY 10021; **Phone:** 212-744-1620; **Board Cert:** Orthopaedic Surgery 1999; **Med School:** Columbia P&S 1974; **Resid:** Surgery, St Lukes Roosevelt Hosp Ctr 1976; Orthopaedic Surgery, Columbia-Presby Med Ctr 1979; **Fellow:** Hand & Microvascular Surgery, Univ Colorado Hosp 1980; **Fac Appt:** Asst Prof OrS, NYU Sch Med

Lenzo, Salvatore MD (HS) - **Spec Exp:** Carpal Tunnel Syndrome; Arthritis Hand Surgery; Hand & Wrist Injuries; **Hospital:** Hosp For Joint Diseases (page 107), NYU Med Ctr (page 102); **Address:** 955 5th Ave, New York, NY 10021; **Phone:** 212-734-9949; **Board Cert:** Orthopaedic Surgery 2000; Hand Surgery 2000; **Med School:** NYU Sch Med 1981; **Resid:** Orthopaedic Surgery, Bellevue Hosp 1986; **Fellow:** Hand Surgery, Bellevue Hosp 1987; **Fac Appt:** Assoc Prof OrS, NYU Sch Med

Melone Jr, Charles P MD (HS) - **Spec Exp:** Arthritis; Wrist Surgery; Fractures; **Hospital:** Beth Israel Med Ctr - Petrie Division (page 90); **Address:** 321 E 34th St, New York, NY 10016; **Phone:** 212-340-0000; **Board Cert:** Orthopaedic Surgery 1976; Hand Surgery 2004; **Med School:** Georgetown Univ 1969; **Resid:** Surgery, Nassau County Med Ctr 1971; Orthopaedic Surgery, Nassau County Med Ctr 1974; **Fellow:** Hand Surgery, NYU Med Ctr 1975; **Fac Appt:** Clin Prof OrS, Albert Einstein Coll Med

Pruzansky, Mark E MD (HS) - **Spec Exp:** Arthritis Hand Surgery; Carpal Tunnel Syndrome; Microsurgery; Wrist Surgery; **Hospital:** Mount Sinai Med Ctr (page 98), Lenox Hill Hosp (page 94); **Address:** 975 Park Ave, New York, NY 10028; **Phone:** 212-249-8700; **Board Cert:** Orthopaedic Surgery 1980; Hand Surgery 2003; **Med School:** Mount Sinai Sch Med 1974; **Resid:** Orthopaedic Surgery, Mount Sinai Med Ctr 1978; **Fellow:** Hand Surgery, South Baptist Hosp 1978; Hand Surgery, Pacific Presby Hosp 1979; **Fac Appt:** Asst Prof OrS, Mount Sinai Sch Med

Raskin, Keith MD (HS) - **Spec Exp:** Wrist/Hand Injuries; Arthritis; Carpal Tunnel Syndrome; **Hospital:** NYU Med Ctr (page 102), Hosp For Joint Diseases (page 107); **Address:** 317 E 34th St, Fl 3, New York, NY 10016; **Phone:** 212-263-4263; **Board Cert:** Orthopaedic Surgery 1991; Hand Surgery 1993; **Med School:** Geo Wash Univ 1983; **Resid:** Orthopaedic Surgery, NYU Med Ctr 1988; **Fellow:** Hand Surgery, Union Mem Hosp 1989; **Fac Appt:** Assoc Clin Prof OrS, NYU Sch Med

Rosenwasser, Melvin MD (HS) - **Spec Exp:** Carpal Tunnel Syndrome; Hand Surgery; Sports Medicine-Hand; **Hospital:** NY-Presby Hosp (page 100); **Address:** 622 W 168th St, PH 11, rm 1119, New York, NY 10032; **Phone:** 212-305-4565; **Board Cert:** Orthopaedic Surgery 1999; Hand Surgery 1999; **Med School:** Columbia P&S 1976; **Resid:** Surgery, Roosevelt Hosp 1979; Orthopaedic Surgery, Columbia Presby Hosp 1982; **Fellow:** Hand Surgery, Columbia Presby Hosp 1983; **Fac Appt:** Prof OrS, Columbia P&S

Strauch, Robert MD (HS) - **Spec Exp:** Hand Reconstruction; Hand & Elbow Nerve Disorders; Hand & Wrist Injuries; **Hospital:** NY-Presby Hosp (page 100); **Address:** 622 W 168th St, rm PH-11, New York, NY 10032; **Phone:** 212-305-4272; **Board Cert:** Orthopaedic Surgery 2005; Hand Surgery 2005; **Med School:** Columbia P&S 1986; **Resid:** Orthopaedic Surgery, Columbia-Presby Hosp 1991; **Fellow:** Hand Surgery, Indiana Hand Center 1992; **Fac Appt:** Assoc Prof OrS, Columbia P&S

Weiland, Andrew J MD (HS) - **Spec Exp:** Wrist/Hand Injuries; Hand Reconstruction; **Hospital:** Hosp For Special Surgery (page 108), NY-Presby Hosp (page 100); **Address:** 535 E 70th St, New York, NY 10021-4872; **Phone:** 212-606-1575; **Board Cert:** Orthopaedic Surgery 1992; Hand Surgery 1989; **Med School:** Wake Forest Univ 1968; **Resid:** Surgery, Univ Michigan Med Ctr 1970; Orthopaedic Surgery, Johns Hopkins Hosp 1975; **Fellow:** Hand Surgery, Kleinert Hosp 1975; **Fac Appt:** Prof OrS, Cornell Univ-Weill Med Coll

Wolfe, Scott W MD (HS) - **Spec Exp:** Wrist Surgery; Nerve Disorders; Fractures; **Hospital:** Hosp For Special Surgery (page 108), St Vincent's Med Ctr - Bridgeport; **Address:** Hand & Upper Extremity Surgery, 535 E 70 St, New York, NY 10021-4872; **Phone:** 212-606-1529; **Board Cert:** Orthopaedic Surgery 2003; Hand Surgery 2003; **Med School:** Cornell Univ-Weill Med Coll 1984; **Resid:** Orthopaedic Surgery, Hosp Special Surg 1989; **Fellow:** Hand & Microvascular Surgery, Columbia Presby Med Ctr 1990; **Fac Appt:** Prof OrS, Cornell Univ-Weill Med Coll

Yang, S Steven MD (HS) - **Spec Exp:** Hand Surgery; Shoulder Surgery; **Hospital:** Lenox Hill Hosp (page 94); **Address:** 130 E 77th St Fl 7, New York, NY 10021; **Phone:** 212-744-8114; **Board Cert:** Orthopaedic Surgery 1998; Hand Surgery 2003; **Med School:** Duke Univ 1988; **Resid:** Orthopaedic Surgery, Lenox Hill Hosp 1994; **Fellow:** Hand Surgery, Hosp for Special Surgery 1995

HEMATOLOGY

Aledort, Louis MD (Hem) - **Spec Exp:** Bleeding/Coagulation Disorders; Platelet Disorders; **Hospital:** Mount Sinai Med Ctr (page 98); **Address:** Mount Sinai Med Ctr, Box 1006, New York, NY 10024; **Phone:** 212-241-7971; **Board Cert:** Internal Medicine 1966; Hematology 1972; **Med School:** Albert Einstein Coll Med 1959; **Resid:** Internal Medicine, Univ Va Hlth Sci Ctr 1961; Hematology, Nat Inst Health 1963; **Fellow:** Internal Medicine, Strong Meml Hosp 1964; Hematology, Strong Meml Hosp 1966; **Fac Appt:** Prof Med, Mount Sinai Sch Med

Amorosi, Edward MD (Hem) - **Hospital:** NYU Med Ctr (page 102); **Address:** NYU Clinical Cancer Ctr, 160 E 34th St, New York, NY 10016; **Phone:** 212-731-5187; **Board Cert:** Internal Medicine 1966; Hematology 1972; **Med School:** NYU Sch Med 1959; **Resid:** Internal Medicine, Bellevue Hosp Ctr- NYU 1962; Internal Medicine, Francis Delafield Hosp 1963; **Fellow:** Hematology, NYU Med Ctr 1965; **Fac Appt:** Prof Med, NYU Sch Med

Castro-Malaspina, Hugo MD (Hem) - **Spec Exp:** Myelodysplastic Syndromes; Bone Marrow Failure; Bone Marrow Transplant; Anemia-Aplastic; **Hospital:** Meml Sloan Kettering Cancer Ctr (page 109); **Address:** Meml Sloan Kettering Cancer Ctr, Dept Med, 1275 York Ave, New York, NY 10021; **Phone:** 212-639-8197; **Med School:** Peru 1971; **Resid:** Internal Medicine, St Louis Hosp; **Fellow:** Hematology & Oncology, Andean Biology Inst; Pediatric Hematology-Oncology, St Louis Hosp

Coller, Barry MD (Hem) - **Spec Exp:** Bleeding/Coagulation Disorders; Thrombotic Disorders; Glanzmann's Thrombasthenia; **Hospital:** Rockefeller Univ, Mount Sinai Med Ctr (page 98); **Address:** Rockefeller Univ, 1230 York Ave, New York, NY 10021; **Phone:** 212-327-7490; **Board Cert:** Internal Medicine 1973; Hematology 1975; **Med School:** NYU Sch Med 1970; **Resid:** Internal Medicine, Bellevue Hosp 1972; **Fellow:** Hematology, Natl Inst Hlth Clin Ctr 1974; **Fac Appt:** Clin Prof Med, Mount Sinai Sch Med

Cook, Perry MD (Hem) - **Spec Exp:** Bone Marrow Transplant; Leukemia; Lymphoma; **Hospital:** NYU Med Ctr (page 102); **Address:** 160 E 34th St, New York, NY 10016; **Phone:** 212-731-5184; **Board Cert:** Internal Medicine 1980; Hematology 1982; Medical Oncology 1983; **Med School:** Univ Iowa Coll Med 1977; **Resid:** Internal Medicine, St Luke's-Roosevelt Hosp Ctr 1979; Internal Medicine, Columbia-Presby Med Ctr 1980; **Fellow:** Hematology & Oncology, Columbia-Presby Med Ctr 1983; **Fac Appt:** Assoc Clin Prof Med, NYU Sch Med

Cuttner, Janet MD (Hem) - **Spec Exp:** Leukemia; Lymphoma; **Hospital:** Mount Sinai Med Ctr (page 98); **Address:** 1735 York Ave, Ste P2, New York, NY 10128; **Phone:** 212-860-9055; **Board Cert:** Internal Medicine 1984; Hematology 1986; **Med School:** Med Coll PA Hahnemann 1957; **Resid:** Internal Medicine, Kings County Hosp 1961; **Fellow:** Hematology, Mount Sinai Med Ctr 1963; **Fac Appt:** Prof Med, Mount Sinai Sch Med

De La Fuente, Beatriz MD (Hem) - **Spec Exp:** Bleeding/Coagulation Disorders; Thrombotic Disorders; **Hospital:** St Luke's - Roosevelt Hosp Ctr - Roosevelt Div (page 90); **Address:** 57 W 57th St, Ste 1107, New York, NY 10019; **Phone:** 212-838-9707; **Med School:** Mexico 1973; **Resid:** Internal Medicine, St Barnabas Med Ctr 1978; **Fellow:** Hematology, Univ Conn Hlth Ctr 1980; Thrombosis, Univ Conn Hlth Ctr 1985; **Fac Appt:** Assoc Clin Prof Med, Columbia P&S

Diaz, Michael MD (Hem) - **Spec Exp:** Anemia; Bleeding/Coagulation Disorders; Lymphoma; **Hospital:** Mount Sinai Med Ctr (page 98); **Address:** 1112 Park Ave, New York, NY 10128; **Phone:** 212-876-4500; **Board Cert:** Internal Medicine 1979; Hematology 1986; **Med School:** St Louis Univ 1971; **Resid:** Internal Medicine, Lenox Hill Hosp 1974; **Fellow:** Hematology, Mt Sinai Med Ctr 1976; **Fac Appt:** Asst Clin Prof Med, Mount Sinai Sch Med

Distenfeld, Ariel MD (Hem) - **Spec Exp:** Anemia; Bleeding/Coagulation Disorders; Hematologic Malignancies; **Hospital:** Cabrini Med Ctr (page 374), NYU Med Ctr (page 102); **Address:** 227 E 19th St, New York, NY 10003-2602; **Phone:** 212-995-6695; **Board Cert:** Internal Medicine 1964; Hematology 1974; **Med School:** NYU Sch Med 1957; **Resid:** Internal Medicine, Bellevue Hosp 1960; **Fellow:** Hematology, NYU Med Ctr 1961; **Fac Appt:** Assoc Clin Prof Med, NYU Sch Med

Diuguid, David L MD (Hem) - **Spec Exp:** Bleeding/Coagulation Disorders; **Hospital:** NY-Presby Hosp (page 100); **Address:** 161 Ft Washington Ave, Rm 862, New York, NY 10032; **Phone:** 212-305-0527; **Board Cert:** Internal Medicine 1982; Hematology 1986; Medical Oncology 1985; **Med School:** Cornell Univ-Weill Med Coll 1979; **Resid:** Internal Medicine, Boston Univ Med Ctr 1983; **Fellow:** Hematology & Oncology, New England Med Ctr 1986; **Fac Appt:** Assoc Prof Med, Columbia P&S

Hematology

Fruchtman, Steven M MD (Hem) - **Spec Exp:** Myeloproliferative Disorders; Polycythemia Rubra Vera; Stem Cell Transplant; **Address:** 1111 Park Ave, New York, NY 10029; **Phone:** 212-427-7700; **Board Cert:** Internal Medicine 1980; Hematology 1984; **Med School:** NY Med Coll 1977; **Resid:** Internal Medicine, Univ Hosp/SUNY 1981; **Fellow:** Hematology, Mount Sinai Med Ctr 1984; Hematology, Meml Sloan Kettering Cancer Ctr 1985; **Fac Appt:** Assoc Prof Med, NY Med Coll

Goldenberg, Alec MD (Hem) - **Spec Exp:** Breast Cancer; Lymphoma; Bleeding/Coagulation Disorders; **Hospital:** NYU Med Ctr (page 102); **Address:** 157 E 32nd St Fl 2, New York, NY 10016; **Phone:** 212-689-6791; **Board Cert:** Internal Medicine 1986; Medical Oncology 1987; **Med School:** Johns Hopkins Univ 1980; **Resid:** Internal Medicine, Bellevue Hosp-NYU 1984; **Fellow:** Hematology & Oncology, Meml Sloan Kettering Canc Ctr 1988; **Fac Appt:** Assoc Clin Prof Med, NYU Sch Med

Halperin, Ira MD (Hem) - **Spec Exp:** Leukemia; Myeloproliferative Disorders; **Hospital:** St Vincent Cath Med Ctrs - Manhattan (page 375); **Address:** 2 Fifth Ave, Ste 9, New York, NY 10011-8855; **Phone:** 212-254-5940; **Board Cert:** Internal Medicine 1970; Hematology 1976; Medical Oncology 1979; **Med School:** NYU Sch Med 1962; **Resid:** Internal Medicine, St Vincents Hosp 1966; **Fellow:** Hematology, Mount Sinai Hosp 1969

Hymes, Kenneth MD (Hem) - **Spec Exp:** Bleeding/Coagulation Disorders; Lymphoma; Leukemia; **Hospital:** NYU Med Ctr (page 102); **Address:** NYU Clinical Cancer Center, 160 E 34th St, New York, NY 10016-6402; **Phone:** 212-731-5189; **Board Cert:** Internal Medicine 1978; Hematology 1980; Medical Oncology 1981; **Med School:** SUNY Upstate Med Univ 1975; **Resid:** Internal Medicine, Barnes Hosp 1978; **Fellow:** Hematology, NYU Med Ctr 1980; Medical Oncology, NYU Med Ctr 1981; **Fac Appt:** Assoc Prof Med, NYU Sch Med

Kempin, Sanford Jay MD (Hem) - **Spec Exp:** Bleeding/Coagulation Disorders; Leukemia; Lymphoma; **Hospital:** St Vincent Cath Med Ctrs - Manhattan (page 375); **Address:** St Vincents Cancer Ctr, 325 W 15th St, Ground Fl, New York, NY 10011; **Phone:** 212-604-6010; **Board Cert:** Internal Medicine 1976; Medical Oncology 1977; Hematology 1978; **Med School:** Belgium 1971; **Resid:** Internal Medicine, Lemuel Shattuck Hosp 1972; **Fellow:** Hematology, St Jude Chldns Hosp 1975; Medical Oncology, Meml Sloan Kettering Cancer Ctr 1976

Leonard, John P MD (Hem) - **Spec Exp:** Lymphoma; Multiple Myeloma; Hematologic Malignancies; **Hospital:** NY-Presby Hosp (page 100); **Address:** NY Presby Hosp-NY Weill Cornell Med Ctr, 525 E 68 St, Box 403, New York, NY 10021; **Phone:** 212-746-2932; **Board Cert:** Internal Medicine 1993; Hematology 1996; Medical Oncology 1997; **Med School:** Univ VA Sch Med 1990; **Resid:** Internal Medicine, NY Hosp-Cornell Med Ctr 1993; **Fellow:** Hematology & Oncology, NY Hosp-Cornell Med Ctr 1996; **Fac Appt:** Assoc Prof Med, Cornell Univ-Weill Med Coll

Levine, Randy MD (Hem) - **Spec Exp:** Hematologic Malignancies; AIDS Related Cancers; **Hospital:** Lenox Hill Hosp (page 94); **Address:** 4 E 76th St, New York, NY 10021; **Phone:** 212-717-1020; **Board Cert:** Internal Medicine 1982; Hematology 1984; Blood Banking 1985; **Med School:** SUNY Buffalo 1979; **Resid:** Internal Medicine, Montefiore Hosp Med Ctr 1982; **Fellow:** Hematology, Montefiore Hosp Med Ctr 1983; Blood Banking, Mt Sinai Hosp 1984

Mears, John Gregory MD (Hem) - **Spec Exp:** Lymphoma; Leukemia; Multiple Myeloma; Breast Cancer; **Hospital:** NY-Presby Hosp (page 100); **Address:** 161 Ft Washington Ave, New York, NY 10032-3713; **Phone:** 212-305-3506; **Board Cert:** Internal Medicine 1976; Hematology 1978; **Med School:** Columbia P&S 1973; **Resid:** Internal Medicine, Boston Univ Med Ctr 1975; **Fellow:** Hematology & Oncology, Columbia-Presby Med Ctr 1978; **Fac Appt:** Clin Prof Med, Columbia P&S

Moskovits, Tibor MD (Hem) - **Spec Exp:** Lymphoma; Breast Cancer; Lung Cancer; **Hospital:** NYU Med Ctr (page 102), NY Downtown Hosp; **Address:** NYU Clinical Cancer Ctr, 160 E 34th St, New York, NY 10016; **Phone:** 212-731-5191; **Board Cert:** Internal Medicine 1988; Hematology 2003; Medical Oncology 1993; **Med School:** SUNY Downstate 1985; **Resid:** Internal Medicine, Beth Israel Med Ctr 1989; **Fellow:** Hematology & Oncology, NYU Med Ctr 1992; **Fac Appt:** Asst Clin Prof Med, NYU Sch Med

Nimer, Stephen D MD (Hem) - **Spec Exp:** Bone Marrow Transplant; Anemia-Aplastic; Leukemia; Stem Cell Transplant; **Hospital:** Meml Sloan Kettering Cancer Ctr (page 109); **Address:** Memorial Sloan Kettering Cancer Ctr, 1275 York Ave, Box 575, New York, NY 10021; **Phone:** 212-639-7871; **Board Cert:** Internal Medicine 1982; Hematology 1986; Medical Oncology 1985; **Med School:** Univ Chicago-Pritzker Sch Med 1979; **Resid:** Internal Medicine, UCLA Med Ctr 1982; **Fellow:** Hematology & Oncology, UCLA Med Ctr 1986; **Fac Appt:** Assoc Prof Med, Cornell Univ-Weill Med Coll

Raphael, Bruce MD (Hem) - **Spec Exp:** Lymphoma; Leukemia; Multiple Myeloma; **Hospital:** NYU Med Ctr (page 102), NY Downtown Hosp; **Address:** 160 E 34th Street Ave Fl 7, NYU Clinical Cancer Ctr, New York, NY 10016-6402; **Phone:** 212-731-5185; **Board Cert:** Internal Medicine 1978; Hematology 1980; Medical Oncology 1981; **Med School:** McGill Univ 1975; **Resid:** Internal Medicine, Jewish Genl Hosp 1977; **Fellow:** Medical Oncology, Meml Sloan Kettering Cancer Ctr 1978; Hematology, NYU Med Ctr 1980; **Fac Appt:** Assoc Prof Med, NYU Sch Med

Savage, David G MD (Hem) - **Spec Exp:** Stem Cell Transplant; Multiple Myeloma; Lymphoma; **Hospital:** NY-Presby Hosp (page 100); **Address:** 177 Fort Washington Ave, rm 6-435, New York, NY 10032; **Phone:** 212-305-9783; **Board Cert:** Internal Medicine 1977; Hematology 1982; Medical Oncology 1985; **Med School:** Columbia P&S 1971; **Resid:** Internal Medicine, Harlem Hosp/Columbia Presby Med Ctr 1975; **Fellow:** Hematology & Oncology, Harlem Hosp/Columbia Presby Med Ctr 1977; **Fac Appt:** Assoc Prof Med, Columbia P&S

Schuster, Michael MD (Hem) - **Spec Exp:** Bone Marrow Transplant; **Hospital:** NY-Presby Hosp (page 100); **Address:** NY Weill Cornell Medical Ctr, 525 E 68th St, Starr 341, New York, NY 10021; **Phone:** 212-746-2119; **Board Cert:** Internal Medicine 1984; Hematology 1986; **Med School:** Dartmouth Med Sch 1980; **Resid:** Internal Medicine, New England Deaconess Hosp 1983; **Fellow:** Hematology & Oncology, Beth Israel Med Ctr 1987; **Fac Appt:** Assoc Prof Med, Cornell Univ-Weill Med Coll

Scigliano, Eileen MD (Hem) - **Spec Exp:** Bone Marrow Transplant; **Hospital:** Mount Sinai Med Ctr (page 98); **Address:** 19 E 98th St, Box 1410, New York, NY 10029-6501; **Phone:** 212-241-6021; **Board Cert:** Internal Medicine 1984; Hematology 1988; **Med School:** Israel 1981; **Resid:** Internal Medicine, Kings County Hosp 1984; **Fellow:** Medical Oncology, VA Med Ctr 1985; Hematology, Mount Sinai 1988; **Fac Appt:** Asst Prof Med, Mount Sinai Sch Med

Troy, Kevin MD (Hem) - **Spec Exp:** Leukemia; Lymphoma; Multiple Myeloma; **Hospital:** Mount Sinai Med Ctr (page 98); **Address:** 1735 York Ave, Ste P2, New York, NY 10128; **Phone:** 212-860-9055; **Board Cert:** Internal Medicine 1982; Hematology 1984; **Med School:** Univ Conn 1979; **Resid:** Internal Medicine, Lenox Hill Hosp 1982; **Fellow:** Hematology, Mount Sinai Hosp 1984; **Fac Appt:** Assoc Clin Prof Med, Mount Sinai Sch Med

Waxman, Samuel MD (Hem) - **Spec Exp:** Lymphoma; Breast Cancer; **Hospital:** Mount Sinai Med Ctr (page 98); **Address:** 1150 5th Ave, Ste 1A, New York, NY 10128-0724; **Phone:** 212-289-2828; **Board Cert:** Internal Medicine 1971; Hematology 1972; **Med School:** SUNY Downstate 1963; **Resid:** Internal Medicine, Mount Sinai Hosp 1966; **Fellow:** Hematology, Mount Sinai Hosp 1970; **Fac Appt:** Clin Prof Med, Mount Sinai Sch Med

Wisch, Nathaniel MD (Hem) - **Spec Exp:** Lymphoma; Breast Cancer; Leukemia; **Hospital:** Lenox Hill Hosp (page 94), Mount Sinai Med Ctr (page 98); **Address:** 12 E 86th St, New York, NY 10028-0506; **Phone:** 212-861-6660; **Board Cert:** Internal Medicine 1965; Hematology 1972; Medical Oncology 1977; **Med School:** Northwestern Univ 1958; **Resid:** Internal Medicine, VA Hosp 1960; Internal Medicine, Montefiore Hosp 1961; **Fellow:** Hematology, Mount Sinai Hosp 1962; **Fac Appt:** Assoc Prof Med, Mount Sinai Sch Med

Zalusky, Ralph MD (Hem) - **Spec Exp:** Anemia; Leukemia; Lymphoma; **Hospital:** Beth Israel Med Ctr - Petrie Division (page 90); **Address:** Beth Israel Med Ctr, First Ave at 16th St, New York, NY 10003; **Phone:** 212-420-4185; **Board Cert:** Internal Medicine 1964; Hematology 1972; **Med School:** Boston Univ 1957; **Resid:** Internal Medicine, Duke Univ Med Ctr 1962; **Fellow:** Hematology, Boston Med Ctr/Harvard 1961; **Fac Appt:** Prof Med, Albert Einstein Coll Med

INFECTIOUS DISEASE

Badshah, Cyrus S MD/PhD (Inf) - **Spec Exp:** Tuberculosis; AIDS/HIV; **Hospital:** Harlem Hosp Ctr, Montefiore Med Ctr; **Address:** Harlem Hospital, MLK Bldg, 506 Lenox Ave, rm 3101A, New York, NY 10037; **Phone:** 212-939-2310; **Board Cert:** Internal Medicine 1999; Infectious Disease 2001; **Med School:** India 1986; **Resid:** Internal Medicine, Montefiore -Weiler Einstein Med Ctr 1999; **Fellow:** Infectious Disease, Cornell Univ/Meml Sloan-Kettering Cancer Ctr

Baum, Stephen MD (Inf) - **Spec Exp:** Viral Infections; AIDS/HIV; **Hospital:** Beth Israel Med Ctr - Petrie Division (page 90); **Address:** Beth Israel Med Ctr, Dept Medicine, 1st Ave & 16th St, New York, NY 10003-2929; **Phone:** 212-420-4059; **Board Cert:** Internal Medicine 1972; Infectious Disease 1972; **Med School:** NYU Sch Med 1962; **Resid:** Internal Medicine, Boston City Hosp 1964; **Fellow:** Infectious Disease, Nat Inst Hlth 1967; **Fac Appt:** Prof Med, Albert Einstein Coll Med

Bell, Evan MD (Inf) - **Spec Exp:** Travel Medicine; AIDS/HIV; **Hospital:** Lenox Hill Hosp (page 94); **Address:** 110 E 59th St, Ste 10B, New York, NY 10022; **Phone:** 212-583-2828; **Board Cert:** Internal Medicine 1983; Infectious Disease 1986; **Med School:** Univ Pennsylvania 1980; **Resid:** Internal Medicine, Lenox Hill Hosp 1983; **Fellow:** Infectious Disease, Lenox Hill Hosp 1985

Blaser, Martin J MD (Inf) - **Spec Exp:** Fevers of Unknown Origin; Infections-Gastrointestinal; Diarrheal Diseases; **Hospital:** NYU Med Ctr (page 102), Bellevue Hosp Ctr; **Address:** 550 1st Ave, OBV-A606, New York, NY 10016; **Phone:** 212-263-6394; **Board Cert:** Internal Medicine 1977; Infectious Disease 1980; **Med School:** NYU Sch Med 1973; **Resid:** Internal Medicine, Univ Colorado Med Ctr 1977; **Fellow:** Infectious Disease, Univ Colorado Med Ctr 1979; **Fac Appt:** Prof Med, NYU Sch Med

New York (Manhattan)

Brause, Barry MD (Inf) - **Spec Exp:** Bone/Joint Infections; Skin/Soft Tissue Infection; Infections in Prosthetic Devices; **Hospital:** Hosp For Special Surgery (page 108), NY-Presby Hosp (page 100); **Address:** 535 E 70th St, New York, NY 10021-5718; **Phone:** 212-570-6122; **Board Cert:** Internal Medicine 1973; Infectious Disease 1976; **Med School:** Univ Pittsburgh 1970; **Resid:** Internal Medicine, New York Hosp 1973; **Fellow:** Infectious Disease, New York Hosp 1975; **Fac Appt:** Clin Prof Med, Cornell Univ-Weill Med Coll

Brown, Arthur E MD (Inf) - **Spec Exp:** Infections in Cancer Patients; Fungal Infections; Infections in Immunocompromised Patients; **Hospital:** Meml Sloan Kettering Cancer Ctr (page 109); **Address:** 1275 York Ave, New York, NY 10021; **Phone:** 212-639-8475; **Med School:** Jefferson Med Coll 1971; **Resid:** Internal Medicine, Roosevelt Hosp 1972; Internal Medicine, USPHS Hosp-Staten Island NY & USPHS Hosp 1974; **Fellow:** Internal Medicine, Roosevelt Hosp 1976; Infectious Disease, Mem Sloan Kettering Cancer Ctr 1978; **Fac Appt:** Clin Prof Med, Cornell Univ-Weill Med Coll

Busillo, Christopher MD (Inf) - **Spec Exp:** AIDS/HIV; Travel Medicine; Lyme Disease; **Hospital:** NY Downtown Hosp; **Address:** 170 William St, FL 7, New York, NY 10038-2668; **Phone:** 212-238-0102; **Board Cert:** Internal Medicine 2000; Infectious Disease 2000; **Med School:** Italy 1986; **Resid:** Internal Medicine, Cabrini Med Ctr 1989; **Fellow:** Infectious Disease, Cabrini Med Ctr 1991

Greene, Jeffrey MD (Inf) - **Spec Exp:** AIDS/HIV; **Hospital:** NYU Med Ctr (page 102); **Address:** 104 E 40th St, Ste 603, New York, NY 10016; **Phone:** 212-375-2940; **Board Cert:** Internal Medicine 1979; Infectious Disease 1982; **Med School:** NYU Sch Med 1976; **Resid:** Internal Medicine, Bellevue Hosp 1979; **Fellow:** Infectious Disease, Bellevue Hosp 1982; **Fac Appt:** Assoc Clin Prof Med, NYU Sch Med

Gumprecht, Jeffrey Paul MD (Inf) - **Spec Exp:** AIDS/HIV; Travel Medicine; Infections-Surgical; **Hospital:** Mount Sinai Med Ctr (page 98); **Address:** 1100 Park Ave, New York, NY 10128; **Phone:** 212-427-9550; **Board Cert:** Internal Medicine 1987; Infectious Disease 1990; **Med School:** Albany Med Coll 1983; **Resid:** Internal Medicine, Mount Sinai Hosp 1987; Internal Medicine, Mount Sinai Hosp 1990; **Fellow:** Infectious Disease, Montefiore Med Ctr 1990; **Fac Appt:** Prof Med, Mount Sinai Sch Med

Hammer, Glenn MD (Inf) - **Spec Exp:** AIDS/HIV; Hospital Acquired Infections; Infections-Surgical; **Hospital:** Mount Sinai Med Ctr (page 98); **Address:** 1100 Park Ave, New York, NY 10128; **Phone:** 212-427-9550; **Board Cert:** Infectious Disease 1974; Internal Medicine 1973; **Med School:** NYU Sch Med 1969; **Resid:** Internal Medicine, Mount Sinai Hosp 1972; **Fellow:** Infectious Disease, Mount Sinai Hosp 1974; **Fac Appt:** Asst Clin Prof Med, Mount Sinai Sch Med

Hammer, Scott M MD (Inf) - **Spec Exp:** AIDS/HIV; **Hospital:** NY-Presby Hosp (page 100); **Address:** 622 W 168th St, Bldg PH - rm 876 West, New York, NY 10032; **Phone:** 212-305-7185; **Board Cert:** Internal Medicine 1975; Infectious Disease 1980; **Med School:** Columbia P&S 1972; **Resid:** Internal Medicine, Columbia-Presby Hosp 1975; Internal Medicine, Stanford Univ Hosp 1976; **Fellow:** Infectious Disease, Mass Genl Hosp 1981; **Fac Appt:** Prof Med, Columbia P&S

Hartman, Barry Jay MD (Inf) - **Spec Exp:** Endocarditis; Infections-Surgical; Parasitic Infections; **Hospital:** NY-Presby Hosp (page 100); **Address:** 407 E 70th St, Fl 4, New York, NY 10021-5302; **Phone:** 212-744-4882; **Board Cert:** Internal Medicine 1976; Infectious Disease 1980; **Med School:** Penn State Univ-Hershey Med Ctr 1973; **Resid:** Internal Medicine, New York Hosp /Cornell Med Ctr 1976; **Fellow:** Infectious Disease, New York Hosp/ Cornell Med Ctr 1981; **Fac Appt:** Clin Prof Med, Cornell Univ-Weill Med Coll

Helfgott, David MD (Inf) - **Spec Exp:** Infections in Immunocompromised Patients; Travel Medicine; **Hospital:** NY-Presby Hosp (page 100); **Address:** 212 E 68th St, New York, NY 10021; **Phone:** 212-879-6004; **Board Cert:** Internal Medicine 1986; Infectious Disease 1988; **Med School:** Yale Univ 1983; **Resid:** Internal Medicine, NY Hosp/Cornell Med Ctr 1986; **Fellow:** Infectious Disease, NY Hosp/Cornell Med Ctr 1989; **Fac Appt:** Asst Clin Prof Med, Cornell Univ-Weill Med Coll

Jacobs, Jonathan MD (Inf) - **Spec Exp:** AIDS/HIV; **Hospital:** NY-Presby Hosp (page 100); **Address:** 449 E 68th St, Ground Fl, New York, NY 10021; **Phone:** 212-734-1365; **Board Cert:** Internal Medicine 1983; Infectious Disease 1986; **Med School:** Yale Univ 1980; **Resid:** Internal Medicine, New York Hosp/Cornell Med Ctr 1983; **Fellow:** Infectious Disease, New York Hosp/Cornell Med Ctr 1986; **Fac Appt:** Clin Prof Med, Cornell Univ-Weill Med Coll

Johnson, Warren MD (Inf) - **Spec Exp:** Travel Medicine; Parasitic Infections; **Hospital:** NY-Presby Hosp (page 100); **Address:** 1300 York Ave, Ste A-421, New York, NY 10021-4805; **Phone:** 212-746-6320; **Board Cert:** Internal Medicine 1971; Infectious Disease 1974; **Med School:** Columbia P&S 1962; **Resid:** Internal Medicine, NY Hosp-Cornell Med Ctr 1964; Internal Medicine, NY Hosp-Cornell Med Ctr 1969; **Fellow:** Infectious Disease, NY Hosp-Cornell Med Ctr 1968; **Fac Appt:** Prof Med, Cornell Univ-Weill Med Coll

Klotman, Mary E MD (Inf) - **Spec Exp:** AIDS/HIV Related Kidney Disease; **Hospital:** Mount Sinai Med Ctr (page 98); **Address:** Mt Sinai Medical Ctr, One Gustave L Levy Pl, Box 1090, New York, NY 10029; **Phone:** 212-241-2950; **Board Cert:** Internal Medicine 1984; Infectious Disease 1986; **Med School:** Duke Univ 1980; **Resid:** Internal Medicine, Duke Univ Med Ctr 1983; **Fellow:** Infectious Disease, Duke Univ Med Ctr 1985; **Fac Appt:** Prof Med, Mount Sinai Sch Med

Lerner, Chester MD (Inf) - **Spec Exp:** AIDS/HIV; Travel Medicine; **Hospital:** NY Downtown Hosp; **Address:** 170 William St Fl 7, New York, NY 10038-2612; **Phone:** 212-238-0106; **Board Cert:** Internal Medicine 1981; Infectious Disease 1984; **Med School:** Univ Pittsburgh 1978; **Resid:** Internal Medicine, Lenox Hill Hosp 1981; **Fellow:** Infectious Disease, Lenox Hill Hosp 1983; **Fac Appt:** Asst Clin Prof Med, NYU Sch Med

Louie, Eddie MD (Inf) - **Spec Exp:** Lyme Disease; AIDS/HIV; Hospital Acquired Infections; **Hospital:** NYU Med Ctr (page 102); **Address:** 345 E 37th St, New York, NY 10016-3256; **Phone:** 212-682-9202; **Board Cert:** Internal Medicine 1982; Infectious Disease 1986; **Med School:** NYU Sch Med 1979; **Resid:** Internal Medicine, Kings County Hosp 1983; **Fellow:** Infectious Disease, NYU Med Ctr 1985; **Fac Appt:** Assoc Clin Prof Med, NYU Sch Med

McMeeking, Alexander MD (Inf) - **Spec Exp:** AIDS/HIV; Hepatitis B & C; Herpes Simplex; Antibiotic Resistance; **Hospital:** NYU Med Ctr (page 102); **Address:** 104 E 40th St, Ste 507, New York, NY 10016; **Phone:** 212-375-2560; **Board Cert:** Internal Medicine 1985; Infectious Disease 1988; **Med School:** UMDNJ-NJ Med Sch, Newark 1982; **Resid:** Internal Medicine, St Luke's-Roosevelt Hosp 1985; **Fellow:** Infectious Disease, Bellvue/NYU Med Ctr 1986

Mildvan, Donna MD (Inf) - **Spec Exp:** AIDS/HIV; Clinical Trials; **Hospital:** Beth Israel Med Ctr - Petrie Division (page 90); **Address:** Beth Israel Med Ctr, Div Infectious Dis, 1st Ave at 16th St, 19BH17, New York, NY 10003; **Phone:** 212-420-4005; **Board Cert:** Internal Medicine 1972; Infectious Disease 1972; **Med School:** Johns Hopkins Univ 1967; **Resid:** Internal Medicine, Mount Sinai Hosp 1970; **Fellow:** Infectious Disease, Mount Sinai Hosp 1972; **Fac Appt:** Prof Med, Albert Einstein Coll Med

Miller, Dennis K MD (Inf) - **Spec Exp:** Lyme Disease; AIDS/HIV; **Hospital:** Lenox Hill Hosp (page 94); **Address:** 4 E 76th St, New York, NY 10021-1811; **Phone:** 212-472-1237; **Board Cert:** Internal Medicine 1985; Infectious Disease 1988; **Med School:** Rush Med Coll 1982; **Resid:** Internal Medicine, Lenox Hill Hosp 1985; **Fellow:** Infectious Disease, Lenox Hill Hosp 1987

Mullen, Michael MD (Inf) - **Spec Exp:** Osteomyelitis; AIDS/HIV; Infectious Disease; **Hospital:** Mount Sinai Med Ctr (page 98); **Address:** Mount Sinai Medical Ctr, 5 E 98th St Fl 11, New York, NY 10029; **Phone:** 212-241-3150; **Board Cert:** Internal Medicine 1985; Infectious Disease 1986; **Med School:** Spain 1981; **Resid:** Internal Medicine, Jewish Hosp Med Ctr 1984; **Fellow:** Infectious Disease, Cabrini Med Ctr 1986; **Fac Appt:** Asst Clin Prof Med, Mount Sinai Sch Med

Neibart, Eric MD (Inf) - **Spec Exp:** Travel Medicine; AIDS/HIV; Fungal Infections; **Hospital:** Mount Sinai Med Ctr (page 98); **Address:** 1100 Park Ave, New York, NY 10128-1202; **Phone:** 212-427-9550; **Board Cert:** Internal Medicine 1983; Infectious Disease 1986; **Med School:** UMDNJ-NJ Med Sch, Newark 1980; **Resid:** Internal Medicine, Mount Sinai 1983; **Fellow:** Infectious Disease, Mount Sinai 1986; **Fac Appt:** Asst Prof Med, Mount Sinai Sch Med

Perlman, David MD (Inf) - **Spec Exp:** AIDS/HIV; Lyme Disease; Travel Medicine; **Hospital:** Beth Israel Med Ctr - Petrie Division (page 90), Lenox Hill Hosp (page 94); **Address:** Beth Israel Med Ctr, 1st Ave at 16th St, New York, NY 10003; **Phone:** 212-420-4470; **Board Cert:** Internal Medicine 1986; Infectious Disease 1988; **Med School:** Albert Einstein Coll Med 1983; **Resid:** Internal Medicine, New York Hosp/Meml Sloan Kettering 1986; **Fellow:** Infectious Disease, Montefiore Hosp 1988; **Fac Appt:** Prof Med, Albert Einstein Coll Med

Polsky, Bruce MD (Inf) - **Spec Exp:** AIDS/HIV; Viral Infections; Infections in Cancer Patients; AIDS Related Cancers; **Hospital:** St Luke's - Roosevelt Hosp Ctr - Roosevelt Div (page 90); **Address:** 1111 Amsterdam Ave, New York, NY 10025; **Phone:** 212-523-2525; **Board Cert:** Internal Medicine 1983; Infectious Disease 1986; **Med School:** Wayne State Univ 1980; **Resid:** Internal Medicine, Montefiore Hosp 1983; **Fellow:** Infectious Disease, Meml Sloan Kettering Cancer Ctr 1986; **Fac Appt:** Prof Med, Columbia P&S

Press, Robert MD (Inf) - **Spec Exp:** Surgical Infections; Hospital Acquired Infections; **Hospital:** NYU Med Ctr (page 102), Manhattan Eye, Ear & Throat Hosp; **Address:** 530 1st Ave, Ste 4G, New York, NY 10016-6402; **Phone:** 212-263-7229; **Board Cert:** Internal Medicine 1976; Infectious Disease 1999; **Med School:** NYU Sch Med 1973; **Resid:** Internal Medicine, Beth Israel Hosp 1975; Internal Medicine, Bellevue Hosp 1976; **Fellow:** Infectious Disease, Montefiore Hosp Med Ctr 1978; **Fac Appt:** Assoc Clin Prof Med, NYU Sch Med

Romagnoli, Mario MD (Inf) - **Spec Exp:** AIDS/HIV; Bone/Joint Infections; **Hospital:** NY-Presby Hosp (page 100); **Address:** 903 Park Ave, New York, NY 10021; **Phone:** 212-396-3390; **Board Cert:** Internal Medicine 1979; Infectious Disease 1982; **Med School:** Columbia P&S 1976; **Resid:** Internal Medicine, Columbia-Presby Med Ctr 1979; **Fellow:** Infectious Disease, Harvard Beth Israel Med Ctr 1981; **Fac Appt:** Assoc Prof Med, Columbia P&S

Sanjana, Veeraf MD/PhD (Inf) - **Spec Exp:** AIDS/HIV; **Hospital:** Cabrini Med Ctr (page 374); **Address:** 310 E 14th St, New York, NY 10003-4201; **Phone:** 212-473-8088; **Board Cert:** Internal Medicine 1981; Infectious Disease 2002; **Med School:** Univ Miami Sch Med 1977; **Resid:** Internal Medicine, Albert Einstein 1978; Internal Medicine, Cabrini Med Ctr 1979; **Fellow:** Infectious Disease, Cabrini Med Ctr 1989

Sepkowitz, Kent MD (Inf) - **Spec Exp:** Tuberculosis; Infections in Cancer Patients; Fungal Infections; **Hospital:** Meml Sloan Kettering Cancer Ctr (page 109); **Address:** 1275 York Ave, New York, NY 10021-0033; **Phone:** 212-639-2441; **Board Cert:** Internal Medicine 1983; Infectious Disease 2000; **Med School:** Univ Okla Coll Med 1980; **Resid:** Internal Medicine, Roosevelt Hosp 1984; **Fellow:** Infectious Disease, Meml Sloan Kettering Cancer Ctr 1991; **Fac Appt:** Prof Med, Cornell Univ-Weill Med Coll

Simberkoff, Michael S MD (Inf) - **Spec Exp:** AIDS/HIV; Pneumonia; **Hospital:** VA Med Ctr - Manhattan, NYU Med Ctr (page 102); **Address:** 423 E 23rd St, New York, NY 10010; **Phone:** 212-951-3417; **Board Cert:** Internal Medicine 1969; Infectious Disease 1972; **Med School:** NYU Sch Med 1962; **Resid:** Internal Medicine, Bellevue Hosp 1967; **Fellow:** Infectious Disease, New York Univ Med Ctr 1969; **Fac Appt:** Assoc Prof Med, NYU Sch Med

Soave, Rosemary MD (Inf) - **Spec Exp:** Infections-Transplant; Parasitic Infections; Infections in Immunocompromised Patients; **Hospital:** NY-Presby Hosp (page 100); **Address:** 1300 York Ave, rm A-421, Box 125, New York, NY 10021-4805; **Phone:** 212-746-6319; **Board Cert:** Internal Medicine 1979; Infectious Disease 1984; **Med School:** Cornell Univ-Weill Med Coll 1976; **Resid:** Internal Medicine, New York Hosp 1979; Internal Medicine, Meml Sloan Kettering Cancer Ctr 1980; **Fellow:** Infectious Disease, New York Hosp/Cornell Med Ctr 1982; **Fac Appt:** Assoc Prof Med, Cornell Univ-Weill Med Coll

Turett, Glenn MD (Inf) - **Spec Exp:** AIDS/HIV; Hospital Acquired Infections; **Hospital:** St Vincent Cath Med Ctrs - Manhattan (page 375); **Address:** 153 W 11th St, Cronin Bldg, rm 1003, New York, NY 10011; **Phone:** 212-604-8328; **Board Cert:** Internal Medicine 1988; Infectious Disease 1992; **Med School:** Mount Sinai Sch Med 1985; **Resid:** Internal Medicine, Mt Sinai Med Ctr 1988; **Fellow:** Infectious Disease, Montefiore Hosp Med Ctr 1992; **Fac Appt:** Assoc Clin Prof Med, NY Med Coll

Wallach, Frances MD (Inf) - **Spec Exp:** AIDS/HIV; HIV & Blood Transfusions; **Hospital:** Mount Sinai Med Ctr (page 98); **Address:** Mount Sinai Medical Ctr, One Gustave L Levy Pl, Box 1009, New York, NY 10029; **Phone:** 212-241-6492; **Board Cert:** Internal Medicine 1989; Infectious Disease 1992; **Med School:** Albany Med Coll 1985; **Resid:** Internal Medicine, Montefiore Medical Ctr 1989; **Fellow:** Nuclear Medicine, Albert Einstein Medical Ctr 1990; Infectious Disease, NY Hosp-Cornel Medical Ctr 1992; **Fac Appt:** Asst Prof Med, Mount Sinai Sch Med

Wetherbee, Roger MD (Inf) - **Spec Exp:** Infections-Transplant; **Hospital:** NYU Med Ctr (page 102); **Address:** 530 1st Ave, Ste 4C, New York, NY 10016; **Phone:** 212-263-7243; **Board Cert:** Internal Medicine 1974; Infectious Disease 1997; **Med School:** NYU Sch Med 1969; **Resid:** Internal Medicine, Bellevue Hosp 1974; Internal Medicine, VA Hosp 1974; **Fellow:** Infectious Disease, Natl Inst Hlth 1972; Infectious Disease, VA Hosp 1975; **Fac Appt:** Assoc Clin Prof Med, NYU Sch Med

Yancovitz, Stanley MD (Inf) - **Spec Exp:** Lyme Disease; AIDS/HIV; **Hospital:** Beth Israel Med Ctr - Petrie Division (page 90); **Address:** 1st Ave at 16th St, Ste17 BH10, New York, NY 10003; **Phone:** 212-420-2600; **Board Cert:** Internal Medicine 1973; Infectious Disease 1976; **Med School:** SUNY Downstate 1967; **Resid:** Internal Medicine, Metropolitan Hosp 1969; Internal Medicine, Beth Israel Med Ctr 1972; **Fellow:** Infectious Disease, Mount Sinai Hosp 1975; **Fac Appt:** Assoc Prof Med, Albert Einstein Coll Med

INTERNAL MEDICINE

Adler, Mitchell MD (IM) `PCP` - **Spec Exp:** Sports Medicine; Geriatric Rehabilitation; **Hospital:** NYU Med Ctr (page 102); **Address:** 317 E 34th St Fl 10, New York, NY 10016; **Phone:** 212-726-7499; **Board Cert:** Internal Medicine 1983; **Med School:** NYU Sch Med 1980; **Resid:** Internal Medicine, Bellevue Hosp 1984; **Fac Appt:** Asst Clin Prof Med, NYU Sch Med

Aronne, Louis J MD (IM) - **Spec Exp:** Obesity; Diabetes; **Hospital:** NY-Presby Hosp (page 100); **Address:** 1165 York Ave, New York, NY 10021; **Phone:** 212-583-1000; **Board Cert:** Internal Medicine 1984; **Med School:** Johns Hopkins Univ 1981; **Resid:** Internal Medicine, Bronx Muni Hosp 1984; **Fellow:** Internal Medicine, New York Hosp 1986; **Fac Appt:** Assoc Clin Prof Med, Cornell Univ-Weill Med Coll

Ascheim, Robert MD (IM) - **Spec Exp:** Coronary Artery Disease; Congestive Heart Failure; **Hospital:** NY-Presby Hosp (page 100); **Address:** CO Executive Office, 10 Rockefellar Plaza Fl 4, New York, NY 10020; **Phone:** 212-332-3774; **Board Cert:** Internal Medicine 1969; **Med School:** Tufts Univ 1962; **Resid:** Internal Medicine, Bellevue Hosp 1968; Cardiovascular Disease, Mem Sloan-Kettering Med Ctr 1967; **Fellow:** Cardiovascular Disease, NY Hosp 1970; **Fac Appt:** Assoc Prof Med, Cornell Univ-Weill Med Coll

Baskin, David MD (IM) `PCP` - **Spec Exp:** Preventive Medicine; Cholesterol/Lipid Disorders; **Hospital:** St Luke's - Roosevelt Hosp Ctr - Roosevelt Div (page 90); **Address:** 185 W End Ave, Ste 1M, New York, NY 10023-5540; **Phone:** 212-595-7701; **Board Cert:** Internal Medicine 1985; **Med School:** Boston Univ 1982; **Resid:** Internal Medicine, St Lukes Roosevelt Hosp Ctr 1985; **Fac Appt:** Asst Clin Prof Med, Columbia P&S

Benovitz, Harvey MD (IM) `PCP` - **Spec Exp:** Diabetes; Thyroid Disorders; Polycystic Ovarian Syndrome; **Hospital:** St Luke's - Roosevelt Hosp Ctr - Roosevelt Div (page 90), Lenox Hill Hosp (page 94); **Address:** 115 Central Park West, New York, NY 10023-4153; **Phone:** 212-877-2100; **Board Cert:** Internal Medicine 1972; **Med School:** Albert Einstein Coll Med 1962; **Resid:** Internal Medicine, Univ Pittsburgh Med Ctr 1964; Internal Medicine, Univ Pittsburgh Med Ctr 1967; **Fellow:** Endocrinology, Diabetes & Metabolism, St Lukes Hosp 1970; **Fac Appt:** Asst Clin Prof Med, Columbia P&S

Berk, Paul D MD (IM) - **Spec Exp:** Liver Disease; Polycythemia Rubra Vera; Myeloproliferative Disorders; **Hospital:** NY-Presby Hosp (page 100); **Address:** Herbert Irving Pavilion, 161 Fort Washington Ave, Ste 301, New York, NY 10032; **Phone:** 212-342-3719; **Board Cert:** Internal Medicine 1971; Hematology 1972; **Med School:** Columbia P&S 1964; **Resid:** Internal Medicine, Columbia-Presby Med Ctr 1966; Hematology, Nat Inst Hlth 1969; **Fellow:** Hematology, Columbia-Presby Med Ctr 1970; Hepatology, Royal Free Hosp

Bruno, Peter MD (IM) - **Spec Exp:** Primary Care Sports Medicine; **Hospital:** Lenox Hill Hosp (page 94), Beth Israel Med Ctr - Petrie Division (page 90); **Address:** Madison Medical, 110 E 59th St, Ste 9A, New York, NY 10022-1304; **Phone:** 212-583-2898; **Board Cert:** Internal Medicine 1979; **Med School:** Hahnemann Univ 1975; **Resid:** Internal Medicine, Lenox Hill Hosp 1979; **Fac Appt:** Assoc Prof Med, NYU Sch Med

Burke, Gary R MD (IM) `PCP` - **Spec Exp:** Preventive Medicine; **Hospital:** St Luke's - Roosevelt Hosp Ctr - Roosevelt Div (page 90); **Address:** 1090 Amsterdam Ave Fl 4, New York, NY 10025; **Phone:** 212-961-5500 x3; **Board Cert:** Internal Medicine 1976; **Med School:** Univ Minn 1973; **Resid:** Internal Medicine, UC Davis Med Ctr 1976; **Fac Appt:** Asst Clin Prof Med, Columbia P&S

Bush, Michael MD (IM) PCP - **Spec Exp:** Preventive Medicine; **Hospital:** Lenox Hill Hosp (page 94); **Address:** 115 E 57th St, Ste 630, New York, NY 10022; **Phone:** 212-583-2990; **Board Cert:** Internal Medicine 1981; **Med School:** SUNY Downstate 1978; **Resid:** Internal Medicine, Lenox Hill Hosp 1982; **Fac Appt:** Asst Clin Prof Med, NYU Sch Med

Carmichael, L David MD (IM) PCP - **Spec Exp:** Preventive Medicine; Travel Medicine; **Hospital:** NY-Presby Hosp (page 100); **Address:** 903 Park Ave, New York, NY 10021; **Phone:** 212-639-9850; **Board Cert:** Internal Medicine 1979; Geriatric Medicine 1994; **Med School:** Albert Einstein Coll Med 1976; **Resid:** Internal Medicine, Bronx Lebanon Hosp 1979Columbia Sch Pub Health 1983; **Fellow:** Internal Medicine, Columbia Presby Med Ctr 1980; **Fac Appt:** Assoc Clin Prof Med, Columbia P&S

Case, David B MD (IM) PCP - **Spec Exp:** Hypertension; Preventive Cardiology; **Hospital:** NY-Presby Hosp (page 100), NY-Presby Hosp (page 100); **Address:** 635 Madison Ave Fl 7, New York, NY 10022-1009; **Phone:** 212-857-4660; **Board Cert:** Internal Medicine 1974; **Med School:** Columbia P&S 1968; **Resid:** Internal Medicine, Johns Hopkins Hosp 1970; **Fellow:** Cardiovascular Disease, Columbia-Presby Med Ctr 1972; **Fac Appt:** Assoc Clin Prof Med, Cornell Univ-Weill Med Coll

Charap, Mitchell MD (IM) - **Hospital:** NYU Med Ctr (page 102); **Address:** 530 1st Ave, Ste 7B, New York, NY 10016; **Phone:** 212-263-7442; **Board Cert:** Internal Medicine 2002; **Med School:** NYU Sch Med 1977; **Resid:** Internal Medicine, NYU Med Ctr 1981; **Fac Appt:** Assoc Clin Prof Med, NYU Sch Med

Charap, Peter MD (IM) PCP - **Spec Exp:** Preventive Medicine; **Hospital:** Mount Sinai Med Ctr (page 98), Lenox Hill Hosp (page 94); **Address:** 234 Central Park West, New York, NY 10024; **Phone:** 212-579-2200; **Board Cert:** Internal Medicine 1987; **Med School:** Mount Sinai Sch Med 1984; **Resid:** Internal Medicine, Mount Sinai Hosp 1987; **Fellow:** Public Health & Genl Preventive Med, Mount Sinai Hosp 1988; **Fac Appt:** Asst Clin Prof Med, Mount Sinai Sch Med

Cimino, James J MD (IM) PCP - **Hospital:** NY-Presby Hosp (page 100); **Address:** 622 W 168th St Bldg VC Fl 2 - rm 224, New York, NY 10032-3720; **Phone:** 212-305-6262; **Board Cert:** Internal Medicine 1984; **Med School:** NY Med Coll 1981; **Resid:** Internal Medicine, St Vincent's Hosp & Med Ctr 1984; **Fellow:** Neuronal Plasticity, Mass Genl Hosp 1988; **Fac Appt:** Assoc Prof Med, Columbia P&S

Cohen, Michael H MD (IM) - **Spec Exp:** Congestive Heart Failure; Coronary Artery Disease; Hypertension; **Hospital:** NY-Presby Hosp (page 100); **Address:** 161 Fort Washington Ave, rm 328, New York, NY 10032-3713; **Phone:** 212-305-5440; **Board Cert:** Internal Medicine 1971; **Med School:** Johns Hopkins Univ 1965; **Resid:** Internal Medicine, Columbia-Presby Med Ctr 1971; **Fellow:** Cardiovascular Disease, Columbia-Presby Med Ctr 1970; **Fac Appt:** Clin Prof Med, Columbia P&S

Cohen, Richard P MD (IM) PCP - **Spec Exp:** Complex Diagnosis; Infectious Disease; **Hospital:** NY-Presby Hosp (page 100); **Address:** 235 E 67th St, New York, NY 10021-6040; **Phone:** 212-734-6464; **Board Cert:** Internal Medicine 1978; **Med School:** Cornell Univ-Weill Med Coll 1975; **Resid:** Internal Medicine, New York Hosp 1978; **Fellow:** Infectious Disease, New York Hosp/Cornell Med Ctr 1979; **Fac Appt:** Prof Med, Cornell Univ-Weill Med Coll

Cohen, Robert L MD (IM) - **Hospital:** St Vincent Cath Med Ctrs - Manhattan (page 375); **Address:** 314 W 14th St, FL 5, New York, NY 10014-5002; **Phone:** 212-620-0144; **Board Cert:** Internal Medicine 1978; **Med School:** Rush Med Coll 1975; **Resid:** Internal Medicine, Cook County Hosp 1979; **Fac Appt:** Asst Prof Med, Albert Einstein Coll Med

Collens, Richard MD (IM) `PCP` - **Hospital:** St Luke's - Roosevelt Hosp Ctr - Roosevelt Div (page 90); **Address:** 697 West End Ave, New York, NY 10025; **Phone:** 212-222-7071; **Board Cert:** Internal Medicine 1973; Cardiovascular Disease 1973; **Med School:** NY Med Coll 1966; **Resid:** Internal Medicine, Bronx Muni Hosp Ctr 1970; **Fellow:** Cardiovascular Disease, Mount Sinai Hosp 1971; **Fac Appt:** Assoc Clin Prof Med, Columbia P&S

Constantiner, Arturo MD (IM) `PCP` - **Spec Exp:** Hypertension; Kidney Disease; Kidney Stones; **Hospital:** NY Downtown Hosp; **Address:** 19 Beekman St, Fl 6, New York, NY 10038-1522; **Phone:** 212-349-8455; **Board Cert:** Internal Medicine 1979; Nephrology 1996; **Med School:** Mexico 1975; **Resid:** Internal Medicine, Elmhurst Hosp 1979; **Fellow:** Nephrology, Mount Sinai Hosp 1981; **Fac Appt:** Asst Clin Prof Med, NYU Sch Med

Cunningham-Rundles, Ward MD (IM) `PCP` - **Spec Exp:** Allergy & Immunology; **Hospital:** Mount Sinai Med Ctr (page 98), Beth Israel Med Ctr - Petrie Division (page 90); **Address:** 240 E 68th St, New York, NY 10021-6001; **Phone:** 212-737-8973; **Board Cert:** Internal Medicine 1976; **Med School:** NYU Sch Med 1971; **Resid:** Internal Medicine, Bellevue Hosp 1973; **Fellow:** Immunology, Meml Sloan Kettering Cancer Ctr 1975; Medical Oncology, Meml Sloan Kettering Cancer Ctr 1976; **Fac Appt:** Asst Clin Prof Med, Mount Sinai Sch Med

Ehrlich, Martin MD (IM) `PCP` - **Spec Exp:** Complementary Medicine; Preventive Medicine; Acupuncture; **Hospital:** Beth Israel Med Ctr - Petrie Division (page 90); **Address:** 245 Fifth Ave Fl 2, New York, NY 10016; **Phone:** 646-935-2220; **Board Cert:** Internal Medicine 1988; **Med School:** Columbia P&S 1985; **Resid:** Internal Medicine, Harlem Hosp 1989; **Fac Appt:** Asst Prof Med, Albert Einstein Coll Med

El-Sadr, Wafaa MD (IM) - **Spec Exp:** AIDS/HIV; **Hospital:** Harlem Hosp Ctr; **Address:** Harlem Hospital, 506 Lenox Ave, rm 3101A, New York, NY 10037; **Phone:** 212-939-2936; **Board Cert:** Internal Medicine 1986; **Med School:** Egypt 1974; **Resid:** Internal Medicine, Columbia-Presby Med Ctr 1982; **Fellow:** Infectious Disease, VA Medical Ctr 1983

Etingin, Orli MD (IM) `PCP` - **Spec Exp:** Preventive Medicine; Bleeding/Coagulation Disorders; Women's Health; **Hospital:** NY-Presby Hosp (page 100); **Address:** 425 E 61st St Fl 11, New York, NY 10021-4870; **Phone:** 212-746-2066; **Board Cert:** Internal Medicine 1984; Hematology 1988; **Med School:** Albert Einstein Coll Med 1980; **Resid:** Internal Medicine, NY Hosp-Cornell Med Ctr 1983; **Fellow:** Hematology & Oncology, NY Hosp-Cornell Med Ctr 1986; **Fac Appt:** Clin Prof Med, Cornell Univ-Weill Med Coll

Faust, Michael MD (IM) - **Spec Exp:** Gastrointestinal Disorders; **Hospital:** NYU Med Ctr (page 102); **Address:** 345 E 37th St, Ste 207, New York, NY 10016-3256; **Phone:** 212-986-3330; **Board Cert:** Internal Medicine 1981; Gastroenterology 1983; Geriatric Medicine 1988; **Med School:** NYU Sch Med 1978; **Resid:** Internal Medicine, Bellevue Hosp/NYU Med Ctr 1981; **Fellow:** Gastroenterology, Bellevue Hosp/NYU Med Ctr 1983; **Fac Appt:** Asst Prof Med, NYU Sch Med

Feltheimer, Seth MD (IM) `PCP` - **Spec Exp:** Preventive Medicine; Perioperative Medical Care; **Hospital:** NY-Presby Hosp (page 100); **Address:** 161 Ft Washington Ave, Ste 336, New York, NY 10032; **Phone:** 212-305-8669; **Board Cert:** Internal Medicine 1984; **Med School:** Spain 1981; **Resid:** Internal Medicine, Interfaith Med Ctr 1984; **Fellow:** Internal Medicine, Columbia-Presby Med Ctr 1985; **Fac Appt:** Assoc Clin Prof Med, Columbia P&S

Feuer, Martin MD (IM) `PCP` - **Spec Exp:** Bronchitis; Asthma; Emphysema; **Hospital:** Beth Israel Med Ctr - Petrie Division (page 90), Mount Sinai Med Ctr (page 98); **Address:** 899 Lexington Ave, New York, NY 10021-6103; **Phone:** 212-744-5433; **Board Cert:** Internal Medicine 1966; Pulmonary Disease 1972; **Med School:** NYU Sch Med 1959; **Resid:** Internal Medicine, Mount Sinai Hosp 1962; **Fellow:** Pulmonary Disease, Montefiore Med Ctr 1963; **Fac Appt:** Asst Clin Prof Med, Albert Einstein Coll Med

Fiedler, Robert MD (IM) `PCP` - **Spec Exp:** Thyroid Disorders; Diabetes; **Hospital:** Mount Sinai Med Ctr (page 98); **Address:** 1175 Park Ave, New York, NY 10128-1211; **Phone:** 212-289-6500; **Board Cert:** Endocrinology 1972; Internal Medicine 1970; **Med School:** Albert Einstein Coll Med 1964; **Resid:** Internal Medicine, DC Gen Hosp 1966; Internal Medicine, VA Med Ctr 1967; **Fellow:** Endocrinology, Mount Sinai Med Ctr 1969; **Fac Appt:** Assoc Clin Prof Med, Mount Sinai Sch Med

Fisch, Morton MD (IM) - **Spec Exp:** Diabetes; Hypertension; **Hospital:** Lenox Hill Hosp (page 94); **Address:** 800A 5th Ave, Ste 301, New York, NY 10021-7215; **Phone:** 212-755-7711; **Board Cert:** Internal Medicine 1967; **Med School:** SUNY Hlth Sci Ctr 1957; **Resid:** Internal Medicine, Lenox Hill Hosp 1963

Fisher, Laura MD (IM) - **Spec Exp:** Preventive Medicine; Lyme Disease; **Hospital:** NY-Presby Hosp (page 100); **Address:** 1385 York Ave, New York, NY 10021; **Phone:** 212-717-5920; **Board Cert:** Internal Medicine 1987; **Med School:** Brown Univ 1984; **Resid:** Internal Medicine, NY Hosp-Cornell Med Ctr 1987; **Fellow:** Infectious Disease, Mass Genl Hosp 1989; **Fac Appt:** Asst Clin Prof Med, Cornell Univ-Weill Med Coll

Fishman, Donald MD (IM) `PCP` - **Spec Exp:** Asthma; Chronic Obstructive Lung Disease (COPD); Bronchoscopy; **Hospital:** St Luke's - Roosevelt Hosp Ctr - Roosevelt Div (page 90), Lenox Hill Hosp (page 94); **Address:** 200 W 57th St, Ste 1201, New York, NY 10019; **Phone:** 212-765-5151; **Board Cert:** Internal Medicine 1976; Pulmonary Disease 1978; **Med School:** Univ Pennsylvania 1973; **Resid:** Internal Medicine, Univ Mich Med Ctr 1976; **Fellow:** Pulmonary Disease, NYU Med Ctr 1978; **Fac Appt:** Asst Clin Prof Med, Columbia P&S

Fried, Richard MD (IM) `PCP` - **Spec Exp:** Lyme Disease; Fevers of Unknown Origin; Infectious Disease; **Hospital:** St Luke's - Roosevelt Hosp Ctr - Roosevelt Div (page 90); **Address:** 15 W 72nd St, Ste 1N, New York, NY 10023; **Phone:** 212-580-4840; **Board Cert:** Internal Medicine 1972; Infectious Disease 1974; **Med School:** Columbia P&S 1968; **Resid:** Internal Medicine, St Lukes Hosp 1972; **Fellow:** Infectious Disease, Stanford Med Ctr 1974; **Fac Appt:** Assoc Clin Prof Med, Columbia P&S

Friedman, Jeffrey Paul MD (IM) `PCP` - **Spec Exp:** Preventive Medicine; Travel Medicine; **Hospital:** NYU Med Ctr (page 102); **Address:** 317 E 34th St Fl 10, New York, NY 10016; **Phone:** 212-726-7440; **Board Cert:** Internal Medicine 1986; **Med School:** NYU Sch Med 1983; **Resid:** Internal Medicine, Bellevue Hosp 1987; **Fac Appt:** Prof Med, NYU Sch Med

Galland, Leopold MD (IM) - **Spec Exp:** Nutrition; Chronic Disease; **Address:** 133 E 73rd St, Ste 308, New York, NY 10021-3556; **Phone:** 212-772-3077; **Board Cert:** Internal Medicine 1973; **Med School:** NYU Sch Med 1968; **Resid:** Internal Medicine, Bellevue Hosp 1972; **Fellow:** Behavioral Medicine, Univ Conn Hlth Ctr 1981

Golden, Flavia MD (IM) `PCP` - **Spec Exp:** Women's Health; **Hospital:** NY-Presby Hosp (page 100); **Address:** 310 E 72nd St Fl 2, New York, NY 10021; **Phone:** 212-396-3016; **Board Cert:** Internal Medicine 2003; **Med School:** NYU Sch Med 1990; **Resid:** Internal Medicine, NY Hosp-Cornell Med Ctr 1993

Goldstein, Marvin MD (IM) `PCP` - **Spec Exp:** Hypertension; Kidney Disease; Heart Disease; **Hospital:** Mount Sinai Med Ctr (page 98); **Address:** 1225 Park Ave, Ste 1E, New York, NY 10128-1758; **Phone:** 212-410-7100; **Board Cert:** Nephrology 1976; Internal Medicine 1987; **Med School:** Med Coll VA 1957; **Resid:** Internal Medicine, Mount Sinai Med Ctr 1961; **Fellow:** Nephrology, Mount Sinai Med Ctr 1963; **Fac Appt:** Clin Prof Med, Mount Sinai Sch Med

Goldstein, Paul H MD (IM) `PCP` - **Spec Exp:** Preventive Medicine; **Hospital:** St Vincent Cath Med Ctrs - Manhattan (page 375), NY Downtown Hosp; **Address:** 80 5th Ave, Ste 1601, New York, NY 10011; **Phone:** 212-645-8500; **Board Cert:** Internal Medicine 1985; **Med School:** NY Med Coll 1982; **Resid:** Internal Medicine, St Vincent's Hosp & Med Ctr 1985; **Fac Appt:** Assoc Prof Med, NY Med Coll

Greaney, Edward J MD (IM) `PCP` - **Hospital:** NYU Med Ctr (page 102); **Address:** 317 E 34th St, New York, NY 10016; **Phone:** 212-726-7488; **Board Cert:** Internal Medicine 1998; **Med School:** NYU Sch Med 1995; **Resid:** Internal Medicine, NYU Med Ctr-Bellevue Hosp 1999

Grieco, Anthony MD (IM) - **Spec Exp:** Homocystinuria; **Hospital:** NYU Med Ctr (page 102); **Address:** 530 1st Ave, Ste 4H, New York, NY 10016; **Phone:** 212-263-7272; **Board Cert:** Internal Medicine 1977; **Med School:** NYU Sch Med 1963; **Resid:** Internal Medicine, NYU Med Ctr 1968; **Fac Appt:** Prof Med, NYU Sch Med

Haber, Stuart MD (IM) `PCP` - **Spec Exp:** AIDS/I IIV, Travel Medicine; Infectious Disease; **Hospital:** St Vincent Cath Med Ctrs - Manhattan (page 375); **Address:** 12-A Sheridan Square, New York, NY 10014; **Phone:** 212-929-2370; **Board Cert:** Internal Medicine 1986; Infectious Disease 2000; **Med School:** NYU Sch Med 1983; **Resid:** Internal Medicine, Emory U Hosp 1986; **Fellow:** Infectious Disease, Emory U Hosp 1989

Hart, Catherine MD (IM) `PCP` - **Spec Exp:** Infectious Disease; **Hospital:** NY-Presby Hosp (page 100); **Address:** 310 E 72nd St, Fl 2, New York, NY 10021; **Phone:** 212-396-3272; **Board Cert:** Internal Medicine 1984; Infectious Disease 1986; **Med School:** Univ Pennsylvania 1980; **Resid:** Internal Medicine, New York Hosp-Cornell Med Ctr 1983; **Fellow:** Infectious Disease, New York Hosp-Cornell Med Ctr 1985; **Fac Appt:** Asst Clin Prof Med, Cornell Univ-Weill Med Coll

Hauptman, Allen S MD (IM) `PCP` - **Spec Exp:** Preventive Medicine; **Hospital:** NYU Med Ctr (page 102); **Address:** 317 E 34th St, New York, NY 10016-4974; **Phone:** 212-726-7494; **Board Cert:** Internal Medicine 1981; **Med School:** NYU Sch Med 1978; **Resid:** Internal Medicine, Bellevue Hosp 1982; **Fac Appt:** Asst Clin Prof Med, NYU Sch Med

Hoffman, Ira MD (IM) `PCP` - **Spec Exp:** Geriatric Medicine; **Hospital:** Lenox Hill Hosp (page 94); **Address:** 800A 5th Ave, New York, NY 10021-7215; **Phone:** 212-755-7711; **Board Cert:** Internal Medicine 1969; **Med School:** SUNY Downstate 1956; **Resid:** Internal Medicine, Long Island Coll Hosp 1960; Internal Medicine, Lenox Hill Hosp 1961; **Fac Appt:** Clin Prof Med, NYU Sch Med

Horbar, Gary MD (IM) `PCP` - **Hospital:** Lenox Hill Hosp (page 94); **Address:** 6 E 85th St, New York, NY 10028; **Phone:** 212-570-9119; **Board Cert:** Internal Medicine 1979; **Med School:** NY Med Coll 1976; **Resid:** Internal Medicine, Lenox Hill Hosp 1980; **Fac Appt:** Asst Clin Prof Med, NYU Sch Med

Horovitz, Len MD (IM) `PCP` - **Spec Exp:** Bronchoscopy; Asthma; Emphysema; **Hospital:** Lenox Hill Hosp (page 94), Manhattan Eye, Ear & Throat Hosp; **Address:** 47 E 77th St, Ste 201, New York, NY 10021; **Phone:** 212-744-3001; **Board Cert:** Internal Medicine 1980; Pulmonary Disease 1984; **Med School:** NYU Sch Med 1976; **Resid:** Internal Medicine, Lenox Hill Hosp 1980; **Fellow:** Pulmonary Disease, Lenox Hill Hosp 1982

Joy, Mark MD (IM) `PCP` - **Spec Exp:** Diabetes; Thyroid Disorders; **Hospital:** NY Downtown Hosp; **Address:** 170 William St Fl 7, New York, NY 10038; **Phone:** 212-238-0100; **Board Cert:** Internal Medicine 1983; **Med School:** W VA Univ 1979; **Resid:** Internal Medicine, Mercy Hospital 1982; **Fac Appt:** Asst Clin Prof Med, NY Med Coll

Kaminsky, Donald MD (IM) - **Spec Exp:** AIDS/HIV; Tropical Diseases; Travel Medicine; **Hospital:** Beth Israel Med Ctr - Petrie Division (page 90); **Address:** 10 Union Square East, Ste 5M-1, New York, NY 10003-3314; **Phone:** 212-253-6800; **Board Cert:** Internal Medicine 1982; **Med School:** Geo Wash Univ 1979; **Resid:** Internal Medicine, Beth Israel Hosp 1982; **Fellow:** Infectious Disease, Beth Israel Hosp 1984; **Fac Appt:** Asst Clin Prof Med, Albert Einstein Coll Med

Karp, Adam MD (IM) `PCP` - **Spec Exp:** Geriatric Medicine; **Hospital:** Hosp For Joint Diseases (page 107), NYU Med Ctr (page 102); **Address:** 301 E 17th St, rm 208A, New York, NY 10003; **Phone:** 212-598-6738; **Board Cert:** Internal Medicine 1999; Geriatric Medicine 1992; **Med School:** Albert Einstein Coll Med 1987; **Resid:** Internal Medicine, Maimonides Med Ctr 1990; **Fellow:** Geriatric Medicine, Bellevue Hosp/NYU 1992; **Fac Appt:** Asst Prof Med, NYU Sch Med

Kaufman, David L MD (IM) `PCP` - **Spec Exp:** AIDS/HIV; Hepatitis C; **Hospital:** St Vincent Cath Med Ctrs - Manhattan (page 375), St. Vincent's Midtown; **Address:** 37 Washington Square W, New York, NY 10011; **Phone:** 212-982-4070; **Board Cert:** Internal Medicine 1980; **Med School:** NY Med Coll 1977; **Resid:** Internal Medicine, St Vincents Hosp & Med Ctr 1980; **Fac Appt:** Asst Clin Prof Med, NY Med Coll

Kennedy, James MD (IM) `PCP` - **Spec Exp:** Thyroid Disorders; Diabetes; **Hospital:** NYU Med Ctr (page 102); **Address:** 650 1st Ave, Fl 4th, New York, NY 10016; **Phone:** 212-689-7768; **Board Cert:** Internal Medicine 1978; **Med School:** NYU Sch Med 1972; **Resid:** Internal Medicine, Bellevue Hosp 1977; **Fac Appt:** Assoc Prof Med, NYU Sch Med

Kennish, Arthur MD (IM) `PCP` - **Spec Exp:** Mitral Valve Disease; Coronary Artery Disease; **Hospital:** Mount Sinai Med Ctr (page 98); **Address:** 108 E 96th St, New York, NY 10128-6217; **Phone:** 212-410-6610; **Board Cert:** Internal Medicine 1980; Cardiovascular Disease 1983; **Med School:** Albert Einstein Coll Med 1977; **Resid:** Internal Medicine, Mount Sinai Hosp 1980; **Fellow:** Cardiovascular Disease, Mount Sinai Hosp 1982; **Fac Appt:** Asst Clin Prof Med, Mount Sinai Sch Med

Lamm, Steven MD (IM) `PCP` - **Spec Exp:** Obesity; Sexual Dysfunction; Preventive Medicine; **Hospital:** NYU Med Ctr (page 102), Lenox Hill Hosp (page 94); **Address:** 12 E 86th St, New York, NY 10028-0506; **Phone:** 212-988-1146; **Board Cert:** Internal Medicine 1977; **Med School:** NYU Sch Med 1974; **Resid:** Internal Medicine, NYU Med Ctr 1979; **Fellow:** Rheumatology, NYU Med Ctr 1978; **Fac Appt:** Asst Clin Prof Med, NYU Sch Med

Lebowitz, Arthur MD (IM) `PCP` - **Spec Exp:** Hypertension; Osteoporosis; Cholesterol/Lipid Disorders; **Hospital:** NYU Med Ctr (page 102), Bellevue Hosp Ctr; **Address:** 404 Park Ave S, New York, NY 10016; **Phone:** 212-725-1474; **Board Cert:** Internal Medicine 1970; **Med School:** NYU Sch Med 1965; **Resid:** Internal Medicine, N Carolina Meml Hosp 1967; Infectious Disease, Bellevue Hosp 1968; **Fellow:** Infectious Disease, Bellevue Hosp 1970; **Fac Appt:** Asst Clin Prof Med, NYU Sch Med

Lee, Roberta A MD (IM) - **Spec Exp:** Complementary Medicine; **Hospital:** Beth Israel Med Ctr - Petrie Division (page 90); **Address:** Center for Health & Healing, 245 Fifth Ave Fl 2, New York, NY 10016; **Phone:** 646-935-2265; **Board Cert:** Internal Medicine 1996; **Med School:** Geo Wash Univ 1985; **Resid:** Internal Medicine, Washington Hosp Ctr 1988; **Fellow:** Complementary Medicine, Univ Arizona Med Ctr 1999

Legato, Marianne J MD (IM) - **Spec Exp:** Cardiovascular Disease; Women's Health; Gender Specific Medicine; **Hospital:** NY-Presby Hosp (page 100), St Luke's - Roosevelt Hosp Ctr - Roosevelt Div (page 90); **Address:** 962 Park Ave, New York, NY 10028-2433; **Phone:** 212-737-5663; **Board Cert:** Internal Medicine 2003; **Med School:** NYU Sch Med 1962; **Resid:** Internal Medicine, Columbia-Presby Med Ctr 1965; **Fellow:** Cardiovascular Disease, Columbia-Presby Med Ctr 1968; **Fac Appt:** Prof Emeritus Med, Columbia P&S

Lewin, Margaret MD (IM) PCP - **Spec Exp:** Women's Health; Breast Cancer; Preventive Medicine; **Hospital:** NY-Presby Hosp (page 100), Hosp For Special Surgery (page 108); **Address:** 650 First Ave Fl 7th, New York, NY 10016; **Phone:** 212-888-8810; **Board Cert:** Internal Medicine 1980; Hematology 1982; Medical Oncology 1983; **Med School:** Case West Res Univ 1977; **Resid:** Internal Medicine, NY Hosp/Cornell Med Ctr 1980; **Fellow:** Hematology & Oncology, NY Hosp/Cornell Med Ctr 1983; **Fac Appt:** Assoc Clin Prof Med, Cornell Univ-Weill Med Coll

Lewin, Sharon MD (IM) PCP - **Spec Exp:** AIDS/HIV; Travel Medicine; Women's Health; **Hospital:** St Luke's - Roosevelt Hosp Ctr - Roosevelt Div (page 90); **Address:** 139 W 82nd St, New York, NY 10024-5544; **Phone:** 212-496-7200; **Board Cert:** Internal Medicine 1978; Infectious Disease 1980; **Med School:** Univ Toronto 1975; **Resid:** Internal Medicine, Wadsworth VA Hosp 1978; Infectious Disease, Bellevue Hosp/NYU Med Ctr 1980; **Fac Appt:** Asst Clin Prof Med, Columbia P&S

Liguori, Michael MD (IM) PCP - **Spec Exp:** Geriatric Rehabilitation; AIDS/HIV; **Hospital:** St Vincent Cath Med Ctrs - Manhattan (page 375); **Address:** 80 5th Ave, Ste 1601, New York, NY 10011-8002; **Phone:** 212-645-8500; **Board Cert:** Internal Medicine 1985; **Med School:** Mount Sinai Sch Med 1981; **Resid:** Internal Medicine, St Vincents Hosp 1984; **Fac Appt:** Asst Clin Prof Med, NY Med Coll

Lipton, Mark Scott MD (IM) PCP - **Spec Exp:** Preventive Cardiology; Coronary Artery Disease; Non-Invasive Cardiology; **Hospital:** NYU Med Ctr (page 102); **Address:** 635 Madison Ave Fl 3, New York, NY 10022-1009; **Phone:** 212-570-2077; **Board Cert:** Internal Medicine 1981; Cardiovascular Disease 1985; **Med School:** NYU Sch Med 1978; **Resid:** Internal Medicine, Bellevue Hosp 1981; **Fellow:** Cardiovascular Disease, NYU Med Ctr 1985; **Fac Appt:** Assoc Clin Prof Med, NYU Sch Med

Liu, George CK MD (IM) PCP - **Spec Exp:** Endocrinology; Chinese Community Health; Diabetes; **Hospital:** NY Downtown Hosp, NYU Med Ctr (page 102); **Address:** 185 Canal St Fl 6, New York, NY 10013-4513; **Phone:** 212-343-7323; **Board Cert:** Internal Medicine 1983; **Med School:** Cornell Univ-Weill Med Coll 1978; **Resid:** Internal Medicine, NYU Med Ctr-Manhattan VA Hosp 1981; **Fellow:** Endocrinology, Stanford Univ Med Ctr 1983; **Fac Appt:** Asst Clin Prof Med, NYU Sch Med

Lodge Jr, Henry S MD (IM) PCP - **Hospital:** NY-Presby Hosp (page 100); **Address:** 635 Madison Ave, New York, NY 10022-1009; **Phone:** 212-857-4555; **Board Cert:** Internal Medicine 1988; Geriatric Medicine 1992; **Med School:** Columbia P&S 1985; **Resid:** Internal Medicine, Columbia-Presby Hosp 1988; **Fac Appt:** Asst Clin Prof Med, Columbia P&S

Logan, Bruce MD (IM) `PCP` - **Spec Exp:** Cholesterol/Lipid Disorders; Preventive Medicine; Lyme Disease; **Hospital:** NY Downtown Hosp; **Address:** 19 Beekman St, Fl 6, New York, NY 10038; **Phone:** 212-608-6634; **Board Cert:** Internal Medicine 1978; **Med School:** Columbia P&S 1971; **Resid:** Internal Medicine, Harlem Hosp Ctr 1978; **Fac Appt:** Assoc Clin Prof Med, NYU Sch Med

Mackenzie, C Ronald MD (IM) `PCP` - **Spec Exp:** Complementary Medicine; **Hospital:** Hosp For Special Surgery (page 108), NY-Presby Hosp (page 100); **Address:** 535 E 70th St, New York, NY 10021; **Phone:** 212-606-1669; **Board Cert:** Internal Medicine 1981; Rheumatology 1991; **Med School:** Univ Calgary 1977; **Resid:** Family Medicine, Calgary Gen Hosp 1978; Internal Medicine, Univ Manitoba Hosp 1981; **Fellow:** Internal Medicine, New York Hosp/Cornell 1983; Rheumatology, Hosp For Spec Surg 1992; **Fac Appt:** Assoc Clin Prof Med, Cornell Univ-Weill Med Coll

McGinn, Thomas MD (IM) `PCP` - **Spec Exp:** Pain-Back; **Hospital:** Mount Sinai Med Ctr (page 98); **Address:** 1470 Madison Ave, New York, NY 10029-6542; **Phone:** 212-241-5451; **Board Cert:** Internal Medicine 1993; **Med School:** SUNY Downstate 1989; **Resid:** Internal Medicine, Albert Einstein Coll Med 1993; **Fac Appt:** Asst Prof Med, Albert Einstein Coll Med

Meyer, Richard MD (IM) - **Spec Exp:** Lymphoma; Head & Neck Cancer; **Hospital:** Mount Sinai Med Ctr (page 98); **Address:** 1111 Park Ave, New York, NY 10128-1234; **Phone:** 212-427-7700; **Board Cert:** Internal Medicine 1975; Hematology 1978; Medical Oncology 1979; **Med School:** Mount Sinai Sch Med 1972; **Resid:** Internal Medicine, Mt Sinai Hosp 1975; Hematology, Mt Sinai Hosp 1977; **Fellow:** Medical Oncology, Mt Sinai Hosp 1977; **Fac Appt:** Assoc Clin Prof Med, Mount Sinai Sch Med

Minkowitz, Susan MD (IM) `PCP` - **Spec Exp:** Asthma; Emphysema; Hypertension; **Hospital:** St Vincent Cath Med Ctrs - Manhattan (page 375); **Address:** 260 E Broadway, Ste 4, New York, NY 10002; **Phone:** 212-475-4093; **Board Cert:** Internal Medicine 1988; Pulmonary Disease 1990; **Med School:** NY Med Coll 1984; **Resid:** Internal Medicine, Metropolitan Hosp Ctr 1987; **Fellow:** Pulmonary Disease, Montefiore Hosp Med Ctr 1989; **Fac Appt:** Asst Prof Med, NY Med Coll

Nelson, Deena MD (IM) `PCP` - **Spec Exp:** Cancer Survivors; Cancer Prevention; **Hospital:** NY-Presby Hosp (page 100), Meml Sloan Kettering Cancer Ctr (page 109); **Address:** 635 Madison Ave, New York, NY 10022-1009; **Phone:** 212-857-4670; **Board Cert:** Internal Medicine 1980; **Med School:** Albert Einstein Coll Med 1977; **Resid:** Internal Medicine, New York Hosp 1979; Internal Medicine, Barnes Hosp 1980; **Fac Appt:** Asst Clin Prof Med, Cornell Univ-Weill Med Coll

Olichney, John MD (IM) - **Hospital:** St Luke's - Roosevelt Hosp Ctr - Roosevelt Div (page 90); **Address:** 350 W 58th St, FL 1, New York, NY 10019-1804; **Phone:** 212-246-9101; **Board Cert:** Internal Medicine 1974; **Med School:** Albany Med Coll 1969; **Resid:** Internal Medicine, Roosevelt Hosp 1972; **Fellow:** Hematology, St Luke's-Roosevelt Hosp Ctr 1973; **Fac Appt:** Clin Prof Med, Columbia P&S

Orsher, Stuart MD (IM) `PCP` - **Spec Exp:** Sports Medicine; **Hospital:** Lenox Hill Hosp (page 94); **Address:** 9 E 79th St, New York, NY 10021-0123; **Phone:** 212-535-7763; **Board Cert:** Internal Medicine 1983; **Med School:** Hahnemann Univ 1975; **Resid:** Internal Medicine, Lenox Hill Hosp 1978

Pecker, Mark S MD (IM) - **Spec Exp:** Hypertension; Cardiology; **Hospital:** NY-Presby Hosp (page 100); **Address:** NY-Cornell Medical Ctr, Hypertension Ctr, 525 E 68th St, Ste 1-L, New York, NY 10021; **Phone:** 212-746-2210; **Board Cert:** Internal Medicine 1980; **Med School:** NYU Sch Med 1977; **Resid:** Internal Medicine, Univ Texas SW Affil Hosps 1980; **Fac Appt:** Clin Prof Med, Cornell Univ-Weill Med Coll

Perla, Elliott MD (IM) `PCP` - **Spec Exp:** Asthma; **Hospital:** Metropolitan Hosp Ctr - NY; **Address:** 1901 1st Ave, New York, NY 10029-7404; **Phone:** 212-423-6771; **Board Cert:** Internal Medicine 1977; Pulmonary Disease 1980; **Med School:** NY Med Coll 1974; **Resid:** Internal Medicine, Mount Sinai Med Ctr 1977; **Fellow:** Pulmonary Disease, Metropolitan Hosp Ctr 1979; **Fac Appt:** Clin Prof Med, NY Med Coll

Postley, John E MD (IM) `PCP` - **Spec Exp:** Preventive Vascular Disease; **Hospital:** NY-Presby Hosp (page 100); **Address:** 635 Madison Ave, New York, NY 10022; **Phone:** 212-317-4646; **Board Cert:** Internal Medicine 1973; **Med School:** Columbia P&S 1968; **Resid:** Internal Medicine, Columbia-Presby Med Ctr 1969; Internal Medicine, Columbia-Presby Med Ctr 1973; **Fac Appt:** Asst Clin Prof Med, Columbia P&S

Reidenberg, Marcus MD (IM) - **Spec Exp:** Clinical Pharmacology; **Hospital:** NY-Presby Hosp (page 100); **Address:** 1300 York Ave, New York, NY 10021-4805; **Phone:** 212-746-6227; **Board Cert:** Internal Medicine 1967; **Med School:** Temple Univ 1958; **Resid:** Internal Medicine, Temple Univ Hosp 1965; **Fellow:** Pharmacology, Temple Univ Hosp 1960; **Fac Appt:** Prof Med, Cornell Univ-Weill Med Coll

Rendel, Michael T MD (IM) `PCP` - **Spec Exp:** Infectious Disease; AIDS/HIV; Travel Medicine; **Hospital:** St Luke's - Roosevelt Hosp Ctr - Roosevelt Div (page 90); **Address:** 139 W 82nd St, New York, NY 10024; **Phone:** 212-496-7200; **Board Cert:** Internal Medicine 1987; Infectious Disease 2001; **Med School:** Univ MD Sch Med 1984; **Resid:** Internal Medicine, Med Coll Penn 1987; **Fellow:** Infectious Disease, NYU Med Ctr 1990; **Fac Appt:** Asst Clin Prof Med, Columbia P&S

Rivlin, Richard S MD (IM) - **Spec Exp:** Cancer Prevention; Nutrition & Cancer Prevention; Endocrinology & Thyroid Disease; **Hospital:** NY-Presby Hosp (page 100); **Address:** Strang Cancer Prevention Ctr,Rockefeller Univ, 1230 York Ave, Box 231, New York, NY 10021; **Phone:** 212-734-1436; **Board Cert:** Internal Medicine 1969; **Med School:** Harvard Med Sch 1959; **Resid:** Internal Medicine, Bellevue Hosp 1960; Internal Medicine, Johns Hopkins Hosp 1961; **Fellow:** Endocrinology, Diabetes & Metabolism, Natl Inst Hlth 1963; Biochemistry, Johns Hopkins Hosp 1966; **Fac Appt:** Prof Med, Cornell Univ-Weill Med Coll

Rodman, John MD (IM) - **Spec Exp:** Kidney Stones; Hypertension; **Hospital:** NY-Presby Hosp (page 100), Lenox Hill Hosp (page 94); **Address:** 435 E 57th St, Ste 1A, New York, NY 10022; **Phone:** 212-752-3043; **Board Cert:** Internal Medicine 1975; Nephrology 1976; **Med School:** Columbia P&S 1970; **Resid:** Internal Medicine, New York Hosp 1972; **Fellow:** Nephrology, New York Hosp 1976; **Fac Appt:** Asst Clin Prof Med, Cornell Univ-Weill Med Coll

Rogers, Murray MD (IM) `PCP` - **Spec Exp:** Pulmonary Disease; Bronchoscopy; **Hospital:** Lenox Hill Hosp (page 94); **Address:** 800A 5th Ave, Ste 301, New York, NY 10021-7215; **Phone:** 212-755-7711; **Board Cert:** Internal Medicine 1968; Pulmonary Disease 1971; **Med School:** Univ Pennsylvania 1955; **Resid:** Internal Medicine, VA Med Ctr 1958; Internal Medicine, Lenox Hill Hosp 1959; **Fac Appt:** Clin Prof Med, NYU Sch Med

Salsitz, Edwin A MD (IM) - **Spec Exp:** Addiction Medicine; Opiate Addiction; **Hospital:** Beth Israel Med Ctr - Petrie Division (page 90); **Address:** Beth Israel Med Ctr, Bernstein Pavilion, 1st Ave at 16th St, rm 10B-45, New York, NY 10003; **Phone:** 212-420-4400; **Board Cert:** Internal Medicine 1977; Pulmonary Disease 1980; **Med School:** SUNY Buffalo 1972; **Resid:** Obstetrics & Gynecology, Beth Israel Med Ctr 1974; Internal Medicine, Beth Israel Med Ctr 1977; **Fellow:** Pulmonary Disease, Beth Israel Med Ctr; **Fac Appt:** Asst Clin Prof Med, Albert Einstein Coll Med

Schneebaum, Cary MD (IM) PCP - **Spec Exp:** Gastroenterology; **Hospital:** Beth Israel Med Ctr - Petrie Division (page 90); **Address:** 22 W 15th St, New York, NY 10011; **Phone:** 212-741-6100; **Board Cert:** Internal Medicine 1984; **Med School:** SUNY Hlth Sci Ctr 1981; **Resid:** Internal Medicine, Beth Israel Med Ctr 1984; **Fellow:** Gastroenterology, Beth Israel Med Ctr 1986

Schneider, Steven J MD (IM) PCP - **Spec Exp:** Travel Medicine; Occupational Medicine; **Hospital:** Lenox Hill Hosp (page 94), Mount Sinai Med Ctr (page 98); **Address:** 115 E 57th St, Ste 630, New York, NY 10022; **Phone:** 212-583-2880; **Board Cert:** Internal Medicine 1979; **Med School:** Johns Hopkins Univ 1976; **Resid:** Internal Medicine, Presby Med Ctr 1979; **Fac Appt:** Asst Clin Prof Med, Cornell Univ-Weill Med Coll

Seltzer, Terry MD (IM) PCP - **Spec Exp:** Diabetes; Thyroid Disorders; Calcium Disorders; **Hospital:** NYU Med Ctr (page 102); **Address:** 530 1st Ave, Ste 4D, New York, NY 10016-6402; **Phone:** 212-263-8717; **Board Cert:** Internal Medicine 1980; Endocrinology 1983; **Med School:** Harvard Med Sch 1977; **Resid:** Internal Medicine, NYU - Bellevue Hosp 1980; **Fellow:** Endocrinology, Diabetes & Metabolism, NYU- Bellevue Hosp 1982; **Fac Appt:** Asst Clin Prof Med, NYU Sch Med

Shorofsky, Morris MD (IM) PCP - **Hospital:** NY-Presby Hosp (page 100), Beth Israel Med Ctr - Petrie Division (page 90); **Address:** 166 E 61st St, Ste 1C, New York, NY 10021; **Phone:** 212-751-0777; **Board Cert:** Internal Medicine 1978; **Med School:** Switzerland 1959; **Resid:** Internal Medicine, Mount Sinai Med Ctr 1964; Internal Medicine, Beth Israel Med Ctr 1965; **Fac Appt:** Assoc Clin Prof Med, Cornell Univ-Weill Med Coll

Silverman, David MD (IM) PCP - **Spec Exp:** Infectious Disease; Preventive Medicine; Lyme Disease; **Hospital:** NYU Med Ctr (page 102), Mount Sinai Med Ctr (page 98); **Address:** 239 Central Park West, New York, NY 10024; **Phone:** 212-496-1929; **Board Cert:** Internal Medicine 1979; **Med School:** Columbia P&S 1976; **Resid:** Internal Medicine, NYU/Bellevue Hosp 1980; **Fellow:** Infectious Disease, NYU/Bellevue Hosp; **Fac Appt:** Assoc Clin Prof Med, NYU Sch Med

Solomon, Gregory MD (IM) PCP - **Spec Exp:** Preventive Medicine; Hypertension; Cholesterol/Lipid Disorders; **Hospital:** Mount Sinai Med Ctr (page 98); **Address:** 899 Lexington Ave, New York, NY 10021-6103; **Phone:** 212-717-9205; **Board Cert:** Internal Medicine 1995; **Med School:** NYU Sch Med 1991; **Resid:** Internal Medicine, Montefiore Med Ctr 1995; **Fac Appt:** Assoc Clin Prof Med, Mount Sinai Sch Med

Spero, Marc MD (IM) PCP - **Spec Exp:** Pulmonary Disease; Diving Medicine; Asthma; **Hospital:** Lenox Hill Hosp (page 94); **Address:** 654 Madison Ave, FL 6, New York, NY 10021-8404; **Phone:** 212-355-8315; **Board Cert:** Internal Medicine 1977; Pulmonary Disease 1980; **Med School:** Albert Einstein Coll Med 1973; **Resid:** Internal Medicine, St Lukes Hosp 1977; **Fellow:** Pulmonary Disease, St Lukes Hosp 1979

Stein, Richard MD (IM) - **Spec Exp:** Dialysis Care; Kidney Disease; **Hospital:** Mount Sinai Med Ctr (page 98); **Address:** 1 Gustave Levy Pl, Box 1243, New York, NY 10029; **Phone:** 212-241-4060; **Board Cert:** Internal Medicine 1966; Nephrology 1972; **Med School:** SUNY Hlth Sci Ctr 1958; **Resid:** Internal Medicine, Kings Co Hosp 1959; Internal Medicine, Maimonides Med Ctr 1961; **Fellow:** Nephrology, Mount Sinai Med Ctr 1963; **Fac Appt:** Prof Med, Mount Sinai Sch Med

Stein, Sidney MD (IM) PCP - **Spec Exp:** Asthma; Bronchitis; Emphysema; **Hospital:** Beth Israel Med Ctr - Petrie Division (page 90); **Address:** 55 E 34th St Fl 6, New York, NY 10016-4337; **Phone:** 212-879-7777; **Board Cert:** Internal Medicine 1982; Pulmonary Disease 1988; **Med School:** SUNY Hlth Sci Ctr 1979; **Resid:** Internal Medicine, Beth Israel Med Ctr 1982; **Fellow:** Pulmonary Disease, Beth Israel Med Ctr 1984; **Fac Appt:** Asst Clin Prof Med, Albert Einstein Coll Med

Steinberg, Charles MD (IM) PCP - **Hospital:** NY-Presby Hosp (page 100); **Address:** 525 E 68th St, New York, NY 10021-4870; **Phone:** 212-746-4100; **Board Cert:** Internal Medicine 1971; Infectious Disease 1974; **Med School:** Cornell Univ-Weill Med Coll 1964; **Resid:** Internal Medicine, New York Hosp 1966; Internal Medicine, New York Hosp 1969; **Fellow:** Infectious Disease, New York Hosp 1971; **Fac Appt:** Prof Med, Cornell Univ-Weill Med Coll

Strauss, Michael MD (IM) PCP - **Spec Exp:** Acupuncture; **Hospital:** Beth Israel Med Ctr - Petrie Division (page 90), Cabrini Med Ctr (page 374); **Address:** 310 E 14th St North Bldg Fl 3, New York, NY 10003; **Phone:** 212-777-3077; **Board Cert:** Internal Medicine 1983; **Med School:** Belgium 1980; **Resid:** Internal Medicine, Cabrini Med Ctr 1983

Tay, Steven MD (IM) PCP - **Spec Exp:** Geriatric Care; **Hospital:** Beth Israel Med Ctr - Petrie Division (page 90); **Address:** 10 Union Square E, Ste 5M, New York, NY 10003; **Phone:** 212-253-9322; **Board Cert:** Internal Medicine 1977; Geriatric Medicine 1994; **Med School:** SUNY Downstate 1973; **Resid:** Internal Medicine, Kings Co Hosp 1977

Taylor, William C MD (IM) PCP - **Hospital:** NYU Med Ctr (page 102); **Address:** 530 1st Ave, Ste 4H, New York, NY 10016; **Phone:** 212-263-7413; **Board Cert:** Internal Medicine 1976; **Med School:** NYU Sch Med 1957; **Resid:** Internal Medicine, Bellevue Hosp 1964; **Fac Appt:** Assoc Prof Med, NYU Sch Med

Weinstein, Jay MD (IM) PCP - **Hospital:** St Vincent Cath Med Ctrs - Manhattan (page 375); **Address:** St Vincent Cath, Med Assoc, 222 W 14th St Fl Ground, New York, NY 10011; **Phone:** 212-604-1800 x8; **Board Cert:** Internal Medicine 1991; **Med School:** Hahnemann Univ 1987; **Resid:** Internal Medicine, St Vincents Hosp & Med Ctr 1990

Weintraub, Gerald MD (IM) PCP - **Spec Exp:** Irritable Bowel Syndrome; Endoscopy; Malabsorption; **Hospital:** St Luke's - Roosevelt Hosp Ctr - Roosevelt Div (page 90); **Address:** 74 E 90th St, New York, NY 10128-1233; **Phone:** 212-348-4741; **Board Cert:** Internal Medicine 1977; Gastroenterology 1967; **Med School:** NYU Sch Med 1954; **Resid:** Internal Medicine, Roosevelt Hosp 1958; Internal Medicine, Bellevue Hosp Ctr 1959; **Fellow:** Gastroenterology, Mount Sinai Hosp 1960; **Fac Appt:** Assoc Clin Prof Med, Columbia P&S

Weiss, Nancy L MD (IM) PCP - **Hospital:** NYU Med Ctr (page 102); **Address:** 135 E 37th St, New York, NY 10016; **Phone:** 212-683-8105; **Board Cert:** Internal Medicine 2004; **Med School:** Albert Einstein Coll Med 1985; **Resid:** Internal Medicine, Manhattan VA-NYU Med Ctr 1988; **Fellow:** Rheumatology, NYU Med Ctr 1990

Wiseman, Paul MD (IM) PCP - **Spec Exp:** Preventive Medicine; **Hospital:** St Luke's - Roosevelt Hosp Ctr - Roosevelt Div (page 90); **Address:** 101 Central Park West, New York, NY 10023-4204; **Phone:** 212-496-5800; **Board Cert:** Internal Medicine 1987; **Med School:** Albert Einstein Coll Med 1981; **Resid:** Internal Medicine, Montefiore Hosp Med Ctr 1984

Yaffe, Bruce MD (IM) - **Spec Exp:** Gastroscopy; Colonoscopy; **Hospital:** Lenox Hill Hosp (page 94); **Address:** 201 E 65th St, New York, NY 10021-6701; **Phone:** 212-879-4700; **Board Cert:** Internal Medicine 1979; Gastroenterology 1981; **Med School:** Geo Wash Univ 1976; **Resid:** Internal Medicine, Mount Sinai Hosp 1979; Hepatology, Mount Sinai Hosp 1980; **Fellow:** Gastroenterology, Lenox Hill Hosp 1982

Zackson, David A MD (IM) - **Spec Exp:** Osteoporosis; Parathyroid Disorders; **Hospital:** NY-Presby Hosp (page 100); **Address:** Div of Endocrin NY Presby Hosp-Cornell, 525 E 68th St, rm 2019, New York, NY 10021; **Phone:** 212-746-6292; **Board Cert:** Internal Medicine 1964; **Med School:** NYU Sch Med 1957; **Resid:** Internal Medicine, Kingsbridge VA Med Ctr 1960; **Fellow:** Nephrology, Montefiore Hosp Med Ctr 1961

Zeale, Peter MD (IM) `PCP` - **Hospital:** St Vincent Cath Med Ctrs - Manhattan (page 375); **Address:** 275 W 7th Ave Fl 3rd, New York, NY 10011; **Phone:** 646-660-9998; **Board Cert:** Internal Medicine 1982; **Med School:** Georgetown Univ 1979; **Resid:** Internal Medicine, St Vincent's Hosp 1983

INTERVENTIONAL CARDIOLOGY

Garratt, Kirk N MD (IC) - **Spec Exp:** Angioplasty & Stent Placement; **Hospital:** Lenox Hill Hosp (page 94); **Address:** 130 E 77th St Fl 9, New York, NY 10021; **Phone:** 212-434-2606; **Board Cert:** Internal Medicine 1987; Cardiovascular Disease 1989; Interventional Cardiology 2000; **Med School:** UC Irvine 1983; **Resid:** Internal Medicine, Duke Univ Med Ctr 1986; **Fellow:** Cardiovascular Disease, UCLA Med Ctr 1988; Interventional Cardiology, Mayo Clinic 1989; **Fac Appt:** Assoc Prof Med, NYU Sch Med

Leon, Martin MD (IC) - **Hospital:** NY-Presby Hosp (page 100); **Address:** 161 Ft Washington Ave Fl 5, New York, NY 10032; **Phone:** 212-305-7060; **Board Cert:** Internal Medicine 1979; Cardiovascular Disease 1983; Interventional Cardiology 1999; **Med School:** Yale Univ 1975; **Resid:** Internal Medicine, Yale-New Haven Hosp 1978; **Fellow:** Cardiovascular Disease, Yale-New Haven Hosp 1980

Moses, Jeffrey W MD (IC) - **Spec Exp:** Angiography-Coronary; Angioplasty & Stent Placement; Heart Valve Disease; **Hospital:** NY-Presby Hosp (page 100); **Address:** 161 Fort Washington Fl 5, New York, NY 10032; **Phone:** 212-305-7060; **Board Cert:** Internal Medicine 1977; Cardiovascular Disease 1981; Interventional Cardiology 1999; **Med School:** Univ Pennsylvania 1974; **Resid:** Internal Medicine, Presby Univ Med Ctr 1977; **Fellow:** Cardiovascular Disease, Presby Univ Penn Med Ctr 1980

Roubin, Gary MD/PhD (IC) - **Spec Exp:** Coronary Angioplasty/Stents; Carotid Artery Stents; Peripheral Vascular Disease; **Hospital:** Lenox Hill Hosp (page 94); **Address:** 130 E 77th St Fl 9th, New York, NY 10021; **Phone:** 212-434-2606; **Med School:** Australia 1975; **Resid:** Internal Medicine, Royal Prince Albert Hosp 1979; Cardiovascular Disease, Hallstrom Inst of Cardiology 1981; **Fellow:** Cardiology Research, Natl Heart Fdn 1983; Interventional Cardiology, Emory Univ 1985

Sharma, Samin MD (IC) - **Spec Exp:** Angioplasty & Stent Placement; Heart Valve Disease; **Hospital:** Mount Sinai Med Ctr (page 98); **Address:** One Gustave L Levy Pl, Box 1030, Mount Sinai Medical Ctr, New York, NY 10029; **Phone:** 212-241-4021; **Board Cert:** Internal Medicine 1986; Cardiovascular Disease 1989; Interventional Cardiology 1999; **Med School:** India 1978; **Resid:** Internal Medicine, SMS Hosp 1982; Internal Medicine, NYU Downtown Hosp 1986; **Fellow:** Cardiovascular Disease, City Hosp Ctr at Elmhurst 1988; Interventional Cardiology, Mt Sinai Hosp 2000; **Fac Appt:** Prof Med, Mount Sinai Sch Med

New York (Manhattan)

Slater, James MD (IC) - **Spec Exp:** Coronary Angioplasty/Stents; Heart Valve Disease; **Hospital:** NYU Med Ctr (page 102), St Luke's - Roosevelt Hosp Ctr - Roosevelt Div (page 90); **Address:** 425 W 59th St, Ste 8B, New York, NY 10019; **Phone:** 212-293-0643; **Board Cert:** Internal Medicine 1980; Cardiovascular Disease 1985; Interventional Cardiology 1999; **Med School:** Univ Rochester 1977; **Resid:** Internal Medicine, Bellevue Hosp Ctr-NYU 1981; **Fellow:** Cardiovascular Disease, Bellevue Hosp Ctr-NYU 1983; **Fac Appt:** Assoc Prof Med, NYU Sch Med

Stone, Gregg W MD (IC) - **Spec Exp:** Angioplasty & Stent Placement; Coronary Artery Disease; **Hospital:** NY-Presby Hosp (page 100); **Address:** Columbia Univ Med Ctr, 161 Fort Washington Ave, New York, NY 10032; **Phone:** 212-851-9304; **Board Cert:** Internal Medicine 1985; Cardiovascular Disease 1987; Interventional Cardiology 1999; **Med School:** Johns Hopkins Univ 1982; **Resid:** Internal Medicine, NY Hosp-Cornell Medical Ctr 1985; **Fellow:** Cardiovascular Disease, Cedars-Sinai Medical Ctr 1988; Coronary Angioplasty, Mid-America Heart Inst 1989

MATERNAL & FETAL MEDICINE

Berkowitz, Richard MD (MF) - **Spec Exp:** Fetal Therapy; Multiple Gestation; Pregnancy & Hematologic Abnormalities; **Hospital:** NY-Presby Hosp (page 100); **Address:** 16 E 60th St Fl 4, New York, NY 10022; **Phone:** 212-326-8952; **Board Cert:** Obstetrics & Gynecology 1974; Maternal & Fetal Medicine 1979; **Med School:** NYU Sch Med 1965; **Resid:** Obstetrics & Gynecology, NY Hosp-Cornell Univ 1972; **Fac Appt:** Prof ObG, Columbia P&S

Chervenak, Francis A MD (MF) - **Spec Exp:** Ultrasound; Pregnancy-High Risk; **Hospital:** NY-Presby Hosp (page 100); **Address:** 525 E 68th St, Ste J-130, New York, NY 10021-4870; **Phone:** 212-746-3184; **Board Cert:** Obstetrics & Gynecology 1984; Maternal & Fetal Medicine 1985; **Med School:** Jefferson Med Coll 1976; **Resid:** Obstetrics & Gynecology, NY Med Coll-Flower Fifth Ave Hosp 1979; Obstetrics & Gynecology, St Lukes Hosp 1981; **Fellow:** Maternal & Fetal Medicine, Yale-New Haven Hosp 1983; **Fac Appt:** Prof ObG, Cornell Univ-Weill Med Coll

D'Alton, Mary Elizabeth MD (MF) - **Spec Exp:** Pregnancy-High Risk; Multiple Gestation; Prenatal Diagnosis; **Hospital:** NY-Presby Hosp (page 100); **Address:** 622 W 168 St, Ste 16-28, New York, NY 10032; **Phone:** 212-326-8951; **Board Cert:** Obstetrics & Gynecology 2001; Maternal & Fetal Medicine 2001; **Med School:** Ireland 1976; **Resid:** Obstetrics & Gynecology, Univ Ottawa 1982; **Fellow:** Maternal & Fetal Medicine, Tufts-New England Med Ctr 1984; **Fac Appt:** Clin Prof ObG, Columbia P&S

Eddleman, Keith A MD (MF) - **Spec Exp:** Obstetric Ultrasound; Pregnancy-High Risk; Fetal Therapy; **Hospital:** Mount Sinai Med Ctr (page 98); **Address:** Mount Sinai Medical Ctr, 5 E 98th St, Box 1170, New York, NY 10029; **Phone:** 212-241-5681; **Board Cert:** Obstetrics & Gynecology 2005; Maternal & Fetal Medicine 2005; Clinical Genetics 1999; **Med School:** Wake Forest Univ 1985; **Resid:** Obstetrics & Gynecology, George Washington Univ Med Ctr 1989; **Fellow:** Maternal & Fetal Medicine, Mt Sinai Med Ctr 1991; Genetics, Ny-Cornell Med Ctr 1996; **Fac Appt:** Assoc Prof ObG, Mount Sinai Sch Med

Edersheim, Terri MD (MF) - **Spec Exp:** Pregnancy-High Risk; Multiple Gestation; Prenatal Diagnosis; **Hospital:** NY-Presby Hosp (page 100); **Address:** 523 E 72nd St, FL 9, New York, NY 10021; **Phone:** 212-472-5340; **Board Cert:** Obstetrics & Gynecology 1997; Maternal & Fetal Medicine 1997; **Med School:** Albert Einstein Coll Med 1980; **Resid:** Obstetrics & Gynecology, New York Hosp 1984; **Fellow:** Maternal & Fetal Medicine, New York Hosp 1986; **Fac Appt:** Asst Clin Prof ObG, Cornell Univ-Weill Med Coll

Grunebaum, Amos MD (MF) - **Spec Exp:** Pregnancy-High Risk; Amniocentesis; **Hospital:** NY-Presby Hosp (page 100); **Address:** Obstetrics & Gynecology, 525 E 68th St, Ste J-130, New York, NY 10021; **Phone:** 212-746-0714; **Board Cert:** Obstetrics & Gynecology 1996; Maternal & Fetal Medicine 1996; **Med School:** Germany 1974; **Resid:** Anesthesiology, Maimonides Med Ctr 1978; Obstetrics & Gynecology, Downstate Med Ctr 1982; **Fellow:** Maternal & Fetal Medicine, Downstate Med Ctr 1984; **Fac Appt:** Assoc Prof ObG, Columbia P&S

Hutson, J Milton MD (MF) - **Spec Exp:** Multiple Gestation; Pregnancy After Age 35; Amniocentesis; **Hospital:** NY-Presby Hosp (page 100); **Address:** 523 E 72nd St, FL 9, New York, NY 10021-4099; **Phone:** 212-472-5340; **Board Cert:** Obstetrics & Gynecology 1997; Maternal & Fetal Medicine 1997; **Med School:** Univ Ala 1975; **Resid:** Obstetrics & Gynecology, Univ Hosp 1979; **Fellow:** Maternal & Fetal Medicine, Columbia-Presby 1982; **Fac Appt:** Asst Clin Prof ObG, Cornell Univ-Weill Med Coll

Manning, Frank A MD (MF) - **Spec Exp:** Fetal Therapy; Prenatal Diagnosis; **Hospital:** NY Downtown Hosp; **Address:** NYU Downtown Hospital, Dept OB/GYN, 170 William St Fl 8, New York, NY 10038; **Phone:** 212-312-5840; **Board Cert:** Obstetrics & Gynecology 1980; Maternal & Fetal Medicine 1983; **Med School:** Univ Manitoba 1970; **Resid:** Obstetrics & Gynecology, Univ of Manitoba 1974; **Fellow:** Maternal & Fetal Medicine, University Hosp 1976; **Fac Appt:** Prof ObG, Cornell Univ-Weill Med Coll

Patrick, Sharon MD (MF) - **Spec Exp:** Pregnancy-High Risk; Premature Labor; **Hospital:** NY-Presby Hosp (page 100); **Address:** 800-A Fifth Ave, Ste 503, New York, NY 10021; **Phone:** 212-230-1785; **Board Cert:** Obstetrics & Gynecology 1993; Maternal & Fetal Medicine 1995; **Med School:** Case West Res Univ 1986; **Resid:** Obstetrics & Gynecology, Columbia Presby Hosp 1990; **Fellow:** Maternal & Fetal Medicine, Columbia Presby Hosp 1992

Rebarber, Andrei MD (MF) - **Spec Exp:** Pregnancy-High Risk; Ultrasound; **Hospital:** Mount Sinai Med Ctr (page 98), Valley Hosp (page 762); **Address:** 70 E 90th St, New York, NY 10128; **Phone:** 212-722-7409; **Board Cert:** Obstetrics & Gynecology 1998; Maternal & Fetal Medicine 2000; **Med School:** SUNY Hlth Sci Ctr 1991; **Resid:** Obstetrics & Gynecology, Beth Israel Med Ctr 1995; **Fellow:** Maternal & Fetal Medicine, Yale-New Haven Hosp 1997; **Fac Appt:** Assoc Prof ObG, Mount Sinai Sch Med

Roshan, Daniel MD (MF) - **Spec Exp:** Pregnancy-High Risk; Fetal Therapy; Pregnancy Loss; Premature Labor; **Hospital:** NYU Med Ctr (page 102), N Shore Univ Hosp at Manhasset; **Address:** NYU Med Ctr, Div Maternal-Fetal Med, 530 First Ave, Ste 7N, New York, NY 10016; **Phone:** 917-481-5802; **Board Cert:** Obstetrics & Gynecology 1999; Maternal & Fetal Medicine 2001; **Med School:** Israel 1992; **Resid:** Obstetrics & Gynecology, Maimonides Med Ctr 1996; **Fellow:** Maternal & Fetal Medicine, Johns Hopkins Hosp 1998; **Fac Appt:** Asst Prof ObG, NYU Sch Med

MEDICAL ONCOLOGY

Bajorin, Dean MD (Onc) - **Spec Exp:** Genitourinary Cancer; Bladder Cancer; Testicular Cancer; **Hospital:** Meml Sloan Kettering Cancer Ctr (page 109); **Address:** 1275 York Ave, New York, NY 10021-6007; **Phone:** 646-422-4333; **Board Cert:** Internal Medicine 1981; Medical Oncology 1985; **Med School:** NY Med Coll 1978; **Resid:** Internal Medicine, Hartford Hosp 1981; **Fellow:** Medical Oncology, Meml Sloan Kettering Ctr 1985; **Fac Appt:** Prof Med, Cornell Univ-Weill Med Coll

Barbasch, Avi MD (Onc) - **Spec Exp:** Breast Cancer; Colon & Rectal Cancer; Lung Cancer; **Hospital:** Mount Sinai Med Ctr (page 98), Lenox Hill Hosp (page 94); **Address:** 1050 Park Ave, New York, NY 10028-1031; **Phone:** 212-860-3292; **Board Cert:** Internal Medicine 1997; Medical Oncology 2000; **Med School:** Mexico 1975; **Resid:** Internal Medicine, Elmhurst Hosp Ctr 1980; **Fellow:** Medical Oncology, Roswell Park Cancer Inst 1982; **Fac Appt:** Assoc Clin Prof Med, Mount Sinai Sch Med

Berman, Ellin MD (Onc) - **Spec Exp:** Leukemia; Lymphoma; **Hospital:** Meml Sloan Kettering Cancer Ctr (page 109); **Address:** 1275 York Ave, New York, NY 10021; **Phone:** 212-639-7762; **Board Cert:** Internal Medicine 1980; Medical Oncology 1985; Hematology 1984; **Med School:** Harvard Med Sch 1977; **Resid:** Internal Medicine, Boston Univ Med Ctr 1980; **Fellow:** Medical Oncology, Meml Sloan Kettering Cancer Ctr 1983

Blum, Ronald MD (Onc) - **Spec Exp:** Melanoma; Sarcoma; Lung Cancer; **Hospital:** Beth Israel Med Ctr - Petrie Division (page 90); **Address:** 10 Union Square East, Ste 4C, New York, NY 10003-3314; **Phone:** 212-844-8282; **Board Cert:** Internal Medicine 1975; Medical Oncology 1975; **Med School:** SUNY Buffalo 1970; **Resid:** Internal Medicine, Boston City Hosp 1974; **Fellow:** Medical Oncology, Dana Farber Cancer Ctr 1975; **Fac Appt:** Prof Med, Albert Einstein Coll Med

Bosl, George MD (Onc) - **Spec Exp:** Testicular Cancer; Head & Neck Cancer; **Hospital:** Meml Sloan Kettering Cancer Ctr (page 109); **Address:** 1275 York Ave, C1289, New York, NY 10021; **Phone:** 212-639-8473; **Board Cert:** Internal Medicine 1976; Medical Oncology 1979; **Med School:** Creighton Univ 1973; **Resid:** Internal Medicine, New York Hosp 1975; Internal Medicine, Memorial Sloan-Kettering Cancer Ctr 1977; **Fellow:** Medical Oncology, Univ Minn Hosps 1979; **Fac Appt:** Prof Med, Cornell Univ-Weill Med Coll

Brower, Mark MD (Onc) - **Spec Exp:** Breast Cancer; Bleeding Disorders; **Hospital:** NY-Presby Hosp (page 100); **Address:** 310 E 72nd St, New York, NY 10021-4703; **Phone:** 212-717-2995; **Board Cert:** Internal Medicine 1977; Hematology 1982; Medical Oncology 1979; **Med School:** Johns Hopkins Univ 1974; **Resid:** Internal Medicine, NY Hosp/Cornell Med Ctr 1977; **Fellow:** Hematology & Oncology, NY Hosp/Cornell Med Ctr 1980; **Fac Appt:** Assoc Clin Prof Med, Cornell Univ-Weill Med Coll

Brunckhorst, Keith MD (Onc) - **Hospital:** Lenox Hill Hosp (page 94); **Address:** 110 E 59th St, Ste 9B, New York, NY 10022-1304; **Phone:** 212-583-2858; **Board Cert:** Internal Medicine 1979; Hematology 1982; Medical Oncology 1983; **Med School:** NY Med Coll 1976; **Resid:** Internal Medicine, Stamford Hosp 1979; **Fellow:** Hematology & Oncology, Lenox Hill Hosp 1983

Chachoua, Abraham MD (Onc) - **Spec Exp:** Lung Cancer; **Hospital:** NYU Med Ctr (page 102); **Address:** NYU Clinical Cancer Ctr, 160 E 34th St Fl 8, New York, NY 10016; **Phone:** 212-652-1910; **Med School:** Australia 1978; **Resid:** Internal Medicine, Alfred Hosp 1982; **Fellow:** Hematology & Oncology, Alfred Hosp 1985; Hematology & Oncology, NYU Med Ctr 1988; **Fac Appt:** Asst Prof Med, NYU Sch Med

Chapman, Paul MD (Onc) - **Spec Exp:** Melanoma; Immunotherapy; **Hospital:** Meml Sloan Kettering Cancer Ctr (page 109); **Address:** 1275 York Ave, New York, NY 10021; **Phone:** 212-639-5015; **Board Cert:** Internal Medicine 1984; Medical Oncology 1987; **Med School:** Cornell Univ-Weill Med Coll 1981; **Resid:** Internal Medicine, Univ Chicago Hosps 1984; **Fellow:** Medical Oncology, Meml Sloan-Kettering Cancer Ctr 1987; **Fac Appt:** Prof Med, Cornell Univ-Weill Med Coll

Cohen, Seymour M MD (Onc) - **Spec Exp:** Melanoma; Breast Cancer; Lung Cancer; **Hospital:** Mount Sinai Med Ctr (page 98), NY Hosp Queens; **Address:** 1045 5th Ave, New York, NY 10028-0138; **Phone:** 212-249-9141; **Board Cert:** Internal Medicine 1971; Medical Oncology 1973; **Med School:** Univ Pittsburgh 1962; **Resid:** Internal Medicine, Montefiore Med Ctr 1964; Internal Medicine, Mount Sinai Med Ctr 1965; **Fellow:** Hematology, Mount Sinai Med Ctr 1966; Hematology & Oncology, LI Jewish Hosp 1969; **Fac Appt:** Assoc Clin Prof Med, Mount Sinai Sch Med

Coleman, Morton MD (Onc) - **Spec Exp:** Lymphoma; Hodgkin's Disease; Multiple Myeloma; Waldenstrom's Macroglobulinemia; **Hospital:** NY-Presby Hosp (page 100); **Address:** 407 E 70th St, FL 3, New York, NY 10021-5302; **Phone:** 212-517-5900; **Board Cert:** Internal Medicine 1971; Hematology 1972; Medical Oncology 1973; **Med School:** Med Coll VA 1963; **Resid:** Internal Medicine, Grady Meml Hosp-Emory 1965; Internal Medicine, New York Hosp-Cornell 1968; **Fellow:** Hematology & Oncology, New York Hosp-Cornell 1970; **Fac Appt:** Clin Prof Med, Cornell Univ-Weill Med Coll

DeBellis, Robert H MD (Onc) - **Spec Exp:** Breast Cancer; Lymphoma; Sickle Cell Disease; **Hospital:** NY-Presby Hosp (page 100); **Address:** 161 Ft Washington Ave, Ste 349, New York, NY 10032; **Phone:** 212-305-5325; **Med School:** Columbia P&S 1958; **Resid:** Internal Medicine, Bronx Municipal Hosp 1961; **Fellow:** Hematology, Columbia-Presby Hosp 1964; **Fac Appt:** Assoc Clin Prof Med, Columbia P&S

Decter, Julian A MD (Onc) - **Spec Exp:** Leukemia & Lymphoma; Multiple Myeloma; Myelodysplastic Syndromes; **Hospital:** NY-Presby Hosp (page 100), St Barnabas Med Ctr; **Address:** Div of Hem/Onc, 407 E 70th St, New York, NY 10021; **Phone:** 212-517-5900; **Board Cert:** Internal Medicine 1972; Hematology 1974; Medical Oncology 1975; **Med School:** NYU Sch Med 1966; **Resid:** Internal Medicine, Ohio State Hosps 1968; **Fellow:** Hematology, NYU Med Ctr 1970; Medical Oncology, Nat Cancer Inst 1974; **Fac Appt:** Assoc Clin Prof Med, Cornell Univ-Weill Med Coll

Dickler, Maura N MD (Onc) - **Spec Exp:** Breast Cancer; **Hospital:** Meml Sloan Kettering Cancer Ctr (page 109); **Address:** Meml Sloan Kettering Cancer Ctr, 1275 York Ave, New York, NY 10021; **Phone:** 212-639-5456; **Board Cert:** Internal Medicine 1994; Medical Oncology 1998; **Med School:** Univ Chicago-Pritzker Sch Med 1991; **Resid:** Internal Medicine, Univ Chicago Hosps 1994; **Fellow:** Medical Oncology, Meml Sloan Kettering Cancer Ctr 1998; **Fac Appt:** Asst Prof Med, Cornell Univ-Weill Med Coll

Fine, Robert MD (Onc) - **Spec Exp:** Pancreatic Cancer; Drug Development; Brain Tumors; **Hospital:** NY-Presby Hosp (page 100); **Address:** Columbia Univ Comprehensive Cancer Ctr, 650 W 168th St, rm BB 20-05, New York, NY 10032; **Phone:** 212-305-1168; **Board Cert:** Internal Medicine 1983; Medical Oncology 1985; **Med School:** Univ Chicago-Pritzker Sch Med 1979; **Resid:** Internal Medicine, Stanford Univ Med Ctr 1982; **Fellow:** Medical Oncology, National Cancer Inst 1988; **Fac Appt:** Assoc Prof Med, Columbia P&S

Gabrilove, Janice MD (Onc) - **Spec Exp:** Myelodysplastic Syndromes; Leukemia; **Hospital:** Mount Sinai Med Ctr (page 98); **Address:** Mount Sinai Med Ctr, Box 1129, One Gustave Levy Pl, New York, NY 10029-6574; **Phone:** 212-241-9650; **Board Cert:** Internal Medicine 1980; Medical Oncology 1983; **Med School:** Mount Sinai Sch Med 1977; **Resid:** Internal Medicine, Columbia-Presby Med Ctr 1980; **Fellow:** Hematology & Oncology, Meml Sloan-Kettering Cancer Ctr 1983; **Fac Appt:** Prof Med, Mount Sinai Sch Med

New York (Manhattan)

Gaynor, Mitchell MD (Onc) - **Spec Exp:** Breast Cancer; Lung Cancer; Nutrition & Complementary Medicine; **Hospital:** NY-Presby Hosp (page 100); **Address:** 331 E 65th St, New York, NY 10021-4635; **Phone:** 212-410-3820; **Board Cert:** Internal Medicine 1985; Medical Oncology 1987; Hematology 1988; **Med School:** Univ Tex SW, Dallas 1982; **Resid:** Internal Medicine, New York Hosp 1985; **Fellow:** Hematology & Oncology, New York Hosp 1988

Goldberg, Arthur I MD (Onc) - **Spec Exp:** Breast Cancer; Prostate Cancer; Colon & Rectal Cancer; **Hospital:** Lenox Hill Hosp (page 94), Mount Sinai Med Ctr (page 98); **Address:** 121 E 79th St, New York, NY 10021-0320; **Phone:** 212-249-0030; **Board Cert:** Internal Medicine 1974; Medical Oncology 1975; **Med School:** SUNY Hlth Sci Ctr 1969; **Resid:** Internal Medicine, Bellevue/NYU Med Ctr 1973; **Fellow:** Cancer Immunology, Natl Cancer Inst 1972; Medical Oncology, Meml Sloan Kettering Cancer Ctr 1975

Goldsmith, Michael MD (Onc) - **Spec Exp:** Breast Cancer; Colon Cancer; Lung Cancer; **Hospital:** Mount Sinai Med Ctr (page 98), NY Hosp Queens; **Address:** 1045 5th Ave, New York, NY 10028-0138; **Phone:** 212-628-6800; **Board Cert:** Internal Medicine 1976; Medical Oncology 1977; **Med School:** Albert Einstein Coll Med 1971; **Resid:** Internal Medicine, Mount Sinai Hosp 1975; **Fellow:** Medical Oncology, Mount Sinai Hosp 1977; **Fac Appt:** Asst Clin Prof Med, Mount Sinai Sch Med

Grace, William MD (Onc) - **Spec Exp:** Breast Cancer; Liver Cancer; **Hospital:** St Vincent Cath Med Ctrs - Manhattan (page 375); **Address:** 36 7th Ave, Ste 511, New York, NY 10011; **Phone:** 212-675-6826; **Board Cert:** Medical Oncology 1977; Internal Medicine 1976; **Med School:** Boston Univ 1969; **Resid:** Internal Medicine, St Vincent's Hosp & Med Ctr 1971; **Fellow:** Hematology & Oncology, Dartmouth-Hitchcock Med Ctr 1976; **Fac Appt:** Assoc Clin Prof Med, NY Med Coll

Grossbard, Lionel MD (Onc) - **Spec Exp:** Lymphoma; Anemia; Breast Cancer; **Hospital:** NY-Presby Hosp (page 100); **Address:** 161 Fort Washington Ave, New York, NY 10032-3713; **Phone:** 212-305-8399; **Board Cert:** Internal Medicine 1973; Hematology 1974; Medical Oncology 1975; **Med School:** Columbia P&S 1961; **Resid:** Internal Medicine, Columbia-Presby Med Ctr 1964; **Fellow:** Hematology, Columbia-Presby Med Ctr 1968; **Fac Appt:** Clin Prof Med, Columbia P&S

Grossbard, Michael L MD (Onc) - **Spec Exp:** Lymphoma; Breast Cancer; Gastrointestinal Cancer; **Hospital:** St Luke's - Roosevelt Hosp Ctr - Roosevelt Div (page 90), Beth Israel Med Ctr - Petrie Division (page 90); **Address:** 1000 10th Ave Fl 11 - Ste C02, New York, NY 10019; **Phone:** 212-523-5419; **Board Cert:** Internal Medicine 1989; Medical Oncology 2001; **Med School:** Yale Univ 1986; **Resid:** Internal Medicine, Mass Genl Hosp 1989; **Fellow:** Medical Oncology, Dana Farber Cancer Inst 1991; **Fac Appt:** Assoc Clin Prof Med, Columbia P&S

Gruenstein, Steven MD (Onc) - **Spec Exp:** Breast Cancer; Gastrointestinal Cancer; Leukemia & Lymphoma; **Hospital:** Mount Sinai Med Ctr (page 98), Lenox Hill Hosp (page 94); **Address:** 12 E 86th St, New York, NY 10028-0506; **Phone:** 212-861-6660; **Board Cert:** Internal Medicine 1988; Hematology 1994; Medical Oncology 2001; **Med School:** Italy 1984; **Resid:** Internal Medicine, Metropolitan Hosp Ctr 1987; **Fellow:** Hematology & Oncology, Beth Israel Med Ctr 1990; **Fac Appt:** Asst Clin Prof Med, Mount Sinai Sch Med

Gulati, Subhash C MD/PhD (Onc) - **Spec Exp:** Breast Cancer; Lymphoma; Lung Cancer; **Hospital:** NY-Presby Hosp (page 100), Wyckoff Heights Med Ctr; **Address:** 449 E 68th St, Ste 2, New York, NY 10021-6310; **Phone:** 212-535-1514; **Board Cert:** Internal Medicine 1980; Hematology 1986; Medical Oncology 1983; **Med School:** Univ Miami Sch Med 1976; **Resid:** Internal Medicine, Buffalo Genl Hosp 1978; **Fellow:** Hematology & Oncology, Meml Sloan Kettering Cancer Ctr 1980; **Fac Appt:** Clin Prof Med, Cornell Univ-Weill Med Coll

Hirschman, Richard J MD (Onc) - **Spec Exp:** Breast Cancer; Colon Cancer; Lung Cancer; **Hospital:** Cabrini Med Ctr (page 374), Beth Israel Med Ctr - Petrie Division (page 90); **Address:** 247 3rd Ave, Ste 401, New York, NY 10010-7455; **Phone:** 212-228-0471; **Board Cert:** Internal Medicine 1971; Hematology 1972; Medical Oncology 1973; **Med School:** Johns Hopkins Univ 1965; **Resid:** Internal Medicine, Bellevue Hosp Ctr 1967; Internal Medicine, Columbia-Presby Hosp 1970; **Fellow:** Hematology & Oncology, Columbia-Presby Hosp 1971; **Fac Appt:** Assoc Clin Prof Med, Mount Sinai Sch Med

Hirshaut, Yashar MD (Onc) - **Spec Exp:** Breast Cancer; Lung Cancer; Colon Cancer; **Hospital:** Lenox Hill Hosp (page 94), NY-Presby Hosp (page 100); **Address:** 860 5th Ave, New York, NY 10021-5856; **Phone:** 212-861-1799; **Board Cert:** Internal Medicine 1972; Medical Oncology 1975; **Med School:** Albert Einstein Coll Med 1963; **Resid:** Internal Medicine, Montefiore Hosp Med Ctr 1965; **Fellow:** Medical Oncology, Natl Cancer Inst 1968; Medical Oncology, Meml Sloan Kettering Cancer Ctr 1970; **Fac Appt:** Assoc Clin Prof Med, Cornell Univ-Weill Med Coll

Hochster, Howard S MD (Onc) - **Spec Exp:** Gastrointestinal Cancer; Gynecologic Cancer; Colon & Rectal Cancer; **Hospital:** NYU Med Ctr (page 102); **Address:** NYU Cancer Institute, 160 E 34 Fl 9, New York, NY 10016; **Phone:** 212-731-5100; **Board Cert:** Internal Medicine 1983; Medical Oncology 1985; Hematology 1986; **Med School:** Yale Univ 1980; **Resid:** Internal Medicine, NYU Med Ctr 1983; **Fellow:** Hematology & Oncology, NYU Med Ctr 1985; Medical Oncology, Jules Bordet Inst 1986; **Fac Appt:** Prof Med, NYU Sch Med

Holland, James F MD (Onc) - **Spec Exp:** Breast Cancer; Psychiatry in Cancer; **Hospital:** Mount Sinai Med Ctr (page 98); **Address:** Ruttenberg Cancer Ctr, Div Med Oncology, OneL Gustave L Levy Pl, Box 1129, New York, NY 10029-6574; **Phone:** 212-241-4495; **Board Cert:** Internal Medicine 1955; **Med School:** Columbia P&S 1947; **Resid:** Internal Medicine, Columbia-Presby Hosp 1949; **Fellow:** Medical Oncology, Francis Delafield Hosp 1953; **Fac Appt:** Prof Med, Mount Sinai Sch Med

Houghton, Alan N MD (Onc) - **Spec Exp:** Melanoma; Immunotherapy; Cancer Vaccines; **Hospital:** Meml Sloan Kettering Cancer Ctr (page 109); **Address:** 1275 York Ave, Box 465, New York, NY 10021; **Phone:** 212-639-7595; **Board Cert:** Internal Medicine 1977; Medical Oncology 1979; **Med School:** Univ Conn 1974; **Resid:** Internal Medicine, Univ Conn Hlth Ctr 1977; **Fellow:** Medical Oncology, Mem Sloan Kettering Cancer Ctr 1979; **Fac Appt:** Prof Med, Cornell Univ-Weill Med Coll

Hudis, Clifford A MD (Onc) - **Spec Exp:** Breast Cancer; **Hospital:** Meml Sloan Kettering Cancer Ctr (page 109); **Address:** Meml Sloan Kettering Cancer Ctr, 1275 York Ave, Box 206, New York, NY 10021-6007; **Phone:** 212-639-5449; **Board Cert:** Internal Medicine 1986; Medical Oncology 2001; **Med School:** Med Coll PA Hahnemann 1983; **Resid:** Internal Medicine, Hosp Med Coll Penn 1986; **Fellow:** Medical Oncology, Meml Sloan Kettering Cancer Ctr 1991; **Fac Appt:** Assoc Prof Med, Cornell Univ-Weill Med Coll

New York (Manhattan)

Jagannath, Sundar MD (Onc) - **Spec Exp:** Multiple Myeloma; **Hospital:** St Vincent Cath Med Ctrs - Manhattan (page 375); **Address:** 325 W 15th St, New York, NY 10011; **Phone:** 212-604-6068; **Board Cert:** Internal Medicine 1980; Medical Oncology 1985; **Med School:** India 1976; **Resid:** Internal Medicine, Bronx Lebanon Hosp 1979; Internal Medicine, Harper-Grace Hosp 1980; **Fellow:** Medical Oncology, MD Anderson Cancer Ctr 1982; **Fac Appt:** Prof Med, NY Med Coll

Jarowski, Charles MD (Onc) - **Spec Exp:** Breast Cancer; Lung Cancer; Colon Cancer; **Hospital:** NY-Presby Hosp (page 100); **Address:** 400 E 77th St, Ste 1A, New York, NY 10021-2366; **Phone:** 212-794-9500; **Board Cert:** Internal Medicine 1975; Medical Oncology 1977; Hematology 1978; **Med School:** Cornell Univ-Weill Med Coll 1972; **Resid:** Internal Medicine, NY Hosp 1975; **Fellow:** Hematology & Oncology, NY Hosp 1978; **Fac Appt:** Asst Prof Med, Cornell Univ-Weill Med Coll

Kabakow, Bernard MD (Onc) - **Spec Exp:** Breast Cancer; Colon & Rectal Cancer; Lung Cancer; **Hospital:** Beth Israel Med Ctr - Petrie Division (page 90), Cabrini Med Ctr (page 374); **Address:** 308 E 15th St, New York, NY 10003; **Phone:** 212-674-4455; **Board Cert:** Internal Medicine 1961; Medical Oncology 1973; **Med School:** Univ VT Coll Med 1953; **Resid:** Internal Medicine, Kings County Hosp 1955; Internal Medicine, Mount Sinai 1956; **Fellow:** Medical Oncology, Montefiore Hosp Med Ctr 1958; **Fac Appt:** Clin Prof Med, Albert Einstein Coll Med

Kelsen, David MD (Onc) - **Spec Exp:** Gastrointestinal Cancer; Neuroendocrine Tumors; Unknown Primary Cancer; **Hospital:** Meml Sloan Kettering Cancer Ctr (page 109); **Address:** Gastrointestinal Oncology Svc, 1275 York Ave Bldg Howard Fl 9 - rm 918, New York, NY 10021; **Phone:** 212-639-8470; **Board Cert:** Internal Medicine 1976; Medical Oncology 1979; **Med School:** Hahnemann Univ 1972; **Resid:** Internal Medicine, Temple Univ Hosp 1976; **Fellow:** Medical Oncology, Meml Sloan Kettering Cancer Ctr 1978; **Fac Appt:** Prof Med, Cornell Univ-Weill Med Coll

Kemeny, Nancy MD (Onc) - **Spec Exp:** Colon Cancer; Rectal Cancer; Liver Cancer; **Hospital:** Meml Sloan Kettering Cancer Ctr (page 109); **Address:** Meml Sloan Kettering Cancer Ctr, 1275 York Ave, Howard 916, New York, NY 10021; **Phone:** 212-639-8068; **Board Cert:** Internal Medicine 1974; Medical Oncology 1981; **Med School:** UMDNJ-NJ Med Sch, Newark 1971; **Resid:** Internal Medicine, St Luke's Hosp 1974; **Fellow:** Medical Oncology, Mem Sloan Kettering Cancer Ctr 1976; **Fac Appt:** Prof Med, Cornell Univ-Weill Med Coll

Kris, Mark G MD (Onc) - **Spec Exp:** Lung Cancer; Mediastinal Tumors; Thymoma; **Hospital:** Meml Sloan Kettering Cancer Ctr (page 109); **Address:** Memorial Sloan Kettering Cancer Ctr, 1275 York Ave, Howard H1018, New York, NY 10021; **Phone:** 212-639-7590; **Board Cert:** Internal Medicine 1980; Medical Oncology 1983; **Med School:** Cornell Univ-Weill Med Coll 1977; **Resid:** Internal Medicine, New York Hosp 1980; **Fellow:** Medical Oncology, Meml Sloan Kettering Cancer Ctr 1983; **Fac Appt:** Prof Med, Cornell Univ-Weill Med Coll

Krown, Susan MD (Onc) - **Spec Exp:** AIDS/HIV; AIDS-Kaposi's Sarcoma; Melanoma; **Hospital:** Meml Sloan Kettering Cancer Ctr (page 109); **Address:** 1275 York Ave, rm H804, New York, NY 10021; **Phone:** 212-639-7426; **Board Cert:** Internal Medicine 1974; Medical Oncology 1977; **Med School:** SUNY Hlth Sci Ctr 1971; **Resid:** Internal Medicine, Mount Sinai Hosp 1974; **Fellow:** Medical Oncology, Meml Sloan Kettering Cancer Ctr 1977; **Fac Appt:** Prof Med, Cornell Univ-Weill Med Coll

Livingston, Philip MD (Onc) - **Spec Exp:** Melanoma; Cancer Vaccines; Immunotherapy; **Hospital:** Meml Sloan Kettering Cancer Ctr (page 109); **Address:** 1275 York Ave, New York, NY 10021-6007; **Phone:** 212-639-7425; **Board Cert:** Internal Medicine 1980; Allergy & Immunology 1974; Rheumatology 1974; Medical Oncology 1981; **Med School:** Harvard Med Sch 1969; **Resid:** Internal Medicine, N Shore Hosp-Cornell Med Ctr 1971; **Fellow:** Immunology, NYU Med Ctr 1973; **Fac Appt:** Prof Med, Cornell Univ-Weill Med Coll

Macdonald, John S MD (Onc) - **Spec Exp:** Colon Cancer; Gastrointestinal Cancer; Pancreatic Cancer; **Hospital:** St Vincent Cath Med Ctrs - Manhattan (page 375); **Address:** 325 W 15th St, New York, NY 10011-5903; **Phone:** 212-604-6011; **Board Cert:** Internal Medicine 1973; Medical Oncology 1975; **Med School:** Harvard Med Sch 1969; **Resid:** Internal Medicine, Beth Israel Hosp 1971; **Fellow:** Hematology & Oncology, Natl Cancer Inst 1974; **Fac Appt:** Prof Med, NY Med Coll

Malamud, Stephen C MD (Onc) - **Spec Exp:** Lung Cancer; Gastrointestinal Cancer; **Hospital:** Beth Israel Med Ctr - Petrie Division (page 90), Hosp For Joint Diseases (page 107); **Address:** 10 Union Square E, Ste 4A, New York, NY 10003; **Phone:** 212-844-8280; **Board Cert:** Internal Medicine 1981; Medical Oncology 1983; **Med School:** Albert Einstein Coll Med 1978; **Resid:** Internal Medicine, Beth Israel Med Ctr 1981; **Fellow:** Medical Oncology, Mt Sinai Hosp 1983; **Fac Appt:** Assoc Prof Med, Albert Einstein Coll Med

Miller, Vincent A MD (Onc) - **Spec Exp:** Lung Cancer; Drug Development; **Hospital:** Meml Sloan Kettering Cancer Ctr (page 109); **Address:** Memorial Sloan Kettering Cancer Ctr, 1275 York Ave, Howard 10, New York, NY 10021; **Phone:** 212-639-7243; **Board Cert:** Internal Medicine 2002; Medical Oncology 2005; **Med School:** UMDNJ-NJ Med Sch, Newark 1987; **Resid:** Internal Medicine, Thos Jefferson Univ Hosp 1991; **Fellow:** Medical Oncology, Meml Sloan Kettering Cancer Ctr 1994

Milowsky, Matthew I MD (Onc) - **Spec Exp:** Prostate Cancer; Bladder Cancer; Kidney Cancer; Testicular Cancer; **Hospital:** NY-Presby Hosp (page 100); **Address:** NY Cornell Medical Ctr, Medical Oncology, 525 E 68th St, Starr 341, New York, NY 10021; **Phone:** 212-746-6717; **Board Cert:** Internal Medicine 1999; Medical Oncology 2002; Hematology 2002; **Med School:** SUNY Downstate 1996; **Resid:** Internal Medicine, New Eng Med Ctr 1999; **Fellow:** Hematology & Oncology, NY Presby Hosp-Cornell U 2002; **Fac Appt:** Asst Prof U, Cornell Univ-Weill Med Coll

Moore, Anne MD (Onc) - **Spec Exp:** Breast Cancer; **Hospital:** NY-Presby Hosp (page 100); **Address:** New York Presbyterian Hosp, 428 E 72nd St, Ste 300, New York, NY 10021-4873; **Phone:** 212-746-2085; **Board Cert:** Internal Medicine 1973; Hematology 1976; Medical Oncology 1977; **Med School:** Columbia P&S 1969; **Resid:** Internal Medicine, Cornell Univ Med Ctr 1973; **Fellow:** Medical Oncology, Rockefeller Univ 1973; **Fac Appt:** Prof Med, Cornell Univ-Weill Med Coll

Motzer, Robert J MD (Onc) - **Spec Exp:** Kidney Cancer; Testicular Cancer; Prostate Cancer; **Hospital:** Meml Sloan Kettering Cancer Ctr (page 109); **Address:** 1275 York Ave, Box 239, New York, NY 10021; **Phone:** 646-422-4312; **Board Cert:** Internal Medicine 1984; Medical Oncology 1987; **Med School:** Univ Mich Med Sch 1981; **Resid:** Internal Medicine, Meml Sloan Kettering Cancer Ctr 1984; **Fellow:** Medical Oncology, Meml Sloan Kettering Cancer Ctr 1987; **Fac Appt:** Assoc Prof Med, Cornell Univ-Weill Med Coll

Muggia, Franco MD (Onc) - **Spec Exp:** Breast Cancer; Gynecologic Cancer; **Hospital:** NYU Med Ctr (page 102); **Address:** NYU Clinical Cancer Ctr, 160 E 34th St Fl 8, New York, NY 10016; **Phone:** 212-731-5433; **Board Cert:** Internal Medicine 1968; Hematology 1974; Medical Oncology 1973; **Med School:** Cornell Univ-Weill Med Coll 1961; **Resid:** Internal Medicine, Hartford Hosp 1964; Internal Medicine, Francis A Delafield Hosp 1966; **Fac Appt:** Prof Med, NYU Sch Med

Norton, Larry MD (Onc) - **Spec Exp:** Breast Cancer; **Hospital:** Meml Sloan Kettering Cancer Ctr (page 109); **Address:** 205 E 64th St, New York, NY 10021; **Phone:** 212-639-5438; **Board Cert:** Internal Medicine 1975; Medical Oncology 1977; **Med School:** Columbia P&S 1972; **Resid:** Internal Medicine, Bronx Muni Hosp 1974; **Fac Appt:** Prof Med, Cornell Univ-Weill Med Coll

O'Reilly, Eileen M MD (Onc) - **Spec Exp:** Pancreatic Cancer; Clinical Trials; Liver Cancer; Liver & Biliary Cancer; **Hospital:** Meml Sloan Kettering Cancer Ctr (page 109); **Address:** 1275 York Ave, Box 324, New York, NY 10021; **Phone:** 212-639-6672; **Med School:** Ireland 1989; **Resid:** Internal Medicine, St Vincent's Hosp 1994; **Fellow:** Hematology, St Vincent's Hosp 1995; Medical Oncology, Memorial-Sloan Kettering Cancer Ctr 1997; **Fac Appt:** Asst Prof Med, Cornell Univ-Weill Med Coll

Offit, Kenneth MD (Onc) - **Spec Exp:** Cancer Genetics; Breast Cancer; Lymphoma; **Hospital:** Meml Sloan Kettering Cancer Ctr (page 109); **Address:** 1275 York Ave, Box 192, New York, NY 10021-6094; **Phone:** 212-434-5149; **Board Cert:** Internal Medicine 1985; Medical Oncology 1987; **Med School:** Harvard Med Sch 1982; **Resid:** Internal Medicine, Lenox Hill Hosp 1985; **Fellow:** Hematology & Oncology, Meml Sloan Kettering Cancer Ctr 1988; **Fac Appt:** Prof Med, Cornell Univ-Weill Med Coll

Oster, Martin W MD (Onc) - **Spec Exp:** Breast Cancer; Gastrointestinal Cancer; Lung Cancer; **Hospital:** NY-Presby Hosp (page 100); **Address:** NY Presbyterian Hosp - Columbia Presby Med Ctr, 161 Fort Washington Ave, New York, NY 10032-3713; **Phone:** 212-305-8231; **Board Cert:** Internal Medicine 1974; Medical Oncology 1975; **Med School:** Columbia P&S 1971; **Resid:** Internal Medicine, Mass Genl Hosp 1973; **Fellow:** Medical Oncology, Natl Cancer Inst/NIH 1976; **Fac Appt:** Assoc Clin Prof Med, Columbia P&S

Pasmantier, Mark MD (Onc) - **Spec Exp:** Lung Cancer; Ovarian Cancer; **Hospital:** NY-Presby Hosp (page 100); **Address:** 407 E 70th St, FL 3, New York, NY 10021-5302; **Phone:** 212-517-5900; **Board Cert:** Internal Medicine 1972; Hematology 1974; Medical Oncology 1975; **Med School:** NYU Sch Med 1966; **Resid:** Internal Medicine, Harlem Hosp 1970; **Fellow:** Hematology, Montefiore Hosp Med Ctr 1971; Medical Oncology, New York Hosp 1972; **Fac Appt:** Clin Prof Med, Cornell Univ-Weill Med Coll

Petrylak, Daniel P MD (Onc) - **Spec Exp:** Genitourinary Cancer; Prostate Cancer; Bladder Cancer; **Hospital:** NY-Presby Hosp (page 100); **Address:** 161 Fort Washington Ave, New York, NY 10032-3713; **Phone:** 212-305-1731; **Board Cert:** Internal Medicine 2001; Medical Oncology 1993; **Med School:** Case West Res Univ 1985; **Resid:** Internal Medicine, Jacobi Med Ctr 1988; **Fellow:** Oncology, Meml-Sloan Kettering Cancer Ctr 1991; **Fac Appt:** Assoc Prof Med, Columbia P&S

Pfister, David G MD (Onc) - **Spec Exp:** Head & Neck Cancer; Laryngeal Cancer; Thyroid Cancer; **Hospital:** Meml Sloan Kettering Cancer Ctr (page 109); **Address:** Memorial Sloan Kettering Cancer Ctr, 1275 York Ave, Box 188, New York, NY 10021; **Phone:** 212-639-8235; **Board Cert:** Internal Medicine 1985; Medical Oncology 1989; **Med School:** Univ Pennsylvania 1982; **Resid:** Internal Medicine, Hosp Univ Penn 1985; **Fellow:** Epidemiology, Yale New Haven Hosp 1987; Hematology & Oncology, Meml Sloan Kettering Cancer Ctr 1989; **Fac Appt:** Prof Med, Cornell Univ-Weill Med Coll

Portlock, Carol S MD (Onc) - **Spec Exp:** Lymphoma; Hodgkin's Disease; **Hospital:** Meml Sloan Kettering Cancer Ctr (page 109); **Address:** Lymphoma Service, 1275 York Ave, New York, NY 10021-6007; **Phone:** 212-639-8109; **Board Cert:** Internal Medicine 1976; Medical Oncology 1978; **Med School:** Stanford Univ 1971; **Resid:** Internal Medicine, Stanford U Med Ctr 1974; **Fellow:** Medical Oncology, Stanford U Med Ctr 1976; **Fac Appt:** Clin Prof Med, Cornell Univ-Weill Med Coll

Ratner, Lynn MD (Onc) - **Spec Exp:** Breast Cancer; **Hospital:** Mount Sinai Med Ctr (page 98), Lenox Hill Hosp (page 94); **Address:** 112 E 83rd St, New York, NY 10028-0506; **Phone:** 212-396-0400; **Board Cert:** Internal Medicine 1971; Medical Oncology 1973; **Med School:** Albert Einstein Coll Med 1964; **Resid:** Bellevue Hosp 1965Bellevue Hosp; **Fellow:** Meml Sloan Kettering Cancer Ctr

Robson, Mark Emerson MD (Onc) - **Spec Exp:** Breast Cancer; Cancer Genetics; **Hospital:** Meml Sloan Kettering Cancer Ctr (page 109); **Address:** Meml Sloan Kettering Cancer Ctr, 205 E 64th St, Concourse Level, New York, NY 10021; **Phone:** 212-639-5434; **Board Cert:** Internal Medicine 1989; Medical Oncology 2001; Hematology 2002; **Med School:** Univ VA Sch Med 1986

Ruggiero, Joseph MD (Onc) - **Spec Exp:** Colon Cancer; Breast Cancer; **Hospital:** NY-Presby Hosp (page 100); **Address:** 428 E 72nd St, Ste 300, New York, NY 10021-4635; **Phone:** 212-746-2083; **Board Cert:** Internal Medicine 1980; Hematology 1982; Medical Oncology 1983; **Med School:** NYU Sch Med 1977; **Resid:** Internal Medicine, NY Hosp-Cornell Med Ctr 1980; **Fellow:** Hematology & Oncology, NY Hosp-Cornell Med Ctr 1983; **Fac Appt:** Assoc Clin Prof Med, Cornell Univ-Weill Med Coll

Saltz, Leonard B MD (Onc) - **Spec Exp:** Colon & Rectal Cancer; Gastrointestinal Cancer & Rare Tumors; Liver Cancer; **Hospital:** Meml Sloan Kettering Cancer Ctr (page 109); **Address:** Memorial Sloan Kettering Cancer Ctr, 1275 York Ave, Howard 917, New York, NY 10021; **Phone:** 212-639-2501; **Board Cert:** Internal Medicine 1986; Hematology 1988; Medical Oncology 1989; **Med School:** Yale Univ 1983; **Resid:** Internal Medicine, New York Hosp-Cornell Med Ctr 1986; **Fellow:** Hematology & Oncology, New York Hosp-Cornell Med Ctr/Rockefeller Univ 1987; **Fac Appt:** Prof Med, Cornell Univ-Weill Med Coll

Sara, Gabriel MD (Onc) - **Spec Exp:** Breast Cancer; Lung Cancer; Lymphoma; Colon & Rectal Cancer; **Hospital:** St Luke's - Roosevelt Hosp Ctr - Roosevelt Div (page 90); **Address:** 30 W 60th St, New York, NY 10023; **Phone:** 212-977-9292; **Board Cert:** Internal Medicine 1984; Hematology 1986; Medical Oncology 1987; **Med School:** Lebanon 1980; **Resid:** Internal Medicine, SUNY Downstate Med Ctr 1984; **Fellow:** Hematology & Oncology, St Luke's-Roosevelt Med Ctr 1986; Hematology & Oncology, Columbia-Presby Med Ctr 1987; **Fac Appt:** Asst Clin Prof Med, Columbia P&S

Scheinberg, David MD/PhD (Onc) - **Spec Exp:** Leukemia; Immunotherapy; Cancer Vaccines; **Hospital:** Meml Sloan Kettering Cancer Ctr (page 109); **Address:** 1275 York Ave, New York, NY 10021-6007; **Phone:** 212-639-5010; **Board Cert:** Internal Medicine 1986; Medical Oncology 1995; **Med School:** Johns Hopkins Univ 1983; **Resid:** Internal Medicine, New York Hosp/Cornell 1985; **Fellow:** Medical Oncology, Meml Sloan Kettering Cancer Ctr 1987; **Fac Appt:** Prof Med, Cornell Univ-Weill Med Coll

Scher, Howard MD (Onc) - **Spec Exp:** Genitourinary Cancer; Prostate Cancer; Bladder Cancer; **Hospital:** Meml Sloan Kettering Cancer Ctr (page 109); **Address:** 1275 York Ave, New York, NY 10021; **Phone:** 646-422-4330; **Board Cert:** Internal Medicine 1979; Medical Oncology 1985; **Med School:** NYU Sch Med 1976; **Resid:** Internal Medicine, Bellevue Hosp 1980; **Fellow:** Medical Oncology, Meml Sloan Kettering Cancer Ctr 1983; **Fac Appt:** Prof Med, Cornell Univ-Weill Med Coll

Sherman, William H MD (Onc) - **Spec Exp:** Pancreatic Cancer; Multiple Myeloma; **Hospital:** NY-Presby Hosp (page 100); **Address:** 161 Fort Washington Ave, Ste 922, New York, NY 10032; **Phone:** 212-305-3856; **Board Cert:** Internal Medicine 1975; Medical Oncology 1979; **Med School:** Jefferson Med Coll 1969; **Resid:** Internal Medicine, Univ Illinois Hosp 1971; **Fellow:** Medical Oncology, Columbia-Presby Hosp 1977; **Fac Appt:** Assoc Clin Prof Med, Columbia P&S

Silver, Richard MD (Onc) - **Spec Exp:** Leukemia; Myeloproliferative Disorders; Lymphoma; **Hospital:** NY-Presby Hosp (page 100); **Address:** 525 E 68th St, Box 581, New York, NY 10021-2577; **Phone:** 212-746-2855; **Board Cert:** Internal Medicine 1962; Medical Oncology 1973; **Med School:** Cornell Univ-Weill Med Coll 1953; **Resid:** Internal Medicine, New York Hosp 1956; Hematology & Oncology, New York Hosp 1957; **Fellow:** Natl Cancer Inst 1958; **Fac Appt:** Clin Prof Med, Cornell Univ-Weill Med Coll

Sklarin, Nancy MD (Onc) - **Spec Exp:** Breast Cancer; **Hospital:** Meml Sloan Kettering Cancer Ctr (page 109); **Address:** 205 E 64th St, New York, NY 10021; **Phone:** 212-639-5488; **Board Cert:** Internal Medicine 1984; Medical Oncology 1987; **Med School:** Albert Einstein Coll Med 1981; **Resid:** Internal Medicine, LI Jewish Hospital 1984; **Fellow:** Hematology & Oncology, Mount Sinai Hospital 1987; **Fac Appt:** Asst Prof Med, Cornell Univ-Weill Med Coll

Slovin, Susan F MD/PhD (Onc) - **Spec Exp:** Prostate Cancer; Genitourinary Cancer; Immunotherapy; **Hospital:** Meml Sloan Kettering Cancer Ctr (page 109), NY-Presby Hosp (page 100); **Address:** Meml Sloan Kettering Cancer Ctr, Dept Med Onc, 1275 York Ave, New York, NY 10021; **Phone:** 646-422-4470; **Board Cert:** Internal Medicine 1995; Medical Oncology 1999; **Med School:** Jefferson Med Coll 1990; **Resid:** Internal Medicine, Mt Sinai Hosp 1993; **Fellow:** Medical Oncology, Meml Sloan Kettering Cancer Ctr 1996; **Fac Appt:** Asst Prof Med, Cornell Univ-Weill Med Coll

Smith, Julia A MD (Onc) - **Spec Exp:** Breast Cancer; Breast Cancer-High Risk Women; **Hospital:** Bellevue Hosp Ctr, NYU Med Ctr (page 102); **Address:** 530 First Ave, Ste 4-G, NYU Medical Ctr, New York, NY 10016; **Phone:** 212-263-7269; **Board Cert:** Internal Medicine 1985; Medical Oncology 1989; **Med School:** NYU Sch Med 1980; **Resid:** Internal Medicine, Brigham & Womens Hosp 1983; **Fellow:** Hematology & Oncology, Meml Sloan Kettering Cancer Ctr 1986; **Fac Appt:** Asst Clin Prof Med, NYU Sch Med

Speyer, James MD (Onc) - **Spec Exp:** Ovarian Cancer; Breast Cancer; Cardiac Toxicity in Cancer Therapy; **Hospital:** NYU Med Ctr (page 102); **Address:** NYU Clinical Cancer Center, 160 E 34th St, New York, NY 10016-6004; **Phone:** 212-731-5432; **Board Cert:** Internal Medicine 1977; Hematology 1978; Medical Oncology 1979; **Med School:** Johns Hopkins Univ 1974; **Resid:** Internal Medicine, Columbia-Presby Med Ctr 1976; Hematology, Columbia-Presby Med Ctr 1977; **Fellow:** Medical Oncology, Natl Cancer Inst 1979; **Fac Appt:** Clin Prof Med, NYU Sch Med

Spriggs, David MD (Onc) - **Spec Exp:** Ovarian Cancer; Drug Development; Uterine Cancer; **Hospital:** Meml Sloan Kettering Cancer Ctr (page 109); **Address:** 1275 York Ave, Box 67, New York, NY 10021-6007; **Phone:** 212-639-2203; **Board Cert:** Internal Medicine 1981; Medical Oncology 1985; **Med School:** Univ Wisc 1977; **Resid:** Internal Medicine, Columbia-Presby Hosp 1981; **Fellow:** Medical Oncology, Dana-Farber Cancer Inst 1985; **Fac Appt:** Prof Med, Cornell Univ-Weill Med Coll

Stoopler, Mark MD (Onc) - **Spec Exp:** Lung Cancer; Esophageal Cancer; Unknown Primary Cancer; **Hospital:** NY-Presby Hosp (page 100); **Address:** 161 Fort Washington Ave, Ste 936, New York, NY 10032-3713; **Phone:** 212-305-8230; **Board Cert:** Internal Medicine 1978; Medical Oncology 1981; **Med School:** Cornell Univ-Weill Med Coll 1975; **Resid:** Internal Medicine, North Shore Univ Hosp 1978; Internal Medicine, Memorial Hosp 1978; **Fellow:** Medical Oncology, Meml-Sloan Kettering Cancer Ctr 1980; **Fac Appt:** Assoc Clin Prof Med, Columbia P&S

Straus, David J MD (Onc) - **Spec Exp:** Lymphoma; Multiple Myeloma; **Hospital:** Meml Sloan Kettering Cancer Ctr (page 109); **Address:** 1275 York Ave, Box 406, New York, NY 10021-6094; **Phone:** 212-639-8365; **Board Cert:** Internal Medicine 1972; Hematology 1976; Medical Oncology 1977; **Med School:** Marquette Sch Med 1969; **Resid:** Internal Medicine, Montefiore Med Ctr 1972; Medical Oncology, Meml Sloan Kettering Cancer Ctr 1977; **Fellow:** Hematology, Beth Israel Hosp-Harvard 1973; **Fac Appt:** Prof Med, Cornell Univ-Weill Med Coll

Taub, Robert MD (Onc) - **Spec Exp:** Sarcoma; Mesothelioma; Melanoma; Thoracic Cancers; **Hospital:** NY-Presby Hosp (page 100); **Address:** 161 Fort Washington Ave, Ste 922, New York, NY 10032-3713; **Phone:** 212-305-4076; **Board Cert:** Internal Medicine 1973; Hematology 1974; Allergy & Immunology 1975; Medical Oncology 1977; **Med School:** Yale Univ 1961; **Resid:** Hematology, New England Med Ctr 1965; Internal Medicine, New England Med Ctr 1966; **Fellow:** Immunology, Natl Inst Med Rsch 1968; **Fac Appt:** Prof Med, Columbia P&S

Tepler, Jeffrey MD (Onc) - **Spec Exp:** Breast Cancer; Lymphoma; Leukemia; **Hospital:** NY-Presby Hosp (page 100); **Address:** 310 E 72nd St, New York, NY 10021; **Phone:** 212-650-1780; **Board Cert:** Internal Medicine 1985; Medical Oncology 1987; Hematology 1988; **Med School:** Yale Univ 1982; **Resid:** Internal Medicine, New York Hosp 1985; **Fellow:** Hematology & Oncology, New York Hosp 1988; **Fac Appt:** Asst Clin Prof Med, Cornell Univ-Weill Med Coll

Vahdat, Linda MD (Onc) - **Spec Exp:** Breast Cancer; **Hospital:** NY-Presby Hosp (page 100); **Address:** 425 E 61st St Fl 8, New York, NY 10021; **Phone:** 212-821-0644; **Board Cert:** Internal Medicine 1990; Medical Oncology 1995; **Med School:** Mount Sinai Sch Med 1987; **Resid:** Internal Medicine, Mt Sinai Hosp 1990; **Fellow:** Hematology & Oncology, Meml Sloan Kettering Cancer Ctr 1994; **Fac Appt:** Assoc Prof Med, Cornell Univ-Weill Med Coll

Vogel, James M MD (Onc) - **Spec Exp:** Breast Cancer; Colon Cancer; Lymphoma; **Hospital:** Mount Sinai Med Ctr (page 98), Mount Sinai Hosp of Queens (page 98); **Address:** 1125 Park Ave, New York, NY 10128-1243; **Phone:** 212-369-4250; **Board Cert:** Internal Medicine 1969; Hematology 1972; Medical Oncology 1973; **Med School:** Columbia P&S 1962; **Resid:** Internal Medicine, Mount Sinai Hosp 1964; Internal Medicine, Mount Sinai Hosp 1967; **Fellow:** Medical Oncology, Natl Cancer Inst 1966; Hematology, Mount Sinai Hosp 1968; **Fac Appt:** Assoc Prof Med, Mount Sinai Sch Med

Wadler, Scott MD (Onc) - **Spec Exp:** Gastrointestinal Cancer; Liver Cancer; Colon & Rectal Cancer; **Hospital:** NY-Presby Hosp (page 100); **Address:** Cornell Med Onc/Solid Tumor Program, 525 E 68th St, Payson 3- Fl 3, New York, NY 10021; **Phone:** 212-746-2844; **Board Cert:** Internal Medicine 1984; Medical Oncology 1987; **Med School:** NYU Sch Med 1980; **Resid:** Internal Medicine, Bellevue Hosp 1983; **Fellow:** Medical Oncology, Mount Sinai 1984; Medical Oncology, NYU Med Ctr 1985; **Fac Appt:** Prof Med, Cornell Univ-Weill Med Coll

Wolf, David J MD (Onc) - **Spec Exp:** Hematologic Malignancies; **Hospital:** NY-Presby Hosp (page 100); **Address:** 115 E 61st St, New York, NY 10021; **Phone:** 212-688-7100; **Board Cert:** Internal Medicine 1976; Hematology 1978; Medical Oncology 1979; **Med School:** SUNY Hlth Sci Ctr 1973; **Resid:** Internal Medicine, NY Hosp/Meml Hosp 1976; **Fellow:** Hematology, NY Hosp 1976; **Fac Appt:** Asst Clin Prof Med, Cornell Univ-Weill Med Coll

Zelenetz, Andrew D MD/PhD (Onc) - **Spec Exp:** Lymphoma; **Hospital:** Meml Sloan Kettering Cancer Ctr (page 109); **Address:** Meml Sloan-Kettering Cancer Ctr, 1275 York Ave, Box 330, New York, NY 10021; **Phone:** 212-639-2656; **Board Cert:** Internal Medicine 1992; Medical Oncology 1993; **Med School:** Harvard Med Sch 1984; **Resid:** Internal Medicine, Stanford Univ Med Ctr 1986; **Fellow:** Medical Oncology, Stanford Univ Med Ctr 1991; **Fac Appt:** Asst Prof Med, Cornell Univ-Weill Med Coll

NEONATAL–PERINATAL MEDICINE

Auld, Peter MD (NP) - **Hospital:** NY-Presby Hosp (page 100); **Address:** 525 E 68th St, Rm N506, New York, NY 10021; **Phone:** 212-746-3530; **Med School:** McGill Univ 1952; **Resid:** Pediatrics, Chldns Hosp 1954; Pediatrics, Boston Chldns Hosp 1958; **Fellow:** Cardiovascular Disease, Chldns Hosp 1962; Neonatal-Perinatal Medicine, Boston Lying-In Hosp 1986; **Fac Appt:** Prof Ped, Cornell Univ-Weill Med Coll

Bateman, David MD (NP) - **Spec Exp:** Critical Care; **Hospital:** NY-Presby Hosp (page 100); **Address:** 3959 Broadway, CHC 1-115, New York, NY 10037; **Phone:** 212-305-5827; **Board Cert:** Pediatrics 1979; Neonatal-Perinatal Medicine 1981; **Med School:** Tufts Univ 1973; **Resid:** Pediatrics, Lincoln Hosp 1975; Pediatrics, Boston Fltg Hosp 1977; **Fellow:** Neonatal-Perinatal Medicine, Colum-Presby Med Ctr 1982; **Fac Appt:** Assoc Prof Ped, Columbia P&S

Fischer, Rita MD (NP) - **Spec Exp:** Prematurity/Low Birth Weight Infants; **Hospital:** St Vincent Cath Med Ctrs - Manhattan (page 375); **Address:** Dept Peds, 153 W 11th St, rm 841, New York, NY 10011; **Phone:** 212-604-7883; **Board Cert:** Pediatrics 1975; Neonatal-Perinatal Medicine 1979; **Med School:** SUNY Downstate 1970; **Resid:** Pediatrics, Columbia-Presby 1972; Pediatrics, Roosevelt Hosp 1974; **Fac Appt:** Asst Prof Ped, NY Med Coll

Hendricks-Munoz, Karen MD (NP) - **Spec Exp:** Breathing Disorders; Neonatal Neurology; Retinopathy of Prematurity; **Hospital:** NYU Med Ctr (page 102), Bellevue Hosp Ctr; **Address:** NYU Med Ctr, Dept Neonatology, 530 1st Ave, Ste HCC-7A, New York, NY 10016-6402; **Phone:** 212-263-7477; **Board Cert:** Pediatrics 1985; Neonatal-Perinatal Medicine 1987; **Med School:** Yale Univ 1978; **Resid:** Pediatrics, Yale-New Haven Hosp 1981; **Fellow:** Neonatology, Strong Meml Hosp-Univ Rochester 1984; **Fac Appt:** Assoc Prof Ped, NYU Sch Med

Holzman, Ian MD (NP) - **Spec Exp:** Neonatal Nutrition; Necrotizing Enterocolitis; Prematurity/Low Birth Weight Infants; **Hospital:** Mount Sinai Med Ctr (page 98); **Address:** Newborn Assocs, 1 Gustave L Levy Pl, Box 1508, New York, NY 10029-6503; **Phone:** 212-241-5446; **Board Cert:** Pediatrics 1975; Neonatal-Perinatal Medicine 1977; **Med School:** Univ Pittsburgh 1971; **Resid:** Pediatrics, Chldns Hosp 1975; **Fellow:** Neonatal-Perinatal Medicine, Univ Colorado Hosp 1977; **Fac Appt:** Prof Ped, Mount Sinai Sch Med

Krauss, Alfred N MD (NP) - **Hospital:** NY-Presby Hosp (page 100); **Address:** 525 E 68th St, rm N506, New York, NY 10021; **Phone:** 212-746-3530; **Board Cert:** Pediatrics 1968; Neonatal-Perinatal Medicine 1975; **Med School:** Cornell Univ-Weill Med Coll 1963; **Resid:** Pediatrics, NY Hosp 1967; **Fellow:** Pediatrics, Cornell-New York Hosp 1969; **Fac Appt:** Assoc Prof Ped, Cornell Univ-Weill Med Coll

Marron-Corwin, Mary MD (NP) - **Spec Exp:** Neonatal Respiratory Care; Critical Care; Neonatal Liver Disease; **Hospital:** St Vincent Cath Med Ctrs - Manhattan (page 375); **Address:** 170 W 12th St, Smith Pavilion, Rm 839, New York, NY 10011-8305; **Phone:** 212-604-7862; **Board Cert:** Pediatrics 2001; Neonatal-Perinatal Medicine 2001; **Med School:** Philippines 1985; **Resid:** Pediatrics, St Vincents Hosp Med Ctr 1988; **Fellow:** Neonatal-Perinatal Medicine, Babies Hosp/Colum-Presby Med Ctr 1990; **Fac Appt:** Assoc Prof Ped, NY Med Coll

Perlman, Jeffrey M MD (NP) - **Spec Exp:** Neonatal Critical Care; Prematurity/Low Birth Weight Infants; Neonatal Neurology; **Hospital:** NY-Presby Hosp (page 100); **Address:** 525 E 68th St, Ste N 506, New York, NY 10021; **Phone:** 212-746-3530; **Board Cert:** Pediatrics 1983; Neonatal-Perinatal Medicine 1983; **Med School:** South Africa 1974; **Resid:** Pediatrics, Johannesburg Chlds Hosp 1979; Pediatrics, St Louis Chldns Hosp 1981; **Fellow:** Neonatology, St Louis Chldns Hosp 1983; **Fac Appt:** Prof Ped, Cornell Univ-Weill Med Coll

Polin, Richard MD (NP) - **Spec Exp:** Neonatal Infections; **Hospital:** NY-Presby Hosp (page 100); **Address:** Morgan Stanley Chlds Hosp of NY-Presby, 3959 Broadway, CHC 115, New York, NY 10032; **Phone:** 212-305-5827; **Board Cert:** Pediatrics 1975; Neonatal-Perinatal Medicine 1977; **Med School:** Temple Univ 1970; **Resid:** Pediatrics, Chldns Meml Hosp 1972; Pediatrics, Babies Hosp-Columbia Presby 1975; **Fellow:** Neonatal-Perinatal Medicine, Babies Hosp-Columbia Presby 1974; **Fac Appt:** Prof Ped, Columbia P&S

Rosen, Tove S MD (NP) - **Spec Exp:** Neonatology; Substance Abuse Effects in Newborn; Ethics; **Hospital:** NY-Presby Hosp (page 100); **Address:** Morgan Stanley Chldns Hosp of NY-Presby, 3959 Broadway, Box CHN1201, New York, NY 10032-1559; **Phone:** 212-305-8500; **Board Cert:** Pediatrics 1971; Neonatal-Perinatal Medicine 1975; **Med School:** SUNY Hlth Sci Ctr 1965; **Resid:** Pediatrics, St Luke's Hosp 1970; **Fellow:** Neonatal-Perinatal Medicine, Columbia-Presby Med Ctr 1975; **Fac Appt:** Clin Prof Ped, Columbia P&S

Shahrivar, Farrokh MD (NP) - **Spec Exp:** Neonatology; Prematurity/Low Birth Weight Infants; **Hospital:** St Luke's - Roosevelt Hosp Ctr - Roosevelt Div (page 90), Beth Israel Med Ctr - Petrie Division (page 90); **Address:** 1000 10th Ave, New York, NY 10019-1192; **Phone:** 212-523-3760; **Board Cert:** Pediatrics 1974; Neonatal-Perinatal Medicine 1975; **Med School:** Iran 1966; **Resid:** Pediatrics, St Luke's-Roosevelt Hosp Ctr 1971; Pediatrics, St Luke's-Roosevelt Hosp Ctr 1972; **Fellow:** Neonatal-Perinatal Medicine, St Christopher's Hosp 1973; Neonatal-Perinatal Medicine, Albert Einstein 1973; **Fac Appt:** Assoc Clin Prof Ped, Columbia P&S

NEPHROLOGY

Ames, Richard MD (Nep) - **Spec Exp:** Hypertension; Kidney Disease; Dialysis Care; **Hospital:** St Luke's - Roosevelt Hosp Ctr - Roosevelt Div (page 90), St Vincent Cath Med Ctrs - Manhattan (page 375); **Address:** 1886 Broadway, New York, NY 10023; **Phone:** 917-224-4270; **Board Cert:** Internal Medicine 1974; Nephrology 1972; Medical Oncology 1973; Hematology 1974; **Med School:** Columbia P&S 1958; **Resid:** Internal Medicine, Boston Med Ctr 1961; **Fellow:** Nephrology, Columbia-Presby Hosp 1963; **Fac Appt:** Clin Prof Med, Columbia P&S

Appel, Gerald MD (Nep) - **Spec Exp:** Glomerulonephritis; Lupus Nephritis; **Hospital:** NY-Presby Hosp (page 100); **Address:** 622 W 168th St, Ste PH4-124, New York, NY 10032-3720; **Phone:** 212-305-3273; **Board Cert:** Internal Medicine 1975; Nephrology 1978; **Med School:** Albert Einstein Coll Med 1972; **Resid:** Internal Medicine, Columbia Presby Hosp 1975; **Fellow:** Nephrology, Columbia Presby Hosp 1976; Nephrology, Yale-New Haven Hosp 1978; **Fac Appt:** Clin Prof Med, Columbia P&S

August, Phyllis MD (Nep) - **Spec Exp:** Hypertension; Hypertension in Pregnancy; **Hospital:** NY-Presby Hosp (page 100); **Address:** 525 E 68th St, Ste L-100, New York, NY 10021-4870; **Phone:** 212-746-2210; **Board Cert:** Internal Medicine 1980; Nephrology 1982; **Med School:** Yale Univ 1977; **Resid:** Internal Medicine, NY Hosp-Cornell Med Ctr 1980; **Fellow:** Nephrology, NY Hosp-Cornell Med Ctr 1983; **Fac Appt:** Prof Med, Cornell Univ-Weill Med Coll

Blumenfeld, Jon D MD (Nep) - **Spec Exp:** Hypertension; Polycystic Kidney Disease; **Hospital:** NY-Presby Hosp (page 100), Rockefeller Univ; **Address:** The Rogesin Inst, 505 E 70th St, rm HT230, New York, NY 10021; **Phone:** 212-746-1495; **Board Cert:** Internal Medicine 1984; Nephrology 1986; **Med School:** Yale Univ 1981; **Resid:** Internal Medicine, NY Hosp-Cornell Med Ctr 1984; **Fellow:** Nephrology, Brigham & Womens Hosp 1986; **Fac Appt:** Assoc Prof Med, Cornell Univ-Weill Med Coll

Burns, Godfrey MD (Nep) - **Spec Exp:** HIV Related Kidney Disease; **Hospital:** St Vincent Cath Med Ctrs - Manhattan (page 375); **Address:** 130 W 12th St, New York, NY 10011; **Phone:** 212-604-8322; **Board Cert:** Internal Medicine 1972; Nephrology 1976; **Med School:** Howard Univ 1967; **Resid:** Internal Medicine, St Vincent's Cath Med Ctr 1970; **Fellow:** Renal Disease, St Vincent's Cath Med Ctr 1971

Cheigh, Jhoong S MD (Nep) - **Spec Exp:** Kidney Failure; Transplant Medicine-Kidney; Dialysis Care; **Hospital:** NY-Presby Hosp (page 100); **Address:** 525 E 68th St, Box 135, New York, NY 10021; **Phone:** 212-746-3096; **Board Cert:** Internal Medicine 1971; Nephrology 1972; **Med School:** South Korea 1960; **Resid:** Internal Medicine, Mt Sinai Med Ctr 1970; **Fellow:** Nephrology, NY Hosp-Cornell 1972; **Fac Appt:** Clin Prof Med, Cornell Univ-Weill Med Coll

Cohen, David J MD (Nep) - **Spec Exp:** Transplant Medicine-Kidney; Glomerulonephritis; **Hospital:** NY-Presby Hosp (page 100); **Address:** Columbia Univ Med Ctr, 622 W 168th St, rm PH 4-124, New York, NY 10032-3720; **Phone:** 212-305-3273; **Board Cert:** Internal Medicine 1980; Nephrology 1984; **Med School:** Albert Einstein Coll Med 1977; **Resid:** Internal Medicine, Mount Sinai Hosp 1980; **Fellow:** Nephrology, Columbia Presby Med Ctr 1981; Transplant Immunobiology, Brigham & Women's Hosp 1983; **Fac Appt:** Assoc Prof Med, Columbia P&S

De Fabritus, Albert MD (Nep) - **Spec Exp:** Kidney Disease-Chronic; Hypertension; Anemia in Chronic Kidney Disease; **Hospital:** St Vincent Cath Med Ctrs - Manhattan (page 375), Cabrini Med Ctr (page 374); **Address:** 36 7th Ave, Ste 418, New York, NY 10011; **Phone:** 212-807-8817; **Board Cert:** Internal Medicine 1976; Nephrology 1978; **Med School:** NY Med Coll 1973; **Resid:** Internal Medicine, St Vincent's Hosp & Med Ctr 1976; **Fellow:** Nephrology, New York Hosp 1978; **Fac Appt:** Asst Clin Prof Med, NY Med Coll

Feinfeld, Donald A MD (Nep) - **Spec Exp:** Hypertension; Kidney Disease; **Hospital:** Beth Israel Med Ctr - Petrie Division (page 90); **Address:** Beth Israel Med Ctr, Div Neph & Hypertension, 350 E 17th St Fl 18, New York, NY 10003; **Phone:** 212-420-4070; **Board Cert:** Internal Medicine 1974; Nephrology 1978; **Med School:** Columbia P&S 1969; **Resid:** Internal Medicine, Bronx Muni Hosp Ctr 1974; **Fellow:** Nephrology, Albert Einstein Coll Med 1976; **Fac Appt:** Clin Prof Med, Albert Einstein Coll Med

Gardenswartz, Mark MD (Nep) - **Hospital:** Lenox Hill Hosp (page 94); **Address:** 110 E 59th St, Ste 10B, New York, NY 10022; **Phone:** 212-583-2930; **Board Cert:** Internal Medicine 1978; Nephrology 1980; Critical Care Medicine 2002; **Med School:** Univ Colorado 1975; **Resid:** Internal Medicine, Columbia Presby Med Ctr 1978; **Fellow:** Nephrology, Univ Colorado Hosp 1978; **Fac Appt:** Asst Clin Prof Med, NY Med Coll

Garvey, Michael MD (Nep) - **Spec Exp:** Dialysis Care; **Hospital:** St Vincent Cath Med Ctrs - Manhattan (page 375); **Address:** 222 W 14th St, New York, NY 10011; **Phone:** 212-807-7920; **Board Cert:** Internal Medicine 1979; Nephrology 1979; **Med School:** NY Med Coll 1975; **Resid:** Internal Medicine, St Vincent's Hosp & Med Ctr 1979; **Fellow:** Nephrology, NYU Med Ctr 1981

Glabman, Sheldon MD (Nep) - **Spec Exp:** Hypertension; **Hospital:** Mount Sinai Med Ctr (page 98); **Address:** 1175 Park Ave, New York, NY 10128; **Phone:** 212-534-3968; **Board Cert:** Internal Medicine 1964; **Med School:** Univ Hlth Sci/Chicago Med Sch 1957; **Resid:** Internal Medicine, Mount Sinai Hosp 1963; **Fellow:** Nephrology, Mt Sinai Hosp 1964

Kaufman, Allen M MD (Nep) - **Spec Exp:** Diabetic Kidney Disease; Dialysis Care; Hypertension; **Hospital:** Lenox Hill Hosp (page 94), Beth Israel Med Ctr - Petrie Division (page 90); **Address:** 1555 Third Ave, Ste 201, New York, NY 10128; **Phone:** 917-438-6986; **Board Cert:** Internal Medicine 1978; Nephrology 1980; **Med School:** Univ Rochester 1975; **Resid:** Internal Medicine, Mount Sinai Hosp 1978; **Fellow:** Nephrology, Mount Sinai Hosp 1980; **Fac Appt:** Assoc Clin Prof Med, Albert Einstein Coll Med

Klotman, Paul E MD (Nep) - **Spec Exp:** AIDS/HIV Related Kidney Disease; **Hospital:** Mount Sinai Med Ctr (page 98); **Address:** Mt Sinai Medical Ctr, One Gustave L Levy Pl, Box 1118, New York, NY 10029; **Phone:** 212-241-4200; **Board Cert:** Internal Medicine 1979; Nephrology 1984; **Med School:** Indiana Univ 1976; **Resid:** Internal Medicine, Duke Univ Med Ctr 1981; **Fellow:** Nephrology, Duke Univ Med Ctr 1982; **Fac Appt:** Prof Med, Mount Sinai Sch Med

Lowenstein, Jerome MD (Nep) - **Spec Exp:** Hypertension; Glomerulonephritis; Acid-Base Disorders; **Hospital:** NYU Med Ctr (page 102); **Address:** 530 1st Ave, Ste 4D, New York, NY 10016-6402; **Phone:** 212-263-7439; **Board Cert:** Internal Medicine 1964; Nephrology 1976; **Med School:** NYU Sch Med 1957; **Resid:** Internal Medicine, Bellevue Hosp 1963; **Fellow:** Nephrology, Bellevue Hosp 1967; **Fac Appt:** Prof Med, NYU Sch Med

Matalon, Robert MD (Nep) - **Spec Exp:** Dialysis Care; Kidney Failure; **Hospital:** NYU Med Ctr (page 102), NY Downtown Hosp; **Address:** 530 1st Ave, Ste 4A, New York, NY 10016-6402; **Phone:** 212-263-7239; **Board Cert:** Internal Medicine 1970; Nephrology 1974; **Med School:** NYU Sch Med 1964; **Resid:** Internal Medicine, Bellevue Hosp 1967; **Fellow:** Nephrology, NYU Med Ctr 1969; **Fac Appt:** Assoc Prof Med, NYU Sch Med

Michelis, Michael F MD (Nep) - **Spec Exp:** Kidney Disease; Hypertension; Renovascular Disease; **Hospital:** Lenox Hill Hosp (page 94); **Address:** 130 E 77th St, FL 5, New York, NY 10021-1851; **Phone:** 212-988-3506; **Board Cert:** Internal Medicine 1969; Geriatric Medicine 1992; **Med School:** Geo Wash Univ 1963; **Resid:** Internal Medicine, Lenox Hill Hosp 1965; Internal Medicine, Hosp Med Coll Penn 1967; **Fellow:** Renal Disease, Univ Pittsburgh 1970; **Fac Appt:** Clin Prof Med, NYU Sch Med

Saal, Stuart MD (Nep) - **Spec Exp:** Kidney Failure; Critical Care; Cholesterol/Lipid Disorders; **Hospital:** NY-Presby Hosp (page 100); **Address:** 505 E 70th St, rm HT230, New York, NY 10021-4872; **Phone:** 212-746-1553; **Board Cert:** Internal Medicine 1974; **Med School:** NY Med Coll 1971; **Resid:** Internal Medicine, St Luke's-Roosevelt Hosp Ctr 1974; **Fellow:** Nephrology, New York Hosp 1976; **Fac Appt:** Assoc Clin Prof Med, Cornell Univ-Weill Med Coll

Sherman, Raymond MD (Nep) - **Spec Exp:** Glomerulonephritis; Hypertension; Kidney Failure-Chronic; **Hospital:** NY-Presby Hosp (page 100); **Address:** 407 E 70th St Fl 4, New York, NY 10021-5302; **Phone:** 212-879-8245; **Board Cert:** Internal Medicine 1969; Nephrology 1974; **Med School:** SUNY Hlth Sci Ctr 1961; **Resid:** Internal Medicine, St Luke's-Roosevelt Hosp Ctr 1965; Nephrology, Strong Meml Hosp 1967; **Fellow:** Nephrology, NY Hosp/Cornell Med Ctr 1969; **Fac Appt:** Clin Prof Med, Cornell Univ-Weill Med Coll

New York (Manhattan)

Wang, John MD (Nep) - **Spec Exp:** Hypertension; **Hospital:** NY-Presby Hosp (page 100); **Address:** 505 E 70th St, rm 213, New York, NY 10021; **Phone:** 212-746-3097; **Board Cert:** Internal Medicine 1985; Nephrology 1986; **Med School:** Cornell Univ-Weill Med Coll 1979; **Resid:** Internal Medicine, Laguardia Hosp 1982; **Fellow:** Nephrology, NY Hosp 1984

Wasser, Walter MD (Nep) - **Spec Exp:** Hemodialysis; Glomerulonephritis; **Hospital:** N Genl Hosp, Cabrini Med Ctr (page 374); **Address:** 211 W 61st St Fl Level B, New York, NY 10023-7832; **Phone:** 212-977-3100; **Board Cert:** Internal Medicine 1979; Nephrology 1984; **Med School:** Albert Einstein Coll Med 1976; **Resid:** Internal Medicine, Maimonides Medical Ctr 1978; Internal Medicine, Mount Sinai 1979; **Fellow:** Nephrology, Mount Sinai 1981Rockefeller Univ Hosp 1983; **Fac Appt:** Asst Clin Prof Med, Cornell Univ-Weill Med Coll

Weisstuch, Joseph MD (Nep) - **Hospital:** NYU Med Ctr (page 102), Hosp For Joint Diseases (page 107); **Address:** 530 1st Ave, Ste 4B, New York, NY 10016-6402; **Phone:** 212-263-0705; **Board Cert:** Internal Medicine 1988; Nephrology 1992; **Med School:** NYU Sch Med 1985; **Resid:** Internal Medicine, NYU Med Ctr 1989; **Fellow:** Nephrology, Bellevue Hosp 1991; **Fac Appt:** Asst Clin Prof Med, NYU Sch Med

Williams, Gail S MD (Nep) - **Spec Exp:** Kidney Failure-Chronic; Transplant Medicine-Kidney; Critical Care; **Hospital:** NY-Presby Hosp (page 100), NY-Presby Hosp (page 100); **Address:** 161 Fort Washington Ave, Ste 351, New York, NY 10032; **Phone:** 212-305-5376; **Board Cert:** Internal Medicine 1972; Nephrology 1974; **Med School:** Columbia P&S 1968; **Resid:** Internal Medicine, Columbia Presby Hosp 1973; **Fellow:** Nephrology, Columbia Presby Hosp 1974; **Fac Appt:** Assoc Clin Prof Med, Columbia P&S

Winston, Jonathan MD (Nep) - **Spec Exp:** Kidney Disease; HIV Related Kidney Disease; Dialysis Care; **Hospital:** Mount Sinai Med Ctr (page 98); **Address:** 5 E 98th St Fl 11, New York, NY 10029-6501; **Phone:** 212-241-4060; **Board Cert:** Internal Medicine 1980; Nephrology 1984; **Med School:** Geo Wash Univ 1977; **Resid:** Internal Medicine, LI Jewish Med Ctr 1980; **Fellow:** Nephrology, Mount Sinai Hosp 1982; **Fac Appt:** Assoc Prof Med, Mount Sinai Sch Med

Neurological Surgery

Bederson, Joshua MD (NS) - **Spec Exp:** Aneurysm-Cerebral; Brain & Spinal Cord Tumors; Trigeminal Neuralgia; Skull Base Tumors; **Hospital:** Mount Sinai Med Ctr (page 98); **Address:** Mount Sinai Med Ctr, 1 Gustave Levy Pl Box 1136, New York, NY 10029; **Phone:** 212-241-2377; **Board Cert:** Neurological Surgery 1993; **Med School:** UCSF 1984; **Resid:** Neurological Surgery, UCSF Med Ctr 1990; **Fellow:** Neurological Vascular Surgery, Barrow Neur Inst 1990; Neurological Vascular Surgery, Univ Hosp Zurich 1990; **Fac Appt:** Prof NS, Mount Sinai Sch Med

Benjamin, Vallo MD (NS) - **Spec Exp:** Spinal Surgery; Skull Base Surgery; Acoustic Neuroma; **Hospital:** NYU Med Ctr (page 102); **Address:** 530 First Ave, Ste 7W, New York, NY 10016; **Phone:** 212-263-5013 x1; **Board Cert:** Neurological Surgery 1967; **Med School:** Iran 1958; **Resid:** Neurological Surgery, Bellevue Hosp 1964; **Fellow:** Neurological Surgery, NYU Med Ctr 1966; **Fac Appt:** Prof NS, NYU Sch Med

Bilsky, Mark H MD (NS) - **Spec Exp:** Spinal Tumors; Skull Base Tumors; Brain Tumors; Spinal Reconstructive Surgery; **Hospital:** Meml Sloan Kettering Cancer Ctr (page 109), NY-Presby Hosp (page 100); **Address:** Memorial Sloan Kettering Cancer Ctr, 1275 York Ave, rm C705, New York, NY 10021; **Phone:** 212-639-8526; **Board Cert:** Neurological Surgery 1999; **Med School:** Emory Univ 1988; **Resid:** Neurological Surgery, NY Hosp-Cornell Med Ctr 1994; **Fellow:** Neurological Oncology, Louisville Univ Med Ctr 1995; **Fac Appt:** Assoc Prof NS, Cornell Univ-Weill Med Coll

Bruce, Jeffrey MD (NS) - **Spec Exp:** Brain Tumors; Pituitary Tumors; Skull Base Surgery; **Hospital:** NY-Presby Hosp (page 100); **Address:** 710 W 168 St Bldg N1 Fl 4 - rm 434, NY Presby Hosp, Dept Neurosurgery, New York, NY 10032-2603; **Phone:** 212-305-7346; **Board Cert:** Neurological Surgery 1993; **Med School:** UMDNJ-RW Johnson Med Sch 1983; **Resid:** Neurological Surgery, Columbia-Presby Med Ctr 1990; **Fellow:** Neurological Surgery, Nat Inst Health 1985; **Fac Appt:** Prof NS, Columbia P&S

Camins, Martin B MD (NS) - **Spec Exp:** Spinal Surgery; Brain Tumors; Microsurgery; **Hospital:** Mount Sinai Med Ctr (page 98), Lenox Hill Hosp (page 94); **Address:** 205 E 68th St, Ste T1C, New York, NY 10021-5735; **Phone:** 212-570-0100; **Board Cert:** Neurological Surgery 1980; **Med School:** Univ Hlth Sci/Chicago Med Sch 1969; **Resid:** Neurology, Neuro Inst-Columbia-Presby Med Ctr 1971; Neurological Surgery, Neuro Inst-Columbia Presb Med Ctry 1975; **Fellow:** Neurological Surgery, National Hosp 1973; Neurological Surgery, NYU Med Ctr 1977; **Fac Appt:** Clin Prof NS, Mount Sinai Sch Med

Cooper, Paul MD (NS) - **Spec Exp:** Spinal Surgery; Spinal Disc Replacement; Spinal Cord Tumors; **Hospital:** NYU Med Ctr (page 102); **Address:** 550 1st Ave, New York, NY 10016-6402; **Phone:** 212-263-6514; **Board Cert:** Neurological Surgery 1977; **Med School:** Univ VA Sch Med 1966; **Resid:** Surgery, Univ Hosp 1968; Neurological Surgery, NYU Med Ctr 1975; **Fac Appt:** Prof NS, NYU Sch Med

Di Giacinto, George V MD (NS) - **Spec Exp:** Spinal Surgery; Brain Tumors; Pain Management; **Hospital:** St Luke's - Roosevelt Hosp Ctr - Roosevelt Div (page 90); **Address:** 425 W 59th St, Ste 4E, New York, NY 10019; **Phone:** 212-523-8500; **Board Cert:** Neurological Surgery 1981; **Med School:** Harvard Med Sch 1970; **Resid:** Surgery, Roosevelt Hosp 1972; Neurological Surgery, Columbia-Presby Hosp 1978

Feldstein, Neil A MD (NS) - **Spec Exp:** Pediatric Neurosurgery; Chiari's Deformity; Brain Tumors-Pediatric; Spinal Cord Surgery-Pediatric; **Hospital:** NY-Presby Hosp (page 100); **Address:** Neurological Inst, 710 W 168th St Fl 2 - rm 213, New York, NY 10032; **Phone:** 212-305-1396; **Board Cert:** Neurological Surgery 1995; Pediatric Neurological Surgery 1995; **Med School:** NYU Sch Med 1984; **Resid:** Neurological Surgery, Baylor Coll Med 1989; **Fellow:** Pediatric Neurological Surgery, NYU Med Ctr 1991; **Fac Appt:** Asst Prof NS, Columbia P&S

Gamache, Francis MD (NS) - **Spec Exp:** Brain & Spinal Cord Tumors; Spinal Surgery-Neck; Cerebrovascular Neurosurgery; **Hospital:** NY-Presby Hosp (page 100), Hosp For Special Surgery (page 108); **Address:** 523 E 72nd St, FL 7, New York, NY 10021-4099; **Phone:** 212-988-5200; **Board Cert:** Neurological Surgery 1982; **Med School:** Cornell Univ-Weill Med Coll 1971; **Resid:** Surgery, NY Hosp-Cornell Med Ctr 1975; Neurological Surgery, NY Hosp-Cornell Med Ctr 1979; **Fellow:** Trauma, MD Inst Emerg Med Serv 1979; Neurovascular Medicine, Univ West Ontario 1980; **Fac Appt:** Assoc Prof NS, Cornell Univ-Weill Med Coll

Golfinos, John G MD (NS) - **Spec Exp:** Brain Tumors; Acoustic Neuroma; Stereotactic Radiosurgery; **Hospital:** NYU Med Ctr (page 102), Lenox Hill Hosp (page 94); **Address:** Dept Neurosurgery, 530 1st Ave, Ste 8R, New York, NY 10016-6402; **Phone:** 212-263-2950; **Board Cert:** Neurological Surgery 1998; **Med School:** Columbia P&S 1988; **Resid:** Neurological Surgery, Barrow Neuro Inst 1995; **Fac Appt:** Asst Prof NS, NYU Sch Med

Goodman, Robert R MD/PhD (NS) - **Spec Exp:** Parkinson's Disease; Epilepsy; Trigeminal Neuralgia; **Hospital:** NY-Presby Hosp (page 100); **Address:** 710 W 168th St, rm 426, New York, NY 10032-2603; **Phone:** 212-305-3774; **Board Cert:** Neurological Surgery 1993; **Med School:** Johns Hopkins Univ 1982; **Resid:** Neurological Surgery, Columbia-Presby Med Ctr 1989

Gutin, Philip MD (NS) - **Spec Exp:** Brain Tumors; Meningioma; Acoustic Neuroma; **Hospital:** Meml Sloan Kettering Cancer Ctr (page 109), NY-Presby Hosp (page 100); **Address:** Meml Sloan Kettering Cancer Ctr, Dept Neurosurgery, 1275 York Ave, rm C703, New York, NY 10021-6007; **Phone:** 212-639-8556; **Board Cert:** Neurological Surgery 1981; **Med School:** Univ Pennsylvania 1971; **Resid:** Neurological Surgery, UCSF Med Ctr 1979; **Fellow:** Natl Cancer Inst 1976; **Fac Appt:** Prof NS, Cornell Univ-Weill Med Coll

Hirschfeld, Alan MD (NS) - **Spec Exp:** Brain Tumors; **Hospital:** St Vincent Cath Med Ctrs - Manhattan (page 375); **Address:** St Vincent Catholic Medical Ctr, Dept Neurosurgery, 170 W 12th St, rm 8, New York, NY 10011; **Phone:** 212-604-7767; **Board Cert:** Neurological Surgery 1986; **Med School:** NYU Sch Med 1977; **Resid:** Surgery, NYU-Bellevue Hosp 1978; **Fellow:** Neurological Surgery, NYU-Bellevue Hosp 1982; **Fac Appt:** Assoc Prof S, NY Med Coll

Holtzman, Robert N N MD (NS) - **Spec Exp:** Brain & Spinal Cord Tumors; Spinal Surgery; Aneurysm-Cerebral; **Hospital:** Lenox Hill Hosp (page 94), NY-Presby Hosp (page 100); **Address:** 247 3rd Ave, Ste 403, New York, NY 10010-7455; **Phone:** 212-529-3580; **Board Cert:** Neurological Surgery 1980; Neurology 1978; **Med School:** Columbia P&S 1969; **Resid:** Neurology, New York Neurological Inst 1972; Surgery, Harbor Genl Hosp 1973; **Fellow:** Neurological Surgery, New York Neurological Inst 1977; **Fac Appt:** Assoc Clin Prof NS, Columbia P&S

Jafar, Jafar MD (NS) - **Spec Exp:** Aneurysm-Cerebral; Brain Tumors; Skull Base Tumors; **Hospital:** NYU Med Ctr (page 102), Lenox Hill Hosp (page 94); **Address:** 530 1st Ave, Ste 8R, New York, NY 10016-6402; **Phone:** 212-263-6312; **Board Cert:** Neurological Surgery 1984; **Med School:** Iran 1976; **Resid:** Neurological Surgery, Univ Chicago 1982; Neurological Surgery, Natl Hosp for Nervous Disease 1981; **Fac Appt:** Prof NS, NYU Sch Med

Kelly, Patrick J MD (NS) - **Spec Exp:** Brain Tumors; Movement Disorders; Gliomas; **Hospital:** NYU Med Ctr (page 102), Lenox Hill Hosp (page 94); **Address:** NYU Med Ctr, Dept Neurological Surgery, 530 1st Ave, Ste 8R, New York, NY 10016; **Phone:** 212-263-8002; **Board Cert:** Neurological Surgery 1978; **Med School:** SUNY Buffalo 1966; **Resid:** Neurological Surgery, Northwestern Univ Hosp 1972; Neurological Surgery, Univ Texas Med Br Hosp 1974; **Fellow:** Neurological Surgery, St Anne Hosp 1977; **Fac Appt:** Prof NS, NYU Sch Med

Lavyne, Michael H MD (NS) - **Spec Exp:** Spinal Surgery; Spinal Tumors; Spinal Disorders; **Hospital:** NY-Presby Hosp (page 100), Hosp For Special Surgery (page 108); **Address:** 523 E 72nd St, New York, NY 10021-4099; **Phone:** 212-717-0200; **Board Cert:** Neurological Surgery 1982; **Med School:** Cornell Univ-Weill Med Coll 1972; **Resid:** Neurological Surgery, Mass Genl Hosp 1979; **Fellow:** Neurology, Beth Israel Hosp 1974; **Fac Appt:** Clin Prof NS, Cornell Univ-Weill Med Coll

McCormick, Paul C MD (NS) - **Spec Exp:** Spinal Surgery; Spinal Tumors; **Hospital:** NY-Presby Hosp (page 100), Valley Hosp (page 762); **Address:** 710 W 168th St, Ste 406, New York, NY 10032-2603; **Phone:** 212-305-7976; **Board Cert:** Neurological Surgery 1993; **Med School:** Columbia P&S 1982; **Resid:** Neurological Surgery, Columbia Presby Med Ctr 1989; **Fellow:** Neurological Surgery, Natl Inst Hlth 1984; Spinal Surgery, Med Coll Wisconsin 1990; **Fac Appt:** Prof NS, Columbia P&S

Moore, Frank M MD (NS) - **Spec Exp:** Aneurysm; Brain Tumors; Spinal Cord Tumors; **Hospital:** Mount Sinai Med Ctr (page 98), Englewood Hosp & Med Ctr (page 760); **Address:** 1158 5th Ave, New York, NY 10029-6917; **Phone:** 212-410-6990; **Board Cert:** Neurological Surgery 1992; **Med School:** France 1983; **Resid:** Neurological Surgery, Mount Sinai Hosp 1988; **Fac Appt:** Assoc Prof NS, Mount Sinai Sch Med

Perin, Noel I MD (NS) - **Spec Exp:** Spinal Surgery-Minimally Invasive; Spinal Tumors; **Hospital:** St Luke's - Roosevelt Hosp Ctr - Roosevelt Div (page 90), Beth Israel Med Ctr - Petrie Division (page 90); **Address:** Roosevelt Hospital, Dept Neurosurgery, 1000 10th Ave, Ste 5G-80, New York, NY 10019; **Phone:** 212-523-6720; **Board Cert:** Neurological Surgery 1995; **Med School:** Sri Lanka 1973; **Resid:** Neurological Surgery, NYU Med Ctr 1990; **Fellow:** Spinal Surgery, NYU Med Ctr 1991; **Fac Appt:** Assoc Clin Prof NS

Post, Kalmon MD (NS) - **Spec Exp:** Pituitary Tumors; Acoustic Neuroma; Meningioma; **Hospital:** Mount Sinai Med Ctr (page 98); **Address:** 5 E 98th St, Fl 7, New York, NY 10029-6501; **Phone:** 212-241-0933; **Board Cert:** Neurological Surgery 1978; **Med School:** NYU Sch Med 1967; **Resid:** Surgery, Bellevue Hosp 1969; Neurological Surgery, Bellevue Hosp-NYU 1975; **Fac Appt:** Prof NS, Mount Sinai Sch Med

Quest, Donald MD (NS) - **Spec Exp:** Spinal Surgery; Neurovascular Surgery; Carotid Artery Surgery; **Hospital:** NY-Presby Hosp (page 100), Valley Hosp (page 762); **Address:** 710 W 168th St, Ste 440, New York, NY 10032; **Phone:** 212-305-5582; **Board Cert:** Neurological Surgery 1978; **Med School:** Columbia P&S 1970; **Resid:** Surgery, Mass Genl Hosp 1972; Neurological Surgery, Columbia-Presby Hosp 1976; **Fac Appt:** Clin Prof NS, Columbia P&S

Sen, Chandranath MD (NS) - **Spec Exp:** Brain Tumors; Skull Base Tumors; Skull Base Surgery; **Hospital:** St Luke's - Roosevelt Hosp Ctr - Roosevelt Div (page 90); **Address:** St Lukes Roosevelt Hosp Ctr, Dept Neurosurgery, 1000 10th Ave, Ste 5G-80, New York, NY 10019; **Phone:** 212-523-6720; **Board Cert:** Neurological Surgery 1989; **Med School:** India 1976; **Resid:** Surgery, Univ Wisconsin Hosps 1980; Neurological Surgery, Univ Wisconsin Hosps 1985; **Fellow:** Microsurgery, Univ Pittsburgh Med Ctr 1986

Sisti, Michael B MD (NS) - **Spec Exp:** Acoustic Neuroma; Brain Tumors; Stereotactic Radiosurgery; **Hospital:** NY-Presby Hosp (page 100); **Address:** 710 W 168th St, New York, NY 10032-2603; **Phone:** 212-305-1728; **Board Cert:** Neurological Surgery 1991; **Med School:** Columbia P&S 1981; **Resid:** Neurological Surgery, Neuro Inst-Columbia-Presby Med Ctr 1988; **Fellow:** Neurological Surgery, Natl Inst Health 1983; **Fac Appt:** Asst Prof NS, Columbia P&S

Snow, Robert MD (NS) - **Spec Exp:** Spinal Surgery; Pituitary Tumors; Minimally Invasive Surgery; **Hospital:** NY-Presby Hosp (page 100); **Address:** 523 E 72nd St Fl 7, New York, NY 10021-4099; **Phone:** 212-717-0256; **Board Cert:** Neurological Surgery 1989; **Med School:** Stanford Univ 1981; **Resid:** Neurological Surgery, NY Cornell Med Ctr 1986; **Fac Appt:** Prof NS, Cornell Univ-Weill Med Coll

Solomon, Robert A MD (NS) - **Spec Exp:** Aneurysm-Cerebral; Arteriovenous Malformations; **Hospital:** NY-Presby Hosp (page 100); **Address:** 710 W 168th St, Ste 439, New York, NY 10032; **Phone:** 212-305-4118; **Board Cert:** Neurological Surgery 1988; **Med School:** Johns Hopkins Univ 1980; **Resid:** Neurological Surgery, Neuro Inst-Columbia Univ 1986; **Fac Appt:** Prof NS, Columbia P&S

Souweidane, Mark MD (NS) - **Spec Exp:** Pediatric Neurosurgery; Brain & Spinal Cord Tumors; **Hospital:** NY-Presby Hosp (page 100), Meml Sloan Kettering Cancer Ctr (page 109); **Address:** NY Presby Hosp, Dept Neurosurg, 520 E 70th St, rm 651, New York, NY 10021; **Phone:** 212-746-2363; **Board Cert:** Neurological Surgery 1999; Pediatric Neurological Surgery ; **Med School:** Wayne State Univ 1988; **Resid:** Neurological Surgery, NYU Sch Med 1994; **Fellow:** Pediatric Neurological Surgery, Hosp Sick Chldn 1995; **Fac Appt:** Assoc Clin Prof NS, Cornell Univ-Weill Med Coll

Steinberger, Alfred A MD (NS) - **Spec Exp:** Spinal Cord Tumors; Aneurysm; Brain Tumors; **Hospital:** Mount Sinai Med Ctr (page 98), Englewood Hosp & Med Ctr (page 760); **Address:** 1158 5th Ave, New York, NY 10029-6917; **Phone:** 212-410-6990; **Board Cert:** Neurological Surgery 1985; **Med School:** Columbia P&S 1976; **Resid:** Neurological Surgery, Neuro Inst-Columbia-Presby 1982; **Fac Appt:** Asst Clin Prof NS, Mount Sinai Sch Med

Stieg, Philip E MD/PhD (NS) - **Spec Exp:** Cerebrovascular Neurosurgery; Acoustic Neuroma; Skull Base Surgery; Meningioma; **Hospital:** NY-Presby Hosp (page 100); **Address:** 525 E 68th St, STARR 651, New York, NY 10021-9800; **Phone:** 212-746-4684; **Board Cert:** Neurological Surgery 1992; **Med School:** Med Coll Wisc 1983; **Resid:** Neurological Surgery, Dallas Chldns Hosp/Parkland Meml Hosp 1988; **Fellow:** Neurological Biology, Karolinska Inst 1988; **Fac Appt:** Prof NS, Cornell Univ-Weill Med Coll

Wisoff, Jeffrey H MD (NS) - **Spec Exp:** Pediatric Neurosurgery; Brain Tumors-Pediatric; Hydrocephalus; **Hospital:** NYU Med Ctr (page 102), Maimonides Med Ctr (page 96); **Address:** 317 E 34th St, Ste 1002, New York, NY 10016-4974; **Phone:** 212-263-6419; **Board Cert:** Neurological Surgery 1990; Pediatric Neurological Surgery 1996; **Med School:** Geo Wash Univ 1978; **Resid:** Neurological Surgery, NYU Med Ctr/Bellevue Hosp 1984; **Fellow:** Pediatric Neurological Surgery, NYU Med Ctr 1985; **Fac Appt:** Assoc Prof NS, NYU Sch Med

NEUROLOGY

Apatoff, Brian R MD/PhD (N) - **Spec Exp:** Multiple Sclerosis; Neuro-Immunology; Lyme Disease; **Hospital:** NY-Presby Hosp (page 100); **Address:** 525 E 68th St, Starr Pavilion, Ste 607, New York, NY 10021; **Phone:** 212-746-4504; **Board Cert:** Neurology 1991; **Med School:** Univ Chicago-Pritzker Sch Med 1984; **Resid:** Neurology, Columbia Presby Med Ctr 1990; **Fellow:** Multiple Sclerosis, Neuro Inst-Columbia Univ 1992; **Fac Appt:** Assoc Prof N, Cornell Univ-Weill Med Coll

Belok, Lennart MD (N) - **Spec Exp:** Carpal Tunnel Syndrome; **Hospital:** Beth Israel Med Ctr - Petrie Division (page 90), Cabrini Med Ctr (page 374); **Address:** 410 E 20th St, Ste MG, New York, NY 10009-8113; **Phone:** 212-254-9716; **Board Cert:** Neurology 1983; Internal Medicine 1977; **Med School:** NY Med Coll 1973; **Resid:** Internal Medicine, Beth Israel 1976; Nephrology, New York Univ Med Ctr 1979

Block, Jerome M MD (N) - **Spec Exp:** Cerebrovascular Disease; Spinal Cord Disorders; Neurologic Rehabilitation; **Hospital:** Lenox Hill Hosp (page 94); **Address:** 1 E 87th St, New York, NY 10128-0506; **Phone:** 212-289-0540; **Board Cert:** Neurology 1961; **Med School:** Harvard Med Sch 1954; **Resid:** Neurology, Mount Sinai Hosp 1959; **Fellow:** Physical Medicine & Rehabilitation, NYU-Rusk Inst 1962; **Fac Appt:** Clin Prof N, NYU Sch Med

Bressman, Susan MD (N) - **Spec Exp:** Parkinson's Disease; Movement Disorders; Dystonia; **Hospital:** Beth Israel Med Ctr - Petrie Division (page 90); **Address:** 10 Union Square East, Ste 2-Q, New York, NY 10003-3314; **Phone:** 212-844-8379; **Board Cert:** Neurology 1983; **Med School:** Columbia P&S 1977; **Resid:** Internal Medicine, New York Hosp 1978; Neurology, Columbia-Presby Med Ctr 1981; **Fellow:** Movement Disorders, Columbia-Presby Med Ctr 1983; **Fac Appt:** Prof N, Albert Einstein Coll Med

Britton, Carolyn B MD (N) - **Spec Exp:** Neurologic Complications-HIV/Infections; Lyme Disease; Multiple Sclerosis; **Hospital:** NY-Presby Hosp (page 100); **Address:** 710 W 168th St, Ste 232, New York, NY 10032-2603; **Phone:** 212-305-5220; **Board Cert:** Internal Medicine 1979; Neurology 1982; **Med School:** NYU Sch Med 1975; **Resid:** Internal Medicine, Harlem Hosp 1977; Neurology, Columbia-Presby Hosp 1980; **Fellow:** Neurology, Columbia-Presby Hosp 1983; **Fac Appt:** Assoc Prof N, Columbia P&S

Bronster, David MD (N) - **Spec Exp:** Headache; Dizziness; Seizure Disorders; **Hospital:** Mount Sinai Med Ctr (page 98); **Address:** 3 E 83rd St, New York, NY 10028-0459; **Phone:** 212-772-0008; **Board Cert:** Neurology 1984; **Med School:** Mount Sinai Sch Med 1979; **Resid:** Neurology, Mount Sinai Hosp 1983; **Fac Appt:** Assoc Clin Prof N, Mount Sinai Sch Med

Brust, John C M MD (N) - **Spec Exp:** Stroke; Substance Abuse; **Hospital:** Harlem Hosp Ctr, NY-Presby Hosp (page 100); **Address:** 506 Lenox Ave, rm 16-101, New York, NY 10037-1802; **Phone:** 212-939-4244; **Board Cert:** Neurology 1971; **Med School:** Columbia P&S 1962; **Resid:** Internal Medicine, Columbia Presby 1966; Neurology, Columbia Presby 1969; **Fac Appt:** Clin Prof N, Columbia P&S

Cafferty, Maureen MD (N) - **Hospital:** St Luke's - Roosevelt Hosp Ctr - Roosevelt Div (page 90); **Address:** 1090 Amsterdam Ave, Ste 8B, New York, NY 10025-1737; **Phone:** 212-636-4994; **Board Cert:** Internal Medicine 1982; Neurology 1987; **Med School:** Columbia P&S 1979; **Resid:** Internal Medicine, St Luke's-Roosevelt Hosp Ctr 1982; Neurology, Columbia-Presby Hosp 1985; **Fac Appt:** Asst Prof N, Columbia P&S

Caronna, John J MD (N) - **Spec Exp:** Stroke; Cerebrovascular Disease; **Hospital:** NY-Presby Hosp (page 100); **Address:** Cornell Univ, Dept Neurology, 520 E 70th St, Ste 607, New York, NY 10021; **Phone:** 212-746-2304; **Board Cert:** Neurology 1974; **Med School:** Cornell Univ-Weill Med Coll 1965; **Resid:** Internal Medicine, NY Hosp 1967; Neurology, NY Hosp 1971; **Fellow:** Neurology, NY Hosp 1973; **Fac Appt:** Prof N, Cornell Univ-Weill Med Coll

Charney, Jonathan MD (N) - **Spec Exp:** Headache; Stroke; **Hospital:** Mount Sinai Med Ctr (page 98); **Address:** 1111 Park Ave, Ste 1A, New York, NY 10128-1234; **Phone:** 212-831-2886; **Board Cert:** Neurology 1977; **Med School:** NY Med Coll 1969; **Resid:** Neurology, Methodist Hosp-Baylor 1971; Neurology, Columbia-Presby Med Ctr 1973; **Fac Appt:** Asst Prof N, Mount Sinai Sch Med

Coll, Raymond MD (N) - **Hospital:** NY-Presby Hosp (page 100); **Address:** 1365 York Ave, New York, NY 10021-4035; **Phone:** 212-249-0840; **Board Cert:** Neurology 1974; **Med School:** South Africa 1961; **Resid:** Neurology, NY Hosp 1971; **Fac Appt:** Assoc Clin Prof N, Cornell Univ-Weill Med Coll

Danon, Moris Jak MD (N) - **Spec Exp:** Neuromuscular Disorders; **Hospital:** Hosp For Special Surgery (page 108); **Address:** Hospital for Special Surgery, 535 E 70th St, New York, NY 10021; **Phone:** 212-606-1309; **Board Cert:** Neurology 1975; **Med School:** Turkey 1967; **Resid:** Neurology, Northwestern U Med Ctr 1971; Neurology, St Vincents Hosp 1973; **Fellow:** Neurology, McGill U Med Ctr 1975; **Fac Appt:** Clin Prof N, Cornell Univ-Weill Med Coll

Daras, Michael MD (N) - **Spec Exp:** Headache; Neuromuscular Disorders; Drug Abuse; **Hospital:** NY-Presby Hosp (page 100); **Address:** 710 W 168 St, rm 246, New York, NY 10032; **Phone:** 212-305-6876; **Board Cert:** Neurology 1980; **Med School:** Greece 1969; **Resid:** Psychiatry, Elmhurst City Hosp 1976; Neurology, NY Med Coll 1979; **Fellow:** Clinical Neurophysiology, Albert Einstein 1980; **Fac Appt:** Prof N, Columbia P&S

De Angelis, Lisa MD (N) - **Spec Exp:** Neuro-Oncology; **Hospital:** Meml Sloan Kettering Cancer Ctr (page 109); **Address:** 1275 York Ave, New York, NY 10021-6007; **Phone:** 212-639-7123; **Board Cert:** Neurology 1986; **Med School:** Columbia P&S 1980; **Resid:** Neurology, Neuro Inst - Presby Hosp 1984; **Fellow:** Neurological Oncology, Neuro Inst - Presby Hosp 1985; Neurological Oncology, Meml Sloan-Kettering Cancer Ctr 1986; **Fac Appt:** Prof N, Cornell Univ-Weill Med Coll

Devinsky, Orrin MD (N) - **Spec Exp:** Epilepsy; Tuberous Sclerosis; Behavioral Neurology; **Hospital:** NYU Med Ctr (page 102), St Barnabas Med Ctr; **Address:** 403 E 34th St, FL 4, New York, NY 10016-4972; **Phone:** 212-263-8871; **Board Cert:** Neurology 1987; Clinical Neurophysiology 1990; **Med School:** Harvard Med Sch 1982; **Resid:** Neurology, New York Hosp-Cornell Med Ctr 1986; **Fellow:** Epilepsy, Natl Inst Health 1988; **Fac Appt:** Prof N, NYU Sch Med

Fahn, Stanley MD (N) - **Spec Exp:** Movement Disorders; Parkinson's Disease; **Hospital:** NY-Presby Hosp (page 100); **Address:** 710 W 168th St, Fl 3rd - rm 350, New York, NY 10032; **Phone:** 212-305-5277; **Board Cert:** Neurology 1968; **Med School:** UCSF 1958; **Resid:** Neurology, Neuro Inst-Columbia Presby Hosp 1962; **Fac Appt:** Prof N, Columbia P&S

Feinberg, Todd E MD (N) - **Spec Exp:** Alzheimer's Disease; Stroke Rehabilitation; **Hospital:** Beth Israel Med Ctr - Petrie Division (page 90), Hosp For Joint Diseases (page 107); **Address:** Yarmon Neurobehavioral Ctr-Beth Israel Med Ctr, First Ave at 16th St, New York, NY 10003; **Phone:** 212-420-4111; **Board Cert:** Psychiatry 1984; Neurology 1987; **Med School:** Mount Sinai Sch Med 1978; **Resid:** Psychiatry, Mount Sinai 1982; Neurology, Mount Sinai 1984; **Fellow:** Behavioral Neurology, Univ Florida 1986; **Fac Appt:** Clin Prof N, Albert Einstein Coll Med

Fink, Matthew E MD (N) - **Spec Exp:** Cerebrovascular Disease; **Hospital:** NY-Presby Hosp (page 100); **Address:** NY Cornell Med Ctr Dept Neurology, 525 E 68th St, Ste F106, New York, NY 10021; **Phone:** 212-746-4564; **Board Cert:** Internal Medicine 1980; Neurology 1983; **Med School:** Univ Pittsburgh 1976; **Resid:** Internal Medicine, Boston Med Ctr 1980; Neurology, Columbia-Presby Hosp 1982; **Fac Appt:** Prof N, Albert Einstein Coll Med

Foo, Sun-Hoo MD (N) - **Spec Exp:** Stroke; Headache; Chinese Community Health; **Hospital:** NYU Med Ctr (page 102), NY Downtown Hosp; **Address:** 650 1st Ave, FL 4, New York, NY 10016-3240; **Phone:** 212-213-0270; **Board Cert:** Internal Medicine 1976; Neurology 1980; **Med School:** Taiwan 1972; **Resid:** Internal Medicine, St Vincent's Hosp 1976; Neurology, NYU Med Ctr 1979; **Fac Appt:** Prof N, NYU Sch Med

Forster, George MD (N) - **Spec Exp:** Multiple Sclerosis; Parkinson's Disease; **Hospital:** Mount Sinai Med Ctr (page 98); **Address:** 1160 5th Ave, Ste 107, New York, NY 10029; **Phone:** 212-410-6400; **Board Cert:** Neurology 1980; **Med School:** Italy 1971; **Resid:** Internal Medicine, Maimonides Med Ctr 1974; Neurology, Mount Sinai Hosp 1977; **Fac Appt:** Asst Clin Prof N, Mount Sinai Sch Med

Gendelman, Seymour MD (N) - **Spec Exp:** Parkinson's Disease; Dementia; Headache; **Hospital:** Mount Sinai Med Ctr (page 98); **Address:** 5 E 98th St Fl 7, Box 1139, New York, NY 10029-6501; **Phone:** 212-241-8172; **Board Cert:** Neurology 1971; **Med School:** Geo Wash Univ 1964; **Resid:** Neurology, Mount Sinai Hosp 1968; **Fac Appt:** Clin Prof N, Mount Sinai Sch Med

Goodgold, Albert MD (N) - **Spec Exp:** Parkinson's Disease; Spinal Cord Disorders; Multiple Sclerosis; Movement Disorders; **Hospital:** NYU Med Ctr (page 102); **Address:** 530 First Ave Fl 5 - Ste 5A, New York, NY 10016; **Phone:** 212-263-7205; **Med School:** Switzerland 1955; **Resid:** Neurology, Bellevue Hosp 1960; **Fac Appt:** Prof N, NYU Sch Med

Gopinathan, Govindan MD (N) - **Spec Exp:** Headache; Parkinson's Disease; Spinal Disorders; **Hospital:** NYU Med Ctr (page 102); **Address:** 650 1st Ave Fl 4, New York, NY 10016; **Phone:** 212-213-9559; **Board Cert:** Neurology 1980; **Med School:** India 1973; **Resid:** Internal Medicine, Coney Island Hosp 1975; Neurology, NYU Med Ctr 1978; **Fellow:** Neurological Pharmacology, Nat Inst Hlth 1980; **Fac Appt:** Clin Prof N, NYU Sch Med

Green, Mark W MD (N) - **Spec Exp:** Headache; Pain-Facial; **Hospital:** NY-Presby Hosp (page 100); **Address:** 16 E 60th St, Ste 310, New York, NY 10022; **Phone:** 212-326-8456; **Board Cert:** Neurology 1979; **Med School:** Albert Einstein Coll Med 1974; **Resid:** Neurology, Albert Einstein Affil Hosp 1978; **Fac Appt:** Clin Prof N, Columbia P&S

Gruber, Michael L MD (N) - **Spec Exp:** Pain-Back; Headache; Neuro-Oncology; **Hospital:** NYU Med Ctr (page 102), Overlook Hosp (page 88); **Address:** NYU Clinical Cancer Ctr, 160 E 34th St, New York, NY 10016; **Phone:** 212-731-5577; **Board Cert:** Neurology 1975; **Med School:** Temple Univ 1966; **Resid:** Pediatrics, Columbia-Presby Med Ctr 1968; Neurology, Columbia-Presby Med Ctr 1973; **Fellow:** Neurological Oncology, Mass Genl Hosp 1990; **Fac Appt:** Prof N, NYU Sch Med

Harden, Cynthia L MD (N) - **Spec Exp:** Epilepsy/Seizure Disorders; **Hospital:** NY-Presby Hosp (page 100); **Address:** NY Presbyterian-Cornell Medical Ctr, 525 E 68th St, rm K619, New York, NY 10021; **Phone:** 212-746-2346; **Board Cert:** Neurology 1989; **Med School:** Univ Wisc 1983; **Resid:** Internal Medicine, St Luke's Roosevelt Hosp 1985; Neurology, Mt Sinai Hosp 1988; **Fellow:** Clinical Neurophysiology, Albert Einstein Med Coll 1989; **Fac Appt:** Assoc Prof N, Cornell Univ-Weill Med Coll

Herbert, Joseph MD (N) - **Spec Exp:** Multiple Sclerosis; Neuromuscular Disorders; Stroke; **Hospital:** Hosp For Joint Diseases (page 107), NY Downtown Hosp; **Address:** 301 E 17th St, Ste 544, New York, NY 10003; **Phone:** 212-598-6305; **Board Cert:** Neurology 1987; **Med School:** Israel 1974; **Resid:** Neurology, Longwood/Harvard U Sch Med 1983; Neuropathology, Children's Hosp 1984; **Fellow:** Clinical Genetics, Columbia Presby Med Ctr 1986; **Fac Appt:** Assoc Prof N, NYU Sch Med

Herbstein, Diego MD (N) - **Spec Exp:** Parkinson's Disease; Cerebrovascular Disease; **Hospital:** Lenox Hill Hosp (page 94), NY-Presby Hosp (page 100); **Address:** 170 E 77th St, Ste 1-D, New York, NY 10021; **Phone:** 212-794-2281; **Board Cert:** Neurology 1976; **Med School:** Argentina 1968; **Resid:** Internal Medicine, Fernandez 1970; Neurology, Albert Einstein 1973; **Fellow:** Neurology, Jacobi Med Ctr 1974; **Fac Appt:** Asst Clin Prof N, Cornell Univ-Weill Med Coll

Hiesiger, Emile MD (N) - **Spec Exp:** Pain Management; Neuro-Oncology; **Hospital:** NYU Med Ctr (page 102), VA Med Ctr - Manhattan; **Address:** 530 1st Ave, Ste 9S, New York, NY 10016-6402; **Phone:** 212-263-6123; **Board Cert:** Neurology 1983; **Med School:** NY Med Coll 1978; **Resid:** Neurology, NYU Med Ctr 1982; **Fellow:** Neurology, Meml Sloan-Kettering Cancer Ctr 1984; **Fac Appt:** Assoc Clin Prof N, NYU Sch Med

Kolodny, Edwin H MD (N) - **Spec Exp:** Pediatric Neurology; Inherited Disorders of Nervous System; Gaucher Disease; Fabry's Disease; **Hospital:** NYU Med Ctr (page 102), Bellevue Hosp Ctr; **Address:** 403 E 34 St Fl 2, New York, NY 10016-6402; **Phone:** 212-263-8344; **Board Cert:** Neurology 1971; Clinical Genetics 1984; Clinical Biochemical Genetics 1987; **Med School:** NYU Sch Med 1962; **Resid:** Internal Medicine, Bellevue Hosp 1964; Neurology, Mass Genl Hosp 1967; **Fellow:** Neurological Pathology, Mass Genl Hosp 1966; Neurology, Nat Inst Neurol Dis & Stroke 1970; **Fac Appt:** Prof N, NYU Sch Med

Koppel, Barbara MD (N) - **Spec Exp:** Epilepsy; Headache; Stroke; AIDS/HIV; **Hospital:** Metropolitan Hosp Ctr - NY; **Address:** Metropolitan Hospital, 1901 First Ave, rm 1316, New York, NY 10029; **Phone:** 212-423-6676; **Board Cert:** Neurology 1983; **Med School:** Columbia P&S 1978; **Resid:** Internal Medicine, Montefiore Hosp Med Ctr 1979; Neurology, Columbia-Presby Hosp 1982; **Fac Appt:** Prof N, NY Med Coll

Kuzniecky, Ruben MD (N) - **Spec Exp:** Epilepsy/Seizure Disorders; MRI; **Hospital:** NYU Med Ctr (page 102); **Address:** 403 E 34th St Fl 4, New York, NY 10016; **Phone:** 212-263-8870; **Board Cert:** Neurology 1990; **Med School:** Argentina 1980; **Resid:** Neurology, McGill Univ 1986; **Fellow:** Epilepsy, McGill Univ 1988

Labar, Douglas MD/PhD (N) - **Spec Exp:** Epilepsy/Seizure Disorders; **Hospital:** NY-Presby Hosp (page 100); **Address:** NY Weill Cornell Med Ctr, 520 E 70th St, rm K619, New York, NY 10021; **Phone:** 212-746-2359; **Board Cert:** Neurology 1987; **Med School:** Med Coll PA 1982; **Resid:** Neurology, Columbia Presby Med Ctr 1986; **Fellow:** Epilepsy, Columbia Presby Med Ctr 1988; **Fac Appt:** Prof N, Cornell Univ-Weill Med Coll

Lange, Dale J MD (N) - **Spec Exp:** Neuromuscular Disorders; Amyotrophic Lateral Sclerosis (ALS); **Hospital:** Mount Sinai Med Ctr (page 98); **Address:** Mount Sinai Medical Ctr, Annenberg Bldg, One Gustave L. Levy Pl, rm 230, Box 1052, New York, NY 10029; **Phone:** 212-241-8674; **Board Cert:** Neurology 1985; **Med School:** NY Med Coll 1978; **Resid:** Neurology, New England Med Ctr 1982; **Fellow:** Neuromuscular Disease, Columbia-Presby Med Ctr 1983; **Fac Appt:** Assoc Prof N, Mount Sinai Sch Med

Latov, Norman MD/PhD (N) - **Spec Exp:** Peripheral Neuropathy; Neuro-Immunology; **Hospital:** NY-Presby Hosp (page 100); **Address:** 635 Madison Ave, Ste 400, New York, NY 10022; **Phone:** 212-888-8516; **Board Cert:** Neurology 1989; **Med School:** Univ Pennsylvania 1975; **Resid:** Internal Medicine, Boston City Hosp 1976; Neurology, Columbia-Presby Med Ctr 1979; **Fellow:** Immunology, Columbia-Presby Med Ctr 1981; **Fac Appt:** Prof N, Cornell Univ-Weill Med Coll

Levine, David N MD (N) - **Spec Exp:** Dementia; Stroke; Spinal Cord Disorders; **Hospital:** NYU Med Ctr (page 102); **Address:** 400 E 34th St, Ste RIRM- 311, New York, NY 10016-4901; **Phone:** 212-263-7744; **Board Cert:** Neurology 1976; **Med School:** Harvard Med Sch 1968; **Resid:** Neurology, Mass Genl Hosp 1974; **Fellow:** Neurology, Mass Genl Hosp 1976; **Fac Appt:** Prof N, NYU Sch Med

Levine, Steven R MD (N) - **Spec Exp:** Stroke; Cerebrovascular Disease; **Hospital:** Mount Sinai Med Ctr (page 98); **Address:** Mt Sinai Sch Med, Neurology, Stroke Program, 1 Gustave Levy Pl, Box 1137, New York, NY 10029-6574; **Phone:** 212-241-1970; **Board Cert:** Neurology 1986; **Med School:** Med Coll Wisc 1981; **Resid:** Neurology, Univ Mich Hosps 1985; **Fellow:** Cerebrovascular Disease, Henry Ford Hosp 1987; **Fac Appt:** Prof N, Mount Sinai Sch Med

Lublin, Fred MD (N) - **Spec Exp:** Multiple Sclerosis; **Hospital:** Mount Sinai Med Ctr (page 98); **Address:** Dickinson Ctr for Multiple Sclerosis, 5 E 98th St, Box 1138, New York, NY 10029-6574; **Phone:** 212-241-6854; **Board Cert:** Neurology 1977; **Med School:** Jefferson Med Coll 1972; **Resid:** Neurology, NY Hosp/Cornell Med Ctr 1976; **Fac Appt:** Prof N, Mount Sinai Sch Med

Luciano, Daniel J MD (N) - **Spec Exp:** Epilepsy/Seizure Disorders; **Hospital:** NYU Med Ctr (page 102); **Address:** 403 E 34th St Bldg Rivergate Fl 4, New York, NY 10016; **Phone:** 212-263-8853; **Board Cert:** Neurology 1992; Clinical Neurophysiology 1996; **Med School:** UMDNJ-NJ Med Sch, Newark 1984; **Resid:** Neurology, Mt Sinai Med Ctr 1988; **Fellow:** Epilepsy, Mt Sinai Med Ctr 1990

Marder, Karen MD (N) - **Spec Exp:** Huntington's Disease; Alzheimer's Disease; Dementia; **Hospital:** NY-Presby Hosp (page 100); **Address:** Neurological Institute, 710 W 168th St, Ste 104, New York, NY 10032-2603; **Phone:** 212-305-6939; **Board Cert:** Neurology 1989; **Med School:** Cornell Univ-Weill Med Coll 1983; **Resid:** Neurology, Neurological Inst 1987; **Fellow:** Behavioral Neurology, Neurological Inst-Columbia 1989; **Fac Appt:** Assoc Prof N, Columbia P&S

Mauskop, Alexander MD (N) - **Spec Exp:** Headache; Pain Management; **Hospital:** Beth Israel Med Ctr - Petrie Division (page 90), Long Island Coll Hosp (page 90); **Address:** 30 E 76th St, New York, NY 10021; **Phone:** 212-794-3550; **Board Cert:** Neurology 1987; Pain Medicine 1995; **Med School:** Ukraine 1979; **Resid:** Internal Medicine, Brookdale Hosp 1981; Neurology, Univ Hosp 1984; **Fellow:** Pain Management, Meml Sloan Kettering Cancer Ctr 1986; **Fac Appt:** Assoc Clin Prof N, SUNY Downstate

Mayer, Stephan A MD (N) - **Spec Exp:** Neurological Critical Care; Stroke; Coma; **Hospital:** NY-Presby Hosp (page 100); **Address:** 710 W 168th St, Unit 39, New York, NY 10032-2603; **Phone:** 212-305-7236; **Board Cert:** Neurology 1993; **Med School:** Cornell Univ-Weill Med Coll 1988; **Resid:** Neurology, Columbia-Presby Med Ctr 1992; **Fellow:** Critical Care Neurology, Columbia-Presby Med Ctr 1993; **Fac Appt:** Assoc Prof N, Columbia P&S

Mayeux, Richard MD (N) - **Spec Exp:** Alzheimer's Disease; Dementia; **Hospital:** NY-Presby Hosp (page 100); **Address:** 630 W 168th St, PH 19, New York, NY 10032; **Phone:** 212-305-9194; **Board Cert:** Neurology 1978; **Med School:** Univ Okla Coll Med 1972; **Resid:** Internal Medicine, Boston City Hosp 1974; Neurology, Columbia Presby Med Ctr 1977; **Fellow:** Neurology, Boston Univ 1978; **Fac Appt:** Prof N, Columbia P&S

Miller, Aaron MD (N) - **Spec Exp:** Multiple Sclerosis; Alzheimer's Disease; Autoimmune Disease; **Hospital:** Mount Sinai Med Ctr (page 98), Maimonides Med Ctr (page 96); **Address:** Corinne Goldsmith Dickinson Ctr for MS, 5 E 98th St, Box 1138, New York, NY 10029; **Phone:** 212-241-6854; **Board Cert:** Internal Medicine 1972; Neurology 1977; **Med School:** NYU Sch Med 1968; **Resid:** Internal Medicine, Jacobi Med Ctr 1970; Neurology, Albert Einstein 1975; **Fellow:** Neurovirology, Johns Hopkins 1977Albert Einstein 1978; **Fac Appt:** Prof N, Mount Sinai Sch Med

Mitsumoto, Hiroshi MD (N) - **Spec Exp:** Amyotrophic Lateral Sclerosis (ALS); Neuromuscular Disorders; Clinical Trials; **Hospital:** NY-Presby Hosp (page 100); **Address:** Neurological Inst, 710 W 168th St Fl 9 - rm 9001, New York, NY 10032; **Phone:** 212-305-1319; **Board Cert:** Neurology 1978; **Med School:** Japan 1968; **Resid:** Internal Medicine, Toho Univ Hosps 1972; Neurology, Univ Hosps 1976; **Fellow:** Neurological Pathology, Cleveland Clinic 1978; Neuromuscular Disease, Tufts Univ 1981; **Fac Appt:** Prof N, Columbia P&S

Mohr, J P MD (N) - **Spec Exp:** Aphasia; Stroke; Aneurysm-Cerebral; **Hospital:** NY-Presby Hosp (page 100); **Address:** Dept Neur-Neuro Inst, 710 W 168 St, rm 615, New York, NY 10032-2603; **Phone:** 212-305-8033; **Board Cert:** Neurology 1971; **Med School:** Univ VA Sch Med 1963; **Resid:** Neurology, Columbia Presby Med Ctr 1966; Neurology, Mass Genl Hosp 1968; **Fellow:** Neurology, Mass Genl Hosp 1969; **Fac Appt:** Clin Prof N, Columbia P&S

Nealon, Nancy MD (N) - **Spec Exp:** Migraine; Multiple Sclerosis; **Hospital:** NY-Presby Hosp (page 100); **Address:** 425 E 61st St, New York, NY 10021; **Phone:** 212-821-0858; **Board Cert:** Internal Medicine 1978; Neurology 1984; **Med School:** Penn State Univ-Hershey Med Ctr 1975; **Resid:** Neurology, NY Hosp 1981; **Fellow:** Neurological Muscular Disease, Columbia-Presby Med Ctr 1982; Medical Oncology, Meml Sloan Kettering Cancer Ctr 1983; **Fac Appt:** Asst Prof N, Cornell Univ-Weill Med Coll

Newman, Lawrence C MD (N) - **Spec Exp:** Headache; Pain-Facial; **Hospital:** St Luke's - Roosevelt Hosp Ctr - Roosevelt Div (page 90); **Address:** St Luke's-Roosevelt Hosp-Headache Inst, 1000 Tenth Ave, Ste 1C10, New York, NY 10019-1192; **Phone:** 212-523-5869; **Board Cert:** Neurology 2005; **Med School:** Mexico 1983; **Resid:** Internal Medicine, Elmhurst Hosp 1986; Neurology, Albert Einstein 1989; **Fac Appt:** Assoc Prof N, Albert Einstein Coll Med

Olanow, C Warren MD (N) - **Spec Exp:** Parkinson's Disease; Movement Disorders; **Hospital:** Mount Sinai Med Ctr (page 98); **Address:** Dept Neurology, 5 E 98th St Fl 1, New York, NY 10029; **Phone:** 212-241-8435; **Med School:** Univ Toronto 1965; **Resid:** Neurology, Toronto Genl Hosp 1968; Neurology, Columbia Presby Hosp 1970; **Fellow:** Neurological Anatomy, Columbia Presby Hosp 1971; **Fac Appt:** Prof N, Mount Sinai Sch Med

Olarte, Marcelo MD (N) - **Spec Exp:** Myasthenia Gravis; Electrodiagnosis; Headache; **Hospital:** NY-Presby Hosp (page 100), St Luke's - Roosevelt Hosp Ctr - Roosevelt Div (page 90); **Address:** 710 W 168th St, New York, NY 10032; **Phone:** 212-305-1832; **Board Cert:** Neurology 1976; **Med School:** Argentina 1970; **Resid:** Neurology, St Vincent's Hosp 1974; **Fellow:** Neuromuscular Disease, Columbia-Presby Hosp 1975; **Fac Appt:** Assoc Clin Prof N, Columbia P&S

Pacia, Steven MD (N) - **Spec Exp:** Epilepsy/Seizure Disorders; **Hospital:** NYU Med Ctr (page 102); **Address:** 403 E 34th St Fl 4, New York, NY 10016; **Phone:** 212-263-8875; **Board Cert:** Neurology 1992; Clinical Neurophysiology 1996; **Med School:** Yale Univ 1989; **Resid:** Neurology, Yale-New Haven Hosp 1992; **Fellow:** Epilepsy, Yale-New Haven Hosp 1992; **Fac Appt:** Assoc Prof N, NYU Sch Med

Pedley, Timothy A MD (N) - **Spec Exp:** Epilepsy/Seizure Disorders; **Hospital:** NY-Presby Hosp (page 100); **Address:** The Neurological Inst, 710 W 168th St, rm 1406, New York, NY 10032; **Phone:** 212-305-6489; **Board Cert:** Neurology 1975; Clinical Neurophysiology 1993; **Med School:** Yale Univ 1969; **Resid:** Neurology, Stanford Univ Hosp 1973; **Fellow:** Clinical Neurophysiology, Stanford Univ Hosp 1975; **Fac Appt:** Prof N, Columbia P&S

Petito, Frank MD (N) - **Spec Exp:** Multiple Sclerosis; Headache; Lyme Disease; **Hospital:** NY-Presby Hosp (page 100); **Address:** 525 E 68th St, rm *607, New York, NY 10021-4870; **Phone:** 212-746-2309; **Board Cert:** Neurology 1972; **Med School:** Columbia P&S 1967; **Resid:** Neurology, New York Hosp 1971; **Fac Appt:** Prof N, Cornell Univ-Weill Med Coll

Posner, Jerome MD (N) - **Spec Exp:** Neuro-Oncology; Brain Tumors; **Hospital:** Meml Sloan Kettering Cancer Ctr (page 109); **Address:** 1275 York Ave, rm C731, New York, NY 10021-6007; **Phone:** 212-639-7047; **Board Cert:** Neurology 1962; **Med School:** Univ Wash 1955; **Resid:** Neurology, Univ WA Affil Hosp 1959; **Fellow:** Biochemistry, Univ WA Affil Hosp 1963; **Fac Appt:** Prof N, Cornell Univ-Weill Med Coll

Rapoport, Samuel MD (N) - **Spec Exp:** Peripheral Nerve Disorders; Pain-Back & Neck; Electromyography; **Hospital:** NY-Presby Hosp (page 100), Lenox Hill Hosp (page 94); **Address:** 354 E 76th St, New York, NY 10021-2505; **Phone:** 212-570-0642; **Board Cert:** Neurology 1986; **Med School:** Cornell Univ-Weill Med Coll 1976; **Resid:** Neurology, New York Hosp-Cornell 1982; **Fac Appt:** Assoc Prof N, Cornell Univ-Weill Med Coll

Relkin, Norman MD/PhD (N) - **Spec Exp:** Alzheimer's Disease; Dementia; Memory Disorders; **Hospital:** NY-Presby Hosp (page 100); **Address:** Memory Disorders Dept, 525 E 68th St, Ste 500, New York, NY 10021; **Phone:** 212-746-2441; **Board Cert:** Neurology 1992; **Med School:** Albert Einstein Coll Med 1987; **Resid:** Neurology, New York Hosp 1991; **Fellow:** Behavioral Neurology, New York Hosp-Cornell 1992; **Fac Appt:** Asst Prof N, Cornell Univ-Weill Med Coll

Rosenfeld, Steven S MD (N) - **Spec Exp:** Brain Tumors; Gliomas; Neuro-Oncology; **Hospital:** NY-Presby Hosp (page 100); **Address:** Neurological Inst of NY-Brain Tumor Ctr, 710 W 168th St, rm 204, New York, NY 10032; **Phone:** 212-305-1718; **Board Cert:** Neurology 1994; **Med School:** Northwestern Univ 1985; **Resid:** Neurology, Duke Univ Med Ctr 1989; **Fellow:** Neurological Oncology, Duke Univ Med Ctr 1990; **Fac Appt:** Prof N, Columbia P&S

Rowan, A James MD (N) - **Spec Exp:** Epilepsy/Seizure Disorders; Seizure Disorders in the Aging; **Hospital:** Mount Sinai Med Ctr (page 98), VA Med Ctr - Bronx; **Address:** 5 E 98th St, Box 1139, New York, NY 10029-6501; **Phone:** 212-241-7076; **Board Cert:** Neurology 1971; **Med School:** Stanford Univ 1961; **Resid:** Internal Medicine, Boston VA 1963; Neurology, Columbia-Presby 1966; **Fellow:** Electroencephalography, London Hosp 1969; **Fac Appt:** Prof N, Mount Sinai Sch Med

Rowland, Lewis P MD (N) - **Spec Exp:** Neuromuscular Disorders; Amyotrophic Lateral Sclerosis (ALS); Myasthenia Gravis; **Hospital:** NY-Presby Hosp (page 100); **Address:** 710 W 168th St, New York, NY 10032-2603; **Phone:** 212-305-4119; **Board Cert:** Neurology 1955; **Med School:** Yale Univ 1948; **Resid:** Internal Medicine, Yale-New Haven Hosp 1950; Neurology, Columbia-Presby Hosp 1953; **Fac Appt:** Prof N, Columbia P&S

Sacco, Ralph L MD (N) - **Spec Exp:** Stroke; **Hospital:** NY-Presby Hosp (page 100); **Address:** Neurological Institute, 710 W 168th St, rm 640, New York, NY 10032; **Phone:** 212-305-1710; **Board Cert:** Neurology 1989; **Med School:** Boston Univ 1983; **Resid:** Neurology, Columbia-Presby Med Ctr 1987; **Fellow:** Cerebrovascular Disease, Columbia-Presby Med Ctr 1989; **Fac Appt:** Prof N, Columbia P&S

Sander, Howard MD (N) - **Spec Exp:** Electromyography; Peripheral Neuropathy; Neuromuscular Disorders; **Hospital:** NY-Presby Hosp (page 100), Hosp For Special Surgery (page 108); **Address:** 635 Madison Ave, Ste 400, New York, NY 10022; **Phone:** 212-888-8516; **Board Cert:** Neurology 1993; Clinical Neurophysiology 2005; Pain Medicine 2000; **Med School:** SUNY Downstate 1988; **Resid:** Neurology, Albert Einstein Coll of Med 1992; **Fellow:** Electromyography, Mass Genl Hosp 1993; **Fac Appt:** Assoc Prof N, Cornell Univ-Weill Med Coll

Schaefer, John A MD (N) - **Spec Exp:** Spinal Diseases; Multiple Sclerosis; Stroke; Cerebrovascular Disease; **Hospital:** NY-Presby Hosp (page 100), Hosp For Special Surgery (page 108); **Address:** 523 E 72nd St Fl 8, New York, NY 10021-4099; **Phone:** 212-717-0231; **Board Cert:** Neurology 1979; **Med School:** Australia 1968; **Resid:** Neurology, St Vincent's Hosp 1973; **Fellow:** Neurology, NY Hosp 1978; **Fac Appt:** Assoc Clin Prof N, Cornell Univ-Weill Med Coll

Sharma, Chandra MD (N) - **Spec Exp:** Headache; **Hospital:** Cabrini Med Ctr (page 374); **Address:** Dept Neurology, 133 E 73rd St, New York, NY 10021-3556; **Phone:** 212-861-9000; **Board Cert:** Neurology 1976; **Med School:** India 1966; **Resid:** Internal Medicine, New Jersey College of Medicine & Dentistry 1969; Neurology, New York Med Coll 1972; **Fellow:** Neurology, New York Med Coll 1973; **Fac Appt:** Prof N, SUNY Downstate

Simpson, David M MD (N) - **Spec Exp:** Infections-CNS; AIDS-Neurologic Complications; Peripheral Neuropathy; Neuromuscular Disorders; **Hospital:** Mount Sinai Med Ctr (page 98); **Address:** Mt Sinai Medical Ctr, Dept Neurology, 5 E 98th St, Box 1052, New York, NY 10029; **Phone:** 212-241-8748; **Board Cert:** Neurology 1984; Clinical Neurophysiology 1996; **Med School:** SUNY Buffalo 1979; **Resid:** Neurology, New York Hosp-Cornell Med Ctr 1983; **Fellow:** Neurourology, Mass General Hosp 1984; **Fac Appt:** Prof N, Mount Sinai Sch Med

Sivak, Mark A MD (N) - **Spec Exp:** Myasthenia Gravis; Amyotrophic Lateral Sclerosis (ALS); Neuromuscular Disorders; **Hospital:** Mount Sinai Med Ctr (page 98); **Address:** 5 E 98th St Fl 7, New York, NY 10029-6501; **Phone:** 212-241-6719; **Board Cert:** Neurology 1978; Clinical Neurophysiology 1999; **Med School:** Univ Louisville Sch Med 1971; **Resid:** Neurology, Mt Sinai Med Ctr 1975; **Fellow:** Electromyography, Mt Sinai Med Ctr 1976; Clinical Neurophysiology, Uppsala Univ 1986; **Fac Appt:** Asst Prof N, Mount Sinai Sch Med

Smallberg, Gerald MD (N) - **Spec Exp:** Spinal Disorders; **Hospital:** Lenox Hill Hosp (page 94); **Address:** 1010 5th Ave, New York, NY 10028-0130; **Phone:** 212-535-5348; **Board Cert:** Neurology 1977; **Med School:** Yale Univ 1969; **Resid:** Internal Medicine, Univ Mich Med Ctr 1971; Neurology, Hosp Univ Penn 1975; **Fellow:** Neurology, Columbia-Presby Med Ctr 1976; **Fac Appt:** Asst Clin Prof N, NYU Sch Med

Snyder, David MD (N) - **Spec Exp:** Multiple Sclerosis; **Hospital:** NY Hosp Queens, Lenox Hill Hosp (page 94); **Address:** 170 E 77th St, Ste 1D, New York, NY 10021-1913; **Phone:** 212-794-2281; **Board Cert:** Neurology 1975; **Med School:** Univ MD Sch Med 1969; **Resid:** Neurology, Univ Maryland Hosp 1973; **Fellow:** Neuropathology, Albert Einstein Med Ctr 1975; **Fac Appt:** Asst Clin Prof N, Cornell Univ-Weill Med Coll

Stacy, Charles B MD (N) - **Spec Exp:** Stroke; Brain Injury; **Hospital:** Mount Sinai Med Ctr (page 98); **Address:** 1107 5th Ave, New York, NY 10128-0145; **Phone:** 212-876-8614; **Board Cert:** Neurology 1983; **Med School:** Cornell Univ-Weill Med Coll 1977; **Resid:** Internal Medicine, Mount Sinai 1979; Neurology, Mount Sinai 1982; **Fellow:** Neurology, Meml Sloan Kettering 1983

Stubgen, Joerg-Patrick MD (N) - **Spec Exp:** Amyotrophic Lateral Sclerosis (ALS); **Hospital:** NY-Presby Hosp (page 100); **Address:** Dept Neur Starr 607, 525 E 68th St, New York, NY 10021; **Phone:** 212-746-2334; **Board Cert:** Neurology 1996; Clinical Neurophysiology 1999; **Med School:** South Africa 1983; **Resid:** Neurology, Univ Pretoria Med Ctr 1989; Neurology, New York Hosp 1995; **Fellow:** Clinical Neurophysiology, Menl Sloan Kettering Cancer Ctr 1995; **Fac Appt:** Assoc Prof N, Cornell Univ-Weill Med Coll

Tuchman, Alan MD (N) - **Spec Exp:** Epilepsy; Multiple Sclerosis; **Hospital:** Our Lady of Mercy Med Ctr, St Vincent Cath Med Ctrs - Manhattan (page 375); **Address:** 975 Park Ave, New York, NY 10028; **Phone:** 212-772-9305; **Board Cert:** Neurology 1979; **Med School:** Univ Cincinnati 1972; **Resid:** Neurology, Mt Sinai Med Ctr 1976; **Fellow:** Multiple Sclerosis, Albert Einstein Med Ctr 1979; **Fac Appt:** Clin Prof N, NY Med Coll

Waters, Cheryl H MD (N) - **Spec Exp:** Parkinson's Disease; Movement Disorders; **Hospital:** NY-Presby Hosp (page 100); **Address:** 710 W 168th St Fl 3, New York, NY 10032; **Phone:** 212-305-3665; **Board Cert:** Neurology 1986; **Med School:** Univ Toronto 1980; **Resid:** Internal Medicine, Univ Toronto Med Ctr 1982; Neurology, Univ Toronto Med Ctr 1985; **Fellow:** Neurological Pharmacology, Univ Toronto Med Ctr 1987; **Fac Appt:** Prof N, Columbia P&S

Weinberg, Harold MD (N) - **Spec Exp:** Headache; Spinal Disorders; Neuromuscular Disorders; **Hospital:** NYU Med Ctr (page 102); **Address:** 650 1st Ave Fl 4, New York, NY 10016-3240; **Phone:** 212-213-9339; **Board Cert:** Neurology 1983; **Med School:** Albert Einstein Coll Med 1978; **Resid:** Neurology, Columbia-Presby Med Ctr 1982; **Fellow:** Neuromuscular Disease, Columbia-Presby Med Ctr 1982; **Fac Appt:** Clin Prof N, NYU Sch Med

Weinberger, Jesse MD (N) - **Spec Exp:** Stroke; **Hospital:** Mount Sinai Med Ctr (page 98), N Genl Hosp; **Address:** 5 E 98th St, New York, NY 10029-6501; **Phone:** 212-241-4529; **Board Cert:** Neurology 1976; **Med School:** Johns Hopkins Univ 1971; **Resid:** Neurology, Mt Sinai Med Ctr 1975; **Fellow:** Cerebrovascular Disease, Hosp Univ Penn 1978; **Fac Appt:** Prof N, Mount Sinai Sch Med

Weiss, Arthur H MD (N) - **Spec Exp:** Parkinson's Disease; Stroke; **Hospital:** Mount Sinai Med Ctr (page 98), Lenox Hill Hosp (page 94); **Address:** 1056 5th Ave, New York, NY 10028-0112; **Phone:** 212-831-1055; **Board Cert:** Neurology 1964; **Med School:** SUNY Hlth Sci Ctr 1957; **Resid:** Neurology, Mount Sinai 1959; Neurology, Mt Sinai Hosp 1963; **Fellow:** Neurology, Columbia-Presby 1965; **Fac Appt:** Asst Clin Prof N, Mount Sinai Sch Med

NEURORADIOLOGY

Berenstein, Alejandro MD (NRad) - **Spec Exp:** Interventional Neuroradiology; Aneurysm-Cerebral; Endovascular Surgery; **Hospital:** St Luke's - Roosevelt Hosp Ctr - St Luke's Hosp (page 90); **Address:** Hyman-Newman Inst Neurolgy & Neuro Surg, 1000 10th Ave, rm GG16, New York, NY 10019; **Phone:** 212-636-3400; **Board Cert:** Diagnostic Radiology 1976; Neuroradiology 1995; **Med School:** Mexico 1970; **Resid:** Radiology, Mount Sinai Med Ctr 1976; **Fellow:** Neuroradiology, NYU Med Ctr 1978; **Fac Appt:** Prof Rad, NYU Sch Med

Deck, Michael MD (NRad) - **Spec Exp:** Brain Tumors; Spinal Diseases; Brain Imaging; Aneurysm-Cerebral; **Hospital:** NY-Presby Hosp (page 100); **Address:** 525 E 68th St, Starr 630, New York, NY 10021-4870; **Phone:** 212-746-2575; **Board Cert:** Diagnostic Radiology 1969; Neuroradiology 2003; **Med School:** Australia 1961; **Resid:** Radiology, Sydney Hosp 1965; **Fellow:** Neuroradiology, Natl Hosp for Neurology & Neurosurgery 1968; **Fac Appt:** Prof Rad, Cornell Univ-Weill Med Coll

Drayer, Burton P MD (NRad) - **Spec Exp:** Stroke; Parkinson's Disease/Aging Brain; MRI & CT of Brain & Spine; **Hospital:** Mount Sinai Med Ctr (page 98); **Address:** 1 Gustave Levy Pl, Box 1234, New York, NY 10029; **Phone:** 212-241-6403; **Board Cert:** Neurology 1976; Diagnostic Radiology 1978; Neuroradiology 1995; **Med School:** Univ Hlth Sci/Chicago Med Sch 1971; **Resid:** Neurology, Univ Vt Med Ctr 1975; Radiology, Univ Pitt Hlth Ctr 1977; **Fellow:** Neuroradiology, Univ Pitt Hlth Ctr 1978; **Fac Appt:** Prof Rad, Mount Sinai Sch Med

Grossman, Robert I MD (NRad) - **Spec Exp:** Multiple Sclerosis Imaging; Brain Injury; MRI; **Hospital:** NYU Med Ctr (page 102), Bellevue Hosp Ctr; **Address:** NYU Med Ctr, Dept Radiology, 560 First Ave, RUSK 229, New York, NY 10016; **Phone:** 212-263-3269; **Board Cert:** Diagnostic Radiology 1979; Neuroradiology 2005; **Med School:** Univ Pennsylvania 1973; **Resid:** Neurological Surgery, Hosp Univ Penn 1976; Radiology, Hosp Univ Penn 1979; **Fellow:** Neuroradiology, Mass Genl Hosp 1981; **Fac Appt:** Prof Rad, NYU Sch Med

Jahre, Caren MD (NRad) - **Hospital:** Lenox Hill Hosp (page 94); **Address:** Lenox Hill Hosp, Dept Radiology, 100 E 77th St Fl 3, New York, NY 10021; **Phone:** 212-434-2900; **Board Cert:** Diagnostic Radiology 1988; Neuroradiology 1995; **Med School:** Cornell Univ-Weill Med Coll 1982; **Resid:** Radiology, New York Hosp 1988; **Fellow:** Neuroradiology, New York Hosp 1990

Khandji, Alexander G MD (NRad) - **Spec Exp:** Pituitary Disorders; Spinal Diseases; MRI; **Hospital:** NY-Presby Hosp (page 100); **Address:** 177 Ft Washington Ave, Ste 4-156, New York, NY 10032-3173; **Phone:** 212-305-7669; **Board Cert:** Diagnostic Radiology 1985; Neuroradiology 1995; **Med School:** SUNY Downstate 1980; **Resid:** Surgery, MS Hershey Med Ctr 1982; Diagnostic Radiology, Columbia-Presby Med Ctr 1985; **Fellow:** Neuroradiology, Columbia-Presby Med Ctr 1987; **Fac Appt:** Clin Prof Rad, Columbia P&S

Litt, Andrew W MD (NRad) - **Spec Exp:** Vascular Lesions of the CNS; Cerebrovascular Disease; Stroke; **Hospital:** NYU Med Ctr (page 102); **Address:** NYU Medical Ctr, Dept Radiology, 560 1st Ave Rusk Bldg - rm 232, New York, NY 10016-6402; **Phone:** 212-263-8121; **Board Cert:** Diagnostic Radiology 1988; Neuroradiology 1995; **Med School:** NYU Sch Med 1983; **Resid:** Radiology, NYU Med Ctr 1987; **Fellow:** Neuroradiology, NYU Med Ctr 1988; **Fac Appt:** Prof Rad, NYU Sch Med

Meyers, Philip M MD (NRad) - **Spec Exp:** Interventional Neuroradiology; Aneurysm-Cerebral; Arteriovenous Malformations; Brain & Spinal Tumors; **Hospital:** NY-Presby Hosp (page 100); **Address:** Neurological Inst, 710 168th St, rm 404, New York, NY 10032; **Phone:** 212-305-6384; **Board Cert:** Diagnostic Radiology 1997; Neuroradiology 2002; **Med School:** Case West Res Univ 1989; **Resid:** Neurological Surgery, Univ Cincinnati Med Ctr 1990; Radiology, Univ Cincinnati Med Ctr 1997; **Fellow:** Neurological Radiology, Univ Cincinnati Med Ctr 1998; Neurovascular Medicine, UCSF Med Ctr 1999; **Fac Appt:** Assoc Prof Rad, Columbia P&S

Pile-Spellman, John MD (NRad) - **Spec Exp:** Interventional Neuroradiology; Cerebrovascular Disease; Aneurysm, Arteriovenous Malformations; **Hospital:** NY-Presby Hosp (page 100), NY-Presby Hosp (page 100); **Address:** 177 Fort Washington Ave, MHB 8SK, New York, NY 10032-3713; **Phone:** 212-305-6515; **Board Cert:** Diagnostic Radiology 1984; **Med School:** Tufts Univ 1978; **Resid:** Neurological Surgery, New England Med Ctr 1981; Neurological Radiology, Mass Genl Hosp 1984; **Fellow:** Interventional Neuroradiology, NYU Med Ctr 1986; **Fac Appt:** Prof Rad, Columbia P&S

NUCLEAR MEDICINE

Abdel-Dayem, Hussein M MD (NuM) - **Spec Exp:** Nuclear Oncology; Nuclear Cardiology; **Hospital:** St Vincent Cath Med Ctrs - Manhattan (page 375); **Address:** 153 W 11th St, New York, NY 10011; **Phone:** 212-604-8783; **Board Cert:** Radiology 1972; Nuclear Medicine 1972; **Med School:** Egypt 1959; **Resid:** Internal Medicine, Cairo Univ Hosp 1963; Nuclear Medicine, Roswell Park Cancer Inst 1971; **Fellow:** Radiation Oncology, Roswell Park Cancer Inst; **Fac Appt:** Prof Rad, NY Med Coll

Fawwaz, Rashib MD (NuM) - **Spec Exp:** PET Imaging; Brain Imaging; Radioimmunotherapy of Cancer; **Hospital:** NY-Presby Hosp (page 100); **Address:** Columbia Presby Med Ctr, Dept Rad, 177 Ft Washington Ave, MHB 3-202A, New York, NY 10032-3713; **Phone:** 212-305-7138; **Board Cert:** Nuclear Medicine 1975; **Med School:** Amer Univ Beirut 1961; **Resid:** Radiology, American Univ Hosp 1963; **Fellow:** Nuclear Medicine, Donner Lab-UC 1966; **Fac Appt:** Clin Prof Rad, Columbia P&S

Goldfarb, C Richard MD (NuM) - **Spec Exp:** Thyroid Disorders; **Hospital:** Beth Israel Med Ctr - Petrie Division (page 90), St Luke's - Roosevelt Hosp Ctr - Roosevelt Div (page 90); **Address:** Beth Israel Med Ctr, Dept Radiology, 1st Ave at 16th St, New York, NY 10003; **Phone:** 212-420-2339; **Board Cert:** Nuclear Medicine 1974; Diagnostic Radiology 1975; **Med School:** NY Med Coll 1970; **Resid:** Diagnostic Radiology, St Luke's Hosp 1974; **Fellow:** Nuclear Medicine, St Luke's Hosp 1975; **Fac Appt:** Assoc Prof NuM, Albert Einstein Coll Med

Goldsmith, Stanley J MD (NuM) - **Spec Exp:** Thyroid Cancer; Neuroendocrine Tumors; PET Imaging; **Hospital:** NY-Presby Hosp (page 100); **Address:** 520 E 70th St Bldg Starr - rm 221, New York, NY 10021-9800; **Phone:** 212-746-4588; **Board Cert:** Internal Medicine 1969; Nuclear Medicine 1972; Endocrinology 1972; **Med School:** SUNY Downstate 1962; **Resid:** Internal Medicine, Kings Co Hosp 1967; **Fellow:** Endocrinology, Diabetes & Metabolism, Mt Sinai Hosp 1968; Nuclear Medicine, Bronx VA Hosp 1969; **Fac Appt:** Prof Rad, Cornell Univ-Weill Med Coll

Kramer, Elissa MD (NuM) - **Spec Exp:** Cancer Detection & Staging; Lymphedema Imaging; Radioimmunotherapy of Cancer; **Hospital:** NYU Med Ctr (page 102), Bellevue Hosp Ctr; **Address:** 560 1st Ave, rm HW231, New York, NY 10016-6402; **Phone:** 212-263-7410; **Board Cert:** Nuclear Medicine 1982; Diagnostic Radiology 1982; **Med School:** NYU Sch Med 1977; **Resid:** Radiology, Bellevue Hosp/NYU 1980; **Fellow:** Nuclear Medicine, Bellevue Hosp/NYU 1982; **Fac Appt:** Prof Rad, NYU Sch Med

Larson, Steven M MD (NuM) - **Spec Exp:** Thyroid Cancer; PET Imaging; **Hospital:** Meml Sloan Kettering Cancer Ctr (page 109); **Address:** Meml Sloan Kettering Cancer Ctr, Nuc Med, 1275 York Ave, Box 77, New York, NY 10021; **Phone:** 212-639-7373; **Board Cert:** Nuclear Medicine 1972; Internal Medicine 1973; **Med School:** Univ Wash 1965; **Resid:** Internal Medicine, Virginia Mason Hosp 1970; Nuclear Medicine, Natl Inst Hlth 1972; **Fac Appt:** Prof NuM, Cornell Univ-Weill Med Coll

Liebeskind, Arie MD (NuM) - **Hospital:** Gracie Square Hosp; **Address:** 525 Park Ave, New York, NY 10021; **Phone:** 212-888-1000; **Board Cert:** Nuclear Medicine 1972; Radiation Oncology 1970; **Med School:** Albert Einstein Coll Med 1965; **Resid:** Radiology, Albert Einstein 1974; Radiology, Jacobi Med Ctr 1969; **Fellow:** Nuclear Radiology, Albert Einstein 1972; **Fac Appt:** Rad, Albert Einstein Coll Med

Pierson Jr, Richard N. MD (NuM) - **Spec Exp:** Osteoporosis; Obesity; **Hospital:** St Luke's - Roosevelt Hosp Ctr - St Luke's Hosp (page 90); **Address:** 1111 Amsterdam Ave, Scrymser - Basement, rm 1012, New York, NY 10025-1716; **Phone:** 212-523-3385; **Board Cert:** Internal Medicine 1980; Nuclear Medicine 1988; **Med School:** Columbia P&S 1955; **Resid:** Internal Medicine, St Luke's-Roosevelt Hosp Ctr 1956; Internal Medicine, St Luke's-Roosevelt Hosp Ctr 1960; **Fellow:** Cardiovascular Disease, St Luke's-Roosevelt Hosp Ctr 1961; Nuclear Medicine, Univ California-Donner Lab 1971; **Fac Appt:** Prof Med, Columbia P&S

Sanger, Joseph J MD (NuM) - **Spec Exp:** Nuclear Cardiology; **Hospital:** NYU Med Ctr (page 102); **Address:** NYU Medical Ctr, 545 1st Ave, rm SC2-184, New York, NY 10016-6402; **Phone:** 212-263-3434; **Board Cert:** Nuclear Medicine 1981; **Med School:** NYU Sch Med 1977; **Resid:** Radiology, NYU Med Ctr 1979; **Fellow:** Nuclear Medicine, NYU Med Ctr 1981; **Fac Appt:** Assoc Clin Prof Rad, NYU Sch Med

Scharf, Stephen MD (NuM) - **Spec Exp:** Thyroid & Parathyroid Imaging; Kidney Imaging; Bone Imaging; **Hospital:** Lenox Hill Hosp (page 94); **Address:** Lenox Hill Hospital, Dept Nuclear Medicine, 100 E 77th St Fl 3, New York, NY 10021-1803; **Phone:** 212-434-2630; **Board Cert:** Internal Medicine 1977; Nuclear Medicine 1979; **Med School:** Albert Einstein Coll Med 1974; **Resid:** Internal Medicine, Bronx Municipal Hosp 1976; Nuclear Medicine, Albert Einstein 1978; **Fellow:** Nephrology, Albert Einstein 1979; **Fac Appt:** Asst Clin Prof NuM, Albert Einstein Coll Med

Strauss, H William MD (NuM) - **Spec Exp:** Cardiac Imaging in Cancer Therapy; Thyroid Disorders; **Hospital:** Meml Sloan Kettering Cancer Ctr (page 109); **Address:** Meml Sloan Kettering Cancer Ctr, 1275 York Ave, S-212, Box 77, Nw York, NY 10021; **Phone:** 212-639-7238; **Board Cert:** Nuclear Medicine 1972; **Med School:** SUNY Downstate 1965; **Resid:** Internal Medicine, Downstate Med Ctr 1967; Internal Medicine, Bellevue Hosp 1968; **Fellow:** Nuclear Medicine, Johns Hopkins Hosp 1970; **Fac Appt:** Prof Rad, Cornell Univ-Weill Med Coll

Van Heertum, Ronald L MD (NuM) - **Spec Exp:** PET Imaging; PET Imaging in Alzheimer's Disease; **Hospital:** NY-Presby Hosp (page 100); **Address:** NY Presby Hosp, Dept Radiology, 622 W 168th St, Ste HP 3-320, New York, NY 10032; **Phone:** 212-305-7132; **Board Cert:** Radiology 1971; Nuclear Medicine 1973; **Med School:** UMDNJ-NJ Med Sch, Newark 1966; **Resid:** Radiology, St Vincents Hosp 1970; **Fellow:** Radiology, St Vincents Hosp Med Ctr 1971; Nuclear Medicine, SUNY-Upstate Med Ctr 1975; **Fac Appt:** Prof Rad, Columbia P&S

OBSTETRICS & GYNECOLOGY

Allen, Machelle MD (ObG) - **Spec Exp:** AIDS/HIV; Substance Abuse; **Hospital:** Bellevue Hosp Ctr, NYU Med Ctr (page 102); **Address:** 530 1st Ave, Ste 7N, New York, NY 10016-6402; **Phone:** 212-263-7021; **Board Cert:** Obstetrics & Gynecology 1991; **Med School:** UCSF 1975; **Resid:** Radiology, UCSF Med Ctr 1977; Obstetrics & Gynecology, Albert Einstein-Bronx Muni Hosp 1981; **Fellow:** Maternal & Fetal Medicine, Columbia-Presby Med Ctr 1984; **Fac Appt:** Asst Prof ObG, NYU Sch Med

Antoine, Clarel MD (ObG) PCP - **Spec Exp:** Pregnancy-High Risk; Miscarriage-Recurrent; **Hospital:** NYU Med Ctr (page 102), Bellevue Hosp Ctr; **Address:** 530 1st Ave, Ste 10Q, New York, NY 10016; **Phone:** 212-263-6541; **Board Cert:** Obstetrics & Gynecology 1982; Maternal & Fetal Medicine 1983; **Med School:** Columbia P&S 1975; **Resid:** Obstetrics & Gynecology, Columbia-Presby Hosp 1979; **Fellow:** Maternal & Fetal Medicine, NYU Med Ctr 1981; **Fac Appt:** Prof ObG, NYU Sch Med

Bacall, Charles MD (ObG) - **Hospital:** Mount Sinai Med Ctr (page 98); **Address:** 1150 5th Ave, Ste 1B, New York, NY 10128-2920; **Phone:** 212-996-9100; **Board Cert:** Obstetrics & Gynecology 1981; **Med School:** NY Med Coll 1975; **Resid:** Obstetrics & Gynecology, Mt Sinai Hosp 1979; **Fac Appt:** Asst Clin Prof ObG, Mount Sinai Sch Med

Baxi, Laxmi Vibhakar MD (ObG) - **Spec Exp:** Pregnancy-High Risk; Miscarriage-Recurrent; Multiple Gestation; **Hospital:** NY-Presby Hosp (page 100); **Address:** Columbia Presby Med Ctr, Dept OB/GYN, 161 Ft Washington Ave Fl 3 - Ste 408, New York, NY 10032-3713; **Phone:** 212-305-5899; **Board Cert:** Obstetrics & Gynecology 1995; Maternal & Fetal Medicine 1995; **Med School:** India 1972; **Resid:** Obstetrics & Gynecology, King Edward M. Hosp 1969; Obstetrics & Gynecology, St Peter's Med Ctr-Rutgers Univ NJ 1977; **Fellow:** Maternal & Fetal Medicine, Columbia-Presby Med Ctr 1979; **Fac Appt:** Prof ObG, Columbia P&S

Obstetrics & Gynecology

Berman, Alvin MD (ObG) - **Spec Exp:** Menopause Problems; Osteoporosis; **Hospital:** Mount Sinai Med Ctr (page 98); **Address:** 111B E 88th St, New York, NY 10128; **Phone:** 212-722-5757; **Board Cert:** Obstetrics & Gynecology 1978; **Med School:** South Africa 1969; **Resid:** Obstetrics & Gynecology, Mount Sinai Hosp 1976; **Fellow:** Neonatal-Perinatal Medicine, Mount Sinai Hosp 1977; **Fac Appt:** Asst Clin Prof ObG, Mount Sinai Sch Med

Blanco, Jody MD (ObG) - **Spec Exp:** Uro-Gynecology; Uterine Fibroids; Colposcopy; **Hospital:** NY-Presby Hosp (page 100); **Address:** 161 Fort Washington Ave, rm 447, Herbert Irving Pavilion, New York, NY 10032-3713; **Phone:** 212-305-1107; **Board Cert:** Obstetrics & Gynecology 1998; **Med School:** SUNY Hlth Sci Ctr 1981; **Resid:** Obstetrics & Gynecology, Columbia-Presby Med Ctr 1985; **Fellow:** Uro-Gynecology, UC Irvine 1986; **Fac Appt:** Asst Clin Prof ObG, Columbia P&S

Brodman, Michael MD (ObG) - **Spec Exp:** Incontinence-Female; Laparoscopic Surgery; Pelvic Organ Prolapse Repair; **Hospital:** Mount Sinai Med Ctr (page 98); **Address:** Dept of Obstetrics & Gynecology, 1176 Fifth Ave Fl 9, Box 1170, New York, NY 10029; **Phone:** 212-241-7952; **Board Cert:** Obstetrics & Gynecology 2004; **Med School:** Mount Sinai Sch Med 1982; **Resid:** Obstetrics & Gynecology, Mount Sinai Hosp 1986; **Fellow:** Pelvic Surgery, Mount Sinai Hosp 1987; **Fac Appt:** Assoc Prof ObG, Mount Sinai Sch Med

Brustman, Lois MD (ObG) - **Spec Exp:** Prematurity/Low Birth Weight Infants; Diabetes in Pregnancy; Preconception Planning; Maternal & Fetal Medicine; **Hospital:** St Luke's - Roosevelt Hosp Ctr - Roosevelt Div (page 90); **Address:** 1000 Tenth Ave, Ste 11A61, New York, NY 10019-1147; **Phone:** 212-523-7579; **Board Cert:** Obstetrics & Gynecology 1996; Maternal & Fetal Medicine 1996; **Med School:** NY Med Coll 1979; **Resid:** Obstetrics & Gynecology, Montefiore Med Ctr 1984; **Fellow:** Maternal & Fetal Medicine, Montefiore Med Ctr 1988; **Fac Appt:** Assoc Prof ObG, NY Med Coll

Buchman, Myron MD (ObG) - **Spec Exp:** Gynecology Only; **Hospital:** NY-Presby Hosp (page 100), Lenox Hill Hosp (page 94); **Address:** 117 E 72nd St, New York, NY 10021-4249; **Phone:** 212-861-1950; **Board Cert:** Obstetrics & Gynecology 2004; **Med School:** Johns Hopkins Univ 1946; **Resid:** Obstetrics & Gynecology, Johns Hopkins Hosp 1947; Obstetrics & Gynecology, New York Lying-In Hosp 1952; **Fac Appt:** Assoc Clin Prof ObG, Cornell Univ-Weill Med Coll

Cherry, Sheldon MD (ObG) - **Spec Exp:** Menopause Problems; Pregnancy-High Risk; Infertility; Cancer Prevention; **Hospital:** Mount Sinai Med Ctr (page 98); **Address:** 1160 Park Ave, New York, NY 10128-1212; **Phone:** 212-860-2600; **Board Cert:** Obstetrics & Gynecology 1981; **Med School:** Columbia P&S 1958; **Resid:** Obstetrics & Gynecology, Columbia-Presby Hosp 1962; **Fac Appt:** Clin Prof ObG, Mount Sinai Sch Med

Chin, Jean MD (ObG) PCP - **Spec Exp:** Menopause Problems; **Hospital:** Mount Sinai Med Ctr (page 98); **Address:** 785 Park Ave, New York, NY 10021; **Phone:** 212-249-7800; **Board Cert:** Obstetrics & Gynecology 1982; **Med School:** Columbia P&S 1976; **Resid:** Obstetrics & Gynecology, Mt Sinai Hosp 1980; **Fac Appt:** Asst Clin Prof ObG, Columbia P&S

Coady, Deborah MD (ObG) - **Spec Exp:** Minimally Invasive Surgery; Vulvar Disease; Pain-Pelvic; Menopause Problems; **Hospital:** NYU Med Ctr (page 102), St Vincent Cath Med Ctrs - Manhattan (page 375); **Address:** 430 West Broadway Fl 2, New York, NY 10012; **Phone:** 212-941-0011; **Board Cert:** Obstetrics & Gynecology 1996; **Med School:** Mount Sinai Sch Med 1980; **Resid:** Obstetrics & Gynecology, NYU-Bellevue Hosp 1984; **Fac Appt:** Asst Clin Prof ObG, NYU Sch Med

Corio, Laura E MD (ObG) **PCP** - **Spec Exp:** Pregnancy-High Risk; Menopause Problems; HPV-Human Papillomavirus; Hysteroscopic Surgery; **Hospital:** Mount Sinai Med Ctr (page 98), NYU Med Ctr (page 102); **Address:** 113 E 64th St, New York, NY 10021; **Phone:** 646-422-0730; **Board Cert:** Obstetrics & Gynecology 1984; **Med School:** UMDNJ-NJ Med Sch, Newark 1978; **Resid:** Obstetrics & Gynecology, Mount Sinai Med Ctr 1982; **Fac Appt:** Clin Prof ObG, Mount Sinai Sch Med

Cox, Kathryn MD (ObG) - **Spec Exp:** Pregnancy After Age 35; Menopause Problems; Gynecologic Surgery; **Hospital:** NY-Presby Hosp (page 100); **Address:** 116 E 66th St, Ste IB, New York, NY 10021; **Phone:** 212-535-2600; **Board Cert:** Obstetrics & Gynecology 1981; **Med School:** Univ Mich Med Sch 1975; **Resid:** Obstetrics & Gynecology, New York Hosp/Cornell 1979

Debrovner, Charles MD (ObG) - **Spec Exp:** Menopause Problems; Infertility; **Hospital:** NYU Med Ctr (page 102), St Luke's - Roosevelt Hosp Ctr - Roosevelt Div (page 90); **Address:** 338 E 30th St, New York, NY 10016; **Phone:** 212-683-0090; **Board Cert:** Obstetrics & Gynecology 1967; **Med School:** NYU Sch Med 1960; **Resid:** Obstetrics & Gynecology, Bellevue Hosp 1965; **Fac Appt:** Clin Prof ObG, NYU Sch Med

Degann, Sona MD (ObG) **PCP** - **Spec Exp:** Gynecologic Surgery; Obstetrics; **Hospital:** NY-Presby Hosp (page 100); **Address:** 408 E 76th St, New York, NY 10021; **Phone:** 212-249-0900; **Board Cert:** Obstetrics & Gynecology 2000; **Med School:** Johns Hopkins Univ 1983; **Resid:** Obstetrics & Gynecology, NY Hosp 1987

Diamond, Sharon MD (ObG) - **Spec Exp:** Menopause Problems; Pap Smear Abnormalities; Gynecology Only; **Hospital:** Mount Sinai Med Ctr (page 98); **Address:** 61 E 86th St, Ste 1, New York, NY 10028-1003; **Phone:** 212-876-2200; **Board Cert:** Obstetrics & Gynecology 2000; **Med School:** Mount Sinai Sch Med 1979; **Resid:** Obstetrics & Gynecology, Mount Sinai Med Ctr 1983; **Fac Appt:** Asst Clin Prof ObG, Mount Sinai Sch Med

Divon, Michael Y MD (ObG) - **Spec Exp:** Maternal & Fetal Medicine; Pregnancy-High Risk; Ultrasound; **Hospital:** Lenox Hill Hosp (page 94); **Address:** 130 E 77th St Fl 2 Black Hall, New York, NY 10021-1851; **Phone:** 212-434-2160; **Board Cert:** Obstetrics & Gynecology 2003; **Med School:** Israel 1979; **Resid:** Obstetrics & Gynecology, Rambam Med Ctr 1983; **Fellow:** Perinatal Medicine, USC 1985; Perinatal Medicine, Albert Einstein 1989; **Fac Appt:** Clin Prof ObG, Albert Einstein Coll Med

Evans, Mark I MD (ObG) - **Spec Exp:** Prenatal Diagnosis; Multiple Gestation; Fetal Therapy; Reproductive Genetics; **Hospital:** Mount Sinai Med Ctr (page 98); **Address:** Comprehensive Genetics, 131 E 65th St, New York, NY 10021; **Phone:** 212-744-2590; **Board Cert:** Obstetrics & Gynecology 2005; Clinical Genetics 1984; **Med School:** SUNY Downstate 1978; **Resid:** Obstetrics & Gynecology, Lying-In Hosp 1982; **Fellow:** Clinical Genetics, Natl Inst Hlth 1984; **Fac Appt:** Prof ObG, Mount Sinai Sch Med

Friedman, Lynn MD (ObG) **PCP** - **Spec Exp:** Miscarriage; Infertility; Pregnancy After Age 35; **Hospital:** Mount Sinai Med Ctr (page 98), Lenox Hill Hosp (page 94); **Address:** 885 Park Ave, Ste 1-D, New York, NY 10021-0325; **Phone:** 212-737-3282; **Board Cert:** Obstetrics & Gynecology 1998; **Med School:** NYU Sch Med 1984; **Resid:** Obstetrics & Gynecology, Mount Sinai Med Ctr 1988; **Fac Appt:** Asst Clin Prof ObG, Mount Sinai Sch Med

Friedman, Ricky MD (ObG) **PCP** - **Spec Exp:** Women's Health; Pap Smear Abnormalities; **Hospital:** Mount Sinai Med Ctr (page 98); **Address:** 47 E 88th St. 1st Fl, New York, NY 10128-1152; **Phone:** 212-534-0200; **Board Cert:** Obstetrics & Gynecology 2000; **Med School:** SUNY Hlth Sci Ctr 1985; **Resid:** Obstetrics & Gynecology, Mount Sinai Hosp 1989; **Fac Appt:** Assoc Clin Prof ObG, Mount Sinai Sch Med

Goldman, Gary MD (ObG) `PCP` - **Spec Exp:** Endometriosis; Laparoscopic Surgery-Complex; Hysterectomy Alternatives; **Hospital:** NY-Presby Hosp (page 100); **Address:** 58 E 66th St, New York, NY 10021-6528; **Phone:** 212-535-6100; **Board Cert:** Obstetrics & Gynecology 2003; **Med School:** SUNY Stony Brook 1986; **Resid:** Obstetrics & Gynecology, New York Hosp 1990; **Fac Appt:** Asst Clin Prof ObG, Cornell Univ-Weill Med Coll

Goldstein, Martin MD (ObG) - **Spec Exp:** Incontinence; Laparoscopic Surgery; Uterine Fibroids; Pelvic Organ Prolapse Repair; **Hospital:** Mount Sinai Med Ctr (page 98); **Address:** 40 E 84th St, New York, NY 10128-1314; **Phone:** 212-472-6500; **Board Cert:** Obstetrics & Gynecology 1980; **Med School:** SUNY Hlth Sci Ctr 1966; **Resid:** Obstetrics & Gynecology, Mount Sinai Hosp 1971; **Fac Appt:** Assoc Clin Prof ObG, Mount Sinai Sch Med

Goldstein, Steven R MD (ObG) - **Spec Exp:** Gynecologic Ultrasound; Menopause Problems; Uterine Fibroids; **Hospital:** NYU Med Ctr (page 102); **Address:** 530 1st Avenue Ste 10N, New York, NY 10016-6402; **Phone:** 212-263-7416; **Board Cert:** Obstetrics & Gynecology 2005; **Med School:** NYU Sch Med 1975; **Resid:** Obstetrics & Gynecology, NYU Affil Hospitals 1980; **Fac Appt:** Prof ObG, NYU Sch Med

Gruss, Leslie MD (ObG) `PCP` - **Hospital:** NYU Med Ctr (page 102); **Address:** 568 Broadway, Ste 304, New York, NY 10012; **Phone:** 212-966-7600; **Board Cert:** Obstetrics & Gynecology 2003; **Med School:** Med Coll PA Hahnemann 1983; **Resid:** Obstetrics & Gynecology, Montefiore Hosp Med Ctr 1987

Hirsch, Lissa MD (ObG) - **Spec Exp:** Menopause Problems; **Hospital:** Lenox Hill Hosp (page 94); **Address:** 755 Park Ave, New York, NY 10021-4255; **Phone:** 212-570-2222; **Board Cert:** Obstetrics & Gynecology 1985; **Med School:** UMDNJ-NJ Med Sch, Newark 1979; **Resid:** Obstetrics & Gynecology, NYU Med Ctr 1983

Holland, Claudia MD (ObG) `PCP` - **Hospital:** St Luke's - Roosevelt Hosp Ctr - Roosevelt Div (page 90); **Address:** 800A 5th Ave, Ste 503, New York, NY 10021; **Phone:** 212-230-1760; **Board Cert:** Obstetrics & Gynecology 1998; **Med School:** Mount Sinai Sch Med 1981; **Resid:** Obstetrics & Gynecology, NYU Med Ctr 1985

Hutcherson, Hilda Y MD (ObG) - **Spec Exp:** Pediatric & Adolescent Gynecology; Sexual Dysfunction; **Hospital:** NY-Presby Hosp (page 100); **Address:** 161 Fort Washington Ave, New York, NY 10032-3713; **Phone:** 212-305-1107; **Board Cert:** Obstetrics & Gynecology 1999; **Med School:** Harvard Med Sch 1980; **Resid:** Internal Medicine, UCSF Med Ctr 1981; Obstetrics & Gynecology, Columbia Presbyterian Hosp 1985; **Fac Appt:** Asst Prof ObG, Columbia P&S

James, David F MD (ObG) `PCP` - **Spec Exp:** Menopause Problems; Women's Health; **Hospital:** Lenox Hill Hosp (page 94), NY-Presby Hosp (page 100); **Address:** 45 E 85th St, New York, NY 10028-0957; **Phone:** 212-535-4611; **Board Cert:** Obstetrics & Gynecology 2003; **Med School:** Scotland 1964; **Resid:** Obstetrics & Gynecology, Lenox Hill Hosp 1969; **Fac Appt:** Asst Clin Prof ObG, Cornell Univ-Weill Med Coll

Kaminsky, Sari J MD (ObG) `PCP` - **Hospital:** Metropolitan Hosp Ctr - NY, Westchester Med Ctr (page 713); **Address:** Metropolitan Hospital, 1901 First Ave, rm 4B5, New York, NY 10029; **Phone:** 212-423-6796; **Board Cert:** Obstetrics & Gynecology 1977; **Med School:** SUNY Hlth Sci Ctr 1971; **Resid:** Obstetrics & Gynecology, Univ Hosp 1975; **Fac Appt:** Assoc Prof ObG, NY Med Coll

Kent, Joan MD (ObG) - **Hospital:** NY-Presby Hosp (page 100); **Address:** 235 E 67th St, rm 204, New York, NY 10021; **Phone:** 212-772-2900; **Board Cert:** Obstetrics & Gynecology 2004; **Med School:** Cornell Univ-Weill Med Coll 1984; **Resid:** Obstetrics & Gynecology, NY Hosp 1988; **Fac Appt:** Assoc Prof ObG, Cornell Univ-Weill Med Coll

Kessler, Alan MD (ObG) - **Spec Exp:** Multiple Gestation; Pregnancy-High Risk; **Hospital:** NY-Presby Hosp (page 100); **Address:** 523 East 72nd St Fl 9, New York, NY 10021-4099; **Phone:** 212-472-5340; **Board Cert:** Obstetrics & Gynecology 1985; **Med School:** Mexico 1978; **Resid:** Obstetrics & Gynecology, NY Hosp 1983; **Fac Appt:** Assoc Prof ObG, Cornell Univ-Weill Med Coll

Kim, Joyce M MD (ObG) PCP - **Spec Exp:** Pregnancy-High Risk; **Hospital:** Mount Sinai Med Ctr (page 98); **Address:** 885 Park Ave, New York, NY 10021; **Phone:** 212-737-3282; **Board Cert:** Obstetrics & Gynecology 2000; **Med School:** Mount Sinai Sch Med 1986; **Resid:** Obstetrics & Gynecology, Mount Sinai Hosp 1990

Krause, Cynthia MD (ObG) PCP - **Spec Exp:** Menopause Problems; Pap Smear Abnormalities; HPV-Human Papillomavirus; Adolescent Gynecology; **Hospital:** Mount Sinai Med Ctr (page 98); **Address:** 1185 Park Ave, Ste 1L, New York, NY 10128; **Phone:** 212-369-0602; **Board Cert:** Obstetrics & Gynecology 2003; **Med School:** Duke Univ 1980; **Resid:** Internal Medicine, Baltimore City Hosp 1982; Obstetrics & Gynecology, Mount Sinai Med Ctr 1986; **Fac Appt:** Asst Prof ObG, Mount Sinai Sch Med

Levine, Richard U MD (ObG) - **Spec Exp:** Uterine Fibroids; Gynecologic Surgery; HPV-Human Papillomavirus; **Hospital:** NY-Presby Hosp (page 100); **Address:** 161 Ft Washington Ave, Ste 436, New York, NY 10032; **Phone:** 212-305-5300; **Board Cert:** Obstetrics & Gynecology 1994; **Med School:** Cornell Univ-Weill Med Coll 1966; **Resid:** Obstetrics & Gynecology, Columbia-Presby Med Ctr 1975; **Fellow:** Obstetrics & Gynecology, Karolinska Inst 1970; **Fac Appt:** Prof ObG, Columbia P&S

Lieberman, Beth MD (ObG) PCP - **Spec Exp:** Menopause Problems; Osteoporosis; Exercise Physiology; **Hospital:** NYU Med Ctr (page 102), Bellevue Hosp Ctr; **Address:** 333 E 30th St, New York, NY 10016; **Phone:** 212-689-4468; **Board Cert:** Obstetrics & Gynecology 1980; **Med School:** NYU Sch Med 1973; **Resid:** Obstetrics & Gynecology, Bellevue Hosp 1977; **Fac Appt:** Asst Clin Prof ObG, NYU Sch Med

Lustig, Ilana MD (ObG) - **Spec Exp:** Pregnancy-High Risk; **Hospital:** NYU Med Ctr (page 102); **Address:** 233 E 31st St, New York, NY 10016-6302; **Phone:** 212-696-9536; **Board Cert:** Obstetrics & Gynecology 1984; Maternal & Fetal Medicine 1989; **Med School:** Geo Wash Univ 1977; **Resid:** Obstetrics & Gynecology, Yale-New Haven 1981; **Fellow:** Maternal & Fetal Medicine, Bellevue Hosp 1983; **Fac Appt:** Assoc Prof ObG, NYU Sch Med

Maggio, John DO (ObG) - **Spec Exp:** Pelvic Reconstruction; Uro-Gynecology; **Hospital:** St Vincent Cath Med Ctrs - Manhattan (page 375), St. Vincent's Midtown; **Address:** 275 E 8th Ave, New York, NY 10011; **Phone:** 212-620-5415; **Board Cert:** Obstetrics & Gynecology 1978; **Med School:** Chicago Coll Osteo Med 1968; **Resid:** Obstetrics & Gynecology, St Clare's Hosp 1974; **Fac Appt:** Assoc Clin Prof ObG, NY Med Coll

Maidman, Jack MD (ObG) PCP - **Spec Exp:** Maternal & Fetal Medicine; Genetic Disorders; Pregnancy-High Risk; **Hospital:** NY-Presby Hosp (page 100); **Address:** 16 E 60th St, Ste 480, New York, NY 10032; **Phone:** 212-326-8951; **Board Cert:** Obstetrics & Gynecology 1970; Maternal & Fetal Medicine 1977; Clinical Genetics 1982; **Med School:** UCSF 1962; **Resid:** Obstetrics & Gynecology, Kings Co Hosp 1968; **Fellow:** Gynecologic Oncology, Kings Co Hosp 1969; Clinical Genetics, Hosp Univ Penn 1970; **Fac Appt:** Assoc Clin Prof ObG, Columbia P&S

McGill, Frances MD (ObG) - **Spec Exp:** Menopause Problems; Women's Health; **Hospital:** St Vincent Cath Med Ctrs - Manhattan (page 375), Beth Israel Med Ctr - Petrie Division (page 90); **Address:** 629 Park Ave, New York, NY 10021; **Phone:** 646-259-0995; **Board Cert:** Obstetrics & Gynecology 1997; **Med School:** Grenada 1981; **Resid:** Obstetrics & Gynecology, Women & Infants Hosp 1985; **Fac Appt:** Assoc Clin Prof ObG, NY Med Coll

Melnick, Hugh MD (ObG) - **Spec Exp:** Infertility-IVF; Infertility-Male; **Hospital:** Lenox Hill Hosp (page 94); **Address:** 1625 3rd Ave, New York, NY 10128-3603; **Phone:** 212-369-8700; **Board Cert:** Obstetrics & Gynecology 1976; **Med School:** Temple Univ 1972; **Resid:** Obstetrics & Gynecology, Lenox Hill Hosp 1976; **Fellow:** Immunology, Univ Birmingham 1969

Moss, Richard MD (ObG) - **Spec Exp:** Colposcopy; Bone Densitometry; Menopause Problems; **Hospital:** Mount Sinai Med Ctr (page 98); **Address:** 1160 Park Ave, New York, NY 10128-1212; **Phone:** 212-860-2600; **Board Cert:** Obstetrics & Gynecology 1979; **Med School:** SUNY Hlth Sci Ctr 1957; **Resid:** Obstetrics & Gynecology, Mount Sinai Hosp 1962; **Fac Appt:** Asst Clin Prof ObG, Mount Sinai Sch Med

Naftolin, Frederick MD/PhD (ObG) - **Spec Exp:** Neuroendocrinology; Reproductive Endocrinology; Menopause Problems; **Hospital:** NYU Med Ctr (page 102); **Address:** NYU Sch of Med, Dept OB/GYN, 550 1st Ave, H528, New York, NY 10016; **Phone:** 203-298-9315; **Board Cert:** Obstetrics & Gynecology 1972; **Med School:** UCSF 1961; **Resid:** Obstetrics & Gynecology, UCLA Med Ctr 1966; **Fellow:** Reproductive Endocrinology, Univ Wash 1968; Neurological Endocrinology, Oxford Univ 1970; **Fac Appt:** Prof ObG, NYU Sch Med

Ordorica, Steven A MD (ObG) - **Spec Exp:** Pregnancy-High Risk; Miscarriage-Recurrent; Maternal & Fetal Medicine; **Hospital:** NYU Med Ctr (page 102); **Address:** NYU Medical Ctr, 530 1st Ave, Ste 10Q, New York, NY 10016-6402; **Phone:** 212-263-5982; **Board Cert:** Obstetrics & Gynecology 2004; Maternal & Fetal Medicine 2004; **Med School:** SUNY Hlth Sci Ctr 1983; **Resid:** Obstetrics & Gynecology, NYU Med Ctr 1987; **Fellow:** Maternal & Fetal Medicine, NYU Med Ctr 1989; **Fac Appt:** Assoc Prof ObG, NYU Sch Med

Panter, Gideon MD (ObG) - **Spec Exp:** Vaginal Surgery; Infertility; Pregnancy-High Risk; **Hospital:** NY-Presby Hosp (page 100); **Address:** 1060 5th Ave, Ste 1B, New York, NY 10021-5954; **Phone:** 212-737-7727; **Board Cert:** Obstetrics & Gynecology 1967; **Med School:** Cornell Univ-Weill Med Coll 1960; **Resid:** Obstetrics & Gynecology, Columbia Presby Med Ctr 1965; **Fac Appt:** Assoc Clin Prof ObG, Cornell Univ-Weill Med Coll

Pascario, Ben MD (ObG) **PCP** - **Spec Exp:** Uterine Fibroids; Laparoscopic Surgery; **Hospital:** Lenox Hill Hosp (page 94), St Luke's - Roosevelt Hosp Ctr - St Luke's Hosp (page 90); **Address:** 8 E 83rd St, New York, NY 10028-0418; **Phone:** 212-628-2400; **Board Cert:** Obstetrics & Gynecology 1977; **Med School:** Romania 1961; **Resid:** Obstetrics & Gynecology, St Luke's Hosp 1975; **Fac Appt:** Asst Prof ObG, Columbia P&S

Post, Robert MD (ObG) **PCP** - **Spec Exp:** Gynecologic Surgery-Benign; **Hospital:** NY-Presby Hosp (page 100); **Address:** 525 E 68th St, rm J130, New York, NY 10021; **Phone:** 212-746-2885; **Board Cert:** Obstetrics & Gynecology 1980; **Med School:** Univ Louisville Sch Med 1958; **Resid:** Obstetrics & Gynecology, Bellevue Hosp 1963; **Fac Appt:** Clin Prof ObG, Cornell Univ-Weill Med Coll

Rehnstrom, Jaana MD (ObG) - **Spec Exp:** Colposcopy; **Hospital:** St Luke's - Roosevelt Hosp Ctr - Roosevelt Div (page 90); **Address:** 103 5th Ave, Fl 3, New York, NY 10003-1009; **Phone:** 212-366-4765; **Board Cert:** Obstetrics & Gynecology 2002; **Med School:** Finland 1979; **Resid:** Obstetrics & Gynecology, St Luke's Hosp 1986

Reiss, Ronald J MD (ObG) **PCP** - **Spec Exp:** Laparoscopic Surgery; Pregnancy-High Risk; Colposcopy; Infertility; **Hospital:** Lenox Hill Hosp (page 94), Greenwich Hosp; **Address:** 124 E 84th St, New York, NY 10028; **Phone:** 212-749-3113; **Board Cert:** Obstetrics & Gynecology 1983; **Med School:** Belgium 1976; **Resid:** Obstetrics & Gynecology, St Luke's-Woman's Hosp 1980

Rodke, Gae MD (ObG) **PCP** - **Spec Exp:** Vulvar Disease; Gynecologic Surgery; **Hospital:** St Luke's - Roosevelt Hosp Ctr - Roosevelt Div (page 90); **Address:** 185 West End Ave, Ste 1D, New York, NY 10023-2005; **Phone:** 212-496-9800; **Board Cert:** Obstetrics & Gynecology 1998; **Med School:** Albert Einstein Coll Med 1981; **Resid:** Family Medicine, Univ Hosp 1982; Obstetrics & Gynecology, Univ Hosp 1986; **Fac Appt:** Asst Clin Prof ObG, Columbia P&S

Rothbard, Malcolm MD (ObG) - **Hospital:** Lenox Hill Hosp (page 94); **Address:** 108 E 66th St, Ste 1B, New York, NY 10021-6543; **Phone:** 212-861-2629; **Board Cert:** Obstetrics & Gynecology 1972; **Med School:** SUNY Downstate 1965; **Resid:** Obstetrics & Gynecology, Kingsbrook Jewish Med Ctr 1970; **Fellow:** Obstetrics & Gynecology, Metropolitan Hosp Ctr 1970

Sadarangani, Balvinder MD (ObG) - **Spec Exp:** Gynecology Only; Minimally Invasive Surgery; **Hospital:** Cabrini Med Ctr (page 374), St Vincent Cath Med Ctrs - Manhattan (page 375); **Address:** 247 3rd Ave, Ste 503, New York, NY 10010; **Phone:** 212-982-4100; **Board Cert:** Obstetrics & Gynecology 1980; **Med School:** India 1968; **Resid:** Obstetrics & Gynecology, St Vincent's Hosp & Med Ctr 1978

Sailon, Peter MD (ObG) - **Spec Exp:** Hysteroscopic Surgery; Laparoscopic Surgery; **Hospital:** Lenox Hill Hosp (page 94); **Address:** 955 Park Ave, New York, NY 10028-0321; **Phone:** 212-879-9191; **Board Cert:** Obstetrics & Gynecology 1982; **Med School:** Italy 1976; **Resid:** Surgery, Univ Hosp Downstate 1977; Obstetrics & Gynecology, St Luke's-Roosevelt Hosp Ctr 1980; **Fellow:** Reproductive Endocrinology, St Luke's-Roosevelt Hosp Ctr 1981

Sandler, Benjamin MD (ObG) - **Spec Exp:** Infertility-IVF; Reproductive Surgery; **Hospital:** Mount Sinai Med Ctr (page 98); **Address:** 635 Madison Ave Fl 10, New York, NY 10022-1009; **Phone:** 212-756-5777; **Board Cert:** Obstetrics & Gynecology 2004; **Med School:** Mexico 1982; **Resid:** Obstetrics & Gynecology, Michael Reese Hosp 1987; **Fellow:** Reproductive Endocrinology, Mount Sinai Hosp 1989; **Fac Appt:** Asst Clin Prof ObG, Mount Sinai Sch Med

Sassoon, Robert I MD (ObG) - **Spec Exp:** Laparoscopic Surgery; Pregnancy-High Risk; Gynecologic Surgery; **Hospital:** NY-Presby Hosp (page 100); **Address:** 449 E 68th St, New York, NY 10021; **Phone:** 212-628-1500; **Board Cert:** Obstetrics & Gynecology 1998; **Med School:** Cornell Univ-Weill Med Coll 1981; **Resid:** Obstetrics & Gynecology, New York Hosp 1985; **Fac Appt:** Clin Prof ObG, Cornell Univ-Weill Med Coll

Scher, Jonathan MD (ObG) - **Spec Exp:** Miscarriage-Recurrent; Pregnancy-High Risk; Infertility-IVF; **Hospital:** Mount Sinai Med Ctr (page 98); **Address:** 1126 Park Ave, New York, NY 10128-1203; **Phone:** 212-427-7400; **Board Cert:** Obstetrics & Gynecology 1981; **Med School:** South Africa 1964; **Resid:** Obstetrics & Gynecology, Groote Schuur Hosp 1970; Obstetrics & Gynecology, Kings College Hosp 1972; **Fac Appt:** Asst Clin Prof ObG, Mount Sinai Sch Med

Schwartz, Judith W MD (ObG) - **Spec Exp:** Gynecologic Surgery; Menopause Problems; **Hospital:** Mount Sinai Med Ctr (page 98); **Address:** 45 E 82nd St Fl 1, New York, NY 10028; **Phone:** 212-879-5959; **Board Cert:** Obstetrics & Gynecology 1998; **Med School:** Mount Sinai Sch Med 1982; **Resid:** Obstetrics & Gynecology, Mount Sinai Hosp 1986; **Fac Appt:** Asst Clin Prof ObG, Mount Sinai Sch Med

Segarra, Pedro R MD (ObG) - **Spec Exp:** Pelvic Organ Prolapse Repair; Incontinence; Gynecologic Surgery; **Hospital:** Lenox Hill Hosp (page 94); **Address:** 1430 2nd Ave, Ste 101, New York, NY 10021; **Phone:** 212-737-0641; **Board Cert:** Obstetrics & Gynecology 2003; **Med School:** NY Med Coll 1983; **Resid:** Obstetrics & Gynecology, Westchester Co Med Ctr 1988

Seiler, Jerome MD (ObG) - **Spec Exp:** Incontinence; Hysteroscopic Surgery; Gynecologic Cancer; **Hospital:** NY-Presby Hosp (page 100); **Address:** 525 E 68th St, Ste J130, New York, NY 10021-6310; **Phone:** 212-746-2885; **Board Cert:** Obstetrics & Gynecology 1991; **Med School:** Univ Hlth Sci/Chicago Med Sch 1964; **Resid:** Obstetrics & Gynecology, Bellevue Hosp 1969; **Fac Appt:** Assoc Clin Prof ObG, Cornell Univ-Weill Med Coll

Sloan, Don MD (ObG) - **Spec Exp:** Psychosomatic Ob/Gyn; Marital Counseling; **Hospital:** Lenox Hill Hosp (page 94), St Barnabas Hosp - Bronx; **Address:** 10 Mitchell Pl, Ste 2-F, New York, NY 10017-1801; **Phone:** 212-371-4482; **Board Cert:** Obstetrics & Gynecology 1981; **Med School:** SUNY Downstate 1963; **Resid:** Obstetrics & Gynecology, Temple Univ Hosp 1967; **Fellow:** Human Sexuality, Masters & Johnson 1973; **Fac Appt:** Assoc Prof ObG, NY Med Coll

Smilen, Scott MD (ObG) - **Spec Exp:** Incontinence; Pelvic Prolapse Repair; Minimally Invasive Surgery; **Hospital:** NYU Med Ctr (page 102); **Address:** NYU Med Ctr, Urogyn, 530 1st Ave, Ste 5F, New York, NY 10016-6497; **Phone:** 212-263-0395; **Board Cert:** Obstetrics & Gynecology 1994; **Med School:** NYU Sch Med 1988; **Resid:** Obstetrics & Gynecology, NYU Med Ctr 1992; **Fellow:** Uro-Gynecology, NYU Med Ctr 1993; **Fac Appt:** Assoc Prof ObG, NYU Sch Med

Snyder, Jon R MD (ObG) - **Spec Exp:** Obstetrics; Menopause Problems; **Hospital:** NYU Med Ctr (page 102), Bellevue Hosp Ctr; **Address:** 530 1st Ave, Ste 10N, New York, NY 10016-6402; **Phone:** 212-263-6356; **Board Cert:** Obstetrics & Gynecology 1978; **Med School:** NYU Sch Med 1972; **Resid:** Obstetrics & Gynecology, Bellevue Hosp 1976; **Fac Appt:** Assoc Clin Prof ObG, NYU Sch Med

Strongin, Michael J MD (ObG) - **Spec Exp:** Gynecologic Surgery; Laparoscopic Surgery; Laser Surgery; **Hospital:** Lenox Hill Hosp (page 94), NY-Presby Hosp (page 100); **Address:** 45 E 85th St, New York, NY 10028; **Phone:** 212-535-4611; **Board Cert:** Obstetrics & Gynecology 2005; **Med School:** Boston Univ 1973; **Resid:** Obstetrics & Gynecology, New York Hosp 1977; **Fac Appt:** Asst Clin Prof ObG, Cornell Univ-Weill Med Coll

Sullum, Stanford MD (ObG) `PCP` - **Spec Exp:** Gynecology Only; **Hospital:** Mount Sinai Med Ctr (page 98); **Address:** 1136 5th Ave, New York, NY 10128-0122; **Phone:** 212-876-4630; **Board Cert:** Obstetrics & Gynecology 1979; **Med School:** Jefferson Med Coll 1973; **Resid:** Obstetrics & Gynecology, Mount Sinai Hosp 1977; **Fac Appt:** Asst Clin Prof ObG, Mount Sinai Sch Med

Van Praagh, Ian MD (ObG) - **Spec Exp:** Vulvar Disease; Colposcopy; Gynecology Only; **Hospital:** Lenox Hill Hosp (page 94), St Luke's - Roosevelt Hosp Ctr - St Luke's Hosp (page 90); **Address:** 103 E 86th St, New York, NY 10028-1058; **Phone:** 212-427-5774; **Board Cert:** Obstetrics & Gynecology 1979; **Med School:** Canada 1955; **Resid:** Obstetrics & Gynecology, Toronto Genl Hosp 1961; Surgery, Toronto Genl-Wellesley Hosp 1959; **Fellow:** Reproductive Medicine, Case Western Res Univ Hospital 1963; Pelvic Surgery, Middlesex Hosp 1963; **Fac Appt:** Asst Clin Prof ObG, Columbia P&S

Yale, Suzanne MD (ObG) - **Hospital:** Lenox Hill Hosp (page 94); **Address:** 768 Park Ave, New York, NY 10021-4114; **Phone:** 212-744-9300; **Board Cert:** Obstetrics & Gynecology 1984; **Med School:** UMDNJ-RW Johnson Med Sch 1977; **Resid:** Obstetrics & Gynecology, Lenox Hill Hosp 1981

Young, Bruce MD (ObG) - **Spec Exp:** Infertility; Minimally Invasive Surgery; Twin to Twin Transfusion Syndrome (TTTS); **Hospital:** NYU Med Ctr (page 102); **Address:** 530 1st Ave, HCC-5th Fl, Ste 5G, New York, NY 10016; **Phone:** 212-263-6359; **Board Cert:** Obstetrics & Gynecology 1970; Maternal & Fetal Medicine 1975; **Med School:** NYU Sch Med 1963; **Resid:** Obstetrics & Gynecology, New York Univ Med Ctr 1968; **Fellow:** Reproductive Endocrinology, New York Univ Med Ctr 1968; **Fac Appt:** Prof ObG, NYU Sch Med

OCCUPATIONAL MEDICINE

Brandt-Rauf, Paul W MD (OM) - **Spec Exp:** Occupational Medicine; Environmental Medicine; **Address:** Columbia Univ Sch Public Hlth, Dept Env Hlth Sci, 60 Haven Ave, Ste B1 - rm 106, New York, NY 10032-2604; **Phone:** 212-305-3464; **Board Cert:** Internal Medicine 1984; Occupational Medicine 1986; **Med School:** Columbia P&S 1979; **Resid:** Pathology, Columbia Presby Hosp 1981; Internal Medicine, Georgetown Univ Hosp 1983; **Fellow:** Occupational Medicine, Columbia Presby Hosp 1984; **Fac Appt:** Prof OM, Columbia P&S

Herbert, Robin MD (OM) - **Spec Exp:** Asbestos-related Diseases; Occupational Lung Disease; Carpal Tunnel Syndrome; Repetetive Strain Injuries; **Hospital:** Mount Sinai Med Ctr (page 98); **Address:** Mt Sinai Div Environmental/Occupational Med, PO Box 1057, New York, NY 10029; **Phone:** 212-241-9059; **Board Cert:** Internal Medicine 1985; **Med School:** SUNY Stony Brook 1982; **Resid:** Internal Medicine, Montefiore Med Ctr 1985; Occupational Medicine, Mt Sinai Med Ctr 1987; **Fellow:** Epidemiology, Mt Sinai Med Ctr 1988; **Fac Appt:** Assoc Prof PrM, Mount Sinai Sch Med

Landrigan, Philip MD (OM) - **Spec Exp:** Environmental Health in Children; **Hospital:** Mount Sinai Med Ctr (page 98); **Address:** Dept of Comm & Prev Med, One Gustave Levy Pl, Box 1057, New York, NY 10029-6500; **Phone:** 212-241-6173; **Board Cert:** Pediatrics 1973; Public Health & Genl Preventive Med 1979; Occupational Medicine 1983; **Med School:** Harvard Med Sch 1967; **Resid:** Internal Medicine, Metro Genl Hosp 1968; Pediatrics, Chldns Hosp 1970; **Fellow:** Epidemiology, Ctrs for Disease Control 1973; Occupational Medicine, Univ London 1977; **Fac Appt:** Prof Ped, Mount Sinai Sch Med

Levin, Stephen M MD (OM) - **Spec Exp:** Asbestos-related Diseases; Occupational Lung Disease; Carpal Tunnel Syndrome; Repetitive Strain Injuries; **Hospital:** Mount Sinai Med Ctr (page 98); **Address:** Mount Sinai Dept Community/Preventive Med, PO Box 1057, New York, NY 10029; **Phone:** 212-241-9059; **Board Cert:** Occupational Medicine 1984; **Med School:** NYU Sch Med ; **Resid:** Occupational Medicine, St Lukes Hosp 1981; **Fac Appt:** Assoc Prof OM, Mount Sinai Sch Med

OPHTHALMOLOGY

Abramson, David H MD (Oph) - **Spec Exp:** Eye Tumors/Cancer; Orbital Tumors/Cancer; Retinoblastoma; Melanoma-Choroidal (eye); **Hospital:** Meml Sloan Kettering Cancer Ctr (page 109); **Address:** 70 E 66th St, New York, NY 10021; **Phone:** 212-744-1700; **Board Cert:** Ophthalmology 1975; **Med School:** Albert Einstein Coll Med 1969; **Resid:** Ophthalmology, Harkness Eye Inst 1974; **Fellow:** Ocular Oncology, Columbia-Presby Med Ctr 1975; **Fac Appt:** Clin Prof Oph, Cornell Univ-Weill Med Coll

Accardi, Frank E MD (Oph) - **Spec Exp:** Cataract Surgery; Refractive Surgery; **Hospital:** New York Eye & Ear Infirm (page 110), Cabrini Med Ctr (page 374); **Address:** 114 E 27th St, New York, NY 10016; **Phone:** 212-481-4000; **Board Cert:** Ophthalmology 1987; **Med School:** Italy 1979; **Resid:** Internal Medicine, Cabrini Med Ctr 1982; Ophthalmology, SUNY-Downstate Med Ctr 1985; **Fellow:** Cornea, SUNY-Downstate Med Ctr 1986; **Fac Appt:** Asst Clin Prof Oph, NY Med Coll

Angioletti, Louis V MD (Oph) - **Spec Exp:** Retinal Disorders; Diabetic Eye Disease/Retinopathy; Macular Degeneration; **Hospital:** New York Eye & Ear Infirm (page 110); **Address:** 7 Gramercy Park, New York, NY 10003-1759; **Phone:** 212-505-8510; **Board Cert:** Ophthalmology 1975; **Med School:** NY Med Coll 1966; **Resid:** Ophthalmology, NY Eye & Ear Infirmary 1973; **Fellow:** Retina, NY Eye & Ear Infirmary 1974; **Fac Appt:** Asst Clin Prof Oph, NY Med Coll

Asbell, Penny MD (Oph) - **Spec Exp:** Corneal Disease & Transplant; LASIK-Refractive Surgery; Cataract Surgery; **Hospital:** Mount Sinai Med Ctr (page 98); **Address:** Mt Sinai Sch Med, 5 E 98th St Fl 7, New York, NY 10029-6501; **Phone:** 212-241-0939; **Board Cert:** Ophthalmology 1980; **Med School:** SUNY Buffalo 1975; **Resid:** Ophthalmology, NYU Med Ctr 1979; **Fellow:** Immunology, NYU Med Ctr 1980; Cornea & Ext Eye Disease, LSU Eye Ctr 1982; **Fac Appt:** Prof Oph, Mount Sinai Sch Med

Barasch, Kenneth MD (Oph) - **Spec Exp:** Corneal Disease; Cataract Surgery; **Hospital:** Manhattan Eye, Ear & Throat Hosp, Lenox Hill Hosp (page 94); **Address:** 115 E 39th St, New York, NY 10016; **Phone:** 212-687-4106; **Board Cert:** Ophthalmology 1968; **Med School:** Cornell Univ-Weill Med Coll 1960; **Resid:** Ophthalmology, New York Hosp-Cornell 1966; **Fac Appt:** Assoc Clin Prof Oph, NYU Sch Med

Barile, Gaetano MD (Oph) - **Spec Exp:** Macular Disease/Degeneration; Retinal Disorders; Diabetic Eye Disease/Retinopathy; **Hospital:** NY-Presby Hosp (page 100); **Address:** Columbia Ophthalmic Consultants, 635 W 165th St, Flanzer Ste, New York, NY 10032; **Phone:** 212-305-9535; **Board Cert:** Ophthalmology 1997; **Med School:** Cornell Univ-Weill Med Coll 1991; **Resid:** Ophthalmology, Manhattan EET Hosp 1995; **Fellow:** Retina/Vitreous, Roosevelt Hosp/Harkness Eye Inst 1997; Retina, Moorfields Eye Hosp 1998; **Fac Appt:** Asst Clin Prof Oph, Columbia P&S

Barker, Barbara Ann MD (Oph) - **Spec Exp:** Glaucoma; Corneal Disease; **Hospital:** New York Eye & Ear Infirm (page 110), Beth Israel Med Ctr - Petrie Division (page 90); **Address:** 11 E 86th St, New York, NY 10028-0501; **Phone:** 212-289-2244; **Board Cert:** Ophthalmology 1981; **Med School:** Mount Sinai Sch Med 1976; **Resid:** Ophthalmology, Mt Sinai Med Ctr 1980; **Fellow:** Glaucoma, Beth Israel 1981; Cornea, Beth Israel 1983; **Fac Appt:** Asst Clin Prof Oph, Mount Sinai Sch Med

Behrens, Myles MD (Oph) - **Spec Exp:** Neuro-Ophthalmology; **Hospital:** NY-Presby Hosp (page 100); **Address:** 635 W 165th St, New York, NY 10032-3701; **Phone:** 212-305-5415; **Board Cert:** Ophthalmology 1971; **Med School:** Columbia P&S 1962; **Resid:** Internal Medicine, Columbia Presby Hosp 1964; Ophthalmology, Columbia Presby Hosp 1970; **Fellow:** Neurological Ophthalmology, UCSF Hosp 1971; **Fac Appt:** Prof Oph, Columbia P&S

Braunstein, Richard E MD (Oph) - **Spec Exp:** LASIK-Refractive Surgery; Corneal Disease & Transplant; Cataract Surgery; **Hospital:** NY-Presby Hosp (page 100), Lenox Hill Hosp (page 94); **Address:** Harkness Eye Inst, 635 W 165th St, Box 39, New York, NY 10032; **Phone:** 212-326-3320; **Board Cert:** Ophthalmology 1995; **Med School:** Columbia P&S 1989; **Resid:** Ophthalmology, Harkness Eye Inst/Columbia Presby Med Ctr 1993; **Fellow:** Cornea & Ext Eye Disease, Wilmer Inst/Johns Hopkins Hosp 1994; **Fac Appt:** Assoc Prof Oph, Columbia P&S

Brown, Alan MD (Oph) - **Hospital:** St Luke's - Roosevelt Hosp Ctr - Roosevelt Div (page 90); **Address:** 205 West End Ave, Ste 1-P, New York, NY 10023-6401; **Phone:** 212-724-4430; **Board Cert:** Ophthalmology 1982; **Med School:** Cornell Univ-Weill Med Coll 1977; **Resid:** Ophthalmology, St Luke's Hosp 1981; **Fellow:** Cornea, Park Ridge Med Ctr 1982

Buxton, Douglas F MD (Oph) - **Spec Exp:** Corneal Disease & Transplant; LASIK-Refractive Surgery; Cataract Surgery-Lens Implant; **Hospital:** New York Eye & Ear Infirm (page 110), Manhattan Eye, Ear & Throat Hosp; **Address:** 310 E 14th St, Ste 403, New York, NY 10003-4201; **Phone:** 212-979-4410; **Board Cert:** Ophthalmology 1987; **Med School:** Cornell Univ-Weill Med Coll 1982; **Resid:** Ophthalmology, New York Eye and Ear Infirmary 1986; **Fellow:** Cornea & Ext Eye Disease, New York Eye and Ear Infirmary 1988; **Fac Appt:** Assoc Clin Prof Oph, NY Med Coll

Campolattaro, Brian MD (Oph) - **Spec Exp:** Pediatric Ophthalmology; Strabismus; Tear Duct Disorders; Eye Muscle Disorders; **Hospital:** New York Eye & Ear Infirm (page 110), Lenox Hill Hosp (page 94); **Address:** 30 E 40th St, Ste 405, New York, NY 10016-3507; **Phone:** 212-684-3980; **Board Cert:** Ophthalmology 1995; **Med School:** UMDNJ-NJ Med Sch, Newark 1990; **Resid:** Ophthalmology, New York Eye & Ear Infirm 1994; **Fellow:** Pediatrics, St Louis Chldns Hosp 1995; **Fac Appt:** Asst Prof Oph, NY Med Coll

Carr, Ronald MD (Oph) - **Spec Exp:** Macular Disease/Degeneration; Retinal Disorders; Electrophysiologic Testing; **Hospital:** NYU Med Ctr (page 102), Bellevue Hosp Ctr; **Address:** 530 1st Ave, Ste 3B, New York, NY 10016-6402; **Phone:** 212-263-7360; **Board Cert:** Ophthalmology 1964; **Med School:** Johns Hopkins Univ 1958; **Resid:** Ophthalmology, Bellevue Hosp-NYU 1963; **Fellow:** Ophthalmology, Natl Inst Hlth 1965; **Fac Appt:** Prof Oph, NYU Sch Med

Casper, Daniel MD/PhD (Oph) - **Spec Exp:** Diabetic Eye Disease; **Hospital:** NY-Presby Hosp (page 100); **Address:** N Berrie Diabetes Ctr, Columbia-Presby Hosp, 1150 St Nicholas Ave Fl 2 - Ste 214, New York, NY 10032; **Phone:** 212-851-5494; **Board Cert:** Ophthalmology 1991; **Med School:** Albany Med Coll 1985; **Resid:** Ophthalmology, Harkness Eye Inst-Columbia 1989; **Fellow:** Oculoplastic Surgery, Harkness Eye Inst-Columbia 1990; **Fac Appt:** Asst Prof Oph, Columbia P&S

Chaiken, Barry MD (Oph) - **Spec Exp:** Cataract Surgery; LASIK-Refractive Surgery; **Hospital:** Manhattan Eye, Ear & Throat Hosp, New York Eye & Ear Infirm (page 110); **Address:** 625 Park Ave, New York, NY 10021-6545; **Phone:** 212-249-1976; **Board Cert:** Ophthalmology 1981; **Med School:** Columbia P&S 1976; **Resid:** Ophthalmology, Mount Sinai Hosp 1980

Chang, Stanley MD (Oph) - **Spec Exp:** Diabetic Eye Disease/Retinopathy; Macular Disease/Degeneration; Retina/Vitreous Surgery; Retinal Disorders; **Hospital:** NY-Presby Hosp (page 100); **Address:** 635 W 165th St, Box 20, New York, NY 10032; **Phone:** 212-305-9535; **Board Cert:** Ophthalmology 1979; **Med School:** Columbia P&S 1974; **Resid:** Ophthalmology, Mass Eye & Ear Infirmary 1978; **Fellow:** Vitreoretinal Surgery, Bascom Palmer Eye Inst 1979; **Fac Appt:** Prof Oph, Columbia P&S

Charles, Norman MD (Oph) - **Spec Exp:** Glaucoma; Eyelid Tumors; Tear Duct Disorders; Eyelid Surgery; **Hospital:** New York Eye & Ear Infirm (page 110), NYU Med Ctr (page 102); **Address:** 620 Park Ave, New York, NY 10021-6591; **Phone:** 212-772-6920; **Board Cert:** Ophthalmology 1971; **Med School:** NYU Sch Med 1963; **Resid:** Ophthalmology, NYU Med Ctr 1970; **Fac Appt:** Clin Prof Oph, NYU Sch Med

Chern, Relly MD (Oph) - **Spec Exp:** Cataract Surgery; Ophthalmic Plastic Surgery; **Hospital:** Montefiore Med Ctr, New York Eye & Ear Infirm (page 110); **Address:** 923 5th Ave, New York, NY 10021; **Phone:** 212-628-0160; **Board Cert:** Ophthalmology 1983; **Med School:** Albert Einstein Coll Med 1976; **Resid:** Ophthalmology, Montefiore Hosp Med Ctr 1980; **Fac Appt:** Asst Clin Prof Oph, Albert Einstein Coll Med

Chu, Wing MD (Oph) - **Spec Exp:** Corneal Disease & Transplant; Cataract Surgery; **Hospital:** Manhattan Eye, Ear & Throat Hosp, St Luke's - Roosevelt Hosp Ctr - Roosevelt Div (page 90); **Address:** 17 E 72nd St, New York, NY 10021; **Phone:** 212-288-3301; **Board Cert:** Ophthalmology 1978; **Med School:** SUNY Hlth Sci Ctr 1972; **Resid:** Internal Medicine, N Shore Univ & Meml Hosp 1974; Ophthalmology, NY Eye & Ear Infirm 1977; **Fellow:** Cornea & Ext Eye Disease, Mass Eye & Ear Infirm 1979; **Fac Appt:** Assoc Clin Prof Oph, Columbia P&S

Cohen, Ben MD (Oph) - **Spec Exp:** Retina/Vitreous Surgery; Macular Degeneration; Diabetic Eye Disease/Retinopathy; **Hospital:** New York Eye & Ear Infirm (page 110), Mount Sinai Med Ctr (page 98); **Address:** 140 E 80th St, FL 1, New York, NY 10021; **Phone:** 212-772-0600; **Board Cert:** Ophthalmology 1981; **Med School:** NY Med Coll 1976; **Resid:** Ophthalmology, Univ Chicago Hosps 1980; **Fellow:** Retina, Manhattan Eye & Ear Infirmary 1981; Retina, Mass Eye & Ear Infirmary 1983

Cohen, Leeber MD (Oph) - **Spec Exp:** Cataract Surgery; AIDS Related Eye Diseases; **Hospital:** New York Eye & Ear Infirm (page 110), St Vincent Cath Med Ctrs - Manhattan (page 375); **Address:** 11 5th Ave, Ste B, New York, NY 10003-4342; **Phone:** 212-777-1644; **Board Cert:** Ophthalmology 1989; **Med School:** SUNY Hlth Sci Ctr 1983; **Resid:** Ophthalmology, Kings Co Hosp/SUNY Downstate 1987; **Fac Appt:** Asst Clin Prof Med, SUNY Downstate

Coleman, D Jackson MD (Oph) - **Spec Exp:** Retina/Vitreous Surgery; Ultrasound; **Hospital:** NY-Presby Hosp (page 100); **Address:** 520 E 70th St, New York, NY 10021; **Phone:** 212-746-5588; **Board Cert:** Ophthalmology 1969; **Med School:** SUNY Buffalo 1960; **Resid:** Ophthalmology, Columbia-Presby Med Ctr 1967; **Fellow:** Retina, Columbia-Presby Med Ctr 1968; **Fac Appt:** Prof Oph, Cornell Univ-Weill Med Coll

Cykiert, Robert MD (Oph) - **Spec Exp:** LASIK-Refractive Surgery; Cataract Surgery; Corneal Disease; **Hospital:** NYU Med Ctr (page 102), New York Eye & Ear Infirm (page 110); **Address:** 345 E 37th St, Ste 210, New York, NY 10016-3217; **Phone:** 212-922-1430; **Board Cert:** Ophthalmology 1981; **Med School:** NY Med Coll 1976; **Resid:** Ophthalmology, Montefiore Hosp Med Ctr 1980; **Fellow:** Cornea, Wills Eye Hosp 1981; **Fac Appt:** Assoc Clin Prof Oph, NYU Sch Med

D'Amico, Robert MD (Oph) - **Spec Exp:** Corneal Disease & Transplant; Cataract Surgery; Glaucoma; **Hospital:** St Vincent Cath Med Ctrs - Manhattan (page 375), St Vincent Cath Med Ctr - Staten Island (page 375); **Address:** 36 Seventh Ave, Ste 506, New York, NY 10011; **Phone:** 212-807-8866; **Board Cert:** Ophthalmology 1964; **Med School:** Georgetown Univ 1955; **Resid:** Ophthalmology, Temple Univ Hosp 1961; **Fellow:** Cornea, Castroviejo Institute 1962; **Fac Appt:** Clin Prof Oph, NYU Sch Med

Del Priore, Lucian MD/PhD (Oph) - **Spec Exp:** Diabetic Eye Disease/Retinopathy; Macular Degeneration; Retinal Detachment; **Hospital:** NY-Presby Hosp (page 100), Manhattan Eye, Ear & Throat Hosp; **Address:** Harkness Eye Inst, 635 W 165th St, New York, NY 10032; **Phone:** 212-305-9535; **Board Cert:** Ophthalmology 1989; **Med School:** Univ Rochester 1982; **Resid:** Ophthalmology, Wilmer Eye Inst/Johns HopkinsHosp 1987; **Fellow:** Glaucoma, Wilmer Eye Inst/Johns Hopkins Hosp 1988; Vitreoretinal Surgery, Wilmer Eye Inst/Johns Hopkins Hosp 1989; **Fac Appt:** Prof Oph, Columbia P&S

Delerme, Milton MD (Oph) - **Hospital:** Harlem Hosp Ctr; **Address:** 75 E 116th St, New York, NY 10029; **Phone:** 212-828-7700; **Board Cert:** Ophthalmology 1987; **Med School:** UMDNJ-NJ Med Sch, Newark 1978; **Resid:** Surgery, UMDNJ-Univ Hosp 1980; Ophthalmology, Harlem Hosp 1984; **Fellow:** Anterior Segment - External Disease, St Francis Hosp 1985

Della Rocca, Robert MD (Oph) - **Spec Exp:** Orbital Tumors/Cancer; Eyelid Tumors/Cancer; Thyroid Eye Disease; Oculoplastic Surgery; **Hospital:** New York Eye & Ear Infirm (page 110), Sound Shore Med Ctr - Westchester (page 711); **Address:** 310 E 14th St, South Bldg, rm 319, New York, NY 10003; **Phone:** 212-979-4575; **Board Cert:** Ophthalmology 1975; **Med School:** Creighton Univ 1967; **Resid:** Ophthalmology, NY Eye & Ear Infirm 1973; **Fellow:** Oculoplastic Surgery, Albany Med Ctr

Dinnerstein, Stephen MD (Oph) - **Spec Exp:** Cataract Surgery; Glaucoma; **Hospital:** New York Eye & Ear Infirm (page 110), Mount Sinai Med Ctr (page 98); **Address:** 36 E 36th St, Ste 1J, New York, NY 10016; **Phone:** 212-889-4944; **Board Cert:** Ophthalmology 1976; **Med School:** NY Med Coll 1970; **Resid:** Ophthalmology, Univ Hosp 1974

Dodick, Jack M MD (Oph) - **Spec Exp:** Cataract Surgery-Lens Implant; Laser Vision Surgery; **Hospital:** Manhattan Eye, Ear & Throat Hosp, NYU Med Ctr (page 102); **Address:** 535 Park Ave, New York, NY 10021-8167; **Phone:** 212-288-7638; **Board Cert:** Ophthalmology 1969; **Med School:** Univ Toronto 1963; **Resid:** Ophthalmology, Manhattan EENT Hosp 1967; **Fellow:** Anterior Segment - External Disease, Westchester Co Med Ctr 1968; **Fac Appt:** Prof Oph, NYU Sch Med

Eggers, Howard M MD (Oph) - **Spec Exp:** Pediatric Ophthalmology; Strabismus; **Hospital:** NY-Presby Hosp (page 100); **Address:** 635 W 165th St, Box 21, New York, NY 10032; **Phone:** 212-305-5409; **Board Cert:** Ophthalmology 1978; **Med School:** Columbia P&S 1971; **Resid:** Ophthalmology, Harkness Inst - Presby Hosp 1975; **Fac Appt:** Prof Oph, Columbia P&S

Eichenbaum, Joseph MD (Oph) - **Spec Exp:** Uveitis; **Hospital:** Mount Sinai Med Ctr (page 98), Manhattan Eye, Ear & Throat Hosp; **Address:** 1050 Park Ave, New York, NY 10028; **Phone:** 212-289-7200; **Board Cert:** Ophthalmology 1980; **Med School:** Yale Univ 1973; **Resid:** Ophthalmology, NYU Med Ctr 1977; **Fac Appt:** Assoc Clin Prof Oph, Mount Sinai Sch Med

Esposito, Donna MD (Oph) - **Spec Exp:** Glaucoma; **Hospital:** St Vincent Cath Med Ctrs - Manhattan (page 375), New York Eye & Ear Infirm (page 110); **Address:** 36 7th Ave, Ste 417, New York, NY 10011-6609; **Phone:** 212-255-4373; **Board Cert:** Ophthalmology 1991; **Med School:** NY Med Coll 1983; **Resid:** Surgery, St Vincent's Hosp & Med Ctr 1985; Ophthalmology, St Vincent's Hosp & Med Ctr 1989; **Fellow:** Glaucoma, NY Hosp 1990

Farris, R Linsy MD (Oph) - **Spec Exp:** Corneal Disease; Contact lenses; **Hospital:** NY-Presby Hosp (page 100), Harlem Hosp Ctr; **Address:** 635 W 165th St, Ste 202, New York, NY 10032-3701; **Phone:** 212-305-9535; **Board Cert:** Ophthalmology 1968; **Med School:** Duke Univ 1961; **Resid:** Ophthalmology, Columbia-Presby Med Ctr 1967; **Fac Appt:** Prof Oph, Columbia P&S

Finger, Paul T MD (Oph) - **Spec Exp:** Eye Tumors/Cancer; Orbital Diseases; **Hospital:** New York Eye & Ear Infirm (page 110), NYU Med Ctr (page 102); **Address:** 115 E 61st St, New York, NY 10021-8183; **Phone:** 212-832-8170; **Board Cert:** Ophthalmology 1990; **Med School:** Tulane Univ 1982; **Resid:** Ophthalmology, Manhattan EET Hosp 1986; **Fellow:** Ocular Oncology, N Shore Univ Hosp-Cornell 1987; **Fac Appt:** Clin Prof Oph, NYU Sch Med

Fisher, Yale MD (Oph) - **Spec Exp:** Retina/Vitreous Surgery; Diabetic Eye Disease; Ultrasound; **Hospital:** Manhattan Eye, Ear & Throat Hosp, NY-Presby Hosp (page 100); **Address:** 460 Park Ave, New York, NY 10022; **Phone:** 212-861-9797; **Board Cert:** Ophthalmology 1973; **Med School:** Cornell Univ-Weill Med Coll 1967; **Resid:** Ophthalmology, Manhattan EET Hosp 1971; **Fac Appt:** Clin Prof Oph, Cornell Univ-Weill Med Coll

Flynn, John T MD (Oph) - **Spec Exp:** Pediatric Ophthalmology; Strabismus; Retinopathy of Prematurity; **Hospital:** NY-Presby Hosp (page 100); **Address:** Harkness Eye Inst, 635 W 165th St, Flanzer Ste, New York, NY 10032; **Phone:** 212-305-3908; **Board Cert:** Ophthalmology 1967; **Med School:** Northwestern Univ 1956; **Resid:** Ophthalmology, New York Hosp 1964; **Fellow:** Strabismus, Natl Inst Hlth 1965; **Fac Appt:** Prof Oph, Columbia P&S

Fong, Raymond MD (Oph) - **Spec Exp:** Cataract Surgery; LASIK-Refractive Surgery; Glaucoma; **Hospital:** Manhattan Eye, Ear & Throat Hosp, NY Downtown Hosp; **Address:** 109 Lafayette St Fl 4, New York, NY 10013-4154; **Phone:** 212-274-1900; **Board Cert:** Ophthalmology 1987; **Med School:** Cornell Univ-Weill Med Coll 1981; **Resid:** Ophthalmology, Manhattan Eye, Ear & Throat Hosp 1985

Fox, Martin L MD (Oph) - **Spec Exp:** LASIK-Refractive Surgery; Cornea Transplant; Corneal Ring Implants; **Hospital:** New York Eye & Ear Infirm (page 110); **Address:** 425 Madison Ave, Ste 1501, New York, NY 10017; **Phone:** 212-838-1053; **Board Cert:** Ophthalmology 1981; **Med School:** Hahnemann Univ 1976; **Resid:** Ophthalmology, Boston Univ Med Ctr 1980; **Fellow:** Ophthalmology, NY Eye & Ear Infirmary 1981

Freilich, Dennis MD (Oph) - **Spec Exp:** Diabetic Eye Disease/Retinopathy; Macular Degeneration; Retinal Disorders; **Hospital:** Mount Sinai Med Ctr (page 98), St Luke's - Roosevelt Hosp Ctr - Roosevelt Div (page 90); **Address:** 14 E 96th St, Ste C, New York, NY 10128; **Phone:** 212-410-5000; **Board Cert:** Ophthalmology 1967; **Med School:** SUNY Downstate 1958; **Resid:** Ophthalmology, St. Luke's-Roosevelt 1964; **Fellow:** Retina, Mass Eye & Ear Infirm 1966; **Fac Appt:** Clin Prof Oph, Mount Sinai Sch Med

Friedman, Alan H MD (Oph) - **Spec Exp:** Uveitis; Eye Tumors/Cancer; Retinal Disorders; **Hospital:** Mount Sinai Med Ctr (page 98), Lenox Hill Hosp (page 94); **Address:** 888 Park Ave, Ste 1A, New York, NY 10021-0235; **Phone:** 212-794-2277; **Board Cert:** Ophthalmology 1971; **Med School:** NYU Sch Med 1963; **Resid:** Ophthalmology, NYU Med Ctr 1970; **Fellow:** Pathology, Hammersmith Hosp 1972; **Fac Appt:** Clin Prof Oph, Mount Sinai Sch Med

Friedman, Alan J MD (Oph) - **Spec Exp:** Glaucoma; Cataract Surgery; Migraine; **Hospital:** New York Eye & Ear Infirm (page 110), NYU Med Ctr (page 102); **Address:** 120 E 36th St, Ste 1C, New York, NY 10016-3423; **Phone:** 212-683-5180; **Board Cert:** Ophthalmology 1965; **Med School:** Harvard Med Sch 1959; **Resid:** Ophthalmology, NYU-Bellevue Hosp 1963; **Fellow:** Glaucoma, NYU-Bellevue Hosp 1964; **Fac Appt:** Assoc Clin Prof Oph, NYU Sch Med

Friedman, Robert MD (Oph) - **Spec Exp:** Laser Refractive Surgery; Cataract Surgery; Retina/Vitreous Surgery; **Hospital:** Lenox Hill Hosp (page 94), Mount Sinai Med Ctr (page 98); **Address:** 1001 Park Ave, New York, NY 10028-0204; **Phone:** 212-772-6202; **Board Cert:** Ophthalmology 1989; **Med School:** Albert Einstein Coll Med 1983; **Resid:** Ophthalmology, Lenox Hill Hosp 1987; **Fellow:** Vitreoretinal Surgery, Manhattan Eye Ear & Throat Hosp 1988

Fromer, Mark D MD (Oph) - **Spec Exp:** Retinal Disorders; Laser Vision Surgery; Cataract Surgery; Diabetic Eye Disease/Retinopathy; **Hospital:** St Vincent Cath Med Ctrs - Manhattan (page 375), Manhattan Eye, Ear & Throat Hosp; **Address:** 550 Park Ave, New York, NY 10021-8183; **Phone:** 212-832-9228; **Board Cert:** Ophthalmology 1989; **Med School:** Rutgers Univ 1984; **Resid:** Ophthalmology, St Vincents Hosp 1988; **Fellow:** Vitreoretinal Surgery, Manhattan Ear, Nose and Throat Hosp 1989; **Fac Appt:** Clin Prof Oph, NY Med Coll

Fuchs, Wayne MD (Oph) - **Spec Exp:** Diabetic Eye Disease/Retinopathy; Macular Disease/Degeneration; Retina/Vitreous Surgery; Retinal Disorders; **Hospital:** Mount Sinai Med Ctr (page 98), Manhattan Eye, Ear & Throat Hosp; **Address:** 121 E 60th St, Ste 5B, New York, NY 10022-1186; **Phone:** 212-319-8205; **Board Cert:** Ophthalmology 1985; **Med School:** Mount Sinai Sch Med 1979; **Resid:** Ophthalmology, Mount Sinai Hosp 1983; **Fellow:** Vitreoretinal Surgery & Disease, New York Hosp/Cornell 1984; **Fac Appt:** Clin Prof Oph, Mount Sinai Sch Med

Gallin, Pamela F MD (Oph) - **Spec Exp:** Strabismus; Amblyopia; Pediatric Ophthalmology; Tear Duct Disorders; **Hospital:** NY-Presby Hosp (page 100), Manhattan Eye, Ear & Throat Hosp; **Address:** Columbia Presby Med Ctr, 635 W 165th St, Ste 224, New York, NY 10032-3701; **Phone:** 212-305-5407; **Board Cert:** Ophthalmology 1983; **Med School:** Washington Univ, St Louis 1978; **Resid:** Ophthalmology, Mount Sinai Med Ctr 1982; **Fellow:** Pediatric Ophthalmology, Chldns Natl Med Ctr 1983; Strabismus, Columbia-Presby Med Ctr 1983; **Fac Appt:** Assoc Prof Oph, Columbia P&S

Gentile, Ronald MD (Oph) - **Spec Exp:** Retina/Vitreous Surgery; Diabetic Eye Disease; Macular Degeneration; **Hospital:** New York Eye & Ear Infirm (page 110); **Address:** 2nd Ave at 14th St, South Bldg - Ste 319, New York, NY 10003-4201; **Phone:** 212-979-4120; **Board Cert:** Ophthalmology 1997; **Med School:** SUNY Downstate 1991; **Resid:** Ophthalmology, New York Eye & Ear Infirm 1995; **Fellow:** Vitreoretinal Surgery & Disease, Kresge Eye Inst 1998; **Fac Appt:** Assoc Prof Oph, NY Med Coll

Gibralter, Richard P MD (Oph) - **Spec Exp:** Cataract Surgery; Corneal Disease & Surgery; **Hospital:** Manhattan Eye, Ear & Throat Hosp; **Address:** 154 E 71st St, New York, NY 10021-5123; **Phone:** 212-628-2202; **Board Cert:** Ophthalmology 1981; **Med School:** Mount Sinai Sch Med 1976; **Resid:** Ophthalmology, Manhattan EE&T Hosp 1980; **Fellow:** Cornea, Manhattan EE&T Hosp 1981; **Fac Appt:** Assoc Prof Oph, Mount Sinai Sch Med

Grayson, Douglas MD (Oph) - **Spec Exp:** Cataract Surgery; Glaucoma; **Hospital:** New York Eye & Ear Infirm (page 110); **Address:** 36 E 36th St, New York, NY 10016-3463; **Phone:** 212-353-0030; **Board Cert:** Ophthalmology 1995; **Med School:** Brown Univ 1989; **Resid:** Ophthalmology, NY Eye & Ear Infirm 1993; **Fellow:** Glaucoma, NY Eye & Ear Infirm 1994; **Fac Appt:** Asst Prof Oph, NY Med Coll

Guillory, Samuel L MD (Oph) - **Spec Exp:** LASIK-Refractive Surgery; Orbital Surgery; Pediatric Ophthalmology; **Hospital:** Mount Sinai Med Ctr (page 98); **Address:** 1103 Park Ave, New York, NY 10128-1236; **Phone:** 212-860-5400; **Board Cert:** Ophthalmology 1980; **Med School:** Mount Sinai Sch Med 1975; **Resid:** Ophthalmology, Mount Sinai Med Ctr 1979; **Fellow:** Ophthalmology, NY Hosp; **Fac Appt:** Assoc Clin Prof Oph, Mount Sinai Sch Med

Haight, David MD (Oph) - **Spec Exp:** Laser Vision Surgery; Cornea Transplant; Cataract Surgery; **Hospital:** Manhattan Eye, Ear & Throat Hosp, NY-Presby Hosp (page 100); **Address:** 155 E 72nd St, New York, NY 10021-4371; **Phone:** 212-772-9474; **Board Cert:** Ophthalmology 1985; **Med School:** Johns Hopkins Univ 1980; **Resid:** Ophthalmology, Manhattan Eye, Ear & Throat Hosp 1984; **Fellow:** Cornea, Manhattan Eye, Ear & Throat Hosp 1985; **Fac Appt:** Clin Prof Oph, NYU Sch Med

Hall, Lisabeth MD (Oph) - **Spec Exp:** Pediatric Ophthalmology; Strabismus; Eye Muscle Disorders; Cataract-Pediatric; **Hospital:** New York Eye & Ear Infirm (page 110), Lenox Hill Hosp (page 94); **Address:** 310 E 14th St South Bldg Fl 2, New York, NY 10003-4201; **Phone:** 212-979-4614; **Board Cert:** Ophthalmology 1998; **Med School:** SUNY Stony Brook 1992; **Resid:** Ophthalmology, Manhattan Eye & Ear Infirm 1996; **Fellow:** Pediatric Ophthalmology, Jules Stein Eye Inst/UCLA 1997; **Fac Appt:** Asst Prof Oph, NY Med Coll

Harmon, Gregory K MD (Oph) - **Spec Exp:** Cataract Surgery; Glaucoma; **Hospital:** NY-Presby Hosp (page 100); **Address:** 520 E 70th St, Starr 823, New York, NY 10021-9800; **Phone:** 212-746-2475; **Board Cert:** Ophthalmology 1991; **Med School:** Mount Sinai Sch Med 1982; **Resid:** Ophthalmology, NY Hosp 1986; **Fellow:** Glaucoma, NY Hosp 1987

Heinemann, Murk-Hein MD (Oph) - **Hospital:** Meml Sloan Kettering Cancer Ctr (page 109), NY-Presby Hosp (page 100); **Address:** 1275 York Ave, A-325, New York, NY 10021; **Phone:** 212-639-7237; **Board Cert:** Ophthalmology 1982; **Med School:** Cornell Univ-Weill Med Coll 1976; **Resid:** Ophthalmology, Yale-New Haven Hosp 1980; **Fellow:** Ophthalmology, New York Hosp 1982; **Fac Appt:** Assoc Prof Oph, Cornell Univ-Weill Med Coll

Hornblass, Albert MD (Oph) - **Spec Exp:** Eyelid Cosmetic & Reconstructive Surgery; Lacrimal Gland Disorders; Orbital Inflammation/Tumors; **Hospital:** Manhattan Eye, Ear & Throat Hosp, Hackensack Univ Med Ctr (page 92); **Address:** 130 E 67th St, New York, NY 10021-6136; **Phone:** 212-879-6824; **Board Cert:** Ophthalmology 1970; **Med School:** Univ Cincinnati 1964; **Resid:** Ophthalmology, SUNY Downstate Med Ctr 1969; **Fellow:** Ophthalmic Plastic Surgery, Manhattan Eye, Ear, & Throat Hosp 1972; **Fac Appt:** Clin Prof Oph, NYU Sch Med

Kazim, Michael MD (Oph) - **Spec Exp:** Thyroid Eye Disease; Oculoplastic Surgery; Orbital Diseases & Tumors; **Hospital:** NY-Presby Hosp (page 100), New York Eye & Ear Infirm (page 110); **Address:** 635 W 165th St, New York, NY 10032-3701; **Phone:** 212-305-5477; **Board Cert:** Ophthalmology 1989; **Med School:** Columbia P&S 1984; **Resid:** Ophthalmology, Columbia-Presby Hosp 1988; **Fellow:** Oculoplastic Surgery, Univ Penn-Childrens Hosp 1989; Orbital Surgery, Allegheny Genl Hosp 1990; **Fac Appt:** Assoc Clin Prof Oph, Columbia P&S

Kelly, Stephen E MD (Oph) - **Spec Exp:** LASIK-Refractive Surgery; Cataract Surgery; Corneal Disease; **Hospital:** New York Eye & Ear Infirm (page 110), Manhattan Eye, Ear & Throat Hosp; **Address:** 154 E 71st St, New York, NY 10021-5125; **Phone:** 212-628-2202; **Board Cert:** Ophthalmology 1976; **Med School:** Washington Univ, St Louis 1970; **Resid:** Ophthalmology, NY Eye & Ear Infirmary 1975; **Fellow:** Cornea, Manhattan EET Hosp 1976

Klapper, Daniel MD (Oph) - **Spec Exp:** Laser-Refractive Surgery; Glaucoma; Cataract Surgery; **Hospital:** Manhattan Eye, Ear & Throat Hosp, New York Eye & Ear Infirm (page 110); **Address:** 7 W 81st St, Ste 1A, New York, NY 10024; **Phone:** 212-874-2726; **Board Cert:** Ophthalmology 1991; **Med School:** Albert Einstein Coll Med 1984; **Resid:** Ophthalmology, Brookdale Univ Hosp 1988

Klein, Noah MD (Oph) - **Spec Exp:** Glaucoma; Cataract Surgery; Diabetic Eye Disease; **Hospital:** Cabrini Med Ctr (page 374), New York Eye & Ear Infirm (page 110); **Address:** 51 E 25th St Fl 3, New York, NY 10010; **Phone:** 212-696-9013; **Board Cert:** Ophthalmology 1985; **Med School:** Albert Einstein Coll Med 1980; **Resid:** Internal Medicine, New York Univ Med Ctr 1981; Ophthalmology, LI Jewish Med Ctr 1984

Koplin, Richard MD (Oph) - **Spec Exp:** Cataract Surgery; Laser Refractive Surgery; Eye Trauma; Eye Infections; **Hospital:** New York Eye & Ear Infirm (page 110), Beth Israel Med Ctr - Petrie Division (page 90); **Address:** 310 E 14th St, Ste 2, New York, NY 10003-4201; **Phone:** 212-979-4428; **Board Cert:** Ophthalmology 1975; **Med School:** NY Med Coll 1969; **Resid:** Ophthalmology, NY Eye & Ear Infirm 1973; **Fac Appt:** Clin Prof Oph, NY Med Coll

Kupersmith, Mark MD (Oph) - **Spec Exp:** Neuro-Ophthalmology; **Hospital:** St Luke's - Roosevelt Hosp Ctr - Roosevelt Div (page 90); **Address:** 1000 10th Ave, rm 1M-11, New York, NY 10128; **Phone:** 212-870-9418; **Board Cert:** Ophthalmology 1981; Neurology 1981; **Med School:** Northwestern Univ 1974; **Resid:** Neurology, NYU Med Ctr 1978; Ophthalmology, NYU Med Ctr 1980; **Fac Appt:** Prof Oph, NYU Sch Med

Lee, Carol MD (Oph) - **Spec Exp:** Retinal/Vitreous Surgery; Diabetic Eye Disease/Retinopathy; **Hospital:** NYU Med Ctr (page 102); **Address:** 161 Madison Ave, rm 5NE, New York, NY 10016-5405; **Phone:** 212-684-2424; **Board Cert:** Ophthalmology 1991; **Med School:** SUNY Downstate 1984; **Resid:** Research, Univ Illinois Eye & Ear Inst 1986; Ophthalmology, NYU Med Ctr 1989; **Fellow:** Vitreoretinal Surgery & Disease, Barnes Hosp-Wash Univ 1991; **Fac Appt:** Clin Prof Oph, NYU Sch Med

Leib, Martin L MD (Oph) - **Spec Exp:** Cataract Surgery; Laser Refractive Surgery; Oculoplastic & Orbital Surgery; **Hospital:** NY-Presby Hosp (page 100), St Luke's - Roosevelt Hosp Ctr - Roosevelt Div (page 90); **Address:** 635 W 165th St, Ste 230, New York, NY 10032; **Phone:** 212-305-2303; **Board Cert:** Ophthalmology 1982; **Med School:** NY Med Coll 1974; **Resid:** Surgery, Mount Sinai Med Ctr 1976; Ophthalmology, McGill Univ Teaching Hosps 1979; **Fellow:** Ophthalmic Plastic Surgery, Columbia-Presby Med Ctr 1980; **Fac Appt:** Clin Prof Oph, Columbia P&S

Lester, Richard MD (Oph) - **Spec Exp:** Diabetic Eye Disease/Retinopathy; Glaucoma; Contact lenses; **Hospital:** St Luke's - Roosevelt Hosp Ctr - Roosevelt Div (page 90), New York Eye & Ear Infirm (page 110); **Address:** 132 E 76th St, Ste 2D, New York, NY 10021; **Phone:** 212-861-4455; **Board Cert:** Ophthalmology 1981; **Med School:** Univ Tex SW, Dallas 1975; **Resid:** Ophthalmology, St Lukes Hosp Ctr 1980; **Fellow:** Retina, Northwestern Univ 1981; **Fac Appt:** Asst Clin Prof Oph, Columbia P&S

Levitzky, Munro MD (Oph) - **Hospital:** NYU Med Ctr (page 102), New York Eye & Ear Infirm (page 110); **Address:** 161 Madison Ave Fl 6W, New York, NY 10016; **Phone:** 212-725-5225; **Board Cert:** Ophthalmology 1970; **Med School:** Columbia P&S 1961; **Resid:** Internal Medicine, Bellevue Hosp 1963; Ophthalmology, Bellevue Hosp 1969; **Fac Appt:** Asst Clin Prof Oph, NYU Sch Med

Lieberman, Theodore MD (Oph) - **Spec Exp:** Neuro-Ophthalmology; **Hospital:** Mount Sinai Med Ctr (page 98); **Address:** 70 E 96th St, New York, NY 10128-0745; **Phone:** 212-722-5477; **Board Cert:** Ophthalmology 1967; **Med School:** Yale Univ 1958; **Resid:** Ophthalmology, Barnes Hosp 1965; **Fellow:** Neurological Ophthalmology, Mount Sinai Hosp 1960; **Fac Appt:** Asst Clin Prof Oph, Mount Sinai Sch Med

Liebmann, Jeffrey MD (Oph) - **Spec Exp:** Glaucoma; Cataract Surgery; **Hospital:** New York Eye & Ear Infirm (page 110), Manhattan Eye, Ear & Throat Hosp; **Address:** 121 E 60th St, New York, NY 10022; **Phone:** 212-477-7540 x330; **Board Cert:** Ophthalmology 1989; **Med School:** Boston Univ 1983; **Resid:** Ophthalmology, SUNY Downstate Med Ctr 1987; **Fellow:** Glaucoma, New York EE Infirmary 1988; **Fac Appt:** Clin Prof Oph, NYU Sch Med

Lisman, Richard D MD (Oph) - **Spec Exp:** Oculoplastic Surgery; Eyelid/Tear Duct Reconstruction; Eyelid Surgery-Cosmetic & Reconstructive; **Hospital:** NYU Med Ctr (page 102), Manhattan Eye, Ear & Throat Hosp; **Address:** 635 Park Ave, New York, NY 10021; **Phone:** 212-585-1405; **Board Cert:** Ophthalmology 1981; **Med School:** NYU Sch Med 1976; **Resid:** Ophthalmology, Manhattan EE Hosp 1980; **Fellow:** Ophthalmic Plastic Surgery, NY Eye & Ear Infirmary 1981; Plastic Surgery, Manhattan EE&T Hosp 1982; **Fac Appt:** Clin Prof Oph, NYU Sch Med

MacKay, Cynthia J MD (Oph) - **Spec Exp:** Diabetic Eye Disease/Retinopathy; Macular Degeneration; Laser Surgery; **Hospital:** NY-Presby Hosp (page 100), Manhattan Eye, Ear & Throat Hosp; **Address:** 46 W 86th St, New York, NY 10024; **Phone:** 212-772-6050; **Board Cert:** Ophthalmology 1982; **Med School:** SUNY Hlth Sci Ctr 1977; **Resid:** Ophthalmology, Columbia-Presby Med Ctr 1981; **Fellow:** Retina, NYU Med Ctr 1982; **Fac Appt:** Clin Prof Oph, Columbia P&S

Magramm, Irene MD (Oph) - **Spec Exp:** Pediatric Ophthalmology; Strabismus; Cataract Surgery; **Hospital:** Manhattan Eye, Ear & Throat Hosp, New York Eye & Ear Infirm (page 110); **Address:** 225 E 64th St, New York, NY 10021; **Phone:** 212-644-5100; **Board Cert:** Ophthalmology 1987; **Med School:** Cornell Univ-Weill Med Coll 1981; **Resid:** Ophthalmology, North Shore Univ Hosp 1985; **Fellow:** Pediatric Ophthalmology, Manhattan Ear, Eye & Throat Hosp 1986; **Fac Appt:** Asst Clin Prof Oph, Cornell Univ-Weill Med Coll

Maher, Elizabeth MD (Oph) - **Spec Exp:** Orbital Surgery; Oculoplastic & Reconstructive Surgery; **Hospital:** New York Eye & Ear Infirm (page 110); **Address:** New York Eye & Ear Infirmary, South Bldg, 310 E 14th St, rm 319, New York, NY 10003; **Phone:** 212-979-4575; **Board Cert:** Ophthalmology 1989; **Med School:** Harvard Med Sch 1984; **Resid:** Ophthalmology, Manhattan EE&T Hosp 1988; **Fellow:** Ophthalmic Plastic & Reconstructive Surgery, Manhattan EE&T Hosp 1990

Mandel, Eric R MD (Oph) - **Spec Exp:** Laser Vision Surgery; Corneal Disease; PRK-Refractive Surgery; LASIK-Refractive Surgery; **Hospital:** New York Eye & Ear Infirm (page 110), Lenox Hill Hosp (page 94); **Address:** 211 E 70th St, New York, NY 10021-5106; **Phone:** 212-734-0111; **Board Cert:** Ophthalmology 1988; **Med School:** SUNY Stony Brook 1982; **Resid:** Ophthalmology, Lenox Hill Hosp 1986; **Fellow:** Cornea & Ext Eye Disease, Mass EE Infirm 1987

Mandelbaum, Sid MD (Oph) - **Spec Exp:** Corneal Disease; LASIK-Refractive Surgery; **Hospital:** New York Eye & Ear Infirm (page 110), Long Island Jewish Med Ctr; **Address:** 178 E 71st St, New York, NY 10021; **Phone:** 212-650-0400; **Board Cert:** Ophthalmology 1982; **Med School:** Yale Univ 1976; **Resid:** Ophthalmology, Los Angeles Chldns Hosp 1981; **Fellow:** Cornea, Bascom Palmer Eye Inst 1982; **Fac Appt:** Assoc Clin Prof Oph, Albert Einstein Coll Med

McDermott, John A MD (Oph) - **Spec Exp:** Glaucoma; Laser Vision Surgery; **Hospital:** New York Eye & Ear Infirm (page 110); **Address:** 310 E 14th St, New York, NY 10003; **Phone:** 212-979-4446; **Board Cert:** Ophthalmology 1982; **Med School:** NY Med Coll 1976; **Resid:** Ophthalmology, NY Eye & Ear Infirm 1981; Ophthalmology; **Fellow:** Glaucoma, Mass Eye & Ear Infirm 1983; **Fac Appt:** Asst Clin Prof Oph, NY Med Coll

McVeigh, Anne Marie MD (Oph) - **Spec Exp:** Retinal Disorders; **Hospital:** St Vincent Cath Med Ctrs - Manhattan (page 375), Cabrini Med Ctr (page 374); **Address:** 36 7th Ave, Ste 519, New York, NY 10011; **Phone:** 212-929-3747; **Board Cert:** Ophthalmology 1989; **Med School:** NY Med Coll 1982; **Resid:** Ophthalmology, St Vincent's Hosp & Med Ctr 1986

Medow, Norman MD (Oph) - **Spec Exp:** Cataract-Pediatric; Glaucoma-Pediatric; Corneal Disease-Pediatric; **Hospital:** Manhattan Eye, Ear & Throat Hosp, NY-Presby Hosp (page 100); **Address:** 225 E 64th St, Ste 6, New York, NY 10021-6690; **Phone:** 212-644-5100; **Board Cert:** Ophthalmology 1975; **Med School:** SUNY Hlth Sci Ctr 1966; **Resid:** Ophthalmology, Manhattan Eye, Ear & Throat Hosp 1972; **Fac Appt:** Assoc Clin Prof Oph, Cornell Univ-Weill Med Coll

Melton, R Christine MD (Oph) - **Hospital:** NY-Presby Hosp (page 100), St Vincent Cath Med Ctrs - Manhattan (page 375); **Address:** 247 3rd Ave, Ste 202, New York, NY 10010-7454; **Phone:** 212-475-3791; **Board Cert:** Ophthalmology 1982; **Med School:** Canada 1977; **Resid:** Ophthalmology, St Vincent's Hosp & Med Ctr 1981; **Fac Appt:** Asst Clin Prof Oph, Cornell Univ-Weill Med Coll

Meltzer, Murray MD (Oph) - **Spec Exp:** Ophthalmic Plastic Surgery; Thyroid Eye Disease; Eyelid Cosmetic Surgery; **Hospital:** Mount Sinai Med Ctr (page 98), Elmhurst Hosp Ctr; **Address:** 5 E 98th St Fl 7, Box 1183, New York, NY 10029-6501; **Phone:** 212-241-6175; **Board Cert:** Ophthalmology 1966; **Med School:** SUNY Downstate 1960; **Resid:** Ophthalmology, Kings County Hosp 1964; **Fellow:** Oculoplastic Surgery, Queen Victoria Hosp 1965; Cornea, Manhattan EET Hosp 1970; **Fac Appt:** Prof Oph, Mount Sinai Sch Med

Merhige, Kenneth MD (Oph) - **Hospital:** St Luke's - Roosevelt Hosp Ctr - Roosevelt Div (page 90); **Address:** St Luke's-Roosevelt Hosp, Div Ophthalmology, 1111 Amsterdam Ave, Stuyvesant 2, rm 4-207, New York, NY 10025; **Phone:** 212-523-2562; **Board Cert:** Ophthalmology 1985; **Med School:** Cornell Univ-Weill Med Coll 1980; **Resid:** Ophthalmology, St Luke's Hosp 1984; **Fellow:** Vitreoretinal Surgery, NY Hosp-Cornell

Merriam, John C MD (Oph) - **Spec Exp:** Cataract Surgery; Refractive Surgery; Reconstructive Surgery; **Hospital:** NY-Presby Hosp (page 100), Manhattan Eye, Ear & Throat Hosp; **Address:** Edward S Harkness Eye Inst, 635 W 165th St, rm 305, New York, NY 10032; **Phone:** 212-305-5402; **Board Cert:** Ophthalmology 1983; **Med School:** Harvard Med Sch 1977; **Resid:** Plastic Surgery, Brigham-Boston Chldns Hosp 1979; Ophthalmology, Mass Eye & Ear Infirm 1982; **Fellow:** Ophthalmology, UCSF Med Ctr 1983; Ophthalmology, Moorefields Eye Hosp; **Fac Appt:** Clin Prof Oph, Columbia P&S

Milite, James MD (Oph) - **Spec Exp:** Oculoplastic Surgery; **Hospital:** New York Eye & Ear Infirm (page 110); **Address:** 36 E 36th St, New York, NY 10016; **Phone:** 212-353-0030; **Board Cert:** Ophthalmology 1995; **Med School:** NYU Sch Med 1990; **Resid:** Ophthalmology, NY Eye and Ear Infirm 1994; **Fellow:** Ocular Pathology, NY Eye and Ear Infirm 1995; Ophthalmology, NY Eye and Ear Infirm 1996; **Fac Appt:** Asst Prof Oph, NY Med Coll

Millman, Arthur MD (Oph) - **Spec Exp:** Oculoplastic Surgery; Cosmetic Surgery-Face; Eyelid Surgery; **Hospital:** Lenox Hill Hosp (page 94), Manhattan Eye, Ear & Throat Hosp; **Address:** 345 E 37th St, Ste 212, New York, NY 10016-3256; **Phone:** 212-697-9797; **Board Cert:** Ophthalmology 1987; **Med School:** Northwestern Univ 1981; **Resid:** Ophthalmology, New York Eye & Ear Infirm 1987; **Fellow:** Oculoplastic Surgery, Illinois Eye & Ear Infirm 1987; Plastic Surgery, New York Eye and Ear Infirm 1988; **Fac Appt:** Asst Prof Oph, NY Med Coll

Mindel, Joel MD/PhD (Oph) - **Spec Exp:** Neuro-Ophthalmology; Ocular Pharmacology; **Hospital:** Mount Sinai Med Ctr (page 98), VA Med Ctr - Bronx; **Address:** 5 E 98th St, Fl 7, Box 1183, New York, NY 10029-6501; **Phone:** 212-241-8800; **Board Cert:** Ophthalmology 1970; **Med School:** Univ MD Sch Med 1964; **Resid:** Ophthalmology, Univ Michigan Med Ctr 1969; **Fellow:** Neurological Ophthalmology, Columbia-Presby Med Ctr 1966; Ocular Pharmacology, Mount Sinai Med Ctr 1973; **Fac Appt:** Prof Oph, Mount Sinai Sch Med

Mitchell, John P MD (Oph) - **Spec Exp:** Neuro-Ophthalmology; Cataract Surgery; Glaucoma; **Hospital:** NY-Presby Hosp (page 100), N Genl Hosp; **Address:** 470 Lenox Ave, Ste 1-R, New York, NY 10037; **Phone:** 212-281-8400; **Board Cert:** Ophthalmology 1978; **Med School:** Cornell Univ-Weill Med Coll 1973; **Resid:** Ophthalmology, Harlem Hosp 1977; **Fellow:** Neurological Ophthalmology, Columbia-Presby Med Ctr 1978; **Fac Appt:** Asst Prof Oph, Columbia P&S

Moskowitz, Bruce K MD (Oph) - **Spec Exp:** Oculoplastic Surgery; Neuro-Ophthalmology; Reconstructive Surgery; **Hospital:** New York Eye & Ear Infirm (page 110); **Address:** 310 E 14th St, Ste 401, New York, NY 10003; **Phone:** 212-979-4586; **Board Cert:** Ophthalmology 1992; **Med School:** SUNY Downstate 1987; **Resid:** Ophthalmology, SUNY Downstate 1991; **Fellow:** Ophthalmology, Kingsbrook Jewish Med Ctr 1992; **Fac Appt:** Asst Clin Prof Oph, SUNY Downstate

Muchnick, Richard MD (Oph) - **Spec Exp:** Pediatric Ophthalmology; Strabismus; **Hospital:** NY-Presby Hosp (page 100); **Address:** 69 E 71st St, New York, NY 10021-4213; **Phone:** 212-744-1726; **Board Cert:** Ophthalmology 1975; **Med School:** Cornell Univ-Weill Med Coll 1967; **Resid:** Ophthalmology, NY Hosp 1973; **Fellow:** Ophthalmic Plastic Surgery, UCSF Med Ctr 1974; Pediatric Ophthalmology, Manhattan Eye, Ear & Throat 1975; **Fac Appt:** Assoc Clin Prof Oph, Cornell Univ-Weill Med Coll

Muldoon, Thomas O MD (Oph) - **Spec Exp:** Retina/Vitreous Surgery; Macular Disease/Degeneration; Diabetic Eye Disease/Retinopathy; **Hospital:** New York Eye & Ear Infirm (page 110); **Address:** 310 E 14th St, Ste 402, New York, NY 10003-4201; **Phone:** 212-979-4595; **Board Cert:** Ophthalmology 1971; **Med School:** Univ Rochester 1962; **Resid:** Surgery, St Lukes Hosp 1966; Ophthalmology, New York EE Infirm 1969; **Fellow:** Retinal Surgery, New York EE Infirm 1970; **Fac Appt:** Assoc Clin Prof Oph, NY Med Coll

Nadel, Alfred MD (Oph) - **Spec Exp:** Macular Degeneration; Diabetic Eye Disease/Retinopathy; **Hospital:** Lenox Hill Hosp (page 94); **Address:** 140 E 80th St, New York, NY 10021; **Phone:** 212-772-0600; **Board Cert:** Ophthalmology 1969; **Med School:** Columbia P&S 1960; **Resid:** Ophthalmology, IL Eye & Ear Infirm 1966; **Fellow:** Ophthalmology, NY Hosp-Cornell 1967

Newton, Michael MD (Oph) - **Spec Exp:** Cornea & Cataract Surgery; Refractive Surgery; Eye Infections; **Hospital:** New York Eye & Ear Infirm (page 110), Mount Sinai Med Ctr (page 98); **Address:** 799 Park Ave, New York, NY 10021-3275; **Phone:** 212-861-0146; **Board Cert:** Ophthalmology 1978; **Med School:** Tufts Univ 1971; **Resid:** Ophthalmology, Mount Sinai Hosp 1977; **Fellow:** Cornea & Ext Eye Disease, AB Nesburn MD 1978; **Fac Appt:** Assoc Clin Prof Oph, Mount Sinai Sch Med

Nightingale, Jeffrey MD (Oph) - **Spec Exp:** LASIK-Refractive Surgery; Cataract Surgery; **Hospital:** New York Eye & Ear Infirm (page 110); **Address:** 211 Central Park West, New York, NY 10024-6020; **Phone:** 212-877-7188; **Board Cert:** Ophthalmology 1977; **Med School:** SUNY Hlth Sci Ctr 1973; **Resid:** Ophthalmology, Bronx Lebanon Hosp 1976; **Fellow:** Oculoplastic Surgery, NY Eye & Ear Infirmary 1977

Noble, Kenneth MD (Oph) - **Spec Exp:** Retinal Disorders; Macular Degeneration; Diabetic Eye Disease/Retinopathy; **Hospital:** NYU Med Ctr (page 102); **Address:** 161 Madison Ave, Ste 5NW, New York, NY 10016-5405; **Phone:** 212-683-2533; **Board Cert:** Ophthalmology 1975; **Med School:** NYU Sch Med 1968; **Resid:** Ophthalmology, NYU Med Ctr 1974; **Fellow:** Retina, NYU Med Ctr 1974; **Fac Appt:** Assoc Prof Oph, NYU Sch Med

Obstbaum, Stephen MD (Oph) - **Spec Exp:** Cataract Surgery; Glaucoma; **Hospital:** Lenox Hill Hosp (page 94), Manhattan Eye, Ear & Throat Hosp; **Address:** 115 E 39th St, New York, NY 10016-0943; **Phone:** 212-687-4106; **Board Cert:** Ophthalmology 1974; **Med School:** NY Med Coll 1967; **Resid:** Ophthalmology, Flower & Fifth Ave Hosp 1972; **Fellow:** Glaucoma, Washington Univ 1973; **Fac Appt:** Clin Prof Oph, NYU Sch Med

Odel, Jeffrey G MD (Oph) - **Spec Exp:** Neuro-Ophthalmology; Retinal Disorders; Optic Nerve Disorders; **Hospital:** NY-Presby Hosp (page 100); **Address:** 635 W 165th St, New York, NY 10032-3701; **Phone:** 212-305-5415; **Board Cert:** Ophthalmology 1981; **Med School:** Univ Rochester 1975; **Resid:** Ophthalmology, Mt Sinai Hosp 1981; **Fellow:** Ophthalmology, Bascom-Palmer Eye Inst 1977; Ophthalmology, Columbia Presby Med Ctr 1982

Podell, Jr, David L MD (Oph) - **Spec Exp:** Cataract Surgery; Glaucoma; Oculoplastic Surgery; **Hospital:** Manhattan Eye, Ear & Throat Hosp, Lenox Hill Hosp (page 94); **Address:** 67 E 78th St, New York, NY 10021-0204; **Phone:** 212-628-2323; **Board Cert:** Ophthalmology 1966; **Med School:** Canada 1957; **Resid:** Ophthalmology, Lenox Hill Hosp 1961

Podos, Steven M MD (Oph) - **Spec Exp:** Glaucoma; **Hospital:** Mount Sinai Med Ctr (page 98); **Address:** One Gustave L Levy Pl, Box 1183, New York, NY 10029; **Phone:** 212-241-6752; **Board Cert:** Ophthalmology 1968; **Med School:** Harvard Med Sch 1962; **Resid:** Ophthalmology, Washington Univ-Barnes Hosp 1967; **Fac Appt:** Prof Oph, Mount Sinai Sch Med

Poole, Thomas MD (Oph) - **Spec Exp:** Retina/Vitreous Surgery; Diabetes; **Hospital:** Manhattan Eye, Ear & Throat Hosp, NY-Presby Hosp (page 100); **Address:** 116 E 63rd St, New York, NY 10021; **Phone:** 212-838-4800; **Board Cert:** Ophthalmology 1974; **Med School:** Harvard Med Sch 1966; **Resid:** Ophthalmology, NY Hosp 1972; **Fellow:** Retina, NY Hosp 1973

Prince, Andrew MD (Oph) - **Spec Exp:** Glaucoma; Cataract Surgery; **Hospital:** New York Eye & Ear Infirm (page 110); **Address:** 178 E 71st St, New York, NY 10021-5119; **Phone:** 212-717-2200; **Board Cert:** Ophthalmology 1987; **Med School:** SUNY Downstate 1981; **Resid:** Ophthalmology, SUNY Downstate Med Ctr 1984; **Fellow:** Glaucoma, NY Eye & Ear Infirmary; **Fac Appt:** Assoc Prof Oph, NYU Sch Med

Raab, Edward L MD (Oph) - **Spec Exp:** Pediatric Ophthalmology; Strabismus; Glaucoma-Pediatric; **Hospital:** Mount Sinai Med Ctr (page 98); **Address:** 5 E 98th St, Fl 7, New York, NY 10029-6501; **Phone:** 212-369-0988; **Board Cert:** Ophthalmology 1966; **Med School:** NYU Sch Med 1958; **Resid:** Ophthalmology, Mount Sinai 1964; **Fellow:** Pediatric Ophthalmology, Chldns Natl Med Ctr 1967; **Fac Appt:** Prof Oph, Mount Sinai Sch Med

Relland, Maureen MD (Oph) - **Spec Exp:** Oculoplastic Surgery; Eyelid Cosmetic Surgery; Cataract Surgery; **Hospital:** St Vincent Cath Med Ctrs - Manhattan (page 375), Cabrini Med Ctr (page 374); **Address:** 36 7th Ave, New York, NY 10011; **Phone:** 212-645-7771; **Board Cert:** Ophthalmology 1971; **Med School:** NY Med Coll 1964; **Resid:** Ophthalmology, St Vincent's Hosp & Med Ctr 1968; **Fac Appt:** Asst Clin Prof Oph, NY Med Coll

Reppucci, Vincent MD (Oph) - **Spec Exp:** Retinal Disorders; Macular Degeneration; Diabetic Eye Disease; **Hospital:** NY-Presby Hosp (page 100), Danbury Hosp; **Address:** 525 E 68th St Bldg Starr - rm 817, New York, NY 10021-4870; **Phone:** 212-746-0777; **Board Cert:** Ophthalmology 1989; **Med School:** Albert Einstein Coll Med 1983; **Resid:** Ophthalmology, Columbia-Presby Med Ctr 1987; **Fellow:** Vitreoretinal Surgery & Disease, New York Hosp-Cornell 1988; **Fac Appt:** Assoc Prof Oph, Cornell Univ-Weill Med Coll

Richards, Renee MD (Oph) - **Spec Exp:** Pediatric Ophthalmology; **Hospital:** Manhattan Eye, Ear & Throat Hosp, New York Eye & Ear Infirm (page 110); **Address:** 220 Madison Ave, New York, NY 10016; **Phone:** 212-683-7330; **Board Cert:** Ophthalmology 1965; **Med School:** Univ Rochester 1959; **Resid:** Ophthalmology, Manhattan EET Hosp 1963; **Fellow:** Ophthalmology, Columbia-Presby Med Ctr 1966

Ritch, Robert MD (Oph) - **Spec Exp:** Glaucoma; **Hospital:** New York Eye & Ear Infirm (page 110); **Address:** 310 E 14th St, rm 304S, New York, NY 10003-4201; **Phone:** 212-477-7540; **Board Cert:** Ophthalmology 1977; **Med School:** Albert Einstein Coll Med 1972; **Resid:** Ophthalmology, Mount Sinai Hosp 1976; **Fellow:** Glaucoma, Mount Sinai Hosp 1978; **Fac Appt:** Clin Prof Oph, NY Med Coll

Roberts, Calvin MD (Oph) - **Spec Exp:** Refractive Surgery; Cataract Surgery; LASIK-Refractive Surgery; **Hospital:** NY-Presby Hosp (page 100); **Address:** 876 Park Ave, New York, NY 10021-1832; **Phone:** 212-734-7788; **Board Cert:** Ophthalmology 1982; **Med School:** Columbia P&S 1978; **Resid:** Ophthalmology, Columbia-Presby Med Ctr 1981; **Fellow:** Cornea, Mass Gen Hosp/Harvard 1982; **Fac Appt:** Clin Prof Oph, Cornell Univ-Weill Med Coll

Rodriguez-Sains, Rene S MD (Oph) - **Spec Exp:** Eyelid Cosmetic & Reconstructive Surgery; Eyelid Tumors/Cancer; Melanoma-Choroidal (eye); Eye Tumors/Cancer; **Hospital:** Manhattan Eye, Ear & Throat Hosp, NYU Med Ctr (page 102); **Address:** 799 Park Ave, New York, NY 10021-3275; **Phone:** 212-535-0315; **Board Cert:** Ophthalmology 1982; **Med School:** NYU Sch Med 1977; **Resid:** Ophthalmology, Manhattan EET Hosp 1981; **Fellow:** Plastic Surgery, Manhattan EET Hosp 1982; **Fac Appt:** Asst Clin Prof Oph, NYU Sch Med

Rosen, Richard MD (Oph) - **Spec Exp:** Diabetic Eye Disease/Retinopathy; Macular Disease/Degeneration; Retinal Detachment; **Hospital:** New York Eye & Ear Infirm (page 110), Beth Israel Med Ctr - Petrie Division (page 90); **Address:** 310 E 14th St, Ste 319, New York, NY 10003-4201; **Phone:** 212-979-4288; **Board Cert:** Ophthalmology 1991; **Med School:** Univ Miami Sch Med 1985; **Resid:** Ophthalmology, New York EE Infirm 1989; **Fellow:** Vitreoretinal Surgery, New York EE Infirm 1991; **Fac Appt:** Assoc Prof Oph, NY Med Coll

Rosenthal, Jeanne L MD (Oph) - **Spec Exp:** Retina/Vitreous Surgery; Macular Degeneration; Diabetic Eye Disease/Retinopathy; **Hospital:** New York Eye & Ear Infirm (page 110); **Address:** 20 E 9th St, New York, NY 10003-5944; **Phone:** 212-674-2970; **Board Cert:** Ophthalmology 1985; **Med School:** SUNY Downstate 1979; **Resid:** Ophthalmology, NY Eye & Ear Infirmary 1983; **Fellow:** Retina, NY Eye & Ear Infirmary 1985; **Fac Appt:** Assoc Clin Prof Oph, NY Med Coll

Rudick, A Joseph MD (Oph) - **Spec Exp:** LASIK-Refractive Surgery; Cataract Surgery; Contact lenses; **Hospital:** New York Eye & Ear Infirm (page 110), NY Downtown Hosp; **Address:** 150 Broadway, Ste 1800, New York, NY 10038; **Phone:** 212-233-2344; **Board Cert:** Ophthalmology 1989; **Med School:** Univ Pennsylvania 1983; **Resid:** Ophthalmology, Manhattan EET Hosp 1988

Schiff, William MD (Oph) - **Spec Exp:** Macular Disease/Degeneration; Diabetic Eye Disease/Retinopathy; Retinal Detachment; **Hospital:** NY-Presby Hosp (page 100), St Luke's - Roosevelt Hosp Ctr - Roosevelt Div (page 90); **Address:** Columbia Ophthalmic Consultants, 635 W 165th St, New York, NY 10032; **Phone:** 212-305-9535; **Board Cert:** Ophthalmology 2006; **Med School:** NYU Sch Med 1988; **Resid:** Ophthalmology, New York Eye & Ear Infirm 1994; **Fellow:** Retina/Vitreous, New York Hosp-Harkness Eye Inst 1996; **Fac Appt:** Asst Clin Prof Oph, Columbia P&S

Schneider, Howard J MD (Oph) - **Spec Exp:** Corneal Disease & Transplant; Glaucoma; Cataract Surgery; **Hospital:** Mount Sinai Med Ctr (page 98); **Address:** 1034 5th Ave, New York, NY 10028; **Phone:** 212-628-2300; **Board Cert:** Ophthalmology 1970; **Med School:** Univ Rochester 1964; **Resid:** Ophthalmology, Northwestern Meml Hosp 1968; Ophthalmology, Chldns Meml Hosp 1968; **Fellow:** Ophthalmology, Ramon Castroveijo 1974; **Fac Appt:** Asst Prof Oph, Mount Sinai Sch Med

Schubert, Hermann MD (Oph) - **Spec Exp:** Diabetic Eye Disease/Retinopathy; Macular Degeneration; Retinal Disorders; Retinal Detachment; **Hospital:** NY-Presby Hosp (page 100), Southampton Hosp; **Address:** 635 W 165th St, Rm 206, New York, NY 10032-3701; **Phone:** 212-305-6534; **Board Cert:** Ophthalmology 1987; Anatomic Pathology 1981; **Med School:** Germany 1974; **Resid:** Pathology, Columbia-Presby Hosp 1979; Ophthalmology, Columbia-Presby Hosp 1985; **Fellow:** Retina, Wills Eye Hosp 1987; **Fac Appt:** Prof Oph, Columbia P&S

Seedor, John A MD (Oph) - **Spec Exp:** Cornea & External Eye Disease; Laser Vision Surgery; **Hospital:** New York Eye & Ear Infirm (page 110); **Address:** 310 E 14th, New York, NY 10003-4201; **Phone:** 212-505-6550; **Board Cert:** Ophthalmology 1987; **Med School:** Hahnemann Univ 1981; **Resid:** Ophthalmology, NY Eye & Ear Infirm 1985; **Fellow:** Cornea, Emory Univ Hosp 1987; **Fac Appt:** Assoc Clin Prof Oph, NY Med Coll

Serle, Janet MD (Oph) - **Spec Exp:** Glaucoma; **Hospital:** Mount Sinai Med Ctr (page 98), N Shore Univ Hosp at Syosset; **Address:** 5 E 98th St Fl 7, Box 1183, New York, NY 10029-6501; **Phone:** 212-241-0939; **Board Cert:** Ophthalmology 1987; **Med School:** Harvard Med Sch 1980; **Resid:** Ophthalmology, Mount Sinai Hosp 1985; **Fellow:** Glaucoma, Mount Sinai Hosp 1982; Glaucoma, Mount Sinai Hosp 1986; **Fac Appt:** Prof Oph, Mount Sinai Sch Med

Shabto, Uri MD (Oph) - **Spec Exp:** Retinopathy of Prematurity; Macular Disease/Degeneration; Diabetic Eye Disease/Retinopathy; **Hospital:** New York Eye & Ear Infirm (page 110), Beth Israel Med Ctr - Petrie Division (page 90); **Address:** 310 E 14th St South Bldg - Ste 419, New York, NY 10003-4201; **Phone:** 212-677-2000; **Board Cert:** Ophthalmology 1991; **Med School:** Harvard Med Sch 1986; **Resid:** Ophthalmology, New York Eye & Ear Infirmary 1990; **Fellow:** Vitreoretinal Surgery, Montefiore Hosp Med Ctr 1991; **Fac Appt:** Asst Prof Oph, NYU Sch Med

Sherman, Spencer MD (Oph) - **Spec Exp:** Cataract Surgery; LASIK-Refractive Surgery; Glaucoma; **Hospital:** Manhattan Eye, Ear & Throat Hosp, Mount Sinai Med Ctr (page 98); **Address:** 166 E 63rd St, New York, NY 10021-7636; **Phone:** 212-753-8300; **Board Cert:** Ophthalmology 1970; **Med School:** Columbia P&S 1962; **Resid:** Ophthalmology, Mount Sinai Hosp 1968; **Fac Appt:** Asst Clin Prof Oph, Mount Sinai Sch Med

Shulman, Julius MD (Oph) - **Spec Exp:** Cataract Surgery; LASIK-Refractive Surgery; Contact lenses; **Hospital:** Mount Sinai Med Ctr (page 98); **Address:** 229 E 79th St, Apt 1L, New York, NY 10021-0866; **Phone:** 212-861-6200; **Board Cert:** Ophthalmology 1976; **Med School:** SUNY Hlth Sci Ctr 1969; **Resid:** Ophthalmology, Mount Sinai Med Ctr 1975; **Fac Appt:** Asst Clin Prof Oph, Mount Sinai Sch Med

Sidoti, Paul MD (Oph) - **Spec Exp:** Glaucoma; **Hospital:** New York Eye & Ear Infirm (page 110), Beth Israel Med Ctr - Petrie Division (page 90); **Address:** New York Eye & Ear Infirmary, 310 E 14th St, Ste 319, New York, NY 10003-4201; **Phone:** 212-979-4590; **Board Cert:** Ophthalmology 1994; **Med School:** Albert Einstein Coll Med 1988; **Resid:** Ophthalmology, New York Eye & Ear Infirm 1992; **Fellow:** Glaucoma, Doheny Eye Inst-USC 1994; **Fac Appt:** Assoc Prof Oph, NY Med Coll

Solomon, Joel MD (Oph) - **Spec Exp:** Cornea & Cataract Surgery; Refractive Surgery; **Hospital:** NYU Med Ctr (page 102), Manhattan Eye, Ear & Throat Hosp; **Address:** 323 E 34th St Fl 4, New York, NY 10016; **Phone:** 212-689-5080; **Board Cert:** Ophthalmology 1987; **Med School:** Cornell Univ-Weill Med Coll 1981; **Resid:** Internal Medicine, Albany Med Ctr 1983; Ophthalmology, NYU Med Ctr 1986; **Fellow:** Cornea & Ext Eye Disease, Med Coll Wisc 1987; **Fac Appt:** Clin Prof Oph, NYU Sch Med

Soloway, Barrie D MD (Oph) - **Spec Exp:** LASIK-Refractive Surgery; Corneal Disease; Glaucoma; **Hospital:** New York Eye & Ear Infirm (page 110), Lenox Hill Hosp (page 94); **Address:** 160 E 56th St, Fl 9th, New York, NY 10022; **Phone:** 212-758-3838; **Board Cert:** Ophthalmology 1987; **Med School:** Penn State Univ-Hershey Med Ctr 1980; **Resid:** Ophthalmology, NY Eye & Ear Infirm 1985; **Fellow:** Cornea, NY Eye & Ear Infirm 1986; **Fac Appt:** Asst Prof Oph, Mount Sinai Sch Med

Spaide, Richard MD (Oph) - **Spec Exp:** Retinal Disorders; Macular Degeneration; Diabetic Eye Disease/Retinopathy; **Hospital:** Manhattan Eye, Ear & Throat Hosp, St Vincent Cath Med Ctrs - Manhattan (page 375); **Address:** 460 Park Ave Fl 5th, New York, NY 10022; **Phone:** 212-861-9797; **Board Cert:** Ophthalmology 1987; **Med School:** Jefferson Med Coll 1981; **Resid:** Ophthalmology, St Vincent's Hosp & Med Ctr 1985; **Fellow:** Vitreoretinal Surgery & Disease, Manhattan EET Hosp 1990; **Fac Appt:** Assoc Clin Prof Oph, NY Med Coll

Starr, Michael MD (Oph) - **Spec Exp:** LASIK-Refractive Surgery; Cornea & Cataract Surgery; Eye Infections; **Hospital:** Lenox Hill Hosp (page 94), Manhattan Eye, Ear & Throat Hosp; **Address:** 67 E 78th St, New York, NY 10021; **Phone:** 212-717-0222; **Board Cert:** Ophthalmology 1978; **Med School:** Mount Sinai Sch Med 1972; **Resid:** Neurology, Mount Sinai 1974; Ophthalmology, Lenox Hill Hosp 1977; **Fellow:** Cornea, UCSF Med Ctr 1979; **Fac Appt:** Assoc Clin Prof Oph, Mount Sinai Sch Med

Steele, Mark MD (Oph) - **Spec Exp:** Pediatric Ophthalmology; Strabismus; Eye Muscle Disorders; **Hospital:** NYU Med Ctr (page 102), New York Eye & Ear Infirm (page 110); **Address:** 40 W 72nd St, New York, NY 10023; **Phone:** 212-981-9800; **Board Cert:** Ophthalmology 1991; **Med School:** NYU Sch Med 1986; **Resid:** Ophthalmology, NYU Med Ctr 1990; **Fellow:** Pediatric Ophthalmology, Wills Eye Hosp 1991; **Fac Appt:** Assoc Clin Prof Oph, NYU Sch Med

Topilow, Harvey MD (Oph) - **Spec Exp:** Retinal Disorders; Macular Degeneration; Retinopathy of Prematurity; **Hospital:** New York Eye & Ear Infirm (page 110), Montefiore Med Ctr; **Address:** 1016 Fifth Ave, New York, NY 10028; **Phone:** 212-288-3860; **Board Cert:** Ophthalmology 1980; **Med School:** Columbia P&S 1975; **Resid:** Ophthalmology, Albert Einstein 1979; **Fellow:** Vitreoretinal Surgery, Mass Eye & Ear Infirmary 1981; **Fac Appt:** Assoc Clin Prof Oph, Albert Einstein Coll Med

Trokel, Stephen MD (Oph) - **Spec Exp:** LASIK-Refractive Surgery; **Hospital:** NY-Presby Hosp (page 100); **Address:** 16 E 60th St, Ste 420, New York, NY 10022; **Phone:** 212-326-3363; **Board Cert:** Ophthalmology 1967; **Med School:** Columbia P&S 1965; **Resid:** Ophthalmology, Columbia-Presby Med Ctr 1966; **Fac Appt:** Prof Oph, Columbia P&S

Tsai, James C MD (Oph) - **Spec Exp:** Glaucoma; **Hospital:** NY-Presby Hosp (page 100); **Address:** Harkness Eye Inst, 635 W 165th St, Box 92, New York, NY 10032; **Phone:** 212-305-9535; **Board Cert:** Ophthalmology 2005; **Med School:** Stanford Univ 1989; **Resid:** Ophthalmology, Doheny Eye Inst/USC 1993; **Fellow:** Glaucoma, Bascom Palmer Eye Inst 1994; Glaucoma, Moorfields Eye Hosp 1995; **Fac Appt:** Assoc Prof Oph, Columbia P&S

Walsh, Joseph MD (Oph) - **Spec Exp:** Diabetic Eye Disease; Macular Degeneration; Retinal Disorders; **Hospital:** New York Eye & Ear Infirm (page 110); **Address:** 310 E 14th St Bldg S Fl 3, New York, NY 10003-4201; **Phone:** 212-979-4500; **Board Cert:** Ophthalmology 2005; **Med School:** Georgetown Univ 1966; **Resid:** Ophthalmology, NY Eye & Ear Infirm 1973; **Fellow:** Retina, Montefiore Hosp Med Ctr 1974; **Fac Appt:** Prof Oph, NY Med Coll

Wang, Frederick MD (Oph) - **Spec Exp:** Pediatric Ophthalmology; Strabismus; Eye Muscle Disorders; **Hospital:** New York Eye & Ear Infirm (page 110), Montefiore Med Ctr; **Address:** 30 E 40th St, Ste 405, New York, NY 10016-1201; **Phone:** 212-684-3980; **Board Cert:** Pediatrics 1978; Ophthalmology 1980; **Med School:** Albert Einstein Coll Med 1972; **Resid:** Pediatrics, Jacobi Med Ctr 1974; Ophthalmology, Albert Einstein 1979; **Fellow:** Pediatric Ophthalmology, Children's Hosp Natl Med Ctr 1980; **Fac Appt:** Clin Prof Oph, Albert Einstein Coll Med

Weiss, Michael J MD/PhD (Oph) - **Spec Exp:** Uveitis; Retinal Disorders; **Hospital:** NY-Presby Hosp (page 100); **Address:** 635 W 165th St, New York, NY 10032-3701; **Phone:** 212-305-9925; **Board Cert:** Ophthalmology 1987; **Med School:** Columbia P&S 1981; **Resid:** Ophthalmology, Columbia-Presby Med Ctr 1985; **Fac Appt:** Assoc Clin Prof Oph, Columbia P&S

Weseley, Peter E MD (Oph) - **Spec Exp:** Retina/Vitreous Surgery; **Hospital:** New York Eye & Ear Infirm (page 110); **Address:** 310 E 14th St, New York, NY 10003; **Phone:** 212-979-4286; **Board Cert:** Ophthalmology 2003; **Med School:** Tulane Univ 1987; **Resid:** Ophthalmology, NY E&E Infirm 1991; **Fellow:** Vitreoretinal Surgery, Devers Eye Inst 1993

Whitmore, Wayne MD (Oph) - **Spec Exp:** Cataract Surgery; Glaucoma; Corneal Disease; **Hospital:** NY-Presby Hosp (page 100), Manhattan Eye, Ear & Throat Hosp; **Address:** 116 E 68th St, New York, NY 10021-5955; **Phone:** 212-249-3030; **Board Cert:** Ophthalmology 1982; **Med School:** Dartmouth Med Sch 1977; **Resid:** Ophthalmology, New York Hosp 1981; **Fellow:** Ophthalmic Oncololgy, New York Hosp 1982; **Fac Appt:** Asst Clin Prof Oph, Cornell Univ-Weill Med Coll

Winterkorn, Jacqueline MD/PhD (Oph) - **Spec Exp:** Neuro-Ophthalmology; Brain Tumors; Eye Muscle Disorders; **Hospital:** NY-Presby Hosp (page 100), St John's Queens Hosp (page 375); **Address:** 520 E 70th St Starr Bldg - rm 607, New York, NY 10021; **Phone:** 212-746-3077; **Board Cert:** Ophthalmology 1989; **Med School:** Cornell Univ-Weill Med Coll 1983; **Resid:** Ophthalmology, Mount Sinai Med Ctr 1987; **Fellow:** Neurological Ophthalmology, Columbia Presby Med Ctr 1988; **Fac Appt:** Clin Prof Oph, Cornell Univ-Weill Med Coll

Wisnicki, H Jay MD (Oph) - **Spec Exp:** Strabismus; Eye Muscle Disorders; Pediatric Ophthalmology; **Hospital:** Beth Israel Med Ctr - Petrie Division (page 90), Mount Sinai Med Ctr (page 98); **Address:** 10 Union Square E, Ste 3B, Phillips Ambulatory Care Ctr, New York, NY 10003; **Phone:** 212-844-8080; **Board Cert:** Ophthalmology 1987; **Med School:** SUNY Hlth Sci Ctr 1981; **Resid:** Ophthalmology, Mount Sinai Med Ctr 1985; **Fellow:** Strabismus, Johns Hopkins Hosp 1986; **Fac Appt:** Assoc Prof Oph, Albert Einstein Coll Med

Wong, Raymond F MD (Oph) - **Spec Exp:** Diabetic Eye Disease/Retinopathy; Retinal Detachment; Macular Disease/Degeneration; **Hospital:** New York Eye & Ear Infirm (page 110), Cabrini Med Ctr (page 374); **Address:** 210 Canal St, Ste 409, New York, NY 10013-4159; **Phone:** 212-227-5451; **Board Cert:** Ophthalmology 1990; **Med School:** SUNY Hlth Sci Ctr 1984; **Resid:** Ophthalmology, Yale-New Haven Hosp 1988; **Fellow:** Retina, USC-Doheny Eye Inst 1990; **Fac Appt:** Asst Clin Prof Oph, NY Med Coll

Yagoda, Arnold MD (Oph) - **Spec Exp:** Macular Degeneration; Laser Vision Surgery; Diabetic Eye Disease/Retinopathy; **Hospital:** Lenox Hill Hosp (page 94), New York Eye & Ear Infirm (page 110); **Address:** 67 E 78th St, New York, NY 10021-0204; **Phone:** 212-744-2513; **Board Cert:** Ophthalmology 1980; **Med School:** Cornell Univ-Weill Med Coll 1975; **Resid:** Ophthalmology, Lenox Hill Hosp 1979; **Fellow:** Retina, Montefiore Hosp Med Ctr 1980; **Fac Appt:** Asst Clin Prof Oph, Albert Einstein Coll Med

Yannuzzi, Lawrence MD (Oph) - **Spec Exp:** Retina/Vitreous Surgery; Macular Disease/Degeneration; Diabetic Eye Disease; **Hospital:** Manhattan Eye, Ear & Throat Hosp; **Address:** 460 Park Ave, Ste 203, New York, NY 10021-4028; **Phone:** 212-861-9797; **Board Cert:** Ophthalmology 1970; **Med School:** Boston Univ 1964; **Resid:** Ophthalmology, Manhattan Eye, Ear & Throat Hosp 1968; **Fellow:** Ophthalmology, Manhattan Eye, Ear & Throat Hosp 1971; **Fac Appt:** Clin Prof Oph, Columbia P&S

Zweifach, Philip MD (Oph) - **Spec Exp:** Cataract Surgery; Neuro-Ophthalmology; Glaucoma; **Hospital:** NY-Presby Hosp (page 100); **Address:** 131 E 69th St, New York, NY 10021-5158; **Phone:** 212-535-1508; **Board Cert:** Ophthalmology 1968; **Med School:** Cornell Univ-Weill Med Coll 1961; **Resid:** Ophthalmology, NY Hosp 1966; Neurology, Boston Med Ctr 1963; **Fellow:** Neurological Ophthalmology, Mass Eye & Ear Infirmary 1967; **Fac Appt:** Clin Prof Oph, Cornell Univ-Weill Med Coll

ORTHOPAEDIC SURGERY

Adler, Edward MD (OrS) - **Spec Exp:** Hip Replacement; Knee Replacement; Foot & Ankle Surgery; **Hospital:** Hosp For Joint Diseases (page 107); **Address:** 1245 Madison Ave, New York, NY 10128-0514; **Phone:** 212-427-3986; **Board Cert:** Orthopaedic Surgery 2002; **Med School:** UMDNJ-NJ Med Sch, Newark 1984; **Resid:** Orthopaedic Surgery, UMDNJ-NJ Med Schl 1989; **Fellow:** Joint Replacement Surgery, Hosp for Joint Dis 1990; **Fac Appt:** Asst Clin Prof OrS, NYU Sch Med

Alexiades, Michael MD (OrS) - **Spec Exp:** Joint Replacement; Sports Medicine; **Hospital:** Lenox Hill Hosp (page 94), Hosp For Special Surgery (page 108); **Address:** 159 E 74th St, FL 2, New York, NY 10021; **Phone:** 212-734-1288; **Board Cert:** Orthopaedic Surgery 2002; **Med School:** Cornell Univ-Weill Med Coll 1983; **Resid:** Orthopaedic Surgery, Lenox Hill Hosp 1988; Surgery, Children's Hosp; **Fellow:** Arthritis Surgery, Hosp for Special Surgery; **Fac Appt:** Asst Prof OrS, Cornell Univ-Weill Med Coll

Bauman, Phillip MD (OrS) - **Spec Exp:** Foot & Ankle Surgery; Knee Surgery; Dance/Sports Medicine; **Hospital:** St Luke's - Roosevelt Hosp Ctr - Roosevelt Div (page 90), NY-Presby Hosp (page 100); **Address:** Orthopaedic Assocs of NY, 343 W 58th St, rm 1, New York, NY 10019; **Phone:** 212-765-2260; **Board Cert:** Orthopaedic Surgery 2001; **Med School:** Columbia P&S 1981; **Resid:** Surgery, St Luke's-Roosevelt Hosp Ctr 1983; Orthopaedic Surgery, Columbia-Presby Med Ctr 1987; **Fac Appt:** Asst Prof OrS, Columbia P&S

Bendo, John A MD (OrS) - **Spec Exp:** Spinal Surgery-Minimally Invasive; Scoliosis; Spinal Disc Replacement; **Hospital:** Hosp For Joint Diseases (page 107), NYU Med Ctr (page 102); **Address:** Hosp for Joint Diseases-Spine Ctr, 301 E 17th St, New York, NY 10003; **Phone:** 212-598-6625; **Board Cert:** Orthopaedic Surgery 1997; **Med School:** Mount Sinai Sch Med 1989; **Resid:** Orthopaedic Surgery, Mt Sinai Hosp 1994; **Fellow:** Spinal Surgery, Hosp Joint Diseases 1996; **Fac Appt:** Asst Prof OrS, NYU Sch Med

Bigliani, Louis MD (OrS) - **Spec Exp:** Shoulder Surgery; Sports Medicine; Arthroscopic Surgery; **Hospital:** NY-Presby Hosp (page 100); **Address:** 622 W 168th St, rm 1130, New York, NY 10032-3720; **Phone:** 212-305-5564; **Board Cert:** Orthopaedic Surgery 1979; **Med School:** Loyola Univ-Stritch Sch Med 1973; **Resid:** Surgery, Roosevelt Hosp 1974; Orthopaedic Surgery, Columbia Presby Med Ctr 1977; **Fac Appt:** Prof OrS, Columbia P&S

Bitan, Fabien D MD (OrS) - **Spec Exp:** Spinal Surgery-Pediatric & Adult; Spinal Disc Replacement; Spinal Deformity & Degeneration; **Hospital:** Lenox Hill Hosp (page 94); **Address:** Phillips Ambulatory Care Ctr, Spine Inst, 130 E 77th St Fl 7, New York, NY 10021; **Phone:** 212-744-8114; **Med School:** France 1981; **Resid:** Orthopaedic Surgery, Hospital Beaujon 1987; Pediatric Orthopaedic Surgery, Hosp des Enfants Malades 1990; **Fellow:** Pediatric Orthopaedic Surgery, Hosp Special Surgery 1997; Spinal Surgery, Beth Israel Med Ctr 1998

Boachie-Adjei, Oheneba MD (OrS) - **Spec Exp:** Spinal Surgery; Scoliosis; **Hospital:** Hosp For Special Surgery (page 108); **Address:** Hospital for Special Surgery, 535 E 70th St, New York, NY 10021; **Phone:** 212-606-1948; **Board Cert:** Orthopaedic Surgery 2000; **Med School:** Columbia P&S 1980; **Resid:** Surgery, St Vincents Hosp 1982; Orthopaedic Surgery, Hosp Spec Surg 1986; **Fellow:** Orthopaedic Pathology, Hosp Spec Surg 1983; Spinal Surgery, Twin Cities Scoliosis Ctr/Minn Spine Ctr 1987; **Fac Appt:** Assoc Clin Prof S, Cornell Univ-Weill Med Coll

Bosco, Joseph MD (OrS) - **Spec Exp:** Sports Medicine; Knee Surgery; Shoulder Surgery; **Hospital:** Hosp For Joint Diseases (page 107), Jamaica Hosp Med Ctr; **Address:** 530 1st Ave, Ste 8U, New York, NY 10016; **Phone:** 212-263-2192; **Board Cert:** Orthopaedic Surgery 1995; **Med School:** Univ VT Coll Med 1986; **Resid:** Orthopaedic Surgery, Univ NC Med Ctr 1991; **Fellow:** Reconstructive Surgery, Univ Ariz Coll Med 1992; **Fac Appt:** Asst Prof OrS, NYU Sch Med

Brisson, Paul M MD (OrS) - **Spec Exp:** Spinal Surgery; **Hospital:** Cabrini Med Ctr (page 374); **Address:** 51 E 25th St Fl 6, New York, NY 10010-2945; **Phone:** 212-813-3632; **Board Cert:** Orthopaedic Surgery 2004; **Med School:** Univ Montreal 1979; **Resid:** Orthopaedic Surgery, McGill Med Ctr 1987; **Fellow:** Spinal Surgery, Hosp Joint Diseases 1988; Spinal Surgery, Buffalo Genl Hosp 1989

Bronson, Michael MD (OrS) - **Spec Exp:** Hip & Knee Replacement; Knee Replacement-Partial; **Hospital:** Mount Sinai Med Ctr (page 98), Lenox Hill Hosp (page 94); **Address:** 159 E 74th St, FL 2, New York, NY 10021-3226; **Phone:** 212-734-2646; **Board Cert:** Orthopaedic Surgery 1984; **Med School:** NY Med Coll 1976; **Resid:** Orthopaedic Surgery, Lenox Hill Hosp 1980; **Fellow:** Hip & Knee Surgery, Columbia-Presby Med Ctr 1981; **Fac Appt:** Assoc Prof OrS, Mount Sinai Sch Med

Buly, Robert L MD (OrS) - **Spec Exp:** Hip Replacement; Minimally Invasive Surgery; Arthritis; **Hospital:** Hosp For Special Surgery (page 108); **Address:** Hospital for Special Surgery, 535 E 70th St, New York, NY 10021; **Phone:** 212-606-1971; **Board Cert:** Orthopaedic Surgery 2004; **Med School:** Cornell Univ-Weill Med Coll 1985; **Resid:** Orthopaedic Surgery, Hosp for Special Surg 1990; **Fellow:** Hip Surgery, Mueller Fdn 1991; Joint Reconstruction, Case Western Res/ Univ Hosp 1992; **Fac Appt:** Asst Prof OrS, Cornell Univ-Weill Med Coll

Burke, Stephen W MD (OrS) - **Spec Exp:** Scoliosis; Clubfoot & Hip Dysplasia; Pediatric Orthopaedic Surgery; Spinal Deformity; **Hospital:** Hosp For Special Surgery (page 108), NY-Presby Hosp (page 100); **Address:** Hosp Special Surg, Dept Ped Orthopaedics, 535 E 70th St, Ste 572, New York, NY 10021-4872; **Phone:** 212-606-1180; **Board Cert:** Orthopaedic Surgery 1977; **Med School:** Cornell Univ-Weill Med Coll 1971; **Resid:** Orthopaedic Surgery, Univ Utah Hosp 1976; **Fellow:** Pediatric Orthopaedic Surgery, LSU Med Ctr 1979; **Fac Appt:** Prof OrS, Cornell Univ-Weill Med Coll

Cammisa Jr, Frank P MD (OrS) - **Spec Exp:** Spinal Surgery; Spinal Disc Replacement; Scoliosis; **Hospital:** Hosp For Special Surgery (page 108), NY-Presby Hosp (page 100); **Address:** 523 E 72nd St, Fl 3, New York, NY 10021; **Phone:** 212-606-1946; **Board Cert:** Orthopaedic Surgery 2001; **Med School:** Columbia P&S 1982; **Resid:** Surgery, Columbia-Presby Hosp 1983; Orthopaedic Surgery, Hosp for Special Surgery 1987; **Fellow:** Spinal Surgery, Jackson Meml Hosp 1988; **Fac Appt:** Assoc Prof OrS, Cornell Univ-Weill Med Coll

Capozzi, James MD (OrS) - **Spec Exp:** Joint Replacement; Fractures in the Elderly; Arthroscopic Surgery; **Hospital:** Mount Sinai Med Ctr (page 98); **Address:** 1065 Park Ave, Fl 2nd, New York, NY 10128-1001; **Phone:** 212-289-0700; **Board Cert:** Orthopaedic Surgery 2000; **Med School:** Mount Sinai Sch Med 1981; **Resid:** Orthopaedic Surgery, Mount Sinai Hosp 1986; **Fellow:** Joint Replacement Surgery, New England Baptist Hosp 1987; **Fac Appt:** Assoc Clin Prof OrS, Mount Sinai Sch Med

Casden, Andrew M MD (OrS) - **Spec Exp:** Spinal Surgery; Spinal Disc Replacement; Minimally Invasive Spinal Surgery; **Hospital:** Beth Israel Med Ctr - Petrie Division (page 90); **Address:** 10 Union Square East, Ste 5P, Spinal Institute, New York, NY 10003-3314; **Phone:** 212-844-8674; **Board Cert:** Orthopaedic Surgery 2001; **Med School:** Cornell Univ-Weill Med Coll 1983; **Resid:** Orthopaedic Surgery, Hosp Joint Diseases 1988; **Fellow:** Spinal Surgery, Rush-Presbyterian Med Ctr 1989; **Fac Appt:** Assoc Prof OrS, Albert Einstein Coll Med

Chorney, Gail MD (OrS) - **Spec Exp:** Pediatric Orthopaedic Surgery; **Hospital:** Hosp For Joint Diseases (page 107), NYU Med Ctr (page 102); **Address:** 301 E 17th St, rm 413, New York, NY 10003-3804; **Phone:** 212-598-6211; **Board Cert:** Orthopaedic Surgery 2000; **Med School:** Boston Univ 1978; **Resid:** Surgery, Baylor Coll Med 1980; Orthopaedic Surgery, Tufts Univ Sch Med 1984; **Fac Appt:** Asst Prof OrS, NYU Sch Med

Cornell, Charles MD (OrS) - **Spec Exp:** Trauma; Joint Replacement; **Hospital:** Hosp For Special Surgery (page 108), NY Hosp Queens; **Address:** 535 E 70th St, New York, NY 10021; **Phone:** 212-606-1414; **Board Cert:** Orthopaedic Surgery 1999; **Med School:** Cornell Univ-Weill Med Coll 1980; **Resid:** Orthopaedic Surgery, Hosp For Special Surg/New York Hosp 1985; **Fellow:** Orthopaedic Surgery, Univ Wash Med Ctr 1986; **Fac Appt:** Clin Prof OrS, Cornell Univ-Weill Med Coll

Craig, Edward V MD (OrS) - **Spec Exp:** Shoulder Arthroscopic Surgery; Shoulder Replacement; Sports Medicine; Elbow Surgery; **Hospital:** Hosp For Special Surgery (page 108); **Address:** 535 E 70th St, New York, NY 10021-4892; **Phone:** 212-606-1966; **Board Cert:** Orthopaedic Surgery 1984; **Med School:** Columbia P&S 1973; **Resid:** Internal Medicine, Columbia-Presby Hosp 1976; Orthopaedic Surgery, Columbia-Presby Hosp 1980; **Fellow:** Shoulder Surgery, Columbia-Presby Hosp 1981; Hand Surgery, Columbia-Presby Hosp 1982; **Fac Appt:** Clin Prof OrS, Cornell Univ-Weill Med Coll

Cuomo, Frances MD (OrS) - **Spec Exp:** Shoulder Surgery; Elbow Surgery; Sports Medicine; **Hospital:** Beth Israel Med Ctr - Petrie Division (page 90); **Address:** Phillips Ambulatory Care Center, 10 Union Square E, Ste 3M, New York, NY 10003; **Phone:** 212-844-6938; **Board Cert:** Orthopaedic Surgery 2002; **Med School:** NYU Sch Med 1983; **Resid:** Surgery, Beth Israel 1984; Orthopaedic Surgery, Lenox Hill Hosp 1988; **Fellow:** Shoulder Surgery, Columbia-Presby 1989; **Fac Appt:** Asst Prof OrS, Albert Einstein Coll Med

Deland, Jonathan T MD (OrS) - **Spec Exp:** Foot & Ankle Surgery; Sports Medicine; Arthritis; **Hospital:** Hosp For Special Surgery (page 108); **Address:** Hosp Spec Surg, Foot & Ankle Service, 535 E 70th St, New York, NY 10021-4099; **Phone:** 212-606-1665; **Board Cert:** Orthopaedic Surgery 1992; **Med School:** Columbia P&S 1980; **Resid:** Orthopaedic Surgery, St Luke's-Rooselvelt Hosp Ctr 1982; Orthopaedic Surgery, Mass Genl Hosp 1987; **Fac Appt:** Asst Prof S, Cornell Univ-Weill Med Coll

Di Cesare, Paul MD (OrS) - **Spec Exp:** Knee Surgery; Hip Replacement; Knee Replacement; **Hospital:** Hosp For Joint Diseases (page 107), NYU Med Ctr (page 102); **Address:** 301 E 17th St, rm 1500, New York, NY 10003-3804; **Phone:** 212-598-6521; **Board Cert:** Orthopaedic Surgery 2004; **Med School:** USC Sch Med 1986; **Resid:** Orthopaedic Surgery, LAC-USC Med Ctr 1991; **Fellow:** Hip Surgery; **Fac Appt:** Prof OrS, NYU Sch Med

Errico, Thomas MD (OrS) - **Spec Exp:** Spinal Surgery; Spinal Disc Replacement; Scoliosis; **Hospital:** NYU Med Ctr (page 102), Hosp For Joint Diseases (page 107); **Address:** 530 1st Ave, Ste 8U, New York, NY 10016-6402; **Phone:** 212-263-7182; **Board Cert:** Orthopaedic Surgery 1986; **Med School:** UMDNJ-NJ Med Sch, Newark 1978; **Resid:** Orthopaedic Surgery, NYU Med Ctr 1983; **Fellow:** Spinal Surgery, Toronto Genl Hosp 1984; **Fac Appt:** Assoc Clin Prof OrS, NYU Sch Med

Fabian, Dennis DO (OrS) - **Spec Exp:** Knee Surgery; Hip Surgery; **Hospital:** St Vincent Cath Med Ctrs - Manhattan (page 375); **Address:** 95 University Pl Fl 8, New York, NY 10003; **Phone:** 212-604-1350; **Board Cert:** Orthopaedic Surgery 1980; **Med School:** Philadelphia Coll Osteo Med 1972; **Resid:** Orthopaedic Surgery, Metropolitan Hosp Ctr 1977; Surgery, St Vincent's Hosp & Med Ctr 1974; **Fellow:** Surgery, Hosp For Special Surg 1978

Farcy, Jean-Pierre MD (OrS) - **Spec Exp:** Spinal Surgery; Spinal Disc Replacement; Sports Medicine; **Hospital:** Hosp For Joint Diseases (page 107); **Address:** 380 2nd Ave Fl 10, New York, NY 10017; **Phone:** 212-534-7758; **Med School:** France 1967; **Resid:** Orthopaedic Surgery, Univ Marseilles Med Ctr 1967; **Fellow:** Orthopaedic Surgery, Columbia Presby Med Ctr 1983; **Fac Appt:** Assoc Clin Prof OrS, NYU Sch Med

Feldman, David S MD (OrS) - **Spec Exp:** Limb Deformities; Spinal Surgery; Pediatric Orthopaedic Surgery; **Hospital:** Hosp For Joint Diseases (page 107), NYU Med Ctr (page 102); **Address:** 67 Irving Pl Fl 8, New York, NY 10003; **Phone:** 212-533-5310; **Board Cert:** Orthopaedic Surgery 1996; **Med School:** Albert Einstein Coll Med 1988; **Resid:** Orthopaedic Surgery, Hosp for Joint Diseases 1993; **Fellow:** Pediatric Surgery, Hosp For Sick Chldn 1994; **Fac Appt:** Asst Prof OrS, NYU Sch Med

Ferriter, Pierce MD (OrS) - **Spec Exp:** Spinal Surgery; **Hospital:** Lenox Hill Hosp (page 94); **Address:** 1421 3rd Ave Fl 5, New York, NY 10028; **Phone:** 212-772-9711; **Board Cert:** Orthopaedic Surgery 1999; **Med School:** UMDNJ-RW Johnson Med Sch 1979; **Resid:** Orthopaedic Surgery, Lenox Hill Hosp 1985; **Fellow:** Spinal Surgery, Buffalo Genl Hosp 1986

Figgie, Mark MD (OrS) - **Spec Exp:** Joint Replacement; Minimally Invasive Surgery; Hip Surgery; Knee Surgery; **Hospital:** Hosp For Special Surgery (page 108), NY-Presby Hosp (page 100); **Address:** 535 E 70th St, Ste 328, New York, NY 10021; **Phone:** 212-606-1932; **Board Cert:** Orthopaedic Surgery 2000; **Med School:** Case West Res Univ 1981; **Resid:** Orthopaedic Surgery, Univ Hosp-Case Western Reserve 1986; **Fellow:** Biomedical Engineering, Hosp For Special Surgery 1987; Joint Replacement Surgery, Hosp For Special Surgery 1988; **Fac Appt:** Assoc Clin Prof OrS, Cornell Univ-Weill Med Coll

Flatow, Evan MD (OrS) - **Spec Exp:** Rotator Cuff Surgery; Shoulder Injuries; Shoulder Replacement; Shoulder Arthroscopic Surgery; **Hospital:** Mount Sinai Med Ctr (page 98); **Address:** 5 E 98th St Fl 9, Box 1188, New York, NY 10029; **Phone:** 212-241-1663; **Board Cert:** Orthopaedic Surgery 2000; **Med School:** Columbia P&S 1981; **Resid:** Surgery, Roosevelt Hosp 1983; Orthopaedic Surgery, Columbia-Presby Med Ctr 1985; **Fellow:** Shoulder Surgery, Columbia-Presby Med Ctr 1987; **Fac Appt:** Prof OrS, Mount Sinai Sch Med

Gilbert, Marvin MD (OrS) - **Spec Exp:** Hemophilia Related Disease; Hip Replacement; Knee Replacement; **Hospital:** Mount Sinai Med Ctr (page 98); **Address:** 1065 Park Ave, New York, NY 10128-1001; **Phone:** 212-289-0700; **Board Cert:** Orthopaedic Surgery 1971; **Med School:** Columbia P&S 1964; **Resid:** Orthopaedic Surgery, Mount Sinai Hosp 1969; **Fac Appt:** Clin Prof OrS, Mount Sinai Sch Med

Gladstone, James MD (OrS) - **Spec Exp:** Shoulder & Knee Surgery; Cartilage Damage; Shoulder Surgery; Sports Medicine; **Hospital:** Mount Sinai Med Ctr (page 98); **Address:** Mt Sinai Med Ctr, 5 E 98th St Fl 9, Box 1188, New York, NY 10029; **Phone:** 212-241-1645; **Board Cert:** Orthopaedic Surgery 1998; **Med School:** Tufts Univ 1990; **Resid:** Orthopaedic Surgery, Columbia-Presby Med Ctr 1995; **Fellow:** Sports Medicine, Am Sports Med Inst 1996; **Fac Appt:** Asst Prof OrS, Mount Sinai Sch Med

Glashow, Jonathan MD (OrS) - **Spec Exp:** Sports Medicine; Shoulder Surgery; Knee Surgery; **Hospital:** Mount Sinai Med Ctr (page 98), Lenox Hill Hosp (page 94); **Address:** 159 E 74th St Fl 1, New York, NY 10021; **Phone:** 212-794-5096; **Board Cert:** Orthopaedic Surgery 2003; **Med School:** Cornell Univ-Weill Med Coll 1984; **Resid:** Orthopaedic Surgery, Lenox Hill Hosp 1989; **Fellow:** Arthroscopic Surgery, S Calif Ortho Inc 1990; Shoulder Surgery, Univ Texas Med Ctr 1990; **Fac Appt:** Assoc Clin Prof OrS, Mount Sinai Sch Med

Goldstein, Jeffrey A MD (OrS) - **Spec Exp:** Spinal Surgery; Minimally Invasive Spinal Surgery; Spinal Disc Replacement; **Hospital:** Hosp For Joint Diseases (page 107), NY Downtown Hosp; **Address:** 19 Beekman St Fl 5, New York, NY 10038; **Phone:** 212-513-7711; **Board Cert:** Orthopaedic Surgery 1998; **Med School:** SUNY Downstate 1990; **Resid:** Orthopaedic Surgery, Case West Univ Med Ctr 1995; **Fellow:** Spinal Surgery, Maryland Spine Fellowship-Johns Hopkins 1996; **Fac Appt:** Asst Clin Prof OrS, NYU Sch Med

Goodwin, Charles MD (OrS) - **Spec Exp:** Spinal Surgery; Sports Medicine; Minimally Invasive Spinal Surgery; **Hospital:** Hosp For Special Surgery (page 108), St Luke's - Roosevelt Hosp Ctr - Roosevelt Div (page 90); **Address:** 635 Madison Ave Fl 7, New York, NY 10022-1009; **Phone:** 212-317-4600; **Board Cert:** Orthopaedic Surgery 1985; **Med School:** Univ Cincinnati 1976; **Resid:** Surgery, St Luke's Roosevelt Hosp Ctr 1979; Orthopaedic Surgery, Columbia-Presby 1982; **Fellow:** Spinal Surgery, Univ of Toronto 1983; **Fac Appt:** Asst Prof OrS, Cornell Univ-Weill Med Coll

Grant, Alfred MD (OrS) - **Spec Exp:** Pediatric Orthopaedic Surgery; Neuromuscular Disorders; Limb Lengthening; Limb Deformities; **Hospital:** Hosp For Joint Diseases (page 107), NYU Med Ctr (page 102); **Address:** 301 E 17th St, Ste 413, New York, NY 10003-3804; **Phone:** 212-598-6605; **Board Cert:** Orthopaedic Surgery 1966; **Med School:** Univ Hlth Sci/Chicago Med Sch 1957; **Resid:** Surgery, Montefiore Med Ctr 1959; Orthopaedic Surgery, Joint Disease Hosp 1962; **Fac Appt:** Clin Prof OrS, NYU Sch Med

Green, Steven MD (OrS) - **Spec Exp:** Hand & Wrist Trauma; Hand & Wrist Reconstruction; Carpal Tunnel Syndrome; **Hospital:** Mount Sinai Med Ctr (page 98), Hosp For Joint Diseases (page 107); **Address:** 2 E 88th St, New York, NY 10128-0555; **Phone:** 212-348-6644; **Board Cert:** Orthopaedic Surgery 1977; Hand Surgery 2000; **Med School:** Albert Einstein Coll Med 1970; **Resid:** Surgery, Georgia Bapt Hosp 1972; Orthopaedic Surgery, Mount Sinai Hosp 1975; **Fellow:** Hand Surgery, Thomas Jefferson Univ Hosp 1978; **Fac Appt:** Assoc Clin Prof OrS, NYU Sch Med

Grelsamer, Ronald P MD (OrS) - **Spec Exp:** Knee-Patella Problems; Sports Medicine; Knee Reconstruction; Hip Reconstruction; **Hospital:** Mount Sinai Med Ctr (page 98); **Address:** Mount Sinai Medical Ctr, Dept Orthopaedics, 5 E 98th St, Box 1188, New York, NY 10029-6574; **Phone:** 212-241-2914; **Board Cert:** Orthopaedic Surgery 1998; **Med School:** Columbia P&S 1979; **Resid:** Surgery, Columbia Presby Med Ctr 1984; **Fellow:** Orthopaedic Surgery, Columbia Presby Med Ctr 1985; **Fac Appt:** Assoc Prof OrS, Mount Sinai Sch Med

Haas, Steven B MD (OrS) - **Spec Exp:** Knee Surgery; Knee Replacement; Minimally Invasive Surgery; **Hospital:** Hosp For Special Surgery (page 108); **Address:** Hospital for Special Surgery, 535 E 70th St, New York, NY 10021; **Phone:** 212-606-1852; **Board Cert:** Orthopaedic Surgery 2004; **Med School:** Univ Rochester 1985; **Resid:** Orthopaedic Surgery, Hosp Special Surgery 1990; **Fellow:** Knee Surgery, Hosp Special Surgery 1991; **Fac Appt:** Assoc Prof OrS, Cornell Univ-Weill Med Coll

Hamilton, William MD (OrS) - **Spec Exp:** Dance Medicine; Foot & Ankle Surgery; Sports Medicine; **Hospital:** St Luke's - Roosevelt Hosp Ctr - Roosevelt Div (page 90); **Address:** 343 W 58th St, New York, NY 10019-1173; **Phone:** 212-765-2260; **Board Cert:** Orthopaedic Surgery 1971; **Med School:** Columbia P&S 1964; **Resid:** Surgery, St Luke's-Roosevelt Hosp Ctr 1966; Orthopaedic Surgery, Columbia-Presby Hosp 1969; **Fellow:** Pediatric Orthopaedic Surgery, Newington Chldrn's Hosp 1970; **Fac Appt:** Clin Prof OrS, Columbia P&S

Hannafin, Jo MD/PhD (OrS) - **Spec Exp:** Sports Medicine-Women; Shoulder Arthroscopic Surgery; Knee Injuries/Ligament Surgery; Ligament Reconstruction; **Hospital:** Hosp For Special Surgery (page 108), NY-Presby Hosp (page 100); **Address:** 535 E 70th St, New York, NY 10021-4872; **Phone:** 212-606-1469; **Board Cert:** Orthopaedic Surgery 1994; **Med School:** Albert Einstein Coll Med 1985; **Resid:** Orthopaedic Surgery, Montefiore Hosp Med Ctr 1990; **Fellow:** Sports Medicine, Hosp Special Surg-Cornell 1992; **Fac Appt:** Assoc Prof OrS, Cornell Univ-Weill Med Coll

Harwin, Steven F MD (OrS) - **Spec Exp:** Hip & Knee Replacement; Arthroscopic Surgery; Shoulder Replacement; **Hospital:** Beth Israel Med Ctr - Petrie Division (page 90); **Address:** Center for Reconstructive Joint Surgery, 910 Park Ave, New York, NY 10021-0255; **Phone:** 212-861-9800; **Board Cert:** Orthopaedic Surgery 1976; **Med School:** SUNY Hlth Sci Ctr 1971; **Resid:** Orthopaedic Surgery, Albert Einstein Coll Med 1975; **Fellow:** Joint Replacement Surgery, Traveling Fellowship 1977; **Fac Appt:** Assoc Clin Prof OrS, Albert Einstein Coll Med

Hausman, Michael R MD (OrS) - **Spec Exp:** Hand Reconstruction; Elbow Reconstruction; Arthroscopic Surgery; **Hospital:** Mount Sinai Med Ctr (page 98); **Address:** 5 E 98th St, Box 1188, New York, NY 10029-6501; **Phone:** 212-241-1658; **Board Cert:** Orthopaedic Surgery 2000; **Med School:** Yale Univ 1979; **Resid:** Surgery, Yale-New Haven Hosp 1981; Orthopaedic Surgery, Yale-New Haven Hosp 1985; **Fellow:** Hand Surgery, Roosevelt Hosp 1987; **Fac Appt:** Assoc Clin Prof OrS, Mount Sinai Sch Med

Healey, John H MD (OrS) - **Spec Exp:** Bone Tumors; Hip & Knee Replacement in Bone Tumors; Prosthetic Reconstruction; Sarcoma-Soft Tissue; **Hospital:** Meml Sloan Kettering Cancer Ctr (page 109), Hosp For Special Surgery (page 108); **Address:** 1275 York Ave, Ste A-342, New York, NY 10021-6007; **Phone:** 212-639-7610; **Board Cert:** Orthopaedic Surgery 2005; **Med School:** Univ VT Coll Med 1978; **Resid:** Orthopaedic Surgery, Hosp Special Surg 1983; **Fellow:** Orthopaedic Oncology, Meml Sloan Kettering Cancer Ctr 1984; Orthopaedic Surgery, Hosp Special Surgery 1984; **Fac Appt:** Prof OrS, Cornell Univ-Weill Med Coll

Helfet, David L MD (OrS) - **Spec Exp:** Fractures-Complex; Fractures-Non Union; Trauma; **Hospital:** Hosp For Special Surgery (page 108), NY-Presby Hosp (page 100); **Address:** 535 E 70th St, New York, NY 10021; **Phone:** 212-606-1888; **Board Cert:** Orthopaedic Surgery 1984; **Med School:** South Africa 1975; **Resid:** Surgery, Edendale Hosp 1977; Orthopaedic Surgery, Johns Hopkins 1981; **Fellow:** Orthopaedic Surgery, Inselspita Hosp 1981; Orthopaedic Surgery, UCLA Med Ctr 1982; **Fac Appt:** Prof OrS, Cornell Univ-Weill Med Coll

Hotchkiss, Robert MD (OrS) - **Spec Exp:** Hand Surgery; Wrist Surgery; Elbow Reconstruction; **Hospital:** Hosp For Special Surgery (page 108), NY-Presby Hosp (page 100); **Address:** 535 E 70th St, New York, NY 10021; **Phone:** 212-606-1964; **Board Cert:** Orthopaedic Surgery 2000; Hand Surgery 2000; **Med School:** Johns Hopkins Univ 1980; **Resid:** Surgery, Johns Hopkins Hosp 1982; Orthopaedic Surgery, Johns Hopkins Hosp 1985; **Fellow:** Hand Surgery, Union Meml Hosp 1987; **Fac Appt:** Assoc Prof OrS, Cornell Univ-Weill Med Coll

Jaffe, Fredrick F MD (OrS) - **Spec Exp:** Hip Replacement; Knee Replacement; **Hospital:** Hosp For Joint Diseases (page 107); **Address:** 301 E 17th St, Ste 213, New York, NY 10003; **Phone:** 212-598-7605; **Board Cert:** Orthopaedic Surgery 1974; **Med School:** Tufts Univ 1968; **Resid:** Surgery, NY Hosp 1970; Orthopaedic Surgery, Hosp for Joint Diseases 1973; **Fellow:** Reconstructive Surgery, Hosp for Joint Diseases 1974; **Fac Appt:** Clin Prof OrS, NYU Sch Med

Jaffe, William MD (OrS) - **Spec Exp:** Hip Replacement; Knee Replacement; Reconstructive Surgery; **Hospital:** Hosp For Joint Diseases (page 107), NYU Med Ctr (page 102); **Address:** 1095 Park Ave, New York, NY 10128-1154; **Phone:** 212-427-7750; **Board Cert:** Orthopaedic Surgery 1972; **Med School:** Temple Univ 1963; **Resid:** Surgery, Hosp For Joint Diseases 1967; Orthopaedic Surgery, Hosp For Joint Diseases 1970; **Fellow:** Hip Surgery, Centre for Hip Surgery 1971; **Fac Appt:** Clin Prof OrS, NYU Sch Med

Kenan, Samuel MD (OrS) - **Spec Exp:** Bone Tumors; Hip Replacement; Knee Replacement; **Hospital:** Hosp For Joint Diseases (page 107), NYU Med Ctr (page 102); **Address:** 317 E 34th St, Fl 9, New York, NY 10016; **Phone:** 212-684-5511; **Med School:** Israel 1976; **Resid:** Orthopaedic Surgery, Hadassah Univ Hosp 1984; **Fellow:** Orthopaedic Pathology, Hosp for Joint Diseases 1987; **Fac Appt:** Prof OrS, NYU Sch Med

Kiernan, Howard MD (OrS) - **Hospital:** NY-Presby Hosp (page 100); **Address:** 161 Fort Washington Ave, rm 249, New York, NY 10032; **Phone:** 212-305-5241; **Board Cert:** Orthopaedic Surgery 1993; **Med School:** NYU Sch Med 1966; **Resid:** Surgery, Bellevue Hosp Ctr-NYU 1970; Orthopaedic Surgery, Columbia-Presby Med Ctr 1974

Kuflik, Paul MD (OrS) - **Spec Exp:** Spinal Surgery; **Hospital:** Beth Israel Med Ctr - Petrie Division (page 90); **Address:** Spine Institute, 10 Union Square East, Ste 5P, New York, NY 10003-3314; **Phone:** 212-844-8688; **Board Cert:** Orthopaedic Surgery 2000; **Med School:** SUNY Hlth Sci Ctr 1981; **Resid:** Orthopaedic Surgery, Hosp Joint Diseases 1986; **Fellow:** Spinal Surgery, Toronto Genl Hosp 1986; **Fac Appt:** Asst Prof OrS, Albert Einstein Coll Med

Lane, Joseph MD (OrS) - **Spec Exp:** Metabolic Bone Disease; Osteoporosis Spinal Fracture; Osteoporosis Spine-Kyphoplasty; Bone Cancer; **Hospital:** Hosp For Special Surgery (page 108), NY-Presby Hosp (page 100); **Address:** Hosp for Special Surgery, 535 E 70th St, New York, NY 10021; **Phone:** 212-606-1172; **Board Cert:** Orthopaedic Surgery 1998; **Med School:** Harvard Med Sch 1965; **Resid:** Surgery, Hosp Univ Penn 1967; Orthopaedic Surgery, Hosp Univ Penn 1973; **Fac Appt:** Prof OrS, Cornell Univ-Weill Med Coll

Laskin, Richard MD (OrS) - **Spec Exp:** Knee Replacement; Minimally Invasive Surgery; **Hospital:** Hosp For Special Surgery (page 108), NY-Presby Hosp (page 100); **Address:** Hosp for Special Surgery, 535 E 70th St, New York, NY 10021-4872; **Phone:** 212-606-1041; **Board Cert:** Orthopaedic Surgery 1997; **Med School:** NYU Sch Med 1964; **Resid:** Surgery, Bronx Muni Hosp 1966; Orthopaedic Surgery, Albert Einstein Affil Hosps 1971; **Fac Appt:** Prof OrS, Cornell Univ-Weill Med Coll

Lehman, Wallace B MD (OrS) - **Spec Exp:** Clubfoot/Foot Deformities in Children; Hip Disorders-Pediatric; Limb Deformities; Blount's Disease; **Hospital:** Hosp For Joint Diseases (page 107), NYU Med Ctr (page 102); **Address:** Hosp Joint Diseases, Dept Ped Orth Surg, 301 E 17th St, Ste 413, New York, NY 10003-3804; **Phone:** 212-598-6403; **Board Cert:** Orthopaedic Surgery 1966; **Med School:** SUNY Hlth Sci Ctr 1958; **Resid:** Orthopaedic Surgery, Hosp Joint Diseases 1963; **Fac Appt:** Prof OrS, NYU Sch Med

Levy, Howard J MD (OrS) - **Spec Exp:** Knee Surgery; Shoulder Surgery; Sports Medicine; Arthroscopic Surgery; **Hospital:** Lenox Hill Hosp (page 94), Beth Israel Med Ctr - Petrie Division (page 90); **Address:** 130 E 77th St, New York, NY 10021; **Phone:** 212-744-8114; **Board Cert:** Orthopaedic Surgery 1993; Hand Surgery 1994; **Med School:** SUNY Hlth Sci Ctr 1983; **Resid:** Orthopaedic Surgery, Univ Miami Hosp 1989; **Fellow:** Sports Medicine, American Sports Med Inst; Hand Surgery, Roosevelt Hosp

Levy, Roger N MD (OrS) - **Spec Exp:** Arthritis; Hip Replacement; Knee Replacement; Arthroscopic Surgery; **Hospital:** Mount Sinai Med Ctr (page 98); **Address:** 5 E 98th St, Box 1188, New York, NY 10029-6501; **Phone:** 212-241-7080; **Board Cert:** Orthopaedic Surgery 1992; **Med School:** SUNY Downstate 1959; **Resid:** Orthopaedic Surgery, Mount Sinai Hosp 1964; **Fellow:** Orthopaedic Surgery, Mount Sinai Hosp 1965; **Fac Appt:** Prof OrS, Mount Sinai Sch Med

Lonner, Baron S MD (OrS) - **Spec Exp:** Spinal Surgery; Scoliosis; Pediatric Orthopaedic Surgery; **Hospital:** Hosp For Joint Diseases (page 107), Long Island Jewish Med Ctr; **Address:** 212 E 69th St, New York, NY 10021; **Phone:** 212-737-5540; **Board Cert:** Orthopaedic Surgery 1997; **Med School:** Boston Univ 1989; **Resid:** Orthopaedic Surgery, Montefiore Med Ctr 1994; **Fellow:** Orthopaedic Surgery, Hosp Special Surgery 1995; **Fac Appt:** Asst Prof OrS, Columbia P&S

Lubliner, Jerry MD (OrS) - **Spec Exp:** Arthroscopic Surgery; Shoulder Surgery; Knee Surgery; **Hospital:** Hosp For Joint Diseases (page 107), Cabrini Med Ctr (page 374); **Address:** 215 E 73rd St, Ste 1C, New York, NY 10021-3653; **Phone:** 212-249-8200; **Board Cert:** Orthopaedic Surgery 1999; **Med School:** SUNY Hlth Sci Ctr 1980; **Resid:** Orthopaedic Surgery, Hosp Joint Diseases 1985; **Fellow:** Sports Medicine, U West Ont Affil Hosps 1985; **Fac Appt:** Assoc Clin Prof S, NYU Sch Med

Lyden, John MD (OrS) - **Spec Exp:** Joint Replacement; Trauma; **Hospital:** Hosp For Special Surgery (page 108), NY-Presby Hosp (page 100); **Address:** 535 E 70th St, rm 355, New York, NY 10021-4892; **Phone:** 212-606-1126; **Board Cert:** Orthopaedic Surgery 1973; **Med School:** Columbia P&S 1965; **Resid:** Surgery, Roosevelt Hosp 1967; Orthopaedic Surgery, Hosp Special Surg 1972; **Fellow:** Hand Surgery, Hosp Special Surg 1973; **Fac Appt:** Assoc Prof OrS, NY Med Coll

McCann, Peter MD (OrS) - **Spec Exp:** Shoulder Surgery; **Hospital:** Beth Israel Med Ctr - Petrie Division (page 90); **Address:** 10 Union Square E, Ste 3M, New York, NY 10003; **Phone:** 212-870-9764; **Board Cert:** Orthopaedic Surgery 1999; **Med School:** Columbia P&S 1980; **Resid:** Surgery, St Vincent's Hosp 1982; Orthopaedic Surgery, Columbia-Presby Med Ctr 1985; **Fellow:** Shoulder Surgery, Columbia-Presby Med Ctr 1986; **Fac Appt:** Asst Prof OrS, Columbia P&S

McClelland, Shearwood J MD (OrS) - **Spec Exp:** Musculoskeletal Trauma; Joint Replacement; **Hospital:** Harlem Hosp Ctr; **Address:** Harlem Hosp Ctr, Dept Ortho Surgery, 506 Lenox Ave, MLK Fl 9 - rm 9122, New York, NY 10037-1889; **Phone:** 212-939-3510; **Board Cert:** Orthopaedic Surgery 2005; **Med School:** Columbia P&S 1974; **Resid:** Surgery, St. Lukes Hosp 1976; Orthopaedic Surgery, NY Ortho Hosp-Columbia 1979; **Fellow:** Joint Arthroplasty, Ohio State Univ Med Ctr 1982; **Fac Appt:** Assoc Prof OrS, Columbia P&S

Menche, David S MD (OrS) - **Spec Exp:** Knee Surgery; Ligament Reconstruction; Cartilage Damage & Transplant; **Hospital:** Hosp For Joint Diseases (page 107), New York Methodist Hosp (page 479); **Address:** 800A 5th Ave, New York, NY 10021-7215; **Phone:** 212-935-1777; **Board Cert:** Orthopaedic Surgery 1998; **Med School:** NYU Sch Med 1979; **Resid:** Orthopaedic Surgery, Hosp For Joint Diseases 1984; **Fellow:** Sports Medicine, Eastern Hosp 1985; **Fac Appt:** Asst Prof OrS, NYU Sch Med

Mendoza, Francis MD (OrS) - **Spec Exp:** Shoulder & Elbow Surgery; Sports Medicine; **Hospital:** Lenox Hill Hosp (page 94); **Address:** 159 E 74th St, New York, NY 10021; **Phone:** 212-628-9600; **Board Cert:** Orthopaedic Surgery 1984; **Med School:** Columbia P&S 1976; **Resid:** Orthopaedic Surgery, Columbia-Presby Hosp 1981; Surgery, St Luke's-Roosevelt Hosp Ctr 1978; **Fellow:** Orthopaedic Surgery, Columbia-Presby Hosp 1982

Moskovich, Ronald MD (OrS) - **Spec Exp:** Scoliosis; Spinal Surgery; Spondylolisthesis; **Hospital:** Hosp For Joint Diseases (page 107), NYU Med Ctr (page 102); **Address:** 301 E 17th St, Ste 400, New York, NY 10003; **Phone:** 212-598-6622; **Board Cert:** Orthopaedic Surgery 2002; **Med School:** South Africa 1978; **Resid:** Surgery, St George's Hosp 1984; Orthopaedic Surgery, Hosp for Joint Diseases 1988; **Fellow:** Spinal Surgery, UC Davis Med Ctr 1989; Neurological Surgery, Natl Hosp 1989; **Fac Appt:** Asst Prof OrS, NYU Sch Med

Neuwirth, Michael MD (OrS) - **Spec Exp:** Scoliosis; Spinal Surgery; **Hospital:** Beth Israel Med Ctr - Petrie Division (page 90); **Address:** Beth Israel Med Ctr - Spine Institute, 10 Union Square E, Ste 5P, New York, NY 10003-3314; **Phone:** 212-844-8692; **Board Cert:** Orthopaedic Surgery 1980; **Med School:** SUNY Hlth Sci Ctr 1974; **Resid:** Orthopaedic Surgery, Hosp for Joint Diseases 1978; **Fellow:** Spinal Surgery, Rush-Presbyterian Med Ctr 1979; **Fac Appt:** Assoc Clin Prof OrS, NYU Sch Med

Nicholas, Stephen J MD (OrS) - **Spec Exp:** Sports Medicine; Shoulder & Knee Surgery; Arthroscopic Surgery; **Hospital:** Lenox Hill Hosp (page 94); **Address:** 130 E 77th St, New York, NY 10021-1803; **Phone:** 212-737-3301; **Board Cert:** Orthopaedic Surgery 2005; **Med School:** NY Med Coll 1986; **Resid:** Orthopaedic Surgery, Hosp for Special Surgery 1991; **Fellow:** Sports Medicine, Lenox Hill Hosp 1992

O'Leary, Patrick MD (OrS) - **Spec Exp:** Spinal Surgery; **Hospital:** Hosp For Special Surgery (page 108); **Address:** 1015 Madison Ave Fl 4, New York, NY 10021; **Phone:** 212-249-8100; **Board Cert:** Orthopaedic Surgery 1983; **Med School:** Ireland 1968; **Resid:** Surgery, Roosevelt Hosp. 1972; Orthopaedic Surgery, Hosp Spec Surg-Cornell 1975; **Fellow:** Spinal Surgery, Univ Toronto Genl Ortho Hosp 1976; **Fac Appt:** Assoc Clin Prof OrS, Cornell Univ-Weill Med Coll

O'Malley, Martin J MD (OrS) - **Spec Exp:** Foot & Ankle Surgery; **Hospital:** Hosp For Special Surgery (page 108), NY-Presby Hosp (page 100); **Address:** 523 E 72nd St Fl 5, New York, NY 10021; **Phone:** 212-606-1579; **Board Cert:** Orthopaedic Surgery 2006; **Med School:** Case West Res Univ 1986; **Resid:** Orthopaedic Surgery, Tufts-New England Med Ctr 1992; **Fellow:** Foot/Ankle Surgery, Hosp for Special Surg 1993; **Fac Appt:** Assoc Prof OrS, Cornell Univ-Weill Med Coll

Pellicci, Paul MD (OrS) - **Spec Exp:** Hip Replacement-Young Adults; Knee Replacement; **Hospital:** Hosp For Special Surgery (page 108), NY-Presby Hosp (page 100); **Address:** 535 E 70th St, New York, NY 10021-4872; **Phone:** 212-606-1010; **Board Cert:** Orthopaedic Surgery 1982; **Med School:** Cornell Univ-Weill Med Coll 1975; **Resid:** Surgery, New York Hosp 1976; Orthopaedic Surgery, Hosp for Special Surgery 1980; **Fellow:** Joint Replacement Surgery, Brigham & Womens Hosp 1981; **Fac Appt:** Prof OrS, Cornell Univ-Weill Med Coll

Pianka, George MD (OrS) - **Spec Exp:** Hand Surgery; Wrist & Upper Extremity Surgery; **Hospital:** Lenox Hill Hosp (page 94), Phelps Meml Hosp Ctr; **Address:** 159 E 74th St, New York, NY 10021-3226; **Phone:** 212-472-5899; **Board Cert:** Orthopaedic Surgery 2003; Hand Surgery 2003; **Med School:** Univ Conn 1984; **Resid:** Orthopaedic Surgery, Lenox Hill Hosp 1989; **Fellow:** Hand Surgery, Hosp For Joint Diseases 1990

Price, Andrew MD (OrS) - **Spec Exp:** Erbs Palsy/Brachial Plexus Injuries; Cerebral Palsy; Fractures-Pediatric; Trauma-Pediatric; **Hospital:** NYU Med Ctr (page 102), St Luke's - Roosevelt Hosp Ctr - Roosevelt Div (page 90); **Address:** 200 W 57th St, Ste 1205, New York, NY 10019; **Phone:** 212-974-7242; **Board Cert:** Orthopaedic Surgery 2001; **Med School:** NYU Sch Med 1980; **Resid:** Orthopaedic Surgery, NYU Med Ctr 1985; **Fellow:** Pediatric Orthopaedic Surgery, Newington Chldns Hosp 1986; **Fac Appt:** Assoc Prof OrS, Columbia P&S

Ranawat, Chitranjan MD (OrS) - **Spec Exp:** Hip Replacement; Knee Replacement; **Hospital:** Lenox Hill Hosp (page 94), Hosp For Special Surgery (page 108); **Address:** 130 E 77th St, FL 11, New York, NY 10021-1851; **Phone:** 212-434-4700; **Board Cert:** Orthopaedic Surgery 1969; **Med School:** India 1958; **Resid:** Surgery, MY Hosp 1963; Orthopaedic Surgery, Albany Med Ctr 1965; **Fellow:** Orthopaedic Surgery, Hosp Special Surg 1969; **Fac Appt:** Prof OrS, Cornell Univ-Weill Med Coll

Rokito, Andrew MD (OrS) - **Spec Exp:** Shoulder & Elbow Surgery; Knee Surgery; Arthroscopic Surgery; Sports Medicine; **Hospital:** Hosp For Joint Diseases (page 107), NYU Med Ctr (page 102); **Address:** 301 E 17th St, Ste 1402, New York, NY 10003; **Phone:** 212-598-6008; **Board Cert:** Orthopaedic Surgery 2005; **Med School:** Boston Univ 1988; **Resid:** Orthopaedic Surgery, Hosp Joint Diseases 1993; **Fellow:** Sports Medicine, Kerlan-Jobe Ortho Clin 1994; **Fac Appt:** Asst Prof OrS, NYU Sch Med

Rose, Donald J MD (OrS) - **Spec Exp:** Dance/Ballet Injuries; Arthroscopic Surgery; Sports Injuries; Hip Surgery; **Hospital:** Hosp For Joint Diseases (page 107), NYU Med Ctr (page 102); **Address:** 1095 Park Ave, New York, NY 10128-1154; **Phone:** 212-427-7750; **Board Cert:** Orthopaedic Surgery 1999; **Med School:** UMDNJ-RW Johnson Med Sch 1980; **Resid:** Surgery, Beth Israel Med Ctr 1981; Orthopaedic Surgery, Hosp for Joint Diseases 1985; **Fellow:** Sports Medicine, Temple Univ Hosp 1986; **Fac Appt:** Assoc Clin Prof OrS, NYU Sch Med

Rose, Howard Anthony MD (OrS) - **Spec Exp:** Sports Medicine; Joint Replacement; **Hospital:** Hosp For Special Surgery (page 108), NY-Presby Hosp (page 100); **Address:** 535 E 70th St, Fl 6th, New York, NY 10021; **Phone:** 212-606-1278; **Board Cert:** Orthopaedic Surgery 1985; **Med School:** Geo Wash Univ 1977; **Resid:** Orthopaedic Surgery, Hosp Special Surg 1982; **Fellow:** Sports Medicine, Brigham & Women's Hospital 1983; Joint Replacement Surgery, Brigham & Women's Hosp 1983; **Fac Appt:** Asst Prof OrS, Cornell Univ-Weill Med Coll

Roye, David MD (OrS) - **Spec Exp:** Pediatric Orthopaedic Surgery; Scoliosis; Hip Disorders-Pediatric; **Hospital:** NY-Presby Hosp (page 100), Greenwich Hosp; **Address:** Morgan Stanley Chlds Hosp NewYork-Presby, 3959 Broadway, 8 North, New York, NY 10032-1559; **Phone:** 212-305-5475; **Board Cert:** Orthopaedic Surgery 1981; **Med School:** Columbia P&S 1975; **Resid:** Orthopaedic Surgery, Columbia-Presby Med Ctr 1979; **Fellow:** Orthopaedic Surgery, Hosp for Sick Chldn 1980; **Fac Appt:** Prof OrS, Columbia P&S

Rozbruch, Jacob D MD (OrS) - **Spec Exp:** Spinal Surgery; Shoulder Surgery; Knee Surgery; **Hospital:** Beth Israel Med Ctr - Petrie Division (page 90); **Address:** 420 E 72nd St, Ste 1J, New York, NY 10021; **Phone:** 212-744-9857; **Board Cert:** Orthopaedic Surgery 1980; Pediatrics 1980; **Med School:** SUNY Buffalo 1973; **Resid:** Surgery, New York Hosp 1976; Orthopaedic Surgery, Hosp for Special Surg 1979; **Fac Appt:** Asst Clin Prof OrS, Albert Einstein Coll Med

Rozbruch, S Robert MD (OrS) - **Spec Exp:** Limb Lengthening; Limb Deformities; Bone Disorders; **Hospital:** Hosp For Special Surgery (page 108), NY-Presby Hosp (page 100); **Address:** 535 E 70th St, New York, NY 10021; **Phone:** 212-606-1415; **Board Cert:** Orthopaedic Surgery 1998; **Med School:** Cornell Univ-Weill Med Coll 1990; **Resid:** Orthopaedic Surgery, Hosp Special Surgery 1995; **Fellow:** Trauma Surgery, Univ Bern Hosp 1997; **Fac Appt:** Asst Prof OrS, Cornell Univ-Weill Med Coll

Salvati, Eduardo A MD (OrS) - **Spec Exp:** Hip Surgery; Hip & Knee Replacement; **Hospital:** Hosp For Special Surgery (page 108); **Address:** Hosp for Spec Surg, 535 E 70th Street, New York, NY 10021-4872; **Phone:** 212-606-1472; **Board Cert:** Orthopaedic Surgery 1972; **Med School:** Argentina 1963; **Resid:** Orthopaedic Surgery, Univ Florence Ortho Clinic 1965; Orthopaedic Surgery, Hosp Buenos Aires 1969; **Fellow:** Hip Surgery, Hosp For Spec Surg 1972; **Fac Appt:** Clin Prof OrS, Cornell Univ-Weill Med Coll

Sandhu, Harvinder S MD (OrS) - **Spec Exp:** Minimally Invasive Surgery; Spinal Disc Replacement; Spinal Surgery; **Hospital:** Hosp For Special Surgery (page 108), NY-Presby Hosp (page 100); **Address:** 535 E 70th St, New York, NY 10021; **Phone:** 212-606-1798; **Board Cert:** Orthopaedic Surgery 1996; **Med School:** Northwestern Univ 1987; **Resid:** Orthopaedic Surgery, Univ Hosp-SUNY Hlth Sci Ctr 1992; **Fellow:** Spinal Surgery, UCLA Med Ctr 1993; **Fac Appt:** Assoc Prof OrS, Cornell Univ-Weill Med Coll

Sands, Andrew MD (OrS) - **Spec Exp:** Foot & Ankle Surgery; Ankle Replacement; Arthroscopic Surgery; Sports Medicine; **Hospital:** St Vincent Cath Med Ctrs - Manhattan (page 375), Kingsbrook Jewish Med Ctr; **Address:** 170 W 12th St, Spellman 7, New York, NY 10011; **Phone:** 212-604-6266; **Board Cert:** Orthopaedic Surgery 2003; **Med School:** NY Med Coll 1985; **Resid:** Orthopaedic Surgery, Lenox Hill Hosp 1990; **Fellow:** Foot/Ankle Surgery, Harborview Med Ctr 1994

Scott, W Norman MD (OrS) - **Spec Exp:** Knee Injuries; Knee Replacement; Sports Medicine; **Hospital:** Lenox Hill Hosp (page 94); **Address:** 210 E 64th St, New York, NY 10021; **Phone:** 212-434-4301; **Board Cert:** Orthopaedic Surgery 1978; **Med School:** Cornell Univ-Weill Med Coll 1972; **Resid:** Surgery, St Luke's-Roosevelt Hosp Ctr 1974; Orthopaedic Surgery, Hosp Special Surg 1977; **Fac Appt:** Clin Prof OrS, Cornell Univ-Weill Med Coll

Scuderi, Giles R MD (OrS) - **Spec Exp:** Knee Replacement; Knee Reconstruction; Knee Injuries/Ligament Surgery; Sports Medicine; **Hospital:** Lenox Hill Hosp (page 94); **Address:** 210 E 64th St Fl 4, New York, NY 10021; **Phone:** 212-434-4310; **Board Cert:** Orthopaedic Surgery 2001; **Med School:** SUNY Downstate 1982; **Resid:** Orthopaedic Surgery, Lenox Hill Hosp 1987; **Fellow:** Knee Surgery, Hosp Special Surgery 1988; **Fac Appt:** Asst Clin Prof OrS, Albert Einstein Coll Med

Sculco, Thomas P MD (OrS) - **Spec Exp:** Hip Replacement; Knee Replacement; Minimally Invasive Surgery; Joint Replacement; **Hospital:** Hosp For Special Surgery (page 108); **Address:** 535 E 70th St, Ste 238, New York, NY 10021-4872; **Phone:** 212-606-1475; **Board Cert:** Orthopaedic Surgery 1976; **Med School:** Columbia P&S 1969; **Resid:** Surgery, Roosevelt Hosp 1971; Orthopaedic Surgery, Hosp For Special Surg 1974; **Fellow:** Orthopaedic Surgery, London Hosp 1975; **Fac Appt:** Prof OrS, Cornell Univ-Weill Med Coll

Sherman, Orrin MD (OrS) - **Spec Exp:** Knee Injuries/ACL; Shoulder Surgery; Sports Medicine; Arthroscopic Surgery; **Hospital:** NYU Med Ctr (page 102), Hosp For Joint Diseases (page 107); **Address:** 530 1st Ave, Ste 8U, New York, NY 10016-6402; **Phone:** 212-263-8961; **Board Cert:** Orthopaedic Surgery 1997; **Med School:** Geo Wash Univ 1978; **Resid:** Orthopaedic Surgery, NYU Med Ctr 1983; **Fellow:** Sports Medicine, So Cal Orthopedic Inst 1984; **Fac Appt:** Assoc Prof OrS, NYU Sch Med

Simon, Sheldon R MD (OrS) - **Spec Exp:** Foot & Ankle Surgery; Pediatric Orthopaedic Surgery; **Hospital:** Beth Israel Med Ctr - Petrie Division (page 90); **Address:** Phillips Ambulatory Care Ctr, 10 Union Square E, Ste 3K, New York, NY 10003; **Phone:** 212-844-6756; **Board Cert:** Orthopaedic Surgery 1966; **Med School:** NYU Sch Med 1966; **Resid:** Surgery, Bellevue Hosp/NYU Med Ctr 1968; Orthopaedic Surgery, Mass General Hosp 1973; **Fac Appt:** Assoc Prof OrS, Albert Einstein Coll Med

Spivak, Jeffrey M MD (OrS) - **Spec Exp:** Spinal Surgery; Scoliosis; Sports Medicine Back Injuries; **Hospital:** Hosp For Joint Diseases (page 107), NYU Med Ctr (page 102); **Address:** Hospital for Joint Diseases, Spine Ctr, 301 E 17th St, Ste 400, New York, NY 10003-3804; **Phone:** 212-598-6696; **Board Cert:** Orthopaedic Surgery 1995; **Med School:** Cornell Univ-Weill Med Coll 1986; **Resid:** Orthopaedic Surgery, Hosp for Joint Diseases 1992; **Fellow:** Spinal Surgery, Thomas Jefferson Univ Hosp 1993; **Fac Appt:** Asst Prof OrS, NYU Sch Med

Strauss, Elton MD (OrS) - **Spec Exp:** Fractures; Hip & Knee Replacement; Osteomyelitis; **Hospital:** Mount Sinai Med Ctr (page 98); **Address:** Mount Sinai Hosp, 5 E 98 St, Box 1188, New York, NY 10029-6501; **Phone:** 212-241-1648; **Board Cert:** Orthopaedic Surgery 1981; **Med School:** Mexico 1974; **Resid:** Orthopaedic Surgery, Albert Einstein Coll Med/Bronx Lebanon Hosp 1979; **Fac Appt:** Assoc Clin Prof OrS, Mount Sinai Sch Med

Strongwater, Allan MD (OrS) - **Spec Exp:** Pediatric Orthopaedic Surgery; Cerebral Palsy; Deformity Reconstruction; **Hospital:** Hosp For Joint Diseases (page 107), Maimonides Med Ctr (page 96); **Address:** 301 E 17th St, New York, NY 10003; **Phone:** 212-598-6190; **Board Cert:** Orthopaedic Surgery 1997; **Med School:** Rush Med Coll 1978; **Resid:** Orthopaedic Surgery, Yale-New Haven Hosp 1983; Pediatric Orthopaedic Surgery, Hosp Joint Diseases 1984; **Fac Appt:** Clin Prof OrS, SUNY Hlth Sci Ctr

Stuchin, Steven MD (OrS) - **Spec Exp:** Hand Surgery; Arthritis; Hip & Knee Replacement; **Hospital:** Hosp For Joint Diseases (page 107), Lenox Hill Hosp (page 94); **Address:** 301 E 17th St, Ste 1402, New York, NY 10003-3804; **Phone:** 212-598-6708; **Board Cert:** Orthopaedic Surgery 1984; **Med School:** Columbia P&S 1976; **Resid:** Surgery, Roosevelt Hosp 1978; Orthopaedic Surgery, Hosp For Special Surg 1981; **Fellow:** Hand Surgery, Thomas Jefferson Univ Hosp 1982; **Fac Appt:** Assoc Prof OrS, NYU Sch Med

Testa, N Noel MD (OrS) - **Spec Exp:** Hip & Knee Replacement; **Hospital:** Bellevue Hosp Ctr, NYU Med Ctr (page 102); **Address:** Dept Orthopaedics, 462 First Ave, NBV21 West 37, New York, NY 10016-9196; **Phone:** 212-263-6391; **Board Cert:** Orthopaedic Surgery 1974; **Med School:** NY Med Coll 1966; **Resid:** Surgery, St Vincents Hosp 1968; Orthopaedic Surgery, NYU Med Ctr 1973; **Fellow:** Orthopaedic Surgery, New England Baptist Hosp 1974; **Fac Appt:** Clin Prof OrS, NY Med Coll

Turtel, Andrew MD (OrS) - **Spec Exp:** Knee Surgery; Shoulder Surgery; Sports Medicine; **Hospital:** Lenox Hill Hosp (page 94), Beth Israel Med Ctr - Petrie Division (page 90); **Address:** 333 E 56th St, New York, NY 10022-3758; **Phone:** 212-319-6500; **Board Cert:** Orthopaedic Surgery 1994; **Med School:** SUNY Upstate Med Univ 1985; **Resid:** Surgery, SUNY Upstate 1987; Orthopaedic Surgery, LI Jewish Med Ctr 1991; **Fellow:** Sports Medicine, NYU Med Ctr 1992; **Fac Appt:** Assoc Clin Prof OrS, Albert Einstein Coll Med

Ulin, Richard MD (OrS) - **Spec Exp:** Scoliosis; Pediatric Orthopaedic Surgery; **Hospital:** Mount Sinai Med Ctr (page 98); **Address:** 1095 Park Ave, New York, NY 10128-1154; **Phone:** 212-860-0905; **Board Cert:** Orthopaedic Surgery 1992; **Med School:** Columbia P&S 1962; **Resid:** Orthopaedic Surgery, Hosp for Joint Diseases 1967; **Fellow:** Orthopaedic Surgery, Rancho Los Amigos Med Ctr 1968; **Fac Appt:** Clin Prof OrS, Mount Sinai Sch Med

Unis, George MD (OrS) - **Spec Exp:** Sports Medicine; Arthroscopic Surgery; **Hospital:** St Luke's - Roosevelt Hosp Ctr - Roosevelt Div (page 90), Lawrence Hosp Ctr; **Address:** 115 E 61st St, FL 8, New York, NY 10021-8101; **Phone:** 212-688-3710; **Board Cert:** Orthopaedic Surgery 1973; **Med School:** UMDNJ-NJ Med Sch, Newark 1965; **Resid:** Surgery, St Lukes Roosevelt Hosp 1967; Orthopaedic Surgery, St Lukes Roosevelt Hosp 1970; **Fac Appt:** Clin Prof OrS, Columbia P&S

Warren, Russell MD (OrS) - **Spec Exp:** Knee Injuries/Ligament Surgery; Shoulder Reconstruction; Shoulder Replacement; Sports Medicine; **Hospital:** Hosp For Special Surgery (page 108), NY-Presby Hosp (page 100); **Address:** 535 E 70th St, New York, NY 10021-4892; **Phone:** 212-606-1178; **Board Cert:** Orthopaedic Surgery 1974; **Med School:** SUNY Upstate Med Univ 1966; **Resid:** Surgery, St Lukes Hosp 1968; Orthopaedic Surgery, Hosp For Special Surgery 1973; **Fellow:** Shoulder Surgery, Columbia-Presby Med Ctr 1977; **Fac Appt:** Prof OrS, Cornell Univ-Weill Med Coll

Weiner, Lon S MD (OrS) - **Spec Exp:** Trauma; Fractures-Adult/Pediatric; **Hospital:** Lenox Hill Hosp (page 94), Mount Sinai Med Ctr (page 98); **Address:** 130 E 77th St Fl 12, New York, NY 10021; **Phone:** 212-434-4880; **Board Cert:** Orthopaedic Surgery 2001; **Med School:** Mount Sinai Sch Med 1982; **Resid:** Orthopaedic Surgery, Mount Sinai 1987; **Fellow:** Pediatric Orthopaedic Surgery, Hosp for Special Surgery 1988

Westrich, Geoffrey H MD (OrS) - **Spec Exp:** Knee Replacement; Hip Replacement; Joint Replacement; **Hospital:** Hosp For Special Surgery (page 108); **Address:** Hospital for Special Surgery, 535 E 70th St, New York, NY 10021; **Phone:** 212-606-1510; **Board Cert:** Orthopaedic Surgery 1998; **Med School:** Tufts Univ 1990; **Resid:** Orthopaedic Surgery, Hosp for Special Surg 1995; **Fellow:** Trauma, Inselspital 1995; Adult Reconstructive Surgery, Hosp for Special Surg 1996; **Fac Appt:** Assoc Prof OrS, Cornell Univ-Weill Med Coll

Wickiewicz, Thomas L MD (OrS) - **Spec Exp:** Shoulder Surgery; Sports Medicine; Knee Surgery; **Hospital:** Hosp For Special Surgery (page 108); **Address:** 535 E 70th St, New York, NY 10021; **Phone:** 212-606-1450; **Board Cert:** Orthopaedic Surgery 1984; **Med School:** UMDNJ-NJ Med Sch, Newark 1976; **Resid:** Orthopaedic Surgery, Hosp for Special Surg 1981; **Fellow:** Sports Medicine, UCLA Med Ctr 1982; **Fac Appt:** Clin Prof OrS, Cornell Univ-Weill Med Coll

Widmann, Roger F MD (OrS) - **Spec Exp:** Pediatric Orthopaedic Surgery; Scoliosis; Limb Lengthening; Limb Deformities; **Hospital:** Hosp For Special Surgery (page 108); **Address:** 535 E 70th St, New York, NY 10021; **Phone:** 212-606-1325; **Board Cert:** Orthopaedic Surgery 1997; **Med School:** Yale Univ 1989; **Resid:** Orthopaedic Surgery, Mass General Hosp 1994; **Fellow:** Pediatric Orthopaedic Surgery, Children's Hosp 1995; **Fac Appt:** Asst Prof OrS, Cornell Univ-Weill Med Coll

Williams, Riley J MD (OrS) - **Spec Exp:** Cartilage Damage & Transplant; Knee Injuries/Ligament Surgery; Shoulder Arthroscopic Surgery; **Hospital:** Hosp For Special Surgery (page 108), NY-Presby Hosp (page 100); **Address:** Hospital For Special Surgery, 535 E 70th St, New York, NY 10021; **Phone:** 212-606-1855; **Board Cert:** Orthopaedic Surgery 2000; **Med School:** Stanford Univ 1992; **Resid:** Orthopaedic Surgery, Hosp for Special Surgery 1997; **Fellow:** Sports Medicine & Shoulder Surgery, Hosp for Special Surgery 1998; **Fac Appt:** Assoc Prof OrS, Cornell Univ-Weill Med Coll

Windsor, Russell MD (OrS) - **Spec Exp:** Knee Replacement; Hip Replacement; Knee Injuries/Ligament Surgery; **Hospital:** Hosp For Special Surgery (page 108), NY-Presby Hosp (page 100); **Address:** Hosp for Special Surgery, 535 E 70th St, New York, NY 10021; **Phone:** 212-606-1166; **Board Cert:** Orthopaedic Surgery 2006; **Med School:** Georgetown Univ 1978; **Resid:** Orthopaedic Surgery, Hosp Univ Penn 1983; **Fellow:** Knee Surgery, Hosp For Special Surg 1984; **Fac Appt:** Prof OrS, Cornell Univ-Weill Med Coll

Zambetti, George J MD (OrS) - **Spec Exp:** Knee Reconstruction; Shoulder Surgery; Sports Medicine; Arthroscopic Surgery; **Hospital:** St Luke's - Roosevelt Hosp Ctr - Roosevelt Div (page 90); **Address:** 343 W 58th St, New York, NY 10019-1173; **Phone:** 212-506-0236; **Board Cert:** Orthopaedic Surgery 1983; **Med School:** Albany Med Coll 1976; **Resid:** Orthopaedic Surgery, Columbia-Presby Med Ctr 1981

Zuckerman, Joseph MD (OrS) - **Spec Exp:** Shoulder Surgery; Hip Replacement; Knee Replacement; Joint Replacement; **Hospital:** Hosp For Joint Diseases (page 107), NYU Med Ctr (page 102); **Address:** Hosp for Joint Diseases, Dept Ortho Surg, 301 E 17th St, Fl 14, New York, NY 10003; **Phone:** 212-598-6674; **Board Cert:** Orthopaedic Surgery 2004; **Med School:** Med Coll Wisc 1978; **Resid:** Orthopaedic Surgery, Univ WA Med Ctr 1983; **Fellow:** Arthritis Surgery, Brigham & Womans Hosp 1984; Shoulder Surgery, Mayo Clinic 1984; **Fac Appt:** Prof OrS, NYU Sch Med

OTOLARYNGOLOGY

Anand, Vijay MD (Oto) - **Spec Exp:** Sinus Disorders/Surgery; Endoscopic Surgery; Laryngeal Laser Surgery; **Hospital:** NY-Presby Hosp (page 100); **Address:** 205 E 64th St, Ste 101, New York, NY 10021-6635; **Phone:** 212-832-3222; **Board Cert:** Otolaryngology 1983; **Med School:** India 1974; **Resid:** Surgery, Our Lady of Mercy Med Ctr 1978; Otolaryngology, Manhattan EE&T Hosp 1982; **Fellow:** Head and Neck Surgery, Mercy Hosp 1983; **Fac Appt:** Assoc Clin Prof Oto, Cornell Univ-Weill Med Coll

Aviv, Jonathan MD (Oto) - **Spec Exp:** Voice Disorders; Swallowing Disorders; Vocal Cord Disorders; Endoscopy; **Hospital:** NY-Presby Hosp (page 100); **Address:** 16 E 60th St, Ste 470, New York, NY 10022-1002; **Phone:** 212-326-8475; **Board Cert:** Otolaryngology 1990; **Med School:** Columbia P&S 1985; **Resid:** Surgery, Mount Sinai Med Ctr 1987; Otolaryngology, Mount Sinai Med Ctr 1990; **Fellow:** Otolaryngology, Mount Sinai Med Ctr 1991; **Fac Appt:** Prof Oto, Columbia P&S

Blaugrund, Stanley MD (Oto) - **Spec Exp:** Thyroid Disorders; Laryngeal Disorders; Head & Neck Surgery; **Hospital:** Lenox Hill Hosp (page 94); **Address:** 787 Park Ave, New York, NY 10021; **Phone:** 212-879-6219; **Board Cert:** Otolaryngology 1964; **Med School:** Univ Tex SW, Dallas 1955; **Resid:** Surgery, Mount Sinai Hosp 1962; Otolaryngology, Mount Sinai Hosp 1963; **Fellow:** Head and Neck Surgery, St Vincent's Hosp & Med Ctr 1965; **Fac Appt:** Clin Prof Oto, NYU Sch Med

Blitzer, Andrew MD/DDS (Oto) - **Spec Exp:** Voice Disorders; Swallowing Disorders; Nasal & Sinus Surgery; Botox Therapy; **Hospital:** St Luke's - Roosevelt Hosp Ctr - Roosevelt Div (page 90), NY-Presby Hosp (page 100); **Address:** 425 W 59th St Fl 10, New York, NY 10019-1104; **Phone:** 212-262-9500; **Board Cert:** Otolaryngology 1977; **Med School:** Mount Sinai Sch Med 1973; **Resid:** Surgery, Beth Israel Med Ctr 1974; Otolaryngology, Mount Sinai Hosp 1977; **Fac Appt:** Clin Prof Oto, Columbia P&S

Branovan, Daniel Igor MD (Oto) - **Spec Exp:** Sinus Disorders/Surgery; Endoscopic Surgery; Thyroid Surgery; **Hospital:** New York Eye & Ear Infirm (page 110), Beth Israel Med Ctr - Petrie Division (page 90); **Address:** NY Eye & Ear Infirm, Dept Otolaryngology, 310 E 14th St Fl 6, New York, NY 10003-4201; **Phone:** 212-979-4200; **Board Cert:** Otolaryngology 1999; **Med School:** Stanford Univ 1992; **Resid:** Otolaryngology, NY E&E Infirm 1996

Brookler, Kenneth MD (Oto) - **Spec Exp:** Hearing Loss/Dizziness; Hearing Disorders; Meniere's Disease; Otology; **Hospital:** Lenox Hill Hosp (page 94); **Address:** 111 E 77th St, New York, NY 10021-1892; **Phone:** 212-861-6900; **Board Cert:** Otolaryngology 1968; **Med School:** Canada 1962; **Resid:** Surgery, Deer Lodge Hospital 1964; Otolaryngology, Mayo Clinic 1967; **Fellow:** Neurotology, Mayo Clinic 1968

Carew, John F MD (Oto) - **Spec Exp:** Head & Neck Surgery; Head & Neck Cancer; **Hospital:** Lenox Hill Hosp (page 94); **Address:** 969 Park Ave, Ste 1BC, New York, NY 10028; **Phone:** 212-744-1941; **Board Cert:** Otolaryngology 1998; **Med School:** Cornell Univ-Weill Med Coll 1991; **Resid:** Otolaryngology, Manhattan EE&T 1997; **Fellow:** Head and Neck Oncology, Meml Sloan Kettering Cancer Ctr 1998

Caruana, Salvatore MD (Oto) - **Spec Exp:** Head & Neck Cancer; Thyroid & Parathyroid Surgery; Nasal & Sinus Disorders; **Hospital:** St Vincent Cath Med Ctrs - Manhattan (page 375), New York Eye & Ear Infirm (page 110); **Address:** 130 W 12th St, Ste 1D, New York, NY 10011; **Phone:** 212-807-7720; **Board Cert:** Otolaryngology 1996; **Med School:** Mount Sinai Sch Med 1989; **Resid:** Otolaryngology, NY EE Infirm 1995; **Fellow:** Head & Neck Surgical Oncology, Meml Sloan-Kettering Canc Ctr 1997; **Fac Appt:** Asst Prof Oto, NY Med Coll

Chandrasekhar, Sujana MD (Oto) - **Spec Exp:** Balance Disorders; Acoustic Neuroma; Ear Disorders; Cochlear Implants; **Hospital:** Mount Sinai Med Ctr (page 98), New York Eye & Ear Infirm (page 110); **Address:** 364 E 69th St, New York, NY 10021; **Phone:** 212-396-4327; **Board Cert:** Otolaryngology 1993; **Med School:** Mount Sinai Sch Med 1986; **Resid:** Surgery, NYU Med Ctr 1988; Otolaryngology, NYU Med Ctr 1992; **Fellow:** Neurotology, House Ear Clin; **Fac Appt:** Assoc Prof Oto, Mount Sinai Sch Med

Cho, Hyun MD (Oto) - **Spec Exp:** Head & Neck Cancer; Laryngeal Cancer; **Hospital:** St Vincent Cath Med Ctrs - Manhattan (page 375); **Address:** St Vincent Catholic Med Ctr, Spellman 5, 170 W 12th St, New York, NY 10011; **Phone:** 212-888-3784; **Board Cert:** Otolaryngology 1982; **Med School:** South Korea 1964; **Resid:** Surgery, Beth Israel Med Ctr 1972; Otolaryngology, Columbia Presby Med Ctr 1982; **Fellow:** Head and Neck Surgery, Beth Israel Med Ctr 1974; **Fac Appt:** Assoc Prof Oto, Albert Einstein Coll Med

Close, Lanny G MD (Oto) - **Spec Exp:** Skull Base Surgery; Head & Neck Cancer; Sinus Disorders/Surgery; **Hospital:** NY-Presby Hosp (page 100); **Address:** 16 E 60th St, Ste 470, New York, NY 10022; **Phone:** 212-326-8475; **Board Cert:** Otolaryngology 1977; **Med School:** Baylor Coll Med 1972; **Resid:** Surgery, Johns Hopkins Hosp 1974; Otolaryngology, Baylor Affil Hosps 1977; **Fellow:** Head and Neck Surgery, MD Anderson Cancer Ctr 1979; **Fac Appt:** Prof Oto, Columbia P&S

Constantinides, Minas MD (Oto) - **Spec Exp:** Cosmetic Surgery-Face; Rhinoplasty; Facial Reconstruction; **Hospital:** NYU Med Ctr (page 102); **Address:** NYU Med Ctr, Div Facial Plastic Surg, 530 First Ave, Ste 7U, New York, NY 10016-6402; **Phone:** 212-263-5882; **Board Cert:** Otolaryngology 1994; Facial Plastic & Reconstructive Surgery 1997; **Med School:** Columbia P&S 1987; **Resid:** Surgery, Harvard Surg Svcs 1989; Otolaryngology, NYU Medical Center 1993; **Fellow:** Facial Plastic Surgery, Univ Toronto 1994; **Fac Appt:** Asst Prof Oto, NYU Sch Med

Costantino, Peter D MD (Oto) - **Spec Exp:** Skull Base Tumors; Head & Neck Cancer; Craniofacial Surgery/Reconstruction; **Hospital:** St Luke's - Roosevelt Hosp Ctr - Roosevelt Div (page 90), NY-Presby Hosp (page 100); **Address:** 1000 W 10th Ave, Ste 5G-80, New York, NY 10019-1104; **Phone:** 212-523-6756; **Board Cert:** Otolaryngology 1990; Facial Plastic & Reconstructive Surgery 2000; **Med School:** Northwestern Univ 1984; **Resid:** Surgery, Northwestern Meml Hosp 1986; Otolaryngology, Northwestern Meml Hosp 1989; **Fellow:** Head and Neck Surgery, Northwestern Meml Hosp 1990; Skull Base Surgery, Univ Pittsburgh 1991; **Fac Appt:** Prof Oto, Columbia P&S

DeLacure, Mark D MD (Oto) - **Spec Exp:** Head & Neck Cancer; Head & Neck Cancer Reconstruction; Reconstructive Microsurgery; **Hospital:** NYU Med Ctr (page 102), VA Med Ctr - Manhattan; **Address:** 160 E 34th St Fl 9, New York, NY 10016; **Phone:** 212-731-5329; **Board Cert:** Otolaryngology 1992; Plastic Surgery 1996; **Med School:** Univ Fla Coll Med 1986; **Resid:** Surgery, Stanford Univ Med Ctr 1988; Otolaryngology, Yale Univ Sch Med 1991; **Fellow:** Head and Neck Oncology, Meml Sloan-Kettering Cancer Ctr 1992; Plastic Reconstructive Surgery, UCLA Med Ctr 1993; **Fac Appt:** Assoc Clin Prof Oto, NYU Sch Med

Dropkin, Lloyd MD (Oto) - **Hospital:** NY-Presby Hosp (page 100); **Address:** 449 E 68th St, Ste 11, New York, NY 10021-6310; **Phone:** 212-535-9191; **Board Cert:** Otolaryngology 1976; **Med School:** Cornell Univ-Weill Med Coll 1970; **Resid:** Otolaryngology, New York Hosp 1976; **Fac Appt:** Assoc Prof Oto, Cornell Univ-Weill Med Coll

Edelstein, David R MD (Oto) - **Spec Exp:** Nasal & Sinus Disorders; Endoscopic Sinus Surgery; Sleep Disorders/Apnea; **Hospital:** Manhattan Eye, Ear & Throat Hosp, Lenox Hill Hosp (page 94); **Address:** 1421 3rd Ave Fl 4, New York, NY 10028; **Phone:** 212-452-1500; **Board Cert:** Otolaryngology 1985; **Med School:** Boston Univ 1980; **Resid:** Otolaryngology, Mount Sinai Hosp 1984; **Fac Appt:** Clin Prof Oto, Cornell Univ-Weill Med Coll

Gold, Scott MD (Oto) - **Spec Exp:** Endoscopic Sinus Surgery; Sinus Disorders/Surgery; **Hospital:** Beth Israel Med Ctr - Petrie Division (page 90), Mount Sinai Med Ctr (page 98); **Address:** 36A E 36th St, Ste 200, New York, NY 10016-3401; **Phone:** 212-889-8575; **Board Cert:** Otolaryngology 1983; **Med School:** Mount Sinai Sch Med 1979; **Resid:** Otolaryngology, Mount Sinai Med Ctr 1983; **Fac Appt:** Asst Clin Prof Oto, Mount Sinai Sch Med

Green, Robert MD (Oto) - **Spec Exp:** Sinus Disorders/Surgery; Hearing Loss/Tinnitus; Throat Disorders; **Hospital:** Mount Sinai Med Ctr (page 98); **Address:** 12 E 87th St, New York, NY 10128-0524; **Phone:** 212-722-5570; **Board Cert:** Otolaryngology 1981; **Med School:** Harvard Med Sch 1977; **Resid:** Surgery, Mount Sinai Hosp 1978; Otolaryngology, Mount Sinai Hosp 1981; **Fac Appt:** Assoc Clin Prof Oto, Mount Sinai Sch Med

Guida, Robert MD (Oto) - **Spec Exp:** Rhinoplasty; Nasal Surgery; Cosmetic Surgery-Face; **Hospital:** NY-Presby Hosp (page 100), Manhattan Eye, Ear & Throat Hosp; **Address:** 8 E 75th St, New York, NY 10021-2641; **Phone:** 212-871-0900; **Board Cert:** Otolaryngology 1989; Facial Plastic & Reconstructive Surgery ; **Med School:** Hahnemann Univ 1983; **Resid:** Surgery, Graduate Hosp 1985; Otolaryngology, NY Eye & Ear Infirm 1989; **Fellow:** Facial Plastic Surgery, Oregon Hlth Sci Ctr 1990; **Fac Appt:** Assoc Prof Oto, Cornell Univ-Weill Med Coll

Hammerschlag, Paul E MD (Oto) - **Spec Exp:** Cochlear Implants; Meniere's Disease; Otosclerosis; Cholesteatoma; **Hospital:** NYU Med Ctr (page 102), Beth Israel Med Ctr - Petrie Division (page 90); **Address:** 650 First Ave, New York, NY 10016-3240; **Phone:** 212-889-2600; **Board Cert:** Otolaryngology 1978; **Med School:** Albert Einstein Coll Med 1972; **Resid:** Surgery, Virginia Mason Hosp 1974; Otolaryngology, Mass Eye & Ear Infirm 1978; **Fellow:** Otolaryngology, Mass Eye & Ear Infirm-Harvard 1978; **Fac Appt:** Assoc Clin Prof Oto, NYU Sch Med

Har-El, Gady MD (Oto) - **Spec Exp:** Head & Neck Cancer; Sinus Disorders/Surgery; Thyroid & Parathyroid Surgery; Skull Base Surgery; **Hospital:** Long Island Coll Hosp (page 90), Lenox Hill Hosp (page 94); **Address:** 110 E 59th St, New York, NY 10022; **Phone:** 212-223-1333; **Board Cert:** Otolaryngology 1992; **Med School:** Israel 1982; **Resid:** Otolaryngology, SUNY Downstate Med Ctr 1991; **Fac Appt:** Prof Oto, SUNY Hlth Sci Ctr

Hoffman, Ronald MD (Oto) - **Spec Exp:** Cochlear Implants; Balance Disorders; Ear Disorders/Surgery; **Hospital:** Beth Israel Med Ctr - Petrie Division (page 90), New York Eye & Ear Infirm (page 110); **Address:** 10 Union Square East, Ste 4H, New York, NY 10003; **Phone:** 212-844-8778; **Board Cert:** Otolaryngology 1976; **Med School:** Jefferson Med Coll 1971; **Resid:** Otolaryngology, NYU Med Ctr 1976; **Fellow:** Otology & Neurotology, Lenox Hill Hosp 1977; **Fac Appt:** Prof Oto, Albert Einstein Coll Med

Jacobs, Joseph MD (Oto) - **Spec Exp:** Nasal Septal Surgery; Endoscopic Sinus Surgery; Laser Surgery; **Hospital:** NYU Med Ctr (page 102); **Address:** 530 1st Ave, Ste 3C, New York, NY 10016-6402; **Phone:** 212-263-7398; **Board Cert:** Otolaryngology 1978; **Med School:** Albert Einstein Coll Med 1974; **Resid:** Otolaryngology, NYU Med Ctr 1978; **Fellow:** Plastic Surgery, UCLA Med Ctr 1979; **Fac Appt:** Prof Oto, NYU Sch Med

Josephson, Jordan S MD (Oto) - **Spec Exp:** Endoscopic Sinus Surgery; Voice Disorders; Rhinoplasty-Nasal Function Correction; **Hospital:** Manhattan Eye, Ear & Throat Hosp, Lenox Hill Hosp (page 94); **Address:** 111 E 77th St, New York, NY 10021-1802; **Phone:** 212-717-1773; **Board Cert:** Otolaryngology 1988; **Med School:** SUNY Downstate 1983; **Resid:** Otolaryngology, LI Jewish Med Ctr 1988; **Fellow:** Sinus Surgery, Johns Hopkins Hosp 1989

Kimmelman, Charles P MD (Oto) - **Spec Exp:** Snoring/Sleep Apnea; Olfactory Disorders; Nasal & Sinus Disorders; **Hospital:** Manhattan Eye, Ear & Throat Hosp, Lenox Hill Hosp (page 94); **Address:** 45 E 72nd St, New York, NY 10021; **Phone:** 212-717-7262; **Board Cert:** Otolaryngology 1979; **Med School:** Temple Univ 1975; **Resid:** Otolaryngology, Univ Penn Med Ctr 1979; **Fac Appt:** Assoc Clin Prof Oto, Cornell Univ-Weill Med Coll

Kohan, Darius MD (Oto) - **Spec Exp:** Cochlear Implants; Acoustic Neuroma; Hearing Disorders; **Hospital:** NYU Med Ctr (page 102), Beth Israel Med Ctr - Petrie Division (page 90); **Address:** 863 Park Ave, Ste 1E, New York, NY 10021; **Phone:** 212-472-1300; **Board Cert:** Otolaryngology 1990; **Med School:** NYU Sch Med 1984; **Resid:** Surgery, Beth Israel Med Ctr 1986; Otolaryngology, NYU Med Ctr 1990; **Fellow:** Otology, NYU Med Ctr 1991; **Fac Appt:** Assoc Prof Oto, NYU Sch Med

Komisar, Arnold MD/DDS (Oto) - **Spec Exp:** Thyroid & Parathyroid Surgery; Salivary Gland Tumors; Nasal & Sinus Surgery; **Hospital:** Lenox Hill Hosp (page 94), Manhattan Eye, Ear & Throat Hosp; **Address:** 1317 3rd Ave Fl 8, New York, NY 10021-2995; **Phone:** 212-861-8888; **Board Cert:** Otolaryngology 1979; **Med School:** Hahnemann Univ 1975; **Resid:** Surgery, Beth Israel Hosp 1976; Otolaryngology, Mount Sinai Med Ctr 1979; **Fac Appt:** Clin Prof Oto, NYU Sch Med

Kraus, Dennis MD (Oto) - **Spec Exp:** Head & Neck Cancer; Skull Base Tumors; Thyroid & Parathyroid Surgery; **Hospital:** Meml Sloan Kettering Cancer Ctr (page 109); **Address:** 1275 York Ave, Box 285, Memorial Sloan Kettering Cancer Ctr, New York, NY 10021-6007; **Phone:** 212-639-5621; **Board Cert:** Otolaryngology 1990; **Med School:** Univ Rochester 1985; **Resid:** Surgery, Cleveland Clinic Hosp 1987; Otolaryngology, Cleveland Clinic Hosp 1990; **Fellow:** Head and Neck Surgery, Meml Sloan Kettering Cancer Ctr 1991; **Fac Appt:** Prof Oto, Cornell Univ-Weill Med Coll

Krespi, Yosef MD (Oto) - **Spec Exp:** Nasal & Sinus Cancer & Surgery; Sleep Disorders/Apnea; Head & Neck Cancer & Surgery; **Hospital:** St Luke's - Roosevelt Hosp Ctr - Roosevelt Div (page 90); **Address:** 425 W 59th St Fl 10, New York, NY 10019-1128; **Phone:** 212-262-4444; **Board Cert:** Otolaryngology 1981; **Med School:** Israel 1973; **Resid:** Surgery, Mount Sinai Hosp 1976; Otolaryngology, Mount Sinai Hosp 1980; **Fellow:** Surgery, Northwestern Meml Hosp 1981; **Fac Appt:** Clin Prof Oto, Columbia P&S

Krevitt, Lane MD (Oto) - **Spec Exp:** Head & Neck Surgery; Endoscopic Sinus Surgery; Voice Disorders/Professional Voice Care; **Hospital:** Beth Israel Med Ctr - Petrie Division (page 90), St Vincent Cath Med Ctrs - Manhattan (page 375); **Address:** 36A E 36th St, New York, NY 10003; **Phone:** 212-889-8575; **Board Cert:** Otolaryngology 1999; **Med School:** Hahnemann Univ 1993; **Resid:** Surgery, Albert Einstein Univ & Affiliated Hosps 1994; Otolaryngology, Albert Einstein Univ & Affiliated Hosps 1998; **Fellow:** Head & Neck Surgical Oncology, Montefiore Med Ctr 1999; **Fac Appt:** Asst Prof Oto, Albert Einstein Coll Med

Kuhel, William MD (Oto) - **Spec Exp:** Head & Neck Surgery; Thyroid Surgery; Parathyroid Surgery; **Hospital:** NY-Presby Hosp (page 100); **Address:** 520 E 70th St, Ste Star 541, New York, NY 10021; **Phone:** 212-746-2220; **Board Cert:** Otolaryngology 1988; **Med School:** Univ Mich Med Sch 1983; **Resid:** Surgery, St Vincent's Hosp & Med Ctr 1985; Otolaryngology, Indiana Univ 1988; **Fellow:** Head and Neck Surgery, MD Anderson Hosp 1989; **Fac Appt:** Assoc Clin Prof Oto, Cornell Univ-Weill Med Coll

Kuriloff, Daniel MD (Oto) - **Spec Exp:** Thyroid Surgery; Parathyroid Surgery; Minimally Invasive Surgery; Head & Neck Surgery; **Hospital:** St Luke's - Roosevelt Hosp Ctr - Roosevelt Div (page 90), NY-Presby Hosp (page 100); **Address:** 425 W 59th St, Fl 10, New York, NY 10019-1104; **Phone:** 212-262-5555; **Board Cert:** Otolaryngology 1988; **Med School:** Mount Sinai Sch Med 1982; **Resid:** Surgery, Beth Israel Hosp 1984; Otolaryngology, NY Eye & Ear Infirmary 1988; **Fellow:** Head & Neck Surgical Oncology, Univ Mich Med Ctr 1990; **Fac Appt:** Assoc Prof Oto, Columbia P&S

Lalwani, Anil Kumar MD (Oto) - **Spec Exp:** Ear Surgery; Facial Nerve Disorders; Pediatric Otology; **Hospital:** NYU Med Ctr (page 102); **Address:** 530 1st Ave, Ste 3C, New York, NY 10016; **Phone:** 212-263-7167; **Board Cert:** Otolaryngology 1992; **Med School:** Univ Mich Med Sch 1985; **Resid:** Surgery, Duke Univ Med Ctr 1987; Otolaryngology, UCSF Med Ctr 1991; **Fellow:** Skull Base Surgery, UCSF Med Ctr 1992; **Fac Appt:** Prof Oto, NYU Sch Med

Lawson, William MD (Oto) - **Spec Exp:** Sinus Disorders/Surgery; Cosmetic Surgery-Face; Head & Neck Cancer; **Hospital:** Mount Sinai Med Ctr (page 98); **Address:** 5 E 98th St Fl 8, Box 1191, New York, NY 10029-6501; **Phone:** 212-241-9410; **Board Cert:** Otolaryngology 1974; **Med School:** NYU Sch Med 1965; **Resid:** Surgery, Bronx VA Hosp 1967; Otolaryngology, Mount Sinai Hosp 1973; **Fellow:** Otolaryngology, Mount Sinai Hosp 1970; **Fac Appt:** Prof Oto, Mount Sinai Sch Med

Lebovics, Robert MD (Oto) - **Spec Exp:** Head & Neck Inflammatory Disorders; Head & Neck Autoimmune Disease; Head & Neck Infectious Disease; **Hospital:** St Luke's - Roosevelt Hosp Ctr - Roosevelt Div (page 90), Lenox Hill Hosp (page 94); **Address:** 425 W 59th St Fl 10, New York, NY 10019; **Phone:** 212-262-2002; **Board Cert:** Otolaryngology 1988; **Med School:** SUNY Downstate 1982; **Resid:** Surgery, Montefiore-Weiler Einstein Div 1983; Otolaryngology, Montefiore-Weiler Einstein Div 1987

Libin, Jeffrey MD (Oto) - **Spec Exp:** Voice Disorders; Throat Disorders; Nasal & Sinus Disorders; **Hospital:** Mount Sinai Med Ctr (page 98); **Address:** 102 E 78th St, New York, NY 10021; **Phone:** 212-628-3800; **Board Cert:** Otolaryngology 1986; **Med School:** Mount Sinai Sch Med 1980; **Resid:** Surgery, Beth Israel Med Ctr 1983; Otolaryngology, NYU Med Ctr 1986; **Fellow:** Facial Plastic Surgery, Mt Sinai Med Ctr 1987

Linstrom, Christopher MD (Oto) - **Spec Exp:** Cochlear Implants; Acoustic Neuroma; Encephalocele; Cholesteatoma; **Hospital:** New York Eye & Ear Infirm (page 110), St Vincent Cath Med Ctrs - Manhattan (page 375); **Address:** NY Eye & Ear Infirmary, Dept Otolaryngology, 310 E 14th St Fl 6, New York, NY 10003-4201; **Phone:** 212-979-4200; **Board Cert:** Otolaryngology 1987; **Med School:** McGill Univ 1982; **Resid:** Surgery, Geo Wash Med Ctr 1984; Otolaryngology, New York Hosp 1987; **Fellow:** Otology & Neurotology, Michigan Ear Inst 1989; **Fac Appt:** Assoc Prof Oto, NY Med Coll

Markowitz, Arlene MD (Oto) - **Hospital:** NY-Presby Hosp (page 100), Lenox Hill Hosp (page 94); **Address:** 133 E 73rd St, New York, NY 10021; **Phone:** 212-861-9000; **Board Cert:** Otolaryngology 1990; **Med School:** Columbia P&S 1984; **Resid:** Otolaryngology, Columbia-Presby Med Ctr 1990

Nass, Richard MD (Oto) - **Spec Exp:** Sinus Disorders/Surgery; Nasal Surgery; Allergy; **Hospital:** NYU Med Ctr (page 102); **Address:** 1430 2nd Ave, Ste 108, New York, NY 10021; **Phone:** 212-734-4515; **Board Cert:** Otolaryngology 1979; **Med School:** NYU Sch Med 1975; **Resid:** Otolaryngology, NYU-Bellevue Hosp 1979; **Fac Appt:** Assoc Clin Prof Oto, NYU Sch Med

Parisier, Simon C MD (Oto) - **Spec Exp:** Cochlear Implants; Hearing Loss; Ear Infections; **Hospital:** New York Eye & Ear Infirm (page 110), Beth Israel Med Ctr - Petrie Division (page 90); **Address:** NY Eye & Ear Infirmary - Otolaryngology, 310 E 14th St, 6th Fl - Window 5, New York, NY 10003-4297; **Phone:** 212-979-4542; **Board Cert:** Otolaryngology 1967; **Med School:** Boston Univ 1961; **Resid:** Otolaryngology, Mount Sinai Hosp 1966; **Fac Appt:** Prof Oto, NY Med Coll

Pastorek, Norman MD (Oto) - **Spec Exp:** Cosmetic Surgery-Face; Rhinoplasty; Eyelid Surgery; **Hospital:** NY-Presby Hosp (page 100), Manhattan Eye, Ear & Throat Hosp; **Address:** 12 E 88th St, New York, NY 10128-0535; **Phone:** 212-987-4700; **Board Cert:** Otolaryngology 1970; Facial Plastic & Reconstructive Surgery 1991; **Med School:** Univ IL Coll Med 1964; **Resid:** Surgery, Hines VA Hosp 1967; Otolaryngology, Univ Illinois Med Ctr 1969; **Fac Appt:** Clin Prof Oto, Cornell Univ-Weill Med Coll

Pearlman, Steven J MD (Oto) - **Spec Exp:** Cosmetic Surgery-Face; Rhinoplasty; Rhinoplasty Revision; Blepharoplasty; **Hospital:** St Luke's - Roosevelt Hosp Ctr - Roosevelt Div (page 90), Manhattan Eye, Ear & Throat Hosp; **Address:** 521 Park Ave, New York, NY 10021-8140; **Phone:** 212-223-8300; **Board Cert:** Otolaryngology 1987; Facial Plastic & Reconstructive Surgery 1991; **Med School:** Mount Sinai Sch Med 1982; **Resid:** Otolaryngology, Mount Sinai Med Ctr 1987; **Fellow:** Facial Plastic Surgery, St Luke's-Roosevelt Hosp 1988; **Fac Appt:** Assoc Clin Prof Oto, Columbia P&S

Persky, Mark S MD (Oto) - **Spec Exp:** Head & Neck Cancer; Skull Base Tumors; Thyroid Cancer; **Hospital:** Beth Israel Med Ctr - Petrie Division (page 90); **Address:** 10 Union Square East, Ste 4J, New York, NY 10003-3314; **Phone:** 212-844-8648; **Board Cert:** Otolaryngology 1976; **Med School:** SUNY Upstate Med Univ 1972; **Resid:** Otolaryngology, Bellevue Hosp 1976; **Fellow:** Head and Neck Surgery, Beth Israel Med Ctr 1977; **Fac Appt:** Clin Prof Oto, Albert Einstein Coll Med

Pincus, Robert MD (Oto) - **Spec Exp:** Sinus Disorders; Voice Disorders; Endoscopic Sinus Surgery; **Hospital:** Beth Israel Med Ctr - Petrie Division (page 90), St Vincent Cath Med Ctrs - Manhattan (page 375); **Address:** 36A E 36th St, Ste 200, New York, NY 10016-3401; **Phone:** 212-889-8575; **Board Cert:** Otolaryngology 1983; **Med School:** Univ Mich Med Sch 1978; **Resid:** Surgery, Lenox Hill Hosp 1979; Otolaryngology, Mount Sinai Med Ctr 1983; **Fac Appt:** Assoc Prof Oto, NY Med Coll

Pollack, Geoffrey MD (Oto) - **Spec Exp:** Head & Neck Surgery; **Hospital:** St Luke's - Roosevelt Hosp Ctr - Roosevelt Div (page 90); **Address:** 211 Central Park West, New York, NY 10024; **Phone:** 212-873-6175; **Board Cert:** Otolaryngology 1984; **Med School:** Columbia P&S 1979; **Resid:** Otolaryngology, Columbia-Presby Med Ctr 1984

Roland Jr, John Thomas MD (Oto) - **Spec Exp:** Acoustic Neuroma; Cochlear Implants; Neuro-Otology; **Hospital:** NYU Med Ctr (page 102); **Address:** 530 First Avenue, Ste 3C, New York, NY 10016; **Phone:** 212-263-5565; **Board Cert:** Otolaryngology 1993; Neurotology 2004; **Med School:** Temple Univ 1983; **Resid:** Otolaryngology, NYU Med Ctr 1992; **Fellow:** Neurotology, NYU Med Ctr 1985; **Fac Appt:** Assoc Prof Oto, NYU Sch Med

Romo III, Thomas MD (Oto) - **Spec Exp:** Cosmetic Surgery-Face; Rhinoplasty; Ear Reconstruction/Microtia; **Hospital:** Lenox Hill Hosp (page 94), Manhattan Eye, Ear & Throat Hosp; **Address:** 135 E 74th St, New York, NY 10021; **Phone:** 212-288-1500; **Board Cert:** Otolaryngology 1985; Facial Plastic & Reconstructive Surgery 1992; **Med School:** Baylor Coll Med 1979; **Resid:** Otolaryngology, Baylor Hosps 1982; Otolaryngology, New York Eye & Ear Infirm 1984; **Fellow:** Facial Plastic Surgery, New York Eye & Ear Infirm 1985; Facial Plastic Surgery, Tampa General Hosp 1987

Rothstein, Stephen G MD (Oto) - **Spec Exp:** Voice Disorders; Swallowing Disorders; Laser Surgery; **Hospital:** NYU Med Ctr (page 102); **Address:** 530 1st Ave, Ste 3C, New York, NY 10016; **Phone:** 212-263-7505; **Board Cert:** Otolaryngology 1988; **Med School:** Univ Hlth Sci/Chicago Med Sch 1982; **Resid:** Surgery, NYU Med Ctr 1984; Otolaryngology, NYU Med Ctr 1987; **Fellow:** Head and Neck Surgery, NYU Med Ctr 1988; **Fac Appt:** Assoc Clin Prof Oto, NYU Sch Med

Sacks, Steven MD (Oto) - **Spec Exp:** Sinus Surgery; Thyroid & Parathyroid Surgery; Parotid Surgery; **Hospital:** Mount Sinai Med Ctr (page 98); **Address:** 12 E 87th St, New York, NY 10128-0524; **Phone:** 212-722-5570; **Board Cert:** Otolaryngology 1981; **Med School:** Washington Univ, St Louis 1977; **Resid:** Otolaryngology, Mount Sinai Hosp 1981; **Fac Appt:** Asst Clin Prof Oto, Mount Sinai Sch Med

Schaefer, Steven D MD (Oto) - **Spec Exp:** Sinus Disorders/Surgery; Head & Neck Surgery; Endoscopic Surgery; **Hospital:** New York Eye & Ear Infirm (page 110), Beth Israel Med Ctr - Petrie Division (page 90); **Address:** NY Eye & Ear Infirm, Dept Otolaryngology, 310 E 14th St, New York, NY 10003-4201; **Phone:** 212-979-4200; **Board Cert:** Otolaryngology 1978; **Med School:** UC Irvine 1972; **Resid:** Surgery, UCLA Med Ctr 1974; Otolaryngology, Stanford Med Ctr 1977; **Fac Appt:** Prof Oto, NY Med Coll

Schantz, Stimson P MD (Oto) - **Spec Exp:** Head & Neck Surgery; Head & Neck Cancer; **Hospital:** New York Eye & Ear Infirm (page 110), Beth Israel Med Ctr - Petrie Division (page 90); **Address:** 310 E 14th St Fl 6N, New York, NY 10003; **Phone:** 212-979-4535; **Board Cert:** Surgery 2006; **Med School:** Univ Cincinnati 1975; **Resid:** Surgery, Georgetown Univ Med Ctr 1982; Otolaryngology, Univ Illinois Eye & Ear Infirm 1980; **Fellow:** Surgical Oncology, MD Anderson Cancer Ctr 1984; **Fac Appt:** Prof Oto, NY Med Coll

Schley, W Shain MD (Oto) - **Spec Exp:** Nasal & Sinus Disorders; Throat Disorders; Voice Disorders; **Hospital:** NY-Presby Hosp (page 100); **Address:** 449 E 68th St Fl 2 - Ste DS 10, New York, NY 10021; **Phone:** 212-746-2223; **Board Cert:** Otolaryngology 1973; **Med School:** Emory Univ 1966; **Resid:** Surgery, St Luke's-Roosevelt Hosp Ctr 1968; Otolaryngology, New York Hosp 1973; **Fac Appt:** Assoc Clin Prof Oto, Cornell Univ-Weill Med Coll

Schneider, Kenneth L MD (Oto) - **Spec Exp:** Snoring/Sleep Apnea; Nasal & Sinus Disorders; Sleep Disorders/Apnea; **Hospital:** NYU Med Ctr (page 102); **Address:** 530 1st Ave, Ste 3C, New York, NY 10016-6402; **Phone:** 212-263-7165; **Board Cert:** Otolaryngology 1982; **Med School:** SUNY Hlth Sci Ctr 1978; **Resid:** Otolaryngology, NYU Med Ctr 1982; **Fellow:** Head and Neck Surgery, Montefiore Hosp Med Ctr 1983; **Fac Appt:** Assoc Clin Prof Oto, NYU Sch Med

Sclafani, Anthony P MD (Oto) - **Spec Exp:** Facial Plastic Surgery; Botox Therapy; Rhinoplasty; **Hospital:** New York Eye & Ear Infirm (page 110), Northern Westchester Hosp; **Address:** 1430 Second Ave, Ste 110, New York, NY 10021; **Phone:** 212-979-4534; **Board Cert:** Otolaryngology 1996; Facial Plastic & Reconstructive Surgery 1999; **Med School:** Univ Pennsylvania 1989; **Resid:** Surgery, Beth Israel Med Ctr 1991; Otolaryngology, NY Eye & Ear Infirm 1995; **Fellow:** Facial Plastic Surgery, St Louis Univ 1996; **Fac Appt:** Prof Oto, NY Med Coll

Selesnick, Samuel H MD (Oto) - **Spec Exp:** Acoustic Neuroma; Cholesteatoma; Otosclerosis; **Hospital:** NY-Presby Hosp (page 100), Meml Sloan Kettering Cancer Ctr (page 109); **Address:** 520 E 70th St, Ste 541, New York, NY 10021; **Phone:** 212-746-2282; **Board Cert:** Otolaryngology 1990; **Med School:** NYU Sch Med 1985; **Resid:** Surgery, St Vincent's Med Ctr 1987; Otolaryngology, Manhattan EE&T Hosp 1990; **Fellow:** Skull Base Surgery, UCSF Med Ctr 1991; **Fac Appt:** Prof Oto, Cornell Univ-Weill Med Coll

Shapshay, Stanley M MD (Oto) - **Spec Exp:** Laryngeal Cancer; Vocal Cord Disorders; **Hospital:** Mount Sinai Med Ctr (page 98); **Address:** Mt Sinai Faculty Practice-Otolaryngology, 5 E 98th St Fl 1, Box 1653, New York, NY 10029; **Phone:** 212-241-9425; **Board Cert:** Otolaryngology 1975; **Med School:** Med Coll VA 1968; **Resid:** Surgery, New England Med Ctr 1971; Otolaryngology, Boston Med Ctr 1975; **Fellow:** Surgery, Serafimer Hosp/Karolinska Med Sch 1972

Shemen, Larry MD (Oto) - **Spec Exp:** Head & Neck Cancer; Thyroid Cancer; Parathyroid Cancer; Parathyroid Surgery; **Hospital:** NY Hosp Queens, Manhattan Eye, Ear & Throat Hosp; **Address:** 233 E 69th St, Ste 1D, New York, NY 10021; **Phone:** 212-472-8882; **Board Cert:** Otolaryngology 1983; **Med School:** Canada 1978; **Resid:** Surgery, Cedar-Sinai Med Ctr 1982; Otolaryngology, St Michael's Med Ctr 1983; **Fellow:** Head and Neck Surgery, Meml Sloan-Kettering Cancer Ctr 1984; **Fac Appt:** Asst Clin Prof Oto, Cornell Univ-Weill Med Coll

Shugar, Joel MD (Oto) - **Spec Exp:** Hearing & Balance Disorders; Head & Neck Surgery; Nasal & Sinus Disorders; **Hospital:** Mount Sinai Med Ctr (page 98), Manhattan Eye, Ear & Throat Hosp; **Address:** 55 E 87th St, Ste 1k, New York, NY 10128-1043; **Phone:** 212-289-1731; **Board Cert:** Otolaryngology 1978; **Med School:** McGill Univ 1972; **Resid:** Surgery, Jewish Genl Hosp 1974; Otolaryngology, Mount Sinai 1978; **Fellow:** Otolaryngology, Mount Sinai 1975; **Fac Appt:** Assoc Clin Prof Oto, Mount Sinai Sch Med

Slavit, David H MD (Oto) - **Spec Exp:** Voice Disorders; Nasal & Sinus Disorders; Head & Neck Surgery; Thyroid & Parathyroid Surgery; **Hospital:** Lenox Hill Hosp (page 94), Manhattan Eye, Ear & Throat Hosp; **Address:** 787 Park Ave, New York, NY 10021-3552; **Phone:** 212-517-9177; **Board Cert:** Otolaryngology 1992; **Med School:** Mount Sinai Sch Med 1986; **Resid:** Otolaryngology, Mayo Clinic 1991; **Fac Appt:** Asst Prof Oto, SUNY Hlth Sci Ctr

Storper, Ian MD (Oto) - **Spec Exp:** Skull Base Surgery; Cochlear Implants; Acoustic Neuroma; **Hospital:** NY-Presby Hosp (page 100); **Address:** 180 Fort Washington Ave, New York, NY 10032-3173; **Phone:** 212-305-1906; **Board Cert:** Otolaryngology 1995; **Med School:** Univ Pennsylvania 1988; **Resid:** Otolaryngology, UCLA Med Ctr 1994; **Fellow:** Otology & Neurotology, Ear Foundation 1995; **Fac Appt:** Asst Prof Oto, Columbia P&S

Turk, Jon B MD (Oto) - **Spec Exp:** Facial Reconstruction; Cosmetic Surgery-Face; Nasal Surgery; Rhinoplasty; **Hospital:** Manhattan Eye, Ear & Throat Hosp, N Shore Univ Hosp at Syosset; **Address:** 800A Fifth Ave, Ste 302, New York, NY 10021; **Phone:** 212-421-4845; **Board Cert:** Otolaryngology 1995; Facial Plastic & Reconstructive Surgery 1996; **Med School:** SUNY Downstate 1988; **Resid:** Surgery, Mt Sinai Hosp 1990; Otolaryngology, Mt Sinai Hosp 1993; **Fellow:** Facial Plastic Surgery, Inselspital-Bern 1994; **Fac Appt:** Assoc Clin Prof Oto, SUNY Downstate

Urken, Mark MD (Oto) - **Spec Exp:** Head & Neck Cancer; Head & Neck Cancer Reconstruction; Thyroid & Parathyroid Cancer & Surgery; Salivary Gland Surgery; **Hospital:** Beth Israel Med Ctr - Petrie Division (page 90); **Address:** Inst for Head, Neck & Thyroid Cancer, 10 Union Square E, Ste 5B, New York, NY 10003; **Phone:** 212-844-8775; **Board Cert:** Otolaryngology 1986; **Med School:** Univ VA Sch Med 1981; **Resid:** Otolaryngology, Mount Sinai Hosp 1986; **Fellow:** Microvascular Surgery, Mercy Hosp 1987; **Fac Appt:** Prof Oto, Albert Einstein Coll Med

Volpi, David MD (Oto) - **Spec Exp:** Sinus Disorders; Sleep Disorders; **Hospital:** Lenox Hill Hosp (page 94), New York Eye & Ear Infirm (page 110); **Address:** 262 Central Park West, Ste 1H, New York, NY 10024; **Phone:** 212-873-6036; **Board Cert:** Otolaryngology 1988; **Med School:** Hahnemann Univ 1982; **Resid:** Otolaryngology, NY Eye & Ear Infirm 1988

Waner, Milton MD (Oto) - **Spec Exp:** Pediatric Facial Plastic Surgery; Hemangiomas; Vascular Malformations; **Hospital:** St Luke's - Roosevelt Hosp Ctr - St Luke's Hosp (page 90), Beth Israel Med Ctr - Petrie Division (page 90); **Address:** 1725 York Ave, Ste 2E, New York, NY 10128; **Phone:** 212-987-0979; **Med School:** South Africa 1977; **Resid:** Surgery, Univ of Witwatersrand 1980; Otolaryngology, Univ of Witwatersrand 1984; **Fellow:** Otolaryngology, Univ Cincinnatti Med Ctr 1985

Woo, Peak MD (Oto) - **Spec Exp:** Voice Disorders; Laryngeal Disorders; Laryngeal Cancer; **Hospital:** Mount Sinai Med Ctr (page 98); **Address:** 5 E 98th St Fl 1, Box 1653, New York, NY 10029-6501; **Phone:** 212-241-9425; **Board Cert:** Otolaryngology 1983; **Med School:** Boston Univ 1978; **Resid:** Otolaryngology, Boston Univ 1983; **Fac Appt:** Prof Oto, Mount Sinai Sch Med

PAIN MEDICINE

Dubois, Michel MD (PM) - **Spec Exp:** Pain-Back; **Hospital:** NYU Med Ctr (page 102), Bellevue Hosp Ctr; **Address:** 317 E 34th St, Ste 902, New York, NY 10016; **Phone:** 212-201-1004; **Board Cert:** Anesthesiology 1985; Pain Medicine 1993; **Med School:** France 1974; **Resid:** Anesthesiology, Georgetown Univ Hosp 1980London Hosp 1976; **Fellow:** Pain Medicine, Georgetown Univ Hosp 1983; **Fac Appt:** Prof Anes, NYU Sch Med

Foley, Kathleen M MD (PM) - **Spec Exp:** Palliative Care; Pain-Cancer; **Hospital:** Meml Sloan Kettering Cancer Ctr (page 109); **Address:** Meml Sloan Kettering Cancer Ctr, Pain Care, 1275 York Ave, Box 52, New York, NY 10021-6007; **Phone:** 212-639-7050; **Board Cert:** Neurology 1977; **Med School:** Cornell Univ-Weill Med Coll 1969; **Resid:** Neurology, New York Hosp 1974; **Fellow:** Clinical Genetics, New York Hosp 1971; **Fac Appt:** Prof N, Cornell Univ-Weill Med Coll

Freedman, Gordon MD (PM) - **Spec Exp:** Pain-Back; Pain-Cancer; Reflex Sympathetic Dystrophy (RSD); **Hospital:** Mount Sinai Med Ctr (page 98), Mount Sinai Hosp of Queens (page 98); **Address:** 1540 York Ave, New York, NY 10028; **Phone:** 212-288-2180; **Board Cert:** Anesthesiology 1992; Pain Medicine 2004; **Med School:** Israel 1985; **Resid:** Anesthesiology, Mt Sinai Hosp 1991; **Fellow:** Pain Medicine, Mt Sinai Hosp 1991; **Fac Appt:** Assoc Prof Anes, Mount Sinai Sch Med

Gharibo, Christopher G MD (PM) - **Hospital:** NYU Med Ctr (page 102); **Address:** 317 E 34th St, Ste 902, New York, NY 10016; **Phone:** 212-201-1004; **Board Cert:** Anesthesiology 1997; Pain Medicine 1998; **Med School:** UMDNJ-NJ Med Sch, Newark 1992; **Resid:** Anesthesiology, NYU Med Ctr 1995; **Fellow:** Pain Medicine, Jefferson Univ Hosp 1997

Gusmorino, Paul MD (PM) - **Spec Exp:** Pain-Chronic; Pain Rehabilitation & Psychiatry; **Hospital:** Hosp For Joint Diseases (page 107); **Address:** 301 E 17th St, New York, NY 10003-3804; **Phone:** 212-598-6204; **Board Cert:** Psychiatry 1980; Child & Adolescent Psychiatry 1982; **Med School:** Italy 1974; **Resid:** Psychiatry, Kings County Hosp 1978; **Fellow:** Child & Adolescent Psychiatry, New York Hosp 1980; **Fac Appt:** Asst Clin Prof Psyc, NYU Sch Med

Jain, Subhash MD (PM) - **Spec Exp:** Pain-Cancer; Pain-Pelvic; Reflex Sympathetic Dystrophy (RSD); **Hospital:** NY-Presby Hosp (page 100); **Address:** 360 S 72nd St, Ste C, New York, NY 10021; **Phone:** 212-439-6100; **Board Cert:** Anesthesiology 1994; Pain Medicine 1998; **Med School:** India 1968; **Resid:** Surgery, St Vincent Med Ctr 1977; Anesthesiology, New York Hosp 1979; **Fellow:** Pain Medicine, New York Hosp/Meml Sloan Kettering Cancer Ctr 1980

Kaplan, Ronald MD (PM) - **Spec Exp:** Pain-Chronic; **Hospital:** Beth Israel Med Ctr - Petrie Division (page 90); **Address:** Pain Medicine & Palliative Care, 10 Union Square E, Ste 4K, New York, NY 10003-3314; **Phone:** 212-844-1305; **Board Cert:** Anesthesiology 2003; Pain Medicine 2003; **Med School:** Univ MD Sch Med 1974; **Resid:** Anesthesiology, Univ Maryland Hosp 1978; **Fellow:** Pediatric Anesthesiology, Childrens Hosp 1979; **Fac Appt:** Clin Prof Anes, Albert Einstein Coll Med

Kreitzer, Joel MD (PM) - **Spec Exp:** Pain-Back; Pain-Cancer; Pain-Neuropathic; **Hospital:** Mount Sinai Med Ctr (page 98), Mount Sinai Hosp of Queens (page 98); **Address:** Upper East Side Pain Medicine, 1540 York Ave, New York, NY 10028; **Phone:** 212-288-2180; **Board Cert:** Anesthesiology 1990; Pain Medicine 2003; **Med School:** Albert Einstein Coll Med 1985; **Resid:** Anesthesiology, Mount Sinai Hosp 1989; **Fellow:** Pain Medicine, Mount Sinai Hosp 1989; **Fac Appt:** Assoc Clin Prof Anes, Mount Sinai Sch Med

Marcus, Norman MD (PM) - **Spec Exp:** Pain-Back; Headache; Sports Injuries; **Hospital:** Lenox Hill Hosp (page 94), NYU Med Ctr (page 102); **Address:** 30 E 40th St, Ste 1100, New York, NY 10016-1201; **Phone:** 212-532-7999; **Board Cert:** Psychiatry 1974; Pain Medicine 1993; **Med School:** SUNY Upstate Med Univ 1967; **Resid:** Psychiatry, Albert Einstein 1971; **Fellow:** Psychosomatic Medicine, Montefiore Hosp Med Ctr 1973; Pain Medicine, Lenox Hill Hosp 1995; **Fac Appt:** Assoc Clin Prof Psyc, NYU Sch Med

Moqtaderi, Farideh MD (PM) - **Spec Exp:** Acupuncture; Pain-Musculoskeletal; Herpetic Neuralgia (Shingles); **Hospital:** Mount Sinai Med Ctr (page 98); **Address:** 520 E 72nd St, Ste 1C, New York, NY 10021-4850; **Phone:** 212-426-9200; **Board Cert:** Anesthesiology 1973; **Med School:** Iran 1966; **Resid:** Anesthesiology, Mount Sinai Hosp 1969; Anesthesiology, Meml Sloan Kettering Hosp 1971; **Fellow:** Pain Medicine, New York Med Coll 1973; **Fac Appt:** Asst Clin Prof Anes, Mount Sinai Sch Med

Ngeow, Jeffrey MD (PM) - **Spec Exp:** Pain-Musculoskeletal-Spine & Neck; Acupuncture; Reflex Sympathetic Dystrophy (RSD); Pain-Neuropathic; **Hospital:** Hosp For Special Surgery (page 108); **Address:** 535 E 70th St, New York, NY 10021-4872; **Phone:** 212-606-1059; **Board Cert:** Anesthesiology 1980; Pain Medicine 2005; **Med School:** England 1971; **Resid:** Anesthesiology, Peter Bent Brigham Hosp 1977; **Fellow:** Pain Medicine, Tufts New England Med Ctr 1978; **Fac Appt:** Assoc Clin Prof Anes, Cornell Univ-Weill Med Coll

Portenoy, Russell MD (PM) - **Spec Exp:** Pain-Cancer; Palliative Care; **Hospital:** Beth Israel Med Ctr - Petrie Division (page 90); **Address:** Beth Israel Med Ctr, Dept Pain Med & Palliative Care, First Ave at 16th St, New York, NY 10003; **Phone:** 212-844-1403; **Board Cert:** Neurology 1985; **Med School:** Univ MD Sch Med 1980; **Resid:** Neurology, Albert Einstein 1984; **Fellow:** Pain Medicine, Meml Sloan-Kettering 1985; **Fac Appt:** Prof N, Albert Einstein Coll Med

Richman, Daniel MD (PM) - **Spec Exp:** Pain-Back & Neck; Complex Regional Pain Syndrome; Reflex Sympathetic Dystrophy (RSD); **Hospital:** Hosp For Special Surgery (page 108); **Address:** 535 E 70th St, New York, NY 10021; **Phone:** 212-606-1768; **Board Cert:** Anesthesiology 1991; Pain Medicine 2005; **Med School:** UMDNJ-NJ Med Sch, Newark 1986; **Resid:** Anesthesiology, Hartford Hosp 1990; **Fellow:** Pain Medicine, Hosp Special Surgery 1991; **Fac Appt:** Assoc Clin Prof Anes, Cornell Univ-Weill Med Coll

Sarno, John E MD (PM) - **Spec Exp:** Pain-Mind/Body Disorder; **Hospital:** NYU Med Ctr (page 102); **Address:** Rusk Institute, Ground Floor, 400 E 34th St, rm 30, New York, NY 10016-4901; **Phone:** 212-263-6035; **Board Cert:** Physical Medicine & Rehabilitation 1965; **Med School:** Columbia P&S 1950; **Resid:** Physical Medicine & Rehabilitation, NYU Med Ctr 1952; Pediatrics, Babies Hosp/Columbia-Presby Med Ctr 1961; **Fellow:** Physical Medicine & Rehabilitation, NYU Med Ctr 1963; **Fac Appt:** Clin Prof PMR, NYU Sch Med

Thomas, Gary MD (PM) - **Spec Exp:** Pain-Neuropathic; Fibromyalgia; Headache; Reflex Sympathetic Dystrophy (RSD); **Hospital:** Cabrini Med Ctr (page 374), New York Methodist Hosp (page 479); **Address:** 233 3rd Ave, Ground FL, New York, NY 10003; **Phone:** 212-995-6495; **Board Cert:** Pain Medicine 1996; Anesthesiology 1996; **Med School:** Mount Sinai Sch Med 1991; **Resid:** Anesthesiology, Mount Sinai Med Ctr 1995; **Fellow:** Pain Medicine, Mount Sinai Med Ctr 1996; **Fac Appt:** Asst Prof Anes, Mount Sinai Sch Med

Waldman, Seth MD (PM) - **Spec Exp:** Pain-Spine; Pain-Neuropathic; Sciatica; **Hospital:** Hosp For Special Surgery (page 108), Burke Rehab Hosp (page 105); **Address:** Hosp For Special Surgery, 535 E 70th St, Ste 640W, New York, NY 10021-4872; **Phone:** 212-606-1686; **Board Cert:** Anesthesiology 1994; Pain Medicine 1994; **Med School:** Albany Med Coll 1988; **Resid:** Internal Medicine, Beth Israel Med Ctr 1990; Anesthesiology, Beth Israel Hosp 1993; **Fellow:** Pain Medicine, Beth Israel Hosp/Mass Genl Hosp 1994; **Fac Appt:** Asst Clin Prof Anes, Cornell Univ-Weill Med Coll

Weinberger, Michael L MD (PM) - **Spec Exp:** Pain-Cancer; Pain-Back; **Hospital:** NY-Presby Hosp (page 100); **Address:** 630 W 168th St, PH5, rm 500, New York, NY 10032-3720; **Phone:** 212-305-7114; **Board Cert:** Internal Medicine 1986; Anesthesiology 1990; Pain Medicine 2003; **Med School:** Columbia P&S 1983; **Resid:** Internal Medicine, St Vincent's Hosp 1986; Anesthesiology, Columbia-Presby Med Ctr 1989; **Fellow:** Pain Medicine, Meml Sloan Kettering Cancer Ctr 1990; **Fac Appt:** Assoc Prof Anes, Colombia

PATHOLOGY

Bleiweiss, Ira J MD (Path) - **Spec Exp:** Breast Pathology; Breast Cancer; **Hospital:** Mount Sinai Med Ctr (page 98); **Address:** Mt Sinai Med Ctr, Dept Pathology, 1 Gustave Levy Pl, Box 1194, New York, NY 10029-6504; **Phone:** 212-241-9159; **Board Cert:** Anatomic & Clinical Pathology 1988; **Med School:** West Indies 1984; **Resid:** Pathology, Mt Sinai Med Ctr 1988; **Fellow:** Surgical Pathology, Mt Sinai Med Ctr 1989; Surgical Pathology, Meml-Sloan Kettering Cancer Ctr 1990; **Fac Appt:** Prof Path, Mount Sinai Sch Med

Bullough, Peter MD (Path) - **Spec Exp:** Bone Pathology; **Hospital:** Hosp For Special Surgery (page 108); **Address:** Hospital for Special Surgery, Dept Pathology, 535 E 70th St, rm 241W, New York, NY 10021-4892; **Phone:** 212-606-1341; **Board Cert:** Anatomic Pathology 1963; **Med School:** England 1956; **Resid:** Pathology, Beth Israel Hosp 1961; **Fac Appt:** Prof Path, Cornell Univ-Weill Med Coll

Chadburn, Amy MD (Path) - **Spec Exp:** Hematopathology; Lymph Node Pathology; Bone Marrow Pathology; **Hospital:** NY-Presby Hosp (page 100); **Address:** Dept Path ST715, 525 E 68th St, New York, NY 10021; **Phone:** 212-746-2442; **Board Cert:** Anatomic Pathology 1988; Clinical Pathology 1988; Hematology 1999; **Med School:** Stanford Univ 1983; **Resid:** Pathology, NY Hosp/Cornell Med Ctr 1988; **Fellow:** Hematology, Columbia-Presby Med Ctr 1989; **Fac Appt:** Prof Path, Cornell Univ-Weill Med Coll

Hoda, Syed A MD (Path) - **Spec Exp:** Breast Cancer; Surgical Pathology; **Hospital:** NY-Presby Hosp (page 100); **Address:** 525 E 68th St, 1028 Starr, New York, NY 10021; **Phone:** 212-746-2700; **Board Cert:** Anatomic & Clinical Pathology 2001; Cytopathology 1991; **Med School:** Pakistan 1984; **Resid:** Anatomic & Clinical Pathology, Tulane Univ Affil Hosps 1990; **Fellow:** Cytopathology, Meml Sloan Kettering Cancer Ctr 1991; Pathology, Meml Sloan Kettering Cancer Ctr 1992; **Fac Appt:** Clin Prof Path, Cornell Univ-Weill Med Coll

Knowles, Daniel MD (Path) - **Spec Exp:** Lymph Node Pathology; Bone Marrow Pathology; Lymphoma; **Hospital:** NY-Presby Hosp (page 100); **Address:** Cornell-Weill Med Coll- Dept Pathology, 1300 York Ave, rm C302, New York, NY 10021; **Phone:** 212-746-6464; **Board Cert:** Anatomic Pathology 1978; Immunopathology 1984; **Med School:** Univ Chicago-Pritzker Sch Med 1973; **Resid:** Anatomic Pathology, Columbia-Presby Med Ctr 1978; **Fellow:** Immunopathology, Rockefeller Univ 1977; **Fac Appt:** Prof Path, Cornell Univ-Weill Med Coll

McCormick, Steven MD (Path) - **Spec Exp:** Ophthalmic Pathology; Head & Neck Pathology; **Hospital:** New York Eye & Ear Infirm (page 110); **Address:** 310 E 14th St, New York, NY 10003; **Phone:** 212-979-4156; **Board Cert:** Anatomic Pathology 1988; **Med School:** W VA Univ 1984; **Resid:** Anatomic Pathology, W Va Univ Hosp 1988; **Fellow:** Ophthalmic Pathology, W Va Univ Hosp 1988; **Fac Appt:** Assoc Prof Path, NY Med Coll

McNutt, N Scott MD (Path) - **Spec Exp:** Dermatopathology; **Hospital:** NY-Presby Hosp (page 100); **Address:** 525 E 68th St, Ste F309, New York, NY 10021-4873; **Phone:** 212-746-6434; **Board Cert:** Anatomic Pathology 1973; Dermatopathology 1979; **Med School:** Harvard Med Sch 1966; **Resid:** Pathology, Mass Genl Hosp 1970; **Fellow:** Pathology, Mass Genl Hosp 1972; **Fac Appt:** Prof Path, Cornell Univ-Weill Med Coll

Melamed, Jonathan MD (Path) - **Spec Exp:** Prostate Cancer; Tumor Banking; **Hospital:** NYU Med Ctr (page 102); **Address:** NYU Medical Ctr, Dept Pathology, TH-461, 560 First Ave, New York, NY 10016; **Phone:** 212-263-8927; **Board Cert:** Anatomic & Clinical Pathology 1992; **Med School:** South Africa 1985; **Resid:** Pathology, Lenox Hill Hosp 1991; **Fellow:** Pathology, Meml Sloan Kettering Cancer Ctr 1992; Urologic Pathology, Meml Sloan Kettering Cancer Ctr 1993; **Fac Appt:** Assoc Prof Path, NYU Sch Med

Rosen, Paul P MD (Path) - **Spec Exp:** Breast Pathology; Breast Cancer; **Hospital:** NY-Presby Hosp (page 100); **Address:** New York Presbyterian, Dept Pathology, 525 E 68th St, Starr 1031, New York, NY 10021-4870; **Phone:** 212-746-6482; **Board Cert:** Anatomic Pathology 1998; **Med School:** Columbia P&S 1964; **Resid:** Pathology, Presby Hosp 1966; Pathology, VA Hosp 1968; **Fellow:** Pathology, Meml Hosp Cancer Ctr 1970; **Fac Appt:** Prof Path, Cornell Univ-Weill Med Coll

Schiller, Alan L MD (Path) - **Spec Exp:** Bone & Joint Pathology; Soft Tissue Pathology; Bone Tumors; **Hospital:** Mount Sinai Med Ctr (page 98); **Address:** Mt Sinai Sch Med, Dept Pathology, 1 Gustave Levy Pl, Box 1194, New York, NY 10029-6500; **Phone:** 212-241-8014; **Board Cert:** Anatomic Pathology 1973; **Med School:** Univ Hlth Sci/Chicago Med Sch 1967; **Resid:** Pathology, Mass Genl Hosp 1972; **Fac Appt:** Prof Path, Mount Sinai Sch Med

Travis, William MD (Path) - **Spec Exp:** Pulmonary Pathology; Lung Cancer; Interstitial Lung Disease; **Hospital:** Meml Sloan Kettering Cancer Ctr (page 109); **Address:** Meml Sloan-Kettering Canc Ctr, Dept Path, 1275 York Ave, New York, NY 10021; **Phone:** 212-639-5905; **Board Cert:** Anatomic & Clinical Pathology 1985; **Med School:** Univ Fla Coll Med 1981; **Resid:** Anatomic Pathology, New England Deaconess Hosp 1983; Clinical Pathology, Mayo Clinic 1985; **Fellow:** Surgical Pathology, Mayo Clinic 1986

Wenig, Bruce M MD (Path) - **Spec Exp:** Head & Neck Pathology; Surgical Pathology; **Hospital:** Beth Israel Med Ctr - Petrie Division (page 90); **Address:** Beth Israel Med Ctr, Dept Pathology, First Ave at 16th St, 11 Silver, Rm 10, New York, NY 10003; **Phone:** 212-420-4031; **Board Cert:** Anatomic Pathology 2003; **Med School:** Israel 1981; **Resid:** Pathology, Mt Sinai Med Ctr 1985; Surgical Pathology, Cedars-Sinai Med Ctr 1986; **Fellow:** Head and Neck Pathology, AFIP 1987

PEDIATRIC ALLERGY & IMMUNOLOGY

Ehrlich, Paul M MD (PA&I) - **Spec Exp:** Asthma; Food Allergy; **Hospital:** NYU Med Ctr (page 102), Beth Israel Med Ctr - Petrie Division (page 90); **Address:** 35 E 35th St, Ste 202, New York, NY 10016-3823; **Phone:** 212-685-4225; **Board Cert:** Pediatrics 1975; Allergy & Immunology 1977; **Med School:** NYU Sch Med 1970; **Resid:** Pediatrics, Bellevue Hosp Ctr 1973; **Fellow:** Allergy & Immunology, Walter Reed Army Med Ctr 1976; **Fac Appt:** Assoc Clin Prof Ped, NYU Sch Med

Rappaport, Irwin MD (PA&I) - **Spec Exp:** Asthma; Food Allergy; Allergic Rhinitis; **Hospital:** NY-Presby Hosp (page 100), Lenox Hill Hosp (page 94); **Address:** 9 E 68th St, Ste 1A, New York, NY 10021; **Phone:** 212-777-8407; **Board Cert:** Pediatrics 1967; Allergy & Immunology 1977; **Med School:** Med Coll VA 1962; **Resid:** Internal Medicine, Bellevue Hosp 1963; Pediatrics, NY Hosp 1965; **Fellow:** Allergy & Immunology, St Vincent's Hosp & Med Ctr 1966; **Fac Appt:** Clin Prof Ped, Cornell Univ-Weill Med Coll

Sampson, Hugh MD (PA&I) - **Spec Exp:** Food Allergy; Drug Sensitivity; Eczema; **Hospital:** Mount Sinai Med Ctr (page 98); **Address:** Mt Sinai Sch Med, Dept Peds, 1 Gustave Levy Pl, Box 1198, New York, NY 10029-6500; **Phone:** 212-241-5548; **Board Cert:** Pediatrics 1980; Allergy & Immunology 1981; **Med School:** SUNY Buffalo 1975; **Resid:** Pediatrics, Chldns Meml Hosp 1979; **Fellow:** Allergy & Immunology, Duke Univ Med Ctr 1980; **Fac Appt:** Prof Ped, Mount Sinai Sch Med

Sicherer, Scott H MD (PA&I) - **Spec Exp:** Food Allergy; Drug Sensitivity; Eczema; **Hospital:** Mount Sinai Med Ctr (page 98); **Address:** 1 Gustave Levy Pl, Box 1198, New York, NY 10029-6500; **Phone:** 212-241-5548; **Board Cert:** Pediatrics 2001; Allergy & Immunology 1997; **Med School:** Johns Hopkins Univ 1990; **Resid:** Pediatrics, Mt Sinai Hosp 1994; **Fellow:** Allergy & Immunology, Johns Hopkins Hosp 1997; **Fac Appt:** Assoc Prof Ped, Mount Sinai Sch Med

PEDIATRIC CARDIOLOGY

Arnon, Rica MD (PCd) - **Spec Exp:** Heart Disease; **Hospital:** Mount Sinai Med Ctr (page 98), Elmhurst Hosp Ctr; **Address:** 1 Gustave Levy Pl, Box 1201, New York, NY 10029-6504; **Phone:** 212-241-7578; **Board Cert:** Pediatrics 1972; Pediatric Cardiology 1973; **Med School:** SUNY Hlth Sci Ctr 1967; **Resid:** Pediatrics, Univ Hosp 1970; **Fellow:** Pediatric Cardiology, Univ Hosp 1973; **Fac Appt:** Assoc Clin Prof Ped, Mount Sinai Sch Med

Barst, Robyn J MD (PCd) - **Spec Exp:** Pulmonary Hypertension; Congenital Heart Disease; **Hospital:** NY-Presby Hosp (page 100); **Address:** Morgan Stanley Chlds Hosp of NY-Presby, 3959 Broadway BH2-255, New York, NY 10032-1551; **Phone:** 212-305-4436; **Board Cert:** Pediatrics 1980; Pediatric Cardiology 1981; **Med School:** Univ NC Sch Med 1976; **Resid:** Pediatrics, Columbia-Presby 1979; **Fellow:** Pediatric Cardiology, Columbia-Presby 1981; Pediatric Pulmonology, Columbia-Presby 1983; **Fac Appt:** Prof Ped, Columbia P&S

Borg, Morton MD (PCd) - **Spec Exp:** Fetal Echocardiography; **Hospital:** Beth Israel Med Ctr - Petrie Division (page 90), Mount Sinai Med Ctr (page 98); **Address:** Phillips Amb Care Ctr, Dept Peds, 10 Union Square E, Ste 2J, New York, NY 10003-3314; **Phone:** 212-844-8313; **Board Cert:** Pediatrics 1986; Pediatric Cardiology 2002; **Med School:** Albert Einstein Coll Med 1981; **Resid:** Pediatrics, Brookdale Hosp 1984; **Fellow:** Pediatric Cardiology, New York Hosp 1986; **Fac Appt:** Asst Prof Ped, Albert Einstein Coll Med

Cooper, Rubin MD (PCd) - **Spec Exp:** Congenital Heart Disease; Rheumatic Heart Disease; Kawasaki Disease; **Hospital:** NY-Presby Hosp (page 100), NY Hosp Queens; **Address:** 525 E 68th St, Ste F695B, New York, NY 10021; **Phone:** 212-746-3561; **Board Cert:** Pediatrics 1976; Pediatric Cardiology 1979; **Med School:** NY Med Coll 1971; **Resid:** Pediatrics, Strong Meml Hosp 1973; **Fellow:** Pediatric Cardiology, Strong Meml Hosp 1975; **Fac Appt:** Prof Ped, Cornell Univ-Weill Med Coll

Gelb, Bruce MD (PCd) - **Spec Exp:** Transplant Medicine-Heart; **Hospital:** Mount Sinai Med Ctr (page 98); **Address:** 1 Gustave Levy Pl, Box 1201, New York, NY 10029; **Phone:** 212-241-3303; **Board Cert:** Pediatric Cardiology 2006; **Med School:** Univ Rochester 1984; **Resid:** Pediatrics, NY Presby Hosp 1987; **Fellow:** Pediatric Cardiology, Baylor College Med 1991; **Fac Appt:** Prof Ped, Mount Sinai Sch Med

Gersony, Welton Mark MD (PCd) - **Spec Exp:** Congenital Heart Disease; Kawasaki Disease; Rheumatic Heart Disease; **Hospital:** NY-Presby Hosp (page 100); **Address:** Morgan Stanley Chlds Hosp of NY-Presby, 3959 Broadway, Babies 2 North, New York, NY 10032; **Phone:** 212-305-3262; **Board Cert:** Pediatrics 1963; Pediatric Cardiology 1966; **Med School:** SUNY Hlth Sci Ctr 1958; **Resid:** Pediatrics, Babies Chldns Hosp 1961; **Fellow:** Pediatric Cardiology, Harvard/Chldns Hosp 1965; **Fac Appt:** Prof Ped, Columbia P&S

Golinko, Richard J MD (PCd) - **Spec Exp:** Congenital Heart Disease-Adult; Echocardiography; **Hospital:** Mount Sinai Med Ctr (page 98); **Address:** One Gustave Levy Pl, Box 1201, New York, NY 10029-6500; **Phone:** 212-241-8665; **Board Cert:** Pediatrics 1961; Pediatric Cardiology 1962; **Med School:** NY Med Coll 1956; **Resid:** Pediatrics, Chldns Hosp 1959; **Fellow:** Pediatric Cardiology, Chldns Hosp 1960; Pediatric Cardiology, Albert Einstein Coll Med 1962; **Fac Appt:** Clin Prof Ped, Mount Sinai Sch Med

Hellenbrand, William E MD (PCd) - **Spec Exp:** Interventional Cardiology; **Hospital:** NY-Presby Hosp (page 100), Robert Wood Johnson Univ Hosp - New Brunswick (page 853); **Address:** Morgan Stanley Chlds Hosp of NY-Presby, 3959 Broadway Fl 2N - Ste 255, New York, NY 10032; **Phone:** 212-305-6069; **Board Cert:** Pediatrics 1975; Pediatric Cardiology 1977; **Med School:** SUNY Downstate 1970; **Resid:** Pediatrics, Yale-New Haven Hosp 1972; **Fellow:** Pediatric Cardiology, Yale-New Haven Hosp 1976; **Fac Appt:** Prof Ped, Columbia P&S

Hordof, Allan MD (PCd) - **Spec Exp:** Arrhythmias; Cardiac Electrophysiology; **Hospital:** NY-Presby Hosp (page 100); **Address:** Morgan Stanley Chlds Hosp of NY-Presby, 3959 Broadway, Ste 255N, New York, NY 10032; **Phone:** 212-305-4432; **Board Cert:** Pediatrics 1971; Pediatric Cardiology 1973; **Med School:** NYU Sch Med 1966; **Resid:** Pediatrics, Chldns Hosp 1968; Pediatrics, Babies Hosp 1969; **Fellow:** Pediatric Cardiology, Babies Hosp 1973; **Fac Appt:** Prof Ped, Columbia P&S

Hsu, Daphne MD (PCd) - **Spec Exp:** Interventional Cardiology; Heart Failure; **Hospital:** NY-Presby Hosp (page 100); **Address:** Morgan Stanley Chldns Hosp NY-Presbyterian, 3959 Broadway Fl 2 - Ste 221N, New York, NY 10032; **Phone:** 212-342-1560; **Board Cert:** Pediatrics 1988; Pediatric Cardiology 2003; **Med School:** Yale Univ 1982; **Resid:** Pediatrics, Babies & Chldns Hosp 1985; **Fellow:** Pediatric Cardiology, Babies & Chldns Hosp 1988; **Fac Appt:** Asst Prof Ped, Columbia P&S

Parness, Ira A MD (PCd) - **Spec Exp:** Echocardiography; Congenital Heart Disease; Fetal Echocardiography; **Hospital:** Mount Sinai Med Ctr (page 98); **Address:** 1 Gustave Levy Pl, Box 1201, New York, NY 10029-6500; **Phone:** 212-241-8662; **Board Cert:** Pediatrics 1984; Pediatric Cardiology 1985; **Med School:** SUNY Downstate 1979; **Resid:** Pediatrics, Brookdale Hosp 1982; **Fellow:** Pediatric Cardiology, Children's Hosp 1985; **Fac Appt:** Assoc Prof Ped, Mount Sinai Sch Med

Schiller, Myles MD (PCd) - **Spec Exp:** Heart Disease-Congenital & Acquired; Interventional Cardiology; **Hospital:** NY-Presby Hosp (page 100), St Barnabas Hosp - Bronx; **Address:** New York Presbyterian Hosp, 525 E 68th St, New York, NY 10021-4885; **Phone:** 212-746-3561; **Board Cert:** Pediatrics 1978; Pediatric Cardiology 1979; **Med School:** Univ Hlth Sci/Chicago Med Sch 1973; **Resid:** Pediatrics, New York Hosp-Cornell 1975; **Fellow:** Pediatric Cardiology, New York Hosp-Cornell 1977; **Fac Appt:** Assoc Clin Prof Ped, Cornell Univ-Weill Med Coll

Sommer, Robert J MD (PCd) - **Spec Exp:** Congenital Heart Disease; Atrial Septal Defect; Cardiac Catheterization; Congenital Heart Disease; **Hospital:** NY-Presby Hosp (page 100), St Joseph's Regl Med Ctr - Paterson; **Address:** 161 Fort Washington Ave, Interventional Cardiology Fl 5, New York, NY 10032; **Phone:** 212-342-0886; **Board Cert:** Pediatric Cardiology 2005; **Med School:** NYU Sch Med 1985; **Resid:** Pediatrics, Mt. Sinai Med Ctr 1988; **Fellow:** Pediatric Cardiology, Mt Sinai Med Ctr 1991; Interventional Cardiology, Childrens Hosp; **Fac Appt:** Assoc Prof Ped, Columbia P&S

Steinfeld, Leonard MD (PCd) - **Spec Exp:** Echocardiography; Rheumatic Fever; **Hospital:** Mount Sinai Med Ctr (page 98), Queens Hosp Ctr - Jamaica; **Address:** 1 Gustave Levy Pl, New York, NY 10029-6500; **Phone:** 212-241-7210; **Board Cert:** Pediatrics 1960; Pediatric Cardiology 1962; **Med School:** SUNY Downstate 1953; **Resid:** Pediatrics, Mount Sinai Hosp 1956; **Fellow:** Pediatric Cardiology, Mount Sinai Hosp 1959; **Fac Appt:** Prof Ped, Mount Sinai Sch Med

Steinherz, Laurel MD (PCd) - **Spec Exp:** Cardiac Effects of Cancer/Cancer Therapy; **Hospital:** Meml Sloan Kettering Cancer Ctr (page 109), NY-Presby Hosp (page 100); **Address:** 1275 York Ave, New York, NY 10021-6007; **Phone:** 212-639-8103; **Board Cert:** Pediatrics 1976; Pediatric Cardiology 1978; **Med School:** Albert Einstein Coll Med 1970; **Resid:** Pediatrics, Childrens Hosp 1972; **Fellow:** Pediatric Cardiology, New York Hosp/Cornell 1975; **Fac Appt:** Assoc Prof Ped, Cornell Univ-Weill Med Coll

PEDIATRIC CRITICAL CARE MEDICINE

Conway Jr, Edward E MD (PCCM) - **Spec Exp:** Neurologic Critical Care; Respiratory Failure; Head Injury; **Hospital:** Beth Israel Med Ctr - Petrie Division (page 90); **Address:** Beth Israel Med Ctr, Dept Peds, 16th St @ 1st Ave, New York, NY 10003; **Phone:** 212-844-1824; **Board Cert:** Pediatrics 2001; Pediatric Critical Care Medicine 2002; **Med School:** SUNY Hlth Sci Ctr 1984; **Resid:** Pediatrics, Montefiore Med Ctr-Albert Einstein 1988; **Fellow:** Pediatric Critical Care Medicine, Montefiore Med Ctr-Albert Einstein 1990; **Fac Appt:** Prof Ped, Albert Einstein Coll Med

Greenwald, Bruce M MD (PCCM) - **Spec Exp:** Respiratory Failure; Cancer Critical Care; Asthma; **Hospital:** NY-Presby Hosp (page 100), Meml Sloan Kettering Cancer Ctr (page 109); **Address:** 525 E 68th St, rm M508, New York, NY 10021; **Phone:** 212-746-3056; **Board Cert:** Pediatrics 1987; Pediatric Critical Care Medicine 1998; **Med School:** NYU Sch Med 1982; **Resid:** Pediatrics, NYU-Bellevue Hosp Ctr 1986; **Fellow:** Pediatric Critical Care Medicine, New York Hosp-Cornell 1988; **Fac Appt:** Clin Prof Ped, Cornell Univ-Weill Med Coll

PEDIATRIC ENDOCRINOLOGY

David, Raphael MD (PEn) - **Spec Exp:** Growth/Development Disorders; Pubertal Disorders; **Hospital:** NYU Med Ctr (page 102), Bellevue Hosp Ctr; **Address:** 530 1st Ave, Ste 3A, New York, NY 10016; **Phone:** 212-263-6462; **Board Cert:** Pediatrics 1965; Pediatric Endocrinology 1978; **Med School:** Switzerland 1954; **Resid:** Pediatrics, Sinai Hosp 1957; Pediatrics, Johns Hopkins Hosp 1958; **Fellow:** Pediatric Endocrinology, Johns Hopkins Hosp 1961; **Fac Appt:** Prof Ped, NYU Sch Med

Fennoy, Ilene MD (PEn) - **Spec Exp:** Growth/Development Disorders; Diabetes; Klinefelter's Syndrome; Obesity; **Hospital:** NY-Presby Hosp (page 100), Harlem Hosp Ctr; **Address:** Chldns Hosp-NY Presby, Div Ped Endo, 630 W 168th St, PH 5E-522, New York, NY 10032; **Phone:** 212-305-6559; **Board Cert:** Pediatrics 1979; Pediatric Endocrinology 1980; **Med School:** UCSF 1973; **Resid:** Pediatrics, Montefiore Hosp Med Ctr 1975; **Fellow:** Nutrition, Columbia-Presby Med Ctr 1977; Endocrinology, Nat Inst Hlth 1979; **Fac Appt:** Assoc Clin Prof Ped, Columbia P&S

Franklin, Bonita MD (PEn) - **Spec Exp:** Diabetes; Growth Disorders; Thyroid Disorders; **Hospital:** NYU Med Ctr (page 102), Mount Sinai Med Ctr (page 98); **Address:** 109 Reade St, New York, NY 10013-3863; **Phone:** 212-732-2401; **Board Cert:** Pediatrics 1982; Pediatric Endocrinology 1983; **Med School:** SUNY Hlth Sci Ctr 1976; **Resid:** Pediatrics, Bronx Muni Hosp 1978; Pediatrics, Mount Sinai Hosp 1979; **Fellow:** Pediatric Endocrinology, Mt Sinai Hosp 1981; **Fac Appt:** Assoc Clin Prof Ped, NYU Sch Med

Greig, Fenella MD (PEn) - **Spec Exp:** Thyroid Disorders; Diabetes; **Hospital:** Mount Sinai Med Ctr (page 98); **Address:** 5 E 98th St Fl 8th, Box 1616, New York, NY 10029; **Phone:** 212-241-6936; **Board Cert:** Pediatrics 1983; Pediatric Endocrinology 1983; **Med School:** Mount Sinai Sch Med 1976; **Resid:** Pediatrics, Beth Israel Med Ctr 1979; Pediatrics, New York Hosp 1980; **Fellow:** Pediatric Endocrinology, New York Hosp 1982; **Fac Appt:** Assoc Prof Ped, Mount Sinai Sch Med

Kohn, Brenda MD (PEn) - **Spec Exp:** Growth Disorders; Pituitary Disorders; Thyroid Disorders; **Hospital:** NYU Med Ctr (page 102), Lenox Hill Hosp (page 94); **Address:** 530 1st Ave, Ste 3A, New York, NY 10016-6402; **Phone:** 212-263-3185; **Board Cert:** Pediatrics 1981; Pediatric Endocrinology 1983; **Med School:** Albert Einstein Coll Med 1976; **Resid:** Pediatrics, NYU Med Ctr 1979; **Fellow:** Endocrinology, Diabetes & Metabolism, NY-Cornell Med Ctr 1983; **Fac Appt:** Assoc Prof Ped, NYU Sch Med

New, Maria I MD (PEn) - **Spec Exp:** Adrenal Disorders; **Hospital:** Mount Sinai Med Ctr (page 98); **Address:** Mount Sinai Medical Ctr, 1 Gustave Levy Pl, Box 1198, New York, NY 10029; **Phone:** 212-241-8210; **Board Cert:** Pediatrics 1960; **Med School:** Univ Pennsylvania 1954; **Resid:** Pediatrics, New York Hosp 1957; **Fellow:** Pediatric Endocrinology, New York Hosp 1958; Endocrinology, Diabetes & Metabolism, New York Hosp 1964; **Fac Appt:** Prof Ped, Cornell Univ-Weill Med Coll

Oberfield, Sharon E MD (PEn) - **Spec Exp:** Adrenal Disorders; Neuroendocrine Growth Disorders; Growth Disorders; **Hospital:** NY-Presby Hosp (page 100); **Address:** 16 E 60th St, Ste PH5E-522, New York, NY 10022; **Phone:** 212-305-6559; **Board Cert:** Pediatrics 1979; Pediatric Endocrinology 2000; **Med School:** Cornell Univ-Weill Med Coll 1974; **Resid:** Pediatrics, NY Hosp-Cornell 1976; **Fellow:** Pediatric Endocrinology, NY Hosp-Cornell 1979; **Fac Appt:** Prof Ped, Columbia P&S

Rapaport, Robert MD (PEn) - **Spec Exp:** Diabetes; Thyroid Disorders; Puberty Disorders; **Hospital:** Mount Sinai Med Ctr (page 98); **Address:** 1468 Madison Ave, Box 1616, New York, NY 10029; **Phone:** 212-241-6936; **Board Cert:** Pediatrics 1980; Pediatric Endocrinology 1983; **Med School:** SUNY Downstate 1974; **Resid:** Pediatrics, LIJ-Hillside Med Ctr 1977; **Fellow:** Pediatric Endocrinology, St Christopher's Hosp 1978; Pediatric Endocrinology, NY Hosp-Cornell Med Ctr 1980; **Fac Appt:** Prof Ped, Mount Sinai Sch Med

Sklar, Charles A MD (PEn) - **Spec Exp:** Cancer Survivors-Late Effects of Therapy; Growth Disorders in Childhood Cancer; Pituitary Disorders; **Hospital:** Meml Sloan Kettering Cancer Ctr (page 109); **Address:** 1275 York Ave, Box 151, New York, NY 10021; **Phone:** 212-639-8138; **Board Cert:** Pediatrics 1979; Pediatric Endocrinology 1980; **Med School:** USC Sch Med 1974; **Resid:** Pediatrics, Childrens Hosp 1976; **Fellow:** Pediatric Endocrinology, UCSF Med Ctr 1979; **Fac Appt:** Assoc Prof Ped, Cornell Univ-Weill Med Coll

PEDIATRIC GASTROENTEROLOGY

Benkov, Keith J MD (PGe) - **Spec Exp:** Inflammatory Bowel Disease/Crohn's; Liver Disease; Celiac Disease; **Hospital:** Mount Sinai Med Ctr (page 98), Englewood Hosp & Med Ctr (page 760); **Address:** 5 E 98th St Fl 8, Box 1656, New York, NY 10029; **Phone:** 212-241-5415; **Board Cert:** Pediatrics 1984; Pediatric Gastroenterology 1998; **Med School:** Mount Sinai Sch Med 1979; **Resid:** Pediatrics, Mount Sinai Hosp 1982; **Fellow:** Pediatric Gastroenterology, Mount Sinai Hosp 1984; **Fac Appt:** Assoc Prof Ped, Mount Sinai Sch Med

Kazlow, Philip MD (PGe) - **Spec Exp:** Inflammatory Bowel Disease; Celiac Disease; Nutrition; **Hospital:** NY-Presby Hosp (page 100), Valley Hosp (page 762); **Address:** Morgan Stanley Chldns Hosp of NY-Presby, 3959 Broadway, rm BHN 702, New York, NY 10032; **Phone:** 212-305-5903; **Board Cert:** Pediatrics 1985; Pediatric Gastroenterology 1998; **Med School:** Mount Sinai Sch Med 1980; **Resid:** Pediatrics, Mt Sinai Hosp 1984; **Fellow:** Pediatric Gastroenterology, Mt Sinai Hosp 1986; **Fac Appt:** Assoc Clin Prof Ped, Columbia P&S

Levy, Joseph MD (PGe) - **Spec Exp:** Celiac Disease; Irritable Bowel Syndrome; Gastroesophageal Reflux Disease (GERD); Nutrition in Autism; **Hospital:** NY-Presby Hosp (page 100); **Address:** Morgan Stanley Chldns Hosp/NY-Presby, 3959 Broadway Bldg BHN - rm 726, New York, NY 10032; **Phone:** 212-305-5693; **Board Cert:** Pediatrics 1979; Pediatric Gastroenterology 1990; **Med School:** Israel 1973; **Resid:** Pediatrics, Beth Israel Med Ctr 1977; **Fellow:** Research, Columbia-Presby Med Ctr 1975; Pediatric Gastroenterology, Columbia-Presby Med Ctr 1979; **Fac Appt:** Prof Ped, Columbia P&S

Lobritto, Steven MD (PGe) - **Spec Exp:** Hepatitis; Liver Disease; Transplant Medicine-Liver; **Hospital:** NY-Presby Hosp (page 100), NY-Presby Hosp (page 100); **Address:** 622 W 168th St, New York, NY 10032; **Phone:** 212-305-0660; **Board Cert:** Pediatrics 2000; Gastroenterology 1995; Pediatric Gastroenterology 1997; **Med School:** NY Med Coll 1988; **Resid:** Pediatrics, New York Hosp 1992; **Fellow:** Pediatric Gastroenterology, Columbia-Presby Med Ctr 1995

Sockolow, Robbyn MD (PGe) - **Spec Exp:** Constipation; Gastroesophageal Reflux Disease (GERD); Inflammatory Bowel Disease/Crohn's; **Hospital:** NY-Presby Hosp (page 100); **Address:** Weill Med Coll, Dept Peds, 525 E 68th St, New York, NY 10021; **Phone:** 212-746-3520; **Board Cert:** Pediatrics 1998; Pediatric Gastroenterology 2002; **Med School:** NY Med Coll 1986; **Resid:** Pediatrics, Albert Einstein 1989; **Fellow:** Pediatric Gastroenterology, Mount Sinai 1990; Pediatric Gastroenterology, Albert Einstein 1992; **Fac Appt:** Asst Prof Ped, Cornell Univ-Weill Med Coll

Spivak, William MD (PGe) - **Spec Exp:** Inflammatory Bowel Disease/Crohn's; Ulcerative Colitis; Gastroesophageal Reflux Disease (GERD); **Hospital:** NY-Presby Hosp (page 100), Lenox Hill Hosp (page 94); **Address:** 177 E 87th St, Ste 305, New York, NY 10128; **Phone:** 212-369-7700; **Board Cert:** Pediatrics 1981; Pediatric Gastroenterology 2005; **Med School:** Albert Einstein Coll Med 1976; **Resid:** Pediatrics, Jacobi Med Ctr 1979; **Fellow:** Gastroenterology, Childrens Hosp 1982; Research, Brigham & Womens Hosp 1982; **Fac Appt:** Clin Prof Ped, Cornell Univ-Weill Med Coll

Suchy, Frederick J MD (PGe) - **Spec Exp:** Liver Disease; **Hospital:** Mount Sinai Med Ctr (page 98); **Address:** Mount Sinai Medical Ctr, 1 Gustave Levy Pl, Box 1198, New York, NY 10029; **Phone:** 212-241-6933; **Board Cert:** Pediatrics 1982; Pediatric Gastroenterology 2004; **Med School:** Univ Cincinnati 1974; **Resid:** Pediatrics, Chidren's Hosp Med Ctr 1978; **Fellow:** Pediatric Gastroenterology, Chidren's Hosp Med Ctr 1981; **Fac Appt:** Prof Ped, Mount Sinai Sch Med

PEDIATRIC HEMATOLOGY-ONCOLOGY

Aledo, Alexander MD (PHO) - **Spec Exp:** Leukemia; Lymphoma; Bone Tumors; **Hospital:** NY-Presby Hosp (page 100), NY Hosp Queens; **Address:** 525 E 68th St, rm P 695, New York, NY 10021-4870; **Phone:** 212-746-3447; **Board Cert:** Pediatrics 2002; Pediatric Hematology-Oncology 1996; **Med School:** NYU Sch Med 1984; **Resid:** Pediatrics, New York Hosp 1987; **Fellow:** Pediatric Hematology-Oncology, Meml Sloan Kettering Cancer Ctr 1990; **Fac Appt:** Assoc Clin Prof Ped, Cornell Univ-Weill Med Coll

Bussel, James MD (PHO) - **Spec Exp:** Autoimmune Disease; Bleeding/Coagulation Disorders; **Hospital:** NY-Presby Hosp (page 100), Lenox Hill Hosp (page 94); **Address:** 525 E 68th St, Ste P-695, New York, NY 10021-4870; **Phone:** 212-746-3474; **Board Cert:** Pediatrics 1979; Pediatric Hematology-Oncology 1981; **Med School:** Columbia P&S 1975; **Resid:** Pediatrics, Chldns Hosp 1978; **Fellow:** Pediatric Hematology-Oncology, NY Hosp 1981; **Fac Appt:** Prof Ped, Cornell Univ-Weill Med Coll

Cairo, Mitchell S MD (PHO) - **Spec Exp:** Bone Marrow Transplant; Leukemia; Lymphoma; **Hospital:** NY-Presby Hosp (page 100); **Address:** Babies/Chldns Hosp, Columbia Presby Med Ctr, 161 Fort Washington Ave Fl 7 - rm 754, New York, NY 10032; **Phone:** 212-305-8316; **Board Cert:** Pediatrics 1980; Pediatric Hematology-Oncology 1982; **Med School:** UCSF 1976; **Resid:** Pediatrics, UCLA Med Ctr 1978; **Fellow:** Pediatric Hematology-Oncology, Indiana Univ Med Ctr 1981; **Fac Appt:** Prof Ped, Columbia P&S

Carroll, William L MD (PHO) - **Spec Exp:** Pediatric Cancers; Leukemia; **Hospital:** NYU Med Ctr (page 102); **Address:** NYU Med Ctr, Div Ped Hem/Onc, 317 E 34th St Fl 8, New York, NY 10016; **Phone:** 212-263-1079; **Board Cert:** Pediatrics 1984; Pediatric Hematology-Oncology 1987; **Med School:** UC Irvine 1978; **Resid:** Pediatrics, Chldns Hosp Med Ctr 1981; **Fellow:** Pediatric Hematology-Oncology, Stanford Univ 1987; **Fac Appt:** Prof Ped, NYU Sch Med

Dunkel, Ira J MD (PHO) - **Spec Exp:** Retinoblastoma; Brain & Spinal Cord Tumors; Brain Cancer; **Hospital:** Meml Sloan Kettering Cancer Ctr (page 109); **Address:** Meml Sloan-Kettering Cancer Ctr, Dept Peds, 1275 York Ave, rm H-1102, New York, NY 10021; **Phone:** 212-639-2153; **Board Cert:** Pediatric Hematology-Oncology 2000; **Med School:** Duke Univ 1985; **Resid:** Pediatrics, Duke Univ Med Ctr 1988; **Fellow:** Pediatric Hematology-Oncology, Memorial-Sloan Kettering 1992; **Fac Appt:** Asst Prof Ped, Cornell Univ-Weill Med Coll

Garvin, James MD/PhD (PHO) - **Spec Exp:** Bone Marrow Transplant; Brain Tumors; Pediatric Cancers; **Hospital:** NY-Presby Hosp (page 100), St Joseph's Regl Med Ctr - Paterson; **Address:** 161 Fort Washington Ave, rm 718, New York, NY 10032; **Phone:** 212-305-8685; **Board Cert:** Pediatrics 1982; Pediatric Hematology-Oncology 1984; **Med School:** Jefferson Med Coll 1976; **Resid:** Pediatrics, Chldns Hosp 1978; Pediatrics, Middlesex Hosp 1979; **Fellow:** Pediatric Hematology-Oncology, Dana Farber Cancer Inst/Childrens Hosp 1982; **Fac Appt:** Clin Prof Ped, Columbia P&S

Giardina, Patricia MD (PHO) - **Spec Exp:** Thalassemia; **Hospital:** NY-Presby Hosp (page 100); **Address:** 525 E 68th St, rm P 695, New York, NY 10021; **Phone:** 212-746-3400; **Board Cert:** Pediatrics 1974; Pediatric Hematology-Oncology 1974; **Med School:** NY Med Coll 1968; **Resid:** Pediatrics, Lenox Hill Hosp; Pediatrics, NY Hosp-Cornell Med Ctr

Karpatkin, Margaret MD (PHO) - **Spec Exp:** Anemia; Thrombotic Disorders; **Hospital:** NYU Med Ctr (page 102), Bellevue Hosp Ctr; **Address:** 550 1st Ave, New York, NY 10016; **Phone:** 212-263-6428; **Board Cert:** Pediatrics 1980; Pediatric Hematology-Oncology 1980; **Med School:** England 1957; **Resid:** St Georges Hosp 1961; **Fellow:** Hematology, St Georges Hosp 1964; **Fac Appt:** Prof Ped, NYU Sch Med

Kernan, Nancy A MD (PHO) - **Spec Exp:** Leukemia; Immune Deficiency; Bone Marrow Transplant; Stem Cell Transplant; **Hospital:** Meml Sloan Kettering Cancer Ctr (page 109), NY-Presby Hosp (page 100); **Address:** Dept Pediatrics, Bone Marrow Transplant Svc, 1275 York Ave, H1402, New York, NY 10021-6007; **Phone:** 212-639-7250; **Board Cert:** Pediatrics 1983; Pediatric Hematology-Oncology 1984; **Med School:** Cornell Univ-Weill Med Coll 1978; **Resid:** Pediatrics, Children's Hosp Natl Med Ctr 1981; **Fellow:** Pediatric Hematology-Oncology, Meml Sloan Kettering Cancer Ctr 1984; **Fac Appt:** Assoc Prof Ped, Cornell Univ-Weill Med Coll

Kushner, Brian H MD (PHO) - **Spec Exp:** Neuroblastoma; Bone Marrow Transplant; Immunotherapy; **Hospital:** Meml Sloan Kettering Cancer Ctr (page 109); **Address:** 1275 York Ave, rm H1113, New York, NY 10021-6007; **Phone:** 212-639-6793; **Board Cert:** Pediatrics 1983; Pediatric Hematology-Oncology 1987; **Med School:** Johns Hopkins Univ 1976; **Resid:** Pediatrics, Columbia-Presby Med Ctr 1978; Pediatrics, New York Hosp 1979; **Fellow:** Pediatric Hematology-Oncology, Boston Chldns Hosp 1980; Pediatric Hematology-Oncology, Meml Sloan Kettering Cancer Ctr 1986; **Fac Appt:** Prof Ped, Cornell Univ-Weill Med Coll

Meyers, Paul MD (PHO) - **Spec Exp:** Pediatric Cancers; Bone Tumors; Sarcoma; **Hospital:** Meml Sloan Kettering Cancer Ctr (page 109), NY-Presby Hosp (page 100); **Address:** 1275 York Ave, Box 471, New York, NY 10021-6007; **Phone:** 212-639-5952; **Board Cert:** Pediatrics 1978; Pediatric Hematology-Oncology 1978; **Med School:** Mount Sinai Sch Med 1973; **Resid:** Pediatrics, Mt Sinai Hosp 1976; **Fellow:** Pediatric Hematology-Oncology, New York Hosp-Cornell 1979; **Fac Appt:** Prof Ped, Cornell Univ-Weill Med Coll

O'Reilly, Richard MD (PHO) - **Spec Exp:** Bone Marrow Transplant; **Hospital:** Meml Sloan Kettering Cancer Ctr (page 109), NY-Presby Hosp (page 100); **Address:** 1275 York Ave, rm H1409, New York, NY 10021; **Phone:** 212-639-5957; **Board Cert:** Pediatrics 1974; **Med School:** Univ Rochester 1968; **Resid:** Pediatrics, Chldrns Hosp 1972; **Fellow:** Infectious Disease, Chldrns Hosp 1973; **Fac Appt:** Prof Ped, Cornell Univ-Weill Med Coll

Rausen, Aaron MD (PHO) - **Spec Exp:** Leukemia & Lymphoma; Bone Tumors; Retinoblastoma; **Hospital:** NYU Med Ctr (page 102), Lenox Hill Hosp (page 94); **Address:** NYU Medical Ctr, 317 E 34th St Fl 8, New York, NY 10016-4974; **Phone:** 212-263-7144; **Board Cert:** Pediatrics 1960; Pediatric Hematology-Oncology 1974; **Med School:** SUNY Downstate 1954; **Resid:** Pediatrics, Bellevue Hosp 1956; Pediatrics, Mount Sinai 1959; **Fellow:** Hematology, Chldns Hosp 1961; **Fac Appt:** Prof Ped, NYU Sch Med

Steinherz, Peter G MD (PHO) - **Spec Exp:** Leukemia & Lymphoma; Pediatric Cancers; Wilms' Tumor; **Hospital:** Meml Sloan Kettering Cancer Ctr (page 109), NY-Presby Hosp (page 100); **Address:** Memorial Sloan Kettering Cancer Ctr, 1275 York Ave, Box 411, New York, NY 10021; **Phone:** 212-639-7951; **Board Cert:** Pediatrics 1973; Pediatric Hematology-Oncology 1978; **Med School:** Albert Einstein Coll Med 1968; **Resid:** Pediatrics, New York Hosp-Cornell 1971; **Fellow:** Pediatric Hematology-Oncology, New York Hosp-Cornell 1975; **Fac Appt:** Prof Ped, Cornell Univ-Weill Med Coll

Truman, John MD (PHO) - **Spec Exp:** Bleeding/Coagulation Disorders; Anemia; **Hospital:** NY-Presby Hosp (page 100); **Address:** Morgan Stanley Chldns Hosp NY-Presbyterian, 3959 Broadway, CHC 114, New York, NY 10032; **Phone:** 212-305-4248; **Board Cert:** Pediatrics 1968; Pediatric Hematology-Oncology 1974; **Med School:** Univ Toronto 1960; **Resid:** Pediatrics, Mass Genl Hosp 1963; **Fellow:** Hematology, Mass Genl Hosp 1965; **Fac Appt:** Prof Ped, Columbia P&S

Weiner, Michael MD (PHO) - **Spec Exp:** Hodgkin's Disease; Lymphoma; Leukemia; **Hospital:** NY-Presby Hosp (page 100), St Joseph's Regl Med Ctr - Paterson; **Address:** 161 Fort Washington Ave, Irving Pavilion-FL 7, New York, NY 10032-3710; **Phone:** 212-305-9770; **Board Cert:** Pediatrics 1980; Pediatric Hematology-Oncology 1980; **Med School:** SUNY Hlth Sci Ctr 1972; **Resid:** Pediatrics, Montefiore Med Ctr 1974; **Fellow:** Pediatric Hematology-Oncology, NYU Med Ctr 1976; Pediatric Hematology-Oncology, Johns Hopkins Hosp 1977; **Fac Appt:** Prof Ped, Columbia P&S

Wexler, Leonard MD (PHO) - **Spec Exp:** Rhabdomyosarcoma; Bone Cancer; Sarcoma-Soft Tissue; Ewing's Sarcoma; **Hospital:** Meml Sloan Kettering Cancer Ctr (page 109); **Address:** 1275 York Ave, Box 210, New York, NY 10021; **Phone:** 212-639-7990; **Board Cert:** Pediatrics 2000; Pediatric Hematology-Oncology 2000; **Med School:** Boston Univ 1985; **Resid:** Pediatrics, Montefiore Med Ctr 1988; **Fellow:** Pediatric Hematology-Oncology, National Cancer Inst 1991; **Fac Appt:** Assoc Prof Ped, Columbia P&S

PEDIATRIC INFECTIOUS DISEASE

Borkowsky, William MD (PInf) - **Spec Exp:** AIDS/HIV; **Hospital:** NYU Med Ctr (page 102), Bellevue Hosp Ctr; **Address:** 550 1st Ave, Dept Pediatrics, New York, NY 10016; **Phone:** 212-263-6513; **Board Cert:** Pediatrics 1979; Infectious Disease 1979; **Med School:** NYU Sch Med 1979; **Resid:** Pediatrics, Bellevue Hosp Ctr 1975; **Fellow:** Infectious Disease, Bellevue Hosp Ctr-NYU 1978; **Fac Appt:** Prof Ped, NYU Sch Med

Gershon, Anne MD (PInf) - **Spec Exp:** Herpes Simplex; Meningitis; **Hospital:** NY-Presby Hosp (page 100); **Address:** 650 W 168th St, Ste BB4-427, New York, NY 10032; **Phone:** 212-305-9445; **Board Cert:** Pediatrics 1992; Pediatric Infectious Disease 2002; **Med School:** Cornell Univ-Weill Med Coll 1964; **Resid:** Pediatrics, New York Hosp 1968; **Fellow:** Infectious Disease, NYU Med Ctr 1970; Infectious Disease, Oxford Univ 1970; **Fac Appt:** Prof Ped, Columbia P&S

Krasinski, Keith M MD (PInf) - **Spec Exp:** AIDS/HIV; Infections-CNS; **Hospital:** Bellevue Hosp Ctr, NYU Med Ctr (page 102); **Address:** NYU Med Ctr, Dept Peds, 550 1st Ave, New York, NY 10016-6497; **Phone:** 212-263-6427; **Board Cert:** Pediatric Infectious Disease 2002; Pediatrics 1980; **Med School:** Univ IL Coll Med 1976; **Resid:** Pediatrics, Children's Hosp 1979; **Fellow:** Pediatric Infectious Disease, Univ Texas SW Med Ctr 1981; **Fac Appt:** Prof Ped, NYU Sch Med

Saiman, Lisa MD (PInf) - **Spec Exp:** Cystic Fibrosis Infection; Fungal Infections; Hospital Acquired Infections; Tuberculosis; **Hospital:** NY-Presby Hosp (page 100); **Address:** 650 W 168th St Fl PH1 W - rm 470, New York, NY 10032; **Phone:** 212-305-9446; **Board Cert:** Pediatrics 1987; Pediatric Infectious Disease 2002; **Med School:** Albert Einstein Coll Med 1983; **Resid:** Pediatrics, Babies Hosp/NY Presbyterian 1986; **Fellow:** Infectious Disease, Babies Hosp/NY Prebyterian 1989; **Fac Appt:** Assoc Clin Prof Ped, Columbia P&S

PEDIATRIC NEPHROLOGY

Johnson, Valerie MD/PhD (PNep) - **Spec Exp:** Nephrotic Syndrome; Hypertension; Glomerulonephritis; **Hospital:** NY-Presby Hosp (page 100); **Address:** 525 E 68th St, rm N-0008, New York, NY 10021; **Phone:** 212-746-3260; **Board Cert:** Pediatrics 2000; Pediatric Nephrology 1985; **Med School:** Cornell Univ-Weill Med Coll 1977; **Resid:** Pediatrics, Mount Sinai Hosp 1979; **Fellow:** Nephrology, Montefiore Med Ctr 1982; **Fac Appt:** Assoc Clin Prof Ped, Cornell Univ-Weill Med Coll

Nash, Martin MD (PNep) - **Spec Exp:** Nephrotic Syndrome; Kidney Failure; Urinary Abnormalities; **Hospital:** NY-Presby Hosp (page 100); **Address:** Morgan Stanley Chlds Hosp of NY-Presby, 3959 Broadway, rm 701, New York, NY 10032-1537; **Phone:** 212-305-5825; **Board Cert:** Pediatrics 1969; Nephrology 1974; **Med School:** Duke Univ 1964; **Resid:** Internal Medicine, Georgetown Univ Hosp 1965; Pediatrics, Columbia-Presbyterian Hosp 1967; **Fellow:** Pediatric Nephrology, Albert Einstein Coll Med 1971; **Fac Appt:** Clin Prof Ped, Columbia P&S

Saland, Jeffrey M MD (PNep) - **Spec Exp:** Transplant Medicine-Kidney; **Hospital:** Mount Sinai Med Ctr (page 98); **Address:** MT Sinai Medical Ctr, Ped Nephrology, 5 E 98th St Fl 8, New York, NY 10029; **Phone:** 212-241-6187; **Board Cert:** Pediatrics 1998; Pediatric Nephrology 2003; **Med School:** Univ New Mexico 1995; **Resid:** Pediatrics, Chldns Hosp Med Ctr 1998; **Fellow:** Pediatric Nephrology, Mount Sinai Med Ctr 2002; **Fac Appt:** Asst Prof Ped, Mount Sinai Sch Med

Satlin, Lisa M MD (PNep) - **Spec Exp:** Kidney Disease-Hereditary; Hypertension; **Hospital:** Mount Sinai Med Ctr (page 98); **Address:** Mount Sinai Med Ctr, Dept Pediatrics, One Gustave L Levy Pl, Box 1664, New York, NY 10029; **Phone:** 212-241-7148; **Board Cert:** Pediatric Nephrology 1985; Pediatrics 1985; **Med School:** Columbia P&S 1979; **Resid:** Pediatrics, Columbia-Presby Med Ctr 1982; **Fellow:** Nephrology, Montefiore Med Ctr 1986; **Fac Appt:** Prof Ped, Mount Sinai Sch Med

Seigle, Robert MD (PNep) - **Spec Exp:** Glomerulonephritis; Kidney Failure; Kidney Disease; **Hospital:** NY-Presby Hosp (page 100); **Address:** Morgan Stanley Chldns Hosp of NY-Presby, 3959 Broadway, rm 701B, New York, NY 10032; **Phone:** 212-305-5825; **Board Cert:** Pediatrics 1980; Pediatric Nephrology 1982; **Med School:** Columbia P&S 1974; **Resid:** Pediatrics, Columbia-Presby Med Ctr 1978; **Fellow:** Pediatric Nephrology, Montefiore Med Ctr 1981; **Fac Appt:** Asst Prof Ped, Columbia P&S

PEDIATRIC OTOLARYNGOLOGY

April, Max M MD (PO) - **Spec Exp:** Sinus Disorders; Sinus Disorders in Cystic Fibrosis; **Hospital:** Lenox Hill Hosp (page 94), Manhattan Eye, Ear & Throat Hosp; **Address:** New York Otolaryngology Inst, 186 E 76th St, Fl 2, New York, NY 10021-2844; **Phone:** 212-327-3000; **Board Cert:** Otolaryngology 1990; **Med School:** Boston Univ 1985; **Resid:** Otolaryngology, Boston Univ Med Ctr 1990; **Fellow:** Pediatric Otolaryngology, Johns Hopkins Hosp 1991; **Fac Appt:** Assoc Clin Prof Oto, NYU Sch Med

New York (Manhattan)

Dolitsky, Jay MD (PO) - **Spec Exp:** Ear Infections; Neck Masses; **Hospital:** New York Eye & Ear Infirm (page 110), St Vincent Cath Med Ctrs - Manhattan (page 375); **Address:** 404 Park Ave S Fl 12, New York, NY 10016; **Phone:** 212-679-3499; **Board Cert:** Otolaryngology 1990; **Med School:** SUNY Downstate 1981; **Resid:** Otolaryngology, Manhattan EE 1990; **Fellow:** Pediatric Otolaryngology, Children's Hosp 1992; **Fac Appt:** Assoc Prof Oto, NY Med Coll

Haddad Jr, Joseph MD (PO) - **Spec Exp:** Ear Infections; Sinus Disorders; Cleft Palate/Lip; **Hospital:** NY-Presby Hosp (page 100); **Address:** Morgan Stanley Chldns Hosp of NY-Presby, 3959 Broadway, Ste 501N, New York, NY 10032-1559; **Phone:** 212-305-8933; **Board Cert:** Otolaryngology 1988; **Med School:** NYU Sch Med 1983; **Resid:** Surgery, Columbia-Presby Hosp 1985; Otolaryngology, Columbia-Presby Hosp 1988; **Fellow:** Pediatric Otolaryngology, Childrens Hosp 1990; **Fac Appt:** Clin Prof Oto, Columbia P&S

Jones, Jacqueline MD (PO) - **Spec Exp:** Sinus Disorders/Surgery; **Hospital:** NY-Presby Hosp (page 100), Lenox Hill Hosp (page 94); **Address:** 1175 Park Ave, Ste 1A, New York, NY 10128; **Phone:** 212-996-2559; **Board Cert:** Otolaryngology 1989; **Med School:** Cornell Univ-Weill Med Coll 1984; **Resid:** Otolaryngology, Hosp Univ Penn 1989; **Fellow:** Pediatric Otolaryngology, Chldns Hosp 1990; **Fac Appt:** Assoc Prof Oto, Cornell Univ-Weill Med Coll

Ward, Robert MD (PO) - **Spec Exp:** Airway Disorders; Sinus Disorders/Surgery; Choanal Atresia; **Hospital:** NY-Presby Hosp (page 100), Manhattan Eye, Ear & Throat Hosp; **Address:** 186 E 76th St Fl 2, New York, NY 10021; **Phone:** 212-327-3000; **Board Cert:** Otolaryngology 1986; **Med School:** Cornell Univ-Weill Med Coll 1981; **Resid:** Surgery, New York Hosp 1983; Otolaryngology, New York Hosp 1986; **Fellow:** Pediatric Otolaryngology, Chldns Hosp 1986; **Fac Appt:** Assoc Clin Prof Oto, Cornell Univ-Weill Med Coll

PEDIATRIC PULMONOLOGY

Bye, Michael R MD (PPul) - **Spec Exp:** Asthma; Pneumonia; Breathing Disorders; **Hospital:** NY-Presby Hosp (page 100); **Address:** Morgan Stanley Chlds Hosp of NY-Presby, 3959 Broadway Bldg CH Fl 7S, New York, NY 10032-1559; **Phone:** 212-305-5122; **Board Cert:** Pediatrics 1980; Pediatric Pulmonology 2003; **Med School:** SUNY Buffalo 1976; **Resid:** Pediatrics, Childrens Hosp 1979; **Fellow:** Pediatric Pulmonology, Children's Hosp 1982; **Fac Appt:** Prof Ped, Columbia P&S

Dimaio, Mary MD (PPul) - **Spec Exp:** Cystic Fibrosis; Asthma; **Hospital:** NY-Presby Hosp (page 100); **Address:** 1440 York Ave, New York, NY 10021; **Phone:** 212-988-5008; **Board Cert:** Pediatrics 1987; Allergy & Immunology 1999; Pediatric Pulmonology 2000; **Med School:** SUNY Hlth Sci Ctr 1981; **Resid:** Pediatrics, Kings Co Hosp/Downstate 1983; Pediatrics, N Shore Univ Hosp 1985; **Fellow:** Pediatric Pulmonology, Mt Sinai Hosp 1988

Kattan, Meyer MD (PPul) - **Spec Exp:** Asthma; Cystic Fibrosis; **Hospital:** Mount Sinai Med Ctr (page 98), Englewood Hosp & Med Ctr (page 760); **Address:** Mount Sinai Medical Ctr, One Gustave Levy Pl, Box 1202B, New York, NY 10029; **Phone:** 212-241-7788; **Board Cert:** Pediatrics 1980; Pediatric Pulmonology 2003; **Med School:** McGill Univ 1973; **Resid:** Pediatrics, Chldns Hosp 1975; Pediatrics, Hosp for Sick Children 1976; **Fellow:** Pulmonary Disease, Hosp for Sick Children 1978; **Fac Appt:** Prof Ped, Mount Sinai Sch Med

Lamm, Carin MD (PPul) - **Spec Exp:** Sleep Disorders; Asthma; **Hospital:** Mount Sinai Med Ctr (page 98); **Address:** 1 Gustave Levy Pl, Box 1202B, New York, NY 10029-6500; **Phone:** 212-241-9787; **Board Cert:** Pediatrics 1987; Pediatric Pulmonology 2003; **Med School:** NYU Sch Med 1975; **Resid:** Pediatrics, Mount Sinai 1979; **Fellow:** Pediatric Pulmonology, Mount Sinai 1981; **Fac Appt:** Assoc Prof Ped, Mount Sinai Sch Med

Loughlin, Gerald M MD (PPul) - **Spec Exp:** Sleep Disorders/Apnea; Swallowing Disorders; Asthma & Chronic Lung Disease; Breathing Disorders; **Hospital:** NY-Presby Hosp (page 100); **Address:** Cornell Med Coll, Dept Peds, 525 E 68th St, rm M-622, New York, NY 10021; **Phone:** 212-746-4111; **Board Cert:** Pediatrics 1993; Pediatric Pulmonology 2003; **Med School:** Univ Rochester 1973; **Resid:** Pediatrics, Univ Ariz Med Ctr 1975; **Fellow:** Pediatric Pulmonology, Univ Ariz Med Ctr 1977; **Fac Appt:** Prof Ped, Cornell Univ-Weill Med Coll

Mellins, Robert MD (PPul) - **Spec Exp:** Asthma; Lung Disease; **Hospital:** NY-Presby Hosp (page 100); **Address:** Morgan Stanley Chlds Hosp of NY-Presby, 3959 Broadway, CHC746, New York, NY 10032-1559; **Phone:** 212-305-5122; **Board Cert:** Pediatrics 1958; Pediatric Pulmonology 1996; **Med School:** Johns Hopkins Univ 1952; **Resid:** Pediatrics, NY Hosp 1956; Pediatrics, Columbia Presby Med Ctr 1957; **Fellow:** Pulmonary Disease, Columbia Presby Med Ctr 1964; **Fac Appt:** Prof Ped, Columbia P&S

Quittell, Lynne MD (PPul) - **Spec Exp:** Cystic Fibrosis; Asthma; **Hospital:** NY-Presby Hosp (page 100); **Address:** Morgan Stanley Chlds Hosp of NY-Presby, 3959 Broadway, CHC 7, New York, NY 10032-1551; **Phone:** 212-305-5122; **Board Cert:** Pediatrics 1986; Pediatric Pulmonology 1997; **Med School:** Israel 1981; **Resid:** Pediatrics, Schneider Chldns Hosp 1984; **Fellow:** Pediatric Pulmonology, St Christopher's Hosp 1988; **Fac Appt:** Assoc Prof Ped, Columbia P&S

Sheares, Beverley J MD (PPul) - **Spec Exp:** Asthma; **Hospital:** NY-Presby Hosp (page 100); **Address:** Morgan Stanley Chlds Hosp NY-Presbyterian, 3959 Broadway Fl 7th, New York, NY 10032; **Phone:** 212-305-5122; **Board Cert:** Pediatrics 1991; Pediatric Pulmonology 2000; **Med School:** Univ NC Sch Med 1986; **Resid:** Pediatrics, Babies Hosp-Columbia Presby Med Ctr 1990; **Fellow:** Pediatric Pulmonology, Columbia Univ Coll Phys & Surg 1996; **Fac Appt:** Asst Prof Ped, Columbia P&S

PEDIATRIC RHEUMATOLOGY

Eichenfield, Andrew MD (PRhu) - **Spec Exp:** Juvenile Arthritis; Lyme Disease; Lupus/SLE; **Hospital:** NY-Presby Hosp (page 100), Blythedale Children's Hosp; **Address:** Morgan Stanley Chlds Hosp, 3959 Broadway, CHN-106, Ped Rheumatology, New York, NY 10032; **Phone:** 212-305-9304; **Board Cert:** Pediatrics 1983; Pediatric Rheumatology 2000; **Med School:** Univ Hlth Sci/Chicago Med Sch 1978; **Resid:** Pediatrics, Mt Sinai Hosp 1982; **Fellow:** Pediatric Rheumatology, Chidren's Hosp 1984; **Fac Appt:** Asst Clin Prof Ped, Columbia P&S

Lehman, Thomas MD (PRhu) - **Spec Exp:** Arthritis; Scleroderma; Lupus/SLE; **Hospital:** Hosp For Special Surgery (page 108), NY-Presby Hosp (page 100); **Address:** 535 E 70th St, New York, NY 10021-4872; **Phone:** 212-606-1151; **Board Cert:** Pediatrics 1979; Pediatric Rheumatology 1999; **Med School:** Jefferson Med Coll 1974; **Resid:** Pediatrics, Chldns Hosp 1976; Pediatrics, UCSF Med Ctr 1977; **Fellow:** Pediatric Rheumatology, Chldns Hosp 1979; Rheumatology, Natl Inst Hlth 1983; **Fac Appt:** Clin Prof Ped, Cornell Univ-Weill Med Coll

Pediatric Surgery

Altman, R Peter MD (PS) - **Spec Exp:** Neonatal Liver Disease; Thoracic Surgery; Cancer Surgery; **Hospital:** NY-Presby Hosp (page 100); **Address:** Morgan Stanley Chldns Hosp of NY-Presbyterian, 3959 Broadway, rm 116 S, New York, NY 10032-1559; **Phone:** 212-305-5804; **Board Cert:** Surgery 1968; Thoracic Surgery 1972; Pediatric Surgery 2003; **Med School:** NY Med Coll 1961; **Resid:** Surgery, Tufts-New England Med Ctr 1967; Thoracic Surgery, Geo Wash Univ Hosp 1968; **Fellow:** Pediatric Surgery, Chldns Hosp 1969; **Fac Appt:** Prof S, Columbia P&S

Beck, A Robert MD (PS) - **Spec Exp:** Neonatal Surgery; Hernia; Undescended Testis; Chest Wall Deformities; **Hospital:** Lenox Hill Hosp (page 94), Beth Israel Med Ctr - Petrie Division (page 90); **Address:** 155 E 76th St, New York, NY 10021; **Phone:** 212-861-0260; **Board Cert:** Surgery 1965; Pediatric Surgery 1995; **Med School:** Albany Med Coll 1958; **Resid:** Surgery, Mount Sinai Hosp 1964; **Fellow:** Pediatric Surgery, Chldns Hosp 1966; **Fac Appt:** Clin Prof S, Mount Sinai Sch Med

Cooper, Arthur MD (PS) - **Spec Exp:** Trauma; **Hospital:** Harlem Hosp Ctr, Metropolitan Hosp Ctr - NY; **Address:** Harlem Hospital, Dept Surgery, 506 Lenox Ave, New York, NY 10037; **Phone:** 212-939-4003; **Board Cert:** Surgery 1992; Surgical Critical Care 1994; Pediatric Surgery 1993; **Med School:** Univ Pennsylvania 1975; **Resid:** Surgery, Hosp Univ Penn 1981; Pediatric Surgery, Childrens Hosp 1984; **Fellow:** Pediatric Nutrition, Columbia P&S-Inst Human Nutrition 1982

Ginsburg, Howard B MD (PS) - **Spec Exp:** Neonatal Surgery; Tumor Surgery; Pediatric Urology; Gastrointestinal Surgery; **Hospital:** NYU Med Ctr (page 102), Bellevue Hosp Ctr; **Address:** 530 1st Ave, Ste 10W, NYU Medical Ctr, Div Pediatric Surgery, New York, NY 10016-6402; **Phone:** 212-263-7391; **Board Cert:** Surgery 1978; Pediatric Surgery 2001; **Med School:** Univ Cincinnati 1972; **Resid:** Surgery, NYU-Bellvue Hosp 1977; Pediatric Surgery, Columbia-Presby Med Ctr 1979; **Fellow:** Pediatric Surgery, Mass Genl Hosp 1980; **Fac Appt:** Assoc Prof S, NYU Sch Med

La Quaglia, Michael MD (PS) - **Spec Exp:** Cancer Surgery; Neuroblastoma; Liver Tumors; Colon & Rectal Cancer; **Hospital:** Meml Sloan Kettering Cancer Ctr (page 109), NY-Presby Hosp (page 100); **Address:** 1275 York Ave, Box 325, New York, NY 10021-6007; **Phone:** 212-639-7002; **Board Cert:** Surgery 2003; Pediatric Surgery 1997; **Med School:** UMDNJ-NJ Med Sch, Newark 1976; **Resid:** Surgery, Mass Genl Hosp 1983; **Fellow:** Cardiothoracic Surgery, Broadgreen Ctr 1984; Pediatric Surgery, Chldns Hosp 1985; **Fac Appt:** Prof S, Cornell Univ-Weill Med Coll

Mosca, Ralph S MD (PS) - **Spec Exp:** Cardiothoracic Surgery; Congenital Heart Surgery; Transplant-Heart; **Hospital:** NY-Presby Hosp (page 100), Robert Wood Johnson Univ Hosp - New Brunswick (page 853); **Address:** Morgan Stanley Chlds Hosp of NY-Presby, 3959 Broadway, rm 274, New York, NY 10032; **Phone:** 212-305-2688; **Board Cert:** Thoracic Surgery 2001; **Med School:** SUNY Upstate Med Univ 1985; **Resid:** Surgery, SUNY Hlth Sci Ctr Syracuse 1990; **Fellow:** Cardiothoracic Surgery, Columbia-Presby Med Ctr 1992; Pediatric Cardiac Surgery, Univ Mich Med Ctr 1993; **Fac Appt:** Assoc Prof TS, Columbia P&S

Quaegebeur, Jan M MD (PS) - **Spec Exp:** Arterial Switch; Heart Valve Surgery; Congenital Heart Surgery; **Hospital:** NY-Presby Hosp (page 100); **Address:** Morgan Stanley Chlds Hosp of NY-Presby, 3959 Broadway, BHN 276, New York, NY 10032; **Phone:** 212-305-5975; **Med School:** Belgium 1969; **Resid:** Surgery, St Michel Clinic 1973; **Fellow:** Thoracic Surgery, Baylor Coll Med 1974; Thoracic Surgery, Univ Hosp 1978; **Fac Appt:** Prof S, Columbia P&S

Stolar, Charles JH MD (PS) - **Spec Exp:** Pediatric Cancers; Neonatal Surgery; Diaphragmatic hernia; **Hospital:** NY-Presby Hosp (page 100); **Address:** Morgan Stanley Chldns Hosp NY-Presby, 3959 Broadway, Fl 2 - rm 215 North, New York, NY 10032; **Phone:** 212-342-8586; **Board Cert:** Surgery 2001; Pediatric Surgery 1996; **Med School:** Georgetown Univ 1974; **Resid:** Surgery, Univ Illinois Hosp 1980; **Fellow:** Pediatric Surgery, Chldns Hosp Natl Med Ctr 1982; **Fac Appt:** Prof S, Columbia P&S

Velcek, Francisca MD (PS) - **Spec Exp:** Anorectal Malformations; Pediatric Gynecology; Neonatal Surgery; Hernia; **Hospital:** Lenox Hill Hosp (page 94), Long Island Coll Hosp (page 90); **Address:** 965 5th Ave, New York, NY 10021; **Phone:** 212-744-9396; **Board Cert:** Surgery 1974; Pediatric Surgery 1997; **Med School:** Philippines 1966; **Resid:** Surgery, St Clares Hosp 1971; Pediatric Surgery, SUNY Downstate Med Ctr 1975; **Fellow:** Pediatric Surgery, SUNY Downstate Med Ctr 1973; **Fac Appt:** Prof S, SUNY Hlth Sci Ctr

PEDIATRICS

Allendorf, Dennis MD (Ped) **PCP** - **Spec Exp:** Congenital Anomalies; **Hospital:** NY-Presby Hosp (page 100), St Luke's - Roosevelt Hosp Ctr - Roosevelt Div (page 90); **Address:** 401 W 118th St, Ste 2, New York, NY 10027-7216; **Phone:** 212-666-4610; **Board Cert:** Pediatrics 1987; **Med School:** NY Med Coll 1970; **Resid:** Pediatrics, St Luke's-Roosevelt Hosp Ctr 1972; Pediatrics, Columbia-Presby Hosp 1973; **Fac Appt:** Asst Clin Prof Ped, Columbia P&S

Arnstein, Ellis MD (Ped) **PCP** - **Spec Exp:** Developmental Disorders; **Hospital:** St Vincent Cath Med Ctrs - Manhattan (page 375), Montefiore Med Ctr; **Address:** Devel Disabilities Clinic, 1249 Fifth Ave, New York, NY 10029; **Phone:** 212-360-3703; **Board Cert:** Pediatrics 1975; Neurodevelopmental Disabilities 2001; **Med School:** SUNY Downstate 1969; **Resid:** Pediatrics, Univ Wash Med Ctr 1973; **Fellow:** Child & Adolescent Psychiatry, Tufts-New England Med Ctr 1974; **Fac Appt:** Asst Prof Ped, NY Med Coll

Arpadi, Stephen MD (Ped) **PCP** - **Spec Exp:** AIDS/HIV; **Hospital:** St Luke's - Roosevelt Hosp Ctr - St Luke's Hosp (page 90); **Address:** 1111 Amsterdam Ave at 114th St, New York, NY 10025; **Phone:** 212-523-3847; **Board Cert:** Pediatrics 1987; **Med School:** Geo Wash Univ 1982; **Resid:** Pediatrics, Chldns Hosp Natl Med Ctr 1985; **Fac Appt:** Assoc Prof Ped, Columbia P&S

Brovender, Bruce J MD (Ped) **PCP** - **Hospital:** Lenox Hill Hosp (page 94), NY-Presby Hosp (page 100); **Address:** 186 E 76th St, New York, NY 10021; **Phone:** 212-585-3329; **Board Cert:** Pediatrics 2004; **Med School:** Italy 1984; **Resid:** Pediatrics, Maimonides Med Ctr 1985; Pediatrics, Lenox Hill Hosp 1987; **Fac Appt:** Asst Prof Ped, Cornell Univ-Weill Med Coll

Burstin, Harris E MD (Ped) **PCP** - **Spec Exp:** Asthma; Allergy; Critical Care; **Hospital:** NYU Med Ctr (page 102); **Address:** 317 E 34th St Fl 3, New York, NY 10016-4974; **Phone:** 212-725-6300; **Board Cert:** Pediatrics 1983; Critical Care Medicine 1998; **Med School:** Mexico 1977; **Resid:** Pediatrics, Bellevue Hosp Ctr 1982; **Fac Appt:** Assoc Prof Ped, NYU Sch Med

Cohen, Michel MD (Ped) **PCP** - **Spec Exp:** Child Development; **Hospital:** St Vincent Cath Med Ctrs - Manhattan (page 375); **Address:** 22 Harrison St, New York, NY 10013; **Phone:** 212-226-7666; **Board Cert:** Pediatrics 1993; **Med School:** France 1989; **Resid:** Pediatrics, New York Univ Med Ctr 1991; Pediatrics, Long Island Hosp 1993

Edelstein, Gary S MD (Ped) `PCP` - **Hospital:** NY-Presby Hosp (page 100); **Address:** Columbia Eastside, Manhattan Pediatrics, 16 E 60th St, Ste 410, New York, NY 10022; **Phone:** 212-326-3351; **Board Cert:** Pediatrics 2001; **Med School:** NYU Sch Med 1990; **Resid:** Pediatrics, Columbia Presbyterian Babies Hosp 1993; **Fellow:** Ambulatory Pediatrics, Columbia Presbyterian Babies Hosp 1995

Ferrier, Genevieve MD (Ped) `PCP` - **Spec Exp:** Developmental & Behavioral Disorders; Adolescent Medicine; **Hospital:** St Vincent Cath Med Ctrs - Manhattan (page 375), NYU Med Ctr (page 102); **Address:** 46 W 11th St, New York, NY 10011-8602; **Phone:** 212-529-4330; **Board Cert:** Pediatrics 2006; **Med School:** Mount Sinai Sch Med 1988; **Resid:** Pediatrics, Children's Hosp 1991; **Fac Appt:** Asst Prof Ped, NY Med Coll

Goldstein, Judith MD (Ped) `PCP` - **Spec Exp:** Newborn Care; Infectious Disease; Adolescent Medicine; **Hospital:** Lenox Hill Hosp (page 94), NY-Presby Hosp (page 100); **Address:** 186 E 76th St, Ground Floor, New York, NY 10021; **Phone:** 212-585-3329; **Board Cert:** Pediatrics 1977; **Med School:** SUNY Hlth Sci Ctr 1972; **Resid:** Pediatrics, Lenox Hill Hosp 1975; **Fac Appt:** Asst Clin Prof Ped, Cornell Univ-Weill Med Coll

Gribetz, Irwin MD (Ped) `PCP` - **Spec Exp:** Asthma; Pulmonary Disease; **Hospital:** Mount Sinai Med Ctr (page 98); **Address:** 1176 5th Ave, Ste 7, New York, NY 10029-6503; **Phone:** 212-876-1855; **Board Cert:** Pediatrics 1961; **Med School:** NY Med Coll 1954; **Resid:** Pediatrics, Mt Sinai Hosp 1957; **Fellow:** Pulmonary Disease, Harvard Med 1958; **Fac Appt:** Prof Ped, Mount Sinai Sch Med

Inamdar, Sarla MD (Ped) `PCP` - **Spec Exp:** Pediatric Rheumatology; **Hospital:** Metropolitan Hosp Ctr - NY; **Address:** 1901 1st Ave, rm 523, New York, NY 10029-7404; **Phone:** 212-423-6228; **Board Cert:** Pediatrics 1974; **Med School:** India 1969; **Resid:** Pediatrics, Metropolitan Hosp Ctr 1972; **Fac Appt:** Clin Prof Ped, NY Med Coll

Kahn, Max MD (Ped) `PCP` - **Hospital:** NYU Med Ctr (page 102), Lenox Hill Hosp (page 94); **Address:** 390 West End Ave, Ste 1E, New York, NY 10024; **Phone:** 212-787-1444; **Board Cert:** Pediatrics 1980; **Med School:** Columbia P&S 1975; **Resid:** Pediatrics, Bronx Muni Hosp 1978; **Fac Appt:** Assoc Clin Prof Ped, NYU Sch Med

Keith, Marie MD (Ped) `PCP` - **Hospital:** NYU Med Ctr (page 102), St Vincent Cath Med Ctrs - Manhattan (page 375); **Address:** 552 Broadway Fl 5, New York, NY 10012; **Phone:** 212-334-3366; **Board Cert:** Pediatrics 1979; **Med School:** Mount Sinai Sch Med 1974; **Resid:** Pediatrics, NY Presby-Columbia Presby Medical Ctr 1978

Kotin, Neal MD (Ped) `PCP` - **Spec Exp:** Asthma; Bronchitis; Sleep Disorders; Pulmonary Disease; **Hospital:** Mount Sinai Med Ctr (page 98), Lenox Hill Hosp (page 94); **Address:** 1125 Park Ave, New York, NY 10128-1243; **Phone:** 212-289-1400; **Board Cert:** Pediatrics 2005; Pediatric Pulmonology 2004; **Med School:** Albany Med Coll 1982; **Resid:** Pediatrics, Johns Hopkins Hosp 1985; **Fellow:** Pediatric Pulmonology, Mt Sinai Med Ctr 1988; **Fac Appt:** Asst Prof Ped, Mount Sinai Sch Med

Laraque, Danielle MD (Ped) `PCP` - **Spec Exp:** Child Abuse; Injury Prevention; Mental Health-Child; **Hospital:** Mount Sinai Med Ctr (page 98); **Address:** Mount Sinai Medical Ctr, Annenberg Bldg, One Gustave L Levy Pl Fl 17 - rm 11, New York, NY 10029; **Phone:** 212-241-5866; **Board Cert:** Pediatrics 1986; **Med School:** UCLA 1981; **Resid:** Pediatrics, Children's Hosp 1984; **Fellow:** Academic Pediatrics, Children's Hosp 1986; **Fac Appt:** Prof Ped, Mount Sinai Sch Med

Larson, Signe S MD (Ped) `PCP` - **Spec Exp:** Pediatric Endocrinology; **Hospital:** Mount Sinai Med Ctr (page 98); **Address:** 1245 Park Ave, New York, NY 10128; **Phone:** 212-427-0540; **Board Cert:** Pediatrics 1984; Pediatric Endocrinology 1989; **Med School:** SUNY Hlth Sci Ctr 1978; **Resid:** Family Medicine, Vancouver Univ Med Ctr 1979; Pediatrics, St Luke's Presby Med Ctr 1982; **Fellow:** Pediatric Endocrinology, Mt Sinai Hosp 1984

Lazarus, George M MD (Ped) `PCP` - **Spec Exp:** Adolescent Medicine; **Hospital:** NY-Presby Hosp (page 100), Lenox Hill Hosp (page 94); **Address:** 106 E 78th Street, New York, NY 10021-0302; **Phone:** 212-744-0840; **Board Cert:** Pediatrics 1976; **Med School:** Columbia P&S 1971; **Resid:** Pediatrics, NY Presby-Columbia Med Ctr 1974; **Fac Appt:** Assoc Clin Prof Ped, Columbia P&S

Lazarus, Herbert MD (Ped) `PCP` - **Spec Exp:** Juvenile Arthritis; Lyme Disease; Pain-Musculoskeletal; **Hospital:** NYU Med Ctr (page 102), Lenox Hill Hosp (page 94); **Address:** 390 West End Ave, rm 1E, New York, NY 10024; **Phone:** 212-787-1444; **Board Cert:** Pediatrics 1987; Pediatric Rheumatology 2000; **Med School:** UMDNJ-NJ Med Sch, Newark 1983; **Resid:** Pediatrics, NYU Med Ctr 1986; **Fellow:** Pediatric Rheumatology, Hosp for Joint Diseases 1987; **Fac Appt:** Asst Clin Prof Ped, NYU Sch Med

Levitzky, Susan MD (Ped) `PCP` - **Spec Exp:** Asthma; Child Development; Adoption & Foster Care; **Hospital:** NYU Med Ctr (page 102), Beth Israel Med Ctr - Petrie Division (page 90); **Address:** 161 Madison Ave, Ste 6W, New York, NY 10016-5405; **Phone:** 212-213-1960; **Board Cert:** Pediatrics 1972; **Med School:** Univ IL Coll Med 1967; **Resid:** Pediatrics, Beth Israel Hosp 1970; **Fac Appt:** Asst Clin Prof Ped, NYU Sch Med

McCarton, Cecelia MD (Ped) - **Spec Exp:** Autism; Learning Disorders; ADD/ADHD; Developmental Disorders; **Hospital:** Montefiore Med Ctr - Weiler-Einstein Div; **Address:** McCarton Ctr for Developmental Pediatrics, 350 E 82nd St, New York, NY 10028; **Phone:** 212-996-9019; **Board Cert:** Pediatrics 1988; **Med School:** Albert Einstein Coll Med 1970; **Resid:** Pediatrics, Bronx Muni Hosp Ctr 1974; **Fellow:** Developmental-Behavioral Pediatrics, Albert Einstein 1977; **Fac Appt:** Prof Ped, Albert Einstein Coll Med

McHugh, Margaret T MD (Ped) - **Spec Exp:** Adolescent Medicine; Child Abuse; **Hospital:** Bellevue Hosp Ctr; **Address:** 462 First Ave New Bellevue, GC65, New York, NY 10016; **Phone:** 212-562-6073; **Board Cert:** Pediatrics 1975; **Med School:** Georgetown Univ 1970; **Resid:** Pediatrics, NY Med Coll 1973; **Fellow:** Ambulatory Pediatrics, Columbia-Presby Med Ctr 1975; **Fac Appt:** Assoc Prof Ped, NYU Sch Med

Monti, Louis G MD (Ped) `PCP` - **Spec Exp:** Infectious Disease; **Hospital:** Mount Sinai Med Ctr (page 98); **Address:** 55 E 87th St, Ste 1G, New York, NY 10128-1049; **Phone:** 212-722-0707; **Board Cert:** Pediatrics 1985; **Med School:** Mount Sinai Sch Med 1980; **Resid:** Pediatrics, Mount Sinai Hosp 1983; **Fellow:** Infectious Disease, Childrens Hosp 1984; **Fac Appt:** Asst Clin Prof Ped, Mount Sinai Sch Med

Murphy, Ramon JC MD (Ped) `PCP` - **Spec Exp:** Adolescent Medicine; Community Medicine; **Hospital:** Mount Sinai Med Ctr (page 98); **Address:** 1245 Park Ave, New York, NY 10128; **Phone:** 212-427-0540; **Board Cert:** Pediatrics 1974; **Med School:** Northwestern Univ 1969; **Resid:** Internal Medicine, Cook Co Hosp 1970; Pediatrics, Childrens Meml Hosp 1971; **Fellow:** Pediatrics, Babies Hospital 1973; Community Medicine, Mount Sinai Med Ctr 1974; **Fac Appt:** Assoc Clin Prof Ped, Mount Sinai Sch Med

Neuspiel, Daniel MD (Ped) PCP - **Spec Exp:** Preventive Medicine; Adoption-International; **Hospital:** Beth Israel Med Ctr - Petrie Division (page 90); **Address:** Phillips Ambulatory Care Ctr, 10 Union Square E, Ste 2J, New York, NY 10003; **Phone:** 212-844-8309; **Board Cert:** Pediatrics 1984; Public Health & Genl Preventive Med 1987; **Med School:** UMDNJ-NJ Med Sch, Newark 1979; **Resid:** Pediatrics, Chldns Hosp 1982; **Fellow:** Cardiovascular Epidemiology, Univ Pittsburgh 1984; **Fac Appt:** Assoc Prof Ped, Albert Einstein Coll Med

Newman-Cedar, Meryl MD (Ped) PCP - **Spec Exp:** Child Development; **Hospital:** NY-Presby Hosp (page 100), Lenox Hill Hosp (page 94); **Address:** 215 E 79th St, Ste 1 C, New York, NY 10021-0848; **Phone:** 212-737-7800; **Board Cert:** Pediatrics 1987; **Med School:** SUNY Downstate 1981; **Resid:** Pediatrics, New York Hosp 1984; **Fellow:** Developmental-Behavioral Pediatrics, New York Hosp 1987

Nicholas, Stephen W MD (Ped) - **Spec Exp:** AIDS/HIV; Asthma; **Hospital:** Harlem Hosp Ctr; **Address:** Harlem Hospital, Director Pediatrics, 506 Lenox Ave, rm MLK 17-104, New York, NY 10037; **Phone:** 212-939-4012; **Board Cert:** Pediatrics 1987; **Med School:** Univ Colorado 1981; **Resid:** Pediatrics, Babies Hosp/Columbia Presby Medical Ctr 1983; Pediatrics, Harlem Hosp 1985; **Fellow:** Pediatrics, Harlem Hosp 1986; Pediatrics, Children's Hosp 1987; **Fac Appt:** Assoc Prof Ped, Columbia P&S

Oeffinger, Kevin MD (Ped) - **Spec Exp:** Cancer Survivors-Late Effects of Therapy; **Hospital:** Meml Sloan Kettering Cancer Ctr (page 109); **Address:** 1275 York Ave, New York, NY 10021; **Phone:** 212-639-8469; **Board Cert:** Family Medicine 2000; **Med School:** Univ Tex, San Antonio 1984; **Resid:** Family Medicine, Baylor Coll Med 1985; **Fellow:** Family Medicine, Fam Practice Faculty Dev Ctr 1999Natl Cancer Inst 2000

Poon, Eric Sin-Kam MD (Ped) PCP - **Spec Exp:** Asthma; Pediatric Cardiology; Developmental Disorders; **Hospital:** NY Downtown Hosp, NY-Presby Hosp (page 100); **Address:** 170 William St Bldg FL 3, New York, NY 10038-2612; **Phone:** 212-312-5350; **Board Cert:** Pediatrics 1988; **Med School:** Mexico 1982; **Resid:** Pediatrics, LI Coll Hosp 1986; **Fellow:** Pediatric Cardiology, NY Hosp-Cornell Med Ctr 1988; **Fac Appt:** Assoc Clin Prof Ped, Cornell Univ-Weill Med Coll

Popper, Laura MD (Ped) PCP - **Spec Exp:** Adolescent Medicine; **Hospital:** Mount Sinai Med Ctr (page 98); **Address:** 116 E 66th St, Ste 1C, New York, NY 10021-6547; **Phone:** 212-794-2136; **Board Cert:** Pediatrics 1981; **Med School:** Columbia P&S 1974; **Resid:** Pediatrics, Babies Hosp 1976; **Fellow:** Pediatrics, Babies Hosp 1977; **Fac Appt:** Asst Clin Prof Ped, NY Coll Osteo Med

Prezioso, Paula MD (Ped) PCP - **Spec Exp:** Behavioral Disorders; Adolescent Medicine; **Hospital:** NYU Med Ctr (page 102); **Address:** 317 E 34th St, Fl 3, New York, NY 10016-4974; **Phone:** 212-725-6300; **Board Cert:** Pediatrics 1999; **Med School:** SUNY Downstate 1987; **Resid:** Pediatrics, NYU-Bellevue Hosp 1991; **Fac Appt:** Asst Clin Prof Ped, NYU Sch Med

Prince, Alice MD (Ped) - **Spec Exp:** AIDS/HIV; **Hospital:** NY-Presby Hosp (page 100); **Address:** 650 W 168th St, New York, NY 10032-3702; **Phone:** 212-305-4193; **Board Cert:** Pediatrics 1979; Pediatric Infectious Disease 2002; **Med School:** Columbia P&S 1975; **Resid:** Pediatrics, Babies Hosp 1978; **Fellow:** Infectious Disease, Columbia Univ 1981; **Fac Appt:** Prof Ped, Columbia P&S

Raucher, Harold S MD (Ped) PCP - **Spec Exp:** Infectious Disease; **Hospital:** Mount Sinai Med Ctr (page 98), Lenox Hill Hosp (page 94); **Address:** 1125 Park Ave, New York, NY 10128-1243; **Phone:** 212-289-1400; **Board Cert:** Pediatrics 1983; Pediatric Infectious Disease 2002; **Med School:** Mount Sinai Sch Med 1978; **Resid:** Pediatrics, Mt Sinai Med Ctr 1980; **Fellow:** Pediatric Infectious Disease, Mt Sinai Med Ctr 1982; **Fac Appt:** Assoc Prof Ped, Mount Sinai Sch Med

Rosello, Lori MD (Ped) PCP - **Hospital:** NYU Med Ctr (page 102), St Vincent Cath Med Ctrs - Manhattan (page 375); **Address:** 46 W 11th St, New York, NY 10011-8602; **Phone:** 212-529-4330; **Board Cert:** Pediatrics 2005; **Med School:** Albert Einstein Coll Med 1987; **Resid:** Pediatrics, Columbia-Presby 1990; **Fac Appt:** Asst Clin Prof Ped, NYU Sch Med

Rosenbaum, Michael MD (Ped) PCP - **Spec Exp:** Nutrition; Growth Disorders; Obesity; **Hospital:** NY-Presby Hosp (page 100); **Address:** 450 West End Ave, New York, NY 10024-5307; **Phone:** 212-769-3070; **Board Cert:** Pediatrics 1988; Pediatric Endocrinology 1991; **Med School:** Cornell Univ-Weill Med Coll 1982; **Resid:** Pediatrics, Columbia-Presby Med Ctr 1985; **Fellow:** Pediatric Endocrinology, New York Hosp 1988; **Fac Appt:** Assoc Prof Ped, Columbia P&S

Rosenfeld, Suzanne MD (Ped) PCP - **Spec Exp:** Developmental Disorders; Adolescent Medicine; Asthma; **Hospital:** NY-Presby Hosp (page 100), Lenox Hill Hosp (page 94); **Address:** 450 West End Ave, New York, NY 10024-5393; **Phone:** 212-769-3070; **Board Cert:** Pediatrics 1986; **Med School:** Columbia P&S 1980; **Resid:** Pediatrics, Columbia-Presby Med Ctr 1983; **Fellow:** Pediatrics, NY Hosp-Cornell Med Ctr 1984

Sacker, Ira MD (Ped) - **Spec Exp:** Eating Disorders; Eating Disorders-Adult/Pediatric; Obesity; **Hospital:** NYU Med Ctr (page 102), Brookdale Univ Hosp Med Ctr; **Address:** 19 W 34th St, Penthouse Fl, New York, NY 10016; **Phone:** 718-240-6451; **Board Cert:** Pediatrics 1982; **Med School:** UCLA 1968; **Resid:** Pediatrics, Bellevue Hosp/NYU Med Ctr 1972; **Fellow:** Adolescent Medicine, Chldns Hosp 1972; **Fac Appt:** Asst Clin Prof Ped, NYU Sch Med

Sanford, Marie MD (Ped) PCP - **Hospital:** Mount Sinai Med Ctr (page 98); **Address:** Westside Pediatrics, Columbus Ave, between 90th & 91st St, New York, NY 10011; **Phone:** 212-874-4500; **Board Cert:** Pediatrics 2002; **Med School:** Mount Sinai Sch Med 1991; **Resid:** Pediatrics, Mount Sina 1995

Saphir, Richard L MD (Ped) PCP - **Spec Exp:** Newborn Care; Adolescent Medicine; Rashes; **Hospital:** Mount Sinai Med Ctr (page 98); **Address:** 55 E 87th St, Ste 1G, New York, NY 10128-1049; **Phone:** 212-722-4950; **Board Cert:** Pediatrics 1963; **Med School:** SUNY Hlth Sci Ctr 1958; **Resid:** Pediatrics, Mount Sinai Hosp 1961; **Fac Appt:** Clin Prof Ped, Mount Sinai Sch Med

Smith, David I MD (Ped) PCP - **Hospital:** NY-Presby Hosp (page 100); **Address:** 186 E 76th St, New York, NY 10021; **Phone:** 212-988-0600; **Board Cert:** Pediatrics 1963; **Med School:** NYU Sch Med 1956; **Resid:** Pediatrics, New York Hosp-Cornell Med Ctr 1961; **Fac Appt:** Clin Prof Ped, Cornell Univ-Weill Med Coll

Softness, Barney MD (Ped) PCP - **Spec Exp:** Diabetes; Growth Disorders; **Hospital:** NY-Presby Hosp (page 100), NY-Presby Hosp (page 100); **Address:** 450 West End Ave, New York, NY 10024-5307; **Phone:** 212-769-3070; **Board Cert:** Pediatrics 1986; Pediatric Endocrinology 1986; **Med School:** Columbia P&S 1980; **Resid:** Pediatrics, Columbia Presby Med Ctr 1983; **Fellow:** Pediatric Endocrinology, NY Cornell Med Ctr 1985; **Fac Appt:** Asst Clin Prof Ped, Columbia P&S

Stein, Barry B MD (Ped) PCP - **Spec Exp:** Developmental & Behavioral Disorders; **Hospital:** Mount Sinai Med Ctr (page 98), Lenox Hill Hosp (page 94); **Address:** 1125 Park Ave, New York, NY 10128-1243; **Phone:** 212-289-1400; **Board Cert:** Pediatrics 1987; **Med School:** South Africa 1980; **Resid:** Pediatrics, Mount Sinai Hosp 1986; **Fac Appt:** Asst Clin Prof Ped, Mount Sinai Sch Med

Stone, Richard K MD (Ped) **PCP** - **Spec Exp:** Behavioral Disorders; **Hospital:** Metropolitan Hosp Ctr - NY; **Address:** 1901 1st Ave, rm 1B4, New York, NY 10029-7418; **Phone:** 212-423-8131; **Board Cert:** Pediatrics 1973; **Med School:** NY Med Coll 1968; **Resid:** Pediatrics, NY Med Coll 1971; **Fac Appt:** Prof Ped, NY Med Coll

Traister, Michael MD (Ped) **PCP** - **Spec Exp:** Adoption & Foster Care; **Hospital:** NYU Med Ctr (page 102), Lenox Hill Hosp (page 94); **Address:** 390 West End Ave, New York, NY 10024; **Phone:** 212-787-1444; **Board Cert:** Pediatrics 1980; **Med School:** NY Med Coll 1975; **Resid:** Pediatrics, Bronx Municipal Hosp 1978; **Fellow:** Ambulatory Pediatrics, Bellevue Hosp 1979; **Fac Appt:** Asst Clin Prof Ped, NYU Sch Med

Weinberger, Sylvain M MD (Ped) **PCP** - **Spec Exp:** Prematurity/Low Birth Weight Infants; **Hospital:** NYU Med Ctr (page 102), Beth Israel Med Ctr - Petrie Division (page 90); **Address:** 51 E 25 St Fl 3, New York, NY 10010; **Phone:** 212-598-0331; **Board Cert:** Pediatrics 1982; Neonatal-Perinatal Medicine 1983; **Med School:** Belgium 1977; **Resid:** Pediatrics, LI Jewish Med Ctr; **Fellow:** Neonatal-Perinatal Medicine, LI Jewish Med Ctr 1981; **Fac Appt:** Asst Clin Prof Ped, NYU Sch Med

Williams Jr, Christine MD (Ped) - **Spec Exp:** Obesity; Cholesterol/Lipid Disorders; Preventive Cardiology; Nutrition; **Hospital:** NY-Presby Hosp (page 100); **Address:** Morgan Stanley Chldns Hosp NY-Presby, 3959 Broadway, BHN7-715, New York, NY 10032; **Phone:** 212-305-5903; **Board Cert:** Pediatrics 1984; Preventive Medicine 1972; **Med School:** Univ Pittsburgh 1967; **Resid:** Preventive Medicine, Johns Hopkins Hosp 1971; Pediatrics, Med Coll Penn Hosp 1973; **Fellow:** Ambulatory Pediatrics, Med Coll Penn 1975; **Fac Appt:** Prof Ped, Columbia P&S

Zimmerman, Sol MD (Ped) **PCP** - **Spec Exp:** Growth/Development Disorders; Behavioral Disorders; Cough-Tic Syndrome; **Hospital:** NYU Med Ctr (page 102); **Address:** 317 E 34th St, New York, NY 10016-4974; **Phone:** 212-725-6300; **Board Cert:** Pediatrics 1977; **Med School:** NYU Sch Med 1972; **Resid:** Pediatrics, Bellevue Hosp Ctr 1975; Pediatrics, Bellevue Hosp/NYU 1978; **Fac Appt:** Assoc Clin Prof Ped, NYU Sch Med

PHYSICAL MEDICINE & REHABILITATION

Ahn, Jung Hwan MD (PMR) - **Spec Exp:** Spinal Cord Injury; Stroke Rehabilitation; Neurologic Rehabilitation; **Hospital:** NYU Med Ctr (page 102); **Address:** 400 E 34th St, rm 421, New York, NY 10016-4901; **Phone:** 212-263-6122; **Board Cert:** Physical Medicine & Rehabilitation 1980; Spinal Cord Injury Medicine 1998; **Med School:** South Korea 1970; **Resid:** Obstetrics & Gynecology, Elmhurst City Hosp - Mt Sinai 1976; Physical Medicine & Rehabilitation, NYU Med Ctr 1979; **Fellow:** Spinal Cord Injury Medicine, NYU Med Ctr 1980; **Fac Appt:** Clin Prof PMR, NYU Sch Med

Brown, Andrew MD (PMR) - **Spec Exp:** Electromyography; **Hospital:** NY Downtown Hosp, Cabrini Med Ctr (page 374); **Address:** 19 Beekman St, New York, NY 10038; **Phone:** 212-513-7711; **Board Cert:** Physical Medicine & Rehabilitation 1988; **Med School:** West Indies 1982; **Resid:** Physical Medicine & Rehabilitation, Mount Sinai 1987

Dillard, James N MD (PMR) - **Spec Exp:** Pain Management; Acupuncture; Complementary Medicine; **Hospital:** NY-Presby Hosp (page 100), Beth Israel Med Ctr - Petrie Division (page 90); **Address:** 200 W 57th St, Ste 608, New York, NY 10019; **Phone:** 212-265-4038; **Board Cert:** Physical Medicine & Rehabilitation 2005; **Med School:** Rush Med Coll 1990; **Resid:** Physical Medicine & Rehabilitation, Columbia-Presby Med Ctr 1994; **Fac Appt:** Asst Clin Prof PMR, Columbia P&S

Feinberg, Joseph Hunt MD (PMR) - **Spec Exp:** Peripheral Nerve Disorders; Spinal Rehabilitation; Electrodiagnosis; Sports Medicine; **Hospital:** Hosp For Special Surgery (page 108), Kessler Inst for Rehab - W Orange; **Address:** 535 E 70th St, New York, NY 10021-4872; **Phone:** 212-606-1568; **Board Cert:** Physical Medicine & Rehabilitation 1991; **Med School:** Albany Med Coll 1983; **Resid:** Surgery, Mt Sinai Hosp 1985; Physical Medicine & Rehabilitation, Rusk Inst Rehab 1990; **Fellow:** Orthopaedic Pathology, Hosp Spec Surg 1986; Orthopaedic Biomechanics, Univ Iowa Hosp & Clins 1987; **Fac Appt:** Assoc Prof PMR, Cornell Univ-Weill Med Coll

Flanagan, Steven Robert MD (PMR) - **Spec Exp:** Brain Injury; **Hospital:** Mount Sinai Med Ctr (page 98); **Address:** 5 E 98th St Fl 6, New York, NY 10029; **Phone:** 212-241-3981; **Board Cert:** Physical Medicine & Rehabilitation 2003; **Med School:** UMDNJ-NJ Med Sch, Newark 1988; **Resid:** Overlook Hosp 1989; Physical Medicine & Rehabilitation, Mt Sinai Hosp 1992; **Fac Appt:** Assoc Prof PMR, Mount Sinai Sch Med

Gold, Joan MD (PMR) - **Spec Exp:** Cerebral Palsy; Spina Bifida; Pediatric Rehabilitation; **Hospital:** NYU Med Ctr (page 102), Hosp For Joint Diseases (page 107); **Address:** 400 E 34th St, Ste 518, New York, Ny 10016-4901; **Phone:** 212-263-6519; **Board Cert:** Pediatrics 1979; Physical Medicine & Rehabilitation 1981; **Med School:** SUNY Downstate 1974; **Resid:** Pediatrics, Beth Israel Med Ctr 1977; Physical Medicine & Rehabilitation, Inst Rehab Med-NYU 1979; **Fac Appt:** Assoc Clin Prof PMR, NYU Sch Med

Goldberg, Robert B DO (PMR) - **Spec Exp:** Pain-Back; Pain-Knee; Sports Medicine; **Hospital:** St Vincent Cath Med Ctrs - Manhattan (page 375); **Address:** 314 W 14th St Fl 2, New York, NY 10014-5002; **Phone:** 212-929-9009; **Board Cert:** Physical Medicine & Rehabilitation 1982; **Med School:** Philadelphia Coll Osteo Med 1977; **Resid:** Physical Medicine & Rehabilitation, St Vincent's Hosp 1980; **Fellow:** Physical Medicine & Rehabilitation, St Vincent's Hosp 1981; **Fac Appt:** Assoc Clin Prof PMR, NY Med Coll

Gotlin, Robert S DO (PMR) - **Spec Exp:** Pain-Knee & Shoulder; Pain-Back; Sports Medicine; **Hospital:** Beth Israel Med Ctr - Petrie Division (page 90); **Address:** 245 Fifth Ave Fl 2, New York, NY 10016; **Phone:** 646-935-2255; **Board Cert:** Physical Medicine & Rehabilitation 1992; **Med School:** Southeastern Univ Coll Osteo Med 1987; **Resid:** Physical Medicine & Rehabilitation, Mount Sinai Hosp 1991; **Fac Appt:** Asst Prof PMR, Albert Einstein Coll Med

Inwald, Gary DO (PMR) - **Spec Exp:** Musculoskeletal Disorders; Pain Management; **Hospital:** St Vincent Cath Med Ctrs - Manhattan (page 375); **Address:** 24 E 12th St, Ste 302, New York, NY 10003; **Phone:** 212-807-6599; **Board Cert:** Physical Medicine & Rehabilitation 1983; **Med School:** Mich State Univ Coll Osteo Med 1976; **Resid:** Physical Medicine & Rehabilitation, St Vincents Hosp 1982

Lachmann, Elisabeth A MD (PMR) - **Spec Exp:** Pain-Back; Sports Medicine; Cancer Rehabilitation; **Hospital:** NY-Presby Hosp (page 100); **Address:** 115 E 64th St, New York, NY 10021; **Phone:** 212-535-3005; **Board Cert:** Physical Medicine & Rehabilitation 1992; **Med School:** Med Coll PA Hahnemann 1987; **Resid:** Physical Medicine & Rehabilitation, NY-Cornell Med Ctr 1991; **Fac Appt:** Assoc Prof PMR, Cornell Univ-Weill Med Coll

Lanyi, Valery MD (PMR) - **Spec Exp:** Arthritis; Stroke Rehabilitation; **Hospital:** NYU Med Ctr (page 102); **Address:** 400 E 34th St, Ste RG33, New York, NY 10016; **Phone:** 212-263-6197; **Board Cert:** Physical Medicine & Rehabilitation 1968; **Med School:** Hungary 1954; **Resid:** Internal Medicine, NYU Med Ctr 1961; **Fac Appt:** Clin Prof PMR, NYU Sch Med

Lee, Mathew H M MD (PMR) - **Spec Exp:** Acupuncture; Pain-Chronic; **Hospital:** NYU Med Ctr (page 102); **Address:** Rusk Institute, 400 E 34th St, rm 600, New York, NY 10016; **Phone:** 212-263-6105; **Board Cert:** Physical Medicine & Rehabilitation 1966; **Med School:** Univ MD Sch Med 1956; **Resid:** Physical Medicine & Rehabilitation, NYU Med Ctr 1964; **Fac Appt:** Clin Prof PMR, NYU Sch Med

Lieberman, James S MD (PMR) - **Spec Exp:** Neurologic Rehabilitation; Pain-Back & Neck; **Hospital:** NY-Presby Hosp (page 100), NY-Presby Hosp (page 100); **Address:** Rehabilitation Med Assoc, 630 W 168th St, Box 38, New York, NY 10032; **Phone:** 212-305-4818; **Board Cert:** Neurology 1971; Physical Medicine & Rehabilitation 1981; **Med School:** UCSF 1963; **Resid:** Neurology, Univ Mich Med Ctr 1965; Neurology, Yale-New Haven Hosp 1967; **Fellow:** Physical Medicine & Rehabilitation, UC Davis 1980; **Fac Appt:** Prof PMR, Columbia P&S

Lutz, Gregory MD (PMR) - **Spec Exp:** Spinal Rehabilitation; Sports Medicine; Pain-Low Back; **Hospital:** Hosp For Special Surgery (page 108), Univ Med Ctr - Princeton; **Address:** 535 E 70th St, New York, NY 10021-4898; **Phone:** 212-606-1648; **Board Cert:** Physical Medicine & Rehabilitation 2003; **Med School:** Georgetown Univ 1988; **Resid:** Physical Medicine & Rehabilitation, Mayo Clinic 1992; **Fellow:** Sports Medicine, Hosp For Spec Surg 1993; **Fac Appt:** Assoc Prof PMR, Cornell Univ-Weill Med Coll

Ma, Dong M MD (PMR) - **Spec Exp:** Electromyography; Musculoskeletal Disorders; **Hospital:** Rusk Inst of Rehab Med (page 111), NYU Med Ctr (page 102); **Address:** 400 E 34th St, rm 211, New York, NY 10016; **Phone:** 212-263-6338; **Board Cert:** Physical Medicine & Rehabilitation 1979; **Med School:** South Korea 1968; **Resid:** Physical Medicine & Rehabilitation, NYU Med Ctr 1975; **Fellow:** Physical Medicine & Rehabilitation, NYU Med Ctr 1977; **Fac Appt:** Clin Prof PMR, NYU Sch Med

Moldover, Jonathan MD (PMR) - **Spec Exp:** Spinal Rehabilitation; Pain-Chronic; **Hospital:** Beth Israel Med Ctr - Petrie Division (page 90), St Luke's - Roosevelt Hosp Ctr - Roosevelt Div (page 90); **Address:** 200 W 57th St, Ste 608, New York, NY 10019; **Phone:** 212-581-4488; **Board Cert:** Physical Medicine & Rehabilitation 1979; Pain Medicine 2002; **Med School:** Columbia P&S 1974; **Resid:** Internal Medicine, Strong Meml Hosp 1976; Physical Medicine & Rehabilitation, Columbia-Presby Med Ctr 1978; **Fac Appt:** Assoc Clin Prof PMR, Albert Einstein Coll Med

Myers, Stanley J MD (PMR) - **Spec Exp:** Muscular Dystrophy; Stroke Rehabilitation; Neuromuscular Disorders; **Hospital:** NY-Presby Hosp (page 100); **Address:** Columbia Presby Rehab Assocs, 180 Fort Washington Ave, HP 1-167, Ste 199, New York, NY 10032-3710; **Phone:** 212-305-3535; **Board Cert:** Physical Medicine & Rehabilitation 1971; **Med School:** SUNY Downstate 1961; **Resid:** Internal Medicine, Maimonides Medical Ctr 1964; Physical Medicine & Rehabilitation, Columbia-Presby Hosp 1969; **Fellow:** Neurological Muscular Disease, Maimonides Medical Ctr 1965; **Fac Appt:** Prof PMR, Columbia P&S

Ragnarsson, Kristjan T MD (PMR) - **Spec Exp:** Spinal Cord Injury; Brain Injury Rehabilitation; Pain-Back & Neck; **Hospital:** Mount Sinai Med Ctr (page 98); **Address:** 5 E 98th St, New York, NY 10029-6501; **Phone:** 212-659-9370; **Board Cert:** Physical Medicine & Rehabilitation 1976; **Med School:** Iceland 1969; **Resid:** Physical Medicine & Rehabilitation, NYU Med Ctr 1974; **Fellow:** Spinal Cord & Brain Injury Rehab, NYU Med Ctr 1975; **Fac Appt:** Prof PMR, Mount Sinai Sch Med

Rho, Dae-Sik MD (PMR) - **Spec Exp:** Sports Medicine; Pain Management; **Hospital:** Lenox Hill Hosp (page 94); **Address:** 100 E 77th St, New York, NY 10021; **Phone:** 212-434-2460; **Board Cert:** Physical Medicine & Rehabilitation 1980; **Med School:** South Korea 1962; **Resid:** Physical Medicine & Rehabilitation, NYU Med Ctr 1975; **Fac Appt:** Asst Clin Prof PMR, Cornell Univ-Weill Med Coll

Ross, Marc MD (PMR) - **Spec Exp:** Sports Medicine; Pain-Back; Gait Disorders; **Hospital:** Cabrini Med Ctr (page 374); **Address:** Cabrini Medical Center, 227 E 19th St, New York, NY 10003-2693; **Phone:** 212-995-6661; **Board Cert:** Physical Medicine & Rehabilitation 2004; **Med School:** NY Med Coll 1989; **Resid:** Physical Medicine & Rehabilitation, Mt Sinai Med Ctr 1993; **Fac Appt:** Asst Prof PMR, Mount Sinai Sch Med

Stein, Adam MD (PMR) - **Spec Exp:** Spinal Cord Injury; Multiple Sclerosis; Stroke Rehabilitation; **Hospital:** Mount Sinai Med Ctr (page 98); **Address:** 5 E 98th St, Fl 6th, New York, NY 10029-6501; **Phone:** 212-241-3981; **Board Cert:** Physical Medicine & Rehabilitation 1992; Spinal Cord Injury Medicine 2003; **Med School:** NYU Sch Med 1987; **Resid:** Physical Medicine & Rehabilitation, Rusk Inst-NYU Med Ctr 1991; **Fac Appt:** Asst Prof PMR, Mount Sinai Sch Med

Vad, Vijay B MD (PMR) - **Spec Exp:** Sports Medicine-Golf & Tennis Injuries; Joint Pain-Minimally Invasive Therapy; Pain-Back; Pain-Knee & Shoulder; **Hospital:** Hosp For Special Surgery (page 108); **Address:** 519 E 72nd St, Ste 203, New York, NY 10021; **Phone:** 212-606-1306; **Board Cert:** Physical Medicine & Rehabilitation 1997; **Med School:** Univ Okla Coll Med 1992; **Resid:** Physical Medicine & Rehabilitation, NY Cornell Med Ctr 1996; **Fellow:** Sports Medicine, Hosp Special Surgery 1997; **Fac Appt:** Asst Prof PMR, Cornell Univ-Weill Med Coll

PLASTIC SURGERY

Ahn, Christina Y MD (PIS) - **Spec Exp:** Breast Reconstruction; Cosmetic Surgery-Face; Cosmetic Surgery-Body; **Hospital:** NYU Med Ctr (page 102), Manhattan Eye, Ear & Throat Hosp; **Address:** 150 E 77th St, New York, NY 10021-1922; **Phone:** 212-717-8860; **Board Cert:** Plastic Surgery 1994; **Med School:** NYU Sch Med 1983; **Resid:** Surgery, Mt Sinai Med Ctr 1988; Plastic Surgery, Univ Pittsburgh Med Ctr 1990; **Fellow:** Microvascular Surgery, UCLA Med Ctr 1991; **Fac Appt:** Assoc Prof S, NYU Sch Med

Almeyda, Elizabeth MD (PIS) - **Spec Exp:** Cosmetic Surgery-Face; Cosmetic Surgery-Breast; Liposuction; **Hospital:** St Luke's - Roosevelt Hosp Ctr - Roosevelt Div (page 90); **Address:** 75 Central Park West, New York, NY 10023-6011; **Phone:** 212-501-0600; **Board Cert:** Plastic Surgery 1988; **Med School:** Univ Rochester 1978; **Resid:** Surgery, Roosevelt Hosp 1983; **Fellow:** Plastic Surgery, New York Hosp 1985

Altchek, Edgar MD (PIS) - **Hospital:** Mount Sinai Med Ctr (page 98), Beth Israel Med Ctr - Petrie Division (page 90); **Address:** 102 E 78th St, New York, NY 10021-0302; **Phone:** 212-734-9266; **Board Cert:** Plastic Surgery 1974; **Med School:** NY Med Coll 1965; **Resid:** Surgery, Beth Israel Hosp 1969; Plastic Surgery, Mount Sinai Hosp 1972; **Fac Appt:** Assoc Clin Prof PIS, Mount Sinai Sch Med

Ascherman, Jeffrey MD (PIS) - **Spec Exp:** Breast Reconstruction; Craniofacial Surgery; Cosmetic Surgery; **Hospital:** NY-Presby Hosp (page 100), New York Eye & Ear Infirm (page 110); **Address:** 161 Ft Washington Ave, Ste 607, New York, NY 10032-3713; **Phone:** 212-305-9612; **Board Cert:** Plastic Surgery 1997; **Med School:** Columbia P&S 1988; **Resid:** Surgery, Columbia-Presby Med Ctr 1991; Plastic Surgery, Columbia-Presby Med Ctr 1994; **Fellow:** Craniofacial Surgery, Hosp Necke-Enfants Malades 1994; Pediatric Plastic Surgery, Hosp St Vincent de Paul 1995; **Fac Appt:** Asst Prof S, Columbia P&S

Aston, Sherrell MD (PIS) - **Spec Exp:** Cosmetic Surgery-Face; Rhinoplasty; Cosmetic Surgery-Breast; Liposuction & Body Contouring; **Hospital:** Manhattan Eye, Ear & Throat Hosp, NYU Med Ctr (page 102); **Address:** 728 Park Ave, New York, NY 10021; **Phone:** 212-249-6000; **Board Cert:** Surgery 1974; Plastic Surgery 1978; **Med School:** Univ VA Sch Med 1968; **Resid:** Surgery, UCLA Med Ctr 1973; Plastic Surgery, New York Univ 1975; **Fellow:** Surgery, Johns Hopkins Hosp 1970; **Fac Appt:** Prof PIS, NYU Sch Med

New York (Manhattan)

Baker, Daniel MD (PlS) - **Spec Exp:** Cosmetic Surgery-Face; Reconstructive Surgery-Face; Rhinoplasty; **Hospital:** Manhattan Eye, Ear & Throat Hosp; **Address:** 65 E 66th St, New York, NY 10021; **Phone:** 212-734-9695; **Board Cert:** Plastic Surgery 1978; **Med School:** Columbia P&S 1968; **Resid:** Surgery, UCSF Med Ctr 1975; Plastic Surgery, NYU Med Ctr 1977; **Fellow:** Head and Neck Surgery, NYU Med Ctr/St Vincents Hosp 1978; **Fac Appt:** Assoc Prof PlS, NYU Sch Med

Beraka, George MD (PlS) - **Spec Exp:** Cosmetic Surgery-Breast; Cosmetic Surgery-Liposuction; Cosmetic Surgery-Face; **Hospital:** Lenox Hill Hosp (page 94), Manhattan Eye, Ear & Throat Hosp; **Address:** 875 Park Ave, New York, NY 10021-0341; **Phone:** 212-288-1122; **Board Cert:** Plastic Surgery 1976; **Med School:** Columbia P&S 1969; **Resid:** Surgery, Johns Hopkins Hosp 1973; Plastic Surgery, New York Hosp-Cornell 1975; **Fac Appt:** Asst Prof PlS, Cornell Univ-Weill Med Coll

Birnbaum, Jay MD (PlS) - **Spec Exp:** Cosmetic Surgery-Face; Breast Cosmetic & Reconstructive Surgery; Liposuction; **Hospital:** Mount Sinai Med Ctr (page 98), Beth Israel Med Ctr - Petrie Division (page 90); **Address:** 74 E 79th St, Ste 1A, New York, NY 10021-0266; **Phone:** 212-472-3040; **Board Cert:** Plastic Surgery 1989; **Med School:** Med Univ SC 1980; **Resid:** Surgery, Mount Sinai Hosp 1983; Plastic Surgery, Mount Sinai Hosp 1986; **Fac Appt:** Assoc Prof S, Mount Sinai Sch Med

Bromley, Gary S MD (PlS) - **Spec Exp:** Cosmetic Surgery; **Hospital:** NY-Presby Hosp (page 100), Jamaica Hosp Med Ctr; **Address:** 5 E 84th St, New York, NY 10028-0407; **Phone:** 212-570-5443; **Board Cert:** Plastic Surgery 1986; Hand Surgery 1996; **Med School:** Cornell Univ-Weill Med Coll 1978; **Resid:** Surgery, New York Hosp 1981; Plastic Surgery, New York Hosp 1983; **Fellow:** Hand Surgery, NYU Med Ctr 1984

Broumand, Stafford MD (PlS) - **Spec Exp:** Eyelid Surgery; Cosmetic Surgery-Face; Breast Surgery; **Hospital:** Mount Sinai Med Ctr (page 98), Englewood Hosp & Med Ctr (page 760); **Address:** 740 Park Ave, New York, NY 10021-4251; **Phone:** 212-879-7900; **Board Cert:** Plastic Surgery 1997; **Med School:** Yale Univ 1985; **Resid:** Surgery, Mt Sinai Med Ctr 1990; **Fellow:** Plastic Surgery, Mass Genl Hosp 1992; Cosmetic Plastic Surgery, Cran Hosp Necker 1993; **Fac Appt:** Asst Clin Prof PlS, Mount Sinai Sch Med

Chiu, David MD (PlS) - **Spec Exp:** Hand & Microvascular Surgery; Cosmetic Surgery-Face; Peripheral Nerve Surgery; **Hospital:** NYU Med Ctr (page 102), Lenox Hill Hosp (page 94); **Address:** 900 Park Ave, New York, NY 10021; **Phone:** 212-879-8880; **Board Cert:** Plastic Surgery 1982; Hand Surgery 2000; **Med School:** Columbia P&S 1973; **Resid:** Surgery, Barnes Jewish Hosp 1977; Plastic Surgery, Columbia-Presby Med Ctr 1979; **Fellow:** Hand Surgery, NYU Med Ctr 1980; **Fac Appt:** Prof S, NYU Sch Med

Colen, Helen S MD (PlS) - **Spec Exp:** Cosmetic Surgery-Face & Nose; Cosmetic Surgery-Breast; Cosmetic Surgery-Liposuction; **Hospital:** NYU Med Ctr (page 102), New York Eye & Ear Infirm (page 110); **Address:** 742 Park Ave, New York, NY 10021-3553; **Phone:** 212-772-1300; **Board Cert:** Plastic Surgery 1983; **Med School:** NYU Sch Med 1972; **Resid:** Surgery, Univ Colorado Med Ctr 1979; Plastic Surgery, St Lukes Hosp 1981; **Fellow:** Microsurgery, NYU Med Ctr 1982; **Fac Appt:** Assoc Clin Prof PlS, NYU Sch Med

Colen, Stephen MD (PlS) - **Spec Exp:** Cosmetic Surgery-Face; Cosmetic Surgery-Breast; Liposuction & Body Contouring; **Hospital:** NYU Med Ctr (page 102), Hackensack Univ Med Ctr (page 92); **Address:** 742 Park Ave, New York, NY 10021; **Phone:** 212-988-8900; **Board Cert:** Plastic Surgery 1983; **Med School:** Hahnemann Univ 1974; **Resid:** Surgery, Univ Colorado Hosp 1979; **Fellow:** Plastic Surgery, NYU Med Ctr 1981; **Fac Appt:** Assoc Prof S, NYU Sch Med

Cordeiro, Peter G MD (PlS) - **Spec Exp:** Reconstructive Surgery; Breast Reconstruction; Facial Plastic & Reconstructive Surgery; **Hospital:** Meml Sloan Kettering Cancer Ctr (page 109), Manhattan Eye, Ear & Throat Hosp; **Address:** Meml Sloan Kettering Cancer Ctr, 1275 York Ave, rm C1193, New York, NY 10021-6007; **Phone:** 212-639-2521; **Board Cert:** Surgery 1998; Plastic Surgery 1994; **Med School:** Harvard Med Sch 1983; **Resid:** Surgery, New Eng Deaconess Hosp-Harvard 1989; Plastic Surgery, NYU Med Ctr 1991; **Fellow:** Microsurgery, Meml Sloan-Kettering Cancer Ctr. 1992; Craniofacial Surgery, Univ Miami 1992; **Fac Appt:** Assoc Prof S, Cornell Univ-Weill Med Coll

Cutting, Court MD (PlS) - **Spec Exp:** Cleft Palate/Lip; Reconstructive Plastic Surgery; Rhinoplasty; Craniofacial Surgery/Reconstruction; **Hospital:** NYU Med Ctr (page 102); **Address:** 333 E 34th St, Ste 1K, New York, NY 10016-6481; **Phone:** 212-447-6229; **Board Cert:** Otolaryngology 1980; Plastic Surgery 1986; **Med School:** Univ Chicago-Pritzker Sch Med 1975; **Resid:** Otolaryngology, Univ Iowa Hosps 1980; Plastic Surgery, NYU Med Ctr 1983; **Fellow:** Craniofacial Surgery, NYU Med Ctr 1984; **Fac Appt:** Prof PlS, NYU Sch Med

Diktaban, Theodore MD (PlS) - **Spec Exp:** Cosmetic Surgery-Liposuction; Cosmetic Surgery-Face; Botox Therapy; Rhinoplasty; **Hospital:** Lenox Hill Hosp (page 94), Manhattan Eye, Ear & Throat Hosp; **Address:** 203 E 69th St, New York, NY 10021-5402; **Phone:** 212-988-5656; **Board Cert:** Otolaryngology 1981; Plastic Surgery 1988; **Med School:** NY Med Coll 1976; **Resid:** Otolaryngology, Mount Sinai Hosp 1981; Plastic Surgery, Lenox Hill Hosp 1983; **Fellow:** Reconstructive Microsurgery, Univ Louisville 1984

Forley, Bryan G MD (PlS) - **Spec Exp:** Cosmetic Surgery; Reconstructive Surgery; **Hospital:** Beth Israel Med Ctr - Petrie Division (page 90), New York Eye & Ear Infirm (page 110); **Address:** 5 E 82nd St, New York, NY 10028-0342; **Phone:** 212-861-3757; **Board Cert:** Plastic Surgery 1997; **Med School:** Mount Sinai Sch Med 1984; **Resid:** Surgery, NYU Med Ctr & Mt Sinai Med Ctr 1989; Plastic Surgery, Saint Francis Meml Hosp 1992; **Fellow:** Craniofacial Surgery, Hosp for Sick Children, Great Ormond St 1993

Foster, Craig A MD (PlS) - **Spec Exp:** Cosmetic Surgery-Face; Cosmetic Surgery-Breast; Nasal Surgery; **Hospital:** Manhattan Eye, Ear & Throat Hosp, Lenox Hill Hosp (page 94); **Address:** 850 Park Ave, Ste 1A, New York, NY 10021-1845; **Phone:** 212-744-5746; **Board Cert:** Otolaryngology 1980; Plastic Surgery 1984; **Med School:** Univ Minn 1974; **Resid:** Otolaryngology, Univ Minn Hosps 1980; Plastic Surgery, NYU Med Ctr 1982; **Fac Appt:** Assoc Prof Oto, NY Med Coll

Freund, Robert M MD (PlS) - **Spec Exp:** Cosmetic Surgery-Face; Breast Augmentation; Liposuction; **Hospital:** Lenox Hill Hosp (page 94), N Shore Univ Hosp at Manhasset; **Address:** 220 E 63rd St, Ste LJ, New York, NY 10021; **Phone:** 212-583-1200; **Board Cert:** Plastic Surgery 1998; **Med School:** Cornell Univ-Weill Med Coll 1987; **Resid:** Surgery, NYU Med Ctr 1993; Plastic Surgery, NYU Med Ctr 1995

Friedman, David Jay MD (PlS) - **Spec Exp:** Cosmetic Surgery-Face; Liposuction & Body Contouring; **Hospital:** Beth Israel Med Ctr - Petrie Division (page 90), Lenox Hill Hosp (page 94); **Address:** 650 Park Ave, New York, NY 10021; **Phone:** 212-439-1600; **Board Cert:** Plastic Surgery 1998; **Med School:** Albany Med Coll 1988; **Resid:** Surgery, Beth Israel Med Ctr 1993; Plastic Surgery, Mt Sinai Med Ctr 1994

Gayle, Lloyd MD (PlS) - **Spec Exp:** Breast Reconstruction & Augmentation; Hand Surgery; Cosmetic Surgery-Body; **Hospital:** NY-Presby Hosp (page 100), NY Hosp Queens; **Address:** 50 E 69th St, New York, NY 10021; **Phone:** 212-452-5121; **Board Cert:** Plastic Surgery 1993; **Med School:** NYU Sch Med 1983; **Resid:** Surgery, NYU Med Ctr 1988; Plastic Surgery, NY Hosp-Cornell Univ 1990; **Fellow:** Hand & Microvascular Surgery, Davies Med Ctr 1991; **Fac Appt:** Assoc Prof S, Cornell Univ-Weill Med Coll

Ginsberg, Gerald D MD (PlS) - **Spec Exp:** Cosmetic Surgery; Reconstructive Plastic Surgery; **Hospital:** NY Downtown Hosp, NYU Med Ctr (page 102); **Address:** 6 E 78th St, New York, NY 10021; **Phone:** 212-452-3421; **Board Cert:** Plastic Surgery 1984; Surgery 1983; **Med School:** Northwestern Univ 1974; **Resid:** Surgery, New York Univ Med Ctr; Plastic Surgery, New York Univ Med Ctr; **Fellow:** Hand Surgery, New York Univ Med Ctr; **Fac Appt:** Assoc Clin Prof PlS, NYU Sch Med

Godfrey, Norman MD (PlS) - **Spec Exp:** Rhinoplasty; Eyelid Surgery; **Hospital:** St Vincent Cath Med Ctrs - Manhattan (page 375), NY Hosp Queens; **Address:** 9 E 93rd St, New York, NY 10128; **Phone:** 212-628-6600; **Board Cert:** Plastic Surgery 1984; **Med School:** Harvard Med Sch 1973; **Resid:** Surgery, Bellevue Hosp 1978; Plastic Surgery, Bellevue Hosp 1980; **Fellow:** Plastic Surgery, Bellevue Hosp 1981; **Fac Appt:** Asst Clin Prof S, Cornell Univ-Weill Med Coll

Godfrey, Philip MD/DMD (PlS) - **Spec Exp:** Cosmetic Surgery-Breast; Abdominoplasty; Liposuction; **Hospital:** St Vincent Cath Med Ctrs - Manhattan (page 375), NY Hosp Queens; **Address:** 9 E 93rd St, New York, NY 10128; **Phone:** 212-628-6600; **Board Cert:** Plastic Surgery 1988; **Med School:** Univ Pennsylvania 1981; **Resid:** Surgery, Hartford Hosp 1984; Plastic Surgery, NY Hosp 1986; **Fellow:** Surgery, Meml Sloan Kettering Cancer Ctr 1987; **Fac Appt:** Asst Clin Prof S, Cornell Univ-Weill Med Coll

Gotkin, Robert MD (PlS) - **Spec Exp:** Cosmetic Surgery-Face; Cosmetic Surgery-Breast; Skin Laser Surgery; **Hospital:** New York Eye & Ear Infirm (page 110), Winthrop - Univ Hosp; **Address:** 625 Park Ave, New York, NY 10021; **Phone:** 212-794-4000; **Board Cert:** Plastic Surgery 1990; **Med School:** Howard Univ 1980; **Resid:** Surgery, SUNY Stony Brook 1985; Plastic Surgery, Georgetown Univ 1988; **Fellow:** Surgical Critical Care, SUNY Stony Brook 1986

Grant, Robert MD (PlS) - **Spec Exp:** Breast Reconstruction; Cosmetic Surgery; Microsurgery; **Hospital:** NY-Presby Hosp (page 100), N Shore Univ Hosp at Manhasset; **Address:** 161 Fort Washington Ave, Ste 601, New York, NY 10032; **Phone:** 212-305-5868; **Board Cert:** Surgery 2001; Plastic Surgery 2003; **Med School:** Albany Med Coll 1983; **Resid:** Surgery, New York Hosp 1988; Plastic Surgery, New York Hosp 1990; **Fellow:** Microvascular Surgery, NYU Med Ctr/Bellevue Hosp 1991; **Fac Appt:** Asst Clin Prof PlS, Columbia P&S

Haher, Jane N. MD (PlS) - **Spec Exp:** Breast Surgery; Liposuction; Cosmetic Surgery-Face & Nose; **Hospital:** St Vincent Cath Med Ctrs - Manhattan (page 375), Cabrini Med Ctr (page 374); **Address:** 5 E 83rd St, New York, NY 10028-0401; **Phone:** 212-744-1828; **Board Cert:** Plastic Surgery 1979; **Med School:** NY Med Coll 1967; **Resid:** Surgery, Kings Co-SUNY Med Ctr 1973; Plastic Surgery, Kings Co-SUNY Med Ctr 1975; **Fac Appt:** Assoc Prof S, NY Med Coll

Hidalgo, David MD (PlS) - **Spec Exp:** Cosmetic Surgery-Face; Cosmetic Surgery-Breast; Rhinoplasty; Reconstructive Surgery; **Hospital:** Manhattan Eye, Ear & Throat Hosp, NY-Presby Hosp (page 100); **Address:** 655 Park Ave Fl 1, New York, NY 10021-5937; **Phone:** 212-517-9777; **Board Cert:** Plastic Surgery 1987; **Med School:** Georgetown Univ 1978; **Resid:** Surgery, NYU Med Ctr 1983; Plastic Surgery, NYU Med Ctr 1985; **Fellow:** Microsurgery, NYU Med Ctr 1986; **Fac Appt:** Clin Prof S, Cornell Univ-Weill Med Coll

Hoffman, Lloyd MD (PlS) - **Spec Exp:** Cosmetic Surgery-Face; Liposuction; Breast Reconstruction; **Hospital:** NY-Presby Hosp (page 100); **Address:** 12 E 68th St, New York, NY 10021; **Phone:** 212-861-1640; **Board Cert:** Plastic Surgery 1989; Hand Surgery 1992; **Med School:** Northwestern Univ 1978; **Resid:** Surgery, New York Hosp 1983; Plastic Surgery, NYU Med Ctr 1986; **Fellow:** Hand Surgery, NYU Med Ctr 1987; **Fac Appt:** Assoc Prof PlS, Cornell Univ-Weill Med Coll

Hoffman, Saul MD (PlS) - **Spec Exp:** Cosmetic Surgery-Face & Breast; Breast Reconstruction; **Hospital:** Mount Sinai Med Ctr (page 98); **Address:** 1125 5th Ave, New York, NY 10128-0143; **Phone:** 212-288-9800; **Board Cert:** Surgery 1963; Plastic Surgery 1964; **Med School:** Univ Alberta 1955; **Resid:** Surgery, Brookdale Hosp 1959; Plastic Surgery, Bronx Muni Hosp Ctr 1961; **Fellow:** Plastic Surgery, Mount Sinai 1963; **Fac Appt:** Clin Prof S, Mount Sinai Sch Med

Hunter, John G MD (PlS) - **Spec Exp:** Cosmetic Surgery-Body; Cosmetic Surgery-Breast; Female Genital Cosmetic Surgery; **Hospital:** NY-Presby Hosp (page 100), New York Methodist Hosp (page 479); **Address:** 47 E 63rd St, New York, NY 10021-7315; **Phone:** 212-751-4444; **Board Cert:** Plastic Surgery 1991; **Med School:** SUNY Downstate 1983; **Resid:** Surgery, Mount Sinai Hosp 1986; **Fellow:** Plastic Surgery, Univ Hosp-SUNY Downstate 1988; **Fac Appt:** Assoc Clin Prof S, Cornell Univ-Weill Med Coll

Imber, Gerald MD (PlS) - **Spec Exp:** Cosmetic Surgery-Face; Eyelid Surgery; **Hospital:** NY-Presby Hosp (page 100); **Address:** 1009 5th Ave, Lower Level, New York, NY 10028; **Phone:** 212-472-1800; **Board Cert:** Plastic Surgery 1976; **Med School:** SUNY Downstate 1966; **Resid:** Surgery, LI Jewish Med Ctr 1972; Plastic Surgery, NY Hosp 1974; **Fac Appt:** Asst Clin Prof S, Cornell Univ-Weill Med Coll

Jacobs, Elliot MD (PlS) - **Spec Exp:** Cosmetic Surgery; Gynecomastia; **Hospital:** New York Eye & Ear Infirm (page 110), Beth Israel Med Ctr - Petrie Division (page 90); **Address:** 815 Park Ave, New York, NY 10021-3276; **Phone:** 212-570-6080; **Board Cert:** Plastic Surgery 1982; **Med School:** Mount Sinai Sch Med 1970; **Resid:** Surgery, Mt Sinai Med Ctr 1974; Plastic Surgery, Mt Sinai Med Ctr 1977

Jelks, Glenn MD (PlS) - **Spec Exp:** Eyelid Surgery; Cosmetic Surgery-Face; Rhinoplasty; **Hospital:** NYU Med Ctr (page 102), Manhattan Eye, Ear & Throat Hosp; **Address:** 875 Park Ave, New York, NY 10021-0341; **Phone:** 212-988-3303; **Board Cert:** Ophthalmology 1979; Plastic Surgery 1982; **Med School:** Mich State Univ 1973; **Resid:** Ophthalmology, UCLA Med Ctr 1978; **Fellow:** Plastic Surgery, New York Univ 1980; **Fac Appt:** Assoc Prof PlS, NYU Sch Med

Karp, Nolan MD (PlS) - **Spec Exp:** Breast Cosmetic & Reconstructive Surgery; Liposuction & Body Contouring; Cosmetic Surgery; **Hospital:** NYU Med Ctr (page 102); **Address:** 530 First Ave, Ste 8Y, New York, NY 10016-6402; **Phone:** 212-263-6004; **Board Cert:** Plastic Surgery 1994; **Med School:** Northwestern Univ 1983; **Resid:** Surgery, NYU Med Ctr 1988; Plastic Surgery, NYU Med Ctr 1991; **Fac Appt:** Assoc Prof PlS, NYU Sch Med

Karpinski, Richard MD (PlS) - **Spec Exp:** Rhinoplasty; Cosmetic Surgery-Liposuction; Cosmetic Surgery-Face; **Hospital:** St Luke's - Roosevelt Hosp Ctr - Roosevelt Div (page 90); **Address:** 200 Central Park South, New York, NY 10019-1436; **Phone:** 212-977-9797; **Board Cert:** Plastic Surgery 1983; **Med School:** Harvard Med Sch 1971; **Resid:** Surgery, Boston City Hosp 1973; Surgery, New England Deaconess 1977; **Fellow:** Plastic Surgery, NYU Med Ctr 1981; **Fac Appt:** Asst Clin Prof PlS, Columbia P&S

Kolker, Adam R MD (PlS) - **Spec Exp:** Cosmetic Surgery; Reconstructive Surgery; Craniofacial Surgery; **Hospital:** St Vincent Cath Med Ctrs - Manhattan (page 375), Mount Sinai Med Ctr (page 98); **Address:** 655 Park Ave, New York, NY 10021; **Phone:** 212-744-6500; **Board Cert:** Surgery 1996; Plastic Surgery 2001; **Med School:** Albany Med Coll 1990; **Resid:** Surgery, St Vincent's Hosp 1995; Plastic Reconstructive Surgery, Beth Israel Med Ctr 1998; **Fellow:** Microsurgery, NYU Med Ctr 1996; Craniofacial Surgery, Univ Melbourne Children's Hosp 2000; **Fac Appt:** Asst Clin Prof S, Mount Sinai Sch Med

Lesesne, Carroll B MD (PlS) - **Spec Exp:** Cosmetic Surgery-Face; Cosmetic Surgery-Liposuction; Rhinoplasty; **Hospital:** Manhattan Eye, Ear & Throat Hosp, Lenox Hill Hosp (page 94); **Address:** 620 Park Ave, New York, NY 10021-6591; **Phone:** 212-570-6318; **Board Cert:** Plastic Surgery 1987; **Med School:** Duke Univ 1980; **Resid:** Surgery, Stanford Univ Med Ctr 1983; Plastic Surgery, NY Hosp-Cornell Med Ctr 1985; **Fellow:** Plastic Surgery, Meml Sloan Kettering Cancer Ctr; **Fac Appt:** Asst Clin Prof PlS, NYU Sch Med

Matarasso, Alan MD (PlS) - **Spec Exp:** Cosmetic Surgery-Face & Eyes; Rhinoplasty; Liposuction & Body Contouring; **Hospital:** Manhattan Eye, Ear & Throat Hosp, New York Eye & Ear Infirm (page 110); **Address:** 1009 Park Ave, New York, NY 10028-0936; **Phone:** 212-249-7500; **Board Cert:** Plastic Surgery 1986; **Med School:** Univ Miami Sch Med 1979; **Resid:** Surgery, Montefiore Med Ctr 1983; Plastic Surgery, Montefiore Med Ctr 1985; **Fellow:** Plastic Surgery, Manhattan EET Hosp/NYU 1985; **Fac Appt:** Assoc Clin Prof PlS, Albert Einstein Coll Med

McCarthy, Joseph G MD (PlS) - **Spec Exp:** Craniofacial Surgery-Pediatric; Reconstructive Surgery-Face; Cosmetic Surgery-Face; **Hospital:** NYU Med Ctr (page 102), Manhattan Eye, Ear & Throat Hosp; **Address:** 722 Park Ave, New York, NY 10021-4954; **Phone:** 212-628-4420; **Board Cert:** Surgery 1972; Plastic Surgery 1974; **Med School:** Columbia P&S 1964; **Resid:** Surgery, Columbia-Presby Med Ctr 1971; Plastic Surgery, NYU Med Ctr 1973; **Fac Appt:** Prof S, NYU Sch Med

Pitman, Gerald H MD (PlS) - **Spec Exp:** Cosmetic Surgery-Face; Liposuction; **Hospital:** Manhattan Eye, Ear & Throat Hosp, NYU Med Ctr (page 102); **Address:** 170 E 73rd St, New York, NY 10021-4352; **Phone:** 212-517-2600; **Board Cert:** Plastic Surgery 1978; **Med School:** Univ Pennsylvania 1968; **Resid:** Surgery, Columbia-Presby Hosp 1975; Plastic Surgery, NYU Med Ctr 1977; **Fellow:** Microsurgery, NYU Med Ctr 1981; **Fac Appt:** Assoc Clin Prof PlS, NYU Sch Med

Razaboni, Rosa MD (PlS) - **Spec Exp:** Cosmetic Surgery; Breast Reconstruction; Liposuction; **Hospital:** Lenox Hill Hosp (page 94), Mount Sinai Med Ctr (page 98); **Address:** 14-A E 68th St, New York, NY 10021-5847; **Phone:** 212-772-0200; **Board Cert:** Plastic Surgery 1993; **Med School:** Brazil 1975; **Resid:** Surgery, St Vincent's Hosp & Med Ctr 1985; Plastic Surgery, New York Univ Med Ctr 1988; **Fellow:** Hosp Trousseau 1986

Reed, Lawrence S MD (PlS) - **Spec Exp:** Cosmetic Surgery-Liposuction; Cosmetic Surgery-Face & Breast; Rhinoplasty; **Hospital:** NY-Presby Hosp (page 100), Manhattan Eye, Ear & Throat Hosp; **Address:** 45 E 85th St, New York, NY 10028-0957; **Phone:** 212-772-8300; **Board Cert:** Plastic Surgery 1978; **Med School:** SUNY Hlth Sci Ctr 1969; **Resid:** Surgery, Einstein Hosp 1972; Surgery, Hosp Univ Penn 1975; **Fellow:** Plastic Surgery, New York Hosp-Cornell Med Ctr 1977; **Fac Appt:** Assoc Prof PlS, Cornell Univ-Weill Med Coll

Romita, Mauro C MD (PlS) - **Spec Exp:** Cosmetic Surgery-Face; Liposuction & Body Contouring; **Hospital:** St Vincent Cath Med Ctrs - Manhattan (page 375), NY Hosp Queens; **Address:** 853 5th Ave, New York, NY 10021; **Phone:** 212-772-3220; **Board Cert:** Plastic Surgery 1983; **Med School:** Univ Miami Sch Med 1973; **Resid:** Surgery, NYU Med Ctr 1978; Plastic Surgery, NYU Med Ctr 1980; **Fac Appt:** Asst Prof S, NY Med Coll

Rosenblatt, William B MD (PlS) - **Spec Exp:** Nasal Surgery; Cosmetic Surgery-Face & Body; Cosmetic Surgery-Breast; Rhinoplasty; **Hospital:** Lenox Hill Hosp (page 94), Manhattan Eye, Ear & Throat Hosp; **Address:** 308 E 79th St, New York, NY 10021; **Phone:** 212-570-6100; **Board Cert:** Otolaryngology 1977; Plastic Surgery 1980; **Med School:** NY Med Coll 1973; **Resid:** Otolaryngology, Metropolitan Hosp 1977; Plastic Surgery, Lenox Hill Hosp 1979

Schulman, Norman MD (PlS) - **Spec Exp:** Cosmetic Surgery-Face & Body; Cosmetic Surgery-Breast; Nasal Surgery; Breast Reconstruction; **Hospital:** Lenox Hill Hosp (page 94), Manhattan Eye, Ear & Throat Hosp; **Address:** 799 Park Ave, New York, NY 10021-3275; **Phone:** 212-861-5004; **Board Cert:** Surgery 1973; Plastic Surgery 1976; **Med School:** Tufts Univ 1965; **Resid:** Surgery, Jacobi Med Ctr 1972; Plastic Surgery, Lenox Hill Hosp 1974; **Fellow:** Plastic Surgery, Roswell Park Cancer Inst 1975

Scott, Susan M MD (PlS) - **Spec Exp:** Cosmetic Surgery-Face; Eyelid Surgery; Hand Reconstruction; **Hospital:** Hosp For Joint Diseases (page 107), Lenox Hill Hosp (page 94); **Address:** 150 E 77th St, New York, NY 10021; **Phone:** 212-288-9922; **Board Cert:** Plastic Surgery 1987; **Med School:** Columbia P&S 1974; **Resid:** Surgery, St Luke's-Roosevelt Hosp Ctr 1979; Plastic Surgery, NYU Med Ctr 1981; **Fellow:** Hand Surgery, St Luke's-Roosevelt Hosp Ctr 1982

Sherman, John E MD (PlS) - **Spec Exp:** Cosmetic Surgery-Face; Cosmetic Surgery-Liposuction; Facial Reconstruction; **Hospital:** NY-Presby Hosp (page 100), Lenox Hill Hosp (page 94); **Address:** 1016 Fifth Ave, Ste 1A, New York, NY 10028; **Phone:** 212-535-2300; **Board Cert:** Plastic Surgery 1984; **Med School:** NY Med Coll 1975; **Resid:** Surgery, Montefiore Hosp Med Ctr 1978; Plastic Surgery, New York Hosp/Meml Sloan Kettering Cancer Ctr 1980; **Fac Appt:** Asst Clin Prof S, Cornell Univ-Weill Med Coll

Siebert, John W MD (PlS) - **Spec Exp:** Facial Reconstruction; Microsurgery; Cosmetic Surgery-Face; **Hospital:** NYU Med Ctr (page 102), Manhattan Eye, Ear & Throat Hosp; **Address:** 50 E 71 St, New York, NY 10021; **Phone:** 212-737-8300; **Board Cert:** Plastic Surgery 1991; **Med School:** Univ Wisc 1981; **Resid:** Surgery, Mass Genl Hosp 1986; Plastic Surgery, NYU Med Ctr 1988; **Fellow:** Microsurgery, NYU Med Ctr 1989; **Fac Appt:** Assoc Prof S, NYU Sch Med

Silich, Robert C MD (PlS) - **Spec Exp:** Cosmetic Surgery-Face & Eyes; Blepharoplasty; Rhinoplasty; Liposuction; **Hospital:** NY-Presby Hosp (page 100), Lenox Hill Hosp (page 94); **Address:** 1009 5th Ave, New York, NY 10028; **Phone:** 212-472-0082; **Board Cert:** Plastic Surgery 2001; **Med School:** Georgetown Univ 1993; **Resid:** Surgery, NY-Cornell Med Ctr 1997; Plastic Surgery, NY-Cornell Med Ctr 1999; **Fac Appt:** Asst Clin Prof PlS, Cornell Univ-Weill Med Coll

Silver, Lester MD (PlS) - **Spec Exp:** Cleft Palate/Lip; Pediatric Plastic Surgery; **Hospital:** Mount Sinai Med Ctr (page 98); **Address:** 5 E 98th St, New York, NY 10029; **Phone:** 212-241-1968; **Board Cert:** Plastic Surgery 1978; **Med School:** Univ Hlth Sci/Chicago Med Sch 1960; **Resid:** Surgery, Albert Einstein 1966; Plastic Surgery, Mt Sinai Med Ctr 1969; **Fac Appt:** Prof PlS, Mount Sinai Sch Med

Skolnik, Richard A MD (PlS) - **Spec Exp:** Cosmetic Surgery-Face; Cosmetic Surgery-Breast; Liposuction & Body Contouring; **Hospital:** Mount Sinai Med Ctr (page 98), Beth Israel Med Ctr - Petrie Division (page 90); **Address:** 21 E 87th St, New York, NY 10128-0506; **Phone:** 212-722-1977; **Board Cert:** Plastic Surgery 1983; **Med School:** Cornell Univ-Weill Med Coll 1976; **Resid:** Surgery, Mount Sinai Hosp 1979; **Fellow:** Plastic Surgery, Mount Sinai Hosp 1982; **Fac Appt:** Assoc Clin Prof PlS, Mount Sinai Sch Med

Spinelli, Henry M MD (PlS) - **Spec Exp:** Cosmetic Surgery; Craniofacial Surgery/Reconstruction; Oculoplastic & Orbital Surgery; **Hospital:** NY-Presby Hosp (page 100), Manhattan Eye, Ear & Throat Hosp; **Address:** 875 Fifth Ave, New York, NY 10021-4952; **Phone:** 212-570-6235; **Board Cert:** Ophthalmology 1987; Plastic Surgery 1993; **Med School:** NYU Sch Med 1981; **Resid:** Ophthalmology, Manhattan EET Hosp 1985; Plastic Reconstructive Surgery, NYU-Bellevue Hosp 1990; **Fellow:** Craniofacial Surgery, NYU Med Ctr 1991; **Fac Appt:** Assoc Prof S, Cornell Univ-Weill Med Coll

New York (Manhattan)

Striker, Paul MD (PlS) - **Spec Exp:** Cosmetic Surgery-Breast; Eyelid Surgery; Rhinoplasty; Laser Surgery; **Hospital:** New York Eye & Ear Infirm (page 110), NY Downtown Hosp; **Address:** 660 Park Ave, New York, NY 10021-5963; **Phone:** 212-744-4265; **Board Cert:** Plastic Surgery 1972; **Med School:** Univ Colorado 1963; **Resid:** Surgery, Bellevue Hosp 1967; Surgery, Columbia-Presby Hosp 1969; **Fellow:** Plastic Surgery, Columbia-Presby Hosp 1971

Sultan, Mark MD (PlS) - **Spec Exp:** Breast Reconstruction; Cosmetic Surgery-Breast; Cosmetic Surgery-Face; **Hospital:** St Luke's - Roosevelt Hosp Ctr - Roosevelt Div (page 90), Beth Israel Med Ctr - Petrie Division (page 90); **Address:** 1100 Park Ave, New York, NY 10128; **Phone:** 212-360-0700; **Board Cert:** Plastic Surgery 1992; **Med School:** Columbia P&S 1982; **Resid:** Surgery, Columbia-Presby Hosp 1987; Plastic Surgery, Columbia-Presby Hosp 1990; **Fellow:** Head and Neck Surgery, Emory Univ Hosp 1989; **Fac Appt:** Assoc Prof S, Columbia P&S

Tabbal, Nicolas MD (PlS) - **Spec Exp:** Rhinoplasty; Cosmetic Surgery-Face; Eyelid Surgery; **Hospital:** Manhattan Eye, Ear & Throat Hosp; **Address:** 521 Park Ave, New York, NY 10021-8140; **Phone:** 212-644-5800; **Board Cert:** Plastic Surgery 1980; **Med School:** Lebanon 1972; **Resid:** Surgery, Am Univ Med Ctr 1976; Plastic Surgery, Akron City Hosp 1979; **Fellow:** Surgery, Upstate Med Ctr 1977; Reconstructive Microsurgery, NYU Med Ctr 1980

Taub, Peter J MD (PlS) - **Spec Exp:** Pediatric Plastic Surgery; Craniofacial Surgery; Cosmetic Surgery; Maxillofacial Surgery; **Hospital:** Mount Sinai Med Ctr (page 98); **Address:** Mount Sinai Medical Ctr, 5 E 98th St Fl 15, New York, NY 10029-6574; **Phone:** 212-241-4410; **Board Cert:** Surgery 2000; Plastic Surgery 2003; **Med School:** Albert Einstein Coll Med 1993; **Resid:** Surgery, Mt Sinai Med Ctr 1999; Plastic Surgery, UCLA Med Ctr 2001; **Fellow:** Craniofacial Surgery, UCLA Med Ctr 2002; **Fac Appt:** Asst Prof PlS, Mount Sinai Sch Med

Thorne, Charles MD (PlS) - **Spec Exp:** Cosmetic Surgery-Face & Breast; Ear Reconstruction/Microtia; Maxillofacial Surgery; Craniofacial Surgery; **Hospital:** NYU Med Ctr (page 102), Manhattan Eye, Ear & Throat Hosp; **Address:** 812 Park Ave, New York, NY 10021-2759; **Phone:** 212-794-0044; **Board Cert:** Plastic Surgery 1991; **Med School:** UCLA 1981; **Resid:** Surgery, Mass Genl Hosp 1986; Plastic Surgery, NYU Med Ctr 1988; **Fellow:** Craniofacial Surgery, NYU Med Ctr 1989; **Fac Appt:** Assoc Prof PlS, NYU Sch Med

Verga, Michele MD (PlS) - **Spec Exp:** Cosmetic Surgery-Face; Liposuction; Body Contouring; **Hospital:** Mount Sinai Med Ctr (page 98); **Address:** 1010 5th Ave, New York, NY 10028-0130; **Phone:** 212-535-0470; **Board Cert:** Plastic Surgery 1984; **Med School:** Italy 1974; **Resid:** Surgery, Mt Sinai Hosp 1978; Surgery, Lutheran Med Ctr 1980; **Fellow:** Plastic Surgery, Mt Sinai Hosp 1983; **Fac Appt:** Asst Clin Prof S, Mount Sinai Sch Med

Vickery, Carlin MD (PlS) - **Spec Exp:** Breast Cosmetic & Reconstructive Surgery; Cosmetic Surgery-Body; Cosmetic Surgery-Face; **Hospital:** Mount Sinai Med Ctr (page 98); **Address:** 1125 5th Ave, New York, NY 10128; **Phone:** 212-288-9800; **Board Cert:** Plastic Surgery 1987; **Med School:** NYU Sch Med 1977; **Resid:** Surgery, New York Univ Med Ctr 1982; **Fellow:** Microsurgery, New York Univ Med Ctr 1985; **Fac Appt:** Assoc Clin Prof S, Mount Sinai Sch Med

Weiss, Paul R MD (PlS) - **Spec Exp:** Breast Cosmetic & Reconstructive Surgery; Cosmetic Surgery-Face; Cosmetic Surgery-Body; **Hospital:** Montefiore Med Ctr, Beth Israel Med Ctr - Petrie Division (page 90); **Address:** 1049 5th Ave, Ste 2D, New York, NY 10028-0115; **Phone:** 212-861-8000; **Board Cert:** Surgery 1975; Plastic Surgery 1977; **Med School:** Tulane Univ 1969; **Resid:** Surgery, Montefiore Hosp Med Ctr/Bronx Muni Hosp 1974; Plastic Surgery, Montefiore Hosp Med Ctr 1976; **Fac Appt:** Clin Prof PlS, Albert Einstein Coll Med

Wells, Scott B MD (PlS) - **Spec Exp:** Cosmetic Surgery-Face; Abdominoplasty; Breast Augmentation; **Hospital:** Winthrop - Univ Hosp; **Address:** 655 Park Ave, New York, NY 10021; **Phone:** 212-794-3900; **Board Cert:** Plastic Surgery 2005; **Med School:** NY Med Coll 1985; **Resid:** Surgery, Beth Israel Med Ctr 1990; Plastic Surgery, SUNY Hlth Sci Ctr 1992

Wood-Smith, Donald MD (PlS) - **Spec Exp:** Rhinoplasty Revision; Cosmetic Surgery-Face; **Hospital:** New York Eye & Ear Infirm (page 110), NY-Presby Hosp (page 100); **Address:** 830 Park Ave, New York, NY 10021-2757; **Phone:** 212-744-2224; **Board Cert:** Plastic Surgery 1970; **Med School:** Australia 1954; **Resid:** Plastic Surgery, NYU Med Ctr 1963; Surgery, Stanford Univ & Santa Clara Valley Med Ctr 1968; **Fellow:** Craniofacial Surgery, NYU Med Ctr 1966; **Fac Appt:** Prof S, Columbia P&S

Zevon, Scott MD (PlS) - **Spec Exp:** Cosmetic Surgery; Breast Surgery; Reconstructive Surgery-Face; **Hospital:** St Luke's - Roosevelt Hosp Ctr - Roosevelt Div (page 90), Long Island Coll Hosp (page 90); **Address:** 75 Central Park West, New York, NY 10023; **Phone:** 212-496-6600; **Board Cert:** Plastic Surgery 1989; **Med School:** Boston Univ 1979; **Resid:** Surgery, St Luke's-Roosevelt Hosp Ctr 1984; Plastic Surgery, Nassau Co Med Ctr 1986; **Fellow:** Craniofacial Surgery, Mayo Clinic 1987

Zide, Barry M MD/DMD (PlS) - **Spec Exp:** Facial Surgery-Chin; Hemangiomas; Facial Reconstruction-Cancer; Craniofacial Surgery-Pediatric; **Hospital:** NYU Med Ctr (page 102), Lenox Hill Hosp (page 94); **Address:** 420 E 55th St, Ste 1D, New York, NY 10022-5140; **Phone:** 212-421-2424; **Board Cert:** Plastic Surgery 1981; **Med School:** Tufts Univ 1973; **Resid:** Surgery, Stanford Med Ctr 1976; Plastic Surgery, U NC Hosp 1978; **Fellow:** Head and Neck Oncology, Roswell Park Cancer Inst 1979; Craniofacial Surgery, NYU Med Ctr 1980; **Fac Appt:** Prof PlS, NYU Sch Med

Preventive Medicine

Cahill, John MD (PrM) - **Spec Exp:** Tropical Diseases; International Health; Disaster Relief Medicine; **Hospital:** St Luke's - Roosevelt Hosp Ctr - Roosevelt Div (page 90), St Luke's - Roosevelt Hosp Ctr - St Luke's Hosp (page 90); **Address:** 425 W 59th St, Ste 8A, New York, NY 10019; **Phone:** 212-492-5500; **Board Cert:** Emergency Medicine 2001; **Med School:** Mount Sinai Sch Med 1996; **Resid:** Emergency Medicine, Rhode Island Hosp 1997; Emergency Medicine, Rhode Island Hosp 2000; **Fellow:** Tropical Medicine, Royal Coll Surgeons 1998; **Fac Appt:** Asst Clin Prof Med, Columbia P&S

Cahill, Kevin M MD (PrM) - **Spec Exp:** Tropical Medicine; International Health; **Hospital:** Lenox Hill Hosp (page 94); **Address:** 850 5th Ave, New York, NY 10021; **Phone:** 212-434-2477; **Board Cert:** Public Health & Genl Preventive Med 1970; **Med School:** Cornell Univ-Weill Med Coll 1961; **Resid:** Internal Medicine, US Navy Med Res Unit 1965; **Fac Appt:** Clin Prof Med, NYU Sch Med

Gemson, Donald H MD (PrM) - **Spec Exp:** Merrill Lynch Employee Health; Occupational Medicine; Tobacco Control; **Address:** Merrill Lynch Hlth Svcs, 4 World Financial Ctr Fl 3, New York, NY 10080; **Phone:** 212-449-9056; **Board Cert:** Internal Medicine 1982; Public Health & Genl Preventive Med 1987; **Med School:** NY Med Coll 1978; **Resid:** Internal Medicine, Roosevelt Hosp 1982; Public Health & Genl Preventive Med, Columbia Univ Sch Public Hlth 1985; **Fac Appt:** Assoc Clin Prof PrM, Columbia P&S

Hoffman, Robert S MD (PrM) - **Spec Exp:** Poison Control; Bioterrorism Preparedness; **Hospital:** NYU Med Ctr (page 102), Bellevue Hosp Ctr; **Address:** NY Poison Control Ctr, 455 1st Ave, rm 123, New York, NY 10016; **Phone:** 212-340-4494; **Board Cert:** Internal Medicine 1987; Emergency Medicine 1995; Medical Toxicology 1999; **Med School:** NYU Sch Med 1984; **Resid:** Internal Medicine, NYU Med Ctr 1987; **Fellow:** Medical Toxicology, NYU Med Ctr 1989; **Fac Appt:** Asst Clin Prof EM, NYU Sch Med

PSYCHIATRY

Alger, Ian MD (Psyc) - **Spec Exp:** Couples Therapy; Psychotherapy; Video-playback Therapy; **Hospital:** NY-Presby Hosp (page 100), NY-Presby Hosp (page 100); **Address:** 500 E 77th St, Ste 132, New York, NY 10162-0021; **Phone:** 212-861-3707; **Med School:** Canada 1949; **Resid:** Psychiatry, Bellevue Hosp 1953; **Fellow:** Psychiatry, NYU Med Ctr 1953; **Fac Appt:** Clin Prof Psyc, Cornell Univ-Weill Med Coll

Alper, Kenneth MD (Psyc) - **Spec Exp:** Psychopharmacology; Neuro-Psychiatry; **Hospital:** NYU Med Ctr (page 102), Bellevue Hosp Ctr; **Address:** 403 E 34th St Fl 4, New York, NY 10016; **Phone:** 212-263-8854; **Board Cert:** Psychiatry 1989; Clinical Neurophysiology 1992; Addiction Psychiatry 1993; **Med School:** Univ Tex, San Antonio 1984; **Resid:** Psychiatry, NYU Med Ctr 1988; **Fellow:** Clinical Neurophysiology, NYU Med Ctr 1990; **Fac Appt:** Assoc Prof Psyc, NYU Sch Med

Arkow, Stan D MD (Psyc) - **Spec Exp:** Psychotherapy; Psychopharmacology; **Hospital:** NY-Presby Hosp (page 100); **Address:** 740 West End Ave, Ste 5-A, New York, NY 10025; **Phone:** 212-663-5185; **Board Cert:** Psychiatry 1985; **Med School:** Columbia P&S 1977; **Resid:** Psychiatry, Columbia-Presby Med Ctr/Psych Inst 1981; **Fac Appt:** Assoc Clin Prof Psyc, Columbia P&S

Aronoff, Michael S MD (Psyc) - **Spec Exp:** Sleep Disorders; Family & Couples Therapy; Forensic/Legal Psychiatry; Stress Management; **Hospital:** Lenox Hill Hosp (page 94); **Address:** 60 Riverside Drive, Ste 16E, New York, NY 10024-6171; **Phone:** 212-799-8257; **Board Cert:** Psychiatry 1977; Forensic Psychiatry 1996; **Med School:** Univ Pennsylvania 1966; **Resid:** Psychiatry, NY State Psych Inst 1972; **Fellow:** Psychoanalysis, Columbia-Presby Hosp 1976; **Fac Appt:** Clin Prof Psyc, NYU Sch Med

Attia, Evelyn MD (Psyc) - **Spec Exp:** Eating Disorders; Mood Disorders; **Hospital:** NY State Psychiatric Inst (page 100), NY-Presby Hosp (page 100); **Address:** 239 Central Park West, New York, NY 10024-6038; **Phone:** 212-721-2850; **Board Cert:** Psychiatry 1992; **Med School:** Columbia P&S 1986; **Resid:** Psychiatry, Hosp Univ Penn 1987; Psychiatry, NY State Psychiatric Inst 1990; **Fac Appt:** Assoc Clin Prof Psyc, Columbia P&S

Auchincloss, Elizabeth MD (Psyc) - **Spec Exp:** Psychoanalysis; **Hospital:** NY-Presby Hosp (page 100); **Address:** 15 W 81st St, New York, NY 10024; **Phone:** 212-874-0070; **Board Cert:** Psychiatry 1982; **Med School:** Columbia P&S 1977; **Resid:** Psychiatry, NY Hosp 1982; **Fellow:** Psychoanalysis, Columbia-Presby Med Ctr 1986; **Fac Appt:** Clin Prof Psyc, Cornell Univ-Weill Med Coll

Barbuto, Joseph MD (Psyc) - **Spec Exp:** Psychiatry of Cancer; Anxiety & Mood Disorders; Personality Disorders; **Hospital:** NY-Presby Hosp (page 100), Meml Sloan Kettering Cancer Ctr (page 109); **Address:** 945 Fifth Ave, New York, NY 10021; **Phone:** 212-724-7366; **Board Cert:** Psychiatry 1983; **Med School:** Albert Einstein Coll Med 1978; **Resid:** Psychiatry, NY Hosp 1982; **Fellow:** Psychiatric Oncology, Meml Sloan Kettering Cancer Ctr 1986; **Fac Appt:** Assoc Clin Prof Psyc, Cornell Univ-Weill Med Coll

Basch, Samuel MD (Psyc) - **Spec Exp:** Psychiatry in Cancer; Psychiatry in Physical Illness; Psychopharmacology; Psychoanalysis; **Hospital:** Mount Sinai Med Ctr (page 98); **Address:** 10 E 85th St, Ste 1B, New York, NY 10028-0778; **Phone:** 212-427-0344; **Board Cert:** Psychiatry 1970; **Med School:** Hahnemann Univ 1961; **Resid:** Psychiatry, Mount Sinai Hosp 1965; **Fellow:** Psychoanalysis, Columbia Presby Hosp 1976; **Fac Appt:** Clin Prof Psyc, Mount Sinai Sch Med

Bone, Stanley MD (Psyc) - **Spec Exp:** Psychotherapy; Psychoanalysis; **Hospital:** NY-Presby Hosp (page 100); **Address:** 1155 Park Ave, New York, NY 10128-1209; **Phone:** 212-831-0917; **Board Cert:** Psychiatry 1979; **Med School:** Mount Sinai Sch Med 1974; **Resid:** Psychiatry, Columbia Presby 1978; **Fellow:** Psychoanalysis, Columbia Univ 1984; **Fac Appt:** Clin Prof Psyc, Columbia P&S

Borbely, Antal MD (Psyc) - **Spec Exp:** Career Related Problems; Relationship Problems; Creativity Enhancement; **Hospital:** Mount Sinai Med Ctr (page 98); **Address:** 675 W End Ave, Ste 1A, New York, NY 10025-7359; **Phone:** 212-222-1678; **Board Cert:** Psychiatry 1976; **Med School:** Switzerland 1968; **Resid:** Psychiatry, NY State Psyc Inst 1972; Psychiatry, Albert Einstein 1973; **Fellow:** Community Psychiatry, Albert Einstein 1975

Breitbart, William MD (Psyc) - **Spec Exp:** Psychiatry in Cancer; AIDS Related Cancers; Pain-Cancer; Palliative Care; **Hospital:** Meml Sloan Kettering Cancer Ctr (page 109); **Address:** Meml Sloan Kettering Cancer Center, 641 Lexington Ave Fl 7, New York, NY 10021; **Phone:** 646-888-0020; **Board Cert:** Internal Medicine 1982; Psychiatry 1986; **Med School:** Albert Einstein Coll Med 1978; **Resid:** Internal Medicine, Bronx Muni Hosp Ctr 1982; Psychiatry, Bronx Muni Hosp Ctr 1984; **Fellow:** Psychiatric Oncology, Meml Sloan Kettering Cancer Ctr 1986; **Fac Appt:** Prof Psyc, Cornell Univ-Weill Med Coll

Brenner, Ronald MD (Psyc) - **Spec Exp:** Depression; Dementia; Panic Disorder; **Hospital:** St John's Epis Hosp - S Shore, Mercy Med Ctr - Rockville Centre; **Address:** 750 Park Ave, New York, NY 10021; **Phone:** 718-869-7248; **Board Cert:** Psychiatry 1979; **Med School:** Spain 1974; **Resid:** Psychiatry, St Luke's-Roosevelt Hosp Ctr 1978St Luke's-Roosevelt Hosp Ctr 1978; **Fellow:** Pharmacology, New York Univ Med Ctr 1979; **Fac Appt:** Clin Prof Psyc, SUNY Hlth Sci Ctr

Brodie, Jonathan D MD (Psyc) - **Spec Exp:** Psychopharmacology; Anxiety & Depression; Neuro-Psychiatry; **Hospital:** NYU Med Ctr (page 102); **Address:** 155 E 38th St, Ste 3L, New York, NY 10016; **Phone:** 212-986-6693; **Board Cert:** Psychiatry 1979; **Med School:** NYU Sch Med 1975; **Resid:** Psychiatry, NYU Med Ctr/Bellevue Hosp 1978; **Fac Appt:** Prof Psyc, NYU Sch Med

Bronheim, Harold MD (Psyc) - **Spec Exp:** Psychotherapy & Psychopharmacology; Psychoanalysis; Medical Illness in Psychiatry; Opiate Addiction; **Hospital:** Mount Sinai Med Ctr (page 98); **Address:** 1155 Park Ave, New York, NY 10128-1209; **Phone:** 212-996-5777; **Board Cert:** Psychiatry 1985; Internal Medicine 1986; Geriatric Psychiatry 2001; **Med School:** SUNY Hlth Sci Ctr 1980; **Resid:** Psychiatry, Mount Sinai Hosp 1984; **Fellow:** Internal Medicine, Beth Israel Hosp 1985; **Fac Appt:** Clin Prof Psyc, Mount Sinai Sch Med

Brown, Richard P MD (Psyc) - **Spec Exp:** Psychopharmacology; Complementary Medicine; **Hospital:** NY-Presby Hosp (page 100); **Address:** 30 East End Ave, Bldg 1B, New York, NY 10028-7053; **Phone:** 212-737-0821; **Board Cert:** Psychiatry 1983; **Med School:** Columbia P&S 1977; **Resid:** Psychiatry, New York Hosp 1982; **Fellow:** Psychopharmacology, New York Hosp 1984; **Fac Appt:** Assoc Prof Psyc, Columbia P&S

Bukberg, Judith MD (Psyc) - **Spec Exp:** Psychotherapy; Psychoanalysis; **Hospital:** St Vincent Cath Med Ctrs - Manhattan (page 375); **Address:** 3 E 10th St, Bldg 1A, New York, NY 10003; **Phone:** 212-614-0312; **Board Cert:** Psychiatry 1979; **Med School:** Mount Sinai Sch Med 1974; **Resid:** Psychiatry, Mount Sinai Hosp 1978; **Fellow:** Liason Psychiatry, Meml Sloan Kettering Cancer Ctr 1980; **Fac Appt:** Assoc Clin Prof Psyc, NY Med Coll

Bulgarelli, Christopher MD (Psyc) - **Spec Exp:** Psychoanalysis; Depression; Anxiety Disorders; **Hospital:** Lenox Hill Hosp (page 94); **Address:** 455 W 23rd St, New York, NY 10011-2148; **Phone:** 212-807-1054; **Board Cert:** Psychiatry 1991; **Med School:** Tufts Univ 1986; **Resid:** Psychiatry, NYU/Bellevue Hosp 1989; **Fac Appt:** Asst Clin Prof Psyc, NYU Sch Med

Call, Pamela MD (Psyc) - **Spec Exp:** Psychiatry of Cancer; **Hospital:** St Vincent Cath Med Ctrs - Manhattan (page 375); **Address:** St Vincents Comp Canc Cntr, 325 W 15th St, New York, NY 10011; **Phone:** 212-604-6023; **Board Cert:** Psychiatry 1989; **Med School:** NY Med Coll 1983; **Resid:** Psychiatry, St Vincent's Hosp & Med Ctr 1987; **Fellow:** Psychiatric Oncology, Meml Sloan Kettering Cancer Ctr; **Fac Appt:** Assoc Prof Psyc, NY Med Coll

Campion, Robert E MD (Psyc) - **Spec Exp:** Forensic Psychiatry; **Hospital:** St. Vincent's Midtown; **Address:** 211 W 56th St, Ste 18M, New York, NY 10019-4312; **Phone:** 212-245-9112; **Board Cert:** Psychiatry 1979; Forensic Psychiatry 1998; Geriatric Psychiatry 2001; **Med School:** Spain 1973; **Resid:** Psychiatry, St Vincent's Hosp & Med Ctr 1977; **Fac Appt:** Asst Clin Prof Psyc, NY Med Coll

Chung, Henry MD (Psyc) - **Spec Exp:** Depression; Anxiety Disorders; **Hospital:** NYU Med Ctr (page 102); **Address:** 726 Broadway, New York, NY 10013; **Phone:** 917-533-6908; **Board Cert:** Psychiatry 2004; **Med School:** SUNY Buffalo 1989; **Resid:** Psychiatry, NY Hosp 1993; **Fellow:** Research, NY Hosp 1995; **Fac Appt:** Assoc Clin Prof Psyc, NYU Sch Med

Cohen, Arnold R MD (Psyc) - **Spec Exp:** Psychotherapy; ADD/ADHD; Autism; **Hospital:** Mount Sinai Med Ctr (page 98); **Address:** 64 E 94th St, Apt 1A, New York, NY 10128; **Phone:** 212-289-6800; **Board Cert:** Psychiatry 1969; **Med School:** SUNY Hlth Sci Ctr 1963; **Resid:** Psychiatry, Mount Sinai Hosp 1966; **Fellow:** Child & Adolescent Psychiatry, Mount Sinai Hosp 1970; **Fac Appt:** Asst Clin Prof Psyc, Mount Sinai Sch Med

Collins, Allen H MD (Psyc) - **Spec Exp:** Anxiety Disorders; Depression; Work Problems; **Hospital:** Lenox Hill Hosp (page 94), NYU Med Ctr (page 102); **Address:** 800A Fifth Ave Fl 3 - Ste 301, New York, NY 10021; **Phone:** 212-588-1205; **Board Cert:** Psychiatry 1975; **Med School:** Tufts Univ 1968; **Resid:** Psychiatry, NYS Psych.Inst./Colum-Presby 1972; Public Health & Genl Preventive Med, Columbia Grad Sch PH 1974; **Fellow:** Psychoanalysis, Wm Alanson White Inst 1980; Psychiatry, NY Academy Med; **Fac Appt:** Clin Prof Psyc, NYU Sch Med

Cordon, David MD (Psyc) - **Spec Exp:** Geriatric Psychiatry; **Hospital:** St Vincent Cath Med Ctrs - Manhattan (page 375); **Address:** 144 W 12th St, New York, NY 10011-8202; **Phone:** 212-604-1525; **Board Cert:** Psychiatry 1990; Geriatric Psychiatry 2003; **Med School:** UMDNJ-RW Johnson Med Sch 1984; **Resid:** Psychiatry, St Vincents Catholic Med Ctr 1988; **Fac Appt:** Assoc Clin Prof Psyc, NY Med Coll

Cournos, Francine MD (Psyc) - **Spec Exp:** Aggression Disorders; Relationship Problems; Psychotherapy; **Hospital:** NY-Presby Hosp (page 100); **Address:** 1051 Riverside Drive, Unit 121, New York, NY 10032; **Phone:** 212-543-6800; **Board Cert:** Psychiatry 1978; **Med School:** NYU Sch Med 1971; **Resid:** Internal Medicine, Montefiore Hosp Med Ctr 1973; Psychiatry, NY State Psyc Inst 1976; **Fac Appt:** Prof Psyc, Columbia P&S

Deutsch, Alexander MD (Psyc) - **Spec Exp:** Psychotherapy; Psychopharmacology; **Hospital:** Cabrini Med Ctr (page 374), NYU Med Ctr (page 102); **Address:** 115 E 82nd St, New York, NY 10028-0831; **Phone:** 212-249-9390; **Board Cert:** Psychiatry 1970; **Med School:** NYU Sch Med 1957; **Resid:** Psychiatry, Yale-New Haven Med Ctr 1964; **Fellow:** Psychiatry, Yale Univ 1965; **Fac Appt:** Assoc Clin Prof Psyc, NYU Sch Med

Douglas, Carolyn MD (Psyc) - **Spec Exp:** Depression; Anxiety Disorders; Relationship Problems; **Hospital:** NY-Presby Hosp (page 100); **Address:** 345 E 84th St, New York, NY 10028-4434; **Phone:** 212-396-9808; **Board Cert:** Psychiatry 1985; **Med School:** Harvard Med Sch 1980; **Resid:** Psychiatry, New York Hosp - Payne Whitney Clinic 1984; **Fac Appt:** Assoc Clin Prof Psyc, Columbia P&S

Druss, Richard MD (Psyc) - **Spec Exp:** Psychotherapy; **Hospital:** NY-Presby Hosp (page 100); **Address:** 180 E End Ave, New York, NY 10128-7763; **Phone:** 212-772-8383; **Board Cert:** Psychiatry 1970; **Med School:** Columbia P&S 1959; **Resid:** Psychiatry, Columbia-Presby Med Ctr 1963; **Fac Appt:** Clin Prof Psyc, Columbia P&S

Eth, Spencer MD (Psyc) - **Spec Exp:** Forensic Psychiatry; Post Traumatic Stress Disorder; **Hospital:** St Vincent Cath Med Ctrs - Manhattan (page 375); **Address:** 144 W 12th St, rm 174, New York, NY 10011-8202; **Phone:** 212-604-8196; **Board Cert:** Child & Adolescent Psychiatry 1982; Geriatric Psychiatry 2000; Forensic Psychiatry 2005; Addiction Psychiatry 1998; **Med School:** UCLA 1976; **Resid:** Psychiatry, NY Cornell Med Ctr 1979; **Fellow:** Child & Adolescent Psychiatry, Cedars -Sinai Med Ctr 1981; **Fac Appt:** Prof Psyc, NY Med Coll

Fabian, Christopher MD (Psyc) - **Hospital:** St Vincent Cath Med Ctrs - Manhattan (page 375); **Address:** 33 5th Ave, New York, NY 10003; **Phone:** 212-673-5230; **Board Cert:** Psychiatry 1989; **Med School:** Georgetown Univ 1983; **Resid:** Psychiatry, St Vincent's Hosp & Med Ctr 1987

Ferran, Ernesto MD (Psyc) - **Spec Exp:** Cultural Psychiatry; **Hospital:** NYU Med Ctr (page 102); **Address:** 15 Charles St, Ste 6H, New York, NY 10014-3024; **Phone:** 212-924-2673; **Board Cert:** Psychiatry 1983; Child & Adolescent Psychiatry 1986; **Med School:** Albert Einstein Coll Med 1976; **Resid:** Psychiatry, Bellevue Hosp/NYU Med Ctr 1979; **Fellow:** Child & Adolescent Psychiatry, Bellevue Hosp/NYU Med Ctr 1981; **Fac Appt:** Clin Prof Psyc, NYU Sch Med

Finkel, Jay MD (Psyc) - **Spec Exp:** Anxiety Disorders; Mood Disorders; **Hospital:** Mount Sinai Med Ctr (page 98); **Address:** 108 E 91st St, New York, NY 10128-1657; **Phone:** 212-289-2077; **Board Cert:** Psychiatry 1985; **Med School:** NY Med Coll 1980; **Resid:** Psychiatry, Mount Sinai Hosp 1984; **Fac Appt:** Asst Clin Prof Psyc, Mount Sinai Sch Med

First, Michael B MD (Psyc) - **Spec Exp:** Psychotherapy; Psychopharmacology; Forensic Psychiatry; **Hospital:** NY-Presby Hosp (page 100); **Address:** NY State Psychiatric Inst, Unit 60, 1051 Riverside Drive, New York, NY 10032; **Phone:** 212-543-5531; **Board Cert:** Psychiatry 1989; **Med School:** Univ Pittsburgh 1983; **Resid:** Psychiatry, NY State Psych Inst 1987; **Fellow:** Psychiatric Research, NY State Psych Inst 1988; **Fac Appt:** Clin Prof Psyc, Columbia P&S

Fleishman, Stewart MD (Psyc) - **Spec Exp:** Palliative Care; **Hospital:** Beth Israel Med Ctr - Petrie Division (page 90); **Address:** 10 Union Square E, New York, NY 10003; **Phone:** 212-844-6295; **Board Cert:** Psychiatry 1985; **Med School:** Mexico 1979; **Resid:** Psychiatry, LI Jewish Med Ctr 1984; **Fellow:** Psychiatric Oncology, Meml Sloan Kettering Cancer Ctr 1986; **Fac Appt:** Assoc Clin Prof Psyc, Albert Einstein Coll Med

Foster, Jeffrey MD (Psyc) - **Spec Exp:** Geriatric Psychiatry; Psychopharmacology; Depression; **Hospital:** NYU Med Ctr (page 102); **Address:** 155 E 29th St, Ste 31D, New York, NY 10016; **Phone:** 212-686-9668; **Board Cert:** Psychiatry 1980; Geriatric Psychiatry 2001; **Med School:** NY Med Coll 1970; **Resid:** Psychiatry, Mount Sinai Hosp 1974; **Fac Appt:** Clin Prof Psyc, NYU Sch Med

Fox, Herbert MD (Psyc) - **Spec Exp:** Electroconvulsive Therapy (ECT); Psychotherapy; Psychopharmacology; **Hospital:** Gracie Square Hosp, Lenox Hill Hosp (page 94); **Address:** 515 E 72nd St, New York, NY 10021-4032; **Phone:** 212-674-8622; **Board Cert:** Psychiatry 1976; Geriatric Psychiatry 1994; **Med School:** Albert Einstein Coll Med 1969; **Resid:** Psychiatry, Albert Einstein 1973; **Fac Appt:** Assoc Prof Psyc, Cornell Univ-Weill Med Coll

Friedman, Richard Alan MD (Psyc) - **Spec Exp:** Psychopharmacology; Anxiety & Mood Disorders; Depression; **Hospital:** NY-Presby Hosp (page 100); **Address:** 525 E 68th St, Box 140, New York, NY 10021-4870; **Phone:** 212-746-5775; **Board Cert:** Psychiatry 1989; **Med School:** UMDNJ-RW Johnson Med Sch 1982; **Resid:** Psychiatry, Mount Sinai 1987; **Fac Appt:** Assoc Clin Prof Psyc, Cornell Univ-Weill Med Coll

Frosch, William MD (Psyc) - **Hospital:** NY-Presby Hosp (page 100); **Address:** 525 E 68th St, Box 170, New York, NY 10021-4870; **Phone:** 212-746-3667; **Board Cert:** Psychiatry 1964; **Med School:** NYU Sch Med 1957; **Resid:** Psychiatry, Bellevue Hosp 1961; **Fac Appt:** Prof Emeritus Psyc, Cornell Univ-Weill Med Coll

Fyer, Abby J MD (Psyc) - **Spec Exp:** Anxiety Disorders; **Hospital:** NY State Psychiatric Inst (page 100); **Address:** 1051 Riverside Dr, Box 82, New York, NY 10032; **Phone:** 212-543-5372; **Board Cert:** Psychiatry 1980; **Med School:** NYU Sch Med 1973

Fyer, Minna R MD (Psyc) - **Spec Exp:** Anxiety Disorders; Mood Disorders; **Hospital:** NY-Presby Hosp (page 100); **Address:** 242 E 72nd St, New York, NY 10021-4574; **Phone:** 212-861-2586; **Board Cert:** Psychiatry 1985; **Med School:** SUNY Hlth Sci Ctr 1980; **Resid:** Psychiatry, NY Hosp/Payne Whitney Cl 1984; **Fellow:** Psychopharmacology, NY State Psych Inst/Columbia 1986; **Fac Appt:** Asst Prof Psyc, Cornell Univ-Weill Med Coll

Gershell, William J MD (Psyc) - **Spec Exp:** Psychopharmacology; Anxiety & Mood Disorders; Neuro-Psychiatry; **Hospital:** Mount Sinai Med Ctr (page 98); **Address:** 1100 Madison Ave, Ste 2C, New York, NY 10028-0338; **Phone:** 212-737-9300; **Board Cert:** Psychiatry 1975; Geriatric Psychiatry 2001; **Med School:** Switzerland 1965; **Resid:** Psychiatry, Mount Sinai 1968; **Fellow:** Child & Adolescent Psychiatry, Mount Sinai 1970; Psychoanalysis, William Alanson White Inst of Psychoanalysis 1977; **Fac Appt:** Asst Clin Prof Psyc, Mount Sinai Sch Med

Glass, Richard MD (Psyc) - **Spec Exp:** Depression; Anxiety Disorders; **Hospital:** NY-Presby Hosp (page 100); **Address:** 65 E 76th St, New York, NY 10021-1844; **Phone:** 212-988-7616; **Board Cert:** Psychiatry 1962; **Med School:** Johns Hopkins Univ 1956; **Resid:** Psychiatry, Jacobi Med Ctr 1959; **Fellow:** Child Psychiatry, Jacobi Med Ctr 1963; **Fac Appt:** Assoc Clin Prof Psyc, Cornell Univ-Weill Med Coll

Glassman, Alexander MD (Psyc) - **Spec Exp:** Depression; Psychopharmacology; **Hospital:** NY State Psychiatric Inst (page 100), NY-Presby Hosp (page 100); **Address:** 161 Fort Washington Ave, New York, NY 10032-1007; **Phone:** 212-543-5750; **Board Cert:** Psychiatry 1975; **Med School:** Univ IL Coll Med 1958; **Resid:** Psychiatry, Jacobi Med Ctr 1962; **Fellow:** Psychiatry, US Public Hlth Service 1964

Goldberger, Marianne MD (Psyc) - **Spec Exp:** Psychoanalysis; Psychotherapy; Child Psychiatry; **Hospital:** NYU Med Ctr (page 102), NY-Presby Hosp (page 100); **Address:** 905 5th Ave, Ste GD, New York, NY 10021; **Phone:** 212-734-3400; **Board Cert:** Psychiatry 1979; Child & Adolescent Psychiatry 1981; **Med School:** NYU Sch Med 1958; **Resid:** Psychiatry, Univ of WI Hosp 1961; **Fellow:** Child & Adolescent Psychiatry, Children's Hosp 1963; **Fac Appt:** Clin Prof Psyc, NYU Sch Med

Goldman, Neil S MD (Psyc) - **Spec Exp:** Mood Disorders; Addiction Psychiatry; Anxiety Disorders; **Hospital:** St Vincent Cath Med Ctrs - Manhattan (page 375); **Address:** 36 7th Ave, Ste 412, New York, NY 10011-6688; **Phone:** 212-929-4395; **Board Cert:** Psychiatry 1981; Addiction Psychiatry 1994; **Med School:** Univ Hlth Sci/Chicago Med Sch 1970; **Resid:** Psychiatry, Brookdale 1974; **Fellow:** Addiction Psychiatry, St Vincent's Hosp & Med Ctr 1979; **Fac Appt:** Asst Prof Psyc, NY Med Coll

Goldstein, Susanna MD (Psyc) - **Spec Exp:** Psychopharmacology; Anxiety Disorders; **Hospital:** Lenox Hill Hosp (page 94), Gracie Square Hosp; **Address:** 65 Central Park West, Ste 1BR, New York, NY 10023; **Phone:** 212-362-6657; **Board Cert:** Geriatric Psychiatry 1996; Psychiatry 1985; **Med School:** Israel 1975; **Resid:** Psychiatry, Rambam Med Ctr 1980; Neurology, Rambam Med Ctr 1981; **Fellow:** Biological Psychiatry, Albert Einstein Hosp 1983; **Fac Appt:** Asst Clin Prof Psyc

Goodman, Berney MD (Psyc) - **Spec Exp:** Psychotherapy & Psychopharmacology; Psychiatry in Physical Illness; Psychosomatic Disorders; **Hospital:** Mount Sinai Med Ctr (page 98), Lenox Hill Hosp (page 94); **Address:** 11 E 68th St, New York, NY 10021-4955; **Phone:** 212-350-0111; **Board Cert:** Psychiatry 1971; Geriatric Psychiatry 1994; **Med School:** South Africa 1957; **Resid:** Internal Medicine, Mount Sinai Hosp 1964; Psychiatry, Bronx Municipal/Montefiore 1969; **Fellow:** Physiology, Mount Sinai 1962; **Fac Appt:** Asst Clin Prof Psyc, Mount Sinai Sch Med

Gorman, Lauren MD (Psyc) - **Spec Exp:** Psychopharmacology; Anxiety & Mood Disorders; **Hospital:** Mount Sinai Med Ctr (page 98); **Address:** 685 West End Ave, Ste 1AF, New York, NY 10025; **Phone:** 212-580-7713; **Board Cert:** Psychiatry 1983; **Med School:** Columbia P&S 1977; **Resid:** Psychiatry, Mount Sinai 1982; **Fellow:** Biological Psychiatry, Montefiore Hosp Med Ctr 1984; **Fac Appt:** Asst Clin Prof Psyc, Mount Sinai Sch Med

Heiman, Peter MD (Psyc) - **Spec Exp:** Medical Illness in Psychiatry; **Hospital:** Montefiore Med Ctr; **Address:** 125 E 84th St, Ste 1A, New York, NY 10028; **Phone:** 212-472-8885; **Board Cert:** Psychiatry 1975; **Med School:** Albert Einstein Coll Med 1968; **Resid:** Psychiatry, Montefiore Hosp Med Ctr 1972; **Fac Appt:** Asst Clin Prof Psyc, Albert Einstein Coll Med

Heller, Stanley MD (Psyc) - **Spec Exp:** Panic Disorder; Depression; **Hospital:** St Luke's - Roosevelt Hosp Ctr - St Luke's Hosp (page 90); **Address:** 62 E 88th St, Ste 205, New York, NY 10128; **Phone:** 212-831-5919; **Board Cert:** Psychiatry 1975; **Med School:** Columbia P&S 1960; **Resid:** Psychiatry, NYS Psyc Inst-Columbia 1966; **Fac Appt:** Assoc Clin Prof Psyc, Columbia P&S

Hoffman, Joel MD (Psyc) - **Spec Exp:** Psychopharmacology; Depression; Treatment Resistant Mental Illness; **Hospital:** Lenox Hill Hosp (page 94), NY-Presby Hosp (page 100); **Address:** 1236 Park Ave, New York, NY 10128-1708; **Phone:** 212-722-3004; **Board Cert:** Psychiatry 1977; **Med School:** Columbia P&S 1963; **Resid:** Internal Medicine, Univ Michigan Med Ctr 1967; Psychiatry, NYS Psychiatric Inst 1972; **Fac Appt:** Asst Clin Prof Psyc, Columbia P&S

Hollander, Eric MD (Psyc) - **Spec Exp:** Obsessive-Compulsive Disorder; Anxiety Disorders; Autism; **Hospital:** Mount Sinai Med Ctr (page 98); **Address:** 300 Central Park West, Ste 1C, New York, NY 10024-1513; **Phone:** 212-873-4051; **Board Cert:** Psychiatry 1987; **Med School:** SUNY Hlth Sci Ctr 1982; **Resid:** Internal Medicine, Mount Sinai Hosp 1983; Psychiatry, Mount Sinai Hosp 1986; **Fellow:** Psychiatry, Columbia-Presby Med Ctr 1988; **Fac Appt:** Prof Psyc, Mount Sinai Sch Med

Isay, Richard A MD (Psyc) - **Spec Exp:** Gay & Lesbian Issues; **Hospital:** NY-Presby Hosp (page 100); **Address:** 55 E End Ave, Ste 1G, New York, NY 10028-7933; **Phone:** 212-535-1863; **Board Cert:** Psychiatry 1969; **Med School:** Univ Rochester 1961; **Resid:** Psychiatry, Yale-New Haven Hosp 1965; **Fac Appt:** Clin Prof Psyc, Cornell Univ-Weill Med Coll

Jacobs, Theodore MD (Psyc) - **Spec Exp:** Adolescent Psychiatry; Creativity Enhancement; **Hospital:** Montefiore Med Ctr; **Address:** 18 E 87th St, New York, NY 10028; **Phone:** 212-879-3002; **Board Cert:** Psychiatry 1968; **Med School:** Univ Chicago-Pritzker Sch Med 1957; **Resid:** Psychiatry, Bronx Municipal Hosp 1961; **Fac Appt:** Clin Prof Psyc, Albert Einstein Coll Med

Kahn, David A MD (Psyc) - **Spec Exp:** Anxiety & Mood Disorders; Psychopharmacology; Psychotherapy; Schizophrenia; **Hospital:** NY-Presby Hosp (page 100); **Address:** 35 E 85th St, New York, NY 10028-0954; **Phone:** 212-472-0100; **Board Cert:** Psychiatry 1984; **Med School:** Columbia P&S 1979; **Resid:** Psychiatry, NY State Psych Inst 1983; **Fellow:** Biological Psychiatry, NY State Psych Inst 1984; **Fac Appt:** Clin Prof Psyc, Columbia P&S

Kalinich, Lila J MD (Psyc) - **Spec Exp:** Psychoanalysis; Psychotherapy; Adolescent Psychiatry; **Hospital:** NY-Presby Hosp (page 100), NY State Psychiatric Inst (page 100); **Address:** 333 Central Park West, Ste 12, New York, NY 10025-7104; **Phone:** 212-866-0200; **Board Cert:** Psychiatry 1975; **Med School:** Northwestern Univ 1969; **Resid:** Psychiatry, Columbia-Presby Hosp 1973; **Fac Appt:** Assoc Clin Prof Psyc, Columbia P&S

Karasu, T Byram MD (Psyc) - **Spec Exp:** Depression; Personality Disorders; Psychotherapy; **Hospital:** Montefiore Med Ctr; **Address:** 2 E 88th St, New York, NY 10128-0555; **Phone:** 212-426-5208; **Board Cert:** Psychiatry 1972; **Med School:** Turkey 1959; **Resid:** Psychiatry, Fairfield Hill Hosp 1967; Psychiatry, Yale-New Haven Hosp 1969; **Fac Appt:** Prof Psyc, Albert Einstein Coll Med

Kass, Frederic MD (Psyc) - **Spec Exp:** Depression; Personality Disorders; Couples Therapy; **Hospital:** NY-Presby Hosp (page 100); **Address:** 1100 Madison Ave, rm 8G, New York, NY 10028; **Phone:** 212-744-4168; **Board Cert:** Psychiatry 1977; **Med School:** Johns Hopkins Univ 1970; **Resid:** Psychiatry, Bronx Muni Hosp 1974; **Fac Appt:** Prof Psyc, Columbia P&S

Kaufmann, Charles A MD (Psyc) - **Spec Exp:** Schizophrenia; Bipolar/Mood Disorders; Genetic Counseling-Psychiatric; **Hospital:** NY-Presby Hosp (page 100), NY State Psychiatric Inst (page 100); **Address:** 161 Fort Washington Ave, New York, NY 10032; **Phone:** 914-238-7909; **Board Cert:** Psychiatry 1982; **Med School:** Columbia P&S 1977; **Resid:** Psychiatry, New York Hosp 1981; **Fellow:** Research, Nat Inst Hlth 1985; Research, Ctr for Neurobio & Behavior 1988; **Fac Appt:** Assoc Prof Psyc, Columbia P&S

Kavey, Neil B MD (Psyc) - **Spec Exp:** Narcolepsy; Sleep Disorders/Apnea; **Hospital:** NY-Presby Hosp (page 100); **Address:** Columbia Presby Med Ctr, Sleep Disorders Ctr, 161 Ft Washington Ave, Fl 3 - rm 346, New York, NY 10032; **Phone:** 212-305-1860; **Board Cert:** Psychiatry 1976; Sleep Medicine 2003; **Med School:** Columbia P&S 1969; **Resid:** Psychiatry, Columbia Presby Med Ctr 1973; **Fac Appt:** Clin Prof Psyc, Columbia P&S

Klein, Donald MD (Psyc) - **Spec Exp:** Psychopharmacology; Depression; Anxiety Disorders; **Hospital:** NY-Presby Hosp (page 100), NY State Psychiatric Inst (page 100); **Address:** NYSPI-Unit 22, 1051 Riverside Dr, New York, NY 10021-0422; **Phone:** 212-543-6249; **Board Cert:** Psychiatry 1959; **Med School:** SUNY Hlth Sci Ctr 1952; **Resid:** Psychiatry, Creedmoor State Hosp 1958; **Fac Appt:** Prof Psyc, Columbia P&S

Kocsis, James MD (Psyc) - **Spec Exp:** Psychopharmacology; Mood Disorders; Anxiety Disorders; **Hospital:** NY-Presby Hosp (page 100); **Address:** 525 E 68th St, Box 140, New York, NY 10021-4885; **Phone:** 212-746-5913; **Board Cert:** Psychiatry 1977; **Med School:** Cornell Univ-Weill Med Coll 1968; **Resid:** Psychiatry, NY Hosp 1975; **Fac Appt:** Prof Psyc, Cornell Univ-Weill Med Coll

Kornfeld, Donald S MD (Psyc) - **Spec Exp:** Liaison Psychiatry; Geriatric Psychiatry; **Hospital:** NY-Presby Hosp (page 100); **Address:** 622 W 168th St Bldg Ph - rm 16C, New York, NY 10032-3702; **Phone:** 212-305-9985; **Board Cert:** Psychiatry 1962; **Med School:** Yale Univ 1954; **Resid:** Psychiatry, Columbia-Presby-NYS Psyc Inst 1960; **Fac Appt:** Prof Psyc, Columbia P&S

Kowallis, George MD (Psyc) - **Spec Exp:** Depression; Anxiety Disorders; ADD/ADHD; **Hospital:** St Vincent Cath Med Ctrs - Manhattan (page 375); **Address:** 162 W 56th St, Ste 407, New York, NY 10019-3831; **Phone:** 212-757-0324; **Board Cert:** Psychiatry 1977; Child & Adolescent Psychiatry 1978; **Med School:** Univ Pennsylvania 1969; **Resid:** Psychiatry, St Luke's-Roosevelt Hosp Ctr 1972; Child & Adolescent Psychiatry, St Luke's-Roosevelt Hosp Ctr 1974; **Fac Appt:** Asst Clin Prof Psyc, NY Med Coll

Kranzler, Elliot MD (Psyc) - **Spec Exp:** Anxiety & Depression; Bereavement/Traumatic Grief; ADD/ADHD; **Hospital:** NY-Presby Hosp (page 100); **Address:** 451 West End Ave, New York, NY 10024-5329; **Phone:** 212-580-9758; **Board Cert:** Psychiatry 1984; Child & Adolescent Psychiatry 1986; **Med School:** Albert Einstein Coll Med 1978; **Resid:** Psychiatry, Payne-Whitney Clinic 1982; **Fellow:** Child & Adolescent Psychiatry, Columbia-Presby 1984; Research, Columbia-Presby/NIMH; **Fac Appt:** Asst Prof Psyc, Columbia P&S

Kremberg, M Roy MD (Psyc) - **Spec Exp:** Mood Disorders; Anxiety Disorders; ADD/ADHD; **Hospital:** St Luke's - Roosevelt Hosp Ctr - Roosevelt Div (page 90), NY-Presby Hosp (page 100); **Address:** 2109 Broadway, Ste 14-54, New York, NY 10023-2106; **Phone:** 212-875-8568; **Board Cert:** Psychiatry 1980; Child & Adolescent Psychiatry 1982; **Med School:** Columbia P&S 1976; **Resid:** Psychiatry, St Luke's-Roosevelt Hosp Ctr 1978; **Fellow:** Child & Adolescent Psychiatry, St Luke's-Roosevelt Hosp Ctr 1980

Lane, Frederick M MD (Psyc) - **Spec Exp:** Psychoanalysis; Psychotherapy; **Address:** 125 E 87th St, Ste 4E, New York, NY 10128; **Phone:** 212-876-0841; **Board Cert:** Psychiatry 1966; **Med School:** Yale Univ 1953; **Resid:** Psychiatry, Yale-New Haven Hosp 1955; Psychiatry, Yale-New Haven Hosp 1958; **Fellow:** Psychiatry, Yale Psych Inst 1959; **Fac Appt:** Clin Prof Psyc, Columbia P&S

Lefer, Jay MD (Psyc) - **Spec Exp:** Psychoanalysis; Somatic Psychiatry; Family Therapy; **Hospital:** Montefiore Med Ctr - Weiler-Einstein Div, Rye Hosp Ctr; **Address:** 200 East End Ave, Ste 9J, New York, NY 10128-7890; **Phone:** 212-427-0427; **Board Cert:** Psychiatry 1962; **Med School:** Switzerland 1955; **Resid:** Psychiatry, Yale-New Haven Hosp; **Fellow:** Psychiatry, Yale-New Haven Hosp 1962; **Fac Appt:** Assoc Clin Prof Psyc, NY Med Coll

Levitan, Stephan MD (Psyc) - **Spec Exp:** Psychotherapy; Psychopharmacology; Couples Therapy; **Hospital:** NY-Presby Hosp (page 100); **Address:** 185 E 85th St, Ste 29J, New York, NY 10028-2143; **Phone:** 212-722-4311; **Board Cert:** Psychiatry 1974; **Med School:** SUNY Buffalo 1965; **Resid:** Psychiatry, Hillside Hosp 1969; **Fellow:** Psychoanalysis, Columbia Psy Anal Ctr 1973; **Fac Appt:** Clin Prof Psyc, Columbia P&S

Lindenmayer, Jean-Pierre MD (Psyc) - **Spec Exp:** Psychopharmacology; Schizophrenia; Bipolar/Mood Disorders; **Hospital:** Gracie Square Hosp; **Address:** 18 E 77th St, Apt B, New York, NY 10021-1700; **Phone:** 212-249-2720; **Board Cert:** Psychiatry 1975; **Med School:** Switzerland 1967; **Resid:** Psychiatry, U Hosp-Geneva Med Sch 1969; Psychiatry, SUNY Downstate Med Ctr 1973; **Fellow:** Research, SUNY Downstate Med Ctr 1975; **Fac Appt:** Clin Prof Psyc, NYU Sch Med

Lipton, Brian MD (Psyc) - **Spec Exp:** Psychotherapy; Psychopharmacology; Psychiatry in Infertility; **Hospital:** Lenox Hill Hosp (page 94); **Address:** 1111 Park Ave, Ste 1A, New York, NY 10128-1234; **Phone:** 212-427-4499; **Board Cert:** Psychiatry 1970; **Med School:** SUNY Hlth Sci Ctr 1964; **Resid:** Psychiatry, Hillside Hosp 1968; **Fac Appt:** Asst Clin Prof Psyc, NYU Sch Med

Mahon, Eugene MD (Psyc) - **Spec Exp:** Psychoanalysis; **Hospital:** NY-Presby Hosp (page 100); **Address:** 6 E 96th St, New York, NY 10128-0706; **Phone:** 212-831-1414; **Med School:** Ireland 1964; **Resid:** Internal Medicine, Brooklyn Hosp 1969; Psychiatry, St Lukes Roosevelt Hosp Ctr 1974; **Fellow:** Psychoanalysis, Columbia Univ Psychoanalytic Ctr 1980

Manevitz, Alan MD (Psyc) - **Spec Exp:** Marital/Family/Sex Therapy; Fibromyalgia Syndrome (FMS); Post Traumatic Stress Disorder; ADD/ADHD; **Hospital:** NY-Presby Hosp (page 100), Lenox Hill Hosp (page 94); **Address:** 60 Sutton Place South, Ste 1CN, New York, NY 10022; **Phone:** 212-751-5072; **Board Cert:** Psychiatry 1987; **Med School:** Columbia P&S 1980; **Resid:** Psychiatry, New York Hosp 1984; **Fellow:** Psychopharmacology, New York Hosp 1985; **Fac Appt:** Assoc Clin Prof Psyc, Cornell Univ-Weill Med Coll

Marcus, Eric R MD (Psyc) - **Spec Exp:** Psychoanalysis; **Hospital:** NY-Presby Hosp (page 100); **Address:** 4 E 89th St, Ste 1D, New York, NY 10128; **Phone:** 212-427-0543; **Board Cert:** Psychiatry 1977; **Med School:** Univ Wisc 1969; **Resid:** Psychiatry, Columbia-Presby Med Ctr 1975; **Fellow:** Psychoanalysis, Columbia Univ 1987; **Fac Appt:** Clin Prof Psyc, Columbia P&S

Marin, Deborah B MD (Psyc) - **Spec Exp:** Alzheimer's Disease; **Hospital:** Mount Sinai Med Ctr (page 98); **Address:** 1 Gustave Levy Pl, Box 1068, Mount Sinai Hospital, New York, NY 10029; **Phone:** 212-241-7139; **Board Cert:** Psychiatry 1990; **Med School:** Mount Sinai Sch Med 1984; **Resid:** Psychiatry, Mount Sinai Hosp 1988; **Fellow:** Psychiatry, New York Hosp-Cornell Med Ctr 1991; **Fac Appt:** Prof Psyc, Mount Sinai Sch Med

Markowitz, John MD (Psyc) - **Spec Exp:** Depression; Post-Traumatic Stress Disorder; Personality Disorders-Borderline; **Hospital:** NY-Presby Hosp (page 100), NY State Psychiatric Inst (page 100); **Address:** 40 E 83rd St, New York, NY 10028; **Phone:** 212-543-6283; **Board Cert:** Psychiatry 1987; **Med School:** Columbia P&S 1982; **Resid:** Psychiatry, Payne Whitney Clin/New York Hosp 1987; **Fac Appt:** Clin Prof Psyc, Cornell Univ-Weill Med Coll

McGowan, James M MD (Psyc) - **Spec Exp:** Alcohol Abuse; Drug Abuse; **Hospital:** NY-Presby Hosp (page 100), St Vincent Cath Med Ctrs - Manhattan (page 375); **Address:** 49 E 78th St, Ste 1-A, New York, NY 10021-0211; **Phone:** 212-517-3888; **Board Cert:** Psychiatry 1974; **Med School:** Univ KY Coll Med 1964; **Resid:** Internal Medicine, Bellevue Hosp 1968; Psychiatry, Albert Einstein Coll Med 1971; **Fellow:** Community Psychiatry, Albert Einstein Coll Med 1972; **Fac Appt:** Asst Clin Prof Psyc, Cornell Univ-Weill Med Coll

McGrath, Patrick J MD (Psyc) - **Spec Exp:** Psychopharmacology; Depression; **Hospital:** NY-Presby Hosp (page 100), NY State Psychiatric Inst (page 100); **Address:** 161 Fort Washington Ave, New York, NY 10032-3713; **Phone:** 212-543-5764; **Board Cert:** Psychiatry 1978; **Med School:** Columbia P&S 1974; **Resid:** Surgery, NY State Psy Inst 1978; **Fac Appt:** Assoc Clin Prof Psyc, Columbia P&S

McMullen, Robert MD (Psyc) - **Spec Exp:** Psychopharmacology; Anxiety & Mood Disorders; Pain-Facial (TMJ); **Hospital:** NY-Presby Hosp (page 100); **Address:** 171 W 79th St, New York, NY 10024-6449; **Phone:** 212-362-9635; **Board Cert:** Psychiatry 1982; **Med School:** Georgetown Univ 1976; **Resid:** Psychiatry, Columbia-Presby Med Ctr 1980; **Fac Appt:** Asst Prof Psyc, Columbia P&S

Mellman, Lisa MD (Psyc) - **Spec Exp:** Anxiety & Depression; Relationship Problems; Work Problems; **Hospital:** NY-Presby Hosp (page 100), NY State Psychiatric Inst (page 100); **Address:** Columbia Univ Med Ctr, 161 Ft Washington Ave, New York, NY 10032; **Phone:** 917-620-6010; **Board Cert:** Psychiatry 1986; **Med School:** Case West Res Univ 1981; **Resid:** Psychiatry, Psych Inst/Columbia-Presby Med Ctr 1985; **Fellow:** Psychoanalysis, Columbia Univ 1991; **Fac Appt:** Assoc Clin Prof Psyc, Columbia P&S

Michels, Robert MD (Psyc) - **Spec Exp:** Psychoanalysis; **Hospital:** NY-Presby Hosp (page 100); **Address:** 418 E 71st St, New York, NY 10021-4894; **Phone:** 212-746-6001; **Board Cert:** Psychiatry 1964; **Med School:** Northwestern Univ 1958; **Resid:** Psychiatry, Columbia-Presby Hosp 1962; **Fac Appt:** Prof Psyc, Cornell Univ-Weill Med Coll

Millman, Robert B MD (Psyc) - **Spec Exp:** Addiction Psychiatry; Psychopharmacology; Psychotherapy; **Hospital:** NY-Presby Hosp (page 100), NY-Presby Hosp (page 100); **Address:** Weill Med Coll/Cornell Univ, 411 E 69th St, New York, NY 10021-5608; **Phone:** 212-746-1248; **Board Cert:** Psychiatry 1978; **Med School:** SUNY Hlth Sci Ctr 1965; **Resid:** Internal Medicine, Bellevue Hosp 1970; Psychiatry, Payne Whitney Psych Clinic 1977; **Fellow:** Metabolic Diseases, Rockefeller Univ Hosp 1971; **Fac Appt:** Prof Psyc, Cornell Univ-Weill Med Coll

Moore, Joanne MD (Psyc) - **Spec Exp:** Depression; Anxiety Disorders; **Hospital:** NY-Presby Hosp (page 100); **Address:** 161 Ft Washington Ave, New York, NY 10032; **Phone:** 212-305-9499; **Board Cert:** Psychiatry 1988; Addiction Psychiatry 1994; **Med School:** Harvard Med Sch 1982; **Resid:** Psychiatry, Columbia-Presby Med Ctr 1987; **Fellow:** Geriatric Psychiatry, Columbia-Presby Med Ctr 1984; **Fac Appt:** Assoc Prof Psyc, Columbia P&S

Muhlbauer, Helen MD (Psyc) - **Spec Exp:** Women's Health-Mental Health; Addiction/Substance Abuse; Psychosomatic Disorders; **Hospital:** NY-Presby Hosp (page 100), Beth Israel Med Ctr - Petrie Division (page 90); **Address:** NY Presbyterian Hosp, 5141 Broadway, New York, NY 10034; **Phone:** 212-932-4642; **Board Cert:** Psychiatry 1991; Addiction Psychiatry 1998; **Med School:** Albert Einstein Coll Med 1977; **Resid:** Psychiatry, Albert Einstein 1981; **Fac Appt:** Asst Prof Psyc, Columbia P&S

Muskin, Philip MD (Psyc) - **Spec Exp:** Psychopharmacology; Anxiety & Depression; Psychiatry in Physical Illness; **Hospital:** NY-Presby Hosp (page 100); **Address:** 1700 York Ave, New York, NY 10128-7820; **Phone:** 212-722-8438; **Board Cert:** Psychiatry 1979; Geriatric Psychiatry 2001; Psychosomatic Medicine 2005; **Med School:** NY Med Coll 1974; **Resid:** Psychiatry, NYS Psych Inst 1978; **Fellow:** Psychosomatic Medicine, Columbia-Presby Hosp 1979; Psychopharmacology, NY State Psych Inst 1979; **Fac Appt:** Prof Psyc, Columbia P&S

Myers, Wayne A MD (Psyc) - **Spec Exp:** Marital/Family/Sex Therapy; Personality Disorders; Psychoanalysis; **Hospital:** NY-Presby Hosp (page 100); **Address:** 60 Sutton Place South, Ste 1CN, New York, NY 10022-4168; **Phone:** 212-838-2325; **Board Cert:** Psychiatry 1959; **Med School:** Columbia P&S 1956; **Resid:** Psychiatry, NY Hosp Med Ctr 1962; **Fac Appt:** Clin Prof Psyc, Cornell Univ-Weill Med Coll

Nersessian, Edward MD (Psyc) - **Hospital:** NY-Presby Hosp (page 100); **Address:** 72 E 91st St, New York, NY 10128-1350; **Phone:** 212-876-1537; **Board Cert:** Psychiatry 1975; **Med School:** Belgium 1970; **Resid:** Psychiatry, Hillside Hosp 1972; Psychiatry, Payne Whitney Clinic 1973; **Fellow:** NY Psychoanalytic Inst 1977; **Fac Appt:** Clin Prof Psyc, Cornell Univ-Weill Med Coll

Nininger, James MD (Psyc) - **Spec Exp:** Psychotherapy; Psychopharmacology; Geriatric Psychiatry; **Hospital:** NY-Presby Hosp (page 100); **Address:** 30 E 76th St, New York, NY 10021; **Phone:** 212-879-8338; **Board Cert:** Psychiatry 1978; Geriatric Psychiatry 1991; **Med School:** Univ Cincinnati 1974; **Resid:** Psychiatry, Mount Sinai 1977; **Fac Appt:** Assoc Clin Prof Psyc, Cornell Univ-Weill Med Coll

Nir, Yehuda MD (Psyc) - **Spec Exp:** Post Traumatic Stress Disorder; Psychotherapy; **Hospital:** NY-Presby Hosp (page 100); **Address:** 903 Park Ave, Ste 11C, New York, NY 10021-0360; **Phone:** 212-744-8615; **Board Cert:** Psychiatry 1979; **Med School:** Israel 1958; **Resid:** Psychiatry, Philadelphia Psych Ctr 1961; Psychiatry, Mt Sinai Hosp 1962; **Fellow:** Child Psychiatry, Jewish Board of Guardians 1964; **Fac Appt:** Assoc Clin Prof Psyc, Cornell Univ-Weill Med Coll

Nunes, Edward MD (Psyc) - **Spec Exp:** Depression; Substance Abuse; **Hospital:** NY State Psychiatric Inst (page 100), NY-Presby Hosp (page 100); **Address:** 1051 Riverside Drive, Mail Unit 51, New York, NY 10032; **Phone:** 212-543-5784; **Board Cert:** Psychiatry 1986; Addiction Psychiatry 1993; **Med School:** Univ Conn 1981; **Resid:** Psychiatry, Columbia-Presby/NYS Psyc Inst 1985; **Fellow:** Psychopharmacology, Columbia-Presby/NYS Psyc Inst 1988; **Fac Appt:** Assoc Clin Prof Psyc, Columbia P&S

Oberfield, Richard MD (Psyc) - **Spec Exp:** Child & Adolescent Psychiatry; Divorce/Family Issues; ADD/ADHD; **Hospital:** NYU Med Ctr (page 102); **Address:** 200 E 33rd St, Ste 2J, New York, NY 10016-4874; **Phone:** 212-684-0148; **Board Cert:** Psychiatry 1979; Child & Adolescent Psychiatry 1980; Forensic Psychiatry 1999; **Med School:** Mount Sinai Sch Med 1974; **Resid:** Psychiatry, Bellevue Hosp 1976; **Fellow:** Child & Adolescent Psychiatry, Bellevue Hosp 1978; **Fac Appt:** Clin Prof Psyc, NYU Sch Med

Olds, David MD (Psyc) - **Spec Exp:** Psychoanalysis; Psychotherapy; **Hospital:** NY-Presby Hosp (page 100); **Address:** 108 E 96th St, Ste 6F, New York, NY 10128; **Phone:** 212-427-9688; **Board Cert:** Psychiatry 1975; **Med School:** Columbia P&S 1967; **Resid:** Psychiatry, NY State Psych Inst 1971; **Fellow:** Columbia-Psych Ctr 1977; **Fac Appt:** Clin Prof Psyc, Columbia P&S

Papp, Laszlo A MD (Psyc) - **Spec Exp:** Anxiety & Mood Disorders; Depression; Phobias; Panic Disorder; **Hospital:** NY-Presby Hosp (page 100), Zucker Hillside Hosp; **Address:** 124 E 84th St, Ste 1B, New York, NY 10028; **Phone:** 212-360-5750; **Board Cert:** Psychiatry 1993; **Med School:** Hungary 1978; **Resid:** Psychiatry, Beth Israel Med Ctr 1986; Endocrinology, Diabetes & Metabolism, Natl Inst of Rheumatology 1981; **Fellow:** Psychopharmacology, Columbia Univ 1989; **Fac Appt:** Assoc Prof Psyc, Columbia P&S

Pawel, Michael A MD (Psyc) - **Spec Exp:** Adolescent Psychiatry; **Hospital:** St Luke's - Roosevelt Hosp Ctr - St Luke's Hosp (page 90); **Address:** 15 W 72nd St, New York, NY 10023; **Phone:** 212-873-9170; **Board Cert:** Psychiatry 1977; **Med School:** Albert Einstein Coll Med 1971; **Resid:** Psychiatry, Montefiore Hosp Med Ctr 1974; **Fac Appt:** Asst Prof Psyc, Columbia P&S

Person, Ethel MD (Psyc) - **Spec Exp:** Psychoanalysis; Sex, Gender, & Relationships; Work Problems; **Hospital:** NY-Presby Hosp (page 100); **Address:** 135 Central Park West, Ste 11 South, New York, NY 10023-2413; **Phone:** 212-873-2700; **Med School:** NYU Sch Med 1960; **Resid:** Psychiatry, NY State Psych Inst 1963; **Fac Appt:** Clin Prof Psyc, Columbia P&S

Pfeffer, Cynthia MD (Psyc) - **Spec Exp:** Child & Adolescent Psychiatry; Bereavement/Traumatic Grief; Anxiety & Depression; ADD/ADHD; **Hospital:** NY-Presby Hosp (page 100), NYU Med Ctr (page 102); **Address:** 1100 Madison Ave, New York, NY 10128-0327; **Phone:** 212-717-2334; **Board Cert:** Psychiatry 1975; Child & Adolescent Psychiatry 1976; **Med School:** NYU Sch Med 1968; **Resid:** Psychiatry, Albert Einstein 1973; **Fellow:** Child & Adolescent Psychiatry, Albert Einstein 1973; **Fac Appt:** Prof Psyc, Cornell Univ-Weill Med Coll

Pines, Jeffrey MD (Psyc) - **Hospital:** NY-Presby Hosp (page 100); **Address:** NY Presbyterian Hosp, 161 Fort Washington Ave, New York, NY 10032; **Phone:** 212-579-1913; **Board Cert:** Psychiatry 1982; **Med School:** Columbia P&S 1973; **Resid:** Internal Medicine, Presbyterian Hosp 1976; Psychiatry, NYState Psych Inst 1980; **Fellow:** Rheumatology, Hosp For Special Surg 1977; Liason Psychiatry, Columbia-Presby Med Ctr 1981; **Fac Appt:** Assoc Clin Prof Psyc, Columbia P&S

Porder, Michael MD (Psyc) - **Spec Exp:** Psychoanalysis; **Hospital:** Mount Sinai Med Ctr (page 98); **Address:** 300 Central Park West, New York, NY 10024; **Phone:** 212-362-1650; **Med School:** Columbia P&S 1958; **Resid:** Psychiatry, Jacobi Med Ctr 1962; **Fac Appt:** Assoc Clin Prof Psyc, Mount Sinai Sch Med

Preven, David MD (Psyc) - **Spec Exp:** Forensic Psychiatry; Psychopharmacology; Psychotherapy; **Hospital:** Montefiore Med Ctr - Weiler-Einstein Div; **Address:** 52 Riverside Drive, New York, NY 10024-6501; **Phone:** 212-799-4907; **Board Cert:** Psychiatry 1969; Forensic Psychiatry 2005; Geriatric Psychiatry 1996; **Med School:** Harvard Med Sch 1963; **Resid:** Psychiatry, Jacobi Hosp/Einstein 1967; **Fellow:** Psychiatry, NIMH-Einstein 1971; **Fac Appt:** Clin Prof Psyc, Albert Einstein Coll Med

Rees, Ellen MD (Psyc) - **Spec Exp:** Psychoanalysis; Psychotherapy; **Hospital:** NY-Presby Hosp (page 100), NY-Presby Hosp (page 100); **Address:** 108 E 96th St, New York, NY 10128-6217; **Phone:** 212-722-5988; **Board Cert:** Psychiatry 1979; **Med School:** Albert Einstein Coll Med 1974; **Resid:** Psychiatry, Mt Sinai Hosp 1977; **Fellow:** Psychiatry, NY Hosp-Cornell 1978; Psychoanalysis, Columbia Univ Ctr Psych Trng 1991; **Fac Appt:** Assoc Clin Prof Psyc, Cornell Univ-Weill Med Coll

Resnick, Richard MD (Psyc) - **Spec Exp:** Marital/Family/Sex Therapy; Anxiety & Depression; Addiction/Substance Abuse; **Hospital:** NYU Med Ctr (page 102), Bellevue Hosp Ctr; **Address:** Ctr for Psychiatry & Family Therapy, 43 W 94th St, New York, NY 10025-7113; **Phone:** 212-678-6949; **Board Cert:** Psychiatry 1965; **Med School:** NY Med Coll 1958; **Resid:** Psychiatry, Hillside Hosp 1961; Psychiatry, Montefiore Hosp 1962; **Fac Appt:** Assoc Clin Prof Psyc, NYU Sch Med

Rice, Emanuel MD (Psyc) - **Hospital:** Mount Sinai Med Ctr (page 98); **Address:** 19 E 88th St, Ste 11C, New York, NY 10128-0538; **Phone:** 212-427-3967; **Board Cert:** Psychiatry 1969; **Med School:** Howard Univ 1961; **Resid:** Psychiatry, Manhattan State Hosp 1965; **Fellow:** Psychiatry, Mount Sinai Hosp; **Fac Appt:** Clin Prof Psyc, Mount Sinai Sch Med

Richards, Arnold D MD (Psyc) - **Hospital:** Mount Sinai Med Ctr (page 98); **Address:** 200 E 89th St, New York, NY 10128; **Phone:** 212-722-0223; **Board Cert:** Psychiatry 1965; **Med School:** SUNY Hlth Sci Ctr 1958; **Resid:** Psychiatry, Menninger Sch Psy-VA Hosp 1963; **Fac Appt:** Asst Clin Prof Psyc, NYU Sch Med

Roose, Steven MD (Psyc) - **Spec Exp:** Depression in the Elderly; **Hospital:** NY-Presby Hosp (page 100); **Address:** NY State Psychiatric Institute, 1051 Riverside Drive, New York, NY 10032; **Phone:** 212-831-8644; **Board Cert:** Psychiatry 1979; **Med School:** Mount Sinai Sch Med 1974; **Resid:** Psychiatry, NY Psychiatric Inst 1978; **Fellow:** Research, Columbia-Presby Med Ctr 1981; **Fac Appt:** Clin Prof Psyc, Columbia P&S

Rosen, Arnold M MD (Psyc) - **Spec Exp:** Depression; Psychopharmacology; **Hospital:** Lenox Hill Hosp (page 94), Lenox Hill Hosp (page 94); **Address:** 200 E 78th St, New York, NY 10021; **Phone:** 212-288-6380; **Board Cert:** Psychiatry 1976; **Med School:** Univ Tex SW, Dallas 1968; **Resid:** Psychiatry, Metropolitan Hosp Ctr 1970; Psychiatry, Metropolitan Hosp Ctr 1974; **Fellow:** Psychiatry, Metropolitan Hosp Ctr 1975

Rosenbloom, Charles MD (Psyc) - **Spec Exp:** Somatic Psychiatry; **Hospital:** Gracie Square Hosp, VA Med Ctr - Bklyn; **Address:** 50 E 86th St, Ste 2A, New York, NY 10028-1067; **Phone:** 212-472-8673; **Board Cert:** Psychiatry 1977; **Med School:** Italy 1964; **Resid:** Psychiatry, St Vincent's Hosp 1967; Psychiatry, Hillside Hosp 1968

Rosenthal, Jesse MD (Psyc) - **Spec Exp:** ADD/ADHD; Anxiety Disorders; Depression; **Hospital:** Beth Israel Med Ctr - Petrie Division (page 90); **Address:** 21 E 93rd St, New York, NY 10128-0609; **Phone:** 212-876-3080; **Board Cert:** Psychiatry 1978; **Med School:** Geo Wash Univ 1973; **Resid:** Psychiatry, Mount Sinai Hosp 1976; **Fac Appt:** Asst Clin Prof Psyc, Mount Sinai Sch Med

Rosenthal, Richard N MD (Psyc) - **Spec Exp:** Anxiety & Mood Disorders; Addiction Psychiatry; **Hospital:** St Luke's - Roosevelt Hosp Ctr - Roosevelt Div (page 90), Beth Israel Med Ctr - Petrie Division (page 90); **Address:** 1090 Amerstdam Ave Fl 16 - Ste G, New York, NY 10025; **Phone:** 212-523-5366; **Board Cert:** Psychiatry 1985; Addiction Psychiatry 2003; **Med School:** SUNY Hlth Sci Ctr 1980; **Resid:** Psychiatry, Mount Sinai Hosp 1984; **Fac Appt:** Prof Psyc, Columbia P&S

Rosner, Richard MD (Psyc) - **Spec Exp:** Adolescent Psychiatry; Forensic Psychiatry; Addiction Medicine; **Hospital:** NYU Med Ctr (page 102), Bellevue Hosp Ctr; **Address:** 140 E 83rd St, Ste 6A, New York, NY 10028-1928; **Phone:** 212-988-6014; **Board Cert:** Psychiatry 1974; Forensic Psychiatry 2004; Addiction Psychiatry ; **Med School:** NYU Sch Med 1966; **Resid:** Psychiatry, Mount Sinai Hosp 1970; **Fac Appt:** Clin Prof Psyc, NYU Sch Med

Rubinstein, Mort MD (Psyc) - **Spec Exp:** Psychopharmacology; **Hospital:** VA Med Ctr - Manhattan; **Address:** 423 E 23rd St, New York, NY 10010-5013; **Phone:** 212-686-7500 x7991; **Board Cert:** Psychiatry 1988; **Med School:** NY Med Coll 1976; **Resid:** Psychiatry, NYU-Bellevue Hosp 1976; **Fellow:** Psychiatry, Mount Sinai 1980; **Fac Appt:** Assoc Clin Prof Psyc, NYU Sch Med

Sacks, Michael MD (Psyc) - **Spec Exp:** Personality Disorders; Relationship Problems; Depression; **Hospital:** NY-Presby Hosp (page 100); **Address:** 525 E 68th St, New York, NY 10021-4870; **Phone:** 212-746-3710; **Board Cert:** Psychiatry 1973; **Med School:** NYU Sch Med 1967; **Resid:** Psychiatry, NY State Psych Inst 1971; **Fellow:** Psychiatry, Natl Inst Mental Health 1973; **Fac Appt:** Prof Psyc, Cornell Univ-Weill Med Coll

Sadock, Benjamin MD (Psyc) - **Spec Exp:** Anxiety Disorders; Depression; Sexual Dysfunction; **Hospital:** NYU Med Ctr (page 102), Lenox Hill Hosp (page 94); **Address:** 4 E 89th St, rm 1E, New York, NY 10128-0656; **Phone:** 212-263-6210; **Board Cert:** Psychiatry 1966; **Med School:** NY Med Coll 1959; **Resid:** Psychiatry, Bellevue Psyc Hosp 1963; **Fac Appt:** Prof Psyc, NYU Sch Med

Sadock, Virginia MD (Psyc) - **Spec Exp:** Psychotherapy; Sexual Dysfunction; Anxiety & Depression; Marital/Family/Sex Therapy; **Hospital:** NYU Med Ctr (page 102); **Address:** 4 E 89th St, Ste 1E, New York, NY 10128; **Phone:** 212-427-0885; **Board Cert:** Psychiatry 1975; **Med School:** NY Med Coll 1970; **Resid:** Psychiatry, Metropolitan Hosp 1973; **Fac Appt:** Clin Prof Psyc, NYU Sch Med

Salkin, Paul MD (Psyc) - **Spec Exp:** Depression; Anxiety Disorders; Post Traumatic Stress Disorder; **Hospital:** Lenox Hill Hosp (page 94), Beth Israel Med Ctr - Petrie Division (page 90); **Address:** 110 East End Ave, New York, NY 10028-7420; **Phone:** 212-737-0136; **Board Cert:** Psychiatry 1962; **Med School:** NYU Sch Med 1956; **Resid:** Psychiatry, Bronx Muni Hosp 1960; **Fac Appt:** Asst Clin Prof Psyc, NY Med Coll

Samberg, Eslee MD (Psyc) - **Spec Exp:** Psychoanalysis; **Hospital:** NY-Presby Hosp (page 100); **Address:** 2211 Broadway, New York, NY 10024-6263; **Phone:** 212-874-7725; **Board Cert:** Psychiatry 1983; **Med School:** Cornell Univ-Weill Med Coll 1978; **Resid:** Psychiatry, NY Hosp-Cornell Med Ctr 1982; **Fac Appt:** Assoc Clin Prof Psyc, Cornell Univ-Weill Med Coll

Sawyer, David MD (Psyc) - **Spec Exp:** Psychoanalysis; Child & Adolescent Psychiatry; **Hospital:** NY-Presby Hosp (page 100); **Address:** 1 W 64th St, Ste 1C, New York, NY 10023; **Phone:** 212-787-8260; **Board Cert:** Psychiatry 1982; Child & Adolescent Psychiatry 1984; **Med School:** NY Med Coll 1977; **Resid:** Psychiatry, NY Hosp-Cornell-Westchester 1980; **Fellow:** Child & Adolescent Psychiatry, NY Hosp-Cornell-Westchester 1982

Scharf, Robert D MD (Psyc) - **Spec Exp:** Psychotherapy; Psychopharmacology; Psychoanalysis; **Hospital:** St Luke's - Roosevelt Hosp Ctr - Roosevelt Div (page 90); **Address:** 207 E 74th St, Ste 1L, New York, NY 10021-3341; **Phone:** 212-988-4145; **Board Cert:** Psychiatry 1976; **Med School:** Albert Einstein Coll Med 1960; **Resid:** Internal Medicine, Straight Ward Med 1960; Psychiatry, Kings Co Hosp 1964; **Fellow:** Psychoanalysis, NY Psychoanalytic Inst 1973; **Fac Appt:** Asst Clin Prof Psyc, Columbia P&S

New York (Manhattan)

Schein, Jonah MD (Psyc) - **Spec Exp:** Depression; Anxiety Disorders; **Hospital:** NY-Presby Hosp (page 100); **Address:** 1349 Lexington Ave, Ste 1E, New York, NY 10128-1514; **Phone:** 212-876-2324; **Board Cert:** Psychiatry 1975; **Med School:** NYU Sch Med 1969; **Resid:** Psychiatry, NY State Psych Inst 1973; **Fac Appt:** Assoc Clin Prof Psyc, Cornell Univ-Weill Med Coll

Schore, Arthur MD (Psyc) - **Spec Exp:** Depression; Sexual Dysfunction; Eating Disorders; **Hospital:** NY-Presby Hosp (page 100); **Address:** 905 5th Ave, New York, NY 10021-4156; **Phone:** 212-535-6070; **Board Cert:** Psychiatry 1979; **Med School:** Univ Hlth Sci/Chicago Med Sch 1965; **Resid:** Columbia-Presby 1969; **Fellow:** NYS Psychiatric Institute 1975; **Fac Appt:** Psyc, Cornell Univ-Weill Med Coll

Shapiro, Peter MD (Psyc) - **Spec Exp:** Depression; Psychiatry in Physical Illness; **Hospital:** NY-Presby Hosp (page 100); **Address:** 239 Central Park West, New York, NY 10024-6038; **Phone:** 212-874-6030; **Board Cert:** Psychiatry 1985; Geriatric Psychiatry 2001; Psychosomatic Medicine 2005; **Med School:** Columbia P&S 1980; **Resid:** Psychiatry, NY State Psych Inst 1984; **Fellow:** Liason Psychiatry, Columbia-Presby Med Ctr 1986; **Fac Appt:** Assoc Prof Psyc, Columbia P&S

Shapiro, Theodore MD (Psyc) - **Spec Exp:** Child & Adolescent Psychiatry; Psychoanalysis; Developmental Disorders; **Hospital:** NY-Presby Hosp (page 100), NY-Presby Hosp (page 100); **Address:** 525 E 68th St, Box 140, New York, NY 10021-4870; **Phone:** 212-746-5713; **Board Cert:** Psychiatry 1965; Child & Adolescent Psychiatry 1970; **Med School:** Cornell Univ-Weill Med Coll 1957; **Resid:** Psychiatry, Bellevue Hosp 1961; **Fellow:** Child & Adolescent Psychiatry, Bellevue Hosp 1963; **Fac Appt:** Prof Emeritus Psyc, Cornell Univ-Weill Med Coll

Shaw, Ronda R MD (Psyc) - **Spec Exp:** Psychoanalysis; Psychotherapy; **Hospital:** Mount Sinai Med Ctr (page 98); **Address:** 35 E 85th St, Profl, Ste 2, New York, NY 10028-0954; **Phone:** 212-772-0321; **Board Cert:** Psychiatry 1977; **Med School:** Wayne State Univ 1966; **Resid:** Psychiatry, Einstein Hosp 1970; **Fac Appt:** Assoc Clin Prof Psyc, Mount Sinai Sch Med

Shear, M Katherine MD (Psyc) - **Spec Exp:** Panic Disorder; Anxiety Disorders; Bereavement/Traumatic Grief; Phobias; **Hospital:** NY-Presby Hosp (page 100); **Address:** 1255 Amsterdam Ave, School of Social Work, MC 4600, New York, NY 10032; **Phone:** 212-851-2122; **Board Cert:** Internal Medicine 1975; Psychiatry 1981; **Med School:** Tufts Univ 1972; **Resid:** Internal Medicine, Mt Sinai Hosp 1976; Psychiatry, Payne Whitney Clin 1979; **Fellow:** Psychosomatic Medicine, Montefiore Hosp 1980; **Fac Appt:** Prof Psyc, Colombia

Shelley, Gabriela MD (Psyc) - **Spec Exp:** Psychotherapy; Psychopharmacology; **Hospital:** Mount Sinai Med Ctr (page 98); **Address:** 40 W 86th St, Ste 1A, New York, NY 10024-3605; **Phone:** 212-769-1646; **Board Cert:** Psychiatry 1996; Geriatric Psychiatry 1996; **Med School:** Albert Einstein Coll Med 1989; **Resid:** Psychiatry, Yale-New Haven Hosp 1993; **Fellow:** Geriatric Psychiatry, McLean Hosp 1994; **Fac Appt:** Asst Prof Psyc, Mount Sinai Sch Med

Shinbach, Kent MD (Psyc) - **Spec Exp:** Depression; Psychopharmacology; Geriatric Psychiatry; **Hospital:** Gracie Square Hosp, Beth Israel Med Ctr - Petrie Division (page 90); **Address:** 435 E 79th St, Ste 1C, New York, NY 10021-1071; **Phone:** 212-744-7100; **Board Cert:** Psychiatry 1970; Geriatric Psychiatry 1992; **Med School:** Jefferson Med Coll 1963; **Resid:** Psychiatry, NY Med Coll 1968; **Fac Appt:** Asst Clin Prof Psyc, Albert Einstein Coll Med

Siever, Larry J MD (Psyc) - **Spec Exp:** Psychopharmacology; Depression; Personality Disorders; **Hospital:** Mount Sinai Med Ctr (page 98), VA Med Ctr - Bronx; **Address:** 1 Gustave Levy Pl, Box 1230, New York, NY 10029-6500; **Phone:** 212-774-1722; **Board Cert:** Psychiatry 1980; **Med School:** Stanford Univ 1975; **Resid:** Psychiatry, McLean Hosp 1978; **Fellow:** Biological Psychiatry, Natl Inst Mntl Hlth 1982; **Fac Appt:** Prof Psyc, Mount Sinai Sch Med

Silver, Jonathan M MD (Psyc) - **Spec Exp:** Neuro-Psychiatry; Psychopharmacology; Brain Injury-Traumatic; **Hospital:** Lenox Hill Hosp (page 94); **Address:** 40 E 83rd St, Ste 1E, New York, NY 10028; **Phone:** 212-874-6453; **Board Cert:** Psychiatry 1984; **Med School:** Albert Einstein Coll Med 1979; **Resid:** Psychiatry, NY State Psych Inst 1983; **Fellow:** Research, NY State Psych Inst 1985; **Fac Appt:** Clin Prof Psyc, NYU Sch Med

Spitz, Henry MD (Psyc) - **Spec Exp:** Family & Couples Therapy; Addiction/Substance Abuse; Anxiety Disorders; **Hospital:** NY-Presby Hosp (page 100); **Address:** 101 Central Park West, Ste 1C, New York, NY 10023-4204; **Phone:** 212-873-1415; **Board Cert:** Psychiatry 1973; **Med School:** NY Med Coll 1965; **Resid:** Psychiatry, NY Med Coll 1969; **Fellow:** NY Med Coll 1970; **Fac Appt:** Clin Prof Psyc, Columbia P&S

Stein, Stefan MD (Psyc) - **Spec Exp:** Couples Therapy; Psychotherapy & Psychopharmacology; **Hospital:** NY-Presby Hosp (page 100); **Address:** 850 Park Ave, Ste 1E, New York, NY 10021; **Phone:** 212-249-0200; **Board Cert:** Psychiatry 1970; **Med School:** NYU Sch Med 1963; **Resid:** Internal Medicine, Boston City Hosp 1964; Psychiatry, Albert Einstein Coll Med 1968; **Fellow:** Psychiatry, Mass Genl Hosp 1965; Psychoanalysis, NY Psychoan Inst 1974; **Fac Appt:** Prof Psyc, Cornell Univ-Weill Med Coll

Steinglass, Peter MD (Psyc) - **Spec Exp:** Family Therapy; Substance Abuse; Alcohol Abuse; **Hospital:** Beth Israel Med Ctr - Petrie Division (page 90); **Address:** Ackerman Institute for the Family, 149 E 78th St, New York, NY 10021-0486; **Phone:** 212-879-4900 x119; **Board Cert:** Psychiatry 1971; **Med School:** Harvard Med Sch 1965; **Resid:** Psychiatry, Jacobi Med Ctr 1969; **Fac Appt:** Clin Prof Psyc, Cornell Univ-Weill Med Coll

Stone, Michael H MD (Psyc) - **Spec Exp:** Personality Disorders; Psychoanalysis; Forensic Psychiatry; **Hospital:** NY-Presby Hosp (page 100); **Address:** 225 Central Park West, Ste 114, New York, NY 10024-6027; **Phone:** 212-758-2000; **Board Cert:** Psychiatry 1971; **Med School:** Cornell Univ-Weill Med Coll 1958; **Resid:** Internal Medicine, Bellevue Hosp 1961; Psychiatry, NYS Psych Inst 1966; **Fellow:** Hematology, Meml Sloan Kettering Cancer Ctr 1962; Medical Oncology, Meml Sloan Kettering Cancer Ctr 1963; **Fac Appt:** Clin Prof Psyc, Columbia P&S

Strain, James MD (Psyc) - **Spec Exp:** Psychiatry in Physical Illness; Psychoanalysis; **Hospital:** Mount Sinai Med Ctr (page 98); **Address:** Mt Sinai Med Ctr, 1 Gustav Levy Pl, Box 1230, New York, NY 10029; **Phone:** 212-659-8728; **Board Cert:** Psychiatry 1969; **Med School:** Case West Res Univ 1962; **Resid:** Psychiatry, Univ Hosps 1966; **Fellow:** Psychiatric Research, Univ Hosps 1967; Psychoanalysis, New York Psychoanal Inst 1972; **Fac Appt:** Prof Psyc, Mount Sinai Sch Med

Sulkowicz, Kerry MD (Psyc) - **Spec Exp:** Psychoanalysis; Psychoanalysis-Corporate; Executive Coaching; **Hospital:** NYU Med Ctr (page 102), Lenox Hill Hosp (page 94); **Address:** 151 E 80th St, Ste 1B, New York, NY 10021-0442; **Phone:** 212-737-1950; **Board Cert:** Psychiatry 1991; **Med School:** Univ Tex Med Br, Galveston 1985; **Resid:** Psychiatry, NYU Med Ctr 1989; **Fellow:** Psychoanalysis, NYS Psychoanalytic Inst 1992; **Fac Appt:** Clin Prof Psyc, NYU Sch Med

Sussman, Norman MD (Psyc) - **Spec Exp:** Psychopharmacology; Anxiety & Mood Disorders; Bipolar/Mood Disorders; **Hospital:** NYU Med Ctr (page 102); **Address:** 150 E 58th St, Fl 27, New York, NY 10155; **Phone:** 212-588-9722; **Board Cert:** Psychiatry 1980; **Med School:** NY Med Coll 1975; **Resid:** Psychiatry, Metropolitan Hosp Ctr 1977; Psychiatry, Westchester Co Med Ctr 1978; **Fac Appt:** Clin Prof Psyc, NYU Sch Med

Swiller, Hillel MD (Psyc) - **Spec Exp:** Psychotherapy; **Hospital:** Mount Sinai Med Ctr (page 98); **Address:** 108 E 96th St, Ste 9F, New York, NY 10128; **Phone:** 212-534-5588; **Board Cert:** Psychiatry 1972; **Med School:** Cornell Univ-Weill Med Coll 1965; **Resid:** Psychiatry, Albert Einstein Coll Med 1969; **Fac Appt:** Clin Prof Psyc, Mount Sinai Sch Med

Tancredi, Laurence R MD (Psyc) - **Spec Exp:** Forensic Psychiatry; Anxiety & Depression; **Hospital:** Lenox Hill Hosp (page 94); **Address:** 129B E 71st St, New York, NY 10021-4201; **Phone:** 212-288-5197; **Board Cert:** Psychiatry 1979; **Med School:** Univ Pennsylvania 1966; **Resid:** Psychiatry, NYS Psych Inst 1975; Psychiatry, Yale-New Haven Hosp 1977; **Fac Appt:** Clin Prof Psyc, NYU Sch Med

Tardiff, Kenneth MD (Psyc) - **Spec Exp:** Psychopharmacology; Forensic Psychiatry; Psychotherapy; **Hospital:** NY-Presby Hosp (page 100); **Address:** Payne Whitney Clinic-NY Hosp, Dept Psyc, 525 E 68th St, Psy Box 140, New York, NY 10021-4870; **Phone:** 212-746-3871; **Board Cert:** Psychiatry 1976; **Med School:** Tulane Univ 1969; **Resid:** Psychiatry, Mass Genl Hosp 1973; **Fac Appt:** Prof Psyc, Cornell Univ-Weill Med Coll

Taylor, Noel MD (Psyc) - **Spec Exp:** Anxiety Disorders; Mood Disorders; **Address:** 150 E 58 St, Fl 27, New York, NY 10155; **Phone:** 212-888-9038; **Board Cert:** Psychiatry 1985; **Med School:** Johns Hopkins Univ 1980; **Resid:** Psychiatry, Johns Hopkins Hosp 1984; **Fellow:** Psychiatry, Beth Israel Med Ctr 1986; **Fac Appt:** Asst Prof Psyc, Albert Einstein Coll Med

Teusink, J Paul MD (Psyc) - **Spec Exp:** Geriatric Psychiatry; Depression; **Hospital:** Beth Israel Med Ctr - Petrie Division (page 90); **Address:** 1st Ave and 16th St, New York, NY 10003; **Phone:** 212-420-4680; **Board Cert:** Psychiatry 1976; Geriatric Psychiatry 2001; **Med School:** Univ Mich Med Sch 1969; **Resid:** Psychiatry, Topeka State Hosp 1971; Psychiatry, Menninger Meml Hosp 1973; **Fac Appt:** Assoc Prof Psyc, Albert Einstein Coll Med

Tolchin, Joan G MD (Psyc) - **Spec Exp:** Child & Adolescent Psychiatry; **Hospital:** NY-Presby Hosp (page 100); **Address:** 35 E 84th St, New York, NY 10028-0871; **Phone:** 212-744-1446; **Board Cert:** Psychiatry 1979; Child & Adolescent Psychiatry 1982; **Med School:** NYU Sch Med 1972; **Resid:** Psychiatry, Jacobi Med Ctr 1975; **Fellow:** Child & Adolescent Psychiatry, NY Hosp-Cornell Med Ctr 1977; **Fac Appt:** Assoc Clin Prof Psyc, Cornell Univ-Weill Med Coll

Wachtel, Alan MD (Psyc) - **Spec Exp:** ADD/ADHD; Mood Disorders; Learning Disorders; **Hospital:** NYU Med Ctr (page 102); **Address:** 201 E 87th St, Ste 16J, New York, NY 10128; **Phone:** 212-348-0175; **Board Cert:** Psychiatry 1977; **Med School:** Mount Sinai Sch Med 1972; **Resid:** Psychiatry, Mt Sinai Hosp 1976; **Fellow:** Liason Psychiatry, NY Hosp-Cornell Med Ctr 1977; **Fac Appt:** Assoc Clin Prof Psyc, NYU Sch Med

Wager, Steven MD (Psyc) - **Spec Exp:** Psychopharmacology; Depression; Anxiety Disorders; **Hospital:** NY-Presby Hosp (page 100); **Address:** 145 W 86th St, Ste 1B, New York, NY 10024-3421; **Phone:** 212-769-9620; **Board Cert:** Psychiatry 1986; **Med School:** Case West Res Univ 1980; **Resid:** Univ Hosp 1981; Psychiatry, Columbia-Presby Med Ctr 1984; **Fellow:** Psychiatry, Columbia-Presby Med Ctr 1986

Wallack, Joel J MD (Psyc) - **Spec Exp:** Psychopharmacology; Psychiatry in Physical Illness; Anxiety & Depression; **Hospital:** Cabrini Med Ctr (page 374), Mount Sinai Med Ctr (page 98); **Address:** 222 E 19th St, Ste 1D, New York, NY 10003-2666; **Phone:** 212-995-7200; **Board Cert:** Psychiatry 1979; **Med School:** UMDNJ-NJ Med Sch, Newark 1974; **Resid:** Psychiatry, St Lukes Hosp 1978; **Fellow:** Liason Psychiatry, Montefiore Hosp Med Ctr 1979; Psychosomatic Medicine, Mount Sinai Hosp 1980; **Fac Appt:** Prof Psyc, Mount Sinai Sch Med

Walsh, B Timothy MD (Psyc) - **Spec Exp:** Eating Disorders; **Hospital:** NY State Psychiatric Inst (page 100), NY-Presby Hosp (page 100); **Address:** NYSPI-Unit 98, 1051 Riverside Dr, New York, NY 10032-2695; **Phone:** 212-543-5316; **Board Cert:** Psychiatry 1978; **Med School:** Harvard Med Sch 1972; **Resid:** Internal Medicine, Dartmouth Affil Hosps 1973; Psychiatry, Bronx Muni Hosp Ctr 1977; **Fac Appt:** Prof Psyc, Columbia P&S

Weill, Terry MD (Psyc) - **Spec Exp:** Bipolar/Mood Disorders; Psychiatry in Physical Illness; **Hospital:** Mount Sinai Med Ctr (page 98); **Address:** 350 Central Park West, New York, NY 10023-6547; **Phone:** 212-316-5818; **Board Cert:** Psychiatry 1985; Geriatric Psychiatry 1992; **Med School:** Hahnemann Univ 1980; **Resid:** Psychiatry, Mount Sinai Med Ctr 1984; **Fellow:** Psychoanalysis, NYS Psyc Inst 1991; **Fac Appt:** Asst Prof Psyc, Mount Sinai Sch Med

Welsh, Howard MD (Psyc) - **Spec Exp:** Psychotherapy; Psychoanalysis; **Hospital:** NYU Med Ctr (page 102); **Address:** 27 W 86th St, Ste C, New York, NY 10024-3615; **Phone:** 212-362-5846; **Board Cert:** Psychiatry 1976; **Med School:** Albert Einstein Coll Med 1971; **Resid:** Psychiatry, Kings Co Hosp 1974; **Fac Appt:** Clin Prof Psyc, NYU Sch Med

Wilner, Philip MD (Psyc) - **Hospital:** NY-Presby Hosp (page 100); **Address:** 525 E 68th St, Box 140, New York, NY 10021; **Phone:** 212-746-3705; **Board Cert:** Psychiatry 1989; **Med School:** Columbia P&S 1983; **Resid:** Psychiatry, NY Hosp 1988; **Fellow:** Psychopharmacology, NY Hosp 1990; **Fac Appt:** Assoc Prof Psyc, Cornell Univ-Weill Med Coll

Winston, Arnold MD (Psyc) - **Spec Exp:** Psychotherapy; Mood Disorders; Psychopharmacology; **Hospital:** Beth Israel Med Ctr - Petrie Division (page 90); **Address:** 317 E 17th St, FL 9, New York, NY 10003-3804; **Phone:** 212-420-2555; **Board Cert:** Psychiatry 1969; **Med School:** SUNY Downstate 1960; **Resid:** Psychiatry, Kings Co Hosp Ctr 1965; **Fac Appt:** Prof Psyc, Albert Einstein Coll Med

Winters, Richard A MD (Psyc) - **Spec Exp:** Psychopharmacology; Crisis Intervention; Psychodynamic Psychotherapy; **Hospital:** Metropolitan Hosp Ctr - NY; **Address:** 35 E 85th St, New York, NY 10028-0954; **Phone:** 212-744-1346; **Board Cert:** Psychiatry 1977; **Med School:** NY Med Coll 1972; **Resid:** Psychiatry, Metropolitan Hosp Ctr 1975; **Fac Appt:** Asst Prof Psyc, NY Med Coll

Zimberg, Sheldon MD (Psyc) - **Spec Exp:** Addiction Psychiatry; Geriatric Psychiatry; Hypnosis; **Hospital:** St Luke's - Roosevelt Hosp Ctr - St Luke's Hosp (page 90), Beth Israel Med Ctr - Petrie Division (page 90); **Address:** 245 A E 61st St, New York, NY 10021-8203; **Phone:** 212-988-5139; **Board Cert:** Psychiatry 1969; Addiction Psychiatry 2004; **Med School:** SUNY Hlth Sci Ctr 1961; **Resid:** Psychiatry, NYS Psych Inst/Colum-Presby Med Ctr 1965; **Fellow:** Community Psychiatry, Columbia Univ Sch Pub Hlth 1966; **Fac Appt:** Clin Prof Psyc, Columbia P&S

PULMONARY DISEASE

Acquista, Angelo MD (Pul) - **Spec Exp:** Asthma; Bioterrorism Preparedness; **Hospital:** Lenox Hill Hosp (page 94); **Address:** Madison Medical, 110 E 59th St, Ste 9C, New York, NY 10022; **Phone:** 212-583-2850; **Board Cert:** Internal Medicine 1984; Pulmonary Disease 1986; **Med School:** NYU Sch Med 1981; **Resid:** Internal Medicine, Lenox Hill Hosp 1984; **Fellow:** Pulmonary Disease, Lenox Hill Hosp 1986

Adams, Francis MD (Pul) - **Spec Exp:** Asthma; Chronic Obstructive Lung Disease (COPD); Sarcoidosis; **Hospital:** NYU Med Ctr (page 102); **Address:** 650 First Ave, Fl 7, New York, NY 10016-3240; **Phone:** 212-447-0088; **Board Cert:** Internal Medicine 1974; Pulmonary Disease 1976; **Med School:** Cornell Univ-Weill Med Coll 1971; **Resid:** Internal Medicine, Georgetown Univ Hosp 1973; **Fellow:** Pulmonary Disease, Bellevue Hosp 1975; **Fac Appt:** Asst Prof Med, NYU Sch Med

Adler, Jack MD (Pul) - **Spec Exp:** Asthma; Chronic Obstructive Lung Disease (COPD); Tuberculosis; **Hospital:** Mount Sinai Med Ctr (page 98), Lenox Hill Hosp (page 94); **Address:** 19 E 80th St, New York, NY 10021-0117; **Phone:** 212-535-3622; **Board Cert:** Internal Medicine 1970; Pulmonary Disease 1971; **Med School:** Univ Chicago-Pritzker Sch Med 1962; **Resid:** Internal Medicine, Philadelphia Genl Hosp 1967; Internal Medicine, Michael Reese Hosp Med Ctr 1968; **Fellow:** Pulmonary Disease, Bronx Municipal Hosp Ctr 1971; **Fac Appt:** Assoc Prof Med, Mount Sinai Sch Med

Arcasoy, Selim M MD (Pul) - **Spec Exp:** Transplant Medicine-Lung; Chronic Obstructive Lung Disease (COPD); Interstitial Lung Disease; **Hospital:** NY-Presby Hosp (page 100); **Address:** Ctr for Advanced Lung Dis/Transplantation, 622 W 168th St, PH, Fl 14E - rm 104, New York, NY 10032-3720; **Phone:** 212-305-6589; **Board Cert:** Internal Medicine 2003; Pulmonary Disease 1996; Critical Care Medicine 1997; **Med School:** Turkey 1990; **Resid:** Internal Medicine, SUNY Downstate Med Ctr 1994; **Fellow:** Pulmonary Critical Care Medicine, Univ Pittsburgh Med Ctr 1998; **Fac Appt:** Assoc Prof Med, Columbia P&S

Baskin, Martin MD (Pul) - **Spec Exp:** Asthma; Pneumonia; Emphysema; **Hospital:** St Luke's - Roosevelt Hosp Ctr - Roosevelt Div (page 90); **Address:** 185 W End Ave, Ste M, New York, NY 10023-5539; **Phone:** 212-595-7701; **Board Cert:** Internal Medicine 1985; Pulmonary Disease 1988; Critical Care Medicine 1989; **Med School:** Mount Sinai Sch Med 1981; **Resid:** Internal Medicine, Beth Israel Med Ctr 1984; **Fellow:** Pulmonary Disease, St Luke's Roosevelt Hosp Ctr 1988; Critical Care Medicine, St Luke's Roosevelt Hosp Ctr 1989; **Fac Appt:** Asst Clin Prof Med, Columbia P&S

Bevelaqua, Frederick MD (Pul) - **Spec Exp:** Asthma; Lung Cancer; Chronic Obstructive Lung Disease (COPD); **Hospital:** NYU Med Ctr (page 102); **Address:** 35 A E 35th St, Ste 204, New York, NY 10016; **Phone:** 212-213-6796; **Board Cert:** Internal Medicine 1978; Pulmonary Disease 1980; **Med School:** NYU Sch Med 1974; **Resid:** Internal Medicine, NYU Med Ctr 1978; **Fellow:** Pulmonary Disease, NYU Med Ctr 1980; **Fac Appt:** Asst Clin Prof Med, NYU Sch Med

Blair, Lester MD (Pul) - **Spec Exp:** Asthma; Sarcoidosis; Bronchitis; **Hospital:** NY Downtown Hosp, Bellevue Hosp Ctr; **Address:** 170 William St, Fl 7, New York, NY 10038-2668; **Phone:** 212-238-0101; **Board Cert:** Internal Medicine 1987; Pulmonary Disease 1980; Critical Care Medicine 1999; **Med School:** Columbia P&S 1974; **Resid:** Internal Medicine, Columbia-Presby Med Ctr 1977; **Fellow:** Pulmonary Disease, Bellevue Hosp 1979; **Fac Appt:** Asst Clin Prof Med, NYU Sch Med

Pulmonary Disease

Cooke, Joseph T MD (Pul) - **Spec Exp:** Asthma; Lung Cancer; Critical Care; **Hospital:** NY-Presby Hosp (page 100); **Address:** Pulmonary and Critical Medicine, 520 E 70th St, Ste 505, New York, NY 10021-9800; **Phone:** 212-746-2250; **Board Cert:** Internal Medicine 1989; Pulmonary Disease 2002; Critical Care Medicine 2002; **Med School:** SUNY Downstate 1985; **Resid:** Internal Medicine, NY Hosp 1988; **Fellow:** Pulmonary Intensive Care, NY Hosp 1991; **Fac Appt:** Assoc Clin Prof Med, Cornell Univ-Weill Med Coll

Eden, Edward MD (Pul) - **Spec Exp:** Emphysema; Asthma; Sarcoidosis; **Hospital:** St Luke's - Roosevelt Hosp Ctr - Roosevelt Div (page 90); **Address:** 425 W 59th St, Ste 8A, New York, NY 10019-1104; **Phone:** 212-523-7090; **Board Cert:** Internal Medicine 1980; Pulmonary Disease 1982; Critical Care Medicine 1997; **Med School:** England 1975; **Resid:** Internal Medicine, Wayne Co Genl Hosp 1978; Internal Medicine, Univ Hosp 1980; **Fellow:** Pulmonary Disease, Mount Sinai Hosp 1982; Pulmonary Disease, Columbia-Presby Med Ctr 1985; **Fac Appt:** Assoc Prof Med, Columbia P&S

Gagliardi, Anthony MD (Pul) - **Spec Exp:** Asthma; Lung Cancer; Tuberculosis; **Hospital:** St Vincent Cath Med Ctrs - Manhattan (page 375); **Address:** 36 7th Ave, Ste 512, New York, NY 10011; **Phone:** 646-336-0924; **Board Cert:** Internal Medicine 1984; Pulmonary Disease 1986; **Med School:** UMDNJ-NJ Med Sch, Newark 1981; **Resid:** Internal Medicine, St Vincent's Hosp & Med Ctr 1984; **Fellow:** Pulmonary Disease, Meml Sloan Kettering Cancer Ctr 1986; **Fac Appt:** Asst Clin Prof Med, NY Med Coll

Garay, Stuart MD (Pul) - **Spec Exp:** Asthma; Chronic Obstructive Lung Disease (COPD); Sleep Apnea; **Hospital:** NYU Med Ctr (page 102); **Address:** 436 3rd Ave Fl 2, New York, NY 10016-6025; **Phone:** 212-685-6001; **Board Cert:** Internal Medicine 1977; Pulmonary Disease 1980; **Med School:** Harvard Med Sch 1974; **Resid:** Internal Medicine, Mt Sinai Hosp 1977; **Fellow:** Pulmonary Disease, Bellevue Hosp 1979; **Fac Appt:** Clin Prof Med, NYU Sch Med

Gribetz, Allen MD (Pul) - **Spec Exp:** Sarcoidosis; Asthma; **Hospital:** Mount Sinai Med Ctr (page 98); **Address:** 927 Park Ave, New York, NY 10028-0250; **Phone:** 212-517-8680; **Board Cert:** Internal Medicine 1974; Pulmonary Disease 1978; **Med School:** NYU Sch Med 1971; **Resid:** Internal Medicine, Mount Sinai Hosp 1974; **Fellow:** Pulmonary Disease, Mount Sinai Hosp 1978; **Fac Appt:** Asst Clin Prof Med, Mount Sinai Sch Med

Kamelhar, David MD (Pul) - **Spec Exp:** Asthma; Mycobacterial Infections; Chronic Obstructive Lung Disease (COPD); Occupational Lung Disease; **Hospital:** NYU Med Ctr (page 102), Cabrini Med Ctr (page 374); **Address:** 404 Park Ave S, Ste 701, New York, NY 10016; **Phone:** 212-685-6611; **Board Cert:** Internal Medicine 1977; Pulmonary Disease 1980; **Med School:** NYU Sch Med 1974; **Resid:** Internal Medicine, VA Hosp 1978; **Fellow:** Pulmonary Disease, Bellevue/NYU Med Ctr 1980; **Fac Appt:** Assoc Prof Med, NYU Sch Med

Klapholz, Ari MD (Pul) - **Spec Exp:** Lung Cancer; Sleep Disorders; Emphysema; **Hospital:** Cabrini Med Ctr (page 374), Beth Israel Med Ctr - Petrie Division (page 90); **Address:** 275 7th St Fl 3, New York, NY 10001; **Phone:** 646-660-9999; **Board Cert:** Internal Medicine 1987; Pulmonary Disease 1990; Critical Care Medicine 1991; **Med School:** NY Med Coll 1984; **Resid:** Internal Medicine, Beth Israel Med Ctr 1987; **Fellow:** Pulmonary Disease, Beth Israel Med Ctr 1989; Critical Care Medicine, Mount Sinai Hosp 1990; **Fac Appt:** Asst Prof Med, Mount Sinai Sch Med

Kolodny, Erwin MD (Pul) - **Spec Exp:** Asthma; Emphysema; Bronchitis; **Hospital:** NYU Med Ctr (page 102); **Address:** 650 1st Ave, New York, NY 10016-3240; **Phone:** 212-213-0090; **Board Cert:** Internal Medicine 1977; Pulmonary Disease 1978; **Med School:** NYU Sch Med 1973; **Resid:** Internal Medicine, Bellevue Hosp 1976; **Fellow:** Pulmonary Disease, NYU Med Ctr 1978; **Fac Appt:** Asst Clin Prof Med, NYU Sch Med

Kutnick, Robert MD (Pul) - **Spec Exp:** Asthma; Sarcoidosis; **Hospital:** Lenox Hill Hosp (page 94); **Address:** 14 E 90th St, Ste 1D, New York, NY 10128; **Phone:** 212-427-4700; **Board Cert:** Internal Medicine 1977; Pulmonary Disease 1980; **Med School:** Albert Einstein Coll Med 1974; **Resid:** Internal Medicine, Montefiore Hosp Med Ctr 1977; **Fellow:** Pulmonary Disease, Montefiore Hosp Med Ctr 1979

Lee, Marjorie MD (Pul) - **Spec Exp:** Asthma; Emphysema; Sarcoidosis; **Hospital:** Cabrini Med Ctr (page 374); **Address:** 222 E 19th St, Ste 1E, New York, NY 10003; **Phone:** 212-533-1185; **Board Cert:** Internal Medicine 1976; Pulmonary Disease 1978; **Med School:** SUNY Hlth Sci Ctr 1973; **Resid:** Internal Medicine, Kaiser Hosp 1976; Pulmonary Disease, Cabrini Hosp 1977; **Fellow:** Pulmonary Disease, Yale-New Haven Hosp 1979; **Fac Appt:** Assoc Clin Prof Med, NY Med Coll

Libby, Daniel MD (Pul) - **Spec Exp:** Asthma; Lung Cancer; Interstitial Lung Disease; **Hospital:** NY-Presby Hosp (page 100); **Address:** 407 E 70th St, New York, NY 10021-5302; **Phone:** 212-628-6611; **Board Cert:** Internal Medicine 1977; Pulmonary Disease 1980; **Med School:** Baylor Coll Med 1974; **Resid:** Internal Medicine, New York Hosp 1977; **Fellow:** Pulmonary Disease, New York Hosp 1979; **Fac Appt:** Clin Prof Med, Cornell Univ-Weill Med Coll

Lowy, Joseph MD (Pul) - **Spec Exp:** Lung Cancer; Asthma; Chronic Obstructive Lung Disease (COPD); **Hospital:** NYU Med Ctr (page 102); **Address:** 436 3rd Ave, New York, NY 10016-6025; **Phone:** 212-685-6660; **Board Cert:** Internal Medicine 1983; Pulmonary Disease 1986; Critical Care Medicine 1997; **Med School:** Univ Rochester 1980; **Resid:** Internal Medicine, Bellevue Hosp 1983; **Fellow:** Pulmonary Disease, UCSD Med Ctr 1986; **Fac Appt:** Asst Prof Med, NYU Sch Med

Marks Jr, Clement E MD (Pul) - **Spec Exp:** Chronic Obstructive Lung Disease (COPD); Asthma; **Hospital:** NYU Med Ctr (page 102); **Address:** 530 1st Ave, Ste 4J, New York, NY 10016; **Phone:** 212-263-7450; **Board Cert:** Internal Medicine 1969; Pulmonary Disease 1974; Geriatric Medicine 1994; **Med School:** Columbia P&S 1962; **Resid:** Internal Medicine, Bellevue Hosp 1969; **Fellow:** Pulmonary Disease, Bellevue Hosp 1973

Maxfield, Roger MD (Pul) - **Spec Exp:** Asthma & Emphysema; Occupational Lung Disease; Lung Cancer; **Hospital:** NY-Presby Hosp (page 100); **Address:** Columbia Presbyterian Eastside, 16 E 60th St, Ste 320, New York, NY 10022-1002; **Phone:** 212-326-8415; **Board Cert:** Internal Medicine 1980; Pulmonary Disease 1986; **Med School:** Brown Univ 1977; **Resid:** Internal Medicine, Georgetown Univ Hosp 1980; **Fellow:** Pulmonary Disease, Bellevue-NYU Med Ctr 1985; **Fac Appt:** Assoc Clin Prof Med, Columbia P&S

Miller, Rachel L MD (Pul) - **Spec Exp:** Asthma; **Hospital:** NY-Presby Hosp (page 100); **Address:** 622 W 168th St - PH8, New York, NY 10032; **Phone:** 212-305-0631; **Board Cert:** Internal Medicine 1993; Pulmonary Disease 1996; Critical Care Medicine 1997; Allergy & Immunology 1999; **Med School:** NYU Sch Med 1990; **Resid:** Internal Medicine, Columbia Presby Medical Ctr 1993; **Fellow:** Pulmonary Critical Care Medicine, Columbia Presby Medical Ctr 1995

Nash, Thomas MD (Pul) - **Spec Exp:** Asthma; Cough; Pneumonia; **Hospital:** NY-Presby Hosp (page 100); **Address:** 310 E 72nd St, New York, NY 10021-4726; **Phone:** 212-734-6612; **Board Cert:** Internal Medicine 1981; Infectious Disease 1984; Pulmonary Disease 1988; **Med School:** NYU Sch Med 1978; **Resid:** Internal Medicine, New York Hosp-Cornell 1981; **Fellow:** Infectious Disease, New York Hosp-Cornell 1985; Pulmonary Disease, Meml Sloan Kettering Cancer Ctr 1985; **Fac Appt:** Assoc Clin Prof Med, NYU Sch Med

Padilla, Maria L MD (Pul) - **Spec Exp:** Lung Disease; Sarcoidosis; Critical Care Medicine; **Hospital:** Mount Sinai Med Ctr (page 98); **Address:** Mt Sinai Med Ctr, Div Pulmonology, One Gustave L Levy Pl, Box 1232, New York, NY 10029-6574; **Phone:** 212-241-5656; **Board Cert:** Internal Medicine 1978; Pulmonary Disease 1980; **Med School:** Mount Sinai Sch Med 1975; **Resid:** Internal Medicine, Mount Sinai Hosp 1986; **Fellow:** Pulmonary Disease, Mount Sinai Hosp 1988; Critical Care Medicine, Mount Sinai Hosp 1990; **Fac Appt:** Assoc Prof Med, Mount Sinai Sch Med

Plottel, Claudia MD (Pul) - **Spec Exp:** Asthma; Chronic Obstructive Lung Disease (COPD); Emphysema; **Hospital:** NYU Med Ctr (page 102); **Address:** NYU Faculty Practice Offices, 530 First Ave, Ste 4D, New York, NY 10016-6402; **Phone:** 212-263-7015; **Board Cert:** Internal Medicine 1987; Pulmonary Disease 2002; **Med School:** Med Coll PA Hahnemann 1984; **Resid:** Internal Medicine, NYU Med Ctr - Bellevue Hosp 1988; **Fellow:** Pulmonary Critical Care Medicine, NYU Med Ctr - Bellevue Hosp 1990; **Fac Appt:** Assoc Clin Prof Med, NYU Sch Med

Posner, David MD (Pul) - **Spec Exp:** Asthma; Lung Cancer; Sarcoidosis; **Hospital:** Lenox Hill Hosp (page 94), NY-Presby Hosp (page 100); **Address:** 178 E 85th St, New York, NY 10028-2119; **Phone:** 212-861-8976; **Board Cert:** Internal Medicine 1984; Pulmonary Disease 1988; **Med School:** NY Med Coll 1981; **Resid:** Internal Medicine, Lenox Hill Hosp 1984; **Fellow:** Pulmonary Disease, LI Jewish Med Ctr 1987; **Fac Appt:** Assoc Clin Prof Med, NYU Sch Med

Prager, Kenneth MD (Pul) - **Spec Exp:** Lung Disease; Asthma; Ethics; **Hospital:** NY-Presby Hosp (page 100); **Address:** 161 Fort Washington Ave, rm 312, New York, NY 10032-3713; **Phone:** 212-305-5535; **Board Cert:** Internal Medicine 1973; **Med School:** Harvard Med Sch 1968; **Resid:** Internal Medicine, Columbia-Presby Med Ctr 1972; Internal Medicine, Billings Hosp 1973; **Fac Appt:** Clin Prof Med, Columbia P&S

Rapoport, David MD (Pul) - **Spec Exp:** Sleep Disorders/Apnea; **Hospital:** Bellevue Hosp Ctr, NYU Med Ctr (page 102); **Address:** 562 1st Ave, rm 7W53, New York, NY 10016; **Phone:** 212-263-6407; **Board Cert:** Internal Medicine 1977; Pulmonary Disease 1980; **Med School:** Albert Einstein Coll Med 1974; **Resid:** Internal Medicine, Roosevelt Hosp 1977; **Fellow:** Pulmonary Disease, NYU/Bellevue Med Ctr 1979; **Fac Appt:** Assoc Prof Med, NYU Sch Med

Raskin, Jonathan MD (Pul) - **Spec Exp:** Asthma; Chronic Obstructive Lung Disease (COPD); Pulmonary Rehabilitation; **Hospital:** Beth Israel Med Ctr - Petrie Division (page 90), Lenox Hill Hosp (page 94); **Address:** 1000 Park Ave, New York, NY 10028-0934; **Phone:** 212-288-4600; **Board Cert:** Internal Medicine 1982; Pulmonary Disease 1985; **Med School:** Mexico 1978; **Resid:** Internal Medicine, Beth Israel Med Ctr 1982; **Fellow:** Pulmonary Disease, Mount Sinai Hosp 1985; **Fac Appt:** Asst Clin Prof Med, Albert Einstein Coll Med

Sanders, Abraham MD (Pul) - **Spec Exp:** Asthma; Bronchitis; **Hospital:** NY-Presby Hosp (page 100), Hosp For Special Surgery (page 108); **Address:** 520 E 70th St, Starr Pavillion, Ste 505, New York, NY 10021-4870; **Phone:** 212-746-2250; **Board Cert:** Internal Medicine 1979; Pulmonary Disease 1983; Critical Care Medicine 1989; **Med School:** SUNY Hlth Sci Ctr 1976; **Resid:** Internal Medicine, Univ Hosp/Kings County Hosp 1980; **Fellow:** Pulmonary Disease, Kings County Hosp 1980; Pulmonary Disease, Royal Postgraduate Sch Med 1981; **Fac Appt:** Assoc Prof Med, Cornell Univ-Weill Med Coll

Schluger, Neil MD (Pul) - **Spec Exp:** Tuberculosis; Pulmonary Infections; Chronic Obstructive Lung Disease (COPD); **Hospital:** NY-Presby Hosp (page 100); **Address:** Div Pulm, Allergy & Crit Care Med, 630 W 168th St, PH-8 East, Rm 101, New York, NY 10032; **Phone:** 212-305-9817; **Board Cert:** Internal Medicine 1988; Pulmonary Disease 2003; **Med School:** Univ Pennsylvania 1985; **Resid:** Internal Medicine, St Lukes Hosp 1989; **Fellow:** Pulmonary Critical Care Medicine, NY Hosp-Cornell 1992; **Fac Appt:** Assoc Prof Med, Columbia P&S

Steiger, David MD (Pul) - **Spec Exp:** Rheumatologic Diseases of the Lung; Asthma; Pulmonary Embolism; Critical Care; **Hospital:** Hosp For Joint Diseases (page 107), NYU Med Ctr (page 102); **Address:** 305 2nd Ave, Ste 16, New York, NY 10003; **Phone:** 212-598-6091; **Board Cert:** Internal Medicine 1987; Pulmonary Disease 2002; Critical Care Medicine 1995; **Med School:** England 1981; **Resid:** Internal Medicine, St Thomas Hosp/Univ Coll Hosp 1984; Internal Medicine, St Lukes Hosp 1989; **Fellow:** Pulmonary Disease, UCSF Med Ctr 1994; **Fac Appt:** Asst Prof Med, NYU Sch Med

Stover-Pepe, Diane E MD (Pul) - **Spec Exp:** Interstitial Lung Disease; Pulmonary Infections; Pulmonary Disease/Immunocompromised; **Hospital:** Meml Sloan Kettering Cancer Ctr (page 109); **Address:** 1275 York Ave, rm H819, New York, NY 10021; **Phone:** 212-639-8380; **Board Cert:** Internal Medicine 1975; Pulmonary Disease 1978; **Med School:** Albert Einstein Coll Med 1970; **Resid:** Internal Medicine, Harlem Hosp Ctr 1972; Internal Medicine, New York Hosp-Cornell 1975; **Fellow:** Pulmonary Disease, Albert Einstein Med Ctr 1977; **Fac Appt:** Prof Med, Cornell Univ-Weill Med Coll

Sukumaran, Muthiah MD (Pul) - **Spec Exp:** Asthma; Chronic Obstructive Lung Disease (COPD); Lung Cancer; **Hospital:** NY Downtown Hosp, St Vincent Cath Med Ctrs - Manhattan (page 375); **Address:** 67 Hudson St, Ste 1B, New York, NY 10013; **Phone:** 212-732-7260; **Board Cert:** Internal Medicine 1976; Pulmonary Disease 1980; **Med School:** India 1973; **Resid:** Internal Medicine, Elmhurst City Hosp 1976; **Fellow:** Pulmonary Disease, Elmhurst City Hosp 1977; **Fac Appt:** Asst Clin Prof Med, NY Med Coll

Teirstein, Alvin MD (Pul) - **Spec Exp:** Sarcoidosis; Interstitial Lung Disease; Lung Cancer; Pulmonary Pathology; **Hospital:** Mount Sinai Med Ctr (page 98), VA Med Ctr - Bronx; **Address:** Mount Sinai Med Ctr, 1 Gustave Levy Pl, Box 1232, New York, NY 10029; **Phone:** 212-241-5656; **Board Cert:** Internal Medicine 1961; Pulmonary Disease 1969; **Med School:** SUNY Downstate 1953; **Resid:** Internal Medicine, Mt Sinai Med Ctr 1957; **Fellow:** Pulmonary Disease, Mt Sinai Med Ctr 1954; Pulmonary Disease, VA Med Ctr 1956; **Fac Appt:** Prof Med, Mount Sinai Sch Med

Thomashow, Byron MD (Pul) - **Spec Exp:** Emphysema; Asthma; Respiratory Failure; Chronic Obstructive Lung Disease (COPD); **Hospital:** NY-Presby Hosp (page 100); **Address:** 161 Fort Washington Ave, rm 311, New York, NY 10032; **Phone:** 212-305-5261; **Board Cert:** Internal Medicine 1977; Pulmonary Disease 1980; **Med School:** Columbia P&S 1974; **Resid:** Internal Medicine, Roosevelt Hosp 1977; Pulmonary Disease, Roosevelt Hosp 1978; **Fellow:** Pulmonary Disease, Harlem Hosp Ctr 1979; **Fac Appt:** Clin Prof Med, Columbia P&S

Villamena, Patricia MD (Pul) - **Spec Exp:** Lung Cancer; Chronic Obstructive Lung Disease (COPD); Critical Care; **Hospital:** Beth Israel Med Ctr - Petrie Division (page 90); **Address:** 1st Ave & 16th St, Dazian Bldg, 7th Fl, Pulmonary Div, New York, NY 10003; **Phone:** 212-420-2377; **Board Cert:** Internal Medicine 1989; Pulmonary Disease 1996; **Med School:** NY Med Coll 1977; **Resid:** Internal Medicine, Metro Hosp Ctr 1980; **Fellow:** Pulmonary Disease, Beth Israel Med Ctr 1986; **Fac Appt:** Asst Prof Med, Albert Einstein Coll Med

Volcovici, Guido MD (Pul) - **Spec Exp:** Asthma; Emphysema; **Hospital:** Saint Joseph's Med Ctr - Yonkers; **Address:** 4915 Broadway, Ste 1A, New York, NY 10034-3119; **Phone:** 914-968-5446; **Board Cert:** Internal Medicine 1985; Pulmonary Disease 1988; **Med School:** Romania 1962; **Resid:** Internal Medicine, Jewish Hosp 1974; **Fellow:** Pulmonary Disease, VA Med Ctr 1976

White, Dorothy MD (Pul) - **Spec Exp:** Lung Cancer; AIDS/HIV; AIDS Related Cancers; **Hospital:** Meml Sloan Kettering Cancer Ctr (page 109); **Address:** 1275 York Ave, rm H803, Box 13, New York, NY 10021; **Phone:** 212-639-8022; **Board Cert:** Internal Medicine 1980; Pulmonary Disease 1984; **Med School:** SUNY Hlth Sci Ctr 1977; **Resid:** Internal Medicine, New York Hosp 1980; Internal Medicine, Meml Sloan Kettering Inst 1981; **Fellow:** Pulmonary Disease, Yale-New Haven Hosp 1984; **Fac Appt:** Prof Med, Cornell Univ-Weill Med Coll

Yip, Chun MD (Pul) - **Spec Exp:** Asthma; Emphysema; Diaphragm Dysfunction; **Hospital:** NY-Presby Hosp (page 100); **Address:** 161 Fort Washington Ave, rm 311, New York, NY 10032-3713; **Phone:** 212-305-8548; **Board Cert:** Internal Medicine 1979; Pulmonary Disease 1984; **Med School:** Albert Einstein Coll Med 1976; **Resid:** Internal Medicine, Columbia-Presby Med Ctr 1979; **Fellow:** Pulmonary Disease, Bellevue Hosp Ctr 1981; **Fac Appt:** Clin Prof Med, Columbia P&S

RADIATION ONCOLOGY

Berson, Anthony M MD (RadRO) - **Spec Exp:** Prostate Cancer; Breast Cancer; Lung Cancer; **Hospital:** St Vincent Cath Med Ctrs - Manhattan (page 375); **Address:** 325 W 15th St, New York, NY 10011-5903; **Phone:** 212-604-6081; **Board Cert:** Radiation Oncology 1990; **Med School:** Hahnemann Univ 1984; **Resid:** Radiation Oncology, UCSF Med Ctr 1989; **Fellow:** Neoplastic Diseases, Lawrence Berkeley Lab 1987; **Fac Appt:** Assoc Prof RadRO, NY Med Coll

Ennis, Ronald D MD (RadRO) - **Spec Exp:** Brachytherapy; Prostate Cancer; Pancreatic Cancer; **Hospital:** St Luke's - Roosevelt Hosp Ctr - Roosevelt Div (page 90), Beth Israel Med Ctr - Petrie Division (page 90); **Address:** St Luke's Roosevelt Hosp, Dept Rad Oncol, 1000 10th Ave, Lower Level, New York, NY 10019; **Phone:** 212-523-7165; **Board Cert:** Radiation Oncology 2005; **Med School:** Yale Univ 1990; **Resid:** Therapeutic Radiology, Yale-New Haven Hosp 1994

Formenti, Silvia C MD (RadRO) - **Spec Exp:** Breast Cancer; Prostate Cancer; Chemo-Radiation Combined Therapy; **Hospital:** NYU Med Ctr (page 102); **Address:** NYU Med Ctr, Dept Radiation Oncology, 566 First Ave, New York, NY 10016-6402; **Phone:** 212-263-2601; **Board Cert:** Radiation Oncology 1991; **Med School:** Italy 1980; **Resid:** Internal Medicine, San Carlo Borromeo Hosp 1983; Medical Oncology, Univ of Pavia Med Ctr 1985; **Fellow:** Radiation Oncology, USC Med Ctr 1990; **Fac Appt:** Asst Prof RadRO, NYU Sch Med

Harrison, Louis MD (RadRO) - **Spec Exp:** Brachytherapy; Head & Neck Cancer; Radiation Therapy-Intraoperative; **Hospital:** Beth Israel Med Ctr - Petrie Division (page 90), St Luke's - Roosevelt Hosp Ctr - Roosevelt Div (page 90); **Address:** Beth Israel Med Ctr, Dept Rad Onc, 10 Union Square East, Ste 4G, New York, NY 10003-3314; **Phone:** 212-844-8087; **Board Cert:** Therapeutic Radiology 1986; **Med School:** SUNY Downstate 1982; **Resid:** Therapeutic Radiology, Yale-New Haven Hosp 1986; **Fac Appt:** Prof RadRO, Albert Einstein Coll Med

Isaacson, Steven MD (RadRO) - **Spec Exp:** Brain Tumors; Neuro-Oncology; **Hospital:** NY-Presby Hosp (page 100); **Address:** Columbia Presby Med Ctr, Dept Rad Oncol, 622 W 168th St, BHN-B11, New York, NY 10032; **Phone:** 212-305-2611; **Board Cert:** Radiation Oncology 1988; Otolaryngology 1978; **Med School:** Jefferson Med Coll 1973; **Resid:** Otolaryngology, Hosp Univ Penn 1978; Radiation Oncology, SUNY Hlth Sci Ctr 1988; **Fac Appt:** Clin Prof RadRO, Columbia P&S

McCormick, Beryl MD (RadRO) - **Spec Exp:** Breast Cancer; Eye Tumors/Cancer; **Hospital:** Meml Sloan Kettering Cancer Ctr (page 109), NY-Presby Hosp (page 100); **Address:** Meml Sloan Kettering - Radiation Oncology, 1275 York Ave, rm SM 04, New York, NY 10021-6007; **Phone:** 212-639-6828; **Board Cert:** Therapeutic Radiology 1977; **Med School:** UMDNJ-NJ Med Sch, Newark 1973; **Resid:** Therapeutic Radiology, Meml Sloan Kettering Cancer Ctr 1977; **Fac Appt:** Prof RadRO, Cornell Univ-Weill Med Coll

Minsky, Bruce MD (RadRO) - **Spec Exp:** Colon & Rectal Cancer; Esophageal Cancer; Gastrointestinal Cancer; **Hospital:** Meml Sloan Kettering Cancer Ctr (page 109); **Address:** Meml Sloan Kettering Cancer Ctr, Dept Rad Onc, 1275 York Ave, New York, NY 10021-6007; **Phone:** 212-639-6817; **Board Cert:** Radiation Oncology 1987; **Med School:** Univ Mass Sch Med 1982; **Resid:** Radiation Oncology, Harvard Jt Ctr Rad Ther 1986; **Fac Appt:** Prof RadRO, Cornell Univ-Weill Med Coll

Ng, John Paul Tracy MD (RadRO) - **Spec Exp:** Prostate Cancer; Head & Neck Cancer; **Hospital:** St Vincent Cath Med Ctrs - Manhattan (page 375); **Address:** 325 W 15th St, New York, NY 10011-5903; **Phone:** 212-604-6083; **Board Cert:** Radiation Oncology 1992; **Med School:** Albert Einstein Coll Med 1988; **Resid:** Radiation Oncology, Meml Sloan Kettering Cancer Ctr 1992; **Fac Appt:** Asst Prof RadRO, NY Med Coll

Nori, Dattatreyudu MD (RadRO) - **Spec Exp:** Breast Cancer; Prostate Cancer; Gynecologic Cancer; **Hospital:** NY-Presby Hosp (page 100), NY Hosp Queens; **Address:** 525 E 68th St, Box 575, New York, NY 10021-4870; **Phone:** 212-746-3679; **Board Cert:** Therapeutic Radiology 1979; **Med School:** India 1970; **Resid:** Radiation Oncology, Meml Sloan Kettering Cancer Ctr 1975; **Fellow:** Radiation Oncology, Meml Sloan Kettering Cancer Ctr 1978; **Fac Appt:** Prof RadRO, Cornell Univ-Weill Med Coll

Rosenbaum, Alfred MD (RadRO) - **Spec Exp:** Breast Cancer; Prostate Cancer; Intensity Modulated Radiotherapy (IMRT); **Hospital:** Mount Sinai Med Ctr (page 98), Lenox Hill Hosp (page 94); **Address:** 945 5th Ave, New York, NY 10021-2655; **Phone:** 212-744-5538; **Board Cert:** Radiology 1973; **Med School:** Germany 1966; **Resid:** Radiology, Maimonides Med Ctr 1969; Radiation Oncology, Mount Sinai Hosp 1972; **Fellow:** Radiology, Montefiore Med Ctr 1973; **Fac Appt:** Asst Clin Prof Rad, Mount Sinai Sch Med

Sadarangani, Gurmukh J MD (RadRO) - **Spec Exp:** Brachytherapy; Prostate Cancer; Breast Cancer; Head & Neck Cancer; **Hospital:** Cabrini Med Ctr (page 374); **Address:** 227 E 19th St, New York, NY 10003; **Phone:** 212-995-6700; **Board Cert:** Therapeutic Radiology 1985; **Med School:** India 1978; **Resid:** Radiation Oncology, Montefiore Hosp Med Ctr 1985

Schiff, Peter B MD/PhD (RadRO) - **Spec Exp:** Prostate Cancer; Gynecologic Cancer; Breast Cancer; **Hospital:** NY-Presby Hosp (page 100); **Address:** Columbia Univ Med Ctr, Dept Rad Oncology, 622 W 168th St, New York, NY 10032-3720; **Phone:** 212-305-2991; **Board Cert:** Radiation Oncology 1990; **Med School:** Albert Einstein Coll Med 1984; **Resid:** Radiation Oncology, Meml Sloan Kettering Cancer Ctr 1988; **Fac Appt:** Prof RadRO, Columbia P&S

Stock, Richard MD (RadRO) - **Spec Exp:** Prostate Cancer; **Hospital:** Mount Sinai Med Ctr (page 98); **Address:** One Gustave L Levy Pl, Box 1236, New York, NY 10029; **Phone:** 212-241-7502; **Board Cert:** Radiation Oncology 1993; **Med School:** Mount Sinai Sch Med 1988; **Resid:** Radiation Oncology, Meml Sloan Kettering Cancer Ctr 1992; **Fac Appt:** Prof Rad, Mount Sinai Sch Med

Vallejo, Alvaro MD (RadRO) - **Hospital:** NY-Presby Hosp (page 100); **Address:** 525 E 68th St, rm NO46, New York, NY 10021; **Phone:** 212-746-3641; **Board Cert:** Therapeutic Radiology 1972; **Med School:** Colombia 1967; **Resid:** Radiation Oncology, Meml Sloan KetteringCancer Ctr 1971; **Fellow:** Radiation Oncology, T Jefferson Univ Hosp 1973; **Fac Appt:** Assoc Prof RadRO, Cornell Univ-Weill Med Coll

Yahalom, Joachim MD (RadRO) - **Spec Exp:** Lymphoma; Hodgkin's Disease; Multiple Myeloma; **Hospital:** Meml Sloan Kettering Cancer Ctr (page 109); **Address:** Meml Sloan Kettering Cancer Ctr, Dept Rad Oncology, 1275 York Ave, New York, NY 10021-6007; **Phone:** 212-639-5999; **Board Cert:** Radiation Oncology 1988; **Med School:** Israel 1976; **Resid:** Internal Medicine, Hadassah Hosp 1979; Radiation Oncology, Hadassah Hosp 1984; **Fellow:** Radiation Oncology, Meml Sloan Kettering Canc Ctr 1986; **Fac Appt:** Prof RadRO, Cornell Univ-Weill Med Coll

Zelefsky, Michael J MD (RadRO) - **Spec Exp:** Prostate Cancer; Brachytherapy; Genitourinary Cancer; **Hospital:** Meml Sloan Kettering Cancer Ctr (page 109); **Address:** Meml Sloan-Kettering Cancer Ctr, 1275 York Ave, New York, NY 10021-6094; **Phone:** 212-639-6802; **Board Cert:** Radiation Oncology 1991; **Med School:** Albert Einstein Coll Med 1986; **Resid:** Radiation Oncology, Meml Sloan Kettering Cancer Ctr 1990; **Fac Appt:** Prof RadRO, Cornell Univ-Weill Med Coll

REPRODUCTIVE ENDOCRINOLOGY

Berkeley, Alan S MD (RE) - **Spec Exp:** Infertility-IVF; Reproductive Surgery; Uterine Fibroids; **Hospital:** NYU Med Ctr (page 102); **Address:** NYU Reproductive Surgery & Infertility, 660 First Ave, Fl 5, New York, NY 10016-3295; **Phone:** 212-263-7629; **Board Cert:** Obstetrics & Gynecology 1980; **Med School:** NY Med Coll 1973; **Resid:** Obstetrics & Gynecology, Yale-New Haven Hosp 1977; **Fellow:** Gynecologic Oncology, Yale-New Haven Hosp 1979; Infertility, Yale-New Haven Hosp 1979; **Fac Appt:** Prof ObG, NYU Sch Med

Cholst, Ina N MD (RE) - **Spec Exp:** Gynecologic Surgery-Laparoscopic; Infertility-IVF; Menopause Problems; **Hospital:** NY-Presby Hosp (page 100); **Address:** Ctr for Reproductive Med & Infertility, 505 E 70th St, Ste 370, New York, NY 10021; **Phone:** 212-746-3025; **Board Cert:** Obstetrics & Gynecology 1984; Reproductive Endocrinology 1985; **Med School:** NYU Sch Med 1977; **Resid:** Obstetrics & Gynecology, Yale-New Haven Hosp 1981; **Fellow:** Reproductive Endocrinology, Columbia-Presby Med Ctr 1983; **Fac Appt:** Assoc Prof ObG, Cornell Univ-Weill Med Coll

Copperman, Alan B MD (RE) - **Spec Exp:** Infertility-IVF; Endometriosis; Laparoscopic Surgery; **Hospital:** Mount Sinai Med Ctr (page 98); **Address:** 635 Madison Ave Fl 10, New York, NY 10022; **Phone:** 212-756-5777; **Board Cert:** Obstetrics & Gynecology 1996; Reproductive Endocrinology 1999; **Med School:** NY Med Coll 1989; **Resid:** Obstetrics & Gynecology, Yale-New Haven Hosp 1993; **Fellow:** Reproductive Endocrinology, Mount Sinai Med Ctr 1995; **Fac Appt:** Assoc Clin Prof ObG, Mount Sinai Sch Med

David, Sami MD (RE) - **Spec Exp:** Infertility; Miscarriage-Recurrent; **Hospital:** Mount Sinai Med Ctr (page 98); **Address:** 1047 Park Ave, New York, NY 10028-1002; **Phone:** 212-831-0430; **Board Cert:** Obstetrics & Gynecology 1980; **Med School:** Columbia P&S 1971; **Resid:** Obstetrics & Gynecology, New York Hosp 1976; **Fellow:** Reproductive Endocrinology, Hosp Univ Penn 1978; **Fac Appt:** Prof ObG, Mount Sinai Sch Med

Davis, Owen MD (RE) - **Spec Exp:** Infertility-IVF; Reproductive Surgery; **Hospital:** NY-Presby Hosp (page 100); **Address:** 505 E 70th St, rm 340, New York, NY 10021-4872; **Phone:** 212-746-1765; **Board Cert:** Obstetrics & Gynecology 2003; Reproductive Endocrinology 2003; **Med School:** Wake Forest Univ 1982; **Resid:** Obstetrics & Gynecology, NY Hosp 1986; **Fellow:** Reproductive Endocrinology, Brigham & Women's Hosp 1988; **Fac Appt:** Assoc Prof ObG, Cornell Univ-Weill Med Coll

Fateh, Majid MD (RE) - **Spec Exp:** Endometriosis; Laparoscopic Surgery; Infertility; **Hospital:** Lenox Hill Hosp (page 94); **Address:** 1016 5th Ave, New York, NY 10028-0132; **Phone:** 212-734-5555; **Board Cert:** Obstetrics & Gynecology 1996; **Med School:** West Indies 1980; **Resid:** Obstetrics & Gynecology, Lenox Hill Hosp 1984; **Fellow:** Reproductive Endocrinology, Hosp Univ Penn 1986

Grifo, James A MD/PhD (RE) - **Spec Exp:** Infertility-IVF; **Hospital:** NYU Med Ctr (page 102), Bellevue Hosp Ctr; **Address:** 660 1st Ave Fl 5, New York, NY 10016; **Phone:** 212-263-7978; **Board Cert:** Obstetrics & Gynecology 2005; Reproductive Endocrinology 2005; **Med School:** Case West Res Univ 1984; **Resid:** Obstetrics & Gynecology, NY Hosp-Cornell Med Ctr 1988; **Fellow:** Reproductive Endocrinology, Yale-New Haven Hosp 1990; **Fac Appt:** Prof ObG, NYU Sch Med

Grunfeld, Lawrence MD (RE) - **Spec Exp:** Infertility-IVF; Hysteroscopic Surgery; Laparoscopic Surgery; **Hospital:** Mount Sinai Med Ctr (page 98), Lenox Hill Hosp (page 94); **Address:** 635 Madison Ave Fl 10, New York, NY 10022-1009; **Phone:** 212-756-5777; **Board Cert:** Obstetrics & Gynecology 1997; Reproductive Endocrinology 1997; **Med School:** Mount Sinai Sch Med 1979; **Resid:** Obstetrics & Gynecology, Albert Einstein Med Ctr 1984; **Fellow:** Reproductive Endocrinology, Albert Einstein Med Ctr 1987; **Fac Appt:** Assoc Clin Prof ObG, Mount Sinai Sch Med

Kelly, Amalia MD (RE) - **Spec Exp:** Laparoscopic Surgery; Infertility; Hysteroscopic Surgery; Miscarriage-Recurrent; **Hospital:** NY-Presby Hosp (page 100); **Address:** 50 E 77th St, New York, NY 10021; **Phone:** 212-639-9122; **Board Cert:** Reproductive Endocrinology 2005; Obstetrics & Gynecology 2005; **Med School:** Tufts Univ 1979; **Resid:** Obstetrics & Gynecology, Columbia-Presby Med Ctr 1983; **Fellow:** Reproductive Endocrinology, Columbia-Presby Med Ctr 1985; **Fac Appt:** Assoc Prof ObG, Columbia P&S

Licciardi, Frederick L MD (RE) - **Spec Exp:** Infertility-IVF; Infertility; Fertility Preservation in Cancer; **Hospital:** NYU Med Ctr (page 102); **Address:** NYU Medical Ctr, 660 First Ave, 5th Fl, New York, NY 10016; **Phone:** 212-263-7754; **Board Cert:** Obstetrics & Gynecology 2005; Reproductive Endocrinology 2005; **Med School:** Rutgers Univ 1986; **Resid:** Obstetrics & Gynecology, St Barnabas Med Ctr 1990; **Fellow:** Reproductive Endocrinology, New York Hosp-Cornell Med Ctr 1992; **Fac Appt:** Assoc Prof ObG, NYU Sch Med

Matera, Cristina MD (RE) - **Spec Exp:** Infertility; Laparoscopic Surgery; **Hospital:** NY-Presby Hosp (page 100); **Address:** 50 E 77th St, New York, NY 10021; **Phone:** 212-639-9122; **Board Cert:** Obstetrics & Gynecology 1994; Reproductive Endocrinology 1996; **Med School:** NYU Sch Med 1986; **Resid:** Obstetrics & Gynecology, Columbia-Presby Hosp 1990; **Fellow:** Reproductive Endocrinology, Columbia-Presby Hosp 1992; **Fac Appt:** Assoc Prof ObG, Columbia P&S

Mukherjee, Tanmoy MD (RE) - **Spec Exp:** Infertility-IVF; **Hospital:** Mount Sinai Med Ctr (page 98); **Address:** 635 Madison Ave Fl 10, New York, NY 10022; **Phone:** 212-756-5777; **Board Cert:** Obstetrics & Gynecology 1997; Reproductive Endocrinology 2000; **Med School:** Albert Einstein Coll Med 1990; **Resid:** Obstetrics & Gynecology, Montefiore Med Ctr 1994; **Fellow:** Reproductive Endocrinology, Mt Sinai Hosp 1996

Noyes, Nicole MD (RE) - **Spec Exp:** Infertility-IVF; Fertility Preservation in Cancer; **Hospital:** NYU Med Ctr (page 102); **Address:** NYU Medical Ctr, 660 First Ave, 5th FL, New York, NY 10016; **Phone:** 212-263-7981; **Board Cert:** Obstetrics & Gynecology 2005; Reproductive Endocrinology 2005; **Med School:** Univ VT Coll Med 1986; **Resid:** Obstetrics & Gynecology, NY Hosp-Cornell Med Ctr 1990; **Fellow:** Reproductive Endocrinology, NY Hosp-Cornell Med Ctr 1992; **Fac Appt:** Assoc Prof ObG, NYU Sch Med

Quagliarello, John MD (RE) - **Spec Exp:** Infertility; Gynecologic Surgery; Uterine Fibroids; **Hospital:** NYU Med Ctr (page 102); **Address:** 530 1st Ave Bldg SKB Fl 10 - Ste Q, New York, NY 10016-6402; **Phone:** 212-263-6358; **Board Cert:** Obstetrics & Gynecology 1979; Reproductive Endocrinology 1981; **Med School:** McGill Univ 1970; **Resid:** Obstetrics & Gynecology, NYU Med Ctr 1977; **Fellow:** Reproductive Endocrinology, NYU Med Ctr 1979; **Fac Appt:** Assoc Prof ObG, NYU Sch Med

Reyniak, J Victor MD (RE) - **Spec Exp:** Endometriosis; Uterine Fibroids; Infertility-IVF; **Hospital:** Mount Sinai Med Ctr (page 98), Lenox Hill Hosp (page 94); **Address:** 1107 5th Ave, New York, NY 10128-0145; **Phone:** 212-410-4080; **Board Cert:** Obstetrics & Gynecology 1999; Reproductive Endocrinology 1999; **Med School:** Poland 1960; **Resid:** Obstetrics & Gynecology, Brooklyn Women's Hosp 1966; **Fellow:** Reproductive Endocrinology, NIH/NY Med Coll; **Fac Appt:** Clin Prof ObG, Mount Sinai Sch Med

Rosenwaks, Zev MD (RE) - **Spec Exp:** Infertility-IVF; Genetic Disorders; Fertility Preservation in Cancer; **Hospital:** NY-Presby Hosp (page 100); **Address:** Ctr For Reproductive Medicine & Infertility, 505 E 70th St, Ste 340, New York, NY 10021-4872; **Phone:** 212-746-1743; **Board Cert:** Obstetrics & Gynecology 1978; Reproductive Endocrinology 1981; **Med School:** SUNY Downstate 1972; **Resid:** Obstetrics & Gynecology, LI Jewish Med Ctr 1976; **Fellow:** Reproductive Endocrinology, Johns Hopkins Hosp 1978; **Fac Appt:** Prof ObG, Cornell Univ-Weill Med Coll

Sauer, Mark MD (RE) - **Spec Exp:** Infertility-IVF; **Hospital:** NY-Presby Hosp (page 100); **Address:** 1790 Broadway Fl 2, New York, NY 10019; **Phone:** 646-756-8282; **Board Cert:** Obstetrics & Gynecology 1996; Reproductive Endocrinology 1996; **Med School:** Univ IL Coll Med 1980; **Resid:** Obstetrics & Gynecology, Univ Illinois Med Ctr 1984; **Fellow:** Reproductive Endocrinology, Harbor-UCLA Med Ctr 1986; **Fac Appt:** Prof ObG, Columbia P&S

Schmidt-Sarosi, Cecilia MD (RE) - **Spec Exp:** Infertility-IVF; Menopause Problems; Polycystic Ovarian Syndrome; **Hospital:** NYU Med Ctr (page 102); **Address:** 51 E 67th St, New York, NY 10021; **Phone:** 212-535-5350; **Board Cert:** Obstetrics & Gynecology 1993; Reproductive Endocrinology 1993; **Med School:** NYU Sch Med 1976; **Resid:** Obstetrics & Gynecology, NYU Med Ctr 1980; **Fellow:** Reproductive Endocrinology, NYU Med Ctr 1982; **Fac Appt:** Prof ObG, NYU Sch Med

Sultan, Khalid MD (RE) - **Spec Exp:** Infertility-IVF; Laparoscopic Surgery; **Hospital:** Lenox Hill Hosp (page 94); **Address:** 1016 5th Ave, New York, NY 10028-0132; **Phone:** 212-734-5555; **Board Cert:** Obstetrics & Gynecology 1995; Reproductive Endocrinology 1997; **Med School:** NY Med Coll 1988; **Resid:** Obstetrics & Gynecology, Lenox Hill Hosp 1992; **Fellow:** Reproductive Endocrinology, NY Hosp 1994; **Fac Appt:** Asst Clin Prof ObG, NYU Sch Med

Warren, Michelle MD (RE) - **Spec Exp:** Menopause Problems; Infertility; Menstrual Disorders; **Hospital:** NY-Presby Hosp (page 100); **Address:** 134 E 73rd St, New York, NY 10021; **Phone:** 212-737-4664; **Board Cert:** Internal Medicine 1972; Endocrinology 1973; **Med School:** Cornell Univ-Weill Med Coll 1965; **Resid:** Internal Medicine, Bellevue Hosp Ctr 1968; Internal Medicine, Meml Sloan Kettering Canc Ctr 1968; **Fellow:** Endocrinology, Columbia P&S 1971; **Fac Appt:** Prof ObG, Columbia P&S

RHEUMATOLOGY

Abramson, Steven B MD (Rhu) - **Spec Exp:** Arthritis; Inflammatory Muscle Disease; **Hospital:** Hosp For Joint Diseases (page 107), NYU Med Ctr (page 102); **Address:** Hosp for Joint Diseases, 301 E 17th St, rm 1410, New York, NY 10003; **Phone:** 212-598-6110; **Board Cert:** Internal Medicine 1977; Rheumatology 1980; **Med School:** Harvard Med Sch 1974; **Resid:** Internal Medicine, Bellevue Hosp/NYU Med Ctr 1978; **Fellow:** Rheumatology, Bellevue Hosp/NYU Med Ctr 1983; **Fac Appt:** Prof Med, NYU Sch Med

Adlersberg, Jay MD (Rhu) - **Spec Exp:** Rheumatoid Arthritis; Osteoarthritis; Psoriatic Arthritis; **Hospital:** Lenox Hill Hosp (page 94), Hosp For Joint Diseases (page 107); **Address:** 220 E 69th St, New York, NY 10021-5737; **Phone:** 212-570-1800; **Board Cert:** Internal Medicine 1972; Rheumatology 1980; **Med School:** Univ Pennsylvania 1969; **Resid:** Internal Medicine, Bellevue Hosp 1972; **Fellow:** Rheumatology, Bellevue Hosp 1974; **Fac Appt:** Asst Prof Med, Mount Sinai Sch Med

Agus, Bertrand MD (Rhu) - **Spec Exp:** Lupus/SLE; Rheumatoid Arthritis; Sarcoidosis; **Hospital:** NYU Med Ctr (page 102); **Address:** 251 E 33rd St, Fl 4, New York, NY 10016-4804; **Phone:** 212-779-8421; **Board Cert:** Internal Medicine 1972; Rheumatology 1972; **Med School:** NYU Sch Med 1965; **Resid:** Internal Medicine, NYU Med Ctr 1970; **Fellow:** Rheumatology, NYU Med Ctr 1972; **Fac Appt:** Assoc Clin Prof Med, NYU Sch Med

Argyros, Thomas MD (Rhu) - **Spec Exp:** Lyme Disease; Lupus/SLE; **Hospital:** Lenox Hill Hosp (page 94); **Address:** 122 E 76th St, New York, NY 10021-2833; **Phone:** 212-988-7680; **Board Cert:** Internal Medicine 1961; **Med School:** NYU Sch Med 1954; **Resid:** Internal Medicine, Lenox Hill Hosp 1958; **Fellow:** Rheumatology, Lenox Hill Hosp 1957; Rheumatology, New York Univ Med Ctr 1965; **Fac Appt:** Clin Prof Med, NYU Sch Med

Bauer, Bertha MD (Rhu) - **Spec Exp:** Fibromyalgia; Osteoporosis; **Hospital:** NYU Med Ctr (page 102); **Address:** 108 E 96th St, New York, NY 10128-6217; **Phone:** 212-828-7933; **Board Cert:** Internal Medicine 1980; Rheumatology 1996; **Med School:** Columbia P&S 1977; **Resid:** Internal Medicine, New England Deaconess Hosp 1980; **Fellow:** Rheumatology, Yale-New Haven Hosp 1982; **Fac Appt:** Asst Clin Prof Med, Columbia P&S

Belmont, Howard Michael MD (Rhu) - **Spec Exp:** Lupus/SLE; Rheumatoid Arthritis; Scleroderma; **Hospital:** Hosp For Joint Diseases (page 107), NYU Med Ctr (page 102); **Address:** 305 2nd Ave, Ste 16, New York, NY 10003-2739; **Phone:** 212-598-6516; **Board Cert:** Internal Medicine 1983; Rheumatology 1986; **Med School:** Univ Pittsburgh 1980; **Resid:** Internal Medicine, Mt Sinai Hosp 1983; **Fellow:** Rheumatology, NYU/Bellevue Hosp Ctr 1985; **Fac Appt:** Assoc Prof Med, NYU Sch Med

Blume, Ralph S MD (Rhu) - **Spec Exp:** Vasculitis; Lupus/SLE; Rheumatoid Arthritis; **Hospital:** NY-Presby Hosp (page 100); **Address:** 161 Fort Washington Ave, Ste 537, New York, NY 10032-3713; **Phone:** 212-305-5512; **Board Cert:** Internal Medicine 1972; Rheumatology 1974; **Med School:** Columbia P&S 1964; **Resid:** Internal Medicine, Columbia-Presby Hosp 1966; Internal Medicine, Columbia-Presby Hosp 1969; **Fellow:** Rheumatology, Columbia P&S 1970; **Fac Appt:** Clin Prof Med, Columbia P&S

Buyon, Jill P MD (Rhu) - **Spec Exp:** Lupus/SLE in Pregnancy; Lupus/SLE in Menopause; **Hospital:** Hosp For Joint Diseases (page 107), NYU Med Ctr (page 102); **Address:** 256 E 20th St, New York, NY 10003; **Phone:** 212-598-6516; **Board Cert:** Internal Medicine 1981; Rheumatology 1984; **Med School:** Albert Einstein Coll Med 1978; **Resid:** Internal Medicine, Albert Einstein 1981; **Fellow:** Rheumatology, NYU Med Ctr 1983; **Fac Appt:** Prof Med, NYU Sch Med

Crane, Richard MD (Rhu) - **Spec Exp:** Rheumatoid Arthritis; Gout; Osteoarthritis; Arthritis; **Hospital:** Mount Sinai Med Ctr (page 98); **Address:** 1088 Park Ave, New York, NY 10128-1132; **Phone:** 212-860-4000; **Board Cert:** Internal Medicine 1984; Rheumatology 1986; **Med School:** Mount Sinai Sch Med 1981; **Resid:** Internal Medicine, Mount Sinai Hosp 1984; **Fellow:** Rheumatology, Mount Sinai Hosp 1986

Faller, Jason MD (Rhu) - **Spec Exp:** Lyme Disease; Rheumatoid Arthritis; Gout; Lupus/SLE; **Hospital:** St Luke's - Roosevelt Hosp Ctr - Roosevelt Div (page 90); **Address:** 333 W 57th St, Ste 104, New York, NY 10019-3115; **Phone:** 212-307-6880; **Board Cert:** Internal Medicine 1980; Rheumatology 1982; **Med School:** Univ Pennsylvania 1977; **Resid:** Internal Medicine, Rush Presby St Lukes Hosp 1980; **Fellow:** Rheumatology, Univ Mich 1982; **Fac Appt:** Asst Clin Prof Med, Columbia P&S

Fields, Theodore MD (Rhu) - **Spec Exp:** Gout; Rheumatoid Arthritis; Osteoarthritis; **Hospital:** Hosp For Special Surgery (page 108), NY-Presby Hosp (page 100); **Address:** Hosp Special Surg-Faculty Practice, 535 E 70th St Fl 7 - Ste 719, New York, NY 10021-4872; **Phone:** 212-606-1286; **Board Cert:** Internal Medicine 1979; Rheumatology 1982; **Med School:** SUNY Downstate 1976; **Resid:** Internal Medicine, Nassau Co Med Ctr 1979; **Fellow:** Rheumatology, Univ Hosp 1982; **Fac Appt:** Assoc Clin Prof Med, Cornell Univ-Weill Med Coll

Fischer, Harry MD (Rhu) - **Spec Exp:** Lupus/SLE; Rheumatoid Arthritis; **Hospital:** Beth Israel Med Ctr - Petrie Division (page 90); **Address:** 10 Union Square East, Ste 3D, New York, NY 10003-3314; **Phone:** 212-844-8101; **Board Cert:** Internal Medicine 1983; Rheumatology 2000; **Med School:** Mount Sinai Sch Med 1979; **Resid:** Internal Medicine, Beth Israel Med Ctr 1983; **Fellow:** Rheumatology, Hosp Joint Diseases 1985; **Fac Appt:** Assoc Clin Prof Med, Albert Einstein Coll Med

Gibofsky, Allan MD (Rhu) - **Spec Exp:** Rheumatic Fever; Rheumatoid Arthritis; **Hospital:** Hosp For Special Surgery (page 108), NY-Presby Hosp (page 100); **Address:** Hospital for Special Surgery, 535 E 70th St, New York, NY 10021; **Phone:** 212-606-1423; **Board Cert:** Internal Medicine 1977; Rheumatology 1980; **Med School:** Cornell Univ-Weill Med Coll 1973; **Resid:** Internal Medicine, NY-Cornell Med Ctr 1977; **Fellow:** Rheumatology/Immunology, Hosp for Special Surgery 1979; **Fac Appt:** Prof Med, Cornell Univ-Weill Med Coll

Goodman, Susan MD (Rhu) - **Spec Exp:** Lupus Nephritis; **Hospital:** Hosp For Special Surgery (page 108), NY-Presby Hosp (page 100); **Address:** 535 E 70th St Fl 6, New York, NY 10021; **Phone:** 212-606-1163; **Board Cert:** Internal Medicine 1980; Rheumatology 1982; **Med School:** Univ Cincinnati 1977; **Resid:** Internal Medicine, Lenox Hill Hosp 1980; **Fellow:** Rheumatology, Columbia-Presby Med Ctr 1983

Gorevic, Peter D MD (Rhu) - **Spec Exp:** Drug Sensitivity; Amyloidosis/Joint Disease; Cryoglobulinemia; **Hospital:** Mount Sinai Med Ctr (page 98); **Address:** Mount Sinai Medical Ctr, 1 Gustave L Levy Pl, New York, NY 10029; **Phone:** 212-241-1671; **Board Cert:** Allergy & Immunology 1977; Rheumatology 1976; Diagnostic Lab Immunology 1986; Geriatric Medicine 1996; **Med School:** NYU Sch Med 1970; **Resid:** Internal Medicine, NYU Med Ctr 1974; **Fellow:** Rheumatology, NYU Med Ctr 1976; Allergy & Immunology, NYU Med Ctr 1977; **Fac Appt:** Prof Med, Mount Sinai Sch Med

Greisman, Stewart MD (Rhu) - **Spec Exp:** Lupus/SLE; Rheumatoid Arthritis; **Hospital:** St Luke's - Roosevelt Hosp Ctr - Roosevelt Div (page 90), Hosp For Special Surgery (page 108); **Address:** 457 W 57th St, Ste 106, New York, NY 10019; **Phone:** 212-265-1471; **Board Cert:** Rheumatology 1986; Internal Medicine 1984; **Med School:** Yale Univ 1981; **Resid:** Internal Medicine, Yale-New Haven Hosp 1984; **Fellow:** Rheumatology, Hosp For Special Surg 1986; **Fac Appt:** Assoc Clin Prof Med, Columbia P&S

Honig, Stephen MD (Rhu) - **Spec Exp:** Osteoporosis; Rheumatoid Arthritis; Osteoarthritis; Lupus/SLE; **Hospital:** Hosp For Joint Diseases (page 107), NYU Med Ctr (page 102); **Address:** 301 E 17th St, Ste 1101, New York, NY 10003-2739; **Phone:** 212-598-6367; **Board Cert:** Internal Medicine 1975; Rheumatology 1978; **Med School:** Univ Tenn Coll Med, Memphis 1972; **Resid:** Internal Medicine, St Vincent's Hosp Med Ctr 1975; **Fellow:** Rheumatology, NYU Med Ctr 1977; **Fac Appt:** Asst Clin Prof Med, NYU Sch Med

Horowitz, Mark D MD (Rhu) - **Spec Exp:** Lupus/SLE; Rheumatoid Arthritis; Fibromyalgia; **Hospital:** Mount Sinai Med Ctr (page 98); **Address:** 21 E 90th St, Ground Fl, New York, NY 10128-0654; **Phone:** 212-860-3077; **Board Cert:** Internal Medicine 1986; Rheumatology 2000; **Med School:** NE Ohio Univ 1983; **Resid:** Internal Medicine, Mt Sinai Med Ctr 1986; **Fellow:** Rheumatology, Mt Sinai Med Ctr 1989

Kerr, Leslie D MD (Rhu) - **Spec Exp:** Rheumatoid Arthritis; Scleroderma; Lupus/SLE; **Hospital:** Mount Sinai Med Ctr (page 98); **Address:** Mount Sinai Medical Ctr, 1 Gustave Levy Pl, Box 1244, New York, NY 10029; **Phone:** 212-241-1671; **Board Cert:** Internal Medicine 1983; Rheumatology 1986; **Med School:** Columbia P&S 1980; **Resid:** Internal Medicine, Mt. Sinai Hospital 1983; **Fellow:** Rheumatology, Mt. Sinai Hospital 1985; **Fac Appt:** Assoc Prof Med, Mount Sinai Sch Med

Lee, Sicy H MD (Rhu) - **Spec Exp:** Rheumatoid Arthritis; Osteoarthritis; Lupus/SLE; **Hospital:** Hosp For Joint Diseases (page 107), NYU Med Ctr (page 102); **Address:** 305 2nd Ave, Ste 16, New York, NY 10003; **Phone:** 212-598-6516; **Board Cert:** Internal Medicine 1982; Rheumatology 1984; **Med School:** Univ Cincinnati 1979; **Resid:** Internal Medicine, Good Samaritan 1982; **Fellow:** Rheumatology, Hosp for Joint Diseases 1984; **Fac Appt:** Asst Clin Prof Med, NYU Sch Med

Lockshin, Michael D MD (Rhu) - **Spec Exp:** Lupus/SLE; Antiphospholipid Syndrome (APS); Pregnancy & Rheumatic Disease; Lupus/SLE in Pregancy; **Hospital:** Hosp For Special Surgery (page 108), NY-Presby Hosp (page 100); **Address:** 535 E 70th St Bldg Hosp Fl 6W - rm 661, New York, NY 10021-4872; **Phone:** 212-606-1461; **Board Cert:** Internal Medicine 1969; Rheumatology 1972; **Med School:** Harvard Med Sch 1963; **Resid:** Internal Medicine, Bellevue Hosp 1968; **Fellow:** Rheumatology, Columbia-Presby Hosp 1970; **Fac Appt:** Prof Med, Cornell Univ-Weill Med Coll

Magid, Steven K. MD (Rhu) - **Spec Exp:** Rheumatoid Arthritis; Osteoarthritis; Lyme Disease; Polymyalgia Rheumatica; **Hospital:** Hosp For Special Surgery (page 108), NY-Presby Hosp (page 100); **Address:** 535 E 70th St West Bldg Fl 7 - rm 778, New York, NY 10021; **Phone:** 212-606-1060; **Board Cert:** Internal Medicine 1979; Rheumatology 1984; **Med School:** Cornell Univ-Weill Med Coll 1976; **Resid:** Internal Medicine, New York Hosp 1979; **Fellow:** Rheumatology, Hosp For Special Surgery 1981; **Fac Appt:** Assoc Clin Prof Med, Cornell Univ-Weill Med Coll

Markenson, Joseph A MD (Rhu) - **Spec Exp:** Rheumatoid Arthritis; Lupus/SLE; Osteoarthritis; **Hospital:** Hosp For Special Surgery (page 108), NY-Presby Hosp (page 100); **Address:** Hosp for Special Surgery, 535 S 70th St, rm 676, New York, NY 10021-4892; **Phone:** 212-606-1261; **Board Cert:** Internal Medicine 1976; Rheumatology 1978; **Med School:** SUNY Downstate 1970; **Resid:** Internal Medicine, New York Hosp-Cornell 1975; **Fellow:** Rheumatology, Hosp For Special Surg 1976; **Fac Appt:** Clin Prof Med, Cornell Univ-Weill Med Coll

Meed, Steven D MD (Rhu) - **Spec Exp:** Lyme Disease; Chronic Fatigue Syndrome; Acupuncture; Fibromyalgia; **Hospital:** Lenox Hill Hosp (page 94), St Luke's - Roosevelt Hosp Ctr - Roosevelt Div (page 90); **Address:** 150 E 58th St Fl 18, New York, NY 10023; **Phone:** 212-583-2960; **Board Cert:** Internal Medicine 1979; Rheumatology 1986; **Med School:** NYU Sch Med 1975; **Resid:** Internal Medicine, Brookdale Hosp 1977; Internal Medicine, Barnes Hosp-Wash Univ 1978; **Fellow:** Rheumatology, Barnes Hosp-Wash Univ 1979; Rheumatology, NYU Med Ctr 1987; **Fac Appt:** Asst Clin Prof Med, NYU Sch Med

Mitnick, Hal J MD (Rhu) - **Spec Exp:** Rheumatoid Arthritis; Psoriatic Arthritis; Osteoporosis; **Hospital:** NYU Med Ctr (page 102); **Address:** 333 E 34th St, Ste 1C, New York, NY 10016-4956; **Phone:** 212-889-7217; **Board Cert:** Internal Medicine 1976; Rheumatology 1978; **Med School:** NYU Sch Med 1972; **Resid:** Internal Medicine, Bellevue Hosp 1976; **Fellow:** Rheumatology, NYU Med Ctr 1978; **Fac Appt:** Clin Prof Med, NYU Sch Med

Nickerson, Katherine MD (Rhu) - **Hospital:** NY-Presby Hosp (page 100); **Address:** 161 Fort Washington Ave, Irving Bldg, rm 221, New York, NY 10032-3713; **Phone:** 212-305-8039; **Board Cert:** Internal Medicine 1984; Rheumatology 1986; **Med School:** UCSF 1981; **Resid:** Internal Medicine, Beth Israel Hosp 1984; **Fellow:** Rheumatology, Columbia-Presby Med Ctr 1986

Paget, Stephen MD (Rhu) - **Spec Exp:** Rheumatoid Arthritis; Lupus/SLE; **Hospital:** Hosp For Special Surgery (page 108); **Address:** 535 E 70th St, rm 721, New York, NY 10021; **Phone:** 212-606-1845; **Board Cert:** Internal Medicine 1974; Rheumatology 1976; **Med School:** SUNY Downstate 1971; **Resid:** Internal Medicine, Johns Hopkins Hosp 1973; **Fellow:** Rheumatology, Hosp Special Surg 1975; **Fac Appt:** Clin Prof Med, Cornell Univ-Weill Med Coll

Parrish, Edward MD (Rhu) - **Spec Exp:** Immune Deficiency; **Hospital:** Hosp For Special Surgery (page 108), NY-Presby Hosp (page 100); **Address:** 535 E 70th St Fl 6, New York, NY 10021; **Phone:** 212-606-1743; **Board Cert:** Internal Medicine 1983; Rheumatology 1986; **Med School:** Wake Forest Univ 1980; **Resid:** Internal Medicine, Columbia-Presby Med Ctr 1983; **Fellow:** Rheumatology, Columbia-Presby Med Ctr 1985

Rackoff, Paula MD (Rhu) - **Spec Exp:** Osteoporosis; Sjogren's Syndrome; Inflammatory Arthritis; **Hospital:** Beth Israel Med Ctr - Petrie Division (page 90); **Address:** 10 Union Square East, Ste 3D, New York, NY 10003-3314; **Phone:** 212-844-8101; **Board Cert:** Internal Medicine 1986; Rheumatology 2003; **Med School:** Yale Univ 1986; **Resid:** Internal Medicine, Yale-New Haven Hosp 1989; **Fellow:** Rheumatology, Yale-New Haven Hosp 1992; **Fac Appt:** Asst Prof Med, Albert Einstein Coll Med

Radin, Allen MD (Rhu) - **Spec Exp:** Lupus/SLE; Rheumatoid Arthritis; Osteoarthritis; **Hospital:** Lenox Hill Hosp (page 94), NY-Presby Hosp (page 100); **Address:** 50 E 81st St, Ste 1, New York, NY 10028; **Phone:** 212-289-6855; **Board Cert:** Internal Medicine 1980; Rheumatology 1982; **Med School:** NYU Sch Med 1977; **Resid:** Internal Medicine, Univ Hosp 1980; **Fellow:** Rheumatology, NYU Med Ctr 1982

Salmon, Jane MD (Rhu) - **Spec Exp:** Lupus/SLE; Rheumatoid Arthritis; Antiphospholipid Syndrome (APS); **Hospital:** Hosp For Special Surgery (page 108), NY-Presby Hosp (page 100); **Address:** 535 E 70th St, New York, NY 10021-4872; **Phone:** 212-606-1671; **Board Cert:** Internal Medicine 1981; Rheumatology 1984; **Med School:** Columbia P&S 1978; **Resid:** Internal Medicine, NY Hosp 1981; **Fellow:** Rheumatology, Hosp For Special Surg 1983; **Fac Appt:** Prof Med, Cornell Univ-Weill Med Coll

Schwartzman, Sergio MD (Rhu) - **Spec Exp:** Arthritis; Lupus/SLE; Uveitis; **Hospital:** Hosp For Special Surgery (page 108); **Address:** 535 E 70 St, New York, NY 10021-4892; **Phone:** 212-606-1557; **Board Cert:** Internal Medicine 1985; Rheumatology 1988; **Med School:** Mount Sinai Sch Med 1982; **Resid:** Internal Medicine, LI Jewish Med Ctr 1985; **Fellow:** Rheumatology, Hosp Spec Surgery 1987

Solitar, Bruce M MD (Rhu) - **Spec Exp:** Arthritis; Fibromyalgia; Reiter's Syndrome; **Hospital:** NYU Med Ctr (page 102); **Address:** 333 E 34th St, New York, NY 10016; **Phone:** 212-889-7217; **Board Cert:** Internal Medicine 2001; Rheumatology 2004; **Med School:** NYU Sch Med 1988; **Resid:** Internal Medicine, NYU/Bellevue Med Ctr 1992; **Fellow:** Rheumatology, NYU/Bellevue Med Ctr 1994; **Fac Appt:** Asst Clin Prof Med, NYU Sch Med

Solomon, Gary MD (Rhu) - **Spec Exp:** Psoriatic Arthritis; Rheumatoid Arthritis; Autoimmune Disease; **Hospital:** Hosp For Joint Diseases (page 107), NYU Med Ctr (page 102); **Address:** Hosp Joint Diseases, Dept Rheumatology, 305 2nd Ave, Ste 16, New York, NY 10003; **Phone:** 212-598-6516; **Board Cert:** Internal Medicine 1980; Rheumatology 1982; **Med School:** Mount Sinai Sch Med 1977; **Resid:** Internal Medicine, Mount Sinai Med Ctr 1980; **Fellow:** Rheumatology, Albert Einstein Coll Med 1982; **Fac Appt:** Assoc Clin Prof Med, NYU Sch Med

Spiera, Harry MD (Rhu) - **Spec Exp:** Lupus/SLE; Scleroderma; Vasculitis; **Hospital:** Mount Sinai Med Ctr (page 98), NY-Presby Hosp (page 100); **Address:** 1088 Park Ave, New York, NY 10128-1132; **Phone:** 212-860-4000 x36; **Board Cert:** Internal Medicine 1965; Rheumatology 1972; **Med School:** NYU Sch Med 1958; **Resid:** Internal Medicine, VA Med Ctr 1960; Internal Medicine, Mount Sinai Hosp 1961; **Fellow:** Rheumatology, Columbia-Presby Med Ctr 1963; **Fac Appt:** Clin Prof Med, Mount Sinai Sch Med

Spiera, Robert MD (Rhu) - **Spec Exp:** Vasculitis; Lupus/SLE; Scleroderma; **Hospital:** Hosp For Special Surgery (page 108), Mount Sinai Med Ctr (page 98); **Address:** 1088 Park Ave, New York, NY 10128-1132; **Phone:** 212-860-2100; **Board Cert:** Internal Medicine 2002; Rheumatology 2004; **Med School:** Yale Univ 1989; **Resid:** Internal Medicine, New York Hosp 1992; **Fellow:** Rheumatology, Hosp Special Surg 1995; **Fac Appt:** Assoc Clin Prof Med, Albert Einstein Coll Med

Stern, Richard MD (Rhu) - **Spec Exp:** Rheumatoid Arthritis; Osteoporosis; Osteoarthritis; **Hospital:** Hosp For Special Surgery (page 108), NY-Presby Hosp (page 100); **Address:** 475 E 72nd St, New York, NY 10021-4458; **Phone:** 212-879-2282; **Board Cert:** Internal Medicine 1973; Rheumatology 1976; **Med School:** Tufts Univ 1970; **Resid:** Internal Medicine, NY Hosp 1973; **Fellow:** Immunology, Rockefeller Univ Hosp 1975; **Fac Appt:** Assoc Clin Prof Med, Cornell Univ-Weill Med Coll

Yee, Arthur M F MD/PhD (Rhu) - **Spec Exp:** Sarcoidosis; Lupus/SLE; **Hospital:** Hosp For Special Surgery (page 108), NY-Presby Hosp (page 100); **Address:** Hosp for Special Surgery, 535 E 70th St, New York, NY 10021; **Phone:** 212-606-1171; **Board Cert:** Internal Medicine 1994; Rheumatology 1996; **Med School:** NYU Sch Med 1991; **Resid:** Internal Medicine, NY Hosp-Cornell Med Ctr 1993; **Fellow:** Rheumatology, NY Hosp-Cornell Med Ctr 1995; **Fac Appt:** Asst Prof Med, Cornell Univ-Weill Med Coll

SPORTS MEDICINE

Altchek, David MD (SM) - **Spec Exp:** Shoulder Surgery; Elbow Surgery; Knee Surgery; Arthroscopic Surgery; **Hospital:** Hosp For Special Surgery (page 108), NY-Presby Hosp (page 100); **Address:** 535 E 70 St, New York, NY 10021; **Phone:** 212-606-1909; **Board Cert:** Orthopaedic Surgery 2001; **Med School:** Cornell Univ-Weill Med Coll 1982; **Resid:** Orthopaedic Surgery, Hosp for Special Surg 1987; **Fellow:** Sports Medicine, Hosp for Special Surg 1988; **Fac Appt:** Assoc Prof OrS, Cornell Univ-Weill Med Coll

Callahan, Lisa MD (SM) - **Spec Exp:** Primary Care Sports Medicine; **Hospital:** Hosp For Special Surgery (page 108), NY-Presby Hosp (page 100); **Address:** 535 E 70th St, New York, NY 10021; **Phone:** 212-606-1532; **Board Cert:** Family Medicine 2004; Sports Medicine 2004; **Med School:** E Carolina Univ 1987; **Resid:** Family Medicine, San Jose Med Ctr/Stanford U 1990; **Fellow:** Sports Medicine, San Jose Med Ctr/Stanford U 1991; **Fac Appt:** Asst Prof FMed, Cornell Univ-Weill Med Coll

Hamner, Daniel MD (SM) - **Spec Exp:** Running Injuries; Acupuncture; Primary Care Sports Medicine; **Address:** 3 E 71st St, New York, NY 10021-4154; **Phone:** 212-737-1991; **Board Cert:** Physical Medicine & Rehabilitation 1986; **Med School:** NY Med Coll 1976; **Resid:** Physical Medicine & Rehabilitation, New York Hosp-Cornell Med Ctr 1979; **Fellow:** Cardiac Rehabilitation, Emory Med Ctr 1980

Hershman, Elliott MD (SM) - **Spec Exp:** Knee Injuries; Knee Surgery; Arthroscopic Surgery; **Hospital:** Lenox Hill Hosp (page 94); **Address:** 130 E 77th St Fl 7, New York, NY 10021-1851; **Phone:** 212-744-8114; **Board Cert:** Orthopaedic Surgery 1998; **Med School:** Univ Rochester 1979; **Resid:** Orthopaedic Surgery, Lenox Hill Hosp 1984; **Fellow:** Sports Medicine, Cleveland Clinic 1985

Krinick, Ronald M MD (SM) - **Spec Exp:** Knee Injuries; Shoulder Injuries; **Hospital:** NY Downtown Hosp; **Address:** 19 Beekman St Fl 5, New York, NY 10038; **Phone:** 212-513-7711; **Board Cert:** Orthopaedic Surgery 1997; **Med School:** NYU Sch Med 1979; **Resid:** Orthopaedic Surgery, NYU/Bellvue Med Ctr 1984; **Fellow:** Sports Medicine, NYU Med Ctr 1985; **Fac Appt:** Assoc Clin Prof OrS, NYU Sch Med

Levine, William MD (SM) - **Spec Exp:** Arthroscopic Surgery; Shoulder & Knee Injuries; **Hospital:** NY-Presby Hosp (page 100); **Address:** 622 W 168th St Fl PH11 East Wing, New York, NY 10032; **Phone:** 212-305-0762; **Board Cert:** Orthopaedic Surgery 1999; **Med School:** Case West Res Univ 1990; **Resid:** Surgery, Beth Israel Hosp 1991; Orthopaedic Surgery, New Eng Med Ctr Hosps 1995; **Fellow:** Shoulder Surgery, Columbia-Presby Med Ctr 1996; Sports Medicine, Univ MD Med Ctr 1998; **Fac Appt:** Assoc Prof OrS, Columbia P&S

Maharam, Lewis G MD (SM) - **Spec Exp:** Running Injuries; Primary Care Sports Medicine; Knee Injuries; Shoulder Injuries; **Hospital:** Hosp For Joint Diseases (page 107); **Address:** 24 W 57th St, New York, NY 10019; **Phone:** 212-765-5763; **Med School:** Emory Univ 1985; **Resid:** Internal Medicine, Danbury Hosp 1987; Internal Medicine, NY Infirm/Beekman Downtown 1989; **Fellow:** Sports Medicine, Pascack Valley Hosp 1990; **Fac Appt:** Asst Clin Prof OrS, NYU Sch Med

Metzl, Jordan D MD (SM) - **Spec Exp:** Pediatric Sports Medicine; **Hospital:** Hosp For Special Surgery (page 108); **Address:** Hospital for Special Surgery,Sports Med, 535 E 70 St, New York, NY 10021; **Phone:** 212-606-1678; **Board Cert:** Pediatrics 2005; Sports Medicine 2001; **Med School:** Univ MO-Columbia Sch Med 1993; **Resid:** Pediatrics, New England Med Ctr 1996; **Fellow:** Sports Medicine, Vanderbilt Univ Med Ctr 1996; Sports Medicine, Hosp Special Surgery 1997; **Fac Appt:** Asst Prof Ped, Cornell Univ-Weill Med Coll

Nisonson, Barton MD (SM) - **Spec Exp:** Knee Injuries; Shoulder & Knee Surgery; **Hospital:** Lenox Hill Hosp (page 94); **Address:** 130 E 77th St, New York, NY 10021-1851; **Phone:** 212-570-9120; **Board Cert:** Orthopaedic Surgery 1974; **Med School:** Columbia P&S 1966; **Resid:** Surgery, Columbia-Presby Med Ctr 1968; Orthopaedic Surgery, Columbia-Presby Med Ctr 1973

Plancher, Kevin D MD (SM) - **Spec Exp:** Shoulder Surgery; Elbow Surgery; Cartilage Damage & Transplant; Shoulder Replacement; **Hospital:** Beth Israel Med Ctr - Petrie Division (page 90), NY Westchester Sq Med Ctr; **Address:** 1160 Park Ave, New York, NY 10128; **Phone:** 212-876-5200; **Board Cert:** Orthopaedic Surgery 2004; Hand Surgery 2005; **Med School:** Georgetown Univ 1986; **Resid:** Orthopaedic Surgery, Mass Genl Hosp/Brigham & Womens Hosp 1991; **Fellow:** Hand Surgery, Indiana Hand Ctr 1993; Sports Medicine, Steadman-Hawkins Clinic 1994; **Fac Appt:** Assoc Clin Prof OrS, Albert Einstein Coll Med

Surgery

Amory, Spencer E MD (S) - **Spec Exp:** Laparoscopic Surgery; Gastrointestinal Surgery; Hernia; **Hospital:** NY-Presby Hosp (page 100); **Address:** 5141 Broadway, Fl 3 - rm 178, New York, NY 10034; **Phone:** 212-932-5221; **Board Cert:** Surgery 2000; Surgical Critical Care 1993; **Med School:** Johns Hopkins Univ 1983; **Resid:** Surgery, Columbia Presby Med Ctr 1989; **Fellow:** Emergency Medicine, Peninsula Hosp 1990; **Fac Appt:** Assoc Clin Prof S, Columbia P&S

Antonacci, Anthony MD (S) - **Hospital:** Lenox Hill Hosp (page 94), NY-Presby Hosp (page 100); **Address:** 350 E 17 St, New York, NY 10003; **Phone:** 212-420-4465; **Board Cert:** Surgery 2005; **Med School:** Geo Wash Univ 1977; **Resid:** Surgery, NY Hosp 1980; Surgery, NY Hosp 1980; **Fellow:** Immunology, Mem Sloan Kettering Canc Ctr 1982; **Fac Appt:** Assoc Clin Prof S, Cornell Univ-Weill Med Coll

Attiyeh, Fadi F MD (S) - **Spec Exp:** Colon & Rectal Cancer; Hepatobiliary Surgery; Pancreatic Surgery; **Hospital:** St Luke's - Roosevelt Hosp Ctr - Roosevelt Div (page 90); **Address:** 425 W 59th St, Ste 8B-1, New York, NY 10019; **Phone:** 212-307-1144; **Board Cert:** Surgery 1975; Colon & Rectal Surgery 1982; **Med School:** Lebanon 1969; **Resid:** Surgery, Amer Univ Hosp 1973; **Fellow:** Surgical Oncology, Meml Sloan Kettering Canc Ctr 1976; **Fac Appt:** Assoc Clin Prof S, Columbia P&S

Axelrod, Deborah MD (S) - **Spec Exp:** Breast Cancer; Breast Disease; **Hospital:** NYU Med Ctr (page 102), St Vincent Cath Med Ctrs - Manhattan (page 375); **Address:** NYU Clinical Cancer Ctr, 160 E 34th St, New York, NY 10016; **Phone:** 212-731-5366; **Board Cert:** Surgery 1998; **Med School:** Israel 1982; **Resid:** Surgery, Beth Israel Med Ctr 1988; **Fellow:** Surgical Oncology, Meml Sloan Kettering Cancer Ctr 1986; **Fac Appt:** Assoc Prof S, NYU Sch Med

Barie, Philip MD (S) - **Spec Exp:** Trauma; Critical Care; Hernia; **Hospital:** NY-Presby Hosp (page 100); **Address:** Weill Med Coll, 525 E 68th St, Ste P713A, New York, NY 10021-4873; **Phone:** 212-746-5401; **Board Cert:** Surgery 2004; Surgical Critical Care 1996; **Med School:** Boston Univ 1977; **Resid:** Surgery, NY Hosp-Cornell Med Ctr 1984; **Fellow:** Trauma, Albany Med Coll 1981; **Fac Appt:** Prof S, Cornell Univ-Weill Med Coll

Bauer, Joel MD (S) - **Spec Exp:** Colon & Rectal Surgery; Inflammatory Bowel Disease; Laparoscopic Surgery; **Hospital:** Mount Sinai Med Ctr (page 98); **Address:** 25 E 69th St, New York, NY 10021-4925; **Phone:** 212-517-8600; **Board Cert:** Surgery 1974; **Med School:** NYU Sch Med 1967; **Resid:** Surgery, Mount Sinai Hosp 1973; **Fac Appt:** Clin Prof S, Mount Sinai Sch Med

Bebawi, Magdi MD (S) - **Spec Exp:** Hernia; Lower Limb Ulcers; Breast Surgery; **Hospital:** N Genl Hosp, St Luke's - Roosevelt Hosp Ctr - St Luke's Hosp (page 90); **Address:** 1824 Madison Ave, New York, NY 10035-3899; **Phone:** 212-876-8655; **Board Cert:** Surgery 1997; **Med School:** Egypt 1963; **Resid:** Surgery, North Genl Hosp 1986; **Fac Appt:** Asst Clin Prof S, Mount Sinai Sch Med

Bernik, Stephanie F MD (S) - **Spec Exp:** Breast Cancer; Breast Disease; Sentinel Node Surgery; **Hospital:** St Vincent Cath Med Ctrs - Manhattan (page 375); **Address:** St Vincent's Comprehensive Breast Ctr, 325 W 15th St, New York, NY 10011; **Phone:** 212-604-6006; **Board Cert:** Surgery 2001; **Med School:** Yale Univ 1993; **Resid:** Surgery, St Vincents Hosp 1999; **Fellow:** Breast Surgery, Memorial Sloan Kettering Cancer Ctr 2000

Bessey, Palmer Q MD (S) - **Spec Exp:** Burn Care; Wound Healing/Care; Nutrition; **Hospital:** NY-Presby Hosp (page 100); **Address:** William Randolph Hearst Burn Center, 525 E 68th St, Box 137, New York, NY 10021; **Phone:** 212-746-0242; **Board Cert:** Surgery 2000; Surgical Critical Care 1994; **Med School:** Univ VT Coll Med 1975; **Resid:** Surgery, Univ Alabama Hosp 1981; **Fellow:** Metabolism, Brigham & Women's Hosp 1983; **Fac Appt:** Prof S, Cornell Univ-Weill Med Coll

Bessler, Marc MD (S) - **Spec Exp:** Obesity/Bariatric Surgery; Laparoscopic Surgery; **Hospital:** NY-Presby Hosp (page 100); **Address:** NY Presby Med Ctr, Dept of Surgery, 161 Fort Washington Ave, rm 620, New York, NY 10032; **Phone:** 212-305-9506; **Board Cert:** Surgery 1997; **Med School:** NYU Sch Med 1989; **Resid:** Surgery, Columbia Presby Med Ctr 1995; **Fac Appt:** Asst Prof S, Columbia P&S

Bloom, Norman MD (S) - **Spec Exp:** Breast Cancer; Sarcoma; Cancer Surgery; **Hospital:** Beth Israel Med Ctr - Petrie Division (page 90), Cabrini Med Ctr (page 374); **Address:** The Gramercy, 61 Irving Pl @ 18th St, New York, NY 10003; **Phone:** 212-505-6167; **Board Cert:** Surgery 1999; **Med School:** SUNY Downstate 1974; **Resid:** Surgery, Maimonides Med Ctr 1978; **Fellow:** Surgical Oncology, Meml Sloan Kettering Canc Ctr 1979; **Fac Appt:** Clin Prof S, NY Med Coll

Blumgart, Leslie H MD (S) - **Spec Exp:** Liver & Biliary Cancer; Pancreatic Cancer; Hepatobiliary Surgery; **Hospital:** Meml Sloan Kettering Cancer Ctr (page 109); **Address:** 1275 York Ave, rm C891, New York, NY 10021-6007; **Phone:** 212-639-5526; **Med School:** England 1964; **Resid:** Surgery, United Sheffield Hosp 1966; Surgery, Nottingham Genl Hosp 1970; **Fac Appt:** Prof S, Cornell Univ-Weill Med Coll

Borgen, Patrick I MD (S) - **Spec Exp:** Breast Cancer; **Hospital:** Meml Sloan Kettering Cancer Ctr (page 109); **Address:** 205 E 64th St, New York, NY 10021-6635; **Phone:** 212-639-5248; **Board Cert:** Surgery 1991; **Med School:** Louisiana State Univ 1984; **Resid:** Surgery, Ochsner Fdn Hosp 1989; **Fellow:** Surgical Oncology, Meml Sloan Kettering Canc Ctr 1990; **Fac Appt:** Prof S, Cornell Univ-Weill Med Coll

Brem, Harold MD (S) - **Spec Exp:** Wound Healing/Care; Lower Limb Ulcers; **Hospital:** NY-Presby Hosp (page 100); **Address:** 5141 Broadway, Allen Pavilion, rm 3-020, New York, NY 10034; **Phone:** 212-932-5094; **Board Cert:** Surgery 1996; **Med School:** McGill Univ 1987; **Resid:** Surgery, Ohio State Univ Hosp 1989; **Fellow:** Surgical Research, Harvard Med Sch 1992; **Fac Appt:** Asst Prof S, Columbia P&S

Brennan, Murray MD (S) - **Spec Exp:** Sarcoma; Pancreatic Cancer; Cancer Surgery; **Hospital:** Meml Sloan Kettering Cancer Ctr (page 109); **Address:** 1275 York Ave, rm C1272, New York, NY 10021; **Phone:** 212-639-6586; **Board Cert:** Surgery 1975; **Med School:** New Zealand 1964; **Resid:** Surgery, Univ Otago Hosp 1969; **Fellow:** Surgery, Harvard Med Sch 1972; Surgery, Peter Bent Brigham Hosp 1975; **Fac Appt:** Prof S, Cornell Univ-Weill Med Coll

Bromberg, Jonathan S MD/PhD (S) - **Spec Exp:** Transplant-Kidney; Transplant-Pancreas; **Hospital:** Mount Sinai Med Ctr (page 98); **Address:** Mount Sinai Medical Ctr, One Gustave Levy Pl, Box 1104, New York, NY 10029; **Phone:** 212-659-8008; **Board Cert:** Surgery 1997; Surgical Critical Care 1993; **Med School:** Harvard Med Sch 1983; **Resid:** Surgery, Univ Washington Med Ctr 1988; **Fellow:** Transplant Surgery, Hosp U Penn 1990; **Fac Appt:** Prof S, Mount Sinai Sch Med

Cammarata, Angelo MD (S) - **Spec Exp:** Breast Surgery; Breast Disease; Breast Cancer; **Hospital:** Cabrini Med Ctr (page 374); **Address:** 55 E 87th St, Ste 1, New York, NY 10128-1043; **Phone:** 212-427-2131; **Board Cert:** Surgery 1968; **Med School:** NY Med Coll 1962; **Resid:** Surgery, Metropolitan Hosp Ctr 1967; **Fellow:** Surgery, NY Meml Cancer Hosp 1968; **Fac Appt:** Asst Clin Prof S, NY Med Coll

Cassell, Lauren MD (S) - **Spec Exp:** Breast Surgery; Breast Cancer; **Hospital:** Lenox Hill Hosp (page 94); **Address:** 114A E 78th St, New York, NY 10021-0302; **Phone:** 212-535-4040; **Board Cert:** Surgery 2003; **Med School:** NY Med Coll 1977; **Resid:** Surgery, Lenox Hill Hosp 1982

Chabot, John A MD (S) - **Spec Exp:** Liver & Biliary Surgery; Pancreatic Cancer; Thyroid & Parathyroid Surgery; **Hospital:** NY-Presby Hosp (page 100), Lawrence Hosp Ctr; **Address:** 161 Ft Washington Ave, Fl 8, New York, NY 10032; **Phone:** 212-305-9468; **Board Cert:** Surgery 2000; **Med School:** Dartmouth Med Sch 1983; **Resid:** Surgery, Columbia-Presby Med Ctr 1990; **Fac Appt:** Assoc Prof S, Columbia P&S

Cioroiu, Michael MD (S) - **Spec Exp:** Breast Disease; Wound Healing/Care; Endoscopy; **Hospital:** Cabrini Med Ctr (page 374), Mount Sinai Hosp of Queens (page 98); **Address:** 247 3rd Ave, Ste L 3, New York, NY 10010-7453; **Phone:** 212-995-8099; **Board Cert:** Surgery 2004; **Med School:** Romania 1971; **Resid:** Surgery, Cabrini Med Ctr 1985; **Fac Appt:** Assoc Clin Prof S, Mount Sinai Sch Med

Clarke, James MD (S) - **Spec Exp:** Hernia; Gallbladder Surgery; **Hospital:** NY-Presby Hosp (page 100); **Address:** 310 E 72nd St, New York, NY 10021; **Phone:** 212-737-2050; **Board Cert:** Surgery 1987; **Med School:** Cornell Univ-Weill Med Coll 1981; **Resid:** Surgery, NY Hosp-Cornell Med Ctr 1986

Cleary, Joseph MD (S) - **Spec Exp:** Breast Surgery; **Hospital:** Beth Israel Med Ctr - Petrie Division (page 90); **Address:** 133 E 73rd St, New York, NY 10021; **Phone:** 212-570-0133; **Board Cert:** Surgery 1979; **Med School:** NY Med Coll 1973; **Resid:** Surgery, NY Med Coll Affil Hosps 1978; Hand Surgery, St Luke's Roosevelt Hosp Ctr; **Fellow:** Surgical Oncology, NY Med Coll Affil Hosps 1976; Plastic Surgery, Columbia Presby Med Ctr 1980; **Fac Appt:** Asst Clin Prof S, NY Med Coll

Coit, Daniel G MD (S) - **Spec Exp:** Melanoma; Pancreatic Cancer; Stomach Cancer; **Hospital:** Meml Sloan Kettering Cancer Ctr (page 109); **Address:** 1275 York Ave, New York, NY 10021-6007; **Phone:** 212-639-8411; **Board Cert:** Surgery 2004; **Med School:** Univ Cincinnati 1976; **Resid:** Internal Medicine, New England Deaconess Hosp 1978; Surgery, New England Deaconess Hosp 1983; **Fellow:** Surgical Oncology, Meml Sloan Kettering Canc Ctr 1985; **Fac Appt:** Assoc Prof S, Cornell Univ-Weill Med Coll

Corvalan, Jose MD (S) - **Spec Exp:** Laparoscopic Surgery; Abdominal Surgery; **Hospital:** St. Vincent's Midtown, St Vincent Cath Med Ctrs - Manhattan (page 375); **Address:** 535 W 110th St, Ste 1H, New York, NY 10025-4145; **Phone:** 212-222-4700; **Board Cert:** Surgery 2001; **Med School:** Argentina 1965; **Resid:** Surgery, Albert Einstein 1975; **Fellow:** Surgery, Albert Einstein 1976; **Fac Appt:** Assoc Prof S, NYU Sch Med

Daliana, Maurizio MD (S) - **Spec Exp:** Gastrointestinal Cancer; Breast Surgery; Vascular Surgery; **Hospital:** Cabrini Med Ctr (page 374), Beth Israel Med Ctr - Petrie Division (page 90); **Address:** 247 3rd Ave, Ste 504, New York, NY 10010-7456; **Phone:** 212-995-9790; **Board Cert:** Surgery 1969; **Med School:** Italy 1961; **Resid:** Surgery, Columbus Hosp 1968; **Fac Appt:** Asst Clin Prof S, Mount Sinai Sch Med

Edye, Michael MD (S) - **Spec Exp:** Laparoscopic Abdominal Surgery; Obesity/Bariatric Surgery; Transplant-Living Kidney Donor; Gastroesophageal Reflux Disease (GERD); **Hospital:** Mount Sinai Med Ctr (page 98), Westchester Med Ctr (page 713); **Address:** 1060 Fifth Ave, New York, NY 10128; **Phone:** 212-426-9614; **Med School:** Australia 1977; **Resid:** Surgery, St Vincents Hosp 1980; Surgery, Royal N Shore Hosp 1984; **Fellow:** Laparoscopic Surgery, Univ Bordeaux 1992; **Fac Appt:** Assoc Clin Prof S, Mount Sinai Sch Med

El-Tamer, Mahmoud B MD (S) - **Spec Exp:** Breast Cancer; **Hospital:** NY-Presby Hosp (page 100); **Address:** Columbia Univ, Dept Surg, 161 Fort Washington Ave Fl 10 - Ste 1003, New York, NY 10032; **Phone:** 212-305-0728; **Board Cert:** Surgery 2001; **Med School:** Lebanon 1981; **Resid:** Surgery, American Univ Hosp 1985; Surgery, SUNY Hlth Sci Ctr 1992; **Fellow:** Surgical Oncology, Meml Sloan Kettering Cancer Ctr 1989; **Fac Appt:** Assoc Prof S, Columbia P&S

Emond, Jean C MD (S) - **Spec Exp:** Transplant-Liver; Liver Cancer; **Hospital:** NY-Presby Hosp (page 100); **Address:** 622 W 168th St, PH - Fl 14, New York, NY 10032; **Phone:** 212-305-0914; **Board Cert:** Surgery 1994; **Med School:** Univ Chicago-Pritzker Sch Med 1979; **Resid:** Surgery, Cook Cty Hosp 1984; **Fellow:** Surgery, Hopital P Brousse/Univ de Paris Sud 1985; Transplant Surgery, Univ Chicago Hosps 1987; **Fac Appt:** Prof S, Columbia P&S

Emre, Sukru MD (S) - **Spec Exp:** Transplant-Liver-Adult & Pediatric; Pulmonary Hypertension; **Hospital:** Mount Sinai Med Ctr (page 98); **Address:** Mount Sinai Medical Ctr, 19 E 98 St, Box 1104, New York, NY 10029; **Phone:** 212-241-6766; **Med School:** Turkey 1977; **Resid:** Surgery, Univ Istanbul 1982; **Fellow:** Hepatobiliary Surgery, Univ Istanbul 1988; Transplant Surgery, Mount Sinai Med Ctr 1994; **Fac Appt:** Prof S, Mount Sinai Sch Med

Eng, Kenneth MD (S) - **Spec Exp:** Colon & Rectal Cancer & Surgery; Pancreatic Cancer; Inflammatory Bowel Disease; **Hospital:** NYU Med Ctr (page 102); **Address:** 530 1st Ave, Ste 6B, New York, NY 10016-6402; **Phone:** 212-263-7301; **Board Cert:** Surgery 1982; **Med School:** NYU Sch Med 1967; **Resid:** Surgery, NYU Med Ctr 1972; **Fac Appt:** Prof S, NYU Sch Med

Enker, Warren MD (S) - **Spec Exp:** Gastrointestinal Surgery; Colon & Rectal Cancer; Liver Tumors; **Hospital:** Beth Israel Med Ctr - Petrie Division (page 90); **Address:** 350 E 17th St, Baird Hall 1622, New York, NY 10003; **Phone:** 212-420-3960; **Board Cert:** Surgery 1973; **Med School:** SUNY Downstate 1967; **Resid:** Surgery, Univ Chicago Hosps 1972; **Fellow:** Cancer Immunology, Univ Chicago Hosps 1973; Cancer Immunology, Univ Minnesota Med Ctr 1974; **Fac Appt:** Prof S, Albert Einstein Coll Med

Estabrook, Alison MD (S) - **Spec Exp:** Breast Cancer; Breast Disease; Breast Cancer-High Risk Women; **Hospital:** St Luke's - Roosevelt Hosp Ctr - Roosevelt Div (page 90); **Address:** 425 W 59th St, Ste 7A, New York, NY 10019-1104; **Phone:** 212-523-7500; **Board Cert:** Surgery 2004; **Med School:** NYU Sch Med 1978; **Resid:** Surgery, Columbia Presby Med Ctr 1984; **Fellow:** Surgical Oncology, Columbia Presby Med Ctr 1982; **Fac Appt:** Prof S, Columbia P&S

Fahey III, Thomas J MD (S) - **Spec Exp:** Endocrine Surgery; Pheochromocytoma; Pancreatic Cancer; **Hospital:** NY-Presby Hosp (page 100), Meml Sloan Kettering Cancer Ctr (page 109); **Address:** NY Presby Cornell Med Ctr, Dept Surgery, 525 E 68 St, rm F2024, New York, NY 10021; **Phone:** 212-746-5130; **Board Cert:** Surgery 2002; **Med School:** Cornell Univ-Weill Med Coll 1986; **Resid:** Surgery, New York Hosp 1992; **Fellow:** Surgery, Royal North Shore Hosp 1993; **Fac Appt:** Assoc Prof S, Cornell Univ-Weill Med Coll

Feldman, Sheldon M MD (S) - **Spec Exp:** Breast Surgery; Breast Cancer; Complementary Medicine; **Hospital:** Beth Israel Med Ctr - Petrie Division (page 90); **Address:** Phillips Ambulatory Care Ctr, 10 Union Square, Ste 4E, New York, NY 10003; **Phone:** 212-844-8959; **Board Cert:** Surgery 2000; **Med School:** NYU Sch Med 1975; **Resid:** Surgery, NYU-Bellevue Med Ctr 1980; **Fellow:** Peripheral Vascular Surgery, Beth Israel Med Ctr 1981; **Fac Appt:** Prof S, Albert Einstein Coll Med

Fielding, George MD (S) - **Spec Exp:** Obesity/Bariatric Surgery; **Hospital:** NYU Med Ctr (page 102); **Address:** 530 First Ave, Ste 10S, New York, NY 10016; **Phone:** 212-263-3166; **Med School:** Australia 1980; **Resid:** Surgery, Royal Brisbane Hosp 1982; Surgery, Berne 1988

Fong, Yuman MD (S) - **Spec Exp:** Pancreatic Cancer; Liver & Biliary Cancer; Stomach Cancer; **Hospital:** Meml Sloan Kettering Cancer Ctr (page 109), NY-Presby Hosp (page 100); **Address:** Memorial Sloan-Kettering Cancer Ctr, 1275 York Ave, New York, NY 10021; **Phone:** 212-639-2016; **Board Cert:** Surgery 2002; **Med School:** Cornell Univ-Weill Med Coll 1986; **Resid:** Surgery, New York Hosp-Cornell Med Ctr 1992; **Fellow:** Surgical Oncology, Meml Sloan-Kettering Cancer Ctr 1994; **Fac Appt:** Prof S, Cornell Univ-Weill Med Coll

Fowler, Dennis MD (S) - **Spec Exp:** Minimally Invasive Surgery; **Hospital:** NY-Presby Hosp (page 100), NY-Presby Hosp (page 100); **Address:** 622 W 168th St Fl PH 12 - rm 126, New York, NY 10032; **Phone:** 212-305-0577; **Board Cert:** Surgery 1998; **Med School:** Univ Kans 1973; **Resid:** Surgery, St Lukes Hosp 1979; **Fellow:** Endoscopy, Mass Genl Hosp 1980; **Fac Appt:** Prof S, Columbia P&S

Gagner, Michel MD (S) - **Spec Exp:** Obesity/Bariatric Surgery; Adrenal Surgery; Pancreatic Surgery; **Hospital:** NY-Presby Hosp (page 100); **Address:** NY Presby-NY Weill Cornell Med Ctr, 525 E 68th St, Box 294, New York, NY 10021; **Phone:** 212-746-5294; **Board Cert:** Surgery 2003; **Med School:** Canada 1982; **Resid:** Surgery, Royal Victoria Hosp/McGill 1988; **Fellow:** Hepatobiliary Surgery, Hosp Paul-Brousse 1989; Hepatobiliary Surgery, Lahey Clinic 1990; **Fac Appt:** Prof S, Cornell Univ-Weill Med Coll

Geller, Peter MD (S) - **Spec Exp:** Gastrointestinal Surgery; Hernia; Breast Cancer; Sentinel Node Surgery; **Hospital:** NY-Presby Hosp (page 100); **Address:** 161 Ft Washington Ave, rm 822, New York, NY 10032-3713; **Phone:** 212-305-6657; **Board Cert:** Surgery 1994; Surgical Critical Care 1989; **Med School:** Columbia P&S 1980; **Resid:** Surgery, Columbia-Presby Med Ctr 1985; **Fellow:** Vascular Surgery, Columbia-Presby Med Ctr 1986; **Fac Appt:** Assoc Prof S, Columbia P&S

Goodman, Elliot R MD (S) - **Spec Exp:** Obesity/Bariatric Surgery; **Hospital:** Beth Israel Med Ctr - Petrie Division (page 90), Holy Name Hosp (page 761); **Address:** First Ave @ 16th St, Dept Surg, Beth Israel Med Ctr-Petrie Div, New York, NY 10003; **Phone:** 212-844-1575; **Board Cert:** Surgery 1997; **Med School:** England 1988; **Resid:** Surgery, Maimonides Med Ctr 1996; **Fac Appt:** Asst Prof S, Albert Einstein Coll Med

Gouge, Thomas MD (S) - **Spec Exp:** Esophageal Cancer; Pancreatic Cancer; **Hospital:** NYU Med Ctr (page 102); **Address:** 530 1st Ave, Ste 6B, New York, NY 10016; **Phone:** 212-263-7301; **Board Cert:** Surgery 1997; **Med School:** Yale Univ 1970; **Resid:** Surgery, NYU Med Ctr 1975; **Fac Appt:** Prof S, NYU Sch Med

Hardy, Mark MD (S) - **Spec Exp:** Transplant-Kidney; Parathyroid Surgery; Islet Cell Transplant; Immunotherapy; **Hospital:** NY-Presby Hosp (page 100); **Address:** 177 Fort Washington Ave, New York, NY 10032; **Phone:** 212-305-5502; **Board Cert:** Surgery 1972; **Med School:** Albert Einstein Coll Med 1962; **Resid:** Surgery, Strong Meml Hosp 1964; Surgery, Bronx Muni Hosp Ctr/Einstein 1971; **Fellow:** Transplant Surgery, Harvard Med Sch 1969; **Fac Appt:** Prof S, Columbia P&S

Harris, Matthew N MD (S) - **Spec Exp:** Cancer Surgery; Melanoma; Breast Cancer; **Hospital:** NYU Med Ctr (page 102), Bellevue Hosp Ctr; **Address:** 160 E 34th St Fl 3, New York, NY 10016-6402; **Phone:** 212-731-5413; **Board Cert:** Surgery 1964; **Med School:** Univ Hlth Sci/Chicago Med Sch 1956; **Resid:** Surgery, Bellevue Hosp-NYU 1963; **Fellow:** Surgical Oncology, NYU Hosp 1963; **Fac Appt:** Prof S, NYU Sch Med

Harris, Michael MD (S) - **Spec Exp:** Gastrointestinal Surgery; Inflammatory Bowel Disease; **Hospital:** Mount Sinai Med Ctr (page 98); **Address:** Mt Sinai Medical Ctr, Dept Surgery, 5 E 98th St, Box 1259, New York, NY 10029; **Phone:** 212-241-1763; **Board Cert:** Surgery 2003; **Med School:** Columbia P&S 1988; **Resid:** Surgery, Mt Sinai Med Ctr 1994; **Fac Appt:** Assoc Clin Prof S, Mount Sinai Sch Med

Heerdt, Alexandra S MD (S) - **Spec Exp:** Breast Cancer; **Hospital:** Meml Sloan Kettering Cancer Ctr (page 109); **Address:** 205 E 64th St, Lower Concourse, New York, NY 10021; **Phone:** 212-639-5253; **Board Cert:** Surgery 2002; **Med School:** Jefferson Med Coll 1987; **Resid:** Surgery, NY Hosp-Cornell Med Ctr 1992; **Fellow:** Surgical Oncology, Meml Sloan Kettering Cancer Ctr 1993

Herron, Daniel M MD (S) - **Spec Exp:** Obesity/Bariatric Surgery; Laparoscopic Surgery; **Hospital:** Mount Sinai Med Ctr (page 98); **Address:** Mt Sinai Med Ctr, 5 E 98th St, Box 1103, New York, NY 10029; **Phone:** 212-241-3699; **Board Cert:** Surgery 1999; **Med School:** Univ Pennsylvania 1992; **Resid:** Surgery, New England Med Ctr 1998; **Fellow:** Laparoscopic Surgery, Oregon U Hlth Sci Ctr 1999; **Fac Appt:** Asst Prof S, Mount Sinai Sch Med

Hofstetter, Steven MD (S) - **Spec Exp:** Laparoscopic Abdominal Surgery; Gastrointestinal Cancer; Hernia; **Hospital:** NYU Med Ctr (page 102); **Address:** 530 1st Ave, Ste 6C, New York, NY 10016-6402; **Phone:** 212-263-7302; **Board Cert:** Surgery 2000; **Med School:** SUNY Hlth Sci Ctr 1971; **Resid:** Surgery, Bellevue Hosp/NYU Med Ctr 1976; **Fac Appt:** Assoc Prof S, NYU Sch Med

Inabnet, William B MD (S) - **Spec Exp:** Thyroid Surgery; Adrenal Surgery; Pancreatic Surgery; Minimally Invasive Surgery; **Hospital:** NY-Presby Hosp (page 100); **Address:** Columbia Univ Med Ctr, 161 Fort Washington Ave, New York, NY 10032; **Phone:** 212-305-0444; **Board Cert:** Surgery 1998; **Med School:** Univ NC Sch Med 1991; **Resid:** Surgery, Rush Presby-St Lukes Med Ctr 1996; **Fellow:** Endocrinology, Cochin Hosp 1997; **Fac Appt:** Asst Prof S, Columbia P&S

Katz, L Brian MD (S) - **Spec Exp:** Abdominal Surgery-Laparoscopic; Esophageal Surgery; Gallbladder Surgery-Laparoscopic; **Hospital:** Mount Sinai Med Ctr (page 98); **Address:** 1010 Fifth Ave, New York, NY 10028; **Phone:** 212-879-6677; **Board Cert:** Surgery 2001; **Med School:** South Africa 1975; **Resid:** Surgery, Mount Sinai Hosp 1982; **Fac Appt:** Assoc Clin Prof S, Mount Sinai Sch Med

Kaufman, Howard L MD (S) - **Spec Exp:** Cancer Surgery; Vaccine Therapy; Melanoma; Immunotherapy; **Hospital:** NY-Presby Hosp (page 100); **Address:** Columbia University, MHB-7SK, 177 Fort Washington Ave, New York, NY 10032; **Phone:** 212-342-6042; **Board Cert:** Surgery 1996; **Med School:** Loyola Univ-Stritch Sch Med 1986; **Resid:** Surgery, Boston Univ Hosp 1995; **Fellow:** Surgical Oncology, Natl Cancer Inst 1996; **Fac Appt:** Assoc Prof S, Columbia P&S

Kimmelstiel, Fred MD (S) - **Spec Exp:** Laparoscopic Surgery; Breast Surgery; Cancer Surgery; **Hospital:** St Luke's - Roosevelt Hosp Ctr - Roosevelt Div (page 90); **Address:** 225 W 71st St, New York, NY 10024; **Phone:** 212-362-6060; **Board Cert:** Surgery 1995; **Med School:** NY Med Coll 1980; **Resid:** Surgery, St Lukes Roosevelt Hosp Ctr 1985; **Fellow:** Transplant Surgery, Univ Hosp 1986; **Fac Appt:** Asst Clin Prof S, Columbia P&S

Liang, Howard MD (S) - **Spec Exp:** Laparoscopic Abdominal Surgery; Gastrointestinal Cancer; Hernia; **Hospital:** NYU Med Ctr (page 102); **Address:** 530 1st Ave, Ste 6C, New York, NY 10016; **Phone:** 212-263-7302; **Board Cert:** Surgery 1997; **Med School:** Washington Univ, St Louis 1974; **Resid:** Surgery, NYU Med Ctr 1982; **Fac Appt:** Asst Prof S, NYU Sch Med

Lieberman, Michael MD (S) - **Spec Exp:** Gastrointestinal Cancer; Colon & Rectal Surgery; Hepatobiliary Surgery; Pancreatic Cancer; **Hospital:** NY-Presby Hosp (page 100); **Address:** NY Presbyterian Hospital, 525 E 68th St, New York, NY 10021; **Phone:** 212-746-5434; **Board Cert:** Surgery 2003; **Med School:** UMDNJ-NJ Med Sch, Newark 1985; **Resid:** Surgery, Hosp U Penn 1992; **Fellow:** Surgical Oncology, Hosp U Penn 1990; Surgical Oncology, Meml Sloan-Kettering Cancer Ctr 1994; **Fac Appt:** Assoc Prof S, Cornell Univ-Weill Med Coll

Michelassi, Fabrizio MD (S) - **Spec Exp:** Gastrointestinal Cancer; Inflammatory Bowel Disease/Crohn's; Pancreatic Cancer; Ulcerative Colitis; **Hospital:** NY-Presby Hosp (page 100); **Address:** Weill Med College, Dept Surgery, 525 E 68th St, rm F-739, New York, NY 10021; **Phone:** 212-746-6006; **Board Cert:** Surgery 2002; **Med School:** Italy 1975; **Resid:** Surgery, NYU Med Ctr 1981; **Fellow:** Research, Mass Genl Hosp-Harvard 1983; **Fac Appt:** Prof S, Cornell Univ-Weill Med Coll

Mills, Christopher B MD (S) - **Spec Exp:** Breast Surgery; Gastrointestinal Surgery; Colon & Rectal Surgery; **Hospital:** St Vincent Cath Med Ctrs - Manhattan (page 375); **Address:** 88 University Pl Fl 9, New York, NY 10003; **Phone:** 646-486-0001; **Board Cert:** Surgery 1999; **Med School:** UMDNJ-NJ Med Sch, Newark 1973; **Resid:** Surgery, St Vincent's Hosp & Med Ctr 1978; **Fellow:** Nutrition & Metabolism, Ravenswood Hosp Med Ctr 1979; **Fac Appt:** Asst Prof S, NY Med Coll

Mizrachy, Benjamin MD (S) - **Spec Exp:** Breast Surgery; **Hospital:** Mount Sinai Med Ctr (page 98); **Address:** 1735 York Ave, rm 201, New York, NY 10128; **Phone:** 212-410-1110; **Board Cert:** Surgery 1967; **Med School:** South Africa 1958; **Resid:** Surgery, Jacoby Hosp 1962; Surgery, Mount Sinai Hosp 1966; **Fellow:** Surgery, Mount Sinai Hosp 1972; **Fac Appt:** Asst Clin Prof Med, Mount Sinai Sch Med

Moore, Eric MD (S) - **Spec Exp:** Breast Surgery; **Hospital:** St Luke's - Roosevelt Hosp Ctr - Roosevelt Div (page 90); **Address:** 30 W 60th St, rm 1H, New York, NY 10023; **Phone:** 212-247-6575; **Board Cert:** Surgery 2001; **Med School:** Columbia P&S 1975; **Resid:** Surgery, St Luke's-Roosevelt Hosp Ctr 1980; **Fellow:** Surgical Oncology, Meml Sloan Kettering Cancer Ctr 1982; Vascular Surgery, Newark Beth Israel Med Ctr 1983; **Fac Appt:** Asst Prof S, Columbia P&S

Morrissey, Kevin MD (S) - **Spec Exp:** Colon & Rectal Surgery; Gastrointestinal Surgery; **Hospital:** NY-Presby Hosp (page 100); **Address:** 50 E 69th St, New York, NY 10021-5016; **Phone:** 212-744-0060; **Board Cert:** Surgery 1972; **Med School:** Cornell Univ-Weill Med Coll 1965; **Resid:** Surgery, NY Hosp 1971; **Fellow:** Gastroenterology, NY Hosp 1973

Newman, Elliot MD (S) - **Spec Exp:** Gastrointestinal Cancer; Pancreatic Cancer; Liver Cancer; Colon & Rectal Cancer; **Hospital:** NYU Med Ctr (page 102); **Address:** NYU Medical Ctr, 530 1st Ave, Ste 6C, New York, NY 10016; **Phone:** 212-263-7302; **Board Cert:** Surgery 2004; **Med School:** NYU Sch Med 1986; **Resid:** Surgery, NYU Med Ctr 1989; Surgery, NYU Med Ctr 1993; **Fellow:** Research, Meml Sloan Kettering Cancer Ctr 1991; Surgical Oncology, Meml Sloan Kettering Cancer Ctr 1995; **Fac Appt:** Assoc Prof S, NYU Sch Med

Nowak, Eugene MD (S) - **Spec Exp:** Breast Cancer; Hernia; Gastrointestinal Disorders; **Hospital:** NY-Presby Hosp (page 100); **Address:** 325 E 79th St, New York, NY 10021-0954; **Phone:** 212-517-6693; **Board Cert:** Surgery 2003; **Med School:** UMDNJ-NJ Med Sch, Newark 1975; **Resid:** Surgery, New York Hosp- Cornell Med Ctr 1980; **Fac Appt:** Assoc Prof S, Cornell Univ-Weill Med Coll

Nunez, Domingo MD (S) - **Spec Exp:** Endoscopic Surgery; Gastrointestinal Surgery; Breast Surgery; **Hospital:** Lenox Hill Hosp (page 94); **Address:** 132 E 76th St, Ste 2A, New York, NY 10021; **Phone:** 212-879-5559; **Board Cert:** Surgery 1995; **Med School:** Columbia P&S 1980; **Resid:** Surgery, Lenox Hill Hosp 1985; **Fellow:** Endoscopy, Toronto Genl Hosp 1986

Nussbaum, Moses MD (S) - **Spec Exp:** Thyroid & Parathyroid Surgery; Head & Neck Cancer; **Hospital:** Beth Israel Med Ctr - Petrie Division (page 90); **Address:** 350 E 17th St Fl 16, New York, NY 10003; **Phone:** 212-844-6648; **Board Cert:** Surgery 1963; **Med School:** NYU Sch Med 1955; **Resid:** Surgery, Bellevue Hosp 1957; Surgery, Beth Israel Hosp 1962; **Fellow:** Head and Neck Surgery, Beth Israel Hosp 1963; **Fac Appt:** Prof S, Albert Einstein Coll Med

Osborne, Michael P MD (S) - **Spec Exp:** Breast Cancer; Breast Cancer-High Risk Women; Breast Disease; **Hospital:** NY-Presby Hosp (page 100); **Address:** 425 E 61 St Fl 8, New York, NY 10021-8722; **Phone:** 212-821-0828; **Med School:** England 1970; **Resid:** Surgery, Charing Cross Hosp 1977; Surgery, Royal Marsden Hosp 1980; **Fellow:** Surgical Oncology, Meml Sloan-Kettering Canc Ctr 1981; **Fac Appt:** Prof S, Cornell Univ-Weill Med Coll

Pachter, H Leon MD (S) - **Spec Exp:** Adrenal Surgery; Gastrointestinal Surgery; Pancreatic Cancer; **Hospital:** NYU Med Ctr (page 102), Bellevue Hosp Ctr; **Address:** 530 1st Ave, Ste 6C, New York, NY 10016; **Phone:** 212-263-7302; **Board Cert:** Surgery 2000; **Med School:** NYU Sch Med 1971; **Resid:** Surgery, NYU Med Ctr 1976; **Fac Appt:** Prof S, NYU Sch Med

Paty, Philip B MD (S) - **Spec Exp:** Colon & Rectal Cancer; Pelvic Tumors; Appendix Cancer; **Hospital:** Meml Sloan Kettering Cancer Ctr (page 109); **Address:** Memorial Sloan Kettering Cancer Ctr, 1275 York Ave, rm C1081, New York, NY 10021-6007; **Phone:** 212-639-6703; **Board Cert:** Surgery 2001; **Med School:** Stanford Univ 1983; **Resid:** Surgery, UCSF Med Ctr 1990; **Fellow:** Surgical Oncology, Memorial Sloan Kettering Cancer Ctr 1992; **Fac Appt:** Prof S, Cornell Univ-Weill Med Coll

Pertsemlidis, Demetrius MD (S) - **Spec Exp:** Endocrine Surgery; Biliary Surgery; **Hospital:** Mount Sinai Med Ctr (page 98); **Address:** 1199 Park Ave, Ste 1A, New York, NY 10128-1712; **Phone:** 212-860-1056; **Board Cert:** Surgery 1966; **Med School:** Germany 1959; **Resid:** Surgery, Mount Sinai Hosp 1965; **Fellow:** Surgery, Mount Sinai Hosp 1966; **Fac Appt:** Clin Prof S, Mount Sinai Sch Med

Pomp, Alfons MD (S) - **Spec Exp:** Obesity/Bariatric Surgery; Abdominal Surgery-Laparoscopic; Hernia; **Hospital:** NY-Presby Hosp (page 100); **Address:** Weill Cornell College of Medicine, 525 E 68th St, Box 294, New York, NY 10021; **Phone:** 212-746-5294; **Board Cert:** Surgery 1999; **Med School:** Univ Sherbrooke 1980; **Resid:** Surgery, Univ Montreal Med Ctr 1985; **Fellow:** Nutrition, Rhode Island Hosp 1988; **Fac Appt:** Assoc Prof S, Cornell Univ-Weill Med Coll

Ratner, Lloyd Evan MD (S) - **Spec Exp:** Transplant-Kidney; Transplant-Pancreas; Pancreatic Surgery; **Hospital:** NY-Presby Hosp (page 100); **Address:** Columbia University, PH 14-408, 622 W 168th St, New York, NY 10032; **Phone:** 212-305-6469; **Board Cert:** Surgery 1998; **Med School:** Hahnemann Univ 1983; **Resid:** Surgery, LIJ Med Ctr 1988; **Fellow:** Transplant Surgery, Barnes Jewish Hosp 1990; **Fac Appt:** Assoc Prof S, Columbia P&S

Reader, Robert MD (S) - **Spec Exp:** Breast Surgery; Hernia; Gastrointestinal Surgery; **Hospital:** NYU Med Ctr (page 102), NY Downtown Hosp; **Address:** 530 First Ave, Ste 6E, New York, NY 10016-6402; **Phone:** 212-263-8008; **Board Cert:** Surgery 2002; **Med School:** Univ Pennsylvania 1975; **Resid:** Surgery, NYU Med Ctr 1980; **Fac Appt:** Clin Prof S, NYU Sch Med

Reiner, Mark MD (S) - **Spec Exp:** Laparoscopic Surgery-Gastrointestinal; Hernia; **Hospital:** Mount Sinai Med Ctr (page 98), Lenox Hill Hosp (page 94); **Address:** 1010 5th Ave, New York, NY 10028-0130; **Phone:** 212-879-6677; **Board Cert:** Surgery 2001; **Med School:** SUNY Downstate 1974; **Resid:** Surgery, Mount Sinai Hosp 1979; **Fac Appt:** Clin Prof S, Mount Sinai Sch Med

Ren, Christine J MD (S) - **Spec Exp:** Obesity/Bariatric Surgery; Laparoscopic Surgery; **Hospital:** NYU Med Ctr (page 102); **Address:** NYU Med Ctr, 530 First Ave, Ste 10S, New York, NY 10016; **Phone:** 212-263-3166; **Board Cert:** Surgery 2000; **Med School:** Tufts Univ 1993; **Resid:** Surgery, NYU Med Ctr 1999; **Fellow:** Bariatric Surgery, NYU Med Ctr 2000; **Fac Appt:** Asst Prof S, NYU Sch Med

Rosenberg, Vladimiro MD (S) - **Spec Exp:** Breast Cancer; Melanoma; Thyroid & Parathyroid Surgery; Sarcoma-Soft Tissue; **Hospital:** Mount Sinai Med Ctr (page 98), Lenox Hill Hosp (page 94); **Address:** 1440 York Ave, Ste P-10, New York, NY 10021; **Phone:** 212-772-0010; **Med School:** Argentina 1965; **Resid:** Surgery, Mount Sinai Hosp 1977; **Fellow:** Surgical Oncology, MD Anderson Canc Ctr 1978; **Fac Appt:** Asst Clin Prof S, Mount Sinai Sch Med

Roses, Daniel F MD (S) - **Spec Exp:** Breast Cancer; Melanoma; Thyroid Cancer; Parathyroid Surgery; **Hospital:** NYU Med Ctr (page 102); **Address:** 530 First Ave, Ste 6E, New York, NY 10016-6402; **Phone:** 212-263-7329; **Board Cert:** Surgery 1975; **Med School:** NYU Sch Med 1969; **Resid:** Surgery, NYU-Bellevue Hosp 1974; **Fellow:** Surgical Oncology, NYU-Bellevue Hosp 1978; **Fac Appt:** Prof Surg & Onc, NYU Sch Med

Roslin, Mitchell S MD (S) - **Spec Exp:** Obesity/Bariatric Surgery; Minimally Invasive Surgery; Robotic Surgery; **Hospital:** Lenox Hill Hosp (page 94); **Address:** 110 E 59th St, Ste AA, New York, NY 10022; **Phone:** 212-434-3285; **Board Cert:** Surgery 2002; **Med School:** NYU Sch Med 1987; **Resid:** Surgery, Maimonides Med Ctr 1993; **Fellow:** Surgery, Univ of Michigan 1994

Rosser Jr, James C MD (S) - **Spec Exp:** Minimally Invasive Surgery; Obesity/Bariatric Surgery; **Hospital:** Beth Israel Med Ctr - Petrie Division (page 90); **Address:** Beth Israel Med Ctr, Dept Surgery, 350 E 17th St, Ste 16BH, New York, NY 10003; **Phone:** 212-420-4337; **Board Cert:** Surgery 2001; **Med School:** Univ Miss 1980; **Resid:** Surgery, Akron Gen Med Hosp 1986; **Fac Appt:** Prof S, Albert Einstein Coll Med

Surgery

Salky, Barry A MD (S) - **Spec Exp:** Laparoscopic Surgery-Gastrointestinal; Gastroesophageal Reflux Disease (GERD); Pancreatic Surgery; **Hospital:** Mount Sinai Med Ctr (page 98); **Address:** Mt Sinai Med Ctr, Div of Laparoscopic Surg, 5 E 98th St, Box 1259, New York, NY 10029; **Phone:** 212-241-5339; **Board Cert:** Surgery 1998; **Med School:** Univ Tenn Coll Med, Memphis 1970; **Resid:** Surgery, Mount Sinai Hosp 1973; Surgery, Mount Sinai Hosp 1978; **Fac Appt:** Prof S, Mount Sinai Sch Med

Scarpinato, Vincent M MD (S) - **Spec Exp:** Breast Surgery; Gastrointestinal Surgery; **Hospital:** St Vincent Cath Med Ctrs - Manhattan (page 375); **Address:** 88 University Pl, Fl 9, New York, NY 10003-4513; **Phone:** 646-486-0001; **Board Cert:** Surgery 2005; **Med School:** NY Med Coll 1987; **Resid:** Surgery, St Vincent's Med Ctr 1992; **Fac Appt:** Asst Clin Prof S, NY Med Coll

Schnabel, Freya MD (S) - **Spec Exp:** Breast Cancer; Breast Cancer-High Risk Women; **Hospital:** NY-Presby Hosp (page 100), South Nassau Comm Hosp; **Address:** 161 Fort Washington Ave Fl 10 - Ste 1011, New York, NY 10032; **Phone:** 212-305-1534; **Board Cert:** Surgery 1998; **Med School:** NYU Sch Med 1982; **Resid:** Surgery, NYU Med Ctr 1987; **Fellow:** Research, SUNY Hlth Sci Ctr 1988; **Fac Appt:** Assoc Clin Prof S, Columbia P&S

Schwartz, Myron MD (S) - **Spec Exp:** Liver Cancer; Hepatobiliary Surgery; Transplant-Liver; **Hospital:** Mount Sinai Med Ctr (page 98); **Address:** Recananti-Miller Transplantation Inst, 19 E 98th St, Box 1104, New York, NY 10029; **Phone:** 212-241-2891; **Board Cert:** Surgery 1998; **Med School:** Jefferson Med Coll 1976; **Resid:** Surgery, Mt Sinai Hosp 1986; Vascular Surgery, Mt Sinai Hosp 1987; **Fac Appt:** Prof S, Mount Sinai Sch Med

Sekons, David MD (S) - **Spec Exp:** Palmar Hyperhidrosis; Endoscopy; Laparoscopic Surgery; **Hospital:** Beth Israel Med Ctr - Petrie Division (page 90), St Vincent Cath Med Ctrs - Manhattan (page 375); **Address:** 41 5th Ave, New York, NY 10003-4319; **Phone:** 212-228-3001; **Board Cert:** Surgery 2003; **Med School:** Israel 1976; **Resid:** Surgery, Beth Israel 1978; Surgery, Beth Israel 1982; **Fellow:** Beth Israel 1983; **Fac Appt:** Asst Clin Prof S, Albert Einstein Coll Med

Shah, Jatin P MD (S) - **Spec Exp:** Head & Neck Cancer; Thyroid Cancer; Skull Base Tumors; **Hospital:** Meml Sloan Kettering Cancer Ctr (page 109); **Address:** 1275 York Ave, Ste C1061, New York, NY 10021-6007; **Phone:** 212-639-7604; **Board Cert:** Surgery 1975; **Med School:** India 1964; **Resid:** Surgery, SSG Hosp 1967; Surgery, New York Infirm 1974; **Fellow:** Head & Neck Surgical Oncology, Meml Sloan-Kettering Hosp 1972; **Fac Appt:** Prof S, Cornell Univ-Weill Med Coll

Shaha, Ashok MD (S) - **Spec Exp:** Head & Neck Cancer; Thyroid Cancer; Parathyroid Cancer; **Hospital:** Meml Sloan Kettering Cancer Ctr (page 109); **Address:** 1275 York Ave, New York, NY 10021-6007; **Phone:** 212-639-7649; **Board Cert:** Surgery 1992; **Med School:** India 1970; **Resid:** Surgery, Downstate Med Ctr 1981; **Fellow:** Surgical Oncology, Meml Sloan Kettering Cancer Ctr 1976; Head and Neck Surgery, Meml Sloan Kettering Cancer Ctr 1982; **Fac Appt:** Prof S, Cornell Univ-Weill Med Coll

Shamamian, Peter MD (S) - **Spec Exp:** Pancreatic Surgery; Pancreatic Cancer; **Hospital:** NYU Med Ctr (page 102); **Address:** 530 1st Ave, Ste 6B, New York, NY 10016-6481; **Phone:** 212-263-7301; **Board Cert:** Surgery 1996; **Med School:** Robert W Johnson Med Sch 1989; **Resid:** Surgery, NYU Med Ctr 1995; **Fellow:** Surgical Oncology, Natl Inst Hlth 1993; **Fac Appt:** Assoc Prof S, NYU Sch Med

Shapiro, Richard L MD (S) - **Spec Exp:** Breast Cancer; Melanoma; Thyroid & Parathyroid Surgery; Cancer Surgery; **Hospital:** NYU Med Ctr (page 102), Bellevue Hosp Ctr; **Address:** NYU Medical Ctr, 160 E 34th St, New York, NY 10016; **Phone:** 212-731-5347; **Board Cert:** Surgery 2004; **Med School:** NYU Sch Med 1988; **Resid:** Surgery, NYU Med Ctr 1993; **Fellow:** Surgical Oncology, NYU Med Ctr 1995; **Fac Appt:** Assoc Prof S, NYU Sch Med

Simmons, Rache M MD (S) - **Spec Exp:** Breast Cancer & Surgery; Breast Disease; **Hospital:** NY-Presby Hosp (page 100); **Address:** Weill Cornell Breast Ctr, 425 E 61st St Fl 8, New York, NY 10021; **Phone:** 212-821-0853; **Board Cert:** Surgery 1996; **Med School:** Duke Univ 1988; **Resid:** Surgery, Univ NC Hosp 1993; **Fellow:** Surgical Oncology, NY Hosp-Cornell Hosp 1994; **Fac Appt:** Assoc Prof S, Cornell Univ-Weill Med Coll

Singer, Samuel MD (S) - **Spec Exp:** Sarcoma-Soft Tissue; **Hospital:** Meml Sloan Kettering Cancer Ctr (page 109); **Address:** Meml Sloan Kettering Cancer Ctr, 1275 York Ave, rm 1210, New York, NY 10021; **Phone:** 212-639-2940; **Board Cert:** Surgery 1998; **Med School:** Harvard Med Sch 1982; **Resid:** Surgery, Brigham & Women's Hosp 1988; **Fellow:** Surgical Oncology, Dana Farber Cancer Inst 1990; **Fac Appt:** Assoc Prof S, Cornell Univ-Weill Med Coll

Skinner, Kristin A MD (S) - **Spec Exp:** Breast Cancer; Gastrointestinal Cancer; Melanoma; **Hospital:** NYU Med Ctr (page 102); **Address:** NYU Clinical Cancer, 160 E 34th St Fl 3, New York, NY 10016; **Phone:** 212-731-5367; **Board Cert:** Surgery 1996; **Med School:** Johns Hopkins Univ 1988; **Resid:** Surgery, UCLA Med Ctr 1995; **Fellow:** Surgical Oncology, UCLA Med Ctr 1994; **Fac Appt:** Assoc Prof S, NYU Sch Med

Slater, Gary MD (S) - **Spec Exp:** Gastrointestinal Surgery; Laparoscopic Surgery; Hernia; **Hospital:** Mount Sinai Med Ctr (page 98); **Address:** 5 E 98th St, New York, NY 10029-6501; **Phone:** 212-241-7646; **Board Cert:** Surgery 1975; **Med School:** NYU Sch Med 1968; **Resid:** Surgery, Mount Sinai Hosp 1974; **Fac Appt:** Prof S, Mount Sinai Sch Med

Stone, Alex MD (S) - **Spec Exp:** Adrenal Surgery; Hernia; Breast Surgery; Gastrointestinal Surgery; **Hospital:** Bellevue Hosp Ctr; **Address:** NYU School of Medicine, Dept Surgery, 530 First Ave, NBV 15 South 5, New York, NY 10016; **Phone:** 212-562-3921; **Board Cert:** Surgery 1972; **Med School:** NYU Sch Med 1966; **Resid:** Surgery, Bellevue Hosp-NYU 1971; **Fac Appt:** Prof S, NYU Sch Med

Strong, Leslie MD (S) - **Spec Exp:** Breast Surgery; Breast Cancer; **Hospital:** Beth Israel Med Ctr - Petrie Division (page 90); **Address:** 28 W 12th St, New York, NY 10011; **Phone:** 212-645-0052; **Board Cert:** Surgery 1975; **Med School:** UCLA 1967; **Resid:** Surgery, Harlem Hosp 1969; Surgery, Kings County Hosp 1973; **Fac Appt:** Prof S, Albert Einstein Coll Med

Swistel, Alexander MD (S) - **Spec Exp:** Breast Cancer; Breast Disease; Sentinal Node Surgery; **Hospital:** NY-Presby Hosp (page 100), St Luke's - Roosevelt Hosp Ctr - Roosevelt Div (page 90); **Address:** 425 E 61st St Fl 8, New York, NY 10021; **Phone:** 212-821-0602; **Board Cert:** Surgery 2005; **Med School:** Brown Univ 1975; **Resid:** Surgery, St Luke's Roosevelt Hosp Ctr 1981; **Fellow:** Surgical Oncology, Meml Sloan Kettering Canc Ctr 1983; **Fac Appt:** Asst Prof S, Cornell Univ-Weill Med Coll

Tartter, Paul MD (S) - **Spec Exp:** Breast Cancer; Breast Cancer in Elderly; Sentinel Node Surgery; **Hospital:** St Luke's - Roosevelt Hosp Ctr - Roosevelt Div (page 90), Mount Sinai Med Ctr (page 98); **Address:** 425 W 59th St, Ste 7A, New York, NY 10019; **Phone:** 212-523-7500; **Board Cert:** Surgery 2003; **Med School:** Brown Univ 1977; **Resid:** Surgery, Mount Sinai Hosp 1982; **Fac Appt:** Assoc Prof S, Columbia P&S

Teperman, Lewis W MD (S) - **Spec Exp:** Transplant-Liver; Transplant-Kidney; Liver Tumors; **Hospital:** NYU Med Ctr (page 102); **Address:** 403 E 34th St Fl 3, New York, NY 10016; **Phone:** 212-263-8134; **Board Cert:** Surgery 1997; **Med School:** Mount Sinai Sch Med 1981; **Resid:** Surgery, Columbia Presby Med Ctr 1984; Surgery, LI Jewish Med Ctr 1986; **Fellow:** Transplant Surgery, Univ Pittsburgh 1988; **Fac Appt:** Assoc Prof S, NYU Sch Med

Wallack, Marc MD (S) - **Spec Exp:** Melanoma; Breast Surgery; **Hospital:** Metropolitan Hosp Ctr - NY; **Address:** 1901 1st Ave, rm 12A-1, New York, NY 10029; **Phone:** 212-423-6614; **Board Cert:** Surgery 2001; **Med School:** Univ Pittsburgh 1970; **Resid:** Surgery, Hosp Univ Penn 1977; **Fellow:** Medical Oncology, Wistar Inst Anatomy & Biology 1977; **Fac Appt:** Prof S, NY Med Coll

Wedderburn, Raymond MD (S) - **Hospital:** St Luke's - Roosevelt Hosp Ctr - Roosevelt Div (page 90); **Address:** 1111 Amsterdam Ave, Muhlenber Bldg, Fl 2 - Ste 208N, New York, NY 10025; **Phone:** 212-523-5295; **Board Cert:** Surgery 1992; Surgical Critical Care 1993; **Med School:** Cornell Univ-Weill Med Coll 1986; **Resid:** Surgery, St Luke's-Roosevelt Hosp Ctr 1991; **Fellow:** Surgical Critical Care, Jackson Meml Hosp 1993

Yurt, Roger MD (S) - **Spec Exp:** Burn Care; Wound Healing/Care; Hyperbaric Medicine; **Hospital:** NY-Presby Hosp (page 100); **Address:** 525 E 68th St, rm L706, New York, NY 10021-4885; **Phone:** 212-746-5410; **Board Cert:** Surgery 1999; **Med School:** Univ Miami Sch Med 1972; **Resid:** Surgery, Parkland Meml Hosp 1974; Surgery, New York Hosp-Cornell Med Ctr 1980; **Fellow:** Internal Medicine, Brigham & Womens Hosp 1978; **Fac Appt:** Prof S, Cornell Univ-Weill Med Coll

THORACIC SURGERY

Adams, David H MD (TS) - **Spec Exp:** Mitral Valve Surgery; Heart Valve Surgery; **Hospital:** Mount Sinai Med Ctr (page 98); **Address:** Mt Sinai Hosp, Cardiac & Thoracic Surg, Box 1028, 1190 Fifth Ave, New York, NY 10029; **Phone:** 212-659-6800; **Board Cert:** Surgery 1992; Thoracic Surgery 1994; **Med School:** Duke Univ 1983; **Resid:** Surgery, Brigham & Women's Hosp; Thoracic Surgery, Brigham & Women's Hosp; **Fac Appt:** Prof TS, Mount Sinai Sch Med

Altorki, Nasser MD (TS) - **Spec Exp:** Esophageal Cancer; Lung Cancer; Gastroesophageal Reflux Disease (GERD); **Hospital:** NY-Presby Hosp (page 100); **Address:** 525 E 68th St, New York, NY 10021-4870; **Phone:** 212-746-5156; **Board Cert:** Surgery 1996; Thoracic Surgery 1998; **Med School:** Egypt 1978; **Resid:** Surgery, Univ Chicago Hosps 1985; **Fellow:** Cardiothoracic Surgery, Univ Chicago Hosps 1987; **Fac Appt:** Prof S, Cornell Univ-Weill Med Coll

Argenziano, Michael MD (TS) - **Spec Exp:** Robotic Heart Surgery; Coronary Artery Robotic Surgery; Maze Procedure for Atrial Fibrillation; **Hospital:** NY-Presby Hosp (page 100); **Address:** Columbia Presby Med Ctr, Milstein Bldg, 177 Fort Washington Ave, rm 7-435, New York, NY 10032; **Phone:** 212-305-5888; **Board Cert:** Surgery 1999; Thoracic Surgery 2002; **Med School:** Columbia P&S 1992; **Resid:** Surgery, Columbia Presby Med Ctr 1998; **Fellow:** Cardiothoracic Surgery, Columbia Presby Med Ctr 1999; **Fac Appt:** Asst Prof S, Columbia P&S

Bains, Manjit MD (TS) - **Spec Exp:** Cardiothoracic Surgery; Esophageal Cancer; Lung Cancer; **Hospital:** Meml Sloan Kettering Cancer Ctr (page 109); **Address:** 1275 York Ave, rm C-861, New York, NY 10021; **Phone:** 212-639-7450; **Board Cert:** Surgery 1971; Thoracic Surgery 1972; **Med School:** India 1963; **Resid:** Surgery, Rochester Genl Hosp 1970; **Fellow:** Thoracic Surgery, Sloan Kettering Cancer Ctr 1972; **Fac Appt:** Clin Prof S, Cornell Univ-Weill Med Coll

New York (Manhattan)

Camunas, Jorge L MD (TS) - **Spec Exp:** Pacemakers; Defibrillators; Lung Cancer; **Hospital:** Mount Sinai Med Ctr (page 98), VA Med Ctr - Bronx; **Address:** 1190 5th Ave, GP-2W, New York, NY 10029-6501; **Phone:** 212-659-6800; **Board Cert:** Thoracic Surgery 2002; **Med School:** Georgetown Univ 1970; **Resid:** Surgery, Harlem Hosp 1976; Cardiothoracic Surgery, Mount Sinai Hosp 1980; **Fellow:** Cardiothoracic Surgery, St Lukes-Roosevelt Med Ctr 1978

Chen, Jonathan M MD (TS) - **Spec Exp:** Pediatric Cardiothoracic Surgery; **Hospital:** NY-Presby Hosp (page 100); **Address:** NY Presbyterian-Weill Cornell Medical Ctr, 525 E 68th St, rm F695B, New York, NY 10021; **Phone:** 212-746-5014; **Board Cert:** Surgery 2001; Thoracic Surgery 2003; **Med School:** Columbia P&S 1994; **Resid:** Surgery, NY Columbia Presby Hosp 2000; **Fellow:** Cardiothoracic Surgery, NY Columbia Presby Hosp 2001; **Fac Appt:** Asst Prof S, Columbia P&S

Colvin, Stephen MD (TS) - **Spec Exp:** Minimally Invasive Cardiac Surgery; Robotic Heart Surgery; Heart Valve Surgery; **Hospital:** NYU Med Ctr (page 102), Bellevue Hosp Ctr; **Address:** 530 1st Ave, Ste 9V, New York, NY 10016; **Phone:** 212-263-6384; **Board Cert:** Thoracic Surgery 1993; **Med School:** Albert Einstein Coll Med 1969; **Resid:** Surgery, NYU/Bellevue Hosp 1971; Thoracic Surgery, NYU/Bellevue Hosp 1978; **Fellow:** Cardiothoracic Surgery, Natl Heart & Lung Inst 1973; **Fac Appt:** Assoc Clin Prof S, NYU Sch Med

Connery, Cliff MD (TS) - **Spec Exp:** Thoracic Cancers; Mediastinal Tumors; Minimally Invasive Surgery; **Hospital:** St Luke's - Roosevelt Hosp Ctr - Roosevelt Div (page 90), Beth Israel Med Ctr - Petrie Division (page 90); **Address:** 1000 Tenth Ave, Ste 2B-05, New York, NY 10019; **Phone:** 212-523-7475; **Board Cert:** Thoracic Surgery 1993; Critical Care Medicine 1993; Surgery 2000; **Med School:** Eastern VA Med Sch 1984; **Resid:** Surgery, Univ Hosp 1989; Thoracic Surgery, Strong Meml Hosp 1992; **Fac Appt:** Asst Prof S, Columbia P&S

Crawford, Bernard MD (TS) - **Spec Exp:** Lung Cancer; Minimally Invasive Surgery; Esophageal Tumors; **Hospital:** NYU Med Ctr (page 102), NY Downtown Hosp; **Address:** 160 E 34th St, New York, NY 10016; **Phone:** 212-731-5580; **Board Cert:** Thoracic Surgery 1999; **Med School:** Geo Wash Univ 1980; **Resid:** Surgery, NYU Med Ctr 1985; **Fellow:** Cardiothoracic Surgery, NYU Med Ctr 1987; **Fac Appt:** Asst Prof TS, NYU Sch Med

Filsoufi, Farzan MD (TS) - **Spec Exp:** Mitral Valve Surgery; Minimally Invasive Heart Valve Surgery; Heart Valve Surgery; Robotic Heart Surgery; **Hospital:** Mount Sinai Med Ctr (page 98), Elmhurst Hosp Ctr; **Address:** Mt Sinai Med Ctr, Dept Cardiothoracic Surg, 1190 5th Ave, Box 1028, New York, NY 10029; **Phone:** 212-659-6813; **Med School:** France 1991; **Resid:** Surgery, Univ Paris Hosps 1994; Thoracic Surgery, Hospital Broussais/U of Paris 1995; **Fellow:** Cardiothoracic Surgery, Hospital Broussais/U of Paris 1996; Heart Valve Surgery, Brigham & Women's Hosp 2000; **Fac Appt:** Asst Prof TS, Mount Sinai Sch Med

Galloway, Aubrey MD (TS) - **Spec Exp:** Minimally Invasive Heart Valve Surgery; Coronary Artery Surgery; Aneurysm-Thoracic Aortic; **Hospital:** NYU Med Ctr (page 102), Bellevue Hosp Ctr; **Address:** 530 1st Ave, Ste 9V, New York, NY 10016-6402; **Phone:** 212-263-7185; **Board Cert:** Thoracic Surgery 1996; **Med School:** Tulane Univ 1978; **Resid:** Surgery, Univ Colo Hlth Sci Ctr 1983; Cardiovascular Surgery, NYU Med Ctr 1985; **Fellow:** Research, Boston Children's Hosp 1981; Cardiothoracic Surgery, NYU Med Ctr 1985; **Fac Appt:** Prof TS, NYU Sch Med

Ginsburg, Mark MD (TS) - **Spec Exp:** Lung Cancer; Transplant-Lung; **Hospital:** NY-Presby Hosp (page 100), Good Samaritan Hosp - Suffern; **Address:** 161 Ft Washington Ave, rm 310, New York, NY 10032; **Phone:** 212-305-3408; **Board Cert:** Surgery 1996; Thoracic Surgery 1996; **Med School:** Tufts Univ 1980; **Resid:** Surgery, Strong Meml Hosp 1985; **Fellow:** Thoracic Surgery, Strong Meml Hosp 1987; **Fac Appt:** Asst Clin Prof S, Columbia P&S

Girardi Jr, Leonard N MD (TS) - **Spec Exp:** Aneurysm-Aortic; Cardiac Surgery; **Hospital:** NY-Presby Hosp (page 100); **Address:** 525 E 68th St, M404, New York, NY 10021; **Phone:** 212-746-5194; **Board Cert:** Surgery 1995; Thoracic Surgery 1998; **Med School:** Cornell Univ-Weill Med Coll 1989; **Resid:** Surgery, NY Presby Hosp 1994; **Fellow:** Cardiac Surgery, NY Presby Hosp 1996; Cardiovascular Surgery, Baylor Coll Med 1997; **Fac Appt:** Assoc Prof TS, Cornell Univ-Weill Med Coll

Griepp, Randall MD (TS) - **Spec Exp:** Aneurysm-Abdominal Aortic; Aneurysm-Thoracic Aortic; Endovascular Surgery; **Hospital:** Mount Sinai Med Ctr (page 98); **Address:** Mt Sinai Med Ctr, Dept Cardiothoracic Surg, 1 Gustave L Levy Pl, Box 1028, New York, NY 10029; **Phone:** 212-659-9495; **Board Cert:** Thoracic Surgery 1997; **Med School:** Stanford Univ 1967; **Resid:** Surgery, Stanford Univ Hosp 1973; **Fellow:** Cardiothoracic Surgery, Stanford Univ Hosp 1972; **Fac Appt:** Prof TS, Mount Sinai Sch Med

Grossi, Eugene A MD (TS) - **Spec Exp:** Minimally Invasive Cardiac Surgery; Mitral Valve Surgery; Cardiac Tumors, Myxomas; **Hospital:** NYU Med Ctr (page 102); **Address:** NYU Med Ctr, 530 1st Ave, Ste 9V, New York, NY 10016-6402; **Phone:** 212-263-7452; **Board Cert:** Thoracic Surgery 2002; **Med School:** Columbia P&S 1981; **Resid:** Surgery, NYU Med Ctr 1987; Thoracic Surgery, NYU Med Ctr 1991; **Fac Appt:** Assoc Prof S, NYU Sch Med

Isom, O Wayne MD (TS) - **Spec Exp:** Cardiac Surgery; Coronary Artery Surgery; Heart Valve Surgery; **Hospital:** NY-Presby Hosp (page 100), NY Hosp Queens; **Address:** 525 E 68th St, rm M-404, New York, NY 10021; **Phone:** 212-746-5151; **Board Cert:** Surgery 1971; Thoracic Surgery 1972; **Med School:** Univ Tex, Houston 1965; **Resid:** Surgery, Parkland Meml Hosp 1970; **Fellow:** Thoracic Surgery, NYU Med Ctr 1972; **Fac Appt:** Prof TS, Cornell Univ-Weill Med Coll

Ko, Wilson MD (TS) - **Spec Exp:** Coronary Artery Surgery; Heart Valve Surgery; Lung Surgery; **Hospital:** NY-Presby Hosp (page 100), NY Hosp Queens; **Address:** Cardiothoracic Surg, New York Hosp-Cornell, 525 E 68th St, Ste M-4, New York, NY 10021; **Phone:** 212-746-5141; **Board Cert:** Surgery 2003; Thoracic Surgery 2004; **Med School:** Univ Hlth Sci/Chicago Med Sch 1988; **Resid:** Surgery, New York Hosp 1993; **Fellow:** Cardiothoracic Surgery, New York Hosp-Cornell 1995; Thoracic Surgery, New York Hosp/Meml Sloan Kettering Cancer Ctr 1995; **Fac Appt:** Assoc Prof S, Cornell Univ-Weill Med Coll

Krellenstein, Daniel J MD (TS) - **Spec Exp:** Lung Cancer; Minimally Invasive Thoracic Surgery; **Hospital:** Mount Sinai Med Ctr (page 98), Lenox Hill Hosp (page 94); **Address:** 16 E 98th St, Ste 1F, New York, NY 10029-6545; **Phone:** 212-423-9311; **Board Cert:** Surgery 1974; Thoracic Surgery 1977; **Med School:** SUNY Buffalo 1964; **Resid:** Surgery, SUNY Downstate Med Ctr 1972; **Fac Appt:** Assoc Clin Prof TS, Mount Sinai Sch Med

Krieger, Karl MD (TS) - **Spec Exp:** Heart Valve Surgery; Coronary Artery Surgery; Robotic Heart Surgery; **Hospital:** NY-Presby Hosp (page 100), NY Hosp Queens; **Address:** Cardiothoracic Surgery Dept, 525 E 68th St, Ste M404, New York, NY 10021-4873; **Phone:** 212-746-5152; **Board Cert:** Thoracic Surgery 1994; **Med School:** Johns Hopkins Univ 1975; **Resid:** Surgery, Johns Hopkins 1976; Bellevue Hosp 1979; **Fellow:** Thoracic Surgery, NYU Med Ctr 1981; **Fac Appt:** Prof S, Cornell Univ-Weill Med Coll

Lang, Samuel MD (TS) - **Spec Exp:** Minimally Invasive Cardiac Surgery; Heart Valve Surgery; **Hospital:** St Vincent Cath Med Ctrs - Manhattan (page 375); **Address:** 170 W 12th St, Spellman-6, New York, NY 10011; **Phone:** 212-604-2488; **Board Cert:** Thoracic Surgery 1996; **Med School:** Univ Ala 1978; **Resid:** Surgery, UCLA Med Ctr 1982; Thoracic Surgery, NYU Med Ctr 1983; **Fellow:** Cardiothoracic Surgery, UCLA Med Ctr 1985; Pediatric Cardiac Surgery, Hosp for Sick Chldn 1986

Loulmet, Didier MD (TS) - **Spec Exp:** Heart Valve Surgery; Robotic Heart Surgery; Minimally Invasive Cardiac Surgery; **Hospital:** Lenox Hill Hosp (page 94); **Address:** Lenox Hill Hosp, William Black Hall, 130 E 77th St, Fl 4, New York, NY 10021-1851; **Phone:** 212-434-3000; **Med School:** France 1984; **Resid:** Cardiothoracic Surgery, Paris Univ Hosp 1990; Cardiothoracic Surgery, Brigham & Women's Hosp 1991; **Fellow:** Pediatric Cardiac Surgery, Chldn's Hosp, Harvard Univ 1992

Naka, Yoshifumi MD/PhD (TS) - **Spec Exp:** Transplant-Heart & Lung; Ventricular Assist Device (LVAD); Heart Failure & Ventricular Containment; Mitral Valve Surgery; **Hospital:** NY-Presby Hosp (page 100); **Address:** 177 Fort Washington Ave, MHB 7-435, New York, NY 10032; **Phone:** 212-305-0828; **Med School:** Japan 1984; **Resid:** Surgery, Osaka Police Hosp 1991; **Fellow:** Cardiovascular Surgery, Osaka Police Hosp 1993; Cardiothoracic Surgery, Columbia Univ 1998; **Fac Appt:** Asst Prof S, Columbia P&S

Nguyen, Khanh H MD (TS) - **Spec Exp:** Pediatric Cardiothoracic Surgery; **Hospital:** Mount Sinai Med Ctr (page 98); **Address:** Mount Sinai Medical Ctr, One Gustave Levy Pl, Box 1028, New York, NY 10029; **Phone:** 212-659-9472; **Board Cert:** Thoracic Surgery 1997; **Med School:** UC Irvine 1985; **Resid:** Surgery, Flushing Hosp 1992; Thoracic Surgery, Mt Sinai Med Ctr 1995

Oz, Mehmet C MD (TS) - **Spec Exp:** Transplant-Heart; Heart Valve Surgery; Minimally Invasive Cardiac Surgery; **Hospital:** NY-Presby Hosp (page 100); **Address:** NY Presby Hosp, Dept Cardiothoracic Surg, 177 Ft Washington Ave, MHB- Rm 7, GN435, New York, NY 10032; **Phone:** 212-305-4434; **Board Cert:** Thoracic Surgery 1994; **Med School:** Univ Pennsylvania 1986; **Resid:** Surgery, Columbia Presby Med Ctr 1991; **Fellow:** Cardiothoracic Surgery, Columbia Presby Med Ctr 1993; **Fac Appt:** Prof S, Columbia P&S

Pass, Harvey MD (TS) - **Spec Exp:** Lung Cancer; Mesothelioma; Clinical Trials; **Hospital:** NYU Med Ctr (page 102); **Address:** NYU Cancer Ctr, 160 E 34th St, New York, NY 10016; **Phone:** 212-731-5414; **Board Cert:** Thoracic Surgery 2001; **Med School:** Duke Univ 1973; **Resid:** Surgery, Duke Univ Med Ctr 1975; Surgery, Univ Miss Med Ctr 1980; **Fellow:** Cardiothoracic Surgery, MUSC Med Ctr 1982; **Fac Appt:** Prof S, NYU Sch Med

Plestis, Konstadinos MD (TS) - **Spec Exp:** Aneurysm-Thoracic Aortic; Heart Valve Surgery; Cardiac Surgery; Aneurysm-Abdominal Aortic; **Hospital:** Mount Sinai Med Ctr (page 98); **Address:** Mt Sinai Med Ctr, Dept Cardiothoracic Surg, 1190 5th Ave, Box 1028, New York, NY 10029; **Phone:** 212-241-8181; **Board Cert:** Surgery 2003; Vascular Surgery 1997; Thoracic Surgery 2000; **Med School:** Greece 1987; **Resid:** Surgery, Brooklyn Hosp Ctr 1993; Vascular Surgery, Baylor Univ Med Ctr 1995; **Fellow:** Cardiothoracic Surgery, Montefiore Med Ctr 1999; **Fac Appt:** Asst Prof S, Mount Sinai Sch Med

Rose, Eric A MD (TS) - **Spec Exp:** Transplant-Heart; Cardiothoracic Surgery; Ventricular Assist Device (LVAD); **Hospital:** NY-Presby Hosp (page 100), Saint Michael's Med Ctr; **Address:** 177 Fort Washington Ave, Ste 7-435, New York, NY 10032; **Phone:** 212-305-6380; **Board Cert:** Thoracic Surgery 2003; **Med School:** Columbia P&S 1975; **Resid:** Surgery, Columbia Presby Med Ctr 1979; Cardiothoracic Surgery, Columbia Presby Med Ctr 1981; **Fac Appt:** Prof S, Columbia P&S

Smith, Craig R MD (TS) - **Spec Exp:** Mitral Valve Surgery; Transplant-Heart; Minimally Invasive Cardiac Surgery; Robotic Heart Surgery; **Hospital:** NY-Presby Hosp (page 100); **Address:** 177 Fort Washington Ave, Ste 7-435, Columbia Presbyterian Med Ctr, New York, NY 10032; **Phone:** 212-305-8312; **Board Cert:** Thoracic Surgery 1996; **Med School:** Case West Res Univ 1977; **Resid:** Surgery, Strong Meml Hosp 1982; **Fellow:** Cardiothoracic Surgery, Columbia Presby Med Ctr 1984; **Fac Appt:** Prof S, Columbia P&S

Sonett, Joshua R MD (TS) - **Spec Exp:** Minimally Invasive Thoracic Surgery; Transplant-Lung; Thoracic Cancers; **Hospital:** NY-Presby Hosp (page 100); **Address:** 622 W 168th St Bldg PH Fl 14 - rm 104, New York, NY 10032; **Phone:** 212-305-8086; **Board Cert:** Surgery 1994; Thoracic Surgery 1997; **Med School:** E Carolina Univ 1988; **Resid:** Surgery, Univ Mass Med Ctr 1993; **Fellow:** Cardiothoracic Surgery, Univ Pittsburgh Med Ctr 1994; Thoracic Surgery, Meml Sloan Kettering Cancer Ctr; **Fac Appt:** Assoc Prof S, Columbia P&S

Spotnitz, Henry MD (TS) - **Spec Exp:** Pacemakers/Defibrillators; Heart Valve Surgery; **Hospital:** NY-Presby Hosp (page 100); **Address:** 622 W 168th St, rm 103, New York, NY 10032; **Phone:** 212-305-6191; **Board Cert:** Surgery 1974; Thoracic Surgery 1994; **Med School:** Columbia P&S 1966; **Resid:** Surgery, Columbia-Presby Med Ctr 1973; Thoracic Surgery, Columbia-Presby Med Ctr 1975; **Fellow:** Research, Natl Inst Hlth 1969; **Fac Appt:** Prof S, Columbia P&S

Steinglass, Kenneth MD (TS) - **Spec Exp:** Lung Cancer; Esophageal Cancer; Chest Wall Tumors; Thoracic Surgery; **Hospital:** NY-Presby Hosp (page 100), Nyack Hosp; **Address:** 161 Fort Washington Ave Fl 3 - Ste 322, New York, NY 10032-3713; **Phone:** 212-305-3408; **Board Cert:** Thoracic Surgery 1999; **Med School:** Harvard Med Sch 1972; **Resid:** Surgery, Columbia-Presby 1977; **Fellow:** Thoracic Surgery, Mayo Clinic 1979; **Fac Appt:** Clin Prof S, Columbia P&S

Stelzer, Paul MD (TS) - **Spec Exp:** Heart Valve Surgery; Aneurysm-Thoracic Aortic; Ross Procedure for Aortic Valve Disease; **Hospital:** Beth Israel Med Ctr - Petrie Division (page 90); **Address:** 317 E 17th St Fl 11, New York, NY 10003-3804; **Phone:** 212-420-2584; **Board Cert:** Surgery 1979; Thoracic Surgery 2002; **Med School:** Columbia P&S 1972; **Resid:** Surgery, St Luke's Roosevelt Hosp 1977; Thoracic Surgery, NY Hosp 1981; **Fac Appt:** Assoc Clin Prof TS, Albert Einstein Coll Med

Subramanian, Valavanur MD (TS) - **Spec Exp:** Minimally Invasive Cardiac Surgery; Coronary Artery Robotic Surgery; Cardiothoracic Surgery; **Hospital:** Lenox Hill Hosp (page 94); **Address:** 130 E 77th St, Fl 4, New York, NY 10021; **Phone:** 212-434-3000; **Board Cert:** Surgery 1972; Thoracic Surgery 1974; **Med School:** India 1962; **Resid:** Surgery, NY Hosp-Cornell 1972

Swanson, Scott J MD (TS) - **Spec Exp:** Lung Cancer; Video Assisted Thoracic Surgery (VATS); Esophageal Cancer; **Hospital:** Mount Sinai Med Ctr (page 98); **Address:** 1190 Fifth Ave GP2W Box 1028, New York, NY 10029-6503; **Phone:** 212-659-6815; **Board Cert:** Surgery 1991; Thoracic Surgery 1996; **Med School:** Harvard Med Sch 1985; **Resid:** Surgery, Brigham & Womens Hosp 1990; **Fellow:** Cardiothoracic Surgery, Brigham & Womens Hosp 1994

Swistel, Daniel MD (TS) - **Spec Exp:** Coronary Artery Surgery; Minimally Invasive Surgery; Heart Valve Surgery; **Hospital:** St Luke's - Roosevelt Hosp Ctr - Roosevelt Div (page 90); **Address:** 1111 Amsterdam Ave, MU2 Section A, New York, NY 10025-8106; **Phone:** 212-523-2705; **Board Cert:** Thoracic Surgery 1998; **Med School:** UMDNJ-RW Johnson Med Sch 1979; **Resid:** Surgery, St Lukes-Roosevelt Hosp 1984; Cardiothoracic Surgery, Montefiore Med Ctr 1986; **Fac Appt:** Assoc Clin Prof TS, Columbia P&S

Tortolani, Anthony J MD (TS) - **Spec Exp:** Transfusion Free Cardiac Surgery; Heart Valve Surgery; Coronary Artery Surgery; **Hospital:** NY-Presby Hosp (page 100), New York Methodist Hosp (page 479); **Address:** NY Presby Hosp, Dept Cardiothoracic Surg, 525 E 68th St, rm M-404, New York, NY 10021-4870; **Phone:** 212-746-5155; **Board Cert:** Surgery 1975; Thoracic Surgery 1999; **Med School:** Geo Wash Univ 1969; **Resid:** Surgery, N Shore Univ Hosp 1974; **Fellow:** Cardiothoracic Surgery, NYU Med Ctr 1978

Tranbaugh, Robert MD (TS) - **Spec Exp:** Coronary Artery Surgery; Heart Valve Surgery; Aneurysm; **Hospital:** Beth Israel Med Ctr - Petrie Division (page 90); **Address:** 317 E 17th St Fl 11, New York, NY 10003; **Phone:** 212-420-2584; **Board Cert:** Thoracic Surgery 2005; **Med School:** Univ Pennsylvania 1976; **Resid:** Surgery, UCSF Med Ctr 1983; Cardiothoracic Surgery, UCSF Med Ctr 1985; **Fac Appt:** Assoc Prof TS, Albert Einstein Coll Med

Waters, Paul F MD (TS) - **Spec Exp:** Lung Cancer; Esophageal Surgery; Thoracic Cancers; Transplant-Lung; **Hospital:** St Vincent Cath Med Ctrs - Manhattan (page 375), Greenwich Hosp; **Address:** St Vincent Hosp Med Ctr, 170 W 12th St Cronin Bldg - rm 817, New York, NY 10011; **Phone:** 212-604-7179; **Board Cert:** Surgery 2004; **Med School:** Univ Toronto 1974; **Resid:** Surgery, Univ Toronto Med Ctr 1979; Thoracic Surgery, Univ Toronto Med Ctr 1980; **Fellow:** Esophageal Surgery, Univ Chicago Hosps 1981

UROLOGY

Armenakas, Noel MD (U) - **Spec Exp:** Genitourinary Reconstruction; Erectile Dysfunction; **Hospital:** Lenox Hill Hosp (page 94), NY-Presby Hosp (page 100); **Address:** 880 5th Ave, New York, NY 10021-4951; **Phone:** 212-535-1950; **Board Cert:** Urology 1994; **Med School:** Greece 1985; **Resid:** Urology, Lenox Hill Hosp 1991; **Fellow:** Trauma, UCSF Med Ctr 1992; **Fac Appt:** Assoc Clin Prof U, Cornell Univ-Weill Med Coll

Bar-Chama, Natan MD (U) - **Spec Exp:** Infertility-Male; Erectile Dysfunction; Microsurgery; **Hospital:** Mount Sinai Med Ctr (page 98); **Address:** 5 E 98th St, Box 1272, New York, NY 10029-6501; **Phone:** 212-241-7443; **Board Cert:** Urology 1996; **Med School:** Albert Einstein Coll Med 1987; **Resid:** Urology, Montefiore/Albert Einstein 1993; **Fellow:** Urology, Baylor Coll Med 1994; **Fac Appt:** Assoc Prof U, Mount Sinai Sch Med

Benson, Mitchell C MD (U) - **Spec Exp:** Prostate Cancer/Robotic Surgery; Bladder Cancer; Kidney Cancer; **Hospital:** NY-Presby Hosp (page 100); **Address:** NY Presby Hosp-Columbia, Dept Urology, 161 Ft Washington Ave Fl 11 - rm 1102, New York, NY 10032-3713; **Phone:** 212-305-5201; **Board Cert:** Urology 1984; **Med School:** Columbia P&S 1977; **Resid:** Surgery, Mount Sinai Med Ctr 1979; Urology, Columbia-Presby Hosp 1982; **Fellow:** Oncology, Johns Hopkins Hosp 1984; **Fac Appt:** Prof U, Columbia P&S

Berman, Steven MD (U) - **Spec Exp:** Prostate Cancer; Kidney Stones; **Hospital:** Beth Israel Med Ctr - Petrie Division (page 90), St Vincent Cath Med Ctrs - Manhattan (page 375); **Address:** 55 E 9th St, New York, NY 10003-6399; **Phone:** 212-673-7300; **Board Cert:** Urology 1998; **Med School:** SUNY Downstate 1981; **Resid:** Urology, Montefiore Hosp Med Ctr 1981

Birkhoff, John MD (U) - **Spec Exp:** Urologic Cancer; Kidney Stones; **Hospital:** NY-Presby Hosp (page 100); **Address:** 161 Fort Washington Ave, rm 347, New York, NY 10032-3713; **Phone:** 212-305-5421; **Board Cert:** Urology 1976; **Med School:** Columbia P&S 1969; **Resid:** Urology, Columbia-Presby 1975; **Fac Appt:** Asst Clin Prof Med, Columbia P&S

Birns, Douglas MD (U) - **Spec Exp:** Prostate Cancer; Kidney Cancer; Bladder Cancer; **Hospital:** Mount Sinai Med Ctr (page 98), Beth Israel Med Ctr - Petrie Division (page 90); **Address:** 157 E 72nd St, New York, NY 10021-4331; **Phone:** 212-744-8700; **Board Cert:** Urology 1998; **Med School:** SUNY Downstate 1981; **Resid:** Surgery, Mount Sinai Hosp 1982; Urology, Mount Sinai Hosp 1986; **Fac Appt:** Asst Clin Prof U, Mount Sinai Sch Med

Blaivas, Jerry G MD (U) - **Spec Exp:** Uro-Gynecology; Urology-Female; Neurogenic Bladder; Incontinence after Prostate Cancer; **Hospital:** NY-Presby Hosp (page 100), Lenox Hill Hosp (page 94); **Address:** 445 E 77th St, New York, NY 10021; **Phone:** 212-772-3900; **Board Cert:** Urology 1978; **Med School:** Tufts Univ 1964; **Resid:** Surgery, Boston Med Ctr 1971; Urology, New England Med Ctr 1976; **Fac Appt:** Clin Prof U, Cornell Univ-Weill Med Coll

Boczko, Stanley MD (U) - **Spec Exp:** Prostate Cancer; Impotence; Prostate Disease; **Hospital:** Montefiore Med Ctr, Lenox Hill Hosp (page 94); **Address:** 23 E 79th St, New York, NY 10021; **Phone:** 212-628-1800; **Board Cert:** Urology 1980; **Med School:** Albert Einstein Coll Med 1973; **Resid:** Urology, Montefiore Med Ctr 1979; **Fellow:** Transplant Surgery, Montefiore Med Ctr 1975

Brodherson, Michael MD (U) - **Spec Exp:** Urologic Cancer; Kidney Stones; **Hospital:** Lenox Hill Hosp (page 94), Cabrini Med Ctr (page 374); **Address:** 4 E 76th St, New York, NY 10021-2611; **Phone:** 212-794-2749; **Board Cert:** Urology 1981; **Med School:** SUNY Downstate 1973; **Resid:** Internal Medicine, Lenox Hill Hosp 1976; Urology, Lenox Hill Hosp 1979

Davis, Joseph E MD (U) - **Spec Exp:** Prostate Surgery; Minimally Invasive Surgery; **Hospital:** Cabrini Med Ctr (page 374); **Address:** 120 E 34th St Fl 1, New York, NY 10022-1663; **Phone:** 212-686-1140; **Board Cert:** Urology 1964; **Med School:** NY Med Coll 1953; **Resid:** Surgery, Flower Fifth Ave Hosps 1955; Urology, Bellevue Hosp 1960; **Fac Appt:** Clin Prof U, NYU Sch Med

Dillon, Robert MD (U) - **Spec Exp:** Kidney Stones; Urologic Cancer; Urology-Female; **Hospital:** Mount Sinai Med Ctr (page 98), Lenox Hill Hosp (page 94); **Address:** 58-A E 79th St, New York, NY 10021-4331; **Phone:** 212-794-9000; **Board Cert:** Urology 1980; **Med School:** NY Med Coll 1973; **Resid:** Surgery, Mt Sinai Hosp 1975; Urology, Mt Sinai Hosp 1978; **Fac Appt:** Asst Clin Prof U, Mount Sinai Sch Med

Droller, Michael J MD (U) - **Spec Exp:** Urologic Cancer; Bladder Cancer; Prostate Cancer; Kidney Cancer; **Hospital:** Mount Sinai Med Ctr (page 98); **Address:** 5 E 98th St Fl 6th, Box 1272, New York, NY 10029-6501; **Phone:** 212-241-3868; **Board Cert:** Urology 2001; **Med School:** Harvard Med Sch 1968; **Resid:** Surgery, Peter Bent Brigham Hosp 1970; Urology, Stanford Univ Med Ctr 1976; **Fellow:** Immunology, Univ Stockholm 1977; **Fac Appt:** Prof U, Mount Sinai Sch Med

Eid, Jean Francois MD (U) - **Spec Exp:** Erectile Dysfunction; Urological Prosthesis; Incontinence; **Hospital:** NY-Presby Hosp (page 100); **Address:** 50 E 69th St, New York, NY 10021; **Phone:** 212-535-6690; **Board Cert:** Urology 1999; **Med School:** Cornell Univ-Weill Med Coll 1982; **Resid:** Surgery, New York Hosp-Cornell Med Ctr 1984; Urology, New York Hosp-Cornell Med Ctr 1988; **Fac Appt:** Assoc Clin Prof U, Cornell Univ-Weill Med Coll

Fine, Eugene M MD (U) - **Spec Exp:** Prostate Cancer; Kidney Stones; Erectile Dysfunction; **Hospital:** Mount Sinai Med Ctr (page 98), Beth Israel Med Ctr - Petrie Division (page 90); **Address:** 12 E 86th St, New York, NY 10028; **Phone:** 212-517-9555; **Board Cert:** Urology 1997; **Med School:** Mexico 1978; **Resid:** Surgery, Univ Hosp 1981; Urology, Mount Sinai Hosp 1985; **Fac Appt:** Asst Clin Prof U, Mount Sinai Sch Med

Fisch, Harry MD (U) - **Spec Exp:** Infertility-Male; Microsurgery; Vasectomy Reversal; **Hospital:** NY-Presby Hosp (page 100), Mount Sinai Med Ctr (page 98); **Address:** 944 Park Ave, Ste 1C, New York, NY 10028; **Phone:** 212-879-0800; **Board Cert:** Urology 1999; **Med School:** Mount Sinai Sch Med 1983; **Resid:** Surgery, Montefiore Hosp Med Ctr 1985; Urology, Montefiore Hosp Med Ctr 1989; **Fac Appt:** Prof U, Columbia P&S

Fracchia, John MD (U) - **Spec Exp:** Urologic Cancer; **Hospital:** Lenox Hill Hosp (page 94), NY-Presby Hosp (page 100); **Address:** 955 Park Ave, New York, NY 10028; **Phone:** 212-570-6800; **Board Cert:** Urology 1981; **Med School:** UMDNJ-NJ Med Sch, Newark 1973; **Resid:** Urology, NY Hosp-Cornell Med Ctr 1978; **Fac Appt:** Assoc Clin Prof S, Cornell Univ-Weill Med Coll

Furey, Robert J MD (U) - **Spec Exp:** Urologic Cancer; Kidney Stones; Trauma; **Hospital:** St Vincent Cath Med Ctrs - Manhattan (page 375); **Address:** 170 W 12 St, Cronin 205, New York, NY 10011; **Phone:** 212-604-1286; **Board Cert:** Urology 1978; **Med School:** NY Med Coll 1962; **Resid:** Surgery, St Vincent's Hosp 1967; Urology, Roosevelt Hosp 1970; **Fac Appt:** Asst Clin Prof U, NY Med Coll

Georgsson, Sverrir MD (U) - **Hospital:** St Vincent Cath Med Ctrs - Manhattan (page 375); **Address:** 36 7th Ave, Ste 505, New York, NY 10011-6600; **Phone:** 212-675-5828; **Board Cert:** Urology 1972; **Med School:** Iceland 1962; **Resid:** Urology, New York Hosp 1968; Urology, Yale-New Haven Hosp 1969; **Fac Appt:** Assoc Clin Prof U, NY Med Coll

Glassberg, Kenneth MD (U) - **Spec Exp:** Pediatric Urology; Genital Reconstruction; Varicocele in Adolescents; **Hospital:** NY-Presby Hosp (page 100); **Address:** Morgan Stanley Chlds Hosp of NY-Presby, 3959 Broadway, BHN 1116, New York, NY 10032; **Phone:** 212-305-9918; **Board Cert:** Urology 1977; **Med School:** SUNY Downstate 1968; **Resid:** Surgery, Montefiore Hosp Med Ctr 1972; Urology, Univ Hosp 1975; **Fellow:** Pediatric Urology, Adler Hey Chldns Hosp 1976; Pediatric Urology, Hosp For Sick Chldn 1976; **Fac Appt:** Prof U, Columbia P&S

Goldstein, Marc MD (U) - **Spec Exp:** Infertility-Male; Vasectomy Reversal; Varicocele Microsurgery; Vasectomy-Scalpelless; **Hospital:** NY-Presby Hosp (page 100); **Address:** Cornell Inst for Reproductive Med, 525 E 68th St, Box 580, New York, NY 10021; **Phone:** 212-746-5470; **Board Cert:** Urology 1982; **Med School:** SUNY Downstate 1972; **Resid:** Surgery, Columbia-Presby Med Ctr 1974; Urology, SUNY Downstate Med Ctr 1980; **Fellow:** Microsurgery, Rockefeller Univ 1982; **Fac Appt:** Prof U, Cornell Univ-Weill Med Coll

Golimbu, Mircea N MD (U) - **Spec Exp:** Kidney Stones; Prostate Cancer; Prostate Benign Disease; **Hospital:** NYU Med Ctr (page 102), Cabrini Med Ctr (page 374); **Address:** 530 1st Ave, rm 3D, New York, NY 10016; **Phone:** 212-263-7327; **Board Cert:** Urology 1975; **Med School:** Romania 1963; **Resid:** Urology, NYU Med Ctr 1973; **Fellow:** Urology, NY Academy Med 1975; **Fac Appt:** Clin Prof U, NYU Sch Med

Grasso, Michael MD (U) - **Spec Exp:** Urologic Cancer; Laparoscopic Surgery; Kidney Stones; **Hospital:** St Vincent Cath Med Ctrs - Manhattan (page 375); **Address:** 170 W 12th St, Ste 205, Dept Urology - Cronin 205, New York, NY 10011; **Phone:** 212-604-1270; **Board Cert:** Urology 2002; **Med School:** Jefferson Med Coll 1986; **Resid:** Surgery, Jefferson Univ Hosp 1988; Urology, Jefferson Univ Hosp 1992; **Fac Appt:** Prof U, NY Med Coll

Gribetz, Michael MD (U) - **Spec Exp:** Prostate Disease; Urology-Female; Sexual Dysfunction; Kidney Stones; **Hospital:** Mount Sinai Med Ctr (page 98); **Address:** 1155 Park Ave, New York, NY 10128-1209; **Phone:** 212-831-1300; **Board Cert:** Urology 1980; **Med School:** Albert Einstein Coll Med 1973; **Resid:** Surgery, Montefiore Hosp Med Ctr 1975; Urology, Mount Sinai Hosp 1978; **Fac Appt:** Asst Clin Prof U, Mount Sinai Sch Med

Hall, Simon J MD (U) - **Spec Exp:** Urologic Cancer; Minimally Invasive Urologic Surgery; **Hospital:** Mount Sinai Med Ctr (page 98); **Address:** Mount Sinai Medical Ctr, 1 Gustave L Levy Pl, Box 1272, New York, NY 10029; **Phone:** 212-241-8711; **Board Cert:** Urology 1999; **Med School:** Columbia P&S 1988; **Resid:** Surgery, Mt Sinai Med Ctr 1990; Urology, Boston Univ 1994; **Fellow:** Urology, Baylor Coll Med 1996; **Fac Appt:** Assoc Prof U, Mount Sinai Sch Med

Hensle, Terry MD (U) - **Spec Exp:** Pediatric Urology; **Hospital:** NY-Presby Hosp (page 100), Hackensack Univ Med Ctr (page 92); **Address:** Morgan Stanley Chldns Hosp of NY-Presby, 3959 Broadway, Ste 219N, New York, NY 10032; **Phone:** 212-305-8510; **Board Cert:** Urology 1978; **Med School:** Cornell Univ-Weill Med Coll 1968; **Resid:** Surgery, Boston City Hosp 1973; Urology, Mass Genl Hosp 1976; **Fellow:** Pediatric Urology, Mass Genl Hosp 1977; Pediatric Urology, Great Ormond St Hosp 1978; **Fac Appt:** Prof U, Columbia P&S

Herr, Harry W MD (U) - **Spec Exp:** Bladder Cancer; Prostate Cancer; Testicular Cancer; **Hospital:** Meml Sloan Kettering Cancer Ctr (page 109), NY-Presby Hosp (page 100); **Address:** Meml Sloan Kettering Canc Ctr, Dept Urol, 353 E 68th St, New York, NY 10021; **Phone:** 646-422-4411; **Board Cert:** Urology 1976; **Med School:** UCSF 1969; **Resid:** Urology, UC Irvine Med Ctr 1974; **Fellow:** Urology, Meml Sloan Kettering Cancer Ctr 1976; **Fac Appt:** Assoc Prof S, Cornell Univ-Weill Med Coll

Kaminetsky, Jed MD (U) - **Spec Exp:** Sexual Dysfunction; Prostate Cancer; Kidney Stones; **Hospital:** NYU Med Ctr (page 102), St Vincent Cath Med Ctrs - Manhattan (page 375); **Address:** 215 Lexington Ave Fl 20, New York, NY 10016; **Phone:** 212-686-9015; **Board Cert:** Urology 2000; **Med School:** NYU Sch Med 1984; **Resid:** Urology, NYU Med Ctr 1990; **Fac Appt:** Asst Clin Prof U, NYU Sch Med

Kaplan, Steven MD (U) - **Spec Exp:** Urodynamics; Voiding Dysfunction; Incontinence after Prostate Cancer; Incontinence; **Hospital:** NY-Presby Hosp (page 100); **Address:** NY Presbyterian-Weill Cornell Medical Ctr, 525 E 68th St, rm F9West, New York, NY 10021; **Phone:** 212-746-4811; **Board Cert:** Urology 2001; **Med School:** Mount Sinai Sch Med 1982; **Resid:** Surgery, Mount Sinai Hosp 1984; Urology, Columbia Presby Med Ctr 1988; **Fellow:** Urology, Columbia Presby Med Ctr 1990; **Fac Appt:** Prof U, Cornell Univ-Weill Med Coll

Katz, Aaron E MD (U) - **Spec Exp:** Prostate Cancer-Cryosurgery; Kidney Cancer-Cryosurgery; Complementary Medicine; **Hospital:** NY-Presby Hosp (page 100); **Address:** Columbia Presby Med Ctr, Herbert Irving Pav, 161 Ft Washington Ave Fl 11, New York, NY 10032; **Phone:** 212-305-6408; **Board Cert:** Urology 2006; **Med School:** NY Med Coll 1986; **Resid:** Urology, Maimonides Med Ctr 1992; **Fellow:** Urologic Oncology, Columbia Presby Med Ctr 1993; **Fac Appt:** Assoc Clin Prof U, Columbia P&S

Kirschenbaum, Alexander M MD (U) - **Spec Exp:** Prostate Cancer; Bladder Cancer; Kidney Cancer; **Hospital:** Mount Sinai Med Ctr (page 98); **Address:** 58A E 79th St, New York, NY 10021; **Phone:** 646-422-0926; **Board Cert:** Urology 2005; **Med School:** Mount Sinai Sch Med 1980; **Resid:** Surgery, Mount Sinai Hosp 1982; Urology, Mount Sinai Hosp 1985; **Fellow:** Urologic Oncology, Mount Sinai Hosp 1987; **Fac Appt:** Assoc Prof U, Mount Sinai Sch Med

Klein, George MD (U) - **Spec Exp:** Kidney Stones; Sexual Dysfunction; Prostate Cancer; **Hospital:** Mount Sinai Med Ctr (page 98), Lenox Hill Hosp (page 94); **Address:** 157 E 72nd St, Ground Fl, New York, NY 10021; **Phone:** 212-744-8700; **Board Cert:** Urology 1983; **Med School:** Cornell Univ-Weill Med Coll 1976; **Resid:** Surgery, North Shore Univ Hosp 1978; Urology, Mount Sinai Hosp 1981; **Fac Appt:** Asst Prof U, Mount Sinai Sch Med

Landman, Jaime MD (U) - **Spec Exp:** Minimally Invasive Urologic Surgery; Kidney Stones; Urologic Cancer; **Hospital:** NY-Presby Hosp (page 100); **Address:** 161 Fort Washington Ave Fl 11, New York, NY 10032; **Phone:** 212-305-0114; **Board Cert:** Urology 2003; **Med School:** Columbia P&S 1993; **Resid:** Urology, Mount Sinai Hosp 1999; **Fellow:** Urologic Laparoscopic Surgery-Endourology, Wash Univ Med Ctr 2001

Lepor, Herbert MD (U) - **Spec Exp:** Prostate Cancer; **Hospital:** NYU Med Ctr (page 102); **Address:** 150 E 32nd St Fl 2, New York, NY 10016; **Phone:** 646-825-6327; **Board Cert:** Urology 2005; **Med School:** Johns Hopkins Univ 1975; **Resid:** Urology, Johns Hopkins Hosp 1986; **Fac Appt:** Prof U, NYU Sch Med

Lizza, Eli MD (U) - **Spec Exp:** Impotence; Infertility-Male; **Hospital:** Lenox Hill Hosp (page 94), NY-Presby Hosp (page 100); **Address:** 955 Park Ave, New York, NY 10028; **Phone:** 212-772-3686; **Board Cert:** Urology 2006; **Med School:** UMDNJ-NJ Med Sch, Newark 1979; **Resid:** Surgery, Lenox Hill Hosp 1981; Urology, W VA Med Ctr 1984; **Fellow:** Infertility, Columbia Presby Med Ctr 1985; **Fac Appt:** Assoc Clin Prof U, UMDNJ-NJ Med Sch, Newark

Loo, Marcus Hsieu-Hong MD (U) - **Spec Exp:** Prostate Disease; Kidney Stones; Voiding Dysfunction; **Hospital:** NY-Presby Hosp (page 100); **Address:** 254 Canal St, Ste 3001, New York, NY 10013-3501; **Phone:** 212-925-8388; **Board Cert:** Urology 2000; **Med School:** Cornell Univ-Weill Med Coll 1981; **Resid:** Surgery, NY Hosp-Cornell Med Ctr 1983; Urology, NY Hosp-Cornell Med Ctr 1988; **Fellow:** Urology, NY Hosp-Cornell Med Ctr 1984; **Fac Appt:** Clin Prof U, Cornell Univ-Weill Med Coll

Lowe, Franklin MD (U) - **Spec Exp:** Prostate Disease; Complementary Medicine; Prostate Cancer; **Hospital:** St Luke's - Roosevelt Hosp Ctr - Roosevelt Div (page 90), NY-Presby Hosp (page 100); **Address:** 425 W 59th St, Ste 3A, New York, NY 10019; **Phone:** 212-523-7790; **Board Cert:** Urology 2005; **Med School:** Columbia P&S 1979; **Resid:** Surgery, Johns Hopkins Hosp 1981; Urology, Johns Hopkins Hosp 1984; **Fac Appt:** Clin Prof U, Columbia P&S

Marans, Hillel MD (U) - **Spec Exp:** Urologic Cancer; Urinary Tract Infections; Prostate Disease; **Hospital:** St Vincent Cath Med Ctrs - Manhattan (page 375), Beth Israel Med Ctr - Petrie Division (page 90); **Address:** 36 Seventh Ave, Ste 514, New York, NY 10011-6609; **Phone:** 212-206-9130; **Board Cert:** Urology 1998; **Med School:** Cornell Univ-Weill Med Coll 1980; **Resid:** Surgery, St Vincent's Hosp 1982; Urology, Albert Einstein-Montefiore Hosp 1985; **Fac Appt:** Asst Clin Prof U, NY Med Coll

Marks, Jon O MD (U) - **Spec Exp:** Kidney Stones; Interstitial Cystitis; **Hospital:** Beth Israel Med Ctr - Petrie Division (page 90); **Address:** 55 E 9th St, New York, NY 10003; **Phone:** 212-673-7300; **Board Cert:** Urology 1983; **Med School:** NY Med Coll 1976; **Resid:** Urology, Lenox Hill Hosp 1981

McGovern, Thomas P MD (U) - **Spec Exp:** Bladder Cancer; Prostate Cancer; **Hospital:** NY-Presby Hosp (page 100), Lenox Hill Hosp (page 94); **Address:** 927 5th Ave, New York, NY 10021; **Phone:** 212-772-7411; **Board Cert:** Urology 1983; **Med School:** Cornell Univ-Weill Med Coll 1974; **Resid:** Surgery, Mass Genl Hosp 1976; Urology, New York Hosp 1980; **Fac Appt:** Asst Clin Prof U, Cornell Univ-Weill Med Coll

McKiernan, James M MD (U) - **Spec Exp:** Urologic Cancer; Bladder Cancer; Prostate Cancer; **Hospital:** NY-Presby Hosp (page 100); **Address:** Dept Urology, 161 Fort Washington Ave Fl 11, New York, NY 10032; **Phone:** 212-305-0114; **Board Cert:** Urology 2003; **Med School:** Columbia P&S 1993; **Resid:** Surgery, Columbia Presby Med Ctr 1995; Urology, Columbia Presby Med Ctr 1999; **Fellow:** Urologic Oncology, Meml Sloan-Kettering Cancer Ctr 2001; **Fac Appt:** Asst Prof U, Columbia P&S

Mulhall, John P MD (U) - **Spec Exp:** Erectile Dysfunction; Peyronie's Disease; Penile Prostheses; **Hospital:** NY-Presby Hosp (page 100), Meml Sloan Kettering Cancer Ctr (page 109); **Address:** Weill Cornell Medical Ctr, 525 E 68th St, Box 94, New York, NY 10021; **Phone:** 212-746-5653; **Board Cert:** Urology 1999; **Med School:** Ireland 1985; **Resid:** Urology, Univ Conn Health Ctr 1994; **Fellow:** Urology, Boston Univ Med Ctr 1996; **Fac Appt:** Assoc Prof U, Cornell Univ-Weill Med Coll

Nagler, Harris M MD (U) - **Spec Exp:** Vasectomy Reversal; Infertility-Male; Varicocele Microsurgery; Erectile Dysfunction; **Hospital:** Beth Israel Med Ctr - Petrie Division (page 90); **Address:** Beth Israel Med Ctr, Dept Urology, 10 Union Square E, Ste 3A, New York, NY 10003; **Phone:** 212-844-8700; **Board Cert:** Urology 1982; **Med School:** Temple Univ 1975; **Resid:** Urology, Columbia Presby Hosp 1980; **Fellow:** Reproductive Medicine, Columbia Presby Hosp 1981; **Fac Appt:** Prof U, Albert Einstein Coll Med

Nitti, Victor MD (U) - **Spec Exp:** Urology-Female; Incontinence-Male & Female; Urodynamics; Voiding Dysfunction; **Hospital:** NYU Med Ctr (page 102); **Address:** 150 E 32nd St, Ste 200, New York, NY 10016; **Phone:** 646-825-6324; **Board Cert:** Urology 2002; **Med School:** UMDNJ-NJ Med Sch, Newark 1985; **Resid:** Surgery, Univ Hosp 1987; Urology, Univ Hosp 1991; **Fellow:** Urology, UCLA Med Ctr 1992; **Fac Appt:** Assoc Prof U, NYU Sch Med

Peng, Benjamin MD (U) - **Spec Exp:** Prostate Disease; Kidney Stones; Urologic Cancer; **Hospital:** NY Downtown Hosp, St Vincent Cath Med Ctrs - Manhattan (page 375); **Address:** 168 Canal St, Ste 510, New York, NY 10013-4503; **Phone:** 212-226-2200; **Board Cert:** Urology 2001; **Med School:** Columbia P&S 1984; **Resid:** Surgery, Mount Sinai Hosp 1986; Urology, Columbia-Presby Hosp 1990; **Fac Appt:** Asst Clin Prof U, NYU Sch Med

Poppas, Dix P MD (U) - **Spec Exp:** Genital Reconstruction-Pediatric; Robotic Surgery-Pediatric; Minimally Invasive Surgery-Pediatric; **Hospital:** NY-Presby Hosp (page 100); **Address:** Inst for Ped Urol, NYPresby Hosp/Weill Cornell, 525 E 68th St, Box 94, New York, NY 10021-4870; **Phone:** 212-746-5337; **Board Cert:** Urology 1999; **Med School:** Eastern VA Med Sch 1988; **Resid:** Urology, New York Hosp-Cornell Med Ctr 1994; **Fellow:** Pediatric Urology, Children's Hosp 1996; **Fac Appt:** Assoc Prof U, Cornell Univ-Weill Med Coll

Provet, John MD (U) - **Spec Exp:** Urologic Cancer; Kidney Stones; Prostate Disease; **Hospital:** NYU Med Ctr (page 102); **Address:** 215 Lexington Ave, FL 20, New York, NY 10016; **Phone:** 212-686-9015; **Board Cert:** Urology 2000; **Med School:** NYU Sch Med 1983; **Resid:** Surgery, NYU/VA Med Ctr/Bellvue Hosp 1985; Urology, NYU/VA Med Ctr/Bellvue Hosp 1989; **Fellow:** Urologic Oncology, NY Academy Med 1990; **Fac Appt:** Assoc Clin Prof U, NYU Sch Med

Reckler, Jon M MD (U) - **Hospital:** NY-Presby Hosp (page 100), Lenox Hill Hosp (page 94); **Address:** 880 5th Ave, New York, NY 10021; **Phone:** 212-535-1950; **Board Cert:** Urology 1976; **Med School:** Harvard Med Sch 1966; **Resid:** Surgery, Univ Hosp 1968; Urology, Peter Bent Brigham Hosp 1974; **Fac Appt:** Clin Prof U, Cornell Univ-Weill Med Coll

Romas, Nicholas A MD (U) - **Spec Exp:** Prostate Disease; Prostate Cancer; Erectile Dysfunction; **Hospital:** St Luke's - Roosevelt Hosp Ctr - Roosevelt Div (page 90), NY-Presby Hosp (page 100); **Address:** 425 W 59th St, Ste 3A, New York, NY 10019-1104; **Phone:** 212-523-7788; **Board Cert:** Urology 1974; **Med School:** Columbia P&S 1962; **Resid:** Surgery, New York Hosp-Cornell 1964; Urology, Columbia-Presby Med Ctr 1968; **Fac Appt:** Clin Prof U, Columbia P&S

Russo, Paul MD (U) - **Spec Exp:** Kidney Cancer; Prostate Cancer; Penile Cancer; **Hospital:** Meml Sloan Kettering Cancer Ctr (page 109); **Address:** 1275 York Ave, New York, NY 10021; **Phone:** 646-422-4391; **Board Cert:** Urology 2004; **Med School:** Columbia P&S 1979; **Resid:** Urology, Barnes Hosp-Wash Univ 1984; **Fellow:** Urologic Oncology, Mem Sloan Kettering Cancer Ctr 1988; **Fac Appt:** Assoc Prof U, Cornell Univ-Weill Med Coll

Scardino, Peter T MD (U) - **Spec Exp:** Prostate Cancer; **Hospital:** Meml Sloan Kettering Cancer Ctr (page 109); **Address:** 1275 York Ave, Box 27, New York, NY 10021; **Phone:** 646-422-4329; **Board Cert:** Urology 1981; **Med School:** Duke Univ 1971; **Resid:** Surgery, Mass Genl Hosp 1973; Urology, UCLA Med Ctr 1979; **Fellow:** Urology, Natl Cancer Inst 1976; **Fac Appt:** Prof U, Cornell Univ-Weill Med Coll

Scherr, Douglas S MD (U) - **Spec Exp:** Prostate Cancer; **Hospital:** NY-Presby Hosp (page 100); **Address:** NY Cornell Medical Ctr, Dept Urology, 525 E 68th St Starr 900, New York, NY 10021; **Phone:** 212-746-5788; **Board Cert:** Urology 2003; **Med School:** Duke Univ 1994; **Resid:** Urology, NY Hosp-Cornell Med Ctr 1999; **Fellow:** Urologic Oncology, Meml Sloan-Kettering Canc Ctr 2002; **Fac Appt:** Asst Prof U, Cornell Univ-Weill Med Coll

Schiff, Howard MD (U) - **Spec Exp:** Incontinence-Female; Prostate Cancer & Disease; Kidney Stones; Minimally Invasive Surgery; **Hospital:** Mount Sinai Med Ctr (page 98), NY-Presby Hosp (page 100); **Address:** 1120 Park Ave, Ste 1E, New York, NY 10128-1242; **Phone:** 212-996-6660; **Board Cert:** Urology 1982; **Med School:** W VA Univ 1975; **Resid:** Surgery, Montefiore Hosp Med Ctr 1977; Urology, Mount Sinai Hosp 1980; **Fac Appt:** Asst Clin Prof U, Mount Sinai Sch Med

Schlegel, Peter MD (U) - **Spec Exp:** Prostate Cancer; Infertility-Male; Fertility Preservation in Cancer; **Hospital:** NY-Presby Hosp (page 100); **Address:** 525 E 68th St, Starr 900, New York, NY 10021-4870; **Phone:** 212-746-5491; **Board Cert:** Urology 2001; **Med School:** Univ Mass Sch Med 1983; **Resid:** Surgery, Johns Hopkins Hosp 1985; Urology, Johns Hopkins Hosp 1989; **Fellow:** Medical Oncology, Johns Hopkins Hosp 1987; Male Reproduction, New York Hosp-Cornell Med Ctr 1991; **Fac Appt:** Prof U, Cornell Univ-Weill Med Coll

Schlussel, Richard MD (U) - **Spec Exp:** Pediatric Urology; Hypospadias; Urologic Surgery; **Hospital:** NY-Presby Hosp (page 100), Englewood Hosp & Med Ctr (page 760); **Address:** Morgan Stanley Chldns Hosp of NY-Presby, 3959 Broadway, Urology, rm 1118, New York, NY 10032; **Phone:** 212-305-1114; **Board Cert:** Urology 1996; **Med School:** Albert Einstein Coll Med 1986; **Resid:** Urology, Mt Sinai Med Ctr 1992; **Fellow:** Urology, Harvard Univ/Chldns Hosp 1994; **Fac Appt:** Asst Prof U, Mount Sinai Sch Med

Shabsigh, Ridwan MD (U) - **Spec Exp:** Impotence; **Hospital:** NY-Presby Hosp (page 100); **Address:** 161 Fort Washington Ave, Ste 1123, New York, NY 10032; **Phone:** 212-305-0123; **Board Cert:** Urology 1992; **Med School:** Syria 1976; **Resid:** Urology, Baylor Med Ctr 1987; **Fellow:** Urology, Baylor Med Ctr 1990

Shapiro, Ellen MD (U) - **Spec Exp:** Pediatric Urology; **Hospital:** NYU Med Ctr (page 102), Hackensack Univ Med Ctr (page 92); **Address:** 150 E 32nd St Fl 2, New York, NY 10016; **Phone:** 646-825-6326; **Board Cert:** Urology 1998; **Med School:** Univ Nebr Coll Med 1978; **Resid:** Surgery, Johns Hopkins Hosp 1980; Urology, Johns Hopkins Hosp 1986; **Fellow:** Pediatric Urology, Chldns Hosp Michigan 1987; **Fac Appt:** Prof U, NYU Sch Med

Sheinfeld, Joel MD (U) - **Spec Exp:** Testicular Cancer; Bladder Cancer; Fertility Preservation in Cancer; **Hospital:** Meml Sloan Kettering Cancer Ctr (page 109); **Address:** Meml Sloan Kettering Canc Ctr-Kimmel Ctr, 1275 York Ave, New York, NY 10021-6007; **Phone:** 646-422-4311; **Board Cert:** Urology 2000; **Med School:** Univ Fla Coll Med 1981; **Resid:** Urology, Strong Meml Hosp 1986; **Fellow:** Urologic Oncology, Meml Sloan Kettering Cancer Ctr 1989; **Fac Appt:** Assoc Prof U, Cornell Univ-Weill Med Coll

Silva, Jose V MD (U) - **Spec Exp:** Urologic Cancer; **Hospital:** St Luke's - Roosevelt Hosp Ctr - Roosevelt Div (page 90), Montefiore Med Ctr; **Address:** 425 W 59th St Fl 3, New York, NY 10019; **Phone:** 212-582-3421; **Board Cert:** Urology 1983; **Med School:** India 1970; **Resid:** Surgery, Beth Israel Med Ctr 1978; Urology, St Luke's-Roosevelt Hosp Ctr 1981; **Fellow:** Surgery, Meml Sloan Kettering Cancer Ctr 1982

Sogani, Pramod MD (U) - **Spec Exp:** Prostate Cancer; Testicular Cancer; Bladder Cancer; Kidney Cancer; **Hospital:** Meml Sloan Kettering Cancer Ctr (page 109); **Address:** 1275 York Ave, New York, NY 10021-6007; **Phone:** 646-422-4395; **Board Cert:** Urology 1976; **Med School:** India 1960; **Resid:** Urology, NYU Med Ctr 1969; Urology, Geo Wash Univ Med Ctr 1971; **Fellow:** Surgical Oncology, Meml Sloan Kettering Cancer Ctr 1973; **Fac Appt:** Prof U, Cornell Univ-Weill Med Coll

Sosa, R Ernest MD (U) - **Spec Exp:** Kidney Stones; Laparoscopic Surgery; Adrenal Surgery; **Hospital:** NY-Presby Hosp (page 100), Lenox Hill Hosp (page 94); **Address:** 880 5th Ave, New York, NY 10021; **Phone:** 212-570-6800; **Board Cert:** Urology 2006; **Med School:** Cornell Univ-Weill Med Coll 1978; **Resid:** Surgery, New York Hosp-Cornell 1980; Urology, New York Hosp-Cornell 1984; **Fellow:** Renal Physiology, New York Hosp-Cornell 1986; **Fac Appt:** Assoc Clin Prof U, Cornell Univ-Weill Med Coll

Sperber, Alan B MD (U) - **Spec Exp:** Prostate Disease; Urinary Tract Infections; Urologic Cancer; **Hospital:** NYU Med Ctr (page 102), Cabrini Med Ctr (page 374); **Address:** 161 Madison Ave, Ste 7-SW, New York, NY 10016; **Phone:** 212-889-5256; **Board Cert:** Urology 1977; **Med School:** NYU Sch Med 1967; **Resid:** Surgery, Albert Einstein 1969; Urology, NYU Med Ctr 1975; **Fac Appt:** Assoc Clin Prof U, NYU Sch Med

Staskin, David R MD (U) - **Spec Exp:** Incontinence-Female; Urology-Female; Uro-Gynecology; **Hospital:** NY-Presby Hosp (page 100); **Address:** NY Presbyterian-NY Weill Cornell Med Ctr, 525 E 68th St, Ste F918, New York, NY 10021; **Phone:** 212-746-5414; **Board Cert:** Urology 1997; **Med School:** Hahnemann Univ 1979; **Resid:** Urology, Hosp U Penn 1984; **Fellow:** Female Urology, UCLA Medical Ctr 1985; **Fac Appt:** Assoc Prof U, Cornell Univ-Weill Med Coll

Taneja, Samir S MD (U) - **Spec Exp:** Kidney Cancer; Prostate Cancer; Urologic Cancer; Laparoscopic Surgery; **Hospital:** NYU Med Ctr (page 102); **Address:** 150 E 32nd St, Ste 200, New York, NY 10016; **Phone:** 646-825-6321; **Board Cert:** Urology 1999; **Med School:** Northwestern Univ 1990; **Resid:** Urology, UCLA Med Ctr 1996; **Fac Appt:** Assoc Prof U, NYU Sch Med

Te, Alexis E MD (U) - **Spec Exp:** Prostate Benign Disease; Prostate Surgery; Incontinence; **Hospital:** NY-Presby Hosp (page 100); **Address:** Weill Medical College, 525 E 68th St, Box 261, New York, NY 10021; **Phone:** 212-746-4811; **Board Cert:** Urology 1998; **Med School:** Cornell Univ-Weill Med Coll 1988; **Resid:** Urology, Ny Presbyterian-Columbia Presby Med Ctr 1993; **Fellow:** Urodynamics, NY Presbyterian-Columbia Presby Med Ctr 1994; **Fac Appt:** Assoc Prof U, Cornell Univ-Weill Med Coll

Tewari, Ashutosh MD (U) - **Spec Exp:** Prostate Cancer/Robotic Surgery; **Hospital:** NY-Presby Hosp (page 100); **Address:** Weill Cornell Brady Urologic Health Ct, 525 E 68th St, Starr 916, New York, NY 10021; **Phone:** 212-746-5638; **Med School:** India 1983; **Resid:** Surgery, GSVM Medical College 1990; Urology, Henry Ford Hosp 2003; **Fellow:** Transplant Surgery, Liverpool 1993; Urologic Oncology, Shands Healthcare 1995; **Fac Appt:** Assoc Prof U, Cornell Univ-Weill Med Coll

Vapnek, Jonathan M MD (U) - **Spec Exp:** Incontinence; Urology-Female; Neurogenic Bladder; **Hospital:** Mount Sinai Med Ctr (page 98); **Address:** 229 E 79th St, New York, NY 10021; **Phone:** 212-717-9500; **Board Cert:** Urology 2005; **Med School:** UCSD 1986; **Resid:** Surgery, UCSD Med Ctr 1988; Urology, UCSF 1992; **Fellow:** Urology, UC Davis 1993; **Fac Appt:** Assoc Clin Prof U, Mount Sinai Sch Med

Vaughan, Edwin D MD (U) - **Spec Exp:** Urologic Cancer; Adrenal Tumors; Prostate Disease; **Hospital:** NY-Presby Hosp (page 100), Meml Sloan Kettering Cancer Ctr (page 109); **Address:** New York Presby Hosp, Dept Urology, 525 E 68th St, Starr 900, Box 94, New York, NY 10021-4870; **Phone:** 212-746-5480; **Board Cert:** Urology 1986; **Med School:** Univ VA Sch Med 1965; **Resid:** Surgery, Vanderbilt Univ Med Ctr 1967; Urology, Univ Virginia Hosp 1971; **Fellow:** Internal Medicine, Columbia Univ 1973; **Fac Appt:** Prof U, Cornell Univ-Weill Med Coll

Williams, John J MD (U) - **Spec Exp:** Genitourinary Cancer; Prostate Disease; Kidney Stones; **Hospital:** NY-Presby Hosp (page 100), Lenox Hill Hosp (page 94); **Address:** 820 Park Ave, New York, NY 10021; **Phone:** 212-861-1100; **Board Cert:** Urology 1976; **Med School:** Georgetown Univ 1966; **Resid:** Surgery, Strong Meml Hosp 1968; Urology, NY Hosp 1974

Young, George Pei Herng MD (U) - **Spec Exp:** Incontinence-Female; Reconstructive Urology-Female; Urologic Cancer; Female Urology; **Hospital:** Lenox Hill Hosp (page 94), N Shore Univ Hosp at Manhasset; **Address:** 1060 Fifth Ave, New York, NY 10128; **Phone:** 212-876-9811; **Board Cert:** Urology 1997; **Med School:** Brazil 1983; **Resid:** Surgery, Staten Island Univ Hosp 1989; Urology, New York Hosp-Cornell 1993; **Fellow:** Microsurgery, Population Council, Rockefeller Univ 1985; Female Urology, UCLA Med Ctr 1994; **Fac Appt:** Assoc Prof U, Cornell Univ-Weill Med Coll

VASCULAR & INTERVENTIONAL RADIOLOGY

Brown, Karen T MD (VIR) - **Spec Exp:** Liver Cancer Chemoembolization; Uterine Fibroid Embolization; **Hospital:** Meml Sloan Kettering Cancer Ctr (page 109); **Address:** Memorial Sloan-Kettering Cancer Ctr, 1275 York Ave, rm H201, New York, NY 10021; **Phone:** 212-639-5882; **Board Cert:** Diagnostic Radiology 1984; Vascular & Interventional Radiology 2004; **Med School:** Boston Univ 1979; **Resid:** Radiology, Mass General Hosp 1984; **Fellow:** Vascular & Interventional Radiology, Mass General Hosp 1985; **Fac Appt:** Assoc Prof Rad, Cornell Univ-Weill Med Coll

Haskal, Ziv MD (VIR) - **Spec Exp:** Uterine Fibroid Embolization; Vascular Malformations; Liver Cancer/Chemoembolization; **Hospital:** NY-Presby Hosp (page 100); **Address:** Director, Div Interventional Radiology, 177 Fort Washington Ave, Ste 4-100, New York, NY 10032; **Phone:** 212-305-8070; **Board Cert:** Diagnostic Radiology 1991; Vascular & Interventional Radiology 1999; **Med School:** Boston Univ 1986; **Resid:** Diagnostic Radiology, UCSF Med Ctr 1991; **Fellow:** Vascular & Interventional Radiology, UCSF Med Ctr 1992; **Fac Appt:** Prof Rad, Columbia P&S

Neff, Richard A MD (VIR) - **Hospital:** St Vincent Cath Med Ctrs - Manhattan (page 375), Cabrini Med Ctr (page 374); **Address:** St Vincent Cath Med, Dep Interventional Radiology, 170 W 12th St, New York, NY 10011-8305; **Phone:** 212-604-8752; **Board Cert:** Diagnostic Radiology 1981; Vascular & Interventional Radiology 1997; **Med School:** Univ IL Coll Med 1977; **Resid:** Radiology, Columbia-Presby Med Ctr 1981; **Fellow:** Interventional Radiology, Columbia-Presby Med Ctr 1982

Rosen, Robert J MD (VIR) - **Spec Exp:** Vascular Malformations; **Hospital:** Lenox Hill Hosp (page 94); **Address:** 130 E 77th St Fl 9, New York, NY 10021; **Phone:** 212-434-2606; **Board Cert:** Diagnostic Radiology 1980; Vascular & Interventional Radiology 1996; **Med School:** Hahnemann Univ 1976; **Resid:** Diagnostic Radiology, Hahnemann Med Coll 1979; **Fellow:** Vascular & Interventional Radiology, Hosp U Penn 1980; **Fac Appt:** Assoc Prof Rad, NYU Sch Med

Weintraub, Joshua L MD (VIR) - **Hospital:** Mount Sinai Med Ctr (page 98); **Address:** Mount Sinai Medical Ctr, Dept Radiology, One Gustave L Levy Pl, Box 1234, New York, NY 10029; **Phone:** 212-241-7409; **Board Cert:** Diagnostic Radiology 1996; Vascular & Interventional Radiology 1998; **Med School:** Wayne State Univ 1991; **Resid:** Diagnostic Radiology, Beth Israel Hosp 1996; **Fellow:** Vascular & Interventional Radiology, Hosp U Penn 1997

VASCULAR SURGERY

Adelman, Mark MD (VascS) - **Spec Exp:** Carotid Artery Surgery; Aneurysm-Abdominal Aortic; Vein Disorders; Endovascular Surgery; **Hospital:** NYU Med Ctr (page 102), Bellevue Hosp Ctr; **Address:** 530 1st Ave, Ste 6F, New York, NY 10016-6402; **Phone:** 212-263-7311; **Board Cert:** Surgery 1999; Vascular Surgery 2001; **Med School:** NYU Sch Med 1985; **Resid:** Surgery, NYU Med Ctr 1990; **Fellow:** Vascular Surgery, NYU Med Ctr 1991; **Fac Appt:** Assoc Prof VascS, NYU Sch Med

Ahmed, Maher MD (VascS) - **Spec Exp:** Endovascular Surgery; Carotid Artery Surgery; Aneurysm-Aortic; **Hospital:** Lenox Hill Hosp (page 94); **Address:** 110 E 59th St, Ste 10C, New York, NY 10022; **Phone:** 212-583-2910; **Board Cert:** Surgery 1999; Vascular Surgery 2001; **Med School:** Egypt 1970; **Resid:** Surgery, Lenox Hill Hosp 1978; **Fellow:** Thoracic Surgery, St Vicents Hosp 1979; Vascular Surgery, Brooklyn Hosp 1980; **Fac Appt:** Asst Clin Prof S, SUNY Downstate

Benvenisty, Alan I MD (VascS) - **Spec Exp:** Peripheral Vascular Surgery; Endovascular Surgery; Transplant-Kidney; **Hospital:** St Luke's - Roosevelt Hosp Ctr - St Luke's Hosp (page 90), St Luke's - Roosevelt Hosp Ctr - Roosevelt Div (page 90); **Address:** 1090 Amsterdam Ave Fl 12, New York, NY 10025; **Phone:** 212-523-4706; **Board Cert:** Surgery 2004; Vascular Surgery 1999; **Med School:** Columbia P&S 1978; **Resid:** Surgery, Columbia-Presby Med Ctr 1983; **Fellow:** Vascular Surgery, Columbia-Presby Med Ctr 1984; Transplant Surgery, Columbia-Presby Med Ctr 1984; **Fac Appt:** Clin Prof S, Columbia P&S

Blumenthal, Jesse MD (VascS) - **Spec Exp:** Varicose Veins; Arterial Disease; **Hospital:** St Vincent Cath Med Ctrs - Manhattan (page 375); **Address:** 170 W 12th St Cronin Bldg - rm 811, New York, NY 10011-6609; **Phone:** 212-337-0600; **Board Cert:** Surgery 1967; **Med School:** Columbia P&S 1960; **Resid:** Surgery, St Luke's-Roosevelt Hosp Ctr 1965; Vascular Surgery, St Luke's-Roosevelt Hosp Ctr 1968; **Fac Appt:** Asst Clin Prof S, Mount Sinai Sch Med

Chideckel, Norman MD (VascS) - **Spec Exp:** Vein Disorders; Wound Healing/Care; **Hospital:** Beth Israel Med Ctr - Petrie Division (page 90); **Address:** 41 Fifth Ave, New York, NY 10003-4319; **Phone:** 212-473-1877; **Board Cert:** Surgery 1998; **Med School:** SUNY Downstate 1979; **Resid:** Surgery, Beth Israel Med Ctr 1984; **Fellow:** Vascular Surgery, Lutheran Med Ctr 1985; **Fac Appt:** Asst Clin Prof S, Albert Einstein Coll Med

Fantini, Gary A MD (VascS) - **Spec Exp:** Spinal Access Surgery; Vein Disorders; Wound Healing/Care; **Hospital:** Hosp For Special Surgery (page 108), NY-Presby Hosp (page 100); **Address:** 635 Madison Ave Fl 7, New York, NY 10022; **Phone:** 212-317-4550; **Board Cert:** Surgery 1999; Vascular Surgery 2000; **Med School:** Albert Einstein Coll Med 1983; **Resid:** Surgery, New York Hosp-Cornell Med Ctr 1989; **Fellow:** Vascular Surgery, UCSF Med Ctr 1990; **Fac Appt:** Assoc Prof S, Cornell Univ-Weill Med Coll

Giangola, Gary MD (VascS) - **Spec Exp:** Carotid Artery Surgery; Aneurysm-Aortic; Diabetic Leg/Foot; **Hospital:** Lenox Hill Hosp (page 94); **Address:** Dept Vascular Surg, 130 E 77th St, Black Hall Fl 13, New York, NY 10021; **Phone:** 212-434-4230; **Board Cert:** Surgery 1996; Vascular Surgery 1998; **Med School:** NYU Sch Med 1980; **Resid:** Surgery, NYU Med Ctr 1985; **Fellow:** Vascular Surgery, NYU Med Ctr 1986; **Fac Appt:** Assoc Clin Prof S, Columbia P&S

Green, Richard M MD (VascS) - **Spec Exp:** Aneurysm-Abdominal Aortic; Carotid Artery Surgery; Percutaneous Vascular Interventions; **Hospital:** Lenox Hill Hosp (page 94); **Address:** 130 E 77th St Fl 13, New York, NY 10021; **Phone:** 212-434-3420; **Board Cert:** Surgery 1993; Vascular Surgery 2003; **Med School:** Univ Rochester 1970; **Resid:** Surgery, Strong Meml Hosp 1976

Grossi, Robert MD (VascS) - **Spec Exp:** Carotid Artery Surgery; Aneurysm; Wound Healing/Care; **Hospital:** Cabrini Med Ctr (page 374), St Vincent Cath Med Ctrs - Manhattan (page 375); **Address:** 20 W 13th St, New York, NY 10011; **Phone:** 212-838-3055; **Board Cert:** Surgery 1995; Vascular Surgery 1996; **Med School:** UMDNJ-NJ Med Sch, Newark 1981; **Resid:** Surgery, St Vincent's Hosp 1986; **Fellow:** Vascular Surgery, Temple Univ Hosp 1987

Haimov, Moshe MD (VascS) - **Spec Exp:** Aneurysm-Aortic; Carotid Artery Surgery; Arterial Bypass Surgery; **Hospital:** Mount Sinai Med Ctr (page 98); **Address:** 12 E 97th St, Ste 1C, New York, NY 10029-6918; **Phone:** 212-289-3180; **Board Cert:** Surgery 1969; Vascular Surgery 1983; **Med School:** Israel 1962; **Resid:** Surgery, Mount Sinai 1968; **Fac Appt:** Clin Prof S, Mount Sinai Sch Med

Harrington, Elizabeth MD (VascS) - **Spec Exp:** Carotid Artery Surgery; Aneurysm-Aortic; Arterial Bypass Surgery-Leg; **Hospital:** Mount Sinai Med Ctr (page 98), Lenox Hill Hosp (page 94); **Address:** 1225 Park Ave, Ste 1D, New York, NY 10128-1758; **Phone:** 212-876-7400; **Board Cert:** Surgery 1999; Vascular Surgery 1997; **Med School:** NY Med Coll 1975; **Resid:** Surgery, Mount Sinai Hosp 1980; **Fellow:** Vascular Surgery, Mount Sinai Hosp 1981; **Fac Appt:** Assoc Prof VascS, Mount Sinai Sch Med

Harrington, Martin MD (VascS) - **Spec Exp:** Carotid Artery Surgery; Aneurysm-Aortic; Arterial Bypass Surgery-Leg; **Hospital:** Mount Sinai Med Ctr (page 98), Lenox Hill Hosp (page 94); **Address:** 1225 Park Ave, Ste 1D, New York, NY 10128-1758; **Phone:** 212-876-7400; **Board Cert:** Internal Medicine 1978; Hematology 1980; Surgery 1994; Vascular Surgery 1998; **Med School:** Harvard Med Sch 1975; **Resid:** Internal Medicine, St Luke's Roosevelt Hosp Ctr 1979; Surgery, Mt Sinai Hosp 1984; **Fellow:** Surgical Oncology, Meml Sloan Kettering Cancer Ctr 1986; Vascular Surgery, Mt Sinai Hosp 1989

Haveson, Stephen MD (VascS) - **Hospital:** Beth Israel Med Ctr - Petrie Division (page 90); **Address:** 306 E 15th St, New York, NY 10003; **Phone:** 212-529-2407; **Board Cert:** Surgery 1973; **Med School:** Albert Einstein Coll Med 1965; **Resid:** Surgery, Beth Israel Med Ctr 1972; **Fellow:** Vascular Surgery, NYU Med Ctr 1973; **Fac Appt:** Asst Clin Prof S, Albert Einstein Coll Med

Jacobowitz, Glenn R MD (VascS) - **Spec Exp:** Vein Disorders; Aneurysm-Abdominal Aortic; Lower Limb Arterial Disease; **Hospital:** NYU Med Ctr (page 102), Bellevue Hosp Ctr; **Address:** Schwartz Health Care Ctr, 530 First Ave, Ste 6F, New York, NY 10016; **Phone:** 212-263-7311; **Board Cert:** Surgery 1996; Vascular Surgery 1998; **Med School:** NYU Sch Med 1989; **Resid:** Surgery, NYU Med Ctr 1995; **Fellow:** Vascular Surgery, NYU Med Ctr 1996; **Fac Appt:** Assoc Prof VascS, NYU Sch Med

Kent, K Craig MD (VascS) - **Spec Exp:** Carotid Artery Surgery; Aneurysm-Abdominal Aortic; Lower Limb Arterial Disease; **Hospital:** NY-Presby Hosp (page 100), NY-Presby Hosp (page 100); **Address:** 530 E 70th St, rm M-014, New York, NY 10021-9800; **Phone:** 212-746-5192; **Board Cert:** Surgery 1997; Vascular Surgery 1998; **Med School:** UCSF 1981; **Resid:** Surgery, UCSF Med Ctr 1986; **Fellow:** Vascular Surgery, Brigham & Women's Hosp 1988; **Fac Appt:** Prof S, Cornell Univ-Weill Med Coll

Marin, Michael L MD (VascS) - **Spec Exp:** Aneurysm-Aortic; Carotid Artery Surgery; Limb Salvage; **Hospital:** Mount Sinai Med Ctr (page 98); **Address:** Mount Sinai Medical Ctr, 5 E 98th St, Box 1273, New York, NY 10029; **Phone:** 212-241-5392; **Board Cert:** Surgery 1999; **Med School:** Mount Sinai Sch Med 1984; **Resid:** Surgery, Columbia-Presby Med Ctr 1990; **Fellow:** Transplant Surgery, Columbia-Presby Med Ctr 1988; Vascular Surgery, Montefiore Med Ctr 1992; **Fac Appt:** Prof S, Mount Sinai Sch Med

Mendes, Donna MD (VascS) - **Spec Exp:** Limb Salvage; Varicose Veins; Aneurysm-Aortic; **Hospital:** St Luke's - Roosevelt Hosp Ctr - Roosevelt Div (page 90), Lenox Hill Hosp (page 94); **Address:** 1090 Amsterdam Ave, Ste 8F, New York, NY 10025; **Phone:** 212-636-4990; **Board Cert:** Surgery 2004; Vascular Surgery 1999; **Med School:** Columbia P&S 1977; **Resid:** Surgery, St Luke's-Roosevelt Hosp Ctr 1982; **Fellow:** Vascular Surgery, Englewood Hosp 1984; **Fac Appt:** Asst Clin Prof S, Columbia P&S

Nowygrod, Roman MD (VascS) - **Spec Exp:** Aneurysm; Carotid Artery Surgery; Endovascular Surgery; **Hospital:** NY-Presby Hosp (page 100); **Address:** 161 Ft Washington Ave, Irving Pavilion, New York, NY 10032-3713; **Phone:** 212-305-5374; **Board Cert:** Surgery 1998; Vascular Surgery 2002; **Med School:** Columbia P&S 1970; **Resid:** Surgery, Columbia-Presby Med Ctr 1976; **Fellow:** Vascular Surgery, Columbia-Presby Med Ctr 1978; **Fac Appt:** Prof S, Columbia P&S

Riles, Thomas MD (VascS) - **Spec Exp:** Aneurysm-Abdominal Aortic; Carotid Artery Surgery; **Hospital:** NYU Med Ctr (page 102); **Address:** NYU Med Ctr, Univ Vascular Assoc, 530 1st Ave, Ste 6F, New York, NY 10016; **Phone:** 212-263-6360; **Board Cert:** Vascular Surgery 2003; **Med School:** Baylor Coll Med 1969; **Resid:** Surgery, NYU Med Ctr 1976; **Fellow:** Vascular Surgery, NYU Med Ctr 1977; **Fac Appt:** Prof S, NYU Sch Med

Schanzer, Harry MD (VascS) - **Spec Exp:** Arterial Bypass Surgery-Leg; Vein Disorders; Carotid Artery Surgery; **Hospital:** Mount Sinai Med Ctr (page 98), Lenox Hill Hosp (page 94); **Address:** 993 Park Ave, New York, NY 10028-0809; **Phone:** 212-396-1254; **Board Cert:** Surgery 1988; Vascular Surgery 1994; **Med School:** Chile 1968; **Resid:** Surgery, Mount Sinai Hosp 1976; **Fellow:** Transplant Surgery, Mount Sinai Hosp 1974; **Fac Appt:** Clin Prof S, Mount Sinai Sch Med

Stein, Jeffrey S MD (VascS) - **Spec Exp:** Aneurysm-Aortic; Arterial Disease; Varicose Veins; **Hospital:** Mount Sinai Med Ctr (page 98), Lenox Hill Hosp (page 94); **Address:** 993 Park Ave, New York, NY 10028; **Phone:** 212-396-0500; **Board Cert:** Surgery 1997; Vascular Surgery 2002; Surgical Critical Care 2001; **Med School:** Washington Univ, St Louis 1982; **Resid:** Surgery, Mount Sinai Hosp 1988; **Fellow:** Surgical Critical Care, Mount Sinai Hosp 1989; Vascular Surgery, Mount Sinai Hosp 1990; **Fac Appt:** Asst Clin Prof S, Mount Sinai Sch Med

Todd, George MD (VascS) - **Spec Exp:** Minimally Invasive Vascular Surgery; Aneurysm-Abdominal Aortic; Carotid Artery Surgery; **Hospital:** St Luke's - Roosevelt Hosp Ctr - Roosevelt Div (page 90); **Address:** St Luke's-Roosevelt Hosp Ctr, Dept Surgery, 1000 10th Ave, rm 5G77, New York, NY 10019; **Phone:** 212-523-7481; **Board Cert:** Surgery 2000; Vascular Surgery 1995; **Med School:** Penn State Univ-Hershey Med Ctr 1974; **Resid:** Surgery, Columbia-Presby Med Ctr 1979; **Fellow:** Vascular Surgery, Columbia-Presby Med Ctr 1980; **Fac Appt:** Prof S, Columbia P&S

Regional Medical Centers
New York (Manhattan)

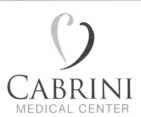

Cabrini Medical Center

227 East 19th Street
(between 2nd & 3rd Avenues)
New York, N.Y. 10003
212-995-6000

CABRINI
MEDICAL CENTER

CABRINI CARDIOVASCULAR DIVISION

INTEGRATED CARDIOVASCULAR IMAGING

Cabrini Medical Center has one of the most advanced and comprehensive integrated cardiovascular imaging programs in the nation. Using state-of-the-art cardiac magnetic resonance imaging (MRI) and computed tomography (CAT Scan) in conjunction with nuclear medicine and ultrasound, Cabrini physicians are able to accurately diagnose and treat many cardiovascular and pulmonary diseases in the most timely and efficient manner.

CLINICAL RESEARCH

Clinical trials of several innovative treatments of high blood pressure and early detection of coronary artery disease are currently underway. Cabrini is also actively involved with Chase Medical in the development of an endoventricular shaper (TRISVR) for performing surgical reshaping of the heart in patients with end stage ischemic cardiomyopathy.

TECHNOLOGY DEVELOPMENT

Advanced cardiac imaging software and protocols are currently being developed at Cabrini in collaboration with Siemens, Terarecon, and Chase Medical, Inc.

CLINICAL SERVICE

The Cardiology program at Cabrini Medical Center is actively involved in a collaborative effort with Mount Sinai School of Medicine in providing a full array of cardiology services to the community, including early and acute diagnosis of coronary artery disease using advanced imaging methods, rapid assessment and specialized treatment of congestive heart failure, the use of drug-eluting stents, implantable pacemakers and defibrillators, and chronic infusion therapy for severe pulmonary hypertension. The ongoing collaborations include the development of clinical and research programs in advanced cardiac imaging, atherosclerosis, congestive heart failure, implantable device-therapy, and pulmonary hypertension. The Cardiologists speak fluent Cantonese, Mandarin, Fuchow, Spanish and Ukranian.

Call us at 212-995-6865 to speak to a patient representative.

752

PHYSICIAN LEADERSHIP

Cabrini Medical Center is in the forefront of the New York metropolitan area for the early diagnosis and treatment of heart and vascular disease. Cabrini Medical Center physicians Michael Poon, MD, Director of Cardiology, Jurij Stecko, MD and Rose Marie Carrera, MD bring world-class cardiac diagnostic and treatment.

Dr. Poon is a leading expert in non-invasive cardiovascular magnetic resonance MRI and computed tomography (CT) imaging and in the treatment of coronary artery disease and pulmonary hypertension.

Dr. Stecko is a recognized expert in Cardiac CT imaging. Dr. Carrera specializes in cardiovascular ultra-sound imaging. Both Dr. Stecko and Dr. Carrera are experts in nuclear cardiology imaging.

For more information, visit our website at www. cabrininy.org

Saint Vincent Catholic Medical Centers

With a tradition of excellence that has spanned more than 150 years, we offer primary and preventive care as well as many of the finest specialty services in the city. We are committed to providing exceptional medical care while honoring the cultural diversity and dignity of our patients.

Academic Affiliation: We serve as the academic medical center for New York Medical College in New York City.

Our Hospitals: St. Vincent's Hospital Manhattan (212-604-7000) St. Vincent's Hospital Westchester (914-967-6500) **Affiliate:** St. Vincent's Midtown Hospital (212-459-8000)

Cancer Services: Our outpatient center offers IGRT, IMRT, HDR Brachytherapy, Respiratory Gating, Stereotactic Radiosurgery and seed implantation. We offer the latest in chemotherapy and drug treatments and have clinical trials available. Our treatment unit operates 24/7. We offer on-site PET/CT scans and the new SuperDimension/Bronchus System (SDBS) and Autoflorescence Bronchoscopy for earlier and safer diagnosis of lung cancer.

Cardiovascular Care: With several catheterization suites, a new electrophysiology laboratory, and new telemetry beds, our specialists work with the most advanced equipment. They routinely perform highly sophisticated procedures that produce long-lasting beneficial results. Because the symptoms for heart disease can be different for women than for men, our Women's Heart Program offers free education and screenings throughout the year.

Orthopedic Services: We offer one of the most highly advanced orthopedic programs in the city and treat the full spectrum of musculoskeletal problems, including arthritis, fractures and dislocations, hip and knee replacement, spine and sports injuries, and many more conditions.

Behavioral Health: We deliver inpatient and ambulatory services through our hospitals and outpatient facilities in Manhattan, Westchester and the Bronx. We offer one of the few inpatient programs for children in the city, a geriatric program that offers medical care and treatment for mental illness, inpatient and outpatient substance-abuse programs, and a bilingual, bicultural Latino treatment program.

Additional Centers of Excellence:

* Cystic Fibrosis * Emergency * Obstetrics and Gynecology * HIV/AIDS *
* Physical Medicine & Rehabilitation * Neonatology * Neurosurgery *
* General & Same-Day Surgery * Urology *

Outpatient Care: Our outpatient sites deliver medical, psychiatric and substance abuse services.

Home Health Agency: Traditional and long-term home healthcare throughout all five boroughs and in Westchester and Nassau Counties. Call 1-866-NURSE-28 for information or a referral.

Saint Vincent Catholic Medical Centers
1-800-CARE-421 www.svcmc.org

Bronx

Bronx County

ADDICTION PSYCHIATRY

Smith, Michael O MD (AdP) - **Spec Exp:** Addiction Medicine; Acupuncture; **Hospital:** Lincoln Med & Mental Hlth Ctr; **Address:** 349 E 140th St, Bronx, NY 10454; **Phone:** 718-993-3100 x113; **Med School:** UCSF 1968; **Resid:** Psychiatry, Albert Einstein Med Ctr 1972; **Fac Appt:** Assoc Prof Psyc, Cornell Univ-Weill Med Coll

ADOLESCENT MEDICINE

Alderman, Elizabeth MD (AM) - **Spec Exp:** Adolescent Gynecology; Eating Disorders; **Hospital:** Montefiore Med Ctr; **Address:** 111 E 210th St, rm NW 674, Adolescent Med, Bronx, NY 10467-2401; **Phone:** 718-920-6614; **Board Cert:** Pediatrics 2004; Adolescent Medicine 2002; **Med School:** SUNY Stony Brook 1987; **Resid:** Pediatrics, Einstein Coll Med/Montefiore Med Ctr 1990; **Fellow:** Adolescent Medicine, Montefiore Hosp Med Ctr 1992; **Fac Appt:** Clin Prof Ped, Albert Einstein Coll Med

Coupey, Susan MD (AM) - **Spec Exp:** Pediatric & Adolescent Gynecology; Eating Disorders; **Hospital:** Montefiore Med Ctr; **Address:** 111 E 210th St, Adolescent Med, Bronx, NY 10467-2490; **Phone:** 718-920-6781; **Board Cert:** Pediatrics 1979; Adolescent Medicine 2002; **Med School:** Canada 1975; **Resid:** Pediatrics, Chldns Hosp 1978; **Fellow:** Adolescent Medicine, Montefiore Hosp Med Ctr 1979; **Fac Appt:** Prof Ped, Albert Einstein Coll Med

ALLERGY & IMMUNOLOGY

Kaufman, Alan MD (A&I) - **Spec Exp:** Asthma; Sinus Disorders; Urticaria; **Hospital:** Our Lady of Mercy Med Ctr, Lawrence Hosp Ctr; **Address:** 3626 E Tremont Ave, Bronx, NY 10465-2030; **Phone:** 718-597-9000; **Board Cert:** Internal Medicine 1988; Allergy & Immunology 1999; **Med School:** West Indies 1984; **Resid:** Internal Medicine, Metropolitan Hosp Ctr 1987; **Fellow:** Allergy & Immunology, Albert Einstein Coll Med 1989

Lehach, Joan MD (A&I) - **Spec Exp:** Asthma; **Hospital:** St Barnabas Hosp - Bronx, Montefiore Med Ctr - Weiler-Einstein Div; **Address:** 1488 Metropolitan Ave, Ste 12, Bronx, NY 10462; **Phone:** 718-918-1991; **Board Cert:** Internal Medicine 2000; **Med School:** Chile 1985; **Resid:** Internal Medicine, St Barnabas Med Ctr 1988; **Fellow:** Allergy & Immunology, Albert Einstein Med Ctr 1990

Resnick, David MD (A&I) - **Spec Exp:** Asthma; Eczema; Nasal Allergies; **Hospital:** NY-Presby Hosp (page 100); **Address:** 3333 Henry Hudson Pkwy, Ste 1A, Riverdale, NY 10463; **Phone:** 718-796-9393; **Board Cert:** Allergy & Immunology 2001; Pediatrics 1998; **Med School:** SUNY Hlth Sci Ctr 1986; **Resid:** Pediatrics, Brookdale 1989; **Fellow:** Allergy & Immunology, Columbia-Presby 1991; **Fac Appt:** Assoc Clin Prof Ped, Columbia P&S

Rosenstreich, David MD (A&I) - **Spec Exp:** Urticaria; Sinusitis; Atopic Dermatitis; **Hospital:** Montefiore Med Ctr; **Address:** 1515 Blondell Ave, Fl 2 - Ste 220, Bronx, NY 10461; **Phone:** 866-633-8255; **Board Cert:** Internal Medicine 1972; Allergy & Immunology 1975; Clinical & Laboratory Immunology 1990; **Med School:** NYU Sch Med 1967; **Resid:** Internal Medicine, Albert Einstein Med Ctr 1969; **Fellow:** Allergy & Immunology, Natl Inst Hlth 1972; **Fac Appt:** Prof Med, Albert Einstein Coll Med

Rubinstein, Arye MD/PhD (A&I) - **Spec Exp:** Immune Deficiency; Asthma; Allergy; **Hospital:** Montefiore Med Ctr, Montefiore Med Ctr - Weiler-Einstein Div; **Address:** 1180 Morris Park Ave, Bronx, NY 10461-1925; **Phone:** 718-863-8465; **Board Cert:** Pediatrics 1976; Allergy & Immunology 1977; **Med School:** Switzerland 1962; **Resid:** Pediatrics, Tel Hashom Hosp 1967; **Fellow:** Allergy & Immunology, Univ Bern 1969; Allergy & Immunology, Harvard Med Sch 1973; **Fac Appt:** Prof Ped, Albert Einstein Coll Med

CARDIAC ELECTROPHYSIOLOGY

Fisher, John D MD (CE) - **Spec Exp:** Arrhythmias; Defibrillators; **Hospital:** Montefiore Med Ctr - Weiler-Einstein Div, N Central Bronx Hosp; **Address:** Arrhythmia Service, 111 E 210th St, Bronx, NY 10467; **Phone:** 718-920-4291; **Board Cert:** Internal Medicine 1972; Cardiovascular Disease 1975; Cardiac Electrophysiology 2002; **Med School:** Wayne State Univ 1969; **Resid:** Internal Medicine, Boston City Hosp 1971; Internal Medicine, NY Hosp-Cornell Med Ctr 1972; **Fellow:** Cardiovascular Disease, Montefiore Med Ctr 1975; Cardiovascular Disease, Hammersmith Hosp 1974; **Fac Appt:** Prof Med, Albert Einstein Coll Med

CARDIOVASCULAR DISEASE

Gordon, Garet M MD (Cv) - **Spec Exp:** Echocardiography; **Hospital:** Montefiore Med Ctr; **Address:** Montefiore Med Ctr, 111 E 210th St, Bronx, NY 10467-2401; **Phone:** 718-920-7638; **Board Cert:** Internal Medicine 1965; Cardiovascular Disease 1968; **Med School:** SUNY Hlth Sci Ctr 1958; **Resid:** Internal Medicine, Montefiore Med Ctr 1961; **Fellow:** Cardiovascular Disease, Montefiore Med Ctr 1962; **Fac Appt:** Assoc Prof, Albert Einstein Coll Med

Greenberg, Mark MD (Cv) - **Spec Exp:** Interventional Cardiology; Cardiac Catheterization; Cardiac Consultation; Ischemic Heart Disease; **Hospital:** Montefiore Med Ctr; **Address:** 111 E 210th St, 2nd Fl-Silver Zone, Bronx, NY 10467; **Phone:** 718-920-4212; **Board Cert:** Internal Medicine 1973; Cardiovascular Disease 1979; Interventional Cardiology 1999; **Med School:** Univ IL Coll Med 1973; **Resid:** Internal Medicine, Montefiore Hosp Med Ctr 1976; **Fellow:** Cardiovascular Disease, Montefiore Hosp Med Ctr 1978; **Fac Appt:** Clin Prof Med, Albert Einstein Coll Med

Keller, Peter Karl MD (Cv) - **Spec Exp:** Congestive Heart Failure; Coronary Artery Disease; **Hospital:** Montefiore Med Ctr - Weiler-Einstein Div, NY Westchester Sq Med Ctr; **Address:** 1578 Williamsbridge Rd, Bronx, NY 10461-6265; **Phone:** 718-892-7817; **Board Cert:** Internal Medicine 1988; Cardiovascular Disease 2001; **Med School:** Mount Sinai Sch Med 1985; **Resid:** Internal Medicine, Bronx Municipal Hosp 1988; **Fellow:** Cardiovascular Disease, Bronx Municipal Hosp 1991; **Fac Appt:** Assoc Clin Prof Med, Albert Einstein Coll Med

Kitsis, Richard N MD (Cv) - **Spec Exp:** Coronary Heart Disease; Heart Failure; **Hospital:** Montefiore Med Ctr - Weiler-Einstein Div; **Address:** Albert Einstein Coll Med, Div Cardiology, 1300 Morris Park Ave, rm G-46, Bronx, NY 10461-1926; **Phone:** 718-430-2609; **Board Cert:** Internal Medicine 1986; Cardiovascular Disease 1991; **Med School:** UCSF 1980; **Resid:** Internal Medicine, Mass Genl Hosp 1981; Internal Medicine, Boston VA Med Ctr 1987; **Fellow:** Cardiovascular Disease, Montefiore Med Ctr-WEiler Einstein Div 1991; **Fac Appt:** Prof Med, Albert Einstein Coll Med

Lucariello, Richard MD (Cv) - **Spec Exp:** Congestive Heart Failure; Angina; Hypertension; **Hospital:** Our Lady of Mercy Med Ctr; **Address:** 600 E 233 St, Bronx, NY 10466; **Phone:** 718-920-9256; **Board Cert:** Internal Medicine 1987; Cardiovascular Disease 2000; **Med School:** NY Med Coll 1984; **Resid:** Internal Medicine, Westchester Med Ctr 1987; **Fellow:** Cardiovascular Disease, St Vincent's Hosp & Med Ctr 1989; Cardiovascular Disease, Westchester Med Ctr 1990; **Fac Appt:** Assoc Clin Prof Med, NY Med Coll

Menegus, Mark MD (Cv) - **Spec Exp:** Coronary Angioplasty/Stents; Cardiac Catheterization; Interventional Cardiology; Cardiac Consultation; **Hospital:** Montefiore Med Ctr; **Address:** Montefiore Med Ctr, Dept Cardiology, 111 E 210th St, Bronx, NY 10467-2401; **Phone:** 718-920-5528; **Board Cert:** Internal Medicine 1984; Cardiovascular Disease 1987; Interventional Cardiology 1999; **Med School:** UMDNJ-RW Johnson Med Sch 1981; **Resid:** Internal Medicine, Montefiore Hosp Med Ctr 1984; **Fellow:** Cardiovascular Disease, Montefiore Hosp Med Ctr 1987; **Fac Appt:** Assoc Prof Med, Albert Einstein Coll Med

Monrad, E Scott MD (Cv) - **Spec Exp:** Coronary Artery Disease; Heart Valve Disease; Cardiac Catheterization; **Hospital:** Montefiore Med Ctr - Weiler-Einstein Div, Jacobi Med Ctr; **Address:** 1825 Eastchester Ave, Bronx, NY 10461; **Phone:** 718-904-2927; **Board Cert:** Internal Medicine 1982; Cardiovascular Disease 1985; Interventional Cardiology 1999; **Med School:** McGill Univ 1979; **Resid:** Internal Medicine, New England Med Ctr 1982; **Fellow:** Cardiovascular Disease, Beth Israel Med Ctr 1985; **Fac Appt:** Clin Prof Med, Albert Einstein Coll Med

Phillips, Malcolm MD (Cv) - **Spec Exp:** Preventive Cardiology; Echocardiography; Cardiac Stress Testing; **Hospital:** St Barnabas Hosp - Bronx; **Address:** 4422 3rd Ave, Bronx, NY 10457-2545; **Phone:** 718-960-6205; **Board Cert:** Internal Medicine 1980; Cardiovascular Disease 1982; **Med School:** Columbia P&S 1976; **Resid:** Internal Medicine, New York Hosp 1978; **Fellow:** Cardiovascular Disease, New York Hosp 1980; **Fac Appt:** Asst Clin Prof Med, Cornell Univ-Weill Med Coll

Scheuer, James MD (Cv) - **Spec Exp:** Coronary Artery Disease; Congestive Heart Failure; **Hospital:** Montefiore Med Ctr, Montefiore Med Ctr - Weiler-Einstein Div; **Address:** 111 E 210th St, N2, Bronx, NY 10467; **Phone:** 718-920-5979; **Board Cert:** Internal Medicine 1963; Cardiovascular Disease 1974; **Med School:** Yale Univ 1956; **Resid:** Internal Medicine, Bellevue Hosp 1957; Internal Medicine, Mount Sinai 1958; **Fellow:** Cardiovascular Disease, Mount Sinai 1959; Cardiovascular Disease, NY Hosp 1963; **Fac Appt:** Prof Med, Albert Einstein Coll Med

Schick, David MD (Cv) - **Hospital:** Montefiore Med Ctr; **Address:** 3201 Grand Concourse, Ste 1J, Bronx, NY 10468-1226; **Phone:** 718-933-2244; **Board Cert:** Internal Medicine 1972; Cardiovascular Disease 1975; **Med School:** Albert Einstein Coll Med 1966; **Resid:** Internal Medicine, Montefiore Hosp 1971; Cardiovascular Disease, Montefiore Hosp 1973; **Fac Appt:** Asst Clin Prof Med, Albert Einstein Coll Med

Silverman, Rubin MD (Cv) - **Spec Exp:** Echocardiography; Pacemakers; **Hospital:** Montefiore Med Ctr - Weiler-Einstein Div, St Barnabas Hosp - Bronx; **Address:** 1180 Morris Park Ave, FL 2, Bronx, NY 10461-1925; **Phone:** 718-409-3335; **Board Cert:** Internal Medicine 1981; Cardiovascular Disease 1983; **Med School:** Albert Einstein Coll Med 1978; **Resid:** Internal Medicine, Jacobi Med Ctr 1981; **Fellow:** Cardiovascular Disease, Montefiore Hosp Med Ctr 1983; **Fac Appt:** Asst Prof Med, Albert Einstein Coll Med

Sonnenblick, Edmund MD (Cv) - **Spec Exp:** Hypertension; Congestive Heart Failure; Coronary Artery Disease; **Hospital:** Montefiore Med Ctr - Weiler-Einstein Div, Mount Sinai Med Ctr (page 98); **Address:** Montefiore Med Ctr-Weiler-Einstein Div, Cardiology, 1825 Eastchester Rd, Bronx, NY 10461-2301; **Phone:** 718-904-2932; **Board Cert:** Internal Medicine 1968; **Med School:** Harvard Med Sch 1958; **Resid:** Internal Medicine, Columbia-Presby Med Ctr 1963; **Fellow:** Cardiovascular Disease, Natl Heart Inst 1967; **Fac Appt:** Prof Med, Albert Einstein Coll Med

Stampfer, Morris MD (Cv) - **Spec Exp:** Echocardiography; Cardiac Stress Testing; **Hospital:** Jacobi Med Ctr; **Address:** Jacobi Med Ctr, Cardiology Div, 1400 Pelham Pkwy S Bldg 1 - rm 5E-2, Bronx, NY 10461; **Phone:** 718-918-5900; **Board Cert:** Internal Medicine 1970; Cardiovascular Disease 1975; **Med School:** Albert Einstein Coll Med 1963; **Resid:** Internal Medicine, Jacobi Med Ctr 1965; **Fellow:** Cardiovascular Disease, Nat Inst Health 1968

CHILD NEUROLOGY

Rapin, Isabelle MD (ChiN) - **Spec Exp:** Autism; Developmental Disorders; Hearing Loss; **Hospital:** Montefiore Med Ctr - Weiler-Einstein Div; **Address:** 1515 Blondell Ave, Ste 220, Bronx, NY 10461-2601; **Phone:** 718-405-8140; **Board Cert:** Neurology 1960; Child Neurology 1968; Neurodevelopmental Disabilities 2001; **Med School:** Switzerland 1952; **Resid:** Neurology, Columbia-Presby Med Ctr 1957; **Fellow:** Child Neurology, Columbia-Presby Med Ctr 1958; **Fac Appt:** Prof N, Albert Einstein Coll Med

Shinnar, Shlomo MD/PhD (ChiN) - **Spec Exp:** Epilepsy/Seizure Disorders; Headache; **Hospital:** Montefiore Med Ctr; **Address:** Montefiore Medical Ctr, Pediatric Neurology, 111 E 210th St, Blue Zone, Ground Fl, Bronx, NY 10467-2401; **Phone:** 718-920-4378; **Board Cert:** Neurology 1984; Pediatrics 1984; Clinical Neurophysiology 1996; **Med School:** Albert Einstein Coll Med 1978; **Resid:** Pediatrics, Johns Hopkins Hosp 1980; Neurology, Johns Hopkins Hosp 1983; **Fac Appt:** Prof N, Albert Einstein Coll Med

CLINICAL GENETICS

Gross, Susan MD (CG) - **Spec Exp:** Prenatal Diagnosis; Prenatal Ultrasound; Reproductive Genetics; **Hospital:** Montefiore Med Ctr; **Address:** 1695 Eastchester Rd, Ste 301, Bronx, NY 10461; **Phone:** 718-405-8150; **Board Cert:** Clinical Genetics 1996; Obstetrics & Gynecology 1995; **Med School:** Univ Toronto 1985; **Resid:** Obstetrics & Gynecology, Univ Toronto Hosp 1991; **Fellow:** Maternal & Fetal Medicine, UNIv Toronto 1992; Clinical Genetics, Univ Tenn 1994; **Fac Appt:** Asst Prof CG, Albert Einstein Coll Med

Lieber, Ernest MD (CG) - **Spec Exp:** Neurofibromatosis; Marfan's Syndrome; **Hospital:** Lincoln Med & Mental Hlth Ctr, New York Methodist Hosp (page 479); **Address:** Lincoln Hosp - Dept Pediatrics, 234 S 149th St Fl 4 - rm 420, Bronx, NY 10451; **Phone:** 718-579-4695; **Board Cert:** Clinical Genetics 1984; **Med School:** Austria 1963; **Resid:** VA Med Ctr 1966; **Fellow:** Clinical Genetics, Mount Sinai Hosp 1969; Clinical Genetics, UCSF Med Ctr 1970; **Fac Appt:** Assoc Prof Ped, SUNY Hlth Sci Ctr

Marion, Robert MD (CG) - **Spec Exp:** Spina Bifida; Williams Syndrome; Marfan's Syndrome; Down Syndrome; **Hospital:** Montefiore Med Ctr, Blythedale Children's Hosp; **Address:** Montefiore Med Ctr, Dept Pediatrics, 111 E 210th St, Bronx, NY 10467-2401; **Phone:** 718-741-2323; **Board Cert:** Pediatrics 1985; Clinical Genetics 1987; **Med School:** Albert Einstein Coll Med 1979; **Resid:** Pediatrics, Montefiore Med Ctr 1982; **Fellow:** Clinical Genetics, Montefiore Med Ctr 1984; **Fac Appt:** Prof Ped, Albert Einstein Coll Med

CRITICAL CARE MEDICINE

Siegel, Robert MD (CCM) - **Spec Exp:** Pneumonia; Infectious Disease; **Hospital:** VA Med Ctr - Bronx, Mount Sinai Med Ctr (page 98); **Address:** 130 W Kingsbridge Rd, Ste 8C, Bronx, NY 10468-3992; **Phone:** 718-584-9000 x6723; **Board Cert:** Internal Medicine 1982; Pulmonary Disease 1986; Critical Care Medicine 1998; **Med School:** Columbia P&S 1979; **Resid:** Internal Medicine, St Luke's Hosp 1982; **Fellow:** Pulmonary Disease, Bronx Municipal Hosp 1985; **Fac Appt:** Assoc Clin Prof Med, Mount Sinai Sch Med

DERMATOLOGY

Burk, Peter MD (D) - **Spec Exp:** Pediatric Dermatology; Geriatric Dermatology; **Hospital:** Montefiore Med Ctr, Montefiore Med Ctr - Weiler-Einstein Div; **Address:** 2600 Netherland Ave, Ste 112, Riverdale, NY 10463; **Phone:** 718-543-7711; **Board Cert:** Dermatology 1974; **Med School:** Duke Univ 1966; **Resid:** Dermatology, Medical Coll oPenn 1968; Dermatology, Mass Genl Hosp 1973; **Fellow:** Dermatology, Natl Cancer Inst, NIH 1971; **Fac Appt:** Assoc Clin Prof Med, Albert Einstein Coll Med

Cohen, Steven R MD (D) - **Spec Exp:** Occupational Dermatology; Contact Dermatitis; Dermatologic Pharmacology; Psoriasis; **Hospital:** Montefiore Med Ctr; **Address:** 111 E 210 St, Bronx, NY 10467; **Phone:** 718-409-8923; **Board Cert:** Dermatology 1978; **Med School:** Univ Pennsylvania 1971; **Resid:** Dermatology, Yale-New Haven Hosp 1977; **Fac Appt:** Prof D, Albert Einstein Coll Med

Katz, Susan MD (D) - **Spec Exp:** Psoriasis; Skin Cancer & Moles; Cutaneous Lymphoma; **Hospital:** Montefiore Med Ctr; **Address:** 1578 Williamsbridge Rd, Bronx, NY 10461-6265; **Phone:** 718-518-8888; **Board Cert:** Dermatology 1983; **Med School:** NYU Sch Med 1977; **Resid:** Internal Medicine, Roosevelt Hosp 1979; Dermatology, Montefiore Hosp Med Ctr 1983; **Fac Appt:** Asst Clin Prof D, Albert Einstein Coll Med

Liteplo, Ronald MD (D) - **Spec Exp:** Melanoma; Skin Diseases-Immunologic; **Hospital:** Montefiore Med Ctr; **Address:** 3176 Bainbridge Ave, Bronx, NY 10467-3980; **Phone:** 718-515-0200; **Board Cert:** Internal Medicine 1975; Dermatology 1978; **Med School:** NYU Sch Med 1972; **Resid:** Internal Medicine, Univ Hosp 1975; Dermatology, Univ Hosp 1978; **Fellow:** Immunology, Univ Hosp 1976; **Fac Appt:** Asst Clin Prof Med, Albert Einstein Coll Med

O'Connor, Kathleen MD (D) - **Spec Exp:** Skin Cancer; Eczema; **Hospital:** Montefiore Med Ctr, Montefiore Med Ctr - Weiler-Einstein Div; **Address:** 1578 Williamsbridge Rd, Bronx, NY 10461; **Phone:** 718-518-8888; **Board Cert:** Dermatology 1975; **Med School:** Ireland 1965; **Resid:** Internal Medicine, Elmhurst Hosp 1968; Dermatology, Bronx Muni Hosp-Einstein 1974; **Fac Appt:** Asst Clin Prof D, Albert Einstein Coll Med

Rosen, Douglas MD (D) - **Spec Exp:** Skin Cancer; Hair Removal-Laser; Acne; **Hospital:** NY Westchester Sq Med Ctr; **Address:** 3620 E Tremont Ave, FL 2, Bronx, NY 10465-2022; **Phone:** 718-792-4700; **Board Cert:** Dermatology 1984; **Med School:** Albert Einstein Coll Med 1980; **Resid:** Dermatology, Montefiore Hosp Med Ctr 1984; **Fac Appt:** Assoc Prof D, Albert Einstein Coll Med

Rudikoff, Donald MD (D) - **Spec Exp:** AIDS Related Skin Disorders; Skin Infections; Smallpox; **Hospital:** Bronx Lebanon Hosp Ctr; **Address:** 1650 Selwyn Ave, Bronx, NY 10457; **Phone:** 718-960-1328; **Board Cert:** Internal Medicine 1980; Dermatology 1983; **Med School:** NY Med Coll 1973; **Resid:** Internal Medicine, Beth Israel Med Ctr 1980; Dermatology, Mount Sinai Hosp 1982; **Fac Appt:** Assoc Prof D, Mount Sinai Sch Med

DIAGNOSTIC RADIOLOGY

Amis Jr, E Stephen MD (DR) - **Spec Exp:** Urologic Imaging; **Hospital:** Montefiore Med Ctr; **Address:** Montefiore Med Ctr, Dept Radiology, 111 E 210th St, Bronx, NY 10467; **Phone:** 718-920-5113; **Board Cert:** Urology 1975; Diagnostic Radiology 1979; **Med School:** Northwestern Univ 1967; **Resid:** Urology, US Naval Hosp 1972; Diagnostic Radiology, US Naval Hosp 1978; **Fellow:** Urologic Radiology, Mass General Hosp 1981; **Fac Appt:** Prof Rad, Albert Einstein Coll Med

Friedman, Stanley N MD (DR) - **Hospital:** NY Westchester Sq Med Ctr; **Address:** NY Westchester Sq Med Ctr, Dept Rad, 2475 St Raymond Ave, Bronx, NY 10461-3124; **Phone:** 718-430-7321; **Board Cert:** Radiology 1974; **Med School:** NY Med Coll 1968; **Resid:** Radiology, Mt Sinai Hosp 1970; Radiation Oncology, Albert Einstein 1972; **Fellow:** Radiology, Mt Sinai Hosp 1973; **Fac Appt:** Asst Clin Prof Rad, Cornell Univ-Weill Med Coll

Haramati, Linda B MD (DR) - **Spec Exp:** AIDS/HIV; Lung Cancer; **Hospital:** Montefiore Med Ctr, Jacobi Med Ctr; **Address:** Montefiore Med Ctr, Dept Radiology, 111 E 210th St, Bronx, NY 10467-2401; **Phone:** 718-920-7458; **Board Cert:** Diagnostic Radiology 1990; **Med School:** Albert Einstein Coll Med 1985; **Resid:** Diagnostic Radiology, Montefiore Med Ctr 1990; **Fellow:** Thoracic Radiology, Columbia-Presby 1991; **Fac Appt:** Prof Rad, Albert Einstein Coll Med

Haramati, Nogah MD (DR) - **Spec Exp:** Orthopaedic Imaging; Rheumatology; Musculoskeletal Imaging; **Hospital:** Montefiore Med Ctr, Jacobi Med Ctr; **Address:** 1825 Eastchester Rd, rm 3-006, Bronx, NY 10461; **Phone:** 718-904-2965; **Board Cert:** Diagnostic Radiology 1990; **Med School:** SUNY Hlth Sci Ctr 1985; **Resid:** Radiology, Montefiore Hosp Med Ctr 1990; **Fellow:** Musculoskeletal Imaging, Columbia-Presby Med Ctr 1991; **Fac Appt:** Clin Prof Rad, Albert Einstein Coll Med

Koenigsberg, Mordecai MD (DR) - **Spec Exp:** Ultrasound; **Hospital:** Montefiore Med Ctr - Weiler-Einstein Div; **Address:** Montefiore Med Ctr-Weiler Einstein,Dept Rad, 1825 Eastchester Rd Fl 3, Bronx, NY 10461; **Phone:** 718-904-2322; **Board Cert:** Pediatrics 1970; Nuclear Medicine 1973; Diagnostic Radiology 1974; **Med School:** Albert Einstein Coll Med 1963; **Resid:** Pediatrics, Jacobi Med Ctr 1966; Diagnostic Radiology, Jacobi Med Ctr 1974; **Fac Appt:** Prof Rad, Albert Einstein Coll Med

Laks, Mitchell MD (DR) - **Spec Exp:** MRI; Ultrasound; **Hospital:** Montefiore Med Ctr; **Address:** Montefiore Med Ctr, Dept Rad, 111 E 210th St, Bronx, NY 10467; **Phone:** 718-920-4396; **Board Cert:** Diagnostic Radiology 1990; **Med School:** Harvard Med Sch 1985; **Resid:** Radiology, Albert Einstein 1990; **Fellow:** Magnetic Resonance Imaging, Brigham Women's Hosp 1991; **Fac Appt:** Asst Prof Rad, Albert Einstein Coll Med

Morehouse, Helen MD (DR) - **Spec Exp:** Genitourinary Imaging; MRI; Mammography; **Hospital:** Bronx Lebanon Hosp Ctr; **Address:** Bronx Lebanon Hosp, Dept Radiology, 1650 Grand Concourse, Bronx, NY 10457-7606; **Phone:** 718-518-5272; **Board Cert:** Diagnostic Radiology 1976; **Med School:** Univ KY Coll Med 1971; **Resid:** Internal Medicine, Rochester Genl Hosp 1972; Diagnostic Radiology, Rochester Genl Hosp 1975; **Fellow:** Radiology, Downstate Med Ctr 1976; **Fac Appt:** Prof Rad, Albert Einstein Coll Med

Rozenblit, Alla MD (DR) - **Spec Exp:** Liver Disease; CT Scan-Body; **Hospital:** Montefiore Med Ctr; **Address:** 111 E 210th St, Bronx, NY 10467-2401; **Phone:** 718-920-4396; **Board Cert:** Diagnostic Radiology 1984; **Med School:** Russia 1971; **Resid:** Diagnostic Radiology, Queens Hosp Ctr 1984; **Fellow:** Ultrasound/CT, LI Jewish Med Ctr 1985; **Fac Appt:** Clin Prof Rad, Albert Einstein Coll Med

Spindola-Franco, Hugo MD (DR) - **Spec Exp:** Cardiac Radiology; Congenital Heart Disease; Thoracic Radiology; **Hospital:** Montefiore Med Ctr; **Address:** 111 E 210th St, Bronx, NY 10467-2401; **Phone:** 718-920-4872; **Board Cert:** Radiology 1970; **Med School:** Mexico 1962; **Resid:** Radiology, Montefiore Hosp Med Ctr 1970; **Fellow:** Cardiovascular Radiology, Peter Bent Brigham Hosp/Harvard Med Sch 1971; **Fac Appt:** Prof Rad, Albert Einstein Coll Med

Stern, Harvey MD (DR) - **Spec Exp:** Nuclear Medicine; **Hospital:** Bronx Lebanon Hosp Ctr; **Address:** 1650 Grand Concourse, Bronx, NY 10457-7606; **Phone:** 718-518-5030; **Board Cert:** Radiology 1975; Nuclear Radiology 1978; **Med School:** Albert Einstein Coll Med 1971; **Resid:** Diagnostic Radiology, Bronx Municipal Hosp 1975; **Fac Appt:** Asst Prof Rad, Albert Einstein Coll Med

Swirsky, Michael MD (DR) - **Spec Exp:** Mammography; Gastrointestinal Imaging; **Hospital:** Our Lady of Mercy Med Ctr, White Plains Hosp Ctr (page 714153); **Address:** Our Lady of Mercy Med Ctr, Dept Rad, 600 E 233rd St, Bronx, NY 10466; **Phone:** 718-920-9188; **Board Cert:** Diagnostic Radiology 1979; **Med School:** Case West Res Univ 1975; **Resid:** Diagnostic Radiology, Strong Meml Hosp 1979; **Fac Appt:** Assoc Prof Rad, NY Med Coll

Wolf, Ellen L MD (DR) - **Spec Exp:** Gastrointestinal Imaging; **Hospital:** Montefiore Med Ctr; **Address:** 111 E 210th St, Bronx, NY 10467; **Phone:** 718-920-4851; **Board Cert:** Radiology 1976; **Med School:** Mount Sinai Sch Med 1972; **Resid:** Diagnostic Radiology, Columbia-Presby 1974; Diagnostic Radiology, Johns Hopkins 1976; **Fellow:** Pediatric Radiology, Columbia-Presby 1977; **Fac Appt:** Clin Prof Rad, Albert Einstein Coll Med

Zelefsky, Melvin MD (DR) - **Spec Exp:** Chest Radiology; Cardiac Radiology; **Hospital:** Jacobi Med Ctr; **Address:** 1400 Pelham Pkwy South, Ste 4N15, Bronx, NY 10461; **Phone:** 718-918-4595; **Board Cert:** Radiology 1965; Nuclear Medicine 1974; **Med School:** Albert Einstein Coll Med 1960; **Resid:** Radiology, Jacobi Med Ctr 1963; **Fellow:** Diagnostic Radiology, Jacobi Med Ctr 1963; **Fac Appt:** Prof Rad, Albert Einstein Coll Med

Endocrinology, Diabetes & Metabolism

Allen, Carol B MD (EDM) - **Spec Exp:** Diabetes; **Hospital:** VA Med Ctr - Bronx; **Address:** 130 W Kingsbridge Rd, Ste A, MC-00AM, Bronx, NY 10468-3904; **Phone:** 718-584-9000 x3777; **Board Cert:** Internal Medicine 1982; **Med School:** Univ Pennsylvania 1979; **Resid:** Internal Medicine, VA Med Ctr 1982; **Fellow:** Endocrinology, Diabetes & Metabolism, VA Med Ctr 1984

Cohen, Charmian MD (EDM) - **Spec Exp:** Diabetes; Thyroid Disorders; **Hospital:** Montefiore Med Ctr - Weiler-Einstein Div, NY Westchester Sq Med Ctr; **Address:** 1200 Waters Pl, Ste M105, Bronx, NY 10461; **Phone:** 718-892-7033; **Board Cert:** Internal Medicine 1987; Endocrinology, Diabetes & Metabolism 1989; **Med School:** South Africa 1977; **Resid:** Internal Medicine, G Schuer Hosp 1984; **Fellow:** Endocrinology, Diabetes & Metabolism, Albert Einstein 1986; **Fac Appt:** Asst Prof Med, Albert Einstein Coll Med

Fleischer, Norman MD (EDM) - **Spec Exp:** Thyroid Disorders; Adrenal Disorders; **Hospital:** Montefiore Med Ctr - Weiler-Einstein Div; **Address:** 1575 Blondell Ave, Ste 200, Bronx, NY 10461-2601; **Phone:** 718-405-8260; **Board Cert:** Internal Medicine 1968; Endocrinology, Diabetes & Metabolism 1973; **Med School:** Vanderbilt Univ 1961; **Resid:** Internal Medicine, Bronx Muni Hosp Ctr 1964; **Fellow:** Endocrinology, Diabetes & Metabolism, Vanderbilt Univ 1966; **Fac Appt:** Prof Med, Albert Einstein Coll Med

Freeman, Ruth MD (EDM) - **Spec Exp:** Osteoporosis; Hormonal Disorders; Thyroid Disorders; Pituitary Disorders; **Hospital:** Montefiore Med Ctr - Weiler-Einstein Div, Jacobi Med Ctr; **Address:** 1695 Eastchester Rd, Ste L2, Bronx, NY 10461; **Phone:** 718-405-8206; **Board Cert:** Internal Medicine 1967; Endocrinology 1972; **Med School:** Albert Einstein Coll Med 1960; **Resid:** Internal Medicine, Flower & Fifth Ave Hosp 1964; **Fellow:** Endocrinology, Mount Sinai 1965; Endocrinology, Emory Univ 1967; **Fac Appt:** Prof Med, Albert Einstein Coll Med

Guzman, Rodolfo MD (EDM) - **Spec Exp:** Endocrinology; Diabetes; Thyroid Disorders; **Hospital:** Bronx Lebanon Hosp Ctr; **Address:** 860 Grand Concourse, Ste 1K, Bronx, NY 10451; **Phone:** 718-585-5060; **Board Cert:** Internal Medicine 2000; Endocrinology, Diabetes & Metabolism 2000; **Med School:** Dominican Republic 1979; **Resid:** Internal Medicine, Bronx Lebanon Hosp 1990; **Fellow:** Endocrinology, Diabetes & Metabolism, Lincoln Med Ctr 1992

Schwartz, Ernest MD (EDM) - **Spec Exp:** Thyroid Disorders; Diabetes; Metabolic Bone Disease; **Hospital:** Our Lady of Mercy Med Ctr, VA Med Ctr - Bronx; **Address:** Our Lady of Mercy Med Ctr, Dept Med, 600 E 233rd St, Bronx, NY 10466-2604; **Phone:** 718-220-2188; **Board Cert:** Internal Medicine 1957; Endocrinology, Diabetes & Metabolism 1972; **Med School:** Columbia P&S 1951; **Resid:** Internal Medicine, UCSF Med Ctr 1953; Internal Medicine, Wadsworth VA Med Ctr 1954; **Fellow:** Endocrinology, Diabetes & Metabolism, Meml Sloan Kettering Cancer Ctr 1957; **Fac Appt:** Assoc Clin Prof Med, Cornell Univ-Weill Med Coll

Shamoon, Harry MD (EDM) - **Hospital:** Montefiore Med Ctr - Weiler-Einstein Div; **Address:** 1575 Blondell Ave, Ste 200, Bronx, NY 10461-2601; **Phone:** 718-405-8260; **Board Cert:** Internal Medicine 1977; Endocrinology, Diabetes & Metabolism 1979; **Med School:** Yale Univ 1974; **Resid:** Internal Medicine, Jacobi Med Ctr 1977; **Fellow:** Endocrinology, Diabetes & Metabolism, Yale-New Haven Hosp 1979; **Fac Appt:** Prof Med, Albert Einstein Coll Med

Surks, Martin MD (EDM) - **Spec Exp:** Thyroid Disorders; **Hospital:** Montefiore Med Ctr, N Central Bronx Hosp; **Address:** 111 E 210th St, Bronx, NY 10467-2401; **Phone:** 866-633-8255; **Board Cert:** Internal Medicine 1967; Endocrinology, Diabetes & Metabolism 1977; **Med School:** NYU Sch Med 1960; **Resid:** Internal Medicine, Montefiore Hosp Med Ctr 1962; Internal Medicine, VA Hosp 1964; **Fellow:** Research, Natl Inst Arthritis-Metabolic Disease 1964; **Fac Appt:** Prof Med, Albert Einstein Coll Med

Zonszein, Joel MD (EDM) - **Spec Exp:** Thyroid Disorders; Diabetes; **Hospital:** Montefiore Med Ctr; **Address:** 1575 Blondell Ave, Ste 200, Bronx, NY 10461; **Phone:** 718-405-8260; **Board Cert:** Nuclear Medicine 1976; Internal Medicine 1977; Endocrinology 1977; **Med School:** Mexico 1969; **Resid:** Internal Medicine, Maimonides Med Ctr 1972; Internal Medicine, Jacobi Med Ctr 1973; **Fellow:** Endocrinology, Northwestern Univ Med Sch 1974; Endocrinology, Georgetown Univ Hosp 1975; **Fac Appt:** Assoc Prof Med, Albert Einstein Coll Med

FAMILY MEDICINE

Biagiotti, Wendy MD (FMed) `PCP` - **Hospital:** NY Westchester Sq Med Ctr; **Address:** 3101 E Tremont Ave, Bronx, NY 10461; **Phone:** 718-863-7925; **Board Cert:** Family Medicine 1995; **Med School:** Mexico 1988; **Resid:** Family Medicine, St Joseph's Hosp&Med Ctr 1994

Cahill, John MD (FMed) `PCP` - **Hospital:** NY Westchester Sq Med Ctr; **Address:** 4000 Seton Ave, Bronx, NY 10466; **Phone:** 718-324-5408; **Board Cert:** Family Medicine 2002; **Med School:** Georgetown Univ 1960; **Resid:** Family Medicine, Kings County Hosp 1961

Cordero, Evelyn MD (FMed) `PCP` - **Hospital:** Our Lady of Mercy Med Ctr, NY Westchester Sq Med Ctr; **Address:** 941 Castle Hill Ave, Bronx, NY 10473; **Phone:** 718-792-3117; **Board Cert:** Family Medicine 2003; **Med School:** SUNY Hlth Sci Ctr 1979; **Resid:** Family Medicine, St Joseph's Hosp&Med Ctr 1982

De Blasio, Maria-Pia MD (FMed) PCP - **Spec Exp:** Diabetes; Hypertension; Thyroid Disorders; **Hospital:** Our Lady of Mercy Med Ctr, St Barnabas Hosp - Bronx; **Address:** 3065 Grand Concourse, Bronx, NY 10468; **Phone:** 718-295-3898; **Med School:** Italy 1967; **Resid:** Surgery, Misericordia Hosp; Clinical Pathology, Misericordia Hosp; **Fellow:** Ophthalmology, Misericordia Hosp

Delaney, Brian MD (FMed) PCP - **Spec Exp:** Geriatric Care; **Hospital:** Montefiore Med Ctr, St Barnabas Hosp - Bronx; **Address:** 2371 Arthur Ave, Bronx, NY 10458; **Phone:** 718-364-6199; **Board Cert:** Family Medicine 2000; Geriatric Medicine 2002; **Med School:** Albert Einstein Coll Med 1983; **Resid:** Family Medicine, Montefiore Med Ctr 1986; **Fac Appt:** Asst Prof FMed, Albert Einstein Coll Med

Dietrich, Marianne DO (FMed) PCP - **Hospital:** Montefiore Med Ctr; **Address:** 1 Fordham Plaza, Bronx, NY 10458; **Phone:** 718-405-4010; **Board Cert:** Family Medicine 1992; **Med School:** NY Coll Osteo Med 1988; **Resid:** Family Medicine, Peninsula Hosp Ctr 1991

Franzetti, Carl DO (FMed) PCP - **Hospital:** Saint Joseph's Med Ctr - Yonkers, NY-Presby Hosp (page 100); **Address:** 3125 Tibbett Ave, Bronx, NY 10463-3897; **Phone:** 718-543-2700; **Board Cert:** Family Medicine 1999; **Med School:** NY Coll Osteo Med 1984; **Resid:** Family Medicine, Warren Hosp 1987

Maselli, Frank MD (FMed) PCP - **Spec Exp:** Diving Medicine; Hyperbaric Medicine; **Hospital:** Saint Joseph's Med Ctr - Yonkers, NY-Presby Hosp (page 100); **Address:** 3125 Tibbett Ave, Bronx, NY 10463; **Phone:** 718-543-2700; **Board Cert:** Family Medicine 1998; **Med School:** Israel 1983; **Resid:** Family Medicine, Univ Hosp 1986; **Fac Appt:** Asst Prof FMed, SUNY Downstate

Morrow, Robert MD (FMed) PCP - **Spec Exp:** Preventive Medicine; Geriatric Medicine; **Hospital:** Saint Joseph's Med Ctr - Yonkers, Montefiore Med Ctr; **Address:** 5997 Riverdale Ave, Bronx, NY 10471-1602; **Phone:** 718-884-9803; **Board Cert:** Family Medicine 2002; Geriatric Medicine 1998; **Med School:** Mount Sinai Sch Med 1974; **Resid:** Family Medicine, Montefiore Hosp Med Ctr 1977; **Fac Appt:** Assoc Clin Prof FMed, Albert Einstein Coll Med

Soloway, Bruce MD (FMed) PCP - **Spec Exp:** AIDS/HIV; **Hospital:** Bronx Lebanon Hosp Ctr; **Address:** 1276 Fulton Ave, Fl 3, Bronx, NY 10456-3500; **Phone:** 718-901-8236; **Board Cert:** Family Medicine 2000; **Med School:** Albert Einstein Coll Med 1985; **Resid:** Family Medicine, Montefiore Hosp Med Ctr 1988; **Fac Appt:** Assoc Prof FMed, Albert Einstein Coll Med

GASTROENTEROLOGY

Abelow, Arthur MD (Ge) - **Spec Exp:** Endoscopy; Nutrition; **Hospital:** Montefiore Med Ctr - Weiler-Einstein Div, NY Westchester Sq Med Ctr; **Address:** 1625 Saint Peters Ave, Bronx, NY 10461-3000; **Phone:** 718-863-7397; **Board Cert:** Internal Medicine 1983; Gastroenterology 1985; **Med School:** Albert Einstein Coll Med 1980; **Resid:** Internal Medicine, Bronx Muni Hosp Ctr 1983; **Fellow:** Gastroenterology, Montefiore Med Ctr 1985; **Fac Appt:** Asst Clin Prof Med, Albert Einstein Coll Med

Antony, Michael MD (Ge) - **Spec Exp:** Colonoscopy; Endoscopy; Liver Disease; **Hospital:** Montefiore Med Ctr - Weiler-Einstein Div, NY Westchester Sq Med Ctr; **Address:** 1840 Williamsbridge Rd, Bronx, NY 10461; **Phone:** 718-828-0100; **Board Cert:** Internal Medicine 1985; Gastroenterology 1989; **Med School:** SUNY Hlth Sci Ctr 1982; **Resid:** Internal Medicine, Bronx Muni Hosp 1985; **Fellow:** Gastroenterology, Montefiore Hosp Med Ctr 1988; **Fac Appt:** Assoc Clin Prof Med, Albert Einstein Coll Med

Brandt, Lawrence MD (Ge) - **Spec Exp:** Geriatric Gastroenterology; Ischemic Bowel Disease; Inflammatory Bowel Disease; **Hospital:** Montefiore Med Ctr; **Address:** 3400 Bainbridge Ave Fl 2, Bronx, NY 10467-2401; **Phone:** 866-633-8255; **Board Cert:** Internal Medicine 1972; Gastroenterology 1975; **Med School:** SUNY Downstate 1968; **Resid:** Internal Medicine, Mount Sinai Hosp 1972; **Fellow:** Gastroenterology, Mount Sinai Hosp 1972; **Fac Appt:** Prof Med, Albert Einstein Coll Med

Frager, Joseph MD (Ge) - **Spec Exp:** Colon Cancer; Endoscopy; Laser Surgery; **Hospital:** Montefiore Med Ctr, NY Hosp Queens; **Address:** 277 Van Cortlandt Ave E, Bronx, NY 10467-3011; **Phone:** 718-798-8867; **Board Cert:** Internal Medicine 1983; Gastroenterology 1985; **Med School:** Univ Pennsylvania 1980; **Resid:** Internal Medicine, Montefiore Med Ctr 1983; **Fellow:** Gastroenterology, Montefiore Med Ctr 1985; **Fac Appt:** Asst Clin Prof Med, Albert Einstein Coll Med

Greenwald, David A MD (Ge) - **Spec Exp:** Endoscopy; Gastroesophageal Reflux Disease (GERD); Peptic Ulcer Disease; **Hospital:** Montefiore Med Ctr, Montefiore Med Ctr - Weiler-Einstein Div; **Address:** Montefiore Med Ctr, Div Gastroenterology, 111 E 210th St, Bronx, NY 10467; **Phone:** 718-920-4846; **Board Cert:** Internal Medicine 1989; Gastroenterology 1993; **Med School:** Albert Einstein Coll Med 1986; **Resid:** Internal Medicine, Columbia Presby Med Ctr 1989; **Fellow:** Gastroenterology, Columbia Presby Med Ctr 1993; **Fac Appt:** Assoc Prof Med, Albert Einstein Coll Med

Gupta, Sanjeev MD (Ge) - **Spec Exp:** Hepatitis; Liver Disease; **Hospital:** Montefiore Med Ctr, Jacobi Med Ctr; **Address:** 1515 Blondell Ave, Ste 220, Bronx, NY 10461-2601; **Phone:** 718-405-8300 x2107; **Board Cert:** Internal Medicine 1989; Gastroenterology 1993; **Med School:** India 1977; **Resid:** Internal Medicine, PGIMER 1981; Internal Medicine, Hammersmith Hosp 1982; **Fellow:** Gastroenterology, Hammersmith Hosp 1985; Hepatology, LAC-USC Med Ctr 1987; **Fac Appt:** Prof Med, Albert Einstein Coll Med

Gutwein, Isadore Phillip MD (Ge) - **Spec Exp:** Pancreatic/Biliary Endoscopy (ERCP); Colonoscopy; Hepatitis; **Hospital:** Montefiore Med Ctr, NY-Presby Hosp (page 100); **Address:** 3765 Riverdale Ave, Bronx, NY 10463-1807; **Phone:** 718-549-4267; **Board Cert:** Internal Medicine 1976; Gastroenterology 1979; **Med School:** Albert Einstein Coll Med 1973; **Resid:** Internal Medicine, Montefiore Hosp Med Ctr 1976; **Fellow:** Gastroenterology, St Luke's Hosp 1978; **Fac Appt:** Asst Prof Med, Albert Einstein Coll Med

Hertan, Hilary MD (Ge) - **Spec Exp:** Endoscopic Ultrasound; **Hospital:** Our Lady of Mercy Med Ctr; **Address:** Dept Gastroenterology, 600 E 233rd St, Bronx, NY 10466; **Phone:** 718-920-9887; **Board Cert:** Internal Medicine 1986; Gastroenterology 1989; **Med School:** NY Med Coll 1982; **Resid:** Internal Medicine, North Shore Univ Hosp 1985; **Fellow:** Gastroenterology, Our Lady of Mercy Med Ctr 1990; **Fac Appt:** Asst Prof Med, NY Med Coll

Korsten, Mark A MD (Ge) - **Spec Exp:** Constipation; Motility Disorders; **Hospital:** Mount Sinai Med Ctr (page 98), VA Med Ctr - Bronx; **Address:** 130 W Kingsbridge Rd, Bronx, NY 10468-3904; **Phone:** 718-584-9000 x6753; **Board Cert:** Internal Medicine 1973; Gastroenterology 1975; **Med School:** Yale Univ 1970; **Resid:** Internal Medicine, Mt Sinai Hosp 1973; **Fellow:** Gastroenterology, Mt Sinai Hosp 1975; **Fac Appt:** Prof Med, Mount Sinai Sch Med

Mehta, Rekha MD (Ge) - **Spec Exp:** Palliative Care; **Hospital:** Calvary Hosp (page 106); **Address:** 1740 Eastchester Rd, Bronx, NY 10461; **Phone:** 718-518-2208; **Board Cert:** Internal Medicine 1984; Gastroenterology 1987; **Med School:** India 1972; **Resid:** Internal Medicine, New Rochelle Med Ctr 1977; **Fellow:** Gastroenterology, Univ of South Carolina 1981; Nutrition, Univ of Pitt Sch of Med 1989; **Fac Appt:** Asst Clin Prof Med, NY Med Coll

Remy, Prospere MD (Ge) - **Spec Exp:** Liver Disease; **Hospital:** Bronx Lebanon Hosp Ctr; **Address:** 860 Grand Concourse, Ste 1A, Bronx, NY 10451-2815; **Phone:** 718-585-5060; **Board Cert:** Internal Medicine 2004; Gastroenterology 2004; Geriatric Medicine 1996; **Med School:** Mexico 1984; **Resid:** Internal Medicine, Bronx Lebanon Hosp 1990; **Fellow:** Gastroenterology, Bronx Lebanon Hosp 1992; **Fac Appt:** Asst Prof Med, Albert Einstein Coll Med

Sable, Robert MD (Ge) - **Spec Exp:** Hepatitis C; Gastroesophageal Reflux Disease (GERD); Inflammatory Bowel Disease; **Hospital:** Montefiore Med Ctr, NY-Presby Hosp (page 100); **Address:** 3765 Riverdale Ave, Ste 7, Bronx, NY 10463-1845; **Phone:** 718-549-4267; **Board Cert:** Internal Medicine 1987; Gastroenterology 2000; Geriatric Medicine 2000; **Med School:** Albert Einstein Coll Med 1973; **Resid:** Internal Medicine, Montefiore Hosp Med Ctr 1976; **Fellow:** Gastroenterology, NY Med Coll 1978; **Fac Appt:** Asst Clin Prof Med, Albert Einstein Coll Med

Schweitzer, Philip E MD (Ge) - **Spec Exp:** Liver Disease; Gastrointestinal Disorders; Esophageal Disorders; **Hospital:** Montefiore Med Ctr, Our Lady of Mercy Med Ctr; **Address:** 3184 Grand Concourse, Ste 2D, Bronx, NY 10458-1031; **Phone:** 718-584-0404; **Board Cert:** Internal Medicine 1972; Gastroenterology 1977; **Med School:** Cornell Univ-Weill Med Coll 1967; **Resid:** Internal Medicine, St Luke's-Roosevelt Hosp Ctr 1972; **Fellow:** Gastroenterology, Mount Sinai Hosp 1974

Sherman, Howard MD (Ge) - **Spec Exp:** Colonoscopy; Biliary Disease; **Hospital:** Montefiore Med Ctr - Weiler-Einstein Div, NY Westchester Sq Med Ctr; **Address:** 1625 St Peters Ave, Bronx, NY 10461-3000; **Phone:** 718-863-7397; **Board Cert:** Internal Medicine 1976; Gastroenterology 1979; **Med School:** Albert Einstein Coll Med 1973; **Resid:** Internal Medicine, Emory Univ Hosp 1976; **Fellow:** Gastroenterology, Emory Univ Hosp 1978; **Fac Appt:** Assoc Clin Prof Med, Albert Einstein Coll Med

Stein, David F MD (Ge) - **Spec Exp:** Liver Disease; Hepatitis B & C; HIV & Hepatitis coinfection; Endoscopy; **Hospital:** St Barnabas Hosp - Bronx, Montefiore Med Ctr; **Address:** 3765 Riverdale Ave, Ste 7, Bronx, NY 10463; **Phone:** 718-549-4267; **Board Cert:** Internal Medicine 1994; Gastroenterology 1997; **Med School:** SUNY Downstate 1990; **Resid:** Internal Medicine, NYU/Bellvue Med Ctr/VA Med Ctr 1994; **Fellow:** Gastroenterology, NYU Med Ctr/Bellevue Med Ctr/VA Med Ctr 1996; **Fac Appt:** Asst Clin Prof Med, Albert Einstein Coll Med

Geriatric Medicine

Dharmarajan, Thiruvinvamvalai MD (Ger) - **Spec Exp:** Kidney Disease; **Hospital:** Our Lady of Mercy Med Ctr; **Address:** 4141 Carpenter Ave, Level C, Bronx, NY 10466-2600; **Phone:** 718-920-9041; **Board Cert:** Internal Medicine 1977; Geriatric Medicine 1998; Nephrology 1980; **Med School:** India 1967; **Resid:** Internal Medicine, Misericordia Hosp 1977; **Fellow:** Nephrology, Misericordia Hosp 1979; **Fac Appt:** Prof Med, NY Med Coll

Goldberg, Roy J MD (Ger) **PCP** - **Spec Exp:** Long Term Care; Medications in the Elderly; Palliative Care; **Hospital:** Montefiore Med Ctr - Weiler-Einstein Div, Sound Shore Med Ctr - Westchester (page 711); **Address:** Director-Kings Harbor Multicare Ctr, 2000 E Gunhill Rd, Bronx, NY 10469; **Phone:** 718-405-3535; **Board Cert:** Internal Medicine 1985; Geriatric Medicine 2002; **Med School:** Albert Einstein Coll Med 1982; **Resid:** Internal Medicine, Montefiore Med Ctr 1985; **Fac Appt:** Asst Clin Prof Med, Albert Einstein Coll Med

Jacobs, Laurie MD (Ger) **PCP** - **Spec Exp:** Stroke; Preventive Medicine; Osteoporosis; **Hospital:** Montefiore Med Ctr; **Address:** Montefiore Med Ctr, Dept Geriatrics, 111 E 210th St, Bronx, NY 10467-2401; **Phone:** 866-633-8255; **Board Cert:** Internal Medicine 1988; Geriatric Medicine 2001; **Med School:** Columbia P&S 1985; **Resid:** Internal Medicine, Montefiore Med Ctr 1988; **Fellow:** Geriatric Medicine, Montefiore Med Ctr 1990; **Fac Appt:** Clin Prof Med, Albert Einstein Coll Med

Russell, Robin MD (Ger) - **Spec Exp:** Kidney Failure; Kidney Disease; Dialysis Care; **Hospital:** Our Lady of Mercy Med Ctr; **Address:** 4141 Carpenter Ave, Renal Unit, Bronx, NY 10466-2600; **Phone:** 718-920-9041; **Board Cert:** Internal Medicine 1974; Nephrology 1980; Geriatric Medicine 2002; **Med School:** Univ New Mexico 1971; **Resid:** Internal Medicine, Harlem Hosp 1974; **Fellow:** Nephrology, Harlem Hosp 1976; **Fac Appt:** Asst Prof Med, NY Med Coll

GERIATRIC PSYCHIATRY

Kennedy, Gary MD (GerPsy) - **Spec Exp:** Alzheimer's Disease; Dementia; Depression; **Hospital:** Montefiore Med Ctr; **Address:** Dept Psyc & Behav Sci, 111 E 210th St, Bronx, NY 10467-2401; **Phone:** 718-920-4236; **Board Cert:** Psychiatry 1980; Geriatric Psychiatry 2000; Psychosomatic Medicine 2005; **Med School:** Univ Tex, San Antonio 1975; **Resid:** Psychiatry, VA Hosp-Univ Texas 1979; **Fellow:** Geriatric Psychiatry, Montefiore Hosp 1984; **Fac Appt:** Prof Psyc, Albert Einstein Coll Med

Weisblatt, Steven MD (GerPsy) - **Spec Exp:** Mental Retardation; Bipolar/Mood Disorders; Psychopharmacology; **Hospital:** SUNY Downstate Med Ctr; **Address:** 2445 Woodhull Ave, Bronx, NY 10469-6209; **Phone:** 718-405-0494; **Board Cert:** Psychiatry 1989; Geriatric Psychiatry 1996; **Med School:** SUNY Hlth Sci Ctr 1984; **Resid:** Psychiatry, Albert Einstein 1988

GYNECOLOGIC ONCOLOGY

Goldberg, Gary L MD (GO) - **Spec Exp:** Ovarian Cancer; Uterine Cancer; **Hospital:** Montefiore Med Ctr - Weiler-Einstein Div; **Address:** 1695 Eastchester Rd, Ste L2, Bronx, NY 10461; **Phone:** 718-405-8200; **Board Cert:** Obstetrics & Gynecology 1988; Gynecologic Oncology 1996; **Med School:** South Africa 1975; **Resid:** Obstetrics & Gynecology, Groote Schuur Hosp 1981; **Fellow:** Gynecologic Oncology, Groote Schuur Hosp 1983; **Fac Appt:** Asst Prof ObG, Albert Einstein Coll Med

HAND SURGERY

Kulick, Roy G MD (HS) - **Spec Exp:** Carpal Tunnel Syndrome; Arthritis; Tendon Surgery; **Hospital:** Montefiore Med Ctr - Weiler-Einstein Div, Westchester Med Ctr (page 713); **Address:** The Tower at Montefiore Medical Park, 1695 Eastchester Rd, Bronx, NY 10461; **Phone:** 718-405-8430; **Board Cert:** Orthopaedic Surgery 1980; Hand Surgery 2001; **Med School:** Cornell Univ-Weill Med Coll 1973; **Resid:** Surgery, St Lukes-Roosevelt Hosp 1975; Orthopaedic Surgery, Columbia Presbyterian Hosp 1978; **Fellow:** Hand Surgery, Hosp for Special Surgery 1979; **Fac Appt:** Assoc Prof OrS, Albert Einstein Coll Med

HEMATOLOGY

Billett, Henny MD (Hem) - **Spec Exp:** Bleeding/Coagulation Disorders; Thrombotic Disorders; Platelet Disorders; **Hospital:** Montefiore Med Ctr - Weiler-Einstein Div, Montefiore Med Ctr; **Address:** 1515 Blondell Ave, Ste 220, Bronx, NY 10461-2601; **Phone:** 718-405-8323; **Board Cert:** Internal Medicine 1979; Hematology 1982; **Med School:** Mount Sinai Sch Med 1974; **Resid:** Internal Medicine, Montefiore Hosp Med Ctr 1979; **Fellow:** Tropical Medicine, London Sch Hygiene/Trop Med 1977; Hematology, Montefiore Hosp Med Ctr 1981; **Fac Appt:** Prof Med, Albert Einstein Coll Med

Landau, Leon MD (Hem) - **Hospital:** Montefiore Med Ctr, Comm Hosp - Dobbs Ferry; **Address:** 75 E Gun Hill Rd, Bronx, NY 10467-2103; **Phone:** 718-655-3932; **Board Cert:** Internal Medicine 1977; Hematology 1978; Medical Oncology 1981; **Med School:** Albert Einstein Coll Med 1971; **Resid:** Internal Medicine, Montefiore Med Ctr 1973; Internal Medicine, Metropolitan Hosp Ctr 1974; **Fellow:** Medical Oncology, Montefiore Med Ctr 1976; Hematology, Montefiore Med Ctr 1978; **Fac Appt:** Asst Prof Med, Albert Einstein Coll Med

Nagel, Ronald MD (Hem) - **Spec Exp:** Sickle Cell Disease; Anemia; **Hospital:** Montefiore Med Ctr - Weiler-Einstein Div, Montefiore Med Ctr; **Address:** 1300 Morris Park Ave, Ullmann Bldg, Ste 921, Bronx, NY 10461; **Phone:** 718-430-2186; **Med School:** Chile 1960; **Resid:** Internal Medicine, JJ Aguirre 1961; **Fellow:** Hematology, Albert Einstein 1966; **Fac Appt:** Prof Med, Albert Einstein Coll Med

Rand, Jacob H MD (Hem) - **Spec Exp:** Bleeding/Coagulation Disorders; Pregnancy-Hematologic Complications; Thrombotic Disorders; **Hospital:** Montefiore Med Ctr; **Address:** Montefiore Medical Ctr, 111 E 210th St, N8 Silverzone, Bronx, NY 10467; **Phone:** 718-920-4481; **Board Cert:** Internal Medicine 1977; Hematology 1978; **Med School:** Albert Einstein Coll Med 1973; **Resid:** Internal Medicine, Mount Sinai Hosp 1976; **Fellow:** Hematology, Montefiore Med Ctr 1978; **Fac Appt:** Prof Med, Albert Einstein Coll Med

Schreiber, Zwi MD (Hem) - **Spec Exp:** Lymphoma; Anemia; **Hospital:** Bronx Lebanon Hosp Ctr, NY Westchester Sq Med Ctr; **Address:** 1650 Grand Concourse Fl 4, Bronx, NY 10457-7606; **Phone:** 718-239-8321; **Board Cert:** Internal Medicine 1974; Hematology 1976; **Med School:** Israel 1962; **Resid:** Internal Medicine, Bronx Lebanon Hosp 1974; **Fellow:** Hematology, Maimonides Med Ctr 1969

INFECTIOUS DISEASE

Berger, Judith MD (Inf) - **Spec Exp:** AIDS/HIV; Travel Medicine; **Hospital:** St Barnabas Hosp - Bronx; **Address:** 4422 Third Ave, Bronx, NY 10457; **Phone:** 718-960-6205; **Board Cert:** Internal Medicine 1984; Infectious Disease 1986; **Med School:** Mount Sinai Sch Med 1980; **Resid:** Internal Medicine, Brookdale Hosp 1984; **Fellow:** Infectious Disease, Downstate Med Ctr 1986; **Fac Appt:** Asst Clin Prof Med, Cornell Univ-Weill Med Coll

Casey, Joan MD (Inf) - **Spec Exp:** Infections in Diabetes; **Hospital:** Montefiore Med Ctr; **Address:** 111 E 210th St, Bronx, NY 10467-2401; **Phone:** 718-920-7700; **Board Cert:** Internal Medicine 1971; Infectious Disease 1972; **Med School:** Canada 1966; **Resid:** Internal Medicine, Boston City Hosp 1970; **Fellow:** Infectious Disease, Boston City Hosp 1969; **Fac Appt:** Prof Med, Albert Einstein Coll Med

Corpuz, Marilou MD (Inf) - **Spec Exp:** Hospital Acquired Infections; **Hospital:** Our Lady of Mercy Med Ctr; **Address:** Our Lady of Mercy Med Ctr, Dept Medicine, 600 E 233rd St, Bronx, NY 10466-2604; **Phone:** 718-920-9889; **Board Cert:** Internal Medicine 1988; Infectious Disease 2002; **Med School:** Philippines 1985; **Resid:** Internal Medicine, Griffin Hosp 1988; **Fellow:** Infectious Disease, LI Jewish Med Ctr 1991; **Fac Appt:** Assoc Prof Med, NY Med Coll

Robbins, Noah MD (Inf) - **Spec Exp:** AIDS/HIV; Sexually Transmitted Diseases; **Hospital:** Montefiore Med Ctr; **Address:** 3400 Bainbridge Ave Fl 8, Bronx, NY 10467; **Phone:** 718-920-8888; **Board Cert:** Internal Medicine 1974; Infectious Disease 1980; **Med School:** McGill Univ 1969; **Resid:** Internal Medicine, Albany Med Ctr 1975; **Fellow:** Infectious Disease, Montefiore Hosp Med Ctr 1976; **Fac Appt:** Assoc Prof Med, Albert Einstein Coll Med

Saltzman, Simone MD (Inf) - **Hospital:** Montefiore Med Ctr - Weiler-Einstein Div; **Address:** 1575 Blondell Ave, Ste 200, Bronx, NY 10461-1915; **Phone:** 866-633-8255; **Board Cert:** Internal Medicine 1977; Infectious Disease 1980; **Med School:** SUNY Downstate 1973; **Resid:** Internal Medicine, Montefiore Hosp Med Ctr 1976; **Fellow:** Infectious Disease, Montefiore Hosp Med Ctr 1979; **Fac Appt:** Asst Prof Med, Albert Einstein Coll Med

Tanowitz, Herbert B MD (Inf) - **Spec Exp:** Parasitic Infections; Tropical Diseases; **Hospital:** Montefiore Med Ctr - Weiler-Einstein Div, Jacobi Med Ctr; **Address:** 1300 Morris Park Ave Bldg F - rm 504, Bronx, NY 10461-1926; **Phone:** 718-430-3342; **Board Cert:** Internal Medicine 1974; Infectious Disease 1976; **Med School:** Albert Einstein Coll Med 1967; **Resid:** Internal Medicine, Lincoln Hosp 1971; **Fellow:** Infectious Disease, Albert Einstein 1973; **Fac Appt:** Prof Med, Albert Einstein Coll Med

Telzak, Edward E MD (Inf) - **Spec Exp:** AIDS/HIV; Tuberculosis; Infections-Opportunistic; **Hospital:** Bronx Lebanon Hosp Ctr; **Address:** 1650 Grand Concourse, Fl 8, Bronx, NY 10457-7606; **Phone:** 718-960-1212; **Board Cert:** Internal Medicine 1983; Infectious Disease 1988; **Med School:** Albert Einstein Coll Med 1980; **Resid:** Internal Medicine, New England Med Ctr 1983; **Fellow:** Infectious Disease, Brigham & Women's Hosp 1985; Tropical Medicine, New England Med Ctr 1986; **Fac Appt:** Prof Med, Albert Einstein Coll Med

Weiss, Louis MD (Inf) - **Spec Exp:** Parasitic Infections; AIDS/HIV; **Hospital:** Montefiore Med Ctr - Weiler-Einstein Div; **Address:** 1575 Blondell Ave, Ste 200, Bronx, NY 10461; **Phone:** 718-405-8311; **Board Cert:** Internal Medicine 1985; Infectious Disease 1988; **Med School:** Johns Hopkins Univ 1982; **Resid:** Internal Medicine, Univ Chicago 1985; **Fellow:** Infectious Disease, Montefiore Hosp Med Ctr 1989; **Fac Appt:** Prof Med, Albert Einstein Coll Med

INTERNAL MEDICINE

Berger, Matthew MD (IM) `PCP` - **Hospital:** Montefiore Med Ctr - Weiler-Einstein Div, Montefiore Med Ctr; **Address:** 1575 Blondell Ave, Ste 200, Bronx, NY 10461; **Phone:** 718-405-8311; **Board Cert:** Internal Medicine 1986; **Med School:** Univ Pennsylvania 1982; **Resid:** Internal Medicine, Jacobi Med Ctr 1986; **Fac Appt:** Assoc Prof Med, Albert Einstein Coll Med

Buatti, Elizabeth MD (IM) `PCP` - **Hospital:** Montefiore Med Ctr; **Address:** 111 E 210th St, Bronx, NY 10467-2401; **Phone:** 718-920-5866; **Board Cert:** Internal Medicine 1981; **Med School:** Georgetown Univ 1978; **Resid:** Internal Medicine, St Vincent's Hosp 1981; **Fac Appt:** Assoc Prof Med, Albert Einstein Coll Med

Chernaik, Richard MD (IM) `PCP` - **Spec Exp:** Diabetes; Cholesterol/Lipid Disorders; **Hospital:** Montefiore Med Ctr; **Address:** 100 Elgar Pl, Bronx, NY 10475-5002; **Phone:** 718-320-2188; **Board Cert:** Internal Medicine 1968; **Med School:** Jefferson Med Coll 1960; **Resid:** Internal Medicine, Jersey City Med Ctr 1965; Internal Medicine, Brooklyn VA Hosp 1967; **Fac Appt:** Asst Clin Prof Med, Albert Einstein Coll Med

Cimino, James E MD (IM) - **Spec Exp:** Palliative Care; Nutrition; **Hospital:** Calvary Hosp (page 106); **Address:** 1740 Eastchester Rd, Bronx, NY 10461-2392; **Phone:** 718-518-2147; **Board Cert:** Internal Medicine 1977; Nephrology 1972; **Med School:** NYU Sch Med 1954; **Resid:** Internal Medicine, EJ Meyer Meml Hosp 1957; **Fellow:** Physiology, SUNY-Buffalo Hosp 1958; **Fac Appt:** Clin Prof Med, NY Med Coll

Bronx

Comfort, Christopher P MD (IM) PCP - **Spec Exp:** Palliative Care; Geriatric Care; **Hospital:** Calvary Hosp (page 106), Montefiore Med Ctr - Weiler-Einstein Div; **Address:** 1740 Eastchester Rd, Bronx, NY 10461; **Phone:** 718-518-2210; **Board Cert:** Internal Medicine 1986; Geriatric Medicine 1993; **Med School:** St Louis Univ 1982; **Resid:** Internal Medicine, Montefiore Med Ctr 1988

Ernst, Jerome MD (IM) PCP - **Spec Exp:** AIDS/HIV; **Hospital:** Bronx Lebanon Hosp Ctr; **Address:** 1770 Grand Concourse, Ste 2G, Bronx, NY 10457; **Phone:** 718-518-5581; **Board Cert:** Internal Medicine 1978; Pulmonary Disease 1982; **Med School:** Israel 1969; **Resid:** Internal Medicine, Montefiore Hosp Med Ctr 1972; **Fellow:** Pulmonary Disease, Montefiore Hosp Med Ctr 1977; **Fac Appt:** Assoc Prof Med, Albert Einstein Coll Med

Fojas, Antonio MD (IM) PCP - **Hospital:** Our Lady of Mercy Med Ctr; **Address:** 4234 Bronx Blvd, Bronx, NY 10466; **Phone:** 347-341-4300; **Board Cert:** Internal Medicine 2003; **Med School:** Philippines 1984; **Resid:** Internal Medicine, Our Lady of Mercy Med Ctr 1987; **Fellow:** Internal Medicine, Our Lady of Mercy Med Ctr 1988; **Fac Appt:** Asst Prof Med, NY Med Coll

Grajower, Martin MD (IM) PCP - **Spec Exp:** Diabetes; Endocrinology; Osteoporosis; **Hospital:** Montefiore Med Ctr; **Address:** 3736 Henry Hudson Pkwy, Riverdale, NY 10463; **Phone:** 718-549-6268; **Board Cert:** Internal Medicine 1987; Endocrinology, Diabetes & Metabolism 1981; **Med School:** Albert Einstein Coll Med 1973; **Resid:** Internal Medicine, Montefiore Hosp Med Ctr 1975; Internal Medicine, Boston Med Ctr 1976; **Fellow:** Endocrinology, Diabetes & Metabolism, Montefiore Hosp Med Ctr 1978; **Fac Appt:** Asst Prof Med, Albert Einstein Coll Med

Kelly, Carol MD (IM) PCP - **Hospital:** Montefiore Med Ctr - Weiler-Einstein Div, NY Westchester Sq Med Ctr; **Address:** 1180 Morris Park Ave, Bronx, NY 10461-1925; **Phone:** 718-863-8465; **Board Cert:** Internal Medicine 1982; Geriatric Medicine 1984; **Med School:** Brown Univ 1979; **Resid:** Internal Medicine, Duke Univ Med Ctr 1982

Mojtabai, Shaparak MD (IM) PCP - **Spec Exp:** Women's Health-Geriatric; Diabetes; Hypertension; **Hospital:** St Barnabas Hosp - Bronx; **Address:** 2016 Bronxdale Ave, Ste 302, Bronx, NY 10462; **Phone:** 718-822-1515; **Board Cert:** Internal Medicine 1989; Geriatric Medicine 1994; **Med School:** Iran 1982; **Resid:** Internal Medicine, St Barnabas 1988; **Fellow:** Internal Medicine, St Barnabas 1989

Nyer, Kenneth MD (IM) - **Spec Exp:** Cardiology; Diabetes; **Hospital:** Montefiore Med Ctr - Weiler-Einstein Div, NY Westchester Sq Med Ctr; **Address:** 1610 Williamsbridge Rd, Bronx, NY 10461-1604; **Phone:** 718-409-6400; **Board Cert:** Internal Medicine 1988; Geriatric Medicine 2004; **Med School:** Albert Einstein Coll Med 1984; **Resid:** Internal Medicine, N Shore Univ Hosp 1987; **Fac Appt:** Asst Clin Prof Med, Albert Einstein Coll Med

Sander, Norbert MD (IM) PCP - **Spec Exp:** Preventive Medicine; Sports Medicine; **Hospital:** Sound Shore Med Ctr - Westchester (page 711); **Address:** 340 City Island Ave, Bronx, NY 10464; **Phone:** 718-885-0333; **Board Cert:** Internal Medicine 1981; **Med School:** Albert Einstein Coll Med 1971; **Resid:** Internal Medicine, Metropolitan Hosp Ctr 1974

Selwyn, Peter MD (IM) - **Spec Exp:** AIDS/HIV; Addiction/Substance Abuse; Palliative Care; **Hospital:** Montefiore Med Ctr; **Address:** Montfiore Med Ctr, 111 E 210th St, Bronx, NY 10467; **Phone:** 718-920-4678; **Board Cert:** Family Medicine 1998; **Med School:** Harvard Med Sch 1981; **Resid:** Family Medicine, Montefiore Hosp 1984; **Fac Appt:** Prof Med, Albert Einstein Coll Med

Teffera, Fassil MD (IM) **PCP** - **Spec Exp:** Diabetes; Hypertension; Preventive Medicine; **Hospital:** Our Lady of Mercy Med Ctr, Montefiore Med Ctr; **Address:** 140-1 Darrow Pl, Bronx, NY 10475; **Phone:** 718-320-2326; **Board Cert:** Internal Medicine 1993; **Med School:** Ethiopia 1976; **Resid:** Internal Medicine, Our Lady of Mercy Med Ctr 1993; **Fac Appt:** Asst Clin Prof Med, NY Med Coll

MATERNAL & FETAL MEDICINE

Merkatz, Irwin R MD (MF) - **Spec Exp:** Maternal & Fetal Medicine; **Hospital:** Montefiore Med Ctr - Weiler-Einstein Div; **Address:** 1300 Morris Park Ave Belfer Bldg - rm B502, Bronx, NY 10461; **Phone:** 718-430-4192; **Board Cert:** Obstetrics & Gynecology 1967; Maternal & Fetal Medicine 1998; **Med School:** Cornell Univ-Weill Med Coll 1958; **Resid:** Obstetrics & Gynecology, NY Hosp 1962; **Fac Appt:** ObG, Albert Einstein Coll Med

MEDICAL ONCOLOGY

Camacho, Fernando J MD (Onc) - **Spec Exp:** Breast Cancer; Lymphoma; Bladder Cancer; **Hospital:** Montefiore Med Ctr, Saint Joseph's Med Ctr - Yonkers; **Address:** 60 E 208th St, Bronx, NY 10467; **Phone:** 718-405-1700; **Board Cert:** Internal Medicine 1976; Hematology 1978; Medical Oncology 1981; **Med School:** SUNY Buffalo 1973; **Resid:** Internal Medicine, Montefiore Med Ctr 1976; Hematology, Montefiore Hosp Med Ctr 1977; **Fellow:** Medical Oncology, Sloan-Kettering Cancer Ctr 1979; **Fac Appt:** Asst Clin Prof Med

Dutcher, Janice P MD (Onc) - **Spec Exp:** Kidney Cancer; Melanoma; Breast Cancer; **Hospital:** Our Lady of Mercy Med Ctr; **Address:** Our Lady of Mercy Cancer Ctr, 600 E 233rd St, 6 South, Bronx, NY 10466-2697; **Phone:** 718-304-7219; **Board Cert:** Internal Medicine 1978; Medical Oncology 1983; **Med School:** UC Davis 1975; **Resid:** Internal Medicine, Rush Presbyterian 1978; **Fellow:** Medical Oncology, National Cancer Inst 1981; **Fac Appt:** Prof Med, NY Med Coll

Fuks, Joachim MD (Onc) - **Spec Exp:** Lung Cancer; Breast Cancer; Colon Cancer; **Hospital:** NY Westchester Sq Med Ctr, Our Lady of Mercy Med Ctr; **Address:** 1578 Williamsbridge Rd Fl 2, Bronx, NY 10461-6265; **Phone:** 718-931-2290; **Board Cert:** Internal Medicine 1981; Medical Oncology 1983; **Med School:** Spain 1975; **Resid:** Internal Medicine, Mount Sinai Hosp 1978; **Fellow:** Medical Oncology, Nat'l Cancer Center 1981; **Fac Appt:** Asst Clin Prof Med, Albert Einstein Coll Med

Hoffman, Anthony MD (Onc) - **Spec Exp:** Breast Cancer; Multiple Myeloma; **Hospital:** Montefiore Med Ctr - Weiler-Einstein Div, NY Westchester Sq Med Ctr; **Address:** 2330 Eastchester Rd, Bronx, NY 10469; **Phone:** 718-732-4000; **Board Cert:** Internal Medicine 2003; Medical Oncology 1997; **Med School:** Geo Wash Univ 1989; **Resid:** Internal Medicine, Albert Einstein 1992; **Fellow:** Medical Oncology, Meml Sloan Kettering Cancer Ctr 1995

Perez-Soler, Roman MD (Onc) - **Spec Exp:** Lung Cancer; Mesothelioma; **Hospital:** Montefiore Med Ctr - Weiler-Einstein Div, Montefiore Med Ctr; **Address:** Montefiore Medical Ctr, Dept Oncology, 111 E 210th St, Hoffheimer Bldg, rm 100, Bronx, NY 10467; **Phone:** 718-920-4001; **Board Cert:** Internal Medicine 1987; Medical Oncology 1989; **Med School:** Spain 1977; **Resid:** Internal Medicine, Univ Autonoma Med Ctr 1982; **Fellow:** Medical Oncology, MD Anderson Hosp 1985; **Fac Appt:** Prof Med, Albert Einstein Coll Med

Ramirez, Mark A MD (Onc) - **Spec Exp:** Non-Hodgkin's Lymphoma; Breast Cancer; **Hospital:** Montefiore Med Ctr, Saint Joseph's Med Ctr - Yonkers; **Address:** 60 E 208th St, Bronx, NY 10467; **Phone:** 718-405-1700; **Board Cert:** Internal Medicine 1985; Medical Oncology 1989; **Med School:** Cornell Univ-Weill Med Coll 1982; **Resid:** Internal Medicine, Montefiore Hosp Med Ctr 1985; **Fellow:** Hematology & Oncology, Montefiore Hosp Med Ctr 1988; **Fac Appt:** Asst Clin Prof Med, Albert Einstein Coll Med

Reed, Mary K MD (Onc) - **Spec Exp:** Breast Cancer; AIDS/HIV; Pain-Cancer; **Hospital:** Bronx Lebanon Hosp Ctr; **Address:** 1650 Grand Concourse, 8th Fl, Bronx, NY 10457; **Phone:** 718-960-1437; **Board Cert:** Internal Medicine 1984; Medical Oncology 2000; Hematology 2004; **Med School:** Boston Univ 1980; **Resid:** Internal Medicine, Henry Ford Hosp 1983; **Fellow:** Hematology & Oncology, LI Jewish Med Ctr 1988; **Fac Appt:** Asst Prof Med, Albert Einstein Coll Med

Sparano, Joseph A MD (Onc) - **Spec Exp:** Breast Cancer; Lymphoma; **Hospital:** Montefiore Med Ctr - Weiler-Einstein Div; **Address:** 1825 Eastchester Rd, Ste 2S-47, Bronx, NY 10461; **Phone:** 718-904-2555; **Board Cert:** Internal Medicine 1986; Medical Oncology 1989; **Med School:** NY Med Coll 1982; **Resid:** Internal Medicine, St Vincents Hosp 1986; **Fellow:** Medical Oncology, Montefiore Med Ctr 1988; **Fac Appt:** Prof Med, Albert Einstein Coll Med

Stein, Cy A MD/PhD (Onc) - **Spec Exp:** Prostate Cancer; Bladder Cancer; **Hospital:** Montefiore Med Ctr; **Address:** Montefiore Med Ctr, Dept Oncology, 111 E 210 St, Hofheimer 100, Bronx, NY 10467; **Phone:** 718-920-8980; **Board Cert:** Internal Medicine 1986; Medical Oncology 1987; **Med School:** Albert Einstein Coll Med 1982; **Resid:** Internal Medicine, NY Hosp-Cornell Med Ctr 1985; **Fellow:** Medical Oncology, Natl Cancer Inst 1988; **Fac Appt:** Prof Med, Albert Einstein Coll Med

Vogl, Steven Edward MD (Onc) - **Spec Exp:** Breast Cancer; Lung Cancer; **Hospital:** Montefiore Med Ctr - Weiler-Einstein Div, NY Westchester Sq Med Ctr; **Address:** 2220 Tiemann Ave, Bronx, NY 10469; **Phone:** 718-519-7774; **Board Cert:** Internal Medicine 1975; Medical Oncology 1975; **Med School:** Cornell Univ-Weill Med Coll 1970; **Resid:** Internal Medicine, Jacobi Med Ctr 1972; **Fellow:** Medical Oncology, Mount Sinai 1975

NEONATAL-PERINATAL MEDICINE

Brion, Luc MD (NP) - **Spec Exp:** Kidney Disease; Growth/Development Disorders; **Hospital:** Montefiore Med Ctr - Weiler-Einstein Div, Montefiore Med Ctr; **Address:** 1825 Eastchester Road, Ste 725, Bronx, NY 10461-1101; **Phone:** 718-904-4105; **Board Cert:** Pediatrics 1987; Neonatal-Perinatal Medicine 1987; **Med School:** Belgium 1976; **Resid:** Pediatrics, Hosp St Pierre 1981; Pediatrics, Albert Einstein Coll Med 1986; **Fellow:** Neonatal-Perinatal Medicine, Hosp For Sick Chldn 1982; Neonatal-Perinatal Medicine, Albert Einstein Coll Med 1985; **Fac Appt:** Prof Ped, Albert Einstein Coll Med

Campbell, Deborah MD (NP) - **Spec Exp:** Prematurity/Low Birth Weight Infants; Neurodevelopmental Disabilities; Nutrition; **Hospital:** Montefiore Med Ctr - Weiler-Einstein Div; **Address:** 1825 Eastchester Rd, Ste 725, Bronx, NY 10461-2301; **Phone:** 718-904-4105; **Board Cert:** Pediatrics 1983; Neonatal-Perinatal Medicine 1985; **Med School:** SUNY Buffalo 1978; **Resid:** Pediatrics, Montefiore Med Ctr 1981; **Fellow:** Neonatal-Perinatal Medicine, Montefiore Med Ctr 1983; **Fac Appt:** Clin Prof Ped, Albert Einstein Coll Med

Katzenstein, Martin MD (NP) - **Spec Exp:** Neonatal Nutrition; Ethics; Neonatal Respiratory Care; **Hospital:** Our Lady of Mercy Med Ctr; **Address:** 600 E 233rd St, Bronx, NY 10466-2604; **Phone:** 718-920-9541; **Board Cert:** Pediatrics 2004; Neonatal-Perinatal Medicine 1999; **Med School:** NY Med Coll 1978; **Resid:** Pediatrics, NY Hosp-Cornell Med Ctr 1980; **Fellow:** Neonatal-Perinatal Medicine, NY Hosp-Cornell Med Ctr 1981; Neonatal-Perinatal Medicine, Westchester County Med Ctr 1984; **Fac Appt:** Asst Clin Prof Ped, NY Med Coll

Reinersman, Gerald MD (NP) - **Spec Exp:** Nutrition; **Hospital:** Montefiore Med Ctr - Weiler-Einstein Div, Montefiore Med Ctr; **Address:** 1825 Eastchester Rd, Rm 725, Bronx, NY 10461; **Phone:** 718-904-4105; **Board Cert:** Pediatrics 1980; Neonatal-Perinatal Medicine 1985; **Med School:** Univ KY Coll Med 1974; **Resid:** Pediatrics, Oregon Hlth Sci Univ Hosp 1979; **Fellow:** Neonatal-Perinatal Medicine, Univ Utah Hosp 1985; **Fac Appt:** Asst Prof Ped, Albert Einstein Coll Med

Nephrology

Charytan, Chaim MD (Nep) - **Spec Exp:** Hypertension; Diabetic Kidney Disease; Kidney Stones; **Hospital:** NY Hosp Queens, Montefiore Med Ctr - Weiler-Einstein Div; **Address:** 1874 Pelham Pkwy South, Bronx, NY 10461-3733; **Phone:** 718-931-5800; **Board Cert:** Internal Medicine 1969; Nephrology 1974; **Med School:** Albert Einstein Coll Med 1964; **Resid:** Internal Medicine, Bronx Municipal Hosp 1967; **Fellow:** Nephrology, Boston Univ Hosp 1968; **Fac Appt:** Clin Prof Med, Cornell Univ-Weill Med Coll

Coco, Maria MD (Nep) - **Spec Exp:** Hypertension; Kidney Disease; **Hospital:** Montefiore Med Ctr; **Address:** 111 E 210th St, Bronx, NY 10467-2401; **Phone:** 718-920-4136; **Board Cert:** Internal Medicine 1985; Nephrology 1988; **Med School:** Italy 1982; **Resid:** Internal Medicine, Bronx Lebanon Hosp 1985; **Fellow:** Nephrology, Montefiore Hosp Med Ctr 1988; **Fac Appt:** Assoc Prof Med, Albert Einstein Coll Med

Croll, James MD (Nep) - **Spec Exp:** Dialysis Care; Hypertension; **Hospital:** St Barnabas Hosp - Bronx; **Address:** 4422 3rd Ave, Bronx, NY 10457; **Phone:** 718-960-6295; **Board Cert:** Internal Medicine 1978; Nephrology 1982; **Med School:** Belgium 1975; **Resid:** Internal Medicine, Genesee Hosp 1978; **Fellow:** Nephrology, VA Med Ctr 1981

Dave, Mahendraray MD (Nep) - **Spec Exp:** Dialysis Care; **Hospital:** Bronx Lebanon Hosp Ctr; **Address:** Bronx Lebanon Hosp Ctr - Nephrology, 1650 Grand Concourse Fl 10, Bronx, NY 10457-7606; **Phone:** 718-518-5232; **Board Cert:** Internal Medicine 1979; Nephrology 1982; **Med School:** India 1971; **Resid:** Internal Medicine, Bronx Lebanon Hosp 1978; **Fellow:** Nephrology, Bronx-Lebanon Hosp Ctr 1980; **Fac Appt:** Assoc Prof Med, Albert Einstein Coll Med

Gorkin, Janet U MD (Nep) - **Spec Exp:** Hypertension; Diabetic Kidney Disease; Kidney Failure; **Hospital:** Montefiore Med Ctr; **Address:** 3327 Bainbridge Ave, Bronx, NY 10467; **Phone:** 718-881-5100; **Board Cert:** Internal Medicine 1976; Nephrology 1980; **Med School:** Mount Sinai Sch Med 1973; **Resid:** Internal Medicine, Mt Sinai Hosp 1976; **Fellow:** Nephrology, Mt Sinai Hosp 1978; **Fac Appt:** Prof Med, Albert Einstein Coll Med

Laitman, Robert MD (Nep) - **Spec Exp:** Diabetic Kidney Disease; Cholesterol/Lipid Disorders; **Hospital:** Montefiore Med Ctr - Weiler-Einstein Div; **Address:** 1521 Jarett Pl, Bronx, NY 10461-2606; **Phone:** 718-518-1276; **Board Cert:** Internal Medicine 1986; Nephrology 1988; Geriatric Medicine 2000; **Med School:** Washington Univ, St Louis 1983; **Resid:** Internal Medicine, Jacobi Med Ctr 1986; **Fellow:** Nephrology, Montefiore Hosp Med Ctr 1988

Lief, Philip MD (Nep) - **Spec Exp:** Hypertension; Kidney Disease; **Hospital:** Montefiore Med Ctr, Montefiore Med Ctr - Weiler-Einstein Div; **Address:** 1575 Blondell Ave, Ste 200, Bronx, NY 10461; **Phone:** 718-405-8377; **Board Cert:** Internal Medicine 1974; Nephrology 1974; **Med School:** Univ Pennsylvania 1965; **Resid:** Internal Medicine, Montefiore Medical Center 1968; **Fellow:** Nephrology, New England Medical Center 1970; **Fac Appt:** Prof Med, Albert Einstein Coll Med

Lynn, Robert MD (Nep) - **Spec Exp:** Hypertension; Dialysis Care; **Hospital:** Montefiore Med Ctr - Weiler-Einstein Div, Sound Shore Med Ctr - Westchester (page 711); **Address:** 1200 Waters Pl, Ste M104, Bronx, NY 10461; **Phone:** 718-794-1200; **Board Cert:** Internal Medicine 1977; Nephrology 1980; **Med School:** Columbia P&S 1974; **Resid:** Internal Medicine, Columbia-Presby Med Ctr 1977; **Fellow:** Nephrology, Yale-New Haven Hosp 1979; **Fac Appt:** Assoc Prof Med, Albert Einstein Coll Med

Schuster, Victor L MD (Nep) - **Hospital:** Montefiore Med Ctr - Weiler-Einstein Div, Montefiore Med Ctr; **Address:** 1300 Morris Park Ave, Belfer 1008, Bronx, NY 10461; **Phone:** 718-430-8560; **Board Cert:** Internal Medicine 1980; Nephrology 1984; **Med School:** Washington Univ, St Louis 1977; **Resid:** Internal Medicine, Univ Wash Med Ctr 1981; **Fellow:** Nephrology, Univ Texas SW Med Ctr 1983; **Fac Appt:** Prof Med, Albert Einstein Coll Med

Uday, Kalpana MD (Nep) - **Spec Exp:** Hypertension; **Hospital:** Bronx Lebanon Hosp Ctr; **Address:** 1650 Grand Concourse, FL 10, Bronx, NY 10457-7606; **Phone:** 718-518-5232; **Board Cert:** Internal Medicine 1989; Nephrology 1992; **Med School:** India 1980; **Resid:** Internal Medicine, Jamaica Med Ctr 1989; **Fellow:** Nephrology, Montefiore Med Ctr 1991; **Fac Appt:** Asst Prof Med, Albert Einstein Coll Med

Weiner, Bernard M MD (Nep) - **Hospital:** Montefiore Med Ctr, NY Westchester Sq Med Ctr; **Address:** 1180 Morris Park Ave, Bronx, NY 10461-1925; **Phone:** 718-863-8465; **Board Cert:** Internal Medicine 1976; Nephrology 1978; **Med School:** Albert Einstein Coll Med 1973; **Resid:** Internal Medicine, Jacobi Med Ctr/Albert Einstein Coll Med 1974; Internal Medicine, Jacobi Med Ctr/Albert Einstein Coll Med 1976; **Fellow:** Renal Physiology, Hosp Univ Penn 1978; **Fac Appt:** Asst Clin Prof Med, Albert Einstein Coll Med

Yoo, Jinil MD (Nep) - **Spec Exp:** Kidney Disease; Hypertension; Diabetes; **Hospital:** Our Lady of Mercy Med Ctr, Westchester Med Ctr (page 713); **Address:** 4234 Bronx Blvd, Bronx, NY 10466-2656; **Phone:** 347-341-4300; **Board Cert:** Internal Medicine 1974; Nephrology 1976; **Med School:** South Korea 1967; **Resid:** Internal Medicine, Lahay Clinic 1972; Internal Medicine, Metropolitan Hosp Ctr 1974; **Fellow:** Internal Medicine, Joslin Diabetes Center 1973; Nephrology, NY Med Coll/Metro Hosp 1976; **Fac Appt:** Assoc Clin Prof Med, NY Med Coll

NEUROLOGICAL SURGERY

Flamm, Eugene MD (NS) - **Spec Exp:** Aneurysm-Cerebral; Brain Tumors; Cerebrovascular Neurosurgery; **Hospital:** Montefiore Med Ctr; **Address:** Montefiore Med Ctr, 111 E 210th St, Bronx, NY 10467-2841; **Phone:** 718-920-2339; **Board Cert:** Neurological Surgery 1973; **Med School:** SUNY Buffalo 1962; **Resid:** Surgery, New York Hosp 1964; Neurological Surgery, NYU Med Ctr 1970; **Fellow:** Neurological Surgery, Univ Zurich 1971; **Fac Appt:** Prof NS, Albert Einstein Coll Med

Goodrich, James T MD (NS) - **Spec Exp:** Craniofacial Surgery/Reconstruction; Spina Bifida; Brain Tumors-Pediatric; **Hospital:** Montefiore Med Ctr, Jacobi Med Ctr; **Address:** Montefiore Med Ctr, Dept Ped Neurosurgery, 111 E 210th St, Bronx, NY 10467-2401; **Phone:** 718-920-4197; **Board Cert:** Neurological Surgery 1989; Pediatric Neurological Surgery 1996; **Med School:** Columbia P&S 1980; **Resid:** Neurological Surgery, NY Neurological Inst 1986; **Fac Appt:** Prof NS, Albert Einstein Coll Med

LaSala, Patrick MD (NS) - **Spec Exp:** Brain Tumors; **Hospital:** Montefiore Med Ctr; **Address:** Dept Neurosurgery, 3316 Rochambeau Ave, Bronx, NY 10467-2803; **Phone:** 718-920-7466; **Board Cert:** Neurological Surgery 1991; **Med School:** Columbia P&S 1980; **Resid:** Neurological Surgery, Columbia-Presby Med Ctr 1987; **Fac Appt:** Assoc Prof NS, Albert Einstein Coll Med

Tabaddor, Kamran MD (NS) - **Spec Exp:** Brain Tumors; Spinal Surgery; Epilepsy; **Hospital:** Our Lady of Mercy Med Ctr, Montefiore Med Ctr; **Address:** 4170 Bronx Blvd, Bronx, NY 10466; **Phone:** 718-655-9111; **Board Cert:** Neurological Surgery 1979; **Med School:** Iran 1967; **Resid:** Neurological Surgery, Johns Hopkins Hosp 1971; Neurological Surgery, Einstein Hosp 1976; **Fac Appt:** Clin Prof NS, Albert Einstein Coll Med

Torres-Gluck, Jose MD (NS) - **Spec Exp:** Brain Tumors; Stereotactic Radiosurgery; **Hospital:** Jacobi Med Ctr; **Address:** Jacobi Medical Ctr, 1400 Pelham Pkwy S, rm 3 West 5, Bronx, NY 10461; **Phone:** 718-918-6220; **Board Cert:** Neurological Surgery 1998; **Med School:** Columbia P&S 1987; **Resid:** Neurological Surgery, Albert Einstein Coll Med 1993; **Fellow:** Neurological Oncology, Meml Sloan Kettering Cancer Ctr 1995

NEUROLOGY

Cohen, Joel S MD (N) - **Spec Exp:** Epilepsy; Headache; Stroke; Parkinson's Disease; **Hospital:** Montefiore Med Ctr, Montefiore Med Ctr - Weiler-Einstein Div; **Address:** 1610 Williamsbridge Rd Fl 2, Bronx, NY 10461-2601; **Phone:** 718-597-8000; **Board Cert:** Neurology 1992; **Med School:** Albert Einstein Coll Med 1983; **Resid:** Neurology, Albert Einstein 1987; **Fellow:** Neurology, Albert Einstein 1988; **Fac Appt:** Assoc Prof N, Albert Einstein Coll Med

Elkin, Rene MD (N) - **Spec Exp:** Multiple Sclerosis; **Hospital:** Bronx Lebanon Hosp Ctr, White Plains Hosp Ctr (page 714); **Address:** 1650 Selwyn Ave, Ste 11F, Bronx, NY 10457-7663; **Phone:** 718-960-1335; **Board Cert:** Neurology 1994; **Med School:** South Africa 1975; **Resid:** Neurology, Groote Schuur Hosp 1980; Neurology, Albert Einstein Med Ctr 1992; **Fac Appt:** Asst Prof N, Albert Einstein Coll Med

Freddo, Lorenza MD (N) - **Spec Exp:** Pain Management; Multiple Sclerosis; Peripheral Neuropathy; **Hospital:** St Barnabas Hosp - Bronx; **Address:** 2371 Arthur Ave, Bronx, NY 10458-8113; **Phone:** 718-364-6199; **Board Cert:** Neurology 1992; **Med School:** Italy 1980; **Resid:** Neurology, Italy 1984; Neurology, Columbia Presby Hosp 1990; **Fellow:** Columbia Presby Hosp 1986

Grenell, Steven MD (N) - **Spec Exp:** Pain Management; Headache; **Hospital:** Montefiore Med Ctr; **Address:** 3975 Sedgewick Ave, Ste 1-F, Bronx, NY 10463; **Phone:** 718-796-6055; **Board Cert:** Neurology 1989; **Med School:** Rutgers Univ 1977; **Resid:** Internal Medicine, Montefiore Hosp 1979; Neurology, Montefiore Hosp 1982; **Fellow:** Internal Medicine, Montefiore Hosp; **Fac Appt:** Asst Prof N, Albert Einstein Coll Med

Herskovitz, Steven MD (N) - **Spec Exp:** Electromyography; Neuromuscular Disorders; **Hospital:** Montefiore Med Ctr; **Address:** 111 E 210th St, Bronx, NY 10467-2401; **Phone:** 718-920-4930; **Board Cert:** Internal Medicine 1983; Neurology 1987; Clinical Neurophysiology 1996; **Med School:** Cornell Univ-Weill Med Coll 1980; **Resid:** Internal Medicine, Montefiore Med Ctr 1983; Neurology, Montefiore Med Ctr 1986; **Fellow:** Electromyography, Montefiore Med Ctr 1987; **Fac Appt:** Prof N, Albert Einstein Coll Med

Hughes, John T MD (N) - **Spec Exp:** Migraine; Epilepsy/Seizure Disorders; **Hospital:** Our Lady of Mercy Med Ctr, Phelps Meml Hosp Ctr; **Address:** Department of Neurology, 4170 Bronx Boulevard, Bronx, NY 10466; **Phone:** 718-652-0509; **Board Cert:** Neurology 1993; Clinical Neurophysiology 1996; **Med School:** NY Med Coll 1982; **Resid:** Internal Medicine, Naval Regl Med Ctr 1986; Neurology, NYU Med Ctr 1992; **Fellow:** Epilepsy, NYU Med Ctr 1993; Clinical Neurophysiology, NYU Med Ctr 1994; **Fac Appt:** Asst Prof N, NY Med Coll

Kaplan, Jerry MD (N) - **Spec Exp:** Electromyography; **Hospital:** Montefiore Med Ctr; **Address:** 1610 Williamsbridge Rd, Bronx, NY 10461; **Phone:** 718-794-2505; **Board Cert:** Neurology 1980; Clinical Neurophysiology 1996; **Med School:** Albert Einstein Coll Med 1975; **Resid:** Neurology, Albert Einstein 1979; **Fellow:** Clinical Neurophysiology, Mass Genl Hosp 1981; Clinical Neurophysiology, Columbia Presby Med Ctr 1982; **Fac Appt:** Assoc Prof N, Albert Einstein Coll Med

Kaufman, David Myland MD (N) - **Spec Exp:** Movement Disorders; **Hospital:** Montefiore Med Ctr; **Address:** 3400 Bainbridge Ave, Main Fl, Bronx, NY 10467; **Phone:** 718-920-4730; **Board Cert:** Internal Medicine 1972; Neurology 1976; **Med School:** Univ Chicago-Pritzker Sch Med 1968; **Resid:** Internal Medicine, Montefiore Hosp Med 1971; Neurology, Albert Einstein Coll Hosp 1974; **Fac Appt:** Prof N, Albert Einstein Coll Med

Miller, Ann Marie MD (N) - **Spec Exp:** Headache; Parkinson's Disease; Multiple Sclerosis; **Hospital:** Montefiore Med Ctr; **Address:** 111 S 210th St, rm NW844, Bronx, NY 10467; **Phone:** 718-920-5412; **Board Cert:** Neurology 1986; **Med School:** SUNY Downstate 1981; **Resid:** Neurology, Albert Einstein 1985; **Fac Appt:** Assoc Clin Prof N, Albert Einstein Coll Med

Moshe, Solomon L MD (N) - **Spec Exp:** Epilepsy-Pediatric; Seizure Disorders-Pediatric; **Hospital:** Montefiore Med Ctr; **Address:** 1515 Blondell Ave, Ste 220, Bronx, NY 10461; **Phone:** 718-405-8140; **Board Cert:** Neurology 1979; Child Neurology 1979; Clinical Neurophysiology 1996; **Med School:** Greece 1972; **Resid:** Pediatrics, Univ MD Hosp 1975; Neurology, Albert Einstein 1978; **Fellow:** Neurology, Albert Einstein 1979; **Fac Appt:** Prof N, Albert Einstein Coll Med

Smith, Charles R MD (N) - **Spec Exp:** Multiple Sclerosis; Headache; Spinal Cord Injury; **Hospital:** Bronx Lebanon Hosp Ctr, White Plains Hosp Ctr (page 714); **Address:** 1770 Grand Concourse Fl 2, Bronx, NY 10457; **Phone:** 718-518-5581; **Board Cert:** Neurology 1984; **Med School:** Univ Toronto 1976; **Resid:** Internal Medicine, Toronto Western Hosp 1978; Neurology, Toronto Genl Hosp 1981; **Fellow:** Neurological Immunology, Albert Einstein Coll Med 1983; **Fac Appt:** Asst Prof N, Albert Einstein Coll Med

Sparr, Steven MD (N) - **Hospital:** Montefiore Med Ctr; **Address:** Montefiore Med Ctr, Stern Stroke Ctr, 111 E 210th St, Bronx, NY 10467; **Phone:** 718-920-6402; **Board Cert:** Internal Medicine 1984; Neurology 1987; **Med School:** SUNY Buffalo 1980; **Resid:** Internal Medicine, Boston City Hosp 1983; Neurology, Albert Einstein 1986; **Fellow:** Neurological Rehabilitation, Burke Rehabilitation Hosp 1987; **Fac Appt:** Assoc Prof N, Albert Einstein Coll Med

Swerdlow, Michael MD (N) - **Spec Exp:** Myasthenia Gravis; Spinal Disorders; Multiple Sclerosis; **Hospital:** Montefiore Med Ctr; **Address:** 3400 Bainbridge Ave, Ste 5A, Bronx, NY 10467-2401; **Phone:** 718-920-4178; **Board Cert:** Neurology 1975; **Med School:** Univ Pennsylvania 1967; **Resid:** Internal Medicine, Mount Sinai Hosp 1969; Neurology, Albert Einstein Coll 1972; **Fellow:** Neurology, Natl Inst Hlth 1974; **Fac Appt:** Prof N, Albert Einstein Coll Med

NEURORADIOLOGY

Bello, Jacqueline A MD (NRad) - **Spec Exp:** Aneurysm-Cerebral; Pain-Back; **Hospital:** Montefiore Med Ctr; **Address:** 111 E 210th St, Bronx, NY 10467; **Phone:** 718-920-4030; **Board Cert:** Diagnostic Radiology 1984; Neuroradiology 1997; **Med School:** Columbia P&S 1980; **Resid:** Radiology, Columbia-PresbyMed Ctr 1984; **Fellow:** Neuroradiology, Neuro Inst/Columbia-Presby Med Ctr 1986; **Fac Appt:** Prof Rad, Albert Einstein Coll Med

NUCLEAR MEDICINE

Blaufox, M Donald MD/PhD (NuM) - **Spec Exp:** Hypertension; Kidney Disease; PET Imaging; **Hospital:** Montefiore Med Ctr - Weiler-Einstein Div, Montefiore Med Ctr; **Address:** Montefiore Medical Park, Dept Nuclear Med, 1695A Eastchester Rd, Bronx, NY 10469-1642; **Phone:** 718-405-8454; **Board Cert:** Internal Medicine 1966; Nuclear Medicine 1972; **Med School:** SUNY Hlth Sci Ctr 1959; **Resid:** Internal Medicine, Mayo Clinic 1964; **Fellow:** Nephrology, Peter Bent Brigham Hosp/Harvard 1966; **Fac Appt:** Prof NuM, Albert Einstein Coll Med

Freeman, Leonard M MD (NuM) - **Spec Exp:** Nuclear Oncology; Gastrointestinal Disorders; PET Imaging; CT Scan; **Hospital:** Montefiore Med Ctr; **Address:** 111 E 210th St, Bronx, NY 10467-2401; **Phone:** 718-920-6060; **Board Cert:** Radiology 1966; Nuclear Medicine 1972; Nuclear Radiology 1974; **Med School:** Univ Hlth Sci/Chicago Med Sch 1961; **Resid:** Radiology, Bronx Municipal Hosp 1965; **Fac Appt:** Prof NuM, Albert Einstein Coll Med

Milstein, David MD (NuM) - **Hospital:** Montefiore Med Ctr - Weiler-Einstein Div, Montefiore Med Ctr; **Address:** 1825 Eastchester Rd, Bronx, NY 10461; **Phone:** 718-904-4058; **Board Cert:** Nuclear Medicine 1972; Diagnostic Radiology 1972; **Med School:** Albert Einstein Coll Med 1967; **Resid:** Radiology, Bronx Muni Hosp Ctr 1972; **Fellow:** Diagnostic Radiology, Bronx Muni Hosp Ctr 1972; **Fac Appt:** Prof NuM, Albert Einstein Coll Med

OBSTETRICS & GYNECOLOGY

Adachi, Akinori MD (ObG) PCP - **Spec Exp:** Cancer Screening; Uterine Fibroids; Pelvic Reconstruction; **Hospital:** Montefiore Med Ctr; **Address:** 3332 Rochambeau Ave, Box 18, Bronx, NY 10467; **Phone:** 718-920-5157; **Board Cert:** Obstetrics & Gynecology 1980; **Med School:** Japan 1963; **Resid:** Obstetrics & Gynecology, Jewish Meml Hosp 1968; **Fellow:** Gynecologic Oncology, NY Med Coll 1969; Reproductive Endocrinology, NY Med Coll/Metropolitan Hosp 1971; **Fac Appt:** Assoc Prof ObG, Albert Einstein Coll Med

Afif, Juan Simon MD (ObG) PCP - **Spec Exp:** Laparoscopic Surgery; **Hospital:** NY Westchester Sq Med Ctr, Our Lady of Mercy Med Ctr; **Address:** 1214 Pelham Pkwy South, Bronx, NY 10461; **Phone:** 718-824-2200; **Board Cert:** Obstetrics & Gynecology 1979; **Med School:** Argentina 1970; **Resid:** Surgery, Albert Einstein 1974; Obstetrics & Gynecology, Misericordia Hosp 1977

Duvivier, Roger MD (ObG) PCP - **Spec Exp:** Colposcopy; Laparoscopy/Hysteroscopy; Preventive Medicine; Women's Health; **Hospital:** Montefiore Med Ctr - Weiler-Einstein Div; **Address:** 1621 Eastchester Rd, Bronx, NY 10461; **Phone:** 718-405-8040; **Board Cert:** Obstetrics & Gynecology 2003; **Med School:** Albert Einstein Coll Med 1974; **Resid:** Obstetrics & Gynecology, Bronx Muni Hosp-Albert Einstein 1978; **Fac Appt:** Assoc Prof ObG, Albert Einstein Coll Med

Henderson, Cassandra E MD (ObG) - **Spec Exp:** Pregnancy-High Risk; **Hospital:** Our Lady of Mercy Med Ctr, Montefiore Med Ctr; **Address:** 600 E 233rd St, Bronx, NY 10466; **Phone:** 718-920-9647; **Board Cert:** Obstetrics & Gynecology 1995; Maternal & Fetal Medicine 1995; **Med School:** Loyola Univ-Stritch Sch Med 1980; **Resid:** Obstetrics & Gynecology, Univ Chicago Hosp 1984; **Fellow:** Maternal & Fetal Medicine, Albert Einstein 1986; **Fac Appt:** Assoc Prof ObG, NY Med Coll

Katz, Nadine MD (ObG) - **Hospital:** Montefiore Med Ctr - Weiler-Einstein Div; **Address:** 1695 Eastchester Rd, Ste L2, Bronx, NY 10461; **Phone:** 718-405-8200; **Board Cert:** Obstetrics & Gynecology 1998; **Med School:** Albert Einstein Coll Med 1987; **Resid:** Obstetrics & Gynecology, Jacobi Med Ctr 1991

Lafontant, Jennifer MD (ObG) **PCP** - **Spec Exp:** Menopause Problems; Pain-Pelvic; Uterine Fibroids; **Hospital:** St Barnabas Hosp - Bronx, NY-Presby Hosp (page 100); **Address:** 2016 Bronxdale Ave Fl 2 - Ste 201, Bronx, NY 10462-3309; **Phone:** 718-823-1010; **Board Cert:** Obstetrics & Gynecology 1985; **Med School:** West Indies 1976; **Resid:** Obstetrics & Gynecology, St Luke's-Roosevelt Hosp Ctr 1980; Obstetrics & Gynecology, Metropolitan Hosp Ctr 1982; **Fac Appt:** Asst Clin Prof ObG, Columbia P&S

Levy, Judith MD (ObG) **PCP** - **Spec Exp:** Diabetes in Pregnancy; **Hospital:** Montefiore Med Ctr - Weiler-Einstein Div; **Address:** 1695 Eastchester Rd, Ste L2, Bronx, NY 10461; **Phone:** 718-405-8200; **Board Cert:** Obstetrics & Gynecology 1998; **Med School:** Albert Einstein Coll Med 1981; **Resid:** Obstetrics & Gynecology, Albert Einstein-Bronx Muni Hosp 1985; **Fac Appt:** Asst Prof ObG, Albert Einstein Coll Med

Mastrantonio, John MD (ObG) - **Hospital:** Montefiore Med Ctr - Weiler-Einstein Div; **Address:** 1578 Williamsbridge Rd, Bronx, NY 10461; **Phone:** 914-961-0201; **Board Cert:** Obstetrics & Gynecology 1974; **Med School:** SUNY Hlth Sci Ctr 1967; **Resid:** Obstetrics & Gynecology, Bronx Muni Hosp 1972

Muscillo, George MD (ObG) - **Spec Exp:** Menopause Problems; **Hospital:** Montefiore Med Ctr - Weiler-Einstein Div, NY Westchester Sq Med Ctr; **Address:** 1072 Esplanade Ave, Bronx, NY 10461-1208; **Phone:** 718-829-6335; **Board Cert:** Obstetrics & Gynecology 1966; **Med School:** NY Med Coll 1958; **Resid:** Obstetrics & Gynecology, Metropolitan Hosp Ctr 1963; **Fac Appt:** Asst Clin Prof ObG, Albert Einstein Coll Med

Reilly, Kevin D MD (ObG) **PCP** - **Spec Exp:** Menopause Problems; **Hospital:** Our Lady of Mercy Med Ctr; **Address:** 600 E 233rd St, Bronx, NY 10466-2604; **Phone:** 718-920-9647; **Board Cert:** Obstetrics & Gynecology 1976; **Med School:** Univ Mich Med Sch 1969; **Resid:** Obstetrics & Gynecology, St Vincent's Hosp & Med Ctr 1974; **Fac Appt:** Assoc Prof ObG, NY Med Coll

OPHTHALMOLOGY

Chess, Jeremy MD (Oph) - **Spec Exp:** Retina/Vitreous Surgery; **Hospital:** Montefiore Med Ctr - Weiler-Einstein Div, Saint Joseph's Med Ctr - Yonkers; **Address:** 2221 Boston Rd, Bronx, NY 10467; **Phone:** 718-798-3030; **Board Cert:** Ophthalmology 1977; **Med School:** Boston Univ 1970; **Resid:** Ophthalmology, Boston Univ Med Ctr 1974; **Fellow:** Vitreoretinal Surgery, Boston Univ Med Ctr 1983; **Fac Appt:** Assoc Clin Prof Oph, Albert Einstein Coll Med

Dankner, Richard MD (Oph) - **Spec Exp:** Laser Refractive Surgery; Cataract Surgery; **Hospital:** NY Westchester Sq Med Ctr; **Address:** 1625 Saint Peters Ave, Bronx, NY 10461; **Phone:** 718-823-9227; **Board Cert:** Ophthalmology 1977; **Med School:** SUNY Upstate Med Univ 1967; **Resid:** Ophthalmology, NYU Med Ctr 1973

Engel, Harry MD (Oph) - **Spec Exp:** Retinal Disorders; **Hospital:** Montefiore Med Ctr; **Address:** Montefiore Med Ctr, Dept Ophthalmology, 111 E 210th St, Bronx, NY 10467; **Phone:** 718-920-2020; **Board Cert:** Ophthalmology 1981; **Med School:** NY Med Coll 1976; **Resid:** Ophthalmology, U Michigan Med Ctr 1980; **Fellow:** Eye Pathology, Wilmer Inst 1981; Retina/Vitreous, Barnes Jewish Hosp 1982; **Fac Appt:** Assoc Prof Oph, Albert Einstein Coll Med

Gurland, Judith MD (Oph) - **Spec Exp:** Pediatric Ophthalmology; Eye Muscle Disorders; **Hospital:** Montefiore Med Ctr, Bronx Lebanon Hosp Ctr; **Address:** 3400 Bainbridge Ave, Bronx, NY 10467-2404; **Phone:** 718-920-2020; **Board Cert:** Ophthalmology 1974; **Med School:** SUNY Downstate 1968; **Resid:** Ophthalmology, SUNY Downstate 1972; **Fellow:** Neurological Ophthalmology, Kingsbrook Jewish Med Ctr 1973; Pediatric Ophthalmology, Columbia-Presby Hosp 1973; **Fac Appt:** Assoc Prof Oph, Albert Einstein Coll Med

Hayworth, Robin MD (Oph) - **Spec Exp:** Cataract Surgery; Glaucoma; **Hospital:** Manhattan Eye, Ear & Throat Hosp, Montefiore Med Ctr - Weiler-Einstein Div; **Address:** 787 Lydig Ave, Bronx, NY 10462-2144; **Phone:** 718-863-7774; **Board Cert:** Ophthalmology 1985; **Med School:** Cornell Univ-Weill Med Coll 1978; **Resid:** Surgery, NY Hosp 1980; Ophthalmology, Manhattan EET Hosp 1983

Mayers, Martin MD (Oph) - **Spec Exp:** Cataract Surgery; Cornea Transplant; **Hospital:** Bronx Lebanon Hosp Ctr, Montefiore Med Ctr; **Address:** Bronx Lebanon Hosp Ctr, Dept Ophthalmology, 1650 Grand Concourse, Milstein, Ste 1C, Bronx, NY 10457; **Phone:** 718-960-2044; **Board Cert:** Ophthalmology 1985; **Med School:** Albert Einstein Coll Med 1979; **Resid:** Ophthalmology, SUNY Downstate Med Ctr 1983; **Fellow:** Cornea, Proctor Fdn-UCSF 1984; **Fac Appt:** Assoc Prof Oph, Albert Einstein Coll Med

Palmer, Edward MD (Oph) - **Spec Exp:** Cataract Surgery; Glaucoma; **Hospital:** Montefiore Med Ctr; **Address:** 100 Casals Pl, Bronx, NY 10475-3002; **Phone:** 718-671-8888; **Board Cert:** Ophthalmology 1972; **Med School:** Meharry Med Coll 1964; **Resid:** Ophthalmology, Bronx Eye & Ear Infirmary 1970; **Fellow:** Ophthalmology, Mt Sinai Sch Med 1972; **Fac Appt:** Assoc Prof Oph, Albert Einstein Coll Med

Rosenbaum, Pearl MD (Oph) - **Spec Exp:** Cataract Surgery; Glaucoma; Eye Tumors/Cancer; Diabetic Eye Disease; **Hospital:** Montefiore Med Ctr, Bronx Lebanon Hosp Ctr; **Address:** 3333 Henry Hudson Pkwy, Riverdale, NY 10471; **Phone:** 718-548-5800; **Board Cert:** Ophthalmology 1988; **Med School:** Albert Einstein Coll Med 1982; **Resid:** Ophthalmology, Albert Einstein 1986; **Fellow:** Ophthalmological Pathology, Baylor Col of Med 1987; Ophthalmic Oncololgy, Baylor Col of Med 1988

Slamovits, Thomas MD (Oph) - **Spec Exp:** Neuro-Ophthalmology; Optic Nerve Disorders; Vision Loss-Unexplained Loss; Diabetic Eye Disease/Retinopathy; **Hospital:** Montefiore Med Ctr, Hackensack Univ Med Ctr (page 92); **Address:** 1250 Pelham Pkwy S, Bronx, NY 10461; **Phone:** 718-794-1500; **Board Cert:** Ophthalmology 1980; **Med School:** Ohio State Univ 1975; **Resid:** Ophthalmology, Univ Pitts Eye & Ear 1979; **Fellow:** Neurological Ophthalmology, Washington Univ-Barnes Hosp 1980; **Fac Appt:** Prof Oph, Albert Einstein Coll Med

Tiwari, Ram MD (Oph) - **Spec Exp:** Diabetic Eye Disease/Retinopathy; Glaucoma; Cataract Surgery; **Hospital:** Our Lady of Mercy Med Ctr, NY-Presby Hosp (page 100); **Address:** 1739 Williamsbridge Rd, Bronx, NY 10461-6203; **Phone:** 718-824-1560; **Board Cert:** Ophthalmology 1977; **Med School:** India 1966; **Resid:** Ophthalmology, Maulana Azad Med Coll 1971; **Fellow:** Retina, Columbia-Presby 1978; **Fac Appt:** Asst Clin Prof Oph, Columbia P&S

Weiss, Daniel I MD (Oph) - **Spec Exp:** Glaucoma; **Hospital:** Montefiore Med Ctr; **Address:** 3755 Henry Hudson Pkwy, Ste 1C, Bronx, NY 10463-1535; **Phone:** 718-549-0123; **Board Cert:** Ophthalmology 1963; **Med School:** SUNY Downstate 1955; **Resid:** Ophthalmology, Willis Eye Hosp 1961; **Fellow:** Ophthalmology, Natl Inst Hlth 1962; **Fac Appt:** Assoc Clin Prof Oph, Albert Einstein Coll Med

Wolf, Kenneth MD (Oph) - **Spec Exp:** Diabetic Eye Disease/Retinopathy; Cataract Surgery; **Hospital:** Montefiore Med Ctr - Weiler-Einstein Div; **Address:** 1180 Morris Park Ave, FL 2, Bronx, NY 10461-1925; **Phone:** 718-892-6110; **Board Cert:** Ophthalmology 1980; **Med School:** Albert Einstein Coll Med 1974; **Resid:** Ophthalmology, Montefiore Hosp Med Ctr 1978; **Fac Appt:** Asst Clin Prof Oph, Albert Einstein Coll Med

ORTHOPAEDIC SURGERY

Cobelli, Neil MD (OrS) - **Spec Exp:** Knee Replacement; Hip Replacement; **Hospital:** Montefiore Med Ctr - Weiler-Einstein Div; **Address:** Montefiore Med Ctr, Dept Orthopaedics, 1695 Eastchester Rd Fl 2, Bronx, NY 10461; **Phone:** 718-405-8430; **Board Cert:** Orthopaedic Surgery 1985; **Med School:** Dartmouth Med Sch 1976; **Resid:** Orthopaedic Surgery, Montefiore Med Ctr 1983; **Fac Appt:** Assoc Prof OrS, Albert Einstein Coll Med

Hirsh, David M MD (OrS) - **Spec Exp:** Knee Replacement; Hip Replacement; **Hospital:** Montefiore Med Ctr - Weiler-Einstein Div, Westchester Med Ctr (page 713); **Address:** Montefiore Med Ctr, Dept Orthopaedics, 1695 Eastchester Rd Fl 2, Bronx, NY 10461; **Phone:** 718-405-8430; **Board Cert:** Orthopaedic Surgery 1970; **Med School:** Albert Einstein Coll Med 1963; **Resid:** Orthopaedic Surgery, Albert Einstein Med Ctr 1968; **Fac Appt:** Assoc Clin Prof OrS, Albert Einstein Coll Med

Kleinman, Paul MD (OrS) - **Spec Exp:** Pediatric Orthopaedic Surgery; Hand Surgery; Trauma; **Hospital:** St Barnabas Hosp - Bronx; **Address:** 2016 Bronxdale Ave, Ste 202, Bronx, NY 10462-3365; **Phone:** 718-863-8695; **Board Cert:** Orthopaedic Surgery 1998; **Med School:** Stanford Univ 1979; **Resid:** Surgery, St Luke's Hosp 1981; Orthopaedic Surgery, Columbia-Presby Hosp 1985; **Fellow:** Hand Surgery, Allegheny Genl Hosp; Pediatric Orthopaedic Surgery, Hosp Joint Dis 1990

Levy, I Martin MD (OrS) - **Hospital:** Montefiore Med Ctr - Weiler-Einstein Div; **Address:** Montefiore Med Ctr, Dept Orthopaedics, 1695 Eastchester Rd Fl 2, Bronx, NY 10461; **Phone:** 718-405-8430; **Board Cert:** Orthopaedic Surgery 1982; **Med School:** NY Med Coll 1976; **Resid:** Orthopaedic Surgery, Bronx Municipal Hosps 1982; Orthopaedic Surgery, Hosp for Special Surgery

Olsewski, John M MD (OrS) - **Spec Exp:** Spinal Reconstructive Surgery; Scoliosis; Spinal Surgery-Neck; **Hospital:** Montefiore Med Ctr - Weiler-Einstein Div, Sound Shore Med Ctr - Westchester (page 711); **Address:** 2157 Tomlinson Ave, Bronx, NY 10461; **Phone:** 718-794-2501; **Board Cert:** Orthopaedic Surgery 2004; **Med School:** SUNY Buffalo 1986; **Resid:** Orthopaedic Surgery, SUNY Buffalo 1992; **Fellow:** Spinal Surgery, Twin Cities Scoliosis/Spine Ctr 1994; **Fac Appt:** Assoc Clin Prof OrS, Albert Einstein Coll Med

Tindel, Nathaniel L MD (OrS) - **Spec Exp:** Spinal Surgery; Osteoporosis Spine-Kyphoplasty; Osteoporosis Spinal Fracture; Scoliosis; **Hospital:** Montefiore Med Ctr - Weiler-Einstein Div, St Catherine's of Siena Med Ctr; **Address:** 1695 Eastchester Ave Fl 2, Bronx, NY 10461; **Phone:** 718-405-8129; **Board Cert:** Orthopaedic Surgery 1998; **Med School:** Univ Pennsylvania 1989; **Resid:** Orthopaedic Surgery, Lenox Hill Hosp 1994; **Fellow:** Spinal Surgery, Univ Miami-Jackson Meml Hosp 1995; **Fac Appt:** Asst Prof OrS, Albert Einstein Coll Med

Wilson, Arnold B MD (OrS) - **Spec Exp:** Hip Replacement; Knee Replacement; Knee Injuries/ACL; **Hospital:** Montefiore Med Ctr, Our Lady of Mercy Med Ctr; **Address:** 75 E Gun Hill Rd, Central Bronx Orthopedic Group, Bronx, NY 10467-2103; **Phone:** 718-798-1000; **Board Cert:** Orthopaedic Surgery 1996; **Med School:** UMDNJ-Univ Med Dent NJ 1987; **Resid:** Orthopaedic Surgery, Catholic Med Ctr of Brooklyn & Queens 1993; **Fellow:** Sports Medicine/Knee Surgery, Beth Israel Med Ctr 1994

OTOLARYNGOLOGY

Berkower, Alan MD/PhD (Oto) - **Spec Exp:** Sinus Surgery; Head & Neck Surgery; Vocal Cord Disorders; **Hospital:** Our Lady of Mercy Med Ctr; **Address:** 4141 Carpenter Ave Fl 3 - rm 312, Bronx, NY 10466; **Phone:** 718-920-9933; **Board Cert:** Otolaryngology 1990; **Med School:** Columbia P&S 1984; **Resid:** Surgery, Mount Sinai Hosp Med Ctr 1986; Otolaryngology, Mount Sinai Hosp Med Ctr 1989; **Fac Appt:** Asst Prof Oto, NY Med Coll

Feghali, Joseph G MD (Oto) - **Spec Exp:** Ear Disorders/Surgery; Acoustic Neuroma; Hearing Disorders; **Hospital:** Montefiore Med Ctr; **Address:** 182 E 210th St, Bronx, NY 10467; **Phone:** 718-881-3277; **Board Cert:** Otolaryngology 1990; **Med School:** Lebanon 1978; **Resid:** Otolaryngology, American Univ Beirut 1982; Otolaryngology, Montefiore Med Ctr 1990; **Fellow:** Otology & Neurotology, House Ear Inst 1983; Neurological Surgery, Meml Sloan Kettering Cancer Ctr 1984; **Fac Appt:** Clin Prof Oto, Albert Einstein Coll Med

Fried, Marvin P MD (Oto) - **Spec Exp:** Endoscopic Sinus Surgery; Head & Neck Tumors; Laryngeal & Voice Disorders; **Hospital:** Montefiore Med Ctr, Montefiore Med Ctr - Weiler-Einstein Div; **Address:** 3400 Bainbridge Ave Fl 3, Bronx, NY 10467; **Phone:** 718-920-4646; **Board Cert:** Otolaryngology 1975; **Med School:** Tufts Univ 1969; **Resid:** Surgery, Jewish Hosp 1971; Otolaryngology, Barnes Hosp 1975; **Fellow:** Stroke, Washington Univ 1976; **Fac Appt:** Prof Oto, Albert Einstein Coll Med

Goldstein, Steven I MD (Oto) - **Spec Exp:** Sinus Surgery; Nasal Surgery; **Hospital:** NY Westchester Sq Med Ctr, St John's Riverside Hosp; **Address:** 1200 Waters Pl, Bronx, NY 10461; **Phone:** 718-863-4366; **Board Cert:** Otolaryngology 1987; **Med School:** SUNY Buffalo 1982; **Resid:** Surgery, NYU Med Ctr 1984; Otolaryngology, NYU Med Ctr 1987; **Fellow:** Facial Plastic Surgery, Mt Sinai Hosp 1988

Ruben, Robert MD (Oto) - **Spec Exp:** Pediatric Otolaryngology; Hearing Disorders; Speech Disorders; **Hospital:** Montefiore Med Ctr, Montefiore Med Ctr - Weiler-Einstein Div; **Address:** 3400 Bainbridge Ave, Fl 3, Bronx, NY 10467-2401; **Phone:** 718-920-2484; **Board Cert:** Otolaryngology 1965; **Med School:** Johns Hopkins Univ 1959; **Resid:** Surgery, Baltimore City Hosps 1963; Otolaryngology, Johns Hopkins Hosp 1964; **Fellow:** Otolaryngology, Johns Hopkins Hosp 1966; **Fac Appt:** Prof Oto, Albert Einstein Coll Med

Smith, Richard V MD (Oto) - **Spec Exp:** Head & Neck Cancer; Thyroid & Parathyroid Surgery; Salivary Gland Tumors; **Hospital:** Montefiore Med Ctr, Montefiore Med Ctr - Weiler-Einstein Div; **Address:** 3400 Bainbridge Rd, MAP Bldg Fl 3, Bronx, NY 10467; **Phone:** 718-920-4646; **Board Cert:** Otolaryngology 1996; **Med School:** Univ VT Coll Med 1990; **Resid:** Otolaryngology, Georgetown Univ Hosp 1995; **Fac Appt:** Assoc Clin Prof Oto, Albert Einstein Coll Med

Yankelowitz, Stanley MD (Oto) - **Spec Exp:** Nasal & Sinus Surgery; Pediatric Otolaryngology; **Hospital:** Montefiore Med Ctr, NY Westchester Sq Med Ctr; **Address:** 1200 Waters Pl, Bronx, NY 10461; **Phone:** 718-863-4366; **Med School:** South Africa 1974; **Resid:** Otolaryngology, Univ Stellenbosch 1985; Otolaryngology, Univ Cape Town 1987; **Fellow:** Pediatric Otolaryngology, Albert Einstein 1988

PATHOLOGY

Dorfman, Howard D MD (Path) - **Spec Exp:** Bone Tumors; Soft Tissue Tumors; Joint Pathology; **Hospital:** Montefiore Med Ctr, Montefiore Med Ctr - Weiler-Einstein Div; **Address:** Orthopaedic Pathology Div, 111 E 210th St, Bronx, NY 10467-2401; **Phone:** 718-920-5622; **Board Cert:** Anatomic Pathology 1958; **Med School:** SUNY Downstate 1951; **Resid:** Pathology, Mt Sinai Hosp 1953; Surgical Pathology, Columbia-Presby Med Ctr 1958; **Fellow:** Pathology, Mt Sinai Med Ctr 1954; **Fac Appt:** Prof Path, Albert Einstein Coll Med

PEDIATRIC CARDIOLOGY

Walsh, Christine A MD (PCd) - **Spec Exp:** Arrhythmias; Congenital Heart Disease; Syncope; **Hospital:** Montefiore Med Ctr, Montefiore Med Ctr - Weiler-Einstein Div; **Address:** 3415 Bainbridge Ave, Bronx, NY 10467-2401; **Phone:** 718-741-2310; **Board Cert:** Pediatrics 1978; Pediatric Cardiology 1983; Pediatric Critical Care Medicine 2003; **Med School:** Yale Univ 1973; **Resid:** Pediatrics, Columbia-Presby Med Ctr 1976; **Fellow:** Pediatric Cardiology, Columbia-Presby Med Ctr 1980; **Fac Appt:** Prof Ped, Albert Einstein Coll Med

PEDIATRIC CRITICAL CARE MEDICINE

Singer, Lewis MD (PCCM) - **Spec Exp:** Respiratory Failure; Airway Disorders; **Hospital:** Montefiore Med Ctr; **Address:** 111 E 210th St, Bronx, NY 10467-2490; **Phone:** 718-741-2477; **Board Cert:** Pediatrics 1981; Pediatric Critical Care Medicine 2005; Neonatal-Perinatal Medicine 1983; **Med School:** UMDNJ-NJ Med Sch, Newark 1977; **Resid:** Pediatrics, Montefiore Hosp Med Ctr 1981; **Fellow:** Neonatology, Montefiore Hosp Med Ctr 1983; Neonatal-Perinatal Medicine; **Fac Appt:** Prof Ped, Albert Einstein Coll Med

Ushay, H Michael MD/PhD (PCCM) - **Spec Exp:** Respiratory Failure; Cancer Critical Care; Critical Care; **Hospital:** Montefiore Med Ctr; **Address:** CHAM, Div Critical Care Med, 3415 Bainbridge Ave, Bronx, NY 10467; **Phone:** 718-741-2440; **Board Cert:** Pediatrics 1998; Pediatric Critical Care Medicine 2002; **Med School:** UMDNJ-NJ Med Sch, Newark 1986; **Resid:** Pediatrics, Montefiore/Bronx Muni Hosp 1989; **Fellow:** Pediatric Pulmonology, Montefiore Med Ctr 1991; Pediatric Critical Care Medicine, NY Hosp-Cornell Univ Med Ctr 1993; **Fac Appt:** Assoc Clin Prof Ped, Albert Einstein Coll Med

Weingarten, Jacqueline MD (PCCM) - **Spec Exp:** Heart Disease; Lung Disease; Nutrition; **Hospital:** Montefiore Med Ctr; **Address:** Rosenthal 4 / Chlds Hosp @ Montefiore, 111 E 210th St, Bronx, NY 10467; **Phone:** 718-741-2440; **Board Cert:** Pediatrics 2003; Pediatric Critical Care Medicine 2003; **Med School:** Cornell Univ-Weill Med Coll 1986; **Resid:** Pediatrics, Columbia-Presbyterian 1989; Pediatrics, Columbia-Presbyterian 1990; **Fellow:** Pediatric Critical Care Medicine, Cornell0New York Hospital 1996; **Fac Appt:** Assoc Prof Ped, Albert Einstein Coll Med

PEDIATRIC ENDOCRINOLOGY

Aranoff, Gaya S MD (PEn) - **Spec Exp:** Growth/Development Disorders; Pubertal Disorders; Hormonal Disorders; **Hospital:** NY-Presby Hosp (page 100); **Address:** 3755 Henry Hudson Pkwy, Ste 1-D, Riverdale, NY 10463; **Phone:** 718-543-4800; **Board Cert:** Pediatrics 1980; Pediatric Endocrinology 1986; **Med School:** Albert Einstein Coll Med 1975; **Resid:** Pediatrics, Roosevelt Hosp 1978; **Fellow:** Pediatric Endocrinology, NYU Med Ctr 1980; Pediatric Endocrinology, Columbia-Presby Med Ctr 1985; **Fac Appt:** Assoc Clin Prof Ped, Columbia P&S

PEDIATRIC HEMATOLOGY-ONCOLOGY

Dasgupta, Indira MD (PHO) - **Spec Exp:** Sickle Cell Disease; Anemia; **Hospital:** Our Lady of Mercy Med Ctr; **Address:** 600 E 233rd St, Fl 4, Bronx, NY 10466-2697; **Phone:** 718-920-9014; **Board Cert:** Pediatrics 1981; Pediatric Hematology-Oncology 1984; **Med School:** India 1966; **Resid:** Pediatrics, New York Methodist Hosp 1974; **Fellow:** Pediatric Hematology-Oncology, Meml Sloan Kettering Cancer Ctr 1979; Pediatric Hematology-Oncology, Mount Sinai Hosp 1980; **Fac Appt:** Assoc Clin Prof Ped

Moulton, Thomas MD (PHO) - **Spec Exp:** Sickle Cell Disease; **Hospital:** Montefiore Med Ctr; **Address:** Chldns Hosp, Dept Ped Hem/Onc, 3415 Bainbridge Ave, Bronx, NY 10467; **Phone:** 718-741-2342; **Board Cert:** Pediatric Hematology-Oncology 2005; **Med School:** Loyola Univ-Stritch Sch Med 1984; **Resid:** Pediatrics, Rainbow-Babies Chldns Hosp 1987; **Fellow:** Pediatric Hematology-Oncology, Babies Hosp 1990; **Fac Appt:** Asst Prof Ped, Albert Einstein Coll Med

Radel, Eva MD (PHO) - **Spec Exp:** Pediatric Cancer; Bleeding/Coagulation Disorders; Hematologic Disorders; **Hospital:** Montefiore Med Ctr; **Address:** Childrens Hosp at Montefiore, 3415 Bainbridge Ave, Bronx, NY 10467-2401; **Phone:** 718-741-2342; **Board Cert:** Pediatrics 1964; Pediatric Hematology-Oncology 1974; **Med School:** NYU Sch Med 1958; **Resid:** Pediatrics, Jacobi Med Ctr 1961; **Fellow:** Pediatric Hematology-Oncology, Albert Einstein 1963; **Fac Appt:** Prof Ped, Albert Einstein Coll Med

PEDIATRIC INFECTIOUS DISEASE

Litman, Nathan MD (PInf) - **Spec Exp:** Infections in Immunocompromised Patients; Hospital Acquired Infections; **Hospital:** Montefiore Med Ctr; **Address:** Montefiore Med Ctr, Div Ped Infectious Dis, 111 E 210th St Bldg Rosen Fl 4, Bronx, NY 10467-2401; **Phone:** 718-741-2470; **Board Cert:** Pediatrics 1978; Pediatric Infectious Disease 2001; **Med School:** Albert Einstein Coll Med 1971; **Resid:** Pediatrics, Montefiore Hosp Med Ctr 1974; **Fellow:** Infectious Disease, Montefiore Hosp Med Ctr 1978; **Fac Appt:** Prof Ped, Albert Einstein Coll Med

PEDIATRIC NEPHROLOGY

Flynn, Joseph T MD (PNep) - **Spec Exp:** Hypertension; **Hospital:** Montefiore Med Ctr; **Address:** Montefiore Med Ctr, Div Ped Nephrology, 111 E 210th St, Bronx, NY 10467; **Phone:** 718-655-1120; **Board Cert:** Pediatrics 2001; Pediatric Nephrology 2001; **Med School:** SUNY Upstate Med Univ 1987; **Resid:** Pediatrics, St Christophers Hosp 1990; **Fellow:** Pediatric Nephrology, St Christophers Hosp 1993; **Fac Appt:** Prof Ped, Albert Einstein Coll Med

Kaskel, Frederick J MD/PhD (PNep) - **Spec Exp:** Transplant Medicine-Kidney; Nephrotic Syndrome; Chronic Kidney Disease; Dialysis Care; **Hospital:** Montefiore Med Ctr, Bronx Lebanon Hosp Ctr; **Address:** Children's Hosp at Montefiore, 111 E 210th St, Bronx, NY 10467-2401; **Phone:** 718-655-1120; **Board Cert:** Pediatrics 1980; Nephrology 1982; **Med School:** Univ Cincinnati 1975; **Resid:** Pediatrics, Montefiore Hosp Med Ctr 1977; **Fellow:** Pediatric Nephrology, Albert Einstein 1981; **Fac Appt:** Prof Ped, Albert Einstein Coll Med

PEDIATRIC PULMONOLOGY

Arens, Raanan MD (PPul) - Spec Exp: Sleep Disorders/Apnea; **Hospital:** Montefiore Med Ctr - Weiler-Einstein Div; **Address:** Chldns Hosp at Montefiore, Resp & Sleep Med, 3415 Bainbridge Ave, Bronx, NY 10467; **Phone:** 718-741-2450; **Board Cert:** Pediatrics 2003; Pediatric Pulmonology 2004; **Med School:** Israel 1986; **Resid:** Pediatrics, Shera Med Ctr 1990; Pediatrics, Chldns Hosp 1995; **Fellow:** Pediatric Pulmonology, Chldns Hosp 1994; **Fac Appt:** Assoc Prof Ped, Albert Einstein Coll Med

PEDIATRIC RHEUMATOLOGY

Ilowite, Norman T MD (PRhu) - Spec Exp: Juvenile Arthritis; Lyme Disease; Lupus/SLE; **Hospital:** Montefiore Med Ctr; **Address:** Montefiore Children's Hosp, Rheumatology, 3415 Bainbridge Ave, Bronx, NY 10467; **Phone:** 718-741-2456; **Board Cert:** Pediatrics 1985; Clinical & Laboratory Immunology 1990; Pediatric Rheumatology 2000; **Med School:** SUNY Downstate 1979; **Resid:** Pediatrics, Chldns Hosp Natl Med Ctr 1982; **Fellow:** Pediatric Rheumatology, Univ WA Med Ctr 1984; **Fac Appt:** Prof Ped, Albert Einstein Coll Med

PEDIATRIC SURGERY

Harris, Burton H MD (PS) - Spec Exp: Birth Defects; Inflammatory Bowel Disease; Trauma; **Hospital:** Montefiore Med Ctr; **Address:** 111 E 210th St, Bronx, NY 10461; **Phone:** 718-920-7200; **Board Cert:** Surgery 1973; Pediatric Surgery 1995; **Med School:** SUNY Downstate 1965; **Resid:** Surgery, SUNY-Kings Co Hosp 1971; Pediatric Surgery, Chldns Hosp 1973; **Fac Appt:** Prof S, Albert Einstein Coll Med

Weinberg, Gerard MD (PS) - Spec Exp: Abdominal Wall Reconstruction; Trauma; Neonatal Surgery; **Hospital:** Montefiore Med Ctr; **Address:** 3355 Bainbridge Ave, Bronx, NY 10467; **Phone:** 718-920-7200; **Board Cert:** Surgery 1998; Pediatric Surgery 2000; **Med School:** Albert Einstein Coll Med 1973; **Resid:** Surgery, Albert Einstein Affil Hosps 1976; Pediatric Surgery, Childrens Hosp 1977; **Fellow:** Pediatric Surgery, Univ of Miami Hosps 1979; **Fac Appt:** Prof S, Albert Einstein Coll Med

PEDIATRICS

Andrade, Joseph MD (Ped) PCP - Spec Exp: Asthma; **Hospital:** Our Lady of Mercy Med Ctr; **Address:** 1163 Manor Ave, Bronx, NY 10472; **Phone:** 718-589-3501; **Board Cert:** Pediatrics 2000; Internal Medicine 2001; **Med School:** Ecuador 1981; **Resid:** Internal Medicine, Our Lady of Mercy 1988; Pediatrics, Our Lady of Mercy 1986

Balk, Sophie MD (Ped) PCP - Spec Exp: Environmental Medicine; Adolescent Medicine; **Hospital:** Montefiore Med Ctr; **Address:** 1621 Eastchester Road, Bronx, NY 10461-2604; **Phone:** 718-405-8040; **Board Cert:** Pediatrics 1979; **Med School:** Albert Einstein Coll Med 1974; **Resid:** Pediatrics, Montefiore Hosp Med Ctr 1977; **Fac Appt:** Assoc Prof Ped, Albert Einstein Coll Med

Bloomfield, Diane MD (Ped) PCP - **Hospital:** Montefiore Med Ctr; **Address:** 3444 Kossuth Ave, DTC Bldg, FL 1B, Bronx, NY 10467-2461; **Phone:** 718-920-5873; **Board Cert:** Pediatrics 1987; **Med School:** Cornell Univ-Weill Med Coll 1982; **Resid:** Pediatrics, NY Hosp 1985; **Fellow:** Ambulatory Pediatrics, NY Hosp 1986; **Fac Appt:** Asst Prof Ped, Cornell Univ-Weill Med Coll

Cohen, Herbert J MD (Ped) - **Spec Exp:** Developmental & Behavioral Disorders; Developmental Delay; **Hospital:** Montefiore Med Ctr - Weiler-Einstein Div, Jacobi Med Ctr; **Address:** Children's Evaluation Rehab Ctr, 1410 Pelham Pkwy S, Ste 237, Bronx, NY 10461-1116; **Phone:** 718-430-8522; **Board Cert:** Pediatrics 1964; **Med School:** SUNY Hlth Sci Ctr 1959; **Resid:** Pediatrics, New York Hosp 1962; **Fellow:** Developmental-Behavioral Pediatrics, Albert Einstein 1966; **Fac Appt:** Prof Ped, Albert Einstein Coll Med

Easton, Lon MD (Ped) PCP - **Spec Exp:** Sports Medicine; **Hospital:** Montefiore Med Ctr, Montefiore Med Ctr - Weiler-Einstein Div; **Address:** 3594 E Tremont Ave, Bronx, NY 10465-2032; **Phone:** 718-863-1050; **Board Cert:** Pediatrics 1983; **Med School:** NY Med Coll 1978; **Resid:** Pediatrics, Metropolitan Hosp 1981; **Fac Appt:** Asst Clin Prof Ped, Albert Einstein Coll Med

Esteban-Cruciani, Nora MD (Ped) PCP - **Spec Exp:** Chronic Illness; Foster Care; **Hospital:** Montefiore Med Ctr, Montefiore Med Ctr - Weiler-Einstein Div; **Address:** 1621 Eastchester Rd - Pediatrics, Bronx, NY 10461; **Phone:** 718-405-8090; **Board Cert:** Pediatrics 2001; **Med School:** Argentina 1979; **Resid:** Pediatrics, Italian Hosp 1983; Pediatrics, Albert Einstein College of Med 1993; **Fellow:** Research, Nat Inst Hlth 1991; Research, Albert Einstein College Med 2005; **Fac Appt:** Assoc Prof Ped, Albert Einstein Coll Med

Haber, Patricia MD (Ped) PCP - **Hospital:** Montefiore Med Ctr; **Address:** 1500 Astor Ave Fl 2, Bronx, NY 10469-5900; **Phone:** 718-881-0100; **Board Cert:** Pediatrics 1981; Pediatric Rheumatology 2004; **Med School:** Johns Hopkins Univ 1976; **Resid:** Pediatrics, Johns Hopkins Hosp 1979; **Fellow:** Immunology, Univ Alabama Hosp 1982; Pediatric Rheumatology, Univ Alabama Hosp 1984; **Fac Appt:** Asst Prof Ped, Albert Einstein Coll Med

Hand, Ivan MD (Ped) - **Spec Exp:** Respiratory Distress Syndrome; Prematurity/Low Birth Weight Infants; Neonatal Infections; **Hospital:** Jacobi Med Ctr, N Central Bronx Hosp; **Address:** 1400 Pelham Pkwy S, rm 803, Bronx, NY 10461-1138; **Phone:** 718-918-6975; **Board Cert:** Pediatrics 1986; Neonatal-Perinatal Medicine 2004; **Med School:** Albert Einstein Coll Med 1982; **Resid:** Pediatrics, Montefiore Med Ctr 1985; Pediatrics, Bronx Lebanon Hosp 1986; **Fellow:** Neonatal-Perinatal Medicine, New York Hosp-Cornell Univ 1988; **Fac Appt:** Assoc Prof Ped, Albert Einstein Coll Med

Hirschman, Alan MD (Ped) PCP - **Spec Exp:** Asthma; **Hospital:** Montefiore Med Ctr; **Address:** 3765 Riverdale Ave, Ste 4, Bronx, NY 10463-1845; **Phone:** 718-548-7300; **Board Cert:** Pediatrics 1981; **Med School:** UMDNJ-NJ Med Sch, Newark 1976; **Resid:** Pediatrics, Montefiore Hosp Med Ctr 1979; **Fellow:** Montefiore Hosp Med Ctr 1980; **Fac Appt:** Asst Clin Prof, Albert Einstein Coll Med

Igel, Gerard MD (Ped) PCP - **Spec Exp:** Chronic Disease; Behavioral Disorders; Developmental Disorders; Foster Care; **Hospital:** Montefiore Med Ctr, Jacobi Med Ctr; **Address:** 1613 Tenbroeck Ave, Bronx, NY 10461-2007; **Phone:** 718-828-9060; **Board Cert:** Pediatrics 1986; **Med School:** Israel 1981; **Resid:** Pediatrics, Jacobi Med Ctr 1984; **Fac Appt:** Asst Clin Prof Ped, Albert Einstein Coll Med

London, Ronald MD (Ped) PCP - **Hospital:** Montefiore Med Ctr, Montefiore Med Ctr - Weiler-Einstein Div; **Address:** 3594 E Tremont Ave, Bronx, NY 10465; **Phone:** 718-863-1050; **Board Cert:** Pediatrics 2003; **Med School:** Israel 1984; **Resid:** Pediatrics, Montefiore Hosp Med Ctr 1987; **Fellow:** Child Development, Albert Einstein 1988

Mayers, Marguerite MD (Ped) `PCP` - **Spec Exp:** Tuberculosis; AIDS/HIV; Travel Medicine; **Hospital:** Montefiore Med Ctr; **Address:** 111 E 210th St, Bronx, NY 10467-2401; **Phone:** 718-920-5871; **Board Cert:** Pediatrics 1977; Pediatric Infectious Disease 2002; **Med School:** Albert Einstein Coll Med 1971; **Resid:** Pediatrics, Montefiore Hosp Med Ctr 1974; **Fellow:** Infectious Disease, Montefiore Hosp Med Ctr 1976; **Fac Appt:** Clin Prof Ped, Albert Einstein Coll Med

Okun, Alex MD (Ped) `PCP` - **Spec Exp:** Chronic Illness; Palliative Care; **Hospital:** Montefiore Med Ctr; **Address:** 1621 Eastchester Rd, Bronx, NY 10461-2604; **Phone:** 718-405-8040; **Board Cert:** Pediatrics 1987; **Med School:** Columbia P&S 1983; **Resid:** Pediatrics, Columbia-Presby Med Ctr 1986; **Fellow:** Child & Adolescent Psychiatry, Jacobi Med Ctr - Albert Einstein Coll Med 1990; **Fac Appt:** Assoc Clin Prof Ped, Albert Einstein Coll Med

Oppedisano, Carlyn MD (Ped) `PCP` - **Spec Exp:** Parenting Issues; **Hospital:** NY-Presby Hosp (page 100); **Address:** 2600 Netherland Ave, Ste 120, Bronx, NY 10463-4813; **Phone:** 718-796-3580; **Board Cert:** Pediatrics 1986; **Med School:** Columbia P&S 1981; **Resid:** Pediatrics, Babies Hosp 1985; **Fac Appt:** Assoc Clin Prof Ped, Columbia P&S

Ozuah, Philip MD (Ped) - **Hospital:** Montefiore Med Ctr; **Address:** 305 E 161 St, Bronx, NY 10451; **Phone:** 718-579-2500; **Board Cert:** Pediatrics 2000; **Med School:** Nigeria 1985; **Resid:** Pediatrics, Montefiore Hosp Med Ctr; **Fellow:** USC Med Ctr; **Fac Appt:** Assoc Prof Ped, Albert Einstein Coll Med

Schechter, Miriam MD (Ped) `PCP` - **Spec Exp:** Teenage Mothers; **Hospital:** Montefiore Med Ctr; **Address:** 1621 Eastchester Rd, Bronx, NY 10461; **Phone:** 718-405-8040; **Board Cert:** Pediatrics 2000; **Med School:** NYU Sch Med 1989; **Resid:** Pediatrics, Mount Sinai 1992; Pediatrics, Mount Sinai 1993; **Fac Appt:** Asst Prof Ped, Albert Einstein Coll Med

Stein, Ruth E.K. MD (Ped) `PCP` - **Spec Exp:** Chronic Illness; Developmental & Behavioral Disorders; **Hospital:** Montefiore Med Ctr; **Address:** 111 E 210th St, Bronx, NY 10467-2401; **Phone:** 718-920-7932; **Board Cert:** Pediatrics 1971; Developmental-Behavioral Pediatrics 2004; **Med School:** Albert Einstein Coll Med 1966; **Resid:** Pediatrics, Bronx Muni Hosp 1968; Pediatrics, Chldns Hosp Natl Med Ctr 1969; **Fellow:** Community Medicine, Chldns Hosp Natl Med Ctr 1969; **Fac Appt:** Prof Ped, Albert Einstein Coll Med

Strassberg, Barbara E MD (Ped) `PCP` - **Spec Exp:** Developmental Disorders; **Hospital:** NY-Presby Hosp (page 100); **Address:** 2600 Netherland Ave, Ste 120, Bronx, NY 10463-4813; **Phone:** 718-796-3580; **Board Cert:** Pediatrics 1986; **Med School:** SUNY Upstate Med Univ 1981; **Resid:** Pediatrics, Columbia-Presby Hosp 1984; **Fac Appt:** Assoc Clin Prof Ped

Tolchin, Deborah MD (Ped) `PCP` - **Spec Exp:** Preventive Medicine; Adolescent Medicine; **Hospital:** Montefiore Med Ctr, Montefiore Med Ctr - Weiler-Einstein Div; **Address:** 1500 Astor Ave Fl 2, Bronx, NY 10469-5900; **Phone:** 718-881-0100; **Board Cert:** Pediatrics 2002; **Med School:** SUNY Hlth Sci Ctr 1966; **Resid:** Pediatrics, Jacobi Med Ctr 1969; **Fac Appt:** Clin Prof Ped, Albert Einstein Coll Med

Uy, Rodolfo MD (Ped) `PCP` - **Hospital:** Our Lady of Mercy Med Ctr; **Address:** 711 Nereid Ave, Bronx, NY 10466; **Phone:** 718-994-6755; **Board Cert:** Pediatrics 1997; **Med School:** Philippines 1979; **Resid:** Pediatrics, Our Lady Mercy Med Ctr 1986

Weiner, Richard L MD (Ped) **PCP** - **Spec Exp:** Adolescent Medicine; **Hospital:** Montefiore Med Ctr, Montefiore Med Ctr - Weiler-Einstein Div; **Address:** 1500 Astor Ave, Bronx, NY 10469-5938; **Phone:** 718-881-0100; **Board Cert:** Pediatrics 1991; **Med School:** Albert Einstein Coll Med 1975; **Resid:** Pediatrics, Jacobi Med Ctr 1978; **Fac Appt:** Assoc Prof Ped, Albert Einstein Coll Med

Wong, Martha Shih MD (Ped) **PCP** - **Spec Exp:** Sickle Cell Disease; Hemophilia; **Hospital:** Bronx Lebanon Hosp Ctr; **Address:** 1770 Grand Concourse, Ste 2, Bronx, NY 10457; **Phone:** 718-901-8101; **Board Cert:** Pediatrics 1972; Pediatric Hematology-Oncology 1978; **Med School:** Taiwan 1966; **Resid:** Pediatrics, Kings County Hosp 1970; **Fellow:** Pediatric Hematology-Oncology, Albert Einstein 1972

Zoltan, Irving MD (Ped) **PCP** - **Spec Exp:** Diagnostic Problems; Asthma; **Hospital:** Montefiore Med Ctr, Montefiore Med Ctr - Weiler-Einstein Div; **Address:** 1613 Tenbroeck Ave, Bronx, NY 10461; **Phone:** 718-828-9060; **Board Cert:** Pediatrics 1979; **Med School:** Albert Einstein Coll Med 1974; **Resid:** Pediatrics, Jacobi Med Ctr 1978; **Fac Appt:** Asst Prof Ped, Albert Einstein Coll Med

PHYSICAL MEDICINE & REHABILITATION

De Araujo, Maria MD (PMR) - **Spec Exp:** Arthritis; Pain-Low Back; Electromyography; **Hospital:** Our Lady of Mercy Med Ctr; **Address:** 600 E 233rd St, Our Lady of Mercy Med Ctr, Dept of Phy Med & Rehab, Bronx, NY 10466-2604; **Phone:** 718-920-9171; **Board Cert:** Physical Medicine & Rehabilitation 1989; **Med School:** Brazil 1972; **Resid:** Physical Medicine & Rehabilitation, St Vincent's Hosp & Med Ctr 1981; **Fellow:** Physical Medicine & Rehabilitation, Westchester Med Ctr 1989; **Fac Appt:** Assoc Prof PMR, NY Med Coll

Fast, Avital MD (PMR) - **Spec Exp:** Pain-Back; **Hospital:** Montefiore Med Ctr, Montefiore Med Ctr - Weiler-Einstein Div; **Address:** 150 E 210th St, Bronx, NY 10467; **Phone:** 718-920-2751; **Board Cert:** Physical Medicine & Rehabilitation 1978; **Med School:** Israel 1972; **Resid:** Physical Medicine & Rehabilitation, Montefiore Med Ctr 1976

Gladstone, Lenore MD (PMR) - **Spec Exp:** Musculoskeletal Disorders; Sports Medicine; Geriatric Rehabilitation; **Hospital:** Montefiore Med Ctr, St Barnabas Hosp - Bronx; **Address:** 3435 Dekalb Ave, Bronx, NY 10467-2301; **Phone:** 718-547-8899; **Board Cert:** Physical Medicine & Rehabilitation 1975; **Med School:** South Africa 1956; **Resid:** Physical Medicine & Rehabilitation, Montefiore Hosp Med Ctr 1971; Physical Medicine & Rehabilitation, Columbia-Presby 1973; **Fac Appt:** Asst Prof PMR, Albert Einstein Coll Med

Levin, Sheryl MD (PMR) - **Spec Exp:** Neurorehabilitation; Pain-Musculoskeletal; Arthritis; **Hospital:** Montefiore Med Ctr; **Address:** 3435 Dekalb Ave, Bronx, NY 10467-2301; **Phone:** 718-547-8899; **Board Cert:** Physical Medicine & Rehabilitation 1989; **Med School:** Cornell Univ-Weill Med Coll 1984; **Resid:** Physical Medicine & Rehabilitation, NY Hosp 1988; **Fac Appt:** Assoc Clin Prof PMR, Albert Einstein Coll Med

PLASTIC SURGERY

Dolich, Barry MD (PlS) - **Spec Exp:** Cosmetic Surgery; Hand Surgery; Breast Reconstruction; **Hospital:** Montefiore Med Ctr - Weiler-Einstein Div, New York Eye & Ear Infirm (page 110); **Address:** Hutchinson Metro Center, 1200 Waters Place, Ste M106, Bronx, NY 10461-6265; **Phone:** 718-430-0942; **Board Cert:** Plastic Surgery 1975; **Med School:** SUNY Upstate Med Univ 1966; **Resid:** Surgery, Albert Einstein 1970; Plastic Surgery, Albert Einstein 1973; **Fellow:** Hand Surgery 1973; **Fac Appt:** Assoc Clin Prof PlS, Albert Einstein Coll Med

Goldstein, Robert MD (PlS) - **Spec Exp:** Breast Surgery; Nasal Surgery; Abdominoplasty; **Hospital:** Montefiore Med Ctr - Weiler-Einstein Div, Montefiore Med Ctr; **Address:** 2425 Eastchester Rd, Bronx, NY 10469; **Phone:** 718-405-7500; **Board Cert:** Plastic Surgery 1985; Hand Surgery 1990; **Med School:** Penn State Univ-Hershey Med Ctr 1977; **Resid:** Surgery, Montefiore Med Ctr 1981; Plastic Surgery, Montefiore Med Ctr 1984; **Fellow:** Hand Surgery, Montefiore Med Ctr-Einstein Div 1982; **Fac Appt:** Assoc Clin Prof PlS, Albert Einstein Coll Med

Greenstein, Bruce MD (PlS) - **Hospital:** Jacobi Med Ctr, N Central Bronx Hosp; **Address:** Jacobi Med Ctr, Dept Plastic Surgery, 1400 Pelham Pkwy S, Bronx, NY 10461; **Phone:** 718-918-5970; **Board Cert:** Plastic Surgery 1984; **Med School:** SUNY Upstate Med Univ 1975; **Resid:** Surgery, Montefiore Hosp Med Ctr 1980; Plastic Surgery, Montefiore Hosp Med Ctr 1982; **Fellow:** Hand Surgery, Montefiore Hosp Med Ctr 1983; **Fac Appt:** Asst Prof PlS, Albert Einstein Coll Med

Liebling, Ralph MD (PlS) - **Spec Exp:** Reconstructive Surgery; Microsurgery; Hand Surgery; Burn Care; **Hospital:** Jacobi Med Ctr; **Address:** Jacobi Med Ctr, Dept Plastic Recons Surg, 1400 Pelham Parkway South, Bronx, NY 10461; **Phone:** 718-918-7000; **Board Cert:** Plastic Surgery 1988; **Med School:** Albert Einstein Coll Med 1977; **Resid:** Surgery, Albert Einstein Coll Med 1981; Plastic Surgery, Albert Einstein Coll Med 1983; **Fellow:** Reconstructive Microsurgery, NYU/Bellevue Hosp Ctr; **Fac Appt:** Asst Prof PlS, Albert Einstein Coll Med

Ofodile, Ferdinand MD (PlS) - **Spec Exp:** Liposuction; Rhinoplasty; Breast Surgery; **Hospital:** St Luke's - Roosevelt Hosp Ctr - Roosevelt Div (page 90), Harlem Hosp Ctr; **Address:** 40-48 Junction Blvd, Corona, NY 10461; **Phone:** 718-651-2843; **Board Cert:** Surgery 1974; Plastic Surgery 1976; **Med School:** Northwestern Univ 1968; **Resid:** Surgery, Harlem Hosp/Columbia-Presby Hosp 1973; Plastic Surgery, Harlem Hosp/Columbia Presby Hosp 1975; **Fellow:** Plastic Surgery, Mayo Clinic 1976; **Fac Appt:** Clin Prof S, Columbia P&S

Rubinstein, Joshua MD (PlS) - **Spec Exp:** Breast Surgery; Cosmetic Surgery-Face; **Hospital:** Bronx Lebanon Hosp Ctr; **Address:** 1650 Selwyn Ave, Bronx, NY 10457; **Phone:** 718-960-2004; **Board Cert:** Plastic Surgery 1995; Hand Surgery 1996; **Med School:** Case West Res Univ 1984; **Resid:** Surgery, Univ Hosp 1989; Plastic Surgery, UMDNJ-Univ Hosp 1991; **Fellow:** Hand Surgery, NYU Med Ctr 1992; **Fac Appt:** Asst Prof S, Albert Einstein Coll Med

Staffenberg, David A MD (PlS) - **Spec Exp:** Craniofacial Surgery/Reconstruction; Pediatric Plastic Surgery; Facial Plastic & Reconstructive Surgery; Cosmetic Surgery-Face; **Hospital:** Montefiore Med Ctr; **Address:** 3353 Bainbridge Ave, Bronx, NY 10467; **Phone:** 718-920-4462; **Board Cert:** Plastic Surgery 1999; **Med School:** NY Med Coll 1989; **Resid:** Surgery, Maimonides Med Ctr 1995; Plastic Surgery, Emory Univ Med Ctr 1997; **Fellow:** Craniofacial Surgery, UCLA Med Ctr 1998; **Fac Appt:** Assoc Prof PlS, Albert Einstein Coll Med

PSYCHIATRY

Asnis, Gregory MD (Psyc) - **Spec Exp:** Psychopharmacology; Mood Disorders; Anxiety Disorders; **Hospital:** Montefiore Med Ctr, Phelps Meml Hosp Ctr; **Address:** 111 E 210th St, Bronx, NY 10467-2401; **Phone:** 718-920-4287; **Board Cert:** Psychiatry 1978; Geriatric Medicine 1996; **Med School:** Hahnemann Univ 1972; **Resid:** Psychiatry, Mount Sinai Hosp 1976; **Fellow:** Psychiatry, Columbia-Presby Med Ctr 1981; **Fac Appt:** Prof Psyc, Albert Einstein Coll Med

Gelfand, Janice MD (Psyc) - **Spec Exp:** Depression; Anxiety Disorders; **Hospital:** NY-Presby Hosp (page 100); **Address:** 3765 Riverdale Ave, Bronx, NY 10463-1845; **Phone:** 718-361-3482; **Board Cert:** Psychiatry 1990; **Med School:** NYU Sch Med 1985; **Resid:** Psychiatry, NYU Med Ctr 1989; **Fellow:** Psychiatry, Beth Israel Med Ctr 1991; **Fac Appt:** Asst Prof Psyc, Columbia P&S

Gerbino-Rosen, Ginny MD (Psyc) - **Spec Exp:** Child & Adolescent Psychiatry; Aggression Disorders; **Hospital:** Bronx Children's Psych Ctr; **Address:** 1000 Waters Pl, Bronx, NY 10461-2701; **Phone:** 718-239-3699; **Board Cert:** Psychiatry 1981; Child & Adolescent Psychiatry 1987; Forensic Psychiatry 1999; **Med School:** Creighton Univ 1976; **Resid:** Psychiatry, NYU Bellevue Med 1979; **Fellow:** Child & Adolescent Psychiatry, NYU Bellevue Med 1981; **Fac Appt:** Asst Prof Psyc, Albert Einstein Coll Med

Lebinger, Martin MD (Psyc) - **Spec Exp:** Depression; Anxiety Disorders; Panic Disorder; **Hospital:** Bronx Psych Ctr; **Address:** 1540 Pelham Pkwy South, Ste 1A, Bronx, NY 10461-1130; **Phone:** 718-518-0222; **Board Cert:** Psychiatry 1980; **Med School:** Albert Einstein Coll Med 1976; **Resid:** Psychiatry, Montefiore Hosp Med Ctr 1979; **Fellow:** Psychiatry, LI Jewish-Hillside Med Ctr 1981; **Fac Appt:** Asst Clin Prof Psyc, Albert Einstein Coll Med

Lomonaco, Salvatore MD (Psyc) - **Hospital:** Montefiore Med Ctr - Weiler-Einstein Div; **Address:** Jack & Pearl Resnick Campus, 1300 Morris Park Ave, Belfer Bldg - rm 405, Bronx, NY 10461; **Phone:** 914-834-0085; **Board Cert:** Psychiatry 1976; **Med School:** SUNY Hlth Sci Ctr 1966; **Resid:** Psychiatry, Montefiore Med Ctr 1971; Child & Adolescent Psychiatry, Montefiore Med Ctr 1972; **Fac Appt:** Assoc Prof Psyc, Albert Einstein Coll Med

Osei-Tutu, John MD (Psyc) - **Spec Exp:** Addiction Psychiatry; Anxiety & Depression; **Hospital:** Bronx Lebanon Hosp Ctr, Brunswick Hall Psych Hosp; **Address:** 1276 Fulton Ave, Bronx, NY 10456; **Phone:** 718-901-6133; **Board Cert:** Psychiatry 1990; Addiction Psychiatry 2003; **Med School:** Ghana 1976; **Resid:** Psychiatry, Bronx Lebanon Hosp 1983; **Fac Appt:** Asst Prof Psyc, Albert Einstein Coll Med

Schwartz, Bruce MD (Psyc) - **Spec Exp:** Depression; Bipolar/Mood Disorders; Schizophrenia; Anxiety Disorders; **Hospital:** Montefiore Med Ctr; **Address:** Montefiore Medical Ctr, Dept Psychiatry, 111 E 210th St, Bronx, NY 10467-2490; **Phone:** 718-920-4040; **Board Cert:** Psychiatry 1980; **Med School:** SUNY Downstate 1975; **Resid:** Psychiatry, Bronx Muni Hosp 1979; **Fac Appt:** Assoc Clin Prof Psyc, Albert Einstein Coll Med

PULMONARY DISEASE

Aldrich, Thomas K MD (Pul) - **Spec Exp:** Respiratory Failure; Asthma; Chronic Obstructive Lung Disease (COPD); **Hospital:** Montefiore Med Ctr; **Address:** Montefiore Med Ctr, Pulmonary Div, 111 E 210th St, Bronx, NY 10467-2401; **Phone:** 718-920-6087; **Board Cert:** Critical Care Medicine 2001; Pulmonary Disease 1980; Internal Medicine 1978; **Med School:** Univ Minn 1975; **Resid:** Internal Medicine, UC Irvine Med Ctr 1978; **Fellow:** Pulmonary Disease, Univ Virginia Med Ctr 1980; Physiology, Univ Penn 1982; **Fac Appt:** Prof Med, Albert Einstein Coll Med

Appel, David MD (Pul) - **Spec Exp:** Asthma; Sleep Disorders/Apnea; Smoking Cessation; **Hospital:** Montefiore Med Ctr; **Address:** 111 E 210th St, Pulmonary Div, Bronx, NY 10467; **Phone:** 718-920-6055; **Board Cert:** Internal Medicine 1976; **Med School:** Albert Einstein Coll Med 1973; **Resid:** Internal Medicine, Bronx Municipal Hosp 1976; **Fellow:** Pulmonary Disease, Bronx Municipal Hosp; **Fac Appt:** Assoc Prof Med, Albert Einstein Coll Med

Casper, Theodore MD (Pul) - **Spec Exp:** Critical Care Medicine; **Hospital:** NY Westchester Sq Med Ctr, Montefiore Med Ctr - Weiler-Einstein Div; **Address:** 1180 Morris Park Ave, Bronx, NY 10461; **Phone:** 718-892-1200; **Board Cert:** Internal Medicine 1983; Pulmonary Disease 1986; Critical Care Medicine 1999; **Med School:** Columbia P&S 1980; **Resid:** Internal Medicine, St Luke's Hosp 1983; **Fellow:** Pulmonary Disease, St Luke's Hosp

Klapper, Philip MD (Pul) - **Spec Exp:** Asthma; Emphysema; **Hospital:** Montefiore Med Ctr, Lawrence Hosp Ctr; **Address:** 3322 Bainbridge Ave, Bronx, NY 10467; **Phone:** 718-884-2000; **Board Cert:** Internal Medicine 1986; Pulmonary Disease 2000; **Med School:** Albert Einstein Coll Med 1983; **Resid:** Internal Medicine, Montefiore Hosp Med Ctr 1986; **Fellow:** Pulmonary Disease, Univ Hosp 1990; Critical Care Medicine, Montefiore Hosp Med Ctr 1991; **Fac Appt:** , Albert Einstein Coll Med

Marino, William MD (Pul) - **Spec Exp:** Respiratory Failure; Asthma; Bronchoscopy; **Hospital:** Our Lady of Mercy Med Ctr; **Address:** 4234 Bronx Blvd Fl 2, Bronx, NY 10466; **Phone:** 347-341-4340; **Board Cert:** Internal Medicine 1980; Pulmonary Disease 1984; Critical Care Medicine 1997; **Med School:** Albert Einstein Coll Med 1977; **Resid:** Internal Medicine, Montefiore Hosp Med Ctr 1980; **Fellow:** Pulmonary Disease, Columbia-Presby 1982; **Fac Appt:** Assoc Clin Prof Med, NY Med Coll

Menon, Latha MD (Pul) - **Spec Exp:** Asthma; Critical Care; Breathing Disorders; **Hospital:** Bronx Lebanon Hosp Ctr; **Address:** 1770 Grand Concourse, Ste 2G, Bronx, NY 10457-5528; **Phone:** 718-518-5420; **Board Cert:** Internal Medicine 1978; Pulmonary Disease 1980; Geriatric Medicine 1992; Critical Care Medicine 2002; **Med School:** India 1972; **Resid:** Internal Medicine, Flushing Hosp 1978; **Fellow:** Pulmonary Disease, Albert Einstein 1981; **Fac Appt:** Assoc Prof Med, Albert Einstein Coll Med

Pinsker, Kenneth MD (Pul) - **Spec Exp:** Asthma; Lung Cancer; Sarcoidosis; **Hospital:** Montefiore Med Ctr; **Address:** 111 E 210th St, Bronx, NY 10467-2490; **Phone:** 718-920-6095; **Board Cert:** Internal Medicine 1972; Pulmonary Disease 1976; **Med School:** Univ Hlth Sci/Chicago Med Sch 1968; **Resid:** Internal Medicine, Montefiore Hosp Med Ctr 1970; Internal Medicine, Jacobi Med Ctr 1971; **Fellow:** Pulmonary Disease, Montefiore Hosp Med Ctr 1972; Pulmonary Disease, Montefiore Hosp Med Ctr 1975; **Fac Appt:** Prof Med, Albert Einstein Coll Med

Prezant, David MD (Pul) - **Spec Exp:** Asthma; **Hospital:** Montefiore Med Ctr; **Address:** 111 E 210th St, Ste 423, Bronx, NY 10467-2401; **Phone:** 718-920-6054; **Board Cert:** Internal Medicine 1984; Pulmonary Disease 1986; **Med School:** Albert Einstein Coll Med 1981; **Resid:** Internal Medicine, Harlem Hosp 1984; **Fellow:** Pulmonary Disease, Montefiore Hosp Med Ctr 1985; **Fac Appt:** Assoc Prof Med, Albert Einstein Coll Med

Pulle, Dunstan MD (Pul) - **Spec Exp:** Asthma; Hypertension; **Hospital:** Our Lady of Mercy Med Ctr, Comm Hosp - Dobbs Ferry; **Address:** 2410 Barker Ave, Ste 1-G, Bronx, NY 10467; **Phone:** 718-547-5880; **Board Cert:** Internal Medicine 1970; Pulmonary Disease 1971; **Med School:** Sri Lanka 1962; **Resid:** Internal Medicine, VA Med Ctr 1969; **Fellow:** Pulmonary Disease, VA Hosp/LI Coll Hosp 1971

Sender, Joel MD (Pul) - **Spec Exp:** Asthma; Sarcoidosis; **Hospital:** St Barnabas Hosp - Bronx; **Address:** 2016 Bronxdale Ave, Ste 301, Bronx, NY 10462-3300; **Phone:** 718-409-2222; **Board Cert:** Internal Medicine 1978; Pulmonary Disease 1980; Geriatric Medicine 1994; **Med School:** Albany Med Coll 1975; **Resid:** Internal Medicine, Mount Sinai Hosp 1978; **Fellow:** Pulmonary Disease, Mount Sinai Hosp 1980

RADIATION ONCOLOGY

Bodner, William MD (RadRO) - **Spec Exp:** Brachytherapy; **Hospital:** Our Lady of Mercy Med Ctr; **Address:** 600 E 233rd St, Bronx, NY 10466; **Phone:** 718-920-9204; **Board Cert:** Radiation Oncology 1996; **Med School:** Wake Forest Univ 1987; **Resid:** Radiation Oncology, NY Med Coll 1995; **Fac Appt:** Assoc Prof Rad, NY Med Coll

Hilaris, Basil MD (RadRO) - **Spec Exp:** Prostate Cancer; Gynecologic Cancer; Brain Cancer; Breast Cancer; **Hospital:** Our Lady of Mercy Med Ctr; **Address:** 600 E 233rd St, Bronx, NY 10466-2604; **Phone:** 718-920-9750; **Board Cert:** Radiation Oncology 1961; **Med School:** Greece 1955; **Resid:** Radiation Oncology, Meml-Sloan Kettering Cancer Ctr 1959; **Fellow:** Radiation Oncology, Mem-Sloan Kettering Cancer Ctr 1964; **Fac Appt:** Prof RadRO, NY Med Coll

RHEUMATOLOGY

Fomberstein, Barry MD (Rhu) - **Hospital:** Our Lady of Mercy Med Ctr; **Address:** 600 E 233rd St, Our Lady of Mercy Medical Ctr, Bronx, NY 10466-2697; **Phone:** 718-920-9168; **Board Cert:** Internal Medicine 1979; Rheumatology 1982; **Med School:** Albert Einstein Coll Med 1976; **Resid:** Internal Medicine, Long Island Jewish 1979; **Fellow:** Rheumatology, Long Island Jewish 1981; **Fac Appt:** Assoc Clin Prof Med, NY Med Coll

Keiser, Harold MD (Rhu) - **Hospital:** Montefiore Med Ctr, Jacobi Med Ctr; **Address:** 1515 Blondell Ave, Ste 220, Bronx, NY 10461-2662; **Phone:** 718-405-8323; **Board Cert:** Internal Medicine 1972; Rheumatology 1972; **Med School:** NYU Sch Med 1964; **Resid:** Internal Medicine, Clevelnd Metro Genl Hosp 1968; **Fellow:** Rheumatology, Albert Einstein Coll Med 1972; **Fac Appt:** Prof Med, Albert Einstein Coll Med

Weinstein, Joshua MD (Rhu) - **Hospital:** Montefiore Med Ctr - Weiler-Einstein Div, NY Hosp Queens; **Address:** 1554 Astor Ave, Bronx, NY 10469; **Phone:** 718-994-8900; **Board Cert:** Internal Medicine 1975; Rheumatology 1978; **Med School:** SUNY Downstate 1972; **Resid:** Internal Medicine, Maimonides Med Ctr 1975; **Fellow:** Rheumatology, Montefiore Med Ctr 1977; **Fac Appt:** Asst Prof Med, Albert Einstein Coll Med

SURGERY

Agarwal, Nanakram MD (S) - **Spec Exp:** Breast Surgery; Colon & Rectal Surgery; **Hospital:** Our Lady of Mercy Med Ctr, Westchester Med Ctr (page 713); **Address:** 600 E 233rd St Fl 4, Bronx, NY 10466; **Phone:** 718-920-9143; **Board Cert:** Surgery 1982; Critical Care Medicine 1987; **Med School:** India 1973; **Resid:** Surgery, Our Lady of Mercy Medical Center 1981; **Fellow:** Critical Care Medicine, Westchester County Medical Center 1982; **Fac Appt:** Prof S, NY Med Coll

Balsano, Nicholas MD (S) - **Spec Exp:** Colon & Rectal Surgery; Vascular Surgery; **Hospital:** Our Lady of Mercy Med Ctr; **Address:** 600 E 233rd St, Bronx, NY 10466-2604; **Phone:** 718-920-9522; **Board Cert:** Surgery 1972; **Med School:** Geo Wash Univ 1965; **Resid:** Surgery, Our Lady of Mercy Med Ctr 1969; **Fellow:** Vascular Surgery, Our Lady of Mercy Med Ctr 1970

Barone, James MD (S) - **Spec Exp:** Abdominal Surgery; Trauma; Critical Care; **Hospital:** Lincoln Med & Mental Hlth Ctr; **Address:** Lincoln Medical & Mental Health Ctr, 234 E 149th St, rm 620, Bronx, NY 10451; **Phone:** 718-579-5900; **Board Cert:** Surgery 2005; Surgical Critical Care 2005; **Med School:** Jefferson Med Coll 1971; **Resid:** Surgery, St Vincent's Hosp & Med Ctr 1976; **Fac Appt:** Clin Prof S, Cornell Univ-Weill Med Coll

Berlin, Arnold MD (S) - **Spec Exp:** Rehabilitation-Geriatric; Colon & Rectal Surgery; **Hospital:** Montefiore Med Ctr; **Address:** 3400 Bainbridge Ave Fl 4, Bronx, NY 10467-2401; **Phone:** 718-920-4800; **Board Cert:** Surgery 1998; **Med School:** NYU Sch Med 1972; **Resid:** Surgery, Montefiore Hosp Med Ctr 1974; Surgery, Univ Conn Hlth Ctr 1978; **Fac Appt:** , Albert Einstein Coll Med

Cayten, C Gene MD (S) - **Spec Exp:** Breast Surgery; Biliary Surgery; **Hospital:** Our Lady of Mercy Med Ctr; **Address:** 600 E 233rd St, Fl 4, Bronx, NY 10466; **Phone:** 718-920-9522; **Board Cert:** Surgery 1975; **Med School:** NY Med Coll 1967; **Resid:** Surgery, Hosp Univ Penn 1973; **Fac Appt:** Prof S, NY Med Coll

Greenstein, Stuart MD (S) - **Spec Exp:** Transplant-Kidney; Dialysis Access Surgery; **Hospital:** Montefiore Med Ctr; **Address:** 111 E 210th St, Bronx, NY 10467; **Phone:** 718-920-6157; **Board Cert:** Surgery 2003; **Med School:** Harvard Med Sch 1979; **Resid:** Surgery, UMDNJ Med Ctr 1984; **Fellow:** Vascular Surgery, Hosp Univ Penn 1985; Transplant Surgery, SUNY Downstate 1986; **Fac Appt:** Prof S, Albert Einstein Coll Med

Gumbs, Milton MD (S) - **Spec Exp:** Breast Surgery; Gastrointestinal Surgery; Hernia; **Hospital:** Bronx Lebanon Hosp Ctr; **Address:** 1276 Fulton Ave, Bronx, NY 10457-7606; **Phone:** 718-960-1256; **Board Cert:** Surgery 1974; **Med School:** Italy 1967; **Resid:** Surgery, Bronx Lebanon Hosp 1973; **Fac Appt:** Prof Med, Albert Einstein Coll Med

Hodgson, W John B MD (S) - **Spec Exp:** Proctology; Hemorrhoids; Anal Disorders & Reconstruction; **Hospital:** Montefiore Med Ctr - Weiler-Einstein Div, Montefiore Med Ctr; **Address:** 1575 Blondell Ave, Ste 125, Montefiore Med Ctr, Dept of Surgery, Bronx, NY 10461; **Phone:** 718-405-8239; **Board Cert:** Surgery 1975; **Med School:** England 1964; **Resid:** Surgery, Univ of London Hosps 1972; **Fellow:** Colon & Rectal Surgery, Mount Sinai Med Ctr 1974; **Fac Appt:** Prof S, Albert Einstein Coll Med

Kaleya, Ronald MD (S) - **Spec Exp:** Pancreatic Cancer; Breast Cancer; Colon & Rectal Cancer; **Hospital:** Montefiore Med Ctr; **Address:** 3400 Bainbridge Ave, 4th fl, Dept Surgery, Bronx, NY 10467-2490; **Phone:** 718-920-4800; **Board Cert:** Surgery 1996; **Med School:** Cornell Univ-Weill Med Coll 1980; **Resid:** Surgery, Albert Einstein Med Ctr 1985; **Fellow:** Surgical Oncology, Meml Sloan Kettering Cancer Ctr 1987; **Fac Appt:** Assoc Prof S, Albert Einstein Coll Med

Sas, Norman MD (S) - **Spec Exp:** Breast Cancer; Laparoscopic Surgery; Hernia; **Hospital:** Montefiore Med Ctr, Saint Joseph's Med Ctr - Yonkers; **Address:** 3220 Fairfield Ave, Riverdale, NY 10463-3240; **Phone:** 718-549-0700; **Board Cert:** Surgery 1999; **Med School:** NY Med Coll 1974; **Resid:** Surgery, Montefiore Med Ctr 1978; **Fac Appt:** Asst Clin Prof S, Albert Einstein Coll Med

Schechner, Richard MD (S) - **Spec Exp:** Transplant-Kidney; Laparoscopic Surgery; Breast Surgery; **Hospital:** Montefiore Med Ctr, Montefiore Med Ctr - Weiler-Einstein Div; **Address:** Transplant Surgery Department, 111 E 210th St, Bronx, NY 10467-2401; **Phone:** 718-920-6157; **Board Cert:** Surgery 2001; **Med School:** NY Med Coll 1983; **Resid:** Surgery, Montefiore Hosp Med Ctr 1988; **Fellow:** Pancreas & Intestinal Transplant, University Hosp 1989; **Fac Appt:** Asst Prof S, Albert Einstein Coll Med

Tellis, Vivian MD (S) - **Spec Exp:** Transplant-Kidney; Dialysis Access Surgery; **Hospital:** Montefiore Med Ctr; **Address:** 111 E 210th St, Fl 4, Bronx, NY 10467-2490; **Phone:** 718-920-6158; **Board Cert:** Surgery 1969; **Med School:** India 1960; **Resid:** Surgery, Jersey City Med Ctr 1965; Surgery, Montefiore Hosp Med Ctr 1968; **Fellow:** Transplant Surgery, Montefiore Hosp Med Ctr 1970; **Fac Appt:** Prof S, Albert Einstein Coll Med

Wilbanks, Tyr MD (S) - **Spec Exp:** Pediatric Surgery; Minimally Invasive Surgery; Vascular Surgery; **Hospital:** Stamford Hosp; **Address:** Lincoln Med & Mental Hlth Ctr, Dept of Surgery, 234 E 149th St, Ste 620, Bronx, NY 10451; **Phone:** 718-579-5900; **Board Cert:** Surgery 2003; **Med School:** Cornell Univ-Weill Med Coll 1983; **Resid:** Surgery, Columbia-Presby Med Ctr 1990; **Fellow:** Research, Columbia-Presby Med Ctr 1987; **Fac Appt:** Asst Clin Prof S, Columbia P&S

THORACIC SURGERY

Keller, Steven M MD (TS) - **Spec Exp:** Lung Cancer; Esophageal Cancer; Palmar Hyperhidrosis; **Hospital:** Montefiore Med Ctr; **Address:** Greene Medical Arts Pavilion, 3400 Bainbridge Ave, Ste 5B, Bronx, NY 10467-2404; **Phone:** 718-920-7580; **Board Cert:** Surgery 1996; Thoracic Surgery 1996; **Med School:** Albany Med Coll 1977; **Resid:** Surgery, Mount Sinai Hosp 1985; Thoracic Surgery, Mem Sloan Kettering Cancer Ctr 1987; **Fellow:** Surgical Oncology, NIH/National Cancer Inst 1983; **Fac Appt:** Prof TS, Albert Einstein Coll Med

Merav, Avraham MD (TS) - **Spec Exp:** Cardiac Surgery-Adult; Lung Surgery; Esophageal Surgery; **Hospital:** Montefiore Med Ctr, Englewood Hosp & Med Ctr (page 760); **Address:** 3316 Rochambeau Ave Fl 2, Bronx, NY 10467-2804; **Phone:** 718-652-0100; **Board Cert:** Surgery 1974; Thoracic Surgery 1995; **Med School:** Switzerland 1964; **Resid:** Surgery, Montefiore Hosp Med Ctr 1973; **Fellow:** Cardiothoracic Surgery, Montefiore Hosp Med Ctr 1975; **Fac Appt:** Assoc Prof TS, Albert Einstein Coll Med

Michler, Robert MD (TS) - **Spec Exp:** Heart Valve Surgery; Coronary Artery Surgery; Ventricular Assist Device (LVAD); Pediatric Cardiothoracic Surgery; **Hospital:** Montefiore Med Ctr; **Address:** Dept Cardiothoracic Surg, 3400 Bainbridge Ave Fl 5, Bronx, NY 10467; **Phone:** 718-920-2100; **Board Cert:** Surgery 1990; Thoracic Surgery 2000; **Med School:** Dartmouth Med Sch 1981; **Resid:** Surgery, Columbia Presby Med Ctr 1987; **Fellow:** Cardiothoracic Surgery, Columbia Presby Med Ctr 1989; Pediatric Surgery, Boston Children's Hosp 1990; **Fac Appt:** Prof S, Albert Einstein Coll Med

UROLOGY

Geisler, Edward MD (U) - **Spec Exp:** Urologic Cancer; Impotence; **Hospital:** Bronx Lebanon Hosp Ctr; **Address:** 1770 Grand Concourse, Ste 1F, Bronx, NY 10457-5524; **Phone:** 718-901-8173; **Board Cert:** Urology 1987; **Med School:** Jefferson Med Coll 1978; **Resid:** Surgery, Beth Israel 1980; Urology, NYU 1984; **Fac Appt:** Asst Prof U, Albert Einstein Coll Med

Gentile, Ralph MD (U) - **Spec Exp:** Prostate Cancer; Impotence; **Hospital:** Montefiore Med Ctr, Our Lady of Mercy Med Ctr; **Address:** 3130 Grand Concourse, Ste 1S, Bronx, NY 10458-1290; **Phone:** 718-295-9400; **Board Cert:** Urology 1964; **Med School:** Columbia P&S 1956; **Resid:** Urology, Columbia-Presby 1959; Urology, Montefiore Hosp Med Ctr 1960; **Fac Appt:** Assoc Clin Prof, Albert Einstein Coll Med

Kahan, Norman MD (U) - **Spec Exp:** Prostate Cancer; **Hospital:** Montefiore Med Ctr, Comm Hosp - Dobbs Ferry; **Address:** Urology Faculty Practice, 3400 Bainbridge Ave, Ste 5C, Bronx, NY 10467-2404; **Phone:** 718-920-4031; **Med School:** NYU Sch Med 1966; **Resid:** Surgery, Montefiore Hosp Med Ctr 1968; Urology, Montefiore Hosp Med Ctr 1973

Melman, Arnold MD (U) - **Spec Exp:** Erectile Dysfunction; Prostate Disease (Thermodilation); Prostate Cancer; **Hospital:** Montefiore Med Ctr; **Address:** 3400 Bainbridge Ave Fl 5th, Bronx, NY 10467; **Phone:** 212-639-1561; **Board Cert:** Urology 1976; **Med School:** Univ Rochester 1966; **Resid:** Urology, Strong Meml Hosp 1968; Urology, UCLA Med Ctr 1974; **Fellow:** Nephrology, Cedars-Sinai Med Ctr 1972; **Fac Appt:** Prof U, Albert Einstein Coll Med

Stein, Mark MD (U) - **Spec Exp:** Incontinence; Impotence; **Hospital:** NY Westchester Sq Med Ctr, Beth Israel Med Ctr - Petrie Division (page 90); **Address:** 3594 E Tremont Ave, Ste 320, Bronx, NY 10465; **Phone:** 718-518-9300; **Board Cert:** Urology 2000; **Med School:** Yale Univ 1984; **Resid:** Urology, Montefiore Med Ctr 1990; **Fac Appt:** Asst Clin Prof U, NY Med Coll

Stone, Peter L MD (U) - **Spec Exp:** Prostate Cancer; Kidney Stones; Erectile Dysfunction; **Hospital:** Montefiore Med Ctr, NY Westchester Sq Med Ctr; **Address:** 1578 Williamsbridge Rd, FL 2, Bronx, NY 10461-6268; **Phone:** 718-892-2100; **Board Cert:** Urology 1996; **Med School:** NY Med Coll 1979; **Resid:** Surgery, Montefiore Hosp Med Ctr 1981; Urology, Montefiore Hosp Med Ctr 1984; **Fac Appt:** Asst Clin Prof U, Albert Einstein Coll Med

VASCULAR & INTERVENTIONAL RADIOLOGY

Cynamon, Jacob MD (VIR) - **Hospital:** Montefiore Med Ctr; **Address:** Montefiore Med Ctr, Dept Interventional Radiology, 111 E 210th St, Bronx, NY 10467; **Phone:** 718-920-5729; **Board Cert:** Diagnostic Radiology 1987; Vascular & Interventional Radiology 2004; **Med School:** Albert Einstein Coll Med 1983; **Resid:** Surgery, Montefiore Hosp Med Ctr 1984; Radiology, Montefiore Hosp Med Ctr 1987; **Fellow:** Vascular & Interventional Radiology, New York Hosp-Cornell 1988; **Fac Appt:** Assoc Prof Rad, Albert Einstein Coll Med

VASCULAR SURGERY

Ohki, Takao MD (VascS) - **Spec Exp:** Endovascular Surgery; Aneurysm-Abdominal Aortic; Carotid Artery Surgery; **Hospital:** Montefiore Med Ctr; **Address:** Montefiore Med Ctr, Div Vascular Surgery, 111 E 210th St, Bronx, NY 10467; **Phone:** 718-920-4707; **Med School:** Japan 1987; **Resid:** Vascular Surgery, Jikei Hospital 1991; **Fac Appt:** Prof S, Albert Einstein Coll Med

Rivers, Steven P MD (VascS) - **Spec Exp:** Limb Salvage; Vein Disorders; Carotid Artery Surgery; **Hospital:** Montefiore Med Ctr - Weiler-Einstein Div, Northern Westchester Hosp; **Address:** 2425 Eastchester Rd, Bronx, NY 10469; **Phone:** 718-405-5900; **Board Cert:** Surgery 1992; Vascular Surgery 1996; **Med School:** Univ MD Sch Med 1975; **Resid:** Surgery, Oregon Hlth Sci Univ Hosp 1983; **Fellow:** Vascular Surgery, Montefiore Hosp Med Ctr 1984; **Fac Appt:** Assoc Prof S, Albert Einstein Coll Med

Suggs, William D MD (VascS) - **Spec Exp:** Vein Disorders; Wound Healing/Care; Carotid Artery Surgery; **Hospital:** Montefiore Med Ctr; **Address:** 111 E 210th St, Bronx, NY 10467; **Phone:** 718-920-6338; **Board Cert:** Surgery 1990; Vascular Surgery 2002; **Med School:** Wake Forest Univ 1983; **Resid:** Surgery, Geo Wash Univ Med Ctr 1989; **Fellow:** Vascular Surgery, Emory Univ Hosp 1991; **Fac Appt:** Assoc Prof VascS, Albert Einstein Coll Med

Kings (Brooklyn)

Kings (Brooklyn)

ADOLESCENT MEDICINE

Hayes-McKenzie, Leslie MD (AM) PCP - **Spec Exp:** Nutrition; Adolescent Gynecology; **Hospital:** Brooklyn Hosp Ctr-Downtown; **Address:** The Brooklyn Hospital Center, 121 DeKalb Ave, Brooklyn, NY 11201; **Phone:** 718-250-6968; **Board Cert:** Pediatrics 2000; Adolescent Medicine 1997; **Med School:** Mount Sinai Sch Med 1986; **Resid:** Pediatrics, Children's Hosp Natl Med Ctr 1989; **Fellow:** Adolescent Medicine, UMDNJ Med Ctr 1991

ALLERGY & IMMUNOLOGY

Greeley, Norman MD (A&I) - **Spec Exp:** Asthma; **Hospital:** Long Island Coll Hosp (page 90); **Address:** 140 Clinton St, FL 1, Brooklyn, NY 11201-4701; **Phone:** 718-624-4465; **Board Cert:** Internal Medicine 1985; Allergy & Immunology 1987; Clinical & Laboratory Immunology 1988; **Med School:** Mexico 1980; **Resid:** Internal Medicine, Long Island Coll Hosp 1985; **Fellow:** Allergy & Immunology, Downstate Med Ctr 1987

Klein, Norman MD (A&I) - **Spec Exp:** Asthma; Food Allergy; Hay Fever; Immune Deficiency; **Hospital:** Brookdale Univ Hosp Med Ctr, Brooklyn Hosp Ctr-Downtown; **Address:** 1648 E 14th St, Brooklyn, NY 11229-1175; **Phone:** 718-627-0183; **Board Cert:** Pediatrics 1981; Allergy & Immunology 1983; **Med School:** SUNY Hlth Sci Ctr 1976; **Resid:** Pediatrics, Brookdale 1979; **Fellow:** Allergy & Immunology, Albert Einstein 1980; **Fac Appt:** Asst Prof Ped, SUNY Hlth Sci Ctr

Schneider, Arlene MD (A&I) - **Spec Exp:** Asthma; Sinusitis; Food Allergy; **Hospital:** Long Island Coll Hosp (page 90); **Address:** Allergy & Asthma Care Ctr, 159 Clinton St, Brooklyn, NY 11201-4601; **Phone:** 718-624-6495; **Board Cert:** Pediatrics 1974; Allergy & Immunology 1989; **Med School:** SUNY Downstate 1968; **Resid:** Pediatrics, LI Coll Hosp 1972; **Fellow:** Allergy & Immunology, LI Coll Hosp 1974; **Fac Appt:** Asst Clin Prof Ped, SUNY Hlth Sci Ctr

Spina, Christopher MD (A&I) - **Spec Exp:** Rhinitis; **Hospital:** Brooklyn Hosp Ctr-Downtown, Winthrop - Univ Hosp; **Address:** 1 Hanson Pl #2304, Brooklyn, NY 11243-2909; **Phone:** 718-875-2820; **Board Cert:** Internal Medicine 1963; Allergy & Immunology 1974; **Med School:** Columbia P&S 1956; **Resid:** Internal Medicine, Brooklyn Hosp 1959; **Fellow:** Allergy & Immunology, Roosevelt Hosp 1960

CARDIAC ELECTROPHYSIOLOGY

Turitto, Gioia MD (CE) - **Spec Exp:** Pacemakers; Defibrillators; Arrhythmias; **Hospital:** New York Methodist Hosp (page 479); **Address:** NY Methodist Hosp, Dept Cardiology, 506 Sixth St, Brooklyn, NY 11215; **Phone:** 718-780-3626; **Board Cert:** Internal Medicine 2002; Cardiovascular Disease 2003; Cardiac Electrophysiology 2004; **Med School:** Italy 1981; **Resid:** Internal Medicine, SUNY Downstate Med Ctr 1992; **Fellow:** Cardiovascular Disease, SUNY Downstate Med Ctr 1993; **Fac Appt:** Assoc Prof Med, SUNY Downstate

Wilbur, Sabrina L MD (CE) - **Spec Exp:** Arrhythmias; Pacemakers/Defibrillators; **Hospital:** Long Island Coll Hosp (page 90), Beth Israel Med Ctr - Petrie Division (page 90); **Address:** LI Coll Hosp, Dept Cardiology, 339 Hicks St, Brooklyn, NY 11201; **Phone:** 718-780-4841; **Board Cert:** Cardiovascular Disease 2005; Cardiac Electrophysiology 1999; **Med School:** Dominican Republic 1987; **Resid:** Internal Medicine, Episcopal Hosp 1991; **Fellow:** Cardiovascular Disease, Episcopal Hosp 1994; Cardiac Electrophysiology, Hosp Univ Penn 1995

CARDIOVASCULAR DISEASE

Buscaino, Giacomo J MD (Cv) - **Spec Exp:** Congestive Heart Failure; Angina; Cholesterol/Lipid Disorders; **Hospital:** Lutheran Med Ctr - Brooklyn, Victory Memorial Hosp - Bklyn; **Address:** 9001 3rd Ave, Brooklyn, NY 11209-5707; **Phone:** 718-748-2900; **Board Cert:** Internal Medicine 1981; Cardiovascular Disease 1983; **Med School:** SUNY Downstate 1978; **Resid:** Internal Medicine, Kings Co-Downstate Med Ctr 1981; **Fellow:** Cardiovascular Disease, Kings Co-Downstate Med Ctr 1983

Charnoff, Judah MD (Cv) - **Spec Exp:** Coronary Artery Disease; Congestive Heart Failure; Cholesterol/Lipid Disorders; **Hospital:** Beth Israel Med Ctr- Kings Hwy Div (page 90), Maimonides Med Ctr (page 96); **Address:** 1262 Ocean Pkwy, Brooklyn, NY 11230-5102; **Phone:** 718-859-5843; **Board Cert:** Internal Medicine 1987; Cardiovascular Disease 1995; **Med School:** NYU Sch Med 1984; **Resid:** Internal Medicine, Brookdale Hosp Med Ctr 1987; **Fellow:** Cardiovascular Disease, Maimonides Med Ctr 1989

Clark, Luther T MD (Cv) - **Spec Exp:** Hypertension; Cholesterol/Lipid Disorders; Preventive Cardiology; **Hospital:** SUNY Downstate Med Ctr; **Address:** SUNY Hlth Sci Ctr, 450 Clarkson Ave, Box 1199, Brooklyn, NY 11203-2056; **Phone:** 718-270-1568; **Board Cert:** Internal Medicine 1978; Cardiovascular Disease 1981; **Med School:** Harvard Med Sch 1975; **Resid:** Internal Medicine, St Luke's-Roosevelt Hosp 1979; Cardiovascular Disease, St Luke's-Roosevelt Hosp 1980; **Fac Appt:** Clin Prof Med, SUNY Hlth Sci Ctr

Feit, Alan MD (Cv) - **Spec Exp:** Interventional Cardiology; **Hospital:** SUNY Downstate Med Ctr; **Address:** SUNY, Dept Cardiology, 450 Clarkson Ave, Box 1199, Brooklyn, NY 11203-2012; **Phone:** 718-270-2631; **Board Cert:** Internal Medicine 1978; Cardiovascular Disease 1981; Interventional Cardiology 1999; **Med School:** Columbia P&S 1975; **Resid:** Internal Medicine, Roosevelt Hosp 1978; **Fellow:** Cardiovascular Disease, Roosevelt Hosp Ctr 1980; **Fac Appt:** Prof Med, SUNY Downstate

Gelbfish, Joseph MD (Cv) - **Spec Exp:** Chest Pain; Preventive Cardiology; Heart Valve Disease; **Hospital:** New York Methodist Hosp (page 479), NY-Presby Hosp (page 100); **Address:** 2500 Avenue I, Brooklyn, NY 11210; **Phone:** 718-951-0100; **Board Cert:** Internal Medicine 1986; Cardiovascular Disease 1990; **Med School:** NYU Sch Med 1980; **Resid:** Surgery, Maimonides Medical Ctr 1984; Internal Medicine, Maimonides Medical Ctr 1985; **Fellow:** Cardiovascular Disease, Maimonides Medical Ctr 1988; Cardiovascular Disease, Beth Israel 1989

Gelles, Jeremiah MD (Cv) - **Spec Exp:** Heart Failure; Heart Attack; Arrhythmias; **Hospital:** New York Methodist Hosp (page 479), Maimonides Med Ctr (page 96); **Address:** 263 7th Ave, Ste 5H, Brooklyn, NY 11215-3690; **Phone:** 718-832-1818; **Board Cert:** Internal Medicine 1972; Cardiovascular Disease 1975; **Med School:** NYU Sch Med 1966; **Resid:** Internal Medicine, Mount Sinai Hosp 1970; **Fellow:** Cardiovascular Disease, Mount Sinai Hosp 1971; Cardiac Electrophysiology, Columbia Presby Med Ctr 1973; **Fac Appt:** Asst Clin Prof Med, Cornell Univ-Weill Med Coll

Greengart, Alvin MD (Cv) - **Spec Exp:** Echocardiography; Non-Invasive Cardiology; **Hospital:** Maimonides Med Ctr (page 96); **Address:** Maimonides Medical Ctr, Dept Cardiology, 4802 Tenth Ave, Brooklyn, NY 11219; **Phone:** 718-283-7489; **Board Cert:** Internal Medicine 1977; Cardiovascular Disease 1979; **Med School:** Mount Sinai Sch Med 1974; **Resid:** Internal Medicine, Brookdale Hosp Med Ctr 1977; **Fellow:** Cardiovascular Disease, Brookdale Hosp Med Ctr 1979

Gupta, Prem MD (Cv) - **Spec Exp:** Cholesterol/Lipid Disorders; Mitral Valve Prolapse; Arrhythmias; **Hospital:** Maimonides Med Ctr (page 96); **Address:** 4709 Fort Hamilton Pkwy, Brooklyn, NY 11219-2927; **Phone:** 718-633-4244; **Board Cert:** Internal Medicine 1971; Cardiovascular Disease 1973; **Med School:** India 1964; **Resid:** Internal Medicine, VA Med Ctr 1968; Internal Medicine, VA Med Ctr 1969; **Fellow:** Cardiovascular Disease, VA Med Ctr 1971; **Fac Appt:** Clin Prof Med, Mount Sinai Sch Med

Hanley, Gerard MD (Cv) - **Spec Exp:** Invasive Cardiology; **Hospital:** Beth Israel Med Ctr- Kings Hwy Div (page 90), New York Methodist Hosp (page 479); **Address:** 1219 Quentin Rd, University Heart Assoc, Brooklyn, NY 11229; **Phone:** 718-253-9511; **Board Cert:** Internal Medicine 1989; Cardiovascular Disease 2001; **Med School:** SUNY Stony Brook 1984; **Resid:** Internal Medicine, Univ Hosp 1987; **Fellow:** Cardiovascular Disease, Univ Hosp 1990; Cardiovascular Disease, Westchester 1991; **Fac Appt:** Asst Prof, SUNY Downstate

Hollander, Gerald MD (Cv) - **Spec Exp:** Coronary Artery Disease; Heart Failure; **Hospital:** Maimonides Med Ctr (page 96); **Address:** 4802 10th Ave, Professional Bldg, Div Cardiology, Brooklyn, NY 11219-2844; **Phone:** 718-283-7643; **Board Cert:** Internal Medicine 1976; Cardiovascular Disease 1979; **Med School:** SUNY Downstate 1973; **Resid:** Internal Medicine, Brookdale Hosp 1976; **Fellow:** Cardiovascular Disease, Brookdale Hosp 1978; **Fac Appt:** Assoc Clin Prof Med, SUNY Hlth Sci Ctr

Kang, Pritpal S MD (Cv) - **Hospital:** Victory Memorial Hosp - Bklyn; **Address:** 705 86th St, Brooklyn, NY 11228-3625; **Phone:** 718-836-0600; **Board Cert:** Internal Medicine 1979; Cardiovascular Disease 1981; **Med School:** India 1972; **Resid:** Internal Medicine, Metro Hosp Ctr 1978; **Fellow:** Cardiovascular Disease, VA Med Ctr 1980

Kantrowitz, Niki E MD (Cv) - **Spec Exp:** Interventional Cardiology; Congestive Heart Failure; **Hospital:** Long Island Coll Hosp (page 90), Beth Israel Med Ctr - Petrie Division (page 90); **Address:** 339 Hicks St, Brooklyn, NY 11201; **Phone:** 718-780-4626; **Board Cert:** Internal Medicine 1981; Cardiovascular Disease 1987; Interventional Cardiology 1999; **Med School:** Wayne State Univ 1977; **Resid:** Internal Medicine, Columbia-Presby Med Ctr 1980; **Fellow:** Cardiovascular Disease, Stanford Univ Med Ctr 1983; **Fac Appt:** Assoc Clin Prof Med, NY Med Coll

Kerstein, Joshua MD (Cv) - **Spec Exp:** Atrial Fibrillation; Coronary Artery Disease; Nuclear Cardiology; **Hospital:** Maimonides Med Ctr (page 96); **Address:** Maimonides Medical Ctr, Div Cardiology, 4802 10th Ave Fl 4, Brooklyn, NY 11219; **Phone:** 718-283-8614; **Board Cert:** Internal Medicine 1992; Cardiovascular Disease 2005; **Med School:** SUNY Downstate 1989; **Resid:** Internal Medicine, Maimonides Med Ctr 1992; **Fellow:** Cardiovascular Disease, Maimonides Med Ctr 1995; **Fac Appt:** Asst Prof Med, SUNY Downstate

Kleeman, Harris J MD (Cv) - **Spec Exp:** Chest Pain; Hypertension; Coronary Artery Disease; **Hospital:** Maimonides Med Ctr (page 96); **Address:** 1660 E 14th St, Ste LL3, Brooklyn, NY 11229-1171; **Phone:** 718-375-6969; **Board Cert:** Internal Medicine 1982; Cardiovascular Disease 1985; **Med School:** SUNY Hlth Sci Ctr 1979; **Resid:** Internal Medicine, Staten Island Hosp 1983; **Fellow:** Cardiovascular Disease, Maimonides Med Ctr 1985

Leff, Sanford MD (Cv) - **Spec Exp:** Heart Failure; Hypertension; Coronary Artery Disease; **Hospital:** New York Methodist Hosp (page 479), Interfaith Med Ctr - St John's Episcopal Hosp; **Address:** 47 Plaza St W, Brooklyn, NY 11217; **Phone:** 718-789-4332; **Board Cert:** Internal Medicine 1974; Cardiovascular Disease 1979; **Med School:** SUNY Buffalo 1968; **Resid:** Internal Medicine, USPHS Hosp 1971; Internal Medicine, Lincoln Hosp 1974; **Fellow:** Cardiovascular Disease, Roosevelt Hosp 1976; **Fac Appt:** Clin Prof Med, SUNY Downstate

Lichstein, Edgar MD (Cv) - **Spec Exp:** Heart Failure; Coronary Artery Disease; Cholesterol/Lipid Disorders; **Hospital:** Maimonides Med Ctr (page 96); **Address:** Maimonides Med Ctr, Dept Medicine, 4802 10th Ave, Brooklyn, NY 11219; **Phone:** 718-283-7074; **Board Cert:** Internal Medicine 1969; Cardiovascular Disease 1973; **Med School:** SUNY Hlth Sci Ctr 1961; **Resid:** Internal Medicine, Lenox Hill Hosp 1963; Internal Medicine, NYU Med Ctr 1964; **Fellow:** Cardiovascular Disease, NYU Med Ctr 1966; **Fac Appt:** Prof Med, Mount Sinai Sch Med

Lotongkhum, Vichai MD (Cv) - **Spec Exp:** Arrhythmias; **Hospital:** Wyckoff Heights Med Ctr; **Address:** 361 Stockholm St, Brooklyn, NY 11237; **Phone:** 718-381-2121; **Board Cert:** Cardiovascular Disease 1977; Internal Medicine 1975; **Med School:** Thailand 1970; **Resid:** Internal Medicine, Wyckoff Heights Hosp 1974; **Fellow:** Cardiovascular Disease, Cumberland Med Ctr 1976

Moskovits, Norbert MD (Cv) - **Spec Exp:** Heart Failure; Coronary Artery Disease; **Hospital:** Maimonides Med Ctr (page 96); **Address:** Maimonides Medical Ctr, Div Cardiology, 4802 Tenth Ave, Brooklyn, NY 11219; **Phone:** 718-283-7948; **Board Cert:** Internal Medicine 2002; Cardiovascular Disease 1995; **Med School:** Germany 1986; **Resid:** Internal Medicine, Maimonides Med Ctr 1993; **Fellow:** Cardiovascular Disease, Beth Israel Med Ctr 1995; **Fac Appt:** Asst Prof Med, SUNY Downstate

Nacht, Robert MD (Cv) - **Spec Exp:** Heart Failure; Arrhythmias; Coronary Artery Disease; **Hospital:** SUNY Downstate Med Ctr; **Address:** 450 Clarkson Ave, Box 57, Brooklyn, NY 11203-2056; **Phone:** 718-270-3128; **Board Cert:** Internal Medicine 1972; Cardiovascular Disease 1975; **Med School:** SUNY Downstate 1964; **Resid:** Internal Medicine, Kings Co-SUNY Downstate 1966; Internal Medicine, Kngs Co-SUNY Downstate 1969; **Fellow:** Cardiovascular Disease, SUNY Downstate 1971; **Fac Appt:** Assoc Clin Prof Med, SUNY Downstate

Paiusco, A Dino MD (Cv) - **Hospital:** Beth Israel Med Ctr- Kings Hwy Div (page 90), Kingsbrook Jewish Med Ctr; **Address:** Univ Heart Assocs, 3131 Kings Hwy, Ste B1, Brooklyn, NY 11234; **Phone:** 718-253-9512; **Board Cert:** Internal Medicine 1989; **Med School:** Mexico 1984; **Resid:** Cardiovascular Disease, Univ Hosp 1991

Reddy, Chatla MD (Cv) - **Spec Exp:** Cardiac Catheterization; Coronary Angioplasty/Stents; Peripheral Vascular Disease; Interventional Cardiology; **Hospital:** New York Methodist Hosp (page 479), NY-Presby Hosp (page 100); **Address:** 8714 5th Ave, Brooklyn, NY 11209; **Phone:** 718-836-3333; **Board Cert:** Internal Medicine 1972; Cardiovascular Disease 1975; Interventional Cardiology 1999; **Med School:** India 1966; **Resid:** Internal Medicine, Misericordia Hosp 1972; **Fellow:** Cardiovascular Disease, Misericordia Hosp 1974; **Fac Appt:** Assoc Clin Prof Med, Cornell Univ-Weill Med Coll

Sacchi, Terrence J MD (Cv) - **Spec Exp:** Arrhythmias; Cardiac Catheterization; Coronary Angioplasty/Stents; **Hospital:** New York Methodist Hosp (page 479), Maimonides Med Ctr (page 96); **Address:** 506 6th St, Brooklyn, NY 11215; **Phone:** 718-780-7830; **Board Cert:** Internal Medicine 1979; Cardiovascular Disease 1981; Interventional Cardiology 1999; **Med School:** Albany Med Coll 1976; **Resid:** Internal Medicine, St Vincents Hosp 1979; **Fellow:** Cardiovascular Disease, Georgetown Univ Hosp 1981; Interventional Cardiology, Mercy Hospital 1986; **Fac Appt:** Assoc Clin Prof Med, SUNY Downstate

Traube, Charles MD (Cv) - **Hospital:** Beth Israel Med Ctr- Kings Hwy Div (page 90), Brookdale Univ Hosp Med Ctr; **Address:** 2270 Kimball St, Ste 210, Brooklyn, NY 11234; **Phone:** 718-692-2700; **Board Cert:** Internal Medicine 1978; Cardiovascular Disease 1981; Geriatric Medicine 1992; **Med School:** Albert Einstein Coll Med 1975; **Resid:** Internal Medicine, Brookdale Hosp 1978; **Fellow:** Cardiovascular Disease, Brookdale Hosp 1980; **Fac Appt:** Asst Clin Prof Med, Albert Einstein Coll Med

Vasavada, Balendu MD (Cv) - **Spec Exp:** Echocardiography; **Hospital:** Long Island Coll Hosp (page 90); **Address:** 339 Hicks St, Brooklyn, NY 11201-5514; **Phone:** 718-780-2944; **Board Cert:** Internal Medicine 1977; Cardiovascular Disease 1979; **Med School:** India 1972; **Resid:** Internal Medicine, Lincoln Med Ctr 1977; **Fellow:** Cardiovascular Disease, Brooklyn Hosp 1979; **Fac Appt:** Asst Clin Prof Med, SUNY Downstate

Wein, Paul MD (Cv) - **Spec Exp:** Preventive Cardiology; **Hospital:** Beth Israel Med Ctr - Petrie Division (page 90), St Francis Hosp - The Heart Ctr (page 112); **Address:** 3131 Kings Hwy, Ste D6, Brooklyn, NY 11234-2642; **Phone:** 718-338-2283; **Board Cert:** Internal Medicine 1977; Cardiovascular Disease 1983; **Med School:** SUNY Hlth Sci Ctr 1976; **Resid:** Internal Medicine, Norwalk Hosp 1979; **Fellow:** Cardiovascular Disease, LI Jewish Medical Ctr 1981

Zaloom, Robert MD (Cv) - **Spec Exp:** Cardiac Catheterization; Angiography-Coronary; **Hospital:** Lutheran Med Ctr - Brooklyn, Lenox Hill Hosp (page 94); **Address:** 217 Ovington Ave, Brooklyn, NY 11209-1204; **Phone:** 718-238-0098; **Board Cert:** Internal Medicine 1986; Cardiovascular Disease 1989; **Med School:** France 1983; **Resid:** Internal Medicine, Lutheran Med Ctr 1986; **Fellow:** Cardiovascular Disease, Univ Hosp 1988

CHILD & ADOLESCENT PSYCHIATRY

Engel, Lenore MD (ChAP) - **Hospital:** Kings County Hosp Ctr, SUNY Downstate Med Ctr; **Address:** 115 Henry St, Ste 1G, Brooklyn, NY 11201-2562; **Phone:** 718-855-8911; **Board Cert:** Psychiatry 1983; Child & Adolescent Psychiatry 1985; Forensic Psychiatry 1998; **Med School:** SUNY Downstate 1978; **Resid:** Psychiatry, SUNY Kings County Hosp 1982; **Fellow:** Child Psychiatry, SUNY Kings County Hosp 1984; **Fac Appt:** Asst Clin Prof Psyc, SUNY Downstate

Holzer, Barry D MD (ChAP) - **Spec Exp:** ADD/ADHD; Behavioral Disorders; Bipolar/Mood Disorders; **Hospital:** Long Island Jewish Med Ctr; **Address:** 2692 Batchelder St, Brooklyn, NY 11235; **Phone:** 718-743-7600; **Board Cert:** Psychiatry 1990; Child & Adolescent Psychiatry 1995; **Med School:** Albert Einstein Coll Med 1984; **Resid:** Internal Medicine, Maimonides Med Ctr 1985; **Fellow:** Psychiatry, Hillside Hosp-LIJ 1988; Child & Adolescent Psychiatry, Schneider Chldns Hosp-LIJ 1990

Shabry, Fryderyka MD (ChAP) - **Spec Exp:** ADD/ADHD; Anxiety Disorders; Depression; **Hospital:** Coney Island Hosp; **Address:** 1014 E 24th St, Brooklyn, NY 11210-3640; **Phone:** 718-377-5383; **Board Cert:** Psychiatry 1983; Pediatrics 1970; Child & Adolescent Psychiatry 1986; **Med School:** Poland 1963; **Resid:** Pediatrics, Brookdale Hosp Med Ctr 1968; Psychiatry, Brookdale Hosp Med Ctr 1980; **Fellow:** Child & Adolescent Psychiatry, Brookdale Hosp Med Ctr 1979; **Fac Appt:** Asst Clin Prof Psyc, SUNY Downstate

Vera, Reinaldo MD (ChAP) - **Hospital:** Maimonides Med Ctr (page 96); **Address:** Community Mental Health Center, 920 48th St Fl 1st, Brooklyn, NY 11219-3133; **Phone:** 718-283-8128; **Board Cert:** Psychiatry 1980; Child & Adolescent Psychiatry 1987; **Med School:** Ecuador 1967; **Resid:** Psychiatry, Maimonides Med Ctr 1972; **Fellow:** Child & Adolescent Psychiatry, Maimonides Med Ctr 1974

CHILD NEUROLOGY

Bender-Cracco, Joan MD (ChiN) - **Spec Exp:** Spina Bifida; Epilepsy; Neurophysiology; **Hospital:** SUNY Downstate Med Ctr, Kings County Hosp Ctr; **Address:** SUNY Downstate Med Ctr, 450 Clarkson Ave, Box 118, Brooklyn, NY 11203-2056; **Phone:** 718-270-2042; **Board Cert:** Pediatrics 1969; Neurology 1972; Clinical Neurophysiology 2001; **Med School:** UMDNJ-NJ Med Sch, Newark 1963; **Resid:** Pediatrics, Mayo Clinic 1966; Neurology, Thomas Jefferson Univ Hosp 1969; **Fac Appt:** Prof N, SUNY Hlth Sci Ctr

Rose, Arthur L MD (ChiN) - **Spec Exp:** Developmental Disorders; **Hospital:** SUNY Downstate Med Ctr, Kings County Hosp Ctr; **Address:** SUNY-Hlth Sci Ctr at Brooklyn, 450 Clarkson Ave, Box 1118 B4-330, Brooklyn, NY 11203-0118; **Phone:** 718-270-2042; **Board Cert:** Pediatrics 1963; Neurology 1969; Child Neurology 1973; **Med School:** England 1957; **Resid:** Pediatrics, Queen Elizabeth Hosp Chldn 1960; Pediatrics, Boston City Hosp 1961; **Fellow:** Child Neurology, Chldns Hosp 1963; Neurological Pathology, Columbia P&S 1967; **Fac Appt:** Prof N, SUNY Downstate

COLON & RECTAL SURGERY

Fleischer, Marian MD (CRS) - **Spec Exp:** Colonoscopy; Colon & Rectal Cancer; Pelvic & Perineal Surgery; **Hospital:** Maimonides Med Ctr (page 96), Beth Israel Med Ctr- Kings Hwy Div (page 90); **Address:** 9707 4th Ave, Brooklyn, NY 11209-8129; **Phone:** 718-836-3603; **Board Cert:** Colon & Rectal Surgery 1984; **Med School:** Italy 1972; **Resid:** Surgery, Maimonides Medical Ctr 1981; Colon & Rectal Surgery, Baltimore Med Ctr 1982

Lacqua, Frank MD (CRS) - **Spec Exp:** Colonoscopy; Colon Cancer; Anal Disorders & Reconstruction; **Hospital:** Victory Memorial Hosp - Bklyn; **Address:** 7513 Ft Hamilton Pkwy, Brooklyn, NY 11228; **Phone:** 718-680-6604; **Board Cert:** Colon & Rectal Surgery 2003; **Med School:** SUNY Buffalo 1985; **Resid:** Surgery, St Lukes-Roosevelt Hosp; **Fellow:** Colon & Rectal Surgery, Univ Tex Hlth Sci Ctr

DERMATOLOGY

Baldwin, Hilary MD (D) - **Spec Exp:** Acne & Rosacea; Cosmetic Dermatology; **Hospital:** SUNY Downstate Med Ctr, Kings County Hosp Ctr; **Address:** 450 Clarkson Ave, Box 46, Brooklyn, NY 11203; **Phone:** 718-270-1230; **Board Cert:** Dermatology 1988; **Med School:** Boston Univ 1984; **Resid:** Dermatology, NYU Med Ctr 1988; **Fac Appt:** Assoc Prof D, SUNY Downstate

Berry, Richard MD (D) - **Spec Exp:** Skin Cancer; Hair Removal-Laser; Botox Therapy; **Hospital:** SUNY Downstate Med Ctr; **Address:** 2820 Ocean Pkwy, Brooklyn, NY 11235-7958; **Phone:** 718-996-3000; **Board Cert:** Dermatology 1978; **Med School:** SUNY Hlth Sci Ctr 1974; **Resid:** Internal Medicine, Roosevelt Hosp 1975; Dermatology, SUNY Downstate Med Ctr 1978; **Fac Appt:** Asst Clin Prof D, SUNY Hlth Sci Ctr

Biro, David MD/PhD (D) - **Spec Exp:** Mohs' Surgery; Skin Laser Surgery; Cosmetic Dermatology; **Hospital:** Lutheran Med Ctr - Brooklyn, Maimonides Med Ctr (page 96); **Address:** 9921 4th Ave Fl 1, Brooklyn, NY 11209-8347; **Phone:** 718-833-7616; **Board Cert:** Dermatology 1995; **Med School:** Columbia P&S 1991; **Resid:** Dermatology, Suny Hlth Sci Ctr 1995; **Fac Appt:** Asst Clin Prof D, SUNY Hlth Sci Ctr

Biro, Laszlo MD (D) - **Spec Exp:** Skin Cancer; Cosmetic Dermatology; **Hospital:** Victory Memorial Hosp - Bklyn, Lutheran Med Ctr - Brooklyn; **Address:** 9921 4th Ave, Brooklyn, NY 11209-8347; **Phone:** 718-833-7616; **Board Cert:** Dermatology 1963; **Med School:** Hungary 1953; **Resid:** Dermatology, Bellevue Hosp 1960; **Fac Appt:** Clin Prof D, SUNY Hlth Sci Ctr

Brancaccio, Ronald R MD (D) - **Spec Exp:** Contact Dermatitis; Skin Laser Surgery; Cosmetic Dermatology; **Hospital:** Lutheran Med Ctr - Brooklyn, NYU Med Ctr (page 102); **Address:** 7901 4th Ave, Brooklyn, NY 11209-3957; **Phone:** 718-491-5800; **Board Cert:** Dermatology 1977; **Med School:** Geo Wash Univ 1972; **Resid:** Dermatology, Univ Oregon Hlth Sci Ctr 1976; **Fac Appt:** Clin Prof D, NYU Sch Med

Danziger, Stephen MD (D) - **Spec Exp:** Skin Cancer & Moles; Acne & Rosacea; Psoriasis/Eczema; Warts; **Hospital:** New York Methodist Hosp (page 479), Long Island Coll Hosp (page 90); **Address:** 1 Hanson Pl, Brooklyn, NY 11243; **Phone:** 718-638-3640; **Board Cert:** Dermatology 1975; **Med School:** SUNY Downstate 1968; **Resid:** Dermatology, SUNY Hlth Sci Ctr 1974; **Fac Appt:** Asst Clin Prof D, SUNY Downstate

Deitz, Marcia MD (D) - **Spec Exp:** Acne; Psoriasis; Warts; Eczema; **Hospital:** Coney Island Hosp; **Address:** 1486 Ocean Pkwy, Brooklyn, NY 11230-6453; **Phone:** 718-627-3024; **Board Cert:** Dermatology 1984; **Med School:** SUNY Downstate 1980; **Resid:** Internal Medicine, Brookdale 1981; Dermatology, NY Med Coll 1984; **Fac Appt:** Asst Clin Prof Med, NY Coll Osteo Med

Feldman, Philip MD (D) - **Spec Exp:** Acne; Eczema; Skin Tumors; **Hospital:** Long Island Coll Hosp (page 90), Brooklyn Hosp Ctr-Downtown; **Address:** 142 Joralemon St, Ste 4B, Brooklyn, NY 11201-4709; **Phone:** 718-237-0404; **Board Cert:** Dermatology 1970; **Med School:** Switzerland 1963; **Resid:** Dermatology, Columbia-Presby Med Ctr 1967; **Fac Appt:** Asst Clin Prof D, SUNY Downstate

Felman, Yehudi M. MD (D) - **Spec Exp:** Sexually Transmitted Diseases; **Hospital:** SUNY Downstate Med Ctr, Maimonides Med Ctr (page 96); **Address:** 8100 Bay Pkwy, Brooklyn, NY 11214; **Phone:** 718-256-2600; **Board Cert:** Dermatology 1968; **Med School:** Albert Einstein Coll Med 1963; **Resid:** Dermatology, Colum Presby Hosp 1967; **Fac Appt:** Clin Prof D, SUNY Hlth Sci Ctr

Milburn, Peter MD (D) - **Spec Exp:** Skin Cancer; Cosmetic Dermatology; **Hospital:** Lutheran Med Ctr - Brooklyn, St Luke's - Roosevelt Hosp Ctr - Roosevelt Div (page 90); **Address:** 8026 5th Ave, Brooklyn, NY 11209; **Phone:** 718-680-2800; **Board Cert:** Dermatology 1981; **Med School:** Albert Einstein Coll Med 1977; **Resid:** Dermatology, Columbia-Presby Med Ctr 1981; **Fac Appt:** Asst Clin Prof D, Columbia P&S

Shalita, Alan MD (D) - **Spec Exp:** Acne; Rosacea; **Hospital:** SUNY Downstate Med Ctr; **Address:** Downstate Derm Assoc, 450 Clarkson Ave, Box 46, Brooklyn, NY 11203-2012; **Phone:** 718-270-1230; **Board Cert:** Dermatology 1971; **Med School:** Wake Forest Univ 1964; **Resid:** Dermatology, NYU Med Ctr 1970; **Fellow:** Dermatologic Research, NYU Med Ctr 1973; **Fac Appt:** Prof D, SUNY Downstate

Simon, Steven MD (D) - **Spec Exp:** Skin Cancer; Acne; Hair Removal-Laser; **Hospital:** Beth Israel Med Ctr-Kings Hwy Div (page 90); **Address:** 2270 Kimball St, Brooklyn, NY 11234-5139; **Phone:** 718-253-4550; **Board Cert:** Dermatology 1981; **Med School:** Mexico 1975; **Resid:** Internal Medicine, Brookdale Hosp 1978; Dermatology, Downstate Med Ctr 1981; **Fac Appt:** Assoc Clin Prof D, SUNY Hlth Sci Ctr

Weinstein, Alan S MD (D) - **Hospital:** NYU Med Ctr (page 102); **Address:** 1122 Ocean Ave, Brooklyn, NY 11230-1975; **Phone:** 718-434-5600; **Board Cert:** Dermatology 1969; **Med School:** Univ Hlth Sci/Chicago Med Sch 1960; **Resid:** Dermatology, NYU Med Ctr 1967; **Fac Appt:** Assoc Clin Prof D, NYU Sch Med

Westfried, Morris MD (D) - **Spec Exp:** Laser Surgery; Hair Loss; Psoriasis; **Hospital:** Maimonides Med Ctr (page 96), Brooklyn Hosp Ctr-Downtown; **Address:** 532 Neptune Ave, Ste 209, Brooklyn, NY 11224-4006; **Phone:** 718-449-8860; **Board Cert:** Dermatology 1980; **Med School:** Yale Univ 1975; **Resid:** Pathology, Maimonides Med Ctr 1977; Dermatology, Univ Hosp 1980; **Fellow:** Mohs Surgery, Henry Ford Hosp

DIAGNOSTIC RADIOLOGY

Garner, Steven MD (DR) - **Spec Exp:** Mammography; Trauma Radiology; Nuclear Terrorism Preparedness; **Hospital:** New York Methodist Hosp (page 479); **Address:** NY Methodist Hosp, Dept Radiology, 506 6th St, Brooklyn, NY 11215; **Phone:** 718-780-5870; **Board Cert:** Diagnostic Radiology 1984; Emergency Medicine 1998; **Med School:** Univ Hlth Sci/Chicago Med Sch 1976; **Resid:** Radiology, Mount Sinai Hosp 1983; **Fac Appt:** Asst Prof Rad, NY Med Coll

Lerman, Jay E MD (DR) - **Spec Exp:** Urologic Imaging; Musculoskeletal Imaging; **Address:** Lerman Diagnostic Imaging, 6511 Fort Hamilton Pkwy, Brooklyn, NY 11219; **Phone:** 718-491-4545; **Board Cert:** Diagnostic Radiology 1991; **Med School:** Albert Einstein Coll Med 1986; **Resid:** Radiology, Montefiore Med Ctr 1991; **Fellow:** Cross Sectional Imaging, Thom Jefferson Hosp 1992

Ramanathan, Kumudha MD (DR) - **Spec Exp:** Mammography; Women's Imaging; **Address:** 161 Atlantic Ave, Brooklyn, NY 11201; **Phone:** 718-624-2222; **Board Cert:** Diag Rad with Spec Comp in Nuc Rad 1982; **Med School:** India 1976; **Resid:** Radiology, LI Coll Hosp 1983

Yaghoobian, Jahangui MD (DR) - **Spec Exp:** Ultrasound; **Hospital:** Victory Memorial Hosp - Bklyn; **Address:** 699 92nd St, Brooklyn, NY 11228-3619; **Phone:** 718-567-1245; **Board Cert:** Radiology 1974; **Med School:** Iran 1966; **Resid:** Radiology, LI Coll Hosp 1969

ENDOCRINOLOGY, DIABETES & METABOLISM

Brickman, Alan MD (EDM) - **Spec Exp:** Diabetes; Thyroid Disorders; Cholesterol/Lipid Disorders; Calcium Disorders; **Hospital:** Maimonides Med Ctr (page 96); **Address:** 1318 52nd St, Brooklyn, NY 11219-3802; **Phone:** 718-436-9898; **Board Cert:** Internal Medicine 1979; Endocrinology, Diabetes & Metabolism 1981; **Med School:** Albert Einstein Coll Med 1976; **Resid:** Internal Medicine, Maimonides Medical Ctr 1979; **Fellow:** Endocrinology, Diabetes & Metabolism, Yale-New Haven Hosp 1981

Giegerich, Edmund W MD (EDM) - **Spec Exp:** Thyroid Disorders; **Hospital:** Long Island Coll Hosp (page 90); **Address:** 339 Hicks St, Brooklyn, NY 11201-5509; **Phone:** 718-780-4797; **Board Cert:** Internal Medicine 1980; Endocrinology, Diabetes & Metabolism 1983; **Med School:** SUNY Downstate 1977; **Resid:** Internal Medicine, Rhode Island Hosp 1980; **Fellow:** Endocrinology, Diabetes & Metabolism, Mount Sinai Hosp 1982; **Fac Appt:** Assoc Clin Prof Med, SUNY Hlth Sci Ctr

Goldman, Joel M MD (EDM) - **Spec Exp:** Thyroid Disorders; Diabetes; **Hospital:** Brookdale Univ Hosp Med Ctr, Beth Israel Med Ctr- Kings Hwy Div (page 90); **Address:** 555 Rockaway Pkwy, rm 101a SBSI, Brooklyn, NY 11212-3132; **Phone:** 718-240-5378; **Board Cert:** Internal Medicine 1976; Endocrinology, Diabetes & Metabolism 1979; **Med School:** Univ Ariz Coll Med 1973; **Resid:** Internal Medicine, UMDNJ-Newark Affil Hosps 1975; Internal Medicine, Albert Einstein Coll of Med 1976; **Fellow:** Endocrinology, Diabetes & Metabolism, NIAMDD-Natl Inst Hlth 1979; **Fac Appt:** Assoc Prof Med, SUNY Downstate

Khan, Farida MD (EDM) - **Spec Exp:** Diabetes; Thyroid Disorders; Reproductive Endocrinology; **Hospital:** New York Methodist Hosp (page 479); **Address:** 506 6th St, Brooklyn, NY 11215-3609; **Phone:** 718-246-8600; **Board Cert:** Internal Medicine 1977; Endocrinology 1981; **Med School:** India 1962; **Resid:** Internal Medicine, Jewish Hosp & Med Ctr 1973; **Fellow:** Endocrinology, Diabetes & Metabolism, Jewish Hosp & Med Ctr 1973; **Fac Appt:** Assoc Prof Med, Cornell Univ-Weill Med Coll

Mann, David MD (EDM) - **Spec Exp:** Thyroid Disorders; Endocrinology; **Hospital:** Long Island Coll Hosp (page 90); **Address:** 142 Joralemon St, Ste 11D, Brooklyn, NY 11201-4709; **Phone:** 718-855-8860; **Board Cert:** Internal Medicine 1980; Endocrinology, Diabetes & Metabolism 1983; **Med School:** Cornell Univ-Weill Med Coll 1977; **Resid:** Internal Medicine, Beth Israel Med Ctr 1980; **Fellow:** Endocrinology, Diabetes & Metabolism, Montefiore Hosp Med Ctr 1983; **Fac Appt:** Asst Prof Med, SUNY Hlth Sci Ctr

Saxena, Anil MD (EDM) - **Spec Exp:** Diabetes; Thyroid Disorders; Osteoporosis; **Hospital:** Kingsbrook Jewish Med Ctr, Beth Israel Med Ctr- Kings Hwy Div (page 90); **Address:** 1700 Flatbush Ave, Brooklyn, NY 11210-3943; **Phone:** 718-951-6495; **Board Cert:** Internal Medicine 1975; Endocrinology, Diabetes & Metabolism 1977; **Med School:** India 1971; **Resid:** Internal Medicine, St Clare's Hosp 1973; Internal Medicine, Kingsbrook Jewish Med Ctr 1975; **Fellow:** Endocrinology, Diabetes & Metabolism, Univ Hosp 1977

Schmidt, Philip MD (EDM) - **Spec Exp:** Diabetes; Thyroid Disorders; Osteoporosis; **Hospital:** Beth Israel Med Ctr- Kings Hwy Div (page 90), New York Methodist Hosp (page 479); **Address:** 3043 Ocean Ave Bldg 102, Brooklyn, NY 11235-3400; **Phone:** 718-648-9200; **Board Cert:** Internal Medicine 1977; Endocrinology, Diabetes & Metabolism 1998; **Med School:** Albert Einstein Coll Med 1960; **Resid:** Internal Medicine, Jewish Hosp 1962; Internal Medicine, Jewish Hosp 1965; **Fellow:** Endocrinology, Diabetes & Metabolism, Jewish Hosp 1966; **Fac Appt:** Asst Clin Prof Med, SUNY Downstate

Schussler, George MD (EDM) - **Spec Exp:** Thyroid Disorders; Parathyroid Disorders; Calcium Disorders; **Hospital:** SUNY Downstate Med Ctr, Kings County Hosp Ctr; **Address:** 450 Clarkson Ave, Box 57, Brooklyn, NY 11203-2098; **Phone:** 718-270-2159; **Board Cert:** Internal Medicine 1963; Endocrinology, Diabetes & Metabolism 1973; **Med School:** Cornell Univ-Weill Med Coll 1956; **Resid:** Internal Medicine, Univ Hosp 1958; **Fellow:** Endocrinology, Diabetes & Metabolism, Boston Med Ctr 1960; **Fac Appt:** Prof Med, SUNY Hlth Sci Ctr

Silverberg, Arnold MD (EDM) - **Spec Exp:** Thyroid Disorders; Osteoporosis; Diabetes; **Hospital:** Maimonides Med Ctr (page 96); **Address:** 908 48th St Fl 1, Brooklyn, NY 11219-2918; **Phone:** 718-283-6200; **Board Cert:** Internal Medicine 1968; Endocrinology 1977; **Med School:** Albert Einstein Coll Med 1961; **Resid:** Internal Medicine, Montefiore Hosp Med Ctr 1965; **Fellow:** Internal Medicine, Mount Sinai Hosp 1964; Endocrinology, Diabetes & Metabolism, Mount Sinai Hosp 1968; **Fac Appt:** Assoc Clin Prof Med, Mount Sinai Sch Med

Spergel, Gabriel MD (EDM) - **Spec Exp:** Diabetes; Thyroid Disorders; **Hospital:** New York Comm Hosp; **Address:** 135 Ocean Pkwy, Brooklyn, NY 11218; **Phone:** 718-853-3702; **Med School:** Albert Einstein Coll Med 1961; **Resid:** Internal Medicine, Kings Co Hosp 1964; **Fellow:** Endocrinology, Diabetes & Metabolism, Kings County Hosp 1965; Endocrinology, Diabetes & Metabolism, Jewish Med Ctr 1967; **Fac Appt:** Assoc Clin Prof Med, Cornell Univ-Weill Med Coll

FAMILY MEDICINE

Athanail, Steven MD (FMed) `PCP` - **Spec Exp:** Sports Medicine; **Hospital:** Lutheran Med Ctr - Brooklyn; **Address:** 268 Bay Ridge Pkwy, Ste 1B, Brooklyn, NY 11209; **Phone:** 718-748-7272; **Board Cert:** Family Medicine 2001; **Med School:** Howard Univ 1979; **Resid:** Family Medicine, Montefiore Hosp Med Ctr 1983

Gradler, Thomas MD (FMed) `PCP` - **Spec Exp:** Asthma & Allergy; Sports Medicine; **Hospital:** Lutheran Med Ctr - Brooklyn; **Address:** 234 Ovington Ave, Brooklyn, NY 11209; **Phone:** 718-745-0309; **Board Cert:** Family Medicine 1999; **Med School:** SUNY Hlth Sci Ctr 1973; **Resid:** Family Medicine, Lutheran Med Ctr 1976; **Fac Appt:** Asst Clin Prof FMed, SUNY Hlth Sci Ctr

Krotowski, Mark MD (FMed) `PCP` - **Spec Exp:** Caribbean Health Care; Hypertension; Diabetes; **Hospital:** Brookdale Univ Hosp Med Ctr, SUNY Downstate Med Ctr; **Address:** Brookdale Hosp, Dept Family Practice, 8923 Avenue A, Brooklyn, NY 11236-1206; **Phone:** 718-385-8181; **Board Cert:** Family Medicine 2001; **Med School:** Israel 1976; **Resid:** Pediatrics, Brookdale Univ Hosp 1977; Family Medicine, Brookdale Univ Hosp 1979; **Fac Appt:** Assoc Clin Prof FMed, SUNY Downstate

Lopez, Clark MD (FMed) `PCP` - **Spec Exp:** Geriatrics; **Hospital:** New York Methodist Hosp (page 479), Lutheran Med Ctr - Brooklyn; **Address:** 60 Plaza St E, Brooklyn, NY 11238; **Phone:** 718-783-3919; **Board Cert:** Family Medicine 2003; **Med School:** SUNY Downstate 1972; **Resid:** Internal Medicine, Kings County Hosp 1974; Family Medicine, Kings County Hosp 1977; **Fellow:** Obstetrics & Gynecology, Kings County Hosp 1997; **Fac Appt:** Asst Prof FMed, SUNY Downstate

Moskowitz, George MD (FMed) `PCP` - **Spec Exp:** Geriatric Medicine; Obesity; Preventive Medicine; **Hospital:** Maimonides Med Ctr (page 96), Beth Israel Med Ctr- Kings Hwy Div (page 90); **Address:** 1318 42nd St, Brooklyn, NY 11219-1405; **Phone:** 718-436-2496; **Board Cert:** Family Medicine 1998; **Med School:** Belgium 1973; **Resid:** Family Medicine, St Vincents Hosp 1976; Family Medicine, Med Univ S Carolina 1978

Sadovsky, Richard MD (FMed) `PCP` - **Spec Exp:** Preventive Medicine; Diabetes; Hepatitis; Thyroid Disorders; **Hospital:** SUNY Downstate Med Ctr; **Address:** 450 Clarkson Ave, Ste B, Brooklyn, NY 11203-2012; **Phone:** 718-270-2697; **Board Cert:** Family Medicine 1996; **Med School:** SUNY Hlth Sci Ctr 1974; **Resid:** Family Medicine, SUNY Hosp 1977; **Fac Appt:** Assoc Prof FMed, SUNY Hlth Sci Ctr

Schiowitz, Emanuel DO (FMed) `PCP` - **Hospital:** Maimonides Med Ctr (page 96), New York Methodist Hosp (page 479); **Address:** 1701 59th St, Brooklyn, NY 11204-2254; **Phone:** 718-259-0222; **Board Cert:** Family Medicine 1968; **Med School:** Philadelphia Coll Osteo Med 1963; **Resid:** Family Medicine, Interboro Med Ctr 1964; **Fac Appt:** Asst Clin Prof FMed, NY Coll Osteo Med

Scott, Norman MD (FMed) `PCP` - **Hospital:** Brookdale Univ Hosp Med Ctr; **Address:** 1381B Linden Blvd, Brooklyn, NY 11212; **Phone:** 718-498-3104; **Board Cert:** Family Medicine 2000; Emergency Medicine 2003; **Med School:** Tulane Univ 1976; **Resid:** Family Medicine, Brookdale 1979

Sheridan, Bernadette MD (FMed) `PCP` - **Spec Exp:** Geriatric Cardiology; Adolescent Medicine; Women's Health; **Hospital:** Brookdale Univ Hosp Med Ctr, New York Methodist Hosp (page 479); **Address:** 1222 East 96 St Fl 2, Brooklyn, NY 11236; **Phone:** 718-257-3355; **Board Cert:** Family Medicine 2004; **Med School:** SUNY Buffalo 1979; **Resid:** Family Medicine, Brookdale Hosp Med Ctr 1982

Vincent, Miriam MD/PhD (FMed) [PCP] - **Spec Exp:** Diabetes; Arthritis; Preventive Medicine; **Hospital:** SUNY Downstate Med Ctr, Kings County Hosp Ctr; **Address:** 470 Clarkson Ave, Box 67, Brooklyn, NY 11203-2012; **Phone:** 718-270-2697; **Board Cert:** Family Medicine 2001; **Med School:** SUNY Hlth Sci Ctr 1985; **Resid:** Family Medicine, Univ Hosp 1988; **Fac Appt:** Prof FMed, SUNY Hlth Sci Ctr

GASTROENTEROLOGY

Arya, Yashpal MD (Ge) - **Spec Exp:** Colonoscopy; Peptic Ulcer Disease; **Hospital:** Wyckoff Heights Med Ctr, St John's Queens Hosp (page 375); **Address:** Gastrointestinal Diagnostic, 129 St. Nicolas Ave, Fl 1, Brooklyn, NY 11237-4039; **Phone:** 718-821-0643; **Board Cert:** Internal Medicine 1972; Gastroenterology 1999; **Med School:** India 1966; **Resid:** Internal Medicine, Wyckoff Heights Hosp 1969; Internal Medicine, Jewish Hosp 1971; **Fellow:** Gastroenterology, Queens Hosp Ctr 1973

Bigajer, Charles MD (Ge) - **Spec Exp:** Endoscopy; Liver Disease; **Hospital:** Brookdale Univ Hosp Med Ctr, Beth Israel Med Ctr- Kings Hwy Div (page 90); **Address:** 1 Brookdale Plaza Katz Bldg - rm 323, Brooklyn, NY 11212-3139; **Phone:** 718-240-6385; **Board Cert:** Internal Medicine 1977; Gastroenterology 1981; Geriatric Medicine 1992; **Med School:** Albert Einstein Coll Med 1974; **Resid:** Internal Medicine, Brookdale Hosp 1977; **Fellow:** Gastroenterology, NYU Med Ctr 1980; **Fac Appt:** Asst Clin Prof Med, SUNY Downstate

Cerulli, Maurice A MD (Ge) - **Spec Exp:** Gastric & Colonic Disorders; Liver Disease; Gastroesophageal Reflux Disease (GERD); Nutrition; **Hospital:** New York Methodist Hosp (page 479); **Address:** 263 7th Ave Fl 5 - rm A, Brooklyn, NY 11215; **Phone:** 718-246-8600; **Board Cert:** Internal Medicine 1975; Gastroenterology 1977; **Med School:** SUNY Hlth Sci Ctr 1972; **Resid:** Internal Medicine, Kings County Hosp 1975; **Fellow:** Gastroenterology, Johns Hopkins Hosp 1977; **Fac Appt:** Assoc Prof Med, Cornell Univ-Weill Med Coll

Cohen, Paul MD (Ge) - **Spec Exp:** Gastroesophageal Reflux Disease (GERD); Gastroparesis; Colonoscopy; **Hospital:** SUNY Downstate Med Ctr; **Address:** 1310 President St, Brooklyn, NY 11213; **Phone:** 718-221-0415; **Board Cert:** Internal Medicine 1989; Gastroenterology 1991; **Med School:** Grenada 1986; **Resid:** Internal Medicine, Kings County Hosp 1989; **Fellow:** Gastroenterology, Kings County Hosp 1991; **Fac Appt:** Assoc Clin Prof Med, SUNY Hlth Sci Ctr

Erber, William MD (Ge) - **Spec Exp:** Endoscopy; Inflammatory Bowel Disease/Crohn's; Gastrointestinal Cancer; **Hospital:** Maimonides Med Ctr (page 96), Beth Israel Med Ctr - Petrie Division (page 90); **Address:** 591 Ocean Pkwy, Brooklyn, NY 11218-5913; **Phone:** 718-972-8500; **Board Cert:** Internal Medicine 1975; Gastroenterology 1979; **Med School:** Univ Hlth Sci/Chicago Med Sch 1967; **Resid:** Internal Medicine, Maimonides Med Ctr 1969; Internal Medicine, Maimonides Med Ctr 1973; **Fellow:** Research, Hadassah Hosp 1972; Gastroenterology, Albert Einstein 1975; **Fac Appt:** Asst Clin Prof Med, SUNY Downstate

Gettenberg, Gary MD (Ge) - **Spec Exp:** Gastrointestinal Cancer; Colon Cancer Screening; Gastroesophageal Reflux Disease (GERD); **Hospital:** Maimonides Med Ctr (page 96); **Address:** 1630 E 14th St, Brooklyn, NY 11229; **Phone:** 718-339-0391; **Board Cert:** Internal Medicine 1987; Gastroenterology 1989; **Med School:** NY Med Coll 1983; **Resid:** Internal Medicine, Maimonides Med Ctr 1986; **Fellow:** Gastroenterology, Maimonides Med Ctr 1988

Grosman, Irwin MD (Ge) - **Spec Exp:** Colon Cancer Screening; Irritable Bowel Syndrome; Liver Disease; **Hospital:** Long Island Coll Hosp (page 90); **Address:** 339 Hicks St, Brooklyn, NY 11201-5514; **Phone:** 718-780-1468; **Board Cert:** Internal Medicine 1987; Gastroenterology 1989; **Med School:** SUNY Stony Brook 1984; **Resid:** Internal Medicine, Montefiore Hosp Med Ctr 1987; **Fellow:** Gastroenterology, Montefiore Hosp Med Ctr 1989; **Fac Appt:** Asst Prof Med, SUNY Hlth Sci Ctr

Gusset, George MD (Ge) - **Spec Exp:** Colonoscopy; Gastroscopy; Liver Disease; **Hospital:** Beth Israel Med Ctr- Kings Hwy Div (page 90), New York Comm Hosp; **Address:** 2815 Ocean Pkwy, Brooklyn, NY 11235-7839; **Phone:** 718-769-9595; **Board Cert:** Internal Medicine 1975; Gastroenterology 1979; **Med School:** Univ Louisville Sch Med 1960; **Resid:** Internal Medicine, VA Med Ctr 1962; Internal Medicine, Brooklyn Jewish Hosp & Med Ctr 1963; **Fellow:** Gastroenterology, Brooklyn Jewish Hosp & Med Ctr 1964

Iswara, Kadirawel MD (Ge) - **Spec Exp:** Pancreatic/Biliary Endoscopy (ERCP); Colonoscopy; Endoscopy; Hepatitis; **Hospital:** Maimonides Med Ctr (page 96), Coney Island Hosp; **Address:** 2560 Ocean Ave, Ste 3A, Brooklyn, NY 11229-4521; **Phone:** 718-615-0400; **Board Cert:** Internal Medicine 1980; Gastroenterology 1975; **Med School:** Sri Lanka 1968; **Resid:** Internal Medicine, Coney Island Hosp 1972; Internal Medicine, Bronx VA Hosp 1973; **Fellow:** Gastroenterology, Maimonides Med Ctr 1976; **Fac Appt:** Asst Clin Prof Med, Mount Sinai Sch Med

Leb, Alvin MD (Ge) - **Spec Exp:** Gastrointestinal Disorders; Endoscopy; **Hospital:** Beth Israel Med Ctr- Kings Hwy Div (page 90), Brookdale Univ Hosp Med Ctr; **Address:** 2985 Quentin Rd, Brooklyn, NY 11229; **Phone:** 718-336-2218; **Board Cert:** Gastroenterology 1989; Internal Medicine 1985; **Med School:** SUNY Downstate 1982; **Resid:** Internal Medicine, Brookdale 1985; **Fellow:** Gastroenterology, Brookdale 1988

Levendoglu, Hulya MD (Ge) - **Spec Exp:** Endoscopy; Motility Disorders; Hepatitis C; **Hospital:** Brookdale Univ Hosp Med Ctr; **Address:** 1 Brookdale Plaza, Katz Pavilion, rm 337, Brooklyn, NY 11212-3198; **Phone:** 718-240-6025; **Board Cert:** Internal Medicine 1976; Gastroenterology 1979; **Med School:** Turkey 1972; **Resid:** Internal Medicine, Cook Co Hosp 1976; **Fellow:** Gastroenterology, Cook Co Hosp 1978; **Fac Appt:** Assoc Prof Med, SUNY Hlth Sci Ctr

Maizel, Barry MD (Ge) - **Spec Exp:** Endoscopy; Inflammatory Bowel Disease; Liver Disease; **Hospital:** New York Methodist Hosp (page 479), NY Hosp Queens; **Address:** 90 8th Ave, Brooklyn, NY 11215-1553; **Phone:** 718-622-8255; **Board Cert:** Internal Medicine 1979; Gastroenterology 1981; **Med School:** Italy 1975; **Resid:** Internal Medicine, Jewish Hosp 1978; **Fellow:** Gastroenterology, NY Med Coll-Metropolitan Hosp 1980

Mayer, Ira E MD (Ge) - **Spec Exp:** Inflammatory Bowel Disease/Crohn's; Gastroesophageal Reflux Disease (GERD); Motility Disorders; **Hospital:** Maimonides Med Ctr (page 96); **Address:** 2560 Ocean Ave, Ste 2A, Brooklyn, NY 11229-4521; **Phone:** 718-891-0100; **Board Cert:** Internal Medicine 1978; Gastroenterology 1981; **Med School:** NY Med Coll 1975; **Resid:** Internal Medicine, Metropolitan Hosp Ctr 1978; **Fellow:** Gastroenterology, Emory Univ Hosp 1980

Notar-Francesco, Vincent J MD (Ge) - **Hospital:** New York Methodist Hosp (page 479); **Address:** 263 7th Ave, Ste 5A, Brooklyn, NY 11215; **Phone:** 718-246-8600; **Board Cert:** Internal Medicine 1989; Gastroenterology 2001; **Med School:** Mount Sinai Sch Med 1986; **Resid:** Internal Medicine, Stony Brook Univ Hosp 1989; **Fellow:** Gastroenterology, SUNY Downstate Med Ctr 1991

Piccione, Paul MD (Ge) - **Hospital:** Lutheran Med Ctr - Brooklyn, Victory Memorial Hosp - Bklyn; **Address:** 560 Bay Ridge Pkwy, Brooklyn, NY 11209-2702; **Phone:** 718-748-5219; **Board Cert:** Internal Medicine 1985; Gastroenterology 1987; **Med School:** Italy 1981; **Resid:** Internal Medicine, Lutheran Med Ctr 1985; **Fellow:** Gastroenterology, St Luke's-Roosevelt Hosp 1986

Safier, Henry L MD (Ge) - **Spec Exp:** Gastric & Esophageal Disorders; Liver & Biliary Disease; **Hospital:** Queens Hosp Ctr - Jamaica; **Address:** 126 Greenpoint Ave, Brooklyn, NY 11222; **Phone:** 718-389-0100; **Board Cert:** Internal Medicine 1976; Gastroenterology 1979; **Med School:** Switzerland 1960; **Resid:** Internal Medicine, VA Med Ctr 1964; Internal Medicine, Jewish Hosp 1965; **Fellow:** Gastroenterology, VA Med Ctr 1966; Hepatology, VA Med Ctr 1971

Sorra, Toomas MD (Ge) - **Spec Exp:** Colon & Rectal Cancer; Hepatitis; Gastroesophageal Reflux Disease (GERD); **Hospital:** Long Island Coll Hosp (page 90); **Address:** 166 Clinton St, Brooklyn, NY 11201-4618; **Phone:** 718-834-0100; **Board Cert:** Internal Medicine 1981; Gastroenterology 1983; **Med School:** Mexico 1975; **Resid:** Internal Medicine, LI Coll Hosp 1980; **Fellow:** Gastroenterology, LI Coll Hosp 1982; **Fac Appt:** Asst Prof Med, SUNY Downstate

Tracer, Robert MD (Ge) - **Hospital:** Brookdale Univ Hosp Med Ctr, Beth Israel Med Ctr- Kings Hwy Div (page 90); **Address:** Brookdale Univ Hosp, 1 Brookdale Plaza, Brooklyn, NY 11212; **Phone:** 718-377-9011; **Board Cert:** Internal Medicine 1983; Gastroenterology 1987; **Med School:** SUNY Hlth Sci Ctr 1980; **Resid:** Internal Medicine, Kings Coun 1983; **Fellow:** Gastroenterology, Brookdale 1985; **Fac Appt:** , SUNY Hlth Sci Ctr

Tutino, Jody MD (Ge) - **Spec Exp:** Hepatitis; Colonoscopy; **Hospital:** New York Methodist Hosp (page 479), Beth Israel Med Ctr- Kings Hwy Div (page 90); **Address:** 10 Plaza St East, Brooklyn, NY 11238-4955; **Phone:** 718-636-2050; **Board Cert:** Internal Medicine 1982; Geriatric Medicine 1996; **Med School:** Italy 1977; **Resid:** Internal Medicine, Mount Sinai Hosp 1980; **Fellow:** Gastroenterology, Univ Hosp 1983

Wolfson, David MD (Ge) - **Spec Exp:** Colonoscopy; Inflammatory Bowel Disease; Gastroesophageal Reflux Disease (GERD); **Hospital:** Maimonides Med Ctr (page 96), New York Methodist Hosp (page 479); **Address:** 801 Avenue N, Brooklyn, NY 11230-5717; **Phone:** 718-627-6800; **Board Cert:** Internal Medicine 1979; Gastroenterology 1981; **Med School:** Harvard Med Sch 1976; **Resid:** Internal Medicine, Mount Sinai Hosp 1979; **Fellow:** Gastroenterology, Mount Sinai Hosp 1981

Zimbalist, Eliot MD (Ge) - **Spec Exp:** Colon Cancer Screening; Hepatitis C; Irritable Bowel Syndrome; **Hospital:** Maimonides Med Ctr (page 96); **Address:** 452 77th St, Brooklyn, NY 11209-3206; **Phone:** 718-921-5548; **Board Cert:** Internal Medicine 1983; Gastroenterology 1985; **Med School:** Mount Sinai Sch Med 1980; **Resid:** Internal Medicine, Maimonides Med Ctr 1983; **Fellow:** Gastroenterology, Meml Sloan Kettering Cancer Ctr 1985; **Fac Appt:** Assoc Prof Med, Mount Sinai Sch Med

GERIATRIC MEDICINE

Ahmad, Mahnaz MD (Ger) PCP - **Spec Exp:** Dementia; Geriatric Functional Assessment; **Hospital:** Brooklyn Hosp Ctr-Downtown; **Address:** Brooklyn Hosp Ctr, 121 Dekalb Ave, Maynard Bldg, rm 7F, Brooklyn, NY 11201; **Phone:** 718-250-6100; **Board Cert:** Internal Medicine 2000; Geriatric Medicine 2001; **Med School:** Bangladesh 1992; **Resid:** Internal Medicine, Legacy Portland Hosp 2000; **Fellow:** Geriatric Medicine, NY Hosp/Weill Cornell Med Ctr 2001

Ahronheim, Judith MD (Ger) PCP - **Spec Exp:** Memory Disorders; **Hospital:** SUNY Downstate Med Ctr; **Address:** SUNY-Downstate Medical Center, 450 W Clarkson Ave, Box 50, Brooklyn, NY 11203; **Phone:** 718-270-3323; **Board Cert:** Internal Medicine 1979; Geriatric Medicine 1998; **Med School:** Univ IL Coll Med 1976; **Resid:** Internal Medicine, SUNY-Brooklyn-Kings Co Hosp 1979; **Fellow:** Geriatric Medicine, Parker Geriatric Inst 1980; **Fac Appt:** Prof Med, SUNY Downstate

Baccash, Emil MD (Ger) PCP - **Hospital:** New York Methodist Hosp (page 479); **Address:** 20 8th Ave, Brooklyn, NY 11217-3766; **Phone:** 718-622-7000; **Board Cert:** Internal Medicine 1981; Geriatric Medicine 2005; **Med School:** Italy 1978; **Resid:** Internal Medicine, NY Methodist Hosp 1981

Paris, Barbara MD (Ger) - **Spec Exp:** Preventive Medicine; Abuse/Neglect; **Hospital:** Maimonides Med Ctr (page 96), Mount Sinai Med Ctr (page 98); **Address:** Maimonides Med Ctr, Dept Medicine, 4802 10th Ave, Brooklyn, NY 11219; **Phone:** 718-283-7071; **Board Cert:** Internal Medicine 1982; Geriatric Medicine 1998; **Med School:** SUNY Downstate 1977; **Resid:** Internal Medicine, St Vincents Hosp 1981; **Fellow:** Geriatric Medicine, Mount Sinai Hosp 1986; **Fac Appt:** Clin Prof Med, Mount Sinai Sch Med

GERIATRIC PSYCHIATRY

Amin, Ravindra MD (GerPsy) - **Spec Exp:** Alzheimer's Disease; Anxiety Disorders; Depression; Memory Disorders; **Hospital:** Long Island Coll Hosp (page 90), Mount Sinai Med Ctr (page 98); **Address:** 97 Amity St Fl 6, Brooklyn, NY 11201; **Phone:** 718-780-1070; **Board Cert:** Psychiatry 1993; Geriatric Psychiatry 1994; Addiction Psychiatry 1996; **Med School:** India 1985; **Resid:** Psychiatry, Elmhurst Hosp/Mt Sinai 1992; **Fellow:** Geriatric Psychiatry, Mt Sinai Med Ctr 1994

Cohen, Carl MD (GerPsy) - **Spec Exp:** Alzheimer's Disease; **Hospital:** SUNY Downstate Med Ctr; **Address:** SUNY Health Science Center Assocs, 370 Lenox Rd, Brooklyn, NY 11226-2206; **Phone:** 718-287-4806; **Board Cert:** Psychiatry 1977; Geriatric Psychiatry 2001; **Med School:** SUNY Buffalo 1971; **Resid:** Psychiatry, Bellevue Hosp 1974; **Fellow:** Community Psychiatry, NYU Med Ctr 1975; **Fac Appt:** Prof Psyc, SUNY Hlth Sci Ctr

Rosen, Evelyn MD (GerPsy) - **Hospital:** New York Methodist Hosp (page 479); **Address:** 583 5th St, Brooklyn, NY 11215-3503; **Phone:** 212-813-9410; **Board Cert:** Psychiatry 1992; Geriatric Psychiatry 1994; **Med School:** Mexico 1986; **Resid:** Psychiatry, Univ Hosp 1991; **Fellow:** Geriatric Psychiatry, Univ Hosp 1992

Samuelly, Israel MD (GerPsy) - **Hospital:** Maimonides Med Ctr (page 96); **Address:** 928 Albemarle Rd, Brooklyn, NY 11218-2708; **Phone:** 718-282-1981; **Board Cert:** Psychiatry 1969; Geriatric Psychiatry 1996; **Med School:** Israel 1961; **Resid:** Psychiatry, Brooklyn State Hosp 1965; **Fac Appt:** Asst Clin Prof Psyc, SUNY Downstate

GYNECOLOGIC ONCOLOGY

Chambers, Joseph MD/PhD (GO) - **Spec Exp:** Uterine Cancer; Pelvic Surgery; **Hospital:** Long Island Coll Hosp (page 90); **Address:** Long Island College Hosp, Dept Ob/Gyn, 339 Hicks St, rm H325, Brooklyn, NY 11201; **Phone:** 718-780-1647; **Board Cert:** Obstetrics & Gynecology 1997; Gynecologic Oncology 1997; **Med School:** Georgetown Univ 1977; **Resid:** Obstetrics & Gynecology, Univ Virginia Hosp 1981; **Fellow:** Gynecologic Oncology, Yale-New Haven Hosp 1984; **Fac Appt:** Clin Prof ObG, Columbia P&S

Economos, Katherine MD (GO) - **Spec Exp:** Ovarian Cancer; Cervical Cancer; Uterine Cancer; **Hospital:** New York Methodist Hosp (page 479); **Address:** New York Methodist Hosp, East Pavilion, 506 6th St Fl 1, Brooklyn, NY 11215; **Phone:** 718-780-3090; **Board Cert:** Gynecologic Oncology 1998; Obstetrics & Gynecology 1996; **Med School:** SUNY Downstate 1986; **Resid:** Obstetrics & Gynecology, Maimonides Medical Ctr 1990; **Fellow:** Gynecologic Oncology, Univ Texas SW Med Ctr 1993; **Fac Appt:** Assoc Clin Prof ObG, Cornell Univ-Weill Med Coll

Khulpateea, Neekianund MD (GO) - **Spec Exp:** Hysterectomy Alternatives; Laser Surgery; Gynecologic Cancer; **Hospital:** Maimonides Med Ctr (page 96), Coney Island Hosp; **Address:** Maimonides Med Ctr, Div Gyn, 953 49th St, Brooklyn, NY 11219-2923; **Phone:** 718-283-7370; **Board Cert:** Obstetrics & Gynecology 1981; **Med School:** Israel 1972; **Resid:** Obstetrics & Gynecology, Meth Hosp 1976; **Fellow:** Gynecologic Oncology, Univ Hosp Downstate 1978; **Fac Appt:** Asst Clin Prof ObG, Mount Sinai Sch Med

Serur, Eli MD (GO) - **Spec Exp:** Nutrition & Cancer; Laparoscopic Surgery; **Hospital:** Brooklyn Hosp Ctr-Downtown, St Vincent Cath Med Ctr - Staten Island (page 375); **Address:** 121 Dekalb Ave, Brooklyn, NY 11201; **Phone:** 718-250-8106; **Board Cert:** Obstetrics & Gynecology 1992; Gynecologic Oncology 1997; **Med School:** NYU Sch Med 1985; **Resid:** Obstetrics & Gynecology, Kings County Hosp 1989; **Fellow:** Gynecologic Oncology, SUNY Downstate Med Ctr 1991; **Fac Appt:** Assoc Prof ObG, Cornell Univ-Weill Med Coll

Vardi, Joseph R MD (GO) - **Spec Exp:** Ovarian Cancer; Uterine Cancer; **Hospital:** New York Methodist Hosp (page 479), Maimonides Med Ctr (page 96); **Address:** 941 48th St, Brooklyn, NY 11219-2919; **Phone:** 718-871-3737; **Board Cert:** Obstetrics & Gynecology 1976; Gynecologic Oncology 1979; **Med School:** Israel 1967; **Resid:** Obstetrics & Gynecology, UC Davis Med Ctr 1974; **Fellow:** Gynecologic Oncology, New England Med Ctr 1979; **Fac Appt:** Clin Prof ObG, SUNY Downstate

HAND SURGERY

Edelstein, S Leonard MD (HS) - **Hospital:** Beth Israel Med Ctr- Kings Hwy Div (page 90), Maimonides Med Ctr (page 96); **Address:** 2382 E 13th St, Brooklyn, NY 11229; **Phone:** 718-646-8787; **Board Cert:** Orthopaedic Surgery 1984; Hand Surgery 2005; **Med School:** SUNY Downstate 1972; **Resid:** Orthopaedic Surgery, Brookdale Med Ctr 1976; **Fellow:** Hand Surgery, Harper Grace Hosp 1977

Monsanto, Enrique MD (HS) - **Spec Exp:** Nerve Disorders; Arthritis; Rotator Cuff Surgery; **Hospital:** New York Methodist Hosp (page 479), Cabrini Med Ctr (page 374); **Address:** 263 7th Ave, Fl 2, Brooklyn, NY 11215; **Phone:** 718-771-1765; **Board Cert:** Orthopaedic Surgery 1998; **Med School:** Columbia P&S 1978; **Resid:** Orthopaedic Surgery, Columbia-Presby Hosp 1983; **Fellow:** Hand Surgery, Columbia-Presby Hosp 1984; **Fac Appt:** Assoc Prof OrS, SUNY Downstate

Patel, Mukund MD (HS) - **Spec Exp:** Arthritis; Carpal Tunnel Syndrome; Fractures; **Hospital:** Victory Memorial Hosp - Bklyn, St Vincent Cath Med Ctr - Staten Island (page 375); **Address:** Comprehensive Hand Surg, 4901 Fort Hamilton Pkwy, Brooklyn, NY 11219; **Phone:** 718-435-4944; **Board Cert:** Orthopaedic Surgery 1972; Hand Surgery 2000; **Med School:** India 1967; **Resid:** Orthopaedic Surgery, Maimonides Med Ctr 1970; **Fellow:** Hand Surgery, Mass Genl Hosp 1971; **Fac Appt:** Assoc Clin Prof S, SUNY Hlth Sci Ctr

Solomon, Ronald MD (HS) - **Hospital:** Long Island Coll Hosp (page 90), Brooklyn Hosp Ctr-Downtown; **Address:** 142 Joraleman St, Ste 12A, Brooklyn, NY 11201-4742; **Phone:** 718-625-4975; **Board Cert:** Surgery 1996; Hand Surgery 1994; **Med School:** Univ Rochester 1972; **Resid:** Surgery, Univ Hosp 1979; Surgery, Metropolit; **Fellow:** Hand Surgery, NY Med Col

HEMATOLOGY

Dosik, Harvey MD (Hem) - **Spec Exp:** Leukemia & Lymphoma; Anemia; Multiple Myeloma; **Hospital:** New York Methodist Hosp (page 479); **Address:** 506 6th St, Brooklyn, NY 11215-3609; **Phone:** 718-780-5240; **Board Cert:** Internal Medicine 1970; Hematology 1976; **Med School:** NYU Sch Med 1963; **Resid:** Internal Medicine, Kings County Hosp 1967; **Fellow:** Hematology, Maimonides Medical Ctr 1969; **Fac Appt:** Prof Med, Cornell Univ-Weill Med Coll

Hyde, Phyllis MD (Hem) - **Hospital:** Long Island Coll Hosp (page 90); **Address:** 46 Livingston St, Brooklyn, NY 11201; **Phone:** 718-855-1124; **Board Cert:** Internal Medicine 1983; Hematology 1986; Medical Oncology 1987; **Med School:** SUNY Downstate 1980; **Resid:** Internal Medicine, Columbia-Presby 1983; Medical Oncology, New York Univ Med Ctr 1986

Kopel, Samuel MD (Hem) - **Spec Exp:** Hematologic Malignancies; Solid Tumors; **Hospital:** Maimonides Med Ctr (page 96); **Address:** MMC Hemoto/Oncol, 6300 8th Ave, Brooklyn, NY 11220; **Phone:** 718-765-2600; **Board Cert:** Internal Medicine 1975; Hematology 1978; Medical Oncology 1979; **Med School:** Italy 1972; **Resid:** Internal Medicine, Jewish Hosp 1975; **Fellow:** Hematology & Oncology, Mt Sinai Med Ctr 1978; **Fac Appt:** Asst Prof Med, SUNY Downstate

Rieder, Ronald F MD (Hem) - **Spec Exp:** Sickle Cell Disease; Thalassemia; Anemia; **Hospital:** Kings County Hosp Ctr, SUNY Downstate Med Ctr; **Address:** SUNY Downstate Med Ctr, Hem-Onc, 450 Clarkson Ave, Box 20, Brooklyn, NY 11203-2012; **Phone:** 718-270-1520; **Board Cert:** Internal Medicine 1972; Hematology 1972; **Med School:** NYU Sch Med 1958; **Resid:** Internal Medicine, Bellevue Hosp 1960; Internal Medicine, Bellevue Hosp 1965; **Fellow:** Hematology, Johns Hopkins Hosp 1964; **Fac Appt:** Prof Med, SUNY Hlth Sci Ctr

INFECTIOUS DISEASE

Asnis, Deborah MD (Inf) - **Spec Exp:** West Nile Virus; AIDS/HIV; Meningitis; **Hospital:** Flushing Hosp Med Ctr, NY Hosp Queens; **Address:** 90 Brighton 11th St, Brooklyn, NY 11235; **Phone:** 718-332-7770; **Board Cert:** Internal Medicine 1985; Infectious Disease 1988; **Med School:** Northwestern Univ 1981; **Resid:** Ophthalmology, LI Jewish Hosp 1983; Internal Medicine, LI Jewish Hosp 1985; **Fellow:** Infectious Disease, LI Jewish Hosp 1987; **Fac Appt:** Asst Clin Prof Med, Cornell Univ-Weill Med Coll

Berkowitz, Leonard B MD (Inf) - **Spec Exp:** AIDS/HIV; **Hospital:** Brooklyn Hosp Ctr-Downtown; **Address:** 121 DeKalb Ave, Brooklyn, NY 11201-5425; **Phone:** 718-250-6922; **Board Cert:** Internal Medicine 1980; Infectious Disease 1984; **Med School:** SUNY Downstate 1977; **Resid:** Internal Medicine, Univ Hosp, Kings Co Med Ctr 1981; **Fellow:** Infectious Disease, Univ Hosp, Kings Co Med Ctr 1983; **Fac Appt:** Asst Clin Prof Med, SUNY Hlth Sci Ctr

Chapnick, Edward MD (Inf) - **Spec Exp:** AIDS/HIV; Travel Medicine; **Hospital:** Maimonides Med Ctr (page 96), Lutheran Med Ctr - Brooklyn; **Address:** Maimonides Medical Ctr, Infectious Disease, 4802 10th Ave, Brooklyn, NY 11219-2844; **Phone:** 718-283-7492; **Board Cert:** Internal Medicine 1988; Infectious Disease 2002; **Med School:** SUNY Downstate 1985; **Resid:** Internal Medicine, Maimonides Med Ctr 1989; **Fellow:** Infectious Disease, Maimonides Med Ctr 1991; **Fac Appt:** Assoc Prof Med, Mount Sinai Sch Med

Cofsky, Richard MD (Inf) - **Hospital:** Brookdale Univ Hosp Med Ctr; **Address:** Brookdale Univ Hospital, 1 Brookdale Plaza Fl 5 - rm 598, Brooklyn, NY 11212-3139; **Phone:** 718-240-5096; **Board Cert:** Internal Medicine 1981; Infectious Disease 1984; **Med School:** Univ MD Sch Med 1978; **Resid:** Internal Medicine, Maimonides Med Ctr 1981; **Fellow:** Infectious Disease, Downstate Med Ctr 1984

Cortes, Hiram MD (Inf) - **Spec Exp:** Lyme Disease; AIDS/HIV; Hepatitis C; **Hospital:** New York Methodist Hosp (page 479); **Address:** 460 13th St, Brooklyn, NY 11215-3710; **Phone:** 718-369-3555; **Board Cert:** Internal Medicine 1997; **Med School:** West Indies 1984; **Resid:** Internal Medicine, NY Methodist Hosp 1988; Infectious Disease, Cabrini Med Ctr 1990

Jonas, Murray MD (Inf) - **Hospital:** Beth Israel Med Ctr- Kings Hwy Div (page 90), New York Methodist Hosp (page 479); **Address:** 1569 E 18th St, Brooklyn, NY 11230-7201; **Phone:** 718-375-6500; **Board Cert:** Internal Medicine 1985; Infectious Disease 1996; **Med School:** SUNY Downstate 1977; **Resid:** Internal Medicine, Metropolitan Hosp Ctr 1978; Internal Medicine, Nassau County Med Ctr 1980; **Fellow:** Infectious Disease, Winthrop Univ Hosp 1983

Lutwick, Larry Irwin MD (Inf) - **Spec Exp:** Hepatitis; Infectious Mononucleosis; Epstein-Barr Virus; **Hospital:** VA Med Ctr - Bklyn, Maimonides Med Ctr (page 96); **Address:** Brooklyn VA Medical Ctr, 800 Poli Pl, rm 12-125, Brooklyn, NY 11209; **Phone:** 718-765-4979; **Board Cert:** Internal Medicine 1975; Infectious Disease 1976; **Med School:** SUNY Downstate 1972; **Resid:** Internal Medicine, Barnes Hosp-Washington Univ 1974; **Fellow:** Infectious Disease, Barnes Hosp-Washington Univ 1976; **Fac Appt:** Prof Med, SUNY Downstate

McCormack, William M MD (Inf) - **Spec Exp:** Vaginitis; Vulvar Disease; Sexually Transmitted Diseases; Urinary Tract Infections; **Hospital:** SUNY Downstate Med Ctr; **Address:** 450 Clarkson Ave, Box 56, Brooklyn, NY 11203; **Phone:** 718-270-1432; **Board Cert:** Internal Medicine 1971; Infectious Disease 1972; **Med School:** SUNY Downstate 1963; **Resid:** Internal Medicine, Columbia-Presby Hosp 1965; Internal Medicine, Mass Genl Hosp 1969; **Fellow:** Infectious Disease, Boston City Hosp 1971; **Fac Appt:** Prof Med, SUNY Downstate

Pujol-Morato, Fernando MD (Inf) - **Spec Exp:** AIDS/HIV; **Hospital:** New York Methodist Hosp (page 479); **Address:** 263 7th Ave, Ste 5A, Meth Hosp, Brooklyn, NY 11215; **Phone:** 718-246-8600; **Board Cert:** Internal Medicine 1986; Infectious Disease 1988; **Med School:** Dominican Republic 1979; **Resid:** Internal Medicine, LI College Hosp 1985; **Fellow:** Infectious Disease, LI College Hosp 1987; **Fac Appt:** Asst Prof Med, Cornell Univ-Weill Med Coll

Sepkowitz, Douglas MD (Inf) - **Spec Exp:** AIDS/HIV; Tuberculosis; **Hospital:** Long Island Coll Hosp (page 90); **Address:** 349 Henry St, Brooklyn, NY 11201; **Phone:** 718-797-4684; **Board Cert:** Internal Medicine 1982; Infectious Disease 1986; **Med School:** Univ Okla Coll Med 1979; **Resid:** Internal Medicine, Maimonides Medical Ctr 1982; **Fellow:** Infectious Disease, Long Island Coll Hosp 1986

Stein, Alan J MD (Inf) - **Spec Exp:** AIDS/HIV; Travel Medicine; **Hospital:** New York Methodist Hosp (page 479), Brooklyn Hosp Ctr-Downtown; **Address:** 348 13th St, Ste 101, Brooklyn, NY 11215; **Phone:** 718-369-4850; **Board Cert:** Internal Medicine 1976; Infectious Disease 1978; **Med School:** NY Med Coll 1972; **Resid:** Internal Medicine, Lenox Hill Hosp 1974; Internal Medicine, Metro Hosp Ctr 1976; **Fellow:** Infectious Disease, NYU Med Ctr 1978; **Fac Appt:** Assoc Clin Prof Med, NYU Sch Med

INTERNAL MEDICINE

Behm, Dutsi MD (IM) PCP - **Spec Exp:** Geriatric Rehabilitation; **Hospital:** New York Methodist Hosp (page 479), Maimonides Med Ctr (page 96); **Address:** 421 Ocean Pkwy, Brooklyn, NY 11218-2408; **Phone:** 718-438-8585; **Med School:** Ukraine 1973; **Resid:** Internal Medicine, NY Methodist Hosp 1983

Berman, Sandra MD (IM) PCP - **Hospital:** Long Island Coll Hosp (page 90); **Address:** 96 Joralemon St, Brooklyn, NY 11201-4032; **Phone:** 718-797-5339; **Board Cert:** Internal Medicine 1996; **Med School:** Mexico 1979; **Resid:** Internal Medicine, LI Jewish Med Ctr

Bharathan, Thayyullathil MD (IM) PCP - **Spec Exp:** Geriatric Medicine; Palliative Care; Alzheimer's Disease; **Hospital:** New York Methodist Hosp (page 479); **Address:** 263 7th Ave, Ste 5A, Brooklyn, NY 11215-3691; **Phone:** 718-246-8600; **Board Cert:** Internal Medicine 1976; Geriatric Medicine 1998; **Med School:** India 1962; **Resid:** Internal Medicine, New York Methodist Hosp 1972; **Fac Appt:** Asst Clin Prof Med, Cornell Univ-Weill Med Coll

Brown, Lawrence S MD (IM) PCP - **Spec Exp:** Addiction Medicine; AIDS/HIV; **Hospital:** NY-Presby Hosp (page 100), Rockefeller Univ; **Address:** 22 Chapel St, Brooklyn, NY 11201; **Phone:** 718-260-2917; **Med School:** NYU Sch Med 1979; **Resid:** Internal Medicine, Harlem Hosp 1982; **Fellow:** Endocrinology, Columbia-Presby Med Ctr 1986; **Fac Appt:** Assoc Clin Prof Public Hlth, Columbia P&S

Butt, Ahmar A MD (IM) PCP - **Spec Exp:** Stroke; Hypertension; Congestive Heart Failure; **Hospital:** Brooklyn Hosp Ctr-Downtown; **Address:** 240 Willoughby St Fl 10 - Ste F, Brooklyn, NY 11201-5465; **Phone:** 718-250-6120; **Board Cert:** Internal Medicine 1995; **Med School:** Pakistan 1983; **Resid:** Internal Medicine, Brooklyn Hospital 1994; **Fac Appt:** Asst Clin Prof Med, Cornell Univ-Weill Med Coll

Cohen, Barry A MD (IM) PCP - **Hospital:** New York Comm Hosp, New York Methodist Hosp (page 479); **Address:** 151A West End Ave, Brooklyn, NY 11235-4808; **Phone:** 718-934-1222; **Board Cert:** Internal Medicine 1986; **Med School:** Dominican Republic 1982; **Resid:** Internal Medicine, City Hosp Ctr/Mt Sinai 1986

Cohn, Steven MD (IM) PCP - **Spec Exp:** Hypertension; Erectile Dysfunction; Perioperative Medical Care; **Hospital:** SUNY Downstate Med Ctr, New York Methodist Hosp (page 479); **Address:** 470 Clarkson Ave, Ste A, Box 68, Brooklyn, NY 11203-2012; **Phone:** 718-270-1531; **Board Cert:** Internal Medicine 1983; **Med School:** Mexico 1978; **Resid:** Internal Medicine, SUNY Downstate-Kings Co Hosp 1982; **Fac Appt:** Clin Prof Med, SUNY Downstate

Ditchek, Alan MD (IM) PCP - **Spec Exp:** Chronic Fatigue Syndrome; Diabetes; Hypertension; **Hospital:** Beth Israel Med Ctr- Kings Hwy Div (page 90), Lutheran Med Ctr - Brooklyn; **Address:** 2516 Ocean Ave, Brooklyn, NY 11229-3916; **Phone:** 718-769-0444; **Board Cert:** Internal Medicine 1986; Infectious Disease 1995; **Med School:** Mexico 1981; **Resid:** Internal Medicine, Luthern Med Ctr 1985; **Fellow:** Infectious Disease, Nassau County Med Ctr 1986; Infectious Disease, SUNY Downstate 1994; **Fac Appt:** Asst Clin Prof Med, SUNY Hlth Sci Ctr

Ellis, Earl A MD (IM) PCP - **Spec Exp:** Geriatric Rehabilitation; **Hospital:** Brooklyn Hosp Ctr-Downtown, SUNY Downstate Med Ctr; **Address:** 66 Rutland Rd, Brooklyn, NY 11225-5313; **Phone:** 718-282-4412; **Board Cert:** Internal Medicine 1984; Geriatric Medicine 2000; **Med School:** Howard Univ 1980; **Resid:** Internal Medicine, Elmhurst Hosp 1983

Grunzweig, Milton MD (IM) `PCP` - **Hospital:** Brookdale Univ Hosp Med Ctr, Beth Israel Med Ctr - Petrie Division (page 90); **Address:** 2560 Ocean Ave, Brooklyn, NY 11229; **Phone:** 718-769-7900; **Board Cert:** Internal Medicine 1989; **Med School:** SUNY Hlth Sci Ctr 1986; **Resid:** Internal Medicine, Brookdale Hosp 1989

Gupta, Jagdish MD (IM) - **Spec Exp:** Colon Cancer; Hepatitis; Peptic Ulcer Disease; **Hospital:** Long Island Coll Hosp (page 90); **Address:** 28 8th Ave, Brooklyn, NY 11217; **Phone:** 718-638-3150; **Board Cert:** Internal Medicine 1975; Gastroenterology 1977; **Med School:** India 1970; **Resid:** Internal Medicine, LI Coll Hosp 1977; **Fellow:** Gastroenterology, LI Coll Hosp 1975; **Fac Appt:** Asst Clin Prof Med, SUNY Downstate

Hsuih, Terence CH MD (IM) - **Hospital:** Lutheran Med Ctr - Brooklyn; **Address:** 775 57th St, Brooklyn, NY 11220; **Phone:** 718-439-6163; **Board Cert:** Internal Medicine 1998; **Med School:** Mount Sinai Sch Med 1995; **Resid:** Internal Medicine, New York Hosp 1998

Jones, Vann MD (IM) `PCP` - **Hospital:** Brooklyn Hosp Ctr-Downtown; **Address:** 121 DeKalb Ave, Maynard 7F, Brooklyn, NY 11201-5425; **Phone:** 718-250-6100; **Board Cert:** Internal Medicine 1972; **Med School:** Howard Univ 1966; **Resid:** Internal Medicine, Kings County 1968; Internal Medicine, Montefiore Hosp Med Ctr 1970

Kaiser, Stephen MD (IM) `PCP` - **Spec Exp:** Diabetes; Hypertension; **Hospital:** Maimonides Med Ctr (page 96); **Address:** 465 Ocean Pkwy, Brooklyn, NY 11218-5152; **Phone:** 718-941-5600; **Board Cert:** Internal Medicine 1972; **Med School:** SUNY Buffalo 1964; **Resid:** Internal Medicine, Kings County Hosp 1967; **Fellow:** Hematology, Maimonides Med Ctr 1969

Katzenelenbogen, Moshe MD (IM) `PCP` - **Spec Exp:** Geriatric Medicine; **Hospital:** Beth Israel Med Ctr-Kings Hwy Div (page 90); **Address:** 3901 Nostrand Ave, Brooklyn, NY 11235; **Phone:** 718-646-1422; **Board Cert:** Internal Medicine 1984; Geriatric Medicine 1992; **Med School:** Romania 1980; **Resid:** Internal Medicine, Coney Island Hosp 1984

Kazdin, Hal MD (IM) `PCP` - **Spec Exp:** Osteoarthritis; Rheumatoid Arthritis; Pain Management; **Hospital:** New York Comm Hosp, Beth Israel Med Ctr- Kings Hwy Div (page 90); **Address:** 90 Brighton 11th St, Brooklyn, NY 11235-5304; **Phone:** 718-332-7770; **Board Cert:** Internal Medicine 1982; **Med School:** Philippines 1977; **Resid:** Internal Medicine, Elmhurst Hosp 1979; Internal Medicine, Elmhurst HHosp 1981; **Fellow:** Rheumatology, Long Island Jewish 1983

Konka, Sudarsanam MD (IM) - **Hospital:** Long Island Coll Hosp (page 90), Long Island Jewish Med Ctr; **Address:** 100 Clinton St, Brooklyn, NY 11201; **Phone:** 718-935-9837; **Board Cert:** Internal Medicine 1974; Cardiovascular Disease 1977; **Med School:** India 1970; **Resid:** Internal Medicine, Long Island Coll Hosp 1974; **Fellow:** Cardiovascular Disease, Nassau County Med Ctr 1975; Cardiovascular Disease, Long Island Coll Hosp 1976

Kurz, Larry MD (IM) `PCP` - **Hospital:** New York Methodist Hosp (page 479); **Address:** 10 Plaza St, Brooklyn, NY 11238; **Phone:** 718-638-2551; **Board Cert:** Internal Medicine 1977; **Med School:** Washington Univ, St Louis 1970; **Resid:** Internal Medicine, Downstate Med Ctr 1977

Kings (Brooklyn)

Levey, Robert MD (IM) `PCP` - **Spec Exp:** Chronic Obstructive Lung Disease (COPD); Alzheimer's Disease; **Hospital:** Long Island Coll Hosp (page 90); **Address:** 8672 Bay Pkwy, Brooklyn, NY 11214-4102; **Phone:** 718-372-2234; **Board Cert:** Internal Medicine 1977; **Med School:** Univ Mich Med Sch 1970; **Resid:** Internal Medicine, Long Island Hosp 1977

Levin, Nathan MD/PhD (IM) `PCP` - **Spec Exp:** Obesity; Osteoarthritis; Diabetes; **Hospital:** New York Methodist Hosp (page 479), New York Comm Hosp; **Address:** 500 Brightwater Ct, Brooklyn, NY 11235-7154; **Phone:** 718-743-7700; **Board Cert:** Internal Medicine 1993; **Med School:** Ukraine 1960; **Resid:** Internal Medicine, St Vincent's Hosp & Med Ctr 1990

Lifshitz, Benjamin MD (IM) `PCP` - **Hospital:** Maimonides Med Ctr (page 96); **Address:** 3043 Ocean Ave, Brooklyn, NY 11235; **Phone:** 718-856-8600; **Board Cert:** Internal Medicine 1988; **Med School:** Cornell Univ-Weill Med Coll 1985; **Resid:** Internal Medicine, Maimonides Med Ctr 1988

Lu, Bing MD (IM) `PCP` - **Spec Exp:** Chinese Community Health; **Hospital:** Maimonides Med Ctr (page 96); **Address:** Maimonides Primary Health Services, 4711 8th Ave, Brooklyn, NY 11220; **Phone:** 718-633-0300; **Board Cert:** Internal Medicine 1997; **Med School:** China 1982; **Resid:** Internal Medicine, Miriam Hosp 1997; **Fac Appt:** Asst Prof Med, SUNY Hlth Sci Ctr

Malik, Asim MD (IM) `PCP` - **Spec Exp:** Peptic Ulcer Disease; **Hospital:** New York Methodist Hosp (page 479), Kingsbrook Jewish Med Ctr; **Address:** 1224 8th Ave, Brooklyn, NY 11215; **Phone:** 718-788-5588; **Board Cert:** Internal Medicine 1994; Gastroenterology 1997; **Med School:** Pakistan 1976; **Resid:** Surgery, New York Methodist Hosp 1978; Internal Medicine, New York Methodist Hosp 1981; **Fellow:** Gastroenterology, Wayne Cnty Genl Hosp 1983

Marush, Arthur MD (IM) `PCP` - **Spec Exp:** Cardiology; **Hospital:** Brookdale Univ Hosp Med Ctr; **Address:** 2270 Kimball St, Ste 101, Brooklyn, NY 11234-5139; **Phone:** 718-692-2700; **Board Cert:** Internal Medicine 1981; **Med School:** Albert Einstein Coll Med 1978; **Resid:** Internal Medicine, Brookdale

Massad, Susan MD (IM) `PCP` - **Spec Exp:** Chronic Illness; **Hospital:** Long Island Coll Hosp (page 90); **Address:** 175 Rensen St, Ste 525, Brooklyn, NY 11201; **Phone:** 718-222-2600; **Board Cert:** Internal Medicine 1973; **Med School:** UCSF 1962; **Resid:** Internal Medicine, Bellevue Hosp 1964; Internal Medicine, VA Med Ctr 1968; **Fellow:** UCSF Med Ctr 1970

Prabhu, H. Sudhakar MD (IM) - **Hospital:** Victory Memorial Hosp - Bklyn, Long Island Coll Hosp (page 90); **Address:** 9920 4th Ave, Ste 315, Brooklyn, NY 11209; **Phone:** 718-833-2620; **Board Cert:** Internal Medicine 1978; Cardiovascular Disease 1981; **Med School:** India 1971; **Resid:** Internal Medicine, LI Coll Hosp 1976; **Fellow:** Cardiovascular Disease, LI Coll Hosp 1978

Romanelli, John MD (IM) `PCP` - **Spec Exp:** Hypertension; Heart Disease; Diabetes; **Hospital:** Long Island Coll Hosp (page 90); **Address:** 554 Henry St, Brooklyn, NY 11231-2705; **Phone:** 718-625-5453; **Board Cert:** Internal Medicine 1995; **Med School:** Italy 1981; **Resid:** Internal Medicine, LI Coll Hosp 1984

Sherman, Frederic MD (IM) `PCP` - **Spec Exp:** Cardiovascular Disease; Alzheimer's Disease; **Hospital:** Long Island Coll Hosp (page 90), Victory Memorial Hosp - Bklyn; **Address:** 8672 Bay Pkwy, Brooklyn, NY 11214-4102; **Phone:** 718-372-2234; **Board Cert:** Internal Medicine 1976; Geriatric Medicine 1988; **Med School:** NY Med Coll 1972; **Resid:** Internal Medicine, Mount SinaiLong Island Coll Hosp 1976; **Fellow:** Cardiovascular Disease, Long Island Coll Hosp 1977

Tal, Avraham MD (IM) `PCP` - **Spec Exp:** Hypertension; Cholesterol/Lipid Disorders; Diabetes; **Hospital:** Coney Island Hosp; **Address:** 2601 Ocean Pkwy, Ste 4N38, Brooklyn, NY 11235-7745; **Phone:** 718-616-3783; **Board Cert:** Internal Medicine 1983; **Med School:** Italy 1975; **Resid:** Internal Medicine, Kingsbrook Jewish Med Ctr 1979

Vieira, Jeffery MD (IM) `PCP` - **Spec Exp:** Infectious Disease; AIDS/HIV; Chronic Fatigue Syndrome; **Hospital:** Long Island Coll Hosp (page 90), New York Methodist Hosp (page 479); **Address:** One Prospect Park W, Brooklyn, NY 11215; **Phone:** 718-857-3237; **Board Cert:** Internal Medicine 1980; **Med School:** NY Med Coll 1977; **Resid:** Internal Medicine, St Elizabeth's Med Ctr 1980; **Fellow:** Infectious Disease, Univ Hosp 1982; **Fac Appt:** Assoc Prof Med, SUNY Downstate

Ziemba, David MD (IM) `PCP` - **Hospital:** Long Island Coll Hosp (page 90); **Address:** 1458 47th St, Brooklyn, NY 11219-2634; **Phone:** 718-438-0600; **Board Cert:** Internal Medicine 1983; **Med School:** SUNY Downstate 1979; **Resid:** Internal Medicine, Coney Island Hosp 1983

INTERVENTIONAL CARDIOLOGY

Shani, Jacob MD (IC) - **Spec Exp:** Cardiac Catheterization; Angioplasty & Stent Placement; Percutaneous Valvuloplasty; **Hospital:** Maimonides Med Ctr (page 96); **Address:** Maimonides Med Ctr, Cardiac Cath Lab, 4802 10th Ave, Brooklyn, NY 11219-2844; **Phone:** 718-283-7480; **Board Cert:** Internal Medicine 1981; Cardiovascular Disease 1983; Interventional Cardiology 1999; **Med School:** Israel 1977; **Resid:** Internal Medicine, Maimonides Med Ctr 1981; **Fellow:** Cardiovascular Disease, Beth Israel Hosp-Harvard 1983; **Fac Appt:** Prof Med, Mount Sinai Sch Med

MATERNAL & FETAL MEDICINE

Bush, Jacqueline MD (MF) - **Spec Exp:** Pregnancy-High Risk; Diabetes in Pregnancy; **Hospital:** New York Methodist Hosp (page 479); **Address:** 263 7th Ave, Ste 3A, Brooklyn, NY 11215; **Phone:** 718-246-8500; **Board Cert:** Obstetrics & Gynecology 1998; **Med School:** SUNY Stony Brook 1989; **Resid:** Obstetrics & Gynecology, Univ Hosp-SUNY Hlth Scis Ctr; Obstetrics & Gynecology, Kings Co Hosp Ctr

Cabbad, Michael MD (MF) - **Spec Exp:** Pregnancy-High Risk; **Hospital:** Brooklyn Hosp Ctr-Downtown, Lutheran Med Ctr - Brooklyn; **Address:** Dept Ob/Gyn, 240 Willoughby St, Fl 3 - Ste E, Brooklyn, NY 11201; **Phone:** 718-250-8322; **Board Cert:** Obstetrics & Gynecology 1998; Maternal & Fetal Medicine 1998; **Med School:** Mexico 1979; **Resid:** Obstetrics & Gynecology, Brookyn Hospital Center 1984; **Fellow:** Maternal & Fetal Medicine, Univ Hosp 1986; **Fac Appt:** Assoc Clin Prof ObG, Cornell Univ-Weill Med Coll

Kofinas, Alexander MD (MF) - **Spec Exp:** Pregnancy-High Risk; Ultrasound; Pregnancy Loss; **Hospital:** New York Methodist Hosp (page 479), N Shore Univ Hosp at Manhasset; **Address:** Kofinas Perinatal, 506 6th St Bldg KP Fl 4, Brooklyn, NY 11215; **Phone:** 718-780-5610; **Board Cert:** Obstetrics & Gynecology 2006; Maternal & Fetal Medicine 2006; **Med School:** Greece 1976; **Resid:** Obstetrics & Gynecology, Brooklyn Hosp Ctr 1985; **Fellow:** Maternal & Fetal Medicine, Wake Forest Univ 1987; **Fac Appt:** Assoc Clin Prof ObG, Cornell Univ-Weill Med Coll

Shiffman, Rebecca L MD (MF) - **Spec Exp:** Miscarriage-Recurrent; Cervical Incompetence; Lupus/SLE in Pregnancy; Diabetes in Pregnancy; **Hospital:** New York Methodist Hosp (page 479); **Address:** 506 6th St, Brooklyn, NY 11215; **Phone:** 718-780-3272; **Board Cert:** Obstetrics & Gynecology 1995; Maternal & Fetal Medicine 1995; **Med School:** Belgium 1980; **Resid:** Obstetrics & Gynecology, Jewish Hosp 1984; **Fellow:** Maternal & Fetal Medicine, Nassau County Med Ctr 1986; **Fac Appt:** Assoc Clin Prof ObG, Cornell Univ-Weill Med Coll

MEDICAL ONCOLOGY

Ahmed, Fakhiuddin MD (Onc) - **Spec Exp:** Breast Cancer; Lung Cancer; Colon Cancer; **Hospital:** Brookdale Univ Hosp Med Ctr, New York Methodist Hosp (page 479); **Address:** 2558 E 18th St, Brooklyn, NY 11235; **Phone:** 718-616-0801; **Board Cert:** Internal Medicine 1972; Hematology 1974; Medical Oncology 1975; **Med School:** India 1966; **Resid:** Internal Medicine, Brookdale Hosp 1970; **Fellow:** Hematology & Oncology, Brookdale Hosp 1973; **Fac Appt:** Assoc Prof Med, SUNY Hlth Sci Ctr

Astrow, Alan MD (Onc) - **Spec Exp:** Ovarian Cancer; Breast Cancer; Lymphoma; **Hospital:** Maimonides Med Ctr (page 96), St Vincent Cath Med Ctrs - Manhattan (page 375); **Address:** MMC Hematology/Oncology, 6300 8th Ave, Brooklyn, NY 11220; **Phone:** 718-765-2653; **Board Cert:** Internal Medicine 1983; Hematology 1986; Medical Oncology 1987; **Med School:** Yale Univ 1980; **Resid:** Internal Medicine, Boston City Hosp 1983; **Fellow:** Hematology & Oncology, NYU Med Ctr 1986; **Fac Appt:** Assoc Clin Prof Med, NY Med Coll

Bashevkin, Michael MD (Onc) - **Spec Exp:** Solid Tumors; Bleeding/Coagulation Disorders; Hematologic Malignancies; **Hospital:** Maimonides Med Ctr (page 96); **Address:** 1660 E 14st St, Ste 501, Brooklyn, NY 11229; **Phone:** 718-382-8500 x501; **Board Cert:** Internal Medicine 1976; Hematology 1978; Medical Oncology 1979; **Med School:** SUNY Downstate 1973; **Resid:** Internal Medicine, VA Med Ctr 1976; Hematology & Oncology, Maimonides Med Ctr 1979

Bruckner, Howard W MD (Onc) - **Spec Exp:** Pancreatic Cancer; **Hospital:** Lutheran Med Ctr - Brooklyn; **Address:** Lutheran Med Ctr, 150 55th St, rm 5111, Brooklyn, NY 11220; **Phone:** 718-630-6580; **Board Cert:** Internal Medicine 1972; Medical Oncology 1973; **Med School:** Albert Einstein Coll Med 1966; **Resid:** Internal Medicine, Montefiore/Weiler-Einstein Div 1970; **Fellow:** Medical Oncology, Yale-New Haven Hosp 1971

Chandra, Pradeep MD (Onc) - **Spec Exp:** Gastrointestinal Cancer; Colon Cancer; Breast Cancer; **Hospital:** Wyckoff Heights Med Ctr; **Address:** Wycoff Heights Medical Ctr, Dept Medicine, 374 Stockholm St, Brooklyn, NY 11237-4006; **Phone:** 718-963-7585; **Board Cert:** Internal Medicine 1980; Hematology 1974; Medical Oncology 1983; **Med School:** India 1966; **Resid:** Internal Medicine, Wyckoff Heights Hosp 1969; Internal Medicine, Bronx Lebanon Hosp 1971; **Fellow:** Hematology, Long Jewish Med Ctr 1973; **Fac Appt:** Clin Prof Med, Cornell Univ-Weill Med Coll

Colella, Frank MD (Onc) - **Spec Exp:** Hematologic Disorders; **Hospital:** New York Methodist Hosp (page 479); **Address:** 9920 Fourth Ave, Ste 311, Brooklyn, NY 11209; **Phone:** 718-921-1672; **Board Cert:** Internal Medicine 1985; Hematology 1992; Medical Oncology 1989; **Med School:** Italy 1978; **Resid:** Internal Medicine, NY Methodist Hosp 1981; **Fellow:** Hematology & Oncology, Hahnemann Hosp 1984

Daya, Rami MD (Onc) - **Spec Exp:** Breast Cancer; Ovarian Cancer; **Hospital:** New York Methodist Hosp (page 479), Lutheran Med Ctr - Brooklyn; **Address:** 9920 4th Ave, Ste 311, Brooklyn, NY 11209-8332; **Phone:** 718-921-1672; **Board Cert:** Internal Medicine 1987; Medical Oncology 1991; Hematology 1997; **Med School:** Syria 1981; **Resid:** Internal Medicine, NY Methodist Hosp 1986; **Fellow:** Hematology & Oncology, UMDNJ Med Ctr 1989; **Fac Appt:** Assoc Clin Prof Med, UMDNJ-NJ Med Sch, Newark

Dosik, David MD (Onc) - **Spec Exp:** Breast Cancer; Lung Cancer; Colon Cancer; **Hospital:** New York Methodist Hosp (page 479), N Central Bronx Hosp; **Address:** NY Methodist Hosp - Dept Medicine, 506 Sixth St, Brooklyn, NY 11215; **Phone:** 718-780-5240; **Board Cert:** Internal Medicine 1993; Hematology 1996; Medical Oncology 1997; **Med School:** SUNY Downstate 1990; **Resid:** Internal Medicine, Staten Island Univ Hosp 1993; **Fellow:** Hematology & Oncology, NYU Med Ctr 1996

Geraghty, Michael MD (Onc) - **Hospital:** Long Island Coll Hosp (page 90); **Address:** 9920 4th Ave, Brooklyn, NY 11209-8333; **Phone:** 718-833-0215; **Board Cert:** Internal Medicine 1972; Hematology 1974; Medical Oncology 1999; **Med School:** Georgetown Univ 1966; **Resid:** Internal Medicine, Bellevue Hosp 1971; **Fellow:** Hematology, Bellevue Hosp 1973; **Fac Appt:** Asst Clin Prof Med, SUNY Hlth Sci Ctr

Lebowicz, Joseph MD (Onc) - **Spec Exp:** Lung Cancer; Breast Cancer; Gastrointestinal Cancer; **Hospital:** Maimonides Med Ctr (page 96); **Address:** 1660 E 14th St, Ste 501, Brooklyn, NY 11229; **Phone:** 718-382-8500; **Board Cert:** Internal Medicine 1978; Hematology 1980; Medical Oncology 1981; **Med School:** Albert Einstein Coll Med 1975; **Resid:** Internal Medicine, Maimonides Med Ctr 1978; **Fellow:** Hematology & Oncology, Maimonides Med Ctr 1981

Lichter, Stephen M MD (Onc) - **Spec Exp:** Breast Cancer; Lung Cancer; Gastrointestinal Cancer; **Hospital:** Beth Israel Med Ctr- Kings Hwy Div (page 90), Brookdale Univ Hosp Med Ctr; **Address:** 2558 E 18th St, Brooklyn, NY 11235; **Phone:** 718-616-0801; **Board Cert:** Internal Medicine 1978; Medical Oncology 1981; **Med School:** Univ Hlth Sci/Chicago Med Sch 1975; **Resid:** Internal Medicine, Brookdale Hosp 1978; **Fellow:** Medical Oncology, Brookdale Hosp 1980; **Fac Appt:** Asst Clin Prof Med, SUNY Hlth Sci Ctr

Nayak, Asha D MD (Onc) - **Hospital:** Brooklyn Hosp Ctr-Downtown, New York Methodist Hosp (page 479); **Address:** 263 7th Ave, Ste 5F, Brooklyn, NY 11215-3690; **Phone:** 718-246-8600; **Board Cert:** Medical Oncology 1981; Hematology 1978; Internal Medicine 1977; **Med School:** India 1970; **Resid:** Internal Medicine, Booth Memorial Med Ctr 1976; Hematology, Coney Island Hosps 1978; **Fellow:** Medical Oncology, Brooklyn/Caledonian Hosps 1979; **Fac Appt:** Asst Clin Prof Med, Cornell Univ-Weill Med Coll

Solomon, William MD (Onc) - **Spec Exp:** Breast Cancer; Prostate Cancer; **Hospital:** SUNY Downstate Med Ctr; **Address:** SUNY Downstate Med Ctr, 450 Clarkson Ave, Box 20, Brooklyn, NY 11203-2012; **Phone:** 718-270-2785; **Board Cert:** Internal Medicine 1978; Hematology 1982; Medical Oncology 1985; **Med School:** Columbia P&S 1975; **Resid:** Internal Medicine, Montefiore Hosp Med Ctr 1978; **Fellow:** Hematology, Beth Israel Hosp 1981; **Fac Appt:** Assoc Prof Med, SUNY Downstate

NEONATAL-PERINATAL MEDICINE

Grieg, Adolfo DO (NP) - **Spec Exp:** Neonatal Neurology; **Hospital:** Wyckoff Heights Med Ctr; **Address:** Chldns Medical Group, 365 Stockholm St Fl 1, Brooklyn, NY 11237; **Phone:** 718-366-4460; **Board Cert:** Pediatrics 1999; Neonatal-Perinatal Medicine 2003; **Med School:** NY Coll Osteo Med 1987; **Resid:** Pediatrics, Brookdale 1991; **Fellow:** Neonatal-Perinatal Medicine, Montefiore Hosp Med Ctr 1994; **Fac Appt:** Asst Clin Prof Ped, Cornell Univ-Weill Med Coll

Gudavalli, Madhu R MD (NP) - **Spec Exp:** Prematurity/Low Birth Weight Infants; **Hospital:** New York Methodist Hosp (page 479); **Address:** New York Methodist Hosp, Dept Pediatrics, 506 6th St, Brooklyn, NY 11215; **Phone:** 718-780-3727; **Board Cert:** Pediatrics 1980; Neonatal-Perinatal Medicine 1983; **Med School:** India 1972; **Resid:** Pediatrics, New York Infirmary 1976; Pediatrics, Booth Meml Hosp 1977; **Fellow:** Neonatal-Perinatal Medicine, Bellevue Hosp 1979

Koenig, Eli MD (NP) - **Hospital:** Long Island Coll Hosp (page 90); **Address:** 339 Hicks St, Brooklyn, NY 11201-5509; **Phone:** 718-780-1025; **Board Cert:** Pediatrics 1986; Neonatal-Perinatal Medicine 1999; **Med School:** Italy 1979; **Resid:** Pediatrics, Bronx Lebanon Hosp 1980; Pediatrics, Beth Israel 1982; **Fellow:** Neonatal-Perinatal Medicine, Babies Hosp 1984; **Fac Appt:** Asst Prof Ped, SUNY Downstate

Parekh, Aruna MD (NP) - **Hospital:** Long Island Coll Hosp (page 90); **Address:** 97 Amity St, Brooklyn, NY 11201-5514; **Phone:** 718-780-1025; **Board Cert:** Pediatrics 1976; Neonatal-Perinatal Medicine ; **Med School:** India 1970; **Resid:** Pediatrics, LI Coll Ho 1974; **Fellow:** Neonatal-Perinatal Medicine, N Shore Univ Hosp 1977

Sokal, Myron MD (NP) - **Spec Exp:** Neonatal Care; **Hospital:** Brookdale Univ Hosp Med Ctr; **Address:** 1 Brookdale Plaza, Brooklyn, NY 11212; **Phone:** 718-240-5629; **Board Cert:** Pediatrics 1972; Neonatal-Perinatal Medicine 1975; **Med School:** Albert Einstein Coll Med 1967; **Resid:** Pediatrics, Yale-New Haven Hosp 1969; **Fellow:** Neonatal-Perinatal Medicine, Columbia-Presby 1971; **Fac Appt:** Prof Ped, SUNY Hlth Sci Ctr

NEPHROLOGY

Chou, Shyan-yih MD (Nep) - **Spec Exp:** Kidney Disease; Hypertension; Dialysis Care; **Hospital:** Brookdale Univ Hosp Med Ctr; **Address:** 1 Brookdale Plaza Ste 169CHC Bldg, Brooklyn, NY 11212-3139; **Phone:** 718-240-5615; **Board Cert:** Internal Medicine 1972; Nephrology 1974; **Med School:** Taiwan 1966; **Resid:** Internal Medicine, Brookdale Hosp Med Ctr 1969; Internal Medicine, Brookdale Hosp Med Ctr 1970; **Fellow:** Nephrology, Brookdale Hosp Med Ctr 1973; **Fac Appt:** Prof Med, SUNY Downstate

Del Monte, Mary MD (Nep) - **Spec Exp:** Kidney Disease; Hypertension; **Hospital:** Brooklyn Hosp Ctr-Downtown; **Address:** 121 Dekalb Ave, Brooklyn, NY 11201; **Phone:** 718-250-8160; **Board Cert:** Internal Medicine 1980; Nephrology 1972; **Med School:** Boston Univ 1967; **Resid:** Internal Medicine, St Elizabeths Hosp 1971; **Fellow:** Nephrology, St Vincents Hosp 1971; Nephrology, SUNY Hlth Sci Ctr 1973

Delano, Barbara MD (Nep) - **Spec Exp:** Dialysis Care; Kidney Failure-Chronic; **Hospital:** SUNY Downstate Med Ctr, Kings County Hosp Ctr; **Address:** 450 Clarkson Ave, Box 52, Brooklyn, NY 11203-2056; **Phone:** 718-270-1584; **Board Cert:** Internal Medicine 2000; **Med School:** SUNY Hlth Sci Ctr 1965; **Resid:** Internal Medicine, SUNY Downstate Med Ctr 1967; **Fellow:** Nephrology, SUNY Downstate Med Ctr 1969; **Fac Appt:** Prof Med, SUNY Downstate

Friedman, Eli A MD (Nep) - **Spec Exp:** Diabetic Kidney Disease; Transplant Medicine-Kidney; Kidney Disease-Chronic; **Hospital:** SUNY Downstate Med Ctr, Kings County Hosp Ctr; **Address:** SUNY Downstate Med Ctr, 450 Clarkson Ave, Box 52, Brooklyn, NY 11203; **Phone:** 718-270-1584; **Board Cert:** Internal Medicine 1967; Nephrology 1974; **Med School:** SUNY Downstate 1957; **Resid:** Internal Medicine, Peter Bent Brigham Hosp 1960; **Fellow:** Nephrology, Peter Bent Brigham Hosp 1961; **Fac Appt:** Prof Med, SUNY Downstate

Lipner, Henry I MD (Nep) - **Spec Exp:** Kidney Disease; Hypertension; Dialysis Care; **Hospital:** Maimonides Med Ctr (page 96); **Address:** 1435 86th St, Brooklyn, NY 11218; **Phone:** 718-648-0101; **Board Cert:** Internal Medicine 1974; Nephrology 1976; **Med School:** NYU Sch Med 1968; **Resid:** Internal Medicine, Jewish Hosp 1971; **Fellow:** Nephrology, Montefiore Hosp Med Ctr 1972

Louis, Bertin M MD (Nep) - **Spec Exp:** Kidney Disease; Hypertension; Dialysis Care; **Hospital:** Maimonides Med Ctr (page 96); **Address:** Maimonides Med Ctr, Div Nephrology, 4802 10th Ave, Brooklyn, NY 11219; **Phone:** 718-283-7907; **Board Cert:** Internal Medicine 1975; Nephrology 1982; **Med School:** Haiti 1964; **Resid:** Internal Medicine, VA Med Ctr 1970; **Fellow:** Nephrology, Maimonides Med Ctr 1972

Markell, Mariana Sari MD (Nep) - **Spec Exp:** Transplant Medicine-Kidney; **Hospital:** SUNY Downstate Med Ctr; **Address:** 450 Clarkson Ave, Box 52, Brooklyn, NY 11203; **Phone:** 718-270-1584; **Board Cert:** Internal Medicine 1984; Nephrology 1986; **Med School:** NY Med Coll 1981; **Resid:** Internal Medicine, Columbia-Presby 1984; **Fellow:** Nephrology, Columbia-Presby 1985UCLA Med Ctr 1986; **Fac Appt:** Assoc Prof Med, SUNY Hlth Sci Ctr

Mittman, Neal MD (Nep) - **Spec Exp:** Lupus Nephritis; Dialysis Care; Hypertension; **Hospital:** Long Island Coll Hosp (page 90); **Address:** 115 Remsen St, Brooklyn, NY 11201-4212; **Phone:** 718-852-4949; **Board Cert:** Internal Medicine 1980; Nephrology 1982; **Med School:** NY Med Coll 1977; **Resid:** Internal Medicine, Metropolitan Hosp Ctr 1980; **Fellow:** Nephrology, Albert Einstein Coll Med 1982; **Fac Appt:** Assoc Prof Med, SUNY Hlth Sci Ctr

Neelakantappa, Kotresha MD (Nep) - **Spec Exp:** Kidney Disease; Hypertension; **Hospital:** New York Methodist Hosp (page 479); **Address:** 9920 4th Ave, Ste 309, Brooklyn, NY 11209; **Phone:** 718-745-3079; **Board Cert:** Nephrology 1978; Internal Medicine 1977; **Med School:** India 1969; **Resid:** Internal Medicine, NY Methodist Hosp 1974; **Fellow:** Nephrology, NYU Med Ctr 1976; **Fac Appt:** Asst Prof Med, NYU Sch Med

Pannone, John MD (Nep) - **Spec Exp:** Dialysis Care; Hypertension; Dialysis Care; **Hospital:** Lutheran Med Ctr - Brooklyn, Victory Memorial Hosp - Bklyn; **Address:** 61 Oliver St, Ste PR-1, Brooklyn, NY 11209; **Phone:** 718-238-4980; **Board Cert:** Internal Medicine 1978; Nephrology 1980; **Med School:** Italy 1974; **Resid:** Internal Medicine, Lutheran Med Ctr 1977; **Fellow:** Nephrology, Brookdale Hosp Med Ctr 1979; Nephrology, New York Hosp-Cornell Med Ctr 1980

Parnes, Eliezer MD (Nep) - **Spec Exp:** Hypertension; Dialysis Care; Diabetic Kidney Disease; **Hospital:** Beth Israel Med Ctr- Kings Hwy Div (page 90); **Address:** 3131 Kings Hwy, rm D-6, Brooklyn, NY 11234-2643; **Phone:** 718-338-2283; **Board Cert:** Internal Medicine 1989; Nephrology 2003; **Med School:** SUNY Downstate 1986; **Resid:** Internal Medicine, Brookdale Hosp 1989; **Fellow:** Nephrology, Brookdale Hosp 1992

Shapiro, Warren MD (Nep) - **Spec Exp:** Kidney Failure-Chronic; Hypertension; Dialysis Care; **Hospital:** Brookdale Univ Hosp Med Ctr; **Address:** 1 Brookdale Plaza, rm 169, Brooklyn, NY 11212-3139; **Phone:** 718-240-5615; **Board Cert:** Internal Medicine 1972; Nephrology 1974; **Med School:** Univ Hlth Sci/Chicago Med Sch 1966; **Resid:** Internal Medicine, UCSF Med Ctr 1967; Internal Medicine, NY Med Coll 1970; **Fellow:** Nephrology, NY Med Coll 1971; **Fac Appt:** Assoc Clin Prof Med, SUNY Downstate

Kings (Brooklyn)

Shein, Leon MD (Nep) - **Spec Exp:** Hypertension; Diabetic Kidney Disease; Electrolyte Disorders; Nutrition; **Hospital:** New York Methodist Hosp (page 479), Interfaith Med Ctr - Bklyn Jewish Div; **Address:** NY Methodist Hosp, 446 McDonald Ave, Brooklyn, NY 11218; **Phone:** 718-972-4200; **Board Cert:** Internal Medicine 1989; Nephrology 2003; **Med School:** Philippines 1983; **Resid:** Internal Medicine, Woodhull Med Ctr 1986; **Fellow:** Nephrology, Brookdale Hosp 1988

Spitalewitz, Samuel MD (Nep) - **Spec Exp:** Diabetic Kidney Disease; Hypertension; **Hospital:** Brookdale Univ Hosp Med Ctr; **Address:** 1 Brookdale Plaza, Ste 169-CHC, Brooklyn, NY 11212-3139; **Phone:** 718-240-5615; **Board Cert:** Internal Medicine 1978; Nephrology 1980; **Med School:** NYU Sch Med 1975; **Resid:** Internal Medicine, Brookdale Hosp 1978; **Fellow:** Nephrology, Brookdale Hosp 1981; **Fac Appt:** Assoc Clin Prof Med, SUNY Downstate

Stam, Lawrence MD (Nep) - **Spec Exp:** Hemodialysis; Plasmapheresis; **Hospital:** New York Methodist Hosp (page 479); **Address:** 506 6th St, Brooklyn, NY 11215-3609; **Phone:** 718-830-7109; **Board Cert:** Internal Medicine 1982; Nephrology 1984; **Med School:** SUNY Stony Brook 1978; **Resid:** Internal Medicine, St Elizabeth Hosp 1981; **Fellow:** Nephrology, Jewish Hosp 1982; **Fac Appt:** Asst Clin Prof Med, Cornell Univ-Weill Med Coll

NEUROLOGICAL SURGERY

Anant, Ashok MD (NS) - **Spec Exp:** Spinal Surgery; Stereotactic Radiosurgery; Brain Tumors; **Hospital:** Lutheran Med Ctr - Brooklyn, St Vincent Cath Med Ctrs - Manhattan (page 375); **Address:** 8413 13th Ave, Brooklyn, NY 11228-3325; **Phone:** 718-234-0979; **Board Cert:** Neurological Surgery 1984; **Med School:** India 1973; **Resid:** Surgery, Maimonides Medical Ctr 1977; Neurological Surgery, Univ Hosp 1982; **Fac Appt:** Assoc Clin Prof NS, NYU Sch Med

Cardoso, Erico R MD (NS) - **Spec Exp:** Pituitary Tumors; Spinal Cord Disorders; Hydrocephalus; **Hospital:** New York Methodist Hosp (page 479), Brookdale Univ Hosp Med Ctr; **Address:** 263 7th Ave, Ste 4B, Brooklyn, NY 11212-3693; **Phone:** 718-246-8610; **Board Cert:** Neurological Surgery 1994; **Med School:** Brazil 1973; **Resid:** Surgery, Ottawa Civic Hosp 1976; Neurological Surgery, Ottawa Civic Hosp 1980; **Fellow:** Neurological Surgery, Clin Rsch Fellowship Univ Hosp 1981; Neurological Surgery, Inst Neurol Scis 1982; **Fac Appt:** Assoc Prof NS, SUNY Downstate

Miller, John I MD (NS) - **Spec Exp:** Brain Tumors; **Hospital:** Long Island Coll Hosp (page 90); **Address:** LI Coll Hosp, Dept Neurosurgery, 339 Hicks St, Brooklyn, NY 11201; **Phone:** 718-780-1388; **Board Cert:** Neurological Surgery 1992; **Med School:** Georgetown Univ 1979; **Resid:** Neurological Surgery, SUNY Downstate 1987; **Fellow:** Pediatric Neurological Surgery, Chldns Hosp Natl Med Ctr 1982

NEUROLOGY

Azhar, Salman MD (N) - **Spec Exp:** Stroke; Headache; Parkinson's Disease; Seizure Disorders; **Hospital:** Lutheran Med Ctr - Brooklyn; **Address:** Lutheran Med Ctr, Stroke Ctr, 150 55th St, Ste 3-31, Brooklyn, NY 11220; **Phone:** 718-630-7316; **Board Cert:** Neurology 1999; **Med School:** Med Coll VA 1993; **Resid:** Neurology, Med Coll Va Hosp 1995; Neurology, Mt Sinai Med Ctr 1997; **Fellow:** Research, NINDS/NIH 1999

Bodis-Wollner, Ivan MD (N) - **Spec Exp:** Parkinson's Disease; Neuro-Ophthalmology; **Hospital:** SUNY Downstate Med Ctr, Kings County Hosp Ctr; **Address:** 470 Clarkson Ave, Brooklyn, NY 11203; **Phone:** 718-270-2502; **Board Cert:** Neurology 1977; Clinical Neurophysiology 1994; **Med School:** Austria 1965; **Resid:** Neurology, Mount Sinai Hosp 1974; **Fellow:** Mass Genl Hosp; **Fac Appt:** Prof N, SUNY Downstate

Crystal, Howard MD (N) - **Spec Exp:** Alzheimer's Disease; Dementia; **Hospital:** SUNY Downstate Med Ctr, Kings County Hosp Ctr; **Address:** 450 Clarkson Ave, Box 25, Brooklyn, NY 11203-2056; **Phone:** 718-270-6388; **Board Cert:** Neurology 1981; **Med School:** Univ Pennsylvania 1976; **Resid:** Neurology, Albert Einstein Med Ctr 1980; **Fellow:** Neurological Pathology, Albert Einstein Coll Med 1982; **Fac Appt:** Prof N, SUNY Downstate

Drexler, Ellen MD (N) - **Spec Exp:** Headache; **Hospital:** Maimonides Med Ctr (page 96); **Address:** 883 65th St, Brooklyn, NY 11210; **Phone:** 718-283-7470; **Board Cert:** Neurology 1983; **Med School:** SUNY Downstate 1978; **Resid:** Neurology, Montefiore Med Ctr 1982; **Fac Appt:** Assoc Prof N, Mount Sinai Sch Med

Gropen, Toby I MD (N) - **Spec Exp:** Stroke; **Hospital:** Long Island Coll Hosp (page 90); **Address:** Long Island Coll Hosp, Dept Neurology, 339 Hicks St, Brooklyn, NY 11201; **Phone:** 718-780-1124; **Board Cert:** Neurology 1993; **Med School:** Univ Tex, San Antonio 1987; **Resid:** Neurology, Neuro Inst/Columbia-Presby Med Ctr 1991; **Fellow:** Neurology, Neuro Inst/Columbia-Presby Med Ctr 1993; **Fac Appt:** Asst Prof N, SUNY Hlth Sci Ctr

Kay, Arthur MD (N) - **Spec Exp:** Alzheimer's Disease; Parkinson's Disease; Dementia; **Hospital:** Brookdale Univ Hosp Med Ctr, Flushing Hosp Med Ctr; **Address:** 1 Brookdale Plaza St, Ste 400, Brooklyn, NY 11212-3139; **Phone:** 718-240-5622; **Board Cert:** Neurology 1983; **Med School:** SUNY Downstate 1978; **Resid:** Internal Medicine, Brookdale Hosp 1979; Neurology, Mount Sinai Hosp 1982; **Fellow:** Natl Inst Hlth 1984; **Fac Appt:** Assoc Prof N, SUNY Downstate

Keilson, Marshall MD (N) - **Spec Exp:** Alzheimer's Disease; Epilepsy; **Hospital:** Maimonides Med Ctr (page 96); **Address:** 4802 10th Ave, Brooklyn, NY 11219-2844; **Phone:** 718-283-7470; **Board Cert:** Neurology 1982; **Med School:** Albert Einstein Coll Med 1977; **Resid:** Internal Medicine, Montefiore Hosp Med Ctr 1978; Neurology, Albert Einstein 1981; **Fellow:** Clinical Neurophysiology, Univ Hosp 1983

Maccabee, Paul J MD (N) - **Spec Exp:** Neuromuscular Disorders; Electromyography; **Hospital:** SUNY Downstate Med Ctr; **Address:** SUNY Downstate Med Ctr, 450 Clarkson Ave, Box 35, Brooklyn, NY 11203; **Phone:** 718-270-2502; **Board Cert:** Neurology 1977; Clinical Neurophysiology 2003; **Med School:** Boston Univ 1970; **Resid:** Neurology, Boston Univ Med Ctr 1976; **Fellow:** Clinical Neurophysiology, Mass Genl Hosp 1978; Clinical Neurophysiology, Mt Sinai Hosp 1979; **Fac Appt:** Prof N, SUNY Hlth Sci Ctr

Maniscalco, Anthony MD (N) - **Spec Exp:** Movement Disorders; Cerebrovascular Disease; Neuromuscular Disorders; **Hospital:** Maimonides Med Ctr (page 96), St Vincent Cath Med Ctrs - Manhattan (page 375); **Address:** Bklyn Neurology, 117 70th St, Brooklyn, NY 11209-1113; **Phone:** 718-836-8800; **Board Cert:** Internal Medicine 1982; Neurology 1988; **Med School:** Italy 1978; **Resid:** Internal Medicine, Maimonides Medical Ctr 1981; Neurology, St Vincent's Hosp & Med Ctr 1984; **Fac Appt:** Assoc Clin Prof N, SUNY Downstate

Nouri, Shahin MD (N) - **Spec Exp:** Epilepsy/Seizure Disorders; **Hospital:** New York Methodist Hosp (page 479); **Address:** NY Methodist Hosp, Dept Neurology, 506 Sixth St, Brooklyn, NY 11215; **Phone:** 718-246-8614; **Board Cert:** Neurology 2004; Clinical Neurophysiology 2005; **Med School:** Germany 1994; **Resid:** Internal Medicine, Staten Island Univ Hosp 1998; Neurology, Georgetown Univ Med Ctr 2001; **Fellow:** Clinical Neurophysiology, NYU Med Ctr 2002

Pitem, Michael DO (N) - **Spec Exp:** Headache; Epilepsy; Pain Management; **Hospital:** Brookdale Univ Hosp Med Ctr; **Address:** Brookdale Hospital, 1 Brookdale Plaza Snapper Bldg - rm 422, Brooklyn, NY 11212-3124; **Phone:** 718-209-9639; **Board Cert:** Neurology 1990; **Med School:** NY Coll Osteo Med 1985; **Resid:** Neurology, Albert Einstein 1989; **Fac Appt:** Asst Clin Prof N, SUNY Downstate

Roohi, Fereydoon MD (N) - **Spec Exp:** Electromyography; Peripheral Nerve Disorders; **Hospital:** Long Island Coll Hosp (page 90); **Address:** 339 Hicks St, Ste 333, Brooklyn, NY 11201-5509; **Phone:** 718-624-3166; **Board Cert:** Neurology 1980; Clinical Neurophysiology 1989; **Med School:** Iran 1967; **Resid:** Neurology, Kings Co Hosp 1975; **Fellow:** Neurology, Presby Hosp 1976; **Fac Appt:** Assoc Prof N, SUNY Downstate

Rosenbaum, Daniel MD (N) - **Spec Exp:** Stroke; **Hospital:** SUNY Downstate Med Ctr; **Address:** SUNY Downstate, Dept Neurology, 450 Clarkson Ave, Brooklyn, NY 11203; **Phone:** 718-270-2051; **Board Cert:** Neurology 1988; **Med School:** Albert Einstein Coll Med 1982; **Resid:** Internal Medicine, Brookdale Hosp 1983; Neurology, Albert Einstein 1986; **Fellow:** Stroke, Univ Tex Med Sch 1988; **Fac Appt:** Prof N, SUNY Downstate

Rudolph, Steven MD (N) - **Spec Exp:** Stroke; Neuro-Ophthalmology; **Hospital:** Maimonides Med Ctr (page 96), Mount Sinai Med Ctr (page 98); **Address:** 948 48th St, Brooklyn, NY 11219; **Phone:** 718-283-7670; **Board Cert:** Neurology 1981; **Med School:** SUNY Hlth Sci Ctr 1976; **Resid:** Neurology, Mount Sinai Hosp 1980; **Fellow:** Neurological Ophthalmology, Mount Sinai Hosp 1982; **Fac Appt:** Asst Clin Prof N, Mount Sinai Sch Med

Salgado, Miran MD (N) - **Spec Exp:** Movement Disorders; Parkinson's Disease; Botox Therapy; Headache; **Hospital:** New York Methodist Hosp (page 479); **Address:** Center for Neurology, 263 7th Ave, Ste 5C, Brooklyn, NY 11215; **Phone:** 718-246-8614; **Board Cert:** Neurology 1995; **Med School:** Sri Lanka 1990; **Resid:** Neurology, SUNY Downstate Med Ctr 1994; **Fellow:** Movement Disorders, Columbia Presby Med Ctr 1995

Slotwiner, Paul MD (N) - **Hospital:** St Vincent Cath Med Ctrs - Manhattan (page 375), Beth Israel Med Ctr-Kings Hwy Div (page 90); **Address:** Neurology Associates, 117 70th St, Brooklyn, NY 11209-1113; **Phone:** 718-836-8800; **Board Cert:** Neurology 1968; **Med School:** Univ Chicago-Pritzker Sch Med 1959; **Resid:** Neurology, Mount Sinai 1963

Sobol, Norman MD (N) - **Spec Exp:** Headache; Stroke; Parkinson's Disease; **Hospital:** Beth Israel Med Ctr-Kings Hwy Div (page 90), Maimonides Med Ctr (page 96); **Address:** 3131 Kings Hwy, Ste C7, Brooklyn, NY 11234-2642; **Phone:** 718-677-0009; **Board Cert:** Neurology 1980; **Med School:** Univ Chicago-Pritzker Sch Med 1974; **Resid:** SUNY Downstate 1976; Neurology, SUNY Downstate 1978; **Fellow:** Clinical Neurophysiology, SUNY Downstate 1980; **Fac Appt:** Asst Prof N, SUNY Downstate

Somasundaram, Mahendra MD (N) - **Spec Exp:** Stroke; Epilepsy; Movement Disorders; **Hospital:** SUNY Downstate Med Ctr, Kings County Hosp Ctr; **Address:** Downstate Neurological Assocs, 450 Clarkson Ave, Brooklyn, NY 11203-2098; **Phone:** 718-270-2502; **Board Cert:** Neurology 1975; **Med School:** Sri Lanka 1959; **Resid:** Neurology, St James Hosp 1965; Neurology, New York Hosp 1973; **Fellow:** Electroencephalography, Univ Wash Med Ctr 1968; **Fac Appt:** Prof N, SUNY Hlth Sci Ctr

Vas, George A MD (N) - **Spec Exp:** Stroke; Multiple Sclerosis; **Hospital:** SUNY Downstate Med Ctr; **Address:** 450 Clarkson Ave, Ste A, Brooklyn, NY 11203-2056; **Phone:** 718-270-2502; **Board Cert:** Internal Medicine 1973; Neurology 1977; Clinical Neurophysiology 2002; **Med School:** Univ Pittsburgh 1970; **Resid:** Internal Medicine, New York Hosp 1972; Neurology, New York Hosp 1975; **Fac Appt:** Prof N, SUNY Downstate

Yellin, Joseph DO (N) - **Spec Exp:** Headache; Memory Disorders; Peripheral Neuropathy; **Hospital:** New York Methodist Hosp (page 479), New York Comm Hosp; **Address:** 2502 Kings Hwy, Brooklyn, NY 11229; **Phone:** 718-377-2223; **Board Cert:** Neurology 1988; **Med School:** Univ Osteo Med & Hlth Sci, Des Moines 1978; **Resid:** Neurology, Kings County Hosp 1982

NUCLEAR MEDICINE

Gerard, Perry MD (NuM) - **Spec Exp:** PET Imaging; Nuclear Cardiology; Ultrasound; Vascular Ultrasound; **Hospital:** Maimonides Med Ctr (page 96); **Address:** 4802 10th Ave, Brooklyn, NY 11219; **Phone:** 718-283-8355; **Board Cert:** Diagnostic Radiology 1987; Nuclear Radiology 1989; **Med School:** Dominica 1980; **Resid:** Diagnostic Radiology, Maimonides Med Ctr 1984; **Fellow:** Diagnostic Imaging, Maimonides Med Ctr 1985; **Fac Appt:** Asst Clin Prof Rad, SUNY Downstate

Strashun, Arnold M MD (NuM) - **Spec Exp:** Neurologic Imaging; Nuclear Cardiology; Thyroid Disorders; PET Imaging-Brain; **Hospital:** SUNY Downstate Med Ctr, Kings County Hosp Ctr; **Address:** 450 Clarkson Ave Fl 2, Box 1210, Brooklyn, NY 11203; **Phone:** 718-245-3692; **Board Cert:** Internal Medicine 1977; Nuclear Medicine 1979; **Med School:** Baylor Coll Med 1974; **Resid:** Internal Medicine, Baylor Med Ctr 1975; Internal Medicine, Texas Med Ctr 1977; **Fellow:** Nuclear Medicine, VA Med Ctr 1978; Nuclear Medicine, Mount Sinai Hosp 1979; **Fac Appt:** Prof Rad, SUNY Downstate

OBSTETRICS & GYNECOLOGY

Barzegar, Hooshang MD (ObG) PCP - **Hospital:** Brookdale Univ Hosp Med Ctr, Long Island Coll Hosp (page 90); **Address:** 1636 E 14th St, Ste 124, Brooklyn, NY 11229-1100; **Phone:** 718-998-3500; **Board Cert:** Obstetrics & Gynecology 1999; **Med School:** Iran 1960; **Resid:** Obstetrics & Gynecology, Brooklyn Cumberland Hosp 1968; Obstetrics & Gynecology, Montefiore Hosp Med Ctr 1970; **Fac Appt:** Asst Clin Prof ObG, SUNY Downstate

Brennan, John P MD (ObG) PCP - **Spec Exp:** Uterine Fibroids; Menopause Problems; Hysteroscopic Surgery; **Hospital:** Long Island Coll Hosp (page 90), Lenox Hill Hosp (page 94); **Address:** 153 Clinton St, Brooklyn, NY 11201-4601; **Phone:** 718-222-3636; **Board Cert:** Obstetrics & Gynecology 2003; **Med School:** Columbia P&S 1985; **Resid:** Obstetrics & Gynecology, Albert Einstein 1989; **Fac Appt:** Asst Prof ObG, SUNY Downstate

Camilien, Louis MD (ObG) - **Spec Exp:** Colposcopy; **Hospital:** New York Methodist Hosp (page 479); **Address:** 506 6th St, Brooklyn, NY 11215; **Phone:** 718-780-3272; **Board Cert:** Obstetrics & Gynecology 1997; **Med School:** Haiti 1977; **Resid:** Pathology, Kings County Hosp 1983; Obstetrics & Gynecology, Kings County Hosp 1986; **Fac Appt:** Clin Prof ObG, Cornell Univ-Weill Med Coll

Chandra Jr, Prasanta C MD (ObG) PCP - **Spec Exp:** Pregnancy-High Risk; Premature Labor; Pregnancy-Teenage; **Hospital:** Wyckoff Heights Med Ctr; **Address:** Wyckoff Heights Medical Ctr, Dept Ob/Gyn, 374 Stockholm St, Brooklyn, NY 11237; **Phone:** 718-963-7168; **Board Cert:** Obstetrics & Gynecology 1979; Maternal & Fetal Medicine 1980; **Med School:** India 1969; **Resid:** Surgery, Bronx Muni Hosp 1972; Obstetrics & Gynecology, Bronx Muni Hosp 1976; **Fellow:** Maternal & Fetal Medicine, Bronx Muni Hosp 1978

Comrie, Millicent MD (ObG) **PCP** - **Spec Exp:** Menopause Problems; Uterine Fibroids; **Hospital:** Long Island Coll Hosp (page 90); **Address:** 148 Pierrepont St, Brooklyn, NY 11201; **Phone:** 718-852-9180; **Board Cert:** Obstetrics & Gynecology 1983; **Med School:** SUNY Hlth Sci Ctr 1976; **Resid:** Obstetrics & Gynecology, Long Island Coll Hosp 1980; **Fellow:** Public Health, Columbia Univ 1981; **Fac Appt:** Asst Clin Prof ObG, SUNY Hlth Sci Ctr

Dor, Nathan MD (ObG) - **Spec Exp:** Pregnancy-High Risk; **Hospital:** Maimonides Med Ctr (page 96); **Address:** 943 48th St, Brooklyn, NY 11219-2919; **Phone:** 718-853-1535; **Board Cert:** Obstetrics & Gynecology 2004; Maternal & Fetal Medicine 2004; **Med School:** Israel 1973; **Resid:** Obstetrics & Gynecology, Montefiore Med Ctr 1977; **Fellow:** Perinatal Medicine, Westchester Co Med Ctr 1979; **Fac Appt:** Asst Prof ObG, SUNY Downstate

Gallousis, Spiro MD (ObG) - **Spec Exp:** Gynecologic Cancer; Laser Surgery; Laparoscopic Surgery; **Hospital:** Long Island Coll Hosp (page 90); **Address:** 9 Pierrepont St, Brooklyn, NY 11201-3302; **Phone:** 718-852-5810; **Board Cert:** Obstetrics & Gynecology 1969; **Med School:** Switzerland 1962; **Resid:** Obstetrics & Gynecology, Long Island Coll Hosp 1967; **Fellow:** Gynecologic Oncology, Univ Hosp 1968; **Fac Appt:** Assoc Clin Prof ObG, SUNY Downstate

Guirguis, Fayez MD (ObG) - **Spec Exp:** Obstetrics; Laparoscopic Surgery; **Hospital:** New York Methodist Hosp (page 479); **Address:** 464 77th St, Brooklyn, NY 11209; **Phone:** 718-768-8500; **Board Cert:** Obstetrics & Gynecology 2000; **Med School:** Egypt 1969; **Resid:** Obstetrics & Gynecology, Brooklyn Hosp 1983

Kerr, Angela MD (ObG) - **Spec Exp:** Colposcopy; **Hospital:** Brooklyn Hosp Ctr-Downtown; **Address:** 240 Willoughby St, Ste 3A, Brooklyn, NY 11201; **Phone:** 718-250-8318; **Board Cert:** Obstetrics & Gynecology 1999; **Med School:** SUNY Downstate 1983; **Resid:** Obstetrics & Gynecology, Kings County Hosp 1987

Lamarque, Madeleine MD (ObG) - **Spec Exp:** Maternal & Fetal Medicine; Adolescent Gynecology; **Hospital:** SUNY Downstate Med Ctr, Kings County Hosp Ctr; **Address:** 601 E 18th St, Ste 109, Brooklyn, NY 11226; **Phone:** 718-434-5373; **Board Cert:** Obstetrics & Gynecology 1983; **Med School:** Haiti 1970; **Resid:** Surgery, Brookdale Hosp 1973; Obstetrics & Gynecology, Catholic Med Ctr 1979; **Fac Appt:** Asst Clin Prof ObG, SUNY Downstate

Lederman, Sanford MD (ObG) - **Spec Exp:** Pregnancy-High Risk; Ultrasound; **Hospital:** Long Island Coll Hosp (page 90); **Address:** 9 Pierrepont St, Brooklyn, NY 11201-3302; **Phone:** 718-852-5810; **Board Cert:** Obstetrics & Gynecology 1982; **Med School:** Mexico 1973; **Resid:** Obstetrics & Gynecology, Long Island Coll Hosp 1979; **Fellow:** Maternal & Fetal Medicine, UC-Irvine Memorial Hosp 1981; **Fac Appt:** Assoc Clin Prof ObG, SUNY Downstate

Minkoff, Howard L MD (ObG) - **Spec Exp:** AIDS/HIV in Pregnancy; **Hospital:** Maimonides Med Ctr (page 96); **Address:** Maimonides Med Ctr, Dept Ob-Gyn, 4802 Tenth Ave, Brooklyn, NY 11219; **Phone:** 718-283-7973; **Board Cert:** Obstetrics & Gynecology 1995; Maternal & Fetal Medicine 1995; **Med School:** Penn State Univ-Hershey Med Ctr 1975; **Resid:** Obstetrics & Gynecology, Kings Co Hosp Ctr 1979; Obstetrics & Gynecology, SUNY Hlth Sci Ctr 1981; **Fellow:** Maternal & Fetal Medicine, Kings Co Hosp Ctr 1981; **Fac Appt:** Prof ObG, SUNY Hlth Sci Ctr

Pili, Manuel MD (ObG) - **Hospital:** Jamaica Hosp Med Ctr, New York Comm Hosp; **Address:** 1331 E 19th St, Brooklyn, NY 11230-6103; **Phone:** 718-998-3038; **Board Cert:** Obstetrics & Gynecology 1973; **Med School:** Philippines 1965; **Resid:** Obstetrics & Gynecology, Kings Co-Downstate Med Ctr 1971; **Fellow:** Gynecologic Oncology, Kings Co-Downstate Med Ctr 1973; **Fac Appt:** Asst Clin Prof ObG, SUNY Hlth Sci Ctr

Reizis, Igal MD (ObG) - **Hospital:** Maimonides Med Ctr (page 96); **Address:** 5925 15th Ave, Brooklyn, NY 11219-5009; **Phone:** 718-972-2700; **Board Cert:** Obstetrics & Gynecology 1984; **Med School:** Israel 1977; **Resid:** Obstetrics & Gynecology, Maimonides Med Ctr

Rubenstein, Janet MD (ObG) - **Hospital:** Maimonides Med Ctr (page 96); **Address:** 4506 12th Ave, Brooklyn, NY 11219; **Phone:** 718-633-3131; **Board Cert:** Obstetrics & Gynecology 1996; **Med School:** Med Coll PA Hahnemann 1978; **Resid:** Obstetrics & Gynecology, Maimonides Medical Ctr 1982

Weinstock, Judith MD (ObG) - **Spec Exp:** Menopause Problems; Adolescent Gynecology; **Hospital:** Long Island Coll Hosp (page 90); **Address:** Brooklyn Women's Hlthcare, 9 Pierrpont St, Brooklyn, NY 11201-3396; **Phone:** 718-852-5810; **Board Cert:** Obstetrics & Gynecology 1997; **Med School:** Baylor Coll Med 1982; **Resid:** Obstetrics & Gynecology, Long Island Coll Hosp 1986; **Fac Appt:** Asst Clin Prof ObG, SUNY Downstate

OPHTHALMOLOGY

Ackerman, Jacob MD (Oph) - **Spec Exp:** Cataract Surgery-Lens Implant; Glaucoma; Laser Surgery; **Hospital:** Brookdale Univ Hosp Med Ctr, New York Comm Hosp; **Address:** 1901 Utica Ave Fl 1, Brooklyn, NY 11234-3213; **Phone:** 718-968-8700; **Board Cert:** Ophthalmology 1976; **Med School:** Albert Einstein Coll Med 1971; **Resid:** Ophthalmology, LI Jewish/Hillside Med Ctr 1975; **Fac Appt:** Asst Prof Oph, SUNY Hlth Sci Ctr

Berman, David H MD (Oph) - **Spec Exp:** Retinal Detachment; Diabetic Eye Disease/Retinopathy; Macular Degeneration; **Hospital:** Brooklyn Hosp Ctr-Downtown; **Address:** 185 Montague St, Ste PH, Brooklyn, NY 11201; **Phone:** 718-222-3050; **Board Cert:** Ophthalmology 1989; **Med School:** SUNY Downstate 1982; **Resid:** Internal Medicine, Kings Co Hosp 1984; Ophthalmology, Kings Co Hosp 1987; **Fellow:** Ophthalmology, Kings Co Hosp 1988; Ophthalmology, Hermann Eye Ctr 1989; **Fac Appt:** Assoc Clin Prof Oph, SUNY Downstate

Brecher, Rubin MD (Oph) - **Spec Exp:** Diabetic Eye Disease/Retinopathy; Macular Degeneration; **Hospital:** Maimonides Med Ctr (page 96), Montefiore Med Ctr; **Address:** 736 Ocean Pkwy, Brooklyn, NY 11230-1116; **Phone:** 718-851-1186; **Board Cert:** Ophthalmology 1991; **Med School:** Albert Einstein Coll Med 1984; **Resid:** Ophthalmology, Montefiore Med Ctr 1988; **Fellow:** Medical Retina, Moorefields Eye Hosp 1989

Deutsch, James A MD (Oph) - **Spec Exp:** Strabismus; Cataract Surgery; **Hospital:** Long Island Coll Hosp (page 90); **Address:** 110 Remsen St, Brooklyn, NY 11201-4261; **Phone:** 718-855-8700; **Board Cert:** Ophthalmology 1989; **Med School:** NYU Sch Med 1984; **Resid:** Ophthalmology, Mt Sinai Hosp 1988; **Fellow:** Pediatric Ophthalmology, Wills Eye Hosp 1989; **Fac Appt:** Asst Clin Prof Oph, Mount Sinai Sch Med

Dolan, Rory MD (Oph) - **Spec Exp:** Cataract Surgery; Glaucoma; **Hospital:** Brooklyn Hosp Ctr-Downtown; **Address:** 11 Plaza St, Brooklyn, NY 11217; **Phone:** 718-638-2020; **Board Cert:** Ophthalmology 1975; **Med School:** NY Med Coll 1969; **Resid:** Ophthalmology, Downstate 1973; **Fellow:** Ophthalmology, Downstate 1974; **Fac Appt:** Assoc Prof Oph, SUNY Downstate

Dweck, Monica MD (Oph) - **Spec Exp:** Eyelid Surgery; Lacrimal Gland Disorders; Orbital Diseases; **Hospital:** SUNY Downstate Med Ctr, Long Island Coll Hosp (page 90); **Address:** SUNY-Downstate Med Ctr, 450 Clarkson Ave, Box 58, Brooklyn, NY 11203-2056; **Phone:** 718-780-1260; **Board Cert:** Ophthalmology 2005; **Med School:** SUNY Downstate 1986; **Resid:** Ophthalmology, NY Eye & Ear Infirm 1990; **Fellow:** Oculoplastic Surgery, The Cleveland Clinic 1991; **Fac Appt:** Asst Prof Oph, SUNY Hlth Sci Ctr

Feinstein, Neil MD (Oph) - **Spec Exp:** Cataract Surgery; Glaucoma; Diabetic Eye Disease/Retinopathy; **Hospital:** Maimonides Med Ctr (page 96); **Address:** 919 48th St, Brooklyn, NY 11219-2919; **Phone:** 718-435-1800; **Board Cert:** Ophthalmology 1979; **Med School:** Albert Einstein Coll Med 1974; **Resid:** Ophthalmology, SUNY Downstate Med Ctr 1978

Freedman, Jeffrey MD/PhD (Oph) - **Spec Exp:** Glaucoma; Uveitis; Cornea Transplant; **Hospital:** Long Island Coll Hosp (page 90), Interfaith Med Ctr - Bklyn Jewish Div; **Address:** 161 Atlantic Ave, Ste 203, Brooklyn, NY 11201-6720; **Phone:** 718-596-9086; **Board Cert:** Ophthalmology 1975; **Med School:** South Africa 1964; **Resid:** Internal Medicine, Baragwanat Genl Hosp 1966; Ophthalmology, Transvaal General Hosp 1967; **Fellow:** Ophthalmology, SUNY Downstate Med Ctr; **Fac Appt:** Prof Oph, SUNY Downstate

Hyman, George MD (Oph) - **Spec Exp:** Laser Vision Surgery; Corneal Disease; Cornea & Cataract Surgery; **Hospital:** Brookdale Univ Hosp Med Ctr; **Address:** 2460 Flatbush Ave, Ste 4, Brooklyn, NY 11234-5000; **Phone:** 718-252-1200; **Board Cert:** Ophthalmology 1976; **Med School:** Univ MD Sch Med 1968; **Resid:** Ophthalmology, Univ Hosp/Downstate Med Ctr 1974; **Fellow:** Anterior Segment - External Disease, Univ Witwatersrand 1975; **Fac Appt:** Asst Prof Oph, SUNY Hlth Sci Ctr

Jaffe, Herbert MD (Oph) - **Spec Exp:** Cataract Surgery; Glaucoma; **Hospital:** Beth Israel Med Ctr- Kings Hwy Div (page 90), SUNY Downstate Med Ctr; **Address:** 2128 Ocean Ave, Brooklyn, NY 11229-1406; **Phone:** 718-339-7469; **Board Cert:** Ophthalmology 1983; **Med School:** Belgium 1968; **Resid:** Ophthalmology, SUNY Downstate Med CtrCtr 1972

Lazzaro, E Clifford MD (Oph) - **Spec Exp:** Glaucoma; Neuro-Ophthalmology; **Hospital:** Lutheran Med Ctr - Brooklyn; **Address:** 7901 4th Ave, Ste A4, Brooklyn, NY 11209; **Phone:** 718-748-1334; **Board Cert:** Ophthalmology 1973; **Med School:** SUNY Hlth Sci Ctr 1965; **Resid:** Ophthalmology, Brooklyn Eye & Ear Hosp 1971

Lebowitz, Mark MD (Oph) - **Spec Exp:** LASIK-Refractive Surgery; Cataract Surgery; Corneal Surgery; **Hospital:** Manhattan Eye, Ear & Throat Hosp; **Address:** 1301 Avenue J, Brooklyn, NY 11230-3605; **Phone:** 718-284-1921; **Board Cert:** Ophthalmology 1987; **Med School:** NYU Sch Med 1982; **Resid:** Ophthalmology, SUNY Downstate 1986; **Fellow:** Cornea, Manhattan EET 1987

Lieberman, David M MD (Oph) - **Spec Exp:** Contact lenses; **Hospital:** New York Methodist Hosp (page 479); **Address:** 9 Prospect Park West, Ste 1-B, Brooklyn, NY 11215; **Phone:** 718-622-8900; **Board Cert:** Ophthalmology 1973; **Med School:** SUNY Downstate 1965; **Resid:** Ophthalmology, Univ Hosp 1970

Lombardo, James MD (Oph) - **Spec Exp:** Cataract Surgery; Diabetic Eye Disease/Retinopathy; Glaucoma; **Hospital:** New York Eye & Ear Infirm (page 110), Victory Memorial Hosp - Bklyn; **Address:** 7801 4th Ave, Brooklyn, NY 11209-3701; **Phone:** 718-836-6661; **Board Cert:** Ophthalmology 1982; **Med School:** NYU Sch Med 1976; **Resid:** Internal Medicine, St Vincent's Hosp & Med Ctr 1977; Ophthalmology, NY Eye & Ear Infirmary 1980

Lombardo, John MD (Oph) - **Spec Exp:** Cornea & Cataract Surgery; Glaucoma; Laser-Refractive Surgery; **Hospital:** New York Eye & Ear Infirm (page 110), Victory Memorial Hosp - Bklyn; **Address:** 7801 4th Ave, Brooklyn, NY 11209-3701; **Phone:** 718-836-6661; **Board Cert:** Psychiatry 1981; Ophthalmology 1983; **Med School:** Columbia P&S 1973; **Resid:** Psychiatry, Columbia-Presby Hosp 1977; Ophthalmology, Manhattan Eye, Ear & Throat Hosp 1982

Pearlstein, Eric MD (Oph) - **Spec Exp:** Cataract Surgery; Corneal Disease; LASIK-Refractive Surgery; **Hospital:** Long Island Coll Hosp (page 90), New York Eye & Ear Infirm (page 110); **Address:** 8721 4th Ave, Brooklyn, NY 11209-5195; **Phone:** 718-680-1500; **Board Cert:** Ophthalmology 1988; **Med School:** SUNY Hlth Sci Ctr 1983; **Resid:** Ophthalmology, LI Jewish Med Ctr 1987; **Fellow:** Cornea & Ext Eye Disease, Univ Minn-Duluth Sch Med 1988

Reich, Raymond MD (Oph) - **Spec Exp:** Cataract Surgery; Ophthalmic Plastic Surgery; Laser Refractive Surgery; **Hospital:** Long Island Coll Hosp (page 90), Maimonides Med Ctr (page 96); **Address:** 118 West End Ave, Brooklyn, NY 11235; **Phone:** 718-332-6200; **Board Cert:** Ophthalmology 1978; **Med School:** Albert Einstein Coll Med 1973; **Resid:** Ophthalmology, Univ Hosp 1977; **Fellow:** Ophthalmic Plastic Surgery, Harvard-Mass EE Infirm 1978; **Fac Appt:** Asst Prof Oph, SUNY Hlth Sci Ctr

Saffra, Norman MD (Oph) - **Spec Exp:** Microsurgery; Retinal Disorders; **Hospital:** Maimonides Med Ctr (page 96), New York Eye & Ear Infirm (page 110); **Address:** 902 49th St, Brooklyn, NY 11219-2922; **Phone:** 718-283-8000; **Board Cert:** Ophthalmology 1994; **Med School:** Albert Einstein Coll Med 1988; **Resid:** Ophthalmology, Albert Einstein 1992; **Fellow:** Retina, SUNY Hlth Sci Ctr 1993; **Fac Appt:** Assoc Clin Prof Oph, Mount Sinai Sch Med

Sciortino, Patrick MD (Oph) - **Spec Exp:** LASIK-Refractive Surgery; Cataract Surgery; **Hospital:** New York Comm Hosp, Long Island Coll Hosp (page 90); **Address:** 914 Bay Ridge Pkwy, Brooklyn, NY 11228-2302; **Phone:** 718-748-5700; **Board Cert:** Ophthalmology 1998; **Med School:** NY Med Coll 1978; **Resid:** Ophthalmology, St Vincents Hosp 1980; Ophthalmology, Catholic Med Ctr; **Fellow:** Ophthalmology, Univ Hosp 1984

Seidman, Mitchell DO (Oph) - **Spec Exp:** Cataract Surgery; **Hospital:** New York Methodist Hosp (page 479); **Address:** 501 Brightwater Ct, Brooklyn, NY 11235; **Phone:** 718-332-2020; **Board Cert:** Ophthalmology 1979; **Med School:** Philadelphia Coll Osteo Med 1974; **Resid:** Ophthalmology, Temple Univ Hosp 1978; **Fellow:** Anterior Segment - External Disease 1979

Sherman, Steven I DO (Oph) - **Spec Exp:** Cataract Surgery; Glaucoma; **Hospital:** New York Methodist Hosp (page 479), Interfaith Med Ctr - St John's Episcopal Hosp; **Address:** 2303 Avenue Z, Brooklyn, NY 11235-2805; **Phone:** 718-934-6600; **Board Cert:** Ophthalmology 1989; **Med School:** Univ Osteo Med & Hlth Sci, Des Moines 1977; **Resid:** Ophthalmology, USPHS Hosp 1982; **Fellow:** Glaucoma, SUNY Downstate 1983; **Fac Appt:** Asst Clin Prof Oph, NY Coll Osteo Med

Silberman, Deborah MD (Oph) - **Spec Exp:** Laser Vision Surgery; Cataract Surgery; **Hospital:** Brookdale Univ Hosp Med Ctr, Maimonides Med Ctr (page 96); **Address:** 1335 Linden Blvd, Brooklyn, NY 11212-4751; **Phone:** 718-240-5557; **Board Cert:** Ophthalmology 1990; **Med School:** SUNY Buffalo 1984; **Resid:** Internal Medicine, St Luke's-Roosevelt Hosp Ctr 1985; Ophthalmology, Brookdale Hosp Med Ctr 1988

Smith, Edward MD (Oph) - **Spec Exp:** Cataract Surgery; **Hospital:** SUNY Downstate Med Ctr, Kingsbrook Jewish Med Ctr; **Address:** Downstate Ophthalmology Assocs, 11 Plaza St West, Brooklyn, NY 11217; **Phone:** 718-638-2020; **Board Cert:** Ophthalmology 1989; **Med School:** SUNY Downstate 1984; **Resid:** Ophthalmology, Univ Hosp 1988; **Fellow:** Neurological Ophthalmology, Univ Hosp 1989; **Fac Appt:** Asst Prof Oph, SUNY Downstate

Stein, Arnold MD (Oph) - **Spec Exp:** Retinal Disorders; Glaucoma; Cataract Surgery; Laser Surgery; **Hospital:** Beth Israel Med Ctr- Kings Hwy Div (page 90), Long Island Jewish Med Ctr; **Address:** 1000 Ocean Pky, Ste LA1, Brooklyn, NY 11230-3417; **Phone:** 718-692-0400; **Board Cert:** Ophthalmology 1987; **Med School:** SUNY Downstate 1982; **Resid:** Brookdale 1983; Ophthalmology, LI Jewish Med Ctr 1986; **Fac Appt:** Asst Clin Prof Oph, Albert Einstein Coll Med

Unterricht, Sam MD (Oph) - **Spec Exp:** Macular Disease/Degeneration; Retinal Disorders; Optic Nerve Disorders; **Hospital:** New York Methodist Hosp (page 479), SUNY Downstate Med Ctr; **Address:** 20 Plaza St, Brooklyn, NY 11238; **Phone:** 718-622-5800; **Board Cert:** Ophthalmology 1982; **Med School:** SUNY Downstate 1976; **Resid:** Ophthalmology, Univ Hosp 1980; **Fellow:** Neurological Ophthalmology, Kingsbrook Jewish MC 1981; Retina/Vitreous, Univ Hosp 1982; **Fac Appt:** Asst Clin Prof Oph, SUNY Hlth Sci Ctr

Wolintz, Arthur H MD (Oph) - **Spec Exp:** Neuro-Ophthalmology; Headache; Vision Loss-Unexplained Loss; **Hospital:** Kingsbrook Jewish Med Ctr, SUNY Downstate Med Ctr; **Address:** 100 Ocean Pkwy, Brooklyn, NY 11218-1755; **Phone:** 718-854-7360; **Board Cert:** Neurology 1970; Ophthalmology 1973; **Med School:** SUNY Downstate 1962; **Resid:** Neurology, Natl Inst Hlth 1966; Ophthalmology, SUNY Downstate Med Ctr 1971; **Fellow:** Neuropathology, Columbia-Presby Hosp 1968; **Fac Appt:** Prof Oph, SUNY Downstate

Zellner, James H MD (Oph) - **Spec Exp:** Laser Refractive Surgery; Cataract Surgery; **Hospital:** New York Eye & Ear Infirm (page 110); **Address:** 454 Bay Ridge Pkwy, Brooklyn, NY 11209-2702; **Phone:** 718-748-2020; **Board Cert:** Ophthalmology 1982; **Med School:** Albert Einstein Coll Med 1977; **Resid:** Ophthalmology, Kings County Hosp Ctr 1981

ORTHOPAEDIC SURGERY

Feliccia, Joseph MD (OrS) - **Hospital:** Maimonides Med Ctr (page 96); **Address:** 355 Ovington Ave, Ste 202, Brooklyn, NY 11209-1453; **Phone:** 718-238-6400; **Board Cert:** Orthopaedic Surgery 1982; **Med School:** Hahnemann Univ 1974; **Resid:** Surgery, Maimonides Med Ctr 1976; Orthopaedic Surgery, Maimonides Med Ctr 1979

Gordon, Stanley L MD (OrS) - **Spec Exp:** Hand Surgery; **Hospital:** SUNY Downstate Med Ctr, Kings County Hosp Ctr; **Address:** 450 Clarkson Ave, Box 30, Brooklyn, NY 11203-0030; **Phone:** 718-270-6317; **Board Cert:** Orthopaedic Surgery 1984; **Med School:** Univ Pittsburgh 1964; **Resid:** Orthopaedic Surgery, Univ Pittsburgh 1971; **Fellow:** Hand Surgery 1977; Hand Surgery 1978; **Fac Appt:** Prof OrS, SUNY Downstate

Mani, John MD (OrS) - **Spec Exp:** Hip Replacement; Knee Replacement; **Hospital:** Long Island Coll Hosp (page 90); **Address:** 161 Atlantic Ave, Brooklyn, NY 11201-6720; **Phone:** 718-855-0088; **Board Cert:** Orthopaedic Surgery 1977; **Med School:** India 1970; **Resid:** Orthopaedic Surgery, Brookdale Hosp 1976; **Fellow:** Orthopaedic Surgery, Hosp for Special Surgery 1978; **Fac Appt:** Assoc Clin Prof OrS, SUNY Hlth Sci Ctr

Menezes, Placido MD (OrS) - **Spec Exp:** Hip Replacement; Knee Replacement; Fractures; **Hospital:** New York Methodist Hosp (page 479), Brooklyn Hosp Ctr-Downtown; **Address:** 543 2nd St, Brooklyn, NY 11215-2607; **Phone:** 718-788-7600; **Board Cert:** Orthopaedic Surgery 1980; **Med School:** India 1970; **Resid:** Surgery, NY Methodist Hosp 1975; Orthopaedic Surgery, Brooklyn Jewish Hosp & Med Ctr 1978; **Fac Appt:** Asst Clin Prof OrS, SUNY Downstate

Merola, Andrew A MD (OrS) - **Spec Exp:** Spinal Surgery; Scoliosis; **Hospital:** Long Island Coll Hosp (page 90), New York Methodist Hosp (page 479); **Address:** 55 8th Ave, Brooklyn, NY 11217; **Phone:** 718-783-5542; **Board Cert:** Orthopaedic Surgery 1998; **Med School:** Hong Kong 1990; **Resid:** Orthopaedic Surgery, Kings City Hosp 1995; **Fellow:** Orthopaedic Surgery, Univ Colorado Med Ctr 1996

Morgan, Daniel J MD (OrS) - **Spec Exp:** Sports Medicine; Joint Replacement; Hip Fracture; **Hospital:** Beth Israel Med Ctr- Kings Hwy Div (page 90); **Address:** 3131 Kings Highway, Ste C11, Brooklyn, NY 11234; **Phone:** 718-258-2588; **Board Cert:** Orthopaedic Surgery 2000; **Med School:** Univ MD Sch Med 1985; **Resid:** Surgery, Beth Israel Med Ctr 1989; Orthopaedic Surgery, Kingsbrook Jewish Med Ctr 1991

Soifer, Todd MD (OrS) - **Spec Exp:** Shoulder & Knee Reconstruction; Foot & Ankle Surgery; Hip Fracture; **Hospital:** Beth Israel Med Ctr- Kings Hwy Div (page 90), Kingsbrook Jewish Med Ctr; **Address:** 3131 Kings Highway, Ste C11, Brooklyn, NY 11234-2643; **Phone:** 718-258-2588; **Board Cert:** Orthopaedic Surgery 1996; **Med School:** Mount Sinai Sch Med 1989; **Resid:** Orthopaedic Surgery, Beth Israel Med Ctr/Kingsbrook Jewish Med Ctr 1994

Splain, Shepard DO (OrS) - **Spec Exp:** Arthroscopic Surgery; Shoulder & Knee Reconstruction; Sports Medicine; **Hospital:** Brookdale Univ Hosp Med Ctr, Long Island Coll Hosp (page 90); **Address:** Linden Blvd & Rockaway Pkwy, Brooklyn, NY 11212; **Phone:** 718-240-5888; **Board Cert:** Orthopaedic Surgery 1980; **Med School:** Mich State Univ Coll Osteo Med 1973; **Resid:** Orthopaedic Surgery, Brookdale Hosp 1978; **Fellow:** Sports Medicine, Oklahoma Hlth Scis Ctr 1979; **Fac Appt:** Asst Clin Prof OrS, SUNY Downstate

Teicher, Joel MD (OrS) - **Spec Exp:** Sports Medicine; Fractures; Joint Replacement; **Hospital:** Brookdale Univ Hosp Med Ctr; **Address:** 1 Brookdale Plaza, Ste 145, Brooklyn, NY 11212; **Phone:** 718-240-5441; **Board Cert:** Orthopaedic Surgery 1969; **Med School:** NYU Sch Med 1960; **Resid:** Surgery, VA Med Ctr 1962; Orthopaedic Surgery, Mount Sinai 1967; **Fac Appt:** Asst Clin Prof OrS, SUNY Downstate

Tepler, Melvin MD (OrS) - **Hospital:** Maimonides Med Ctr (page 96); **Address:** 1252 E 9th St, Brooklyn, NY 11230-5180; **Phone:** 718-677-6000; **Board Cert:** Orthopaedic Surgery 1999; **Med School:** NY Med Coll 1980; **Resid:** Orthopaedic Surgery, Maimonides Med Ctr 1985

Tischler, Henry MD (OrS) - **Spec Exp:** Hip Replacement; Knee Replacement; Joint Reconstruction; **Hospital:** New York Methodist Hosp (page 479), St Vincent Cath Med Ctrs - Manhattan (page 375); **Address:** Brooklyn Spine & Arthritis Ctr, 263 7th Ave, Ste 2B, Brooklyn, NY 11215; **Phone:** 718-246-8700; **Board Cert:** Orthopaedic Surgery 1995; **Med School:** SUNY Downstate 1985; **Resid:** Orthopaedic Surgery, SUNY Downstate Med Ctr 1990; **Fellow:** Orthopaedic Surgery, Tampa Gen Hosp/Fla Osteo Inst 1991; **Fac Appt:** Asst Prof OrS, SUNY Hlth Sci Ctr

Walsh, Raymond MD (OrS) - **Hospital:** Lutheran Med Ctr - Brooklyn, Maimonides Med Ctr (page 96); **Address:** 355 Ovington Ave, Brooklyn, NY 11209-1453; **Phone:** 718-238-6400; **Board Cert:** Orthopaedic Surgery 1981; **Med School:** England 1974; **Resid:** Surgery, Maimonides Med Ctr 1976; Orthopaedic Surgery, Maimonides Med Ctr 1979

Wert, Sanford MD (OrS) - **Hospital:** New York Comm Hosp; **Address:** 3075 Brighton 13th St, Brooklyn, NY 11235-5607; **Phone:** 718-332-4747; **Board Cert:** Orthopaedic Surgery 1985; **Med School:** Mexico 1974; **Resid:** Orthopaedic Surgery, Long Islan 1979Maimonides 1975

Wolpin, Martin MD (OrS) - **Spec Exp:** Spinal Surgery; Spinal Diseases; Scoliosis; **Hospital:** Maimonides Med Ctr (page 96); **Address:** 1301 57th St, Brooklyn, NY 11219-4636; **Phone:** 718-438-6400; **Board Cert:** Orthopaedic Surgery 1971; **Med School:** SUNY Hlth Sci Ctr 1963; **Resid:** Surgery, Mather AFB Hosp 1966; Orthopaedic Surgery, Univ Hosp 1969; **Fac Appt:** Asst Prof, SUNY Downstate

OTOLARYNGOLOGY

Chaudhry, M Rashid MD (Oto) - **Spec Exp:** Cosmetic Surgery-Face; Sinus Surgery; **Hospital:** Brookdale Univ Hosp Med Ctr; **Address:** 1 Brookdale Plaza, Ste 157 CHC, Brooklyn, NY 11212; **Phone:** 718-240-6366; **Board Cert:** Otolaryngology 1978; **Med School:** Pakistan 1969; **Resid:** Otolaryngology, Univ Hosp 1978; **Fac Appt:** Asst Prof Oto, SUNY Downstate

Habib, Mohsen MD (Oto) - **Spec Exp:** Head & Neck Surgery; Facial Plastic/Reconstructive Surgery; Sleep Disorders/Apnea; **Hospital:** New York Methodist Hosp (page 479), Victory Memorial Hosp - Bklyn; **Address:** 7333 6th Ave, Brooklyn, NY 11209-2607; **Phone:** 718-833-0515; **Board Cert:** Otolaryngology 1983; **Med School:** Egypt 1969; **Resid:** Otolaryngology, NY Eye & Ear Infirm 1980; **Fellow:** Head and Neck Surgery, Lenox Hill Hosp 1980; **Fac Appt:** Assoc Prof Oto, NY Med Coll

Lucente, Frank MD (Oto) - **Spec Exp:** Nasal & Sinus Disorders; Ear Disorders; **Hospital:** Long Island Coll Hosp (page 90), SUNY Downstate Med Ctr; **Address:** 134 Atlantic Ave, Brooklyn, NY 11201; **Phone:** 718-780-1498; **Board Cert:** Otolaryngology 1974; **Med School:** Yale Univ 1968; **Resid:** Otolaryngology, Barnes Hosp

Mendelsohn, Michael MD (Oto) - **Spec Exp:** Pediatric Otolaryngology; **Address:** 8622 Bay Pkwy, rm 2D, Brooklyn, NY 11214; **Phone:** 718-372-8402; **Board Cert:** Otolaryngology 1999; **Med School:** Boston Univ 1990; **Resid:** Otolaryngology, LI Jewish Med Ctr 1995; **Fellow:** Pediatric Otolaryngology, Univ Virginia Med Ctr 1996

Shulman, Abraham MD (Oto) - **Spec Exp:** Hearing Disorders; Hearing Loss; Vertigo; Otology; **Hospital:** SUNY Downstate Med Ctr, Kings County Hosp Ctr; **Address:** 450 Clarkson Ave, Box 1239, Brooklyn, NY 11203-2056; **Phone:** 718-773-8888; **Board Cert:** Otolaryngology 1962; **Med School:** Switzerland 1955; **Resid:** Otolaryngology, Kings County Hosp 1960; Surgery, Lempert Inst of Otology 1960; **Fac Appt:** Prof Oto, SUNY Hlth Sci Ctr

Sperling, Neil M MD (Oto) - **Spec Exp:** Otosclerosis; Hearing Loss; Meniere's Disease; **Hospital:** Long Island Coll Hosp (page 90), New York Eye & Ear Infirm (page 110); **Address:** University Otolaryngologists, 134 Atlantic Ave, Brooklyn, NY 11201; **Phone:** 718-780-1498; **Board Cert:** Otolaryngology 1990; **Med School:** NY Med Coll 1985; **Resid:** Surgery, Beth Israel Med Ctr 1986; Otolaryngology, New York Eye & Ear Infirmary 1990; **Fellow:** Otology, Minnesota Ear Clinic 1991; **Fac Appt:** Assoc Prof Oto, SUNY Downstate

Vastola, A Paul MD (Oto) - **Spec Exp:** Throat Disorders; **Hospital:** Maimonides Med Ctr (page 96), St Vincent Cath Med Ctrs - Manhattan (page 375); **Address:** 919 49th St, Brooklyn, NY 11219-2916; **Phone:** 718-283-6260; **Board Cert:** Internal Medicine 1990; Otolaryngology 1995; **Med School:** Boston Univ 1988; **Resid:** Otolaryngology, Manhattan Eye, Ear & Throat Hospital 1993; **Fellow:** Texas Children's Hosp 1994; **Fac Appt:** Asst Clin Prof Oto, SUNY Hlth Sci Ctr

Weiss, Michael H MD (Oto) - **Spec Exp:** Head & Neck Cancer; **Hospital:** Maimonides Med Ctr (page 96), Lutheran Med Ctr - Brooklyn; **Address:** 919 49th St, Brooklyn, NY 11219-2923; **Phone:** 718-283-6260; **Board Cert:** Otolaryngology 1987; **Med School:** Albert Einstein Coll Med 1982; **Resid:** Otolaryngology, New York Univ Med Ctr 1989; **Fac Appt:** Assoc Prof Oto, SUNY Downstate

PAIN MEDICINE

Lefkowitz, Mathew MD (PM) - **Spec Exp:** Pain-Low Back; Pain after Spinal Surgery; Sciatica; **Hospital:** Long Island Coll Hosp (page 90); **Address:** 185 Montague St, Brooklyn, NY 11201; **Phone:** 718-625-4244; **Board Cert:** Pain Medicine 2005; Anesthesiology 1993; **Med School:** Belgium 1983; **Resid:** Anesthesiology, Mount Sinai Hosp 1986; **Fellow:** Pain Medicine, Mount Sinai Hosp 1987

PATHOLOGY

Mirra, Suzanne S MD (Path) - **Spec Exp:** Neuropathology; Alzheimer's Disease; **Hospital:** SUNY Downstate Med Ctr, Kings County Hosp Ctr; **Address:** SUNY Health Science Ctr, Dept Pathology, 450 Clarkson Ave, Box 25, Brooklyn, NY 11203; **Phone:** 718-270-4599; **Board Cert:** Anatomic Pathology 1973; Neuropathology 1973; **Med School:** SUNY Downstate 1967; **Resid:** Anatomic Pathology, Kings Co Hosp 1970; Neuropathology, Montefiore Med Ctr 1971; **Fellow:** Neuropathology, Yale Univ 1973; **Fac Appt:** Prof Path, SUNY Downstate

Vigorita, Vincent J MD (Path) - **Spec Exp:** Bone Pathology; **Hospital:** Maimonides Med Ctr (page 96), SUNY Downstate Med Ctr; **Address:** 4802 Tenth Ave, Brooklyn, NY 11219; **Phone:** 718-283-7025; **Board Cert:** Anatomic Pathology 1980; **Med School:** NY Med Coll 1976; **Resid:** Pathology, Johns Hopkins Hosp 1978; **Fellow:** Pathology, Meml Sloan Kettering Cancer Ctr 1979; **Fac Appt:** Prof Path, SUNY Downstate

PEDIATRIC CARDIOLOGY

Kaplovitz, Harry MD (PCd) - **Spec Exp:** Heart Murmurs; Heart Disease-Congenital; Arrhythmias; **Hospital:** Maimonides Med Ctr (page 96), Lutheran Med Ctr - Brooklyn; **Address:** Maimonides Med Ctr, Div Pediatric Cardiology, 4802 10th Ave, Ste K-106, Brooklyn, NY 11219-2844; **Phone:** 718-283-7501; **Board Cert:** Pediatrics 1988; Pediatric Cardiology 2000; **Med School:** Albert Einstein Coll Med 1981; **Resid:** Pediatrics, N Shore Univ Hosp 1984; **Fellow:** Pediatric Cardiology, New York Univ Med Ctr 1986; **Fac Appt:** Asst Prof Ped, Mount Sinai Sch Med

Presti, Salvatore MD (PCd) - **Spec Exp:** Fetal Echocardiography; Congenital Heart Disease; Kawasaki Disease; **Hospital:** Lenox Hill Hosp (page 94), Long Island Coll Hosp (page 90); **Address:** 25 Schermerhorn St, Brooklyn, NY 11201-4824; **Phone:** 718-923-1123; **Board Cert:** Pediatrics 1984; Pediatric Cardiology 2003; **Med School:** Italy 1978; **Resid:** Pediatrics, Lenox Hill Hosp 1982; **Fellow:** Pediatric Cardiology, NYU Med Ctr 1984; **Fac Appt:** Assoc Clin Prof Ped, NYU Sch Med

Ramaswamy, Prema MD (PCd) - **Spec Exp:** Fetal Echocardiography; Heart Disease-Congenital; **Hospital:** Maimonides Med Ctr (page 96); **Address:** 4802 10th Ave, Brooklyn, NY 11219-2844; **Phone:** 718-283-7501; **Board Cert:** Pediatrics 1994; Pediatric Cardiology 1996; **Med School:** India 1986; **Resid:** Pediatrics, M.Y.Hosp 1990; Pediatrics, Montefiore Med Ctr 1993; **Fellow:** Pediatric Cardiology, NY Hosp-Cornell 1996; **Fac Appt:** Asst Prof Ped, Mount Sinai Sch Med

Steinberg, L Gary MD (PCd) - **Spec Exp:** Echocardiography; Heart Murmurs; Heart Disease-Congenital; **Hospital:** Brooklyn Hosp Ctr-Downtown, New York Methodist Hosp (page 479); **Address:** Brooklyn Hosp Ctr, 121 Dekalb Ave, Maynard Bldg, Ste 11-G, Brooklyn, NY 11201; **Phone:** 718-250-6919; **Board Cert:** Pediatrics 1999; Pediatric Cardiology 1998; **Med School:** Philippines 1985; **Resid:** Pediatrics, Elmhurst Hosp 1989; **Fellow:** Pediatric Cardiology, Mount Sinai Hosp 1992

PEDIATRIC ENDOCRINOLOGY

Agdere, Levon MD (PEn) - **Spec Exp:** Diabetes; Short Stature in Children; Thyroid Disorders; **Hospital:** Brooklyn Hosp Ctr-Downtown, St Vincent Cath Med Ctr - Staten Island (page 375); **Address:** Brooklyn Hosp Ctr, 121 DeKalb Ave Maynard Bldg Fl 9 - rm 9K, Brooklyn, NY 11201; **Phone:** 718-250-8017; **Board Cert:** Pediatrics 1999; Pediatric Endocrinology 1999; **Med School:** Turkey 1981; **Resid:** Pediatrics, Lutheran Med Ctr 1986; **Fellow:** Pediatric Endocrinology, NY Hosp-Cornell Med Ctr 1989

Avruskin, Theodore W MD (PEn) - **Spec Exp:** Growth Disorders; Diabetes; Thyroid Disorders; **Hospital:** Brookdale Univ Hosp Med Ctr; **Address:** 1 Brookdale Plaza, Aaron Bldg, Ste 222, Brooklyn, NY 11212; **Phone:** 718-240-5960; **Board Cert:** Pediatrics 1965; **Med School:** Univ Toronto 1960; **Resid:** Pediatrics, Montreal Chldns Hosp 1962; Pediatrics, Chldns Hosp Med Ctr 1964; **Fellow:** Pediatric Endocrinology, Chldns Hosp Med Ctr 1968; **Fac Appt:** Prof Ped, SUNY Downstate

PEDIATRIC GASTROENTEROLOGY

Jelin, Abraham MD (PGe) - **Spec Exp:** Nutrition; Breast Feeding Problems; **Hospital:** Brooklyn Hosp Ctr-Downtown, St Vincent Cath Med Ctr - Staten Island (page 375); **Address:** Bklyn Hosp Ctr, Dept Peds, 121 Dekalb Ave, Brooklyn, NY 11201-5425; **Phone:** 718-250-6277; **Board Cert:** Pediatrics 1977; Pediatric Gastroenterology 1997; **Med School:** NYU Sch Med 1972; **Resid:** Pediatrics, Grady Mem 1973; Pediatrics, Montefiore Hosp Med Ctr 1974; **Fellow:** Pediatric Gastroenterology, Emory U Hosp 1977; **Fac Appt:** Asst Clin Prof Ped, NYU Sch Med

McFarlane-Ferreira, Yvonne B MD (PGe) - **Hospital:** New York Methodist Hosp (page 479); **Address:** NY Methodist Hosp, Dept Pediatrics, 506 6th St, Brooklyn, NY 11215; **Phone:** 718-780-5225; **Board Cert:** Pediatrics 2005; Pediatric Gastroenterology 2003; **Med School:** West Indies 1983; **Resid:** Pediatrics, Brooklyn Hosp 1989; **Fellow:** Pediatric Gastroenterology, Mt Sinai Hosp 1992; **Fac Appt:** Asst Clin Prof Ped, Mount Sinai Sch Med

Schwarz, Steven M MD (PGe) - **Spec Exp:** Gastroesophageal Reflux Disease (GERD); Nutrition; Endoscopy; **Hospital:** Long Island Coll Hosp (page 90), Beth Israel Med Ctr - Petrie Division (page 90); **Address:** LI Coll Hosp - Dept of Pediatrics, 339 Hicks St, Brooklyn, NY 11201-5514; **Phone:** 718-780-1146; **Board Cert:** Pediatrics 1979; Pediatric Gastroenterology 1998; **Med School:** Columbia P&S 1974; **Resid:** Pediatrics, Columbia-Presby Med Ctr 1977; **Fellow:** Pediatric Gastroenterology, Stanford Univ Med Ctr 1978; Pediatric Gastroenterology, Columbia-Presby Med Ctr 1980; **Fac Appt:** Prof Ped, SUNY Downstate

Treem, William R MD (PGe) - **Spec Exp:** Liver Disease; Inflammatory Bowel Disease; Crohn's Disease; **Hospital:** SUNY Downstate Med Ctr; **Address:** SUNY Downstate Med Ctr, Dept Peds, 445 Lennox Rd, Box 49, Brooklyn, NY 11203; **Phone:** 718-270-4714; **Board Cert:** Pediatrics 1981; Pediatric Gastroenterology 1997; **Med School:** Stanford Univ 1977; **Resid:** Pediatrics, Children's Hosp 1980; **Fellow:** Pediatric Gastroenterology, Children's Hosp 1985; **Fac Appt:** Prof Ped, SUNY Downstate

Wetzler, Graciela MD (PGe) - **Spec Exp:** Peptic Ulcer Disease; Gastroesophageal Reflux Disease (GERD); **Hospital:** Maimonides Med Ctr (page 96); **Address:** Maimonides Med Ctr, Dept Peds GE, 977 48th St, Brooklyn, NY 11219; **Phone:** 718-283-7329; **Board Cert:** Pediatrics 2000; Pediatric Gastroenterology 2003; **Med School:** Argentina 1984; **Resid:** Pediatrics, Montefiore Med Ctr 1992; **Fellow:** Pediatric Gastroenterology, New York Hosp-Cornell Med Ctr 1995

PEDIATRIC HEMATOLOGY-ONCOLOGY

Guarini, Ludovico MD (PHO) - **Spec Exp:** Leukemia; Solid Tumors; Sickle Cell Disease; **Hospital:** Maimonides Med Ctr (page 96); **Address:** 977 48th St, Brooklyn, NY 11220; **Phone:** 718-283-8260; **Board Cert:** Pediatrics 1984; Pediatric Hematology-Oncology 2000; **Med School:** Italy 1974; **Resid:** Pediatrics, Beth Israel Hosp 1981; **Fellow:** Pediatric Hematology-Oncology, Columbia-Presby Med Ctr 1984; **Fac Appt:** Assoc Prof Ped, Mount Sinai Sch Med

Kulpa, Jolanta MD (PHO) - **Spec Exp:** Sickle Cell Disease; Leukemia; Transfusion Free Medicine; **Hospital:** Long Island Coll Hosp (page 90), Beth Israel Med Ctr - Petrie Division (page 90); **Address:** 340 Henry St, Brooklyn, NY 11201-5514; **Phone:** 718-780-1025; **Board Cert:** Pediatrics 1983; Pediatric Hematology-Oncology 1984; **Med School:** Med Coll PA 1972; **Resid:** Pediatrics, Lenox Hill Hosp 1975; **Fellow:** Blood Banking Transfusion Medicine, NY Blood Center 1977; Pediatric Hematology-Oncology, NY Hosp/Cornell/Sloan Kettering 1979; **Fac Appt:** Asst Clin Prof Ped, SUNY Hlth Sci Ctr

Miller, Scott T MD (PHO) - **Spec Exp:** Sickle Cell Disease; Bone Tumors; Solid Tumors; **Hospital:** SUNY Downstate Med Ctr, Kings County Hosp Ctr; **Address:** Univ Hosp Brooklyn, 450 Clarkson Ave, Box 49, Brooklyn, NY 11203-2056; **Phone:** 718-270-4714; **Board Cert:** Pediatrics 1981; Pediatric Hematology-Oncology 1982; **Med School:** Albert Einstein Coll Med 1976; **Resid:** Pediatrics, Montefiore Hosp Med Ctr 1979; **Fellow:** Pediatric Hematology-Oncology, Cornell/Meml Sloan Kettering 1981; **Fac Appt:** Prof Ped, SUNY Downstate

Sadanandan, Swayam MD (PHO) - **Spec Exp:** Sickle Cell Disease; **Hospital:** Brooklyn Hosp Ctr-Downtown; **Address:** 121 Dekalb Ave, Brooklyn, NY 11201; **Phone:** 718-250-6074; **Board Cert:** Pediatrics 1980; Pediatric Hematology-Oncology 1984; **Med School:** India 1972; **Resid:** Pediatrics, St Vincent's Hosp & Med Ctr 1979; **Fellow:** Pediatric Hematology-Oncology, New York Univ Med Ctr 1981; **Fac Appt:** Asst Clin Prof Ped, NYU Sch Med

Sundaram, Revathy MD (PHO) - **Spec Exp:** Thalassemia; Sickle Cell Disease; Leukemia; **Hospital:** Long Island Coll Hosp (page 90), Beth Israel Med Ctr - Petrie Division (page 90); **Address:** 339 Hicks St, Brooklyn, NY 11201-5509; **Phone:** 718-780-1025; **Board Cert:** Pediatrics 1980; Pediatric Hematology-Oncology 1984; **Med School:** India 1973; **Resid:** Pediatrics, Long Island Hosp 1980; Pediatrics, Rutgers Univ Hosp 1978; **Fellow:** Pediatric Hematology-Oncology, Long Island Hosp 1983; **Fac Appt:** Asst Prof Ped, SUNY Hlth Sci Ctr

Viswanathan, Kusum MD (PHO) - **Spec Exp:** Sickle Cell Disease; Pediatric Cancer; Anemia; **Hospital:** Brookdale Univ Hosp Med Ctr; **Address:** 1 Brookdale Plaza, Ste 346, Brooklyn, NY 11212-3139; **Phone:** 718-240-5904; **Board Cert:** Pediatrics 1986; Pediatric Hematology-Oncology 1987; **Med School:** India 1980; **Resid:** Pediatrics, LI Coll Hosp 1984; **Fellow:** Pediatric Hematology-Oncology, LI Coll Hosp 1986; **Fac Appt:** Assoc Clin Prof Ped, SUNY Hlth Sci Ctr

PEDIATRIC INFECTIOUS DISEASE

Gesner, Matthew MD (PInf) - **Spec Exp:** AIDS/HIV; Kawasaki Disease; **Hospital:** Kings County Hosp Ctr, SUNY Downstate Med Ctr; **Address:** Kings Co Hosp, 451 Clarkson Ave, Box 294, Brooklyn, NY 11203; **Phone:** 718-245-4486; **Board Cert:** Pediatrics 2006; Pediatric Infectious Disease 2002; **Med School:** SUNY Downstate 1988; **Resid:** Pediatrics, Chldns Hosp 1991; **Fellow:** Pediatric Infectious Disease, Bellevue Hosp Ctr/NYU Sch Med 1994; **Fac Appt:** Asst Prof Ped, SUNY Downstate

PEDIATRIC NEPHROLOGY

Kaplan, Matthew MD (PNep) - **Spec Exp:** Hypertension; Glomerulonephritis; **Hospital:** Long Island Coll Hosp (page 90); **Address:** 97 Amity St Fl 2, Brooklyn, NY 11201; **Phone:** 718-780-1025; **Board Cert:** Pediatrics 1974; Pediatric Nephrology 1976; **Med School:** SUNY Downstate 1968; **Resid:** Pediatrics, NY Hosp-Cornell Med Ctr 1972; **Fellow:** Pediatric Nephrology, NY Hosp-Cornell Med Ctr 1976; **Fac Appt:** Assoc Clin Prof Ped, SUNY Downstate

Schoeneman, Morris J MD (PNep) - **Spec Exp:** Hypertension; Kidney Failure-Chronic; Urinary Tract Infection; Dialysis Care; **Hospital:** SUNY Downstate Med Ctr, St Vincent Cath Med Ctr - Staten Island (page 375); **Address:** SUNY Downstate Med Ctr, 450 Clarkson Ave, Box 49, Brooklyn, NY 11203; **Phone:** 718-270-1626; **Board Cert:** Pediatrics 1974; Pediatric Nephrology 1974; **Med School:** Georgetown Univ 1969; **Resid:** Pediatrics, U NC Hosp 1970; Pediatrics, U MD Hosp 1972; **Fellow:** Pediatric Nephrology, Albert Ein 1975; **Fac Appt:** Prof Ped, SUNY Hlth Sci Ctr

PEDIATRIC OTOLARYNGOLOGY

Rosenfeld, Richard M MD (PO) - **Spec Exp:** Sinus Disorders/Surgery; Head & Neck Surgery; Cochlear Implants; Ear Disorders/Surgery; **Hospital:** Long Island Coll Hosp (page 90), SUNY Downstate Med Ctr; **Address:** Univ Otolaryngologists, 134 Atlantic Ave, Brooklyn, NY 11201; **Phone:** 718-780-1498; **Board Cert:** Otolaryngology 1989; **Med School:** SUNY Buffalo 1984; **Resid:** Otolaryngology, Mount Sinai Med Ctr 1989; **Fellow:** Pediatric Otolaryngology, Chldn's Hosp 1991; **Fac Appt:** Prof Oto, SUNY Downstate

PEDIATRIC PULMONOLOGY

Emre, Umit Berk MD (PPul) - **Spec Exp:** Asthma; Sleep Disorders/Apnea; **Hospital:** Long Island Coll Hosp (page 90); **Address:** 97 Amity St Fl 2, Brooklyn, NY 11201; **Phone:** 718-780-1025; **Board Cert:** Pediatrics 2001; Pediatric Pulmonology 2004; **Med School:** Turkey 1984; **Resid:** Pediatrics, Univ Hosp 1986; **Fellow:** Pediatric Pulmonology, Univ Hosp 1987; **Fac Appt:** Asst Prof Ped, SUNY Downstate

Giusti, Robert MD (PPul) - **Spec Exp:** Cystic Fibrosis; Asthma; Cough-Chronic; **Hospital:** Long Island Coll Hosp (page 90), NYU Med Ctr (page 102); **Address:** 97 Amity St, Brooklyn, NY 11201-6004; **Phone:** 718-780-1025; **Board Cert:** Pediatrics 1987; Pediatric Pulmonology 2004; **Med School:** SUNY Downstate 1981; **Resid:** Pediatrics, Bellevue Hosp 1985; **Fac Appt:** Asst Prof Ped, SUNY Downstate

Narula, Pramod MD (PPul) - **Spec Exp:** Asthma; Chronic Lung Disease; **Hospital:** New York Methodist Hosp (page 479), Brooklyn Hosp Ctr-Downtown; **Address:** 506 6th St, Brooklyn, NY 11215-9008; **Phone:** 718-780-3066; **Board Cert:** Pediatrics 1998; Pulmonary Disease 2002; **Med School:** India 1977; **Resid:** Pediatrics, Winthrop Univ Hosp 1989; **Fellow:** Pediatric Pulmonology, Columbia-Presby Med Ctr 1994; **Fac Appt:** Assoc Clin Prof Ped, Cornell Univ-Weill Med Coll

Rao, Madu MD (PPul) - **Spec Exp:** Lung Disease; Asthma; **Hospital:** SUNY Downstate Med Ctr; **Address:** 450 Clarkson Ave, Box 49, Brooklyn, NY 11203-2056; **Phone:** 718-270-1524; **Board Cert:** Pediatrics 1968; Pediatric Pulmonology 2000; **Med School:** India 1961; **Resid:** Pediatrics, Kings County Hosp 1967; **Fellow:** Pediatric Pulmonology, Kings County Hosp 1969; **Fac Appt:** Prof Ped, SUNY Hlth Sci Ctr

PEDIATRIC SURGERY

Garrow, Eugene MD (PS) - **Hospital:** SUNY Downstate Med Ctr, Kings County Hosp Ctr; **Address:** 450 Clarkson Ave, Brooklyn, NY 11203; **Phone:** 718-270-1386; **Board Cert:** Surgery 1964; Pediatric Surgery 1993; **Med School:** SUNY Hlth Sci Ctr 1958; **Resid:** Surgery, Montefiore Hosp Med Ctr 1963; Pediatric Surgery, Michigan Chldns Hosp 1964; **Fac Appt:** Assoc Clin Prof S, UMDNJ-NJ Med Sch, Newark

Shlasko, Edward MD (PS) - **Spec Exp:** Laparoscopic Surgery; Robotic Surgery; **Hospital:** Maimonides Med Ctr (page 96), Mount Sinai Med Ctr (page 98); **Address:** Dept Ped Surg, 921 49th St, Brooklyn, NY 11219-2923; **Phone:** 718-283-7384; **Board Cert:** Surgery 1999; Pediatric Surgery 1994; **Med School:** Columbia P&S 1985; **Resid:** Surgery, Mount Sinai Hosp 1991; **Fellow:** Surgical Oncology, NIH-NCI Surg Branch 1989; Pediatric Surgery, SUNY Hlth Sci Ctr 1993; **Fac Appt:** Asst Prof S, Mount Sinai Sch Med

PEDIATRICS

Ajl, Stephen MD (Ped) PCP - **Hospital:** Brooklyn Hosp Ctr-Downtown; **Address:** 120 Dekalb Ave, Brooklyn, NY 11201; **Phone:** 718-250-8764; **Board Cert:** Pediatrics 1980; **Med School:** Temple Univ 1975; **Resid:** Pediatrics, NY Hosp 1978; **Fellow:** Ambulatory Pediatrics, Mount Sinai Hosp 1979; **Fac Appt:** Assoc Clin Prof Ped, SUNY Downstate

Fernandes, David R MD (Ped) PCP - **Hospital:** Long Island Coll Hosp (page 90); **Address:** 126 95th St, Brooklyn, NY 11209-7203; **Phone:** 718-238-7842; **Board Cert:** Pediatrics 1980; **Med School:** SUNY Downstate 1972; **Resid:** Pediatrics, Kings County Hosp 1974; Pediatrics, N Shore Univ Hosp 1976; **Fellow:** Ambulatory Pediatrics, NYU-Bellevue Hosp 1977; **Fac Appt:** Asst Clin Prof Ped, SUNY Downstate

Gately, Adrian MD (Ped) PCP - **Hospital:** New York Methodist Hosp (page 479); **Address:** 300 Park Pl, Brooklyn, NY 11238; **Phone:** 718-622-0469; **Board Cert:** Pediatrics 1983; **Med School:** Albert Einstein Coll Med 1975; **Resid:** Pediatrics, Jacobi Med Ctr 1978

Glaser, Amy MD (Ped) PCP - **Spec Exp:** Adolescent Medicine; **Hospital:** Long Island Coll Hosp (page 90), NYU Med Ctr (page 102); **Address:** 33 8th Ave, Brooklyn, NY 11217-3902; **Phone:** 718-636-0999; **Board Cert:** Pediatrics 1985; **Med School:** Mount Sinai Sch Med 1979; **Resid:** Pediatrics, Montefiore Hosp Med Ctr; **Fellow:** Adolescent Medicine, Mt Sinai Hospital 1983

Jackson, Rosemary MD (Ped) PCP - **Spec Exp:** Diabetes; Obesity; **Hospital:** SUNY Downstate Med Ctr, Long Island Coll Hosp (page 90); **Address:** 86 E 49th St, Ste G, Brooklyn, NY 11203; **Phone:** 718-363-6646; **Board Cert:** Pediatrics 2001; **Med School:** SUNY Upstate Med Univ 1985; **Resid:** Pediatrics, Downstate Med Ctr 1988; **Fac Appt:** Asst Clin Prof Ped, SUNY Downstate

Krieger, Ben-Zion MD (Ped) PCP - **Spec Exp:** Allergy & Immunology; **Hospital:** Maimonides Med Ctr (page 96); **Address:** 571 McDonald Ave, Brooklyn, NY 11218; **Phone:** 718-435-6700; **Board Cert:** Pediatrics 1986; **Med School:** Italy 1978; **Resid:** Pediatrics, Maimonides Med Ctr 1983; **Fellow:** Allergy & Immunology, Albert Einstein Med Ctr 1985; **Fac Appt:** Assoc Clin Prof Ped, Mount Sinai Sch Med

Mezey, Andrew MD (Ped) PCP - **Spec Exp:** Special Healthcare Needs; Behavioral Disorders; **Hospital:** Maimonides Med Ctr (page 96); **Address:** 1301 57th St, Brooklyn, NY 11219; **Phone:** 718-283-3650; **Board Cert:** Pediatrics 1966; **Med School:** NYU Sch Med 1960; **Resid:** Pediatrics, Jacobi Med Ctr 1964; **Fac Appt:** Prof Ped, Albert Einstein Coll Med

Oghia, Hady MD (Ped) PCP - **Spec Exp:** Newborn Care; **Hospital:** St Vincent Cath Med Ctr - Staten Island (page 375), Victory Memorial Hosp - Bklyn; **Address:** 8411 13th Ave, Brooklyn, NY 11228-3301; **Phone:** 718-331-3166; **Med School:** Mexico 1979; **Resid:** Pediatrics, St Vincent's Hosp & Med Ctr 1983

Preis, Oded MD (Ped) PCP - **Spec Exp:** Prematurity/Low Birth Weight Infants; **Hospital:** Maimonides Med Ctr (page 96), New York Methodist Hosp (page 479); **Address:** 1729 E 12th St, Brooklyn, NY 11229; **Phone:** 718-339-4919; **Board Cert:** Pediatrics 1978; Neonatal-Perinatal Medicine 1981; **Med School:** Israel 1971; **Resid:** Pediatrics, Maimonides Med Ctr 1975; **Fellow:** Neonatal-Perinatal Medicine, SUNY - Downstate Med Ctr 1977; **Fac Appt:** Assoc Clin Prof Ped, SUNY Downstate

Rajagopal, Venktesalu MD (Ped) - **Hospital:** SUNY Downstate Med Ctr, Kings County Hosp Ctr; **Address:** University Hospital of Brooklyn SUNY HSC Brooklyn, 451 Clarkson Ave, rm B-6202, Brooklyn, NY 11203; **Phone:** 718-245-4105; **Board Cert:** Pediatrics 1967; **Med School:** India 1962; **Resid:** Pediatrics, Norwalk Hosp 1964Kings Co Hosp 1966; **Fac Appt:** Clin Prof Ped, SUNY Hlth Sci Ctr

Santilli, Veronica MD (Ped) PCP - **Spec Exp:** Adolescent Medicine; Chronic Disease; Special Healthcare Needs; **Hospital:** Maimonides Med Ctr (page 96), Lutheran Med Ctr - Brooklyn; **Address:** 2462 65th St, Brooklyn, NY 11204-4150; **Phone:** 718-376-6600; **Board Cert:** Pediatrics 1972; **Med School:** Med Coll PA Hahnemann 1966; **Resid:** Pediatrics, Maimonides Med Ctr 1969

Schaeffer, Henry MD (Ped) PCP - **Hospital:** Maimonides Med Ctr (page 96), Coney Island Hosp; **Address:** Maimonides Medical Ctr, Dept Pediatrics, 4802 10th Ave, Brooklyn, NY 11219-2844; **Phone:** 718-283-8918; **Board Cert:** Pediatrics 1969; **Med School:** NYU Sch Med 1963; **Resid:** Pediatrics, Bellevue Hosp/NYU Med Ctr 1968; **Fac Appt:** Clin Prof Ped, Mount Sinai Sch Med

Sen, Dilip MD (Ped) PCP - **Hospital:** New York Methodist Hosp (page 479), SUNY Downstate Med Ctr; **Address:** 6 Sutter Ave, Brooklyn, NY 11212-3838; **Phone:** 718-756-1355; **Board Cert:** Pediatrics 2002; **Med School:** India 1966; **Resid:** Pediatrics, New York Methodist Hospital 1981; **Fellow:** Pediatrics, Downstate Med Center 1983; **Fac Appt:** Asst Prof Ped, SUNY Downstate

Sergiou, Harry MD (Ped) PCP - **Hospital:** Long Island Coll Hosp (page 90); **Address:** 554 Henry St, Brooklyn, NY 11231; **Phone:** 718-625-5591; **Board Cert:** Pediatrics 2004; **Med School:** Greece 1979; **Resid:** Pediatrics, Long Island Coll Hosp 1985

Shelov, Steven MD (Ped) PCP - **Spec Exp:** Behavioral Disorders; **Hospital:** Maimonides Med Ctr (page 96), Lutheran Med Ctr - Brooklyn; **Address:** Dept Pediatrics, 4802 10th Ave, Brooklyn, NY 11219-2844; **Phone:** 718-283-6150; **Board Cert:** Pediatrics 1976; **Med School:** Med Coll Wisc 1971; **Resid:** Pediatrics, Montefiore Med Ctr 1975; **Fac Appt:** Prof Ped, Mount Sinai Sch Med

Trainin, Eugene MD (Ped) PCP - **Hospital:** New York Methodist Hosp (page 479), Maimonides Med Ctr (page 96); **Address:** 1909 Quentin Rd, Brooklyn, NY 11229-2370; **Phone:** 718-627-1999; **Board Cert:** Pediatrics 1975; Pediatric Nephrology ; **Med School:** SUNY Hlth Sci Ctr 1970; **Resid:** Pediatrics, Kings Coun 1973; **Fellow:** Pediatric Nephrology, Albert Ein 1976

Wu, Jason J MD/PhD (Ped) `PCP` - **Spec Exp:** Chinese Community Health; **Hospital:** Maimonides Med Ctr (page 96); **Address:** Pediatrics at 8th Ave, 4711 8th Ave, Brooklyn, NY 11220; **Phone:** 718-633-0300; **Board Cert:** Pediatrics 2002; **Med School:** China 1982; **Resid:** Pediatrics, Maimonides Med Ctr 2001; **Fac Appt:** Asst Clin Prof Ped, Mount Sinai Sch Med

PHYSICAL MEDICINE & REHABILITATION

Atakent, Pinar MD (PMR) - **Spec Exp:** Pain Management; Stroke Rehabilitation; Electrodiagnosis; Acupuncture; **Hospital:** Long Island Coll Hosp (page 90); **Address:** LI Coll Hosp, 339 Hicks St, Brooklyn, NY 11201-5509; **Phone:** 718-780-4685; **Board Cert:** Physical Medicine & Rehabilitation 1982; **Med School:** Turkey 1971; **Resid:** Physical Medicine & Rehabilitation, Jacobi Med Ctr 1981; **Fac Appt:** Asst Clin Prof PMR, SUNY Hlth Sci Ctr

Gifford, Irina MD (PMR) - **Spec Exp:** Musculoskeletal Disorders; Neurological Disorders; Rehabilitation-Pediatric; **Hospital:** Kingsbrook Jewish Med Ctr; **Address:** 585 Schenectady Ave, Ste 333, Brooklyn, NY 11203-1822; **Phone:** 718-604-5369; **Board Cert:** Physical Medicine & Rehabilitation 1990; **Med School:** Romania 1960; **Resid:** Physical Medicine & Rehabilitation, Mount Sinai Hosp 1989; **Fellow:** Physical Medicine & Rehabilitation, Albert Einstein 1990

Stein, Perry MD (PMR) - **Spec Exp:** Pain Management; **Hospital:** Mercy Med Ctr - Rockville Centre, Maimonides Med Ctr (page 96); **Address:** 383 Ocean Pkwy, Brooklyn, NY 11218; **Phone:** 718-941-6000; **Board Cert:** Physical Medicine & Rehabilitation 1991; **Med School:** Mexico 1985; **Resid:** Physical Medicine & Rehabilitation, Univ Hosp 1990

Vallarino, Ramon MD (PMR) - **Spec Exp:** Pain Management; Functional Ability Loss; Electromyography; **Hospital:** New York Methodist Hosp (page 479); **Address:** 816 8th Ave, Brooklyn, NY 11215; **Phone:** 718-788-5762; **Board Cert:** Physical Medicine & Rehabilitation 1977; **Med School:** Peru 1966; **Resid:** Physical Medicine & Rehabilitation, Mount Sinai Hosp 1968; **Fellow:** Rheumatology, Mount Sinai Hosp 1968; **Fac Appt:** Asst Clin Prof PMR, SUNY Hlth Sci Ctr

PLASTIC SURGERY

Feldman, David L MD (PlS) - **Spec Exp:** Cosmetic Surgery; Laser Surgery; **Hospital:** Maimonides Med Ctr (page 96), Lutheran Med Ctr - Brooklyn; **Address:** 925 49th St, Brooklyn, NY 11219; **Phone:** 718-283-7022; **Board Cert:** Plastic Surgery 1994; **Med School:** Duke Univ 1984; **Resid:** Surgery, St Luke's/Roosevelt 1989; Plastic Surgery, Duke Univ Med Ctr 1992; **Fellow:** Hand Surgery, Kleinert Inst for Hand/Microsurg; **Fac Appt:** Asst Prof PlS, Mount Sinai Sch Med

Roth, Malcolm Z MD (PlS) - **Spec Exp:** Cosmetic Surgery-Liposuction; Cosmetic Surgery-Breast; Cosmetic Surgery-Face & Eyelid; Body Contouring after Weight Loss; **Hospital:** Maimonides Med Ctr (page 96), Beth Israel Med Ctr - Petrie Division (page 90); **Address:** 925 49th St, Brooklyn, NY 11219; **Phone:** 718-283-7022; **Board Cert:** Plastic Surgery 1991; **Med School:** NY Med Coll 1982; **Resid:** Surgery, Beth Israel Med Ctr 1985; Plastic Surgery, NY Hosp 1987; **Fellow:** Hand Surgery, Hosp Special Surg 1988; **Fac Appt:** Asst Clin Prof PlS, SUNY Hlth Sci Ctr

Kings (Brooklyn)

PREVENTIVE MEDICINE

Imperato, Pascal James MD (PrM) - **Spec Exp:** Infectious Disease; Tropical Diseases; **Hospital:** SUNY Downstate Med Ctr, Kings County Hosp Ctr; **Address:** 450 Clarkson Ave, Box 43, Brooklyn, NY 11203-2056; **Phone:** 718-270-1056; **Board Cert:** Public Health & Genl Preventive Med 1972; **Med School:** SUNY Hlth Sci Ctr 1962; **Resid:** Internal Medicine, Long Island College Hosp 1965; **Fellow:** Tropical Medicine, Tulane Univ Sch Pub Hlth 1966; **Fac Appt:** Prof PrM, SUNY Downstate

PSYCHIATRY

Berkowitz, Howard MD (Psyc) - **Spec Exp:** Anxiety Disorders; Depression; Geriatric Psychiatry; **Hospital:** Maimonides Med Ctr (page 96); **Address:** 4715 Fort Hamilton Pkwy, Brooklyn, NY 11219-2927; **Phone:** 718-633-2025; **Board Cert:** Psychiatry 1977; Geriatric Psychiatry 2004; **Med School:** Albert Einstein Coll Med 1972; **Resid:** Internal Medicine, Beth Israel Hosp 1973; Psychiatry, Kings County Hosp 1976; **Fellow:** Consultation Psychiatry, Kings County Hosp 1977; **Fac Appt:** Assoc Clin Prof Psyc, SUNY Downstate

Coplan, Jeremy MD (Psyc) - **Spec Exp:** Anxiety Disorders; Psychosomatic Disorders; Bipolar/Mood Disorders; **Hospital:** SUNY Downstate Med Ctr; **Address:** 450 Clarkson Ave, Box 1203, Brooklyn, NY 11203; **Phone:** 718-270-2023; **Board Cert:** Psychiatry 1990; **Med School:** South Africa 1983; **Resid:** Psychiatry, SUNY-Downstate Med Ctr 1989; **Fellow:** Biological Psychiatry, Columbia-Presby Med Ctr; **Fac Appt:** Prof Psyc, SUNY Downstate

Eitan, Noam MD (Psyc) - **Spec Exp:** Anxiety Disorders; Depression; Gay & Lesbian Issues; **Hospital:** Woodhull Med & Mental Hlth Ctr; **Address:** 760 Broadway, Brooklyn, NY 11206; **Phone:** 718-963-5793; **Board Cert:** Psychiatry 1998; **Med School:** Israel 1986; **Resid:** Psychiatry, Shalvata Hosp 1991; **Fellow:** Psychoanalysis, Sackler Sch Med 1995

Goldberg, Jeffrey DO (Psyc) - **Spec Exp:** Geriatric Psychiatry; Anxiety & Depression; **Hospital:** Maimonides Med Ctr (page 96); **Address:** 5025 Ft Hamilton Pkwy, Brooklyn, NY 11219; **Phone:** 718-633-8183; **Board Cert:** Psychiatry 1986; Geriatric Psychiatry 1996; **Med School:** NY Coll Osteo Med 1981; **Resid:** Psychiatry, Maimonides Med Ctr 1985; **Fac Appt:** Asst Clin Prof Psyc, SUNY Downstate

Idupuganti, Sudharam MD (Psyc) - **Spec Exp:** Depression; Electroconvulsive Therapy (ECT); Panic Disorder; **Hospital:** Maimonides Med Ctr (page 96), Victory Memorial Hosp - Bklyn; **Address:** 585 Bayridge Pkwy, Brooklyn, NY 11209; **Phone:** 718-921-1001; **Board Cert:** Psychiatry 1981; **Med School:** India 1974; **Resid:** Psychiatry, Maimonides Med Ctr 1979; **Fac Appt:** Asst Prof Psyc, SUNY Downstate

Levy, Norman B MD (Psyc) - **Spec Exp:** Eating Disorders; Somatic Psychiatry; Psychiatry in Physical Illness; **Hospital:** Kingsboro Psyc Ctr; **Address:** 169 Westminster Rd, Brooklyn, NY 11218-3445; **Phone:** 718-693-6280; **Board Cert:** Psychiatry 1967; **Med School:** SUNY Downstate 1956; **Resid:** Internal Medicine, Univ Pittsburgh 1958; Psychiatry, Kings Co/Downstate Med Ctr 1963; **Fellow:** Psychosomatic Medicine, Kings Co/Downstate Med Ctr 1965; **Fac Appt:** Prof Psyc, SUNY Downstate

Licht, Arnold MD (Psyc) - **Spec Exp:** Geriatric Psychiatry; Mood Disorders; Addiction Psychiatry; **Hospital:** Long Island Coll Hosp (page 90); **Address:** LI Coll Hosp, Dept Psych, 339 Hicks St Fl 6, Brooklyn, NY 11201-5509; **Phone:** 718-935-0986; **Board Cert:** Psychiatry 1975; Geriatric Psychiatry 2001; Addiction Psychiatry 1996; **Med School:** SUNY Hlth Sci Ctr 1969; **Resid:** Psychiatry, Albert Einstein 1973; **Fac Appt:** Asst Prof Psyc, SUNY Downstate

Lipkowitz, Marvin MD (Psyc) - **Spec Exp:** Depression; **Hospital:** Maimonides Med Ctr (page 96); **Address:** Maimonides Mntl Hlth Ctr, 920 48th St, Brooklyn, NY 11219; **Phone:** 718-283-8163; **Board Cert:** Psychiatry 1963; **Med School:** Temple Univ 1956; **Resid:** Psychiatry, Kings Co Hosp 1960; **Fac Appt:** Clin Prof Psyc, SUNY Downstate

Nayak, Devdutt MD (Psyc) - **Spec Exp:** Psychopharmacology; Electroconvulsive Therapy (ECT); Medical Illness in Psychiatry; **Hospital:** New York Methodist Hosp (page 479); **Address:** 517 6th St, Brooklyn, NY 11215-3608; **Phone:** 718-780-3771; **Board Cert:** Psychiatry 1977; Geriatric Psychiatry 1992; Addiction Psychiatry 1993; Forensic Psychiatry 1996; **Med School:** India 1969; **Resid:** Psychiatry, LI Jewish Med Ctr 1976; **Fac Appt:** Assoc Clin Prof Psyc, Cornell Univ-Weill Med Coll

Segura-Bustamante, Alina MD (Psyc) - **Spec Exp:** Chronic Illness; Child & Adolescent Psychiatry; **Hospital:** Long Island Coll Hosp (page 90); **Address:** 97 Amity St, Brooklyn Heights, NY 11201; **Phone:** 718-780-1070; **Board Cert:** Psychiatry 1989; Child & Adolescent Psychiatry 1997; **Med School:** Spain 1979; **Resid:** Psychiatry, Univ Hosp 1983; **Fellow:** Psychiatry, Univ Hosp 1985; **Fac Appt:** Psyc, SUNY Downstate

Sultan, Joseph A. MD (Psyc) - **Hospital:** Maimonides Med Ctr (page 96); **Address:** 913 49th St, Brooklyn, NY 11219-2923; **Phone:** 718-851-1144; **Board Cert:** Psychiatry 1977; **Med School:** Albert Einstein Coll Med 1968; **Resid:** Psychiatry, Montefiore Hosp Med Ctr 1972; Psychiatry, Bronx Psychiatric Ctr 1974; **Fac Appt:** Asst Clin Prof Psyc, SUNY Downstate

Viswanathan, Ramaswamy MD (Psyc) - **Spec Exp:** Depression; Anxiety Disorders; **Hospital:** SUNY Downstate Med Ctr, Kings County Hosp Ctr; **Address:** 450 Clarkson Ave, Ste B5-350, Brooklyn, NY 11203-2098; **Phone:** 718-270-2352; **Board Cert:** Psychiatry 1978; Internal Medicine 1989; Addiction Psychiatry 2003; Geriatric Psychiatry 2002; **Med School:** India 1972; **Resid:** Internal Medicine, Qns Hosp Ctr 1974; Psychiatry, SUNY Hlth Sci Ctr 1977; **Fellow:** Psychiatry, SUNY Hlth Sci Ctr 1978; **Fac Appt:** Assoc Clin Prof Psyc, SUNY Hlth Sci Ctr

Weiden, Peter MD (Psyc) - **Spec Exp:** Schizophrenia; Psychopharmacology; **Hospital:** SUNY Downstate Med Ctr; **Address:** Univ Hosp, Dept Psyc, 450 Clarkson Ave, Box 1203, Brooklyn, NY 11203; **Phone:** 718-270-4483; **Board Cert:** Psychiatry 1986; **Med School:** SUNY Stony Brook 1981; **Resid:** Psychiatry, NY Hosp 1985; **Fac Appt:** Assoc Prof Psyc, SUNY Downstate

Pulmonary Disease

Abott, Michael MD (Pul) - **Spec Exp:** Asthma; Emphysema; **Hospital:** New York Methodist Hosp (page 479), Maimonides Med Ctr (page 96); **Address:** 7124 18th Ave, Brooklyn, NY 11204-5203; **Phone:** 718-234-3333; **Board Cert:** Internal Medicine 1983; Pulmonary Disease 1986; Critical Care Medicine 1991; Geriatric Medicine 1994; **Med School:** Mexico 1978; **Resid:** Internal Medicine, Coney Island Hosp 1982; **Fellow:** Pulmonary Disease, Albert Einstein Coll Med 1984

Akerman, Michael MD (Pul) - **Spec Exp:** Asthma; Pulmonary Disease; **Hospital:** SUNY Downstate Med Ctr; **Address:** 450 Clarkson Ave, Box 19, Brooklyn, NY 11203-2056; **Phone:** 718-270-4247; **Board Cert:** Internal Medicine 1984; Pulmonary Disease 1986; Geriatric Medicine 1994; Critical Care Medicine 1999; **Med School:** Univ Rochester 1981; **Resid:** Internal Medicine, Brookdale Med Ctr 1985; **Fellow:** Pulmonary Disease, SUNY Downstate-Hlth Sci Ctr 1986; **Fac Appt:** Assoc Prof Med, SUNY Downstate

Amin, Hossam H MD (Pul) - **Spec Exp:** Asthma & Allergy; Critical Care; **Hospital:** Metropolitan Hosp Ctr - NY, New York Methodist Hosp (page 479); **Address:** 370 Bay Ridge Pkwy, Ste G, Brooklyn, NY 11209; **Phone:** 718-238-6161; **Board Cert:** Internal Medicine 1996; Pulmonary Disease 1998; Critical Care Medicine 1999; **Med School:** Egypt 1988; **Resid:** Internal Medicine, Interfaith Med Ctr 1993; **Fellow:** Pulmonary Disease, Interfaith Med Ctr 1998; Critical Care Medicine, Mt Sinai Med Ctr 1990; **Fac Appt:** Assoc Prof Med, NY Med Coll

Bakoss, Imad John MD (Pul) - **Spec Exp:** Asthma & Chronic Lung Disease; Lung Cancer; Sleep Disorders; **Hospital:** Lutheran Med Ctr - Brooklyn, New York Methodist Hosp (page 479); **Address:** 2165 71st St Fl 1, Brooklyn, NY 11204; **Phone:** 718-621-7100; **Board Cert:** Internal Medicine 1977; Pulmonary Disease 1980; **Med School:** Iraq 1972; **Resid:** Internal Medicine, LI Coll Hosp 1977; **Fellow:** Pulmonary Disease, LI Coll Hosp 1978; Pulmonary Disease, NY Hosp-Cornell Med Ctr 1979

Bergman, Michael I MD (Pul) - **Spec Exp:** Asthma; Bronchitis; Respiratory Failure; Pneumonia; **Hospital:** Long Island Coll Hosp (page 90); **Address:** 339 Hicks St, Brooklyn, NY 11201; **Phone:** 718-780-1416; **Board Cert:** Internal Medicine 1981; Pulmonary Disease 1984; Critical Care Medicine 1997; **Med School:** Albert Einstein Coll Med 1978; **Resid:** Internal Medicine, Brookdale Hosp 1981; **Fellow:** Pulmonary Disease, Mount Sinai Hosp 1984; **Fac Appt:** Asst Prof Med, SUNY Hlth Sci Ctr

Bernstein, Chaim MD (Pul) - **Spec Exp:** Asthma; Emphysema; Lung Cancer; **Hospital:** Beth Israel Med Ctr-Kings Hwy Div (page 90), New York Comm Hosp; **Address:** 3131 Kings Hwy, Ste D10, Brooklyn, NY 11234-2643; **Phone:** 718-252-3590; **Board Cert:** Internal Medicine 1977; Pulmonary Disease 1982; Critical Care Medicine 1997; **Med School:** NYU Sch Med 1974; **Resid:** Internal Medicine, Brookdale Med Ctr 1977; Pulmonary Disease, Manhattan VA Hosp; **Fellow:** Pulmonary Disease, Bellevue Hosp-NYU 1979

Bernstein, Martin MD (Pul) - **Spec Exp:** Asthma; Chronic Obstructive Lung Disease (COPD); Lung Cancer; **Hospital:** Maimonides Med Ctr (page 96), Beth Israel Med Ctr- Kings Hwy Div (page 90); **Address:** 2107 Avenue N, Brooklyn, NY 11210-5041; **Phone:** 718-434-3320; **Board Cert:** Internal Medicine 1963; Pulmonary Disease 1974; **Med School:** SUNY Hlth Sci Ctr 1956; **Resid:** Internal Medicine, Maimonides Med Ctr 1958; Internal Medicine, Maimonides Med Ctr 1959; **Fellow:** Pulmonary Disease, Kings County Hosp; Pulmonary Disease, Columbia-Presby; **Fac Appt:** Asst Clin Prof Med, SUNY Downstate

Bondi, Elliott MD (Pul) - **Spec Exp:** Asthma; Tuberculosis; Pneumonia; **Hospital:** Brookdale Univ Hosp Med Ctr; **Address:** Brookdale Hospital, Pulmonary Medicine, 1 Brookdale Plaza, Brooklyn, NY 11212; **Phone:** 718-240-5236; **Board Cert:** Internal Medicine 1982; Pulmonary Disease 1987; **Med School:** Univ MD Sch Med 1971; **Resid:** Internal Medicine, Maimonides Medical Ctr 1973; Internal Medicine, Bronx Municipal Hosp 1974; **Fellow:** Pulmonary Disease, Bronx Municipal Hosp 1976; **Fac Appt:** Assoc Clin Prof Med, SUNY Downstate

Demetis, Spiro MD (Pul) - **Spec Exp:** Sarcoidosis; Lung Cancer; Asthma & Emphysema; **Hospital:** SUNY Downstate Med Ctr, Lutheran Med Ctr - Brooklyn; **Address:** 450 Clarkson Ave, Box 19, Brooklyn, NY 11203; **Phone:** 718-270-1821; **Board Cert:** Internal Medicine 1989; **Med School:** Mexico 1983; **Resid:** Internal Medicine, Univ Hosp 1988; **Fellow:** Pulmonary Disease, Univ Hosp 1990; Critical Care Medicine, Univ Hosp 1991; **Fac Appt:** Assoc Prof Med, SUNY Hlth Sci Ctr

Dhar, Santi MD (Pul) - **Spec Exp:** Asthma; Lung Cancer; Tuberculosis; **Hospital:** Coney Island Hosp; **Address:** 2601 Ocean Pkwy, Brooklyn, NY 11235-7745; **Phone:** 718-616-3171; **Board Cert:** Internal Medicine 1972; Pulmonary Disease 1974; Critical Care Medicine 2001; **Med School:** India 1958; **Resid:** Internal Medicine, Polyclinic Hosp 1968; Internal Medicine, NY Med Coll 1971; **Fellow:** Pulmonary Disease, Albert Einstein Coll Med 1973; **Fac Appt:** Assoc Clin Prof Med, SUNY Downstate

Groopman, Jacob MD (Pul) - **Spec Exp:** Asthma; Emphysema; **Hospital:** Maimonides Med Ctr (page 96); **Address:** Pulmonary & Critical Care Medicine, 953 49th St Fl 5, Brooklyn, NY 11219-2923; **Phone:** 718-283-8380; **Board Cert:** Internal Medicine 1979; Pulmonary Disease 1980; **Med School:** SUNY Hlth Sci Ctr 1974; **Resid:** Internal Medicine, Maimonides Med Ctr 1978; **Fellow:** Pulmonary Disease, NYU Med Ctr 1980; **Fac Appt:** Asst Prof Med, Mount Sinai Sch Med

Gulrajani, Ramesh MD (Pul) - **Spec Exp:** Asthma; Sarcoidosis; Lung Cancer; **Hospital:** Brooklyn Hosp Ctr-Downtown; **Address:** 121 Dekalb Ave, Ste 7F, Brooklyn, NY 11201-5425; **Phone:** 718-250-6950; **Board Cert:** Internal Medicine 1979; Pulmonary Disease 1984; **Med School:** India 1974; **Resid:** Internal Medicine, Brooklyn Cumberland Med Ctr 1979; **Fellow:** Pulmonary Disease, Brooklyn Cumberland Med Ctr 1981; **Fac Appt:** Assoc Clin Prof Med, Cornell Univ-Weill Med Coll

Hammer, Arthur MD (Pul) - **Spec Exp:** Asthma; Sleep Disorders; Pulmonary Fibrosis; **Hospital:** Beth Israel Med Ctr- Kings Hwy Div (page 90), New York Comm Hosp; **Address:** 3131 Kings Hwy, Ste D10, Brooklyn, NY 11234-2643; **Phone:** 718-252-3590; **Board Cert:** Internal Medicine 1996; Pulmonary Disease 1998; **Med School:** Mexico 1970; **Resid:** Internal Medicine, Brookdale Hosp 1974; **Fellow:** Pulmonary Disease, NYU Med Sch 1976

Kupfer, Yizhak MD (Pul) - **Spec Exp:** Sleep & Snoring Disorders; Cough; Mechanical Ventilation; **Hospital:** Maimonides Med Ctr (page 96); **Address:** Div Pulmonary & Critical Care Medicine, 953 49th St Fl 5 - Ste 511, Brooklyn, NY 11219-2923; **Phone:** 718-283-8380; **Board Cert:** Internal Medicine 1989; Pulmonary Disease 2000; Critical Care Medicine 2000; **Med School:** SUNY Downstate 1986; **Resid:** Internal Medicine, Maimonides Med Ctr 1989; **Fellow:** Pulmonary Disease, Maimonides Med Ctr 1991; Critical Care Medicine, Maimonides Med Ctr 1992; **Fac Appt:** Assoc Clin Prof Med, SUNY Downstate

Lombardo, Gerard MD (Pul) - **Spec Exp:** Sleep Apnea; Sleep & Snoring Disorders; **Hospital:** New York Methodist Hosp (page 479); **Address:** Ctr for Sleep Disorders, Med & Research, 519 Sixth St, Brooklyn, NY 11215-3609; **Phone:** 718-780-3017; **Board Cert:** Internal Medicine 1984; Pulmonary Disease 1986; Critical Care Medicine 1989; Sleep Medicine 1994; **Med School:** Grenada 1981; **Resid:** Internal Medicine, NY Methodist Hosp 1982; Internal Medicine, NY Methodist Hosp 1984; **Fellow:** Pulmonary Disease, NY Methodist Hosp 1986; **Fac Appt:** Assoc Clin Prof Med, Cornell Univ-Weill Med Coll

Miarrostami, Rameen M. MD (Pul) - **Spec Exp:** Asthma; Chronic Obstructive Lung Disease (COPD); Emphysema; **Hospital:** New York Methodist Hosp (page 479), Victory Memorial Hosp - Bklyn; **Address:** 7124 18th Ave Fl 2, Brooklyn, NY 11204-5203; **Phone:** 718-234-3333; **Board Cert:** Internal Medicine 2001; Pulmonary Disease 2004; **Med School:** Dominican Republic 1985; **Resid:** Internal Medicine, Lincoln Med Ctr 1991; **Fellow:** Pulmonary Disease, LI Coll Hosp 1993

Raoof, Suhail MD (Pul) - **Spec Exp:** Critical Care Medicine; Lung Cancer; Chronic Obstructive Lung Disease (COPD); **Hospital:** New York Methodist Hosp (page 479); **Address:** New York Methodist Hosp, Pulmonary Med, 506 6th St, Brooklyn, NY 11215; **Phone:** 718-780-5835; **Board Cert:** Internal Medicine 2002; Pulmonary Disease 2003; Critical Care Medicine 2004; **Med School:** India 1982; **Resid:** Internal Medicine, LIJ Med Ctr 1989; Internal Medicine, Nassau County Med Ctr 1991; **Fellow:** Pulmonary Critical Care Medicine, Stony Brook Affil Hosps 1992; **Fac Appt:** Assoc Prof Med, SUNY Stony Brook

Saleh, Anthony MD (Pul) - **Spec Exp:** Asthma; Interstitial Lung Disease; Lung Cancer; **Hospital:** New York Methodist Hosp (page 479); **Address:** 7206 7th Ave, Brooklyn, NY 11209; **Phone:** 718-745-1200; **Board Cert:** Internal Medicine 1988; Pulmonary Disease 2000; **Med School:** Grenada 1985; **Resid:** Internal Medicine, New York Methodist Hosp 1988; **Fellow:** Pulmonary Disease, New York Methodist Hosp 1990; **Fac Appt:** Asst Clin Prof Med, Cornell Univ-Weill Med Coll

Smith, Peter R MD (Pul) - **Spec Exp:** Asthma; Chronic Obstructive Lung Disease (COPD); Smoking Cessation; Pneumonia; **Hospital:** Long Island Coll Hosp (page 90); **Address:** Long Island Coll Hosp, Div Pulmonology, 339 Hicks St, Brooklyn, NY 11201-5514; **Phone:** 718-780-2905; **Board Cert:** Internal Medicine 1973; Pulmonary Disease 1974; Critical Care Medicine 1997; **Med School:** Columbia P&S 1968; **Resid:** Internal Medicine, Downstate Med Ctr 1970; Internal Medicine, Jacobi Med Ctr 1971; **Fellow:** Pulmonary Disease, Downstate Med Ctr 1974; **Fac Appt:** Clin Prof Med, SUNY Hlth Sci Ctr

Tessler, Sidney MD (Pul) - **Spec Exp:** Cough; Asthma; Mechanical Ventilation; **Hospital:** Maimonides Med Ctr (page 96); **Address:** 953 49th St Fl 5 - rm 511, Div Pul & Critical Care Med, Brooklyn, NY 11219-2923; **Phone:** 718-283-8380; **Board Cert:** Internal Medicine 1977; Pulmonary Disease 1980; Critical Care Medicine 1997; **Med School:** SUNY Hlth Sci Ctr 1970; **Resid:** Internal Medicine, Coney Island Hosp 1972; Internal Medicine, Maimonides Med Ctr 1976; **Fellow:** Pulmonary Disease, Maimonides Med Ctr 1977; **Fac Appt:** Clin Prof Med, SUNY Hlth Sci Ctr

RADIATION ONCOLOGY

Ashamalla, Hani MD (RadRO) - **Spec Exp:** Brain Tumors; Prostate Cancer; Gastrointestinal Cancer; **Hospital:** New York Methodist Hosp (page 479); **Address:** Dept Radiation Oncology, 506 6th St, Brooklyn, NY 11215; **Phone:** 718-780-3677; **Board Cert:** Radiation Oncology 2004; **Med School:** Egypt 1983; **Resid:** Radiation Oncology, NY Methodist Hosp 1994; **Fellow:** Radiation Oncology, NY Methodist Hosp 1995; Radiation Oncology, Children's Hosp 1995; **Fac Appt:** Asst Clin Prof Rad, Cornell Univ-Weill Med Coll

Cooper, Jay MD (RadRO) - **Spec Exp:** Head & Neck Cancer; Skin Cancer; Chemo-Radiation Combined Therapy; **Hospital:** Maimonides Med Ctr (page 96); **Address:** Maimonides Cancer Ctr, 6300 8th Ave, Brooklyn, NY 11220; **Phone:** 718-765-2700; **Board Cert:** Therapeutic Radiology 1977; **Med School:** NYU Sch Med 1973; **Resid:** Radiation Oncology, NYU Med Ctr 1977

Donahue, Bernadine R MD (RadRO) - **Spec Exp:** Brain Tumors; **Hospital:** Maimonides Med Ctr (page 96); **Address:** Maimonides Med Ctr, Dept Radiation Oncology, 6300 8th Ave, Lower Level, New York, NY 11220; **Phone:** 718-765-2700; **Board Cert:** Internal Medicine 1987; Radiation Oncology 1991; **Med School:** Boston Univ 1984; **Resid:** Internal Medicine, Boston Univ Med Ctr 1987; **Fellow:** Radiation Oncology, NYU Med Ctr 1990

Gliedman, Paul MD (RadRO) - **Spec Exp:** Breast Cancer; Prostate Cancer; Brain Tumors; **Hospital:** St Luke's - Roosevelt Hosp Ctr - Roosevelt Div (page 90), Beth Israel Med Ctr - Petrie Division (page 90); **Address:** Brooklyn Radiation Oncology, 2101 Avenue X, Brooklyn, NY 11235; **Phone:** 718-891-6800; **Board Cert:** Radiation Oncology 1987; **Med School:** Columbia P&S 1983; **Resid:** Radiation Oncology, NYU Med Ctr 1987

Huh, Sun MD (RadRO) - **Spec Exp:** Prostate Cancer; **Hospital:** Brooklyn Hosp Ctr-Downtown, Kingsbrook Jewish Med Ctr; **Address:** 121 Dekalb Ave, Brooklyn, NY 11201; **Phone:** 718-250-8248; **Board Cert:** Radiation Oncology 1974; **Med School:** South Korea 1964; **Resid:** Surgery, Jamaica Med Ctr 1971; Radiation Oncology, Meml Sloan-Kettering 1974; **Fellow:** Radiation Oncology, Meml Sloan Kettering Cancer Ctr 1975; **Fac Appt:** Asst Prof Rad, Mount Sinai Sch Med

Rafla, Sameer Demetrious MD (RadRO) - **Spec Exp:** Head & Neck Cancer; Urologic Cancer; Brachytherapy; **Hospital:** New York Methodist Hosp (page 479), St Vincent Cath Med Ctrs - Manhattan (page 375); **Address:** 506 6th St, Brooklyn, NY 11215-3609; **Phone:** 718-780-3677; **Board Cert:** Therapeutic Radiology 1976; **Med School:** Egypt 1954; **Resid:** Radiology, Cairo Univ Hosp 1956; Radiation Oncology, Royal Marsden Hosp 1965; **Fellow:** Radiology, Royal Marsden Hosp 1967; **Fac Appt:** Clin Prof RadRO, Cornell Univ-Weill Med Coll

Rotman, Marvin MD (RadRO) - **Spec Exp:** Bladder Cancer; Gynecologic Cancer; Breast Cancer; Prostate Cancer; **Hospital:** SUNY Downstate Med Ctr, Long Island Coll Hosp (page 90); **Address:** 450 Clarkson Ave, Box 1211, Brooklyn, NY 11203-2056; **Phone:** 718-270-2181; **Board Cert:** Radiology 1966; Radiation Oncology 1999; **Med School:** Jefferson Med Coll 1958; **Resid:** Internal Medicine, Albert Einstein Med Ctr 1960; Radiation Oncology, Montefiore Hosp Med Ctr 1965; **Fac Appt:** Prof RadRO, SUNY Downstate

REPRODUCTIVE ENDOCRINOLOGY

Grazi, Richard MD (RE) - **Spec Exp:** Infertility-IVF; Preimplantation Genetic Diagnosis (PGD); **Hospital:** Maimonides Med Ctr (page 96), St Vincent Cath Med Ctr - Staten Island (page 375); **Address:** 1355 84th St, Brooklyn, NY 11228-3030; **Phone:** 718-283-8600; **Board Cert:** Obstetrics & Gynecology 1997; Reproductive Endocrinology 1997; **Med School:** SUNY Buffalo 1981; **Resid:** Obstetrics & Gynecology, NYU Med Ctr 1985; **Fellow:** Reproductive Endocrinology, New Jersey Med Sch 1987; **Fac Appt:** Assoc Clin Prof ObG, Mount Sinai Sch Med

Kofinas, George MD (RE) - **Spec Exp:** Infertility-IVF; Laparoscopic Surgery; Uterine Fibroids; **Hospital:** New York Methodist Hosp (page 479); **Address:** Fertility Inst, New York Meth Hosp, 506 6th St, Fl 4, Brooklyn, NY 11215-9008; **Phone:** 718-780-5065; **Board Cert:** Obstetrics & Gynecology 1998; Reproductive Endocrinology 1998; **Med School:** Greece 1975; **Resid:** Obstetrics & Gynecology, NY Methodist Hosp 1982; Obstetrics & Gynecology, Brooklyn Hosp 1984; **Fellow:** Reproductive Endocrinology, Univ Hosp 1986; **Fac Appt:** Asst Prof ObG, SUNY Hlth Sci Ctr

Seifer, David B MD (RE) - **Spec Exp:** Infertility; Infertility-Advanced Maternal Age; Fertility Preservation in Cancer; **Hospital:** Maimonides Med Ctr (page 96); **Address:** 1355 84th St, Brooklyn, NY 11228; **Phone:** 718-283-8600; **Board Cert:** Obstetrics & Gynecology 1998; Reproductive Endocrinology 1998; **Med School:** Univ IL Coll Med 1981; **Resid:** Obstetrics & Gynecology, Stanford Univ Hosp 1985; **Fellow:** Reproductive Endocrinology, Yale-New Haven Hosp 1991; **Fac Appt:** Prof ObG, Mount Sinai Sch Med

RHEUMATOLOGY

Bernstein, Lawrence J MD (Rhu) - **Spec Exp:** Rheumatoid Arthritis; Polymyositis; Scleroderma; **Hospital:** Brookdale Univ Hosp Med Ctr; **Address:** 1 Brookdale Plaza, rm 344 CHC, Dept Rehab Medicine, Brooklyn, NY 11212; **Phone:** 718-240-6126; **Board Cert:** Internal Medicine 1965; Physical Medicine & Rehabilitation 1968; Rheumatology 1972; Geriatric Medicine 1990; **Med School:** NYU Sch Med 1958; **Resid:** Internal Medicine, Bellevue Hosp 1961; **Fellow:** Rheumatology, New York Univ Med Ctr 1962

Bienenstock, Harry MD (Rhu) - **Spec Exp:** Rheumatoid Arthritis; Musculoskeletal Disorders; **Hospital:** Hosp For Special Surgery (page 108), Long Island Coll Hosp (page 90); **Address:** 4015 Avenue U, Brooklyn, NY 11234-5117; **Phone:** 718-252-8181; **Board Cert:** Internal Medicine 1965; **Med School:** Univ Hlth Sci/Chicago Med Sch 1957; **Resid:** Internal Medicine, VA Med Ctr 1960; **Fellow:** Rheumatology, Hosp For Special Surgery 1962; **Fac Appt:** Assoc Clin Prof Med, Cornell Univ-Weill Med Coll

Garner, Bruce MD (Rhu) - **Spec Exp:** Lupus/SLE; Rheumatoid Arthritis; Osteoarthritis; **Hospital:** Lutheran Med Ctr - Brooklyn; **Address:** 7901 4th Ave, Ste A5, Brooklyn, NY 11209-3915; **Phone:** 718-921-5239; **Board Cert:** Internal Medicine 1987; Rheumatology 1988; **Med School:** Mexico 1981; **Resid:** Internal Medicine, Lutheran Med Ctr 1985; **Fellow:** Rheumatology, Washington Hosp Ctr 1987; **Fac Appt:** Asst Clin Prof Med, SUNY Downstate

Ginzler, Ellen MD (Rhu) - **Spec Exp:** Lupus/SLE; **Hospital:** SUNY Downstate Med Ctr, Kings County Hosp Ctr; **Address:** SUNY Downstate, Dept Rheumatology, 450 Clarkson Ave, Box 42, Brooklyn, NY 11203-0042; **Phone:** 718-270-1662; **Board Cert:** Internal Medicine 1972; Rheumatology 1974; **Med School:** Case West Res Univ 1969; **Resid:** Internal Medicine, Kings Co Hosp 1971; Internal Medicine, Bellevue Hosp 1972; **Fellow:** Rheumatology, Univ Hosp 1974; **Fac Appt:** Prof Med, SUNY Downstate

Golden, Brian D MD (Rhu) - **Spec Exp:** Spinal Rehabilitation; **Hospital:** Hosp For Joint Diseases (page 107); **Address:** 186 Joralemon St Fl 8, Brooklyn, NY 11201; **Phone:** 718-858-3263; **Board Cert:** Internal Medicine 1994; Rheumatology 1996; **Med School:** Mount Sinai Sch Med 1991; **Resid:** Internal Medicine, Mount Sinai Hosp 1994; **Fellow:** Rheumatology, Hosp for Joint Diseases 1996

Green, Stuart MD (Rhu) - **Spec Exp:** Rheumatoid Arthritis; Osteoporosis; Lupus/SLE; **Hospital:** Brooklyn Hosp Ctr-Downtown; **Address:** 121 Dekalb Ave Fl 7, Brooklyn, NY 11201-5425; **Phone:** 718-250-6921; **Board Cert:** Internal Medicine 1982; Rheumatology 1986; **Med School:** Georgetown Univ 1979; **Resid:** Internal Medicine, St Luke's Roosevelt Hosp Ctr 1982; **Fellow:** Rheumatology, Downstate Univ Hosp 1985; **Fac Appt:** Asst Clin Prof Med, NYU Sch Med

Lesser, Robert MD (Rhu) - **Spec Exp:** Polymyalgia Rheumatica; Rheumatoid Arthritis; Lupus/SLE; **Hospital:** Beth Israel Med Ctr- Kings Hwy Div (page 90); **Address:** 4015 Avenue U, Brooklyn, NY 11234-5117; **Phone:** 718-252-5151; **Board Cert:** Internal Medicine 1985; Rheumatology 1988; **Med School:** Univ Hlth Sci/Chicago Med Sch 1982; **Resid:** Internal Medicine, Hahnemann Univ Hosp 1985; **Fellow:** Rheumatology, Hahnemann Univ Hosp 1987; **Fac Appt:** Assoc Clin Prof Med, SUNY Hlth Sci Ctr

Patel, Jitendra K MD (Rhu) - **Spec Exp:** Arthritis; Fibromyalgia; Pain-Back; **Hospital:** Kingsbrook Jewish Med Ctr, Beth Israel Med Ctr- Kings Hwy Div (page 90); **Address:** 3420 Ave N, Brooklyn, NY 11234-2607; **Phone:** 718-258-7019; **Board Cert:** Internal Medicine 1979; Rheumatology 1982; **Med School:** India 1975; **Resid:** Internal Medicine, Mem U Newfoundland 1979; **Fellow:** Rheumatology, Georgetown Univ Hosp 1982

Ricciardi, Daniel D MD (Rhu) - **Spec Exp:** Rheumatoid Arthritis; Osteoporosis; Osteoarthritis; **Hospital:** Long Island Coll Hosp (page 90), New York Methodist Hosp (page 479); **Address:** 100 Clinton St, Brooklyn, NY 11201-4618; **Phone:** 718-834-0070; **Board Cert:** Internal Medicine 1998; **Med School:** Grenada 1981; **Resid:** Internal Medicine, LI Coll Hosp 1984; **Fellow:** Rheumatology, LI Coll Hosp 1986; **Fac Appt:** Assoc Clin Prof Med, SUNY Downstate

Schiff, Carl MD (Rhu) - **Spec Exp:** Rheumatoid Arthritis; Osteoporosis; **Hospital:** Maimonides Med Ctr (page 96); **Address:** Maimonides Med Ctr, 4802 10th Ave, Ste 352, Brooklyn, NY 11219-2916; **Phone:** 718-283-8519; **Board Cert:** Internal Medicine 1983; Rheumatology 1986; **Med School:** Yale Univ 1980; **Resid:** Internal Medicine, Mt Sinai Hosp 1983; **Fellow:** Rheumatology, Columbia-Presby Med Ctr 1986; **Fac Appt:** Asst Clin Prof Med, SUNY Hlth Sci Ctr

SURGERY

Adler, Harry MD (S) - **Spec Exp:** Biliary Surgery; Laparoscopic Surgery; **Hospital:** Maimonides Med Ctr (page 96); **Address:** 958 48th St Fl 3, Brooklyn, NY 11219; **Phone:** 718-283-7952; **Board Cert:** Surgery 2006; Surgical Critical Care 1998; **Med School:** NYU Sch Med 1980; **Resid:** Surgery, Bellevue Hosp/NYU Med Ctr 1985; **Fellow:** Surgery, Maimonides Medical Ctr 1986; **Fac Appt:** Asst Clin Prof, SUNY Downstate

Alfonso, Antonio MD (S) - **Spec Exp:** Breast Cancer; Head & Neck Surgery; **Hospital:** Long Island Coll Hosp (page 90), SUNY Downstate Med Ctr; **Address:** Long Island Coll Hosp, 339 Hicks St, Brooklyn, NY 11201-6005; **Phone:** 718-875-3244; **Board Cert:** Surgery 1973; **Med School:** Philippines 1968; **Resid:** Surgery, Temple Univ Hosp 1972; **Fellow:** Surgical Oncology, Meml Sloan Kettering Cancer Ctr 1974; **Fac Appt:** Prof S, SUNY Downstate

Amiruddin, Qamar MD (S) - **Spec Exp:** Breast Cancer; **Hospital:** Coney Island Hosp, Maimonides Med Ctr (page 96); **Address:** 2601 Ocean Pkwy, Brooklyn, NY 11235-7745; **Phone:** 718-616-3440; **Board Cert:** Surgery 1998; **Med School:** Pakistan 1966; **Resid:** Surgery, Maimonides Med Ctr 1977; **Fellow:** Surgical Oncology, Kings County Hosp 1977

Asarian, Armand MD (S) - **Spec Exp:** Colon Cancer; Breast Cancer; **Hospital:** Brooklyn Hosp Ctr-Downtown; **Address:** 121 Dekalb Ave, Brooklyn Hospital Ctr, Dept Surgery, Brooklyn, NY 11201; **Phone:** 718-250-6088; **Board Cert:** Surgery 2006; Colon & Rectal Surgery 1998; **Med School:** SUNY Downstate 1991; **Resid:** Surgery, Brooklyn Hosp Ctr 1996; **Fellow:** Colon & Rectal Surgery, Baylor Univ Med Ctr 1997; **Fac Appt:** Asst Clin Prof S, Cornell Univ-Weill Med Coll

Bernstein, Michael O MD (S) - **Spec Exp:** Hernia; Biliary Surgery; Breast Disease; **Hospital:** Long Island Coll Hosp (page 90); **Address:** 350 Henry St, Brooklyn, NY 11201; **Phone:** 718-780-1563; **Board Cert:** Surgery 1997; Surgical Critical Care 1998; **Med School:** Penn State Univ-Hershey Med Ctr 1983; **Resid:** Surgery, SUNY-Kings Co Hosp 1988; **Fac Appt:** Asst Prof S, SUNY Downstate

Borriello, Raffaele MD (S) - **Spec Exp:** Breast Surgery; Hernia; **Hospital:** Long Island Coll Hosp (page 90); **Address:** 350 Henry St Fl 2, Brooklyn, NY 11201; **Phone:** 718-780-1562; **Board Cert:** Surgery 1996; Surgical Critical Care 1999; **Med School:** SUNY Downstate 1981; **Resid:** Surgery, Kings County Hosp 1986; **Fac Appt:** Assoc Prof S, SUNY Downstate

Kings (Brooklyn)

Choe, Dai-sun MD (S) - **Spec Exp:** Breast Surgery; Hernia; Gallbladder Surgery; **Hospital:** Victory Memorial Hosp - Bklyn, Lutheran Med Ctr - Brooklyn; **Address:** 7501 4th Ave, Brooklyn, NY 11209-3201; **Phone:** 718-238-6116; **Board Cert:** Surgery 1974; **Med School:** South Korea 1958; **Resid:** Surgery, Lutheran Med Ctr 1971; **Fellow:** Surgery, Lahey Clinic 1973

Dresner, Lisa MD (S) - **Spec Exp:** Trauma; Critical Care; Breast Surgery; **Hospital:** SUNY Downstate Med Ctr, Kings County Hosp Ctr; **Address:** SUNY HSC, Dept Surg, 450 Clarkson Ave, Box 40, Brooklyn, NY 11203-2056; **Phone:** 718-270-3287; **Board Cert:** Surgery 2001; Surgical Critical Care 2003; **Med School:** SUNY Downstate 1985; **Resid:** Surgery, Kings Co Hosp Ctr 1992; **Fellow:** Surgical Critical Care, Jackson Meml Hosp 1993; **Fac Appt:** Assoc Prof S, SUNY Downstate

Fahoum, Bashar MD (S) - **Spec Exp:** Laparoscopic Surgery; Critical Care; **Hospital:** New York Methodist Hosp (page 479); **Address:** 506 6th St, Brooklyn, NY 11215; **Phone:** 718-780-3288; **Board Cert:** Surgery 2003; **Med School:** Syria 1987; **Resid:** Surgery, New York Methodist Hosp 1993

Fogler, Richard MD (S) - **Spec Exp:** Breast Surgery; Colon & Rectal Surgery; Gastrointestinal Surgery; **Hospital:** Brookdale Univ Hosp Med Ctr; **Address:** 1 Brookdale Plz, Rm 122, Brooklyn, NY 11212-3139; **Phone:** 718-240-5437; **Board Cert:** Surgery 1975; **Med School:** NY Med Coll 1968; **Resid:** Surgery, Brookdale Hosp 1973; **Fac Appt:** Clin Prof S, SUNY Hlth Sci Ctr

Genato, Romulo MD (S) - **Spec Exp:** Breast Surgery; Laparoscopic Surgery; Hernia; **Hospital:** Brooklyn Hosp Ctr-Downtown; **Address:** Brooklyn Hospital, 121 Dekalb Ave, Brooklyn, NY 11201-5425; **Phone:** 718-250-8970; **Board Cert:** Surgery 1999; **Med School:** Philippines 1972; **Resid:** Surgery, Brooklyn Hosp 1979; **Fac Appt:** Asst Clin Prof S, Cornell Univ-Weill Med Coll

Glass, David MD (S) - **Spec Exp:** Vascular Surgery; Laparoscopic Surgery; Endovascular Surgery; **Hospital:** New York Methodist Hosp (page 479), Brooklyn Hosp Ctr-Downtown; **Address:** 2989 Ocean Pkwy, Brooklyn, NY 11235-8386; **Phone:** 718-996-4400; **Board Cert:** Surgery 1996; Vascular Surgery 2003; **Med School:** Belgium 1978; **Resid:** Surgery, Beth Israel Hosp 1983; **Fellow:** Vascular Surgery, Newark Beth Israel Med Ctr 1985

Gorecki, Piotr J MD (S) - **Spec Exp:** Laparoscopic Surgery; Obesity/Bariatric Surgery; **Hospital:** New York Methodist Hosp (page 479); **Address:** NY Methodist Hospital, Dept Surgery, 506 Sixth St, Brooklyn, NY 11215; **Phone:** 718-246-8600; **Board Cert:** Surgery 1999; **Med School:** Poland 1991; **Resid:** Surgery, NY Methodist Hosp 1998; **Fellow:** Laparoscopic Surgery, Mayo Clinic 1999

Hedayati, Hossein MD (S) - **Spec Exp:** Breast Disease; Thyroid Surgery; Gallbladder Surgery; **Hospital:** New York Methodist Hosp (page 479); **Address:** 9920 4th Ave Fl 3 - Ste 311, Brooklyn, NY 11209-8333; **Phone:** 718-833-2600; **Board Cert:** Surgery 1969; **Med School:** Iran 1962; **Resid:** Pathology, DE Paul Hosp 1968; Surgery, Methodist Hosp 1968; **Fellow:** Surgery, SUNY Downstate 1970; **Fac Appt:** Asst Clin Prof S, Cornell Univ-Weill Med Coll

Hong, Joon Ho MD (S) - **Spec Exp:** Transplant-Kidney; Vascular Access; **Hospital:** SUNY Downstate Med Ctr; **Address:** SUNY Downstate Med Ctr, 450 Clarkson Ave, Box 40, Brooklyn, NY 11203; **Phone:** 718-270-1898; **Board Cert:** Surgery 1998; **Med School:** South Korea 1967; **Resid:** Surgery, Downstate Med Ctr 1979; **Fac Appt:** Prof S, SUNY Downstate

Horovitz, Joel MD (S) - **Hospital:** Maimonides Med Ctr (page 96); **Address:** 4802 10th Ave Bldg Admin Fl 4, Brooklyn, NY 11219-2916; **Phone:** 718-283-8461; **Board Cert:** Surgery 1974; Surgical Critical Care 2001; **Med School:** McGill Univ 1967; **Resid:** Surgery, Jewish Genl Hosp 1973; **Fellow:** Surgery, Parkland Meml Hosp 1972; **Fac Appt:** Assoc Clin Prof S, SUNY Hlth Sci Ctr

Khafif, Rene MD (S) - **Spec Exp:** Breast Cancer; Head & Neck Surgery; Skin Cancer; **Hospital:** Lutheran Med Ctr - Brooklyn, Maimonides Med Ctr (page 96); **Address:** 2219 Ocean Ave, Brooklyn, NY 11229-2303; **Phone:** 718-376-6580; **Board Cert:** Surgery 1964; **Med School:** France 1956; **Resid:** Surgery, Maimonides Medical Ctr 1962; **Fellow:** Surgical Research, USPHS Hosp 1960; **Fac Appt:** Clin Prof S, SUNY Downstate

Kumar, Sampath MD (S) - **Spec Exp:** Laparoscopic Surgery; Breast Surgery; **Hospital:** Lutheran Med Ctr - Brooklyn, Victory Memorial Hosp - Bklyn; **Address:** 7517 6th Ave, Brooklyn, NY 11209; **Phone:** 718-630-5777; **Board Cert:** Surgery 1983; Vascular Surgery 1983; **Med School:** India 1975; **Resid:** Surgery, Lutheran Med Ctr 1981; **Fellow:** Vascular Surgery, Lutheran Med Ctr 1983

Lois, William A MD (S) - **Spec Exp:** Dialysis Access Surgery; Vascular Surgery; **Hospital:** Beth Israel Med Ctr-Kings Hwy Div (page 90), Kingsbrook Jewish Med Ctr; **Address:** 5723 Avenue N, Brooklyn, NY 11234-4026; **Phone:** 718-251-1111; **Board Cert:** Surgery 1999; **Med School:** Spain 1982; **Resid:** Surgery, Interfaith Med Ctr 1987

Lutchman, Gordon MD (S) - **Spec Exp:** Wound Healing/Care; Vein Disorders; Laser Surgery; **Hospital:** Coney Island Hosp, Maimonides Med Ctr (page 96); **Address:** Dept of Surgery, 2601 Ocean Pkwy, Brooklyn, NY 11235; **Phone:** 718-616-3440; **Board Cert:** Surgery 1998; **Med School:** Jamaica 1976; **Resid:** Surgery, Royal United Hosp 1982; Surgery, Maimonides Med Ctr 1987; **Fellow:** Vascular Surgery, Maimonides Med Ctr 1988; Surgery, Royal Col of Surgeons of England 2004

Rajpal, Sanjeev MD (S) - **Spec Exp:** Cancer Surgery; Laparoscopic Surgery; Breast Surgery; **Hospital:** Beth Israel Med Ctr- Kings Hwy Div (page 90), Brookdale Univ Hosp Med Ctr; **Address:** 1663 Remsen Ave, Brooklyn, NY 11236-5233; **Phone:** 718-251-1212; **Board Cert:** Surgery 1982; **Med School:** India 1975; **Resid:** Surgery, Brookdale Hosp Med Ctr 1980; **Fellow:** Surgical Oncology, Roswell Park Meml Can Inst 1982; **Fac Appt:** Asst Prof S, SUNY Downstate

Raju, Ramanathan MD (S) - **Spec Exp:** Breast Surgery; Laparoscopic Surgery; **Hospital:** Coney Island Hosp; **Address:** Coney Island Hosp, 2601 Ocean Pkwy, Brooklyn, NY 11235; **Phone:** 718-616-5380; **Board Cert:** Surgery 1997; **Med School:** India 1976; **Resid:** Surgery, Lutheran Med Ctr 1987; Vascular Surgery, Lutheran Med Ctr 1988; **Fellow:** Royal Coll Surgeons; **Fac Appt:** Asst Clin Prof S, SUNY Hlth Sci Ctr

Rao, Addagada MD (S) - **Spec Exp:** Laparoscopic Cholecystectomy; Colon Surgery; **Hospital:** Wyckoff Heights Med Ctr; **Address:** 145 Saint Nicholas Ave, Brooklyn, NY 11237-4439; **Phone:** 718-418-5900; **Board Cert:** Surgery 1974; **Med School:** India 1965; **Resid:** Surgery, Wyckoff Heights Hosp 1972

Rucinski, James MD (S) - **Spec Exp:** Laparoscopic Surgery; **Hospital:** New York Methodist Hosp (page 479); **Address:** NY Methodist Hosp, Dept Surg, 506 6th St, Brooklyn, NY 11215; **Phone:** 718-780-3288; **Board Cert:** Surgery 2003; Emergency Medicine 2000; **Med School:** Univ Mich Med Sch 1979; **Resid:** Surgery, Lenox Hill 1992; **Fac Appt:** Asst Prof S, Cornell Univ-Weill Med Coll

Sapala, James A MD (S) - **Spec Exp:** Obesity/Bariatric Surgery; **Hospital:** St Vincent Cath Med Ctrs - Manhattan (page 375); **Address:** 8714 5th Ave, Brooklyn, NY 11209; **Phone:** 212-966-7007; **Board Cert:** Surgery 1997; **Med School:** Univ Mich Med Sch 1970; **Resid:** Surgery, Henry Ford Hosp 1975

Schwartzman, Alexander MD (S) - **Hospital:** SUNY Downstate Med Ctr; **Address:** 450 Clarkson Ave, Box 40, Brooklyn, NY 11203; **Phone:** 718-270-1791; **Board Cert:** Surgery 1998; **Med School:** Dominican Republic 1983; **Resid:** Surgery, Brooklyn Hosp 1988

Steiner, Henry MD (S) - **Spec Exp:** Breast Surgery; **Hospital:** Maimonides Med Ctr (page 96), Peninsula Hosp Ctr; **Address:** 8105 Bay Pkwy, Brooklyn, NY 11214; **Phone:** 718-331-7314; **Board Cert:** Surgery 2001; **Med School:** SUNY Downstate 1976; **Resid:** Surgery, Maimonides Med Ctr 1980; **Fellow:** Vascular Surgery, Maimonides Med Ctr 1981

Tanchajja, Supoj MD (S) - **Hospital:** Long Island Coll Hosp (page 90), Victory Memorial Hosp - Bklyn; **Address:** 239 82nd St, Brooklyn, NY 11209-3810; **Phone:** 718-748-4603; **Board Cert:** Surgery 2000; **Med School:** Thailand 1972; **Resid:** Surgery, NY Methodist hosp 1977; Surgery, Long Island Coll Hosp 1980

Wright, Albert MD (S) - **Spec Exp:** Breast Disease; Colon & Rectal Surgery; Thyroid Surgery; **Hospital:** Interfaith Med Ctr - St John's Episcopal Hosp, New York Methodist Hosp (page 479); **Address:** 1 Plaza St, Ste 1B, Brooklyn, NY 11217; **Phone:** 718-638-1971; **Board Cert:** Surgery 1999; **Med School:** England 1970; **Resid:** Surgery, Mt Sinai Hosp 1977; **Fac Appt:** Asst Clin Prof S, Cornell Univ-Weill Med Coll

Zenilman, Michael MD (S) - **Spec Exp:** Pancreatic Surgery; Gastrointestinal Surgery; Laparoscopic Surgery; **Hospital:** SUNY Downstate Med Ctr, Long Island Coll Hosp (page 90); **Address:** SUNY Downstate Med Ctr, 450 Clarkson Ave, Box 40, Brooklyn, NY 11203-2056; **Phone:** 718-270-1421; **Board Cert:** Surgery 2003; **Med School:** SUNY Downstate 1980; **Resid:** Surgery, Barnes Jewish Hosp 1991; **Fac Appt:** Prof S, SUNY Downstate

THORACIC SURGERY

Abrol, Sunil MD (TS) - **Spec Exp:** Cardiac Surgery; Robotic Heart Surgery; **Hospital:** Maimonides Med Ctr (page 96); **Address:** Maimonides Med Ctr, Cardiothoracic Surgery, 4802 10th Ave, Brooklyn, NY 11219; **Phone:** 718-283-7686; **Board Cert:** Surgery 1999; Thoracic Surgery 2002; **Med School:** India 1987; **Resid:** Surgery, Maimonides Med Ctr 1998; **Fellow:** Thoracic Surgery, SUNY Hlth Sci Ctr 2001

Acinapura, Anthony MD (TS) - **Spec Exp:** Cardiothoracic Surgery; Vascular Surgery; Endovascular Surgery; **Hospital:** Lutheran Med Ctr - Brooklyn, Maimonides Med Ctr (page 96); **Address:** Lutheran Med Ctr, 150 55th St, Ste 3524, Brooklyn, NY 11220; **Phone:** 718-630-7351; **Board Cert:** Surgery 1971; Thoracic Surgery 1972; **Med School:** Georgetown Univ 1963; **Resid:** Surgery, Bellevue Hosp/NYU Med Ctr 1969; Thoracic Surgery, Bellevue Hosp/NYU Med Ctr 1971; **Fellow:** Surgery, Duke Univ Med Ctr 1966; **Fac Appt:** Prof S, NY Med Coll

Burack, Joshua H MD (TS) - **Spec Exp:** Cardiothoracic Surgery; **Hospital:** SUNY Downstate Med Ctr, Kings County Hosp Ctr; **Address:** SUNY Hlth Sci Ctr, Dept Cardiothor Surg, 450 Clarkson Ave, Box 40, Brooklyn, NY 11203; **Phone:** 718-270-1981; **Board Cert:** Surgery 1999; Thoracic Surgery 1999; **Med School:** Albert Einstein Coll Med 1982; **Resid:** Surgery, Albert Einstein 1987; **Fellow:** Cardiothoracic Surgery, Univ Hosp 1989; **Fac Appt:** Assoc Prof S, SUNY Downstate

Cunningham Jr, Joseph N MD (TS) - **Spec Exp:** Coronary Artery Surgery; Heart Valve Surgery; **Hospital:** Maimonides Med Ctr (page 96); **Address:** Maimonides Med Ctr, Cardiothoracic Dept, 4802 10th Ave, rm 4D, Brooklyn, NY 11219; **Phone:** 718-283-8302; **Board Cert:** Surgery 1973; Thoracic Surgery 1975; **Med School:** Univ Ala 1966; **Resid:** Surgery, Parkland Meml Hosp 1972; **Fellow:** Cardiovascular Disease, NYU Med Ctr 1974; **Fac Appt:** Prof S, SUNY Downstate

Lazzaro, Richard MD (TS) - **Spec Exp:** Minimally Invasive Surgery; Obesity/Bariatric Surgery; **Hospital:** Maimonides Med Ctr (page 96); **Address:** 948 48th St Fl 2nd, Dept Surgery, Brooklyn, NY 11219; **Phone:** 718-283-7602; **Board Cert:** Surgery 1996; Thoracic Surgery 1999; **Med School:** Albany Med Coll 1988; **Resid:** Surgery, North Shore Univ Hosp 1993; **Fellow:** Cardiothoracic Surgery, Maimonedes Med Ctr 1997

Okadigwe, Chukuma MD (TS) - **Spec Exp:** Lung Cancer; Thoracic Surgery; Minimally Invasive Surgery; **Hospital:** New York Methodist Hosp (page 479), Brookdale Univ Hosp Med Ctr; **Address:** 191 Ocean Ave, Brooklyn, NY 11225-4701; **Phone:** 718-287-0505; **Board Cert:** Surgery 1975; Thoracic Surgery 1997; **Med School:** Univ Colorado 1968; **Resid:** Surgery, Kings County Hosp 1974; Thoracic Surgery, Univ Hosp-SUNY Downstate 1976; **Fac Appt:** Asst Prof S, SUNY Downstate

UROLOGY

Florio, Francis MD (U) - **Spec Exp:** Incontinence; Prostate Disease; Prostate Cancer; **Hospital:** New York Methodist Hosp (page 479), Long Island Coll Hosp (page 90); **Address:** 355 Ovington Ave, Ste 200, Brooklyn, NY 11209-1483; **Phone:** 718-238-1818; **Board Cert:** Urology 1983; **Med School:** NY Med Coll 1975; **Resid:** Urology, NYU Med Ctr 1981

Friedman, Steven C MD (U) - **Spec Exp:** Pediatric Urology; Urinary Tract Infection; Robotic Urologic Surgery; **Hospital:** Maimonides Med Ctr (page 96), Schneider Chldn's Hosp; **Address:** 909 49th St, Brooklyn, NY 11219; **Phone:** 718-283-7743; **Board Cert:** Urology 2000; **Med School:** SUNY Downstate 1983; **Resid:** Surgery, Beth Israel 1985; Urology, Maimonides Medical Ctr 1988; **Fellow:** Children's Hosp 1991

Godec, Circil MD (U) - **Spec Exp:** Prostate Cancer; Erectile Dysfunction; **Hospital:** Long Island Coll Hosp (page 90), SUNY Downstate Med Ctr; **Address:** LI Coll Hosp, Dept Urology, 339 Hicks St Fl 7, Brooklyn, NY 11201-6004; **Phone:** 718-780-1520; **Board Cert:** Urology 1979; **Med School:** Slovenia 1983; **Resid:** Urology, Univ Minn Med Ctr 1976; **Fac Appt:** Clin Prof U, SUNY Downstate

Grunberger, Ivan MD (U) - **Spec Exp:** Prostate Cancer & Disease; Impotence; Minimally Invasive Surgery; Kidney Stones; **Hospital:** Long Island Coll Hosp (page 90), SUNY Downstate Med Ctr; **Address:** Long Island College Hospital, 339 Hicks St Fl 7, Brooklyn, NY 11201-5509; **Phone:** 718-780-1520; **Board Cert:** Urology 1998; **Med School:** NYU Sch Med 1980; **Resid:** Surgery, North Shore Univ Hosp 1982; Urology, NYU Med Ctr 1986; **Fac Appt:** Assoc Clin Prof U, SUNY Hlth Sci Ctr

Irwin, Mark MD (U) - **Spec Exp:** Prostate Disease; Erectile Dysfunction; Kidney Stones; **Hospital:** Long Island Coll Hosp (page 90); **Address:** 339 Hicks St, Brooklyn, NY 11201; **Phone:** 718-780-1520; **Board Cert:** Urology 1991; **Med School:** Med Coll Wisc 1982; **Resid:** Urology, Kings County Hosp 1988; **Fac Appt:** Asst Prof U, SUNY Downstate

Kim, Hong MD (U) - **Hospital:** Brookdale Univ Hosp Med Ctr; **Address:** Brookdale Hospital, 1 Brookdale Plaza, Ste 5C4, Brooklyn, NY 11212; **Phone:** 718-240-5323; **Board Cert:** Urology 1976; **Med School:** South Korea 1965; **Resid:** Surgery, Brookdale Hosp 1971; Urology, Univ Nebraska Med Ctr 1974; **Fac Appt:** Assoc Clin Prof U, SUNY Downstate

Lindsay, Gaius K MD (U) - **Hospital:** Coney Island Hosp, Maimonides Med Ctr (page 96); **Address:** 1616-B Voorhies Ave, Brooklyn, NY 11235; **Phone:** 718-769-5158; **Board Cert:** Urology 1976; **Med School:** India 1967; **Resid:** Surgery, NY Methodist Hosp 1970; Urology, Maimonides Med Ctr 1973; **Fac Appt:** Asst Clin Prof U, SUNY Downstate

Macchia, Richard MD (U) - **Spec Exp:** Prostate Disease; Prostate Cancer; Voiding Dysfunction; **Hospital:** SUNY Downstate Med Ctr; **Address:** SUNY Downstate Med School, Dept Urology, 445 Lenox Rd, Box 79, Brooklyn, NY 11203-2098; **Phone:** 718-270-2554; **Board Cert:** Urology 1977; **Med School:** NY Med Coll 1969; **Resid:** Surgery, St Vincent's Hosp 1971; Urology, SUNY Downstate Med Ctr 1974; **Fellow:** Urologic Oncology, Meml Sloan Kettering Cancer Ctr 1976; **Fac Appt:** Prof U, SUNY Downstate

Mandel, Edmund MD (U) - **Spec Exp:** Incontinence; Prostate Cancer; Infertility-Male; **Hospital:** New York Comm Hosp, Mount Sinai Med Ctr (page 98); **Address:** 2460 Flatbush Ave, Ste 8, Brooklyn, NY 11234-5000; **Phone:** 718-692-0020; **Board Cert:** Urology 1988; **Med School:** Temple Univ 1981; **Resid:** Urology, Mount Sinai Hosp 1986; **Fac Appt:** Asst Clin Prof U, Mount Sinai Sch Med

Mazzarino, Aldo MD (U) - **Spec Exp:** Pediatric Urology; **Hospital:** Lutheran Med Ctr - Brooklyn, New York Methodist Hosp (page 479); **Address:** 9000 Shore Rd, Brooklyn, NY 11209-3206; **Phone:** 718-745-0771; **Board Cert:** Urology 1968; **Med School:** Italy 1959; **Resid:** Urology, NY Methodist Hosp 1961; Urology, NY Med Coll 1964; **Fac Appt:** Asst Clin Prof U, SUNY Hlth Sci Ctr

Meisenberg, Gene MD (U) - **Spec Exp:** Prostate Disease; Kidney Stones; Impotence; **Hospital:** NY-Presby Hosp (page 100), Long Island Coll Hosp (page 90); **Address:** 1523 Voorhies Ave, Brooklyn, NY 11235; **Phone:** 718-743-2200; **Board Cert:** Urology 2001; **Med School:** Russia 1981; **Resid:** Surgery, Beth Israel Hosp 1993; Urology, RW Johnson Univ Hosp 1997

Rosenthal, Sheldon MD (U) - **Spec Exp:** Kidney Stones; Prostate Disease; **Hospital:** Wyckoff Heights Med Ctr, St John's Queens Hosp (page 375); **Address:** 220A Saint Nicholas Ave, Brooklyn, NY 11237-4024; **Phone:** 718-821-3200; **Board Cert:** Urology 1977; **Med School:** Univ Hlth Sci/Chicago Med Sch 1967; **Resid:** Surgery, Albert Einstein 1970; Urology, NY Med Coll 1973

Saada, Simon MD (U) - **Spec Exp:** Kidney Stones; Prostate Cancer; Kidney Cancer; **Hospital:** Victory Memorial Hosp - Bklyn, NY-Presby Hosp (page 100); **Address:** 705 86th St, Bldg M2, Brooklyn, NY 11228-3219; **Phone:** 718-238-1075; **Board Cert:** Urology 1981; **Med School:** Egypt 1970; **Resid:** Urology, Charlston Area Med Ctr 1977; Surgery, Long Island Hosp 1974; **Fac Appt:** U, Columbia P&S

Silver, David A. MD (U) - **Spec Exp:** Laparoscopic Surgery; Urologic Cancer; **Hospital:** Maimonides Med Ctr (page 96), Lutheran Med Ctr - Brooklyn; **Address:** 6323 7th Ave, Brooklyn, NY 11220; **Phone:** 718-283-7153; **Board Cert:** Urology 1999; **Med School:** Albert Einstein Coll Med 1989; **Resid:** Surgery, Maimonides Med Ctr 1995; **Fellow:** Urology, Meml Sloan-Kettering Canc Ctr 1997

Wainstein, Sasha MD (U) - **Spec Exp:** Impotence; Voiding Dysfunction; Endourology; **Hospital:** Maimonides Med Ctr (page 96), Victory Memorial Hosp - Bklyn; **Address:** 4711 12th Ave, Brooklyn, NY 11219-2500; **Phone:** 718-436-3900; **Board Cert:** Urology 1977; **Med School:** Colombia 1969; **Resid:** Urology, Maimonides Medical Ctr 1975

Wise, Gilbert J MD (U) - **Spec Exp:** Prostate Cancer & Disease; Voiding Dysfunction; Kidney Stones; **Hospital:** Maimonides Med Ctr (page 96); **Address:** Maimonides Med Ctr, Dept Urology, 4802 Tenth Ave, Brooklyn, NY 11219-2916; **Phone:** 718-283-7742; **Board Cert:** Urology 1969; **Med School:** Johns Hopkins Univ 1957; **Resid:** Urology, Univ Hosp 1959; Urology, Montefiore Med Ctr 1965; **Fac Appt:** Prof U, SUNY Downstate

VASCULAR & INTERVENTIONAL RADIOLOGY

Sclafani, Salvatore MD (VIR) - **Spec Exp:** Uterine Fibroid Embolization; Vascular Malformations; **Hospital:** SUNY Downstate Med Ctr, Kings County Hosp Ctr; **Address:** Kings County Hosp, B Bldg, 451 Clarkson Ave, rm B3301, Brooklyn, NY 11203; **Phone:** 718-245-4447; **Board Cert:** Diagnostic Radiology 1976; Vascular & Interventional Radiology 1997; **Med School:** SUNY Upstate Med Univ 1972; **Resid:** Radiology, Univ Hosp-SUNY 1976; **Fac Appt:** Prof Rad, SUNY Downstate

VASCULAR SURGERY

Ascher, Enrico MD (VascS) - **Spec Exp:** Carotid Artery Surgery; Aneurysm; Limb Salvage; **Hospital:** Maimonides Med Ctr (page 96), Lutheran Med Ctr - Brooklyn; **Address:** Maimonides Med Ctr, Dept Vascular Surg, 4802 10th Ave Fl 4, Brooklyn, NY 11219-2844; **Phone:** 718-283-7957; **Board Cert:** Vascular Surgery 1995; **Med School:** Brazil 1974; **Resid:** Surgery, NY Med Coll 1981; **Fellow:** Vascular Surgery, Montefiore Hosp Med Ctr 1982; **Fac Appt:** Prof S, SUNY Downstate

D'Ayala, Marcus D MD (VascS) - **Spec Exp:** Endovascular Surgery; Aneurysm-Abdominal Aortic; **Hospital:** New York Methodist Hosp (page 479); **Address:** NY Methodist Hospital, Dept Surgery, 506 Sixth St, Brooklyn, NY 11215; **Phone:** 718-780-3288; **Board Cert:** Surgery 1998; Vascular Surgery 2000; **Med School:** Univ Wisc 1992; **Resid:** Surgery, Montefiore Med Ctr 1997; **Fellow:** Vascular Surgery, Mt Sinai Med Ctr 1998; **Fac Appt:** Asst Prof S, Mount Sinai Sch Med

Flores, Lucio MD (VascS) - **Hospital:** Brookdale Univ Hosp Med Ctr; **Address:** 2035 Ralph Ave, Ste B5, Brooklyn, NY 11234; **Phone:** 718-209-1400; **Board Cert:** Surgery 1995; Vascular Surgery 1998; **Med School:** Peru 1968; **Resid:** Surgery, Jewish Hosp Med Ctr 1975

Ilkhani, Rahman MD (VascS) - **Spec Exp:** Vein Disorders; Aneurysm; Carotid Artery Surgery; **Hospital:** New York Methodist Hosp (page 479), Metropolitan Hosp Ctr - NY; **Address:** 263 7th Ave, Ste 5E, Brooklyn, NY 11215-3704; **Phone:** 718-768-3560; **Board Cert:** Surgery 2006; **Med School:** Iran 1974; **Resid:** Surgery, NY Methodist Hosp 1982; **Fellow:** Vascular Surgery, Texas Heart Inst 1983

Shin, Choon S MD (VascS) - **Spec Exp:** Angioplasty & Stent Placement; Video Assisted Thoracic Surgery (VATS); Arterial Bypass Surgery; **Hospital:** New York Comm Hosp, New York Methodist Hosp (page 479); **Address:** 3619 Bedford Ave, Ste 1K, Brooklyn, NY 11229; **Phone:** 718-692-5315; **Board Cert:** Surgery 1972; Thoracic Surgery 2004; Vascular Surgery 1996; **Med School:** South Korea 1965; **Resid:** Surgery, Methodist Hosp 1970; **Fellow:** Cardiovascular Surgery, Brooklyn Jewish Hosp & Med Ctr 1972; **Fac Appt:** Clin Prof S, Cornell Univ-Weill Med Coll

Weiser, Robert MD (VascS) - **Spec Exp:** Lower Limb Arterial Disease; Carotid Artery Surgery; Lower Limb Ulcers; **Hospital:** Long Island Coll Hosp (page 90); **Address:** 107 Joralemon St Fl 1, Brooklyn, NY 11201-4066; **Phone:** 718-797-1101; **Board Cert:** Surgery 1994; **Med School:** Albert Einstein Coll Med 1977; **Resid:** Surgery, Montefiore-Einstein Med Ctr 1982; **Fellow:** Vascular Surgery, Montefiore-Einstein Med Ctr 1983

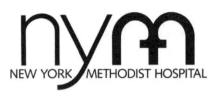

NEW YORK METHODIST HOSPITAL

506 Sixth Street, Brooklyn, N.Y. 11215
Phone (718) 780-3000, Fax (718) 780-3770
http://www.nym.org

Sponsorship	Voluntary, Not-for-Profit
Beds	570; 42 bassinets
Accreditation	Joint Commission on Accreditation of Healthcare Organizations (JCAHO), Council on Graduate Medical Education

GENERAL DESCRIPTION

New York Methodist Hospital (NYM), a member of the New York Presbyterian Healthcare System, has served the neighborhoods of Brooklyn for over 125 years. NYM's medical programs have recently expanded significantly and the hospital's campus facilities in Park Slope have been extensively renovated. In addition, New York Methodist maintains satellite outpatient health centers throughout Brooklyn.

MEDICAL STAFF

NYM has about 1,000 physicians on staff; 90% are board certified or board eligible. Many physicians at NYM are known for the impressive and outstanding work they have done in their individual fields. New York Methodist Hospital offers medical residency programs in internal medicine, surgery, pediatrics, obstetrics/gynecology, radiation oncology, nuclear medicine, anesthesiology, emergency medicine, podiatry and dentistry. The Hospital also offers fellowships in several medical subspecialties.

SPECIAL PROGRAMS

Emergency Medicine: A newly renovated, expanded Emergency Department houses a pediatric emergency room and private rooms for obstetrics/gynecology patients. The Hospital is a State-designated Stroke Center an AHA Heart Center and EMS 911 Receiving Hospital. 718 780-3136.

Institute for Cancer Care: 866-411-ONCO.

Institute for Cardiology and Cardiac Surgery: See Centers of Excellence Section. 866 84-HEART.

Institute for Orthopedic Medicine and Surgery: See Centers of Excellence Section. 866 ORTHO-11.

Institute for Asthma and Lung Diseases: See Centers of Excellence Section. 866 ASK-LUNG.

Institute for Neurosciences: See Centers of Excellence Section. 866 DO-NEURO.

Institute for Digestive and Liver Disorders: See Centers of Excellence Section.866 DIGEST-1.

Institute for Vascular Medicine and Surgery: 866 438-VEIN.

Institute for Diabetes and Other Endocrine Disorders: 866-4-GLAND-2.

Birthing Center: Spacious, beautifully appointed rooms allow women to experience a "home-like" birth with the reassurance that high-tech medical equipment and specialists are instantly accessible if needed. Full-time lactation services are available for new mothers.

Physician Referral: The Hospital has a free seven-day, 24-hour telephone and computer on-line physician referral service. To find a doctor in any specialty with a convenient office location, area of specialization and insurance and billing policies, call 718 499-CARE or go to http://www.nym.org. 742

Queens

Queens

ALLERGY & IMMUNOLOGY

Bernstein, Larry MD (A&I) - **Spec Exp:** Asthma; Immune Deficiency; Sinus Disorders; Food Allergy; **Hospital:** Montefiore Med Ctr, NY Hosp Queens; **Address:** 110-55 72nd Rd, Ste L-1, Forest Hills, NY 11375-5481; **Phone:** 718-544-6641; **Board Cert:** Allergy & Immunology 1985; Pediatrics 1981; **Med School:** Albert Einstein Coll Med 1977; **Resid:** Pediatrics, Jacobi Med Ctr 1981; **Fellow:** Allergy & Immunology, Albert Einstein 1983; **Fac Appt:** Assoc Clin Prof Ped, Albert Einstein Coll Med

Fine, Stanley MD (A&I) - **Spec Exp:** Asthma; Drug Sensitivity; Latex Allergy; **Hospital:** NY Hosp Queens, Flushing Hosp Med Ctr; **Address:** 37-31 149th St, Flushing, NY 11354-4841; **Phone:** 718-358-5565; **Board Cert:** Internal Medicine 1964; Allergy & Immunology 1972; **Med School:** Columbia P&S 1957; **Resid:** Internal Medicine, Jacobi Med Ctr 1959; Internal Medicine, Montefiore Hosp Med Ctr 1962; **Fellow:** Allergy & Immunology, St Luke's-Roosevelt Hosp Ctr 1963; **Fac Appt:** Asst Clin Prof Med, Cornell Univ-Weill Med Coll

Menchell, David MD (A&I) - **Spec Exp:** Asthma; Nasal & Sinus Disorders; **Hospital:** NY Hosp Queens, St John's Queens Hosp (page 375); **Address:** 73-03 198th St, Fresh Meadows, NY 11366-1818; **Phone:** 718-465-4100; **Board Cert:** Internal Medicine 1980; Allergy & Immunology 1983; **Med School:** NYU Sch Med 1977; **Resid:** Internal Medicine, NY Hosp Med Ctr 1980; **Fellow:** Allergy & Immunology, NY Hosp Med Ctr 1983

CARDIAC ELECTROPHYSIOLOGY

Suri, Ranjit MD (CE) - **Spec Exp:** Arrhythmias; **Hospital:** NY Hosp Queens; **Address:** 56-45 Main St, Ste 3S, Flushing, NY 11355; **Phone:** 718-661-7400; **Board Cert:** Internal Medicine 1994; Cardiovascular Disease 2006; Pulmonary Disease 1996; Cardiovascular Disease 2001; **Med School:** India 1986; **Resid:** Internal Medicine, Univ Conn Sch Med 1994; Pulmonary Critical Care Medicine, Univ Conn Sch Med 1990; **Fellow:** Cardiovascular Disease, Univ Conn Sch Med 1993; Cardiac Electrophysiology, Mass Genl Hosp 2000; **Fac Appt:** Asst Clin Prof Med, Cornell Univ-Weill Med Coll

CARDIOVASCULAR DISEASE

Akinboboye, Olakunle MD (Cv) - **Spec Exp:** Diabetes & Heart Disease; Nuclear Stress Test; Hypertension; Coronary Heart Disease; **Address:** Laurelton Heart Specialists, 224-14 Merrick Blvd, Laurelton, NY 11413; **Phone:** 718-949-9400; **Board Cert:** Internal Medicine 2005; Cardiovascular Disease 2005; **Med School:** Nigeria 1984; **Resid:** Internal Medicine, Nassau County Med Ctr 1991; **Fellow:** Cardiovascular Disease, Columbia Presby Med Ctr 1995; Nuclear Cardiology, Columbia Presby Med Ctr 1994; **Fac Appt:** Assoc Prof Med, SUNY Stony Brook

Hsueh, John Tzu-Lang MD (Cv) - **Spec Exp:** Coronary Artery Disease; Heart Valve Disease; **Hospital:** NY Hosp Queens, Flushing Hosp Med Ctr; **Address:** 43-45 Parsons Blvd, Flushing, NY 11355-2164; **Phone:** 718-886-6400; **Board Cert:** Internal Medicine 1987; Cardiovascular Disease 1979; **Med School:** Taiwan 1970; **Resid:** Internal Medicine, Flushing Hosp Med Ctr 1976; **Fellow:** Cardiovascular Disease, Wayne State Univ 1978

Robbins, Michael MD (Cv) - **Spec Exp:** Cardiac Consultation; Echocardiography; **Hospital:** Mount Sinai Med Ctr (page 98), St John's Queens Hosp (page 375); **Address:** 94-36 58th Ave, Ste G4, Rego Park, NY 11373; **Phone:** 718-760-0011; **Board Cert:** Internal Medicine 1984; Cardiovascular Disease 1987; **Med School:** Cornell Univ-Weill Med Coll 1981; **Resid:** Internal Medicine, Bronx Muni Hosp Ctr/Albert Einstein 1985; **Fellow:** Cardiovascular Disease, Mount Sinai Hosp 1987; **Fac Appt:** Assoc Clin Prof Med, Mount Sinai Sch Med

Rosenberg, Peter MD (Cv) - **Hospital:** NY Hosp Queens, N Shore Univ Hosp at Manhasset; **Address:** 26-19 212th St, Bayside, NY 11360; **Phone:** 718-224-2022; **Board Cert:** Internal Medicine 1977; Cardiovascular Disease 1979; **Med School:** SUNY Hlth Sci Ctr 1974; **Resid:** Internal Medicine, Bronx Muni Hosp Ctr 1977; **Fellow:** Cardiovascular Disease, Montefiore Hosp Med Ctr 1979

Rydzinski, Mayer MD (Cv) - **Hospital:** Parkway Hosp, N Shore Univ Hosp at Forest Hills; **Address:** 70-31 108th St, Ste 7, Forest Hills, NY 11375-4450; **Phone:** 718-268-7633; **Board Cert:** Internal Medicine 1979; Cardiovascular Disease 1981; **Med School:** Albert Einstein Coll Med 1976; **Resid:** Internal Medicine, Metropolitan Hosp Ctr 1977; Internal Medicine, Montefiore Hosp Med Ctr 1979; **Fellow:** Cardiovascular Disease, LI Jewish Hosp 1981

Siskind, Steven Jay MD (Cv) - **Spec Exp:** Angina; Congenital Heart Disease; **Hospital:** NY Hosp Queens, NY-Presby Hosp (page 100); **Address:** 56-45 Main St Fl 2, Flushing, NY 11355; **Phone:** 718-670-1234; **Board Cert:** Internal Medicine 1979; Cardiovascular Disease 1981; **Med School:** Albert Einstein Coll Med 1976; **Resid:** Internal Medicine, Jacobi Med Ctr 1979; **Fellow:** Cardiovascular Disease, Albert Einstein 1981; **Fac Appt:** Asst Prof, Cornell Univ-Weill Med Coll

Tenet, William MD (Cv) - **Spec Exp:** Congestive Heart Failure; Coronary Artery Disease; **Hospital:** NY Hosp Queens, NY-Presby Hosp (page 100); **Address:** 44-01 Francis Lewis Blvd, Bayside, NY 11361; **Phone:** 718-423-3355; **Board Cert:** Internal Medicine 1983; Cardiovascular Disease 1987; **Med School:** Italy 1980; **Resid:** Internal Medicine, Booth Meml Med Ctr 1984; **Fellow:** Cardiovascular Disease, Univ Conn Hlth Ctr 1986; **Fac Appt:** Asst Clin Prof Med, Cornell Univ-Weill Med Coll

Visco, Ferdinand MD (Cv) - **Spec Exp:** Nuclear Cardiology; Echocardiography; Congestive Heart Failure; **Hospital:** St John's Queens Hosp (page 375), Mary Immaculate Hosp; **Address:** St Johns Queens Hosp, 90-02 Queens Blvd, Elmhurst, NY 11373-4941; **Phone:** 718-558-1830; **Board Cert:** Internal Medicine 1973; Cardiovascular Disease 1977; **Med School:** Italy 1969; **Resid:** Internal Medicine, Queens Hosp Ctr 1972; **Fellow:** Cardiovascular Disease, Nassau County Med Ctr 1974; **Fac Appt:** Asst Clin Prof Med, NY Med Coll

CHILD & ADOLESCENT PSYCHIATRY

Perlmutter, Ilisse MD (ChAP) - **Spec Exp:** Disaster Psychiatry; Post Traumatic Stress Disorder; **Hospital:** Elmhurst Hosp Ctr; **Address:** Elmhurst Hosp Ctr, Dept Psychiatry, 79-01 Broadway, Elmhurst, NY 11373; **Phone:** 718-334-3273; **Board Cert:** Psychiatry 1989; Child & Adolescent Psychiatry 1991; **Med School:** Geo Wash Univ 1984; **Resid:** Psychiatry, Mt Sinai Med Ctr 1987; **Fellow:** Child & Adolescent Psychiatry, Columbia-Presby Med Ctr 1989

COLON & RECTAL SURGERY

Tiszenkel, Howard MD (CRS) - **Spec Exp:** Colon Cancer; **Hospital:** NY Hosp Queens; **Address:** NY Hospital Medical Ctr of Queens, 56-45 Main St, rm M204, Flushing, NY 11355-5000; **Phone:** 718-445-0220; **Board Cert:** Surgery 1996; Colon & Rectal Surgery 1988; **Med School:** NY Med Coll 1981; **Resid:** Surgery, St Luke's Hosp 1986; Colon & Rectal Surgery, Carle Clinic 1987

DERMATOLOGY

Beyda, Bernadette MD (D) - **Hospital:** NY Hosp Queens; **Address:** 141-23 59th Ave, Flushing, NY 11355-5304; **Phone:** 718-445-0566; **Board Cert:** Dermatology 1982; **Med School:** France 1976; **Resid:** Pathology, Booth Meml Med Ctr 1979; Dermatology, New York Hosp 1982

Gladstein, Michael MD (D) - **Hospital:** Mount Sinai Hosp of Queens (page 98); **Address:** 3062 36th Street, Astoria, NY 11103-4798; **Phone:** 718-728-8979; **Board Cert:** Dermatology 1987; **Med School:** NYU Sch Med 1979; **Resid:** Dermatology, NYU Med Ctr 1985

Pereira, Frederick MD (D) - **Spec Exp:** Skin Cancer; Geriatric Dermatology; Psoriasis; **Hospital:** NY Hosp Queens; **Address:** 51-14 Kissena Blvd, Flushing, NY 11355-4163; **Phone:** 718-359-4425; **Board Cert:** Dermatology 1975; **Med School:** UMDNJ-NJ Med Sch, Newark 1968; **Resid:** Dermatology, Mount Sinai Hosp 1974; Dermatology, Metropolitan Hosp 1975

DIAGNOSTIC RADIOLOGY

Mollin, Joel MD (DR) - **Spec Exp:** Ultrasound; CT Scan; **Hospital:** Elmhurst Hosp Ctr; **Address:** 79-01 Broadway, E1-18, Radiology, Elmhurst, NY 11373; **Phone:** 718-334-2052; **Board Cert:** Diagnostic Radiology 1985; Psychiatry 1976; **Med School:** SUNY Downstate 1969; **Resid:** Diagnostic Radiology, USPHS Hosp-Staten Island 1981; Diagnostic Radiology, Mt Sinai Hosp 1983; **Fac Appt:** Asst Clin Prof Rad, Mount Sinai Sch Med

Sprecher, Stanley MD (DR) - **Hospital:** Peninsula Hosp Ctr; **Address:** Peninsula Radiology Assocs, 51-15 Beach Channel Drive, Far Rockaway, NY 11691-1042; **Phone:** 718-734-2616; **Board Cert:** Diagnostic Radiology 1982; Nuclear Radiology 1983; **Med School:** Albert Einstein Coll Med 1977; **Resid:** Radiology, Univ Hosp 1979; Nuclear Medicine, St Vincent's Hosp & Med Ctr 1980

Tartell, Jay MD (DR) - **Hospital:** Mount Sinai Hosp of Queens (page 98); **Address:** 89-40 56th Ave, Elmhurst, NY 11373-4943; **Phone:** 718-335-5532; **Board Cert:** Radiology 1987; **Med School:** NY Med Coll 1982; **Resid:** Diagnostic Radiology, Bronx Muni Hosp/Albert Einstein 1986; **Fellow:** Ultrasound/CT/MRI, North Shore Univ Hosp 1987

Youner, Craig MD (DR) - **Hospital:** Mount Sinai Hosp of Queens (page 98); **Address:** 29-16 Astoria Blvd, Astoria, NY 11102-1742; **Phone:** 718-204-5800; **Board Cert:** Diagnostic Radiology 1978; **Med School:** Albany Med Coll 1973; **Resid:** Internal Medicine, North Shore Univ Hosp 1975; Diagnostic Radiology, North Shore Univ Hosp 1978; **Fac Appt:** Asst Clin Prof Rad, Cornell Univ-Weill Med Coll

ENDOCRINOLOGY, DIABETES & METABOLISM

Kukar, Narinder MD (EDM) - **Spec Exp:** Diabetes; Thyroid Disorders; Osteoporosis; **Hospital:** Wyckoff Heights Med Ctr, Jamaica Hosp Med Ctr; **Address:** 68-71 Grand Ave, Maspeth, NY 11378; **Phone:** 718-507-4400; **Board Cert:** Internal Medicine 1977; Endocrinology, Diabetes & Metabolism 1981; **Med School:** India 1960; **Resid:** Internal Medicine, Wycoff Heights Hosp 1969; **Fellow:** Endocrinology, Diabetes & Metabolism, SUNY Downstate 1971; **Fac Appt:** Asst Prof Med, SUNY Hlth Sci Ctr

Leder, Marvin MD (EDM) - **Spec Exp:** Diabetes; Cholesterol/Lipid Disorders; Hypertension; Thyroid Disorders; **Hospital:** NY Hosp Queens; **Address:** 69-15 Yellowstone Blvd, Forest Hills, NY 11375-3753; **Phone:** 718-268-4500; **Board Cert:** Internal Medicine 1974; **Med School:** SUNY Upstate Med Univ 1957; **Resid:** Internal Medicine, Manhattan VA Hosp 1959; Internal Medicine, Montefiore Hosp 1961; **Fellow:** Endocrinology, US Naval Hosp 1963

Lorber, Daniel MD (EDM) - **Spec Exp:** Diabetes; **Hospital:** NY Hosp Queens, Flushing Hosp Med Ctr; **Address:** 59-45 161st St, Flushing, NY 11365; **Phone:** 718-762-3111; **Board Cert:** Internal Medicine 1975; Endocrinology, Diabetes & Metabolism 1977; **Med School:** Albert Einstein Coll Med 1972; **Resid:** Internal Medicine, Jacobi Med Ctr 1975; **Fellow:** Endocrinology, Diabetes & Metabolism, Vanderbilt Univ Hosp 1977; **Fac Appt:** Assoc Clin Prof Med, Cornell Univ-Weill Med Coll

Resta, Christine MD (EDM) - **Spec Exp:** Diabetes; Thyroid Disorders; Osteoporosis; **Hospital:** NY Hosp Queens, Flushing Hosp Med Ctr; **Address:** 5945 161st St, Flushing, NY 11365; **Phone:** 718-762-3111; **Board Cert:** Internal Medicine 2002; Endocrinology, Diabetes & Metabolism 2005; **Med School:** Albert Einstein Coll Med 1989; **Resid:** Internal Medicine, Montefiore Med Ctr 1992; **Fellow:** Endocrinology, Diabetes & Metabolism, Montefiore Med Ctr 1995; **Fac Appt:** Asst Clin Prof Med, Albert Einstein Coll Med

Rosman, Lawrence MD (EDM) - **Spec Exp:** Thyroid Disorders; Osteoporosis; Diabetes; **Hospital:** Parkway Hosp, NY Hosp Queens; **Address:** 112-03 Queens Blvd, Ste 207, Flushing, NY 11375-5550; **Phone:** 718-263-3718; **Board Cert:** Internal Medicine 1978; Endocrinology 1983; **Med School:** NYU Sch Med 1975; **Resid:** Internal Medicine, NYU Med Ctr 1978; **Fellow:** Endocrinology, Diabetes & Metabolism, NYU Med Ctr 1980; **Fac Appt:** Asst Clin Prof Med, NYU Sch Med

Tibaldi, Joseph MD (EDM) - **Spec Exp:** Diabetes; Thyroid Disorders; Geriatric Endocrinology; **Hospital:** Flushing Hosp Med Ctr, NY Hosp Queens; **Address:** 59-45 161st St, Flushing, NY 11365-1414; **Phone:** 718-762-3111; **Board Cert:** Internal Medicine 1982; Endocrinology, Diabetes & Metabolism 1985; **Med School:** Mount Sinai Sch Med 1979; **Resid:** Internal Medicine, Nassau County Med Ctr 1981; Internal Medicine, Mount Sinai Hosp 1982; **Fellow:** Endocrinology, Montefiore Hosp Med Ctr 1983; **Fac Appt:** Asst Clin Prof Med, Albert Einstein Coll Med

FAMILY MEDICINE

Di Scala, Reno MD (FMed) PCP - **Hospital:** Mount Sinai Hosp of Queens (page 98), NY Hosp Queens; **Address:** 46-04 31st Ave, Long Island City, NY 11103; **Phone:** 718-545-2100; **Board Cert:** Family Medicine 2001; **Med School:** Italy 1982; **Resid:** Family Medicine, Community Hosp 1987; Surgery, Catholic Med Ctr 1985

Douglas, Montgomery MD (FMed) PCP - **Spec Exp:** Obstetrics; Geriatric Medicine; **Hospital:** Mary Immaculate Hosp, St John's Queens Hosp (page 375); **Address:** 114-49 Sutphin Blvd, Jamaica, NY 11434; **Phone:** 718-558-7160; **Board Cert:** Family Medicine 2001; Geriatric Medicine 2003; **Med School:** Cornell Univ-Weill Med Coll 1986; **Resid:** Family Medicine, Highland Hosp 1989; **Fac Appt:** Assoc Prof FMed, NY Med Coll

Fisher, George C MD (FMed) PCP - **Spec Exp:** Preventive Medicine; Hypertension; Cholesterol/Lipid Disorders; Diabetes; **Hospital:** Mount Sinai Hosp of Queens (page 98), Mount Sinai Med Ctr (page 98); **Address:** 22-33 33rd St, Astoria, NY 11105; **Phone:** 718-726-1000; **Board Cert:** Family Medicine 2000; **Med School:** England 1979; **Resid:** Family Medicine, St Joseph Med Ctr 1993

Istrico, Richard A DO (FMed) PCP - **Spec Exp:** Sports Injuries; Nutrition; Preventive Medicine; **Hospital:** Long Island Jewish Med Ctr, Parkway Hosp; **Address:** 158-01 Crossbay Blvd, Jamaica, NY 11414-3137; **Phone:** 718-738-9115; **Board Cert:** Family Medicine 1981; Sports Medicine 1995; **Med School:** Philadelphia Coll Osteo Med 1978; **Resid:** Family Medicine, Interboro Hosp 1979; Sports Medicine, Baptist Med Ctr 1980

Molnar, Thomas MD (FMed) PCP - **Spec Exp:** Hypertension; Diabetes; **Hospital:** NY Hosp Queens, Flushing Hosp Med Ctr; **Address:** 83-39 Daniels St, Jamaica, NY 11435-1208; **Phone:** 718-291-5151; **Board Cert:** Family Medicine 2002; **Med School:** Hungary 1982; **Resid:** Surgery, Flushing Hosp 1985; Family Medicine, Univ Hosp 1988

Reddy, Mallikarjuna MD (FMed) PCP - **Spec Exp:** Geriatric Care; **Hospital:** NY Hosp Queens, St John's Queens Hosp (page 375); **Address:** 72-18 164th St, Flushing, NY 11365-4222; **Phone:** 718-969-6640; **Board Cert:** Family Medicine 1996; Geriatric Medicine 1996; **Med School:** India 1982; **Resid:** Family Medicine, Catholic Med Ctr 1990

Roth, Alan DO (FMed) PCP - **Spec Exp:** Preventive Medicine; Diabetes; Hypertension; **Hospital:** Jamaica Hosp Med Ctr, Parkway Hosp; **Address:** 11940 Metropolitan Ave, Kew Gardens, NY 11415; **Phone:** 718-849-0624; **Board Cert:** Family Medicine 2002; **Med School:** NY Coll Osteo Med 1986; **Resid:** Family Medicine, Jamaica Hosp Med Ctr 1989; **Fac Appt:** Asst Clin Prof FMed, Mount Sinai Sch Med

GASTROENTEROLOGY

Harooni, Robert MD (Ge) - **Spec Exp:** Colonoscopy; Peptic Ulcer Disease; **Hospital:** NY Hosp Queens; **Address:** 55-16 Main St, Flushing, NY 11355-5044; **Phone:** 718-461-6161; **Board Cert:** Internal Medicine 1981; Gastroenterology 1985; **Med School:** Iran 1973; **Resid:** Internal Medicine, Booth Mem 1982; Internal Medicine, Booth Mem 1983; **Fellow:** Gastroenterology, Booth Mem 1984; Gastroenterology; **Fac Appt:** Med, Cornell Univ-Weill Med Coll

Klingenstein, Jeffrey MD (Ge) - **Spec Exp:** Hepatitis C; Colon Cancer; **Hospital:** Mount Sinai Med Ctr (page 98), NY Hosp Queens; **Address:** 36-01 31st Ave, Astoria, NY 11106; **Phone:** 718-626-2337; **Board Cert:** Internal Medicine 1978; Gastroenterology 1981; **Med School:** Boston Univ 1975; **Resid:** Internal Medicine, Boston VA 1978; **Fellow:** Gastroenterology, Mount Sinai 1981

Martin, George MD (Ge) - **Hospital:** NY Hosp Queens; **Address:** 56-28 Main St, Flushing, NY 11355-5046; **Phone:** 718-939-1800; **Board Cert:** Internal Medicine 1974; Gastroenterology 1977; Geriatric Medicine 1988; **Med School:** NYU Sch Med 1971; **Resid:** Internal Medicine, Bellevue Hosp 1975; **Fellow:** Gastroenterology, Peter Bent Brigham Hosp 1976Bellevue Hosp 1977; **Fac Appt:** Assoc Prof Med, Cornell Univ-Weill Med Coll

Moskowitz, Sam MD (Ge) - **Spec Exp:** Colitis; Hepatitis; **Hospital:** Beth Israel Med Ctr- Kings Hwy Div (page 90), Brookdale Univ Hosp Med Ctr; **Address:** 107-21 Queens Blvd, Ste 4, Forest Hills, NY 11375; **Phone:** 718-520-0857; **Board Cert:** Internal Medicine 1979; Gastroenterology 1981; **Med School:** Albert Einstein Coll Med 1976; **Resid:** Internal Medicine, Brookdale 1979; **Fellow:** Gastroenterology, VA Med Ctr 1981; **Fac Appt:** Asst Clin Prof, SUNY Downstate

Nussbaum, Michel E MD (Ge) - **Spec Exp:** Endoscopy & Colonoscopy; Colon Cancer; Inflammatory Bowel Disease; **Hospital:** NY Hosp Queens, Flushing Hosp Med Ctr; **Address:** 142-43 Booth Memorial Ave, Flushing, NY 11355-5343; **Phone:** 718-886-1919; **Board Cert:** Internal Medicine 1981; Gastroenterology 1983; **Med School:** Belgium 1977; **Resid:** Internal Medicine, NY Hosp-Queens 1980; **Fellow:** Gastroenterology, NY Hosp-Queens 1982; **Fac Appt:** Asst Clin Prof Med, Cornell Univ-Weill Med Coll

Ramgopal, Mekala MD (Ge) - **Spec Exp:** Peptic Acid Disorders; Gastroesophageal Reflux Disease (GERD); Endoscopy; **Hospital:** St John's Epis Hosp - S Shore, Peninsula Hosp Ctr; **Address:** 21-24 Camp Rd, Far Rockaway, NY 11691; **Phone:** 718-327-0207; **Board Cert:** Internal Medicine 1978; Gastroenterology 1979; Geriatric Medicine 1988; **Med School:** India 1974; **Resid:** Internal Medicine, Jersey City Med Ctr 1976; Internal Medicine, VA Med Ctr 1977; **Fellow:** Gastroenterology, Univ of Med/Dentistry 1979

Rand, James MD (Ge) - **Spec Exp:** Colonoscopy; **Hospital:** NY Hosp Queens, N Shore Univ Hosp at Manhasset; **Address:** 200-12 44th Ave, Bayside, NY 11361; **Phone:** 718-224-7454; **Board Cert:** Internal Medicine 1978; Gastroenterology 1981; **Med School:** Albert Einstein Coll Med 1975; **Resid:** Internal Medicine, Strong Meml Hosp 1977; Internal Medicine, Columbia-Presby 1978; **Fellow:** Gastroenterology, Montefiore Hosp Med Ctr 1980

Rosman, Sidney MD (Ge) - **Spec Exp:** Endoscopy; Liver Disease; **Hospital:** Parkway Hosp, N Shore Univ Hosp at Forest Hills; **Address:** 112-03 Queens Blvd, Ste 207, Forest Hills, NY 11375; **Phone:** 718-544-7077; **Board Cert:** Gastroenterology 1985; Internal Medicine 1980; **Med School:** Albert Einstein Coll Med 1976; **Resid:** Internal Medicine, VA Med Ctr 1978; Internal Medicine, VA Medical Ctr/NYU/Bellevue 1980; **Fellow:** Gastroenterology, VA Med Ctr 1982

Vogelman, Arthur MD (Ge) - **Spec Exp:** Colon Cancer; Peptic Ulcer Disease; Gastroesophageal Reflux Disease (GERD); **Hospital:** Parkway Hosp, NY Hosp Queens; **Address:** 7146 110th St, Forest Hills, NY 11375-4842; **Phone:** 718-261-2500; **Board Cert:** Internal Medicine 1979; Gastroenterology 1981; **Med School:** Univ Pittsburgh 1975; **Resid:** Internal Medicine, Mt Sinai Hosp 1978; **Fellow:** Gastroenterology, Mt Sinai Hosp 1980

Weg, Arnold MD (Ge) - **Spec Exp:** Endoscopy; Inflammatory Bowel Disease/Crohn's; **Hospital:** NY-Presby Hosp (page 100); **Address:** 71-36 110th St, Ste 1G, Forest Hills, NY 11375-4836; **Phone:** 718-520-2210; **Board Cert:** Internal Medicine 1985; Gastroenterology 1987; **Med School:** NYU Sch Med 1982; **Resid:** Gastroenterology, Columbia-Presby 1985; **Fellow:** Gastroenterology, NY Hosp

GERIATRIC MEDICINE

Brody, Samuel MD (Ger) - **Hospital:** N Shore Univ Hosp at Forest Hills; **Address:** 69-15 Yellowstone Blvd, Forest Hills, NY 11375; **Phone:** 718-268-4500; **Board Cert:** Internal Medicine 1980; Gastroenterology 1983; Geriatric Medicine 1998; **Med School:** Vanderbilt Univ 1977; **Resid:** Internal Medicine, Vanderbilt Med Ctr 1980; **Fellow:** Gastroenterology, Temple Univ Hosp 1982

GERIATRIC PSYCHIATRY

Greenwald, Blaine MD (GerPsy) - **Spec Exp:** Depression; Dementia; **Hospital:** Long Island Jewish Med Ctr; **Address:** 75-59 263rd St, Div Geriatric Psychiatry, Glen Oaks, NY 11004; **Phone:** 718-470-8159; **Board Cert:** Psychiatry 1983; Geriatric Psychiatry 2001; **Med School:** NY Med Coll 1978; **Resid:** Psychiatry, Mount Sinai Hosp 1982; **Fellow:** Geriatric Psychiatry, Mount Sinai Hosp/Bronx VA Hosp 1983; **Fac Appt:** Assoc Prof Psyc, Albert Einstein Coll Med

GYNECOLOGIC ONCOLOGY

Jacobs, Allan J MD (GO) - **Spec Exp:** Gynecologic Cancer; **Hospital:** Flushing Hosp Med Ctr; **Address:** 146-01 45th Ave, Flushing, NY 11355; **Phone:** 718-670-5792; **Board Cert:** Obstetrics & Gynecology 1994; Gynecologic Oncology 1983; **Med School:** USC Sch Med 1972; **Resid:** Obstetrics & Gynecology, Parkland Meml Hosp 1976; **Fellow:** Gynecologic Oncology, Mt Sinai Hosp 1980; **Fac Appt:** Prof ObG, NYU Sch Med

Welshinger, Marie MD (GO) - **Spec Exp:** Gynecologic Cancer; **Hospital:** NY Hosp Queens; **Address:** 163-03 Horace Harding Expy Fl 3 - Ste 300, Fresh Meadows, NY 11365-1449; **Phone:** 718-670-1170; **Board Cert:** Obstetrics & Gynecology 2004; Gynecologic Oncology 2004; **Med School:** Univ Minn 1988; **Resid:** Obstetrics & Gynecology, SUNY Stony Brook Hosp 1992; **Fellow:** Gynecologic Oncology, Meml Sloan Kett Cancer Ctr 1996; **Fac Appt:** Asst Clin Prof ObG, UMDNJ-RW Johnson Med Sch

HAND SURGERY

Roger, Ignatius Daniel MD (HS) - **Spec Exp:** Wrist/Hand Injuries; Carpal Tunnel Syndrome; Reconstructive Surgery; Tendon Surgery; **Hospital:** St John's Queens Hosp (page 375), Mary Immaculate Hosp; **Address:** 91-31 Queens Blvd, Ste 301, Elmhurst, NY 11373-5540; **Phone:** 718-205-2100; **Board Cert:** Plastic Surgery 1993; Hand Surgery 1995; **Med School:** Mount Sinai Sch Med 1980; **Resid:** Surgery, Staten Island Hosp 1984; Surgery, Catholic Med Ctr 1985; **Fellow:** Plastic Surgery, Albany Med Ctr 1987

INFECTIOUS DISEASE

Landesman, Sheldon MD (Inf) - **Hospital:** SUNY Downstate Med Ctr; **Address:** SUNY Downstate, 450 Clarkson Ave, Box 9, Brooklyn, NY 11415; **Phone:** 718-270-3034; **Board Cert:** Internal Medicine 1976; **Med School:** SUNY Downstate 1972; **Resid:** Interventional Cardiology, Tufts-New England Med Ctr 1976; **Fellow:** Research, Baltimore Cancer Rsrch Inst/NCI 1975; Infectious Disease, Tufts-New England Med Ctr 1977

Masci, Joseph MD (Inf) - **Spec Exp:** AIDS/HIV; Tropical Diseases; Bioterrorism Preparedness; **Hospital:** Elmhurst Hosp Ctr; **Address:** Elmhurst Hosp, Dept Med, 79-01 Broadway, rm C 6-10, Elmhurst, NY 11373; **Phone:** 718-334-3446; **Board Cert:** Internal Medicine 1979; Infectious Disease 1982; **Med School:** NYU Sch Med 1976; **Resid:** Internal Medicine, Boston City Hosp 1979; **Fellow:** Infectious Disease, Mt Sinai Hosp 1982; **Fac Appt:** Prof Med, Mount Sinai Sch Med

Rahal, James MD (Inf) - **Spec Exp:** West Nile Virus; Antibiotic Resistance; Hospital Acquired Infections; **Hospital:** NY Hosp Queens; **Address:** NY Hosp Queens, Div Infectious Disease, 56-45 Main St, Flushing, NY 11355-5095; **Phone:** 718-670-1525; **Board Cert:** Internal Medicine 1967; Infectious Disease 1972; **Med School:** Tufts Univ 1959; **Resid:** Internal Medicine, Bellevue Hosp Ctr 1961; Internal Medicine, New England Ctr Hosp 1964; **Fellow:** Infectious Disease, New England Ctr Hosp 1965; **Fac Appt:** Prof Med, Cornell Univ-Weill Med Coll

INTERNAL MEDICINE

Amin, Mahendra MD (IM) **PCP** - **Hospital:** NY Hosp Queens, Long Island Jewish Med Ctr; **Address:** 89-02 Springfield Blvd, Queens Village, NY 11427-2514; **Phone:** 718-776-4444; **Board Cert:** Internal Medicine 1984; **Med School:** India 1978; **Resid:** Internal Medicine, Metropolitan Hosp Ctr 1982; **Fellow:** Internal Medicine, Metropolitan Hosp Ctr 1985

Beyda, Allan MD (IM) **PCP** - **Spec Exp:** Preventive Medicine; **Hospital:** NY Hosp Queens; **Address:** 141-23 59th Ave, Flushing, NY 11355-5304; **Phone:** 718-359-7406; **Board Cert:** Internal Medicine 1979; **Med School:** France 1976; **Resid:** Internal Medicine, New York Hosp Med Ctr 1979

Blum, Daniel N MD (IM) **PCP** - **Spec Exp:** Geriatrics; Hypertension; Diabetes; **Hospital:** NY Hosp Queens; **Address:** 13806 Jewel Ave, Flushing, NY 11367-1933; **Phone:** 718-520-0248; **Board Cert:** Internal Medicine 1984; **Med School:** Albert Einstein Coll Med 1980; **Resid:** Internal Medicine, NY Hosp of Queens 1984

Brewer, Marlon MD (IM) - **Spec Exp:** Diabetes; Hypertension; **Hospital:** Elmhurst Hosp Ctr; **Address:** 79-01 Broadway, Rm D124, Elmhurst, NY 11373; **Phone:** 718-334-2490; **Board Cert:** Internal Medicine 1994; **Med School:** Spain 1986; **Resid:** Internal Medicine, Elmhurst Hosp 1992; **Fac Appt:** Asst Clin Prof Med, Mount Sinai Sch Med

Fukilman, Oscar J MD (IM) **PCP** - **Hospital:** Mount Sinai Hosp of Queens (page 98); **Address:** 25-31 30th Road, Ste 1A, Astoria, NY 11102; **Phone:** 718-267-1102; **Board Cert:** Internal Medicine 1979; **Med School:** Argentina 1968; **Resid:** Internal Medicine, Elmhurst Hosp/Mt Sinai Hosp Svc 1972

Joseph, John MD (IM) **PCP** - **Spec Exp:** Rheumatology; Osteoporosis; Arthritis; **Hospital:** Parkway Hosp, NY Hosp Queens; **Address:** 66-20 108th St, Forest Hills, NY 11375; **Phone:** 718-896-8920; **Board Cert:** Internal Medicine 1983; **Med School:** Mexico 1977; **Resid:** Internal Medicine, Coney Island Hosp 1982; **Fellow:** Rheumatology, Long Island Coll Hosp 1984

Lempel, Herbert MD (IM) **PCP** - **Hospital:** NY Hosp Queens; **Address:** 112-47 Queens Blvd, rm 109, Forest Hills, NY 11375-5554; **Phone:** 718-544-9023; **Board Cert:** Internal Medicine 1984; **Med School:** NY Med Coll 1981; **Resid:** Internal Medicine, Booth Meml Med Ctr 1984

Messana, Ida MD (IM) **PCP** - **Hospital:** Long Island Jewish Med Ctr, N Shore Univ Hosp at Manhasset; **Address:** 109-33 71st Rd, Ste 2E, Forest Hills, NY 11375; **Phone:** 718-263-4345; **Board Cert:** Internal Medicine 1988; **Med School:** SUNY Stony Brook 1984; **Resid:** Internal Medicine, Montefiore Med Ctr 1987; **Fellow:** Geriatric Medicine, Montefiore Med Ctr 1989

Mohrer, Jonathan MD (IM) **PCP** - **Spec Exp:** Cardiovascular Disease; Diabetes; **Hospital:** NY Hosp Queens, Parkway Hosp; **Address:** 114-06 Queens Blvd, Ste A-8, Forest Hills, NY 11375; **Phone:** 718-575-9787; **Board Cert:** Internal Medicine 1983; **Med School:** Univ Conn 1980; **Resid:** Internal Medicine, LI Jewish Med Ctr 1983

Qadir, Shuja MD (IM) PCP - **Spec Exp:** Heart Failure; Arrhythmias; Syncope; **Hospital:** Mary Immaculate Hosp, N Shore Univ Hosp at Manhasset; **Address:** 85-04 67th Rd, Rego Park, NY 11374; **Phone:** 718-275-6061; **Board Cert:** Internal Medicine 1984; Cardiovascular Disease 1987; **Med School:** Pakistan 1977; **Resid:** Internal Medicine, Catholic Med Ctr 1985; **Fellow:** Cardiovascular Disease, Catholic Med Ctr 1987; **Fac Appt:** Asst Prof Med, NY Med Coll

Reilly, Thomas MD (IM) PCP - **Hospital:** St John's Queens Hosp (page 375), St Vincent Cath Med Ctrs - Manhattan (page 375); **Address:** 86-27 Forest Pkwy, Woodhaven, NY 11421-1132; **Phone:** 718-805-2404; **Board Cert:** Internal Medicine 1984; **Med School:** SUNY Hlth Sci Ctr 1979; **Resid:** Internal Medicine, Staten Island Hosp 1982; **Fellow:** Hematology, St Vincent's Hosp & Med Ctr 1985; **Fac Appt:** Asst Clin Prof Med, NY Med Coll

Reuben, Stephen MD (IM) PCP - **Spec Exp:** Hypertension; Diabetes; Cholesterol/Lipid Disorders; **Hospital:** NY Hosp Queens; **Address:** 6142 Maspeth Ave, Maspeth, NY 11378; **Phone:** 718-326-1933; **Board Cert:** Internal Medicine 1996; **Med School:** Vanderbilt Univ 1977; **Resid:** Internal Medicine, Lenox Hill Hosp 1980

Sciales, John MD (IM) PCP - **Spec Exp:** Preventive Medicine; Geriatric Rehabilitation; Mood Disorders; **Hospital:** NY Hosp Queens; **Address:** 163-03 Oak Ave, Flushing, NY 11358-3796; **Phone:** 718-445-2298; **Board Cert:** Internal Medicine 1987; Geriatric Medicine 1994; **Med School:** SUNY Hlth Sci Ctr 1984; **Resid:** Internal Medicine, Booth Meml Med Ctr 1987

INTERVENTIONAL CARDIOLOGY

Papadakos, Stylianos P MD (IC) - **Spec Exp:** Cardiac Catheterization; Percutaneous Myocardial Revasc (PMR); **Hospital:** NY Hosp Queens; **Address:** NY Hosp Med Ctr Queens, Cardiac Cath, 56-45 Main St Fl 3, Flushing, NY 11355; **Phone:** 718-670-1000; **Board Cert:** Cardiovascular Disease 2004; Interventional Cardiology 1999; **Med School:** Greece 1985; **Resid:** Internal Medicine, Booth Meml Med Ctr 1989; Internal Medicine, Mt Sinai Hosp 1990; **Fellow:** Cardiovascular Disease, Univ Conn Hosp 1994

MATERNAL & FETAL MEDICINE

Inglis, Steven R MD (MF) - **Spec Exp:** Pregnancy-High Risk; Premature Labor; **Hospital:** Jamaica Hosp Med Ctr; **Address:** Jamaica Hospital, Dept OB/GYN, 89-06 135th St, Ste 6A, Jamaica, NY 11418; **Phone:** 718-206-6808; **Board Cert:** Obstetrics & Gynecology 2004; Maternal & Fetal Medicine 2004; **Med School:** NY Med Coll 1986; **Resid:** Obstetrics & Gynecology, Albany Med Ctr 1990; **Fellow:** Maternal & Fetal Medicine, NY Hosp-Cornell Med Ctr 1992; **Fac Appt:** Assoc Prof ObG, Cornell Univ-Weill Med Coll

Skupski, Daniel MD (MF) - **Spec Exp:** Fetal Therapy; **Hospital:** NY Hosp Queens, NY-Presby Hosp (page 100); **Address:** 56-45 Main St, Flushing, NY 11355-5060; **Phone:** 718-670-1534; **Board Cert:** Obstetrics & Gynecology 2001; Maternal & Fetal Medicine 2001; **Med School:** Univ Mich Med Sch 1985; **Resid:** Obstetrics & Gynecology, Hurley Med Ctr 1989; **Fellow:** Maternal & Fetal Medicine, NY Hosp Cornell Med Ctr 1994; **Fac Appt:** Assoc Prof ObG, Cornell Univ-Weill Med Coll

MEDICAL ONCOLOGY

Benisovich, Vladimir I MD (Onc) - **Spec Exp:** Breast Cancer; Lung Cancer; Colon Cancer; **Hospital:** Elmhurst Hosp Ctr, Mount Sinai Med Ctr (page 98); **Address:** 79-01 Broadway, Ste H2-04, Elmhurst, NY 11373-1329; **Phone:** 718-334-3723; **Board Cert:** Internal Medicine 1982; Hematology 1984; Medical Oncology 1985; **Med School:** Russia 1966; **Resid:** Internal Medicine, Bronx Lebanon Med Ctr 1980; **Fellow:** Hematology, NYU Med Ctr 1982; Medical Oncology, Mt Sinai Med Ctr 1983

Cortes, Engracio P MD (Onc) - **Spec Exp:** Breast Cancer; Gastrointestinal Cancer; Lung Cancer; **Hospital:** NY Hosp Queens, Long Island Jewish Med Ctr; **Address:** 200-20 44th Ave, Bayside, NY 11361; **Phone:** 718-279-9101; **Board Cert:** Internal Medicine 1976; Medical Oncology 1977; **Med School:** Philippines 1964; **Resid:** Internal Medicine, Lemuel Shattuck Hosp 1968; **Fellow:** Medical Oncology, Roswell Park Cancer Inst 1971; **Fac Appt:** Assoc Clin Prof Med, Cornell Univ-Weill Med Coll

Daly, Jane MD (Onc) - **Hospital:** St John's Queens Hosp (page 375), NY Hosp Queens; **Address:** 87-23 Myrtle Ave, Glendale, NY 11385-7431; **Phone:** 718-441-5581; **Board Cert:** Internal Medicine 1978; Hand Surgery 1980; Medical Oncology 1981; **Med School:** NY Med Coll 1975; **Resid:** Internal Medicine, Kings County Hosp 1978; **Fellow:** Hematology, LI Jewish Med Ctr 1980; Medical Oncology, Albert Einstein 1981

Greenberg, Howard MD (Onc) - **Spec Exp:** Breast Cancer; **Hospital:** Mount Sinai Hosp of Queens (page 98), Mount Sinai Med Ctr (page 98); **Address:** 25-75 34th St, Astoria, NY 11103; **Phone:** 718-278-3569; **Board Cert:** Internal Medicine 1976; Hematology 1978; Medical Oncology 1979; **Med School:** SUNY Downstate 1973; **Resid:** Internal Medicine, Mt Sinai Hosp 1976; **Fellow:** Hematology, Mt Sinai Hosp 1978; Medical Oncology, Meml Sloan Kettering Cancer Ctr 1978; **Fac Appt:** Asst Clin Prof Med, Mount Sinai Sch Med

Kaplan, Barry MD/PhD (Onc) - **Spec Exp:** Lung Cancer; Leukemia; Breast Cancer; **Hospital:** NY Hosp Queens; **Address:** 59-16 174th St, Fresh Meadows, NY 11365-1539; **Phone:** 718-460-2300; **Board Cert:** Internal Medicine 1970; Hematology 1972; Medical Oncology 1975; **Med School:** Johns Hopkins Univ 1962; **Resid:** Internal Medicine, Bronx Municipal Hosp 1967; **Fellow:** Hematology, Bronx Municipal Hosp/Einstein 1968; **Fac Appt:** Assoc Clin Prof Med, Cornell Univ-Weill Med Coll

Shum, Kee MD (Onc) - **Spec Exp:** Breast Cancer; Lung Cancer; Colon Cancer; **Hospital:** NY Hosp Queens, Flushing Hosp Med Ctr; **Address:** 136-25 Maple Ave, Ste 205, Flushing, NY 11355-3891; **Phone:** 718-463-2245; **Board Cert:** Internal Medicine 1984; Medical Oncology 1987; **Med School:** Cornell Univ-Weill Med Coll 1981; **Resid:** Internal Medicine, Kings County Hosp 1985; **Fellow:** Medical Oncology, Meml Sloan Kettering Cancer Ctr 1987

NEPHROLOGY

Galler, Marilyn MD (Nep) - **Spec Exp:** Hypertension; Kidney Disease; **Hospital:** NY Hosp Queens, Montefiore Med Ctr - Weiler-Einstein Div; **Address:** 56-45 Main St, Flushing, NY 11355; **Phone:** 718-670-1151; **Board Cert:** Internal Medicine 1980; Nephrology 1984; **Med School:** NYU Sch Med 1975; **Resid:** Internal Medicine, Bronx Municipal Hosp 1979; **Fellow:** Nephrology, Albert Einstein 1981; **Fac Appt:** Asst Clin Prof Med, Cornell Univ-Weill Med Coll

Kostadaras, Ari MD (Nep) - **Spec Exp:** Hypertension; Dialysis Care; Kidney Stones; **Hospital:** Mount Sinai Hosp of Queens (page 98), NY Hosp Queens; **Address:** 23-18 31st St, Astoria, NY 11105; **Phone:** 718-721-4440; **Board Cert:** Internal Medicine 1993; Nephrology 1998; **Med School:** Grenada 1989; **Resid:** Internal Medicine, LaGuardia Hosp 1992; **Fellow:** Nephrology, Nassau County Med Ctr 1994

Mattoo, Nirmal MD (Nep) - **Hospital:** Wyckoff Heights Med Ctr, N Shore Univ Hosp at Forest Hills; **Address:** 25-11 Astoria Blvd, Astoria, NY 11102; **Phone:** 718-545-3617; **Board Cert:** Internal Medicine 1974; Nephrology 1978; **Med School:** India 1967; **Resid:** Internal Medicine, Queens Hosp Ctr 1971; Internal Medicine, Catholic Med Ctr 1972; **Fellow:** Nephrology, Elmhurst Hosp Ctr 1975

Rascoff, Joel MD (Nep) - **Spec Exp:** Hypertension; Kidney Disease; Kidney Stones; **Hospital:** NY Hosp Queens, Montefiore Med Ctr - Weiler-Einstein Div; **Address:** 56-45 Main St, Flushing, NY 11355-5045; **Phone:** 718-670-1151; **Board Cert:** Internal Medicine 1973; Nephrology 1976; **Med School:** Columbia P&S 1968; **Resid:** Internal Medicine, Bronx Muni Hosp-Einstein 1973; **Fellow:** Nephrology, Hosp Univ Penn 1975; **Fac Appt:** Assoc Clin Prof Med, Cornell Univ-Weill Med Coll

Scott III, David MD (Nep) - **Spec Exp:** Hypertension; Kidney Disease; Diabetes; **Hospital:** NY Hosp Queens, Mary Immaculate Hosp; **Address:** 134-35 Springfield Blvd, Springfield Gardens, NY 11413; **Phone:** 718-276-4750; **Board Cert:** Internal Medicine 2003; Nephrology 1994; **Med School:** Tufts Univ 1985; **Resid:** Internal Medicine, Harlem Hosp 1988; **Fellow:** Nephrology, Harlem Hosp 1990

Spinowitz, Bruce MD (Nep) - **Spec Exp:** Kidney Disease-Diabetic; Hypertension; Kidney Stones; **Hospital:** NY Hosp Queens, Montefiore Med Ctr - Weiler-Einstein Div; **Address:** 56-45 Main St, Flushing, NY 11355-5045; **Phone:** 718-670-1151; **Board Cert:** Internal Medicine 1976; Nephrology 1978; **Med School:** NYU Sch Med 1973; **Resid:** Internal Medicine, Bellevue Hosp 1976; **Fellow:** Nephrology, Bellevue Hosp 1978; **Fac Appt:** Assoc Clin Prof Med, Cornell Univ-Weill Med Coll

NEUROLOGY

Casson, Ira MD (N) - **Spec Exp:** Sports Neurology; Headache; Head Injury; **Hospital:** Parkway Hosp, Long Island Jewish Med Ctr; **Address:** 112-03 Queens Blvd, Forest Hills, NY 11375-5550; **Phone:** 718-544-6633; **Board Cert:** Neurology 1980; **Med School:** NYU Sch Med 1975; **Resid:** Neurology, NYU Med Ctr 1979; **Fac Appt:** Asst Prof N, Albert Einstein Coll Med

Schaul, Neil MD (N) - **Spec Exp:** Epilepsy/Seizure Disorders; Electrodiagnosis; **Hospital:** NY Hosp Queens; **Address:** Comprehensive Epilepsy Center, 56-45 Main St Fl 6 South, Flushing, NY 11355-5045; **Phone:** 718-670-2900; **Board Cert:** Neurology 1976; **Med School:** SUNY Hlth Sci Ctr 1966; **Resid:** Internal Medicine, DC General Hosp 1968; Neurology, Montreal Neur Inst 1974; **Fellow:** Neurological Physiology, Montreal Neur Inst 1977; **Fac Appt:** Assoc Prof Med, Cornell Univ-Weill Med Coll

OBSTETRICS & GYNECOLOGY

Benedicto, Milagros A MD (ObG) - **Hospital:** Wyckoff Heights Med Ctr; **Address:** 58-10 Catalpa Ave, Flushing, NY 11385-5032; **Phone:** 718-381-7016; **Board Cert:** Obstetrics & Gynecology 2004; **Med School:** Philippines 1964; **Resid:** Obstetrics & Gynecology, Wyckoff Heights Hosp 1969; **Fellow:** Obstetrics & Gynecology, Wyckoff Heights Hosp 1971

Concannon, Patrick MD (ObG) **PCP** - **Spec Exp:** Menopause Problems; Osteoporosis; **Hospital:** N Shore Univ Hosp at Manhasset, Flushing Hosp Med Ctr; **Address:** 140-55 34th Ave, Flushing, NY 11354-3055; **Phone:** 718-445-1716; **Board Cert:** Obstetrics & Gynecology 1978; **Med School:** NYU Sch Med 1955; **Resid:** Obstetrics & Gynecology, Naval Hosp-St Albans 1958; Obstetrics & Gynecology, Flushing Hosp 1962; **Fac Appt:** Asst Clin Prof ObG, Cornell Univ-Weill Med Coll

Guarnaccia, Gary MD (ObG) - **Spec Exp:** Laparoscopic Surgery; **Hospital:** Parkway Hosp, Long Island Jewish Med Ctr; **Address:** 112-03 Queens Blvd, Ste 200, Forest Hills, NY 11375-5550; **Phone:** 718-268-8383; **Board Cert:** Obstetrics & Gynecology 1980; **Med School:** UMDNJ-NJ Med Sch, Newark 1974; **Resid:** Obstetrics & Gynecology, Bellevue Hosp/NYU Med Ctr 1978

Mandeville, Edgar MD (ObG) - **Hospital:** NY Hosp Queens; **Address:** 177-14 Wexford Terr, Jamaica Estates, NY 11432; **Phone:** 718-523-4422; **Board Cert:** Obstetrics & Gynecology 1976; **Med School:** Meharry Med Coll 1967; **Resid:** Obstetrics & Gynecology, Harlem Hosp Ctr 1974

Pellettieri, John MD (ObG) **PCP** - **Hospital:** Flushing Hosp Med Ctr; **Address:** 30-49 36th St, Long Island City, NY 11103-4704; **Phone:** 718-278-2126; **Board Cert:** Obstetrics & Gynecology 1970; **Med School:** NY Med Coll 1963; **Resid:** Obstetrics & Gynecology, St Vincent's Hosp Med Ctr 1968

Schuster, Stephen MD (ObG) - **Spec Exp:** Infectious Disease OB/GYN; **Hospital:** NY Hosp Queens, Flushing Hosp Med Ctr; **Address:** 58-34 Main St, Flushing, NY 11355-5336; **Phone:** 718-939-0111; **Board Cert:** Obstetrics & Gynecology 1998; **Med School:** NYU Sch Med 1967; **Resid:** Obstetrics & Gynecology, NYU Med Ctr 1972; **Fac Appt:** Asst Clin Prof ObG, Cornell Univ-Weill Med Coll

Tsin, Daniel MD (ObG) - **Spec Exp:** Gynecologic Surgery-Laparoscopic; Colposcopy; **Hospital:** Mount Sinai Hosp of Queens (page 98); **Address:** 82-11 37th Ave Fl 5th, Jackson Heights, NY 11372; **Phone:** 718-899-7878; **Board Cert:** Obstetrics & Gynecology 1976; **Med School:** Argentina 1965; **Resid:** Obstetrics & Gynecology, Roosevelt Hosp 1974

Younus, Bazaga MD (ObG) **PCP** - **Hospital:** St John's Queens Hosp (page 375), Mary Immaculate Hosp; **Address:** 42-66 Kissena Blvd, Flushing, NY 11355; **Phone:** 718-353-1223; **Board Cert:** Obstetrics & Gynecology 1985; **Med School:** India 1978; **Resid:** Obstetrics & Gynecology, Catholic Med Ctr 1979

OPHTHALMOLOGY

Aharon, Raphael MD (Oph) - **Hospital:** Parkway Hosp, NY Hosp Queens; **Address:** 108-37 71st Ave, Forest Hills, NY 11375-4566; **Phone:** 718-268-6120; **Board Cert:** Ophthalmology 1987; **Med School:** Albert Einstein Coll Med 1980; **Resid:** Internal Medicine, Brookdale Hosp 1981; Ophthalmology, Albert Einstein Coll Med 1984; **Fac Appt:** Asst Clin Prof Oph, Albert Einstein Coll Med

Boniuk, Vivien MD (Oph) - **Spec Exp:** Diagnostic Problems; **Hospital:** Long Island Jewish Med Ctr, N Shore Univ Hosp at Forest Hills; **Address:** Queens Hosp Ctr, Dept Oph, 82-68 164th St, Jamaica, NY 11432-1140; **Phone:** 718-883-2020; **Board Cert:** Ophthalmology 1969; **Med School:** Dalhousie Univ 1964; **Resid:** Ophthalmology, Barnes Hosp-Washington Univ 1967; **Fellow:** Ophthalmological Pathology, Baylor Coll Med 1968; **Fac Appt:** Assoc Prof Oph, Albert Einstein Coll Med

Fishman, Allen J. MD (Oph) - **Spec Exp:** Cataract Surgery-Lens Implant; LASIK-Refractive Surgery; **Hospital:** Parkway Hosp; **Address:** 92-29 Queens Blvd, Ste 21, Rego Park, NY 11374; **Phone:** 71 -261-7007; **Board Cert:** Ophthalmology 1981; **Med School:** Univ Hlth Sci/Chicago Med Sch 1976; **Resid:** Surgery, Beth Israel Hospital 1977; Ophthalmology, Brookdale Hospital 1980

Goldberg, Robert T MD (Oph) - **Spec Exp:** Glaucoma; Diabetic Eye Disease/Retinopathy; **Hospital:** NY Hosp Queens, Long Island Jewish Med Ctr; **Address:** 142-10 Roosevelt Ave, Ste B, Flushing, NY 11354-6046; **Phone:** 718-539-2992; **Board Cert:** Ophthalmology 1964; **Med School:** NYU Sch Med 1956; **Resid:** Ophthalmology, NYU Med Ctr 1960; Ophthalmology, SUNY Downstate Med Ctr 1963; **Fellow:** Strabismus, NYU Med Ctr 1965; **Fac Appt:** Assoc Clin Prof Oph, NYU Sch Med

Grasso, Cono M MD (Oph) - **Spec Exp:** Cataract Surgery; Glaucoma; Oculoplastic Surgery; **Hospital:** St John's Queens Hosp (page 375), Manhattan Eye, Ear & Throat Hosp; **Address:** 83-05 Grand Ave, Elmhurst, NY 11373-4104; **Phone:** 718-429-0300; **Board Cert:** Ophthalmology 1979; **Med School:** NYU Sch Med 1974; **Resid:** Ophthalmology, Wills Eye 1978; **Fac Appt:** Assoc Prof Oph, NY Med Coll

Ko, Wilson MD (Oph) - **Spec Exp:** Cataract Surgery; Chinese Eye Care; Anterior Segment Surgery; **Hospital:** Flushing Hosp Med Ctr; **Address:** 136-25 Maple Ave, Ste 202, Flushing, NY 11355; **Phone:** 718-358-5900; **Board Cert:** Ophthalmology 1989; **Med School:** Columbia P&S 1983; **Resid:** Ophthalmology, NYU M ' Ctr 1987; **Fellow:** Cornea & Ext Eye Disease, Wills Eye Hosp 1988

Mackool, Richard MD (Oph) - **Spec Exp:** Cataract Surgery; LASIK-Refractive Surgery; Lens Implants-Multifocal (Restor); Corneal Disease & Surgery; **Hospital:** New York Eye & Ear Infirm (page 110); **Address:** 31-27 41st St, Astoria, NY 11103; **Phone:** 718-728-3400; **Board Cert:** Ophthalmology 1975; **Med School:** Boston Univ 1968; **Resid:** Ophthalmology, New York EE Infirm 1973; **Fac Appt:** Asst Clin Prof Oph, NY Med Coll

Seidenfeld, Andrew MD (Oph) - **Spec Exp:** Cataract Surgery; LASIK-Refractive Surgery; **Hospital:** New York Eye & Ear Infirm (page 110), Wyckoff Heights Med Ctr; **Address:** 73-09 Myrtle Ave, Glendale, NY 11385-7431; **Phone:** 718-456-9500; **Board Cert:** Ophthalmology 1982; **Med School:** Univ Hlth Sci/Chicago Med Sch 1976; **Resid:** Ophthalmology, NY EE Infirmary 1980

ORTHOPAEDIC SURGERY

Besser, Walter MD (OrS) - **Spec Exp:** Joint Replacement; **Hospital:** Mount Sinai Hosp of Queens (page 98), Hosp For Joint Diseases (page 107); **Address:** 30-71 29th St, Astoria, NY 11102; **Phone:** 718-204-7752; **Board Cert:** Orthopaedic Surgery 1977; **Med School:** Spain 1968; **Resid:** Orthopaedic Surgery, LI Jewish Hosp 1971; Orthopaedic Surgery, Brooklyn Jewish Hosp 1974; **Fellow:** Orthopaedic Surgery, Hosp Special Surg 1977

Denton, John MD (OrS) - **Hospital:** Mary Immaculate Hosp; **Address:** 88-25 153rd St, Ste 1S, Jamaica, NY 11432-3748; **Phone:** 718-558-7241; **Board Cert:** Orthopaedic Surgery 1973; **Med School:** Univ Ala 1967; **Resid:** Surgery, Roosevelt Hosp 1969; Orthopaedic Surgery, NY Orthopaedic Hosp 1972; **Fellow:** Orthopaedic Surgery, NY Orthopaedic Hosp 1973

Eswar, Sounder MD (OrS) - **Spec Exp:** Hand Surgery; Arthroscopic Surgery; Joint Replacement; **Hospital:** Mary Immaculate Hosp, Wyckoff Heights Med Ctr; **Address:** 157-48 85th St, Howard Beach, NY 11414-2619; **Phone:** 718-738-6223; **Board Cert:** Orthopaedic Surgery 1975; **Med School:** India 1966; **Resid:** Surgery, NY Methodist Hosp 1970; Orthopaedic Surgery, CMC-Mary Immac Hosp 1973; **Fellow:** Hand Surgery, Hosp for Joint Diseases 1974

Giannaris, Theodore MD (OrS) - **Spec Exp:** Arthroscopic Surgery; Hip & Knee Replacement; **Hospital:** St. Vincent's Midtown, Mount Sinai Hosp of Queens (page 98); **Address:** 2747 Cresent St, Astoria, NY 11102; **Phone:** 718-278-1855; **Board Cert:** Orthopaedic Surgery 1977; **Med School:** Greece 1965; **Resid:** Orthopaedic Surgery, St Vincent's Hosp & Med Ctr 1974; Orthopaedic Surgery, NY Polyclinic Hosp 1972; **Fellow:** Pediatric Orthopaedic Surgery, St Giles Hosp 1976; **Fac Appt:** Asst Prof OrS, NY Med Coll

Goldman, Arnold MD (OrS) - **Spec Exp:** Arthroscopic Surgery; Sports Medicine; Foot & Ankle Surgery; **Hospital:** Parkway Hosp, NY Hosp Queens; **Address:** 113-13 76th Rd, Forest Hills, NY 11375-6528; **Phone:** 718-263-7300; **Board Cert:** Orthopaedic Surgery 2001; **Med School:** SUNY Upstate Med Univ 1981; **Resid:** Orthopaedic Surgery, NYU Med Ctr 1986; **Fellow:** Sports Medicine, NYU Med Ctr; Foot/Ankle Surgery, NYU Med Ctr

Schwartz, Evan MD (OrS) - **Spec Exp:** Sports Medicine; Shoulder Surgery; Knee Surgery; **Hospital:** St John's Queens Hosp (page 375); **Address:** 90-02 Queens Blvd, Elmhurst, NY 11373-4941; **Phone:** 718-558-1975; **Board Cert:** Orthopaedic Surgery 2000; **Med School:** SUNY Buffalo 1981; **Resid:** Orthopaedic Surgery, Einstein/Montefiore Med Ctr 1986; **Fellow:** Sports Medicine, Hosp For Special Surgery 1987; **Fac Appt:** Asst Prof OrS, NY Med Coll

Toriello, Edward MD (OrS) - **Spec Exp:** Arthritis; Sports Medicine; Osteoporosis; **Hospital:** Wyckoff Heights Med Ctr, St John's Queens Hosp (page 375); **Address:** 78-15 Eliot Ave, Middle Village, NY 11379-1300; **Phone:** 718-458-8944; **Board Cert:** Orthopaedic Surgery 1997; **Med School:** SUNY Buffalo 1980; **Resid:** Orthopaedic Surgery, Downstate Med Ctr 1985

OTOLARYNGOLOGY

La Marca, Charles MD (Oto) - **Hospital:** St John's Queens Hosp (page 375); **Address:** 75-06 Eliot Ave, Middle Village, NY 11379-1207; **Phone:** 718-335-2224; **Board Cert:** Otolaryngology 1984; **Med School:** Mexico 1977; **Resid:** Otolaryngology, Downstate Med Ctr 1982

Snyder, Gary M MD (Oto) - **Spec Exp:** Cosmetic Surgery-Face; Endoscopic Sinus Surgery; Voice Disorders; **Hospital:** Flushing Hosp Med Ctr, N Shore Univ Hosp at Plainview; **Address:** 26-01 Corporal Kennedy St, FL 1, Bayside, NY 11360-2452; **Phone:** 718-423-4091; **Board Cert:** Otolaryngology 1983; **Med School:** NY Med Coll 1979; **Resid:** Surgery, North Shore Univ Hosp 1980; Otolaryngology, Manhattan EET Hosp 1983

PEDIATRIC CARDIOLOGY

Rutkovsky, Lisa Rosner MD (PCd) - **Spec Exp:** Congenital Heart Disease; Arrhythmias; **Hospital:** NY Hosp Queens; **Address:** 56-34 Main St, Flushing, NY 11355; **Phone:** 718-670-1945; **Board Cert:** Pediatrics 2000; Pediatric Cardiology 2000; **Med School:** NYU Sch Med 1986; **Resid:** Pediatrics, N Shore Univ Hosp 1989; **Fellow:** Pediatric Cardiology, NYU-Bellevue Hosp 1989; **Fac Appt:** Asst Clin Prof Ped, NYU Sch Med

PEDIATRIC ENDOCRINOLOGY

Speiser, Phyllis W MD (PEn) - **Spec Exp:** Pubertal Disorders; Growth/Development Disorders; Adrenal Disorders; Thyroid Disorders; **Hospital:** Schneider Chldn's Hosp, N Shore Univ Hosp at Manhasset; **Address:** Schneider Chldns Hosp, Div Ped Endo, 269-01 76th Ave, New Hyde Park, NY 11040-1433; **Phone:** 718-470-3290; **Board Cert:** Pediatrics 1984; Pediatric Endocrinology 1986; **Med School:** Columbia P&S 1979; **Resid:** Pediatrics, Jacobi Med Ctr-Albert Einstein 1982; **Fellow:** Pediatric Endocrinology, New York Hosp-Cornell 1984; **Fac Appt:** Prof Ped, NYU Sch Med

PEDIATRIC GASTROENTEROLOGY

Bangaru, Babu MD (PGe) - **Spec Exp:** Ulcerative Colitis/Crohn's; Liver Disease; Nutritional Disorders; Endoscopy; **Hospital:** NYU Med Ctr (page 102), Flushing Hosp Med Ctr; **Address:** 94-22 59th Ave, Ste E1, Elmhurst, NY 11373; **Phone:** 718-592-7797; **Board Cert:** Pediatrics 1978; Pediatric Gastroenterology 1998; **Med School:** India 1970; **Resid:** Pediatrics, St Luke's Hosp 1976; **Fellow:** Hepatology, Albert Einstein Coll Med 1978; Pediatric Gastroenterology, Emory Univ Sch Med 1979; **Fac Appt:** Assoc Clin Prof Ped, NYU Sch Med

PEDIATRIC OTOLARYNGOLOGY

Goldsmith, Ari J MD (PO) - **Spec Exp:** Voice Disorders; Airway Disorders; Hearing Loss; Sleep Apnea; **Hospital:** Schneider Chldn's Hosp; **Address:** 212-45 26th Ave, Ste 1, Bayside, NY 11360; **Phone:** 718-631-8899; **Board Cert:** Otolaryngology 1994; **Med School:** Albert Einstein Coll Med 1988; **Resid:** Otolaryngology, LI Jewish Hosp 1993; **Fellow:** Pediatric Otolaryngology, Children's Hospital/Harvard 1994; **Fac Appt:** Assoc Prof Oto, SUNY Hlth Sci Ctr

PEDIATRICS

Abularrage, Joseph J MD (Ped) [PCP] - **Hospital:** NY Hosp Queens; **Address:** 56-45 Main St, Flushing, NY 11355-5045; **Phone:** 718-670-1033; **Board Cert:** Pediatrics 1981; **Med School:** NYU Sch Med 1975; **Resid:** Pediatrics, NYU-Bellevue Hosp 1979; **Fellow:** Public Health & Genl Preventive Med, Columbia-Presby Med Ctr 1981; **Fac Appt:** Assoc Prof Ped, Cornell Univ-Weill Med Coll

Eden, Alvin N MD (Ped) [PCP] - **Spec Exp:** Obesity; Breast Feeding Problems; Behavioral Disorders; **Hospital:** Wyckoff Heights Med Ctr, Long Island Jewish Med Ctr; **Address:** 107-21 Queens Blvd, Ste 7, Forest Hills, NY 11375-4451; **Phone:** 718-261-8989; **Board Cert:** Pediatrics 1957; **Med School:** Boston Univ 1952; **Resid:** Pediatrics, Univ Hosp-Bellevue Med Ctr 1955; **Fac Appt:** Clin Prof Ped, Cornell Univ-Weill Med Coll

Goldstein, Steven J MD (Ped) [PCP] - **Spec Exp:** Nutrition; Asthma; **Hospital:** Long Island Jewish Med Ctr, NY Hosp Queens; **Address:** 141-49 70th Rd, Flushing, NY 11367; **Phone:** 718-268-5282; **Board Cert:** Pediatrics 1981; Pediatric Endocrinology 1983; **Med School:** SUNY Hlth Sci Ctr 1978; **Resid:** Pediatrics, LI Jewish Med Ctr 1981

Reddy, Gaddam D MD (Ped) [PCP] - **Spec Exp:** Pediatric Cardiology; **Hospital:** St John's Queens Hosp (page 375), Mary Immaculate Hosp; **Address:** 43-43 Kissena Blvd, Ste 1, Flushing, NY 11355; **Phone:** 718-886-5680; **Board Cert:** Pediatrics 1971; **Med School:** Turkey 1963; **Resid:** Pediatrics, Chldns Hosp 1969; **Fellow:** Cardiovascular Disease, LI Jewish Med Ctr

Yadoo, Moshe MD (Ped) [PCP] - **Hospital:** St Mary's Hosp for Chldn, Winthrop - Univ Hosp; **Address:** St Mary's Hosp for Children, 29-01 216 St, Bayside, NY 11360; **Phone:** 718-880-8525; **Board Cert:** Pediatrics 1987; **Med School:** SUNY Hlth Sci Ctr 1983; **Resid:** Pediatrics, Brookdale Hosp 1986; **Fellow:** Neonatal-Perinatal Medicine, LI Jewish Med Ctr/Schneider 1988

PHYSICAL MEDICINE & REHABILITATION

Gasalberti, Richard MD (PMR) - **Spec Exp:** Pain Management; Sports Medicine; **Hospital:** Parkway Hosp, St. Vincent's Midtown; **Address:** 111-20 Queens Blvd, Forest Hills, NY 11375-6343; **Phone:** 718-544-7700; **Board Cert:** Physical Medicine & Rehabilitation 1994; **Med School:** West Indies 1984; **Resid:** Physical Medicine & Rehabilitation, Mount Sinai Hosp 1988; Surgery, New York Hosp Med Ctr 1986; **Fellow:** Sports Medicine, Hosp for Joint Diseases 1989

PLASTIC SURGERY

Kraft, Robert L MD (PlS) - **Spec Exp:** Cosmetic Surgery-Breast; Liposuction; Cosmetic Surgery-Face; **Hospital:** NY Hosp Queens, N Shore Univ Hosp at Manhasset; **Address:** 112-03 Queens Blvd, Ste 205, Forest Hills, NY 11375-5550; **Phone:** 718-263-6868; **Board Cert:** Plastic Surgery 1987; **Med School:** Yale Univ 1978; **Resid:** Surgery, Montefiore Med Ctr 1982; Plastic Surgery, Montefiore Med Ctr 1984

PSYCHIATRY

Mendelowitz, Alan MD (Psyc) - **Spec Exp:** Schizophrenia; Psychopharmacology; **Hospital:** Zucker Hillside Hosp; **Address:** 75-59 263rd St, Rm 209, Glen Oaks, NY 11004; **Phone:** 718-470-8397; **Board Cert:** Psychiatry 1992; Geriatric Psychiatry 1994; Addiction Psychiatry 1996; **Med School:** Rutgers Univ 1987; **Resid:** Psychiatry, Long Island Jewish Med Ctr 1991; **Fac Appt:** Asst Prof Psyc, Albert Einstein Coll Med

Nayak, Kumbla MD (Psyc) - **Spec Exp:** Eating Disorders; **Hospital:** Coney Island Hosp; **Address:** 151-33 78th St, Howard Beach, NY 11414; **Phone:** 718-616-5434; **Board Cert:** Psychiatry 1983; Forensic Psychiatry 1994; Geriatric Psychiatry 1995; Addiction Psychiatry 1996; **Med School:** India 1970; **Resid:** Psychiatry, Elmhurst City Hosp 1977; Psychiatry, Chicago VA Hosp 1978

Rifkin, Arthur MD (Psyc) - **Spec Exp:** Mood Disorders; Anxiety Disorders; Psychopharmacology; **Hospital:** Long Island Jewish Med Ctr; **Address:** 75-59 263rd St, Glen Oaks, NY 11004; **Phone:** 718-470-8075; **Board Cert:** Psychiatry 1968; **Med School:** SUNY Downstate 1961; **Resid:** Psychiatry, Hillside Hosp 1965; **Fellow:** Psychiatry, SUNY Downstate Med Ctr 1969; **Fac Appt:** Prof Psyc, Albert Einstein Coll Med

Selzer, Jeffrey A MD (Psyc) - **Spec Exp:** Addiction Psychiatry; Mood Disorders/Depression; **Hospital:** Zucker Hillside Hosp; **Address:** 75-59 263rd St, Glen Oaks, NY 11004-1150; **Phone:** 718-470-8023; **Board Cert:** Psychiatry 1985; Addiction Psychiatry 2003; Geriatric Psychiatry 1995; **Med School:** Univ Mich Med Sch 1979; **Resid:** Psychiatry, UCLA Med Ctr 1983; **Fac Appt:** Asst Prof Psyc, Albert Einstein Coll Med

Siris, Samuel G MD (Psyc) - **Spec Exp:** Schizophrenia; Depression in Schizophrenia; Panic Disorder in Schizophrenia; **Hospital:** Zucker Hillside Hosp; **Address:** 75-59 263rd St, Glen Oaks, NY 11004-1150; **Phone:** 718-470-8138; **Board Cert:** Psychiatry 1976; **Med School:** Columbia P&S 1970; **Resid:** Psychiatry, NY State Psychiatric Inst 1974; **Fellow:** Biological Psychiatry, Nat Inst Mental Hlth 1976; Psychoanalysis, Columbia Univ 1982; **Fac Appt:** Prof Psyc, Albert Einstein Coll Med

Sullivan, Ann Marie MD (Psyc) - **Spec Exp:** Psychotherapy; Psychopharmacology; **Hospital:** Elmhurst Hosp Ctr, Mount Sinai Med Ctr (page 98); **Address:** Elmhurst Hosp, 79-01 Broadway, Elmhurst, NY 11373; **Phone:** 718-334-1141; **Board Cert:** Psychiatry 1978; **Med School:** NYU Sch Med 1974; **Resid:** Psychiatry, Bellevue Hosp 1978; **Fac Appt:** Assoc Prof Psyc, Mount Sinai Sch Med

Vivek, Seeth MD (Psyc) - **Spec Exp:** Depression; Panic Disorder; Obsessive-Compulsive Disorder; **Hospital:** Jamaica Hosp Med Ctr, Flushing Hosp Med Ctr; **Address:** 75-58 113th St, Ste 1A, Forest Hills, NY 11375-7429; **Phone:** 718-268-9595; **Board Cert:** Psychiatry 1980; Geriatric Psychiatry 1994; Forensic Psychiatry 1994; Psychosomatic Medicine 2005; **Med School:** India 1972; **Resid:** Psychiatry, Natl Inst Mental Hlth 1976; Psychiatry, Mount Sinai Hosp 1979; **Fellow:** Liason Psychiatry, Montefiore Hosp 1981

PULMONARY DISEASE

Ankobiah, William MD (Pul) - **Spec Exp:** Chronic Obstructive Lung Disease (COPD); Tuberculosis; Pulmonary Disease; **Hospital:** Franklin Hosp Med Ctr, St John's Epis Hosp - S Shore; **Address:** 253-02 147th Ave, Jamaica, NY 11422-2541; **Phone:** 718-341-3535; **Board Cert:** Internal Medicine 2003; Pulmonary Disease 2002; **Med School:** Ghana 1978; **Resid:** Internal Medicine, Woodhull Med Ctr 1987; **Fellow:** Pulmonary Disease, Univ Hosp 1989; **Fac Appt:** Asst Prof Med, SUNY Downstate

Chadha, Jang B S MD (Pul) - **Spec Exp:** Sleep Disorders; Asthma; Emphysema; Critical Care Medicine; **Hospital:** Parkway Hosp, N Shore Univ Hosp at Forest Hills; **Address:** 11203 Queens Blvd, Ste 201, Forest Hills, NY 11375; **Phone:** 718-544-6660; **Board Cert:** Internal Medicine 1982; Pulmonary Disease 1984; Critical Care Medicine 1997; Geriatric Medicine 2004; **Med School:** India 1976; **Resid:** Internal Medicine, Lincoln Hosp 1982; **Fellow:** Pulmonary Disease, NY Med Coll 1984

Donath, Joseph MD (Pul) - **Spec Exp:** Asthma; Lung Cancer; **Hospital:** St John's Queens Hosp (page 375), Parkway Hosp; **Address:** 112-41 Queens Blvd, Forest Hills, NY 11375-5564; **Phone:** 718-380-1553; **Board Cert:** Internal Medicine 1980; Pulmonary Disease 1982; Critical Care Medicine 1999; **Med School:** Hungary 1972; **Resid:** Internal Medicine, VA Med Ctr 1980; **Fellow:** Pulmonary Disease, Mount Sinai Hosp 1982; **Fac Appt:** Asst Clin Prof Med, NY Med Coll

Fleischman, Jean K MD (Pul) - **Hospital:** Queens Hosp Ctr - Jamaica; **Address:** Queens Hosp Ctr, Dept Medicine, 82-68 164th St N Bldg Fl 7, Jamaica, NY 11432; **Phone:** 718-883-4050; **Board Cert:** Internal Medicine 1985; Pulmonary Disease 1988; **Med School:** NYU Sch Med 1982; **Resid:** Internal Medicine, Manhattan VA/NYU Med Ctr 1985; **Fellow:** Pulmonary Disease, NYU Med Ctr 1987; **Fac Appt:** Asst Prof Med, Mount Sinai Sch Med

Karbowitz, Stephen MD (Pul) - **Spec Exp:** Asthma; Lung Cancer; Chronic Obstructive Lung Disease (COPD); **Hospital:** NY Hosp Queens; **Address:** 56-45 Main St, Ste WA-100, Flushing, NY 11355-5045; **Phone:** 718-670-1405; **Board Cert:** Pulmonary Disease 1976; Internal Medicine 1974; **Med School:** Albert Einstein Coll Med 1971; **Resid:** Internal Medicine, Montefiore Hosp Med Ctr 1974; **Fellow:** Pulmonary Disease, Montefiore Hosp Med Ctr 1976; **Fac Appt:** Asst Prof Med, Cornell Univ-Weill Med Coll

Kassapidis, Sotirios MD (Pul) - **Hospital:** Mount Sinai Hosp of Queens (page 98), N Shore Univ Hosp at Manhasset; **Address:** 22-31 33rd Street, Astoria, NY 11105; **Phone:** 718-278-6595; **Board Cert:** Pulmonary Disease 1997; Critical Care Medicine 1998; **Med School:** Grenada 1987; **Resid:** Internal Medicine, SUNY Hlth Sci Ctr 1993; **Fellow:** Pulmonary Disease, SUNY Hlth Sci Ctr 1995; Critical Care Medicine, SUNY Hlth Sci Ctr 1996

Mehra, Sunil MD (Pul) - **Spec Exp:** Asthma; Emphysema; Lung Cancer; **Hospital:** St John's Queens Hosp (page 375), Mount Sinai Hosp of Queens (page 98); **Address:** 84-04 Penelope Ave, Middle Village, NY 11379-2433; **Phone:** 718-894-8500; **Board Cert:** Internal Medicine 1982; Pulmonary Disease 1986; Critical Care Medicine 1998; Geriatric Medicine 1992; **Med School:** India 1977; **Resid:** Internal Medicine, Kingsbrook Jewish MC 1982; **Fellow:** Pulmonary Disease, LI Jewish Med Ctr 1984; **Fac Appt:** Assoc Prof Med, NY Med Coll

Miller, Albert MD (Pul) - **Spec Exp:** Asthma-Occupational; Sarcoidosis; Lung Cancer; **Hospital:** Mary Immaculate Hosp; **Address:** 88-25 153rd St, Ste 3J, Jamaica, NY 11432; **Phone:** 718-558-7227; **Board Cert:** Internal Medicine 1966; Pulmonary Disease 1972; **Med School:** Univ Wisc 1959; **Resid:** Internal Medicine, VA Med Ctr 1962; Internal Medicine, Mt Sinai Med Ctr 1965; **Fellow:** Pulmonary Disease, Mt Sinai Med Ctr 1961; **Fac Appt:** Prof Med, NY Med Coll

Multz, Alan S MD (Pul) - **Spec Exp:** Sepsis; Respiratory Distress Syndrome; **Hospital:** Long Island Jewish Med Ctr, N Shore Univ Hosp at Manhasset; **Address:** 270-05 76th Ave, New Hyde Park, NY 11040-1433; **Phone:** 718-470-7270; **Board Cert:** Internal Medicine 1988; Pulmonary Disease 2000; Critical Care Medicine 2000; **Med School:** Boston Univ 1985; **Resid:** Internal Medicine, Montefiore Hosp Med Ctr 1988; **Fellow:** Pulmonary Disease, Albert Einstein 1990; Critical Care Medicine, Montefiore Hosp Med Ctr 1991; **Fac Appt:** Assoc Prof Med, Albert Einstein Coll Med

Nath, Sunil MD (Pul) - **Spec Exp:** Asthma; Emphysema; Lung Cancer; **Hospital:** NY Hosp Queens; **Address:** 55-14 Main St, Flushing, NY 11355-5044; **Phone:** 718-359-3131; **Board Cert:** Internal Medicine 1980; Pulmonary Disease 1982; **Med School:** India 1976; **Resid:** Internal Medicine, NY Hosp Med Ctr 1980; **Fellow:** Pulmonary Disease, NY Hosp Med Ctr 1982

Silverman, Joel MD (Pul) - **Spec Exp:** Emphysema; Asthma; Pulmonary Rehabilitation; **Hospital:** Parkway Hosp; **Address:** 111-20 Queens Blvd, Forest Hills, NY 11375; **Phone:** 718-544-4224; **Board Cert:** Internal Medicine 1977; Pulmonary Disease 1979; Critical Care Medicine 1989; **Med School:** Univ Okla Coll Med 1974; **Resid:** Internal Medicine, N Shore Univ Hosp 1977; **Fellow:** Pulmonary Disease, Bellevue Hosp 1979

RADIATION ONCOLOGY

Dalton, Jack F MD (RadRO) - **Spec Exp:** Brain Tumors; Head & Neck Cancer; Breast Cancer; **Hospital:** Mount Sinai Med Ctr (page 98), Lenox Hill Hosp (page 94); **Address:** 106-14 70th Ave, Forest Hills, NY 11375-4253; **Phone:** 718-520-6620; **Board Cert:** Internal Medicine 1974; Hematology 1976; Medical Oncology 1981; Therapeutic Radiology 1983; **Med School:** Univ Pittsburgh 1970; **Resid:** Hematology, Mt Sinai Hosp 1975; Radiology, Mt Sinai Hosp 1981; **Fac Appt:** Asst Clin Prof Med, Mount Sinai Sch Med

Lipsztein, Roberto MD (RadRO) - **Hospital:** Lenox Hill Hosp (page 94), Mount Sinai Med Ctr (page 98); **Address:** 106-14 70th Ave, Forest Hills, NY 11375-4253; **Phone:** 718-520-6620; **Board Cert:** Therapeutic Radiology 1982; **Med School:** Brazil 1974; **Resid:** Internal Medicine, Mount Sinai Hosp 1979; **Fellow:** Radiation Oncology, Mount Sinai Hosp 1981

Varsos, George MD (RadRO) - **Hospital:** Mount Sinai Hosp of Queens (page 98); **Address:** 23-22 30th Ave, Astoria, NY 11102; **Phone:** 718-267-2763; **Board Cert:** Radiation Oncology 1992; **Med School:** Mount Sinai Sch Med 1986; **Resid:** Surgery, Univ Hosp-SUNY 1987; Radiation Oncology, SUNY Hlth Science Ctr 1991; **Fellow:** Radiation Oncology, Memorial Sloan-Kettering 1992; **Fac Appt:** Asst Clin Prof RadRO, SUNY Downstate

RHEUMATOLOGY

Sonpal, Girish MD (Rhu) - **Spec Exp:** Osteoporosis; Rheumatoid Arthritis; Lupus/SLE; **Hospital:** Flushing Hosp Med Ctr, NY Hosp Queens; **Address:** 149-65 24th Ave, Flushing, NY 11357-3646; **Phone:** 718-445-0500; **Board Cert:** Internal Medicine 1974; Rheumatology 1976; **Med School:** India 1969; **Resid:** Internal Medicine, Catholic Med Ctr 1974; **Fellow:** Rheumatology, Worcester City Hosp 1975; **Fac Appt:** Asst Prof Med, Cornell Univ-Weill Med Coll

SPORTS MEDICINE

Silverman, Marc MD (SM) - **Spec Exp:** Shoulder Injuries; Knee Injuries; **Hospital:** Hosp For Joint Diseases (page 107), St Barnabas Hosp - Bronx; **Address:** 97-17 64th Rd, Rego Park, NY 11374; **Phone:** 718-575-9896; **Board Cert:** Orthopaedic Surgery 2005; **Med School:** Albert Einstein Coll Med 1985; **Resid:** Orthopaedic Surgery, NY Med Coll 1990; **Fellow:** Spinal Surgery, Univ Toronto; Sports Medicine, Hosp for Joint Diseases

SURGERY

Kemeny, Mary Margaret MD (S) - **Spec Exp:** Liver Cancer; Pancreatic Cancer; Colon & Rectal Cancer; **Hospital:** Queens Hosp Ctr - Jamaica, N Shore Univ Hosp at Manhasset; **Address:** Queens Cancer Ctr at Queens Hosp, 82-68 164th St, Jamaica, NY 11432-1140; **Phone:** 718-883-4031; **Board Cert:** Surgery 2004; **Med School:** Columbia P&S 1972; **Resid:** Surgery, Columbia-Presby Hosp 1974; Surgery, Univ Colorado Med Ctr 1976; **Fellow:** Surgery, Meml Sloan Kettering Cancer Ctr 1977; Surgical Oncology, National Cancer Inst 1981; **Fac Appt:** Prof S, Mount Sinai Sch Med

Manolas, Panagiotis MD (S) - **Spec Exp:** Breast Cancer; Laparoscopic Surgery; Colon Cancer; **Hospital:** Mount Sinai Hosp of Queens (page 98), Mount Sinai Med Ctr (page 98); **Address:** 30-16 30th Drive, Astoria, NY 11102-1855; **Phone:** 718-626-0707; **Board Cert:** Surgery 1999; **Med School:** Greece 1982; **Resid:** Surgery, NY Methodist Hosp 1989; **Fac Appt:** Asst Clin Prof S, Mount Sinai Sch Med

Pace, Benjamin MD (S) - **Spec Exp:** Breast Surgery; Breast Cancer; **Hospital:** Queens Hosp Ctr - Jamaica; **Address:** Department of Surgery, 82-68 164th St, rm A-365, Jamaica, NY 11432-1140; **Phone:** 718-883-4640; **Board Cert:** Surgery 2004; **Med School:** Mexico 1977; **Resid:** Surgery, LI Jewish Med Ctr 1983; **Fac Appt:** Assoc Clin Prof S, Mount Sinai Sch Med

Rifkind, Kenneth M MD (S) - **Spec Exp:** Breast Cancer; Breast Surgery; Melanoma; **Hospital:** NY Hosp Queens; **Address:** 56-45 Main St Fl 2, Flushing, NY 11355; **Phone:** 718-445-0220; **Board Cert:** Surgery 1995; Surgical Critical Care 2001; **Med School:** NYU Sch Med 1969; **Resid:** Surgery, NYU Med Ctr 1975; **Fac Appt:** Asst Clin Prof S, NYU Sch Med

Siegel, Beth MD (S) - **Spec Exp:** Breast Cancer; Breast Disease; **Hospital:** South Nassau Comm Hosp; **Address:** 55-12 Main St, Lower Level, Flushing, NY 11355; **Phone:** 718-460-3547; **Board Cert:** Surgery 2002; **Med School:** Dominica 1982; **Resid:** Surgery, NY Hosp Med Ctr 1988

Sung, Kap-jae MD (S) - **Spec Exp:** Breast Cancer; Laparoscopic Surgery; **Hospital:** St John's Queens Hosp (page 375), NY Hosp Queens; **Address:** 68-07 Eliot Ave, Middle Village, NY 11379-1130; **Phone:** 718-651-2929; **Board Cert:** Surgery 1995; **Med School:** South Korea 1973; **Resid:** Surgery, Wyckoff Heights Hosp 1986; **Fac Appt:** Asst Prof S, NY Med Coll

Turner, James MD (S) - **Spec Exp:** Esophageal Surgery; Laparoscopic Surgery; Carotid Artery Surgery; **Hospital:** NY Hosp Queens; **Address:** 56-45 Main St, Fl 2, Flushing, NY 11355; **Phone:** 718-445-0220; **Board Cert:** Surgery 1995; Surgical Critical Care 1995; **Med School:** Eastern VA Med Sch 1970; **Resid:** Surgery, NYU Med Ctr 1975; **Fac Appt:** Assoc Clin Prof S, Cornell Univ-Weill Med Coll

Zeitlin, Alan MD (S) - **Spec Exp:** Vascular Surgery; Breast Cancer; Abdominal Surgery; **Hospital:** Parkway Hosp, Lenox Hill Hosp (page 94); **Address:** 69-60 108th St, Forest Hills, NY 11375-4323; **Phone:** 718-544-0442; **Board Cert:** Surgery 2002; **Med School:** Univ Miami Sch Med 1974; **Resid:** Surgery, Albert Einstein 1979; **Fac Appt:** Asst Clin Prof S, Mount Sinai Sch Med

THORACIC SURGERY

Lee, Paul C MD (TS) - **Spec Exp:** Lung Cancer; Esophageal Cancer; Gastroesophageal Reflux Disease (GERD); Minimally Invasive Thoracic Surgery; **Hospital:** NY Hosp Queens, NY-Presby Hosp (page 100); **Address:** 56-45 Main St, Ste WA-100, Flushing, NY 11355; **Phone:** 718-670-2707; **Board Cert:** Surgery 2002; Thoracic Surgery 2004; **Med School:** Johns Hopkins Univ 1995; **Resid:** Surgery, Univ Pittsburgh Med Ctr 1998; Cardiothoracic Surgery, NY Presby Hosp-Cornell 2003; **Fellow:** Thoracic Surgery, Meml Sloan Kettering Cancer Ctr 2003; Thoracic Surgery, Univ Pittsburgh 2003; **Fac Appt:** Asst Prof S, Cornell Univ-Weill Med Coll

Moideen, Ahamed S MD (TS) - **Spec Exp:** Vascular Surgery; Critical Care; **Hospital:** Flushing Hosp Med Ctr; **Address:** 146-01 45th Ave, Ste 406, Flushing, NY 11355-2280; **Phone:** 718-670-5473; **Board Cert:** Thoracic Surgery 2001; Surgical Critical Care 1995; **Med School:** India 1964; **Resid:** Surgery, Flushing Hosp 1979; Thoracic Surgery, Wayne Co Genl Hosp 1981; **Fac Appt:** Assoc Prof S, SUNY Hlth Sci Ctr

Slovin, Alvin MD (TS) - **Spec Exp:** Carotid Artery Surgery; Thoracic Cancers; Lung Surgery; **Hospital:** Peninsula Hosp Ctr, South Nassau Comm Hosp; **Address:** 5115 Beach Channel Drive, Far Rockaway, NY 11691; **Phone:** 718-734-2300; **Board Cert:** Thoracic Surgery 1971; Surgery 1970; **Med School:** SUNY Downstate 1963; **Resid:** Surgery, SUNY Brooklyn 1970; Thoracic Surgery, Kings County Hosp 1970; **Fac Appt:** Asst Prof S, Albert Einstein Coll Med

UROLOGY

Caponegro, Robert MD (U) - **Hospital:** Wyckoff Heights Med Ctr, St. John's Episcopal Hosp-Queens; **Address:** 68-10 Forest Ave, Ridgewood, NY 11385; **Phone:** 718-497-3503; **Board Cert:** Urology 1969; **Med School:** Creighton Univ 1958; **Resid:** Surgery, St Catherine's Hosp 1962; Urology, Kings County Hosp 1965

Farrell, Robert MD (U) - **Spec Exp:** Endourology; Pediatric Urology; Urologic Cancer; **Hospital:** NY Hosp Queens, Flushing Hosp Med Ctr; **Address:** 58-42 Main St, Flushing, NY 11355; **Phone:** 718-539-3312; **Board Cert:** Urology 1976; **Med School:** Cornell Univ-Weill Med Coll 1966; **Resid:** Surgery, New York Hosp 1968; Urology, New York Hosp 1974

Sandhaus, Jeffrey MD (U) - **Spec Exp:** Prostate Cancer; Minimally Invasive Surgery; Vasectomy-Scalpelless; **Hospital:** Mount Sinai Hosp of Queens (page 98), NY-Presby Hosp (page 100); **Address:** 36-01 31st Ave Fl 1, Astoria, NY 11106-1051; **Phone:** 718-932-3535; **Board Cert:** Urology 1976; **Med School:** NY Med Coll 1966; **Resid:** Urology, Univ Hosp 1973; **Fellow:** Nephrology, Univ Hosp 1970; **Fac Appt:** Asst Clin Prof U, Mount Sinai Sch Med

Tarasuk, Albert MD (U) - **Spec Exp:** Prostate Disease; Bladder Surgery; Kidney Stones; **Hospital:** NY Hosp Queens, Flushing Hosp Med Ctr; **Address:** 58-42 Main St, Flushing, NY 11355-5336; **Phone:** 718-353-3710; **Board Cert:** Urology 1972; **Med School:** Geo Wash Univ 1964; **Resid:** Urology, Beth Israel Med Ctr 1969

Weber, Michael MD (U) - **Spec Exp:** Prostate Disease; Bladder Cancer; **Hospital:** NY Hosp Queens, Long Island Jewish Med Ctr; **Address:** 106-15 Queens Blvd LL Bldg, Forest Hills, NY 11375-4365; **Phone:** 718-544-1474; **Board Cert:** Urology 1995; **Med School:** Mexico 1977; **Resid:** Urology, Montefiore Med Ctr 1982; **Fac Appt:** Asst Prof U, Mexico

VASCULAR SURGERY

Kaynan, Arieh MD (VascS) - **Spec Exp:** Carotid Artery Surgery; Lower Limb Arterial Disease; **Hospital:** Mount Sinai Hosp of Queens (page 98), NY Hosp Queens; **Address:** 188-15 Radnor Rd, Hollis, NY 11423-1018; **Phone:** 718-479-0582; **Board Cert:** Vascular Surgery 2001; **Med School:** Israel 1966; **Resid:** Surgery, Mount Sinai Hosp 1974; **Fellow:** Vascular Surgery, Mount Sinai Hosp 1975; **Fac Appt:** Assoc Clin Prof S, Mount Sinai Sch Med

Yatco, Ruben MD (VascS) - **Spec Exp:** Arterial Bypass Surgery-Leg; Dialysis Access Surgery; **Hospital:** Mary Immaculate Hosp, Jamaica Hosp Med Ctr; **Address:** 177-06 Wexford Ter, Jamaica, NY 11432-2927; **Phone:** 718-262-9456; **Board Cert:** Surgery 1997; **Med School:** Philippines 1972; **Resid:** Surgery, Catholic Med Ctr 1979; Surgery, NY Methodist Hosp 1982; **Fellow:** Cardiac Surgery, Arizonia Heart Inst 1983

Richmond
(Staten Island)

Richmond (Staten Island)

ADOLESCENT MEDICINE

Lee, April MD (AM) `PCP` - **Hospital:** Staten Island Univ Hosp-North Site; **Address:** Staten Island Univ Hosp, Dept Adol Med, 475 Seaview Ave, Staten Island, NY 10305; **Phone:** 718-226-6294; **Board Cert:** Pediatrics 1986; Adolescent Medicine 2002; **Med School:** NYU Sch Med 1980; **Resid:** Pediatrics, NYU Med Ctr 1983; **Fellow:** Adolescent Medicine, Brookdale Hosp 1986; **Fac Appt:** Asst Clin Prof Ped, SUNY Hlth Sci Ctr

ALLERGY & IMMUNOLOGY

Rao, Yalamanchi K MD (A&I) - **Hospital:** Staten Island Univ Hosp-North Site; **Address:** 896 Targee St, Staten Island, NY 10304; **Phone:** 718-816-8200; **Board Cert:** Pediatrics 1978; Allergy & Immunology 1989; **Med School:** India 1968; **Resid:** Pediatrics, Long Island Coll Hosp 1977; **Fellow:** Allergy & Immunology, Long Island Coll Hosp 1979; **Fac Appt:** Asst Clin Prof Med, SUNY Downstate

CARDIOVASCULAR DISEASE

Besser, Louis MD (Cv) - **Spec Exp:** Coronary Artery Disease; Arrhythmias; **Hospital:** St Vincent Cath Med Ctr - Staten Island (page 375), Staten Island Univ Hosp-North Site; **Address:** 11 Ralph Pl, ste 310, Staten Island, NY 10304-4419; **Phone:** 718-442-1777; **Board Cert:** Internal Medicine 1988; Cardiovascular Disease 1989; **Med School:** Mexico 1981; **Resid:** Internal Medicine, St Vincent's Hosp & Med Ctr 1986; **Fellow:** Cardiovascular Disease, St Vincent's Hosp & Med Ctr 1988; **Fac Appt:** Asst Clin Prof Med, NY Med Coll

Bloomfield, Dennis A MD (Cv) - **Spec Exp:** Cardiac Catheterization; Hypertension; Pulmonary Embolism; Coronary Artery Disease; **Hospital:** St Vincent Cath Med Ctr - Staten Island (page 375), St Vincent Cath Med Ctrs - Manhattan (page 375); **Address:** 1102 Victory Blvd, Staten Island, NY 10301; **Phone:** 718-442-5230; **Med School:** Australia 1956; **Resid:** Internal Medicine, Royal Perth Hosp 1960; Internal Medicine, Royal Prince Alfred Hosp 1961; **Fellow:** Cardiovascular Disease, Hallstrom Inst Cardiology 1962; Cardiovascular Disease, Vanderbilt Univ Med Ctr 1965; **Fac Appt:** Clin Prof Med, NY Med Coll

Bogin, Marc MD (Cv) - **Spec Exp:** Echocardiography; Cardiac Catheterization; **Hospital:** St Vincent Cath Med Ctr - Staten Island (page 375), Staten Island Univ Hosp-North Site; **Address:** 501 Seaview Ave, Ste 200, Staten Island, NY 10305; **Phone:** 718-663-6400; **Board Cert:** Internal Medicine 1989; Cardiovascular Disease 1993; **Med School:** Mexico 1985; **Resid:** Internal Medicine, Booth Meml Hosp 1989; Internal Medicine, Booth Meml Hosp 1990; **Fellow:** Cardiovascular Disease, St Vincent's Hosp & Med Ctr 1993; **Fac Appt:** Asst Clin Prof Med, NY Med Coll

Costantino, Thomas MD (Cv) - **Spec Exp:** Congestive Heart Failure; Cholesterol/Lipid Disorders; **Hospital:** Staten Island Univ Hosp-North Site; **Address:** 501 Seaview Ave, Ste 300, Staten Island, NY 10305; **Phone:** 718-663-7000; **Board Cert:** Internal Medicine 1973; Cardiovascular Disease 1973; **Med School:** Georgetown Univ 1966; **Resid:** Internal Medicine, Georgetown Univ Hosp 1969; Internal Medicine, New York Hosp 1970; **Fellow:** Cardiovascular Disease, Georgetown Univ Hosp 1972; **Fac Appt:** Asst Clin Prof Med, SUNY Downstate

Grodman, Richard MD (Cv) - **Spec Exp:** Echocardiography; Cardiac Catheterization; **Hospital:** St Vincent Cath Med Ctr - Staten Island (page 375); **Address:** SVCMC-Staten Island, Div Cardiology, 355 Bard Ave, Staten Island, NY 10310-1664; **Phone:** 718-818-4642; **Board Cert:** Internal Medicine 1976; Cardiovascular Disease 1979; **Med School:** SUNY Downstate 1973; **Resid:** Internal Medicine, SUNY Downstate 1976; Critical Care Medicine, SUNY Downstate 1977; **Fellow:** Cardiovascular Disease, Rhode Island Hosp 1979; **Fac Appt:** Assoc Clin Prof Med, NY Med Coll

Richmond (Staten Island)

Homayuni, Ali MD (Cv) - **Spec Exp:** Interventional Cardiology; Coronary Angioplasty/Stents; Carotid Artery Stents; **Hospital:** Staten Island Univ Hosp-North Site, St Vincent Cath Med Ctrs - Manhattan (page 375); **Address:** 501 Seaview Ave, Staten Island, NY 10305; **Phone:** 718-663-7093; **Board Cert:** Internal Medicine 1988; Cardiovascular Disease 2001; Interventional Cardiology 1999; **Med School:** SUNY Downstate 1985; **Resid:** Internal Medicine, Staten Island Hosp 1988; **Fellow:** Cardiovascular Disease, St Vincent's Hosp & Med Ctr 1991; **Fac Appt:** Assoc Clin Prof Med, SUNY Downstate

Lafferty, James MD (Cv) - **Spec Exp:** Electrophysiologic Testing; **Hospital:** Staten Island Univ Hosp-North Site; **Address:** 501 Seaview Ave Fl 3, Staten Island, NY 10305; **Phone:** 718-351-3111; **Board Cert:** Internal Medicine 1985; Cardiovascular Disease 1987; Cardiac Electrophysiology 1996; **Med School:** SUNY Hlth Sci Ctr 1982; **Resid:** Internal Medicine, Staten Island Hosp 1985; **Fellow:** Cardiovascular Disease, Univ Hosp 1987; **Fac Appt:** Assoc Prof Med, SUNY Downstate

Malpeso, James MD (Cv) - **Spec Exp:** Cardiac Catheterization; Angioplasty; **Hospital:** Staten Island Univ Hosp - South Site, St Vincent Cath Med Ctr - Staten Island (page 375); **Address:** 501 Seaview Ave, Ste 300, Staten Island, NY 10306; **Phone:** 718-663-7000; **Board Cert:** Internal Medicine 1979; Cardiovascular Disease 1981; **Med School:** Albert Einstein Coll Med 1975; **Resid:** Internal Medicine, Kings County Hosp 1978; **Fellow:** Cardiovascular Disease, St Vincent's Hosp & Med Ctr 1980; **Fac Appt:** Asst Prof Med, SUNY Downstate

Schwartz, Charles A MD (Cv) - **Spec Exp:** Cardiac Stress Testing; Cardiac Catheterization; Echocardiography; **Hospital:** Staten Island Univ Hosp-North Site; **Address:** 501 Seaview Ave, Ste 300, Staten Island, NY 10312-3836; **Phone:** 718-663-7000; **Board Cert:** Internal Medicine 1983; Cardiovascular Disease 1985; **Med School:** SUNY Downstate 1980; **Resid:** Internal Medicine, Staten Island Hosp 1983; **Fellow:** Cardiovascular Disease, St Vincent's Hosp & Med Ctr 1985; **Fac Appt:** Asst Clin Prof Med, SUNY Downstate

Swamy, Samala MD (Cv) - **Spec Exp:** Preventive Cardiology; Invasive Cardiology; Interventional Cardiology; Nuclear Cardiology; **Hospital:** St Vincent Cath Med Ctr - Staten Island (page 375), Staten Island Univ Hosp - South Site; **Address:** 1366 Victory Blvd, Ste B, Staten Island, NY 10301-3907; **Phone:** 718-442-8351; **Board Cert:** Internal Medicine 1977; Cardiovascular Disease 1979; Interventional Cardiology 2004; **Med School:** India 1972; **Resid:** Internal Medicine, St Vincent's Hosp 1977; **Fellow:** Cardiovascular Disease, Cook Co Hosp 1978; Cardiovascular Disease, St Vincent's Hosp 1979; **Fac Appt:** Asst Prof Med, NY Med Coll

Vazzana, Thomas MD (Cv) - **Spec Exp:** Invasive Cardiology; Non-Invasive Cardiology; Interventional Cardiology; **Hospital:** Staten Island Univ Hosp-North Site, St Vincent Cath Med Ctr - Staten Island (page 375); **Address:** 501 Seaview Ave, Ste 200, Staten Island, NY 10305; **Phone:** 718-447-7899; **Board Cert:** Internal Medicine 1989; Cardiovascular Disease 2001; Interventional Cardiology 2002; **Med School:** Grenada 1985; **Resid:** Internal Medicine, St Joseph's Hosp & Med Ctr 1989; **Fellow:** Cardiovascular Disease, St Vincent's Hosp & Med Ctr 1991; **Fac Appt:** Asst Prof Med, NY Med Coll

Winter, Steven MD (Cv) - **Spec Exp:** Cholesterol/Lipid Disorders; Preventive Cardiology; Non-Invasive Cardiology; **Hospital:** Staten Island Univ Hosp - South Site, St Vincent Cath Med Ctr - Staten Island (page 375); **Address:** 2627 Hylan Blvd, Bldg B, Staten Island, NY 10306-4339; **Phone:** 718-351-5600; **Board Cert:** Internal Medicine 1979; Cardiovascular Disease 1981; **Med School:** UMDNJ-NJ Med Sch, Newark 1976; **Resid:** Internal Medicine, N Shore Univ Hosp 1979; Internal Medicine, Meml Sloan Kettering Cancer Ctr 1979; **Fellow:** Cardiovascular Disease, Rhode Island Hosp-Brown Univ 1981; **Fac Appt:** Asst Clin Prof Med, SUNY Hlth Sci Ctr

CHILD NEUROLOGY

De Carlo, Regina MD (ChiN) - **Spec Exp:** Autism; Headache; Learning Disorders; Developmental Disorders; **Hospital:** St Vincent Cath Med Ctr - Staten Island (page 375), NYU Med Ctr (page 102); **Address:** 2550 Victory Blvd, Staten Island, NY 10314-6610; **Phone:** 718-983-0923; **Board Cert:** Pediatrics 1984; Child Neurology 1984; **Med School:** UMDNJ-NJ Med Sch, Newark 1977; **Resid:** Pediatrics, NYU Med Ctr 1979; Neurology, NYU Med Ctr 1981; **Fellow:** Child Neurology, NYU Med Ctr 1982; **Fac Appt:** Asst Clin Prof N, NYU Sch Med

COLON & RECTAL SURGERY

Bopaiah, Vinod MD (CRS) - **Spec Exp:** Rectal Prolapse; Rectal Cancer; Anal Disorders & Reconstruction; **Hospital:** Staten Island Univ Hosp-North Site, St Vincent Cath Med Ctr - Staten Island (page 375); **Address:** 400 Seaview Ave, Ste 7, Staten Island, NY 10305; **Phone:** 718-351-0199; **Board Cert:** Surgery 2003; Colon & Rectal Surgery 1991; **Med School:** India 1976; **Resid:** Surgery, Interfaith Med Ctr 1980; **Fellow:** Colon & Rectal Surgery, Sacred Heart Hosp 1981

DERMATOLOGY

Bernstein, Charles MD (D) - **Hospital:** Staten Island Univ Hosp-North Site, Staten Island Univ Hosp - South Site; **Address:** 3163 Hylan Blvd, Staten Island, NY 10306-4145; **Phone:** 718-980-5767; **Board Cert:** Internal Medicine 1983; Dermatology 1987; **Med School:** SUNY Downstate 1980; **Resid:** Internal Medicine, Staten Island Hosp 1984; Dermatology, Downstate Med Ctr 1987; **Fac Appt:** Assoc Clin Prof D, SUNY Hlth Sci Ctr

Lederman, Josiane MD (D) - **Spec Exp:** Cosmetic Dermatology; Skin Cancer; Laser Surgery; **Hospital:** St Vincent Cath Med Ctr - Staten Island (page 375); **Address:** 116 Lamberts Ln, Staten Island, NY 10314-7210; **Phone:** 718-370-0422; **Board Cert:** Dermatology 1986; **Med School:** France 1981; **Resid:** Dermatology, Saint Louis Hosp 1983; **Fellow:** Dermatology, Mass Genl Hosp-Harvard 1986

McCormack, Patricia MD (D) - **Spec Exp:** Psoriasis; Skin Cancer; Skin Laser Surgery; **Hospital:** St Vincent Cath Med Ctr - Staten Island (page 375); **Address:** 1550 Richmond Ave, Ste 207, Staten Island, NY 10314; **Phone:** 718-698-1616; **Board Cert:** Dermatology 1985; **Med School:** Rutgers Univ 1981; **Resid:** Dermatology, NY Med Coll 1985; **Fac Appt:** Asst Prof D, NY Med Coll

Urbanek, Richard W MD (D) - **Spec Exp:** Liposuction; Laser Surgery; Botox Therapy; **Hospital:** Staten Island Univ Hosp-North Site; **Address:** 1324 Victory Blvd, Staten Island, NY 10314; **Phone:** 718-448-4488; **Board Cert:** Dermatology 1977; **Med School:** Cornell Univ-Weill Med Coll 1972; **Resid:** Dermatology, Temple Univ Hosp 1976; **Fac Appt:** Asst Prof D, NYU Sch Med

DIAGNOSTIC RADIOLOGY

Buchbinder, Shalom MD (DR) - **Spec Exp:** Mammography; Breast Imaging; **Hospital:** Staten Island Univ Hosp-North Site; **Address:** Staten Island Univ Hosp, Heart Tower, 475 Seaview Ave Fl 1, Staten Island, NY 10305; **Phone:** 718-226-9175; **Board Cert:** Diagnostic Radiology 1986; **Med School:** Albert Einstein Coll Med 1981; **Resid:** Radiology, Montefiore-Weiler Einstein Med Ctr 1985; **Fac Appt:** Assoc Prof Rad, Albert Einstein Coll Med

Giaimo, Thomas MD (DR) - **Hospital:** St Vincent Cath Med Ctr - Staten Island (page 375); **Address:** 75 Vanderbilt Ave, Staten Island, NY 10304; **Phone:** 718-818-5734; **Med School:** Italy 1982; **Resid:** Catholic Med Ctr 1984; Radiology, St Vincent's Hosp & Med Ctr 1988

Richmond (Staten Island)

ENDOCRINOLOGY, DIABETES & METABOLISM

Cohen, Neil MD (EDM) - **Spec Exp:** Diabetes; Thyroid Disorders; Osteoporosis; **Hospital:** Staten Island Univ Hosp-North Site, Staten Island Univ Hosp - South Site; **Address:** 1460 Victory Blvd, Staten Island, NY 10301-3914; **Phone:** 718-442-0300; **Board Cert:** Internal Medicine 2003; Endocrinology, Diabetes & Metabolism 1995; **Med School:** Med Coll PA Hahnemann 1990; **Resid:** Internal Medicine, N Shore Univ Hosp 1993; **Fellow:** Endocrinology, Diabetes & Metabolism, Montefiore Med Ctr 1995; **Fac Appt:** Assoc Clin Prof Med, SUNY Downstate

Das, Seshadri MD (EDM) - **Spec Exp:** Diabetes; Thyroid Disorders; **Hospital:** St Vincent Cath Med Ctr - Staten Island (page 375); **Address:** 45 Little Clove Rd, Staten Island, NY 10301; **Phone:** 718-273-5522; **Board Cert:** Internal Medicine 1983; Endocrinology, Diabetes & Metabolism 1997; **Med School:** India 1968; **Resid:** Internal Medicine, North Middlesex Hosp 1975; Internal Medicine, Whittington Hosp 1976; **Fellow:** Endocrinology, Diabetes & Metabolism, SUNY Downstate 1980

Hoffman, Richard S MD (EDM) - **Spec Exp:** Diabetes; Thyroid Disorders; **Hospital:** Staten Island Univ Hosp-North Site; **Address:** 1460 Victory Blvd, Staten Island, NY 10301; **Phone:** 718-442-0300; **Board Cert:** Internal Medicine 1971; Endocrinology, Diabetes & Metabolism 1975; **Med School:** SUNY Hlth Sci Ctr 1965; **Resid:** Internal Medicine, Boston City Hosp 1968; **Fellow:** Endocrinology, Boston City Hosp 1970; **Fac Appt:** Assoc Clin Prof Med, SUNY Downstate

Rothman, Jeffrey MD (EDM) - **Spec Exp:** Diabetes; Osteoporosis; Thyroid Disorders; **Hospital:** Staten Island Univ Hosp-North Site, Staten Island Univ Hosp - South Site; **Address:** 1460 Victory Blvd, Staten Island, NY 10301-3914; **Phone:** 718-442-0300; **Board Cert:** Internal Medicine 1973; Endocrinology, Diabetes & Metabolism 1977; **Med School:** SUNY Buffalo 1970; **Resid:** Internal Medicine, Hosp Univ Penn 1973; **Fellow:** Endocrinology, Diabetes & Metabolism, Hosp Univ Penn 1977; **Fac Appt:** Asst Clin Prof Med, SUNY Downstate

GASTROENTEROLOGY

Bruckstein, Alex MD (Ge) - **Spec Exp:** Colonoscopy; Gastroscopy; Gastroesophageal Reflux Disease (GERD); **Hospital:** St Vincent Cath Med Ctr - Staten Island (page 375), Staten Island Univ Hosp-North Site; **Address:** 2627 Hylan Blvd, Staten Island, NY 10306-4339; **Phone:** 718-667-3200; **Board Cert:** Internal Medicine 1979; Gastroenterology 1983; Geriatric Medicine 1992; **Med School:** Albert Einstein Coll Med 1975; **Resid:** Internal Medicine, Roosevelt Hosp 1977; Internal Medicine, St Luke's Hosp 1978; **Fellow:** Gastroenterology, VA Med Ctr-NYU 1980; **Fac Appt:** Asst Clin Prof Med, SUNY Downstate

Fazio, Richard MD (Ge) - **Spec Exp:** Colonoscopy; Gastroesophageal Reflux Disease (GERD); **Hospital:** St Vincent Cath Med Ctr - Staten Island (page 375); **Address:** 78 Todt Hill Rd, Ste 203, Staten Island, NY 10314-4528; **Phone:** 718-448-1122; **Board Cert:** Internal Medicine 1982; Gastroenterology 1983; **Med School:** Italy 1978; **Resid:** Internal Medicine, Maimonides Med Ctr 1981; **Fellow:** Gastroenterology, St Vincent's Hosp & Med Ctr 1983; **Fac Appt:** Prof Med, SUNY Downstate

Kalman, Jeffery MD (Ge) - **Hospital:** Staten Island Univ Hosp - South Site; **Address:** 129 Slosson Ave, Staten Island, NY 10314; **Phone:** 718-720-5928; **Board Cert:** Internal Medicine 1982; Gastroenterology 1982; **Med School:** SUNY Downstate 1979; **Resid:** Internal Medicine, Staten Island Hosp 1982; **Fellow:** Gastroenterology, Yale Affil Hosps 1984

Megna, Daniel MD (Ge) - **Spec Exp:** Esophageal Disorders; Biliary Disease; Gastric & Colonic Disorders; **Hospital:** Staten Island Univ Hosp-North Site, Staten Island Univ Hosp - South Site; **Address:** 360 Edison St, Staten Island, NY 10306-3041; **Phone:** 718-351-6377; **Board Cert:** Internal Medicine 1975; Gastroenterology 1981; **Med School:** Duke Univ 1969; **Resid:** Internal Medicine, USPHS 1970; **Fellow:** Gastroenterology, Yale-New Haven Hosp 1974; Gastroenterology, USPHS 1975; **Fac Appt:** Assoc Clin Prof Med, SUNY Downstate

Shaps, Jeffrey MD (Ge) - **Spec Exp:** Liver Disease; Colitis; Gastroesophageal Reflux Disease (GERD); **Hospital:** Staten Island Univ Hosp-North Site, Staten Island Univ Hosp - South Site; **Address:** 2285 Victory Blvd, Staten Island, NY 10314; **Phone:** 718-761-9319; **Board Cert:** Internal Medicine 1980; Gastroenterology 1983; **Med School:** SUNY Hlth Sci Ctr 1976; **Resid:** Internal Medicine, Staten Island Univ Hosp; **Fellow:** Gastroenterology, VA Hospital; **Fac Appt:** Asst Clin Prof Med, SUNY Downstate

Wickremesinghe, Prasanna MD (Ge) - **Spec Exp:** Inflammatory Bowel Disease/Crohn's; Hepatitis; Endoscopy; **Hospital:** St Vincent Cath Med Ctr - Staten Island (page 375); **Address:** 481 Bard Ave, Staten Island, NY 10310; **Phone:** 718-448-0865; **Board Cert:** Internal Medicine 1974; Gastroenterology 1975; **Med School:** Sri Lanka 1968; **Resid:** Genl Hosp 1970; Internal Medicine, Coney Island Hosp 1972; **Fellow:** Gastroenterology, Maimonides Medical Ctr 1975; **Fac Appt:** Asst Prof Med, NY Med Coll

GYNECOLOGIC ONCOLOGY

Maiman, Mitchell MD (GO) - **Spec Exp:** Cervical Cancer; Ovarian Cancer; Uterine Cancer; **Hospital:** Staten Island Univ Hosp-North Site; **Address:** 256 Mason Ave, Staten Island, NY 10305-3408; **Phone:** 718-226-6400; **Board Cert:** Obstetrics & Gynecology 1998; Gynecologic Oncology 1998; **Med School:** SUNY Hlth Sci Ctr 1981; **Resid:** Obstetrics & Gynecology, Albert Einstein Coll Med 1985; **Fellow:** Gynecologic Oncology, SUNY Downstate Med CTr 1987; **Fac Appt:** Prof ObG, SUNY Downstate

HEMATOLOGY

Forte, Frank J MD (Hem) - **Spec Exp:** Palliative Care; Pain Management; **Hospital:** Staten Island Univ Hosp-North Site; **Address:** Univ Phys Onc/Hem Grp, 256C Mason Ave, Staten Island, NY 10305; **Phone:** 718-226-6400; **Board Cert:** Internal Medicine 1975; Hematology 1976; Medical Oncology 1979; **Med School:** Creighton Univ 1969; **Resid:** Internal Medicine, Staten Island Hosp 1973; **Fellow:** Hematology, NYU Med Ctr 1975; **Fac Appt:** Assoc Clin Prof Med, SUNY Hlth Sci Ctr

INFECTIOUS DISEASE

Glaser, Jordan MD (Inf) - **Hospital:** Staten Island Univ Hosp - South Site, Staten Island Univ Hosp-North Site; **Address:** 1408 Richmond Rd, Staten Island, NY 10304; **Phone:** 718-816-3362; **Board Cert:** Internal Medicine 1982; Infectious Disease 1984; **Med School:** SUNY Hlth Sci Ctr 1979; **Resid:** Internal Medicine, Staten Island Hosp 1980; Infectious Disease, Staten Island Hosp 1982; **Fellow:** Infectious Disease, Univ Hosp 1984; **Fac Appt:** Assoc Clin Prof Med, SUNY Hlth Sci Ctr

INTERNAL MEDICINE

Di Maso, Gerald MD (IM) PCP - **Hospital:** Staten Island Univ Hosp - South Site; **Address:** 68 Seguine Ave, Staten Island, NY 10309; **Phone:** 718-356-6500; **Board Cert:** Internal Medicine 2001; Geriatric Medicine 2000; **Med School:** SUNY Stony Brook 1986; **Resid:** Internal Medicine, Staten Island Univ Hosp 1989; **Fac Appt:** Asst Prof Med, SUNY Downstate

Fulop, Robert MD (IM) PCP - **Spec Exp:** Diagnostic Problems; Geriatric Medicine; **Hospital:** St Vincent Cath Med Ctr - Staten Island (page 375), Staten Island Univ Hosp-North Site; **Address:** 476 Klondike Ave, Staten Island, NY 10314-6216; **Phone:** 718-761-1156; **Board Cert:** Internal Medicine 1982; Geriatric Medicine 2004; **Med School:** SUNY Upstate Med Univ 1978; **Resid:** Internal Medicine, Brookdale Hosp 1981; **Fac Appt:** Asst Clin Prof Med, NY Med Coll

Gazzara, Paul MD (IM) PCP - **Spec Exp:** Addiction Medicine; Complementary Medicine; Acupuncture; **Hospital:** Staten Island Univ Hosp-North Site, Staten Island Univ Hosp - South Site; **Address:** 3589 Hylan Blvd, Staten Island, NY 10308-3513; **Phone:** 718-966-3700; **Board Cert:** Internal Medicine 1986; **Med School:** SUNY Downstate 1983; **Resid:** Internal Medicine, Staten Island Hosp 1986; **Fac Appt:** Asst Clin Prof Med, SUNY Hlth Sci Ctr

Hendricks, Judith MD (IM) PCP - **Spec Exp:** Hypertension; Cholesterol/Lipid Disorders; **Hospital:** Staten Island Univ Hosp-North Site; **Address:** 1870 Richmond Ave, Staten Island, NY 10306; **Phone:** 718-667-5400; **Board Cert:** Internal Medicine 1978; **Med School:** Univ Okla Coll Med 1975; **Resid:** Internal Medicine, Staten Island Hosp 1978; **Fac Appt:** Asst Clin Prof Med, SUNY Hlth Sci Ctr

Malach, Barbara MD (IM) PCP - **Spec Exp:** Geriatric Medicine; **Hospital:** Staten Island Univ Hosp-North Site; **Address:** 2627B Hylan Blvd, Staten Island, NY 10306-4339; **Phone:** 718-987-6000; **Board Cert:** Internal Medicine 1983; Geriatric Medicine 1998; **Med School:** SUNY Downstate 1979; **Resid:** Internal Medicine, Staten Island Hosp 1982

Santiamo, Joseph MD (IM) PCP - **Spec Exp:** Alzheimer's Disease; **Hospital:** St Vincent Cath Med Ctr - Staten Island (page 375), Staten Island Univ Hosp-North Site; **Address:** 4268 Richmond Ave, Staten Island, NY 10312-6239; **Phone:** 718-967-3000; **Board Cert:** Internal Medicine 1999; **Med School:** Mexico 1981; **Resid:** Internal Medicine, LI Coll Hosp 1986; **Fellow:** Geriatric Medicine, Parker Inst-LI Jewish Med Ctr 1988; **Fac Appt:** Asst Clin Prof Med, NY Med Coll

Seminara, Donna MD (IM) - **Spec Exp:** Geriatric Medicine; **Hospital:** Staten Island Univ Hosp-North Site; **Address:** Island Internists, 420 Lyndale Ave, Staten Island, NY 10312-6131; **Phone:** 718-967-5630; **Board Cert:** Internal Medicine 2000; Geriatric Medicine 2000; **Med School:** Mexico 1986; **Resid:** Internal Medicine, Staten Island Univ Hosp 1990

Strange, Theodore MD (IM) PCP - **Spec Exp:** Geriatric Medicine; **Hospital:** Staten Island Univ Hosp - South Site, Staten Island Univ Hosp-North Site; **Address:** 68 Seguine Ave, Staten Island, NY 10309-3723; **Phone:** 718-356-6500; **Board Cert:** Internal Medicine 2001; Geriatric Medicine 2002; **Med School:** SUNY Hlth Sci Ctr 1985; **Resid:** Internal Medicine, Staten Island Univ Hosp 1988; **Fac Appt:** Assoc Clin Prof Med, SUNY Downstate

Tursi, William MD (IM) PCP - **Hospital:** Staten Island Univ Hosp-North Site, St Vincent Cath Med Ctr - Staten Island (page 375); **Address:** 741 Jewett Ave, Staten Island, NY 10314; **Phone:** 718-816-0101; **Board Cert:** Internal Medicine 1980; Geriatric Medicine 1994; **Med School:** Italy 1977; **Resid:** Internal Medicine, St Barnabas Hosp 1980; Internal Medicine, Meth hosp 1979

MATERNAL & FETAL MEDICINE

Moretti, Michael MD (MF) - **Hospital:** St Vincent Cath Med Ctr - Staten Island (page 375), Lutheran Med Ctr - Brooklyn; **Address:** 355 Bard Ave, Ste 208, Staten Island, NY 10310-1664; **Phone:** 718-818-3287; **Board Cert:** Obstetrics & Gynecology 1998; Maternal & Fetal Medicine 1998; **Med School:** Mexico 1981; **Resid:** Obstetrics & Gynecology, Staten Island Hosp 1986; **Fellow:** Maternal & Fetal Medicine, Univ Tenn Hosp 1988

MEDICAL ONCOLOGY

Forlenza, Thomas MD (Onc) - **Spec Exp:** Hospice-Palliative Care; Ethics; **Hospital:** St Vincent Cath Med Ctr - Staten Island (page 375); **Address:** 102 Hart Blvd, Staten Island, NY 10301-2615; **Phone:** 718-816-4949; **Board Cert:** Internal Medicine 1981; Hematology 1984; Medical Oncology 1985; Geriatric Medicine 1996; **Med School:** Boston Univ 1977; **Resid:** Internal Medicine, Univ Kentucky Med Ctr 1980; **Fellow:** Hematology, NYU Med Ctr 1982; Medical Oncology, Kings County Hosp 1983; **Fac Appt:** Clin Prof Med, NYU Sch Med

Friscia, Philip MD (Onc) - **Spec Exp:** Lung Cancer; Colon Cancer; Hematology; **Hospital:** Staten Island Univ Hosp-North Site, Staten Island Univ Hosp - South Site; **Address:** 256 Mason Ave Bldg C, Staten Island, NY 10305; **Phone:** 718-226-6400; **Board Cert:** Internal Medicine 1978; Medical Oncology 1981; **Med School:** Italy 1972; **Resid:** Internal Medicine, Long Island Coll Hosp 1976; **Fellow:** Hematology & Oncology, Long Island Coll Hosp 1979; **Fac Appt:** Asst Clin Prof Med, SUNY Downstate

NEONATAL-PERINATAL MEDICINE

Harin, Anantham MD (NP) - **Spec Exp:** Neonatal Care; **Hospital:** St Vincent Cath Med Ctr - Staten Island (page 375); **Address:** 355 Bard Ave, Staten Island, NY 10310; **Phone:** 718-818-4310; **Board Cert:** Pediatrics 1975; Neonatal-Perinatal Medicine 1977; **Med School:** Sri Lanka 1970; **Resid:** Pediatrics, Kings County Hosp 1973; **Fellow:** Neonatology, N Shore Univ Hosp 1975; **Fac Appt:** Clin Prof Ped, NYU Sch Med

Roth, Philip MD/PhD (NP) - **Spec Exp:** Neonatal Infections/Immunity; Breast Feeding Problems; **Hospital:** Staten Island Univ Hosp-North Site; **Address:** 475 Seaview Ave Fl 4 East, Staten Island, NY 10305-3436; **Phone:** 718-226-9796; **Board Cert:** Pediatrics 1987; Neonatal-Perinatal Medicine 2004; **Med School:** Columbia P&S 1982; **Resid:** Pediatrics, Chldns Hosp 1986; **Fellow:** Neonatal-Perinatal Medicine, Hosp U Penn 1988; **Fac Appt:** Assoc Prof Ped, SUNY Downstate

Siracuse, Jeffrey F MD (NP) - **Spec Exp:** Necrotizing Enterocolitis; Respiratory Distress Syndrome; Neonatology; **Hospital:** St Vincent Cath Med Ctr - Staten Island (page 375); **Address:** 355 Bard Ave, Staten Island, NY 10310-1664; **Phone:** 718-818-2859; **Board Cert:** Pediatrics 1985; Neonatal-Perinatal Medicine 1985; **Med School:** Italy 1977; **Resid:** Pediatrics, St Vincent's Hosp 1980; **Fellow:** Neonatal-Perinatal Medicine, Columbia-Presb Med Ctr 1982; **Fac Appt:** Asst Prof Ped, NY Med Coll

NEPHROLOGY

Grossman, Susan MD (Nep) - **Hospital:** St Vincent Cath Med Ctr - Staten Island (page 375); **Address:** St Vincent's Med Ctr, Dept Med, 355 Bard Ave, Staten Island, NY 10310; **Phone:** 718-818-2416; **Board Cert:** Internal Medicine 1980; Nephrology 1982; **Med School:** UMDNJ-NJ Med Sch, Newark 1977; **Resid:** Internal Medicine, Univ Hosp 1980; **Fellow:** Nephrology, New England Med Ctr 1982

Richmond (Staten Island)

Kleiner, Morton MD (Nep) - **Spec Exp:** Hypertension; Kidney Disease; **Hospital:** Staten Island Univ Hosp-North Site, Maimonides Med Ctr (page 96); **Address:** 347 Edison St, Staten Island, NY 10306; **Phone:** 718-351-1136; **Board Cert:** Internal Medicine 1977; Nephrology 1982; **Med School:** NY Med Coll 1974; **Resid:** Internal Medicine, N Shore Univ Hosp 1977; **Fellow:** Nephrology, NY Hosp-Cornell Med Ctr 1979; **Fac Appt:** Asst Clin Prof Med, SUNY Downstate

Pepe, John MD (Nep) - **Spec Exp:** Transplant Medicine-Kidney; **Hospital:** St Vincent Cath Med Ctr - Staten Island (page 375), Staten Island Univ Hosp - South Site; **Address:** 1550 Richmond Ave, Ste 205, Staten Island, NY 10314-1519; **Phone:** 718-982-7800; **Board Cert:** Internal Medicine 1978; Nephrology 1980; **Med School:** Med Coll PA Hahnemann 1975; **Resid:** Internal Medicine, Univ Hosp 1978; **Fellow:** Nephrology, Bronx Muni Hosp/ Einstein 1980; **Fac Appt:** Asst Prof Med, NY Med Coll

NEUROLOGY

Jutkowitz, Robert MD (N) - **Spec Exp:** Headache; Seizure Disorders; **Hospital:** St Vincent Cath Med Ctr - Staten Island (page 375); **Address:** 78 Todt Hill Rd, Ste 205, Staten Island, NY 10314-4528; **Phone:** 718-442-7133; **Board Cert:** Neurology 1976; **Med School:** Univ Louisville Sch Med 1968; **Resid:** Internal Medicine, St Viincents Hosp 1970; Neurology, Mount Sinai Hosp 1974

Kulick, Stephen A MD (N) - **Spec Exp:** Electromyography; Parkinson's Disease; Multiple Sclerosis; **Hospital:** Staten Island Univ Hosp-North Site, St Vincent Cath Med Ctr - Staten Island (page 375); **Address:** 1099 Targee St, Staten Island, NY 10304-4310; **Phone:** 718-448-3210; **Board Cert:** Neurology 1969; **Med School:** Boston Univ 1961; **Resid:** Internal Medicine, Boston VA Hosp 1963; Neurology, Mount Sinai Hosp 1966; **Fac Appt:** Asst Clin Prof N, Mount Sinai Sch Med

Perel, Allan MD (N) - **Spec Exp:** Headache; Multiple Sclerosis; Alzheimer's Disease; **Hospital:** Staten Island Univ Hosp-North Site, Staten Island Univ Hosp - South Site; **Address:** Alpha Med Ctr, 27-31 New Dorp Ln, Staten Island, NY 10306; **Phone:** 718-667-3800; **Board Cert:** Neurology 1990; **Med School:** SUNY Downstate 1985; **Resid:** Neurology, Columbia-Presby Med Ctr 1989; **Fac Appt:** Assoc Clin Prof N, SUNY Downstate

OBSTETRICS & GYNECOLOGY

Gonzalez Jr, Orlando MD (ObG) - **Spec Exp:** Hysterectomy Alternatives; Laparoscopic Surgery; **Hospital:** St Vincent Cath Med Ctr - Staten Island (page 375), Staten Island Univ Hosp-North Site; **Address:** 78 Todt Hill Rd, Ste 107, Staten Island, NY 10314; **Phone:** 718-273-6034; **Board Cert:** Obstetrics & Gynecology 1998; **Med School:** Mexico 1982; **Resid:** Obstetrics & Gynecology, St Vincent's Hosp & Med Ctr 1988; **Fellow:** Obstetrics & Gynecology, Meml Sloan Kettering Cancer Ctr 1986; **Fac Appt:** Asst Clin Prof ObG, NY Med Coll

Grecco, Michael MD (ObG) **PCP** - **Hospital:** St Vincent Cath Med Ctr - Staten Island (page 375), Staten Island Univ Hosp-North Site; **Address:** 1984 Richmond Rd, Staten Island, NY 10306; **Phone:** 718-667-1111; **Board Cert:** Obstetrics & Gynecology 2003; **Med School:** West Indies 1982; **Resid:** Obstetrics & Gynecology, Univ Hosp 1989

Perry, Kathleen MD (ObG) - **Spec Exp:** Menopause Problems; Women's Health; Colposcopy; **Hospital:** St Vincent Cath Med Ctr - Staten Island (page 375), St Vincent Cath Med Ctrs - Manhattan (page 375); **Address:** 539 Castleton Ave, Staten Island, NY 10301-2060; **Phone:** 718-727-9700; **Board Cert:** Obstetrics & Gynecology 1977; **Med School:** NY Med Coll 1967; **Resid:** Obstetrics & Gynecology, Staten Island Hosp 1971; **Fellow:** Obstetrics & Gynecology, Staten Island Hosp 1975; **Fac Appt:** Asst Clin Prof ObG, SUNY Downstate

Pillari, Vincent MD (ObG) **PCP** - **Spec Exp:** Uro-Gynecology; Pregnancy-High Risk; **Hospital:** St Vincent Cath Med Ctr - Staten Island (page 375); **Address:** 355 Bard Ave, Staten Island, NY 10310-1664; **Phone:** 718-818-4293; **Board Cert:** Obstetrics & Gynecology 2000; **Med School:** Loyola Univ-Stritch Sch Med 1962; **Resid:** Obstetrics & Gynecology, Nassau County Med Ctr 1964; Obstetrics & Gynecology, Univ Hosp 1966; **Fac Appt:** Prof ObG, NY Med Coll

Rapp, Lynn MD (ObG) - **Spec Exp:** Colposcopy; Obstetrics; Gynecologic Surgery; **Hospital:** Staten Island Univ Hosp-North Site, St Vincent Cath Med Ctr - Staten Island (page 375); **Address:** 2627 Hylan Blvd, Apt Bldg A, Staten Island, NY 10306-4336; **Phone:** 718-351-6265; **Board Cert:** Obstetrics & Gynecology 2003; **Med School:** Italy 1983; **Resid:** Obstetrics & Gynecology, Staten Island Hosp 1988

Reilly, James G DO (ObG) - **Spec Exp:** Colposcopy; Gynecologic Surgery-Laparoscopic; Hysterectomy Alternatives; **Hospital:** St Vincent Cath Med Ctr - Staten Island (page 375), Staten Island Univ Hosp-North Site; **Address:** 668 Castleton Ave, Staten Island, NY 10301; **Phone:** 718-448-4300; **Board Cert:** Obstetrics & Gynecology 1998; **Med School:** NY Coll Osteo Med 1991; **Resid:** Obstetrics & Gynecology, St Vincent Cath Med Ctr 1995; **Fellow:** Gynecologic Oncology, Meml Sloan Kettering Cancer Ctr 1996; **Fac Appt:** Asst Clin Prof ObG, NY Med Coll

OPHTHALMOLOGY

Derespinis, Patrick MD (Oph) - **Spec Exp:** Eye Muscle Disorders; Pediatric Ophthalmology; Eye Disorders-Congenital; **Hospital:** Staten Island Univ Hosp - South Site, UMDNJ-Univ Hosp-Newark; **Address:** 2504 Richmond Rd, Staten Island, NY 10306; **Phone:** 718-667-1010; **Board Cert:** Ophthalmology 1989; **Med School:** Mexico 1981; **Resid:** Internal Medicine, Booth Meml Med Ctr 1983; Ophthalmology, UMDNJ 1987; **Fellow:** Pediatric Ophthalmology, Manhattan Eye, Ear & Throat Hosp 1988; **Fac Appt:** Assoc Clin Prof Oph, UMDNJ-NJ Med Sch, Newark

Kramer, Philip MD (Oph) - **Spec Exp:** Diabetic Eye Disease/Retinopathy; Cataract Surgery; Glaucoma; **Hospital:** Staten Island Univ Hosp - South Site, New York Eye & Ear Infirm (page 110); **Address:** 1460 Victory Blvd, Staten Island, NY 10301-3914; **Phone:** 718-447-0022; **Board Cert:** Ophthalmology 1985; **Med School:** Temple Univ 1980; **Resid:** Ophthalmology, NY Eye & Ear Infirmary 1984

Zerykier, Abraham MD (Oph) - **Spec Exp:** Cataract Surgery; Diabetic Eye Disease/Retinopathy; **Hospital:** Staten Island Univ Hosp - South Site, Beth Israel Med Ctr- Kings Hwy Div (page 90); **Address:** 16 Ross Ave, Staten Island, NY 10306-2216; **Phone:** 718-667-4444; **Board Cert:** Ophthalmology 1980; **Med School:** Hahnemann Univ 1975; **Resid:** Internal Medicine, Brookdale Hosp 1976; Ophthalmology, Jewish Hosp 1979; **Fac Appt:** Asst Clin Prof Oph, SUNY Downstate

ORTHOPAEDIC SURGERY

Accettola, Albert MD (OrS) - **Hospital:** Staten Island Univ Hosp-North Site, Staten Island Univ Hosp - South Site; **Address:** 3311 Hylan Blvd, Staten Island, NY 10306; **Phone:** 718-667-7500; **Board Cert:** Orthopaedic Surgery 1982; **Med School:** Belgium 1974; **Resid:** Surgery, Staten Island Hosp 1976; Orthopaedic Surgery, Bellevue Hosp Ctr-NYU 1979

Drucker, David MD (OrS) - **Spec Exp:** Hip & Knee Replacement; **Hospital:** Staten Island Univ Hosp - South Site, UMDNJ-Univ Hosp-Newark; **Address:** 1460 Victory Blvd, Ste D, Staten Island, NY 10301; **Phone:** 718-447-0182; **Board Cert:** Orthopaedic Surgery 2004; **Med School:** Univ Chicago-Pritzker Sch Med 1983; **Resid:** Orthopaedic Surgery, UNDMJ Univ Hosp 1989; **Fellow:** Indiana Univ 1990; **Fac Appt:** Asst Clin Prof OrS, UMDNJ-NJ Med Sch, Newark

Flynn, Maryirene MD (OrS) - **Spec Exp:** Arthroscopic Surgery; Sports Medicine; **Hospital:** St Vincent Cath Med Ctr - Staten Island (page 375), Staten Island Univ Hosp-North Site; **Address:** 1551 Richmond Rd, Staten Island, NY 10304; **Phone:** 718-351-6500; **Board Cert:** Orthopaedic Surgery 1994; **Med School:** Albert Einstein Coll Med 1986; **Resid:** Orthopaedic Surgery, Montefiore Hosp Med Ctr 1991; **Fellow:** Sports Medicine, Staten Island Hosp 1993

Jayaram, Nadubeethi MD (OrS) - **Spec Exp:** Hand Surgery; **Hospital:** St Vincent Cath Med Ctr - Staten Island (page 375); **Address:** 11 Ralph Pl, Ste 102, Staten Island, NY 10304; **Phone:** 718-447-6545; **Board Cert:** Orthopaedic Surgery 2003; **Med School:** India 1973; **Resid:** Surgery, Univ Hosp 1981; Orthopaedic Surgery, Univ Hosp 1985; **Fellow:** Vascular Surgery, Lutheran Med Ctr 1982; Hand Surgery, Univ Alabama Hosp 1988

Reilly, John MD (OrS) - **Spec Exp:** Sports Medicine; Trauma; **Hospital:** Staten Island Univ Hosp - South Site; **Address:** 3311 Hylan Blvd, Staten Island, NY 10306; **Phone:** 718-667-7500; **Board Cert:** Orthopaedic Surgery 1989; **Med School:** SUNY Hlth Sci Ctr 1981; **Resid:** Orthopaedic Surgery, Lenox Hill Hosp 1986; Orthopaedic Surgery, Children's Hosp; **Fellow:** Orthopaedic Surgery, Univ MD Hosp 1987

Sherman, Mark F MD (OrS) - **Spec Exp:** Sports Medicine; Knee Injuries; **Hospital:** St Vincent Cath Med Ctr - Staten Island (page 375), Staten Island Univ Hosp-North Site; **Address:** 1551 Richmond Rd, Staten Island, NY 10304; **Phone:** 718-351-6500; **Board Cert:** Orthopaedic Surgery 1981; **Med School:** NYU Sch Med 1975; **Resid:** Surgery, Bellevue Hosp 1976; Orthopaedic Surgery, Bellevue Hosp 1979; **Fellow:** Sports Medicine, Hosp for Special Surgery 1980

OTOLARYNGOLOGY

Castellano, Bartolomeo MD (Oto) - **Hospital:** St Vincent Cath Med Ctr - Staten Island (page 375); **Address:** 78 Todt Hill Rd, Ste 204, Staten Island, NY 10314-4528; **Phone:** 718-273-2626; **Board Cert:** Otolaryngology 1985; **Med School:** Mexico 1979; **Resid:** Otolaryngology, NYU Med Ctr 1984; **Fellow:** Plastic Surgery, Mount Sinai Med Ctr 1985; **Fac Appt:** Asst Prof Oto, NYU Sch Med

Sinnreich, Abraham MD (Oto) - **Spec Exp:** Sinus Disorders; Sleep Disorders/Apnea; **Hospital:** Long Island Coll Hosp (page 90), St Vincent Cath Med Ctr - Staten Island (page 375); **Address:** 1887 Richmond Ave, Ste 5, Staten Island, NY 10314; **Phone:** 718-370-0072; **Board Cert:** Otolaryngology 1984; **Med School:** Albert Einstein Coll Med 1979; **Resid:** Otolaryngology, Mount Sinai Hosp 1983; **Fac Appt:** Asst Clin Prof Oto, SUNY Downstate

Wiesenthal, Carl MD (Oto) - **Hospital:** St Vincent Cath Med Ctr - Staten Island (page 375); **Address:** 78 Todt Hill Rd, Ste 204, Staten Island, NY 10314-4528; **Phone:** 718-273-2626; **Board Cert:** Otolaryngology 1978; **Med School:** Italy 1973; **Resid:** Otolaryngology, Columbia Presby Med Ctr 1978

PEDIATRIC ALLERGY & IMMUNOLOGY

Misra, Sabita MD (PA&I) - **Spec Exp:** Food Allergy; Asthma; Allergy & Immunology; **Hospital:** Staten Island Univ Hosp-North Site, St Vincent Cath Med Ctr - Staten Island (page 375); **Address:** 3335 Richmond Rd, Staten Island, NY 10306-1425; **Phone:** 718-667-7617; **Board Cert:** Pediatrics 1998; Allergy & Immunology 1999; **Med School:** India 1981; **Resid:** Pediatrics, Staten Island Univ Hosp 1987; **Fellow:** Allergy & Immunology, LI Coll Hosp 1989; **Fac Appt:** Asst Clin Prof Ped, SUNY Downstate

PEDIATRIC ENDOCRINOLOGY

Torrado-Jule, Carmen MD (PEn) - **Spec Exp:** Diabetes; Thyroid Disorders; Growth Disorders; Obesity; **Hospital:** Staten Island Univ Hosp-North Site, N Shore Univ Hosp at Manhasset; **Address:** 584 Forest Ave, Staten Island, NY 10310-2512; **Phone:** 718-226-5619; **Board Cert:** Pediatrics 2000; Pediatric Endocrinology 2005; **Med School:** Dominican Republic 1983; **Resid:** Pediatrics, Kings County Hosp 1987; **Fellow:** Pediatric Endocrinology, Kings County Hosp 1990; **Fac Appt:** Asst Prof Ped, SUNY Hlth Sci Ctr

PEDIATRIC GASTROENTEROLOGY

Rabinowitz, Simon S MD/PhD (PGe) - **Spec Exp:** Inflammatory Bowel Disease; Hepatitis; Gastroesophageal Reflux Disease (GERD); **Hospital:** St Vincent Cath Med Ctr - Staten Island (page 375); **Address:** St Vincent Catholic Medical Ctr, Pediatrics, 355 Bard Ave, Ste 314, Staten Island, NY 10310-1699; **Phone:** 718-818-4636; **Board Cert:** Pediatrics 1988; Pediatric Gastroenterology 1992; **Med School:** Univ Miami Sch Med 1983; **Resid:** Pediatrics, Mount Sinai Hosp 1985; **Fellow:** Pediatric Gastroenterology, Mount Sinai Hosp 1987; **Fac Appt:** Assoc Clin Prof Ped, SUNY Downstate

PEDIATRIC HEMATOLOGY-ONCOLOGY

Potaznik, Daniel MD (PHO) - **Spec Exp:** Hematology; **Hospital:** Staten Island Univ Hosp-North Site; **Address:** 256 Mason Ave, Staten Island, NY 10305; **Phone:** 718-226-6474; **Board Cert:** Pediatrics 1987; Pediatric Hematology-Oncology 1987; **Med School:** Belgium 1970; **Resid:** Pediatrics, Sheba Med Ctr 1975; **Fellow:** Pediatric Hematology-Oncology, Meml Sloan Kettering Cancer Ctr 1983; **Fac Appt:** Asst Clin Prof Ped, SUNY Hlth Sci Ctr

PEDIATRIC PULMONOLOGY

Marcus, Michael MD (PPul) - **Spec Exp:** Asthma; Sleep Apnea; **Hospital:** Maimonides Med Ctr (page 96), St Vincent Cath Med Ctr - Staten Island (page 375); **Address:** 1491 Richmond Rd, Staten Island, NY 10304; **Phone:** 718-980-5864; **Board Cert:** Pediatrics 1984; Allergy & Immunology 1987; Pediatric Pulmonology 2002; **Med School:** SUNY Stony Brook 1980; **Resid:** Pediatrics, Nassau County Med Ctr 1983; **Fellow:** Pediatric Pulmonology, Chldns Hosp 1985; **Fac Appt:** Asst Clin Prof Ped, SUNY Stony Brook

PEDIATRICS

Bastawros, Mary MD (Ped) PCP - **Hospital:** St Vincent Cath Med Ctr - Staten Island (page 375), Staten Island Univ Hosp-North Site; **Address:** 314 Seaview Ave, Staten Island, NY 10305; **Phone:** 718-668-3417; **Board Cert:** Pediatrics 1985; **Med School:** Egypt 1966; **Resid:** Pediatrics, Methodist Hosp 1974

Richmond (Staten Island)

Duchnowska, Alicja MD (Ped) PCP - **Hospital:** Staten Island Univ Hosp-North Site; **Address:** 934 Ionia Ave, Staten Island, NY 10309-2308; **Phone:** 718-984-5255; **Board Cert:** Pediatrics 1985; **Med School:** Poland 1965; **Resid:** Pediatrics, National Inst of Mother & Child 1970; Pediatrics, Staten Island Hosp 1982; **Fellow:** Pediatrics, Staten Island Hosp 1984

Purow, Henry MD (Ped) PCP - **Spec Exp:** Newborn Care; **Hospital:** Staten Island Univ Hosp-North Site, St Vincent Cath Med Ctr - Staten Island (page 375); **Address:** 1326 Clove Rd, Staten Island, NY 10301; **Phone:** 718-727-7272; **Board Cert:** Pediatrics 1974; Neonatal-Perinatal Medicine 1975; **Med School:** SUNY Buffalo 1968; **Resid:** Pediatrics, Columbia-Presby Hosp 1971; Pediatrics, Staten Island Hosp 1972; **Fellow:** Neonatal-Perinatal Medicine, Downstate Med Ctr 1974

Short, Joan MD (Ped) PCP - **Hospital:** St Vincent Cath Med Ctr - Staten Island (page 375), Staten Island Univ Hosp-North Site; **Address:** 32 2nd St, Staten Island, NY 10306; **Phone:** 718-979-7472; **Board Cert:** Pediatrics 1982; **Med School:** Univ Tenn Coll Med, Memphis 1966; **Resid:** Pediatrics, City of Memphis Hosp; **Fellow:** Pediatric Oncology, St Jude Chldns Hosp

Visconti, Ernest MD (Ped) PCP - **Spec Exp:** Infectious Disease; **Hospital:** Lutheran Med Ctr - Brooklyn, St Vincent Cath Med Ctr - Staten Island (page 375); **Address:** 314 Seaview Ave, Staten Island, NY 10305-2246; **Phone:** 718-668-3417; **Board Cert:** Pediatrics 1992; Pediatric Infectious Disease 2002; **Med School:** SUNY Upstate Med Univ 1971; **Resid:** Pediatrics, NY Hosp 1974; **Fellow:** Infectious Disease, Rhode Island Hosp 1978

PHYSICAL MEDICINE & REHABILITATION

Weinberg, Jeffrey MD (PMR) - **Spec Exp:** Geriatric Rehabilitation; Musculoskeletal Injuries; **Hospital:** Staten Island Univ Hosp-North Site; **Address:** Staten Island Univ Hosp, Dept Rehab Med, 475 Seaview Ave, Staten Island, NY 10305-3436; **Phone:** 718-226-6362; **Board Cert:** Physical Medicine & Rehabilitation 1985; **Med School:** NY Med Coll 1980; **Resid:** Physical Medicine & Rehabilitation, NYU Med Ctr 1983; **Fellow:** Geriatric Medicine, NYU Med Ctr; **Fac Appt:** Asst Clin Prof PMR, NYU Sch Med

PLASTIC SURGERY

Cherofsky, Alan MD (PlS) - **Spec Exp:** Breast Surgery; Pediatric Plastic Surgery; Cosmetic Surgery-Body; **Hospital:** Staten Island Univ Hosp - South Site, St Vincent Cath Med Ctr - Staten Island (page 375); **Address:** 4546 Hylan Blvd, Staten Island, NY 10312-6400; **Phone:** 718-967-3300; **Board Cert:** Plastic Surgery 1993; **Med School:** SUNY Hlth Sci Ctr 1982; **Resid:** Surgery, Staten Island Univ Hosp 1987; Plastic Surgery, Univ Missouri Hosp 1989

Cutolo Jr, Louis Carmine MD (PlS) - **Spec Exp:** Breast Augmentation; Liposuction; Eyelid Surgery; **Hospital:** Staten Island Univ Hosp-North Site, Long Island Coll Hosp (page 90); **Address:** 3710 Richmond Ave, Staten Island, NY 10312; **Phone:** 718-984-8910; **Board Cert:** Plastic Surgery 1995; **Med School:** SUNY Downstate 1985; **Resid:** Surgery, Staten Island Hosp 1990; **Fellow:** Plastic Surgery, Univ Florida/Shands Hosp 1992

Raju, Raghava MD (PlS) - **Hospital:** Staten Island Univ Hosp - South Site, St Vincent Cath Med Ctr - Staten Island (page 375); **Address:** 2131 Richmond Rd, Staten Island, NY 10306; **Phone:** 718-979-5553; **Board Cert:** Plastic Surgery 1983; **Med School:** India 1967; **Resid:** Surgery, New York Methodist Hosp 1976; Plastic Surgery, St Luke's-Roosevelt Hosp Ctr 1979; **Fellow:** Plastic Surgery, Cleveland 1980

PSYCHIATRY

Di Buono, Mark MD (Psyc) - **Spec Exp:** Geriatric Psychiatry; Depression; **Hospital:** Staten Island Univ Hosp - South Site; **Address:** 4349 Hylan Blvd, Staten Island, NY 10312; **Phone:** 718-227-1897; **Board Cert:** Psychiatry 1990; Geriatric Psychiatry 1996; **Med School:** Mexico 1981; **Resid:** Psychiatry, Stony Brook Univ Hosp 1986; **Fac Appt:** Asst Clin Prof Psyc, SUNY Downstate

Lee, Chol MD (Psyc) - **Spec Exp:** Anxiety & Mood Disorders; Schizophrenia; Child Psychiatry; **Hospital:** St Vincent Cath Med Ctr - Staten Island (page 375); **Address:** 1430 Clove Rd, Staten Island, NY 10301; **Phone:** 718-448-0066; **Board Cert:** Psychiatry 1977; **Med School:** South Korea 1960; **Resid:** Psychiatry, Medfield St Hosp 1969; **Fellow:** Child & Adolescent Psychiatry, NYU/Bellevue Med 1971; **Fac Appt:** Asst Clin Prof Psyc, NY Med Coll

Miller, Lawrence MD (Psyc) - **Hospital:** St Vincent Cath Med Ctr - Staten Island (page 375); **Address:** 1430 Clove Rd, Staten Island, NY 10301-4335; **Phone:** 718-816-8322; **Board Cert:** Psychiatry 1963; Child & Adolescent Psychiatry 1965; **Med School:** Switzerland 1955; **Resid:** Child & Adolescent Psychiatry, Mental Health Clinic/USPHS 1961; **Fellow:** Child & Adolescent Psychiatry, Staten Island Hosp 1963; **Fac Appt:** Assoc Prof Psyc, NYU Sch Med

PULMONARY DISEASE

Castellano, Michael A MD (Pul) - **Spec Exp:** Asthma; Emphysema; **Hospital:** Staten Island Univ Hosp-North Site; **Address:** 501 Seaview Ave, Ste 102, Staten Island, NY 10305; **Phone:** 718-980-5700; **Board Cert:** Internal Medicine 1974; Pulmonary Disease 1978; Critical Care Medicine 1997; Geriatric Medicine 1994; **Med School:** Italy 1968; **Resid:** Internal Medicine, Staten Island Hosp 1972; **Fellow:** Pulmonary Disease, NYU-Bellvue Hosp 1974; **Fac Appt:** Asst Prof Med, SUNY Downstate

Maniatis, Theodore MD (Pul) - **Spec Exp:** Asthma; Lung Cancer; Chronic Obstructive Lung Disease (COPD); **Hospital:** Staten Island Univ Hosp-North Site, Staten Island Univ Hosp - South Site; **Address:** 501 Seaview Ave, Ste 102, Staten Island, NY 10305; **Phone:** 718-980-5700; **Board Cert:** Internal Medicine 1983; Pulmonary Disease 1986; Critical Care Medicine 1997; **Med School:** SUNY Hlth Sci Ctr 1980; **Resid:** Internal Medicine, Staten Island Univ Hosp 1983; **Fellow:** Pulmonary Disease, UMDNJ Med Ctr 1985; **Fac Appt:** Asst Clin Prof Med, SUNY Downstate

Martins, Publius MD (Pul) - **Spec Exp:** Asthma; Emphysema; **Hospital:** St Vincent Cath Med Ctr - Staten Island (page 375), Staten Island Univ Hosp - South Site; **Address:** 283 Bard Ave, Staten Island, NY 10310-1664; **Phone:** 718-816-8068; **Board Cert:** Internal Medicine 1984; Pulmonary Disease 1992; **Med School:** Portugal 1975; **Resid:** Internal Medicine, St Vincent's Hosp 1981; **Fellow:** Pulmonary Disease, Meml Hosp 1983; **Fac Appt:** Assoc Clin Prof Med, NY Med Coll

Sasso, Louis MD (Pul) - **Spec Exp:** Asthma; Chronic Obstructive Lung Disease (COPD); Interstitial Lung Disease; **Hospital:** Staten Island Univ Hosp-North Site; **Address:** 501 Seaview Ave, Staten Island, NY 10305; **Phone:** 718-980-5700; **Board Cert:** Internal Medicine 1976; Pulmonary Disease 1978; Critical Care Medicine 2005; Geriatric Medicine 1998; **Med School:** UMDNJ-NJ Med Sch, Newark 1972; **Resid:** Internal Medicine, St Vincent's Hosp & Med Ctr 1974; Internal Medicine, CMDNJ-Martland Hosp 1975; **Fellow:** Pulmonary Disease, Bellevue Hos/NYU Med Ctr 1977; **Fac Appt:** Asst Clin Prof Med, SUNY Downstate

Richmond (Staten Island)

RADIATION ONCOLOGY

Adams, Marc MD (RadRO) - **Spec Exp:** Prostate Cancer; Breast Cancer; **Hospital:** St Vincent Cath Med Ctr - Staten Island (page 375); **Address:** 360 Bard Ave, Staten Island, NY 10310; **Phone:** 718-876-2023; **Board Cert:** Radiation Oncology 1990; **Med School:** Univ Ala 1985; **Resid:** Radiation Oncology, St Barnabas Hosp 1989; **Fac Appt:** Asst Prof Rad, NYU Sch Med

RHEUMATOLOGY

Garjian, Peggy Ann MD (Rhu) - **Hospital:** St Vincent Cath Med Ctr - Staten Island (page 375); **Address:** 71 Todt Hill Rd, Ste 201, Staten Island, NY 10314-4535; **Phone:** 718-720-1030; **Board Cert:** Internal Medicine 1994; Rheumatology 1997; **Med School:** Mexico 1981; **Resid:** Internal Medicine, Lutheran Med Ctr 1985; **Fellow:** Rheumatology, Univ Conn Health Ctr 1987

Goldstein, Mark A MD (Rhu) - **Spec Exp:** Rheumatoid Arthritis; Osteoporosis; Lupus/SLE; **Hospital:** Staten Island Univ Hosp - South Site, St Vincent Cath Med Ctr - Staten Island (page 375); **Address:** 1478 Victory Blvd, Staten Island, NY 10301; **Phone:** 718-447-0055; **Board Cert:** Internal Medicine 1982; Rheumatology 1988; **Med School:** NY Med Coll 1979; **Resid:** Internal Medicine, Montefiore Hosp Med Ctr 1980; Internal Medicine, Montefiore Hosp Med Ctr 1982; **Fellow:** Critical Care Medicine, Montefiore Hosp Med Ctr 1983; Rheumatology, Albert Einstein 1987

Jarrett, Mark MD (Rhu) - **Spec Exp:** Lupus/SLE; Osteoporosis; Rheumatoid Arthritis; **Hospital:** Staten Island Univ Hosp-North Site, Staten Island Univ Hosp - South Site; **Address:** 1478 Victory Blvd, Staten Island, NY 10301; **Phone:** 718-447-0055; **Board Cert:** Internal Medicine 1978; Rheumatology 1980; Geriatric Medicine 1998; **Med School:** NYU Sch Med 1975; **Resid:** Internal Medicine, Montefiore Hosp Med Ctr 1978; **Fellow:** Rheumatology, Montefiore Hosp Med Ctr 1980; **Fac Appt:** Asst Clin Prof Med, SUNY Downstate

SURGERY

Coppa, Gene F MD (S) - **Spec Exp:** Minimally Invasive Surgery; Hepatobiliary Surgery; Gastrointestinal Surgery; Pancreatic Surgery; **Hospital:** Staten Island Univ Hosp-North Site; **Address:** Staten Island Univ Hosp, 256 Mason Ave Bldg B, Staten Island, NY 10305; **Phone:** 718-226-6398; **Board Cert:** Surgery 2000; **Med School:** NYU Sch Med 1974; **Resid:** Surgery, NYU/Bellview Med Ctr 1979; **Fac Appt:** Prof S, SUNY Downstate

D'Anna, John MD (S) - **Spec Exp:** Vascular Surgery; **Hospital:** Staten Island Univ Hosp-North Site, Staten Island Univ Hosp - South Site; **Address:** 256B Mason Ave, Staten Island, NY 10305; **Phone:** 718-226-6398; **Board Cert:** Surgery 2003; **Med School:** Georgetown Univ 1977; **Resid:** Surgery, St Vincent's Hosp Med Ctr 1982; **Fellow:** Vascular Surgery, St Vincent's Hosp Med Ctr 1983; **Fac Appt:** Assoc Clin Prof S, SUNY Downstate

Ferzli, George MD (S) - **Spec Exp:** Laparoscopic Surgery; Obesity/Bariatric Surgery; Endocrine Surgery; **Hospital:** Lutheran Med Ctr - Brooklyn, Staten Island Univ Hosp-North Site; **Address:** 65 Cromwell Ave, Staten Island, NY 10304; **Phone:** 718-667-8100; **Board Cert:** Surgery 2003; Surgical Critical Care 1994; **Med School:** Lebanon 1979; **Resid:** Surgery, Staten Island Univ Hosp 1984; **Fac Appt:** Prof S, SUNY Downstate

Hornyak, Stephen W MD (S) - **Spec Exp:** Breast Surgery; Laparoscopic Surgery; Abdominal Surgery; **Hospital:** Staten Island Univ Hosp-North Site, St Vincent Cath Med Ctr - Staten Island (page 375); **Address:** 1130 Victory Blvd, Staten Island, NY 10301; **Phone:** 718-442-3400; **Board Cert:** Surgery 1999; **Med School:** SUNY Hlth Sci Ctr 1974; **Resid:** Surgery, Kings County Hosp 1979; **Fellow:** Research, Meml Sloan Kettering Cancer Ctr 1980; **Fac Appt:** Asst Clin Prof S, SUNY Downstate

Lansigan, Nicholas MD (S) - **Spec Exp:** Laparoscopic Cholecystectomy; Laparoscopic Surgery-GERD; Obesity/Bariatric Surgery; **Hospital:** St Vincent Cath Med Ctr - Staten Island (page 375), Staten Island Univ Hosp-North Site; **Address:** 1366 Victory Blvd, Staten Island, NY 10301-3907; **Phone:** 718-442-4777; **Board Cert:** Surgery 1997; **Med School:** Philippines 1966; **Resid:** Surgery, St Vincent's Hosp & Med Ctr 1973; Surgery, Philippine Genl Hosp 1969; **Fellow:** Meml Sloan Kettering Cancer Ctr 1974

Pahuja, Murlidhar MD (S) - **Spec Exp:** Breast Cancer; Laparoscopic Surgery; Wound Healing/Care; **Hospital:** Staten Island Univ Hosp-North Site, Victory Memorial Hosp - Bklyn; **Address:** 4287 Richmond Ave, Staten Island, NY 10312; **Phone:** 718-967-6230; **Board Cert:** Surgery 2004; **Med School:** Pakistan 1971; **Resid:** Surgery, Stamford Hosp 1978; Surgery, Staten Island Hosp 1982; **Fellow:** Burn Surgery, New York Hosp 1980

Silich, Robert J MD (S) - **Spec Exp:** Breast Surgery; Colon & Rectal Surgery; Thyroid & Parathyroid Surgery; **Hospital:** Staten Island Univ Hosp-North Site, St Vincent Cath Med Ctr - Staten Island (page 375); **Address:** 1557 Victory Blvd, Staten Island, NY 10314-3528; **Phone:** 718-447-0404; **Board Cert:** Surgery 1973; **Med School:** NY Med Coll 1967; **Resid:** Surgery, Staten Island Hosp 1972; **Fac Appt:** Assoc Clin Prof S, SUNY Hlth Sci Ctr

Steinbruck, Richard MD (S) - **Spec Exp:** Breast Surgery; Laparoscopic Surgery; **Hospital:** St Vincent Cath Med Ctr - Staten Island (page 375), Staten Island Univ Hosp-North Site; **Address:** 1366 Victory Blvd, Ste A, Staten Island, NY 10301; **Phone:** 718-447-5211; **Board Cert:** Surgery 1995; **Med School:** SUNY Upstate Med Univ 1991; **Resid:** Surgery, Univ Hosp - SUNY Downstate Med Ctr 1986

THORACIC SURGERY

McGinn Jr, Joseph MD (TS) - **Spec Exp:** Cardiothoracic Surgery; **Hospital:** Staten Island Univ Hosp-North Site, St Vincent Cath Med Ctr - Staten Island (page 375); **Address:** 475 Seaview Ave, Staten Island, NY 10305; **Phone:** 718-226-1612; **Board Cert:** Surgery 1998; Thoracic Surgery 2003; **Med School:** SUNY Downstate 1981; **Resid:** Surgery, Downstate Med Ctr 1985; Thoracic Surgery, LIJ Med Ctr 1987; **Fellow:** Cardiothoracic Surgery, LIJ Med Ctr 1988; **Fac Appt:** Asst Clin Prof S, SUNY Downstate

UROLOGY

Lessing, Jeffrey MD (U) - **Spec Exp:** Prostate Disease; Impotence; Kidney Stones; **Hospital:** St Vincent Cath Med Ctr - Staten Island (page 375), Staten Island Univ Hosp - South Site; **Address:** 78 Todt Hill Rd, Ste 112, Staten Island, NY 10314-4535; **Phone:** 718-448-3880; **Board Cert:** Urology 1982; **Med School:** NYU Sch Med 1975; **Resid:** Surgery, New York Univ Med Ctr 1977; Urology, Mount Sinai Hosp 1980

Raboy, Adley MD (U) - **Spec Exp:** Prostate Disease; Kidney Stones; Minimally Invasive Surgery; **Hospital:** Staten Island Univ Hosp-North Site, Staten Island Univ Hosp - South Site; **Address:** 1460 Victory Blvd, Staten Island, NY 10301-3914; **Phone:** 718-273-8100; **Board Cert:** Urology 2002; **Med School:** SUNY Downstate 1984; **Resid:** Surgery, Staten Island Hosp 1986; **Fellow:** Urology, Univ Hosp 1990; **Fac Appt:** Asst Clin Prof U, SUNY Downstate

Richmond (Staten Island)

Savino, Michael MD (U) - **Spec Exp:** Minimally Invasive Urologic Surgery; Prostate Cancer; Kidney Stones; **Hospital:** Staten Island Univ Hosp-North Site, St Vincent Cath Med Ctr - Staten Island (page 375); **Address:** 78 Todt Hill Rd, Ste 112, Staten Island, NY 10314-4528; **Phone:** 718-448-3880; **Board Cert:** Urology 1989; **Med School:** Mexico 1979; **Resid:** Surgery, Coney Island Hosp 1982; Urology, Maimonides Med Ctr 1985

VASCULAR SURGERY

Panetta, Thomas F MD (VascS) - **Hospital:** Staten Island Univ Hosp-North Site, St Vincent Cath Med Ctr - Staten Island (page 375); **Address:** Staten Island Univ Hosp, Div Vasc Surg, 256 Mason Ave Bldg B Fl 2, Staten Island, NY 10305; **Phone:** 718-226-6800; **Board Cert:** Surgery 1992; Vascular Surgery 1995; **Med School:** SUNY Downstate 1977; **Resid:** Surgery, Univ Hosp 1982; **Fellow:** Vascular Surgery, Baylor Med 1983

Pomper, Stuart MD (VascS) - **Spec Exp:** Laser Vein Surgery; Carotid Artery Surgery; **Hospital:** Staten Island Univ Hosp-North Site, St Vincent Cath Med Ctr - Staten Island (page 375); **Address:** 3000 Hylan Blvd, Staten Island, NY 10306; **Phone:** 718-979-9100; **Board Cert:** Surgery 1994; **Med School:** SUNY Hlth Sci Ctr 1980; **Resid:** Surgery, Staten Island Hosp 1985; **Fellow:** Vascular Surgery, Maimonides Medical Ctr 1986

Nassau

Nassau

ADOLESCENT MEDICINE

Arden, Martha MD (AM) - **Spec Exp:** Adolescent Gynecology; Nutrition; **Hospital:** Schneider Chldn's Hosp, N Shore Univ Hosp at Manhasset; **Address:** 410 Lakeville Rd, Ste 108, New Hyde Park, NY 11040-1101; **Phone:** 516-465-3270; **Board Cert:** Pediatrics 2002; Adolescent Medicine 2002; **Med School:** Yale Univ 1984; **Resid:** Pediatrics, Babies Hosp 1987; **Fellow:** Adolescent Medicine, Schneider Children's Hosp 1990; **Fac Appt:** Assoc Clin Prof Ped, Albert Einstein Coll Med

Fisher, Martin M MD (AM) - **Spec Exp:** Eating Disorders; **Hospital:** Schneider Chldn's Hosp, N Shore Univ Hosp at Manhasset; **Address:** 410 Lakeville Rd, Ste 108, New Hyde Park, NY 11042-1102; **Phone:** 516-465-3270; **Board Cert:** Pediatrics 1979; Adolescent Medicine 2002; **Med School:** Albert Einstein Coll Med 1975; **Resid:** Pediatrics, LIJ Med Ctr 1978; **Fellow:** Adolescent Medicine, LIJ Med Ctr 1980; **Fac Appt:** Prof Ped, NYU Sch Med

Jacobson, Marc S MD (AM) - **Spec Exp:** Cholesterol/Lipid Disorders; Obesity; Preventive Cardiology; **Hospital:** Schneider Chldn's Hosp, N Shore Univ Hosp at Manhasset; **Address:** 410 Lakeville Rd, Ste 108, New Hyde Park, NY 11040; **Phone:** 516-465-3270; **Board Cert:** Pediatrics 1983; Adolescent Medicine 1994; **Med School:** Univ Kans 1973; **Resid:** Pediatrics, Univ Kansas Med Ctr 1977; **Fellow:** Adolescent Medicine, Univ Maryland Hosp 1979; **Fac Appt:** Prof Ped, Albert Einstein Coll Med

ALLERGY & IMMUNOLOGY

Bonagura, Vincent R MD (A&I) - **Spec Exp:** AIDS/HIV; Immune Deficiency; Pediatric Allergy & Immunology; **Hospital:** Schneider Chldn's Hosp, Long Island Jewish Med Ctr; **Address:** 865 Northern Blvd, rm 101, Great Neck, NY 11021; **Phone:** 516-622-5070; **Board Cert:** Pediatrics 1979; Allergy & Immunology 1981; Clinical & Laboratory Immunology 1986; **Med School:** Columbia P&S 1975; **Resid:** Pediatrics, Columbia Presby Hosp 1978; **Fellow:** Allergy & Immunology, Columbia Presby Hosp 1983; **Fac Appt:** Prof Ped, Albert Einstein Coll Med

Boxer, Mitchell MD (A&I) - **Spec Exp:** Asthma; Drug Sensitivity; Allergic Aspergillosis; **Hospital:** Long Island Jewish Med Ctr; **Address:** 560 Northern Blvd, Ste 209, Great Neck, NY 11021-5100; **Phone:** 516-482-0910; **Board Cert:** Internal Medicine 1984; Allergy & Immunology 1987; **Med School:** NY Med Coll 1981; **Resid:** Internal Medicine, LI Jewish Med Ctr 1984; **Fellow:** Allergy & Immunology, Northwestern Meml Med Ctr 1987; **Fac Appt:** Asst Clin Prof Med, Albert Einstein Coll Med

Corriel, Robert MD (A&I) - **Spec Exp:** Asthma & Allergy; Sinus Disorders; Rhinitis; **Hospital:** N Shore Univ Hosp at Manhasset; **Address:** 2110 Northern Blvd, Ste 210, Manhasset, NY 11030-3500; **Phone:** 516-365-6077; **Board Cert:** Pediatrics 1983; Allergy & Immunology 1985; **Med School:** Wake Forest Univ 1976; **Resid:** Pediatrics, North Shore Univ Hosp 1979; **Fellow:** Allergy & Immunology, Univ Tex Hlth Sci Ctr 1981; **Fac Appt:** Asst Clin Prof Ped, NYU Sch Med

Edwards, Bruce MD (A&I) - **Spec Exp:** Asthma; Sinus Disorders; Food Allergy; **Hospital:** Long Island Jewish Med Ctr, N Shore Univ Hosp at Plainview; **Address:** 700 Old Country Rd, Ste 105, Plainview, NY 11803-4932; **Phone:** 516-933-1125; **Board Cert:** Pediatrics 1998; Allergy & Immunology 1999; **Med School:** Case West Res Univ 1984; **Resid:** Pediatrics, Babies Hosp/Columbia Presby 1987; **Fellow:** Allergy & Immunology, Schneider Chldns Hosp-LIJ 1989

Fonacier, Luz MD (A&I) - **Spec Exp:** Drug Sensitivity; Skin Allergies; Asthma & Allergy; **Hospital:** Winthrop - Univ Hosp; **Address:** 120 Mineola Blvd, Ste 410, Mineola, NY 11501; **Phone:** 516-663-2097; **Board Cert:** Internal Medicine 1989; Allergy & Immunology 2001; **Med School:** Philippines 1978; **Resid:** Dermatology, Univ Philippines 1983; Internal Medicine, Lutheran Med Ctr 1989; **Fellow:** Dermatology, NYU Med Ctr 1986; Allergy & Immunology, NY Hosp-Cornell Med Ctr 1991; **Fac Appt:** Assoc Prof A&I, SUNY Stony Brook

Frieri, Marianne MD/PhD (A&I) - **Spec Exp:** Asthma; Food Allergy; Immune Deficiency; Rhinitis; **Hospital:** N Shore Univ Hosp at Manhasset, Nassau Univ Med Ctr; **Address:** 566 Broadway, Massapequa, NY 11758; **Phone:** 516-541-6262; **Board Cert:** Internal Medicine 1984; Allergy & Immunology 1985; Clinical & Laboratory Immunology 1990; **Med School:** Loyola Univ-Stritch Sch Med 1978; **Resid:** Internal Medicine, St Josephs Hosp 1980; **Fellow:** Allergy & Immunology, NIH/NIAID 1983; **Fac Appt:** Prof Med, SUNY Stony Brook

Goldstein, Stanley MD (A&I) - **Spec Exp:** Asthma; Pulmonary Disease; **Hospital:** Long Island Jewish Med Ctr, Mercy Med Ctr - Rockville Centre; **Address:** 242 Merrick Rd, Ste 401, Rockville Centre, NY 11570; **Phone:** 516-536-7336; **Board Cert:** Pediatrics 1979; Allergy & Immunology 1981; Pediatric Pulmonology 1997; **Med School:** NY Med Coll 1975; **Resid:** Pediatrics, LI Jewish Med Ctr 1978; **Fellow:** Allergy & Immunology, Chldns Hosp 1982

Lang, Paul MD (A&I) - **Spec Exp:** Allergy & Immunology; Asthma; Food Allergy; Insect Allergies; **Hospital:** N Shore Univ Hosp at Manhasset, Winthrop - Univ Hosp; **Address:** One Hollow Lane, Ste 110, New Hyde Park, NY 11042; **Phone:** 516-365-6666; **Board Cert:** Pediatrics 1978; Allergy & Immunology 1979; **Med School:** Cornell Univ-Weill Med Coll 1973; **Resid:** Pediatrics, USC Med Ctr 1975; Allergy & Immunology, Roosevelt Hosp 1977; **Fac Appt:** Assoc Clin Prof Ped, NYU Sch Med

Novick, Brian MD (A&I) - **Spec Exp:** Asthma-Adult & Pediatric; Sinus Disorders; Food Allergy; **Hospital:** Montefiore Med Ctr, Lenox Hill Hosp (page 94); **Address:** 30 Newbridge Rd, East Meadow, NY 11554; **Phone:** 516-731-5740; **Board Cert:** Pediatrics 1984; Allergy & Immunology 1999; **Med School:** Mexico 1978; **Resid:** Pediatrics, Albert Einstein 1982; **Fellow:** Allergy & Immunology, Albert Einstein 1984; **Fac Appt:** Asst Clin Prof A&I, Albert Einstein Coll Med

Sicklick, Marc MD (A&I) - **Spec Exp:** Asthma; Allergy; Immune Deficiency; **Hospital:** N Shore Univ Hosp at Manhasset, South Nassau Comm Hosp; **Address:** 123 Grove Ave, Ste 110, Cedarhurst, NY 11516-2302; **Phone:** 516-569-5550; **Board Cert:** Pediatrics 1979; Allergy & Immunology 1987; **Med School:** Albert Einstein Coll Med 1974; **Resid:** Pediatrics, Bronx Muni Hosp Ctr 1977; **Fellow:** Allergy & Immunology, Albert Einstein Coll Med 1979; **Fac Appt:** Assoc Clin Prof Ped, Albert Einstein Coll Med

Weinstock, Gary MD (A&I) - **Spec Exp:** Asthma; Allergy; Hives; **Hospital:** N Shore Univ Hosp at Manhasset, N Shore Univ Hosp at Glen Cove; **Address:** 310 E Shore Rd, Ste 207, Great Neck, NY 11023-2432; **Phone:** 516-487-1073; **Board Cert:** Internal Medicine 1982; Allergy & Immunology 1985; Pulmonary Disease 1984; **Med School:** Albany Med Coll 1979; **Resid:** Internal Medicine, Cornell Affil Hosp 1982; **Fellow:** Pulmonary Disease, SUNY-Stony Brook 1983; Allergy & Immunology, SUNY-Stony Brook 1986; **Fac Appt:** Asst Clin Prof Med, NYU Sch Med

CARDIAC ELECTROPHYSIOLOGY

Levine, Joseph H MD (CE) - **Spec Exp:** Arrhythmias; Sudden Death Prevention; Pacemakers; Atrial Fibrillation; **Hospital:** St Francis Hosp - The Heart Ctr (page 112), Good Samaritan Hosp Med Ctr - West Islip; **Address:** 100 Port Washington Blvd, Roslyn, NY 11576; **Phone:** 516-622-1011; **Board Cert:** Internal Medicine 1983; Cardiovascular Disease 1987; Cardiac Electrophysiology 2003; **Med School:** Univ Rochester 1980; **Resid:** Internal Medicine, Yale-New Haven Hosp 1983; **Fellow:** Cardiovascular Disease, Johns Hopkins Hosp 1986; Cardiac Electrophysiology, Hosp Univ Penn 1986

CARDIOVASCULAR DISEASE

Anto, Maliakal J MD (Cv) - **Spec Exp:** Hypertension; Coronary Artery Disease; Non-Invasive Cardiology; Congestive Heart Failure; **Hospital:** N Shore Univ Hosp at Syosset, N Shore Univ Hosp at Plainview; **Address:** 8 Greenfield Rd, Syosset, NY 11791; **Phone:** 516-496-7900; **Board Cert:** Internal Medicine 1980; Cardiovascular Disease 1989; **Med School:** India 1974; **Resid:** Internal Medicine, Our Lady of Mercy Med Ctr 1979; **Fellow:** Cardiovascular Disease, Nassau County Med Ctr 1981

Bodenheimer, Monty MD (Cv) - **Hospital:** Long Island Jewish Med Ctr, N Shore Univ Hosp at Manhasset; **Address:** 3003 New Hyde Park Rd, Ste 406, New Hyde Park, NY 11042; **Phone:** 516-719-0102; **Board Cert:** Internal Medicine 1972; Cardiovascular Disease 1975; **Med School:** Univ Manitoba 1969; **Resid:** Internal Medicine, Sinai Hosp 1971; Internal Medicine, Einstein 1972; **Fellow:** Cardiovascular Disease, Mt Sinai Hosp 1973

Breen, William MD (Cv) - **Hospital:** N Shore Univ Hosp at Plainview, St Francis Hosp - The Heart Ctr (page 112); **Address:** 43 Crossways Park Dr, Woodbury, NY 11797; **Phone:** 516-938-3000; **Board Cert:** Internal Medicine 1980; Cardiovascular Disease 1983; **Med School:** NY Med Coll 1977; **Resid:** Internal Medicine, North Shore Univ Hosp 1980; **Fellow:** Cardiovascular Disease, North Shore Univ Hosp 1982; **Fac Appt:** Assoc Prof Med, NYU Sch Med

Budow, Jack MD (Cv) - **Spec Exp:** Coronary Artery Disease; Congestive Heart Failure; **Hospital:** Winthrop - Univ Hosp, N Shore Univ Hosp at Manhasset; **Address:** 711 Stewart Ave, Ste 100, Garden City, NY 11530; **Phone:** 516-222-8680; **Board Cert:** Internal Medicine 1977; Cardiovascular Disease 1973; **Med School:** South Africa 1956; **Resid:** Internal Medicine, Cincinnati Jewish Hosp 1962; **Fellow:** Cardiovascular Disease, New York Heart Assn 1964

Chadda, Kul MD (Cv) - **Spec Exp:** Cardiac Electrophysiology; **Hospital:** South Nassau Comm Hosp; **Address:** South Nassau Comm Hosp - Electrophysiology Svcs, 1 Healthy Way, Oceanside, NY 11572; **Phone:** 516-632-3418; **Board Cert:** Internal Medicine 1974; Cardiovascular Disease 1977; **Med School:** India 1966; **Resid:** Internal Medicine, Elmhurst City Hosp 1972; Cardiovascular Disease, Prebyterian Hosp 1973; **Fac Appt:** Clin Prof Med, SUNY Stony Brook

Chesner, Michael MD (Cv) - **Spec Exp:** Preventive Cardiology; Cholesterol/Lipid Disorders; Cardiac Stress Testing; **Hospital:** Long Beach Med Ctr; **Address:** 325 W Park Ave, Long Beach, NY 11561-3223; **Phone:** 516-432-2004; **Board Cert:** Cardiovascular Disease 1997; **Med School:** Albert Einstein Coll Med 1987; **Resid:** Internal Medicine, Bronx Municipal Hosp/Einstein Co 1990; **Fellow:** Cardiovascular Disease, LI Jewish Hosp 1993; **Fac Appt:** Assoc Prof Med, NY Coll Osteo Med

Cramer, Marvin MD (Cv) - **Spec Exp:** Coronary Artery Disease; Arrhythmias; **Hospital:** N Shore Univ Hosp at Manhasset, St Francis Hosp - The Heart Ctr (page 112); **Address:** 225 Community Drive, Ste 130, Great Neck, NY 11021; **Phone:** 516-504-0474; **Board Cert:** Internal Medicine 1974; Cardiovascular Disease 1977; **Med School:** Jefferson Med Coll 1969; **Resid:** Internal Medicine, St Lukes Med Ctr 1971; Internal Medicine, St Lukes Med Ctr 1974; **Fellow:** Cardiovascular Disease, Columbia-Presby Med Ctr; **Fac Appt:** Assoc Clin Prof Med, NYU Sch Med

D'Agostino, Ronald DO (Cv) - **Spec Exp:** Hypertension; Cholesterol/Lipid Disorders; Mitral Valve Disease; **Hospital:** Long Island Jewish Med Ctr, N Shore Univ Hosp at Manhasset; **Address:** 1129 Northern Blvd, Ste 408, Manhasset, NY 11030-3022; **Phone:** 516-627-2121; **Board Cert:** Internal Medicine 2000; Cardiovascular Disease 2000; **Med School:** NY Coll Osteo Med 1985; **Resid:** Internal Medicine, Long Island Jewish Hosp 1989; Internal Medicine, Long Island Jewish Hosp 1993; **Fellow:** Cardiovascular Disease, Long Island Jewish Hosp 1992; **Fac Appt:** Asst Prof Med, NY Coll Osteo Med

Davison, Edward MD (Cv) - **Spec Exp:** Geriatric Cardiology; **Hospital:** Franklin Hosp Med Ctr, St Francis Hosp - The Heart Ctr (page 112); **Address:** 300 Franklin Ave, Valley Stream, NY 11580; **Phone:** 516-599-8280; **Board Cert:** Internal Medicine 1966; Cardiovascular Disease 1977; **Med School:** Bowman Gray 1959; **Resid:** Internal Medicine, Maimonides Med Ctr 1963; **Fellow:** Cardiovascular Disease, Mt Sinai Hosp 1965

Dresdale, Robert MD (Cv) - **Spec Exp:** Heart Disease in Women; **Hospital:** N Shore Univ Hosp at Manhasset, St Francis Hosp - The Heart Ctr (page 112); **Address:** 225 Community Drive, Ste 130, Great Neck, NY 11021; **Phone:** 516-504-0474; **Board Cert:** Internal Medicine 1975; Cardiovascular Disease 1977; **Med School:** Columbia P&S 1972; **Resid:** Internal Medicine, Columbia-Presby Med Ctr 1974; **Fellow:** Cardiovascular Disease, Columbia-Presby Med Ctr 1976; **Fac Appt:** Assoc Clin Prof Med, NYU Sch Med

Ezratty, Ari M MD (Cv) - **Spec Exp:** Interventional Cardiology; **Hospital:** St Francis Hosp - The Heart Ctr (page 112); **Address:** 1155 Northern Blvd, Ste 120, Manhasset, NY 11030; **Phone:** 516-570-6907; **Board Cert:** Internal Medicine 1988; Cardiovascular Disease 2002; **Med School:** Mount Sinai Sch Med 1985; **Resid:** Internal Medicine, Mt Sinai Hosp 1989; **Fellow:** Cardiovascular Disease, Brigham & Women's Hosp 1992; Interventional Cardiology, Mt Sinai Hosp 1994

Gindea, Aaron MD (Cv) - **Spec Exp:** Heart Valve Disease; Congestive Heart Failure; Heart Disease-Congenital; **Hospital:** St Francis Hosp - The Heart Ctr (page 112), N Shore Univ Hosp at Manhasset; **Address:** 800 Community Drive, Manhasset, NY 11030-3803; **Phone:** 516-627-6622; **Board Cert:** Cardiovascular Disease 1989; Internal Medicine 1985; **Med School:** NYU Sch Med 1982; **Resid:** Internal Medicine, Bellevue Hosp 1985; **Fellow:** Cardiovascular Disease, Bellevue Hosp; **Fac Appt:** Assoc Clin Prof Med, NYU Sch Med

Gleckel, Louis Wade MD (Cv) - **Spec Exp:** Preventive Cardiology; Cardiac Stress Testing; **Hospital:** Long Island Jewish Med Ctr, N Shore Univ Hosp at Forest Hills; **Address:** 2800 Marcus Ave, Lake Success, NY 11042-1052; **Phone:** 516-622-6060; **Board Cert:** Internal Medicine 1986; **Med School:** SUNY Hlth Sci Ctr 1983; **Resid:** Internal Medicine, LI Jewish Hosp 1986; **Fellow:** Cardiovascular Disease, LI Jewish Hosp 1988; **Fac Appt:** Asst Prof Med, Albert Einstein Coll Med

Goldberg, Douglas MD (Cv) - **Hospital:** N Shore Univ Hosp at Manhasset; **Address:** 310 E Shore Rd, Great Neck, NY 11023-2479; **Phone:** 516-829-9550; **Board Cert:** Internal Medicine 1986; **Med School:** SUNY Downstate 1983; **Resid:** Internal Medicine 1986; **Fellow:** Cardiovascular Disease, Mt Sinai Hosp 1989

Goldberg, Steven M MD (Cv) - **Spec Exp:** Cholesterol/Lipid Disorders; Preventive Cardiology; **Hospital:** N Shore Univ Hosp at Manhasset; **Address:** 1010 Northern Blvd, Ste 110, Great Neck, NY 11021-5306; **Phone:** 516-390-2430; **Board Cert:** Internal Medicine 1982; Cardiovascular Disease 1985; **Med School:** Univ Pennsylvania 1979; **Resid:** Internal Medicine, N Shore Univ Hosp 1982; **Fellow:** Cardiovascular Disease, N Shore Univ Hosp 1984; **Fac Appt:** Assoc Prof Med, NYU Sch Med

Goodman, Mark A MD (Cv) - **Spec Exp:** Cholesterol/Lipid Disorders; Hypertension; Heart Failure; **Hospital:** Winthrop - Univ Hosp, N Shore Univ Hosp at Manhasset; **Address:** 975 Stewart Ave, Garden City, NY 11530-4831; **Phone:** 516-222-8610; **Board Cert:** Internal Medicine 1972; Cardiovascular Disease 1973; **Med School:** SUNY Upstate Med Univ 1967; **Resid:** Internal Medicine, Montefiore Hosp Med Ctr 1969; Internal Medicine, Mt Sinai Hosp 1970; **Fellow:** Cardiovascular Disease, Montefiore Hosp Med Ctr 1972; **Fac Appt:** Assoc Clin Prof Med, SUNY Stony Brook

Green, Stephen MD (Cv) - **Spec Exp:** Heart Attack; Angioplasty; Cholesterol/Lipid Disorders; **Hospital:** N Shore Univ Hosp at Manhasset, Long Island Jewish Med Ctr; **Address:** Division Cardiology, 300 Community Drive, Manhasset, NY 11030; **Phone:** 516-562-4100; **Board Cert:** Internal Medicine 1983; Cardiovascular Disease 1985; Interventional Cardiology 1999; **Med School:** Tufts Univ 1980; **Resid:** Internal Medicine, N Shore Univ Hosp 1983; **Fellow:** Cardiovascular Disease, N Shore Univ Hosp 1985; **Fac Appt:** Assoc Clin Prof Med, NYU Sch Med

Greenberg, Steven M MD (Cv) - **Spec Exp:** Pacemakers/Defibrillators; Arrhythmias; Congestive Heart Failure; **Hospital:** St Francis Hosp - The Heart Ctr (page 112), Good Samaritan Hosp Med Ctr - West Islip; **Address:** 100 Port Washington Blvd, Arrhythmia Center, Roslyn, NY 11576; **Phone:** 516-562-6672; **Board Cert:** Internal Medicine 1986; Cardiovascular Disease 1989; **Med School:** Albany Med Coll 1983; **Resid:** Internal Medicine, Bronx Muni Hosp Ctr 1987; **Fellow:** Cardiovascular Disease, Mt Sinai Med Ctr 1990

Gulotta, Stephen J MD (Cv) - **Spec Exp:** Cardiac Catheterization; Cardiac Consultation; **Hospital:** St Francis Hosp - The Heart Ctr (page 112); **Address:** 100 Port Washington Blvd, Roslyn, NY 11576-1353; **Phone:** 516-365-5599; **Board Cert:** Internal Medicine 1965; Cardiovascular Disease 1968; **Med School:** SUNY Hlth Sci Ctr 1958; **Resid:** Internal Medicine, Montefiore Hosp 1961; **Fellow:** Cardiovascular Disease, NY Hosp/Cornell 1962

Hamby, Robert I MD (Cv) - **Spec Exp:** Invasive Cardiology; **Hospital:** St Francis Hosp - The Heart Ctr (page 112), South Nassau Comm Hosp; **Address:** New York Cardiology Group, 100 Port Washington Blvd, Roslyn, NY 11576; **Phone:** 516-365-5000; **Board Cert:** Internal Medicine 1966; Cardiovascular Disease 1967; **Med School:** NYU Sch Med 1959; **Resid:** Internal Medicine, Cleveland 1961; Internal Medicine, LI Jewish Hosp 1964; **Fellow:** Cardiovascular Disease, New York Hosp 1962; Cardiovascular Disease, Mount Sinai Hosp 1963

Hershman, Ronnie MD (Cv) - **Spec Exp:** Invasive Cardiology; **Hospital:** St Francis Hosp - The Heart Ctr (page 112); **Address:** 1 Hollow Ln, Ste 103, Lake Success, NY 11042; **Phone:** 516-869-5400; **Board Cert:** Internal Medicine 1985; Cardiovascular Disease 1987; **Med School:** Mount Sinai Sch Med 1982; **Resid:** Internal Medicine, Mt Sinai Med Ctr 1985; **Fellow:** Cardiovascular Disease, Mt Sinai Med Ctr 1989

Jelveh, Mansoor MD (Cv) - **Hospital:** New Island Hosp, N Shore Univ Hosp at Plainview; **Address:** 875 Old Country Rd, Ste 102, Plainview, NY 11803; **Phone:** 516-935-8877; **Board Cert:** Cardiovascular Disease 1977; Internal Medicine 1975; **Med School:** Iran 1968; **Resid:** Internal Medicine, Nassau County Med Ctr 1975; **Fellow:** Cardiovascular Disease, Beth Israel 1977

Katz, Stanley MD (Cv) - **Spec Exp:** Interventional Cardiology; **Hospital:** N Shore Univ Hosp at Manhasset; **Address:** N Shore Univ Hosp, Div Cardiology, 300 Community Drive, Ste 1 Cohen, Manhasset, NY 11030; **Phone:** 516-562-4101; **Board Cert:** Internal Medicine 1976; Cardiovascular Disease 1979; Interventional Cardiology 1999; **Med School:** South Africa 1970; **Resid:** Pathology, Boston Univ Med Ctr 1974; Internal Medicine, LI Jewish Med Ctr 1976; **Fellow:** Cardiovascular Disease, Montefiore Hosp 1978; **Fac Appt:** Asst Prof Med, SUNY Stony Brook

Kirtane, Sanjay MD (Cv) - **Spec Exp:** Coronary Artery Disease; **Hospital:** St John's Epis Hosp - S Shore, Peninsula Hosp Ctr; **Address:** 135 Rockaway Tpke, Ste 103, Lawrence, NY 11559; **Phone:** 516-239-7812; **Board Cert:** Cardiovascular Disease 1983; Internal Medicine 1980; **Med School:** India 1974; **Resid:** Internal Medicine, St John's 1980; **Fellow:** Cardiovascular Disease, LI Jewish Med Ctr 1982

Kobren, Steven MD (Cv) - **Spec Exp:** Non-Invasive Cardiology; Mitral Valve Prolapse; Nuclear Stress Testing; **Hospital:** St Francis Hosp - The Heart Ctr (page 112), Long Island Jewish Med Ctr; **Address:** Great Neck Med Group, 488 Great Neck Rd, Great Neck, NY 11021-5100; **Phone:** 516-482-6747; **Board Cert:** Internal Medicine 1986; Cardiovascular Disease 1989; Critical Care Medicine 2001; **Med School:** SUNY Downstate 1983; **Resid:** Internal Medicine, LIJ Medical Ctr 1987; **Fellow:** Cardiovascular Disease, LIJ Medical Ctr 1989

Koss, Jerome MD (Cv) - **Spec Exp:** Interventional Cardiology; Heart Valve Disease; Nuclear Cardiology; **Hospital:** Long Island Jewish Med Ctr, NY Hosp Queens; **Address:** 3003 New Hyde Park Rd, Ste 406, New Hyde Park, NY 11042; **Phone:** 516-358-5401; **Board Cert:** Internal Medicine 1977; Cardiovascular Disease 1981; Interventional Cardiology 1999; **Med School:** Albert Einstein Coll Med 1974; **Resid:** Internal Medicine, Jacobi Med Ctr 1978; **Fellow:** Cardiovascular Disease, Montefiore Hosp Med Ctr 1980; **Fac Appt:** Asst Prof Med, Albert Einstein Coll Med

Mieres, Jennifer MD (Cv) - **Hospital:** N Shore Univ Hosp at Manhasset; **Address:** N Shore Univ Hosp, Div Cardiology, 300 Community Drive, Manhasset, NY 11030; **Phone:** 516-562-4100; **Board Cert:** Internal Medicine 1991; Cardiovascular Disease 1997; **Med School:** Boston Univ 1986; **Resid:** Internal Medicine, St Lukes Roosevelt Hosp 1990

Monteleone, Bernard B MD (Cv) - **Hospital:** St Francis Hosp - The Heart Ctr (page 112); **Address:** 100 Port Washington Blvd, Ste G-05, Roslyn, NY 11576; **Phone:** 516-869-6481; **Board Cert:** Internal Medicine 1974; Cardiovascular Disease 1976; **Med School:** Med Coll Wisc 1969; **Resid:** Internal Medicine, Lenox Hill Hosp 1970; Internal Medicine, Bellevue Hosp 1974; **Fellow:** Cardiovascular Disease, Montefiore Hosp Med Ctr 1976

Nejat, Moosa MD (Cv) - **Spec Exp:** Coronary Artery Disease; Heart Failure; Heart Valve Disease; **Hospital:** N Shore Univ Hosp at Manhasset, Beth Israel Med Ctr- Kings Hwy Div (page 90); **Address:** 833 Northern Blvd, Ste 120, Great Neck, NY 11021; **Phone:** 516-829-0066; **Board Cert:** Internal Medicine 1972; Cardiovascular Disease 1975; **Med School:** Iran 1962; **Resid:** Internal Medicine, Presby Hosp 1967; **Fellow:** Cardiovascular Disease, Mount Sinai Hosp 1968; Cardiovascular Disease, Maimonides Med Ctr 1969

Nicosia, Thomas A MD (Cv) - **Spec Exp:** Coronary Artery Disease; Congestive Heart Failure; **Hospital:** St Francis Hosp - The Heart Ctr (page 112), N Shore Univ Hosp at Manhasset; **Address:** 1615 Northern Blvd, Ste 301, Manhasset, NY 11030; **Phone:** 516-627-9355; **Board Cert:** Cardiovascular Disease 1981; Internal Medicine 1978; **Med School:** Univ Cincinnati 1974; **Resid:** Internal Medicine, University Hosp 1978; **Fellow:** Cardiovascular Disease, Bellevue Hosp 1980

Pappas, Thomas W MD (Cv) - **Spec Exp:** Interventional Cardiology; Coronary Angioplasty/Stents; Angiography-Coronary; **Hospital:** St Francis Hosp - The Heart Ctr (page 112); **Address:** 100 Port Washington Blvd, Ste 105, Roslyn, NY 11576-1353; **Phone:** 516-390-9640; **Board Cert:** Internal Medicine 1986; Cardiovascular Disease 1989; Interventional Cardiology 2000; **Med School:** Cornell Univ-Weill Med Coll 1983; **Resid:** Internal Medicine, New York Hosp 1986; **Fellow:** Cardiovascular Disease, New York Hosp-Cornell 1988; Interventional Cardiology, NYU Med Ctr 1990

Ragno, Philip D MD (Cv) - **Spec Exp:** Cholesterol/Lipid Disorders; Congestive Heart Failure; **Hospital:** Winthrop - Univ Hosp, N Shore Univ Hosp at Manhasset; **Address:** 80 E Jericho Tpke, Ste 100, Mineola, NY 11501; **Phone:** 516-877-2626; **Board Cert:** Internal Medicine 1987; Cardiovascular Disease 1989; **Med School:** SUNY Stony Brook 1984; **Resid:** Internal Medicine, Winthrop Univ Hosp 1987; **Fellow:** Cardiovascular Disease, Winthrop Univ Hosp 1989

Rutkovsky, Edward MD (Cv) - **Spec Exp:** Nuclear Stress Testing; Echocardiography; **Hospital:** N Shore Univ Hosp at Manhasset, St Francis Hosp - The Heart Ctr (page 112); **Address:** 2035 Lakeville Rd, Ste 101, New Hyde Park, NY 11040-1661; **Phone:** 516-328-9797; **Board Cert:** Internal Medicine 1987; Cardiovascular Disease 1989; **Med School:** NYU Sch Med 1984; **Resid:** Internal Medicine, NYU Med Ctr 1987; **Fellow:** Cardiovascular Disease, N Shore Univ Hosp 1989; **Fac Appt:** Asst Clin Prof Med, NYU Sch Med

Schreiber, Carl MD (Cv) - **Spec Exp:** Coronary Artery Disease; Nuclear Cardiology; **Hospital:** N Shore Univ Hosp at Glen Cove, N Shore Univ Hosp at Manhasset; **Address:** 70 Glen St, Glen Cove, NY 11542; **Phone:** 516-484-7893; **Board Cert:** Internal Medicine 1982; Cardiovascular Disease 1985; **Med School:** Med Coll GA 1979; **Resid:** Internal Medicine, Columbia-Presby Med Ctr 1982; **Fellow:** Cardiovascular Disease, Westchester Med Ctr 1984

Shlofmitz, Richard A MD (Cv) - **Spec Exp:** Interventional Cardiology; **Hospital:** St Francis Hosp - The Heart Ctr (page 112); **Address:** 100 Port Washington Blvd, Ste 105, Roslyn, NY 11576-1353; **Phone:** 516-390-9640; **Board Cert:** Internal Medicine 1984; Cardiovascular Disease 1987; **Med School:** NYU Sch Med 1980; **Resid:** Internal Medicine, North Shore Univ Hosp 1984; **Fellow:** Cardiovascular Disease, Columbia Presby Med Ctr 1987

Spadaro, Louise A MD (Cv) - **Spec Exp:** Preventive Cardiology; Heart Disease in Women; Cardiac Imaging; **Hospital:** St Francis Hosp - The Heart Ctr (page 112); **Address:** St. Francis Hosp, 100 Port Washington Blvd Bldg VIZZA - rm 101, Roslyn, NY 11576; **Phone:** 516-562-6653; **Board Cert:** Internal Medicine 1987; Cardiovascular Disease 1989; **Med School:** NYU Sch Med 1984; **Resid:** Internal Medicine, Bellevue Hosp 1987; **Fellow:** Cardiovascular Disease, Bellevue Hosp/NYU Med Ctr 1989

Weg, Ira MD (Cv) - **Spec Exp:** Congestive Heart Failure; Coronary Artery Disease; **Hospital:** Long Island Jewish Med Ctr, Mercy Med Ctr - Rockville Centre; **Address:** 158 Hempstead Ave, Lynbrook, NY 11563; **Phone:** 516-593-3541; **Board Cert:** Internal Medicine 1979; Cardiovascular Disease 1981; **Med School:** SUNY Hlth Sci Ctr 1976; **Resid:** Internal Medicine, Kings County Hosp 1979; **Fellow:** Cardiovascular Disease, Montefiore Med Ctr 1981; **Fac Appt:** Asst Prof Med, Albert Einstein Coll Med

Weitzman, Lee MD (Cv) - **Hospital:** Long Beach Med Ctr; **Address:** 325 W Park Ave, Long Beach, NY 11561-3223; **Phone:** 516-432-2004; **Board Cert:** Internal Medicine 1981; Cardiovascular Disease 1983; **Med School:** NYU Sch Med 1978; **Resid:** Internal Medicine, NYU Med Ctr 1981; **Fellow:** Cardiovascular Disease, NYU Med Ctr 1983

Young, Melvin MD (Cv) - **Spec Exp:** Coronary Artery Disease; Cholesterol/Lipid Disorders; **Hospital:** South Nassau Comm Hosp, Long Island Jewish Med Ctr; **Address:** 123 Grove Ave, Ste 216, Cedarhurst, NY 11516; **Phone:** 516-569-5200; **Board Cert:** Internal Medicine 1972; Cardiovascular Disease 1974; **Med School:** Univ Hlth Sci/Chicago Med Sch 1963; **Resid:** Internal Medicine, Kings County Hosp 1965; Internal Medicine, Montefiore Hosp 1966; **Fellow:** Cardiovascular Disease, Montefiore Hosp 1971; Cardiovascular Disease, LI Jewish Hosp 1971; **Fac Appt:** Assoc Prof Med, SUNY Stony Brook

Zeldis, Steven M MD (Cv) - **Spec Exp:** Echocardiography; Cardiac Stress Testing; **Hospital:** Winthrop - Univ Hosp; **Address:** 200 Old Country Rd, Ste 278, Mineola, NY 11501; **Phone:** 516-877-0977; **Board Cert:** Internal Medicine 1975; Cardiovascular Disease 1977; **Med School:** Yale Univ 1972; **Resid:** Internal Medicine, Yale Med Ctr 1975; **Fellow:** Cardiovascular Disease, Hosp Univ Penn 1977; **Fac Appt:** Assoc Prof Med, SUNY Stony Brook

CHILD & ADOLESCENT PSYCHIATRY

Foley, Carmel MD (ChAP) - **Spec Exp:** Mood Disorders; **Hospital:** Schneider Chldn's Hosp; **Address:** Schneider Chldns Hosp, Child & Adolescent Psych, 400 Lakeville Rd, Ste 441A, New Hyde Park, NY 11040; **Phone:** 718-470-3550; **Board Cert:** Psychiatry 1979; Child & Adolescent Psychiatry 1981; Addiction Psychiatry 1997; Forensic Psychiatry 1999; **Med School:** Ireland 1972; **Resid:** Psychiatry, St Patrick's Hosp 1976; Psychiatry, Lafayette Clinic 1977; **Fellow:** Child & Adolescent Psychiatry, Lafayette Clinic 1979; **Fac Appt:** Assoc Prof Psyc, Albert Einstein Coll Med

Fornari, Victor MD (ChAP) - **Spec Exp:** Eating Disorders; Trauma Psychiatry; **Hospital:** N Shore Univ Hosp at Manhasset; **Address:** N Shore Univ Hosp, Dept Psychiatry, 400 Community Drive, Manhasset, NY 11030-3815; **Phone:** 516-562-3051; **Board Cert:** Psychiatry 1984; Child & Adolescent Psychiatry 1985; **Med School:** SUNY Downstate 1979; **Resid:** Psychiatry, Hosp Univ Penn 1982; **Fellow:** Child & Adolescent Psychiatry, LIJ Med Ctr 1984; **Fac Appt:** Assoc Prof Psyc, NYU Sch Med

Williams, Daniel T MD (ChAP) - **Spec Exp:** Neuro-Psychiatry; Psychopharmacology; Psychosomatic Disorders; **Hospital:** NY-Presby Hosp (page 100), Long Island Jewish Med Ctr; **Address:** 3003 New Hyde Park Rd, Ste 204, New Hyde Park, NY 11042; **Phone:** 516-488-3636; **Board Cert:** Psychiatry 1975; Child & Adolescent Psychiatry 1976; **Med School:** Cornell Univ-Weill Med Coll 1969; **Resid:** Psychiatry, Mount Sinai Hosp 1972; **Fellow:** Child & Adolescent Psychiatry, Columbia-Presby Hosp 1974; **Fac Appt:** Clin Prof Psyc, Columbia P&S

CHILD NEUROLOGY

Eviatar, Lydia MD (ChiN) - **Spec Exp:** Headache; Balance Disorders; Tourette's Syndrome; Cerebral Palsy; **Hospital:** Schneider Chldn's Hosp, Blythedale Children's Hosp; **Address:** 269-01 76th Ave, rm 267, New Hyde Park, NY 11040-1433; **Phone:** 718-470-3450; **Board Cert:** Pediatrics 1968; Child Neurology 1977; **Med School:** Israel 1961; **Resid:** Pediatrics, Tel Hashomer Hosp 1966; **Fellow:** Child Neurology, UCLA Med Ctr 1967; Neurology, UCLA Med Ctr 1969; **Fac Appt:** Prof N, Albert Einstein Coll Med

Maytal, Joseph MD (ChiN) - **Spec Exp:** Epilepsy/Seizure Disorders; Migraine; **Hospital:** Schneider Chldn's Hosp; **Address:** 269-01 76th Ave Fl 2nd - rm 267, New Hyde Park, NY 11040-1434; **Phone:** 718-470-3450; **Board Cert:** Pediatrics 1986; Child Neurology 1988; **Med School:** Israel 1978; **Resid:** Pediatrics, Brookdale Hosp 1983; Child Neurology, Albert Einstein Coll Med 1986; **Fellow:** Neurological Physiology, Albert Einstein Med Coll 1987; **Fac Appt:** Clin Prof N, Albert Einstein Coll Med

CLINICAL GENETICS

Angulo, Moris MD (CG) - **Spec Exp:** Endocrinology; Obesity; Prader-Willi Syndrome; **Hospital:** Winthrop - Univ Hosp; **Address:** 120 Mineola Blvd, Ste 210, Mineola, NY 11501-4077; **Phone:** 516-663-3069; **Board Cert:** Pediatrics 1983; Clinical Genetics 1984; Pediatric Endocrinology 1986; **Med School:** El Salvador 1976; **Resid:** Pediatrics, Nassau County Med Ctr 1979; **Fellow:** Clinical Genetics, Nassau County Med Ctr 1984

Bialer, Martin G MD (CG) - **Spec Exp:** Marfan's Syndrome; Neurofibromatosis; Metabolic Genetic Disorders; **Hospital:** Schneider Chldn's Hosp, Long Island Jewish Med Ctr; **Address:** 1554 Northern Blvd, Ste 204, Manhasset, NY 11030; **Phone:** 516-365-3996; **Board Cert:** Clinical Genetics 1990; Clinical Biochemical Genetics 1990; Clinical Molecular Genetics 1990; Pediatrics 1987; **Med School:** Med Univ SC 1983; **Resid:** Pediatrics, N Shore Univ Hosp 1986; **Fellow:** Clinical Genetics, Univ VA Hlth Sci Ctr 1989; **Fac Appt:** Clin Prof Ped, NYU Sch Med

Fox, Joyce MD (CG) - **Hospital:** Long Island Jewish Med Ctr, Schneider Chldn's Hosp; **Address:** Dept Clinical Genetics, 269-01 76th Ave, rm CH009, New Hyde Park, NY 11040; **Phone:** 718-470-3010; **Board Cert:** Clinical Genetics 1987; Pediatrics 1986; **Med School:** Columbia P&S 1980; **Resid:** Pediatrics, Case Western Univ Hosp 1983; **Fellow:** Clinical Genetics, Yale-New Haven Hosp 1986; **Fac Appt:** , Albert Einstein Coll Med

COLON & RECTAL SURGERY

Greenwald, Marc MD (CRS) - **Spec Exp:** Laparoscopic Surgery; Colonoscopy; Anorectal Disorders; Colon & Rectal Cancer; **Hospital:** N Shore Univ Hosp at Manhasset, St Francis Hosp - The Heart Ctr (page 112); **Address:** 310 E Shore Rd, Ste 203, Great Neck, NY 11023-2432; **Phone:** 516-482-8657; **Board Cert:** Surgery 2000; Colon & Rectal Surgery 2003; **Med School:** Albert Einstein Coll Med 1985; **Resid:** Surgery, Montefiore Hosp Med Ctr 1990; **Fellow:** Colon & Rectal Surgery, St Francis Hosp 1991

Kalafatic, Alfredo MD (CRS) - **Spec Exp:** Colonoscopy; Colon & Rectal Cancer; Anorectal Disorders; **Hospital:** New Island Hosp, N Shore Univ Hosp at Plainview; **Address:** 4277 Hempstead Tpke, Ste 203, Bethpage, NY 11714-5706; **Phone:** 516-735-3001; **Board Cert:** Colon & Rectal Surgery 1983; **Med School:** Italy 1970; **Resid:** Surgery, LI Jewish Med Ctr 1979; **Fellow:** Colon & Rectal Surgery, Mid-Island Hosp 1981

Levin, Leroy MD (CRS) - **Spec Exp:** Colon Cancer; Ulcerative Colitis; Crohn's Disease; **Hospital:** Long Island Jewish Med Ctr, N Shore Univ Hosp at Manhasset; **Address:** 1000 Northern Blvd, Ste 130, Great Neck, NY 11021; **Phone:** 516-466-5260; **Board Cert:** Surgery 1970; Colon & Rectal Surgery 1970; **Med School:** SUNY Downstate 1962; **Resid:** Surgery, LI Jewish Med Ctr 1964; Surgery, LI Jewish Med Ctr 1968; **Fellow:** Colon & Rectal Surgery, Cleveland Clinic 1969; **Fac Appt:** Asst Prof S, Albert Einstein Coll Med

Procaccino, John MD (CRS) - **Spec Exp:** Inflammatory Bowel Disease/Crohn's; Colon & Rectal Cancer; Anorectal Disorders; **Hospital:** N Shore Univ Hosp at Manhasset, Long Island Jewish Med Ctr; **Address:** 900 Northern Blvd, Ste 100, Great Neck, NY 11021; **Phone:** 516-730-2100; **Board Cert:** Colon & Rectal Surgery 1992; Surgery 1990; **Med School:** NYU Sch Med 1984; **Resid:** Surgery, N Shore Univ Hosp 1989; **Fellow:** Colon & Rectal Surgery, Cleveland Clinic 1990; **Fac Appt:** Asst Clin Prof S, Cornell Univ-Weill Med Coll

DERMATOLOGY

Aprile, Georgette MD (D) - **Spec Exp:** Acne; Atopic Dermatitis; **Hospital:** N Shore Univ Hosp at Glen Cove; **Address:** 8 Med Plaza, Lower Level, Glen Cove, NY 11542; **Phone:** 516-759-9200; **Board Cert:** Dermatology 1978; **Med School:** NY Med Coll 1974; **Resid:** Dermatology, New York Hosp 1978

Bruckstein, Robert MD (D) - **Spec Exp:** Acne; Skin Cancer; Cosmetic Dermatology; Skin Laser Surgery; **Hospital:** St John's Epis Hosp - S Shore, Peninsula Hosp Ctr; **Address:** 290 Central Ave, Ste 206, Lawrence, NY 11559-8507; **Phone:** 516-239-2332; **Board Cert:** Dermatology 1977; **Med School:** NYU Sch Med 1972; **Resid:** Dermatology, Bellevue Hosp Ctr-NYU 1975; **Fac Appt:** Asst Clin Prof D, NYU Sch Med

De Pietro, William MD (D) - **Spec Exp:** Skin Laser Surgery; Dermatologic Surgery; **Hospital:** N Shore Univ Hosp at Glen Cove; **Address:** 10 Medical Plz, Ste 102, Glen Cove, NY 11542; **Phone:** 516-671-1780; **Board Cert:** Dermatology 1980; **Med School:** Georgetown Univ 1976; **Resid:** Dermatology, St Luke's Hosp 1980

Demento, Frank MD (D) - **Spec Exp:** Dermatologic Surgery; Skin Cancer; **Hospital:** Winthrop - Univ Hosp, Nassau Univ Med Ctr; **Address:** 520 Franklin Ave, Ste 229, Garden City, NY 11530; **Phone:** 516-746-1227; **Board Cert:** Dermatology 1969; **Med School:** UMDNJ-NJ Med Sch, Newark 1964; **Resid:** Dermatology, USPHS Hosp 1966; **Fellow:** Dermatology, Columbia-Presby Hosp 1968

Dolitsky, Charisse MD (D) - **Spec Exp:** Acne; Skin Cancer; Hair Removal-Laser; **Hospital:** Long Beach Med Ctr, South Nassau Comm Hosp; **Address:** 604 E Park Ave, Long Beach, NY 11561; **Phone:** 516-432-0011; **Board Cert:** Dermatology 1989; **Med School:** SUNY Downstate 1985; **Resid:** Dermatology, Univ Hosp 1989

Falcon, Ronald MD (D) - **Spec Exp:** Skin Cancer; Acne; Psoriasis; **Hospital:** Long Beach Med Ctr, South Nassau Comm Hosp; **Address:** 604 E Park Ave, Long Beach, NY 11561-2505; **Phone:** 516-432-0011; **Board Cert:** Dermatology 1989; **Med School:** SUNY Downstate 1985; **Resid:** Dermatology, SUNY Downstate 1989

Franck, Jeanne M MD (D) - **Spec Exp:** Mohs' Surgery; **Hospital:** Winthrop - Univ Hosp; **Address:** 520 Franklin Ave, Ste 207, Garden City, NY 11530; **Phone:** 516-741-1055; **Board Cert:** Dermatology 1995; **Med School:** Columbia P&S 1991; **Resid:** Dermatology, Columbia Presby Med Ctr 1995; **Fellow:** Mohs Surgery, U Minn Med Ctr

Funt, Tina K MD (D) - **Spec Exp:** Pediatric Dermatology; **Hospital:** Winthrop - Univ Hosp, Mercy Med Ctr - Rockville Centre; **Address:** 229 7th St, Ste 105, Garden City, NY 11530; **Phone:** 516-747-7778; **Board Cert:** Dermatology 1989; **Med School:** SUNY Hlth Sci Ctr 1984; **Resid:** Pediatrics, Albert Einstein 1986; Dermatology, NY Med Coll 1989

Hefter, Harold MD (D) - **Spec Exp:** Cosmetic Dermatology; Dermatologic Surgery; Acne; **Hospital:** Franklin Hosp Med Ctr, Jacobi Med Ctr; **Address:** 135 Rockaway Tpke, Ste 100, Lawrence, NY 11559; **Phone:** 516-371-1600; **Board Cert:** Dermatology 1985; **Med School:** Albert Einstein Coll Med 1981; **Resid:** Dermatology, Albert Einstein 1985; **Fac Appt:** Asst Prof D, Albert Einstein Coll Med

Hisler, Barbara MD (D) - **Spec Exp:** Skin Cancer; Acne; Psoriasis; **Hospital:** Long Island Jewish Med Ctr; **Address:** 1300 Union Tpke, Ste 303, New Hyde Park, NY 11040-1759; **Phone:** 516-326-0333; **Board Cert:** Internal Medicine 1986; Dermatology 1989; **Med School:** NY Med Coll 1983; **Resid:** Internal Medicine, LI Jewish Med Ctr 1985; Dermatology, Detroit Med Ctr 1988; **Fac Appt:** Asst Prof Med, Albert Einstein Coll Med

Kristal, Leonard MD (D) - **Spec Exp:** Pediatric Dermatology; **Hospital:** Schneider Chldn's Hosp, Stony Brook Univ Hosp; **Address:** 2001 Marcus Ave, Ste S40, Lake Success, NY 11042; **Phone:** 516-352-6151; **Board Cert:** Pediatrics 2004; Dermatology 2001; **Med School:** Univ Hlth Sci/Chicago Med Sch 1986; **Resid:** Pediatrics, Chldns Hosp 1989; Dermatology, Univ Hosp-SUNY 1993; **Fellow:** Dermatology, Chldns Hosp 1994; **Fac Appt:** Asst Clin Prof Ped, SUNY Stony Brook

Krivo, James MD (D) - **Spec Exp:** Skin Cancer; **Hospital:** Winthrop - Univ Hosp, Franklin Hosp Med Ctr; **Address:** 54 New Hyde Park Rd, Garden City, NY 11530; **Phone:** 516-481-4920; **Board Cert:** Dermatology 1973; **Med School:** Univ Chicago-Pritzker Sch Med 1966; **Resid:** Dermatology, Univ Chicago 1968; Dermatology, NY Med Coll 1972; **Fac Appt:** D, SUNY Stony Brook

Levine, Laurie J MD (D) - **Spec Exp:** Skin Laser Surgery; Botox Therapy; Cosmetic Dermatology; **Hospital:** Winthrop - Univ Hosp; **Address:** 200 Old Country Rd, Ste 140, Mineola, NY 11501-4237; **Phone:** 516-742-6136; **Board Cert:** Dermatology 1988; **Med School:** SUNY Stony Brook 1984; **Resid:** Dermatology, T Jefferson Univ Hosp 1988; **Fellow:** Dermatologic Surgery, T Jefferson Univ Hosp 1989; **Fac Appt:** Asst Clin Prof D, SUNY Stony Brook

Meyers, John H MD (D) - **Hospital:** N Shore Univ Hosp at Glen Cove; **Address:** 10 Medical Plaza, Ste 204, Glen Cove, NY 11542; **Phone:** 516-671-7666; **Board Cert:** Dermatology 1956; **Med School:** Yale Univ 1950; **Resid:** Dermatology, NY Hosp 1953; Dermatology, NY Polyclinic Hosp & Med Coll 1954

Pacernick, Lawrence MD (D) - **Spec Exp:** Acne; Aging Skin; **Hospital:** N Shore Univ Hosp at Plainview, Nassau Univ Med Ctr; **Address:** 700 Old Country Rd, Ste 203, Plainview, NY 11803-4032; **Phone:** 516-822-9730; **Board Cert:** Dermatology 1973; **Med School:** Univ Mich Med Sch 1966; **Resid:** Internal Medicine, Michael Reese Hosp 1968; Dermatology, Univ Chicago Hosps 1973

Paltzik, Robert MD (D) - **Spec Exp:** Pediatric Dermatology; Dermatologic Surgery; **Hospital:** N Shore Univ Hosp at Manhasset, Winthrop - Univ Hosp; **Address:** 2 Hillside Ave, Ste G, Williston Park, NY 11596-2335; **Phone:** 516-747-2230; **Board Cert:** Pediatrics 1976; Dermatology 1977; **Med School:** NYU Sch Med 1971; **Resid:** Pediatrics, Yale-New Haven Hosp 1973; Dermatology, SUNY Downstate Med Ctr 1977; **Fac Appt:** Asst Prof D, NYU Sch Med

Sklar, Jeffrey MD (D) - **Spec Exp:** Liposuction; Cosmetic Dermatology; Botox Therapy; **Hospital:** NY-Presby Hosp (page 100), N Shore Univ Hosp at Syosset; **Address:** 800 Woodbury Rd, Ste A, Woodbury, NY 11797-2503; **Phone:** 516-496-9400; **Board Cert:** Dermatology 1986; **Med School:** Columbia P&S 1982; **Resid:** Dermatology, Columbia Presby Hosp 1986; **Fac Appt:** Asst Clin Prof D, Columbia P&S

Spinowitz, Alan MD (D) - **Spec Exp:** Skin Cancer; Mohs' Surgery; **Hospital:** Franklin Hosp Med Ctr; **Address:** 877 Stewart Ave, Ste 27, Garden City, NY 11530-4803; **Phone:** 516-745-0606; **Board Cert:** Dermatology 1985; **Med School:** SUNY Hlth Sci Ctr 1981; **Resid:** Dermatology, Univ Illinois Med Ctr 1985; **Fellow:** Dermatologic Surgery, Univ Illinois Med Ctr 1987

Walczyk, John MD (D) - **Hospital:** NY-Presby Hosp (page 100), N Shore Univ Hosp at Plainview; **Address:** 1165 Northern Blvd, Ste 405, Manhasset, NY 11030; **Phone:** 516-365-8030; **Board Cert:** Dermatology 2003; **Med School:** Columbia P&S 1990; **Resid:** Internal Medicine, N Shore Univ Hosp 1991; Dermatology, Columbia Presby Hosp 1994

Diagnostic Radiology

Goodman, Ken J MD (DR) - **Spec Exp:** Urologic Imaging; Ultrasound; CT Scan; **Hospital:** St Francis Hosp - The Heart Ctr (page 112); **Address:** 100 Port Washington Blvd, Roslyn, NY 11576-1353; **Phone:** 516-562-6500; **Board Cert:** Diagnostic Radiology 1977; **Med School:** Univ Tex, San Antonio 1972; **Resid:** Diagnostic Radiology, Cornell Med Ctr 1977; **Fellow:** Radiology, Cornell Med Ctr 1978

Hammel, Jay MD (DR) - **Spec Exp:** MRI; **Hospital:** New Island Hosp; **Address:** 4273 Hempstead Tpke, Bethpage, NY 11714; **Phone:** 516-579-5800; **Board Cert:** Diagnostic Radiology 1989; **Med School:** SUNY Upstate Med Univ 1984; **Resid:** Diagnostic Radiology, St Vincent's Med Ctr 1989

Hoffman, Janet C MD (DR) - **Hospital:** Long Island Jewish Med Ctr; **Address:** 270-05 76th Ave, rm C-204, New Hyde Park, NY 11040; **Phone:** 718-470-7181; **Board Cert:** Diagnostic Radiology 1978; **Med School:** SUNY Downstate 1974; **Resid:** Radiology, Colum Presby Hosp 1978; **Fellow:** Ultrasound, NY Hosp-Cornell Med Ctr 1979

Khan, Arfa MD (DR) - **Spec Exp:** Thoracic Radiology; **Hospital:** Long Island Jewish Med Ctr; **Address:** 270-05 76th Ave, rm C204, New Hyde Park, NY 11040; **Phone:** 718-470-7177; **Board Cert:** Radiology 1971; **Med School:** India 1964; **Resid:** Radiology, Queens Hosp 1970; **Fellow:** Radiology, LI Jewish Med Ctr 1971; **Fac Appt:** Assoc Prof Rad, Albert Einstein Coll Med

Lefkowitz, Harvey MD (DR) - **Spec Exp:** Musculoskeletal Imaging; Mammography; Forensic Medicine; **Address:** 4160 Merrick Rd, Massapequa, NY 11758; **Phone:** 516-333-1313; **Board Cert:** Diagnostic Radiology 1975; **Med School:** SUNY Downstate 1969; **Resid:** Internal Medicine, USPHS Hosp 1972; Diagnostic Radiology, SUNY Dwnst Med Ctr 1975

Mendelsohn, Steven MD (DR) - ; **Address:** 680 Old Country Rd, Plainview, NY 11808; **Phone:** 516-798-4242; **Board Cert:** Diagnostic Radiology 1984; **Med School:** Jefferson Med Coll 1979; **Resid:** Diagnostic Radiology, N Shore Univ Hosp 1983

Rossi, Dennis MD (DR) - **Spec Exp:** MRI; **Hospital:** Long Beach Med Ctr, St. John's Episcopal Hosp-Queens; **Address:** 1575 Hillside Ave, Ste 301, New Hyde Park, NY 11040; **Phone:** 516-354-4200; **Board Cert:** Radiology 1973; **Med School:** SUNY Downstate 1968; **Resid:** Radiology, Montefiore Hosp Med Ctr 1972; **Fac Appt:** Assoc Clin Prof Rad, SUNY Stony Brook

Sherman, Scott J MD (DR) - **Spec Exp:** CT Scan; PET Imaging; **Hospital:** St Francis Hosp - The Heart Ctr (page 112); **Address:** 100 Port Washington Blvd, Roslyn, NY 11576; **Phone:** 516-562-6511; **Board Cert:** Nuclear Medicine 1984; Diagnostic Radiology 1983; **Med School:** Northwestern Univ 1979; **Resid:** Radiology, NY Hosp 1983; Nuclear Medicine, NY Hosp 1984; **Fellow:** Ultrasound, NY Hosp 1985

Sitron, Alan MD (DR) - **Spec Exp:** Ultrasound; Interventional Radiology; Nuclear Medicine; **Hospital:** New Island Hosp; **Address:** 4277 Hempstead Tpke, Ste 200, Bethpage, NY 11714-5706; **Phone:** 516-796-4340; **Board Cert:** Diagnostic Radiology 1975; **Med School:** Albany Med Coll 1971; **Resid:** Diagnostic Radiology, Albert Einstein 1975

Weck, Steven MD (DR) - **Spec Exp:** Interventional Radiology; **Hospital:** N Shore Univ Hosp at Glen Cove; **Address:** Dept Radiology, 101 St. Andrew's Ln, Glen Cove, NY 11542; **Phone:** 516-674-7540; **Board Cert:** Diagnostic Radiology 1977; **Med School:** NYU Sch Med 1973; **Resid:** Radiology, NYU Med Ctr 1977

ENDOCRINOLOGY, DIABETES & METABOLISM

Aloia, John MD (EDM) - **Spec Exp:** Osteoporosis; **Hospital:** Winthrop - Univ Hosp; **Address:** 222 Station Plaza North, Ste 350, Mineola, NY 11501; **Phone:** 516-663-3511; **Board Cert:** Internal Medicine 1969; Endocrinology 1972; **Med School:** Creighton Univ 1962; **Resid:** Internal Medicine, Meadowbrook Hosp 1966; Internal Medicine, Harrisburg Hosp 1967; **Fellow:** Endocrinology, Diabetes & Metabolism, Jefferson Univ Med Ctr 1969; **Fac Appt:** Prof Med, SUNY Stony Brook

Bhatt, Anjani MD (EDM) - **Spec Exp:** Thyroid Disorders; Diabetes; **Hospital:** Long Beach Med Ctr; **Address:** 871 E Park Ave, Long Beach, NY 11561; **Phone:** 516-889-8853; **Board Cert:** Internal Medicine 1983; Endocrinology, Diabetes & Metabolism 1985; **Med School:** India 1976; **Resid:** Internal Medicine, Brooklyn Hosp 1981; **Fellow:** Endocrinology, Brooklyn Hosp 1984

Friedman, Seth G MD (EDM) - **Spec Exp:** Thyroid Disorders; Pituitary Disorders; Diabetes; Osteoporosis; **Hospital:** N Shore Univ Hosp at Manhasset, Long Island Jewish Med Ctr; **Address:** 560 Northern Blvd, Ste 207, Great Neck, NY 11021; **Phone:** 516-466-6165; **Board Cert:** Internal Medicine 2002; Endocrinology, Diabetes & Metabolism 2003; **Med School:** Mount Sinai Sch Med 1988; **Resid:** Internal Medicine, LI Jewish Med Ctr 1991; **Fellow:** Endocrinology, Diabetes & Metabolism, Albert Einstein 1993

Gordon, Jeffrey MD (EDM) - **Spec Exp:** Diabetes; Thyroid Disorders; Pituitary Disorders; **Hospital:** St Francis Hosp - The Heart Ctr (page 112), N Shore Univ Hosp at Manhasset; **Address:** 3 School St, Ste 306, Glen Cove, NY 11542-2548; **Phone:** 516-759-2420; **Board Cert:** Internal Medicine 1972; Endocrinology, Diabetes & Metabolism 1973; **Med School:** Cornell Univ-Weill Med Coll 1965; **Resid:** Internal Medicine, Bellevue Hosp 1967; **Fellow:** Endocrinology, Duke Univ Med Ctr 1970; Endocrinology, VA Hosp 1972; **Fac Appt:** Asst Clin Prof Med, NYU Sch Med

Greenfield, Martin MD (EDM) - **Spec Exp:** Diabetes; Thyroid Disorders; Osteoporosis; **Hospital:** Long Island Jewish Med Ctr, N Shore Univ Hosp at Manhasset; **Address:** 560 Northern Blvd, Ste 107, Great Neck, NY 11021-5100; **Phone:** 516-482-3433; **Board Cert:** Internal Medicine 1987; Endocrinology, Diabetes & Metabolism 1979; **Med School:** SUNY Downstate 1968; **Resid:** Internal Medicine, LI Jewish Med Ctr 1971; **Fellow:** Endocrinology, Diabetes & Metabolism, Brigham & Womens Hosp 1975; **Fac Appt:** Asst Clin Prof Med, Albert Einstein Coll Med

Hershon, Kenneth MD (EDM) - **Spec Exp:** Diabetes; Osteoporosis; Cholesterol/Lipid Disorders; **Hospital:** N Shore Univ Hosp at Manhasset, Long Island Jewish Med Ctr; **Address:** 3003 New Hyde Park Rd, Ste 201, New Hyde Park, NY 11042; **Phone:** 516-327-0850; **Board Cert:** Internal Medicine 1979; Endocrinology 1981; **Med School:** Albert Einstein Coll Med 1976; **Resid:** Internal Medicine, Mount Sinai Hosp 1979; **Fellow:** Endocrinology, Diabetes & Metabolism, Univ WA Med Ctr 1981; **Fac Appt:** Clin Prof Med, Albert Einstein Coll Med

Hupart, Kenneth MD (EDM) - **Spec Exp:** Thyroid Disorders; Osteoporosis; Diabetes; Cholesterol/Lipid Disorders; **Hospital:** Nassau Univ Med Ctr; **Address:** 2201 Hempstead Tpke, East Meadow, NY 11554; **Phone:** 516-572-1303; **Board Cert:** Internal Medicine 1985; Endocrinology 1989; **Med School:** SUNY Stony Brook 1982; **Resid:** Internal Medicine, Montefiore Hosp Med Ctr 1986; **Fellow:** Endocrinology, Diabetes & Metabolism, Montefiore Hosp Med Ctr 1988; **Fac Appt:** Assoc Clin Prof Med, Albert Einstein Coll Med

Klass, Evan MD (EDM) - **Spec Exp:** Diabetes; Thyroid Disorders; **Hospital:** N Shore Univ Hosp at Manhasset, Long Island Jewish Med Ctr; **Address:** 2800 Marcus Ave, Ste 200, Lake Success, NY 11042; **Phone:** 516-708-2540; **Board Cert:** Internal Medicine 1979; Endocrinology, Diabetes & Metabolism 1983; **Med School:** NY Med Coll 1976; **Resid:** Internal Medicine, LI Jewish Med Ctr 1979; **Fellow:** Endocrinology, Diabetes & Metabolism, Geo Wash U Med Ctr 1982; **Fac Appt:** Asst Clin Prof Med, Albert Einstein Coll Med

Klein, Irwin MD (EDM) - **Spec Exp:** Thyroid Disorders; Thyroid Cancer; **Hospital:** N Shore Univ Hosp at Manhasset; **Address:** 2800 Marcus Ave, Ste 200, Lake Success, NY 11042; **Phone:** 516-708-2540; **Board Cert:** Internal Medicine 1978; Endocrinology 1985; **Med School:** NYU Sch Med 1973; **Resid:** Internal Medicine, Hosp Univ Penn 1975; **Fellow:** Natl Cancer Inst/NIH 1977; Endocrinology, Diabetes & Metabolism, Univ Miami Hosps 1979; **Fac Appt:** Prof Med, NYU Sch Med

Lomasky, Steven MD (EDM) - **Spec Exp:** Diabetes; Cholesterol/Lipid Disorders; **Hospital:** South Nassau Comm Hosp, Long Island Jewish Med Ctr; **Address:** 242 Merrick Rd, rm 403, Rockville Ctr, NY 11570; **Phone:** 516-536-3700; **Board Cert:** Endocrinology, Diabetes & Metabolism 1989; Internal Medicine 1985; **Med School:** Israel 1982; **Resid:** Internal Medicine, Montefiore Hosp Med Ctr 1986; **Fellow:** Endocrinology, Diabetes & Metabolism, Albert Einstein 1987; **Fac Appt:** Asst Clin Prof Med, Albert Einstein Coll Med

Margulies, Paul MD (EDM) - **Spec Exp:** Thyroid Disorders; Adrenal Disorders; Pituitary Disorders; **Hospital:** N Shore Univ Hosp at Manhasset; **Address:** 444 Community, Ste 312, Manhasset, NY 11030-3820; **Phone:** 516-627-1366; **Board Cert:** Internal Medicine 1975; Endocrinology, Diabetes & Metabolism 1977; **Med School:** Univ Chicago-Pritzker Sch Med 1970; **Resid:** Internal Medicine, New York Hosp 1975; **Fellow:** Endocrinology, Diabetes & Metabolism, New York Hosp 1976; **Fac Appt:** Assoc Prof Med, NYU Sch Med

Rosenthal, David S MD (EDM) - **Spec Exp:** Thyroid Disorders; Pituitary Disorders; Adrenal Disorders; **Hospital:** N Shore Univ Hosp at Plainview, New Island Hosp; **Address:** 4150 Sunrise Hwy, Massapequa, NY 11758-5303; **Phone:** 516-541-1721; **Board Cert:** Internal Medicine 1969; Endocrinology, Diabetes & Metabolism 1972; **Med School:** NYU Sch Med 1963; **Resid:** Internal Medicine, Wilford Hall USAF Med Ctr 1967; **Fellow:** Endocrinology, Diabetes & Metabolism, Boston Univ Med Ctr 1972; Nuclear Medicine, Boston Univ Med Ctr 1972; **Fac Appt:** Asst Prof Med, SUNY Stony Brook

Shapiro, Lawrence MD (EDM) - **Spec Exp:** Thyroid Disorders; **Hospital:** Winthrop - Univ Hosp; **Address:** 222 Station Plaza N, Ste 350, Mineola, NY 11501; **Phone:** 516-663-3511; **Board Cert:** Internal Medicine 1975; Endocrinology 1977; **Med School:** SUNY Hlth Sci Ctr 1971; **Resid:** Internal Medicine, Bellevue Hosp 1974; **Fellow:** Endocrinology, Diabetes & Metabolism, NYU Med Ctr 1975; **Fac Appt:** Prof Med, Cornell Univ-Weill Med Coll

Vaswani, Ashok N MD (EDM) - **Spec Exp:** Osteoporosis; Obesity; **Hospital:** Winthrop - Univ Hosp; **Address:** 520 Franklin Ave, Ste L-2, Garden City, NY 11530; **Phone:** 516-739-0414; **Board Cert:** Endocrinology, Diabetes & Metabolism 1983; Internal Medicine 1977; **Med School:** India 1970; **Resid:** Internal Medicine, Nassau County Med Ctr 1974; **Fac Appt:** Asst Prof Med, SUNY Stony Brook

Weinerman, Stuart MD (EDM) - **Spec Exp:** Osteoporosis; Calcium Disorders; **Hospital:** N Shore Univ Hosp at Manhasset; **Address:** 2800 Marcus Ave, Ste 200, Lake Success, NY 11021-5310; **Phone:** 516-708-2540; **Board Cert:** Internal Medicine 1987; Endocrinology, Diabetes & Metabolism 1989; **Med School:** Albert Einstein Coll Med 1984; **Resid:** Internal Medicine, N Shore Univ Hosp 1987; **Fellow:** Endocrinology, Diabetes & Metabolism, NY Hosp/Meml Sloan Kettering Cancer Ctr 1989; **Fac Appt:** Assoc Prof Med, NYU Sch Med

FAMILY MEDICINE

Arcati, Anthony T MD (FMed) - **Hospital:** Winthrop - Univ Hosp; **Address:** 540 Hicksville Rd, Bethpage, NY 11714; **Phone:** 516-931-4285; **Board Cert:** Family Medicine 2002; **Med School:** Mexico 1975; **Resid:** Family Medicine, Nassau Co Med Ctr 1979

Arcati, Robert J MD (FMed) **PCP** - **Hospital:** Winthrop - Univ Hosp; **Address:** 540 Hicksville Rd, Bethpage, NY 11714; **Phone:** 516-931-4285; **Board Cert:** Family Medicine 2002; **Med School:** Mount Sinai Sch Med 1986; **Resid:** Family Medicine, Somercet Med Ctr 1989

Capobianco, Luigi MD (FMed) **PCP** - **Spec Exp:** Geriatrics; **Hospital:** N Shore Univ Hosp at Glen Cove; **Address:** One School St, Ste 203, Glen Cove, NY 11542; **Phone:** 516-671-9800; **Board Cert:** Geriatric Medicine 1996; Family Medicine 1988; **Med School:** Italy 1984; **Resid:** Family Medicine, N Shore Univ Hosp 1988

Edelstein, Martin MD (FMed) **PCP** - **Spec Exp:** Concierge Medicine; Cholesterol/Lipid Disorders; **Hospital:** N Shore Univ Hosp at Manhasset; **Address:** 11 Beverly Rd, Great Neck, NY 11021-1320; **Phone:** 516-487-1614; **Board Cert:** Family Medicine 2001; **Med School:** McGill Univ 1971; **Resid:** Family Medicine, Jewish Genl Hosp 1973; **Fac Appt:** Asst Clin Prof FMed, NYU Sch Med

Moynihan, Brian DO (FMed) **PCP** - **Spec Exp:** Hypertension; Diabetes; Skin Diseases; **Hospital:** New Island Hosp, N Shore Univ Hosp at Manhasset; **Address:** 2840 Jerusalem Ave, Wantagh, NY 11793-2017; **Phone:** 516-781-1141; **Board Cert:** Family Medicine 1985; **Med School:** NY Coll Osteo Med 1983; **Resid:** Family Medicine, Massapequa Genl Hosp 1984; Family Medicine, Kennedy Meml Hosp 1985; **Fac Appt:** Asst Prof FMed, NY Coll Osteo Med

Muraca, Glenn DO (FMed) **PCP** - **Spec Exp:** Sports Medicine; Nutrition; **Hospital:** Parkway Hosp; **Address:** 86-16 Jamaica Ave, Woodhaven, NY 11563; **Phone:** 718-805-0037; **Board Cert:** Family Medicine 1994; **Med School:** NY Coll Osteo Med 1990; **Resid:** Family Medicine, Peninsula Hosp 1994

Rechter, Lesley MD (FMed) **PCP** - **Spec Exp:** Women's Health; **Hospital:** Stony Brook Univ Hosp; **Address:** 54 Birchwood Park Dr, Jericho, NY 11753-2202; **Phone:** 516-933-6850; **Board Cert:** Family Medicine 2003; **Med School:** NY Med Coll 1976; **Resid:** Family Medicine, Nassau County Med Ctr 1979; **Fac Appt:** Assoc Clin Prof FMed, SUNY Stony Brook

Sklar, Barrett MD (FMed) **PCP** - **Hospital:** Winthrop - Univ Hosp; **Address:** 530 Hicksville Rd, Bethpage, NY 11714; **Phone:** 516-937-5000; **Board Cert:** Family Medicine 1997; **Med School:** Loyola Univ-Stritch Sch Med 1959; **Resid:** Internal Medicine, Meadowbrook Hosp; **Fac Appt:** Asst Prof FMed, SUNY Stony Brook

Soskel, Neil DO (FMed) **PCP** - **Spec Exp:** Sports Medicine; Adolescent Medicine; **Hospital:** South Nassau Comm Hosp; **Address:** 185 Merrick Rd, Lynbrook, NY 11563; **Phone:** 516-887-0077; **Board Cert:** Family Medicine 2004; **Med School:** NY Coll Osteo Med 1986; **Resid:** Family Medicine, S Nassau Comm Hosp 1989; **Fac Appt:** Assoc Prof FMed, NY Coll Osteo Med

GASTROENTEROLOGY

Bank, Simmy MD (Ge) - **Spec Exp:** Pancreatic Disease; Peptic Ulcer Disease; Gastroesophageal Reflux Disease (GERD); Inflammatory Bowel Disease; **Hospital:** Long Island Jewish Med Ctr, N Shore Univ Hosp at Manhasset; **Address:** 270-05 76th Ave, New Hyde Park, NY 11040-1433; **Phone:** 718-470-4692; **Med School:** South Africa 1954; **Resid:** Internal Medicine, Groote Schur Hosp; Internal Medicine, Balham; **Fellow:** Gastroenterology, Groote Schur Hosp; **Fac Appt:** Prof Med, Albert Einstein Coll Med

Bartolomeo, Robert MD (Ge) - **Spec Exp:** Colonoscopy; Inflammatory Bowel Disease; Gastroesophageal Reflux Disease (GERD); Colon Cancer Screening; **Hospital:** Winthrop - Univ Hosp, N Shore Univ Hosp at Manhasset; **Address:** 1103 Stewart Ave, Ste 300, Garden City, NY 11530; **Phone:** 516-248-3737; **Board Cert:** Internal Medicine 1974; Gastroenterology 1977; **Med School:** NY Med Coll 1971; **Resid:** Internal Medicine, Metropolitan Hosp Ctr 1973; Internal Medicine, Beth Israel Hosp 1974; **Fellow:** Gastroenterology, Bridgeport Hosp/Yale Univ 1976

Bernstein, David E MD (Ge) - **Spec Exp:** Liver Disease; Hepatitis; Nutrition; **Hospital:** N Shore Univ Hosp at Manhasset; **Address:** N Shore U Hospital, Div Gastroenterology, 300 Community Drive, Manhasset, NY 11030; **Phone:** 516-562-4281; **Board Cert:** Internal Medicine 2000; Gastroenterology 2003; **Med School:** SUNY Stony Brook 1988; **Resid:** Internal Medicine, Montefiore Med Ctr 1991; **Fellow:** Gastroenterology, Jackson Meml Hosp 1993; **Fac Appt:** Assoc Prof Med, SUNY Stony Brook

Blumstein, Meyer MD (Ge) - **Spec Exp:** Endoscopy; Gastroesophageal Reflux Disease (GERD); Inflammatory Bowel Disease; **Hospital:** Long Island Jewish Med Ctr, South Nassau Comm Hosp; **Address:** 158 Hempstead Ave, Lynnbrook, NY 11563-1605; **Phone:** 516-593-3541; **Board Cert:** Internal Medicine 1989; Gastroenterology 2001; **Med School:** SUNY Hlth Sci Ctr 1986; **Resid:** Internal Medicine, LI Jewish Med Ctr 1989; **Fellow:** Gastroenterology, LI Jewish Med Ctr 1991; **Fac Appt:** Asst Prof Med, Albert Einstein Coll Med

Caccese, William MD (Ge) - **Spec Exp:** Endoscopy; Colon Cancer; **Hospital:** N Shore Univ Hosp at Plainview; **Address:** 700 Old Country Rd, Ste 206, Plainview, NY 11803-4932; **Phone:** 516-681-1200; **Board Cert:** Internal Medicine 1981; Gastroenterology 1983; **Med School:** SUNY Hlth Sci Ctr 1978; **Resid:** Internal Medicine, N Shore Univ Hosp 1981; **Fellow:** Gastroenterology, N Shore Univ Hosp 1983

Cohen, Jacob L MD (Ge) - **Hospital:** Mercy Med Ctr - Rockville Centre; **Address:** 2 Lincoln Ave, Ste 201, Rockville Centre, NY 11570; **Phone:** 516-536-0600; **Board Cert:** Internal Medicine 1968; Gastroenterology 1972; **Med School:** SUNY Upstate Med Univ 1961; **Resid:** Internal Medicine, Maimonides Med Ctr 1963; Internal Medicine, SUNY Upstate 1966; **Fellow:** Gastroenterology, Maimonides Med Ctr 1968

DeVito, Bethany S MD (Ge) - **Spec Exp:** Women's Health; Capsule Endoscopy; **Hospital:** N Shore Univ Hosp at Manhasset; **Address:** N Shore Univ Hospital, 4 Levitt Pavilion, 300 Community Drive, Manhasset, NY 11030; **Phone:** 516-562-4281; **Board Cert:** Internal Medicine 1996; Gastroenterology 1997; **Med School:** SUNY Upstate Med Univ 1992; **Resid:** Internal Medicine, St Vincents Hosp & Med Ctr 1995; **Fellow:** Gastroenterology, NY Hosp of Queens 1997

Farber, Charles MD (Ge) - **Spec Exp:** Colon Cancer; Gastroesophageal Reflux Disease (GERD); **Hospital:** N Shore Univ Hosp at Plainview, New Island Hosp; **Address:** 146A Manetto Hill Rd, Ste 205, Plainveiw, NY 11803; **Phone:** 516-822-4404; **Board Cert:** Gastroenterology 1983; Internal Medicine 1981; **Med School:** SUNY Hlth Sci Ctr 1978; **Resid:** Internal Medicine, N Shore Univ Hosp 1981; **Fellow:** Gastroenterology, Albert Einstein 1983

Goldblum, Lester DO (Ge) - **Spec Exp:** Endoscopy; Colon Cancer; Capsule Endoscopy; **Hospital:** New Island Hosp, N Shore Univ Hosp at Plainview; **Address:** 850 Hicksville Rd, Ste 100, Seaford, NY 11783; **Phone:** 516-796-9000; **Board Cert:** Internal Medicine 1983; Gastroenterology 2001; **Med School:** Coll Osteo Med 1979; **Resid:** Internal Medicine, Nassau County Med Ctr 1983; **Fellow:** Gastroenterology, Nassau County Med Ctr 1985; **Fac Appt:** Asst Clin Prof Med, NY Coll Osteo Med

Goldman, Ira S MD (Ge) - **Spec Exp:** Endoscopy & Colonoscopy; Colon Cancer Screening; **Hospital:** N Shore Univ Hosp at Manhasset, St Francis Hosp - The Heart Ctr (page 112); **Address:** 310 E Shore Rd, Ste 206, Great Neck, NY 11023-2432; **Phone:** 516-487-7677; **Board Cert:** Internal Medicine 1980; Gastroenterology 1983; **Med School:** Columbia P&S 1977; **Resid:** Internal Medicine, Columbia-Presby Med Ctr 1980; **Fellow:** Gastroenterology, UCSF Med Ctr 1983; **Fac Appt:** Assoc Prof Med, NYU Sch Med

Gould, Perry MD (Ge) - **Spec Exp:** Ulcerative Colitis; Colon & Rectal Cancer; **Hospital:** Winthrop - Univ Hosp; **Address:** 1103 Stewart Ave, Garden City, NY 11530; **Phone:** 516-248-3737; **Board Cert:** Internal Medicine 1980; Gastroenterology 1983; **Med School:** NY Med Coll 1977; **Resid:** Internal Medicine, LI Jewish Hosp 1980; Gastroenterology, NY Med Coll 1982

Greenberg, Ronald MD (Ge) - **Spec Exp:** Inflammatory Bowel Disease; Peptic Acid Disorders; **Hospital:** Long Island Jewish Med Ctr; **Address:** 270-05 76th Ave, rm B 202, New Hyde Park, NY 11040; **Phone:** 718-470-7281; **Board Cert:** Internal Medicine 1982; Gastroenterology 1985; **Med School:** Hahnemann Univ 1979; **Resid:** Internal Medicine, Albany Med Ctr 1982; **Fellow:** Gastroenterology, St Luke's Hosp 1985; **Fac Appt:** Assoc Clin Prof Med, Albert Einstein Coll Med

Grendell, James H MD (Ge) - **Spec Exp:** Pancreatic Disease; Nutrition; Liver Disease; **Hospital:** Winthrop - Univ Hosp; **Address:** 222 Station Plaza N, Ste 428, Mineola, NY 11501-3819; **Phone:** 516-663-2066; **Board Cert:** Internal Medicine 1978; Gastroenterology 1981; **Med School:** Ohio State Univ 1975; **Resid:** Internal Medicine, Beth Israel Hosp 1978; **Fellow:** Gastroenterology, UCSF Med Ctr 1981; **Fac Appt:** Prof Med, SUNY Stony Brook

Gutman, David MD (Ge) - **Spec Exp:** Hepatitis C; Gastroesophageal Reflux Disease (GERD); **Hospital:** N Shore Univ Hosp at Plainview, New Island Hosp; **Address:** 200 Old Country Rd, Ste 250, Mineloa, NY 11501; **Phone:** 516-739-4604; **Board Cert:** Gastroenterology 1989; Internal Medicine 1986; **Med School:** Baylor Coll Med 1983; **Resid:** Internal Medicine, Baylor Coll Med 1986; **Fellow:** Gastroenterology, Univ of PA Hosp 1988

Katz, Seymour MD (Ge) - **Spec Exp:** Inflammatory Bowel Disease; Colonoscopy; Endoscopy; **Hospital:** N Shore Univ Hosp at Manhasset, Long Island Jewish Med Ctr; **Address:** 1000 Northern Blvd, Ste 140, Great Neck, NY 11021; **Phone:** 516-466-2340; **Board Cert:** Gastroenterology 1972; Internal Medicine 1971; **Med School:** NYU Sch Med 1964; **Resid:** Internal Medicine, Albert Einstein Sch Med 1966; Internal Medicine, Jacobi Med Ctr 1969; **Fellow:** Gastroenterology, NY Hosp 1971; **Fac Appt:** Asst Clin Prof Med, Cornell Univ-Weill Med Coll

McKinley, Matthew MD (Ge) - **Spec Exp:** Gastroesophageal Reflux Disease (GERD); Barrett's Esophagus; Biliary Disease; **Hospital:** N Shore Univ Hosp at Manhasset; **Address:** 2800 Marcus Ave, Ste 201, Lake Success, NY 11042; **Phone:** 516-622-6076; **Board Cert:** Internal Medicine 1978; Gastroenterology 1981; **Med School:** Creighton Univ 1975; **Resid:** Internal Medicine, N Shore Univ Hosp 1978; Internal Medicine, Meml Sloan Kettering Cancer Ctr 1978; **Fellow:** Gastroenterology, Yale-New Haven Hosp 1980; **Fac Appt:** Assoc Prof Med, NYU Sch Med

Miller, Seth MD (Ge) - **Hospital:** Long Beach Med Ctr; **Address:** 206 West Park Ave, Long Beach, NY 11561; **Phone:** 516-432-8021; **Board Cert:** Internal Medicine 1983; Gastroenterology 1987; **Med School:** Mount Sinai Sch Med 1980; **Resid:** Internal Medicine, Beth Israel Med Ctr 1983; **Fellow:** Gastroenterology, Beth Israel Med Ctr 1985

Milman, Perry MD (Ge) - **Spec Exp:** Gastroesophageal Reflux Disease (GERD); Colon Cancer; Inflammatory Bowel Disease; **Hospital:** Long Island Jewish Med Ctr, N Shore Univ Hosp at Manhasset; **Address:** 2001 Marcus Ave, Ste N18, Lake Success, NY 11042-1035; **Phone:** 516-775-7770; **Board Cert:** Internal Medicine 1976; Gastroenterology 1979; **Med School:** SUNY Downstate 1973; **Resid:** Internal Medicine, LI Jewish Med Ctr 1976; **Fellow:** Gastroenterology, VA Hosp/NYU 1978; **Fac Appt:** Asst Clin Prof Med, Albert Einstein Coll Med

Palmer, Melissa MD (Ge) - **Spec Exp:** Liver Disease; Hepatitis C; **Hospital:** N Shore Univ Hosp at Plainview; **Address:** 1097 Old Country Rd, Ste 104, Plainview, NY 11803-6505; **Phone:** 516-939-2626; **Board Cert:** Internal Medicine 1988; **Med School:** Mount Sinai Sch Med 1985; **Resid:** Internal Medicine, Beth Israel Medical Ctr 1988; **Fellow:** Gastroenterology, Stony Brook Univ Hosp 1990; Hepatology, Mt Sinai Medical Ctr 1991

Schwartz, Gary MD (Ge) - **Spec Exp:** Colon Cancer Screening; Gastroesophageal Reflux Disease (GERD); **Hospital:** Winthrop - Univ Hosp; **Address:** 1103 Stewart Ave, Garden City, NY 11530; **Phone:** 516-248-3737; **Board Cert:** Internal Medicine 1985; Gastroenterology 1987; **Med School:** Mexico 1979; **Resid:** Internal Medicine, Winthrop Univ Hosp 1983; **Fellow:** Gastroenterology, Univ Hosp 1986

Soterakis, Jack MD (Ge) - **Spec Exp:** Liver Disease; Gastrointestinal Endoscopy; Pancreatic Disease; **Hospital:** St Francis Hosp - The Heart Ctr (page 112), N Shore Univ Hosp at Glen Cove; **Address:** 139 Plandome Rd, Manhasset, NY 11030-2331; **Phone:** 516-365-4950; **Board Cert:** Internal Medicine 1975; Gastroenterology 1977; **Med School:** Italy 1968; **Resid:** Internal Medicine, Catholic Med Ctr 1972; Gastroenterology, Lemuel Shattuck Hosp-Tufts 1973; **Fellow:** Gastroenterology, Univ MD Hosp 1974

Talansky, Arthur L MD (Ge) - **Spec Exp:** Crohn's Disease; Ulcerative Colitis; Colonoscopy; **Hospital:** N Shore Univ Hosp at Manhasset, St Francis Hosp - The Heart Ctr (page 112); **Address:** 233 E Shore Rd, Ste 101, Great Neck, NY 11023-2433; **Phone:** 516-487-2444; **Board Cert:** Internal Medicine 1980; Gastroenterology 1983; **Med School:** Mount Sinai Sch Med 1977; **Resid:** Internal Medicine, Meml Sloan Kettering Cancer Ctr 1980; **Fellow:** Gastroenterology, Mount Sinai Hosp 1982; **Fac Appt:** Asst Clin Prof Med, NYU Sch Med

Weissman, Gary MD (Ge) - **Spec Exp:** Gastrointestinal Cancer; Inflammatory Bowel Disease; Esophageal Disorders; **Hospital:** N Shore Univ Hosp at Manhasset; **Address:** 2800 Marcus Ave, Ste 201, Lake Success, NY 11042; **Phone:** 516-622-6076; **Board Cert:** Internal Medicine 1982; Gastroenterology 1983; **Med School:** NY Med Coll 1976; **Resid:** Internal Medicine, North Shore Univ Hosp 1980; **Fellow:** Gastroenterology, Meml Sloan Kettering Cancer Ctr 1982; **Fac Appt:** Assoc Clin Prof Med, NYU Sch Med

GERIATRIC MEDICINE

Gomolin, Irving MD (Ger) - **Spec Exp:** Medications in the Elderly; Geriatric-Acute Hospital Care; Dementia; **Hospital:** Winthrop - Univ Hosp; **Address:** Winthrop Univ Hosp, 222 Station Plaza N Fl 5 - Ste 518, Mineola, NY 11501; **Phone:** 516-663-2588; **Board Cert:** Internal Medicine 1979; Geriatric Medicine 1998; **Med School:** Canada 1976; **Resid:** Internal Medicine, Jewish Genl Hosp-McGill Univ 1978; Internal Medicine, Beth Israel/Harvard 1981; **Fellow:** Clinical Pharmacology, Harvard Med Sch 1980; **Fac Appt:** Clin Prof Med, SUNY Stony Brook

Lanman, Geraldine MD (Ger) PCP - **Hospital:** Long Island Jewish Med Ctr; **Address:** 2800 Marcus Ave, rm 202, New Hyde Park, NY 11042; **Phone:** 516-354-0622; **Board Cert:** Internal Medicine 1983; Geriatric Medicine 1988; **Med School:** Univ Calgary 1980; **Resid:** Internal Medicine, LIJ Med Ctr 1986; **Fellow:** Geriatric Medicine, LIJ Med Ctr 1988; **Fac Appt:** Asst Clin Prof Med, Albert Einstein Coll Med

Macina, Lucy MD (Ger) PCP - **Spec Exp:** Frail Elderly; Dementia; **Hospital:** Winthrop - Univ Hosp; **Address:** 222 Station Plaza N, Ste 518, Mineola, NY 11501-3893; **Phone:** 516-663-2588; **Board Cert:** Internal Medicine 1982; Geriatric Medicine 2002; **Med School:** Loyola Univ-Stritch Sch Med 1978; **Resid:** Internal Medicine, VA Hosp 1980; Internal Medicine, Loyola U-Stritch Sch Med 1982; **Fellow:** Geriatric Medicine, Roger Williams Med Ctr 1985; **Fac Appt:** Asst Clin Prof Med, SUNY Stony Brook

Wolf-Klein, Gisele MD (Ger) PCP - **Spec Exp:** Dementia; Falls in the Elderly; **Hospital:** Long Island Jewish Med Ctr; **Address:** 1 Delaware Drive, Ste 102, Lake Success, NY 11042; **Phone:** 516-586-1700; **Board Cert:** Internal Medicine 1984; Geriatric Medicine 1998; **Med School:** Switzerland 1975; **Resid:** Internal Medicine, Long Island Hosp 1978; **Fellow:** Geriatric Medicine, LI Jewish Med Ctr 1979

GYNECOLOGIC ONCOLOGY

Lovecchio, John MD (GO) - **Spec Exp:** Ovarian Cancer; Uterine Cancer; Cervical Cancer; Vulvar Disease/Cancer; **Hospital:** N Shore Univ Hosp at Manhasset; **Address:** North Shore Hospital, 10 Monti, 300 Community Drive, Manhasset, NY 11030-3876; **Phone:** 516-562-4438; **Board Cert:** Obstetrics & Gynecology 1999; Gynecologic Oncology 1999; **Med School:** SUNY Buffalo 1975; **Resid:** Obstetrics & Gynecology, Univ Hosp Case West Res 1979; **Fellow:** Gynecologic Oncology, Jackson Meml Hosp 1982; **Fac Appt:** Prof ObG, NYU Sch Med

Menzin, Andrew MD (GO) - **Spec Exp:** Uterine Cancer; Ovarian Cancer; Cervical Cancer; **Hospital:** N Shore Univ Hosp at Manhasset; **Address:** North Shore Univ Hosp, Div Gyn Oncology, 300 Community Drive, Manhasset, NY 11030; **Phone:** 516-562-4438; **Board Cert:** Obstetrics & Gynecology 1999; Gynecologic Oncology 1999; **Med School:** NYU Sch Med 1989; **Resid:** Obstetrics & Gynecology, Hosp Univ Penn 1993; **Fellow:** Gynecologic Oncology, Hosp Univ Penn 1995; **Fac Appt:** Assoc Clin Prof ObG, NYU Sch Med

Seltzer, Vicki MD (GO) - **Hospital:** Long Island Jewish Med Ctr, N Shore Univ Hosp at Manhasset; **Address:** LI Jewish Med Ctr, Dept Ob/Gyn, 270-05 76th Ave, Ste 1100, New Hyde Parl, NY 11040; **Phone:** 718-470-7660; **Board Cert:** Obstetrics & Gynecology 1979; Gynecologic Oncology 1982; **Med School:** NYU Sch Med 1973; **Resid:** Obstetrics & Gynecology, Bellevue Hosp 1977; **Fellow:** Gynecologic Oncology, NY Med Coll 1978; Gynecologic Oncology, Meml Sloan Kettering Cancer Ctr 1979; **Fac Appt:** Prof ObG, Albert Einstein Coll Med

Smotkin, David MD (GO) - **Spec Exp:** Gynecologic Cancer; **Hospital:** Long Island Jewish Med Ctr; **Address:** LIJ Medical Ctr, Dept Ob/Gyn, 270-05 76th Ave, rm 1100, New Hyde Park, NY 11040; **Phone:** 718-470-7660; **Board Cert:** Obstetrics & Gynecology 1998; Gynecologic Oncology 1998; **Med School:** Yale Univ 1980; **Fellow:** Gynecologic Oncology, UCLA Med Ctr 1987

HAND SURGERY

Kamler, Kenneth MD (HS) - **Spec Exp:** Carpal Tunnel Syndrome; Arthritis; Fractures; **Hospital:** Long Island Jewish Med Ctr, Winthrop - Univ Hosp; **Address:** 410 Lakeville Rd, Ste 100, New Hyde Park, NY 11042-1102; **Phone:** 516-326-8810; **Med School:** France 1975; **Resid:** Orthopaedic Surgery, LI Jewish Med Ctr 1979; **Fellow:** Hand Surgery, Columbia-Presby Med Ctr 1981

Lane, Lewis B MD (HS) - **Spec Exp:** Carpal Tunnel Syndrome; Arthritis; Sports Injuries; **Hospital:** N Shore Univ Hosp at Manhasset, St Francis Hosp - The Heart Ctr (page 112); **Address:** 600 Northern Blvd, Ste 300, Great Neck, NY 11021; **Phone:** 516-627-8717; **Board Cert:** Orthopaedic Surgery 1981; Hand Surgery 2000; **Med School:** Columbia P&S 1974; **Resid:** Surgery, New York Hosp 1975; Orthopaedic Surgery, Hosp for Special Surg 1979; **Fellow:** Research, Hosp for Special Surg 1976; Hand Surgery, St Luke's-Roosevelt Hosp Ctr 1980; **Fac Appt:** Assoc Clin Prof OrS, Albert Einstein Coll Med

Palmieri, Thomas J MD (HS) - **Spec Exp:** Arthritis; Carpal Tunnel Syndrome; Nerve Compression; **Hospital:** Long Island Jewish Med Ctr, N Shore Univ Hosp at Manhasset; **Address:** 1901 New Hyde Park Rd, New Hyde Park, NY 11040; **Phone:** 516-822-4843; **Board Cert:** Surgery 1971; Hand Surgery 1996; **Med School:** SUNY Hlth Sci Ctr 1964; **Resid:** Internal Medicine, St Luke's-Roosevelt Hosp Ctr 1966; Surgery, LI Jewish Med Ctr 1970; **Fellow:** Hand Surgery, Hosp Joint Diseases; Hand Surgery, Columbia Presby Med Ctr; **Fac Appt:** Assoc Clin Prof S, Albert Einstein Coll Med

HEMATOLOGY

Allen, Steven MD (Hem) - **Spec Exp:** Coagulation Disorders; Leukemia; Multiple Myeloma; **Hospital:** N Shore Univ Hosp at Manhasset, Long Island Jewish Med Ctr; **Address:** Monter Cancer Ctr, 450 Lakeville Rd, Lake Success, NY 11042; **Phone:** 516-734-8959; **Board Cert:** Internal Medicine 1980; Hematology 1982; Medical Oncology 1983; **Med School:** Johns Hopkins Univ 1977; **Resid:** Internal Medicine, New York Hosp-Cornell 1980; **Fellow:** Hematology & Oncology, New York Hosp-Cornell 1983; **Fac Appt:** Assoc Prof Med, NYU Sch Med

Dittmar, Klaus MD (Hem) - **Spec Exp:** Lymphoma; Multiple Myeloma; Anemia; Hematologic Malignancies; **Hospital:** N Shore Univ Hosp at Manhasset, St Francis Hosp - The Heart Ctr (page 112); **Address:** 1201 Northern Blvd, Manhasset, NY 11030-3001; **Phone:** 516-627-1221; **Board Cert:** Internal Medicine 1969; Hematology 1972; Medical Oncology 1979; **Med School:** Germany 1957; **Resid:** Internal Medicine, Mt Sinai Hosp 1964; Hematology, Mt Sinai Hosp 1965; **Fac Appt:** Asst Clin Prof Med, NYU Sch Med

Kolitz, Jonathan E MD (Hem) - **Spec Exp:** Leukemia; Hematologic Malignancies; Hodgkin's Disease; Lymphoma; **Hospital:** N Shore Univ Hosp at Manhasset; **Address:** N Shore Univ Hosp, Monti Bldg, 300 Community Drive Fl 9, Manhasset, NY 11030; **Phone:** 516-562-8970; **Board Cert:** Internal Medicine 1982; Medical Oncology 1985; Hematology 1988; **Med School:** Yale Univ 1979; **Resid:** Internal Medicine, N Shore Univ Hosp 1982; **Fellow:** Hematology & Oncology, Meml Sloan Kettering Cancer Ctr 1985; **Fac Appt:** Assoc Prof Med, NYU Sch Med

Rai, Kanti MD (Hem) - **Spec Exp:** Leukemia; Lymphoma; Multiple Myeloma; **Hospital:** Long Island Jewish Med Ctr; **Address:** 270-05 76th Ave, New Hyde Park, NY 11040-1433; **Phone:** 718-470-7135; **Board Cert:** Pediatrics 1961; **Med School:** India 1955; **Resid:** Pediatrics, Lincoln Hosp 1958; Pediatrics, North Shore Univ Hosp 1959; **Fellow:** Hematology, LI Jewish Med Ctr 1960; **Fac Appt:** Prof Med, Albert Einstein Coll Med

Wang, Jen Chin MD (Hem) - **Hospital:** Long Beach Med Ctr, N Shore Univ Hosp at Manhasset; **Address:** 5 E Walnut St, Long Beach, NY 11561; **Phone:** 516-889-7447; **Board Cert:** Internal Medicine 1976; Hematology 1978; Medical Oncology 1977; **Med School:** Taiwan 1969; **Resid:** Internal Medicine, Brookdale Hosp 1974; Hematology & Oncology, Brookdale Hosp 1976; **Fac Appt:** Assoc Prof Med, Mount Sinai Sch Med

INFECTIOUS DISEASE

Cervia, Joseph MD (Inf) - **Spec Exp:** AIDS/HIV; Travel Medicine; Pediatric Infections; **Hospital:** N Shore Univ Hosp at Manhasset, Schneider Chldn's Hosp; **Address:** North Shore-LIJ Health System, 300 Community Drive, Manhasset, NY 11030; **Phone:** 516-562-4280; **Board Cert:** Internal Medicine 1989; Pediatrics 1989; Infectious Disease 1998; Pediatric Infectious Disease 2002; **Med School:** NY Med Coll 1984; **Resid:** Internal Medicine, Brookdale Hosp 1988; Pediatrics, Brookdale Hosp 1988; **Fellow:** Infectious Disease, New York Hosp/Cornell 1990; **Fac Appt:** Prof Med, Albert Einstein Coll Med

Cunha, Burke A MD (Inf) - **Spec Exp:** Infections in Immunocompromised Patients; Fevers of Unknown Origin; Pneumonia; Chronic Fatigue Syndrome; **Hospital:** Winthrop - Univ Hosp; **Address:** 222 Station Plz N, Ste 432, Mineola, NY 11501; **Phone:** 516-663-2507; **Board Cert:** Internal Medicine 1977; Infectious Disease 1978; **Med School:** Penn State Univ-Hershey Med Ctr 1972; **Resid:** Internal Medicine, Hartford Hosp 1975; **Fellow:** Infectious Disease, Hartford Hosp 1977; **Fac Appt:** Prof Med, SUNY Stony Brook

Farber, Bruce MD (Inf) - **Hospital:** N Shore Univ Hosp at Manhasset; **Address:** N Shore Univ Hosp, Div Infectious Dis, 300 Community Drive Fl 4, Manhasset, NY 11030; **Phone:** 516-562-4280; **Board Cert:** Internal Medicine 1979; Infectious Disease 1984; **Med School:** Northwestern Univ 1976; **Resid:** Internal Medicine, Univ Va Hosp 1979; **Fellow:** Infectious Disease, Mass Genl Hosp 1982

Glatt, Aaron E MD/DDS (Inf) - **Spec Exp:** Antibiotic Resistance; Urinary Tract Infections; Pneumonia; **Hospital:** New Island Hosp; **Address:** New Island Hospital, 4295 Hempstead Tpke, Bethpage, NY 11714; **Phone:** 516-520-2387; **Board Cert:** Internal Medicine 1986; Infectious Disease 1988; **Med School:** Columbia P&S 1983; **Resid:** Internal Medicine, Brookdale Hosp 1986; **Fellow:** Infectious Disease, SUNY Brooklyn Health Sci Ctr 1988

Greenspan, Joel MD (Inf) - **Hospital:** N Shore Univ Hosp at Manhasset; **Address:** 44 S Bayles Ave, Ste 216, Port Washington, NY 11050; **Phone:** 516-767-7771; **Board Cert:** Infectious Disease 1978; Internal Medicine 1973; **Med School:** SUNY Upstate Med Univ 1969; **Resid:** Internal Medicine, Bellevue Hosp 1972; Internal Medicine, Bellevue Hosp 1973; **Fellow:** Infectious Disease, Bellevue Hosp 1977; **Fac Appt:** Asst Clin Prof Med, NYU Sch Med

Hilton, Eileen MD (Inf) - **Spec Exp:** Lyme Disease; Travel Medicine; **Hospital:** Long Island Jewish Med Ctr; **Address:** 225 Community Dr, Ste 100, Great Neck, NY 11021; **Phone:** 516-470-6900; **Board Cert:** Internal Medicine 1981; Infectious Disease 1984; **Med School:** Columbia P&S 1978; **Resid:** Internal Medicine, Bronx Muni Hosp 1981; **Fellow:** Infectious Disease, Montefiore Med Ctr/ Albert Einstein 1983; **Fac Appt:** Prof Med, Albert Einstein Coll Med

Johnson, Diane H MD (Inf) - **Spec Exp:** AIDS/HIV; Sexually Transmitted Diseases; Travel Medicine; **Hospital:** Winthrop - Univ Hosp; **Address:** 222 Satation Plaza N, Ste 432, Mineola, NY 11501; **Phone:** 516-663-2505; **Board Cert:** Internal Medicine 2004; Infectious Disease 2004; **Med School:** Univ VT Coll Med 1989; **Resid:** Internal Medicine, Winthrop Univ Hosp 1992; **Fellow:** Infectious Disease, Winthrop Univ Hosp 1994; **Fac Appt:** Asst Prof Med, SUNY Stony Brook

Klein, Natalie MD (Inf) - **Hospital:** Winthrop - Univ Hosp; **Address:** 222 Station Plaza N, Ste 432, Mineola, NY 11501-3957; **Phone:** 516-663-2507; **Board Cert:** Internal Medicine 1982; Infectious Disease 1984; **Med School:** Jefferson Med Coll 1979; **Resid:** Internal Medicine, Mount Sinai Hosp 1982; **Fellow:** Infectious Disease, Mount Sinai Hosp 1984; **Fac Appt:** Assoc Prof Med, SUNY Stony Brook

Scheer, Max MD (Inf) - **Spec Exp:** Skin/Soft Tissue Infection; Infections-Respiratory; Sexually Transmitted Diseases; **Hospital:** N Shore Univ Hosp at Manhasset; **Address:** 15 Irving Pl, Woodmere, NY 11598-1229; **Phone:** 516-374-6750; **Board Cert:** Internal Medicine 1979; Infectious Disease 1982; **Med School:** SUNY Downstate 1975; **Resid:** Family Medicine, Kings Co Hosp-SUNY 1978; Internal Medicine, Morristown Meml Hosp 1979; **Fellow:** Infectious Disease, Mt Sinai Hosp 1981; **Fac Appt:** Asst Clin Prof Med, NYU Sch Med

Singer, Carol MD (Inf) - **Spec Exp:** Infections in Immunocompromised Patients; Travel Medicine; **Hospital:** Long Island Jewish Med Ctr; **Address:** 270-05 76th Ave, Staff House, Ste 226, New Hyde Park, NY 11040-1433; **Phone:** 718-470-7290; **Board Cert:** Internal Medicine 1973; Infectious Disease 1978; **Med School:** Cornell Univ-Weill Med Coll 1970; **Resid:** Internal Medicine, Univ Michigan Med Ctr 1972; Internal Medicine, NY Hosp 1973; **Fellow:** Infectious Disease, Memorial Hosp 1975; **Fac Appt:** Prof Med, Albert Einstein Coll Med

Smith, Miriam MD (Inf) - **Spec Exp:** Lyme Disease; **Hospital:** Long Island Jewish Med Ctr; **Address:** LIJ Med Ctr, Div Infectious Disease, 270-05 76th Ave, Staff House, Ste 226, New Hyde Park, NY 11040; **Phone:** 718-470-7290; **Board Cert:** Internal Medicine 1982; Infectious Disease 1984; **Med School:** Univ Cincinnati 1979; **Resid:** Internal Medicine, Stanford Univ Hosp 1982; **Fellow:** Infectious Disease, Einstein Montefiore Med Ctr 1985

INTERNAL MEDICINE

Ammazzalorso, Michael MD (IM) **PCP** - **Spec Exp:** Hypertension; Diabetes; **Hospital:** Winthrop - Univ Hosp; **Address:** 222 Station Plz N, Ste 310, Mineola, NY 11501-3893; **Phone:** 516-663-2051; **Board Cert:** Internal Medicine 2000; Geriatric Medicine 2003; **Med School:** SUNY Downstate 1987; **Resid:** Internal Medicine, Staten Island Hosp 1991; **Fac Appt:** Asst Prof Med, SUNY Stony Brook

Ausubel, Herbert MD (IM) **PCP** - **Hospital:** Franklin Hosp Med Ctr, Mercy Med Ctr - Rockville Centre; **Address:** 509 W Merrick Rd, Ste 101, Valley Stream, NY 11580-5236; **Phone:** 516-561-8188; **Board Cert:** Internal Medicine 1961; **Med School:** Harvard Med Sch 1954; **Resid:** Internal Medicine, Bellevue Hosp Ctr 1959; Hematology, Mt Sinai Med Ctr 1960; **Fellow:** Medical Oncology, Meml Sloan Kettering Canc Ctr

Berger, Jeffrey MD (IM) **PCP** - **Spec Exp:** Ethics; Palliative Care; **Hospital:** Winthrop - Univ Hosp; **Address:** 222 Station Plaza North, Ste 518, Mineola, NY 11501-3808; **Phone:** 516-663-2588; **Board Cert:** Internal Medicine 2001; **Med School:** SUNY Stony Brook 1988; **Resid:** Internal Medicine, Winthrop Univ Hosp 1991; **Fac Appt:** Assoc Prof Med, SUNY Stony Brook

Ciccarelli, Ciro MD (IM) - **Spec Exp:** Pulmonary Disease; **Hospital:** South Nassau Comm Hosp; **Address:** Pulmonary & Critical Care Consultants, 444 Merrick Rd, Lynbrook, NY 11563; **Phone:** 516-593-9500; **Board Cert:** Internal Medicine 1989; **Med School:** Italy 1985; **Resid:** Internal Medicine, Mt Sinai-Elmhurst Hosp 1988; **Fellow:** Pulmonary Disease, Mt Sinai-Elmhurst Hosp 1990

Condon, Edward M MD (IM) PCP - **Spec Exp:** Diabetes; Thyroid Disorders; Hypogonadism; Adrenal Disorders; **Hospital:** N Shore Univ Hosp at Manhasset, Long Island Jewish Med Ctr; **Address:** 833 Northern Blvd, Ste 120, Great Neck, NY 11021; **Phone:** 516-487-0167; **Med School:** Mexico 1973; **Resid:** Internal Medicine, Mount Sinai Hosp 1976; **Fellow:** Endocrinology, Diabetes & Metabolism, Mount Sinai Hosp 1978

Corapi, Mark MD (IM) PCP - **Hospital:** Winthrop - Univ Hosp; **Address:** 222 Station Plaza N, Ste 310, Mineola, NY 11501; **Phone:** 516-663-2056; **Board Cert:** Internal Medicine 1985; **Med School:** SUNY Downstate 1982; **Resid:** Internal Medicine, Long Island Jewish Med Ctr 1985; **Fellow:** Internal Medicine, Long Island Jewish Med Ctr 1986; **Fac Appt:** Assoc Prof Med, SUNY Stony Brook

Cusumano, Stephen MD (IM) PCP - **Spec Exp:** Hypertension; Asthma; **Hospital:** New Island Hosp, Winthrop - Univ Hosp; **Address:** 850 Hicksville Rd, Ste 110, Seaford, NY 11783; **Phone:** 516-735-5454; **Board Cert:** Internal Medicine 1988; **Med School:** Univ Hlth Sci/Chicago Med Sch 1985; **Resid:** Internal Medicine, Winthrop Univ Hosp 1988

Federbush, Richard MD (IM) PCP - **Spec Exp:** Hypertension; Cholesterol/Lipid Disorders; Diabetes; **Hospital:** N Shore Univ Hosp at Plainview, N Shore Univ Hosp at Syosset; **Address:** 175 Jericho Tpke, Ste 216, Syosset, NY 11791; **Phone:** 516-364-9800; **Board Cert:** Internal Medicine 2001; **Med School:** Mexico 1985; **Resid:** Internal Medicine, Univ Hosp-SUNY 1989

Foley, Conn J MD (IM) PCP - **Spec Exp:** Alzheimer's Disease; **Hospital:** Long Island Jewish Med Ctr; **Address:** Medical Dept, 271-11 76th Ave, New Hyde Park, NY 11040; **Phone:** 718-289-2277; **Board Cert:** Geriatric Medicine 1988; Internal Medicine 1979; **Med School:** Ireland 1972; **Resid:** Internal Medicine, Oakwood Hosp 1978; **Fellow:** Geriatric Medicine, LI Jewish Med Ctr 1979; **Fac Appt:** Assoc Prof Med, Albert Einstein Coll Med

Gelberg, Burt MD (IM) PCP - **Spec Exp:** Preventive Medicine; Gastrointestinal Endoscopy; **Hospital:** Franklin Hosp Med Ctr, Mercy Med Ctr - Rockville Centre; **Address:** 401 Franklin Ave, Franklin Square, NY 11010-1227; **Phone:** 516-326-2255; **Board Cert:** Internal Medicine 1975; **Med School:** SUNY Hlth Sci Ctr 1972; **Resid:** Internal Medicine, Lenox Hill Hosp 1975; **Fellow:** Gastroenterology, Lenox Hill Hosp 1977

Goodman, Michael MD (IM) - **Hospital:** South Nassau Comm Hosp; **Address:** 2495 Newbridge Rd, Bellmore, NY 11710; **Phone:** 516-826-1200; **Board Cert:** Internal Medicine 1980; **Med School:** Italy 1975; **Resid:** Internal Medicine, Nassau County Med Ctr 1978

Gorski, Lydia E MD (IM) PCP - **Spec Exp:** Women's Health; Geriatric Medicine; Preventive Medicine; **Hospital:** Winthrop - Univ Hosp, N Shore Univ Hosp at Manhasset; **Address:** 820 Jericho Tpke, New Hyde Park, NY 11040-4514; **Phone:** 516-352-0430; **Board Cert:** Internal Medicine 1988; **Med School:** Poland 1982; **Resid:** Internal Medicine, St Vincent's Catholic Med Ctrs 1986

Gottridge, Joanne MD (IM) `PCP` - **Hospital:** N Shore Univ Hosp at Manhasset; **Address:** 865 Northern Blvd, Ste 102, Great Neck, NY 11021; **Phone:** 516-622-5001; **Board Cert:** Internal Medicine 1983; **Med School:** Case West Res Univ 1980; **Resid:** Internal Medicine, N Shore Univ Hosp 1983; **Fac Appt:** Prof Med, NYU Sch Med

Holden, Melvin MD (IM) `PCP` - **Hospital:** N Shore Univ Hosp at Plainview; **Address:** 453 S Oyster Bay Rd, Plainview, NY 11803; **Phone:** 516-433-2922; **Board Cert:** Pulmonary Disease 1971; Internal Medicine 1966; **Med School:** SUNY Downstate 1959; **Resid:** Internal Medicine, Montefiore Hosp Med Ctr 1962; Internal Medicine, VA Med Ctr 1963; **Fac Appt:** Asst Clin Prof Med, SUNY Stony Brook

Hotchkiss, Edward MD (IM) `PCP` - **Hospital:** Long Island Jewish Med Ctr, South Nassau Comm Hosp; **Address:** 158 Hempstead Ave, Lynbrook, NY 11563-1605; **Phone:** 516-593-3541; **Board Cert:** Internal Medicine 1972; **Med School:** SUNY Hlth Sci Ctr 1965; **Resid:** Internal Medicine, LI Jewish Med Ctr 1972; **Fellow:** Psychiatry, Univ Hosp 1971; **Fac Appt:** Assoc Prof Med, Albert Einstein Coll Med

Leong, Pauline MD (IM) `PCP` - **Hospital:** N Shore Univ Hosp at Manhasset; **Address:** 865 Northern Blvd, Ste 102, Great Neck, NY 11021-5310; **Phone:** 516-622-5000; **Board Cert:** Internal Medicine 1988; **Med School:** NYU Sch Med 1983; **Resid:** Internal Medicine, New York Hosp 1988

Pascaru, Adina MD (IM) - **Spec Exp:** Coronary Artery Disease; **Hospital:** N Shore Univ Hosp at Manhasset, St Francis Hosp - The Heart Ctr (page 112); **Address:** 833 Northern Blvd, Ste 120, Great Neck, NY 11021; **Phone:** 516-829-6660; **Board Cert:** Internal Medicine 1983; Cardiovascular Disease 1987; **Med School:** Romania 1964; **Resid:** Internal Medicine, LIJ Med Ctr 1981; **Fellow:** Cardiovascular Disease, LIJ Med Ctr 1983

Pollak, Harvey MD (IM) `PCP` - **Spec Exp:** Hypertension; Heart Disease; Cholesterol/Lipid Disorders; **Hospital:** N Shore Univ Hosp at Manhasset; **Address:** 2800 Marcus Ave, Lake Success, NY 11042; **Phone:** 516-622-6040; **Board Cert:** Internal Medicine 1974; **Med School:** Univ Hlth Sci/Chicago Med Sch 1971; **Resid:** Internal Medicine, N Shore Univ Hosp 1975; **Fac Appt:** Prof Med, NYU Sch Med

Rakowitz, Frederic MD (IM) `PCP` - **Spec Exp:** Preventive Medicine; **Hospital:** N Shore Univ Hosp at Manhasset; **Address:** 295 Northern Blvd, Ste 208, Great Neck, NY 11021; **Phone:** 516-482-4940; **Board Cert:** Internal Medicine 1981; **Med School:** Albany Med Coll 1978; **Resid:** Internal Medicine, North Shore Univ Hosp 1981

Rosenberg, Alan MD (IM) `PCP` - **Spec Exp:** Congestive Heart Failure; Preventive Cardiology; **Hospital:** N Shore Univ Hosp at Manhasset; **Address:** 1010 Northern Blvd, rm 110, Great Neck, NY 11021; **Phone:** 516-390-2410; **Board Cert:** Internal Medicine 1971; **Med School:** Albert Einstein Coll Med 1962; **Resid:** Internal Medicine, Montefiore Hosp Med Ctr 1967; Cardiovascular Disease, Montefiore Hosp Med Ctr 1968; **Fellow:** Cardiovascular Disease, Mount Sinai Hosp 1969; **Fac Appt:** Asst Clin Prof Med, NYU Sch Med

Rubenstein, Jack MD (IM) `PCP` - **Spec Exp:** Complex Diagnosis; Kidney Failure/Pre-Dialysis; Geriatric Care; **Hospital:** N Shore Univ Hosp at Manhasset, Franklin Hosp Med Ctr; **Address:** 70 Glen Cove Rd, Ste 301, Roslyn Heights, NY 11577-1731; **Phone:** 516-621-1502; **Board Cert:** Internal Medicine 1998; Nephrology 1998; Geriatric Medicine 1998; **Med School:** NY Med Coll 1976; **Resid:** Internal Medicine, North Shore Univ Hosp 1979; **Fellow:** Nephrology, North Shore Univ Hosp 1980; Nephrology, NYU Med Ctr 1982; **Fac Appt:** Assoc Clin Prof Med, NYU Sch Med

Rucker, Steve MD (IM) `PCP` - **Spec Exp:** Hypertension; Kidney Disease; Kidney Stones; **Hospital:** St Francis Hosp - The Heart Ctr (page 112), Long Island Jewish Med Ctr; **Address:** 488 Great Neck Rd, Ste 225, Great Neck, NY 11021; **Phone:** 516-482-8880; **Board Cert:** Internal Medicine 1986; Nephrology 1988; **Med School:** Univ Pittsburgh 1983; **Resid:** Internal Medicine, LI Jewish Med Ctr 1986; **Fellow:** Nephrology, Mount Sinai Med Ctr 1988

Smith, Lawrence MD (IM) - **Spec Exp:** Sports Medicine; **Hospital:** N Shore Univ Hosp at Manhasset; **Address:** 125 Community Drive, Great Neck, NY 11021; **Phone:** 516-465-3194; **Board Cert:** Internal Medicine 1979; Critical Care Medicine 1997; **Med School:** NYU Sch Med 1976; **Resid:** Internal Medicine, Strong Meml Hosp 1979; **Fac Appt:** Prof Med, Mount Sinai Sch Med

Taubman, Lowell MD (IM) `PCP` - **Spec Exp:** Dementia; Alzheimer's Disease; **Hospital:** Long Beach Med Ctr; **Address:** 206 Riverside Blvd, Long Beach, NY 11561; **Phone:** 516-432-5670; **Board Cert:** Internal Medicine 1988; **Med School:** Mexico 1980; **Resid:** Internal Medicine, Montefiore Hosp 1983; Internal Medicine, St Clares Hosp 1984; **Fellow:** Geriatric Medicine, Jewish Inst Geriatric Care 1986

Timpone, Leonard MD (IM) `PCP` - **Spec Exp:** Geriatric Medicine; Headache; **Hospital:** Franklin Hosp Med Ctr, Mercy Med Ctr - Rockville Centre; **Address:** 1051 Adams Ave, Franklin Square, NY 11010-2251; **Phone:** 516-354-4858; **Board Cert:** Internal Medicine 2003; **Med School:** France 1984; **Resid:** Internal Medicine, NY Downtown Hosp 1988

Weinstein, Mark MD (IM) `PCP` - **Spec Exp:** Hypertension; Diabetes; Cholesterol/Lipid Disorders; **Hospital:** N Shore Univ Hosp at Plainview, New Island Hosp; **Address:** 4277 Hempsttead Tpke, Ste 209, Bethpage, NY 11714-5706; **Phone:** 516-731-7770; **Board Cert:** Internal Medicine 1978; Infectious Disease 1980; **Med School:** Harvard Med Sch 1975; **Resid:** Internal Medicine, Univ Hosp 1978; **Fellow:** Infectious Disease, Univ Hosp 1980

INTERVENTIONAL CARDIOLOGY

Abittan, Meyer H MD (IC) - **Spec Exp:** Angiography-Coronary; Preventive Cardiology; **Hospital:** St Francis Hosp - The Heart Ctr (page 112); **Address:** St Francis Hosp, The Heart Ctr, 100 Port Washington Blvd, Ste G-03, Roslyn, NY 11576; **Phone:** 516-365-6444; **Board Cert:** Internal Medicine 1989; Cardiovascular Disease 1991; Interventional Cardiology 1999; **Med School:** Mount Sinai Sch Med 1986; **Resid:** Internal Medicine, Brookdale Univ Hosp Med Ctr 1989; **Fellow:** Cardiovascular Disease, Mt Sinai Med Ctr 1990

Berke, Andrew D MD (IC) - **Hospital:** St Francis Hosp - The Heart Ctr (page 112), South Nassau Comm Hosp; **Address:** 100 Port Washington Blvd, Roslyn, NY 11576; **Phone:** 516-365-2211; **Board Cert:** Interventional Cardiology 1999; Cardiovascular Disease 1985; Internal Medicine 1982; **Med School:** Brown Univ 1979; **Resid:** Internal Medicine, Columbia-Presby Med Ctr 1982; **Fellow:** Cardiovascular Disease, Columbia-Presby Med Ctr 1985; **Fac Appt:** Asst Clin Prof Med, Columbia P&S

Lituchy, Andrew MD (IC) - **Spec Exp:** Coronary Artery Disease; Angioplasty & Stent Placement; Congestive Heart Failure; Peripheral Vascular Disease; **Hospital:** St Francis Hosp - The Heart Ctr (page 112), South Nassau Comm Hosp; **Address:** 100 Port Washington Blvd, Roslyn, NY 11576; **Phone:** 516-365-4888; **Board Cert:** Internal Medicine 1991; Cardiovascular Disease 1995; Interventional Cardiology 2000; **Med School:** Hahnemann Univ 1988; **Resid:** Internal Medicine, Bronx Muni/Albert Einstein Med Ctr 1991; **Fellow:** Cardiovascular Disease, NY-Cornell Med Ctr 1994; Interventional Cardiology, NY-Cornell Med Ctr 1995

Petrossian, George A MD (IC) - **Spec Exp:** Carotid Artery Stents; Peripheral Vascular Disease; Coronary Angioplasty/Stents; **Hospital:** St Francis Hosp - The Heart Ctr (page 112), South Nassau Comm Hosp; **Address:** New York Cardiology Group, 100 Port Washington Blvd, Roslyn, NY 11576-1353; **Phone:** 516-365-5000; **Board Cert:** Internal Medicine 1986; Cardiovascular Disease 1989; Interventional Cardiology 2000; **Med School:** Mount Sinai Sch Med 1983; **Resid:** Internal Medicine, Columbia-Presby Med Ctr 1987; **Fellow:** Cardiovascular Disease, Columbia -Presby Med Ctr 1989; Interventional Cardiology, Mass Genl Hosp 1990

MATERNAL & FETAL MEDICINE

Klein, Victor MD (MF) - **Spec Exp:** Multiple Gestation; Pregnancy-High Risk; **Hospital:** N Shore Univ Hosp at Manhasset; **Address:** 900 Northern Blvd, Ste 220, Great Neck, NY 11021-5302; **Phone:** 516-466-0778; **Board Cert:** Obstetrics & Gynecology 1997; Maternal & Fetal Medicine 1997; Clinical Genetics 2002; **Med School:** SUNY Downstate 1980; **Resid:** Internal Medicine, Kings Co Hosp Ctr 1981; Obstetrics & Gynecology, Johns Hopkins 1985; **Fellow:** Clinical Genetics, Univ Texas SW Med Ctr 1988; Maternal & Fetal Medicine, Univ Texas SW Med Ctr 1988; **Fac Appt:** Assoc Prof ObG, NYU Sch Med

Maulik, Dev MD/PhD (MF) - **Spec Exp:** Pregnancy-High Risk; **Hospital:** Winthrop - Univ Hosp; **Address:** Winthrop Univ Hosp, Dept Ob/Gyn, 259 1st St, Mineola, NY 11501; **Phone:** 516-663-2264; **Board Cert:** Maternal & Fetal Medicine 1999; Obstetrics & Gynecology 1999; **Med School:** India 1962; **Resid:** Obstetrics & Gynecology, Truman Hosp 1970; Obstetrics & Gynecology, Charing Cross Hosp 1975; **Fellow:** Maternal & Fetal Medicine, Strong Meml Hosp 1987; **Fac Appt:** Prof ObG, SUNY Stony Brook

Rochelson, Burton MD (MF) - **Spec Exp:** Pregnancy-High Risk; Ultrasound; Prenatal Diagnosis; **Hospital:** N Shore Univ Hosp at Manhasset; **Address:** N Shore Univ Hosp, Dept Maternal/Fetal Med, 300 Community Drive, Manhasset, NY 11030-3876; **Phone:** 516-562-4458; **Board Cert:** Obstetrics & Gynecology 1997; Maternal & Fetal Medicine 1997; **Med School:** Univ Mich Med Sch 1978; **Resid:** Obstetrics & Gynecology, LI Jewish Med Ctr 1982; **Fellow:** Maternal & Fetal Medicine, Univ Hosp 1986; **Fac Appt:** Assoc Clin Prof ObG, NYU Sch Med

MEDICAL ONCOLOGY

Bradley, Thomas P MD (Onc) - **Spec Exp:** Lymphoma; Prostate Cancer; **Hospital:** N Shore Univ Hosp at Manhasset; **Address:** N Shore Univ Hosp-Dept Hem/Oncology, 300 Community Drive-Monti Bldg, Fl9, Manhasset, NY 11030; **Phone:** 516-562-8900; **Board Cert:** Internal Medicine 1987; Medical Oncology 2001; Hematology 2002; **Med School:** Mexico 1982; **Resid:** Internal Medicine, Univ Hosp-SUNY Downstate 1987; **Fellow:** Hematology & Oncology, Univ Hosp-SUNY Downstate 1991; **Fac Appt:** Asst Prof Med, NYU Sch Med

Budman, Daniel MD (Onc) - **Spec Exp:** Breast Cancer; Leukemia; Clinical Pharmacology; **Hospital:** N Shore Univ Hosp at Manhasset; **Address:** North Shore Univ Hosp, Div Med Oncology, 300 Community Dr, Monti Bldg, 9th Fl, Manhasset, NY 11030; **Phone:** 516-562-8958; **Board Cert:** Internal Medicine 1975; Hematology 1978; Medical Oncology 1979; **Med School:** Albert Einstein Coll Med 1972; **Resid:** Internal Medicine, Hosp Univ Penn 1974; Hematology, Natl Inst Hlth 1976; **Fellow:** Medical Oncology, Sloan Kettering Cancer Ctr 1977; Hematology, NYU Med Ctr 1978; **Fac Appt:** Prof Med, NYU Sch Med

Citron, Marc L MD (Onc) - **Spec Exp:** Breast Cancer; Lung Cancer; **Hospital:** Long Island Jewish Med Ctr; **Address:** Pro Hlthcare Assoc, Div Oncology, 2800 Marcus Ave, Ste 205, New Hyde Park, NY 11042-1008; **Phone:** 516-622-6150; **Board Cert:** Internal Medicine 1977; Medical Oncology 1979; **Med School:** Wayne State Univ 1974; **Resid:** Internal Medicine, Georgetown Univ Hosp 1977; **Fellow:** Medical Oncology, Georgetown Univ Hosp 1979; **Fac Appt:** Clin Prof Med, Albert Einstein Coll Med

Kappel, Bruce MD (Onc) - **Spec Exp:** Breast Cancer; Colon Cancer; **Hospital:** N Shore Univ Hosp at Plainview, New Island Hosp; **Address:** 40 Crossways Park Drive, Ste 103, Woodbury, NY 11791; **Phone:** 516-921-5533; **Board Cert:** Internal Medicine 1985; Medical Oncology 1987; Hematology 1988; **Med School:** Emory Univ 1982; **Resid:** Internal Medicine, Emory Univ Hosp 1985; **Fellow:** Medical Oncology, Columbia-Presby Med Ctr 1988

Kessler, Leonard MD (Onc) - **Hospital:** South Nassau Comm Hosp, Mercy Med Ctr - Rockville Centre; **Address:** 242 Merrick Rd, Ste 301, Rockville Centre, NY 11570; **Phone:** 516-536-1455; **Board Cert:** Internal Medicine 1979; Medical Oncology 1981; Hematology 1982; **Med School:** Albert Einstein Coll Med 1975; **Resid:** Internal Medicine, Montefiore Hosp Med Ctr 1977; **Fellow:** Hematology, Montefiore Hosp Med Ctr 1981; Medical Oncology, Meml Sloan Kettering Cancer Ctr 1980

Marino, John MD (Onc) - **Spec Exp:** Breast Cancer; Colon Cancer; Lung Cancer; **Hospital:** N Shore Univ Hosp at Manhasset, St Francis Hosp - The Heart Ctr (page 112); **Address:** 44 S Bayles Ave, Bldg 218, Port Washington, NY 11050-3765; **Phone:** 516-883-0122; **Board Cert:** Internal Medicine 1982; Medical Oncology 1985; **Med School:** NY Med Coll 1979; **Resid:** Internal Medicine, N Shore Univ Hosp 1982; **Fellow:** Medical Oncology, Jacobi Med Ctr 1983; Medical Oncology, N Shore Univ Hosp 1984; **Fac Appt:** Asst Clin Prof Med, NYU Sch Med

Rothman, Ivan MD (Onc) - **Hospital:** South Nassau Comm Hosp, Mercy Med Ctr - Rockville Centre; **Address:** 242 Merrick Rd, Ste 301, Rockville Centre, NY 11570; **Phone:** 516-536-1455; **Board Cert:** Medical Oncology 1977; Hematology 1976; Internal Medicine 1974; **Med School:** NYU Sch Med 1971; **Resid:** Internal Medicine, NC Meml Hosp- UNC 1973; **Fellow:** Hematology, NYU Hosp 1977; **Fac Appt:** Asst Clin Prof Med, SUNY Stony Brook

Schwartz, Paula R MD (Onc) - **Spec Exp:** Breast Cancer; Colon Cancer; **Hospital:** N Shore Univ Hosp at Manhasset, Long Island Jewish Med Ctr; **Address:** 3003 New Hyde Park Rd, Ste 401, New Hyde Park, NY 11042; **Phone:** 516-354-5700; **Board Cert:** Internal Medicine 1986; Hematology 1988; Medical Oncology 1991; **Med School:** SUNY Downstate 1980; **Resid:** Internal Medicine, LI Jewish Med Ctr 1981; Internal Medicine, LI Jewish Med Ctr 1983; **Fellow:** Hematology, Mt Sinai Hosp 1985; Hematology, N Shore Univ Hosp 1989

Stein, Alvin MD (Onc) - **Hospital:** N Shore Univ Hosp at Plainview, New Island Hosp; **Address:** 3601 Hempstead Tpke, Ste 421, Levittown, NY 11756; **Phone:** 516-796-1500; **Board Cert:** Internal Medicine 1971; Medical Oncology 1975; **Med School:** Albert Einstein Coll Med 1961; **Resid:** Internal Medicine, Bellevue Hosp 1964; **Fellow:** Hematology, NYU Med Ctr 1965; Cancer Research, NCI Canc Ctr-Rsch Ctr 1967

Tomao, Frank MD (Onc) - **Spec Exp:** Lung Cancer; Breast Cancer; **Hospital:** N Shore Univ Hosp at Manhasset, St Francis Hosp - The Heart Ctr (page 112); **Address:** 44 S Bayles Ave, Ste 218, Port Washington, NY 11050-3765; **Phone:** 516-883-0122; **Board Cert:** Internal Medicine 1974; Medical Oncology 1975; **Med School:** Cornell Univ-Weill Med Coll 1965; **Resid:** Medical Oncology, Meml Sloan Kettering Cancer Ctr 1967; Medical Oncology, Bellevue Hosp 1968; **Fellow:** Medical Oncology, Meml Sloan Kettering Cancer Ctr 1969

Vinciguerra, Vincent MD (Onc) - **Spec Exp:** Breast Cancer; Gastrointestinal Cancer; Lung Cancer; **Hospital:** N Shore Univ Hosp at Manhasset, N Shore Univ Hosp at Glen Cove; **Address:** 300 Community Drive, Manhasset, NY 11030-3876; **Phone:** 516-562-8954; **Board Cert:** Internal Medicine 1971; Hematology 1974; Medical Oncology 1975; **Med School:** Georgetown Univ 1966; **Resid:** Internal Medicine, New York Hosp-Cornell 1969; Internal Medicine, N Shore Univ Hosp 1971; **Fellow:** Hematology & Oncology, New York Hosp-Cornell 1970; Hematology & Oncology, N Shore Univ Hosp 1974; **Fac Appt:** Prof Med, NYU Sch Med

Weiselberg, Lora MD (Onc) - **Spec Exp:** Breast Cancer; **Hospital:** N Shore Univ Hosp at Manhasset; **Address:** 450 Lakeville Rd, Lake Success, NY 11042; **Phone:** 516-734-8963; **Board Cert:** Internal Medicine 1978; Medical Oncology 1981; Hematology 1982; **Med School:** NY Med Coll 1975; **Resid:** Internal Medicine, Stamford Hosp 1978; **Fellow:** Medical Oncology, N Shore Univ Hosp 1980; Hematology, N Shore Univ Hosp 1981; **Fac Appt:** Assoc Clin Prof Med, NYU Sch Med

Weiss, Rita MD (Onc) - **Hospital:** St Francis Hosp - The Heart Ctr (page 112), N Shore Univ Hosp at Manhasset; **Address:** 107 Northern Blvd, Ste 306, Great Neck, NY 11021-4309; **Phone:** 516-482-0080; **Board Cert:** Internal Medicine 1984; Medical Oncology 1989; **Med School:** Mexico 1977; **Resid:** Internal Medicine, Winthrop Univ Hosp 1980; **Fellow:** Medical Oncology, Mount Sinai 1982; **Fac Appt:** Asst Clin Prof Med, NYU Sch Med

NEONATAL-PERINATAL MEDICINE

Aggarwal, Renu MD (NP) - **Spec Exp:** Neonatal Respiratory Care; **Hospital:** Winthrop - Univ Hosp; **Address:** North Pavilion, Lower Level, 259 1st St, Mineola, NY 11501; **Phone:** 516-663-2288; **Board Cert:** Pediatrics 1978; Neonatal-Perinatal Medicine 1985; **Med School:** India 1970; **Resid:** Pediatrics, Nassau County Med Ctr 1976; **Fellow:** Neonatal-Perinatal Medicine, Nassau County Med Ctr 1978; **Fac Appt:** Asst Prof Ped, SUNY Stony Brook

Boxer, Harriet MD (NP) - **Spec Exp:** Prematurity/Low Birth Weight Infants; Chronic Obstructive Lung Disease (COPD); **Hospital:** Nassau Univ Med Ctr; **Address:** Nassau Univ Med Ctr, Div Neonatology, 2201 Hempstead Tpke, Box 30, East Meadow, NY 11554; **Phone:** 516-572-3319; **Board Cert:** Pediatrics 1977; Neonatal-Perinatal Medicine 1977; **Med School:** SUNY Downstate 1972; **Resid:** Pediatrics, Babies Hosp 1974; Pediatrics, Children's Hosp 1975; **Fellow:** Neonatal-Perinatal Medicine, LI Jewish-Hillside Med Ctr 1977; **Fac Appt:** Asst Prof Ped, SUNY Stony Brook

Davidson, Dennis MD (NP) - **Spec Exp:** Lung Disease in Newborns; **Hospital:** Schneider Chldn's Hosp; **Address:** Schneider Chldns Hosp, Neonatal Div, 269-01 76th Ave, Ste 344, New Hyde Park, NY 11040; **Phone:** 718-470-3440; **Board Cert:** Pediatrics 1980; Neonatal-Perinatal Medicine 1981; **Med School:** Loyola Univ-Stritch Sch Med 1974; **Resid:** Pediatrics, Babies Hosp-Columbia Univ 1978; **Fellow:** Neonatal-Perinatal Medicine, Babies Hosp-Columbia Univ 1981; **Fac Appt:** Assoc Prof Ped, Albert Einstein Coll Med

Davis, Jonathan M MD (NP) - **Spec Exp:** Lung Disease in Newborns; **Hospital:** Winthrop - Univ Hosp; **Address:** Winthrop Univ Hosp - Neonatology, 259 1st St, Mineola, NY 11501-3957; **Phone:** 516-663-3853; **Board Cert:** Pediatrics 1985; Neonatal-Perinatal Medicine 1987; **Med School:** McGill Univ 1981; **Resid:** Pediatrics, Chldns Hosp 1984; **Fellow:** Neonatal-Perinatal Medicine, Chldns Hosp 1986; **Fac Appt:** Prof Ped, SUNY Stony Brook

Schanler, Richard MD (NP) - **Spec Exp:** Nutrition; Breast Feeding Problems; **Hospital:** N Shore Univ Hosp at Manhasset, Schneider Chldn's Hosp; **Address:** Dept Pediatrics, 300 Community Drive, Manhasset, NY 11030; **Phone:** 516-562-4665; **Board Cert:** Pediatrics 1979; Neonatal-Perinatal Medicine 1981; **Med School:** UMDNJ-NJ Med Sch, Newark 1974; **Resid:** Pediatrics, Univ Colorado Hlth Sci Ctr 1977; **Fellow:** Neonatology, Brown Univ; **Fac Appt:** Prof Ped, Albert Einstein Coll Med

Steele, Andrew M MD (NP) - **Spec Exp:** Lung Disease in Newborns; Sudden Infant Death Syndrome (SIDS); **Hospital:** Schneider Chldn's Hosp, N Shore Univ Hosp at Manhasset; **Address:** Schneider Chldns Hosp, 269-01 76th Ave, New Hyde Park, NY 11040-1433; **Phone:** 718-470-3440; **Board Cert:** Pediatrics 1981; Neonatal-Perinatal Medicine 1981; **Med School:** SUNY Hlth Sci Ctr 1976; **Resid:** Pediatrics, LI Jewish Med Ctr 1978; **Fellow:** Neonatal-Perinatal Medicine, LI Jewish Med Ctr 1980; **Fac Appt:** Assoc Prof Ped, Albert Einstein Coll Med

NEPHROLOGY

Bellucci, Alessandro MD (Nep) - **Spec Exp:** Hypertension; Kidney Stones; Kidney Disease; Kidney Failure; **Hospital:** N Shore Univ Hosp at Manhasset; **Address:** 100 Community Drive Fl 2, Great Neck, NY 11021-5501; **Phone:** 516-465-8200; **Board Cert:** Internal Medicine 1979; Nephrology 1982; **Med School:** Italy 1975; **Resid:** Internal Medicine, Cabrini Med Ctr 1979; **Fellow:** Nephrology, N Shore Univ Hosp 1982; **Fac Appt:** Assoc Prof Med, NYU Sch Med

Bourla, Steven MD (Nep) - **Hospital:** N Shore Univ Hosp at Plainview; **Address:** 789 Old Country Rd, Plainview, NY 11803; **Phone:** 516-433-3600; **Board Cert:** Internal Medicine 1979; Nephrology 1982; **Med School:** NY Med Coll 1975; **Resid:** Internal Medicine, LI Jewish Med Ctr 1978; **Fellow:** Nephrology, NYU Med Ctr 1981

Fishbane, Steven MD (Nep) - **Spec Exp:** Kidney Disease-Chronic; Dialysis Care; **Hospital:** Winthrop - Univ Hosp; **Address:** 200 Old Country Rd, Ste 135, Mineola, NY 11501; **Phone:** 516-663-2169; **Board Cert:** Internal Medicine 2001; Nephrology 1994; **Med School:** Albert Einstein Coll Med 1988; **Resid:** Internal Medicine, Montefiore Med Ctr 1991; **Fellow:** Nephrology, Montefiore-Weiler Einstein Med Ctr 1993

Mailloux, Lionel MD (Nep) - **Spec Exp:** Hypertension; Dialysis Care; **Hospital:** N Shore Univ Hosp at Manhasset, N Shore Univ Hosp at Glen Cove; **Address:** 50 Seaview Blvd, Port Washington, NY 11050; **Phone:** 516-484-6093; **Board Cert:** Internal Medicine 1977; Nephrology 1972; **Med School:** Hahnemann Univ 1962; **Resid:** Internal Medicine, Hartford Hosp 1965; **Fellow:** Nephrology, Hahnemann Hosp 1966; **Fac Appt:** Assoc Prof Med, NYU Sch Med

Mattana, Joseph MD (Nep) - **Spec Exp:** Diabetic Kidney Disease; Hypertension; **Hospital:** Long Island Jewish Med Ctr; **Address:** 410 Lakeville Rd, Ste 105, New Hyde Park, NY 11042; **Phone:** 516-465-5260; **Board Cert:** Internal Medicine 2000; Nephrology 1994; **Med School:** SUNY Hlth Sci Ctr 1987; **Resid:** Internal Medicine, LI Jewish Hosp 1990; **Fellow:** Nephrology, LI Jewish Hosp 1993; **Fac Appt:** Assoc Prof Med, Albert Einstein Coll Med

Mossey, Robert MD (Nep) - **Spec Exp:** Dialysis Care; Hypertension; **Hospital:** N Shore Univ Hosp at Manhasset; **Address:** 100 Community Fl 2, Great Neck, NY 11021-5501; **Phone:** 516-465-8200; **Board Cert:** Internal Medicine 1974; Nephrology 1978; **Med School:** St Louis Univ 1969; **Resid:** Internal Medicine, N Shore Univ Hosp 1974; **Fellow:** Nephrology, N Shore Univ Hosp 1976; **Fac Appt:** Assoc Clin Prof Med, NYU Sch Med

Singhal, Pravin C MD (Nep) - **Spec Exp:** Hypertension; Diabetic Kidney Disease; **Hospital:** Long Island Jewish Med Ctr; **Address:** 410 Lakeville Rd, Ste 207, New Hyde Park, NY 11042; **Phone:** 718-470-7360; **Board Cert:** Internal Medicine 1983; Nephrology 1986; **Med School:** India 1970; **Resid:** Internal Medicine, Postgrad Inst Med Ed. 1972; Internal Medicine, Brigham Womens Hosp 1983; **Fellow:** Nephrology, Albert Einstein Coll Med 1985

Wagner, John MD (Nep) - **Spec Exp:** Hypertension; Dialysis Care; Kidney Failure-Chronic; **Hospital:** Long Island Jewish Med Ctr; **Address:** 410 Lakeville, Ste 105, New Hyde Park, NY 11042-1102; **Phone:** 516-465-5260; **Board Cert:** Internal Medicine 1981; Nephrology 1984; **Med School:** Yale Univ 1978; **Resid:** Internal Medicine, Bellevue-NYU 1982; **Fellow:** Nephrology, Bellevue-NYU-VAMC 1984; **Fac Appt:** Assoc Clin Prof Med, Albert Einstein Coll Med

Neurological Surgery

Brown, Jeffrey A MD (NS) - **Spec Exp:** Trigeminal Neuralgia; Pain-Chronic; **Hospital:** N Shore Univ Hosp at Manhasset, Winthrop - Univ Hosp; **Address:** 600 Northern Blvd, Ste 118, Great Neck, NY 11021; **Phone:** 516-478-0008; **Board Cert:** Neurological Surgery 1986; **Med School:** Univ Chicago-Pritzker Sch Med 1976; **Resid:** Surgery, Univ Chicago Hosps 1977; Neurological Surgery, Univ Chicago Hosps 1982

Hollis, Peter H MD (NS) - **Hospital:** N Shore Univ Hosp at Manhasset, Winthrop - Univ Hosp; **Address:** 900 Northern Blvd, Ste 260, Great Neck, NY 11021; **Phone:** 516-773-7737; **Board Cert:** Neurological Surgery 1992; **Med School:** Mount Sinai Sch Med 1981; **Resid:** Neurological Surgery, Mount Sinai Hosp 1986; **Fac Appt:** Asst Clin Prof N, Mount Sinai Sch Med

Levine, Mitchell E MD (NS) - **Spec Exp:** Brain Tumors; **Hospital:** N Shore Univ Hosp at Manhasset, NY Hosp Queens; **Address:** 900 Northern Blvd, Ste 260, Great Neck, NY 11021; **Phone:** 516-773-7737; **Board Cert:** Neurological Surgery 1987; **Med School:** Mount Sinai Sch Med 1977; **Resid:** Surgery, Mt Sinai Hosp 1978; Neurological Surgery, Mt Sinai Hosp 1983

Mechanic, Alan MD (NS) - **Spec Exp:** Brain Tumors; Spinal Diseases; Trigeminal Neuralgia; **Hospital:** N Shore Univ Hosp at Manhasset, Long Island Jewish Med Ctr; **Address:** 410 Lakeville Rd, Ste 204, New Hyde Park, NY 11042; **Phone:** 516-354-3401; **Board Cert:** Neurological Surgery 1992; **Med School:** Emory Univ 1980; **Resid:** Surgery, Beth Israel Med Ctr 1982; Neurological Surgery, Hahnemann Univ 1987; **Fac Appt:** Asst Clin Prof NS, NYU Sch Med

Milhorat, Thomas H MD (NS) - **Spec Exp:** Chiari's Deformity; Syringomyelia & Spinal Cord Diseases; Hydrocephalus; **Hospital:** N Shore Univ Hosp at Manhasset, Schneider Chldn's Hosp; **Address:** N Shore Univ Hosp, Dept Neurosurgery, 300 Community Drive, Ste 2-DSU, Manhasset, NY 11030-3616; **Phone:** 516-562-3020; **Board Cert:** Neurological Surgery 1972; **Med School:** Cornell Univ-Weill Med Coll 1961; **Resid:** Surgery, NY Hosp-Cornel Med Ctr 1963; Neurological Surgery, NY Hosp-Cornel Med Ctr 1969; **Fellow:** Neurological Surgery, Natl Inst Hlth 1965; **Fac Appt:** Prof NS, NYU Sch Med

Overby, M Chris MD (NS) - **Spec Exp:** Spinal Surgery; Spinal Cord Tumors; **Hospital:** N Shore Univ Hosp at Manhasset, Queens Hosp Ctr - Jamaica; **Address:** 900 Northern Blvd, Ste 260, Great Neck, NY 11021; **Phone:** 516-773-7737; **Board Cert:** Neurological Surgery 1990; **Med School:** Tufts Univ 1979; **Resid:** Neurological Surgery, Mount Sinai 1986

NEUROLOGY

Blanck, Richard MD (N) - **Spec Exp:** Multiple Sclerosis; Pain-Back; **Hospital:** N Shore Univ Hosp at Manhasset, St Francis Hosp - The Heart Ctr (page 112); **Address:** 1000 Northern Blvd, Ste 150, Great Neck, NY 11021; **Phone:** 516-466-4700; **Board Cert:** Internal Medicine 1976; Neurology 1980; **Med School:** UMDNJ-NJ Med Sch, Newark 1973; **Resid:** Internal Medicine, N Shore Univ Hosp 1975; Neurology, N Shore Univ Hosp 1977; **Fac Appt:** Assoc Clin Prof N, NYU Sch Med

Ettinger, Alan MD (N) - **Spec Exp:** Epilepsy; Seizure Disorders; **Hospital:** Long Island Jewish Med Ctr, Huntington Hosp; **Address:** Long Island Jewish Med Ctr, EEG Lab, 270-05 76th Ave Bldg Research - rm BC27, New Hyde Park, NY 11040; **Phone:** 718-470-7310; **Board Cert:** Neurology 1989; Clinical Neurophysiology 1997; **Med School:** Boston Univ 1983; **Resid:** Internal Medicine, Hartford Hosp 1985; Neurology, Montefiore Med Ctr 1988; **Fellow:** Neurological Physiology, Montefiore Med Ctr 1989; **Fac Appt:** Assoc Prof N, Albert Einstein Coll Med

Gordon, Marc L MD (N) - **Spec Exp:** Dementia; Headache; Multiple Sclerosis; Alzheimer's Disease; **Hospital:** Long Island Jewish Med Ctr; **Address:** LI Jewish Med Ctr, Dept Neurology, 270-05 76th Ave, Ste 222, New Hyde Park, NY 11040-1433; **Phone:** 718-470-7366; **Board Cert:** Neurology 1990; **Med School:** Columbia P&S 1985; **Resid:** Neurology, Albert Einstein 1989; **Fellow:** Neuropsychopharmacology, Albert Einstein Coll Med 1990; **Fac Appt:** Assoc Clin Prof N, Albert Einstein Coll Med

Haimovic, Itzhak MD (N) - **Spec Exp:** Spinal Diseases; Epilepsy; Headache; **Hospital:** N Shore Univ Hosp at Manhasset, Long Island Jewish Med Ctr; **Address:** 170 Great Neck Rd, Great Neck, NY 11021; **Phone:** 516-487-4464; **Board Cert:** Neurology 1981; Clinical Neurophysiology 1994; **Med School:** NY Med Coll 1975; **Resid:** Neurology, N Shore Univ Hosp 1977; Neurology, NY Hosp-Cornell Univ 1980; **Fellow:** Neurological Physiology, Columbia-Presby 1981; **Fac Appt:** Assoc Clin Prof N, NYU Sch Med

Hainline, Brian MD (N) - **Spec Exp:** Pain-Chronic; Spinal Disorders; Reflex Sympathetic Dystrophy (RSD); **Hospital:** N Shore Univ Hosp at Manhasset; **Address:** 2 Prohealth Plaza, Lake Success, NY 11042; **Phone:** 516-622-6088; **Board Cert:** Neurology 1987; Pain Medicine 2002; **Med School:** Univ Chicago-Pritzker Sch Med 1982; **Resid:** Neurology, NY Hosp 1986; **Fac Appt:** Assoc Clin Prof N, NYU Sch Med

Kanner, Ronald MD (N) - **Spec Exp:** Headache; Pain-Chronic; **Hospital:** Long Island Jewish Med Ctr; **Address:** 270-05 76th Ave, rm 222, New Hyde Park, NY 11040; **Phone:** 718-470-7311; **Board Cert:** Neurology 1980; **Med School:** Spain 1975; **Resid:** Internal Medicine, Philadelphia Genl Hosp 1976; Neurology, Albert Einstein 1979; **Fellow:** Neurology, Meml Sloan Kettering Cancer Ctr 1981; **Fac Appt:** Prof N, Albert Einstein Coll Med

Kelemen, John MD (N) - **Spec Exp:** Electromyography; **Hospital:** N Shore Univ Hosp at Plainview; **Address:** 824 Old Country Rd, Plainview, NY 11803-4935; **Phone:** 516-822-2230; **Board Cert:** Neurology 1979; **Med School:** Georgetown Univ 1974; **Resid:** Internal Medicine, Nassau County Med Ctr 1978; **Fellow:** Neurology, New England Med Ctr 1980; **Fac Appt:** Asst Clin Prof N, NYU Sch Med

Kessler, Jeffrey MD (N) - **Hospital:** N Shore Univ Hosp at Manhasset, St Francis Hosp - The Heart Ctr (page 112); **Address:** 1000 Northern Blvd, Great Neck, NY 11021; **Phone:** 516-466-4700; **Board Cert:** Internal Medicine 1974; Neurology 1976; **Med School:** Cornell Univ-Weill Med Coll 1969; **Resid:** Internal Medicine, New York Hosp-Cornell Med Ctr 1971; **Fellow:** Neurology, New York Hosp-Cornell Med Ctr 1973; **Fac Appt:** Assoc Clin Prof N, NYU Sch Med

Kula, Roger W MD (N) - **Spec Exp:** Neuromuscular Disorders; Myasthenia Gravis; Syringomyelia & Spinal Cord Diseases; **Hospital:** N Shore Univ Hosp at Manhasset, Long Island Jewish Med Ctr; **Address:** 865 Northern Blvd, Ste 302, Great Neck, NY 11021; **Phone:** 516-570-4400; **Board Cert:** Internal Medicine 1975, Neurology 1977; **Med School:** Johns Hopkins Univ 1970; **Resid:** Internal Medicine, New York Hosp 1972; Neurology, UCSF Med Ctr 1974; **Fellow:** Neuromuscular Disease, Natl Inst Hlth 1977; **Fac Appt:** Assoc Prof N, SUNY Hlth Sci Ctr

Levy, Lewis MD (N) - **Spec Exp:** Tourette's Syndrome; Parkinson's Disease; **Hospital:** South Nassau Comm Hosp, Long Beach Med Ctr; **Address:** 777 Sunrise Hwy, Ste 200, Lynbrook, NJ 11563; **Phone:** 516-887-3516; **Board Cert:** Neurology 1979; **Med School:** SUNY Downstate 1973; **Resid:** Neurology, Albert Einstein 1977; **Fac Appt:** Asst Clin Prof N, Albert Einstein Coll Med

Libman, Richard MD (N) - **Spec Exp:** Stroke; **Hospital:** Long Island Jewish Med Ctr; **Address:** 270-05 76th Ave, Ste 222, New Hyde Park, NY 11040-1433; **Phone:** 718-470-7260; **Board Cert:** Neurology 1991; **Med School:** McGill Univ 1986; **Resid:** Albert Einstein 1990; **Fellow:** Columbia-Presby 1993; **Fac Appt:** Assoc Prof N, Albert Einstein Coll Med

Mallin, Jeffrey MD (N) - **Spec Exp:** Stroke; Dementia; **Hospital:** Long Island Jewish Med Ctr, St Francis Hosp - The Heart Ctr (page 112); **Address:** 3003 New Hyde Park Rd, Ste 200, New Hyde Park, NY 11042-1214; **Phone:** 516-488-1888; **Board Cert:** Psychiatry 1989; Neurology 1989; **Med School:** Mexico 1982; **Resid:** Internal Medicine, LI Jewish Med Ctr 1984; Neurology, Albert Einstein 1987

Newman, Stephen MD (N) - **Spec Exp:** Multiple Sclerosis; Migraine; **Hospital:** N Shore Univ Hosp at Plainview; **Address:** 824 Old Country Rd, Plainview, NY 11803; **Phone:** 516-822-2230; **Board Cert:** Neurology 1978; **Med School:** SUNY Buffalo 1972; **Resid:** Neurology, Nassau County Med Ctr 1976

Schlesinger, Irwin MD (N) - **Spec Exp:** Parkinson's Disease; Headache; Electromyography; **Hospital:** N Shore Univ Hosp at Manhasset, Long Island Jewish Med Ctr; **Address:** 170 Great Neck Rd, Great Neck, NY 11021; **Phone:** 516-487-4464; **Board Cert:** Neurology 1971; Clinical Neurophysiology 1994; **Med School:** SUNY Hlth Sci Ctr 1961; **Resid:** Internal Medicine, Bellevue Hosp 1963; Neurology, Bronx Muni Hosp 1968; **Fac Appt:** Assoc Clin Prof N, NYU Sch Med

Turner, Ira MD (N) - **Spec Exp:** Headache; Epilepsy; **Hospital:** N Shore Univ Hosp at Plainview; **Address:** 824 Old Country Rd, Plainview, NY 11803; **Phone:** 516-822-2230; **Board Cert:** Neurology 1978; **Med School:** SUNY Downstate 1972; **Resid:** Neurology, Nassau County Med Ctr

NUCLEAR MEDICINE

Margouleff, Donald MD (NuM) - **Spec Exp:** Thyroid Cancer; PET Imaging; **Hospital:** N S. ore Univ Hosp at Manhasset; **Address:** 300 Community Drive, Manhasset, NY 11030; **Phone:** 516-562-4400; **Board Cert:** Internal Medicine 1965; Nuclear Medicine 1972; **Med School:** Switzerland 1956; **Resid:** Internal Medicine, VA Med Ctr 1959; Internal Medicine, VA Med Ctr 1962; **Fellow:** Nuclear Medicine, LI Jewish Hosp 1964; **Fac Appt:** Clin Prof Med, NYU Sch Med

Palestro, Christopher MD (NuM) - **Spec Exp:** Pain after Joint Replacement; Diabetic Leg/Foot Infections; AIDS Related Infections; **Hospital:** Long Island Jewish Med Ctr; **Address:** Nuclear Medicine, 270-05 76th Ave, New Hyde Park, NY 11040-1496; **Phone:** 718-470-7080; **Board Cert:** Nuclear Medicine 1982; **Med School:** Mexico 1975; **Resid:** Diagnostic Radiology, Roosevelt Hosp 1980; **Fellow:** Nuclear Medicine, Meml Sloan Kettering Cancer Ctr 1982; **Fac Appt:** Prof NuM, Albert Einstein Coll Med

Yung, Elizabeth MD (NuM) - **Spec Exp:** PET Imaging; **Hospital:** Winthrop - Univ Hosp; **Address:** 259 First St, Mineola, NY 11501; **Phone:** 516-663-2778; **Board Cert:** Diagnostic Radiology 1984; Nuclear Radiology 1991; **Med School:** Tufts Univ 1980; **Resid:** Diagnostic Radiology, St Vincent's Hosp & Med Ctr 1984; **Fellow:** Nuclear Medicine, Yale-New Haven Hosp 1991

Zanzi, Italo MD (NuM) - **Spec Exp:** Prostate Imaging; Radioimmunotherapy of Cancer; PET Imaging; **Hospital:** N Shore Univ Hosp at Manhasset; **Address:** 300 Community Drive Bldg Levitt Fl 1, Manhasset, NY 11030-0586; **Phone:** 516-562-4400; **Board Cert:** Nuclear Medicine 1975; **Med School:** Chile 1957; **Resid:** Internal Medicine, Univ Clinic Hosp 1958; Nuclear Medicine, Hammersmith Hosp 1965; **Fellow:** Nassau County Med Ctr 1975; **Fac Appt:** Assoc Prof Med, NYU Sch Med

OBSTETRICS & GYNECOLOGY

Barbaccia, Ann MD (ObG) - **Spec Exp:** Menopause Problems; Gynecologic Surgery; **Hospital:** Mercy Med Ctr - Rockville Centre; **Address:** 2000 N Village Ave, Rockville Centre, NY 11570; **Phone:** 516-678-4222; **Board Cert:** Obstetrics & Gynecology 1980; **Med School:** NY Med Coll 1972; **Resid:** Obstetrics & Gynecology, Nassau County Med Ctr 1978

Bednoff, Stuart MD (ObG) - **Spec Exp:** Menopause Problems; Osteoporosis; Vulvar Disease; **Hospital:** N Shore Univ Hosp at Manhasset, Long Island Jewish Med Ctr; **Address:** 560 Northern Blvd, Ste 103, Great Neck, NY 11021; **Phone:** 516-482-8741; **Board Cert:** Obstetrics & Gynecology 1968; **Med School:** SUNY Downstate 1961; **Resid:** Obstetrics & Gynecology, N Shore Univ Hosp 1966; **Fac Appt:** Assoc Clin Prof ObG, NYU Sch Med

Bernstein, Robert M MD (ObG) - **Spec Exp:** Colposcopy; Minimally Invasive Surgery; **Hospital:** N Shore Univ Hosp at Manhasset; **Address:** 3111 New Hyde Park Rd, New Hyde Park, NY 11042-1217; **Phone:** 516-365-6100; **Board Cert:** Obstetrics & Gynecology 1998; **Med School:** Mexico 1979; **Resid:** Obstetrics & Gynecology, N Shore Univ Hosp 1984; **Fac Appt:** Assoc Clin Prof ObG, NYU Sch Med

Bialkin, Robert MD (ObG) **PCP** - **Spec Exp:** Gynecologic Surgery; **Hospital:** Mercy Med Ctr - Rockville Centre, Franklin Hosp Med Ctr; **Address:** 2000 N Village Ave, Ste 411, Rockville Ctr, NY 11570; **Phone:** 516-764-1344; **Board Cert:** Obstetrics & Gynecology 1979; **Med School:** Univ Pennsylvania 1960; **Resid:** Obstetrics & Gynecology, Bellevue Hosp 1966

Fleischer, Adiel MD (ObG) - **Spec Exp:** Pregnancy-High Risk; Maternal & Fetal Medicine; **Hospital:** Long Island Jewish Med Ctr; **Address:** LIJ Med Ctr, Dept ObGyn, 270-05 76th Ave, rm 471, New Hyde Park, NY 11040; **Phone:** 718-470-7636; **Board Cert:** Obstetrics & Gynecology 1999; Maternal & Fetal Medicine 1999; **Med School:** Romania 1972; **Resid:** Obstetrics & Gynecology, Maimonides Med Ctr 1975; **Fellow:** Maternal & Fetal Medicine, Albert Einstein 1976; **Fac Appt:** Assoc Prof ObG, Albert Einstein Coll Med

Garfinkel, Burton MD (ObG) - **Spec Exp:** Colposcopy; Adolescent Gynecology; Menopause Problems; **Hospital:** N Shore Univ Hosp at Manhasset, Long Island Jewish Med Ctr; **Address:** 560 Northern Blvd, Ste 103, Great Neck, NY 11021-5100; **Phone:** 516-482-8741; **Board Cert:** Obstetrics & Gynecology 1965; **Med School:** Univ Hlth Sci/Chicago Med Sch 1956; **Resid:** Obstetrics & Gynecology, LI Jewish Med Ctr 1960; **Fac Appt:** Assoc Prof ObG, NYU Sch Med

Haselkorn, Joan MD (ObG) **PCP** - **Spec Exp:** Laparoscopic Surgery; Hysteroscopic Surgery; Uterine Fibroids; **Hospital:** South Nassau Comm Hosp, Long Island Jewish Med Ctr; **Address:** 3227 Long Beach Rd, Oceanside, NY 11572; **Phone:** 516-255-2044; **Board Cert:** Obstetrics & Gynecology 1998; **Med School:** Israel 1982; **Resid:** Obstetrics & Gynecology, NYU Med Ctr 1986

Jacob, Jessica MD (ObG) **PCP** - **Spec Exp:** Obstetrics; **Hospital:** N Shore Univ Hosp at Manhasset; **Address:** 3003 New Hyde Park Rd, Ste 407, New Hyde Park, NY 11042-1214; **Phone:** 516-488-8145; **Board Cert:** Obstetrics & Gynecology 1999; **Med School:** NYU Sch Med 1983; **Resid:** Obstetrics & Gynecology, N Shore Univ Hosp 1987; **Fac Appt:** Asst Clin Prof ObG, NYU Sch Med

Khulpateea, Taru MD (ObG) - **Hospital:** New Island Hosp, Winthrop - Univ Hosp; **Address:** 4200 Sunrise Hwy, Massapequa, NY 11758; **Phone:** 516-541-2100; **Board Cert:** Obstetrics & Gynecology 1982; **Med School:** India 1968; **Resid:** Obstetrics & Gynecology, Brooklyn Nair Hosp 1972; Obstetrics & Gynecology, New York Methodist Hosp 1978

Krim, Eileen MD (ObG) - **Spec Exp:** Menopause Problems; Adolescent Gynecology; **Hospital:** N Shore Univ Hosp at Manhasset; **Address:** 3111 New Hyde Rd, North Hills, NY 11040-3500; **Phone:** 516-365-6100; **Board Cert:** Obstetrics & Gynecology 1982; **Med School:** NY Med Coll 1975; **Resid:** Obstetrics & Gynecology, Beth Israel 1979; **Fellow:** Maternal & Fetal Medicine, N Shore Univ Hosp 1981; **Fac Appt:** Assoc Clin Prof ObG, NYU Sch Med

Kuncham, Sudha MD (ObG) - **Hospital:** New Island Hosp, Winthrop - Univ Hosp; **Address:** 2155 Wantagh Ave, Wantagh, NY 11793; **Phone:** 516-221-6500; **Board Cert:** Obstetrics & Gynecology 2003; **Med School:** India 1977; **Resid:** Obstetrics & Gynecology, Beth Israel Med Ctr

Mack, Laurence MD (ObG) **PCP** - **Spec Exp:** Infertility; **Hospital:** N Shore Univ Hosp at Plainview, Winthrop - Univ Hosp; **Address:** 627 Broadway, PO Box 1550, N Massapequa, NY 11758; **Phone:** 516-799-3462; **Board Cert:** Obstetrics & Gynecology 2004; **Med School:** Univ Hlth Sci/Chicago Med Sch 1985; **Resid:** Obstetrics & Gynecology, Brookdale Hosp 1989

Nimaroff, Michael MD (ObG) **PCP** - **Spec Exp:** Laparoscopic Surgery; Hysterectomy Alternatives; Hysteroscopic Surgery; **Hospital:** N Shore Univ Hosp at Manhasset, Long Island Jewish Med Ctr; **Address:** 900 Northern Blvd, Ste 220, Great Neck, NY 11021-5302; **Phone:** 516-466-0778; **Board Cert:** Obstetrics & Gynecology 1993; **Med School:** UMDNJ-NJ Med Sch, Newark 1987; **Resid:** Obstetrics & Gynecology, N Shore Univ Hosp 1991; **Fac Appt:** Asst Clin Prof ObG, NYU Sch Med

Rebold, Bruce MD (ObG) - **Hospital:** N Shore Univ Hosp at Plainview, N Shore Univ Hosp at Syosset; **Address:** 87 Cold Spring Rd, Syosset, NY 11791; **Phone:** 516-921-3168; **Board Cert:** Obstetrics & Gynecology 1984; **Med School:** Mexico 1977; **Resid:** Obstetrics & Gynecology, Nassau County Med Ctr 1982

Rifkin, Terry MD (ObG) PCP - **Spec Exp:** Laparoscopic Surgery; Hysteroscopic Surgery; Menopause Problems; **Hospital:** N Shore Univ Hosp at Manhasset; **Address:** 900 Northern Blvd, Ste 220, Great Neck, NY 11021-5302; **Phone:** 516-466-0778; **Board Cert:** Obstetrics & Gynecology 1997; **Med School:** Columbia P&S 1981; **Resid:** Obstetrics & Gynecology, N Shore Univ Hosp 1985; **Fac Appt:** Asst Clin Prof ObG, NYU Sch Med

Rothbaum, David MD (ObG) PCP - **Spec Exp:** Osteoporosis; Menopause Problems; Uterine Fibroids; **Hospital:** N Shore Univ Hosp at Manhasset; **Address:** 233 E Shore Rd, Ste 109, Great Neck, NY 11023-2433; **Phone:** 516-487-3498; **Board Cert:** Obstetrics & Gynecology 1997; **Med School:** Boston Univ 1982; **Resid:** Obstetrics & Gynecology, North Shore Univ Hosp 1986

Spector, Ira MD (ObG) - **Spec Exp:** Infertility; Menopause Problems; **Hospital:** N Shore Univ Hosp at Manhasset, Winthrop - Univ Hosp; **Address:** 300 Old Country Rd, Ste 201, Mineola, NY 11501; **Phone:** 516-747-4404; **Board Cert:** Obstetrics & Gynecology 1974; **Med School:** SUNY Hlth Sci Ctr 1968; **Resid:** LI Jewish Med Ctr 1972; **Fellow:** LI Jewish Med Ctr 1975; **Fac Appt:** Asst Prof, SUNY Stony Brook

Taubman, Richard MD (ObG) - **Spec Exp:** Laparoscopic Surgery; **Hospital:** Long Island Jewish Med Ctr; **Address:** 900 Northern Blvd, Ste 240, Great Neck, NY 11021; **Phone:** 516-482-4343; **Board Cert:** Obstetrics & Gynecology 1998; **Med School:** SUNY Downstate 1980; **Resid:** Obstetrics & Gynecology, LI Jewish Med Ctr 1984; **Fac Appt:** Assoc Clin Prof ObG, Albert Einstein Coll Med

Toles, Allen MD (ObG) PCP - **Spec Exp:** Pregnancy-High Risk; **Hospital:** Long Island Jewish Med Ctr; **Address:** 1554 Northern Blvd Fl 5, Manhasset, NY 11030; **Phone:** 516-390-9242; **Board Cert:** Obstetrics & Gynecology 1992; **Med School:** Meharry Med Coll 1986; **Resid:** Obstetrics & Gynecology, Howard Univ Hosp 1990; **Fac Appt:** Asst Prof ObG, Albert Einstein Coll Med

Tydings, Lawrence MD (ObG) PCP - **Spec Exp:** Laparoscopic Surgery; Menstrual Disorders; Endometriosis; **Hospital:** N Shore Univ Hosp at Plainview, N Shore Univ Hosp at Manhasset; **Address:** 400 S Oyster Bay Rd, Ste 204, Hicksville, NY 11801-3500; **Phone:** 516-931-4800; **Board Cert:** Obstetrics & Gynecology 1975; **Med School:** SUNY Downstate 1969; **Resid:** Obstetrics & Gynecology, LI Jewish Med Ctr 1973

Vasudeva, Kusum MD (ObG) - **Spec Exp:** Pregnancy-High Risk; **Hospital:** N Shore Univ Hosp at Manhasset; **Address:** 2 Pro Health Plaza, Lake Success, NY 11042; **Phone:** 516-608-6800; **Board Cert:** Obstetrics & Gynecology 1975; **Med School:** India 1968; **Resid:** Obstetrics & Gynecology, N Shore Univ Hosp 1973; **Fellow:** Maternal & Fetal Medicine, N Shore Univ Hosp 1975

Veloso, Manuel MD (ObG) - **Hospital:** Long Beach Med Ctr, South Nassau Comm Hosp; **Address:** 303 E Park Ave, Long Beach, NY 11561; **Phone:** 516-431-2828; **Board Cert:** Obstetrics & Gynecology 1979; **Med School:** Philippines 1966; **Resid:** Obstetrics & Gynecology, Kings Co Hosp 1972

Weiss, Karen MD (ObG) PCP - **Spec Exp:** Menopause Problems; Gynecology Only; **Hospital:** Long Island Jewish Med Ctr, N Shore Univ Hosp at Manhasset; **Address:** 2001 Marcus Ave, Ste N220, Lake Success, NY 11042-1011; **Phone:** 516-354-4364; **Board Cert:** Obstetrics & Gynecology 2000; **Med School:** Univ Colorado 1984; **Resid:** Obstetrics & Gynecology, Long Island Jewish Hosp 1988

OCCUPATIONAL MEDICINE

Mendelsohn, Sara L MD (OM) - **Spec Exp:** Travel Medicine; Occupational Disease & Injury; **Hospital:** Stony Brook Univ Hosp; **Address:** 800 Woodbury Rd, Unit K, Woodbury, NY 11797; **Phone:** 516-682-9142; **Board Cert:** Occupational Medicine 1993; **Med School:** Boston Univ 1988; **Resid:** Occupational Medicine, Univ of Illinois Med Ctr 1991; **Fac Appt:** Asst Clin Prof Med, SUNY Stony Brook

OPHTHALMOLOGY

Berke, Stanley J MD (Oph) - **Spec Exp:** Glaucoma; Cataract Surgery-Lens Implant; Laser Surgery; **Hospital:** Mercy Med Ctr - Rockville Centre; **Address:** 360 Merrick Rd, Lynbrook, NY 11563-1610; **Phone:** 516-593-7709; **Board Cert:** Ophthalmology 1987; **Med School:** SUNY Buffalo 1981; **Resid:** Ophthalmology, Nassau Med Ctr 1985; **Fellow:** Anterior Segment - External Disease, Mass Eye & Ear Infirmary 1986; **Fac Appt:** Assoc Clin Prof Oph, Albert Einstein Coll Med

Broderick, Robert MD (Oph) - **Spec Exp:** LASIK-Refractive Surgery; Cataract Surgery; Glaucoma; **Hospital:** St Francis Hosp - The Heart Ctr (page 112), N Shore Univ Hosp at Manhasset; **Address:** 585 Plandome Rd, Ste 104, Manhasset, NY 11030-1971; **Phone:** 516-627-3232; **Board Cert:** Ophthalmology 1983; **Med School:** NY Med Coll 1977; **Resid:** Ophthalmology, St Vincent's Hosp & Med Ctr 1981; **Fellow:** Ophthalmology, Holy Cross Hosp 1983

Cook, Jack MD (Oph) - **Spec Exp:** Cataract Surgery; Glaucoma; **Hospital:** Winthrop - Univ Hosp; **Address:** 305 Hillside Ave, Williston Park, NY 11596; **Phone:** 516-747-4011; **Board Cert:** Ophthalmology 1980; **Med School:** Albert Einstein Coll Med 1975; **Resid:** Ophthalmology, LI Jewish Med Ctr 1979

D'Aversa, Gerard MD (Oph) - **Spec Exp:** Cataract Surgery; Laser-Refractive Surgery; Cornea Transplant; **Hospital:** Long Island Jewish Med Ctr, Mercy Med Ctr - Rockville Centre; **Address:** 65 Roosevelt Ave, rm 204, Valley Stream, NY 11580-1106; **Phone:** 516-374-4199; **Board Cert:** Ophthalmology 1995; **Med School:** Albert Einstein Coll Med 1989; **Resid:** Ophthalmology, LI Jewish Med Ctr 1993; **Fellow:** Univ Fla Coll Med 1994; **Fac Appt:** Asst Prof Oph, Albert Einstein Coll Med

Donnenfeld, Eric D MD (Oph) - **Spec Exp:** LASIK-Refractive Surgery; Corneal Disease; Cataract Surgery; **Hospital:** Mercy Med Ctr - Rockville Centre, Nassau Univ Med Ctr; **Address:** 2000 N Village Ave, Ste 402, Rockville Centre, NY 11570-1001; **Phone:** 516-766-2519; **Board Cert:** Ophthalmology 1985; **Med School:** Dartmouth Med Sch 1980; **Resid:** Ophthalmology, Manhattan EET Hosp 1984; **Fellow:** Cornea, Wills Eye Hosp 1985; **Fac Appt:** Asst Prof Oph, Cornell Univ-Weill Med Coll

Fastenberg, David M MD (Oph) - **Spec Exp:** Retina/Vitreous Surgery; Macular Degeneration; Diabetic Eye Disease/Retinopathy; **Hospital:** N Shore Univ Hosp at Syosset, Long Island Jewish Med Ctr; **Address:** 600 Northern Blvd, rm 216, Great Neck, NY 11021; **Phone:** 516-466-0390; **Board Cert:** Ophthalmology 1981; **Med School:** NY Med Coll 1976; **Resid:** Ophthalmology, Northwestern Univ Med Ctr 1980; **Fellow:** Retina, USC-Doheny Eye Inst 1982; **Fac Appt:** Assoc Clin Prof Oph, Albert Einstein Coll Med

Ferrone, Philip J MD (Oph) - **Spec Exp:** Retinal Disorders; **Hospital:** Long Island Jewish Med Ctr; **Address:** 600 Northern Blvd, Ste 216, Great Neck, NY 11021; **Phone:** 516-466-0390; **Board Cert:** Ophthalmology 2006; **Med School:** Harvard Med Sch 1989; **Resid:** Ophthalmology, Duke Univ Med Ctr 1993; **Fellow:** Vitreoretinal Surgery, Associated Retinal Consultants

Garber, Perry MD (Oph) - **Spec Exp:** Ophthalmic Plastic Surgery; Blepharoplasty; Lacrimal Gland Disorders; **Hospital:** Long Island Jewish Med Ctr, Winthrop - Univ Hosp; **Address:** 800 Community Drive, Manhasset, NY 11030; **Phone:** 516-627-6630; **Board Cert:** Ophthalmology 1976; **Med School:** SUNY Downstate 1968; **Resid:** Surgery, Mount Sinai Hosp 1970; Ophthalmology, Bellevue Hosp 1975; **Fellow:** Ophthalmic Plastic Surgery, NY Eye & Ear Infirmary 1976; **Fac Appt:** Assoc Clin Prof Oph, Albert Einstein Coll Med

Girardi, Anthony MD (Oph) - **Spec Exp:** Cataract Surgery; Glaucoma; **Hospital:** N Shore Univ Hosp at Glen Cove; **Address:** 8 Medical Plaza Bldg 8, Glen Cove, NY 11542; **Phone:** 516-676-4596; **Board Cert:** Ophthalmology 1985; **Med School:** SUNY Stony Brook 1980; **Resid:** Ophthalmology, Kings Co Hosp 1984; **Fac Appt:** Asst Clin Prof Oph, SUNY Downstate

Goldberg, Leslie MD (Oph) - **Spec Exp:** Cataract Surgery; LASIK-Refractive Surgery; Eyelid Cosmetic Surgery; **Hospital:** St Francis Hosp - The Heart Ctr (page 112), N Shore Univ Hosp at Manhasset; **Address:** 2110 Northern Blvd, Ste 208, Manhasset, NY 11030-3500; **Phone:** 516-627-5113; **Board Cert:** Ophthalmology 1977; **Med School:** Univ Hlth Sci/Chicago Med Sch 1970; **Resid:** Ophthalmology, NYU Med Ctr 1976; **Fac Appt:** Asst Clin Prof Oph, NYU Sch Med

Hatsis, Alexander MD (Oph) - **Spec Exp:** LASIK-Refractive Surgery; Cornea Transplant; Corneal Disease & Surgery; **Hospital:** South Nassau Comm Hosp, Nassau Univ Med Ctr; **Address:** 2 Lincoln Ave, Ste 401, Rockville Centre, NY 11570; **Phone:** 516-763-4106; **Board Cert:** Ophthalmology 1992; **Med School:** Italy 1978; **Resid:** Ophthalmology, Nassau County Med Ctr 1981; **Fellow:** Ophthalmology, Nassau County Med Ctr 1983

Kasper, William MD (Oph) - **Spec Exp:** Cataract Surgery; Glaucoma; Cornea & External Eye Disease; **Hospital:** Winthrop - Univ Hosp, Mercy Med Ctr - Rockville Centre; **Address:** 330 Old Country Rd, Ste 100, Mineola, NY 11501; **Phone:** 516-742-3937; **Board Cert:** Ophthalmology 1974; **Med School:** Belgium 1967; **Resid:** Ophthalmology, Nassau Co Med Ctr 1971; **Fac Appt:** Asst Clin Prof S, SUNY Stony Brook

Klein, Robert J MD (Oph) - **Spec Exp:** Cataract Surgery; Glaucoma; **Hospital:** Long Beach Med Ctr, Long Island Coll Hosp (page 90); **Address:** 202 W Park Ave, Long Beach, NY 11561; **Phone:** 516-431-1101; **Board Cert:** Ophthalmology 1987; **Med School:** SUNY Downstate 1981; **Resid:** Ophthalmology, Univ Hosp 1985

Lopez, Robert MD (Oph) - **Spec Exp:** Diabetic Eye Disease/Retinopathy; Retina/Vitreous Surgery; **Hospital:** NY-Presby Hosp (page 100), Mercy Med Ctr - Rockville Centre; **Address:** 230 Hilton Ave, Ste 118, Hempstead, NY 11550; **Phone:** 516-481-1570; **Board Cert:** Ophthalmology 1987; **Med School:** Harvard Med Sch 1982; **Resid:** Ophthalmology, Columbia-Presby Hosp 1986; **Fellow:** Retinal Surgery, NY Hosp-Cornell 1987; **Fac Appt:** Assoc Prof Oph, Columbia P&S

Marks, Alan MD (Oph) - **Spec Exp:** Cataract Surgery; Laser-Refractive Surgery; Eyelid Surgery-Cosmetic; **Hospital:** St Francis Hosp - The Heart Ctr (page 112), N Shore Univ Hosp at Syosset; **Address:** 2110 Northern Blvd, Ste 208, Manhasset, NY 11030; **Phone:** 516-627-5113; **Board Cert:** Ophthalmology 1983; **Med School:** NY Med Coll 1978; **Resid:** Ophthalmology, N Shore Univ Hosp 1982

Nelson, David B MD (Oph) - **Spec Exp:** Cataract Surgery; Glaucoma; **Hospital:** Mercy Med Ctr - Rockville Centre, South Nassau Comm Hosp; **Address:** 2000 N Village Ave, Ste 402, Rockville Centre, NY 11570-1001; **Phone:** 516-766-2519; **Board Cert:** Ophthalmology 1977; **Med School:** SUNY Hlth Sci Ctr 1972; **Resid:** Ophthalmology, NY Eye & Ear Infirmary 1976; **Fac Appt:** Asst Prof Oph, SUNY Stony Brook

Packer, Samuel MD (Oph) - **Spec Exp:** Cataract Surgery; Ethics; **Hospital:** N Shore Univ Hosp at Manhasset, Long Island Jewish Med Ctr; **Address:** 600 Northern Blvd, Ste 107, Great Neck, NY 11021; **Phone:** 516-465-8400; **Board Cert:** Ophthalmology 1973; **Med School:** SUNY Hlth Sci Ctr 1966; **Resid:** Ophthalmology, Yale-New Haven Hosp 1971; **Fellow:** Yale-New Haven Hosp 1968; **Fac Appt:** Prof Oph, NYU Sch Med

Perry, Henry MD (Oph) - **Spec Exp:** Laser-Refractive Surgery; Cornea Transplant; Cataract Surgery; **Hospital:** Mercy Med Ctr - Rockville Centre, N Shore Univ Hosp at Syosset; **Address:** 2000 N Village Ave, Ste 402, Rockville Centre, NY 11570; **Phone:** 516-766-2519; **Board Cert:** Ophthalmology 1977; **Med School:** Univ Cincinnati 1971; **Resid:** Ophthalmology, Nassau County Med Ctr; Ophthalmology, Hosp Univ Penn 1974; **Fellow:** Cornea, Mass Eye & Ear Infirmary 1977; **Fac Appt:** Assoc Clin Prof Oph, Cornell Univ-Weill Med Coll

Prywes, Arnold MD (Oph) - **Spec Exp:** Glaucoma; Cataract Surgery; **Hospital:** New Island Hosp, N Shore Univ Hosp at Syosset; **Address:** 4212 Hempstead Tpke, Bethpage, NY 11714-5709; **Phone:** 516-731-4800; **Board Cert:** Ophthalmology 1978; **Med School:** Mount Sinai Sch Med 1972; **Resid:** Ophthalmology, Mount Sinai 1977; **Fellow:** Ophthalmology, Mount Sinai 1974; **Fac Appt:** Asst Clin Prof Oph, Albert Einstein Coll Med

Rosenthal, Kenneth J MD (Oph) - **Spec Exp:** Corneal Disease; **Hospital:** N Shore Univ Hosp at Syosset, Long Island Jewish Med Ctr; **Address:** 310 E Shore Rd, rm 102, Great Neck, NY 11023; **Phone:** 516-466-8989; **Board Cert:** Ophthalmology 1986; **Med School:** Albany Med Coll 1978; **Resid:** Ophthalmology, N Shore Univ Hosp 1983

Rubin, Laurence MD (Oph) - **Spec Exp:** Cataract Surgery; Intraocular Lenses; Glaucoma; **Hospital:** New Island Hosp, N Shore Univ Hosp at Syosset; **Address:** 4277 Hempstead Tpke, Ste 109, Bethpage, NY 11714-5706; **Phone:** 516-796-4030; **Board Cert:** Ophthalmology 1987; **Med School:** NY Med Coll 1980; **Resid:** Ophthalmology, New York Eye & Ear Infirm 1984

Rubin, Steven MD (Oph) - **Spec Exp:** Strabismus; Pediatric Ophthalmology; Amblyopia; **Hospital:** N Shore Univ Hosp at Manhasset, Long Island Jewish Med Ctr; **Address:** 600 Northern Blvd, Ste 220, Great Neck, NY 11021-5200; **Phone:** 516-465-8444; **Board Cert:** Ophthalmology 1983; **Med School:** SUNY Downstate 1978; **Resid:** Internal Medicine, Jackson Meml Hosp 1979; Ophthalmology, Univ Penn-Scheie Eye Inst 1982; **Fellow:** Pediatric Ophthalmology, Wills Eye Hosp 1983; **Fac Appt:** Prof Oph, NYU Sch Med

Sturm, Richard MD (Oph) - **Spec Exp:** Glaucoma; Cataract Surgery; **Hospital:** Mercy Med Ctr - Rockville Centre, Long Island Jewish Med Ctr; **Address:** 360 Merrick Rd Fl 3, Lynbrook, NY 11563; **Phone:** 516-593-7709; **Board Cert:** Ophthalmology 1989; **Med School:** NY Med Coll 1983; **Resid:** Ophthalmology, St Luke's-Roosevelt Hosp Ctr 1987; **Fellow:** Glaucoma, Mass Eye & Ear Infirmary 1988

Svitra, Paul MD (Oph) - **Spec Exp:** Diabetic Eye Disease/Retinopathy; Macular Degeneration; **Hospital:** N Shore Univ Hosp at Manhasset; **Address:** 3003 New Hyde Park Rd, Ste 203, New Hyde Park, NY 11042; **Phone:** 516-327-0505; **Board Cert:** Ophthalmology 1990; **Med School:** Cornell Univ-Weill Med Coll 1984; **Resid:** Ophthalmology, Mass Eye & Ear Infirmary 1989; **Fellow:** Retina, Duke Eye Ctr 1990; **Fac Appt:** Asst Prof Oph, Cornell Univ-Weill Med Coll

Udell, Ira J MD (Oph) - **Spec Exp:** Cornea Transplant; Corneal Disease; Eye Infections; **Hospital:** Long Island Jewish Med Ctr, N Shore Univ Hosp at Manhasset; **Address:** LI Jewish Med Ctr, Ophthamololgy Dept, 600 Northern Blvd, Ste 214, Great Neck, NY 11021-5200; **Phone:** 516-470-2020; **Board Cert:** Ophthalmology 1980; **Med School:** Tulane Univ 1974; **Resid:** Ophthalmology, LI Jewish Med Ctr 1979; **Fellow:** Cornea, Mass Eye & Ear/Harvard 1981; **Fac Appt:** Prof Oph, Albert Einstein Coll Med

Weinstein, Joseph MD (Oph) - **Spec Exp:** Cataract Surgery; Refractive Surgery; Contact lenses; **Hospital:** New Island Hosp, Long Island Jewish Med Ctr; **Address:** 4212 Hempstead Tpke, Eye Care Assoc, Bethpage, NY 11714-5712; **Phone:** 516-731-4800; **Board Cert:** Ophthalmology 1982; **Med School:** Albert Einstein Coll Med 1977; **Resid:** Ophthalmology, Long Island Jewish Med Ctr 1981

Younger, Joseph MD (Oph) - **Spec Exp:** Diabetic Eye Disease/Retinopathy; **Hospital:** Winthrop - Univ Hosp; **Address:** 520 Franklin Ave, Ste 101, Garden City, NY 11530; **Phone:** 516-741-4488; **Board Cert:** Ophthalmology 1982; **Med School:** Mexico 1976; **Resid:** Ophthalmology, U Louisville 1980; **Fellow:** Ophthalmology, Joslin Diabetes Center 1981

ORTHOPAEDIC SURGERY

Asnis, Stanley MD (OrS) - **Spec Exp:** Hip Replacement; Knee Replacement; **Hospital:** N Shore Univ Hosp at Manhasset, Hosp For Special Surgery (page 108); **Address:** 600 Northern Blvd, Manhasset, NY 11021; **Phone:** 516-627-8717; **Board Cert:** Orthopaedic Surgery 1976; **Med School:** Washington Univ, St Louis 1968; **Resid:** Surgery, New York Hosp 1971; Orthopaedic Surgery, Hosp for Special Surg 1975; **Fellow:** Research, Hosp for Special Surg 1972; **Fac Appt:** Assoc Clin Prof OrS, Albert Einstein Coll Med

Cataletto, Mauro MD (OrS) - **Spec Exp:** Spinal Surgery; Osteoporosis; **Hospital:** Winthrop - Univ Hosp, Long Island Jewish Med Ctr; **Address:** 200 Old Country Road, Ste 470, Mineola, NY 11501-4282; **Phone:** 516-248-4488; **Board Cert:** Orthopaedic Surgery 2000; **Med School:** Mexico 1978; **Resid:** Orthopaedic Surgery, Maimonides Med Ctr 1984; **Fellow:** Spinal Surgery, Hosp for Special Surg 1985; **Fac Appt:** Asst Clin Prof OrS, SUNY Stony Brook

Corso, Salvatore MD (OrS) - **Hospital:** N Shore Univ Hosp at Plainview, Winthrop - Univ Hosp; **Address:** 205 Froehlich Farm Blvd, Woodbury, NY 11797; **Phone:** 516-364-0070; **Board Cert:** Orthopaedic Surgery 1995; **Med School:** SUNY Hlth Sci Ctr 1987; **Resid:** Orthopaedic Surgery, Long Island Jewish Med Ctr 1992; **Fellow:** Sports Medicine, Orthopaedic Research Virginia 1993

Dines, David M MD (OrS) - **Spec Exp:** Shoulder Surgery; Sports Medicine; Shoulder Replacement; **Hospital:** Long Island Jewish Med Ctr, Hosp For Special Surgery (page 108); **Address:** 935 Northern Blvd, Ste 303, Great Neck, NY 11021-5309; **Phone:** 516-482-1037; **Board Cert:** Orthopaedic Surgery 1980; **Med School:** UMDNJ-NJ Med Sch, Newark 1974; **Resid:** Surgery, NY Hosp-Cornell Med Ctr 1976; Orthopaedic Surgery, Hosp Special Surg 1979; **Fac Appt:** Clin Prof OrS, Albert Einstein Coll Med

Garroway, Robert MD (OrS) - **Spec Exp:** Sports Injuries; Arthroscopic Surgery; Hand Surgery; Knee Surgery; **Hospital:** South Nassau Comm Hosp, Long Island Jewish Med Ctr; **Address:** 64 N Long Beach Rd, Rockville Centre, NY 11570; **Phone:** 516-764-7100; **Board Cert:** Orthopaedic Surgery 1985; **Med School:** Univ Hlth Sci/Chicago Med Sch 1977; **Resid:** Orthopaedic Surgery, Univ Hosp 1982; Arthroscopic Surgery, Ortho Rsch Va 1982; **Fellow:** Hand Surgery, Univ Virginia Hosp 1983; **Fac Appt:** Asst Prof OrS, SUNY Stony Brook

Illman, Arnold MD (OrS) - **Spec Exp:** Sports Medicine; Arthroscopic Surgery; Pediatric Orthopaedic Surgery; **Hospital:** New Island Hosp, N Shore Univ Hosp at Plainview; **Address:** 4180 Sunrise Hwy, Massapequa, NY 11758-5303; **Phone:** 516-541-7500; **Board Cert:** Orthopaedic Surgery 1970; **Med School:** Boston Univ 1960; **Resid:** Surgery, Mass Meml Hosp 1963; Orthopaedic Surgery, Lahey Clinic/Boston City Hosp 1966; **Fac Appt:** Assoc Prof OrS, SUNY Stony Brook

Leppard, John MD (OrS) - **Hospital:** N Shore Univ Hosp at Plainview, Winthrop - Univ Hosp; **Address:** 205 Froehlich Farm Blvd, Woodbury, NY 11797; **Phone:** 516-364-0070; **Board Cert:** Orthopaedic Surgery 1997; Hand Surgery 1995; **Med School:** Bowman Gray 1976; **Resid:** Orthopaedic Surgery, Columbia-Presby; **Fellow:** Hand Surgery, Indiana Hand Center

Lesniewski, Peter J MD (OrS) - **Hospital:** Winthrop - Univ Hosp, N Shore Univ Hosp at Plainview; **Address:** 30 Merrick Ave, East Meadow, NY 11554; **Phone:** 516-794-7010; **Board Cert:** Orthopaedic Surgery 1985; **Med School:** Cornell Univ-Weill Med Coll 1977; **Resid:** Surgery, N Shore Univ Hosp 1980; Orthopaedic Surgery, Bellevue Hosp 1983

Levitz, Craig L MD (OrS) - **Spec Exp:** Sports Medicine; Knee Replacement; **Hospital:** South Nassau Comm Hosp; **Address:** 36 Lincoln Ave Fl 3, Rockville Centre, NY 11570; **Phone:** 516-536-2800; **Board Cert:** Orthopaedic Surgery 2000; **Med School:** Univ Pennsylvania 1992; **Resid:** Orthopaedic Surgery, Hosp Univ Penn 1997; **Fellow:** Sports Medicine, Amer Sports Med Inst 1998

Marcus, Stephen MD (OrS) - **Spec Exp:** Sports Medicine; **Hospital:** South Nassau Comm Hosp, Peninsula Hosp Ctr; **Address:** 657 Central Ave, Cedarhurst, NY 11516; **Phone:** 516-295-0111; **Board Cert:** Orthopaedic Surgery 1973; **Med School:** NY Med Coll 1967; **Resid:** Orthopaedic Surgery, Albert Einstein Affil Hosp 1972

Montero, Carlos Felix MD (OrS) - **Spec Exp:** Hand Surgery; **Hospital:** New Island Hosp, N Shore Univ Hosp at Plainview; **Address:** 2920 Hempstead Tpke, Levittown, NY 11756; **Phone:** 516-735-4048; **Board Cert:** Orthopaedic Surgery 1974; **Med School:** Argentina 1968; **Resid:** Orthopaedic Surgery, Nassau County Med Ctr 1973; **Fellow:** Hand Surgery, Nassau County Med Ctr 1974; **Fac Appt:** Asst Clin Prof OrS, SUNY Stony Brook

Rich, Daniel MD (OrS) - **Spec Exp:** Hip Replacement; Knee Replacement; **Hospital:** N Shore Univ Hosp at Manhasset, Hosp For Special Surgery (page 108); **Address:** 585 Plandome Rd, Ste 103, Manhasset, NY 11030-1971; **Phone:** 516-627-1525; **Board Cert:** Orthopaedic Surgery 1984; **Med School:** Harvard Med Sch 1977; **Resid:** Surgery, St Luke's-Roosevelt Hosp Ctr 1979; Orthopaedic Surgery, Hosp for Special Surgery 1982

Shebairo, Raymond MD (OrS) - **Spec Exp:** Arthroscopic Surgery; Shoulder & Knee Surgery; Joint Replacement; **Hospital:** Long Island Jewish Med Ctr, Mercy Med Ctr - Rockville Centre; **Address:** 1575 Hillside Ave, Ste 303, New Hyde Park, NY 11040; **Phone:** 516-437-5500; **Board Cert:** Orthopaedic Surgery 1982; **Med School:** Med Coll Wisc 1973; **Resid:** Orthopaedic Surgery, LI Jewish Med Ctr 1977

Simonson, Barry G MD (OrS) - **Spec Exp:** Sports Medicine; Arthroscopic Surgery; Shoulder & Knee Reconstruction; **Hospital:** N Shore Univ Hosp at Glen Cove, Long Island Jewish Med Ctr; **Address:** 825 Northern Blvd, Great Neck, NY 11021-5323; **Phone:** 516-773-7500; **Board Cert:** Orthopaedic Surgery 2003; **Med School:** Mount Sinai Sch Med 1984; **Resid:** Orthopaedic Surgery, LI Jewish Med Ctr 1990; **Fellow:** Sports Medicine, New York Univ Med Ctr 1991

OTOLARYNGOLOGY

Abramson, Allan MD (Oto) - **Spec Exp:** Head & Neck Cancer & Surgery; Laryngeal Cancer; Hearing Disorders; **Hospital:** Long Island Jewish Med Ctr; **Address:** LIJ Med Ctr, Dept Otolaryngology, 270-05 76th Ave, Ste 1120, New Hyde Park, NY 11040; **Phone:** 516-470-7555; **Board Cert:** Otolaryngology 1972; **Med School:** SUNY Downstate 1967; **Resid:** Surgery, LI Jewish-Hillside Med Ctr 1969; Otolaryngology, Mount Sinai Med Ctr 1972; **Fac Appt:** Prof Oto, Albert Einstein Coll Med

Draizin, Dennis L MD (Oto) - **Spec Exp:** Hearing Disorders; Nasal & Sinus Disorders; Voice Disorders; **Hospital:** South Nassau Comm Hosp, Winthrop - Univ Hosp; **Address:** 195 N Village Ave, Rockville Centre, NY 11570; **Phone:** 516-536-7777; **Board Cert:** Otolaryngology 1980; **Med School:** Univ VA Sch Med 1975; **Resid:** Surgery, Northshore Univ Hosp 1977; Otolaryngology, Mt Sinai Sch Med 1980

Durante, Anthony MD (Oto) - **Hospital:** Winthrop - Univ Hosp; **Address:** 134 Mineola Blvd, Ste 201, Mineola, NY 11501; **Phone:** 516-294-9363; **Board Cert:** Otolaryngology 1975; **Med School:** Italy 1967; **Resid:** Otolaryngology, Albert Einstein Coll Med. 1975; Otolaryngology, Nassau Hosp. 1970; **Fac Appt:** Asst Clin Prof S, SUNY Stony Brook

Goldofsky, Elliot MD (Oto) - **Spec Exp:** Hearing Loss; Ear Disorders; Vertigo; **Hospital:** Long Island Jewish Med Ctr, N Shore Univ Hosp at Manhasset; **Address:** 600 Northern Blvd, Ste 100, Great Neck, NY 11021-5200; **Phone:** 516-482-3223; **Board Cert:** Otolaryngology 1990; **Med School:** Mount Sinai Sch Med 1984; **Resid:** Otolaryngology, LI Jewish Med Ctr 1989; **Fellow:** Otology & Neurotology, NYU Med Ctr 1990; **Fac Appt:** Assoc Clin Prof Oto, Albert Einstein Coll Med

Gordon, Michael A MD (Oto) - **Spec Exp:** Ear Surgery; Hearing Disorders; Skull Base Surgery; **Hospital:** Long Island Jewish Med Ctr; **Address:** LIJ Med Ctr, Hearing & Speech Center, 270-05 76th Ave, New Hyde Park, NY 11040; **Phone:** 718-470-8922; **Board Cert:** Otolaryngology 1993; **Med School:** Albert Einstein Coll Med 1986; **Resid:** Otolaryngology, Montrfiore Hosp Med Ctr 1992; **Fellow:** Otolaryngology, Ear Research Foundation 1993; **Fac Appt:** Asst Prof Oto, Albert Einstein Coll Med

Grosso, John MD (Oto) - **Spec Exp:** Pediatric Otolaryngology; Otology; **Hospital:** N Shore Univ Hosp at Plainview; **Address:** 875 Old Country Rd, Ste 200, Plainview, NY 11803-4934; **Phone:** 516-931-5552; **Board Cert:** Otolaryngology 1993; **Med School:** SUNY Upstate Med Univ 1986; **Resid:** Otolaryngology, Univ Hosp 1992

Mattucci, Kenneth MD (Oto) - **Spec Exp:** Otology; Neuro-Otology; Nasal & Sinus Disorders; **Hospital:** St Francis Hosp - The Heart Ctr (page 112), N Shore Univ Hosp at Manhasset; **Address:** 333 E Shore Rd, Ste 102, Manhasset, NY 11030-2900; **Phone:** 516-482-8778; **Board Cert:** Otolaryngology 1970; **Med School:** Wake Forest Univ 1964; **Resid:** Surgery, New York Hosp 1966; Otolaryngology, NY Eye & Ear Infirm 1969; **Fellow:** Otolaryngology, New York Hosp 1970; **Fac Appt:** Clin Prof Oto, NY Med Coll

Moisa, Idel MD (Oto) - **Spec Exp:** Thyroid & Parathyroid Surgery; Sinusitis; Snoring/Sleep Apnea; **Hospital:** N Shore Univ Hosp at Glen Cove, Winthrop - Univ Hosp; **Address:** 3 School St, Rm 304, Glen Cove, NY 11542-2548; **Phone:** 516-671-0085; **Board Cert:** Otolaryngology 1988; **Med School:** Albert Einstein Coll Med 1983; **Resid:** Otolaryngology, Montefiore Med Ctr 1988; **Fellow:** Head and Neck Surgery, Montefiore Med Ctr 1990; **Fac Appt:** Asst Clin Prof Oto, Albert Einstein Coll Med

Myssiorek, David MD (Oto) - **Spec Exp:** Thyroid & Parathyroid Surgery; Laryngeal Surgery; Salivary Gland Surgery; **Hospital:** Long Island Jewish Med Ctr, Schneider Chldn's Hosp; **Address:** 270-05 76th Ave, Ste 1120, New Hyde Park, NY 11040-1433; **Phone:** 718-470-7552; **Board Cert:** Otolaryngology 1985; **Med School:** NYU Sch Med 1980; **Resid:** Otolaryngology, Bellevue/NYU/VA Med Ctr 1984; **Fellow:** Head and Neck Oncology, Montefiore Hosp Med Ctr 1985; **Fac Appt:** Assoc Prof Oto, Albert Einstein Coll Med

Rosner, Louis MD (Oto) - **Spec Exp:** Rhinoplasty; Endoscopic Sinus Surgery; Head & Neck Cancer; **Hospital:** South Nassau Comm Hosp, Mercy Med Ctr - Rockville Centre; **Address:** 176 N Village Ave, Ste 1A, Rockville Centre, NY 11570-3800; **Phone:** 516-678-0303; **Board Cert:** Otolaryngology 1982; **Med School:** Univ Hlth Sci/Chicago Med Sch 1978; **Resid:** Otolaryngology, NY Eye & Ear Infirmary 1982

Setzen, Michael MD (Oto) - **Spec Exp:** Nasal & Sinus Surgery; Rhinoplasty; Sleep Disorders/Apnea; Snoring/Sleep Apnea; **Hospital:** N Shore Univ Hosp at Manhasset, St Francis Hosp - The Heart Ctr (page 112); **Address:** 333 E Shore Rd, Ste 102, Manhasset, NY 11030; **Phone:** 516-482-8778; **Board Cert:** Otolaryngology 1982; **Med School:** South Africa 1974; **Resid:** Surgery, Cleveland Clinic Fdn 1978; Otolaryngology, Barnes Jewish Hosp 1982; **Fac Appt:** Assoc Clin Prof Oto, NYU Sch Med

Shikowitz, Mark MD (Oto) - **Hospital:** Long Island Jewish Med Ctr, Schneider Chldn's Hosp; **Address:** LIJ Med Ctr, Dept ENT, 270-05 76th Ave, New Hyde Park, NY 11040; **Phone:** 718-470-7557; **Board Cert:** Otolaryngology 1987; **Med School:** Dominican Republic 1981; **Resid:** Otolaryngology, LI Jewish Med Ctr 1986; **Fac Appt:** Assoc Prof Oto, Albert Einstein Coll Med

Tawfik, Bernard MD (Oto) - **Spec Exp:** Thyroid Disorders; Sinus Disorders; Snoring/Sleep Apnea; Sleep Disorders/Apnea; **Hospital:** N Shore Univ Hosp at Glen Cove, Winthrop - Univ Hosp; **Address:** Three School St, Ste 304, Glen Cove, NY 11542; **Phone:** 516-671-0085; **Board Cert:** Otolaryngology 1977; **Med School:** Johns Hopkins Univ 1971; **Resid:** Otolaryngology, Manhattan Eye & Ear 1977

Youngerman, Jay MD (Oto) - **Spec Exp:** Pediatric Otolaryngology; Head & Neck Surgery; Sleep & Snoring Disorders; **Hospital:** N Shore Univ Hosp at Plainview, Long Island Jewish Med Ctr; **Address:** 875 Old Country Rd, Ste 200, Plainview, NY 11803-4934; **Phone:** 516-931-5552; **Board Cert:** Otolaryngology 1984; **Med School:** Med Coll VA 1979; **Resid:** Otolaryngology, LI Jewish Med Ctr 1983

Zahtz, Gerald MD (Oto) - **Spec Exp:** Sinus Disorders/Surgery; Pediatric Otolaryngology; **Hospital:** Long Island Jewish Med Ctr; **Address:** 270-05 76th Ave, New Hyde Park, NY 11040; **Phone:** 718-470-7554; **Board Cert:** Otolaryngology 1981; **Med School:** St Louis Univ 1977; **Resid:** Surgery, LIJ-Hillside Med Ctr 1978; Otolaryngology, LIJ-Hillside Med Ctr 1981; **Fac Appt:** Assoc Prof Oto, Albert Einstein Coll Med

Zelman, Warren H MD (Oto) - **Spec Exp:** Head & Neck Surgery; Sinus Disorders/Surgery; Pediatric Otolaryngology; **Hospital:** Winthrop - Univ Hosp; **Address:** 975 Franklin Ave Fl 2 - Ste 203B, Garden City, NY 11530; **Phone:** 516-739-3999; **Board Cert:** Otolaryngology 1987; **Med School:** Univ Hlth Sci/Chicago Med Sch 1982; **Resid:** Internal Medicine, Univ Hosp-SUNY 1984; **Fellow:** Otolaryngology, Manhattan EE&T Hosp 1987

PAIN MEDICINE

Pinsky, Steven MD (PM) - **Hospital:** Mercy Med Ctr - Rockville Centre; **Address:** 176 N Village Ave, Ste 2D, Rockville Center, NY 11570; **Phone:** 516-764-4875; **Board Cert:** Anesthesiology 1994; Pain Medicine 2007; **Med School:** Albert Einstein Coll Med 1989; **Resid:** Anesthesiology, SUNY Downstate 1993; **Fellow:** Pain Medicine, St Lukes Roosevelt Med Ctr 1994

PATHOLOGY

Kahn, Leonard B MD (Path) - **Spec Exp:** Bone Pathology; Head & Neck Pathology; Soft Tissue Tumors; **Hospital:** Long Island Jewish Med Ctr, N Shore Univ Hosp at Manhasset; **Address:** 270-05 76th Ave, rm B67, New Hyde Park, NY 11040-1433; **Phone:** 718-470-7491; **Board Cert:** Anatomic Pathology 1980; **Med School:** South Africa 1960; **Resid:** Pathology, Univ Cape Town 1966; **Fellow:** Pathology, Washington Univ Sch Med 1969; **Fac Appt:** Prof Path, Albert Einstein Coll Med

Wasserman, Patricia G MD (Path) - **Spec Exp:** Gynecologic Pathology; **Hospital:** Long Island Jewish Med Ctr; **Address:** Long Island Jewish Med Ctr, Dept Pathology, 270-05 76th Ave, New Hyde Park, NY 11040; **Phone:** 718-470-7490; **Board Cert:** Anatomic & Clinical Pathology 1990; Cytopathology 1994; **Med School:** Argentina 1983; **Resid:** Pathology, Mt Sinai Med Ctr 1989; **Fellow:** Cytopathology, Mt Sinai Med Ctr 1990; **Fac Appt:** Asst Prof Path, Albert Einstein Coll Med

PEDIATRIC ALLERGY & IMMUNOLOGY

Fagin, James MD (PA&I) - **Spec Exp:** Asthma; Ear Infections; Sinus Disorders; **Hospital:** N Shore Univ Hosp at Manhasset, Schneider Chldn's Hosp; **Address:** Schneider Chldns Hosp, Div Allergy/Immun, 865 Northern Blvd, Ste 101, Great Neck, NY 11021-5303; **Phone:** 516-622-5070; **Board Cert:** Pediatrics 1980; Allergy & Immunology 1983; **Med School:** Belgium 1976; **Resid:** Pediatrics, N Shore Univ Hosp 1978; Pediatrics, N Shore Univ Hosp 1979; **Fellow:** Allergy & Immunology, Chldns Hosp of Pittsburgh 1981; **Fac Appt:** Asst Prof Ped, NYU Sch Med

Markovics, Sharon B MD (PA&I) - **Spec Exp:** Allergy; **Hospital:** N Shore Univ Hosp at Manhasset; **Address:** 2110 Northern Blvd, Ste 210, Manhasset, NY 11030-3500; **Phone:** 516-365-6077; **Board Cert:** Pediatrics 1979; Allergy & Immunology 1981; **Med School:** Albert Einstein Coll Med 1975; **Resid:** Pediatrics, NYU-Bellevue Hosp Ctr 1977; **Fellow:** Allergy & Immunology, Montreal Childrens Hosp 1979; **Fac Appt:** Asst Clin Prof Ped, NYU Sch Med

PEDIATRIC CARDIOLOGY

Better, Donna MD (PCd) - **Spec Exp:** Echocardiography; Fetal Echocardiography; **Hospital:** Winthrop - Univ Hosp, NY-Presby Hosp (page 100); **Address:** 200 Old Country Road, Ste 440, Mineola, NY 11501; **Phone:** 516-663-9415; **Board Cert:** Pediatrics 2000; Pediatric Cardiology 2003; **Med School:** Albert Einstein Coll Med 1989; **Resid:** Pediatrics, Mount Sinai Hosp 1992; **Fellow:** Pediatric Cardiology, Columbia-Presby Med Ctr 1995

Bierman, Fredrick MD (PCd) - **Spec Exp:** Fetal Echocardiography; Kawasaki Disease; Congenital Heart Disease; **Hospital:** Schneider Chldn's Hosp; **Address:** Chlds Heart Ctr, Schneider Chlds Hosp, 269-01 76th Ave, New Hyde Park, NY 11040; **Phone:** 718-470-7350; **Board Cert:** Pediatrics 1978; Pediatric Cardiology 1981; **Med School:** SUNY Downstate 1973; **Resid:** Pediatrics, Mount Sinai Med Ctr 1976; **Fellow:** Pediatric Cardiology, Harvard Chldns Hosp 1979; **Fac Appt:** Prof Ped, Albert Einstein Coll Med

Levchuck, Sean G MD (PCd) - **Spec Exp:** Interventional Cardiology; Congenital Heart Disease; Atrial Septal Defect; **Hospital:** St Francis Hosp - The Heart Ctr (page 112), Schneider Chldn's Hosp; **Address:** 100 Port Washington Blvd, Roslyn, NY 11576-1353; **Phone:** 516-365-3340; **Board Cert:** Pediatrics 2001; Pediatric Cardiology 2004; **Med School:** West Indies 1989; **Resid:** Pediatrics, Winthrop Univ Hosp 1992; **Fellow:** Pediatric Cardiology, St Christopher's Hosp 1995

Reitman, Milton MD (PCd) - **Spec Exp:** Cardiac Catheterization; Interventional Cardiology; **Hospital:** St Francis Hosp - The Heart Ctr (page 112), Schneider Chldn's Hosp; **Address:** 100 Port Washington Blvd, Ste 108, Pediatric Cardiology, Roslyn, NY 11576; **Phone:** 516-365-3340; **Board Cert:** Pediatrics 1974; Pediatric Cardiology 1978; **Med School:** NY Med Coll 1969; **Resid:** Pediatrics, Flower Fifth Ave Hosp 1971; **Fellow:** Pediatric Cardiology, Texas Chldns Hosp 1974

Romano, Angela MD (PCd) - **Spec Exp:** Echocardiography; Marfan's Syndrome; Kawasaki Disease; **Hospital:** Schneider Chldn's Hosp, N Shore Univ Hosp at Manhasset; **Address:** Dept Pediatric Cardiology, 26901 76th Ave Fl 1, New Hyde Park, NY 11040; **Phone:** 718-470-7350; **Board Cert:** Pediatrics 1984; Pediatric Cardiology 2003; **Med School:** Columbia P&S 1980; **Resid:** Pediatrics, Babies Hosp/Columbia Univ Med Ctr 1984; **Fellow:** Pediatric Cardiology, Children's Hosp 1987; **Fac Appt:** Asst Prof Ped, Albert Einstein Coll Med

Schiff, Russell MD (PCd) - **Spec Exp:** Echocardiography; Fetal Echocardiography; **Hospital:** Winthrop - Univ Hosp; **Address:** 120 Mineola Blvd, Ste 210, Mineola, NY 11501; **Phone:** 516-663-9415; **Board Cert:** Pediatrics 1986; Pediatric Cardiology 2003; **Med School:** SUNY Stony Brook 1981; **Resid:** Pediatrics, Schneider Children's Hosp 1984; **Fellow:** Pediatric Cardiology, Schneider Children's Hosp 1986; **Fac Appt:** Asst Prof Ped, NYU Sch Med

Shapir, Yehuda MD (PCd) - **Spec Exp:** Heart Disease-Congenital & Acquired; Echocardiography; Fetal Echocardiography; **Hospital:** Schneider Chldn's Hosp; **Address:** 269-01 76th Ave Fl 4, New Hyde Park, NY 11040-1433; **Phone:** 718-470-7350; **Board Cert:** Pediatrics 1998; Pediatric Cardiology 1999; **Med School:** Israel 1977; **Resid:** Pediatrics, Rambam Med Ctr 1981; **Fellow:** Pediatric Cardiology, UCLA Med Ctr 1985; **Fac Appt:** Assoc Prof Ped, Albert Einstein Coll Med

PEDIATRIC CRITICAL CARE MEDICINE

Sagy, Mayer MD (PCCM) - **Spec Exp:** Critical Care; **Hospital:** Long Island Jewish Med Ctr; **Address:** 269-01 76th Ave, New Hyde Park, NY 11040; **Phone:** 718-470-3330; **Board Cert:** Pediatrics 1990; Pediatric Critical Care Medicine 1992; **Med School:** Israel 1972; **Resid:** Pediatrics, Chaim Sheba Med Ctr 1982; **Fellow:** Pediatric Critical Care Medicine, Children's Hosp 1984

PEDIATRIC ENDOCRINOLOGY

Carey, Dennis MD (PEn) - **Spec Exp:** Diabetes; Calcium Disorders; **Hospital:** Schneider Chldn's Hosp; **Address:** Schneider Children's Hosp, Ped Endocrinology, 400 Lake View Rd, Ste 180, New Hyde Park, NY 11042; **Phone:** 718-470-3290; **Board Cert:** Pediatrics 1979; Pediatric Endocrinology 1983; **Med School:** SUNY Downstate 1973; **Resid:** Pediatric Surgery, LI Jewish Med Ctr 1979; **Fellow:** Pediatric Endocrinology, UCSD Med Ctr 1980; **Fac Appt:** Assoc Prof Ped, Albert Einstein Coll Med

Castro-Magana, Mariano MD (PEn) - **Spec Exp:** Growth/Development Disorders; Adrenal Disorders; Sexual Development Problems; **Hospital:** Winthrop - Univ Hosp; **Address:** Winthrop Univ Hosp, Div Ped Endocrinology, 120 Mineola Blvd, Ste 210, Mineola, NY 11501; **Phone:** 516-663-3069; **Board Cert:** Pediatrics 1983; Pediatric Endocrinology 1983; **Med School:** El Salvador 1974; **Resid:** Pediatrics, Nassau County Med Ctr 1980; **Fellow:** Pediatric Endocrinology, Nassau County Med Ctr 1982; **Fac Appt:** Clin Prof Ped, NYU Sch Med

Fort, Pavel MD (PEn) - **Spec Exp:** Diabetes; Growth/Development Disorders; Thyroid Disorders; **Hospital:** Schneider Chldn's Hosp; **Address:** Schneider Chldn's Hosp, Peds Endo, 400 Lakeville Rd, Ste 180, New Hyde Park, NY 11040; **Phone:** 718-470-3290; **Board Cert:** Pediatrics 1976; Pediatric Endocrinology 1978; **Med School:** Czech Republic 1969; **Resid:** Pediatrics, N Shore Univ Hosp 1974; **Fellow:** Pediatric Endocrinology, N Shore Univ Hosp 1976; **Fac Appt:** Assoc Clin Prof Ped, NYU Sch Med

Frank, Graeme MD (PEn) - **Spec Exp:** Pubertal Disorders; Growth/Development Disorders; Diabetes; Thyroid Disorders; **Hospital:** Schneider Chldn's Hosp; **Address:** Schneider Chldn's Hosp, Peds Endo, 400 Lakeville Rd, Ste 180, New Hyde Park, NY 11040; **Phone:** 718-470-3290; **Board Cert:** Pediatrics 1998; Pediatric Endocrinology 1995; **Med School:** South Africa 1982; **Resid:** Pediatrics, LIJ-Schneider Chldns Hosp 1991; **Fellow:** Pediatric Endocrinology, Children's Hosp 1994; **Fac Appt:** Asst Prof Ped, Albert Einstein Coll Med

Kreitzer, Paula MD (PEn) - **Spec Exp:** Diabetes; Growth/Development Disorders; **Hospital:** Schneider Chldn's Hosp, Long Island Jewish Med Ctr; **Address:** Schneider Chldn's Hosp, Dept Ped En, 400 Lakeville Rd, Ste 180, New Hyde Park, NY 11040; **Phone:** 718-470-3292; **Board Cert:** Pediatrics 1987; Pediatric Endocrinology 2004; **Med School:** Univ NC Sch Med 1982; **Resid:** Pediatrics, LIJ-Schneider Chldns Hosp; Pediatric Endocrinology, LIJ-Schneider Chldns Hosp

Slonim, Alfred E MD (PEn) - **Spec Exp:** Muscular Disorders-Metabolic; Inflammatory Bowel Disease/Crohn's; Glycogen Storage Diseases; **Hospital:** NY-Presby Hosp (page 100), Schneider Chldn's Hosp; **Address:** 2001 Marcus Ave, Ste N210, Lake Success, NY 11042; **Phone:** 516-616-0074; **Board Cert:** Pediatrics 1978; Pediatric Endocrinology 1986; **Med School:** Australia 1958; **Resid:** Pediatrics, Royal Chldns Hosp 1963; **Fellow:** Pediatrics, Royal Chldns Hosp 1965; Endocrinology, Hadassah Hosp 1970; **Fac Appt:** Assoc Prof Ped, NYU Sch Med

St Louis, Yolaine MD (PEn) - **Spec Exp:** Diabetes; **Hospital:** Bronx Lebanon Hosp Ctr, Mercy Med Ctr - Rockville Centre; **Address:** 905 Uniondale Ave, Uniondale, NY 11553; **Phone:** 516-485-4630; **Board Cert:** Pediatrics 1986; Pediatric Endocrinology 2001; **Med School:** Hahnemann Univ 1981; **Resid:** Pediatrics, N Shore Univ Hosp 1984; **Fellow:** Pediatric Endocrinology, Montefiore Hosp Med Ctr 1987

PEDIATRIC GASTROENTEROLOGY

Aiges, Harvey MD (PGe) - **Spec Exp:** Crohn's Disease; Liver Disease; Irritable Bowel Syndrome; **Hospital:** Nassau Univ Med Ctr; **Address:** Nassau Univ Med Ctr, Dept Pediatrics, 2201 Hempstead Tpke, East Meadow, NY 11554; **Phone:** 516-572-6177; **Board Cert:** Pediatrics 1976; Pediatric Gastroenterology 1998; **Med School:** NY Med Coll 1971; **Resid:** Pediatrics, Jacobi Med Ctr 1975; **Fellow:** Pediatric Gastroenterology, North Shore Univ Hosp 1979; **Fac Appt:** Prof Ped, NYU Sch Med

Daum, Fredric MD (PGe) - **Spec Exp:** Inflammatory Bowel Disease; Liver Disease; **Hospital:** Winthrop - Univ Hosp; **Address:** 222 Station Plaza N, Ste 408, Mineola, NY 11501; **Phone:** 516-663-8534; **Board Cert:** Pediatrics 1972; Pediatric Gastroenterology 2005; **Med School:** Tufts Univ 1967; **Resid:** Pediatrics, Jacobi Med Ctr 1969; **Fellow:** Clinical Pharmacology, Montefiore Med Ctr 1972

Levine, Jeremiah MD (PGe) - **Spec Exp:** Inflammatory Bowel Disease; Crohn's Disease; Liver Disease; **Hospital:** Schneider Chldn's Hosp, N Shore Univ Hosp at Manhasset; **Address:** Schneider Chldns Hosp, Dept GI & Nutrition, 269-01 76th Ave, rm 161, New Hyde Park, NY 11040-1433; **Phone:** 718-470-3430; **Board Cert:** Pediatrics 1985; Pediatric Gastroenterology 1998; **Med School:** Harvard Med Sch 1980; **Resid:** Pediatrics, Albert Einstein Coll Med Ctr 1983; **Fellow:** Pediatric Gastroenterology, Children's Hosp 1985; **Fac Appt:** Prof Ped, Albert Einstein Coll Med

Markowitz, James MD (PGe) - **Spec Exp:** Inflammatory Bowel Disease/Crohn's; Gastroesophageal Reflux Disease (GERD); **Hospital:** Schneider Chldn's Hosp; **Address:** Schneider Chldns Hosp, Ped GI, 269-01 76th Ave Fl 2 - rm 234, New Hyde Park, NY 11030; **Phone:** 718-470-3430; **Board Cert:** Pediatrics 1981; Pediatric Gastroenterology 1998; **Med School:** Cornell Univ-Weill Med Coll 1977; **Resid:** Pediatrics, NY Hosp 1980; **Fellow:** Pediatric Gastroenterology, N Shore Univ Hosp 1983; **Fac Appt:** Assoc Prof Ped, NYU Sch Med

Pettei, Michael MD/PhD (PGe) - **Spec Exp:** Celiac Disease; Nutrition; Inflammatory Bowel Disease/Crohn's; **Hospital:** Schneider Chldn's Hosp, N Shore Univ Hosp at Manhasset; **Address:** 269-01 76th Ave, rm 234, New Hyde Park, NY 11040-1433; **Phone:** 718-470-3430; **Board Cert:** Pediatrics 1986; Pediatric Gastroenterology 1998; **Med School:** Univ Miami Sch Med 1980; **Resid:** Pediatrics, Mt Sinai Med Ctr 1982; **Fellow:** Pediatric Gastroenterology, Columbia-Presby Med Ctr 1984; **Fac Appt:** Assoc Prof Ped, Albert Einstein Coll Med

Weinstein, Toba MD (PGe) - **Spec Exp:** Inflammatory Bowel Disease/Crohn's; Gastroesophageal Reflux Disease (GERD); Irritable Bowel Syndrome; **Hospital:** Schneider Chldn's Hosp, Long Island Jewish Med Ctr; **Address:** 269-01 76th Ave, New Hyde Park, NY 11040-1433; **Phone:** 718-470-3430; **Board Cert:** Pediatrics 2000; Pediatric Gastroenterology 2000; **Med School:** Columbia P&S 1986; **Resid:** Pediatrics, Children's Hosp Natl MC 1989; **Fellow:** Pediatric Gastroenterology, Schneider Children's Hosp-LIJ 1991; **Fac Appt:** Assoc Prof Ped, Albert Einstein Coll Med

PEDIATRIC HEMATOLOGY-ONCOLOGY

Karayalcin, Gungor MD (PHO) - **Spec Exp:** Sickle Cell Disease; Hodgkin's Disease; Bleeding/Coagulation Disorders; **Hospital:** Schneider Chldn's Hosp, Long Island Jewish Med Ctr; **Address:** 269-01 76th Ave, New Hyde Park, NY 11040-1433; **Phone:** 718-470-3460; **Board Cert:** Pediatrics 1972; Pediatric Hematology-Oncology 1974; **Med School:** Turkey 1959; **Resid:** Pediatrics, Queens Hosp 1965; **Fellow:** Pediatric Hematology-Oncology, Queens Hosp 1966; Pediatric Hematology-Oncology, Queens Hosp; **Fac Appt:** Prof Ped, Albert Einstein Coll Med

Lanzkowsky, Philip MD (PHO) - **Spec Exp:** Solid Tumors; Leukemia; **Hospital:** Schneider Chldn's Hosp, N Shore Univ Hosp at Manhasset; **Address:** 269-01 76th Ave, Ste CH102, New Hyde Park, NY 11040-1434; **Phone:** 718-470-3460; **Board Cert:** Pediatrics 1966; Pediatric Hematology-Oncology 1974; **Med School:** South Africa 1954; **Resid:** Pediatrics, Red Cross War Meml Chldns Hosp 1960; Pediatrics, St Mary's Hosp 1961; **Fellow:** Pediatric Hematology-Oncology, Duke Univ Med Ctr 1962; Pediatric Hematology-Oncology, Univ UT Hosp 1963; **Fac Appt:** Prof Ped, Albert Einstein Coll Med

Lipton, Jeffrey M MD/PhD (PHO) - **Spec Exp:** Bone Marrow Failure; Stem Cell Transplant; Bone Marrow Transplant; **Hospital:** Schneider Chldn's Hosp; **Address:** Div Hem-Onc & Stem Cell Transplant, 269-01 76th Ave, rm 255, MC-07670, New Hyde Park, NY 11040-1433; **Phone:** 718-470-3460; **Board Cert:** Pediatrics 1981; **Med School:** St Louis Univ 1975; **Resid:** Pediatrics, Boston Chldns Hosp 1977; **Fellow:** Pediatric Hematology-Oncology, Boston Chldns Hosp/Dana Farber Cancer Inst 1979; **Fac Appt:** Prof Ped, Albert Einstein Coll Med

Redner, Arlene MD (PHO) - **Spec Exp:** Leukemia; Brain Tumors; Solid Tumors; **Hospital:** Schneider Chldn's Hosp; **Address:** 269-01 76th Ave, rm 255, New Hyde Park, NY 11040-1434; **Phone:** 718-470-3460; **Board Cert:** Pediatrics 1982; Pediatric Hematology-Oncology 1984; **Med School:** Univ Pennsylvania 1977; **Resid:** Pediatrics, Boston Floating Hosp 1980; **Fellow:** Pediatric Hematology-Oncology, Meml Sloan Kettering Hosp 1985; **Fac Appt:** Assoc Clin Prof Ped, Albert Einstein Coll Med

Sabatino, Dominick P MD (PHO) - **Spec Exp:** Cooley's Anemia; Thalassemia; Sickle Cell Disease; **Hospital:** Nassau Univ Med Ctr; **Address:** Nassau Univ Med Ctr, Dept Peds, 2201 Hempstead Tpke, East Meadow, NY 11554; **Phone:** 516-572-6177; **Board Cert:** Pediatrics 1975; Pediatric Hematology-Oncology 1982; **Med School:** Italy 1968; **Resid:** Pediatrics, LI College Hosp 1974; **Fellow:** Pediatric Hematology-Oncology, LI College Hosp 1975; **Fac Appt:** Clin Prof Ped, SUNY Stony Brook

Weinblatt, Mark MD (PHO) - **Spec Exp:** Leukemia; Lymphoma; Bleeding/Coagulation Disorders; **Hospital:** Winthrop - Univ Hosp; **Address:** 200 Old Country Rd, Ste 440, Mineola, NY 11501-4262; **Phone:** 516-663-9400; **Board Cert:** Pediatrics 1980; Pediatric Hematology-Oncology 1982; **Med School:** Albert Einstein Coll Med 1976; **Resid:** Pediatrics, Jacobi Med Ctr 1979; **Fellow:** Pediatric Hematology-Oncology, Children's Hosp 1981; **Fac Appt:** Prof Ped, SUNY Stony Brook

PEDIATRIC INFECTIOUS DISEASE

Krilov, Leonard MD (PInf) - **Spec Exp:** Infections-Respiratory; Infections in Int'l Adopted Children; Chronic Fatigue Syndrome; **Hospital:** Winthrop - Univ Hosp; **Address:** 120 Mineola Blvd, Ste 210, Mineola, NY 11501; **Phone:** 516-663-9570; **Board Cert:** Pediatrics 2001; Pediatric Infectious Disease 2001; **Med School:** Columbia P&S 1978; **Resid:** Pediatrics, Johns Hopkins Hosp 1981; **Fellow:** Pediatric Infectious Disease, Chldns Hosp 1984; **Fac Appt:** Prof Ped, SUNY Stony Brook

Rubin, Lorry MD (PInf) - **Spec Exp:** Kawasaki Disease; Tuberculosis; Fevers of Unknown Origin; **Hospital:** Schneider Chldn's Hosp, N Shore Univ Hosp at Manhasset; **Address:** 269-01 76th Ave, Ste 365, New Hyde Park, NY 11040-1433; **Phone:** 718-470-3480; **Board Cert:** Pediatrics 2002; Pediatric Infectious Disease 2002; **Med School:** Rush Med Coll 1978; **Resid:** Pediatrics, Children's Hosp 1980; **Fellow:** Pediatric Infectious Disease, Johns Hopkins Hosp 1982; **Fac Appt:** Prof Ped, Albert Einstein Coll Med

Sood, Sunil MD (PInf) - **Spec Exp:** Fevers of Unknown Origin; Tuberculosis; Lyme Disease; **Hospital:** N Shore Univ Hosp at Manhasset, Schneider Chldn's Hosp; **Address:** 269-01 76th Ave, New Hyde Park, NY 11040-1433; **Phone:** 718-470-3480; **Board Cert:** Pediatrics 1987; Pediatric Infectious Disease 2002; **Med School:** India 1976; **Resid:** Pediatrics, Baltimore City Hosp 1983; Pediatrics, Georgetown Univ Hosp 1985; **Fellow:** Infectious Disease, Tulane Univ 1988; **Fac Appt:** Assoc Prof Ped, Albert Einstein Coll Med

PEDIATRIC NEPHROLOGY

Trachtman, Howard MD (PNep) - **Spec Exp:** Electrolyte Disorders; Hypertension; Hemolytic Uremic Syndrome; **Hospital:** Long Island Jewish Med Ctr, Schneider Chldn's Hosp; **Address:** 269-01 76th Ave, Ste 365, New Hyde Park, NY 11040-1433; **Phone:** 718-470-3491; **Board Cert:** Pediatrics 1983; Nephrology 2003; **Med School:** Univ Pennsylvania 1978; **Resid:** Pediatrics, New England Med Ctr 1980; Pediatrics, Bronx Muni Hosp Ctr 1981; **Fellow:** Pediatric Nephrology, Albert Einstein 1983; **Fac Appt:** Prof Ped, Albert Einstein Coll Med

PEDIATRIC PULMONOLOGY

Schaeffer, Janis MD (PPul) - **Spec Exp:** Asthma; Cough-Chronic; Lung Disorders-Congenital; **Hospital:** Schneider Chldn's Hosp, N Shore Univ Hosp at Manhasset; **Address:** 3003 New Hyde Park Rd, Ste 204, New Hyde Park, NY 11042-1214; **Phone:** 516-488-7575; **Board Cert:** Pediatrics 1984; Pediatric Pulmonology 2004; **Med School:** SUNY Hlth Sci Ctr 1979; **Resid:** Pediatrics, LI Jewish Med Ctr 1983; **Fellow:** Pediatric Pulmonology, Columbia-Presby 1986; **Fac Appt:** Asst Prof Ped, Albert Einstein Coll Med

PEDIATRIC RHEUMATOLOGY

Gottlieb, Beth MD (PRhu) - **Hospital:** Schneider Chldn's Hosp; **Address:** Schneider Chldns Hosp, Div Rheumatology, 269-01 76th Ave, New Hyde Park, NY 11040; **Phone:** 718-470-3530; **Board Cert:** Pediatrics 2003; Pediatric Rheumatology 1998; **Med School:** Israel 1992; **Resid:** Pediatrics, Schneider Children's Hosp 1995; **Fellow:** Pediatric Rheumatology, Schneider Children's Hosp 1998; **Fac Appt:** Asst Prof Ped, Albert Einstein Coll Med

PEDIATRIC SURGERY

Bohrer, Stuart MD (PS) - **Hospital:** Winthrop - Univ Hosp, NY Hosp Queens; **Address:** 320 Post Avenue, Westbury, NY 11590; **Phone:** 516-766-6606; **Board Cert:** Pediatric Surgery 1995; **Med School:** Baylor Coll Med 1977; **Resid:** Surgery, Johns Hopkins Hosp 1984; Pediatric Surgery, Johns Hopkins Hosp 1986

Coren, Charles MD (PS) - **Hospital:** Winthrop - Univ Hosp, NY Hosp Queens; **Address:** 320 Post Ave, Westbury, NY 11590; **Phone:** 516-997-1199; **Board Cert:** Surgery 1993; Pediatric Surgery 1993; **Med School:** Univ Cincinnati 1978; **Resid:** Surgery, New York Univ Med Ctr 1983; **Fellow:** Pediatric Surgery, Univ Hosp 1985; **Fac Appt:** Asst Prof S, SUNY Hlth Sci Ctr

Dolgin, Stephen MD (PS) - **Spec Exp:** Neonatal Surgery; Ulcerative Colitis; Laparoscopy & Thoracostomy; Inflammatory Bowel Disease/Crohn's; **Hospital:** Schneider Chldn's Hosp, N Shore Univ Hosp at Manhasset; **Address:** Schneider Children's Hosp, Pediatric Surgery, 269-10 76th Ave, New Hyde Park, NY 11040; **Phone:** 718-470-3636; **Board Cert:** Surgery 2000; Pediatric Surgery 2003; Surgical Critical Care 2000; **Med School:** NYU Sch Med 1977; **Resid:** Surgery, Peter Bent Brigham Hosp 1982; Pediatric Surgery, Chldns Meml Hosp 1984

Hong, Andrew MD (PS) - **Spec Exp:** Neonatal Surgery; Minimally Invasive Surgery; **Hospital:** Schneider Chldn's Hosp, N Shore Univ Hosp at Manhasset; **Address:** 269-01 76th Ave, rm CH 158, Schneider Children's Hospital, New Hyde Park, NY 11040; **Phone:** 718-470-3636; **Board Cert:** Surgery 1991; Pediatric Surgery 1996; **Med School:** Univ Wisc 1985; **Resid:** Surgery, Med Ctr Hosp 1990; **Fellow:** Pediatric Surgery, Montreal Chldns Hosp 1992; **Fac Appt:** Asst Prof S, Albert Einstein Coll Med

Kessler, Edmund MD (PS) - **Spec Exp:** Neck Surgery-Pediatric; Tumor Surgery; Gallbladder Surgery-Pediatric; Neonatal Surgery; **Hospital:** Schneider Chldn's Hosp, New York Methodist Hosp (page 479); **Address:** 1000 Northern Blvd, Ste 250, Great Neck, NY 11021; **Phone:** 516-498-9000; **Med School:** South Africa 1968; **Resid:** Surgery, Univ Witwatersrand 1970; **Fellow:** Pediatric Surgery, Univ Witwatersrand 1977; **Fac Appt:** Asst Clin Prof S, Columbia P&S

Kutin, Neil MD (PS) - **Spec Exp:** Hernia; Intestinal Surgery; Undescended Testis; **Hospital:** Schneider Chldn's Hosp, Flushing Hosp Med Ctr; **Address:** 1300 Union Tpke, Ste 107, New Hyde Park, NY 11040-1759; **Phone:** 516-352-5750; **Board Cert:** Surgery 1985; Pediatric Surgery 1997; **Med School:** NYU Sch Med 1970; **Resid:** Surgery, Bellevue-NYU Med Ctr 1975; **Fellow:** Pediatric Surgery, Children's Hosp 1979, **Fac Appt:** Asst Prof S, NYU Sch Med

Parnell, Vincent MD (PS) - **Spec Exp:** Cardiothoracic Surgery; Heart Disease-Congenital; **Hospital:** Schneider Chldn's Hosp, N Shore Univ Hosp at Manhasset; **Address:** Schneider Chldns Hosp, Ped Cardiothor Surg, 26901 76th Ave, New Hyde Park, NY 11040; **Phone:** 718-470-3580; **Board Cert:** Surgery 2003; Thoracic Surgery 2004; **Med School:** SUNY Downstate 1976; **Resid:** Surgery, N Shore Univ Hosp 1981; Thoracic Surgery, Harper Hosp 1983; **Fellow:** Pediatric Cardiac Surgery, Chldns Hosp 1984

Schwartz, David L MD (PS) - **Spec Exp:** Hernia; Intestinal Surgery; Undescended Testis; **Hospital:** Schneider Chldn's Hosp, Flushing Hosp Med Ctr; **Address:** 1300 Union Tpke, Ste 107, New Hyde Park, NY 11040-1759; **Phone:** 516-352-5750; **Board Cert:** Surgery 1971; Pediatric Surgery 1997; **Med School:** Albert Einstein Coll Med 1964; **Resid:** Surgery, Bronx Municipal Hosp 1970; Pediatric Surgery, Johns Hopkins Hosp 1973; **Fellow:** Pediatric Surgery, Johns Hopkins Hosp 1974; **Fac Appt:** Asst Prof S, Albert Einstein Coll Med

Pediatrics

Adesman, Andrew MD (Ped) - **Spec Exp:** Autism; Asperger's Syndrome; Developmental Disorders; Tourette's Syndrome; **Hospital:** Schneider Chldn's Hosp; **Address:** 1983 Marcus Ave, Ste 130, Lake Success, NY 11042; **Phone:** 516-802-6100; **Board Cert:** Pediatrics 1987; Neurodevelopmental Disabilities 2001; Developmental-Behavioral Pediatrics 2001; **Med School:** Univ Pennsylvania 1981; **Resid:** Pediatrics, Chldns Hosp Natl Med Ctr 1984; **Fellow:** Developmental-Behavioral Pediatrics, Children's Hosp 1986; **Fac Appt:** Assoc Prof Ped, Albert Einstein Coll Med

Agulnek, Milton MD (Ped) **PCP** - **Hospital:** Long Island Jewish Med Ctr, N Shore Univ Hosp at Plainview; **Address:** 1021 Old Country Rd, Plainview, NY 11803-4919; **Phone:** 516-935-4343; **Board Cert:** Pediatrics 1962; **Med School:** NYU Sch Med 1956; **Resid:** Pediatrics, Kings County Hosp 1957

Chianese, Maurice MD (Ped) **PCP** - **Spec Exp:** Pediatric Sports Medicine; **Hospital:** N Shore Univ Hosp at Manhasset, Schneider Chldn's Hosp; **Address:** Dept Pediatrics, 2 Pro Health Plaza, Lake Success, NY 11042; **Phone:** 516-622-7337; **Board Cert:** Pediatrics 1997; **Med School:** NY Med Coll 1986; **Resid:** Pediatrics, North Shore Univ Hosp 1990; **Fac Appt:** Asst Prof Ped, NYU Sch Med

Cooper, Seymour MD (Ped) **PCP** - **Hospital:** Winthrop - Univ Hosp, Schneider Chldn's Hosp; **Address:** 173 Mineola Blvd, Ste 100, Mineola, NY 11501-2524; **Phone:** 516-746-2299; **Board Cert:** Pediatrics 1977; **Med School:** NY Med Coll 1972; **Resid:** Pediatrics, Montefiore Hosp Med Ctr 1975

Friedman, Eugene B MD (Ped) PCP - **Hospital:** Long Island Jewish Med Ctr, Winthrop - Univ Hosp; **Address:** 271 Jericho Tpke, Floral Park, NY 11002; **Phone:** 516-354-7575; **Board Cert:** Pediatrics 1973; **Med School:** NY Med Coll 1968; **Resid:** Pediatrics, Metropolitan Hosp Ctr 1971; **Fac Appt:** Asst Clin Prof Ped, Albert Einstein Coll Med

Galinkin, Lawrence MD (Ped) PCP - **Hospital:** N Shore Univ Hosp at Manhasset, Long Island Jewish Med Ctr; **Address:** 700 Old Bethpage Rd, Old Bethpage, NY 11804; **Phone:** 516-293-0666; **Board Cert:** Pediatrics 1976; **Med School:** Tulane Univ 1971; **Resid:** Pediatrics, Bronx Muni Hosp 1974

Gerberg Jr, Lynda Frances MD (Ped) - **Spec Exp:** Sports Medicine; Obesity; **Hospital:** Schneider Chldn's Hosp, Long Island Jewish Med Ctr; **Address:** 410 Lakeville Rd, Ste 108, New Hyde Park, NY 11042; **Phone:** 516-465-4377; **Board Cert:** Pediatrics 1994; **Med School:** Mexico 1987; **Resid:** Pediatrics, Schneider Chldns Hosp 1993; **Fellow:** Pediatrics, Children's Hosp 1994; **Fac Appt:** Asst Prof Ped, Albert Einstein Coll Med

Glatt, Hershel MD (Ped) PCP - **Spec Exp:** Cardiology; Asthma; Obesity; **Hospital:** South Nassau Comm Hosp, Winthrop - Univ Hosp; **Address:** 3051 Long Beach Rd, Ste 1, Oceanside, NY 11572; **Phone:** 516-536-2000; **Board Cert:** Pediatrics 1977; **Med School:** Belgium 1969; **Resid:** Pediatrics, Maimonides Medical Ctr 1972; **Fellow:** Pediatric Cardiology, Maimonides Medical Ctr 1972; **Fac Appt:** Asst Clin Prof Ped, SUNY Stony Brook

Good, Leonard MD (Ped) PCP - **Hospital:** N Shore Univ Hosp at Manhasset, Long Island Jewish Med Ctr; **Address:** 1077 Northern Blvd, Roslyn, NY 11576-1614; **Phone:** 516-365-5500; **Board Cert:** Pediatrics 1985; **Med School:** Albert Einstein Coll Med 1979; **Resid:** Pediatrics, Jacobi Med Ctr 1982

Gould, Eric MD (Ped) PCP - **Spec Exp:** Developmental Disorders; **Hospital:** Long Island Jewish Med Ctr, N Shore Univ Hosp at Manhasset; **Address:** 15 Barstow Rd, Great Neck, NY 11021-2229; **Phone:** 516-829-9409; **Board Cert:** Pediatrics 1976; **Med School:** NY Med Coll 1970; **Resid:** Pediatrics, Bellevue Hosp Ctr/NYU 1974; **Fellow:** Child Development, Montefiore-Weiler Einstein Div 1976

Green, Abraham MD (Ped) PCP - **Spec Exp:** Asthma; Nutrition; **Hospital:** Long Island Jewish Med Ctr, N Shore Univ Hosp at Manhasset; **Address:** 115 Franklin Pl, Woodmere, NY 11598; **Phone:** 516-295-1200; **Board Cert:** Pediatrics 1984; **Med School:** Albert Einstein Coll Med 1979; **Resid:** Pediatrics, Jacobi Med Ctr 1980; Pediatrics, Montefiore Med Ctr 1983

Grijnsztein, Jacob MD (Ped) PCP - **Spec Exp:** Allergy; **Hospital:** Long Island Jewish Med Ctr, N Shore Univ Hosp at Manhasset; **Address:** 107 Northern Blvd, Ste 201, Great Neck, NY 11021; **Phone:** 516-487-6565; **Board Cert:** Pediatrics 1979; **Med School:** NYU Sch Med 1973; **Resid:** Pediatrics, Bellevue Hosp 1976

Hankin, Dorie MD (Ped) - **Spec Exp:** Developmental Disorders; Behavioral Disorders; **Hospital:** Winthrop - Univ Hosp, Schneider Chldn's Hosp; **Address:** 173 Mineola Blvd, Ste 301B, Mineola, NY 11501; **Phone:** 516-739-1936; **Board Cert:** Pediatrics 1980; Neurodevelopmental Disabilities 2001; Developmental-Behavioral Pediatrics 2002; **Med School:** Albert Einstein Coll Med 1974; **Resid:** Pediatrics, Montefiore Hosp Med Ctr 1978; **Fellow:** Child Development, Montefiore-Einstein Med Ctr 1980; **Fac Appt:** Asst Clin Prof Ped, Albert Einstein Coll Med

Levy, Morton MD (Ped) PCP - **Hospital:** N Shore Univ Hosp at Manhasset, Schneider Chldn's Hosp; **Address:** 73 Garden St, Roslyn Heights, NY 11577-1009; **Phone:** 516-621-9360; **Board Cert:** Pediatrics 1966; **Med School:** SUNY Downstate 1961; **Resid:** Pediatrics, Mount Sinai 1964; **Fac Appt:** Asst Clin Prof Ped, NYU Sch Med

Marino, Ronald DO (Ped) PCP - **Spec Exp:** Developmental & Behavioral Disorders; Adolescent Medicine; **Hospital:** Winthrop - Univ Hosp, Good Samaritan Hosp Med Ctr - West Islip; **Address:** 222 Station Plaza North, Ste 611, Mineola, NY 11501-3808; **Phone:** 516-663-2532; **Board Cert:** Pediatrics 1985; **Med School:** Mich State Univ 1978; **Resid:** Pediatrics, Doctors Hosp 1981; **Fellow:** Behavioral Pediatrics, Univ Maryland Med Ctr 1985; **Fac Appt:** Prof Ped, NY Coll Osteo Med

Nerwen, Clifford MD (Ped) PCP - **Hospital:** Schneider Chldn's Hosp, N Shore Univ Hosp at Manhasset; **Address:** Schneider Chldns Hosp, Genl Peds Div, 410 Lakeville Rd, Ste 108, New Hyde Park, NY 11042; **Phone:** 516-465-4377; **Board Cert:** Pediatrics 2003; **Med School:** Univ Conn 1991; **Resid:** Pediatrics, Schneider Chldns Hosp 1994

Rabinowicz, Morris MD (Ped) PCP - **Hospital:** N Shore Univ Hosp at Plainview, Schneider Chldn's Hosp; **Address:** 995 Old Country Rd, Plainview, NY 11803; **Phone:** 516-935-7333; **Board Cert:** Pediatrics 1985; **Med School:** SUNY Downstate 1978; **Resid:** Pediatrics, LI Jewish Med Ctr 1980; Pediatrics, Brookdale Hosp 1983

Resmovits, Marvin MD (Ped) PCP - **Hospital:** Schneider Chldn's Hosp, N Shore Univ Hosp at Manhasset; **Address:** 107 NE Northern Blvd Fl s - Ste 201, Great Neck, NY 11021-1125; **Phone:** 516-487-6565; **Board Cert:** Pediatrics 1984; **Med School:** SUNY Buffalo 1979; **Resid:** Pediatrics, LI Jewish Hosp 1982

PHYSICAL MEDICINE & REHABILITATION

Root, Barry MD (PMR) - **Spec Exp:** Spinal Cord Injury; Electromyography; Spinal Rehabilitation; **Hospital:** N Shore Univ Hosp at Glen Cove; **Address:** Dept Physical Med & Rehab, 101 St Andrews Ln Fl 1, Glen Cove, NY 11542-2254; **Phone:** 516-674-7501; **Board Cert:** Physical Medicine & Rehabilitation 1988; Spinal Cord Injury Medicine 2003; **Med School:** Ohio State Univ 1984; **Resid:** Physical Medicine & Rehabilitation, Nassau County Med Ctr 1987; **Fac Appt:** Asst Clin Prof PMR, Cornell Univ-Weill Med Coll

PLASTIC SURGERY

Breitbart, Arnold MD (PlS) - **Spec Exp:** Cosmetic Surgery-Face & Body; Liposuction; Breast Reconstruction; **Hospital:** N Shore Univ Hosp at Manhasset, NY-Presby Hosp (page 100); **Address:** 1155 Northern Blvd, Ste 110, Manhasset, NY 11030; **Phone:** 516-365-3511; **Board Cert:** Surgery 1992; Plastic Surgery 1996; **Med School:** NYU Sch Med 1985; **Resid:** Surgery, NYU Med Ctr 1991; Plastic Surgery, NYU Med Ctr 1993; **Fellow:** Craniofacial Surgery, NYU Med Ctr 1994; Microsurgery, Meml Sloan Kettering Cancer Ctr 1995; **Fac Appt:** Asst Prof S, Cornell Univ-Weill Med Coll

DeVita, Gregory MD (PlS) - **Spec Exp:** Rhinoplasty; Cosmetic Surgery-Breast; Cosmetic Surgery-Face; Cosmetic Surgery-Body; **Hospital:** St Francis Hosp - The Heart Ctr (page 112), N Shore Univ Hosp at Manhasset; **Address:** 650 Northern Blvd, Great Neck, NY 11021-5204; **Phone:** 516-466-7000; **Board Cert:** Plastic Surgery 1989; **Med School:** SUNY Downstate 1980; **Resid:** Surgery, St Luke's Hosp 1982; Surgery, Jersey City Med Ctr 1983; **Fellow:** Plastic Surgery, New York Methodist Hosp 1984; Plastic Surgery, SUNY Downstate Med Ctr 1986

Di Gregorio, Vincent MD (PlS) - **Spec Exp:** Rhinoplasty Revision; Breast Reconstruction & Augmentation; Blepharoplasty; **Hospital:** Winthrop - Univ Hosp; **Address:** 999 Franklin Ave Fl 4, Garden City, NY 11530; **Phone:** 516-742-3404; **Board Cert:** Plastic Surgery 1978; **Med School:** Albany Med Coll 1968; **Resid:** Surgery, Thomas Jefferson Univ Hosp 1974; Plastic Surgery, Nassau County Med Ctr 1976

Doctor, Naishad MD (PlS) - **Hospital:** Mercy Med Ctr - Rockville Centre, Winthrop - Univ Hosp; **Address:** 2000 N Village Ave, Ste 103, Rockville Centre, NY 11570-1001; **Phone:** 516-678-2517; **Board Cert:** Plastic Surgery 1993; **Med School:** India 1974; **Resid:** Surgery, Univ Hosp 1987; Plastic Surgery, Univ Utah Hosp 1990; **Fellow:** Burn Surgery, Univ Hosp 1988

Duboys, Elliot MD (PlS) - **Spec Exp:** Cosmetic & Reconstructive Surgery; Pediatric Plastic Surgery; Breast Surgery; **Hospital:** N Shore Univ Hosp at Plainview, Stony Brook Univ Hosp; **Address:** 800 Woodbury Rd, Ste G, Woodbury, NY 11797-2503; **Phone:** 516-921-2244; **Board Cert:** Plastic Surgery 1985; **Med School:** Belgium 1977; **Resid:** Surgery, SUNY - Stony Brook Univ Hosp 1982; Plastic Surgery, Nassau County Med Ctr 1984

Feinberg, Joseph MD (PlS) - **Spec Exp:** Cosmetic Surgery-Face; Cosmetic Surgery-Breast; Abdominoplasty; **Hospital:** St Francis Hosp - The Heart Ctr (page 112), N Shore Univ Hosp at Manhasset; **Address:** 1201 Northern Blvd, Ste 202, Manhasset, NY 11030; **Phone:** 516-869-6200; **Board Cert:** Plastic Surgery 1980; **Med School:** Cornell Univ-Weill Med Coll 1973; **Resid:** Surgery, NY Hosp 1976; Plastic Surgery, NY Hosp 1978; **Fellow:** Facial Plastic & Reconstructive Surgery, Meml Sloan Kettering Cancer Ctr; **Fac Appt:** Asst Clin Prof S, Cornell Univ-Weill Med Coll

Funt, David MD (PlS) - **Spec Exp:** Cosmetic Surgery-Face & Body; Liposuction; Botox Therapy; **Hospital:** South Nassau Comm Hosp, N Shore Univ Hosp at Manhasset; **Address:** 19 Irving Pl, Woodmere, NY 11598; **Phone:** 516-295-0404; **Board Cert:** Plastic Surgery 1987; **Med School:** Geo Wash Univ 1979; **Resid:** Plastic Surgery, Montefiore Hosp Med Ctr 1985; Surgery, Montefiore Hosp Med Ctr 1983; **Fac Appt:** Asst Clin Prof PlS, Albert Einstein Coll Med

Gallagher, Pamela M MD (PlS) - **Spec Exp:** Cosmetic Surgery; Cleft Palate/Lip; **Hospital:** Winthrop - Univ Hosp, N Shore Univ Hosp at Manhasset; **Address:** 190 E Jericho Tpke, Mineola, NY 11501; **Phone:** 631-661-2579; **Board Cert:** Plastic Surgery 1980; **Med School:** Univ Chicago-Pritzker Sch Med 1974; **Resid:** Surgery, New York Hosp 1977; Plastic Surgery, New York Hosp 1979

Gold, Alan MD (PlS) - **Spec Exp:** Cosmetic Surgery; Cosmetic Surgery-Face & Eyelid; Nasal Surgery; **Hospital:** N Shore Univ Hosp at Manhasset, N Shore Univ Hosp at Glen Cove; **Address:** 833 Northern Blvd, Ste 240, Great Neck, NY 11021-5308; **Phone:** 516-498-2800; **Board Cert:** Plastic Surgery 1979; **Med School:** SUNY Downstate 1971; **Resid:** Surgery, N Shore Univ Hosp 1975; Plastic Surgery, Kings County-Suny Med Ctr 1978; **Fellow:** Hand Surgery, Nassau County Med Ctr 1976; **Fac Appt:** Assoc Clin Prof S, Cornell Univ-Weill Med Coll

Groeger, William MD (PlS) - **Hospital:** Long Beach Med Ctr, South Nassau Comm Hosp; **Address:** 1800 Rockaway Ave, Ste 210, Hewlett, NY 11557-1645; **Phone:** 516-887-5502; **Board Cert:** Plastic Surgery 1982; **Med School:** SUNY Downstate 1972; **Resid:** Surgery, Beth Israel Hosp 1977; Plastic Surgery, Univ Hosp 1979

Keller, Alex J MD (PlS) - **Spec Exp:** Breast Reconstruction; **Hospital:** Long Island Jewish Med Ctr, N Shore Univ Hosp at Manhasset; **Address:** 900 Northern Blvd, Ste 130, Great Neck, NY 11021; **Phone:** 516-482-1100; **Board Cert:** Plastic Surgery 1984; **Med School:** NYU Sch Med 1975; **Resid:** Surgery, NYU Med Ctr 1978; Surgery, LI Jewish Hosp 1980; **Fellow:** Plastic Surgery, NYU Med Ctr 1982; Microsurgery, NYU Med Ctr 1983; **Fac Appt:** Asst Clin Prof PlS, NYU Sch Med

Kessler, Martin E MD (PlS) - **Spec Exp:** Cosmetic Surgery-Face & Body; Reconstructive Surgery-Face; Breast Reconstruction; Hand Surgery; **Hospital:** South Nassau Comm Hosp, N Shore Univ Hosp at Manhasset; **Address:** The Plastic Surgery Group, 650 Northern Blvd, Great Neck, NY 11021; **Phone:** 516-536-5858; **Board Cert:** Plastic Surgery 1987; Hand Surgery 1995; **Med School:** Cornell Univ-Weill Med Coll 1980; **Resid:** Surgery, NY Hosp 1983; Plastic Surgery, NY Hosp 1985; **Fellow:** Hand Surgery, Cleveland Clinic 1986

Leipziger, Lyle S MD (PlS) - **Spec Exp:** Cosmetic Surgery-Face & Eyes; Breast Reconstruction & Augmentation; Liposuction & Body Contouring; **Hospital:** N Shore Univ Hosp at Manhasset, Long Island Jewish Med Ctr; **Address:** 825 Northern Blvd Fl 3, Great Neck, NY 11021; **Phone:** 516-465-8787; **Board Cert:** Plastic Surgery 1994; **Med School:** Cornell Univ-Weill Med Coll 1985; **Resid:** Plastic Surgery, New York Hosp 1990; **Fellow:** Craniofacial Surgery, Johns Hopkins Hosp 1991; **Fac Appt:** Asst Prof S, Albert Einstein Coll Med

Lukash, Frederick MD (PlS) - **Spec Exp:** Pediatric & Adolescent Plastic Surgery; Cosmetic Surgery-Face; Breast Cosmetic & Reconstructive Surgery; Rhinoplasty; **Hospital:** Long Island Jewish Med Ctr, Schneider Chldn's Hosp; **Address:** 1129 Northern Blvd, Ste 403, Manhasset, NY 11030-3022; **Phone:** 516-365-1040; **Board Cert:** Plastic Surgery 1982; **Med School:** Tulane Univ 1973; **Resid:** Surgery, Emory Univ Hosp 1975; Surgery, Univ Hosp 1980; **Fellow:** Plastic Surgery, Mass Genl Hosp 1981; **Fac Appt:** Asst Prof S, Albert Einstein Coll Med

Silberman, Mark MD (PlS) - **Spec Exp:** Cosmetic Surgery-Face; Cosmetic Surgery-Breast; Liposuction; **Hospital:** N Shore Univ Hosp at Manhasset, Winthrop - Univ Hosp; **Address:** 650 Northern Blvd, Great Neck, NY 11021-5204; **Phone:** 516-466-7000; **Board Cert:** Plastic Surgery 1988; **Med School:** SUNY Downstate 1980; **Resid:** Surgery, Beth Israel Med Ctr 1983; Plastic Surgery, SUNY Downstate Med Ctr 1985

Simpson, Roger MD (PlS) - **Spec Exp:** Eyelid Surgery; Hand Surgery; **Hospital:** Mercy Med Ctr - Rockville Centre, Winthrop - Univ Hosp; **Address:** 999 Franklin Ave, Garden City, NY 11530; **Phone:** 516-742-3404; **Board Cert:** Plastic Surgery 1981; **Med School:** Belgium 1974; **Resid:** Surgery, Nassau Co Med Ctr 1978; Plastic Surgery, Nassau Co Med Ctr 1980; **Fellow:** Hand Surgery, St Luke's-Roosevelt Hosp Ctr 1981; **Fac Appt:** Asst Clin Prof S, SUNY Stony Brook

Sklansky, B Donald MD (PlS) - **Spec Exp:** Cosmetic Surgery; Breast Reconstruction; Skin Cancer; **Hospital:** N Shore Univ Hosp at Manhasset, NY-Presby Hosp (page 100); **Address:** 833 Northern Blvd, Ste 115, Great Neck, NY 11021-5308; **Phone:** 516-504-1800; **Board Cert:** Plastic Surgery 1979; Otolaryngology 1976; **Med School:** SUNY Downstate 1969; **Resid:** Surgery, Hosp Univ Penn 1970; Otolaryngology, Mass Genl Hosp 1976; **Fellow:** Facial Plastic & Reconstructive Surgery, Natl Cancer Inst 1973; Facial Plastic & Reconstructive Surgery, Meml Sloan Kettering Cancer Ctr; **Fac Appt:** Asst Clin Prof S, Cornell Univ-Weill Med Coll

PSYCHIATRY

Bailine, Samuel MD (Psyc) - **Spec Exp:** Depression; Psychopharmacology; Electroconvulsive Therapy (ECT); **Hospital:** Long Island Jewish Med Ctr; **Address:** 5 Ridgeway Rd, Port Washington, NY 11050-2729; **Phone:** 516-883-3304; **Board Cert:** Psychiatry 1970; **Med School:** NYU Sch Med 1964; **Resid:** Psychiatry, Tulane Univ Med Ctr 1968; **Fac Appt:** Asst Prof Psyc, Albert Einstein Coll Med

Behr, Raymond MD (Psyc) - **Spec Exp:** Depression; Bipolar/Mood Disorders; **Hospital:** Long Island Jewish Med Ctr; **Address:** 81-A Arleigh Rd, Great Neck, NY 11021; **Phone:** 516-482-1980; **Board Cert:** Psychiatry 1981; Child & Adolescent Psychiatry 1982; **Med School:** South Africa 1973; **Resid:** Psychiatry, LI Jewish Med Ctr 1978; **Fellow:** Child & Adolescent Psychiatry, LI Jewish Med Ctr 1980; **Fac Appt:** Asst Clin Prof Psyc, Albert Einstein Coll Med

Benjamin, John MD (Psyc) - **Spec Exp:** Depression; Anxiety Disorders; Schizophrenia; **Hospital:** N Shore Univ Hosp at Manhasset; **Address:** 20 Canterbury Rd, Great Neck, NY 11021; **Phone:** 516-482-7797; **Board Cert:** Psychiatry 1983; Geriatric Psychiatry 1992; **Med School:** India 1969; **Resid:** Psychiatry, N Shore Univ Hosp 1981; **Fac Appt:** Asst Clin Prof Psyc, NYU Sch Med

Berman, Sheldon S MD (Psyc) - **Spec Exp:** Psychodynamic Psychotherapy; Psychopharmacology; Psychiatry in Palliative Care; **Address:** 8 Payne Circle, Hewlett Harbor, NY 11557; **Phone:** 516-374-4417; **Board Cert:** Psychiatry 1979; **Med School:** Univ Hlth Sci/Chicago Med Sch 1969; **Resid:** Psychiatry, Brookdale Hosp 1973; **Fac Appt:** Asst Clin Prof Psyc, SUNY Downstate

Bhatt, Ashok MD (Psyc) - **Spec Exp:** Depression; Psychopharmacology; **Hospital:** Long Beach Med Ctr; **Address:** 871 E Park Ave, Long Beach, NY 11561; **Phone:** 516-889-8853; **Board Cert:** Psychiatry 1985; **Med School:** India 1976; **Resid:** Psychiatry, LI Jewish Med Ctr 1981; **Fellow:** Psychiatry, LI Jewish Med Ctr 1983

Budman, Cathy L MD (Psyc) - **Spec Exp:** Tourette's Syndrome; ADD/ADHD; Obsessive-Compulsive Disorder; **Hospital:** N Shore Univ Hosp at Manhasset; **Address:** North Shore-LIJ Health System, Dept Psy & Neur, 400 Community Drive, Manhasset, NY 11030; **Phone:** 516-562-3223; **Board Cert:** Psychiatry 1991; **Med School:** SUNY Buffalo 1984; **Resid:** Psychiatry, Langley Porter Psych Inst/UCSF 1986; Psychiatry, N Shore Univ Hosp 1990; **Fellow:** Family Medicine, Sydney Univ-Royal Price Albert Hosp 1988; Neuropsychiatry, N Shore Univ Hosp 1991; **Fac Appt:** Assoc Prof Psyc, NYU Sch Med

Carone, Patrick F MD (Psyc) - **Spec Exp:** Geriatric Psychiatry; Depression; **Hospital:** Mercy Med Ctr - Rockville Centre; **Address:** 2000 N Village Ave, Ste 305, Rockville Centre, NY 11570-1001; **Phone:** 516-766-2871; **Board Cert:** Psychiatry 1977; **Med School:** Johns Hopkins Univ 1970; **Resid:** Psychiatry, Yale-New Haven Hosp 1976; Public Health & Genl Preventive Med, Yale-New Haven Hosp 1977; **Fac Appt:** Asst Clin Prof Psyc, SUNY Stony Brook

Crasta, Jovita M MD (Psyc) - **Spec Exp:** Anxiety Disorders; Depression; Bipolar/Mood Disorders; **Hospital:** South Nassau Comm Hosp; **Address:** 2277 Grand Ave, Baldwin, NY 11510-3148; **Phone:** 516-771-7509; **Board Cert:** Psychiatry 1991; **Med School:** India 1981; **Resid:** Psychiatry, Nassau County Med Ctr 1987; **Fac Appt:** Asst Prof Psyc, NY Coll Osteo Med

Desai, Rajesh MD (Psyc) - **Spec Exp:** Child & Adolescent Psychiatry; Geriatric Psychiatry; **Hospital:** Long Beach Med Ctr; **Address:** 871 E Park Ave, Long Beach, NY 11561; **Phone:** 516-889-8844; **Board Cert:** Child & Adolescent Psychiatry 1977; Geriatric Psychiatry 2004; Addiction Psychiatry 1996; Forensic Psychiatry 1998; **Med School:** India 1970; **Resid:** Psychiatry, Mt Sinai Hosp 1974; Child & Adolescent Psychiatry, Mt Sinai Hosp 1976

Gurevich, Michael MD (Psyc) - **Spec Exp:** Psychotherapy & Psychopharmacology; Acupuncture; Addiction/Substance Abuse; Complementary Medicine; **Hospital:** N Shore Univ Hosp at Glen Cove; **Address:** 997 Glen Cove Avenue, Glen Head, NY 11545-1584; **Phone:** 516-674-9489; **Board Cert:** Psychiatry 1989; Addiction Psychiatry 1993; **Med School:** Lithuania 1974; **Resid:** Psychiatry, Elmhurst Hosp Ctr 1987; **Fellow:** Child Psychiatry, Elmhurst Hosp Ctr 1989

Katus, Eli MD (Psyc) - **Spec Exp:** Psychopharmacology; Psychotherapy; Child & Adolescent Psychiatry; **Hospital:** N Shore Univ Hosp at Manhasset, Winthrop - Univ Hosp; **Address:** 1035 Route 106, East Norwich, NY 11732-1005; **Phone:** 516-922-5607; **Board Cert:** Psychiatry 1990; Child & Adolescent Psychiatry 1991; **Med School:** Germany 1982; **Resid:** Psychiatry, N Shore Univ Hosp 1986; **Fellow:** Child & Adolescent Psychiatry, N Shore Univ Hosp 1988

Katz, Jack L. MD (Psyc) - **Spec Exp:** Eating Disorders; Mood Disorders; Anxiety Disorders; **Hospital:** N Shore Univ Hosp at Manhasset; **Address:** N Shore Univ Hosp, Dept Psychiatry, 400 Community Drive, Ste 81, Manhasset, NY 11030-3815; **Phone:** 516-562-3201; **Board Cert:** Psychiatry 1968; **Med School:** Albert Einstein Coll Med 1960; **Resid:** Psychiatry, Montefiore Hosp Med Ctr 1966; **Fellow:** Psychiatry, Montefiore Hosp Med Ctr-Einstein 1968; **Fac Appt:** Prof Psyc, NYU Sch Med

Sami, Sherif MD (Psyc) - **Spec Exp:** Depression; Anxiety & Mood Disorders; Geriatric Psychiatry; **Hospital:** Winthrop - Univ Hosp, N Shore Univ Hosp at Manhasset; **Address:** 7 Bond St, Great Neck, NY 11021; **Phone:** 516-487-9191; **Board Cert:** Psychiatry 1973; Geriatric Psychiatry 1996; **Med School:** Egypt 1961; **Resid:** Psychiatry, Cairo Univ Hosp 1966; Psychiatry, Elmhurst Hosp 1969; **Fellow:** Community Psychiatry, Albert Einstein Coll of Med

PULMONARY DISEASE

Blum, Alan MD (Pul) - **Spec Exp:** Cough-Chronic; Asthma; Sleep Disorders; **Hospital:** South Nassau Comm Hosp, Franklin Hosp Med Ctr; **Address:** 444 Merrick Rd Fl Lower Level 1, Lynbrook, NY 11563-2400; **Phone:** 516-593-9500; **Board Cert:** Internal Medicine 1981; Pulmonary Disease 1984; Critical Care Medicine 1997; **Med School:** Mexico 1977; **Resid:** Internal Medicine, Mt Sinai Hosp Ctr 1981; **Fellow:** Pulmonary Disease, Mt Sinai Hosp Ctr 1983

Breidbart, David MD (Pul) - **Spec Exp:** Asthma; Chronic Obstructive Lung Disease (COPD); Sarcoidosis; **Hospital:** N Shore Univ Hosp at Manhasset, St Francis Hosp - The Heart Ctr (page 112); **Address:** 6 Ohio Drive, Ste 201, LSQ Medical Bldg, Lake Success, NY 11042-1129; **Phone:** 516-328-8700; **Board Cert:** Internal Medicine 1982; Pulmonary Disease 1984; **Med School:** SUNY Downstate 1979; **Resid:** Internal Medicine, North Shore Univ Hosp 1982; **Fellow:** Pulmonary Disease, Memorial Sloan-Kettering Hosp 1983; Pulmonary Disease, Montefiore-Albert Einstein Med Ctr 1985; **Fac Appt:** Asst Clin Prof Med, NYU Sch Med

Cohen, Michael L MD (Pul) - **Spec Exp:** Asthma; Bronchitis; Emphysema; **Hospital:** N Shore Univ Hosp at Manhasset; **Address:** N Shore Internal Med Assocs, PC, 560 Northern Blvd, Ste 203, Great Neck, NY 11021-5100; **Phone:** 516-482-0600; **Board Cert:** Internal Medicine 1972; Pulmonary Disease 1974; **Med School:** SUNY Upstate Med Univ 1967; **Resid:** Internal Medicine, Montefiore Hosp Med Ctr 1970; **Fellow:** Pulmonary Disease, Montefiore Hosp Med Ctr 1971; Pulmonary Disease, LI Jewish Med Ctr 1974; **Fac Appt:** Asst Clin Prof Med, NYU Sch Med

Efferen, Linda S MD (Pul) - **Spec Exp:** Sarcoidosis; Tuberculosis; Critical Care Medicine; **Hospital:** Long Island Jewish Med Ctr, N Shore Univ Hosp at Manhasset; **Address:** 270-05 76th Ave, rm B205, New Hyde Park, NY 11040; **Phone:** 718-470-7717; **Board Cert:** Internal Medicine 1988; Pulmonary Disease 2001; Critical Care Medicine 2001; **Med School:** Israel 1983; **Resid:** Internal Medicine, Kings Co Hosp 1987; **Fellow:** Pulmonary Disease, Albert Einstein 1989; Critical Care Medicine, Albert Einstein 1990; **Fac Appt:** Assoc Clin Prof Med, Albert Einstein Coll Med

Fein, Alan MD (Pul) - **Spec Exp:** Chronic Obstructive Lung Disease (COPD); Asthma; Pneumonia; **Hospital:** N Shore Univ Hosp at Manhasset, Long Island Jewish Med Ctr; **Address:** 2800 Marcus Ave, Dept Pulmonary Med, Lake Success, NY 11042; **Phone:** 516-608-2890; **Board Cert:** Internal Medicine 2000; Pulmonary Disease 2000; Critical Care Medicine 1999; **Med School:** SUNY Downstate 1973; **Resid:** Albert Einstein 1976; **Fellow:** Pulmonary Disease, UC San Francisco Med Ctr 1978

Gordon, Richard Eric MD (Pul) - **Spec Exp:** Emphysema; Sleep Disorders; Asthma; **Hospital:** New Island Hosp, N Shore Univ Hosp at Plainview; **Address:** Island Pul Assoc, 4271 Hempstead Tpke, Bethpage, NY 11714-5718; **Phone:** 516-796-3700; **Board Cert:** Internal Medicine 1984; Pulmonary Disease 1986; **Med School:** Mount Sinai Sch Med 1980; **Resid:** Internal Medicine, Beth Israel 1983; **Fellow:** Pulmonary Disease, Queens Hosp Ctr 1985

Greenberg, Harly MD (Pul) - **Spec Exp:** Sleep Disorders/Apnea; Lung Disease; Critical Care; **Hospital:** Long Island Jewish Med Ctr; **Address:** North Shore LIJ Sleep Disorders Ctr, 410 Lakeville Rd, Ste 105, New Hyde Park, NY 11040; **Phone:** 516-465-3899; **Board Cert:** Internal Medicine 1985; Pulmonary Disease 1988; **Med School:** NYU Sch Med 1982; **Resid:** Internal Medicine, North Shore Univ Hosp 1985; **Fellow:** Pulmonary Disease, NYU-Bellevue Hosp Ctr 1987; **Fac Appt:** Assoc Prof Med, Albert Einstein Coll Med

Kamholz, Stephan MD (Pul) - **Spec Exp:** Critical Care; Tuberculosis; Transplant Medicine-Lung; **Hospital:** N Shore Univ Hosp at Manhasset, Long Island Jewish Med Ctr; **Address:** 300 Community Drive, Dept Medicine, 4DSU, Manhasset, NY 11030; **Phone:** 516-562-4310; **Board Cert:** Internal Medicine 1987; Pulmonary Disease 1978; Critical Care Medicine 1997; **Med School:** NY Med Coll 1972; **Resid:** Internal Medicine, Montefiore Hosp Med Ctr 1975; **Fellow:** Pulmonary Disease, Montefiore Hosp Med Ctr 1977; **Fac Appt:** Prof Med, NYU Sch Med

Karp, Jason B MD (Pul) - **Spec Exp:** Asthma; Chronic Obstructive Lung Disease (COPD); Critical Care; **Hospital:** N Shore Univ Hosp at Manhasset, St Francis Hosp - The Heart Ctr (page 112); **Address:** 6 Ohio Drive, Ste 201, LSQ Medical Bldg, Lake Success, NY 10042; **Phone:** 516-328-8700; **Board Cert:** Internal Medicine 2002; Pulmonary Disease 2004; Critical Care Medicine 2000; **Med School:** SUNY Downstate 1988; **Resid:** Internal Medicine, Montefiore Med Ctr 1991; **Fellow:** Pulmonary Disease, NYU Med Ctr

Marcus, Philip MD (Pul) - **Spec Exp:** Asthma-Adult & Pediatric; Chronic Obstructive Lung Disease (COPD); Sarcoidosis; **Hospital:** St Francis Hosp - The Heart Ctr (page 112), N Shore Univ Hosp at Manhasset; **Address:** 233 E Shore Rd, Ste 112, Great Neck, NY 11023-2433; **Phone:** 516-482-7810; **Board Cert:** Internal Medicine 1987; Pulmonary Disease 1978; Critical Care Medicine 1999; **Med School:** SUNY Downstate 1973; **Resid:** Internal Medicine, Long Island Jewish-Hillside Med Ctr 1976; Pulmonary Disease, Queens Hosp Ctr 1977; **Fellow:** Pulmonary Disease, Northport VA Hosp 1978; **Fac Appt:** Prof Med, NY Coll Osteo Med

Mensch, Alan MD (Pul) - **Spec Exp:** Asthma; Chronic Obstructive Lung Disease (COPD); **Hospital:** N Shore Univ Hosp at Plainview, N Shore Univ Hosp at Syosset; **Address:** 453 S Oyster Bay Rd, Plainview, NY 11803-3311; **Phone:** 516-433-2922; **Board Cert:** Internal Medicine 1976; Pulmonary Disease 1978; **Med School:** Univ Hlth Sci/Chicago Med Sch 1973; **Resid:** Internal Medicine, Nassau County Med Ctr 1976; **Fellow:** Pulmonary Disease, Nassau County Med Ctr 1978; **Fac Appt:** Asst Clin Prof Med, SUNY Stony Brook

Mermelstein, Steve MD (Pul) - **Spec Exp:** Asthma; Chronic Obstructive Lung Disease (COPD); Cough-Chronic; **Hospital:** South Nassau Comm Hosp, Franklin Hosp Med Ctr; **Address:** 444 Merrick Rd, Lower Level 1, Lynbrook, NY 11563-2456; **Phone:** 516-593-9500; **Board Cert:** Internal Medicine 1980; Pulmonary Disease 1982; Critical Care Medicine 1997; **Med School:** Albert Einstein Coll Med 1977; **Resid:** Internal Medicine, Metropolitan Hosp Ctr 1980; **Fellow:** Pulmonary Disease, St Luke's-Roosevelt Hosp Ctr 1982

Newmark, Ian H MD (Pul) - **Spec Exp:** Critical Care; Asthma; Lung Cancer; **Hospital:** N Shore Univ Hosp at Plainview, N Shore Univ Hosp at Syosset; **Address:** 8 Greenfield Rd, Syosset, NY 11791-4831; **Phone:** 516-496-7900; **Board Cert:** Internal Medicine 1982; Pulmonary Disease 1986; Critical Care Medicine 2000; **Med School:** SUNY Hlth Sci Ctr 1979; **Resid:** Internal Medicine, Nassau County Med Ctr 1982; **Fellow:** Pulmonary Intensive Care, Nassau County Med Ctr 1984; **Fac Appt:** Asst Clin Prof Med, SUNY Stony Brook

Niederman, Michael MD (Pul) - **Spec Exp:** Infections-Respiratory; Emphysema; Respiratory Failure; Pneumonia; **Hospital:** Winthrop - Univ Hosp; **Address:** 222 Station Plaza N, Ste 400, Mineola, NY 11501-3893; **Phone:** 516-663-2834; **Board Cert:** Internal Medicine 1980; Pulmonary Disease 1983; Critical Care Medicine 1997; **Med School:** Boston Univ 1977; **Resid:** Internal Medicine, Northwestern Univ Med Ctr 1980; **Fellow:** Pulmonary Disease, Yale-New Haven Hosp 1983; **Fac Appt:** Prof Med, SUNY Stony Brook

Rossoff, Leonard MD (Pul) - **Hospital:** Long Island Jewish Med Ctr; **Address:** LIJ Med Ctr, Div Pulmonary Med, 410 Lakeville Rd, Ste 107, New Hyde Park, NY 11040; **Phone:** 516-465-5400; **Board Cert:** Internal Medicine 1978; Pulmonary Disease 1980; **Med School:** McGill Univ 1972; **Resid:** Internal Medicine, McGill Univ 1976; **Fellow:** Pulmonary Critical Care Medicine, Univ Toronto Genl Hosp 1978; Pulmonary Critical Care Medicine, Mt Sinai Hosp 1979; **Fac Appt:** Assoc Prof Med, Albert Einstein Coll Med

Rothman, Nathan MD (Pul) - **Spec Exp:** Asthma; **Hospital:** St John's Epis Hosp - S Shore, South Nassau Comm Hosp; **Address:** 360 Central Ave, Ste 113, Lawrence, NY 11559; **Phone:** 516-569-6966; **Board Cert:** Internal Medicine 1977; Pulmonary Disease 1982; Critical Care Medicine 1998; **Med School:** Albert Einstein Coll Med 1974; **Resid:** Internal Medicine, Montefiore Hosp Med Ctr 1977; **Fellow:** Pulmonary Disease, Montefiore Med Ctr

Rubenstein, Roy MD (Pul) - **Spec Exp:** Asthma; Chronic Obstructive Lung Disease (COPD); Emphysema; **Hospital:** Mercy Med Ctr - Rockville Centre, Franklin Hosp Med Ctr; **Address:** 505 Hempstead Ave, Rockville Centre, NY 11570; **Phone:** 516-766-3343; **Board Cert:** Internal Medicine 1982; Pulmonary Disease 1986; Critical Care Medicine 1999; **Med School:** NYU Sch Med 1978; **Resid:** Internal Medicine, Jacobi Med Ctr 1981; **Fellow:** Pulmonary Disease, Albert Einstein 1983

Schulster, Rita B MD (Pul) - **Spec Exp:** Asthma; Bronchitis; **Hospital:** Long Beach Med Ctr, South Nassau Comm Hosp; **Address:** 442 E Waukena Ave, Oceanside, NY 11572; **Phone:** 516-599-8234; **Board Cert:** Pulmonary Disease 1978; Internal Medicine 1977; **Med School:** Albert Einstein Coll Med 1970; **Resid:** Internal Medicine, Beth Israel 1973; Internal Medicine, Beth Israel 1974; **Fellow:** Pulmonary Disease, LI Jewish Med Ctr 1975; Pulmonary Disease, Beth Israel 1976

Steinberg, Harry MD (Pul) - **Spec Exp:** Asthma; Emphysema; Lung Cancer; **Hospital:** Long Island Jewish Med Ctr, N Shore Univ Hosp at Manhasset; **Address:** LI Jewish Med Ctr, Dept Med, 270-05 76th Ave, New Hyde Park, NY 11040-1496; **Phone:** 718-465-5400; **Med School:** Temple Univ 1966; **Resid:** Internal Medicine, LI Jewish Med Ctr 1969; Pulmonary Critical Care Medicine, LI Jewish Med Ctr 1970; **Fellow:** Pulmonary Disease, Hosp U Penn 1974; **Fac Appt:** Clin Prof Med, Albert Einstein Coll Med

Wyner, Perry A MD (Pul) - **Spec Exp:** Asthma; Cough-Chronic; Emphysema; **Hospital:** Mercy Med Ctr - Rockville Centre, Winthrop - Univ Hosp; **Address:** 2 Lincoln Ave, Ste 201, Rockville Centre, NY 11570-5775; **Phone:** 516-536-0600; **Board Cert:** Internal Medicine 1980; Pulmonary Disease 1982; **Med School:** Cornell Univ-Weill Med Coll 1977; **Resid:** Internal Medicine, Med Coll Virginia Hosps 1980; **Fellow:** Pulmonary Disease, Bellevue Hosp 1982

Yang, Chin-tsun MD (Pul) - **Spec Exp:** Chronic Obstructive Lung Disease (COPD); Asthma; Emphysema; Lung Cancer; **Hospital:** Mercy Med Ctr - Rockville Centre, Franklin Hosp Med Ctr; **Address:** 505 Hempstead Ave, Rockville Centre, NY 11570; **Phone:** 516-766-3343; **Board Cert:** Internal Medicine 1974; Pulmonary Disease 1976; **Med School:** Taiwan 1967; **Resid:** Internal Medicine, Elmhurst - Mt Sinai Hosps 1974; **Fellow:** Pulmonary Disease, Elmhurst - Mt Sinai Hosps 1976

Zupnick, Henry MD (Pul) - **Spec Exp:** Asthma; Bronchitis; Cough; **Hospital:** Long Island Jewish Med Ctr, South Nassau Comm Hosp; **Address:** 158 Hempstead Ave, Lynbrook, NY 11563; **Phone:** 516-593-3541; **Board Cert:** Internal Medicine 1983; Pulmonary Disease 1988; Critical Care Medicine 1998; **Med School:** Albert Einstein Coll Med 1980; **Resid:** Internal Medicine, Brookdale Hosp Med Ctr 1983; **Fellow:** Pulmonary Disease, Columbia-Presby Med Ctr 1985; Critical Care Medicine, Mount Sinai Hosp 1987; **Fac Appt:** Asst Clin Prof Med, SUNY Downstate

RADIATION ONCOLOGY

Ames, John W MD (RadRO) - **Spec Exp:** Prostate Cancer; Brain Tumors; Lymphoma; **Hospital:** St Francis Hosp - The Heart Ctr (page 112), N Shore Univ Hosp at Syosset; **Address:** 6 Ohio Drive, Lake Success, NY 11042; **Phone:** 516-394-8100; **Board Cert:** Radiation Oncology 1996; **Med School:** Geo Wash Univ 1987; **Resid:** Radiation Oncology, Hosp U Penn 1994; **Fac Appt:** Assoc Clin Prof RadRO, NY Coll Osteo Med

Bosworth, Jay L MD (RadRO) - **Spec Exp:** Breast Cancer; Prostate Cancer; Lymphoma; **Hospital:** St Francis Hosp - The Heart Ctr (page 112), N Shore Univ Hosp at Syosset; **Address:** 1129 Northern Blvd, Manhasset, NY 11030-3022; **Phone:** 516-365-6544; **Board Cert:** Therapeutic Radiology 1974; **Med School:** Albert Einstein Coll Med 1970; **Resid:** Radiation Oncology, Bronx Muni Hosp Ctr 1974

Del Rowe, John MD (RadRO) - **Spec Exp:** Lung Cancer; Brain Cancer; **Hospital:** Long Island Jewish Med Ctr; **Address:** LI Jewish Med Ctr, Dept Rad Onc, 270-05 76th Ave, New Hyde Park, NY 11040; **Phone:** 718-470-7733; **Board Cert:** Radiation Oncology 1984; **Med School:** Hahnemann Univ 1979; **Resid:** Radiation Oncology, NYU Med Ctr 1983

Diamond, Ezriel MD (RadRO) - **Hospital:** N Shore Univ Hosp at Plainview, New Island Hosp; **Address:** 688 Old Country Rd, Plainview, NY 11803; **Phone:** 516-932-6007; **Board Cert:** Therapeutic Radiology 1982; **Med School:** NYU Sch Med 1978; **Resid:** Radiation Oncology, NYU Med Ctr 1981; **Fellow:** Radiation Oncology, NY Methodist Hosp 1982

Katz, Alan MD (RadRO) - **Spec Exp:** Brachytherapy; Prostate Cancer; **Hospital:** Winthrop - Univ Hosp, New Island Hosp; **Address:** Winthrop Univ Hosp, Dept Rad Onc, 259 1st St, Mineola, NY 11501; **Phone:** 516-663-2501; **Board Cert:** Therapeutic Radiology 1981; **Med School:** NYU Sch Med 1977; **Resid:** Therapeutic Radiology, NYU Med Ctr 1981

Marin, Lorraine A MD (RadRO) - **Spec Exp:** Breast Cancer; Gynecologic Cancer; Pediatric Cancers; **Hospital:** Long Island Jewish Med Ctr, N Shore Univ Hosp at Glen Cove; **Address:** 270-05 76th Ave, New Hyde Park, NY 11040-1496; **Phone:** 718-470-7194; **Board Cert:** Internal Medicine 1980; Medical Oncology 1983; Therapeutic Radiology 1986; **Med School:** UC Davis 1977; **Resid:** Internal Medicine, UC Davis Med Ctr 1980; **Fellow:** Medical Oncology, Natl Cancer Inst/NIH 1983; Radiation Oncology, Natl Cancer Inst/NIH 1985; **Fac Appt:** Asst Clin Prof RadRO, Albert Einstein Coll Med

Pollack, Jed MD (RadRO) - **Spec Exp:** Head & Neck Cancer; Prostate Cancer; Brain Tumors; **Address:** Long Island Radiation Therapy, 6 Ohio Drive, Ste 103, Lake Success, NY 11042; **Phone:** 516-394-8100; **Board Cert:** Therapeutic Radiology 1985; **Med School:** Univ New Mexico 1981; **Resid:** Therapeutic Radiology, Meml Sloan-Kettering Cancer Ctr 1985; **Fac Appt:** Asst Clin Prof RadRO, Albert Einstein Coll Med

Rush, Stephen MD (RadRO) - **Spec Exp:** Brain Tumors; Gamma Knife Radiosurgery; Head & Neck Cancer; **Hospital:** NYU Med Ctr (page 102); **Address:** LI Rad Therapy Ctr, 700 Stweart Ave Fl 1, Garden City, NY 11530; **Phone:** 516-365-6544; **Board Cert:** Radiation Oncology 1990; **Med School:** Howard Univ 1983; **Resid:** Radiation Oncology, NYU Med Ctr 1989; **Fac Appt:** Asst Clin Prof RadRO, NYU Sch Med

Reproductive Endocrinology

Brenner, Steven H MD (RE) - **Spec Exp:** Infertility-IVF; Polycystic Ovarian Syndrome; **Hospital:** Long Island Jewish Med Ctr, John T Mather Meml Hosp of Port Jefferson; **Address:** 2001 Marcus Ave, Ste N213, Lake Success, NY 11042; **Phone:** 516-358-6363; **Board Cert:** Obstetrics & Gynecology 1985; Reproductive Endocrinology 1987; **Med School:** SUNY Downstate 1978; **Resid:** Obstetrics & Gynecology, Beth Israel Med Ctr 1982; **Fellow:** Reproductive Endocrinology, NYU Med Ctr 1984; **Fac Appt:** Assoc Clin Prof ObG, Albert Einstein Coll Med

Rosenfeld, David MD (RE) - **Spec Exp:** Infertility-IVF; Endometriosis; Uterine Fibroids; **Hospital:** N Shore Univ Hosp at Manhasset; **Address:** Div Human Reproduction, 300 Community Drive Ambulatory Bldg, Manhasset, NY 11030-3801; **Phone:** 516-562-2229; **Board Cert:** Reproductive Endocrinology 1980; Obstetrics & Gynecology 1976; **Med School:** Univ Pennsylvania 1970; **Resid:** Obstetrics & Gynecology, Hosp Univ Penn 1974; **Fellow:** Reproductive Endocrinology, Hosp Univ Penn 1976; **Fac Appt:** Prof ObG, NYU Sch Med

Rheumatology

Belilos, Elise MD (Rhu) - **Spec Exp:** Polymyalgia Rheumatica; Giant Cell Arteritis; Rheumatoid Arthritis; **Hospital:** Winthrop - Univ Hosp; **Address:** Winthrop Univ Hosp, Div Rheum, 120 Mineola Blvd, Ste 410, Mineola, NY 11501; **Phone:** 516-663-2097; **Board Cert:** Internal Medicine 1989; Rheumatology 2004; **Med School:** SUNY Stony Brook 1986; **Resid:** Internal Medicine, Winthrop Univ Hosp 1990; **Fellow:** Rheumatology, Winthrop UnivHosp 1993; **Fac Appt:** Asst Clin Prof Med, SUNY Stony Brook

Blau, Sheldon P MD (Rhu) - **Spec Exp:** Lupus/SLE; Scleroderma; Rheumatoid Arthritis; **Hospital:** Winthrop - Univ Hosp; **Address:** 566 Broadway, Massapequa, NY 11758-5017; **Phone:** 516-541-6262; **Board Cert:** Internal Medicine 1969; Rheumatology 1972; **Med School:** Albert Einstein Coll Med 1961; **Resid:** Internal Medicine, Montefiore Med Ctr 1964; **Fellow:** Rheumatology, Albert Einstein Coll Med 1965; **Fac Appt:** Clin Prof Med, SUNY Stony Brook

Carsons, Steven MD (Rhu) - **Spec Exp:** Rheumatoid Arthritis; Sjogren's Syndrome; **Hospital:** Winthrop - Univ Hosp; **Address:** Div Rheumatology & Allergy, 222 Station Plaza N, Ste 430, Mineola, NY 11501; **Phone:** 516-663-2097; **Board Cert:** Internal Medicine 1978; Rheumatology 1980; Clinical & Laboratory Immunology 1988; **Med School:** NY Med Coll 1975; **Resid:** Internal Medicine, Maimonides Med Ctr 1978; **Fellow:** Rheumatology, SUNY Hosp 1980; **Fac Appt:** Prof Med, SUNY Hlth Sci Ctr

Chiorazzi, Nicholas MD (Rhu) - **Spec Exp:** Rheumatoid Arthritis; Lupus/SLE; **Hospital:** N Shore Univ Hosp at Manhasset; **Address:** 350 Community Drive, Manhasset, NY 11030; **Phone:** 516-562-1085; **Board Cert:** Internal Medicine 1973; Allergy & Immunology 1999; Clinical & Laboratory Immunology 1990; Rheumatology 1996; **Med School:** Georgetown Univ 1970; **Resid:** Internal Medicine, Cornell Co-op Hosps 1974; **Fellow:** Allergy & Immunology, NY Hosp-Cornell 1987; **Fac Appt:** Prof Med, NYU Sch Med

Cohen, Daniel H MD (Rhu) - **Spec Exp:** Osteoporosis; Arthritis; **Hospital:** St John's Epis Hosp - S Shore, Long Beach Med Ctr; **Address:** 1157 Broadway, Hewlett, NY 11557; **Phone:** 516-295-4481; **Board Cert:** Rheumatology 1984; Internal Medicine 1981; **Med School:** NYU Sch Med 1978; **Resid:** Internal Medicine, Columbia-Presby 1981; **Fellow:** Rheumatology, New York Univ Med Ctr 1983

Furie, Richard MD (Rhu) - **Spec Exp:** Lupus/SLE; Vasculitis; Rheumatoid Arthritis; **Hospital:** N Shore Univ Hosp at Manhasset, Hosp For Special Surgery (page 108); **Address:** North Shore Long Island Jewish Health System, 2800 Marcus Ave, Ste 200, Lake Success, NY 11042; **Phone:** 516-708-2550; **Board Cert:** Internal Medicine 1982; Rheumatology 1984; **Med School:** Cornell Univ-Weill Med Coll 1979; **Resid:** Internal Medicine, NY Hosp 1982; **Fellow:** Rheumatology, Hosp For Special Surgery 1984; **Fac Appt:** Assoc Prof, NYU Sch Med

Greenwald, Robert MD (Rhu) - **Spec Exp:** Rheumatoid Arthritis; Psoriatic Arthritis; Osteoarthritis; **Hospital:** Long Island Jewish Med Ctr, N Shore Univ Hosp at Syosset; **Address:** 2800 Marcus Ave, Ste 200, Lake Success, NY 11042; **Phone:** 516-708-2550; **Board Cert:** Internal Medicine 1973; Rheumatology 1974; **Med School:** Johns Hopkins Univ 1967; **Resid:** Internal Medicine, Long Island Jewish-Hillside Med Ctr 1970; **Fellow:** Rheumatology, SUNY Brooklyn Med Ctr 1972; **Fac Appt:** Prof Med, Albert Einstein Coll Med

Hoffman, Michael L MD (Rhu) - **Spec Exp:** Lupus/SLE; Rheumatoid Arthritis; Osteoarthritis; **Hospital:** Long Island Jewish Med Ctr, NY Hosp Queens; **Address:** 277 Northern Blvd, Ste 312, Great Neck, NY 11021; **Phone:** 516-498-3500; **Board Cert:** Internal Medicine 1971; **Med School:** SUNY Downstate 1965; **Resid:** Internal Medicine, Maimonides Med Ctr 1967; Internal Medicine, Jacobi Med Ctr 1968; **Fellow:** Rheumatology, Hosp for Special Surg 1970; **Fac Appt:** Assoc Clin Prof Med, Albert Einstein Coll Med

Lipstein-Kresch, Esther MD (Rhu) - **Spec Exp:** Rheumatoid Arthritis; Osteoarthritis; Osteoporosis; **Hospital:** Long Island Jewish Med Ctr, N Shore Univ Hosp at Manhasset; **Address:** 2800 Marcus Ave, Ste 200-A, Lake Success, NY 11042-1008; **Phone:** 516-622-6090; **Board Cert:** Internal Medicine 1982; Rheumatology 1984; **Med School:** SUNY Hlth Sci Ctr 1979; **Resid:** Internal Medicine, LI Jewish Med Ctr 1982; **Fellow:** Rheumatology, LI Jewish Med Ctr 1984; **Fac Appt:** Asst Prof Med, Mount Sinai Sch Med

Meredith, Gary MD (Rhu) - **Spec Exp:** Gout; Lupus/SLE; Rheumatoid Arthritis; **Hospital:** Mercy Med Ctr - Rockville Centre, Franklin Hosp Med Ctr; **Address:** 242 Merrick Rd, Ste 303, Rockville Centre, NY 11570-5254; **Phone:** 516-536-9424; **Board Cert:** Internal Medicine 1984; Rheumatology 1986; **Med School:** NYU Sch Med 1981; **Resid:** Internal Medicine, Bellevue Hosp 1984; **Fellow:** Rheumatology, NYU Med Ctr 1986; **Fac Appt:** Asst Clin Prof Med, NYU Sch Med

Porges, Andrew MD (Rhu) - **Spec Exp:** Osteoporosis; **Hospital:** N Shore Univ Hosp at Manhasset, N Shore Univ Hosp at Glen Cove; **Address:** 1044 Northern Blvd, Ste 104, Roslyn, NY 11576; **Phone:** 516-484-6880; **Board Cert:** Internal Medicine 1989; Rheumatology 1992; **Med School:** Cornell Univ-Weill Med Coll 1986; **Resid:** Internal Medicine, NY Hosp 1989; **Fellow:** Rheumatology, Hosp Special Surg 1992; **Fac Appt:** Asst Prof Med, Cornell Univ-Weill Med Coll

Sullivan, James MD (Rhu) - **Spec Exp:** Rheumatoid Arthritis; Lupus/SLE; Osteoarthritis; **Hospital:** Winthrop - Univ Hosp; **Address:** 181 E Jericho Tpke, Mineola, NY 11501; **Phone:** 516-248-6262; **Board Cert:** Internal Medicine 1977; Rheumatology 1980; **Med School:** SUNY Hlth Sci Ctr 1974; **Resid:** Internal Medicine, Univ Michigan Med Ctr 1977; **Fellow:** Rheumatology, Univ Michigan Med Ctr 1979

Tiger, Louis MD (Rhu) - **Spec Exp:** Rheumatoid Arthritis; Lupus/SLE; Osteoarthritis; **Hospital:** Winthrop - Univ Hosp, Mercy Med Ctr - Rockville Centre; **Address:** 566 Broadway, Massapequa, NY 11758-5017; **Phone:** 516-541-6262; **Board Cert:** Internal Medicine 1975; Rheumatology 1976; **Med School:** Univ Louisville Sch Med 1967; **Resid:** Internal Medicine, Maimonides Medical Ctr 1970; **Fellow:** Rheumatology, Albert Einstein 1974; **Fac Appt:** Asst Clin Prof Med, SUNY Stony Brook

Sports Medicine

Hershon, Stuart MD (SM) - **Spec Exp:** Sports Medicine; Shoulder Injuries; Knee Injuries; **Hospital:** N Shore Univ Hosp at Manhasset, St Luke's - Roosevelt Hosp Ctr - Roosevelt Div (page 90); **Address:** 333 E Shore Rd, Ste 101, Manhasset, NY 11030; **Phone:** 516-466-3351; **Board Cert:** Orthopaedic Surgery 1973; **Med School:** NY Med Coll 1963; **Resid:** Surgery, Georgetown Univ Hosp 1967; Orthopaedic Surgery, St Luke's-Roosevelt Hosp Ctr 1970; **Fac Appt:** Asst Prof OrS, Cornell Univ-Weill Med Coll

Orlin, Harvey MD (SM) - **Spec Exp:** Sports Injuries; Knee Surgery; Hip Surgery; **Hospital:** South Nassau Comm Hosp; **Address:** 36 Lincoln Ave Fl 3, Rockville Centre, NY 11570; **Phone:** 516-536-2800; **Board Cert:** Orthopaedic Surgery 1968; **Med School:** SUNY Hlth Sci Ctr 1961; **Resid:** Orthopaedic Surgery, Bellevue Hosp 1963; Orthopaedic Surgery, Columbia-Presby Med Ctr 1966

Putterman, Eric A MD (SM) - **Spec Exp:** Arthroscopic Surgery; **Hospital:** N Shore Univ Hosp at Plainview, N Shore Univ Hosp at Glen Cove; **Address:** 651 Old Country Rd, Plainview, NY 11803-4942; **Phone:** 516-681-8822; **Board Cert:** Orthopaedic Surgery 1988; **Med School:** Mount Sinai Sch Med 1980; **Resid:** Orthopaedic Surgery, NYU-Bellevue Med Ctr 1985; **Fellow:** Sports Medicine, NYU-Bellevue Med Ctr 1985

Yerys, Paul MD (SM) - **Spec Exp:** Arthroscopic Surgery; Sports Medicine; Knee Surgery; **Hospital:** N Shore Univ Hosp at Syosset, Winthrop - Univ Hosp; **Address:** 30 Merrick Ave, East Meadow, NY 11554-1580; **Phone:** 516-794-7010; **Board Cert:** Orthopaedic Surgery 1972; **Med School:** SUNY Hlth Sci Ctr 1961; **Resid:** Surgery, Meadowbrook Hosp 1967; **Fellow:** Orthopaedic Surgery, Meadowbrook Hosp 1970; **Fac Appt:** Clin Prof OrS, SUNY Stony Brook

SURGERY

Auguste, Louis J MD (S) - **Spec Exp:** Breast Disease; Melanoma; Thyroid & Parathyroid Surgery; **Hospital:** Long Island Jewish Med Ctr, N Shore Univ Hosp at Manhasset; **Address:** 410 Lakeville Rd, Ste 100, New Hyde Park, NY 11042; **Phone:** 516-775-2070; **Board Cert:** Surgery 2000; **Med School:** Haiti 1973; **Resid:** Surgery, L I Jewish Med Ctr 1980; **Fellow:** Surgical Oncology, Roswell Park Meml Inst 1982; **Fac Appt:** Assoc Clin Prof S, Albert Einstein Coll Med

Blau, Steven MD (S) - **Spec Exp:** Critical Care; Trauma; **Hospital:** N Shore Univ Hosp at Manhasset; **Address:** 300 Community Drive, Manhasset, NY 11030; **Phone:** 516-562-2993; **Board Cert:** Surgery 2001; Surgical Critical Care 1997; **Med School:** Univ Chicago-Pritzker Sch Med 1974; **Resid:** Surgical Oncology, NIH-NCI 1978; Surgery, Tulane Univ 1981; **Fellow:** Trauma, LA State Univ 1982; **Fac Appt:** Assoc Prof S, Albert Einstein Coll Med

Conte, Charles Carmine MD (S) - **Spec Exp:** Cancer Surgery; Breast Cancer; Pancreatic Cancer; **Hospital:** N Shore Univ Hosp at Manhasset, Flushing Hosp Med Ctr; **Address:** 600 Northern Blvd, Ste 111, Great Neck, NY 11021; **Phone:** 516-487-9454; **Board Cert:** Surgery 1995; **Med School:** Dartmouth Med Sch 1981; **Resid:** Surgery, Hartford Hosp 1986; **Fellow:** Surgical Oncology, Roswell Park Cancer Inst 1988

Cosgrove, John M MD (S) - **Spec Exp:** Laparoscopic Surgery; **Hospital:** N Shore Univ Hosp at Manhasset; **Address:** 1919 Marcus Ave, Ste 106C, Lake Success, NY 11042; **Phone:** 516-233-3600; **Board Cert:** Surgery 1998; **Med School:** NY Med Coll 1983; **Resid:** Surgery, Beth Israel Med Ctr 1988; **Fac Appt:** Assoc Prof S, Albert Einstein Coll Med

Datta, Rajiv MD (S) - **Spec Exp:** Head & Neck Cancer; Liver Cancer; Pancreatic Cancer; **Hospital:** South Nassau Comm Hosp; **Address:** South Nassau Cancer Ctr, Surgical Oncology, 1 S Central Ave, Valley Stream, NY 11580; **Phone:** 516-632-3350; **Board Cert:** Surgery 1999; **Med School:** India 1984; **Resid:** Surgery, Maimonides Med Ctr

Denoto, George MD (S) - **Spec Exp:** Laparoscopic Surgery; Hernia; **Hospital:** N Shore Univ Hosp at Manhasset; **Address:** 1919 Marcus Ave, Ste 106C, Lake Success, NY 11042; **Phone:** 516-233-3600; **Board Cert:** Surgery 1994; **Med School:** SUNY Stony Brook 1988; **Resid:** Surgery, Mt Sinai Hosp 1993

DeRisi, Dwight MD (S) - **Spec Exp:** Breast Surgery; Breast Cancer; **Hospital:** N Shore Univ Hosp at Manhasset, St Francis Hosp - The Heart Ctr (page 112); **Address:** 1010 Northern Blvd, Ste 140, Great Neck, NY 11021; **Phone:** 516-487-8888; **Med School:** Georgetown Univ 1973; **Resid:** Surgery, North Shore Univ Hosp 1979; **Fellow:** Pathology, North Shore Univ Hosp 1979; **Fac Appt:** Assoc Prof S, Cornell Univ-Weill Med Coll

Friedman, Steven I MD (S) - **Spec Exp:** Breast Surgery; Laparoscopic Surgery; Vascular Surgery; **Hospital:** South Nassau Comm Hosp; **Address:** 77 N Centre Ave, Ste 207, Rockville Centre, NY 11570-3923; **Phone:** 516-764-6206; **Board Cert:** Surgery 2002; **Med School:** NY Med Coll 1976; **Resid:** Surgery, Bronx Muni Hosp Ctr 1978; Surgery, Nassau County Med Ctr 1981

Garber, Shawn MD (S) - **Spec Exp:** Obesity/Bariatric Surgery; Laparoscopic Abdominal Surgery; **Hospital:** St Francis Hosp - The Heart Ctr (page 112), N Shore Univ Hosp at Manhasset; **Address:** 3003 New Hyde Park Rd, Ste 307, New Hyde Park, NY 11042; **Phone:** 516-616-5500; **Board Cert:** Surgery 1998; **Med School:** NY Med Coll 1992; **Resid:** Surgery, LI Jewish Med Ctr 1997; **Fellow:** Laparoscopic Surgery, George Washington Univ Med Ctr 1998; **Fac Appt:** Asst Clin Prof S, Albert Einstein Coll Med

Gecelter, Gary MD (S) - **Spec Exp:** Pancreatic Cancer; Esophageal Surgery; Laparoscopic Surgery; Biliary Surgery; **Hospital:** Long Island Jewish Med Ctr; **Address:** Long Island Jewish Medical Ctr, 270-05 76th Ave, rm B241, New Hyde Park, NY 11040; **Phone:** 718-470-7389; **Board Cert:** Surgery 1990; **Med School:** South Africa 1981; **Resid:** Surgery, Johannesburg Hosp 1990; **Fellow:** Gastroenterology, Johannesburg Hosp 1992

Goldstein, Jonathan MD (S) - **Spec Exp:** Breast Cancer; Gastrointestinal Surgery; **Hospital:** Mercy Med Ctr - Rockville Centre, South Nassau Comm Hosp; **Address:** 30 Hempstead Ave, Ste 144, Rockville Centre, NY 11570-4034; **Phone:** 516-764-5900; **Board Cert:** Surgery 1971; **Med School:** Cornell Univ-Weill Med Coll 1963; **Resid:** Surgery, Bronx Municipal Hosp 1969; **Fac Appt:** Asst Clin Prof S, SUNY Stony Brook

Gordon, Lawrence A MD (S) - **Spec Exp:** Breast Disease; Hernia; **Hospital:** Long Island Jewish Med Ctr, N Shore Univ Hosp at Manhasset; **Address:** 1300 Union Tpke, Ste 108, New Hyde Park, NY 11040-1759; **Phone:** 516-488-2743; **Board Cert:** Surgery 1971; **Med School:** SUNY Downstate 1964; **Resid:** Surgery, LI Jewish Med Ctr 1969

Grieco, Michael B MD (S) - **Spec Exp:** Breast Surgery; Laparoscopic Abdominal Surgery; Laparoscopic Colon Surgery; **Hospital:** N Shore Univ Hosp at Glen Cove, N Shore Univ Hosp at Manhasset; **Address:** 10 Medical Plaza, Glen Cove, NY 11542; **Phone:** 516-676-1060; **Board Cert:** Surgery 2001; Colon & Rectal Surgery 1982; **Med School:** Albany Med Coll 1974; **Resid:** Surgery, N Shore Univ Hosp 1979; **Fellow:** Surgery, Lahey Clinic 1980; Colon & Rectal Surgery, Greater Baltimore Med Ctr 1981; **Fac Appt:** Asst Clin Prof S, SUNY Stony Brook

Held, Douglas MD (S) - **Spec Exp:** Laparoscopic Surgery; Colon & Rectal Surgery; Hernia; **Hospital:** Long Island Jewish Med Ctr, N Shore Univ Hosp at Manhasset; **Address:** 1300 Union Tpke, Ste 108, New Hyde Park, NY 11040; **Phone:** 516-488-2743; **Board Cert:** Surgery 1995; Colon & Rectal Surgery 2001; **Med School:** SUNY Downstate 1980; **Resid:** Surgery, LI Jewish Med Ctr 1985; **Fellow:** Colon & Rectal Surgery, Lehigh Valley Hosp 1986

Heller, Keith S MD (S) - **Spec Exp:** Head & Neck Tumors; Parathyroid Surgery; Thyroid Surgery; **Hospital:** Long Island Jewish Med Ctr, N Shore Univ Hosp at Manhasset; **Address:** 410 Lakeville Rd, Ste 310, Lake Success, NY 11042; **Phone:** 516-437-1111; **Board Cert:** Surgery 1996; **Med School:** NYU Sch Med 1971; **Resid:** Surgery, NYU-Bellevue Hosp 1976; **Fellow:** Surgical Oncology, Meml Sloan Kettering Cancer Ctr 1978; **Fac Appt:** Clin Prof S, Albert Einstein Coll Med

Katz, Paul MD (S) - **Spec Exp:** Laparoscopic Surgery; Breast Surgery; Hernia; **Hospital:** Long Island Jewish Med Ctr, N Shore Univ Hosp at Manhasset; **Address:** 310 E Shore Rd, Ste 309, Great Neck, NY 11042-1214; **Phone:** 516-352-9682; **Board Cert:** Surgery 2004; **Med School:** Hahnemann Univ 1966; **Resid:** Surgery, Long Island Jewish Med Ctr 1974; **Fac Appt:** Asst Clin Prof S, Albert Einstein Coll Med

Khalife, Michael MD (S) - **Spec Exp:** Laparoscopic Surgery; Breast Surgery; **Hospital:** Winthrop - Univ Hosp, N Shore Univ Hosp at Manhasset; **Address:** 173 Mineola Blvd, Ste 302, Mineola, NY 11501; **Phone:** 516-741-4138; **Board Cert:** Surgery 1995; **Med School:** France 1978; **Resid:** Surgery, Univ Hosp 1979; **Fac Appt:** Asst Clin Prof S, SUNY Stony Brook

Kostroff, Karen MD (S) - **Spec Exp:** Breast Cancer & Surgery; **Hospital:** Long Island Jewish Med Ctr, N Shore Univ Hosp at Manhasset; **Address:** 2001 Marcus Ave, Ste W-270, Lake Success, NY 11042; **Phone:** 516-775-7676; **Board Cert:** Surgery 1985; **Med School:** Boston Univ 1979; **Resid:** Surgery, New York Hosp 1984; **Fellow:** Surgical Oncology, Brigham & Womens Hosp 1985; **Fac Appt:** Asst Clin Prof S, Albert Einstein Coll Med

Kurtz, Lewis MD (S) - **Spec Exp:** Breast Surgery; Gallbladder Surgery; Hernia; **Hospital:** St Francis Hosp - The Heart Ctr (page 112), Long Island Jewish Med Ctr; **Address:** 310 E Shore Rd, Ste 203, Great Neck, NY 11023; **Phone:** 516-352-9682; **Board Cert:** Surgery 2000; **Med School:** Italy 1972; **Resid:** Surgery, Long Island Jewish-Hillside Med Ctr 1977; **Fellow:** Research, Long Island Jewish-Hillside Med Ctr 1978

Mansouri, Hormoz MD (S) - **Spec Exp:** Varicose Veins; **Hospital:** New Island Hosp, N Shore Univ Hosp at Plainview; **Address:** 175 Jericho Tpke, Ste 201, Syosset, NY 11791; **Phone:** 516-682-4800; **Board Cert:** Surgery 1980; **Med School:** Iran 1964; **Resid:** Surgery, Henry Ford Hosp 1969; Surgery, Nassau Co Med Ctr 1971

Mansouri, Mehran MD (S) - **Hospital:** N Shore Univ Hosp at Plainview; **Address:** 1181 Old Country Rd, Plainview, NY 11803; **Phone:** 516-681-6611; **Board Cert:** Surgery 1997; **Med School:** Iran 1978; **Resid:** Surgery, Nassau County Med Ctr 1987; **Fellow:** Vascular Surgery, Winthrop Univ Hosp 1988

Monteleone, Frank MD (S) - **Spec Exp:** Breast Surgery; Laparoscopic Surgery; **Hospital:** Winthrop - Univ Hosp; **Address:** 173 Mineola Blvd, Ste 203, Mineola, NY 11501; **Phone:** 516-741-3560; **Board Cert:** Surgery 1996; **Med School:** Italy 1971; **Resid:** Surgery, Nassau Hosp 1977; Surgery, SUNY Stonybrook Med Ctr 1977; **Fac Appt:** Asst Clin Prof S, SUNY Stony Brook

Pesiri, Vincent MD (S) - **Spec Exp:** Breast Surgery; Colon Surgery; Hernia; **Hospital:** N Shore Univ Hosp at Glen Cove; **Address:** 3 School St, Ste 204, Glen Cove, NY 11542-2548; **Phone:** 516-759-2681; **Board Cert:** Surgery 1993; **Med School:** SUNY Downstate 1978; **Resid:** Surgery, Kings County Hosp 1983; **Fellow:** Vascular Surgery, Kings County Hosp 1984; **Fac Appt:** Asst Prof S, SUNY Stony Brook

Pomeranz, Lee MD (S) - **Spec Exp:** Laparoscopic Cholecystectomy; Colon Surgery; Hernia; **Hospital:** N Shore Univ Hosp at Plainview, New Island Hosp; **Address:** 700 Old Country Rd, Ste 205, Plainview, NY 11803-4932; **Phone:** 516-822-1433; **Board Cert:** Surgery 1995; **Med School:** SUNY Hlth Sci Ctr 1979; **Resid:** Surgery, Albert Einstein Coll Med 1984

Procaccino, Angelo MD (S) - **Spec Exp:** Gastrointestinal Surgery; Hernia; Laparoscopic Surgery; **Hospital:** N Shore Univ Hosp at Manhasset, St Francis Hosp - The Heart Ctr (page 112); **Address:** 310 E Shore Rd, Ste 203, Great Neck, NY 11023; **Phone:** 516-482-8657; **Board Cert:** Surgery 1995; **Med School:** NY Med Coll 1979; **Resid:** Surgery, N Shore Univ Hosp 1984

Reiner, Dan MD (S) - **Spec Exp:** Laparoscopic Surgery; Hernia; Gastrointestinal Surgery; **Hospital:** N Shore Univ Hosp at Manhasset, N Shore Univ Hosp at Syosset; **Address:** 2800 Marcus Ave, Lake Success, NY 11042-1052; **Phone:** 516-622-6120; **Board Cert:** Surgery 2005; Surgical Critical Care 1996; **Med School:** St Louis Univ 1980; **Resid:** Surgery, St Louis Univ-Group Hosps 1985; **Fellow:** Surgical Critical Care, UMDNJ-NJ Hosp 1986; **Fac Appt:** Assoc Clin Prof S, NYU Sch Med

Rochman, Andrew J MD (S) - **Spec Exp:** Laparoscopic Surgery; Colon & Rectal Cancer; Hernia; **Hospital:** N Shore Univ Hosp at Plainview, New Island Hosp; **Address:** 700 Old Country Rd, Ste 205, Plainview, NY 11803-4932; **Phone:** 516-822-1433; **Board Cert:** Surgery 2000; **Med School:** Dominican Republic 1980; **Resid:** Surgery, Maimonides Med Ctr 1987; **Fellow:** Research, Maimonides Med Ctr 1988

Romero, Carlos MD (S) - **Spec Exp:** Laparoscopic Surgery; Head & Neck Surgery; Breast Surgery; **Hospital:** Winthrop - Univ Hosp, Mercy Med Ctr - Rockville Centre; **Address:** 173 Mineola Blvd, Ste 401, Mineola, NY 11501-2555; **Phone:** 516-741-6464; **Board Cert:** Surgery 1996; **Med School:** Argentina 1969; **Resid:** Surgery, Winthrop Univ Hosp 1975; **Fellow:** Surgical Oncology, Med Coll Virginia 1977; **Fac Appt:** Assoc Prof S, SUNY Stony Brook

Salzer, Peter MD (S) - **Spec Exp:** Wound Healing/Care; Hyperbaric Medicine; **Hospital:** New Island Hosp, N Shore Univ Hosp at Plainview; **Address:** 4295 Hempstead Tpke, Bethpage, NY 11714; **Phone:** 516-796-1313; **Board Cert:** Surgery 1996; Undersea & Hyperbaric Medicine 2002; **Med School:** Tufts Univ 1970; **Resid:** Surgery, Nassau County Med Ctr 1975; **Fac Appt:** Asst Clin Prof S, SUNY Stony Brook

Vitale, Gerard MD (S) - **Spec Exp:** Aneurysm; Vascular Surgery; Arterial Bypass Surgery; **Hospital:** N Shore Univ Hosp at Glen Cove; **Address:** 10 Medical Plaza, Ste 305, Glen Cove, NY 11542; **Phone:** 516-759-5559; **Board Cert:** Surgery 1997; **Med School:** SUNY Buffalo 1982; **Resid:** Surgery, N Shore Univ Hosp 1987; **Fellow:** Vascular Surgery, St Vincent's Hosp & Med Ctr 1988

Thoracic Surgery

Barrett, Leonard O MD (TS) - **Spec Exp:** Chest Trauma; Esophageal Tumors; **Hospital:** Nassau Univ Med Ctr; **Address:** Nassau Univ Med Ctr, 2201 Hempstead Tpke Fl 8, East Meadow, NY 11554; **Phone:** 516-572-6705; **Board Cert:** Thoracic Surgery 2005; Surgery 2000; Surgical Critical Care 2001; **Med School:** SUNY Downstate 1983; **Resid:** Surgery, SUNY Stony Brook Med Ctr 1989; Cardiothoracic Surgery, Beth Israel Med Ctr 1993; **Fellow:** Surgical Critical Care, Winthrop Univ Med Ctr 1990

Beil, Arthur MD (TS) - **Hospital:** N Shore Univ Hosp at Manhasset; **Address:** 410 Lakeville Rd, Ste 203, New Hyde Park, NY 11040; **Phone:** 516-470-7520; **Board Cert:** Thoracic Surgery 1967; Surgery 1966; **Med School:** Cornell Univ-Weill Med Coll 1959; **Resid:** Thoracic Surgery, NY Hosp-Cornell Med Ctr 1966

Bercow, Neil R MD (TS) - **Spec Exp:** Arterial Bypass Surgery; Cardiac Surgery; Minimally Invasive Cardiac Surgery; Heart Valve Surgery; **Hospital:** St Francis Hosp - The Heart Ctr (page 112); **Address:** Vizza Bldg, 100 Port Washington Blvd, Ste G-01, Roslyn, NY 11576; **Phone:** 516-627-2173; **Board Cert:** Surgery 1999; Thoracic Surgery 1994; **Med School:** West Indies 1985; **Resid:** Surgery, Brooklyn Hosp 1990; Thoracic Surgery, Univ Hosp 1993

Damus, Paul S MD (TS) - **Spec Exp:** Cardiac Surgery; **Hospital:** St Francis Hosp - The Heart Ctr (page 112); **Address:** 100 Port Washington Blvd, Roslyn, NY 11576; **Phone:** 516-365-8372; **Board Cert:** Surgery 1975; Thoracic Surgery 1998; **Med School:** UCLA 1968; **Resid:** Surgery, UCLA Med Ctr 1975; Thoracic Surgery, Columbia Presby Hosp 1979; **Fellow:** Surgical Research, Harvard Med Sch 1972; Cardiothoracic Surgery, Hosp Sick Chldn 1980

Durban, Lawrence H MD (TS) - **Spec Exp:** Cardiac Surgery; Thoracic Surgery; **Hospital:** St Francis Hosp - The Heart Ctr (page 112); **Address:** 100 Port Washington Blvd, Ste G-01, Roslyn, NY 11576; **Phone:** 516-627-2173; **Board Cert:** Surgery 1999; Thoracic Surgery 1999; **Med School:** Cornell Univ-Weill Med Coll 1982; **Resid:** Surgery, NY Hosp-Cornell Med Ctr 1987; **Fellow:** Cardiothoracic Surgery, NY Hosp-Cornell Med Ctr 1989

Fox, Stewart MD (TS) - **Spec Exp:** Minimally Invasive Thoracic Surgery; Pacemakers; Palmar Hyperhidrosis; **Hospital:** South Nassau Comm Hosp, Franklin Hosp Med Ctr; **Address:** 444 Merrick Rd, Ste 380, Lynbrook, NY 11563; **Phone:** 516-255-5010; **Board Cert:** Thoracic Surgery 2000; Surgery 1990; **Med School:** Med Coll VA 1972; **Resid:** Surgery, Yale-New Haven Hosp 1977; **Fellow:** Thoracic Surgery, MS Hershey Med Ctr 1979

Graver, L Michael MD (TS) - **Spec Exp:** Heart Valve Surgery-Aortic; Coronary Artery Surgery; Atrial Fibrillation; **Hospital:** Long Island Jewish Med Ctr, N Shore Univ Hosp at Manhasset; **Address:** 270-05 76th Ave, New Hyde Park, NY 11040-1433; **Phone:** 718-470-7460; **Board Cert:** Surgery 1993; Thoracic Surgery 1995; **Med School:** Albany Med Coll 1977; **Resid:** Surgery, St Luke's-Roosevelt Hosp Ctr 1982; Cardiovascular Surgery, Deaconness Hosp 1983; **Fellow:** Cardiovascular Pathology, NY Hosp-Cornell Med Ctr 1985; **Fac Appt:** Prof TS, Albert Einstein Coll Med

Hartman, Alan MD (TS) - **Spec Exp:** Minimally Invasive Heart Valve Surgery; Aneurysm-Thoracic Aortic; Coronary Artery Surgery; **Hospital:** N Shore Univ Hosp at Manhasset; **Address:** N Shore Univ Hosp, Div Cardiothoracic Surg, 300 Community Drive, Manhasset, NY 11030; **Phone:** 516-562-4970; **Board Cert:** Surgery 2004; Thoracic Surgery 1996; Surgical Critical Care 2000; **Med School:** Mount Sinai Sch Med 1979; **Resid:** Surgery, Bellevue Hosp/NYU 1984; **Fellow:** Cardiothoracic Surgery, Bellevue Hosp/NYU 1986; **Fac Appt:** Assoc Prof S, SUNY Stony Brook

Kline, Gary MD (TS) - **Spec Exp:** Thoracic Surgery; Lung Cancer; Emphysema; Mediastinal Tumors; **Hospital:** Long Island Jewish Med Ctr, N Shore Univ Hosp at Manhasset; **Address:** LI Jewish Med Ctr-Dept Cardiothoracic Surg, 410 Lakeville Rd, Ste 203, New Hyde Park, NY 11040-1433; **Phone:** 718-470-7460; **Board Cert:** Surgery 2004; Thoracic Surgery 1996; **Med School:** Wayne State Univ 1986; **Resid:** Surgery, Detroit Med Ctr 1991; **Fellow:** Thoracic Surgery, Hosp Univ Penn 1994; **Fac Appt:** Asst Prof S, Albert Einstein Coll Med

La Mendola, Christopher MD (TS) - **Spec Exp:** Coronary Artery Surgery; Minimally Invasive Heart Valve Surgery; Atrial Fibrillation; **Hospital:** St Francis Hosp - The Heart Ctr (page 112); **Address:** 100 Port Washington Blvd, Ste G01, Roslyn, NY 11576-1353; **Phone:** 516-627-2173; **Board Cert:** Surgery 2002; Thoracic Surgery 2003; **Med School:** SUNY Hlth Sci Ctr 1985; **Resid:** Surgery, New York Univ Med Ctr 1992; **Fellow:** Thoracic Surgery, New York Univ Med Ctr 1994

Robinson, Newell B MD (TS) - **Spec Exp:** Minimally Invasive Cardiac Surgery; Maze Procedure for Atrial Fibrillation; **Hospital:** St Francis Hosp - The Heart Ctr (page 112); **Address:** 100 Port Washington Blvd, Vizza Bldg - rm G-01, Roslyn, NY 11576; **Phone:** 516-627-2173; **Board Cert:** Surgery 1995; Thoracic Surgery 1997; **Med School:** Univ Miss 1977; **Resid:** Surgery, NY-Cornell Med Ctr 1984; Surgery, Meml Sloan Kettering Cancer Ctr 1984; **Fellow:** Trauma, Univ Washington Med Ctr 1981; Cardiothoracic Surgery, NY-Cornell Med Ctr 1986

Saha, Chanchal MD (TS) - **Spec Exp:** Lung Cancer; Pacemakers; **Hospital:** N Shore Univ Hosp at Plainview, New Island Hosp; **Address:** 754 Old Country Rd, Plainview, NY 11803; **Phone:** 516-931-0182; **Board Cert:** Thoracic Surgery 2000; **Med School:** India 1964; **Resid:** Thoracic Surgery, Hosp for Joint Diseases 1973; Thoracic Surgery, Huron Road Hosp 1970; **Fellow:** Cardiothoracic Surgery, Mt Sinai Hosp 1976; **Fac Appt:** Assoc Prof S, Cornell Univ-Weill Med Coll

UROLOGY

Alyskewycz, Roman MD (U) - **Hospital:** N Shore Univ Hosp at Glen Cove, N Shore Univ Hosp at Manhasset; **Address:** 10 Medical Plz, Ste 101, Glen Cove, NY 11542; **Phone:** 516-676-4328; **Board Cert:** Urology 2000; **Med School:** Austria 1965; **Resid:** Urology, St Luke's-Roosevelt Hosp Ctr 1972; Vascular Surgery, New York Polyclin Hosp 1967

Ashley, Richard MD (U) - **Hospital:** Winthrop - Univ Hosp; **Address:** 233 7th St, Ste 203, Garden City, NY 11530; **Phone:** 516-294-7666; **Board Cert:** Urology 1980; **Med School:** NY Med Coll 1972; **Resid:** Urology, SUNY 1978; Surgery, St Vincents Hosp 1975; **Fac Appt:** Asst Clin Prof U, SUNY Stony Brook

Badlani, Gopal MD (U) - **Spec Exp:** Incontinence; Prostate Surgery; **Hospital:** Long Island Jewish Med Ctr; **Address:** LIJ Med Ctr, Dept Urology, 270-05 76th Ave, New Hyde Park, NY 11042; **Phone:** 718-470-7220; **Board Cert:** Urology 1982; **Med School:** India 1973; **Resid:** Surgery, St Agnes Hosp 1977; Urology, LI Jewish Hosp 1980; **Fellow:** Urology, Baylor Med Ctr 1983; **Fac Appt:** Prof U, Albert Einstein Coll Med

Brock, William A MD (U) - **Spec Exp:** Pediatric Urology; Varicocele in Adolescents; Undescended Testis; **Hospital:** Long Island Jewish Med Ctr, N Shore Univ Hosp at Manhasset; **Address:** 1999 Marcus Ave, Ste M18, Lake Success, NY 11042; **Phone:** 516-466-6953; **Board Cert:** Urology 1980; **Med School:** Emory Univ 1971; **Resid:** Surgery, NY Hosp 1973; Urology, UCSD Med Ctr 1978; **Fellow:** Pediatric Urology, UCSD Med Ctr 1979; Pediatric Urology, Alder Hey Children's Hosp; **Fac Appt:** Clin Prof U, Albert Einstein Coll Med

Bruno, Anthony MD (U) - **Spec Exp:** Prostate Cancer; Kidney Stones; Voiding Dysfunction; **Hospital:** Winthrop - Univ Hosp, Franklin Hosp Med Ctr; **Address:** 1305 Franklin Ave, Ste 100, Garden City, NY 11530; **Phone:** 516-746-5550; **Board Cert:** Urology 1977; **Med School:** Italy 1968; **Resid:** Surgery, Nassua Hosp. 1972; Urology, Bellevue Hosp. Ctr. 1975; **Fac Appt:** Asst Prof U, SUNY Stony Brook

Buchbinder, Mitchell MD (U) - **Spec Exp:** Prostate Disease; Kidney Stones; **Hospital:** Long Island Jewish Med Ctr, N Shore Univ Hosp at Manhasset; **Address:** 2001 Marcus Ave, rm N-214, Lake Success, NY 11042; **Phone:** 516-437-4228; **Board Cert:** Urology 1976; **Med School:** SUNY Downstate 1969; **Resid:** Surgery, LI Jewish Med Ctr 1971; Urology, LI Jewish Med Ctr 1974; **Fac Appt:** Asst Clin Prof U, Albert Einstein Coll Med

Hanna, Moneer MD (U) - **Spec Exp:** Hydronephrosis; Pediatric Urology; Hypospadias; Bladder Surgery; **Hospital:** NY-Presby Hosp (page 100), Schneider Chldn's Hosp; **Address:** 935 Northern Blvd, Ste 303, Great Neck, NY 11021; **Phone:** 516-466-6950; **Board Cert:** Urology 1978; **Med School:** Egypt 1963; **Resid:** Urology, Univ Affiliated Hosp 1972; Urology, Univ West Ont Affil Hosps 1976; **Fellow:** Pediatric Urology, Hosp For Sick Chldn 1975; **Fac Appt:** Clin Prof U, Cornell Univ-Weill Med Coll

Harris, Steven MD (U) - **Spec Exp:** Impotence; Prostate Disease; Kidney Stones; **Hospital:** Long Beach Med Ctr, South Nassau Comm Hosp; **Address:** 309 W Park Ave, Ste 5, Long Beach, NY 11561-3241; **Phone:** 516-431-9800; **Board Cert:** Urology 1984; **Med School:** Albert Einstein Coll Med 1976; **Resid:** Urology, Mount Sinai Med Ctr 1981; **Fac Appt:** Asst Prof U, NY Coll Osteo Med

Kavoussi, Louis R MD (U) - **Spec Exp:** Laparoscopic Surgery; Endourology; Kidney Stones; **Hospital:** Long Island Jewish Med Ctr; **Address:** 300 Community Dr, 9 Tower, Manhasset, NY 11030; **Phone:** 516-562-2880; **Board Cert:** Urology 1999; **Med School:** SUNY Buffalo 1983; **Resid:** Surgery, Barnes Hosp/Wash Univ 1985; Urology, Barnes Hosp/Wash Univ 1989; **Fac Appt:** Prof U, NYU Sch Med

Layne, Jeffrey MD (U) - **Spec Exp:** Kidney Stones; Incontinence; Impotence; **Hospital:** N Shore Univ Hosp at Plainview, N Shore Univ Hosp at Syosset; **Address:** 1181 Old Country Rd, Ste 1, Plainview, NY 11803; **Phone:** 516-933-6060; **Board Cert:** Urology 1997; **Med School:** SUNY Stony Brook 1989; **Resid:** Surgery, New England Med Ctr 1991; Urology, New England Med Ctr 1995

Leventhal, Arnold MD (U) - **Spec Exp:** Prostate Cancer; Kidney Stones; **Hospital:** Franklin Hosp Med Ctr; **Address:** 1800 Rockaway Ave, Ste 212, Hewlett, NY 11557-1677; **Phone:** 516-593-1838; **Board Cert:** Urology 2002; **Med School:** NYU Sch Med 1984; **Resid:** Surgery, Bellevue Hosp 1986; Urology, Bellevue Hosp 1990

Lieberman, Elliott MD (U) - **Spec Exp:** Urologic Cancer; Interstitial Cystitis; Prostate Disease; **Hospital:** N Shore Univ Hosp at Plainview, N Shore Univ Hosp at Manhasset; **Address:** 875 Old Country Road Rd, Ste 301, Plainview, NY 11803-4934; **Phone:** 516-931-1710; **Board Cert:** Urology 1983; **Med School:** SUNY Downstate 1976; **Resid:** Surgery, Mount Sinai 1978; Urology, SUNY-Downstate 1981

Mellinger, Brett MD (U) - **Spec Exp:** Infertility-Male; Impotence; Andrology; **Hospital:** Winthrop - Univ Hosp, N Shore Univ Hosp at Plainview; **Address:** Urology Inst, 100 Garden City Plaza, Ste 101, Garden City, NY 11530; **Phone:** 516-873-5353; **Board Cert:** Urology 1999; **Med School:** Indiana Univ 1981; **Resid:** Urology, Downstate Med Ctr 1985; Urology, New York Hosp-Cornell 1986; **Fellow:** Male Infertility, New York Hosp-Cornell 1988; **Fac Appt:** Assoc Clin Prof U, Albert Einstein Coll Med

Moldwin, Robert MD (U) - **Spec Exp:** Interstitial Cystitis; Prostate Benign Disease; Urinary Tract Infections; **Hospital:** Long Island Jewish Med Ctr; **Address:** 270-05 76th Ave Bldg Oncology Fl 4, New Hyde Park, NY 11040-1433; **Phone:** 718-470-7223; **Board Cert:** Urology 1993; **Med School:** Univ Chicago-Pritzker Sch Med 1984; **Resid:** Urology, LI Jewish Med Ctr 1990; **Fellow:** Infectious Disease, Thomas Jefferson Univ Hosp 1991; **Fac Appt:** Assoc Clin Prof U, Albert Einstein Coll Med

Shepard, Barry R MD (U) - **Spec Exp:** Kidney Stones; Urologic Cancer; **Hospital:** Mercy Med Ctr - Rockville Centre, Winthrop - Univ Hosp; **Address:** 601 Franklin Ave, Ste 300, Garden City, NY 11530; **Phone:** 516-742-3200; **Board Cert:** Urology 1996; **Med School:** SUNY Downstate 1979; **Resid:** Surgery, LIJ Med Ctr 1981; Urology, Columbia-Presby Med Ctr 1984

Smith, Arthur D MD (U) - **Spec Exp:** Kidney Stones; Laparoscopic Surgery; **Hospital:** Long Island Jewish Med Ctr, N Shore Univ Hosp at Manhasset; **Address:** Long Island Jewish Med Ctr, 270-05 76th Ave, Fl 4th, New Hyde Park, NY 11040; **Phone:** 718-470-7221; **Board Cert:** Urology 1980; **Med School:** South Africa 1962; **Resid:** Surgery, Baragwananath Hosp 1966; Urology, Genl Hosp 1966; **Fellow:** Urology, Johannesburg Hosp 1967; **Fac Appt:** Prof U, Albert Einstein Coll Med

Steckel, Joph MD (U) - **Spec Exp:** Prostate Cancer; Bladder Cancer; Kidney Cancer; **Hospital:** N Shore Univ Hosp at Manhasset; **Address:** 535 Plandome Rd, Ste 3, Manhasset, NY 11030-1961; **Phone:** 516-627-6188; **Board Cert:** Urology 2004; **Med School:** Cornell Univ-Weill Med Coll 1986; **Resid:** Surgery, New York Hosp/Cornell Med Ctr 1991; Urology, Meml Sloan Kett Cancer Ctr 1993; **Fellow:** Urologic Oncology, UCLA Med Ctr 1994

Sunshine, Robert D MD (U) - **Spec Exp:** Urologic Surgery; Sexual Dysfunction; Vasectomy-Scalpelless; Pediatric Urology; **Hospital:** New Island Hosp, N Shore Univ Hosp at Plainview; **Address:** 4230 Hempstead Tpke, Ste 200, Bethpage, NY 11714-5700; **Phone:** 516-796-2222; **Board Cert:** Urology 2005; **Med School:** Mexico 1977; **Resid:** Surgery, Long Island Jewish Hosp 1981; Urology, Mount Sinai Med Ctr 1985

Waldbaum, Robert MD (U) - **Spec Exp:** Prostate Cancer; Prostate Disease; Urologic Cancer; **Hospital:** N Shore Univ Hosp at Manhasset, St Francis Hosp - The Heart Ctr (page 112); **Address:** 535 Plandome Rd, Ste 3, Manhasset, NY 11030-1961; **Phone:** 516-627-6188; **Board Cert:** Urology 1973; **Med School:** Columbia P&S 1962; **Resid:** Surgery, Columbia Presby Med Ctr 1966; Urology, New York Hosp-Cornell 1970; **Fac Appt:** Clin Prof U, Cornell Univ-Weill Med Coll

Ziegelbaum, Michael M MD (U) - **Spec Exp:** Incontinence-Male & Female; Prostate Disease; Kidney Stones; **Hospital:** Long Island Jewish Med Ctr, N Shore Univ Hosp at Manhasset; **Address:** 2001 Marcus Ave, Lake Success, NY 11042; **Phone:** 516-437-4228; **Board Cert:** Urology 1999; **Med School:** Cornell Univ-Weill Med Coll 1982; **Resid:** Urology, Cleveland Clinic 1988; **Fellow:** Stone Disease, Univ Hosp 1989; **Fac Appt:** Asst Clin Prof S, Albert Einstein Coll Med

VASCULAR & INTERVENTIONAL RADIOLOGY

Crystal, Kenneth MD (VIR) - **Spec Exp:** Interventional Radiology; Angioplasty; Uterine Fibroid Embolization; **Hospital:** St Francis Hosp - The Heart Ctr (page 112); **Address:** St Francis Hospital, Dept Radiology, 100 Port Washington Blvd, Roslyn, NY 11576; **Phone:** 516-562-6509; **Board Cert:** Diagnostic Radiology 1986; Vascular & Interventional Radiology 1995; **Med School:** Univ Rochester 1981; **Resid:** Internal Medicine, Beth Israel Med Ctr 1982; Radiology, NYU Med Ctr 1986; **Fellow:** Vascular & Interventional Radiology, NYU Med Ctr 1986; **Fac Appt:** Asst Prof Rad, NYU Sch Med

VASCULAR SURGERY

Berroya, Renato MD (VascS) - **Spec Exp:** Carotid Artery Surgery; Aneurysm-Abdominal Aortic; Endovascular Surgery; **Hospital:** St Francis Hosp - The Heart Ctr (page 112), N Shore Univ Hosp at Manhasset; **Address:** 639 Port Washington Blvd, Port Washington, NY 11050-3733; **Phone:** 516-883-2212; **Board Cert:** Surgery 1969; Vascular Surgery 1974; **Med School:** Philippines 1961; **Resid:** Surgery, Winthrop Univ Hosp 1968; Vascular Surgery, St Francis Hosp 1970

Chang, John MD (VascS) - **Spec Exp:** Carotid Artery Surgery; Endovascular Surgery; Aneurysm-Abdominal Aortic; **Hospital:** Long Island Jewish Med Ctr, St Francis Hosp - The Heart Ctr (page 112); **Address:** 1050 Northern Blvd, Roslyn, NY 11576-1503; **Phone:** 516-484-3430; **Board Cert:** Vascular Surgery 2004; **Med School:** South Korea 1962; **Resid:** Surgery, LI Jewish Med Ctr 1971; Cardiovascular Surgery, LI Jewish Med Ctr 1973; **Fac Appt:** Clin Prof S, Albert Einstein Coll Med

Chaudhry, Saqib S MD (VascS) - **Spec Exp:** Aneurysm-Aortic; Carotid Artery Surgery; Dialysis Access Surgery; **Hospital:** N Shore Univ Hosp at Forest Hills, N Shore Univ Hosp at Manhasset; **Address:** 2001 Marcus Ave, Ste South, Box 50, Lake Success, NY 11042; **Phone:** 516-328-9800; **Board Cert:** Thoracic Surgery 2000; Vascular Surgery 1999; **Med School:** Iraq 1972; **Resid:** Surgery, Flushing Hosp 1974; Thoracic Surgery, Wayne State Univ 1980

Cohen, Jon MD (VascS) - **Spec Exp:** Aneurysm-Abdominal Aortic; Carotid Artery Surgery; **Hospital:** Long Island Jewish Med Ctr; **Address:** LIJ Med Ctr, Vascular Surgery, 270-05 76th Ave, New Hyde Park, NY 11040; **Phone:** 718-470-8787; **Board Cert:** Surgery 2004; Vascular Surgery 1996; **Med School:** Univ Miami Sch Med 1979; **Resid:** Surgery, NY Hosp-Cornell Med Ctr 1984; **Fellow:** Vascular Surgery, Brigham & Women's Hosp 1985; **Fac Appt:** Prof S, Albert Einstein Coll Med

Faust, Glenn MD (VascS) - **Spec Exp:** Carotid Artery Surgery; Diabetic Leg/Foot; Aneurysm-Abdominal Aortic; **Hospital:** Long Island Jewish Med Ctr; **Address:** LIJ Med Ctr, Vascular Surgery, 270-05 76th Ave, New Hyde Park, NY 11040; **Phone:** 718-470-7299; **Board Cert:** Surgery 1993; Vascular Surgery 2004; **Med School:** Yale Univ 1986; **Resid:** Surgery, LI Jewish Med Ctr 1991; **Fellow:** Vascular Surgery, LI Jewish Med Ctr 1992; **Fac Appt:** Asst Prof S, Albert Einstein Coll Med

Garvey, Julius W MD (VascS) - **Spec Exp:** Varicose Veins; Wound Healing/Care; **Hospital:** Long Island Jewish Med Ctr; **Address:** 3003 New Hyde Park Rd, Ste 410, New Hyde Park, NY 11042; **Phone:** 516-326-3255; **Board Cert:** Vascular Surgery 1970; Thoracic Surgery 1970; **Med School:** McGill Univ 1961; **Resid:** Surgery, Harlem Hosp 1968; Thoracic Surgery, Univ Maryland Hosp 1970; **Fac Appt:** Assoc Prof S, Albert Einstein Coll Med

Hines, George L MD (VascS) - **Spec Exp:** Carotid Artery Surgery; Aneurysm-Aortic; **Hospital:** Winthrop - Univ Hosp; **Address:** 120 Mineola Blvd, Ste 300, Mineola, NY 11501-4077; **Phone:** 516-663-4400; **Board Cert:** Thoracic Surgery 1998; Vascular Surgery 1994; **Med School:** Boston Univ 1969; **Resid:** Surgery, Sinai Hosp 1971; Surgery, LI Jewish Med Ctr 1974; **Fellow:** Thoracic Surgery, NYU Med Ctr 1976; **Fac Appt:** Prof S, SUNY Stony Brook

LiCalzi, Luke K MD (VascS) - **Spec Exp:** Carotid Artery Surgery; Aneurysm-Abdominal Aortic; Peripheral Vascular Surgery; **Hospital:** South Nassau Comm Hosp; **Address:** 77 N Centre Ave, Ste 208, Rockville Centre, NY 11570-3923; **Phone:** 516-764-5455; **Board Cert:** Surgery 1999; **Med School:** Albany Med Coll 1975; **Resid:** Surgery, Yale-New Haven Hosp 1980; **Fellow:** Vascular Surgery, NYU Med Ctr 1982; **Fac Appt:** Asst Clin Prof S, SUNY Stony Brook

Smirnov, Viktor MD (VascS) - **Spec Exp:** Peripheral Vascular Surgery; **Hospital:** Winthrop - Univ Hosp, Mercy Med Ctr - Rockville Centre; **Address:** 30 Merrick Ave, Ste 109, East Meadow, NY 11554; **Phone:** 516-794-0444; **Board Cert:** Surgery 1995; Vascular Surgery 1993; **Med School:** Russia 1972; **Resid:** Surgery, Univ Hosp 1985; **Fellow:** Vascular Surgery, Univ Hosp 1987; **Fac Appt:** Asst Clin Prof S, SUNY Stony Brook

Rockland

Rockland

ALLERGY & IMMUNOLOGY

Bosso, John MD (A&I) - **Spec Exp:** Drug Sensitivity; Asthma; Contact Dermatitis; Food Allergy; **Hospital:** Nyack Hosp, Pascack Valley Hosp; **Address:** 2 Crossfield Ave, Ste 406, West Nyack, NY 10994-1313; **Phone:** 845-353-9600; **Board Cert:** Internal Medicine 1988; Allergy & Immunology 2001; **Med School:** SUNY Buffalo 1985; **Resid:** Internal Medicine, Staten Island Univ Hosp 1988; **Fellow:** Allergy & Immunology, Scripps Clinic Reseach Fdn 1990

CARDIOVASCULAR DISEASE

Innerfield, Michael MD (Cv) - **Spec Exp:** Interventional Cardiology; Peripheral Vascular Disease; **Hospital:** Nyack Hosp, Hackensack Univ Med Ctr (page 92); **Address:** 2 Crossfield Ave, Ste 407, West Nyack, NY 10994-2212; **Phone:** 845-353-5050; **Board Cert:** Internal Medicine 1984; Cardiovascular Disease 1987; Interventional Cardiology 1999; **Med School:** NY Med Coll 1981; **Resid:** Internal Medicine, Bronx Muni Hosp 1984; **Fellow:** Cardiovascular Disease, Montefiore Hosp Med Ctr 1986; Cardiovascular Disease, Cooper Hosp 1987; **Fac Appt:** Asst Prof S, Mount Sinai Sch Med

Roth, Richard MD (Cv) - **Spec Exp:** Cholesterol/Lipid Disorders; Non-Invasive Cardiology; **Hospital:** Good Samaritan Hosp - Suffern, Nyack Hosp; **Address:** 222 Route 59, Ste 302, Suffern, NY 10901; **Phone:** 845-368-0100; **Board Cert:** Internal Medicine 1978; Cardiovascular Disease 1981; Critical Care Medicine 1989; **Med School:** Yale Univ 1975; **Resid:** Internal Medicine, Boston Med Ctr 1978; **Fellow:** Cardiovascular Disease, Boston Univ Med Ctr 1980; **Fac Appt:** Asst Clin Prof Med, Columbia P&S

COLON & RECTAL SURGERY

Ozuner, Gokhan MD (CRS) - **Spec Exp:** Inflammatory Bowel Disease; Colon & Rectal Cancer; Rectal Prolapse; Laparoscopic Surgery; **Hospital:** Good Samaritan Hosp - Suffern; **Address:** 100 Route 59, Ste 101, Suffern, NY 10901; **Phone:** 845-357-8800; **Board Cert:** Surgery 2002; Colon & Rectal Surgery 2005; **Med School:** Turkey 1984; **Resid:** Surgery, Staten Island Univ Hosp 1993; **Fellow:** Colon & Rectal Surgery, Cleveland Clin Fdn 1995

DERMATOLOGY

Waldorf, Donald MD (D) - **Spec Exp:** Skin Cancer; Acne; Psoriasis; **Hospital:** Nyack Hosp; **Address:** 57 N Middletown Rd, Nanuet, NY 10954-2312; **Phone:** 845-623-7077; **Board Cert:** Dermatology 1967; **Med School:** Univ Pennsylvania 1962; **Resid:** Dermatology, Hosp Univ Penn 1964; Dermatology, NYU Medical Center 1967; **Fellow:** Dermatology, Natl Cancer Inst 1966

DIAGNOSTIC RADIOLOGY

Bobroff, Lewis M MD (DR) - **Spec Exp:** Mammography; Nuclear Medicine; PET Imaging; **Hospital:** Good Samaritan Hosp - Suffern; **Address:** 255 Lafayette Ave, Suffern, NY 10901-5103; **Phone:** 845-368-5196; **Board Cert:** Diagnostic Radiology 1974; **Med School:** Harvard Med Sch 1969; **Resid:** Diagnostic Radiology, Montefiore Hosp Med Ctr 1973; **Fellow:** Interventional Radiology, Montefiore Hosp Med Ctr 1973

Boltin, Harry MD (DR) - **Hospital:** Good Samaritan Hosp - Suffern; **Address:** 972 Rte 45, Pomona Profl Plaza, Pomona, NY 10970; **Phone:** 845-354-7700; **Board Cert:** Radiology 1968; **Med School:** UMDNJ-RW Johnson Med Sch 1963; **Resid:** Radiology, Montefiore Hosp Med Ctr 1967

Geller, Mark E MD (DR) - **Spec Exp:** MRI; Ultrasound; Nuclear Medicine; **Hospital:** Nyack Hosp; **Address:** 18 Squadron Blvd, New City, NY 10956-5210; **Phone:** 845-634-9729; **Board Cert:** Diagnostic Radiology 1989; **Med School:** SUNY Downstate 1985; **Resid:** Diagnostic Radiology, NY Med Coll 1989; **Fac Appt:** Asst Clin Prof Rad, NY Med Coll

Handler, Elliot MD (DR) - **Spec Exp:** Obstetric Ultrasound; CT Scan; **Hospital:** Nyack Hosp; **Address:** 18 Squadron Blvd, New City, NY 10956-5210; **Phone:** 845-634-9729; **Board Cert:** Diagnostic Radiology 1984; **Med School:** SUNY Downstate 1980; **Resid:** Radiology, Boston Univ Med Ctr 1985; **Fellow:** Ultrasound/CT, Boston Univ Med Ctr 1985

Peck, Harvey MD (DR) - **Hospital:** Good Samaritan Hosp - Suffern; **Address:** 972 Route 45, Pomona Profl Plaza, Pomona, NY 10970; **Phone:** 845-354-7700; **Board Cert:** Radiology 1960; **Med School:** Yale Univ 1953; **Resid:** Radiology, Mt Sinai Hosp 1960; **Fellow:** Radiology, Mt Sinai Hosp 1955

Schwartz, Joel M MD (DR) - **Spec Exp:** Neuroradiology; Head & Neck Imaging; **Hospital:** Nyack Hosp; **Address:** 1609 North Midland Ave, Nyack, NY 10960; **Phone:** 845-348-2450; **Board Cert:** Diagnostic Radiology 1990; Neuroradiology 1996; **Med School:** SUNY Upstate Med Univ 1985; **Resid:** Diagnostic Radiology, NYU Med Ctr 1990; **Fellow:** Neuroradiology, NYU Med Ctr 1991

ENDOCRINOLOGY, DIABETES & METABOLISM

Cosman, Felicia MD (EDM) - **Spec Exp:** Osteoporosis; Bone Densitometry; **Hospital:** Helen Hayes Hosp, NY-Presby Hosp (page 100); **Address:** Helen Hayes Hosp, Reg Bone Ctr, Route 9W, West Haverstraw, NY 10993; **Phone:** 845-786-4318; **Board Cert:** Internal Medicine 1986; Endocrinology, Diabetes & Metabolism 1989; **Med School:** SUNY Stony Brook 1983; **Resid:** Internal Medicine, Columbia Presby Med Ctr 1986; **Fellow:** Endocrinology, Columbia Presby Med Ctr 1988; **Fac Appt:** Assoc Clin Prof Med, Columbia P&S

Josef, Minna MD (EDM) - **Spec Exp:** Thyroid Disorders; Osteoporosis; Diabetes; **Hospital:** Nyack Hosp, Good Samaritan Hosp - Suffern; **Address:** 2 Crosfield Ave, Ste 204, West Nyack, NY 10994-2221; **Phone:** 845-358-6266; **Board Cert:** Internal Medicine 1988; Endocrinology, Diabetes & Metabolism 1991; **Med School:** NYU Sch Med 1985; **Resid:** Internal Medicine, Columbia-Presby Med Ctr 1988; **Fellow:** Endocrinology, Diabetes & Metabolism, Columbia-Presby Med Ctr 1991

FAMILY MEDICINE

Ibelli, Vincent MD (FMed) PCP - **Spec Exp:** Asthma; Hypertension; **Hospital:** Good Samaritan Hosp - Suffern, Nyack Hosp; **Address:** 97 Route 303, Blauvelt, NY 10983; **Phone:** 845-359-5005; **Board Cert:** Family Medicine 2000; **Med School:** Italy 1983; **Resid:** Family Medicine, JFK Med Ctr 1986

Ingrassia, Joseph MD (FMed) PCP - **Hospital:** Good Samaritan Hosp - Suffern; **Address:** 36 College Ave, Nanuet, NY 10954-3093; **Phone:** 845-623-2456; **Board Cert:** Family Medicine 1978; **Med School:** Mexico 1974; **Resid:** Family Medicine, Nassau Co Hosp 1978

GASTROENTEROLOGY

May, Louis MD (Ge) - **Spec Exp:** Hepatitis; Endoscopy; Pancreatic/Biliary Endoscopy (ERCP); **Hospital:** Good Samaritan Hosp - Suffern, Nyack Hosp; **Address:** 500 New Hempstead Rd, New City, NY 10956; **Phone:** 845-362-3200; **Board Cert:** Internal Medicine 1981; Gastroenterology 1983; **Med School:** Univ Miami Sch Med 1978; **Resid:** Internal Medicine, Univ Utah Med Ctr 1981; **Fellow:** Gastroenterology, Univ Utah Med Ctr 1983

HEMATOLOGY

Rader, Michael MD (Hem) - **Spec Exp:** Bleeding/Coagulation Disorders; Breast Cancer; Lung Cancer; **Hospital:** Nyack Hosp, Good Samaritan Hosp - Suffern; **Address:** 500 New Hempstead Rd, New City, NY 10956-1132; **Phone:** 845-362-1750; **Board Cert:** Internal Medicine 1978; Hematology 1980; Medical Oncology 1981; **Med School:** SUNY Downstate 1975; **Resid:** Internal Medicine, SUNY-Kings Co Med Ctr 1978; **Fellow:** Hematology, Montefiore Hosp Med Ctr 1980; Medical Oncology, Memorial Sloan Kettering Cancer Ctr 1981; **Fac Appt:** Asst Clin Prof Med, Columbia P&S

INTERNAL MEDICINE

Friedman, Sam MD (IM) **PCP** - **Spec Exp:** Irritable Bowel Syndrome; Inflammatory Bowel Disease/Crohn's; Esophageal Disorders; **Hospital:** Good Samaritan Hosp - Suffern, Nyack Hosp; **Address:** 1 Medical Park Dr, Pomona, NY 10970-3516; **Phone:** 845-354-9500; **Board Cert:** Internal Medicine 1977; Gastroenterology 1970; **Med School:** SUNY Downstate 1959; **Resid:** Internal Medicine, Montefiore Med Ctr 1962; Gastroenterology, Montefiore Med Ctr 1965

Glassman, Charles F MD (IM) **PCP** - **Spec Exp:** Concierge Medicine; Preventive Medicine; Complementary Medicine; **Hospital:** Good Samaritan Hosp - Suffern, Nyack Hosp; **Address:** 7 Medical Park Drive, Ste C, Pomona, NY 10970; **Phone:** 845-362-1169; **Board Cert:** Internal Medicine 1989; **Med School:** NY Med Coll 1985; **Resid:** Internal Medicine, Westchester County Med Ctr 1988; **Fac Appt:** Asst Clin Prof Med, NY Med Coll

Handelsman, Richard E DO (IM) - **Spec Exp:** Concierge Medicine; Preventive Medicine; **Hospital:** Nyack Hosp; **Address:** 7 Medical Park Drive, Ste C, Pomona, NY 10970-3562; **Phone:** 845-362-1169; **Board Cert:** Internal Medicine 1981; **Med School:** Univ Osteo Med & Hlth Sci, Des Moines 1976; **Resid:** Internal Medicine, UMDNJ Med Ctr 1978; Internal Medicine, Norwalk Hosp 1980; **Fac Appt:** Asst Clin Prof Med, NY Med Coll

Leahy, Mary MD (IM) **PCP** - **Spec Exp:** Preventive Medicine; **Hospital:** Nyack Hosp, Good Samaritan Hosp - Suffern; **Address:** 2 Crosfield Ave, Ste 318, West Nyack, NY 10994; **Phone:** 845-353-5600; **Board Cert:** Internal Medicine 1988; **Med School:** Italy 1983; **Resid:** Internal Medicine, Misericordia Hospital 1986; **Fellow:** Nephrology, Westchester Co Med Ctr 1988

NEONATAL-PERINATAL MEDICINE

Mendoza, Glenn MD (NP) - **Spec Exp:** Perinatal Medicine; Pediatrics; **Hospital:** Good Samaritan Hosp - Suffern; **Address:** Good Samaritan Hosp, Dept Neonatology, 255 Lafayette Ave, Suffern, NY 10901; **Phone:** 845-368-5104; **Board Cert:** Pediatrics 1983; Neonatal-Perinatal Medicine 1985; **Med School:** Philippines 1976; **Resid:** Family Medicine, Elyria Meml Hosp; Pediatrics, Brooklyn Jewish Hosp & Med Ctr 1983; **Fellow:** Neonatal-Perinatal Medicine, Mt Sinai Hosp 1986; **Fac Appt:** Asst Prof Ped, Columbia P&S

Nephrology

Kozin, Arthur MD (Nep) - **Spec Exp:** Hypertension; Kidney Failure-Chronic; Diabetic Kidney Disease; **Hospital:** Nyack Hosp, Good Samaritan Hosp - Suffern; **Address:** 2 Crossfield Ave, Ste 312, West Nyack, NY 10994-2212; **Phone:** 845-358-2400; **Board Cert:** Internal Medicine 1985; Nephrology 1988; Critical Care Medicine 2002; **Med School:** Albert Einstein Coll Med 1982; **Resid:** Internal Medicine, Montefiore Hosp Med Ctr 1985; **Fellow:** Nephrology, Bellevue Hosp 1987

Shapiro, Kenneth MD (Nep) - **Spec Exp:** Hypertension; Kidney Disease-Diabetic; Transplant Medicine-Kidney; **Hospital:** Nyack Hosp, Good Samaritan Hosp - Suffern; **Address:** 2 Crosfield Ave, Ste 312, West Nyack, NY 10994-2220; **Phone:** 845-358-2400; **Board Cert:** Internal Medicine 1978; Nephrology 1980; **Med School:** Rush Med Coll 1975; **Resid:** Internal Medicine, Albany Med Ctr 1978; **Fellow:** Nephrology, New England Med Ctr 1980; **Fac Appt:** Asst Clin Prof Med, NY Med Coll

Yablon, Steven MD (Nep) - **Spec Exp:** Hypertension; Kidney Failure; Dialysis Care; **Hospital:** Nyack Hosp, Good Samaritan Hosp - Suffern; **Address:** 2 Crosfield Ave, Ste 312, West Nyack, NY 10994-2220; **Phone:** 845-358-2400; **Board Cert:** Internal Medicine 1976; Nephrology 1978; **Med School:** UMDNJ-NJ Med Sch, Newark 1973; **Resid:** Internal Medicine, Tuft's New England Med Ctr 1975; **Fellow:** Nephrology, Hosp Univ Penn 1977

Neurological Surgery

Oppenheim, Jeffrey MD (NS) - **Spec Exp:** Spinal Disc Replacement; Brain Tumors; Spinal Surgery; **Hospital:** Nyack Hosp, Good Samaritan Hosp - Suffern; **Address:** Hudson Valley Neurosurgical Assocs, 222 Route 59, Ste 205, Suffern, NY 10901-5204; **Phone:** 845-368-0286; **Board Cert:** Neurological Surgery 1996; **Med School:** Cornell Univ-Weill Med Coll 1988; **Resid:** Neurological Surgery, Mount Sinai Hosp 1994

Spitzer, Daniel MD (NS) - **Spec Exp:** Brain Tumors; Spinal Surgery; Stereotactic Radiosurgery; **Hospital:** Nyack Hosp, Good Samaritan Hosp - Suffern; **Address:** 222 Route 59, Ste 205, Suffern, NY 10901-5206; **Phone:** 845-368-0286; **Board Cert:** Neurological Surgery 1992; **Med School:** NYU Sch Med 1983; **Resid:** Neurological Surgery, Albert Einstein 1989; **Fac Appt:** Asst Clin Prof NS, Columbia P&S

Neurology

Seliger, Glenn MD (N) - **Spec Exp:** Brain Injury; **Hospital:** Helen Hayes Hosp; **Address:** Helen Hayes Hospital, Dept Neurology, Route 9W, West Haverstraw, NY 10993; **Phone:** 845-786-4459; **Board Cert:** Neurology 1988; **Med School:** SUNY Downstate 1983; **Resid:** Neurology, Neurological Inst 1987; **Fellow:** Neurological Rehabilitation, Braintree Hosp 1988; **Fac Appt:** Assoc Clin Prof N, Columbia P&S

Ophthalmology

Weingarten, Phyllis MD (Oph) - **Spec Exp:** Pediatric Ophthalmology; **Hospital:** Good Samaritan Hosp - Suffern; **Address:** 4 Medical Park Dr, Pomona, NY 10970-3516; **Phone:** 845-354-6225; **Board Cert:** Ophthalmology 1991; **Med School:** NY Med Coll 1986; **Resid:** Ophthalmology, Brookdale Hosp Med Ctr 1990; **Fellow:** Strabismus, Downstate Med Ctr 1991; Pediatric Ophthalmology, Johns Hopkins Hosp 1992; **Fac Appt:** Asst Clin Prof Oph, Columbia P&S

ORTHOPAEDIC SURGERY

Kraushaar, Barry S MD (OrS) - **Spec Exp:** Shoulder Arthroscopic Surgery; Hip & Knee Replacement; Knee Injuries/Ligament Surgery; Sports Medicine; **Hospital:** Nyack Hosp, Good Samaritan Hosp - Suffern; **Address:** 2 Medical Park Drive, West Nyack, NY 10994; **Phone:** 845-425-0555; **Board Cert:** Orthopaedic Surgery 1998; **Med School:** Albert Einstein Coll Med 1990; **Resid:** Orthopaedic Surgery, Bronx Lebanon Hosp 1995; **Fellow:** Sports Medicine, Arlington Hosp/Georgetown Univ 1996

OTOLARYNGOLOGY

Sadowski, John MD (Oto) - **Spec Exp:** Nasal & Sinus Disorders; Voice Disorders; Swallowing Disorders; Hearing Disorders; **Hospital:** Good Samaritan Hosp - Suffern; **Address:** 29 N Airmont Rd, Suffern, NY 10901-4242; **Phone:** 845-357-6222; **Board Cert:** Otolaryngology 1967; **Med School:** NY Med Coll 1958; **Resid:** Surgery, VA Hosp 1960; Otolaryngology, NYU Med Ctr 1963; **Fac Appt:** Assoc Clin Prof Oto, NYU Sch Med

PAIN MEDICINE

Burns, Paul MD (PM) - **Hospital:** Good Samaritan Hosp - Suffern; **Address:** Ramapo Anesthesiologists, 133 Lafayette Ave, Suffern, NY 10901-5614; **Phone:** 845-357-5745; **Board Cert:** Anesthesiology 1984; Pain Medicine 1996; **Med School:** SUNY Buffalo 1978; **Resid:** Anesthesiology, NY Hosp 1981

PEDIATRICS

Bernstein, William H MD (Ped) - **Hospital:** Nyack Hosp; **Address:** 100 Phillips Hill Rd, New City, NY 10956-6426; **Phone:** 845-634-8911; **Board Cert:** Pediatrics 1966; **Med School:** Vanderbilt Univ 1960; **Resid:** Pediatrics, Bellevue Hosp 1962; Pediatrics, Mt Sinai Hosp 1965; **Fellow:** Neonatology, Mt Sinai Hosp 1966

Diamant, Esther MD (Ped) PCP - **Hospital:** Hackensack Univ Med Ctr (page 92); **Address:** Refauh Health Center, 728 N Main St, Spring Valley, NY 10977; **Phone:** 845-354-9300; **Board Cert:** Pediatrics 2005; **Med School:** Mount Sinai Sch Med 1987; **Resid:** Pediatrics, Mt. Sinai Hosp 1991; **Fellow:** Pediatrics, Mt. Sinai Hosp 1993

Greenberg, William MD (Ped) PCP - **Spec Exp:** ADD/ADHD; Learning Disorders; **Hospital:** Good Samaritan Hosp - Suffern, Nyack Hosp; **Address:** 4C Medical Park Drive, Pomona, NY 10970-3541; **Phone:** 845-362-0202; **Board Cert:** Pediatrics 1976; **Med School:** Univ Hlth Sci/Chicago Med Sch 1967; **Resid:** Pediatrics, New York Hosp 1970

Puder, Douglas MD (Ped) PCP - **Spec Exp:** Asthma; Developmental Disorders; **Hospital:** Nyack Hosp; **Address:** 35 Smith St, Nanuet, NY 10954; **Phone:** 845-623-7100; **Board Cert:** Pediatrics 1987; **Med School:** NYU Sch Med 1982; **Resid:** Pediatrics, NYU/Bellevue Hosp 1985; **Fellow:** Ambulatory Pediatrics, NYU Med Ctr 1987; **Fac Appt:** Assoc Clin Prof Ped, Columbia P&S

Siegal, Elliot MD (Ped) PCP - **Spec Exp:** Thyroid Disorders; Growth Disorders; **Hospital:** Nyack Hosp; **Address:** 200 E Eckerson Rd, New City, NY 10956-7169; **Phone:** 845-352-5511; **Board Cert:** Pediatrics 1975; Pediatric Endocrinology 1978; **Med School:** Univ Pennsylvania 1968; **Resid:** Pediatrics, NY Hosp 1971; **Fellow:** Pediatric Endocrinology, NY Hosp 1972

PSYCHIATRY

Levy, Michael I MD (Psyc) - **Spec Exp:** Psychopharmacology; Psychiatry-Adult; Geriatric Psychiatry; **Hospital:** Nyack Hosp; **Address:** North Midland Ave, Nyack, NY 10960-2505; **Phone:** 845-348-2116; **Board Cert:** Psychiatry 1982; Geriatric Psychiatry 2001; **Med School:** Albert Einstein Coll Med 1977; **Resid:** Psychiatry, Mount Sinai Hosp 1981; **Fac Appt:** Asst Clin Prof Psyc, NY Med Coll

Schroeder, Karl MD (Psyc) - **Spec Exp:** Addiction/Substance Abuse; Psychiatry in Physical Illness; Post Traumatic Stress Disorder; **Hospital:** Helen Hayes Hosp; **Address:** Helen Hayes Hosp, 104 Montebello Rd, Suffern, NY 10901; **Phone:** 845-357-9367; **Board Cert:** Psychiatry 1980; **Med School:** Columbia P&S 1974; **Resid:** Psychiatry, Columbia-Presby Hosp 1977; **Fac Appt:** Asst Clin Prof Med, Columbia P&S

PULMONARY DISEASE

Harris, Leon MD (Pul) - **Hospital:** Good Samaritan Hosp - Suffern; **Address:** 2 Crosfield Ave, Ste 318, West Nyack, NY 10994-2212; **Phone:** 845-353-5600; **Board Cert:** Internal Medicine 1979; Pulmonary Disease 1982; **Med School:** Mount Sinai Sch Med 1976; **Resid:** Internal Medicine, Mt Sinai Hosp 1979; **Fellow:** Pulmonary Disease, Mass Genl Hosp 1981

Hodes, David MD (Pul) - **Hospital:** Nyack Hosp, Good Samaritan Hosp - Suffern; **Address:** 2 Crosfield Ave, Ste 318, West Nyack, NY 10994; **Phone:** 845-353-5600; **Board Cert:** Internal Medicine 1976; Pulmonary Disease 1978; Critical Care Medicine 1991; **Med School:** NYU Sch Med 1973; **Resid:** Internal Medicine, St Luke's Hosp 1976; **Fellow:** Pulmonary Disease, Bellevue Hosp/NYU 1978

Osei, Clement MD (Pul) - **Spec Exp:** Asthma; Emphysema; Lung Cancer; **Hospital:** Good Samaritan Hosp - Suffern, Nyack Hosp; **Address:** 2 Crosfield Ave, Ste 318, West Nyack, NY 10994; **Phone:** 845-353-5600; **Board Cert:** Internal Medicine 1975; Pulmonary Disease 1978; **Med School:** Germany 1970; **Resid:** Internal Medicine, Elmhurst Hosp Ctr/Mt Sinai 1975; **Fellow:** Pulmonary Disease, Elmhurst Hosp Ctr/Mt Sinai 1977

RHEUMATOLOGY

Becker, Alfred MD (Rhu) - **Hospital:** Good Samaritan Hosp - Suffern, Nyack Hosp; **Address:** 222 Rte 59, Ste 204, Suffern, NY 10901; **Phone:** 845-357-6464; **Board Cert:** Internal Medicine 1969; Rheumatology 1972; **Med School:** Albert Einstein Coll Med 1962; **Resid:** Internal Medicine, Pittsburgh Hlth Ctr 1967; **Fellow:** Rheumatology, Einstein Med Ctr 1968; **Fac Appt:** Asst Clin Prof Med, Columbia P&S

SPORTS MEDICINE

Berezin, Marc MD (SM) - **Spec Exp:** Arthroscopic Surgery; **Hospital:** Nyack Hosp, Good Samaritan Hosp - Suffern; **Address:** 99 Dutch Hill Rd, Orangeburg, NY 10962-2106; **Phone:** 845-359-1877; **Board Cert:** Orthopaedic Surgery 2001; **Med School:** NY Med Coll 1985; **Resid:** Orthopaedic Surgery, NY Med Coll 1990; **Fellow:** Sports Medicine, Arthoscopy Assoc Ortho 1991

Katz, Lawrence MD (SM) - **Hospital:** Good Samaritan Hosp - Suffern; **Address:** 18 College Rd, Monsey, NY 10952-2852; **Phone:** 845-356-2900; **Board Cert:** Orthopaedic Surgery 1974; **Med School:** Temple Univ 1968; **Resid:** Surgery, Royal Victoria Hosp 1970; Orthopaedic Surgery, Columbia Presby 1973

SURGERY

Facelle, Thomas MD (S) - **Spec Exp:** Laparoscopic Surgery; Breast Cancer; Hernia; **Hospital:** Good Samaritan Hosp - Suffern; **Address:** 100 Route 59, Ste 101, Suffern, NY 10901-4927; **Phone:** 845-357-8800; **Board Cert:** Surgery 1993; **Med School:** NY Med Coll 1979; **Resid:** Surgery, New York Hosp 1984

Fleischer, Lee S MD (S) - **Spec Exp:** Breast Disease; Laparoscopic Surgery; Gastrointestinal Surgery; **Hospital:** Good Samaritan Hosp - Suffern, Nyack Hosp; **Address:** 100 Route 59, Ste 101, Suffern, NY 10901-4927; **Phone:** 845-357-8800; **Board Cert:** Surgery 2002; **Med School:** McGill Univ 1987; **Resid:** Surgery, Beth Israel Med Ctr 1992

Simon, Lawrence MD (S) - **Spec Exp:** Breast Surgery; Hernia; Gallbladder Surgery; **Hospital:** Nyack Hosp, Good Samaritan Hosp - Suffern; **Address:** 11 Medical Park Dr, Ste 203, Pomona, NY 10970-3559; **Phone:** 845-354-2241; **Board Cert:** Surgery 1971; **Med School:** SUNY Upstate Med Univ 1965; **Resid:** Surgery, St Lukes Hosp 1970

THORACIC SURGERY

Gorenstein, Lyall MD (TS) - **Spec Exp:** Thoracic Cancers; Esophageal Surgery; Minimally Invasive Thoracic Surgery; Palmar Hyperhidrosis; **Hospital:** Good Samaritan Hosp - Suffern, NY-Presby Hosp (page 100); **Address:** 5A Medical Park Drive, Pomona, NY 10970-3565; **Phone:** 845-362-0075; **Board Cert:** Surgery 1998; Thoracic Surgery 2001; **Med School:** Canada 1983; **Resid:** Radiation Therapy, Univ Toronto 1988; Thoracic Surgery, Univ Toronto 1990; **Fellow:** Thoracic Surgery, MD Anderson Cancer Ctr 1990

UROLOGY

Giella, John MD (U) - **Spec Exp:** Kidney Stones; Prostate Cancer; Hypospadias; **Hospital:** Nyack Hosp, Good Samaritan Hosp - Suffern; **Address:** 6 Medical Park Drive, Pomona, NY 10970-3525; **Phone:** 845-354-5000; **Board Cert:** Urology 2002; **Med School:** Harvard Med Sch 1986; **Resid:** Surgery, St Vincent's Hosp 1988; Urology, Columbia-Presby Med Ctr 1992

Kroll, Richard MD (U) - **Spec Exp:** Prostate Cancer; Bladder Surgery; Bladder Cancer; Prostate Benign Disease; **Hospital:** Good Samaritan Hosp - Suffern, Nyack Hosp; **Address:** 6 Medical Park Dr, Pomona, NY 10970-3525; **Phone:** 845-354-5000; **Board Cert:** Urology 1980; **Med School:** Albany Med Coll 1972; **Resid:** Surgery, St Vincent's Hosp & Med Ctr 1974; Urology, Columbia-Presby Med Ctr 1978

Rudin, Leonard MD (U) - **Spec Exp:** Urologic Cancer; Kidney Stones; **Hospital:** Good Samaritan Hosp - Suffern, Nyack Hosp; **Address:** 6 Medical Park Drive, Pomona, NY 10970-3525; **Phone:** 845-354-5000; **Board Cert:** Urology 1976; **Med School:** SUNY Upstate Med Univ 1966; **Resid:** Urology, Columbia-Presby 1974; Surgery, St Luke's-Roosevelt Hosp Ctr 1968

VASCULAR SURGERY

Schwartz, Michael L MD (VascS) - **Spec Exp:** Carotid Artery Surgery; Aneurysm-Aortic; Limb Salvage; Angioplasty; **Hospital:** Nyack Hosp, Good Samaritan Hosp - Suffern; **Address:** 5A Medical Park Drive, Pomona, NY 10970-3516; **Phone:** 845-362-0075; **Board Cert:** Surgery 1994; Vascular Surgery 2005; **Med School:** Univ S Fla Coll Med 1988; **Resid:** Surgery, Montefiore Med Ctr 1993; **Fellow:** Vascular Surgery, Montefiore Med Ctr 1995

Suffolk

ALLERGY & IMMUNOLOGY

Cancellieri, Russell MD (A&I) - **Spec Exp:** Asthma; **Hospital:** Southampton Hosp; **Address:** 596 Hampton Rd, Southampton, NY 11968; **Phone:** 631-283-3300; **Board Cert:** Allergy & Immunology 1981; Pediatrics 1979; **Med School:** Georgetown Univ 1974; **Resid:** Pediatrics, Georgetown Univ Hosp 1977; Allergy & Immunology, St Luke's-Roosevelt Hosp Ctr 1979

Lusman, Paul MD (A&I) - **Spec Exp:** Asthma; Sinus Disorders; Hives; **Hospital:** John T Mather Meml Hosp of Port Jefferson, St Charles Hosp; **Address:** 120 N Country Rd, Port Jefferson, NY 11777-2120; **Phone:** 631-928-4990; **Board Cert:** Pediatrics 1971; Allergy & Immunology 1974; **Med School:** Albert Einstein Coll Med 1965; **Resid:** Pediatrics, Strong Meml Hosp 1966; Pediatrics, Bellevue Hosp 1968; **Fellow:** Allergy & Immunology, Duke U Med Ctr 1972; **Fac Appt:** Asst Clin Prof Med, SUNY Stony Brook

Mayer, Daniel L MD (A&I) - **Spec Exp:** Asthma; Allergic Rhinitis; Food Allergy; Sinusitis; **Hospital:** Stony Brook Univ Hosp, St Catherine's of Siena Med Ctr; **Address:** 263 E Main St, Smithtown, NY 11787; **Phone:** 631-366-5252; **Board Cert:** Pediatrics 1993; Allergy & Immunology 1999; **Med School:** Italy 1978; **Resid:** Pediatrics, Albany Med Ctr 1985; **Fellow:** Allergy & Immunology, Long Island Hosp 1987; **Fac Appt:** Asst Prof A&I, SUNY Stony Brook

Richheimer, Michael MD (A&I) - **Spec Exp:** Asthma; Skin Allergies; Sinus Disorders; Headache; **Hospital:** New York Methodist Hosp (page 479), Stony Brook Univ Hosp; **Address:** 1855 Union Blvd, Bay Shore, NY 11706; **Phone:** 631-665-6363; **Board Cert:** Internal Medicine 1997; **Med School:** Grenada 1985; **Resid:** Internal Medicine, St. Joseph's Hosp-Seton Hall Univ 1988; **Fellow:** Allergy & Immunology, SUNY Stonybrook Med Ctr 1990; **Fac Appt:** Assoc Clin Prof A&I, SUNY Stony Brook

Satnick, Steven MD (A&I) - **Spec Exp:** Asthma; Urticaria; **Hospital:** Stony Brook Univ Hosp, Mercy Med Ctr - Rockville Centre; **Address:** 900 Main St, Ste 102, Holbrook, NY 11741-1813; **Phone:** 631-588-4486; **Board Cert:** Internal Medicine 1983; Allergy & Immunology 1987; **Med School:** SUNY Downstate 1980; **Resid:** Internal Medicine, Univ Hosp 1984; **Fellow:** Allergy & Immunology, Univ Hosp 1987

CARDIOVASCULAR DISEASE

Altschul, Larry MD (Cv) - **Spec Exp:** Non-Invasive Cardiology; Echocardiography; Nuclear Cardiology; **Hospital:** Good Samaritan Hosp Med Ctr - West Islip, Southside Hosp; **Address:** 540 Union Blvd, West Islip, NY 11795; **Phone:** 631-422-6565; **Board Cert:** Internal Medicine 1980; Cardiovascular Disease 1983; **Med School:** SUNY Buffalo 1977; **Resid:** Infectious Disease, Nassau County Med Ctr 1980; **Fellow:** Cardiovascular Disease, Nassau County Med Ctr 1982

Borek, Mark MD (Cv) - **Spec Exp:** Nuclear Cardiology; Echocardiography; Cardiac Catheterization; **Hospital:** St Catherine's of Siena Med Ctr, John T Mather Meml Hosp of Port Jefferson; **Address:** 496 Smithtown Bypass, Ste 101, Smithtown, NY 11787; **Phone:** 631-979-8880; **Board Cert:** Internal Medicine 1985; Cardiovascular Disease 1987; **Med School:** SUNY Downstate 1981; **Resid:** Internal Medicine, Nassau Co Med Ctr 1984; **Fellow:** Cardiovascular Disease, Long Island Coll Hosp 1987

Chengot, Mathew MD (Cv) - **Spec Exp:** Nuclear Cardiology; Interventional Cardiology; Heart Failure; **Hospital:** Good Samaritan Hosp Med Ctr - West Islip, New Island Hosp; **Address:** Amityville Heart Ctr, 129 Broadway, Amityville, NY 11701-2729; **Phone:** 631-598-3434; **Board Cert:** Internal Medicine 1983; Cardiovascular Disease 1985; **Med School:** India 1976; **Resid:** Internal Medicine, Lincoln Med Ctr 1982; **Fellow:** Cardiovascular Disease, Mt Sinai Hosp 1984

Dervan, John MD (Cv) - **Spec Exp:** Interventional Cardiology; Cholesterol/Lipid Disorders; **Hospital:** Stony Brook Univ Hosp, St Catherine's of Siena Med Ctr; **Address:** 2500-1 Nesconset Hwy, Stony Brook, NY 11790; **Phone:** 631-689-7700; **Board Cert:** Internal Medicine 1979; Cardiovascular Disease 1985; Interventional Cardiology 1999; **Med School:** St Louis Univ 1976; **Resid:** Internal Medicine, Faulkner Hosp 1980; **Fellow:** Cardiovascular Disease, Beth Israel Hosp 1983; **Fac Appt:** Assoc Clin Prof Med, SUNY Stony Brook

Falco, Thomas MD (Cv) - **Hospital:** Peconic Bay Med Ctr, Eastern Long Island Hosp; **Address:** 1279 E Main St, Riverhead, NY 11901; **Phone:** 631-727-2100; **Board Cert:** Internal Medicine 1985; Cardiovascular Disease 1987; **Med School:** Mexico 1980; **Resid:** Internal Medicine, Winthrop Univ Hosp 1984; Cardiovascular Disease, Winthrop Univ Hosp 1985; **Fellow:** Cardiovascular Disease, Albany Med Ctr 1987

Lense, Lloyd MD (Cv) - **Spec Exp:** Cholesterol/Lipid Disorders; Hypertension; Coronary Artery Disease; **Hospital:** John T Mather Meml Hosp of Port Jefferson, Stony Brook Univ Hosp; **Address:** 3400 Nesconset Hwy, Ste 105, E Setauket, NY 11733-3327; **Phone:** 631-689-1400; **Board Cert:** Internal Medicine 1980; Cardiovascular Disease 1983; **Med School:** NYU Sch Med 1977; **Resid:** Internal Medicine, Mount Sinai 1980; **Fellow:** Cardiovascular Disease, Montefiore Hosp Med Ctr 1983; **Fac Appt:** Assoc Clin Prof Med, SUNY Stony Brook

Masciello, Michael MD (Cv) - **Spec Exp:** Coronary Artery Disease; **Hospital:** Southside Hosp, Good Samaritan Hosp Med Ctr - West Islip; **Address:** 540 Union Blvd, West Islip, NY 11795; **Phone:** 631-669-2555; **Board Cert:** Internal Medicine 1983; Cardiovascular Disease 1985; Critical Care Medicine 2003; **Med School:** Univ Miami Sch Med 1980; **Resid:** Cardiovascular Disease, Nassau County Med Ctr 1985; **Fellow:** Cardiovascular Disease, Nassau County Med Ctr 1985

Matilsky, Michael MD (Cv) - **Spec Exp:** Cholesterol/Lipid Disorders; Hypertension; Coronary Artery Disease; **Hospital:** St Charles Hosp, John T Mather Meml Hosp of Port Jefferson; **Address:** 3400 Nesconset Hwy, Ste 105, East Setauket, NY 11733-3327; **Phone:** 631-689-1400; **Board Cert:** Internal Medicine 1985; Cardiovascular Disease 1987; **Med School:** SUNY Stony Brook 1982; **Resid:** Internal Medicine, Mount Sinai Hosp 1985; **Fellow:** Cardiovascular Disease, NY Hosp 1988; **Fac Appt:** Asst Clin Prof Med, SUNY Stony Brook

Vlay, Stephen C MD (Cv) - **Spec Exp:** Arrhythmias & Pacemakers; Congestive Heart Failure; Cardiac Electrophysiology; **Hospital:** Stony Brook Univ Hosp; **Address:** SUNY Hlth Sciences Ctr Rd, Ste T-16 080, Stony Brook, NY 11794-8167; **Phone:** 631-444-1060; **Board Cert:** Internal Medicine 1978; Cardiovascular Disease 1981; Cardiac Electrophysiology 1996; **Med School:** Yale Univ 1975; **Resid:** Internal Medicine, Bellevue Hosp 1978; **Fellow:** Cardiovascular Disease, Johns Hopkins Hosp 1980; **Fac Appt:** Prof Med, SUNY Stony Brook

Weinberg, Marc MD (Cv) - **Hospital:** Huntington Hosp; **Address:** West Carver Med Assocs, 200 W Carver St, Ste 1, Huntington, NY 11743-3303; **Phone:** 631-421-0020; **Board Cert:** Internal Medicine 1976; Cardiovascular Disease 1987; **Med School:** Yale Univ 1973; **Resid:** Internal Medicine, New Haven Hospital 1977; **Fellow:** Cardiovascular Disease, New Haven Hospital 1979

Zema, Michael MD (Cv) - **Spec Exp:** Cholesterol/Lipid Disorders; Hypertension; Non-Invasive Cardiology; **Hospital:** Brookhaven Meml Hosp & Med Ctr, Stony Brook Univ Hosp; **Address:** Brookhaven Memorial Hosp, Dept Cardiology, 101 Hospital Rd, Patchogue, NY 11772-4870; **Phone:** 631-654-7279; **Board Cert:** Internal Medicine 1977; Cardiovascular Disease 1979; **Med School:** Cornell Univ-Weill Med Coll 1974; **Resid:** Internal Medicine, N Shore Univ Hosp/Meml Hosp 1977; Cardiovascular Disease, New York Hosp-Cornell Med Ctr 1978; **Fellow:** Cardiovascular Disease, N Shore Univ Hosp 1979; **Fac Appt:** Clin Prof Med, SUNY Stony Brook

CHILD & ADOLESCENT PSYCHIATRY

Carlson, Gabrielle A MD (ChAP) - **Spec Exp:** Child Psychiatry; Bipolar/Mood Disorders; ADD/ADHD; **Hospital:** Stony Brook Univ Hosp; **Address:** Putnam Hall, South Campus, SUNY-Stony Brook, Stony Brook, NY 11794-8790; **Phone:** 631-632-8840; **Board Cert:** Child & Adolescent Psychiatry 1978; Psychiatry 1975; **Med School:** Cornell Univ-Weill Med Coll 1968; **Resid:** Psychiatry, Barnes Hosp-Washington Univ 1970; Psychiatry, Nat Inst Mental Hlth 1972; **Fellow:** Child & Adolescent Psychiatry, UCLA Med Ctr 1978; **Fac Appt:** Prof Psyc, SUNY Stony Brook

Gandhi, Lajpat MD (ChAP) - **Hospital:** Huntington Hosp; **Address:** 110 E Main St, Ste 5, Huntington, NY 11743; **Phone:** 631-427-6411; **Board Cert:** Psychiatry 1981; Child & Adolescent Psychiatry 1985; **Med School:** India 1975; **Resid:** Psychiatry, Metropolitan Hosp 1979; **Fellow:** Psychiatry, Elmhurst Hosp-Mt Sinai 1980; Child & Adolescent Psychiatry, LI Jewish-Hillside Med Ctr 1981

Greenberg, Judith J MD (ChAP) - **Hospital:** Long Island Jewish Med Ctr, N Shore Univ Hosp at Manhasset; **Address:** 410 E Main St, Centerport, NY 11721; **Phone:** 631-754-4060; **Board Cert:** Psychiatry 1990; Pediatrics 1985; Child & Adolescent Psychiatry 1990; **Med School:** SUNY Downstate 1980; **Resid:** Pediatrics, Children's Meml Hosp 1983; Psychiatry, N Shore Univ Hosp 1987; **Fellow:** Child Psychiatry, Univ Illinois Hosp 1984; Child Psychiatry, N Shore Univ Hosp 1985

Pomeroy, John C MD (ChAP) - **Spec Exp:** Autism; Mental Retardation; Developmental Disorders; **Hospital:** Stony Brook Univ Hosp; **Address:** The Cody Ctr, 5 Medical Drive, Port Jefferson Stn, NY 11776; **Phone:** 631-632-3070; **Board Cert:** Psychiatry 1984; Child & Adolescent Psychiatry 1988; **Med School:** England 1973; **Resid:** Psychiatry, St.Mary's Hosp 1979; **Fellow:** Child & Adolescent Psychiatry, Univ Iowa Hosps 1981; **Fac Appt:** Assoc Prof Psyc, SUNY Stony Brook

Weisbrot, Deborah M MD (ChAP) - **Spec Exp:** Anxiety & Mood Disorders; Epilepsy; Aggression Disorders; Multiple Sclerosis; **Hospital:** Stony Brook Univ Hosp; **Address:** SUNY Stony Brook, Div Child & Adolescent Psychiatry, Putnam Hall, South Campus, Stony Brook, NY 11794-8790; **Phone:** 631-632-8840; **Board Cert:** Psychiatry 1985; Child & Adolescent Psychiatry 1991; **Med School:** SUNY Buffalo 1979; **Resid:** Psychiatry, Yale-New Haven Hosp 1983; **Fellow:** Child Psychiatry, New York Hosp-Payne Whitney Clin 1986; **Fac Appt:** Asst Prof Psyc, SUNY Stony Brook

CHILD NEUROLOGY

Andriola, Mary MD (ChiN) - **Spec Exp:** Epilepsy; ADD/ADHD; Headache; **Hospital:** Stony Brook Univ Hosp; **Address:** SUNY-Stony Brook, Dept Neurology, HSC T12020, Stony Brook, NY 11794-0001; **Phone:** 631-444-2599; **Board Cert:** Pediatrics 1970; Child Neurology 1972; Clinical Neurophysiology 2002; Neurodevelopmental Disabilities 2005; **Med School:** Duke Univ 1965; **Resid:** Pediatrics, Univ Fla Shands Hosp 1967; **Fellow:** Neurology, Univ Fla Shands Hosp 1970; **Fac Appt:** Prof N, SUNY Stony Brook

CLINICAL GENETICS

Hyman, David B MD (CG) - **Spec Exp:** Prenatal Diagnosis; Genetic Disorders; Cancer Risk Assessment; **Hospital:** Stony Brook Univ Hosp, St Catherine's of Siena Med Ctr; **Address:** 48 Route 25-A, Ste 205, Smithtown, NY 11787-1448; **Phone:** 631-862-3620; **Board Cert:** Pediatrics 1983; Clinical Genetics 1984; Clinical Biochemical Genetics 1990; **Med School:** Univ IL Coll Med 1978; **Resid:** Pediatrics, Yale Univ Sch Med 1980; **Fellow:** Clinical Genetics, Yale Univ Sch Med 1983

COLON & RECTAL SURGERY

Leiboff, Arnold MD (CRS) - **Hospital:** John T Mather Meml Hosp of Port Jefferson, St Charles Hosp; **Address:** 3400 Nesconset Hwy, Ste 100, East Setauket, NY 11733; **Phone:** 631-689-2600; **Board Cert:** Surgery 1996; Colon & Rectal Surgery 1999; **Med School:** NY Med Coll 1978; **Resid:** Surgery, SUNY at Stony Brook 1985; **Fellow:** Colon & Rectal Surgery, Carle Foundation Hosp-Univ Ill 1989

Sconzo Jr, Frank MD (CRS) - **Spec Exp:** Colon Cancer; Anorectal Disorders; **Hospital:** Brookhaven Meml Hosp & Med Ctr; **Address:** 286 Sills Rd, Ste 5, East Patchogue, NY 11772-8830; **Phone:** 631-654-3100; **Board Cert:** Colon & Rectal Surgery 1992; **Med School:** NY Med Coll 1983; **Resid:** Surgery, St Barnabas Med Ctr 1988; Colon & Rectal Surgery, Jefferson Med Coll 1989

Smithy, William MD (CRS) - **Spec Exp:** Colon & Rectal Cancer; Anorectal Disorders; Colonoscopy; **Hospital:** Stony Brook Univ Hosp, St Catherine's of Siena Med Ctr; **Address:** 1077 W Jericho Tpke, Smithtown, NY 11787; **Phone:** 631-864-7870; **Board Cert:** Surgery 1997; Colon & Rectal Surgery 1989; **Med School:** Columbia P&S 1981; **Resid:** Surgery, Roosevelt Hosp 1987; **Fellow:** Colon & Rectal Surgery, RWJ Univ Hosp 1988; **Fac Appt:** Asst Clin Prof S, SUNY Stony Brook

DERMATOLOGY

Basuk, Pamela MD (D) - **Spec Exp:** Cosmetic Dermatology; Melanoma; Dermatologic Surgery; **Hospital:** Southside Hosp, Good Samaritan Hosp Med Ctr - West Islip; **Address:** 2011 Union Blvd, Ste 1, Bayshore, NY 11706; **Phone:** 631-666-2900; **Board Cert:** Dermatology 1988; **Med School:** NYU Sch Med 1984; **Resid:** Dermatology, Brown Univ Hosp 1988

Berger, Bernard MD (D) - **Hospital:** Southampton Hosp; **Address:** 319 Hampton Rd, Southampton, NY 11968-5029; **Phone:** 631-283-7722; **Board Cert:** Dermatology 1975; **Med School:** UC Irvine 1963; **Resid:** Dermatology, Mount Sinai Hosp 1971

Clark, Richard MD (D) - **Hospital:** Stony Brook Univ Hosp; **Address:** 181 N Belle Meade Rd, Ste 6, East Setauket, NY 11733; **Phone:** 631-444-4270; **Board Cert:** Dermatology 1980; **Med School:** Univ Rochester 1971; **Resid:** Internal Medicine, Strong Meml Hosp 1973; **Fellow:** Allergy & Immunology, Nat Inst Health 1976; Dermatology, Mass Genl Hosp 1980; **Fac Appt:** Prof D, SUNY Stony Brook

Huh, Julie MD (D) - **Spec Exp:** Acne; Skin Cancer; **Hospital:** Good Samaritan Hosp Med Ctr - West Islip, Southside Hosp; **Address:** 332 E Main St, Bayshore, NY 11706-8404; **Phone:** 631-666-0500; **Board Cert:** Dermatology 1995; **Med School:** Columbia P&S 1991; **Resid:** Dermatology, Columbia-Presby Med Ctr 1995

Miller, Richard L MD (D) - **Spec Exp:** Skin Cancer; Eczema; Psoriasis; **Hospital:** John T Mather Meml Hosp of Port Jefferson, St Charles Hosp; **Address:** 200 Main St, Ste 5, Setauket, NY 11733-2918; **Phone:** 631-751-7070; **Board Cert:** Dermatology 1975; **Med School:** Duke Univ 1968; **Resid:** Dermatology, Naval Reg Med Ctr 1974; **Fac Appt:** Asst Clin Prof D, SUNY Stony Brook

Moynihan, Gavan D MD (D) - **Spec Exp:** Melanoma; Skin Cancer; **Hospital:** Good Samaritan Hosp Med Ctr - West Islip; **Address:** 332 E Main St, Bay Shore, NY 11706-8404; **Phone:** 631-666-0500; **Board Cert:** Dermatology 1977; **Med School:** Howard Univ 1973; **Resid:** Dermatology, USPHS Hosp-Staten Island NY & USPHS Hosp 1976; **Fellow:** Dermatology, Columbia-Presby Med Ctr 1977; **Fac Appt:** Asst Prof D, SUNY Stony Brook

Notaro, Antoinette MD (D) - **Spec Exp:** Skin Cancer; Botox Therapy; Psoriasis; Acne; **Hospital:** Eastern Long Island Hosp, Peconic Bay Med Ctr; **Address:** 13405 Main Rd, Box 93, Mattituck, NY 11952-0093; **Phone:** 631-298-1122; **Board Cert:** Dermatology 1982; **Med School:** SUNY Hlth Sci Ctr 1978; **Resid:** Dermatology, Albert Einstein 1982; **Fac Appt:** Asst Clin Prof D, SUNY Stony Brook

Siegel, Daniel M MD (D) - **Spec Exp:** Mohs' Surgery; Dermatologic Surgery; Skin Cancer; **Hospital:** St Catherine's of Siena Med Ctr, Eastern Long Island Hosp; **Address:** 994 Jericho Tpke, Ste 103, Smithtown, NY 11787; **Phone:** 631-864-6647; **Board Cert:** Dermatology 1985; **Med School:** Albany Med Coll 1981; **Resid:** Dermatology, Parkland Univ Texas SW Med Ctr 1985; **Fellow:** Mohs Surgery, Baylor Coll Med 1986; **Fac Appt:** Assoc Clin Prof D, SUNY Stony Brook

Skrokov, Robert MD (D) - **Spec Exp:** Vascular Malformations/Birthmarks; Psoriasis; Skin Cancer; **Hospital:** Good Samaritan Hosp Med Ctr - West Islip, Southside Hosp; **Address:** 332 E Main St, Bay Shore, NY 11706-8404; **Phone:** 631-666-0500; **Board Cert:** Dermatology 1986; **Med School:** SUNY Downstate 1982; **Resid:** Dermatology, SUNY-Downstate Med Ctr 1986; **Fac Appt:** Asst Clin Prof D, SUNY Stony Brook

Tom, Jack MD (D) - **Spec Exp:** Acne; Geriatric Dermatology; **Hospital:** Mount Sinai Med Ctr (page 98); **Address:** 207 Hallock Rd, Ste 211, Stony Brook, NY 11790-3076; **Phone:** 631-444-0004; **Board Cert:** Dermatology 1986; **Med School:** NYU Sch Med 1982; **Resid:** Internal Medicine, NYU Med Ctr 1983; Dermatology, Mount Sinai Med Ctr 1986

Tonnesen, Marcia MD (D) - **Spec Exp:** Geriatric Dermatology; **Hospital:** Stony Brook Univ Hosp, VA Med Ctr @ Northport; **Address:** 181 N Belle Meade Rd, Ste 6, East Setauket, NY 11733; **Phone:** 631-444-4200; **Board Cert:** Dermatology 1980; **Med School:** Univ Utah 1973; **Resid:** Dermatology, Harvard Affil Hosps 1978; **Fellow:** Dermatology, Brigham Hosp/Harvard 1981; **Fac Appt:** Assoc Prof D, SUNY Stony Brook

DIAGNOSTIC RADIOLOGY

Brancaccio, William R MD (DR) - **Spec Exp:** Abdominal Radiology; Mammography; **Hospital:** Southampton Hosp, Peconic Bay Med Ctr; **Address:** 240 Meeting House Ln, Southampton, NY 11698; **Phone:** 631-726-8411; **Board Cert:** Diagnostic Radiology 1981; **Med School:** Geo Wash Univ 1975; **Resid:** Diagnostic Radiology, Univ Hosp 1979; **Fellow:** Diagnostic Radiology, NYU Med Ctr 1980

Cohen, Harris L MD (DR) - **Spec Exp:** Pediatric Ultrasound/Imaging; Pediatric Radiology; Fetal Ultrasound/Obstetrical Imaging; **Hospital:** Stony Brook Univ Hosp; **Address:** Stony Brook Univ Hosp, Dept Radiology, HCS level 4, rm 120, Stony Brook, NY 11794-8460; **Phone:** 631-444-8193; **Board Cert:** Diagnostic Radiology 1980; Pediatric Radiology 2005; **Med School:** SUNY Downstate 1976; **Resid:** Internal Medicine, Nassau County Med Ctr 1977; Diagnostic Radiology, Univ Hosp 1980; **Fellow:** Pediatric Radiology, Children's Hosp 1981; **Fac Appt:** Prof Rad, SUNY Stony Brook

Laucella, Michael MD (DR) - **Hospital:** Huntington Hosp, Southside Hosp; **Address:** 375 E Main St, Bay Shore, NY 11706; **Phone:** 631-665-2261; **Board Cert:** Diagnostic Radiology 1984; Neuroradiology 1995; **Med School:** Univ Chicago-Pritzker Sch Med 1980; **Resid:** Diagnostic Radiology, Tufts-New England Med Ctr 1984; **Fellow:** Neurological Radiology, Tufts-New England Med Ctr 1986

Mankes, Seth MD (DR) - **Hospital:** Stony Brook Univ Hosp; **Address:** Stony Brook Univ Hosp, HSC, Level 4, rm 120, Stony Brook, NY 11794-8460; **Phone:** 631-444-7224; **Board Cert:** Diagnostic Radiology 1981; Neuroradiology 1995; **Med School:** NYU Sch Med 1976; **Resid:** Diagnostic Radiology, NYU Med Ctr 1981; **Fellow:** Ultrasound, NYU Med Ctr 1982

Rifkin, Matthew MD (DR) - **Spec Exp:** Ultrasound; **Hospital:** Good Samaritan Hosp Med Ctr - West Islip; **Address:** 1000 Montauk Hwy, West Islip, NY 11795; **Phone:** 631-376-4030; **Board Cert:** Diagnostic Radiology 1978; **Med School:** Albert Einstein Coll Med 1974; **Resid:** Diagnostic Radiology, Montefiore Hosp 1978; **Fellow:** Ultrasound/CT, Johns Hopkins Hosp 1979

ENDOCRINOLOGY, DIABETES & METABOLISM

Balkin, Michael MD (EDM) - **Spec Exp:** Diabetes; Thyroid Disorders; Hirsutism (Excessive Body Hair); Osteoporosis; **Hospital:** Huntington Hosp, Nassau Univ Med Ctr; **Address:** 191 E Main St, Huntington, NY 11743-2921; **Phone:** 631-549-2525; **Board Cert:** Internal Medicine 1976; Endocrinology 1977; **Med School:** Mount Sinai Sch Med 1972; **Resid:** Internal Medicine, Kings County Med Ctr 1975; **Fellow:** Endocrinology, Diabetes & Metabolism, Mt Sinai Med Ctr 1977; Endocrinology, Diabetes & Metabolism, Meml Sloan Kettering Cancer Ctr 1980; **Fac Appt:** Asst Clin Prof Med, SUNY Stony Brook

Brand, Howard A MD (EDM) - **Spec Exp:** Thyroid Disorders; Pituitary Disorders; **Hospital:** St Charles Hosp, John T Mather Meml Hosp of Port Jefferson; **Address:** 2500 Nesconset Hwy Bldg 3, Stony Brook, NY 11790; **Phone:** 631-751-2400; **Board Cert:** Internal Medicine 1987; Endocrinology, Diabetes & Metabolism 1991; **Med School:** UMDNJ-RW Johnson Med Sch 1984; **Resid:** Internal Medicine, Mt Sinai Hosp 1987; Internal Medicine, Bronx VA Med Ctr 1988; **Fellow:** Endocrinology, Diabetes & Metabolism, NYU Med Ctr 1990

Carlson, Harold E MD (EDM) - **Spec Exp:** Thyroid Disorders; Pituitary Disorders; Gynecomastia; **Hospital:** Stony Brook Univ Hosp; **Address:** Stony Brook Univ Hosp, Dept Medicine, Div Endocrinology & Metabolism, Stony Brook, NY 11794-8154; **Phone:** 631-444-0580; **Board Cert:** Internal Medicine 1974; Endocrinology 1975; **Med School:** Cornell Univ-Weill Med Coll 1968; **Resid:** Internal Medicine, Barnes Hosp 1970; Internal Medicine, Natl Inst Hlth 1972; **Fellow:** Endocrinology, Wash Univ 1974; **Fac Appt:** Prof Med, SUNY Stony Brook

Gelato, Marie MD (EDM) - **Spec Exp:** Thyroid Disorders; Pituitary Disorders; Adrenal Disorders; **Hospital:** Stony Brook Univ Hosp; **Address:** 26 Research Way, East Setauket, NY 11733; **Phone:** 631-444-0580; **Board Cert:** Internal Medicine 1982; Endocrinology 1985; **Med School:** Mich State Univ 1979; **Resid:** Internal Medicine, Dartmouth Med Ctr 1982; **Fellow:** Endocrinology, Natl Inst Hlth 1985; **Fac Appt:** Prof Med, SUNY Stony Brook

Gioia, Leonard MD (EDM) - **Spec Exp:** Diabetes; Thyroid Disorders; **Hospital:** Southside Hosp, Good Samaritan Hosp Med Ctr - West Islip; **Address:** 200 Howells Rd, Bay Shore, NY 11706-5300; **Phone:** 631-666-6275; **Board Cert:** Internal Medicine 1979; Endocrinology, Diabetes & Metabolism 1981; **Med School:** SUNY Downstate 1976; **Resid:** Internal Medicine, St Vincent's Hosp & Med Ctr 1979; **Fellow:** Endocrinology, Diabetes & Metabolism, Boston Univ Med Ctr 1981

Goldenberg, Alan MD (EDM) - **Spec Exp:** Diabetes; Thyroid Disorders; Hormonal Disorders; **Hospital:** Southampton Hosp, Peconic Bay Med Ctr; **Address:** East End Endocine Assocs, 189 Main Rd, Riverhead, NY 11901; **Phone:** 631-288-7120; **Board Cert:** Internal Medicine 1996; Endocrinology, Diabetes & Metabolism 1998; **Med School:** SUNY Stony Brook 1993; **Resid:** Internal Medicine, Winthrop Univ Hosp 1996; **Fellow:** Endocrinology, Diabetes & Metabolism, Winthrop Univ Hosp 1998

Wexler, Craig B MD (EDM) - **Spec Exp:** Diabetes; Thyroid Disorders; Hormonal Disorders; Cholesterol/Lipid Disorders; **Hospital:** Brookhaven Meml Hosp & Med Ctr; **Address:** 285 Sills Rd, Bldg 15 - Ste D, East Patchogue, NY 11772-8810; **Phone:** 631-758-5858; **Board Cert:** Internal Medicine 1981; Endocrinology, Diabetes & Metabolism 1989; **Med School:** Univ Hlth Sci/Chicago Med Sch 1978; **Resid:** Internal Medicine, LI Jewish-Hillside Med Ctr 1981; **Fellow:** Endocrinology, Diabetes & Metabolism, LI Jewish-Hillside Med Ctr 1989

Wu, Ching-hui MD (EDM) - **Spec Exp:** Thyroid Disorders; Pituitary Disorders; **Hospital:** John T Mather Meml Hosp of Port Jefferson, St Charles Hosp; **Address:** 2500 Nesconset Hwy 12C Bldg, Stony Brook, NY 11790-2555; **Phone:** 631-751-2185; **Board Cert:** Internal Medicine 1970; Endocrinology, Diabetes & Metabolism 1977; **Med School:** Taiwan 1959; **Resid:** Internal Medicine, Metropolitan Hosp Ctr 1964; **Fellow:** Endocrinology, Diabetes & Metabolism, NY Med Coll 1966; **Fac Appt:** Asst Clin Prof Med, SUNY Stony Brook

FAMILY MEDICINE

Aponte, Alex M MD (FMed) `PCP` - **Hospital:** Southampton Hosp; **Address:** Westhampton Primary Care, 80 Old Riverhead Rd, Westhampton Beach, NY 11978; **Phone:** 631-288-7746; **Board Cert:** Family Medicine 2002; **Med School:** SUNY Buffalo 1992; **Resid:** Family Medicine, Overlook Hosp 1995

Bilmes, Ernest MD (FMed) `PCP` - **Hospital:** Brookhaven Meml Hosp & Med Ctr; **Address:** 485 N Ocean Ave, Ste A, Patchogue, NY 11772; **Phone:** 631-475-6900; **Board Cert:** Family Medicine 1996; **Med School:** Univ Hlth Sci/Chicago Med Sch 1959; **Resid:** Internal Medicine, Kings County Hosp 1960

Blyskal, Stanley MD (FMed) `PCP` - **Spec Exp:** Preventive Cardiology; Depression/Mood Disorders; Osteoporosis; **Hospital:** Southside Hosp; **Address:** 126 E Main St, Ste 1, East Islip, NY 11730-2600; **Phone:** 631-581-0090; **Board Cert:** Family Medicine 1997; **Med School:** Albany Med Coll 1974; **Resid:** Family Medicine, Southside Hosp 1977; **Fac Appt:** Asst Clin Prof FMed, SUNY Stony Brook

D'Esposito, Michael MD (FMed) **PCP** - **Hospital:** St Catherine's of Siena Med Ctr; **Address:** 121 E Northport Rd, Kings Park, NY 11754; **Phone:** 631-269-1148; **Board Cert:** Family Medicine 2003; **Med School:** West Indies 1984; **Resid:** Family Medicine, St Mary's Hosp 1987

Ebarb, Raymond MD (FMed) **PCP** - **Hospital:** Southside Hosp, Good Samaritan Hosp Med Ctr - West Islip; **Address:** 213 Montauk Hwy, West Sayville, NY 11796; **Phone:** 631-563-6205; **Board Cert:** Family Medicine 1999; **Med School:** Mexico 1982; **Resid:** Family Medicine, Southside Hosp 1987; **Fac Appt:** Asst Clin Prof FMed, SUNY Stony Brook

Fishkin, Michael DO (FMed) **PCP** - **Hospital:** John T Mather Meml Hosp of Port Jefferson, St Charles Hosp; **Address:** 2500 Nesconset Hwy 7D Bldg, Stony Brook, NY 11790-2552; **Phone:** 631-751-3322; **Board Cert:** Family Medicine 2000; **Med School:** Univ Osteo Med & Hlth Sci, Des Moines 1973; **Resid:** Family Medicine, Nassau County Med Ctr 1976; **Fac Appt:** Assoc Prof FMed, SUNY Stony Brook

Franco, John MD (FMed) **PCP** - **Hospital:** St Catherine's of Siena Med Ctr; **Address:** 9 Brookside Dr, Smithtown, NY 11787; **Phone:** 631-724-1331; **Board Cert:** Family Medicine 2002; Geriatric Medicine 2002; **Med School:** Mexico 1974; **Resid:** Family Medicine, Nassau County Med Ctr 1978

Greenberg, Maury J MD (FMed) **PCP** - **Spec Exp:** Women's Health; Travel Medicine; **Hospital:** Stony Brook Univ Hosp; **Address:** 2500 Nesconset Hwy Bldg 6D, Stony Brook, NY 11790-2559; **Phone:** 631-751-5550; **Board Cert:** Family Medicine 1985; **Med School:** Albert Einstein Coll Med 1982; **Resid:** Family Medicine, Southside Hosp 1985; **Fac Appt:** Assoc Prof FMed, SUNY Stony Brook

Greenblatt, Louis DO (FMed) **PCP** - **Spec Exp:** Preventive Medicine; Geriatric Medicine; **Hospital:** St Catherine's of Siena Med Ctr, Stony Brook Univ Hosp; **Address:** 533 Rte 111, Hauppauge, NY 11788; **Phone:** 631-366-1788; **Board Cert:** Family Medicine 2000; Geriatric Medicine 1996; **Med School:** NY Coll Osteo Med 1983; **Resid:** Family Medicine, Univ Hosp 1986; **Fac Appt:** Asst Clin Prof FMed, SUNY Stony Brook

Klein, Steven MD (FMed) **PCP** - **Spec Exp:** Hypertension; Asthma; **Hospital:** Southside Hosp; **Address:** 19 E Main St, Ste 8, Bay Shore, NY 11706; **Phone:** 631-665-0760; **Board Cert:** Family Medicine 2003; **Med School:** Univ VT Coll Med 1983; **Resid:** Family Medicine, Southside Hosp 1986

Levites, Kenneth MD (FMed) **PCP** - **Spec Exp:** Asthma; Occupational Medicine; Hypertension; Diabetes; **Hospital:** Southside Hosp, Good Samaritan Hosp Med Ctr - West Islip; **Address:** 213 Montauk Hwy, West Sayville, NY 11796-1800; **Phone:** 631-563-6205; **Board Cert:** Family Medicine 2003; **Med School:** Albany Med Coll 1974; **Resid:** Family Medicine, Southside 1977

Roth, Ronald MD (FMed) **PCP** - **Spec Exp:** Sports Medicine; Women's Health; **Hospital:** St Catherine's of Siena Med Ctr; **Address:** 100 Maple Ave, Smithtown, NY 11787; **Phone:** 631-265-7671 x11; **Board Cert:** Family Medicine 2003; **Med School:** NY Med Coll 1973; **Resid:** Family Medicine, Southside 1978; **Fac Appt:** Assoc Prof FMed, SUNY Stony Brook

Schwinn, Hans Dieter MD (FMed) **PCP** - **Hospital:** Southampton Hosp; **Address:** 80 Old Riverhead Rd, Westhampton Beach, NY 11978-1401; **Phone:** 631-288-4004; **Board Cert:** Family Medicine 2000; **Med School:** Germany 1978; **Resid:** Family Medicine, Community Hosp 1981

GASTROENTEROLOGY

Berman, Richard E MD (Ge) - **Hospital:** Brookhaven Meml Hosp & Med Ctr; **Address:** 260 Patchogue Yaphank Rd, Ste C, East Patchogue, NY 11772; **Phone:** 631-289-0300; **Board Cert:** Gastroenterology 1975; Internal Medicine 1973; **Med School:** Univ Rochester 1969; **Resid:** Internal Medicine, Temple Hosp 1972; Gastroenterology, Mount Sinai 1974

Cohn, William J MD (Ge) - **Spec Exp:** Liver Disease; **Hospital:** John T Mather Meml Hosp of Port Jefferson, St Charles Hosp; **Address:** 3400 Nesconset Hwy, Ste 101, Setauket, NY 11733; **Phone:** 631-751-8700; **Board Cert:** Internal Medicine 1975; Gastroenterology 1979; **Med School:** Med Coll VA 1972; **Resid:** Internal Medicine, Med Coll Va 1975; **Fellow:** Gastroenterology, Albert Einstein 1978; **Fac Appt:** Asst Clin Prof Med, SUNY Stony Brook

Duva, Joseph MD (Ge) - **Spec Exp:** Endoscopy & Colonoscopy; Gastroesophageal Reflux Disease (GERD); Irritable Bowel Syndrome; **Hospital:** Peconic Bay Med Ctr; **Address:** 887 Old Country Rd, Ste A, Riverhead, NY 11901-2115; **Phone:** 631-727-6122; **Board Cert:** Internal Medicine 1981; Gastroenterology 1997; **Med School:** Mount Sinai Sch Med 1978; **Resid:** Internal Medicine, Nassau County Med Ctr 1980; **Fellow:** Gastroenterology, Nassau County Med Ctr 1983

Ells, Peter F MD (Ge) - **Spec Exp:** Hepatitis; **Hospital:** Stony Brook Univ Hosp; **Address:** 3 Technology Drive, Ste 700, East Setauket, NY 11733; **Phone:** 631-444-5220; **Board Cert:** Internal Medicine 1977; Gastroenterology 1979; **Med School:** Tufts Univ 1974; **Resid:** Internal Medicine, Univ VA Hlth Sci Ctr 1977; **Fellow:** Gastroenterology, UCSF Med Ctr 1981; **Fac Appt:** Assoc Clin Prof Med, SUNY Stony Brook

Glanzman, Barry MD (Ge) - **Spec Exp:** Colonoscopy; Gastroesophageal Reflux Disease (GERD); Liver Disease; **Hospital:** Huntington Hosp; **Address:** 152 E Main St, Ste C, Huntington, NY 11743; **Phone:** 631-421-2185; **Board Cert:** Gastroenterology 1989; Internal Medicine 1984; **Med School:** SUNY Downstate 1980; **Resid:** Internal Medicine, LI Jewish hosp 1981; Internal Medicine, LI Jewish Hosp 1983; **Fellow:** Gastroenterology, Med Coll of VA 1986

Harrison, Aaron R MD (Ge) - **Spec Exp:** Gastroesophageal Reflux Disease (GERD); Peptic Acid Disorders; Crohn's Disease; **Hospital:** Southside Hosp, Good Samaritan Hosp Med Ctr - West Islip; **Address:** 375 E Main St, Ste 21, Bay Shore, NY 11706; **Phone:** 631-968-8288; **Board Cert:** Internal Medicine 1977; Gastroenterology 1979; **Med School:** Albert Einstein Coll Med 1974; **Resid:** Internal Medicine, Jacobi Med Ctr 1977; **Fellow:** Gastroenterology, UCLA Med Ctr 1979; **Fac Appt:** Asst Clin Prof Med, SUNY Stony Brook

Lazar, Robert MD (Ge) - **Hospital:** St Catherine's of Siena Med Ctr; **Address:** 48 Route 25a, Smithtown, NY 11787-1431; **Phone:** 631-862-3680; **Board Cert:** Internal Medicine 1986; Gastroenterology 2000; **Med School:** Mexico 1982

Naso, Kristin DO (Ge) - **Spec Exp:** Liver Disease; **Hospital:** Southampton Hosp; **Address:** 223 Hampton Rd, Southampton, NY 11968; **Phone:** 631-283-0090; **Board Cert:** Internal Medicine 1989; Gastroenterology 2001; **Med School:** NY Coll Osteo Med 1985; **Resid:** Internal Medicine, LI Coll Hosp 1988; **Fellow:** Gastroenterology, LI Coll Hosp 1990

Spielberg, Alan MD (Ge) - **Spec Exp:** Inflammatory Bowel Disease; Colitis; Colonoscopy; **Hospital:** St Catherine's of Siena Med Ctr, Stony Brook Univ Hosp; **Address:** 48 Route 25A, Ste 203, Smithtown, NY 11787-1448; **Phone:** 631-724-1178; **Board Cert:** Internal Medicine 1977; Gastroenterology 1979; **Med School:** Belgium 1974; **Resid:** Internal Medicine, Albany Med Ctr 1977; **Fellow:** Gastroenterology, Albany Med Ctr 1979

GYNECOLOGIC ONCOLOGY

Chalas, Eva MD (GO) - **Spec Exp:** Gynecologic Cancer; **Hospital:** Stony Brook Univ Hosp, Winthrop - Univ Hosp; **Address:** 1077 W Jericho Tpke, Smithtown, NY 11787; **Phone:** 631-864-5440; **Board Cert:** Obstetrics & Gynecology 2005; Gynecologic Oncology 2005; **Med School:** SUNY Stony Brook 1981; **Resid:** Obstetrics & Gynecology, Univ Hosp 1985; **Fellow:** Gynecologic Oncology, Meml Sloan Kettering Cancer Ctr 1987; **Fac Appt:** Assoc Prof ObG, SUNY Stony Brook

HAND SURGERY

Hurst, Lawrence C MD (HS) - **Spec Exp:** Microvascular Surgery; Nerve Disorders; Dupuytren's Contracture; **Hospital:** Stony Brook Univ Hosp, St Charles Hosp; **Address:** SUNY Stony Brook Med Ctr, Dept Orthopaedics, 100 Nichole Rd, E Setauket, NY 11794; **Phone:** 631-444-3145; **Board Cert:** Orthopaedic Surgery 1980; Hand Surgery 2000; **Med School:** Univ VT Coll Med 1973; **Resid:** Orthopaedic Surgery, N Carolina Meml Hosp 1978; **Fellow:** Hand Surgery, Columbia-Presby Med Ctr 1979; **Fac Appt:** Prof OrS, SUNY Stony Brook

HEMATOLOGY

Avvento, Louis MD (Hem) - **Spec Exp:** Breast Cancer; Lymphoma; **Hospital:** Peconic Bay Med Ctr, Southampton Hosp; **Address:** 1333 E Main St, Riverhead, NY 11901; **Phone:** 631-727-8500; **Board Cert:** Internal Medicine 1985; Medical Oncology 1987; Hematology 1994; **Med School:** Italy 1981; **Resid:** Internal Medicine, Jamaica Med Ctr 1985; **Fellow:** Hematology, Univ Hosp-SUNY 1988

Schulman, Philip MD (Hem) - **Spec Exp:** Leukemia; Lymphoma; Multiple Myeloma; **Hospital:** St Catherine's of Siena Med Ctr; **Address:** Meml Sloan Kettering at Suffolk, 650 Commack Rd, Commack, NY 11725; **Phone:** 631-623-4100; **Board Cert:** Internal Medicine 1977; Medical Oncology 1979; Hematology 1980; **Med School:** SUNY Upstate Med Univ 1974; **Resid:** Internal Medicine, N Shore Univ Hosp 1976; Medical Oncology, Meml Sloan-Kettering 1977; **Fellow:** Medical Oncology, Meml Sloan-Kettering 1978; Hematology, N Shore Univ Hosp 1979; **Fac Appt:** Prof Med, Cornell Univ-Weill Med Coll

INFECTIOUS DISEASE

Collins, Adriane DO (Inf) - **Hospital:** Good Samaritan Hosp Med Ctr - West Islip; **Address:** 786 Montauk Hwy, West Islip, NY 11795; **Phone:** 631-376-6075; **Board Cert:** Internal Medicine 1995; Infectious Disease 1998; **Resid:** Internal Medicine, NYU Med Ctr 1993

Klein, Arthur MD (Inf) - **Spec Exp:** Travel Medicine; Lyme Disease; Bone Infections; **Hospital:** John T Mather Meml Hosp of Port Jefferson, Stony Brook Univ Hosp; **Address:** 14 Technology Drive, Ste 10, East Setauket, NY 11733; **Phone:** 631-689-5400; **Board Cert:** Internal Medicine 1986; Infectious Disease 1988; **Med School:** SUNY Downstate 1983; **Resid:** Internal Medicine, Univ Hosp 1986; **Fellow:** Infectious Disease, Univ Hosp 1989

Nash, Bernard J MD (Inf) - **Hospital:** Good Samaritan Hosp Med Ctr - West Islip, Southside Hosp; **Address:** 500 Montauk Hwy, Ste S, West Islip, NY 11795; **Phone:** 631-587-7733; **Board Cert:** Internal Medicine 1978; Infectious Disease 1982; **Med School:** Georgetown Univ 1975; **Resid:** Internal Medicine, St Elizabeth Hosp 1978; **Fellow:** Infectious Disease, Boston Univ Med Ctr 1981

Sacks-Berg, Anne MD (Inf) - **Spec Exp:** Travel Medicine; **Hospital:** Huntington Hosp; **Address:** 120 New York Ave, Huntington, NY 11743-2743; **Phone:** 631-423-9809; **Board Cert:** Internal Medicine 1986; Infectious Disease 1988; **Med School:** SUNY Hlth Sci Ctr 1983; **Resid:** Internal Medicine, Winthrop Univ Hosp 1986; **Fellow:** Infectious Disease, Winthrop Univ Hosp 1988

Samuels, Steven MD (Inf) - **Spec Exp:** Lyme Disease; AIDS/HIV; **Hospital:** Good Samaritan Hosp Med Ctr - West Islip, Southside Hosp; **Address:** 500 Montauk Hwy, Ste S, West Islip, NY 11795; **Phone:** 631-587-7733; **Board Cert:** Internal Medicine 1977; Infectious Disease 1982; **Med School:** NY Med Coll 1974; **Resid:** Internal Medicine, Nassau County Med Ctr 1977; **Fellow:** Immunopathology, UC Irvine Med Ctr 1979; **Fac Appt:** Asst Prof Med, SUNY Stony Brook

INTERNAL MEDICINE

Balot, Barry DO (IM) `PCP` - **Hospital:** Good Samaritan Hosp Med Ctr - West Islip, Southside Hosp; **Address:** 150 E Sunrise Hwy, Lindenhurst, NY 11757; **Phone:** 631-225-6200; **Board Cert:** Internal Medicine 1989; Geriatric Medicine 1994; **Med School:** NY Coll Osteo Med 1985; **Resid:** Internal Medicine, Univ Hosp 1987; Internal Medicine, Overlook Hosp 1989

Bernard, Robert MD (IM) `PCP` - **Spec Exp:** Heart Disease; Skin Diseases; **Hospital:** Peconic Bay Med Ctr; **Address:** 6144 Rte 25-A C Bldg - Ste 10, Wading River, NY 11792; **Phone:** 631-929-5900; **Board Cert:** Internal Medicine 1989; **Med School:** Grenada 1986; **Resid:** Internal Medicine, St Joseph's Hosp & Med Ctr 1989

Biasetti, John MD (IM) `PCP` - **Hospital:** John T Mather Meml Hosp of Port Jefferson, St Charles Hosp; **Address:** 116 Terryville Rd, Port Jefferson Station, NY 11776-4870; **Phone:** 631-928-2002; **Board Cert:** Internal Medicine 1972; **Med School:** NY Med Coll 1963; **Resid:** Internal Medicine, Nassau County Med Ctr 1970

Chernaik, Robert MD (IM) `PCP` - **Spec Exp:** Lyme Disease; **Hospital:** Brookhaven Meml Hosp & Med Ctr; **Address:** 285 Sills Rd Bldg Ste 4D, Patchogue, NY 11772-4857; **Phone:** 631-654-1800; **Board Cert:** Internal Medicine 1968; **Med School:** UMDNJ-NJ Med Sch, Newark 1961; **Resid:** Internal Medicine, Beth Israel Hosp 1963; Internal Medicine, Montefiore Hosp 1964; **Fellow:** Pathology, Univ Colorado Hosp 1965; **Fac Appt:** Asst Clin Prof Med, SUNY Stony Brook

Covey, Alexander J MD (IM) `PCP` - **Spec Exp:** Aging Skin; Hypertension; **Hospital:** Peconic Bay Med Ctr; **Address:** 445 Main St, Center Moriches, NY 11934; **Phone:** 631-878-9200; **Board Cert:** Internal Medicine 1988; **Med School:** Univ Hlth Sci/Chicago Med Sch 1985; **Resid:** Internal Medicine, Winthrop Univ Hosp 1988

Delman, Michael MD (IM) `PCP` - **Spec Exp:** Addiction Medicine; Gastroenterology; **Hospital:** Southside Hosp; **Address:** 301 E Main St, Bayshore, NY 11706; **Phone:** 631-968-3118; **Board Cert:** Internal Medicine 1972; Gastroenterology 1975; **Med School:** NY Med Coll 1968; **Resid:** Internal Medicine, NY Med-Metro Hosp Ctr 1971; Gastroenterology, NY Med-Metro Hosp Ctr 1972; **Fellow:** Gastroenterology, NY Med-Metro Hosp Ctr 1973; **Fac Appt:** Asst Clin Prof Med, SUNY Stony Brook

Fahey, Julia A MD (IM) `PCP` - **Spec Exp:** Palliative Care; **Hospital:** Brookhaven Meml Hosp & Med Ctr; **Address:** 16 Station Rd, Ste 5 & 6, Bellport, NY 11713; **Phone:** 631-286-3995; **Board Cert:** Pediatrics 2002; Internal Medicine 1995; **Med School:** Mexico 1983; **Resid:** Internal Medicine & Pediatrics, Metropolitan Hosp Ctr 1989

Friedling, Steven MD (IM) `PCP` - **Spec Exp:** Preventive Medicine; Chronic Illness; **Hospital:** St Catherine's of Siena Med Ctr, Stony Brook Univ Hosp; **Address:** 267 E Main St, Ste A, Smithtown, NY 11787-2580; **Phone:** 631-724-2000; **Board Cert:** Internal Medicine 1973; Infectious Disease 1980; **Med School:** SUNY Downstate 1968; **Resid:** Medical Oncology, Natl Cancer Inst 1971; Internal Medicine, Barnes Hosp 1973; **Fellow:** Infectious Disease, Barnes Hosp 1974; **Fac Appt:** Asst Clin Prof Med, SUNY Stony Brook

German, Harold MD (IM) `PCP` - **Spec Exp:** Hematology; Cardiology; **Hospital:** Huntington Hosp; **Address:** 150 Main St, Huntington, NY 11743-6908; **Phone:** 631-271-8700; **Board Cert:** Internal Medicine 1973; Hematology 1978; **Med School:** Columbia P&S 1967; **Resid:** Internal Medicine, Lenox Hill Hosp 1968; Internal Medicine, Columbia Presby Hosp 1972; **Fellow:** Hematology, Columbia Presby Hosp 1973

Goldfarb, Steven MD (IM) `PCP` - **Spec Exp:** Lyme Disease; Preventive Medicine; Concierge Medicine; **Hospital:** Southampton Hosp; **Address:** 365 County Rd 39-A, Ste 12, Southampton, NY 11968; **Phone:** 631-283-5542; **Board Cert:** Internal Medicine 1989; **Med School:** Italy 1983; **Resid:** Internal Medicine, Berkshire Med Ctr-U Mass 1986

Hallal, Edward MD (IM) `PCP` - **Hospital:** Southside Hosp, Good Samaritan Hosp Med Ctr - West Islip; **Address:** 180 E Main St, Bay Shore, NY 11706; **Phone:** 631-665-0027; **Board Cert:** Internal Medicine 1987; **Med School:** Grenada 1984; **Resid:** Internal Medicine, New York Methodist Hosp 1987

Lalli, Corradino MD (IM) `PCP` - **Spec Exp:** Geriatric Medicine; **Hospital:** St Catherine's of Siena Med Ctr; **Address:** 359 Route 111, Smithtown, NY 11787-4739; **Phone:** 631-366-0404; **Board Cert:** Internal Medicine 1979; Geriatric Medicine 1998; **Med School:** Albert Einstein Coll Med 1976; **Resid:** Internal Medicine, Nassau County Med Ctr 1979; **Fellow:** Pulmonary Disease, Nassau County Med Ctr 1980; **Fac Appt:** Asst Clin Prof Med, SUNY Stony Brook

Lerner, Harvey MD (IM) `PCP` - **Spec Exp:** Hypertension; Diabetes; Chronic Fatigue Syndrome; **Hospital:** St Catherine's of Siena Med Ctr, Stony Brook Univ Hosp; **Address:** 215 E Main St, Smithtown, NY 11787-2807; **Phone:** 631-265-5858; **Board Cert:** Internal Medicine 1974; **Med School:** Univ Chicago-Pritzker Sch Med 1957; **Resid:** Montefiore Med Ctr 1959Kings County Hosp 1961

Matkovic, Christopher MD/PhD (IM) - **Spec Exp:** Osteomyelitis; Endocarditis; **Hospital:** St Catherine's of Siena Med Ctr, Stony Brook Univ Hosp; **Address:** 80 Maple Ave, Ste 205, Smithtown, NY 11787-3520; **Phone:** 631-265-0075; **Board Cert:** Internal Medicine 1977; Infectious Disease 1980; **Med School:** Columbia P&S 1974; **Resid:** Internal Medicine, Presby Hosp 1977; **Fellow:** Infectious Disease, Presby Hosp 1979; **Fac Appt:** Asst Clin Prof Med, SUNY Stony Brook

Oppenheimer, John MD (IM) `PCP` - **Spec Exp:** Geriatric Medicine; AIDS/HIV; **Hospital:** Southampton Hosp; **Address:** 60 Bay St, Box 3137, Sag Harbor, NY 11963; **Phone:** 631-725-4600; **Board Cert:** Internal Medicine 1984; **Med School:** Tulane Univ 1981; **Resid:** Internal Medicine, Tulane Univ Hosp 1982; Internal Medicine, Harlem Hosp 1983; **Fac Appt:** Asst Clin Prof Med, SUNY Stony Brook

Romano, Rosario MD (IM) **PCP** - **Hospital:** John T Mather Meml Hosp of Port Jefferson, St Charles Hosp; **Address:** 5225 Nesconset Hwy, Ste 15, Port Jeffrson Station, NY 11776-2054; **Phone:** 631-331-1000; **Board Cert:** Internal Medicine 1977; **Med School:** NY Med Coll 1973; **Resid:** Internal Medicine, Lenox Hill Hosp 1977; **Fac Appt:** Asst Clin Prof Med, SUNY Stony Brook

Simon, Lloyd MD (IM) **PCP** - **Spec Exp:** Addiction Medicine; **Hospital:** Eastern Long Island Hosp; **Address:** 44210 C County Rd, Ste 48, Box 1341, Southold, NY 11971; **Phone:** 631-765-4150; **Board Cert:** Internal Medicine 1983; **Med School:** SUNY Buffalo 1980; **Resid:** Internal Medicine, Univ Mass Med Ctr 1983

INTERVENTIONAL CARDIOLOGY

Brown, David L MD (IC) - **Spec Exp:** Atrial Septal Defect; Angioplasty & Stent Placement; Peripheral Vascular Disease; **Hospital:** Stony Brook Univ Hosp; **Address:** SUNY Stony Brook Sch Med, Div Cardiology, Health Sci Ctr T16-080, Stony Brook, NY 11794; **Phone:** 631-444-1060; **Board Cert:** Internal Medicine 1986; Interventional Cardiology 2001; **Med School:** Baylor Coll Med 1982; **Resid:** Internal Medicine, Baylor Coll Med 1986; Cardiovascular Disease, UCSF Med Ctr 1989; **Fellow:** Interventional Cardiology, Cleveland Clinic 1991; **Fac Appt:** Prof Med, SUNY Stony Brook

MATERNAL & FETAL MEDICINE

Monheit, Alan G MD (MF) - **Hospital:** Stony Brook Univ Hosp; **Address:** SUNY Stony Brook, Health Sci Ctr T-9, rm 030, Stony Brook, NY 11794-8091; **Phone:** 631-444-7650; **Board Cert:** Obstetrics & Gynecology 1982; Maternal & Fetal Medicine 1983; **Med School:** Univ Pennsylvania 1975; **Resid:** Obstetrics & Gynecology, UCSD Med Ctr 1978; **Fellow:** Maternal & Fetal Medicine, UCSD Med Ctr 1981; **Fac Appt:** Assoc Clin Prof ObG, SUNY Stony Brook

MEDICAL ONCOLOGY

Berger, E Roy MD (Onc) - **Spec Exp:** Prostate Cancer; **Hospital:** St Catherine's of Siena Med Ctr, John T Mather Meml Hosp of Port Jefferson; **Address:** North Shore Hem/Onc Assocs, 235 N Belle Meade Rd, East Setauket, NY 11733; **Phone:** 631-751-3000; **Board Cert:** Internal Medicine 1973; Hematology 1976; Medical Oncology 1977; **Med School:** SUNY Downstate 1970; **Resid:** Internal Medicine, Roosevelt Hosp 1973; **Fellow:** Hematology, Roosevelt Hosp 1974; Medical Oncology, Mem Sloan Kettering Cancer Ctr 1975; **Fac Appt:** Asst Clin Prof Med, NY Med Coll

Caruso, Rocco MD (Onc) - **Hospital:** Stony Brook Univ Hosp, St Catherine's of Siena Med Ctr; **Address:** 2500 Nesconset Hway 26B Bldg, Stony Brook, NY 11790; **Phone:** 631-751-8305; **Board Cert:** Internal Medicine 1982; Hematology 1984; Medical Oncology 1995; **Med School:** Univ Pennsylvania 1979; **Resid:** Internal Medicine, St Luke's-Roosevelt Hosp Ctr 1982; **Fellow:** Hematology, NYU Med Ctr 1985; Medical Oncology, LI Jewish Med Ctr 1985; **Fac Appt:** Asst Prof Med, SUNY Stony Brook

Dobbs, Joan MD (Onc) - **Spec Exp:** Stem Cell Transplant; **Hospital:** St Catherine's of Siena Med Ctr, John T Mather Meml Hosp of Port Jefferson; **Address:** 235 N Belle Meade Rd, East Setauket, NY 11733-3456; **Phone:** 631-751-3000; **Board Cert:** Internal Medicine 1971; Hematology 1977; Medical Oncology 1979; **Med School:** SUNY Downstate 1960; **Resid:** Pathology, Stanford Med Ctr 1962; Internal Medicine, Montefiore Hosp Med Ctr 1964; **Fellow:** Hematology, Mount Sinai Hosp 1965; Hematology, Maimonides Medical Ctr 1966; **Fac Appt:** Asst Clin Prof Med, NY Med Coll

Fiore, John J MD (Onc) - **Spec Exp:** Lung Cancer; **Hospital:** St Catherine's of Siena Med Ctr; **Address:** Meml Sloan Kettering at Suffolk, 650 Commack Rd, Commack, NY 11725; **Phone:** 631-623-4100; **Board Cert:** Internal Medicine 1978; Hematology 1982; Medical Oncology 1983; **Med School:** Tufts Univ 1975; **Resid:** Internal Medicine, VA Med Ctr 1979; **Fellow:** Hematology, VA Med Ctr 1981; Medical Oncology, Meml Sloan Kettering Cancer Ctr 1984; **Fac Appt:** Assoc Prof Med, SUNY Stony Brook

Kim, Jung Yong MD (Onc) - **Hospital:** Brookhaven Meml Hosp & Med Ctr; **Address:** 285 Sills Rd Bldg 16, Patchogue, NY 11772; **Phone:** 631-758-7575; **Board Cert:** Internal Medicine 1981; Medical Oncology 1983; **Med School:** South Korea 1973; **Resid:** Internal Medicine, Booth Meml Hosp 1981; **Fellow:** Medical Oncology, Roswell Park Cancer Inst 1983

Madajewicz, Stefan MD/PhD (Onc) - **Spec Exp:** Gastrointestinal Cancer; Brain Tumors; Breast Cancer; **Hospital:** Stony Brook Univ Hosp; **Address:** Stony Brook University Hospital HSC, Tower 17, Rm 080, Stony Brook, NY 11794-8174; **Phone:** 631-444-8382; **Board Cert:** Internal Medicine 1981; Medical Oncology 1983; **Med School:** Poland 1963; **Resid:** Internal Medicine, NY Med Coll 1974; Internal Medicine, SUNY-Buffalo Med Ctr 1979; **Fellow:** Medical Oncology, Roswell Park Cancer Ins 1978; **Fac Appt:** Prof Med, SUNY Stony Brook

Ostrow, Stanley MD (Onc) - **Spec Exp:** Breast Cancer; Lung Cancer; Hematology; Lymphoma; **Hospital:** Stony Brook Univ Hosp, Brookhaven Meml Hosp & Med Ctr; **Address:** 235 N Belle Mead Rd, East Setauket, NY 11733; **Phone:** 631-751-5151; **Board Cert:** Internal Medicine 1978; Medical Oncology 1979; Hematology 1982; **Med School:** SUNY Downstate 1974; **Resid:** Internal Medicine, Jewish Meml Hosp 1976; **Fellow:** Hematology & Oncology, Natl Cancer Inst 1980; **Fac Appt:** Asst Prof Med, SUNY Stony Brook

Rizvi, Hasan MD (Onc) - **Hospital:** Good Samaritan Hosp Med Ctr - West Islip, Southside Hosp; **Address:** 180 E Main St, Bay Shore, NY 11706-8427; **Phone:** 631-666-0262; **Board Cert:** Internal Medicine 1998; Medical Oncology 1999; Hematology 2002; **Med School:** Pakistan 1975; **Resid:** Clinical Pathology, Ellis Hosp 1978; Internal Medicine, Mt Sinai Sch Med 1981; **Fellow:** Hematology & Oncology, Winthrop Univ Hosp 1983; Hematology & Oncology, St Elizabeth Hosp 1984

Strauss, Barry MD (Onc) - **Spec Exp:** Lung Cancer; Breast Cancer; **Hospital:** Southampton Hosp; **Address:** 353 Meeting House Ln, Southampton, NY 11968-5051; **Phone:** 631-283-6611; **Board Cert:** Internal Medicine 1975; Medical Oncology 1975; **Med School:** Geo Wash Univ 1971; **Resid:** Internal Medicine, Beth Israel Hosp 1973; **Fellow:** Medical Oncology, National Cancer Inst 1975

NEONATAL-PERINATAL MEDICINE

Sosulski, Richard MD (NP) - **Spec Exp:** Lung Disease in Newborns; **Hospital:** Stony Brook Univ Hosp, St Catherine's of Siena Med Ctr; **Address:** 269 E Main St, Smithtown, NY 11787-2807; **Phone:** 631-361-2121; **Board Cert:** Pediatrics 1982; Neonatal-Perinatal Medicine 1983; **Med School:** SUNY Downstate 1977; **Resid:** Pediatrics, LI Jewish Med Ctr 1980; **Fellow:** Neonatal-Perinatal Medicine, Chldns Hosp 1982; **Fac Appt:** Assoc Clin Prof Ped, SUNY Stony Brook

NEPHROLOGY

Schwarz, Richard B MD (Nep) - **Spec Exp:** Hypertension; Kidney Disease; **Hospital:** Huntington Hosp; **Address:** 325 Park Ave, Huntington, NY 11743-2798; **Phone:** 631-351-3784; **Board Cert:** Internal Medicine 1983; Geriatric Medicine 2000; Nephrology 2000; **Med School:** NYU Sch Med 1979; **Resid:** Internal Medicine, LAC-USC Med Ctr 1981; Internal Medicine, Kaiser Fdn Hosp 1982; **Fellow:** Nephrology, Kaiser Fdn Hosp 1984; **Fac Appt:** Assoc Clin Prof Med, SUNY Stony Brook

NEUROLOGICAL SURGERY

Davis, Raphael P MD (NS) - **Spec Exp:** Acoustic Neuroma; Skull Base Surgery; Spinal Disc Replacement; **Hospital:** Stony Brook Univ Hosp, St Charles Hosp; **Address:** Stony Brook Univ Hosp, Dept Neurosurgery, HSC - T12. 080, Stony Brook, NY 11794-8122; **Phone:** 631-444-1213; **Board Cert:** Neurological Surgery 1990; **Med School:** Mount Sinai Sch Med 1981; **Resid:** Neurological Surgery, Mount Sinai Med Ctr 1987; **Fac Appt:** Prof NS, SUNY Stony Brook

NEUROLOGY

Chernik, Norman MD (N) - **Spec Exp:** Acupuncture; **Hospital:** Southside Hosp; **Address:** 280 Montauk Hwy, Bay Shore, NY 11706; **Phone:** 631-666-3939; **Board Cert:** Neuropathology 1974; **Med School:** St Louis Univ 1965; **Resid:** Neurology, Mount Sinai 1968; Neuropathology, Kings Co Hosp 1969; **Fellow:** Neurological Oncology, Sloan-Kettering Cancer Ctr 1971; **Fac Appt:** Assoc Clin Prof N, SUNY Stony Brook

Cohen, Daniel MD (N) - **Spec Exp:** Stroke; Neuromuscular Disorders; Multiple Sclerosis; **Hospital:** Good Samaritan Hosp Med Ctr - West Islip, Southside Hosp; **Address:** 370 E Main St, Ste 1, Bay Shore, NY 11706; **Phone:** 631-666-4767; **Board Cert:** Neurology 1986; Clinical Neurophysiology 1985; **Med School:** Univ Miami Sch Med 1980; **Resid:** Neurology, Jackson Meml Hosp 1984

Coyle, Patricia K MD (N) - **Spec Exp:** Multiple Sclerosis; Neuro-Immunology; Lyme Disease; Infections-Neurologic; **Hospital:** Stony Brook Univ Hosp; **Address:** SUNY Stony Brook, Dept Neurology, HSC T12-020, Stony Brook, NY 11794-8121; **Phone:** 631-444-2599; **Board Cert:** Neurology 1978; **Med School:** Johns Hopkins Univ 1974; **Resid:** Neurology, Johns Hopkins Hosp 1978; **Fellow:** Neurological Immunology, Johns Hopkins Hosp 1980; **Fac Appt:** Prof N, SUNY Stony Brook

Gerber, Oded MD (N) - **Spec Exp:** Stroke; Parkinson's Disease; Neuromuscular Disorders; **Hospital:** Stony Brook Univ Hosp; **Address:** SUNY-Stony Brook, Dept Neurology, HSC, T-12-020, Stony Brook, NY 11794-8121; **Phone:** 631-444-2599; **Board Cert:** Neurology 1979; **Med School:** SUNY Downstate 1972; **Resid:** Internal Medicine, Kings County Hosp 1974; Neurology, Mt Sinai Hosp 1977; **Fac Appt:** Asst Clin Prof N, Mount Sinai Sch Med

Mendelsohn, Frederic MD (N) - **Spec Exp:** Headache; Pain-Back & Neck; Brain Injury Rehabilitation; **Hospital:** Stony Brook Univ Hosp; **Address:** 650 Hawkins Ave, Ste 7, Ronkonkoma, NY 11779-4587; **Phone:** 631-737-0055; **Board Cert:** Neurology 1977; **Med School:** Univ Louisville Sch Med 1971; **Resid:** Neurology, Nassau County Med Ctr 1975; **Fac Appt:** Asst Clin Prof N, SUNY Stony Brook

Moreta, Henry MD (N) - **Hospital:** Peconic Bay Med Ctr; **Address:** 280 Montauk Hwy, Box 9182, Bay Shore, NY 11706; **Phone:** 631-666-3939; **Board Cert:** Neurology 1987; **Med School:** Harvard Med Sch 1977; **Resid:** Neurology, New York Hosp 1981

OBSTETRICS & GYNECOLOGY

Baker, David A MD (ObG) - **Spec Exp:** Infectious Disease; Premature Labor; **Hospital:** Stony Brook Univ Hosp; **Address:** Stony Brook Univ Hospital, Dept Ob/Gyn, Nicolls Rd, Stony Brook, NY 11794-8091; **Phone:** 631-444-2729; **Board Cert:** Obstetrics & Gynecology 1979; Maternal & Fetal Medicine 1981; **Med School:** SUNY Hlth Sci Ctr 1973; **Resid:** Obstetrics & Gynecology, Hosp Univ Penn 1977; **Fellow:** Maternal & Fetal Medicine, Med Ctr Hosp 1979; **Fac Appt:** Prof ObG, SUNY Stony Brook

Davenport, Deborah M MD (ObG) - **Spec Exp:** Menopause Problems; **Hospital:** Stony Brook Univ Hosp; **Address:** 100-16 S Jersey Ave, East Setauket, NY 11733-2036; **Phone:** 631-689-6400; **Board Cert:** Obstetrics & Gynecology 1985; **Med School:** Univ Pennsylvania 1975; **Resid:** Obstetrics & Gynecology, Univ Hosp 1983; **Fac Appt:** Asst Clin Prof ObG, SUNY Stony Brook

Gentilesco, Michael MD (ObG) PCP - **Hospital:** St Catherine's of Siena Med Ctr; **Address:** 48 Route 25A, Ste 207, Smithtown, NY 11787; **Phone:** 631-862-3800, **Board Cert:** Obstetrics & Gynecology 1997; **Med School:** Albert Einstein Coll Med 1980; **Resid:** Obstetrics & Gynecology, Columbia-Presby Med Ctr 1984

Giammarino, Anthony MD (ObG) - **Spec Exp:** Menopause Problems; Gynecologic Surgery; **Hospital:** St Charles Hosp, John T Mather Meml Hosp of Port Jefferson; **Address:** 118 N Country Rd, Port Jefferson, NY 11777; **Phone:** 631-473-7171; **Board Cert:** Obstetrics & Gynecology 1969; **Med School:** Italy 1960; **Resid:** Obstetrics & Gynecology, SUNY Downstate 1966

Goldman, Mitchell MD (ObG) - **Spec Exp:** Laparoscopic Surgery; **Hospital:** Southside Hosp, Good Samaritan Hosp Med Ctr - West Islip; **Address:** 971 Montauk Hwy, Oakdale, NY 11769-1434; **Phone:** 631-589-4344; **Board Cert:** Obstetrics & Gynecology 1978; **Med School:** Univ Hlth Sci/Chicago Med Sch 1955; **Resid:** Obstetrics & Gynecology, Kings County Hosp 1960

Hirt, Paula MD (ObG) - **Hospital:** Good Samaritan Hosp Med Ctr - West Islip; **Address:** 83 W Main St, East Islip, NY 11730; **Phone:** 631-277-5800; **Board Cert:** Obstetrics & Gynecology 1985; **Med School:** NYU Sch Med 1979; **Resid:** Obstetrics & Gynecology, NYU Med Ctr 1983

Kramer, Mitchell MD (ObG) - **Spec Exp:** Gynecologic Surgery; Menopause Problems; **Hospital:** Huntington Hosp, N Shore Univ Hosp at Manhasset; **Address:** 202 E Main St, Huntington, NY 11743; **Phone:** 631-271-4330; **Board Cert:** Obstetrics & Gynecology 2001; **Med School:** NY Med Coll 1985; **Resid:** Obstetrics & Gynecology, LI Jewish Med Ctr 1989; **Fac Appt:** Asst Clin Prof ObG, NYU Sch Med

Lee, Douglas S MD (ObG) PCP - **Spec Exp:** Menopause Problems; **Hospital:** John T Mather Meml Hosp of Port Jefferson, St Charles Hosp; **Address:** 118 N Country Rd, Port Jefferson, NY 11776; **Phone:** 631-475-4404; **Board Cert:** Obstetrics & Gynecology 1979; **Med School:** NYU Sch Med 1973; **Resid:** Obstetrics & Gynecology, Albert Einstein 1977; **Fac Appt:** Asst Clin Prof ObG, SUNY Stony Brook

Mann, Charles MD (ObG) PCP - **Hospital:** St Catherine's of Siena Med Ctr, Stony Brook Univ Hosp; **Address:** 48 Route 25-A, Ste 207, Smithtown, NY 11787; **Phone:** 631-862-3800; **Board Cert:** Obstetrics & Gynecology 1979; **Med School:** Creighton Univ 1974; **Resid:** Obstetrics & Gynecology, Barnes Hosp-Washington Univ 1977

Matalon, Martin MD (ObG) - **Hospital:** Southside Hosp, Good Samaritan Hosp Med Ctr - West Islip; **Address:** 375 E Main St, Ste 4, Bay Shore, NY 11706-8418; **Phone:** 631-665-8226; **Board Cert:** Obstetrics & Gynecology 1973; **Med School:** Univ Cincinnati 1966; **Resid:** Obstetrics & Gynecology, Brookdale Univ Med Ctr 1971

Ott, Allen MD (ObG) - **Spec Exp:** Infertility; **Hospital:** Southampton Hosp; **Address:** 595 Hampton Rd, Southampton, NY 11968-3021; **Phone:** 631-283-0918; **Board Cert:** Obstetrics & Gynecology 1979; **Med School:** Boston Univ 1972; **Resid:** Obstetrics & Gynecology, Hosp Univ Penn 1976

Pallotta, John MD (ObG) - **Spec Exp:** Gynecologic Surgery; Vaginal Surgery; Menopause Problems; **Hospital:** Good Samaritan Hosp Med Ctr - West Islip, Southside Hosp; **Address:** 320 Montauk Hwy, West Islip, NY 11795; **Phone:** 631-587-5033 x3; **Board Cert:** Obstetrics & Gynecology 1979; **Med School:** NY Med Coll 1955; **Resid:** Obstetrics & Gynecology, NY Med Coll 1962; **Fac Appt:** Assoc Clin Prof ObG, NY Coll Osteo Med

San Roman, Gerardo MD (ObG) - **Spec Exp:** Obstetrics; **Hospital:** St Charles Hosp, John T Mather Meml Hosp of Port Jefferson; **Address:** 118 N Country Rd, Port Jefferson, NY 11777; **Phone:** 631-473-7171; **Board Cert:** Obstetrics & Gynecology 1997; **Med School:** Johns Hopkins Univ 1981; **Resid:** Obstetrics & Gynecology, NY Hosp 1985

Tesauro, William MD (ObG) - **Spec Exp:** Infertility; Gynecologic Surgery; **Hospital:** Good Samaritan Hosp Med Ctr - West Islip, Southside Hosp; **Address:** 750 Montauk Hwy, West Islip, NY 11795-4411; **Phone:** 631-669-5900; **Board Cert:** Obstetrics & Gynecology 1978; **Med School:** NY Med Coll 1962; **Resid:** Obstetrics & Gynecology, NY Methodist Hosp 1967; **Fac Appt:** Asst Clin Prof ObG, SUNY Stony Brook

OCCUPATIONAL MEDICINE

Hailoo, Wajdy MD (OM) - **Spec Exp:** Environmental Medicine; **Hospital:** Stony Brook Univ Hosp; **Address:** SUNY-Stony Brook Sch Med, Hlth Sci Ctr, L3-086, Stony Brook, NY 11794-8036; **Phone:** 631-444-2196; **Board Cert:** Occupational Medicine 1989; **Med School:** Iraq 1969; **Resid:** Internal Medicine, Port Genl Hosp 1974; Occupational Medicine, Mount Sinai Hosp 1987; **Fellow:** Occupational Medicine, Univ London 1977; Pulmonary Disease, Mount Sinai Hosp 1987; **Fac Appt:** Assoc Prof Med, SUNY Stony Brook

OPHTHALMOLOGY

Aries, Philip MD (Oph) - **Spec Exp:** Cataract Surgery; Glaucoma; **Hospital:** Southside Hosp, Good Samaritan Hosp Med Ctr - West Islip; **Address:** 375 E Main St, Ste 24, Bay Shore, NY 11706; **Phone:** 631-665-1330; **Board Cert:** Ophthalmology 1975; **Med School:** NY Med Coll 1967; **Resid:** Ophthalmology, Nassau County Med Ctr 1973

Bogaty, Stanley MD (Oph) - **Spec Exp:** Cataract Surgery; Glaucoma; **Hospital:** St Charles Hosp, John T Mather Meml Hosp of Port Jefferson; **Address:** 251 E Oakland Ave, Port Jefferson, NY 11777-2170; **Phone:** 631-473-5329; **Board Cert:** Ophthalmology 1974; **Med School:** Univ Hlth Sci/Chicago Med Sch 1966; **Resid:** Ophthalmology, Beth Israel Hosp 1972

Cossari, Alfred MD (Oph) - **Spec Exp:** Pediatric Ophthalmology; Strabismus; **Hospital:** John T Mather Meml Hosp of Port Jefferson, St Charles Hosp; **Address:** 311 Barnum Ave, Port Jefferson, NY 11777-1682; **Phone:** 631-928-6400; **Board Cert:** Ophthalmology 1976; **Med School:** Italy 1969; **Resid:** Ophthalmology, Nassau County Med Ctr 1974; **Fellow:** Retina, Johns Hopkins Hosp 1974; Pediatric Ophthalmology, Children's Natl Med Ctr 1975

Di Leo, Frank MD (Oph) - **Spec Exp:** Cataract Surgery; Oculoplastic Surgery; **Hospital:** Southampton Hosp; **Address:** 365 County Road 39A, Ste 14, Southampton, NY 11968; **Phone:** 631-283-3677; **Board Cert:** Ophthalmology 1987; **Med School:** Albert Einstein Coll Med 1981; **Resid:** Ophthalmology, St Luke's-Roosevelt Hosp Ctr 1985

El Baba, Fadi MD (Oph) - **Spec Exp:** Retinal/Vitreous Surgery; Diabetic Eye Disease/Retinopathy; Macular Degeneration; HIV Retinitis; **Hospital:** Stony Brook Univ Hosp; **Address:** 33 Research Way, East Setauket, NY 11733; **Phone:** 631-444-4090; **Board Cert:** Ophthalmology 2003; **Med School:** Amer Univ Beirut 1982; **Resid:** Ophthalmology, Amer Univ Beirut 1987; Ophthalmology, Doheny Eye Inst/USC Med Ctr 1991; **Fellow:** Eye Pathology, Wilmer Eye Inst/Johns Hopkins 1986; Retina, Oregon Lions Sight & Hearing Inst 1987; **Fac Appt:** Assoc Prof Oph, SUNY Stony Brook

Gordon, Bernard MD (Oph) - **Hospital:** Huntington Hosp; **Address:** 755 Park Ave, Huntington, NY 11743-6918; **Phone:** 631-421-2676; **Board Cert:** Ophthalmology 1977; **Med School:** SUNY Downstate 1966; **Resid:** Ophthalmology, Manhattan Eye Ear Hosp 1976

Martin, Sidney A MD (Oph) - **Spec Exp:** Cataract Surgery; Laser Vision Surgery; **Hospital:** St Catherine's of Siena Med Ctr; **Address:** 260 Middle Country Rd, Ste 201, Smithtown, NY 11787; **Phone:** 631-265-8780; **Board Cert:** Ophthalmology 1963; **Med School:** SUNY Hlth Sci Ctr 1955; **Resid:** Ophthalmology, Baltimore Eye & Ear Hosp 1956

Michalos, Peter MD (Oph) - **Spec Exp:** Cataract Surgery; Tear Duct Disorders; Eyelid Tumors; **Hospital:** Southampton Hosp, NY-Presby Hosp (page 100); **Address:** 365 County Road 39-A, Ste 14, Southampton, NY 11968-5243; **Phone:** 631-283-8604; **Board Cert:** Ophthalmology 1991; **Med School:** SUNY Downstate 1986; **Resid:** Ophthalmology, St Luke's-Roosevelt Hosp Ctr 1990; **Fellow:** Ophthalmic Plastic Surgery, Columbia-Presby Med Ctr 1991; **Fac Appt:** Assoc Clin Prof Oph, Columbia P&S

Morabito, Carmine D MD (Oph) - **Hospital:** Southside Hosp; **Address:** 375 E Main St, Ste 24, Bay Shore, NY 11706; **Phone:** 631-665-1330; **Board Cert:** Ophthalmology 1971; **Med School:** Switzerland 1962; **Resid:** Ophthalmology, Hosp Univ Penn 1969

Morris, Robert P MD (Oph) - **Hospital:** St Catherine's of Siena Med Ctr; **Address:** 222 E Main St, Ste 330, Smithtown, NY 11787; **Phone:** 631-724-4488; **Board Cert:** Ophthalmology 1974; **Med School:** SUNY Upstate Med Univ 1966; **Resid:** Ophthalmology, SUNY Downstate Med Ctr 1972

Nattis, Richard MD (Oph) - **Spec Exp:** Cataract Surgery; Laser Vision Surgery; **Hospital:** Good Samaritan Hosp Med Ctr - West Islip, Southside Hosp; **Address:** 150 East Sunrise Hwy, Ste 105, Lindenhurst, NY 11757; **Phone:** 631-957-3355; **Board Cert:** Ophthalmology 1985; **Med School:** NY Med Coll 1980; **Resid:** Ophthalmology, St Vincent's Hosp 1984; **Fac Appt:** Asst Clin Prof Oph, NY Coll Osteo Med

O'Malley, Grace M MD (Oph) - **Spec Exp:** Cataract Surgery; LASIK-Refractive Surgery; **Hospital:** Southampton Hosp; **Address:** 186 Old Towne Rd, Southampton, NY 11968; **Phone:** 631-283-3533; **Board Cert:** Ophthalmology 1989; **Med School:** NY Med Coll 1981; **Resid:** Ophthalmology, NY Med Coll 1985

Pizzarello, Louis MD (Oph) - **Spec Exp:** Diabetic Eye Disease/Retinopathy; **Hospital:** Southampton Hosp; **Address:** 137 Hampton Rd, Southampton, NY 11968; **Phone:** 631-283-5152; **Board Cert:** Ophthalmology 1980; **Med School:** Univ VA Sch Med 1975; **Resid:** Ophthalmology, Columbia-Presby Med Ctr 1979

Romanelli, John MD (Oph) - **Spec Exp:** Cataract Surgery; Glaucoma; **Hospital:** St Catherine's of Siena Med Ctr, Stony Brook Univ Hosp; **Address:** 222 E Main St, Ste 330, Smithtown, NY 11787-2814; **Phone:** 631-724-4488; **Board Cert:** Ophthalmology 2003; **Med School:** Harvard Med Sch 1987; **Resid:** Ophthalmology, Manhattan EET Hosp 1991; **Fac Appt:** Clin Prof Oph, SUNY Stony Brook

Rothberg, Charles MD (Oph) - **Spec Exp:** Cataract Surgery; Glaucoma; LASIK-Refractive Surgery; **Hospital:** Brookhaven Meml Hosp & Med Ctr; **Address:** 331 East Main Street, Patchogue, NY 11772; **Phone:** 631-758-5300; **Board Cert:** Ophthalmology 1989; **Med School:** SUNY Downstate 1983; **Resid:** Ophthalmology, Univ Hosp 1987

Schneck, Gideon MD (Oph) - **Spec Exp:** Eyelid Cosmetic Surgery; Thyroid Eye Disease; Orbital Surgery; **Hospital:** Stony Brook Univ Hosp, St Charles Hosp; **Address:** 2500 Route 347, Building 17B, Stony Brook, NY 11790; **Phone:** 631-246-9140; **Board Cert:** Ophthalmology 1991; **Med School:** Boston Univ 1986; **Resid:** Ophthalmology, Northwestern Univ Med Sch 1990; **Fellow:** Oculoplastic Surgery, IL Eye & Ear Infirmary 1991; **Fac Appt:** Asst Clin Prof Oph, SUNY Stony Brook

Sibony, Patrick MD (Oph) - **Spec Exp:** Neuro-Ophthalmology; Orbital Diseases; **Hospital:** Stony Brook Univ Hosp; **Address:** Stony Brook Ophthalmology, 33 Research Way, East Setauket, NY 11733; **Phone:** 631-444-4090; **Board Cert:** Ophthalmology 1982; **Med School:** Boston Univ 1977; **Resid:** Ophthalmology, Boston Univ Med Ctr 1981; **Fellow:** Ophthalmology, Eye & Ear Hosp 1982; **Fac Appt:** Prof Oph, SUNY Stony Brook

Stoller, Gerald MD (Oph) - **Spec Exp:** Retinal Disorders; **Hospital:** St Charles Hosp, John T Mather Meml Hosp of Port Jefferson; **Address:** 251 E Oakland Ave, Port Jefferson, NY 11777-2170; **Phone:** 631-473-5329; **Board Cert:** Ophthalmology 1973; **Med School:** Temple Univ 1966; **Resid:** Ophthalmology, Bronx Municipal Hosp 1971

Weber, Pamela MD (Oph) - **Spec Exp:** Retinal Disorders; Macular Degeneration; Diabetic Eye Disease/Retinopathy; **Hospital:** Stony Brook Univ Hosp, St Charles Hosp; **Address:** 1500 William Floyd Pkwy, Ste 304, Shirley, NY 11967; **Phone:** 631-924-4300; **Board Cert:** Ophthalmology 1989; **Med School:** Columbia P&S 1984; **Resid:** Ophthalmology, New York Eye & Ear Infirm 1988; **Fellow:** Vitreoretinal Surgery, Retina Assoc 1990; **Fac Appt:** Asst Prof Oph, SUNY Stony Brook

Zweibel, Lawrence MD (Oph) - **Spec Exp:** LASIK-Refractive Surgery; Cataract Surgery; Glaucoma; **Hospital:** St Catherine's of Siena Med Ctr; **Address:** 260 Middle Country Rd, Ste 201, Smithtown, NY 11787-2982; **Phone:** 631-265-8780; **Board Cert:** Ophthalmology 1977; **Med School:** Albany Med Coll 1972; **Resid:** Ophthalmology, French-Polyclinic Hosp 1976

ORTHOPAEDIC SURGERY

Alpert, Scott W MD (OrS) - **Spec Exp:** Shoulder & Elbow Surgery; Hip Surgery; Knee Surgery; Sports Medicine; **Hospital:** Huntington Hosp; **Address:** 33 Walt Whitman Rd, Ste 200B, Huntington Station, NY 11746-3627; **Phone:** 631-423-4090; **Board Cert:** Orthopaedic Surgery 1997; **Med School:** Harvard Med Sch 1989; **Resid:** Orthopaedic Surgery, Hosp Joint Diseases 1994; **Fellow:** Sports Medicine, Kerlan-Jobe Orth Clinic 1995

Arvan, Glenn Douglas MD (OrS) - **Spec Exp:** Trauma; Pediatric Orthopaedic Surgery; Joint Replacement; Geriatric Orthopaedic Surgery; **Hospital:** Good Samaritan Hosp Med Ctr - West Islip, Southside Hosp; **Address:** 661 Deer Park Ave, Babylon, NY 11702-1314; **Phone:** 631-661-0202; **Board Cert:** Orthopaedic Surgery 1979; **Med School:** Duke Univ 1972; **Resid:** Orthopaedic Surgery, NY Hosp 1974; Orthopaedic Surgery, Case Western Res Med Ctr 1977

Bleifeld, Charles MD (OrS) - **Spec Exp:** Hip Surgery; Knee Surgery; Hip & Knee Replacement; **Hospital:** St Catherine's of Siena Med Ctr; **Address:** 48 Route 25A, Ste 106, Smithtown, NY 11787-1447; **Phone:** 631-863-1007; **Board Cert:** Orthopaedic Surgery 1975; **Med School:** Geo Wash Univ 1968; **Resid:** Surgery, St Luke's Roosevelt Hosp Ctr 1970; Orthopaedic Surgery, Hosp For Special Surg 1973

Dowling, Thomas MD (OrS) - **Spec Exp:** Spinal Surgery; Spinal Deformity; **Hospital:** St Catherine's of Siena Med Ctr, Huntington Hosp; **Address:** 763 Larkfield Rd Fl 2, Commack, NY 11725-2900; **Phone:** 631-462-2225; **Board Cert:** Orthopaedic Surgery 2001; **Med School:** Boston Univ 1981; **Resid:** Surgery, North Shore Univ Hosp 1983; Orthopaedic Surgery, Univ Hosp-SUNY 1987; **Fellow:** Spinal Surgery, N Shore Univ Hosp 1983; Spinal Surgery, Univ Toronto 1988

Dubrow, Eric N MD (OrS) - **Spec Exp:** Hip & Knee Replacement; Sports Medicine; Cerebral Palsy; **Hospital:** St Charles Hosp, John T Mather Meml Hosp of Port Jefferson; **Address:** 6 Technology Drive, East Setauket, NY 11733; **Phone:** 631-698-6698; **Board Cert:** Orthopaedic Surgery 1997; **Med School:** Belgium 1979; **Resid:** Surgery, Nassau Co Med Ctr 1980; Orthopaedic Surgery, Univ Hosp-SUNY 1984; **Fac Appt:** Asst Clin Prof S, SUNY Stony Brook

Kurtz, Neil J MD (OrS) - **Spec Exp:** Hip & Knee Replacement; Arthroscopic Surgery; **Hospital:** St Charles Hosp, John T Mather Meml Hosp of Port Jefferson; **Address:** 6 Technology Drive, Ste 100, East Setauket, NY 11733; **Phone:** 631-689-6698; **Board Cert:** Orthopaedic Surgery 1978; **Med School:** NYU Sch Med 1971; **Resid:** Orthopaedic Surgery, Univ Pittsburgh 1976; **Fellow:** Physical Medicine & Rehabilitation, NYU Med Ctr 1973; **Fac Appt:** Asst Clin Prof OrS, SUNY Stony Brook

Tabershaw, Richard MD (OrS) - **Spec Exp:** Shoulder Surgery; Sports Medicine; **Hospital:** Southside Hosp; **Address:** 375 E Main St, Ste 1, Bay Shore, NY 11706-8418; **Phone:** 631-665-8790; **Board Cert:** Orthopaedic Surgery 1999; **Med School:** Georgetown Univ 1980; **Resid:** Surgery, St Vincent Med Ctr 1983; Orthopaedic Surgery, Columbia-Presby Hosp 1986

OTOLARYNGOLOGY

Caruso, Anthony MD (Oto) - **Spec Exp:** Sinus Disorders/Surgery; Head & Neck Surgery; **Hospital:** Southampton Hosp; **Address:** 580 County Rd, 39A, Southampton, NY 11968; **Phone:** 631-283-4412; **Board Cert:** Otolaryngology 1979; **Med School:** Jefferson Med Coll 1975; **Resid:** Surgery, Mercy Fitzgerald Hosp 1976; Otolaryngology, Thomas Jefferson Univ Hosp 1979

Chitkara, Dev MD (Oto) - **Spec Exp:** Sinus Disorders; Hearing Disorders; Balance Disorders; **Hospital:** St Catherine's of Siena Med Ctr; **Address:** 29 Manor Rd, Smithtown, NY 11787-2714; **Phone:** 631-979-0311; **Board Cert:** Otolaryngology 1967; **Med School:** India 1961; **Resid:** Surgery, LI Coll Hosp 1964; Otolaryngology, Boston Med Ctr 1967; **Fellow:** Otolaryngology, Georgetown Univ Hosp 1970; **Fac Appt:** Asst Clin Prof Oto, SUNY Stony Brook

Dash, Greg MD (Oto) - **Spec Exp:** Ear Surgery; Sinusitis; Airway Disorders; **Hospital:** Good Samaritan Hosp Med Ctr - West Islip, Southside Hosp; **Address:** 1111 Montauk Hwy, Fl 2, West Islip, NY 11795-4910; **Phone:** 631-422-2700; **Board Cert:** Otolaryngology 1987; **Med School:** Columbia P&S 1982; **Resid:** Surgery, St Luke's Hosp 1983; Otolaryngology, NY EE Infirm 1987

Gargano, Robert M MD (Oto) - **Hospital:** Southside Hosp; **Address:** 375 E Main St, Ste 17, Bay Shore, NY 11706; **Phone:** 631-665-2430; **Board Cert:** Otolaryngology 1989; **Med School:** Tufts Univ 1984; **Resid:** Otolaryngology, New England Med Ctr 1989

Katz, Arnold MD (Oto) - **Spec Exp:** Cosmetic Surgery-Face; Pediatric Otolaryngology; **Hospital:** Stony Brook Univ Hosp; **Address:** 37 Research Way, East Setauket, NY 11733; **Phone:** 631-444-4121; **Board Cert:** Otolaryngology 1976; **Med School:** Washington Univ, St Louis 1967; **Resid:** Otolaryngology, Univ IA Hosp 1976; **Fac Appt:** Prof Oto, SUNY Stony Brook

Litman, Richard MD (Oto) - **Spec Exp:** Pediatric Otolaryngology; Head & Neck Surgery; Otology; Sinus Surgery; **Hospital:** John T Mather Meml Hosp of Port Jefferson, St Charles Hosp; **Address:** 251 E Oakland Ave, Port Jefferson, NY 11777; **Phone:** 631-928-0188; **Board Cert:** Otolaryngology 1976; **Med School:** Wake Forest Univ 1971; **Resid:** Surgery, Albert Einstein-Bronx Muni Hosp 1972; Surgery, Long Island Jewish Med Ctr 1973; **Fellow:** Otolaryngology, Albert Einstein-Bronx Muni Hosp 1976; **Fac Appt:** Asst Clin Prof Oto, SUNY Stony Brook

Sampogna, Dominick A MD (Oto) - **Hospital:** Southside Hosp, Good Samaritan Hosp Med Ctr - West Islip; **Address:** 375 E Main St, Ste 17, Bay Shore, NY 11706; **Phone:** 631-665-2430; **Board Cert:** Otolaryngology 1971; **Med School:** Boston Univ 1965; **Resid:** Surgery, Boston Univ Med Ctr 1967; Otolaryngology, Boston Univ Med Ctr 1970

Shindo, Maisie L MD (Oto) - **Spec Exp:** Head & Neck Cancer & Surgery; Thyroid Cancer; Laryngeal Cancer; Parathyroid Surgery; **Hospital:** Stony Brook Univ Hosp; **Address:** Stony Brook Univ Hosp, HSC (T19-090), Stony Brook, NY 11794-8191; **Phone:** 631-444-8242; **Board Cert:** Otolaryngology 1989; **Med School:** Univ Saskatchewan 1984; **Resid:** Otolaryngology, LAC& USC Med Ctr 1989; **Fellow:** Head and Neck Surgery, Northwestern Univ 1991; **Fac Appt:** Assoc Prof Oto, SUNY Stony Brook

PAIN MEDICINE

Agin, Carole MD (PM) - **Spec Exp:** Acupuncture; Complex Regional Pain Syndrome; Pain-Neuropathic; **Hospital:** Stony Brook Univ Hosp; **Address:** 181 Belle Meade Rd, Ste 5, East Setauket, NY 11733; **Phone:** 631-444-4234; **Board Cert:** Anesthesiology 1991; Pain Medicine 2001; **Med School:** Univ Hlth Sci/Chicago Med Sch 1986; **Resid:** Anesthesiology, Beth Israel Med Ctr 1990; **Fellow:** Pain Medicine, Meml Sloan Kettering Cancer Ctr 1991; **Fac Appt:** Assoc Prof Anes, SUNY Stony Brook

Gargiulo, Juan MD (PM) - **Spec Exp:** Pain-Chronic; Pain-Back; Pain-Cancer; **Hospital:** Southampton Hosp; **Address:** 365 County Rd 39A, Ste 15-16, Southampton, NY 11968; **Phone:** 631-702-2300; **Board Cert:** Anesthesiology 1993; Pain Medicine 1997; **Med School:** Uruguay 1984; **Resid:** Anesthesiology, Westchester Med Ctr 1991

Litman, Steven MD (PM) - **Hospital:** Southside Hosp, Good Samaritan Hosp Med Ctr - West Islip; **Address:** 387 E Main St, Ste 104, Bayshore, NY 11706; **Phone:** 631-665-0075; **Board Cert:** Anesthesiology 1992; Pain Medicine 1996; **Med School:** NY Med Coll 1987; **Resid:** Anesthesiology, Westchester Co Med Ctr 1991

Vaillancourt, Philippe D MD (PM) - **Spec Exp:** Headache; Pain-Chronic; **Hospital:** Southampton Hosp; **Address:** 877 E Main St, Ste 106, Riverhead, NY 11901; **Phone:** 631-727-0660; **Board Cert:** Neurology 1986; Pain Medicine 2000; **Med School:** McGill Univ 1978; **Resid:** Neurology, Mount Sinai Med Ctr 1983; **Fac Appt:** Assoc Prof N, SUNY Stony Brook

PATHOLOGY

Tornos, Carmen MD (Path) - **Spec Exp:** Gynecologic Cancer; Breast Cancer; Ovarian Cancer; **Hospital:** Stony Brook Univ Hosp; **Address:** Stony Brook Univ Hospital, Dept Pathology, Level 2, rm 766, Stony Brook, NY 11794-7025; **Phone:** 631-444-2222; **Board Cert:** Anatomic & Clinical Pathology 1997; **Med School:** Spain 1977; **Resid:** Hematology, Ciudad Sanitaria Valle de Hebron 1982; Anatomic & Clinical Pathology, MD Anderson Cancer Ctr 1989; **Fellow:** Surgical Pathology, MD Anderson Cancer Ctr 1990

PEDIATRIC CARDIOLOGY

Biancaniello, Thomas MD (PCd) - **Spec Exp:** Congenital Heart Disease; Fetal Echocardiography; Interventional Cardiology; Cardiac Catheterization; **Hospital:** Stony Brook Univ Hosp; **Address:** Stony Brook Univ Hosp, Dept Pediatrics, 100 Nicholls Rd, Stony Brook, NY 11794-8111; **Phone:** 631-444-5437; **Board Cert:** Pediatrics 1979; Pediatric Cardiology 1981; **Med School:** NY Med Coll 1975; **Resid:** Pediatrics, North Shore Univ Hosp 1977; **Fellow:** Pediatric Cardiology, Cincinnati Chldns Hosp 1980; **Fac Appt:** Prof Ped, SUNY Stony Brook

PEDIATRIC ENDOCRINOLOGY

Wilson, Thomas MD (PEn) - **Spec Exp:** Growth Disorders; Adrenal Disorders; Sexual Differentiation Disorders; Thyroid Disorders; **Hospital:** Stony Brook Univ Hosp; **Address:** SUNY Stony Brook, Dept Pediatrics, HSC T11, rm 080, Stony Brook, NY 11794-8111; **Phone:** 631-444-3429; **Board Cert:** Pediatrics 1983; **Med School:** Univ Pennsylvania 1973; **Resid:** Pediatrics, Children's Hosp 1976; **Fellow:** Pediatric Endocrinology, Univ Virginia Med Ctr 1982; **Fac Appt:** Prof Ped, SUNY Stony Brook

PEDIATRIC GASTROENTEROLOGY

Gold, David MD (PGe) - **Spec Exp:** Gastroesophageal Reflux Disease (GERD); Irritable Bowel Syndrome; Ulcerative Colitis/Crohn's; **Hospital:** Good Samaritan Hosp - Suffern, Schneider Chldn's Hosp; **Address:** 1111 Montauk Hwy Fl 3, West Islip, NY 11795; **Phone:** 631-376-4092; **Board Cert:** Pediatrics 1998; Pediatric Gastroenterology 2003; **Med School:** Albert Einstein Coll Med 1987; **Resid:** Pediatrics, LI Jewish Med Ctr 1990; **Fellow:** Pediatric Gastroenterology, LI Jewish Med Ctr 1993

Kessler, Bradley MD (PGe) - **Spec Exp:** Inflammatory Bowel Disease/Crohn's; Liver Disease; Malabsorption; **Hospital:** Good Samaritan Hosp Med Ctr - West Islip; **Address:** 1111 Montauk Hwy Fl 3, West Islip, NY 11795; **Phone:** 631-376-4092; **Board Cert:** Pediatrics 1988; Pediatric Gastroenterology 2004; **Med School:** SUNY Downstate 1982; **Resid:** Pediatrics, N Shore Univ Hosp 1985; **Fellow:** Pediatric Gastroenterology, Baylor-Tex Chldns Hosp 1988

Lowenheim, Mark Saul MD (PGe) - **Spec Exp:** Inflammatory Bowel Disease/Crohn's; **Hospital:** Stony Brook Univ Hosp; **Address:** Chldn's Med Ctr-Stony Brook, Dept Ped, Fl T-11 - rm 080, Stony Brook, NY 11794-8111; **Phone:** 631-444-8115; **Board Cert:** Pediatrics 1999; Pediatric Gastroenterology 2002; **Med School:** West Indies 1984; **Resid:** Pediatrics, Elmhurst Hosp 1986; **Fellow:** Pediatric Gastroenterology, Mount Sinai Med Ctr 1989; **Fac Appt:** Assoc Prof Ped, SUNY Stony Brook

PEDIATRIC HEMATOLOGY-ONCOLOGY

Parker, Robert MD (PHO) - **Spec Exp:** Pediatric Cancers; Bleeding/Coagulation Disorders; Platelet Disorders; **Hospital:** Stony Brook Univ Hosp; **Address:** Stony Brook Univ Hosp, Dept Peds, HSC T-11, Rm 029, Stony Brook, NY 11794-8111; **Phone:** 631-444-7720; **Board Cert:** Pediatrics 1983; Pediatric Hematology-Oncology 1984; **Med School:** Brown Univ 1976; **Resid:** Internal Medicine, Roger Williams Med Ctr 1977; Pediatrics, Rhode Island Hosp 1979; **Fellow:** Pediatric Hematology-Oncology, Natl Cancer Inst 1981; Hematology, Natl Cancer Inst 1984; **Fac Appt:** Prof Ped, SUNY Stony Brook

PEDIATRIC INFECTIOUS DISEASE

Nachman, Sharon MD (PInf) - **Spec Exp:** Lyme Disease; AIDS/HIV; **Hospital:** Stony Brook Univ Hosp; **Address:** SUNY at Stony Brook, HSC 11, rm 031, Stony Brook, NY 11794-8111; **Phone:** 631-444-7692; **Board Cert:** Pediatrics 1987; Pediatric Infectious Disease 2002; **Med School:** SUNY Stony Brook 1983; **Resid:** Pediatrics, Schneiders Chldns Hosp/LI Jewish 1986; **Fellow:** Pediatric Infectious Disease, NY Med Coll 1987Rockefeller Univ 1989; **Fac Appt:** Prof Ped, SUNY Stony Brook

PEDIATRIC SURGERY

Lee, Thomas Kang-Ming MD (PS) - **Spec Exp:** Minimally Invasive Surgery; **Hospital:** Stony Brook Univ Hosp; **Address:** 37 Research Way, East Setauket, NY 11733; **Phone:** 631-444-4538; **Board Cert:** Surgery 2005; Pediatric Surgery 1998; **Med School:** Univ Chicago-Pritzker Sch Med 1988; **Resid:** Surgery, NY Hosp-Cornell Med Ctr 1995; **Fellow:** Transplant Surgery, Hosps Univ Pittsburgh 1992; Pediatric Surgery, Cardinal Glennon Chldns Hosp/St Louis Univ 1997; **Fac Appt:** Asst Prof S, SUNY Stony Brook

Winick, Martin MD (PS) - **Spec Exp:** Neonatal Surgery; Hernia; Undescended Testis; **Hospital:** Good Samaritan Hosp Med Ctr - West Islip, St Catherine's of Siena Med Ctr; **Address:** 158 E Main St, Huntington, NY 11743; **Phone:** 631-427-1300; **Board Cert:** Surgery 1966; Pediatric Surgery 1995; **Med School:** SUNY Downstate 1960; **Resid:** Surgery, Jewish Hosp 1965; **Fellow:** Pediatric Surgery, St Christopher Hosp 1966; **Fac Appt:** Assoc Clin Prof S, SUNY Stony Brook

PEDIATRICS

Adler, Albert MD (Ped) `PCP` - **Spec Exp:** Mental Retardation; **Hospital:** Stony Brook Univ Hosp, St Catherine's of Siena Med Ctr; **Address:** 1 Teapot Ln, Smithtown, NY 11787; **Phone:** 631-265-7272; **Board Cert:** Pediatrics 1963; **Med School:** Switzerland 1958; **Resid:** Pediatrics, Queens Hosp 1961; **Fellow:** Pediatrics, Queens Hosp; **Fac Appt:** Asst Clin Prof Ped, SUNY Stony Brook

Augustine, Viruppamattan M MD (Ped) PCP - **Spec Exp:** Asthma; **Hospital:** Good Samaritan Hosp Med Ctr - West Islip, Southside Hosp; **Address:** 160 Middle Rd, Ste 2, Sayville, NY 11782; **Phone:** 631-589-5533; **Board Cert:** Pediatrics 1979; Neonatal-Perinatal Medicine 1983; **Med School:** India 1970; **Resid:** Pediatrics, Harlem Hosp Ctr 1976; Neonatal-Perinatal Medicine, Harlem Hosp Ctr 1977; **Fellow:** Neonatal-Perinatal Medicine, Harlem Hosp Ctr 1978

Bernstein, Harvey MD (Ped) PCP - **Hospital:** St Catherine's of Siena Med Ctr; **Address:** Smithtown Pediatric Group, 260 Middle Country Rd, Smithtown, NY 11787; **Phone:** 631-979-7222; **Board Cert:** Pediatrics 1978; **Med School:** Univ Pennsylvania 1973; **Resid:** Pediatrics, Bronx Muni Hosp 1976; **Fac Appt:** Asst Clin Prof Ped, SUNY Stony Brook

Chernobilsky, Lev MD (Ped) PCP - **Spec Exp:** Asthma; **Hospital:** Stony Brook Univ Hosp, St Catherine's of Siena Med Ctr; **Address:** 269-D E Main St, Smithtown, NY 11787; **Phone:** 631-361-2121; **Board Cert:** Pediatrics 1987; **Med School:** Russia 1974; **Resid:** Pediatrics, SUNY Med Ctr 1985; **Fac Appt:** Assoc Clin Prof Ped, SUNY Stony Brook

Cusumano, Barbara MD (Ped) PCP - **Hospital:** Southampton Hosp; **Address:** 325 Meeting House Ln, Southampton, NY 11968-5087; **Phone:** 631-283-7733; **Board Cert:** Pediatrics 2002; **Med School:** Univ Hlth Sci/Chicago Med Sch 1984; **Resid:** Pediatrics, New York Hosp 1987

Festa, Robert S MD (Ped) PCP - **Hospital:** St Charles Hosp, Stony Brook Univ Hosp; **Address:** 911 Montauk Hwy, Shirley, NY 11967; **Phone:** 631-281-2525; **Board Cert:** Pediatrics 1978; Pediatric Hematology-Oncology 1980; **Med School:** SUNY Downstate 1972; **Resid:** Pediatrics, Montefiore Hosp Med Ctr 1975; **Fellow:** Pediatric Hematology-Oncology, Chldns Hosp 1978

Grello, Ciro T MD (Ped) PCP - **Hospital:** Good Samaritan Hosp Med Ctr - West Islip, Southside Hosp; **Address:** 390 Montauk Hwy, West Islip, NY 11795; **Phone:** 631-422-0700; **Board Cert:** Pediatrics 2000; **Med School:** Univ VA Sch Med 1989; **Resid:** Pediatrics, New York Hosp-Cornell 1992

Kaplan, Martin MD (Ped) PCP - **Spec Exp:** Asthma; Developmental Disorders; ADD/ADHD; **Hospital:** St Charles Hosp, Stony Brook Univ Hosp; **Address:** 12 Medical Drive, Port Jefferson Station, NY 11776-1588; **Phone:** 631-331-1710; **Board Cert:** Pediatrics 1977; **Med School:** NYU Sch Med 1972; **Resid:** Pediatrics, Bellevue Hosp 1974; Pediatrics, Duke Univ Med Ctr 1975; **Fac Appt:** Asst Clin Prof Ped, SUNY Stony Brook

Kolker, Harvey A MD (Ped) PCP - **Hospital:** St Charles Hosp, Stony Brook Univ Hosp; **Address:** 111 Sylvan Ave, Miller Place, NY 11764-2420; **Phone:** 631-928-4888; **Board Cert:** Pediatrics 1971; **Med School:** SUNY Downstate 1966; **Resid:** Pediatrics, Madigan Genl Hosp 1969; **Fac Appt:** Assoc Clin Prof Ped, SUNY Stony Brook

Kurfist, Lee MD (Ped) PCP - **Hospital:** Huntington Hosp; **Address:** 205 E Main St, Ste 2-8, Huntington, NY 11743; **Phone:** 631-424-1741; **Board Cert:** Pediatrics 2000; **Med School:** Italy 1985; **Resid:** Pediatrics, Nassau County Med Ctr 1988; **Fellow:** Mt Sinai Hosp 1990

Manners, Richard MD (Ped) PCP - **Hospital:** St Charles Hosp, Stony Brook Univ Hosp; **Address:** 1770 Motor Pkwy, Hauppauge, NY 11749; **Phone:** 631-434-1770; **Board Cert:** Pediatrics 1980; **Med School:** Albert Einstein Coll Med 1975; **Resid:** Pediatrics, Univ MN Med Ctr 1978

Musiker, Seymour MD (Ped) PCP - **Spec Exp:** Breast Feeding Problems; **Hospital:** Stony Brook Univ Hosp, St Charles Hosp; **Address:** 2233 Nesconset Hwy, Ste 106, Lake Grove, NY 11755-1000; **Phone:** 631-585-4440; **Board Cert:** Pediatrics 1966; **Med School:** Univ Hlth Sci/Chicago Med Sch 1961; **Resid:** Pediatrics, Bronx Muni Hosp Ctr 1964; **Fac Appt:** Assoc Clin Prof Ped, SUNY Stony Brook

Parker, Margaret MD (Ped) - **Spec Exp:** Sepsis; Respiratory Failure; Critical Care; **Hospital:** Stony Brook Univ Hosp; **Address:** Stony Brook University, Dept Pediatrics, HSC T-11.040, Stony Brook, NY 11794-8111; **Phone:** 631-444-8211; **Board Cert:** Internal Medicine 1980; Pediatrics 2003; Critical Care Medicine 1997; **Med School:** Brown Univ 1977; **Resid:** Internal Medicine, Roger Williams Med Ctr 1980; **Fellow:** Critical Care Medicine, Nat Inst Hlth 1982; **Fac Appt:** Prof Ped, SUNY Stony Brook

Parles, James G MD (Ped) PCP - **Hospital:** Stony Brook Univ Hosp, St Catherine's of Siena Med Ctr; **Address:** 260 Middle Country Rd, Smithtown, NY 11787; **Phone:** 631-979-7252; **Board Cert:** Pediatrics 2002; **Med School:** NYU Sch Med 1985; **Resid:** Pediatrics, Mount Sinai Hospital 1988; **Fac Appt:** Asst Clin Prof Ped, SUNY Upstate Med Univ

Quinn, Joseph MD (Ped) PCP - **Spec Exp:** ADD/ADHD; **Hospital:** Southampton Hosp; **Address:** 325 Meeting House Ln, Ste C, Southampton, NY 11968; **Phone:** 631-283-7733; **Board Cert:** Pediatrics 1987; **Med School:** Univ VT Coll Med 1981; **Resid:** Pediatrics, New York Hosp 1984

PHYSICAL MEDICINE & REHABILITATION

Rosenberg, Craig H MD (PMR) - **Spec Exp:** Repetitive Strain Injuries; Pain-Back & Neck; **Hospital:** Southside Hosp; **Address:** PO Box 230, Islip, NY 11751; **Phone:** 631-232-0057; **Board Cert:** Physical Medicine & Rehabilitation 1987; **Med School:** Mexico 1981; **Resid:** Physical Medicine & Rehabilitation, NYU Med Ctr/Rusk Inst 1985; **Fac Appt:** Asst Clin Prof PMR, SUNY Stony Brook

PLASTIC SURGERY

Anton, John R MD (PlS) - **Spec Exp:** Cosmetic Surgery-Face; Eyelid Surgery; Liposuction; **Hospital:** Southampton Hosp, Peconic Bay Med Ctr; **Address:** 138 Old Town Rd, Southampton, NY 11968-5011; **Phone:** 631-283-9100; **Board Cert:** Plastic Surgery 1992; **Med School:** Univ VT Coll Med 1981; **Resid:** Surgery, Mass Genl Hosp 1986; Plastic Surgery, Wayne State Univ Med Ctr 1987

Dagum, Alexander B MD (PlS) - **Spec Exp:** Reconstructive Plastic Surgery; Microvascular Surgery; Hand Surgery; **Hospital:** Stony Brook Univ Hosp; **Address:** SUNY Health Science Ctr, T19-060, Box 8191, Stony Brook, NY 11794-8191; **Phone:** 631-444-8210; **Board Cert:** Plastic Surgery 2003; Hand Surgery 2004; **Med School:** Canada 1987; **Resid:** Plastic Surgery, Univ Toronto Med Ctr 1993; **Fellow:** Microsurgery, Univ Toronto Med Ctr 1984; Hand Surgery, Stony Brook Univ Hosp 1995; **Fac Appt:** Assoc Prof S, SUNY Stony Brook

Wise, Arthur MD (PlS) - **Spec Exp:** Cosmetic Surgery; Reconstructive Surgery; Wound Healing/Care; **Hospital:** St Francis Hosp - The Heart Ctr (page 112), N Shore Univ Hosp at Manhasset; **Address:** 1 Expressway Plaza, Roslyn Heights, NY 11977; **Phone:** 516-484-4100; **Board Cert:** Plastic Surgery 1973; Surgery 1971; **Med School:** Hahnemann Univ 1965; **Resid:** Surgery, SUNY Downstate Med Ctr 1967; Surgery, Univ Hlth Ctr-Vermont 1970; **Fellow:** Plastic Surgery, SUNY Downstate Med Ctr 1972; **Fac Appt:** Asst Prof S, SUNY Downstate

PREVENTIVE MEDICINE

Lane, Dorothy S MD (PrM) - **Spec Exp:** Women's Health; Cancer Prevention; Health Promotion & Disease Prevention; **Hospital:** Stony Brook Univ Hosp; **Address:** Stony Brook Univ Sch Med, HSC L4, rm 179, Stony Brook, NY 11794-8437; **Phone:** 631-444-2094; **Board Cert:** Public Health & Genl Preventive Med 1970; Family Medicine 2000; **Med School:** Columbia P&S 1965; **Resid:** Public Health & Genl Preventive Med, NY Health Dept 1968; **Fac Appt:** Prof PrM, SUNY Stony Brook

PSYCHIATRY

Aronson, Thomas MD (Psyc) - **Spec Exp:** Depression; Bipolar/Mood Disorders; **Hospital:** St Catherine's of Siena Med Ctr; **Address:** 9 Brooksite Dr, Smithtown, NY 11787-3400; **Phone:** 631-265-0909; **Board Cert:** Psychiatry 1985; **Med School:** Washington Univ, St Louis 1980; **Resid:** Psychiatry, Hosp Univ Penn 1984; **Fac Appt:** Assoc Clin Prof Psyc, SUNY Stony Brook

Koreen, Amy R MD (Psyc) - ; **Address:** 107 Woodbury Rd, Huntington, NY 11743; **Phone:** 631-423-8368; **Board Cert:** Psychiatry 1993; **Med School:** Mount Sinai Sch Med 1988; **Resid:** Psychiatry, Univ Maryland Med Ctr 1991; Psychiatry, LIJ Med Ctr 1992; **Fellow:** Neuropsychopharmacology, LIJ Med Ctr 1993

Lee, Kwang Soo MD (Psyc) - **Hospital:** Brunswick Gen Hosp; **Address:** Suite 303 22 Broadway, Amityville, NY 11701; **Phone:** 631-789-7448; **Board Cert:** Psychiatry 1979; **Med School:** South Korea 1965; **Resid:** Internal Medicine, Booth Meml Hosp 1967; Psychiatry, Bellevue Hosp 1969; **Fellow:** Psychiatry, Amer Inst Psychoanalysis 1969

Liang, Vera MD (Psyc) - **Spec Exp:** Women's Health-Mental Health; Depression; Anxiety Disorders; **Hospital:** N Shore Univ Hosp at Glen Cove; **Address:** 221 Broadway, Ste 221, Amityville, NY 11701-2700; **Phone:** 631-598-7396; **Board Cert:** Psychiatry 1977; Child & Adolescent Psychiatry 1981; **Med School:** Hong Kong 1969; **Resid:** Psychiatry, LI Jewish Med Ctr 1973; **Fellow:** Child & Adolescent Psychiatry, Albert Einstein Coll Med 1975

Nass, Jack MD (Psyc) - **Spec Exp:** Geriatric Rehabilitation; Bipolar/Mood Disorders; Depression; **Hospital:** S Oaks Hosp; **Address:** 580 Sunrise Hwy, West Babylon, NY 11704; **Phone:** 631-321-7697; **Board Cert:** Psychiatry 1980; Geriatric Psychiatry 1991; **Med School:** Belgium 1975; **Resid:** Psychiatry, LI Jewish Med Ctr 1979

Packard, William MD (Psyc) - **Spec Exp:** Depression; Psychopharmacology; Gender Issues; **Address:** 887 Old Country Rd, Riverhead, NY 11901-2115; **Phone:** 631-727-3596; **Board Cert:** Psychiatry 1981; **Med School:** Cornell Univ-Weill Med Coll 1976; **Resid:** Psychiatry, St Luke's-Roosevelt Hosp Ctr 1980; **Fellow:** Forensic Psychiatry, NYU Med Ctr 1984; **Fac Appt:** Asst Prof Psyc, SUNY Stony Brook

Rosen, Bruce I MD (Psyc) - **Spec Exp:** Depression; Anxiety Disorders; Bipolar/Mood Disorders; Psychopharmacology; **Hospital:** St Catherine's of Siena Med Ctr, Stony Brook Univ Hosp; **Address:** 222 E Middle Country Rd, Ste 210, Smithtown, NY 11787-2814; **Phone:** 631-265-6868; **Board Cert:** Psychiatry 1976; Geriatric Psychiatry 1996; **Med School:** Loyola Univ-Stritch Sch Med 1971; **Resid:** Psychiatry, LI Jewish-Hillside Med Ctr 1974; **Fellow:** Psychiatry, LI Jewish-Hillside Med Ctr 1975; **Fac Appt:** Assoc Clin Prof Psyc, SUNY Stony Brook

Schwartz, Michael MD (Psyc) - **Spec Exp:** Forensic Psychiatry; Psychotherapy & Psychopharmacology; Depression; **Hospital:** Stony Brook Univ Hosp; **Address:** 33 E Carver St, Huntington, NY 11743-3409; **Phone:** 631-385-3313; **Board Cert:** Psychiatry 1984; Forensic Psychiatry 1999; Geriatric Psychiatry 2001; **Med School:** Univ Miami Sch Med 1977; **Resid:** Internal Medicine, Mount Sinai Hosp 1981; **Fellow:** Psychiatry, Natl Inst Aging 1983; **Fac Appt:** Assoc Clin Prof Psyc, SUNY Stony Brook

Upadhyay, Yogendra MD (Psyc) - **Spec Exp:** Child & Adolescent Psychiatry; Bipolar/Mood Disorders; Depression; **Hospital:** S Oaks Hosp; **Address:** 400 Sunrise Hwy, Amityville, NY 11701-2508; **Phone:** 631-608-5215; **Board Cert:** Pediatrics 1967; Psychiatry 1977; Child & Adolescent Psychiatry 1978; **Med School:** India 1962; **Resid:** Psychiatry, Albert Einstein Coll Med 1974; **Fellow:** Child & Adolescent Psychiatry, Johns Hopkins 1972; Child & Adolescent Psychiatry, Albert Einstein Coll Med 1975

PULMONARY DISEASE

Baram, Daniel MD (Pul) - **Spec Exp:** Critical Care Medicine; **Hospital:** Stony Brook Univ Hosp; **Address:** Health Sci Ctr, T-17 - Rm 040, Stony Brook, NY 11794-8122; **Phone:** 631-444-2981; **Board Cert:** Internal Medicine 1993; Critical Care Medicine 1997; Pulmonary Disease 1998; **Med School:** Jefferson Med Coll 1990; **Resid:** Internal Medicine, NY Presby Hosp Cornell 1993; **Fellow:** Critical Care Medicine, National Institute Health 1994

Bernardini, Dennis MD (Pul) - **Spec Exp:** Asthma; Emphysema; Bronchitis; **Hospital:** Huntington Hosp; **Address:** 175 E Main St, Huntington, NY 11743-2939; **Phone:** 631-424-3787; **Board Cert:** Internal Medicine 1986; Pulmonary Disease 1983; Critical Care Medicine 2002; Geriatric Medicine 1996; **Med School:** Johns Hopkins Univ 1980; **Resid:** Internal Medicine, St Luke's Hosp 1983; **Fellow:** Pulmonary Disease, Univ Hospital 1985; Critical Care Medicine, Univ Hospital 1985

Bohensky, Paul MD (Pul) - **Spec Exp:** Asthma-Adult & Pediatric; Bronchitis; Emphysema; Chronic Obstructive Lung Disease (COPD); **Hospital:** Brookhaven Meml Hosp & Med Ctr; **Address:** 286 Sills Rd, Ste 4, Patchogue, NY 11772; **Phone:** 631-654-7800; **Board Cert:** Internal Medicine 1981; Pulmonary Disease 1984; Critical Care Medicine 1987; **Med School:** Jamaica 1977; **Resid:** Internal Medicine, Stony Brook Univ/VA Hosp 1981; **Fellow:** Pulmonary Disease, Stony Brook Univ/VA Hosp 1983

Glaser, Morton MD (Pul) - **Hospital:** John T Mather Meml Hosp of Port Jefferson, St Charles Hosp; **Address:** 60 N Country Rd, Ste 203, Port Jefferson, NY 11777; **Phone:** 631-928-3444; **Board Cert:** Internal Medicine 1980; Pulmonary Disease 1984; Critical Care Medicine 1999; **Med School:** Med Coll Wisc 1976; **Resid:** Internal Medicine, Roger Williams Med Ctr 1979; **Fellow:** Pulmonary Disease, Univ Hosp 1981

Scheuch, Robert MD (Pul) - **Spec Exp:** Asthma; Emphysema; Pneumonia; **Hospital:** Southampton Hosp; **Address:** 50 N Main St, Southampton, NY 11968-5013; **Phone:** 631-283-8008; **Board Cert:** Internal Medicine 1985; Pulmonary Disease 2000; **Med School:** Univ Mass Sch Med 1982; **Resid:** Internal Medicine, St Vincent's Hosp 1984; Internal Medicine, Westchester Med Ctr 1985; **Fellow:** Pulmonary Disease, NY Med Coll 1987

Schneyer, Barton MD (Pul) - **Spec Exp:** Asthma; Emphysema; Lung Cancer; **Hospital:** St Catherine's of Siena Med Ctr; **Address:** 222 E Main St, Ste 200, Smithtown, NY 11787; **Phone:** 631-780-9992; **Board Cert:** Internal Medicine 1975; Pulmonary Disease 1980; Critical Care Medicine 1997; **Med School:** Jefferson Med Coll 1972; **Resid:** Internal Medicine, Montefiore Hosp 1975; **Fellow:** Pulmonary Disease, Montefiore Hosp 1979

Sklarek, Howard MD (Pul) - **Spec Exp:** Asthma; Emphysema; Cough; **Hospital:** Southampton Hosp; **Address:** 50 N Main St, Southampton, NY 11968-3336; **Phone:** 631-283-8008; **Board Cert:** Internal Medicine 1984; Pulmonary Disease 1986; Critical Care Medicine 1998; **Med School:** SUNY Buffalo 1981; **Resid:** Internal Medicine, Winthrop Univ Hosp 1984; **Fellow:** Pulmonary Critical Care Medicine, Winthrop Univ Hosp 1986

Tow, Tony MD (Pul) - **Hospital:** Southside Hosp, Good Samaritan Hosp Med Ctr - West Islip; **Address:** 370 E Main St, Ste 5, Bay Shore, NY 11706-8405; **Phone:** 631-666-5864; **Board Cert:** Internal Medicine 1982; Pulmonary Disease 1984; Critical Care Medicine 1997; **Med School:** Cornell Univ-Weill Med Coll 1979; **Resid:** Internal Medicine, NY Hosp 1982; **Fellow:** Pulmonary Disease, Mount Sinai Med Ctr 1984

Walser, Lawrence MD (Pul) - **Hospital:** Peconic Bay Med Ctr, Eastern Long Island Hosp; **Address:** 185 Old Country Rd, Ste 3, Riverhead, NY 11901; **Phone:** 631-727-2523; **Board Cert:** Internal Medicine 1982; Pulmonary Disease 1997; Critical Care Medicine 1997; **Med School:** SUNY Downstate 1979; **Resid:** Internal Medicine, Berkshire Med Ctr 1982; **Fellow:** Pulmonary Disease, SUNY/Univ Hosp 1984

Weiner, Jerome MD (Pul) - **Hospital:** Good Samaritan Hosp Med Ctr - West Islip, Southside Hosp; **Address:** 370 E Main St, Ste 5, Bay Shore, NY 11706-8418; **Phone:** 631-666-5800; **Board Cert:** Internal Medicine 1980; Pulmonary Disease 1982; Critical Care Medicine 1998; **Med School:** Mount Sinai Sch Med 1977; **Resid:** Internal Medicine, Mount Sinai Med Ctr 1980; **Fellow:** Pulmonary Disease, Montefiore Med Ctr 1982

Wohlberg, Gary MD (Pul) - **Spec Exp:** Sleep Disorders/Apnea; **Hospital:** Southside Hosp, Good Samaritan Hosp Med Ctr - West Islip; **Address:** 370 E Main St, Ste 5, Bay Shore, NY 11706-8405; **Phone:** 631-666-5864; **Board Cert:** Internal Medicine 1985; Pulmonary Disease 1986; Critical Care Medicine 1999; **Med School:** SUNY Hlth Sci Ctr 1981; **Resid:** Internal Medicine, Long Island Hosp 1984; **Fellow:** Pulmonary Disease, Montefiore Hosp Med Ctr 1986

RADIATION ONCOLOGY

Meek, Allen MD (RadRO) - **Spec Exp:** Breast Cancer; Prostate Cancer; Radiation Therapy-Intraoperative; Head & Neck Cancer; **Hospital:** Stony Brook Univ Hosp; **Address:** Stony Brook Univ Hosp, Dept Rad Onc - L2, 100 Nichols Rd, Stony Brook, NY 11794-7028; **Phone:** 631-444-2210; **Board Cert:** Internal Medicine 1979; Therapeutic Radiology 1983; **Med School:** Johns Hopkins Univ 1974; **Resid:** Internal Medicine, Johns Hopkins Hosp 1979; Radiation Oncology, Johns Hopkins Hosp 1982; **Fellow:** Medical Oncology, Johns Hopkins Hosp 1980; **Fac Appt:** Prof RadRO, SUNY Stony Brook

Park, Tae MD (RadRO) - **Spec Exp:** Prostate Cancer; Breast Cancer; Gynecologic Cancer; **Hospital:** Stony Brook Univ Hosp; **Address:** Stony Brook Univ Hosp, Dept Rad Onc, Stony Brook, NY 11794-7028; **Phone:** 631-444-2210; **Board Cert:** Therapeutic Radiology 1984; **Med School:** South Korea 1976; **Resid:** Radiation Oncology, Kings Co Downstate Med Ctr. 1984; **Fellow:** Radiation Oncology, MD Anderson Cancer Ctr 1985; **Fac Appt:** Assoc Clin Prof RadRO, SUNY Stony Brook

REPRODUCTIVE ENDOCRINOLOGY

Kenigsberg, Daniel MD (RE) - **Spec Exp:** Infertility-IVF; Uterine Fibroids; Endometriosis; Reproductive Surgery; **Hospital:** John T Mather Meml Hosp of Port Jefferson, Stony Brook Univ Hosp; **Address:** 625 Belle Terre Rd, Ste 200, Port Jefferson, NY 11777-2318; **Phone:** 631-331-7575; **Board Cert:** Obstetrics & Gynecology 1995; Reproductive Endocrinology 1995; **Med School:** NY Med Coll 1978; **Resid:** Obstetrics & Gynecology, Johns Hopkins 1982; **Fellow:** Reproductive Endocrinology, Natl Inst Hlth 1984; **Fac Appt:** Assoc Prof ObG, SUNY Stony Brook

RHEUMATOLOGY

Bennett, Ronald MD (Rhu) - **Spec Exp:** Rheumatoid Arthritis; Osteoarthritis; Lupus/SLE; **Hospital:** St Charles Hosp, John T Mather Meml Hosp of Port Jefferson; **Address:** 7 Medical Drive, Port Jefferson Station, NY 11777; **Phone:** 631-928-4885; **Board Cert:** Internal Medicine 1975; Rheumatology 1980; **Med School:** SUNY Hlth Sci Ctr 1972; **Resid:** Internal Medicine, Nassau Co Med Ctr 1975; **Fellow:** Rheumatology, Kings Co Hosp 1977; **Fac Appt:** Asst Clin Prof Med, SUNY Stony Brook

Hamburger, Max MD (Rhu) - **Spec Exp:** Rheumatoid Arthritis; Psoriatic Arthritis; Osteoarthritis; **Hospital:** St Catherine's of Siena Med Ctr, John T Mather Meml Hosp of Port Jefferson; **Address:** 1895 Walt Whitman Rd, Melville, NY 11747; **Phone:** 631-249-9525; **Board Cert:** Internal Medicine 1977; Rheumatology 1980; **Med School:** Albert Einstein Coll Med 1973; **Resid:** Internal Medicine, Bellevue Hosp 1976; **Fellow:** Allergy & Immunology, Nat Inst Health 1979; **Fac Appt:** Asst Clin Prof Med, SUNY Stony Brook

Kaell, Alan MD (Rhu) - **Spec Exp:** Geriatric Rheumatology; Vasculitis; Connective Tissue Disorders; Osteoporosis; **Hospital:** St Charles Hosp, John T Mather Meml Hosp of Port Jefferson; **Address:** 315 Middle Country Rd, Smithtown, NY 11787-2817; **Phone:** 631-360-7778; **Board Cert:** Internal Medicine 1981; Rheumatology 1984; Geriatric Medicine 2000; **Med School:** Brown Univ 1978; **Resid:** Internal Medicine, Strong Meml Hosp 1981; **Fellow:** Rheumatology, Hosp For Special Surgery/Cornell 1983; **Fac Appt:** Clin Prof Med, SUNY Stony Brook

Repice, Michael MD (Rhu) - **Spec Exp:** Arthritis; Connective Tissue Disorders; **Hospital:** Huntington Hosp; **Address:** 5 E Main St, Huntington, NY 11743-2812; **Phone:** 631-271-1640; **Board Cert:** Internal Medicine 1976; Rheumatology 1980; **Med School:** Georgetown Univ 1973; **Resid:** Rheumatology, Worcester City Hosp 1977; **Fellow:** Rheumatology, Northwestern Univ 1979; **Fac Appt:** Asst Prof Med, SUNY Stony Brook

Schorn, Karen MD (Rhu) - **Spec Exp:** Lupus Nephritis; Osteoporosis; **Hospital:** N Shore Univ Hosp at Plainview; **Address:** 124 Main St, Ste 10, Huntington, NY 11743; **Phone:** 631-385-5030; **Board Cert:** Internal Medicine 1986; Rheumatology 2003; **Med School:** Mexico 1982; **Resid:** Internal Medicine, Maimonides Medical Ctr 1986; **Fellow:** Rheumatology, Univ Hosp 1988

Tan, Mark MD (Rhu) - **Spec Exp:** Lupus/SLE; Rheumatoid Arthritis; **Hospital:** St Catherine's of Siena Med Ctr, St Charles Hosp; **Address:** 222 Middle Country Rd Fl 3 - Ste 312, Smithtown, NY 11787; **Phone:** 631-724-8900; **Board Cert:** Internal Medicine 1989; Rheumatology 1994; **Med School:** SUNY Buffalo 1983; **Resid:** Internal Medicine, Univ Hosp 1986; **Fellow:** Rheumatology, Johns Hopkins Univ 1989

SURGERY

Busch-Devereaux, Erna MD (S) - **Spec Exp:** Breast Cancer; Breast Surgery; **Hospital:** Huntington Hosp, N Shore Univ Hosp at Manhasset; **Address:** 152 E Main St, Ste A, Huntington, NY 11743; **Phone:** 631-423-1414; **Board Cert:** Surgery 2000; **Med School:** UMDNJ-NJ Med Sch, Newark 1985; **Resid:** Surgery, St Vincents Hosp 1990; **Fellow:** Surgical Oncology, Roswell Park Cancer 1993; **Fac Appt:** Asst Prof S, NYU Sch Med

Capizzi, Anthony J MD (S) - **Spec Exp:** Breast Cancer; Laparoscopic Surgery; Colon & Rectal Surgery; **Hospital:** Good Samaritan Hosp Med Ctr - West Islip; **Address:** 786 Montauk Hwy, West Islip, NY 11795; **Phone:** 631-669-3700; **Board Cert:** Surgery 1989; **Med School:** NY Med Coll 1983; **Resid:** Surgery, Montefiore Med Ctr 1988

Cohen, Bradley MD (S) - **Spec Exp:** Breast Disease; Cancer Surgery; Laparoscopic Surgery; **Hospital:** Good Samaritan Hosp Med Ctr - West Islip, Southside Hosp; **Address:** 111 Carleton Ave, Islip Terrace, NY 11752-2236; **Phone:** 631-581-4400; **Board Cert:** Surgery 1989; **Med School:** Mount Sinai Sch Med 1983; **Resid:** Surgery, Lenox Hill Hosp 1988; **Fellow:** Surgical Oncology, Meml Sloan Kettering Cancer Ctr 1989

Craig, Nicholas MD (S) - **Hospital:** John T Mather Meml Hosp of Port Jefferson, St Charles Hosp; **Address:** 41 N Country Rd, Port Jefferson, NY 11777; **Phone:** 631-928-8300; **Board Cert:** Surgery 2002; **Med School:** Italy 1982; **Resid:** Surgery, Hosp of St Raphael 1988

Francfort, John MD (S) - **Spec Exp:** Breast Surgery; Gastrointestinal Surgery; Vascular Surgery; **Hospital:** Good Samaritan Hosp Med Ctr - West Islip, Southside Hosp; **Address:** 580 Union Blvd, West Islip, NY 11795; **Phone:** 631-321-6801; **Board Cert:** Surgery 1996; Vascular Surgery 1997; **Med School:** UMDNJ-NJ Med Sch, Newark 1980; **Resid:** Surgery, Hosp Univ PA 1986; **Fellow:** Vascular Surgery, Northwesten Univ 1987; **Fac Appt:** Asst Clin Prof S, SUNY Stony Brook

Gallagher, John F MD (S) - **Spec Exp:** Vascular Surgery; **Hospital:** Southside Hosp; **Address:** 580 Union Blvd, West Islip, NY 11795; **Phone:** 631-321-6801; **Board Cert:** Surgery 2003; **Med School:** Univ Chicago-Pritzker Sch Med 1974; **Resid:** Surgery, New York Hosp 1976; Surgery, New York Hosp 1981; **Fellow:** Vascular Surgery, Newark Beth Israel 1982

Green, Stephen MD (S) - **Spec Exp:** Breast Disease; Breast Surgery; **Hospital:** Brookhaven Meml Hosp & Med Ctr; **Address:** 285 Sills Rd, Bldg 2 - Ste A, E Patchogue, NY 11772-4855; **Phone:** 631-475-8846; **Board Cert:** Surgery 1975; **Med School:** NYU Sch Med 1966; **Resid:** Surgery, Bronx Municipal Hosp 1972

Karpeh Jr, Martin S MD (S) - **Spec Exp:** Gastrointestinal Cancer; Esophageal Cancer; Colon & Rectal Cancer; **Hospital:** Stony Brook Univ Hosp; **Address:** Stony Brook Univ Hosp, Hlth Science Ctr, Fl T18 - rm 060, Stony Brook, NY 11794-8191; **Phone:** 631-444-1793; **Board Cert:** Surgery 1998; **Med School:** Penn State Univ-Hershey Med Ctr 1983; **Resid:** Surgery, Hosp Univ Penn 1989; **Fellow:** Surgical Oncology, Memorial Sloan Kettering Cancer Ctr 1991; **Fac Appt:** Prof S, SUNY Stony Brook

Klausner, Stanley MD (S) - **Spec Exp:** Breast Surgery; **Hospital:** Brookhaven Meml Hosp & Med Ctr; **Address:** 285 Sills Rd, Ste 2-A, Patchogue, NY 11772; **Phone:** 631-475-8846; **Board Cert:** Surgery 1975; **Med School:** NYU Sch Med 1967; **Resid:** Surgery, Bronx Muni Hosp 1973

Martin, William MD (S) - **Spec Exp:** Breast Surgery; Laparoscopic Surgery; Vascular Surgery; **Hospital:** Huntington Hosp; **Address:** 325 Park Ave, Huntington, NY 11743-2779; **Phone:** 631-351-3758; **Board Cert:** Surgery 1999; Vascular Surgery 2005; **Med School:** Univ VT Coll Med 1985; **Resid:** Surgery, Mount Sinai Hosp 1990; **Fellow:** Vascular Surgery, Mount Sinai Hosp 1991

McCormick, Ellen MD (S) - **Hospital:** Southside Hosp, Good Samaritan Hosp Med Ctr - West Islip; **Address:** 580 Union Blvd, West Islip, NY 11795; **Phone:** 631-321-6801; **Board Cert:** Surgery 1997; Internal Medicine 1982; **Med School:** Georgetown Univ 1978; **Resid:** Internal Medicine, Vanderbilt Univ Hosp 1981; Surgery, Med Univ SC 1986

O'Hea, Brian MD (S) - **Spec Exp:** Breast Cancer; Sentinel Node Surgery; **Hospital:** Stony Brook Univ Hosp; **Address:** SUNY Stony Brook, Dept Surg, HSC T-18, Rm 060, Stony Brook, NY 11794-8191; **Phone:** 631-444-1795; **Board Cert:** Surgery 1992; **Med School:** Georgetown Univ 1986; **Resid:** Surgery, St Vincent's Hosp 1991; **Fellow:** Breast Disease, Meml Sloan-Kettering Cancer Ctr 1996; **Fac Appt:** Asst Prof S, SUNY Stony Brook

Prichep, Robert MD (S) - **Spec Exp:** Laparoscopic Surgery; Liver Tumors; Vascular Surgery; **Hospital:** Brookhaven Meml Hosp & Med Ctr, St Charles Hosp; **Address:** 286 Sills Rd, Ste 5, East Patchogue, NY 11772; **Phone:** 631-654-9090; **Board Cert:** Surgery 1999; **Med School:** Mexico 1980; **Resid:** Surgery, Maimonides Med Ctr 1986; **Fellow:** Vascular Surgery, Maimonides Med Ctr 1987

Robinson, John C MD (S) - **Spec Exp:** Cancer Surgery; Hernia; **Hospital:** St Catherine's of Siena Med Ctr; **Address:** 48 Route 25A, Ste 102, Smithtown, NY 11787; **Phone:** 631-360-1720; **Board Cert:** Surgery 1998; **Med School:** Washington Univ, St Louis 1970; **Resid:** Surgery, Jewish Hosp 1976; **Fellow:** Surgery, Mass Genl Hosp 1978

Sclafani, Lisa MD (S) - **Spec Exp:** Breast Surgery; Cancer Surgery; **Hospital:** Meml Sloan Kettering Cancer Ctr (page 109); **Address:** Meml Sloan Kettering at Suffolk, 650 Commack Rd, Commack, NY 11725; **Phone:** 631-623-4050; **Board Cert:** Surgery 1997; **Med School:** NYU Sch Med 1982; **Resid:** Surgery, Albert Einstein Coll Med 1987; **Fellow:** Surgical Oncology, Meml Sloan Kettering Cancer Ctr 1989; **Fac Appt:** Assoc Clin Prof S, Cornell Univ-Weill Med Coll

Shapiro, Marc MD (S) - **Spec Exp:** Laparoscopic Surgery; Minimally Invasive Surgery; Burn Care; **Hospital:** Stony Brook Univ Hosp; **Address:** Stony Brook Univ Hosp, Nicolls Rd HSC T-18 Bldg - rm 040, Stony Brook, NY 11794-8191; **Phone:** 631-444-1045; **Board Cert:** Surgery 1994; Surgical Critical Care 1995; **Med School:** Univ Mich Med Sch 1979; **Resid:** Surgery, Henry Ford Hosp 1984; **Fellow:** Critical Care Medicine, Univ Pittsburgh Hosp 1985; **Fac Appt:** Prof S, SUNY Stony Brook

Simon, John MD (S) - **Spec Exp:** Laparoscopic Surgery; **Hospital:** Southside Hosp, Good Samaritan Hosp Med Ctr - West Islip; **Address:** 580 Union Blvd, West Islip, NY 11795; **Phone:** 631-321-6801; **Board Cert:** Surgery 1992; **Med School:** India 1981; **Resid:** Surgery, NY Infirm/Beekman Downtown Hosp 1987

Zingale, Robert MD (S) - **Spec Exp:** Laparoscopic Surgery; Breast Disease; **Hospital:** Huntington Hosp; **Address:** 158 E Main St, Ste 7, Huntington, NY 11743-2988; **Phone:** 631-271-1822; **Board Cert:** Surgery 1998; Surgical Critical Care 1999; **Med School:** SUNY Downstate 1983; **Resid:** Surgery, Maimonides Med Ctr 1988; **Fellow:** Trauma, Coney Island Hosp 1989; **Fac Appt:** Assoc Clin Prof S, NY Med Coll

THORACIC SURGERY

Bilfinger, Thomas MD (TS) - **Spec Exp:** Cardiac Surgery-Adult; Burn Care; Lung Cancer; **Hospital:** Stony Brook Univ Hosp; **Address:** Univ Hosp & Med Ctr-StonyBrook/Div Cardiothoracic Surgery, HSC 19, rm 080, Stony Brook, NY 11794-8191; **Phone:** 631-444-1820; **Board Cert:** Surgery 1996; Thoracic Surgery 1998; Surgical Critical Care 2000; **Med School:** Switzerland 1978; **Resid:** Surgery, Univ Chicago 1982; Surgery, Univ TX Med Branch Hosp 1986; **Fellow:** Thoracic Surgery, Univ TX Med Branch Hosp 1988; **Fac Appt:** Prof S, SUNY Stony Brook

Dranitzke, Richard MD (TS) - **Spec Exp:** Lung Surgery; Vascular Surgery; Endovascular Surgery; **Hospital:** St Charles Hosp, John T Mather Meml Hosp of Port Jefferson; **Address:** 635 Belle Terre Rd, Ste 201, Port Jefferson, NY 11777; **Phone:** 631-473-1602; **Board Cert:** Thoracic Surgery 1995; Surgery 1974; **Med School:** Columbia P&S 1966; **Resid:** Surgery, Bellevue Hosp 1972; Thoracic Surgery, Albany Med Ctr 1975

Palatt, Terry MD (TS) - **Spec Exp:** Lung Disease; **Hospital:** Good Samaritan Hosp Med Ctr - West Islip, Southside Hosp; **Address:** 111 Carleton Ave, Ste 2A, Islip Terrace, NY 11752; **Phone:** 631-581-4400; **Board Cert:** Thoracic Surgery 1999; Surgery 1997; **Med School:** Grenada 1981; **Resid:** Surgery, Maimonides Med Ctr 1986; Thoracic Surgery, Maimonides Medical Ctr 1988

Rubenstein, Richard B MD (TS) - **Spec Exp:** Vascular Surgery; Obesity/Bariatric Surgery; **Hospital:** Brookhaven Meml Hosp & Med Ctr; **Address:** 250 Yaphank Rd, Ste 7, E Patchogue, NY 11772; **Phone:** 631-475-1013; **Board Cert:** Thoracic Surgery 2001; **Med School:** SUNY Downstate 1972; **Resid:** Surgery, Beth Israe Med Ctrl 1977; Thoracic Surgery, Charlotte Meml Hosp 1979; **Fellow:** Cardiothoracic Surgery, Mayo Clinic; **Fac Appt:** Assoc Clin Prof S, SUNY Stony Brook

UROLOGY

Beccia, David MD (U) - **Spec Exp:** Prostate Cancer; Erectile Dysfunction; **Hospital:** Southside Hosp, Good Samaritan Hosp Med Ctr - West Islip; **Address:** 332 E Main St, Bay Shore, NY 11706-8404; **Phone:** 631-665-3737; **Board Cert:** Urology 1979; **Med School:** NY Med Coll 1970; **Resid:** Surgery, Hartford Hosp 1973; Urology, Boston Univ Med Ctr 1977

Cruickshank, David MD (U) - **Spec Exp:** Vasectomy-Scalpelless; Prostate Benign Disease; Kidney Stones; **Hospital:** Southampton Hosp, Eastern Long Island Hosp; **Address:** 315 Meeting House Ln, Box 1523, Southampton, NY 11968-5051; **Phone:** 631-283-0323; **Board Cert:** Urology 1978; **Med School:** SUNY Downstate 1970; **Resid:** Surgery, St Vincent's Hosp 1972; Urology, Kings Co Hosp/SUNY 1976; **Fac Appt:** Asst Clin Prof U, SUNY Stony Brook

Frischer, Zelik MD (U) - **Spec Exp:** Transplant-Kidney; Urologic Cancer; Uro-Gynecology; Reconstructive Surgery; **Hospital:** Stony Brook Univ Hosp, St Catherine's of Siena Med Ctr; **Address:** 2500 Nesconset Hwy, Ste 23B, Stony Brook, NY 11790; **Phone:** 631-444-6270; **Board Cert:** Urology 2000; **Med School:** Russia 1960; **Resid:** Urology, Leningrad Second Mercy Hosp 1969; Urology, Belinson Med Ctr 1978; **Fellow:** Urology, Beth Israel Hosp 1986; **Fac Appt:** Prof U, SUNY Stony Brook

Mills, Carl MD (U) - **Spec Exp:** Urologic Cancer; **Hospital:** St Charles Hosp, Brookhaven Meml Hosp & Med Ctr; **Address:** 250 Yaphank Rd, Ste 15, East Patchogue, NY 11772; **Phone:** 631-475-5051; **Board Cert:** Urology 1984; **Med School:** Geo Wash Univ 1975; **Resid:** Surgery, New York Hosp 1978; Urology, New York Hosp 1982

Pastore, Louis T MD (U) - **Spec Exp:** Urologic Cancer; Kidney Stones; Urology-Female; **Hospital:** Brookhaven Meml Hosp & Med Ctr, John T Mather Meml Hosp of Port Jefferson; **Address:** 250 Yaphank Rd, Ste 15, East Patchogue, NY 11772; **Phone:** 631-475-5051; **Board Cert:** Urology 1974; **Med School:** Canada 1965; **Resid:** Urology, Kings County Hosp 1967

Wasnick, Robert MD (U) - **Spec Exp:** Hypospadias; Undescended Testis; Pediatric Urology; **Hospital:** Stony Brook Univ Hosp, St Charles Hosp; **Address:** Stony Brook Medical Park, 24 Research Way, Ste 500, Setauket, NY 11733; **Phone:** 631-444-6270; **Board Cert:** Urology 1982; **Med School:** Jefferson Med Coll 1974; **Resid:** Surgery, St Vincents Hosp Med Ctr 1977; Urology, Downstate Med Ctr 1980; **Fellow:** Pediatric Urology, Alder Hey Chldns Hosp 1981; **Fac Appt:** Clin Prof U, SUNY Stony Brook

VASCULAR SURGERY

Arnold, Thomas E MD (VascS) - **Spec Exp:** Carotid Artery Surgery; Aneurysm-Abdominal Aortic; Varicose Veins; **Hospital:** John T Mather Meml Hosp of Port Jefferson, St Charles Hosp; **Address:** 5225 Route 347, Ste 60, Port Jefferson, NY 11776; **Phone:** 631-476-9100; **Board Cert:** Surgery 2003; Vascular Surgery 2003; **Med School:** SUNY Downstate 1985; **Resid:** Surgery, Presbyterian Med Ctr/Univ Penn 1987; Surgery, Medical Coll Penn 1991

Gredysa, Leslaw MD (VascS) - **Hospital:** Southampton Hosp, Peconic Bay Med Ctr; **Address:** 234 Hampton Rd, Southampton, NY 11968; **Phone:** 631-287-1433; **Board Cert:** Surgery 1995; **Med School:** Poland 1982; **Resid:** Surgery, Biernacki Med Ctr 1983; Surgery, Wyckoff Heights Hosp 1988; **Fellow:** Vascular Surgery, Nassau County Med Ctr 1992

Pollina, Robert M MD (VascS) - **Spec Exp:** Varicose Veins; Aneurysm; Carotid Artery Surgery; Endovascular Surgery; **Hospital:** John T Mather Meml Hosp of Port Jefferson, St Charles Hosp; **Address:** 5225-60 Rte 347, Port Jefferson, NY 11776; **Phone:** 631-476-9100; **Board Cert:** Surgery 1994; Vascular Surgery 1998; **Med School:** SUNY Hlth Sci Ctr 1988; **Resid:** Surgery, Kings County Hosp 1992; **Fellow:** Vascular Surgery, Maimonides Medical Ctr 1994

Ricotta, John MD (VascS) - **Spec Exp:** Aneurysm; Carotid Artery Surgery; **Hospital:** Stony Brook Univ Hosp; **Address:** SUNY HSC, Dept Surgery, HSC T19, rm 020, Stony Brook, NY 11794-8191; **Phone:** 631-444-7875; **Board Cert:** Surgery 2000; Vascular Surgery 1995; **Med School:** Johns Hopkins Univ 1973; **Resid:** Surgery, Johns Hopkins Hosp 1977; **Fellow:** Vascular Surgery, Johns Hopkins Hosp 1979; **Fac Appt:** Prof S, Johns Hopkins Univ

Westchester

Westchester

ALLERGY & IMMUNOLOGY

Dattwyler, Raymond MD (A&I) - **Spec Exp:** Allergy; Immune Deficiency; Tick-borne Diseases; Lyme Disease; **Hospital:** Westchester Med Ctr (page 713); **Address:** Allergy, Immunology And Rheumatology, NYMC-Munger Pavilion, rm G73, Valhalla, NY 10595; **Phone:** 914-594-4444; **Board Cert:** Internal Medicine 1977; Allergy & Immunology 1979; Clinical & Laboratory Immunology 1986; **Med School:** SUNY Buffalo 1973; **Resid:** Internal Medicine, New England Med Ctr 1977; **Fellow:** Immunology, Mayo Clinic 1976; Clinical Immunology, Mass General Hosp 1978; **Fac Appt:** Prof Med, SUNY Stony Brook

Fusillo, Christine MD (A&I) - **Spec Exp:** Asthma & Allergy; Food Allergy; Drug Sensitivity; **Hospital:** Westchester Med Ctr (page 713); **Address:** 55 S Broadway, Tarrytown, NY 10591-4000; **Phone:** 914-631-3283; **Board Cert:** Pediatrics 1986; Allergy & Immunology 1987; **Med School:** NYU Sch Med 1980; **Resid:** Pediatrics, Bellevue Hosp-NYU 1983; **Fellow:** Allergy & Immunology, St Luke's-Roosevelt Hosp Ctr 1987

Geraci-Ciardullo, Kira MD (A&I) - **Spec Exp:** Asthma; Sinus Disorders; Food Allergy; Insect Allergies; **Hospital:** White Plains Hosp Ctr (page 714), Sound Shore Med Ctr - Westchester (page 711); **Address:** 1600 Harrison Ave, Ste 304, Rockledge Plaza, Mamaroneck, NY 10543-3145; **Phone:** 914-777-1179; **Board Cert:** Pediatrics 1984; Allergy & Immunology 1997; **Med School:** Columbia P&S 1980; **Resid:** Pediatrics, NY-Cornell Hosp 1983; **Fellow:** Allergy & Immunology, NY-Cornell Hosp 1985

Goldman, Neil C MD (A&I) - **Spec Exp:** Asthma; Drug Sensitivity; Sinusitis; **Hospital:** Hudson Valley Hosp Ctr, Phelps Meml Hosp Ctr; **Address:** 35 S Riverside Ave, Ste 106, Croton On Hudson, NY 10520-2653; **Phone:** 914-271-0001; **Board Cert:** Allergy & Immunology 1977; **Med School:** NY Med Coll 1966; **Resid:** Internal Medicine, Beth Israel Hosp 1968; Internal Medicine, Metropolitan Hosp Ctr 1969; **Fellow:** Allergy & Immunology, Jewish Hosp 1970

Mendelsohn, Lois MD (A&I) - **Spec Exp:** Asthma; Hay Fever; Food Allergy; Eczema; **Hospital:** Northern Westchester Hosp; **Address:** 103 S Bedford Rd, Ste 208, Mt Kisco, NY 10549; **Phone:** 914-666-7171; **Board Cert:** Internal Medicine 1989; Allergy & Immunology 2001; **Med School:** NY Med Coll 1986; **Resid:** Internal Medicine, Lenox Hill Hosp 1989; **Fellow:** Allergy & Immunology, Mt Sinai Hosp 1991

Pollowitz, James MD (A&I) - **Spec Exp:** Asthma; Food Allergy; Hives; **Hospital:** White Plains Hosp Ctr (page 714), Lawrence Hosp Ctr; **Address:** 281 Garth Rd, Ste A, Scarsdale, NY 10583-4034; **Phone:** 914-472-3833; **Board Cert:** Pediatrics 1978; Allergy & Immunology 1979; **Med School:** NYU Sch Med 1973; **Resid:** Pediatrics, Bronx Muni Hosp Ctr 1976; **Fellow:** Allergy & Immunology, St Vincent Med Ctr 1978; **Fac Appt:** Asst Clin Prof Ped, NY Med Coll

CARDIAC ELECTROPHYSIOLOGY

Cohen, Martin B MD (CE) - **Spec Exp:** Interventional Cardiology; Pacemakers; Defibrillators; **Hospital:** Westchester Med Ctr (page 713); **Address:** 19 Bradhurst Ave, Ste 700, Hawthorne, NY 10532-2140; **Phone:** 914-593-7800; **Board Cert:** Internal Medicine 1983; Cardiovascular Disease 1985; Cardiac Electrophysiology 1996; Interventional Cardiology 2004; **Med School:** SUNY Downstate 1980; **Resid:** Internal Medicine, Univ Hosp 1983; **Fellow:** Cardiovascular Disease, Univ Hosp 1985; Interventional Cardiology, Westchester Co Med Ctr 1986; **Fac Appt:** Assoc Clin Prof Med, NY Med Coll

Rubin, David Albert MD (CE) - **Spec Exp:** Arrhythmias; Radiofrequency Ablation; Pacemakers/Defibrillators; **Hospital:** NY-Presby Hosp (page 100); **Address:** 222 Westchester Ave, White Plains, NY 10604-2906; **Phone:** 914-428-3888; **Board Cert:** Internal Medicine 1978; Cardiovascular Disease 1981; Cardiac Electrophysiology 2002; **Med School:** Columbia P&S 1975; **Resid:** Internal Medicine, Columbia-Presby Hosp 1978; **Fellow:** Cardiovascular Disease, Mount Sinai Hosp 1980; **Fac Appt:** Clin Prof Med, Columbia P&S

CARDIOVASCULAR DISEASE

Bleiberg, Melvyn MD (Cv) - **Hospital:** Saint Joseph's Med Ctr - Yonkers, Westchester Med Ctr (page 713); **Address:** 127 S Broadway, Yonkers, NY 10701; **Phone:** 914-965-6060; **Board Cert:** Internal Medicine 1978; Cardiovascular Disease 1981; **Med School:** Albert Einstein Coll Med 1974; **Resid:** Internal Medicine, Brookdale Hosp 1977; **Fellow:** Cardiovascular Disease, Brookdale Hosp 1979

Cooper, Jerome MD (Cv) - **Spec Exp:** Coronary Artery Disease; Hypertension; Heart Valve Disease; **Hospital:** Sound Shore Med Ctr - Westchester (page 711), NY-Presby Hosp (page 100); **Address:** 150 Lockwood Ave, Ste 28, New Rochelle, NY 10801; **Phone:** 914-633-7870; **Board Cert:** Internal Medicine 1968; Cardiovascular Disease 1973; **Med School:** SUNY Hlth Sci Ctr 1961; **Resid:** Internal Medicine, Baltimore City Hosps 1963; Cardiovascular Disease, Montefiore Hosp Med Ctr 1964; **Fellow:** Cardiovascular Disease, Johns Hopkins 1966; Cardiovascular Disease, Johns Hopkins 1967; **Fac Appt:** Assoc Clin Prof Med, Columbia P&S

De Martino, Anthony G. MD (Cv) - **Spec Exp:** Heart Disease; Hypertension; Congestive Heart Failure; **Hospital:** Lawrence Hosp Ctr; **Address:** 77 Pondfield Rd, Bronxville, NY 10708-3809; **Phone:** 914-337-2033; **Board Cert:** Internal Medicine 1967; Cardiovascular Disease 1975; **Med School:** SUNY Downstate 1957; **Resid:** Internal Medicine, Kings County Hosp 1962; **Fellow:** Cardiovascular Disease, New York Hosp 1964; **Fac Appt:** Asst Clin Prof Med, NY Med Coll

Epstein, Stanley MD (Cv) - **Spec Exp:** Non-Invasive Cardiology; Preventive Cardiology; Hypertension; Cholesterol/Lipid Disorders; **Hospital:** NY-Presby Hosp (page 100), Lawrence Hosp Ctr; **Address:** 688 White Plains Rd, Scarsdale, NY 10583-5059; **Phone:** 914-722-6300; **Board Cert:** Internal Medicine 1967; Cardiovascular Disease 1975; **Med School:** Univ Hlth Sci/Chicago Med Sch 1958; **Resid:** Internal Medicine, Jewish Hosp 1960; Internal Medicine, San Francisco Genl Hosp 1961; **Fellow:** Cardiovascular Disease, Montefiore Hosp Med Ctr 1967; **Fac Appt:** Clin Prof Med, Columbia P&S

Fass, Arthur MD (Cv) - **Spec Exp:** Preventive Cardiology; Coronary Artery Disease; Hypertension; **Hospital:** Phelps Meml Hosp Ctr, Westchester Med Ctr (page 713); **Address:** 465 N State Rd, Briarcliff Manor, NY 10510; **Phone:** 914-762-5810; **Board Cert:** Internal Medicine 1979; Cardiovascular Disease 1981; **Med School:** NY Med Coll 1976; **Resid:** Internal Medicine, Metro Hosp 1979; **Fellow:** Cardiovascular Disease, Westchester Med Ctr 1981; **Fac Appt:** Assoc Clin Prof Med, NY Med Coll

Feld, Michael MD (Cv) - **Spec Exp:** Pacemakers; Coronary Artery Disease; **Hospital:** Phelps Meml Hosp Ctr, Comm Hosp - Dobbs Ferry; **Address:** 200 S Broadway, Ste E, Tarrytown, NY 10591-4500; **Phone:** 914-631-2895; **Board Cert:** Internal Medicine 1980; Cardiovascular Disease 1983; **Med School:** Penn State Univ-Hershey Med Ctr 1977; **Resid:** Internal Medicine, Montefiore Hosp Med Ctr 1980; **Fellow:** Cardiovascular Disease, Montefiore Hosp Med Ctr 1983; **Fac Appt:** Asst Clin Prof Med, Albert Einstein Coll Med

Fishbach, Mitchell MD (Cv) - **Spec Exp:** Non-Invasive Cardiology; Sports Medicine; **Hospital:** Lawrence Hosp Ctr, Montefiore Med Ctr; **Address:** 688 White Plains Rd, Ste 201, Scarsdale, NY 10583; **Phone:** 914-722-6300; **Board Cert:** Internal Medicine 1980; Cardiovascular Disease 1983; **Med School:** Albert Einstein Coll Med 1977; **Resid:** Internal Medicine, Montefiore Hosp Med Ctr 1978; Internal Medicine, Montefiore Hosp Med Ctr 1980; **Fellow:** Cardiovascular Disease, Montefiore Hosp Med Ctr 1982

Frishman, William MD (Cv) - **Spec Exp:** Coronary Artery Disease; Preventive Cardiology; Hypertension; Heart Failure; **Hospital:** Westchester Med Ctr (page 713); **Address:** NY Med Coll, Dept Med/Westchester Med Ctr, Munger Pavilion, rm 263, Valhalla, NY 10595; **Phone:** 914-594-4383; **Board Cert:** Internal Medicine 1997; Cardiovascular Disease 1997; Geriatric Medicine 2002; **Med School:** Boston Univ 1969; **Resid:** Internal Medicine, Montefiore Hosp Med Ctr 1971; Internal Medicine, Bronx Muni Hosp 1972; **Fellow:** Cardiovascular Disease, New York Hosp 1974; **Fac Appt:** Prof Med, NY Med Coll

Gabelman, Gary MD (Cv) - **Spec Exp:** Non-Invasive Cardiology; Echocardiography; Nuclear Cardiology; **Hospital:** Lawrence Hosp Ctr, NY-Presby Hosp (page 100); **Address:** 688 White Plains Rd, Scarsdale, NY 10583; **Phone:** 914-722-6300; **Board Cert:** Internal Medicine 1988; Cardiovascular Disease 2001; **Med School:** Mount Sinai Sch Med 1985; **Resid:** Internal Medicine, Montefiore Hosp Med Ctr 1989; **Fellow:** Cardiovascular Disease, Montefiore Hosp Med Ctr 1991; **Fac Appt:** Assoc Clin Prof Med, Columbia P&S

Gitler, Bernard MD (Cv) - **Spec Exp:** Heart Valve Disease; Sports Medicine-Cardiology; Nuclear Stress Testing; Coronary Artery Disease; **Hospital:** Sound Shore Med Ctr - Westchester (page 711), NY-Presby Hosp (page 100); **Address:** 150 Lockwood Ave, Ste 28, New Rochelle, NY 10801-4913; **Phone:** 914-633-7870; **Board Cert:** Internal Medicine 1998; Cardiovascular Disease 1998; Critical Care Medicine 1999; **Med School:** Cornell Univ-Weill Med Coll 1976; **Resid:** Internal Medicine, Jacobi Med Ctr 1979; **Fellow:** Cardiovascular Disease, Montefiore Hosp Med Ctr 1981; **Fac Appt:** Assoc Clin Prof Med, Albert Einstein Coll Med

Golier, Francis MD (Cv) - **Spec Exp:** Transesophageal Echocardiography; Stress Echocardiography; **Hospital:** Phelps Meml Hosp Ctr, Montefiore Med Ctr; **Address:** 200 S Broadway, Tarrytown, NY 10591-4500; **Phone:** 914-631-2895; **Board Cert:** Internal Medicine 1972; Cardiovascular Disease 1978; **Med School:** Med Coll Wisc 1969; **Resid:** Internal Medicine, Lenox Hill Hosp 1972; **Fellow:** Cardiovascular Disease, Montefiore Hosp Med Ctr 1974; **Fac Appt:** Asst Clin Prof Med, Albert Einstein Coll Med

Greif, Richard MD (Cv) - **Hospital:** Saint Joseph's Med Ctr - Yonkers; **Address:** 127 S Broadway, Yonkers, NY 10701; **Phone:** 914-378-7584; **Board Cert:** Internal Medicine 1978; Cardiovascular Disease 1981; **Med School:** NY Med Coll 1975; **Resid:** Internal Medicine, Metropolitan Hosp 1978; **Fellow:** Cardiovascular Disease, St Vincents Hosp 1981; **Fac Appt:** Assoc Clin Prof Med, NY Med Coll

Kay, Richard H MD (Cv) - **Spec Exp:** Preventive Cardiology; Congestive Heart Failure; Non-Invasive Cardiology; **Hospital:** Westchester Med Ctr (page 713); **Address:** 19 Bradhurst Ave, Ste 700, Hawthorne, NY 10532-2140; **Phone:** 914-593-7800; **Board Cert:** Internal Medicine 1979; Cardiovascular Disease 1981; **Med School:** Johns Hopkins Univ 1976; **Resid:** Internal Medicine, Columbia-Presby Med Ctr 1979; **Fellow:** Cardiovascular Disease, Mount Sinai Hosp 1981; **Fac Appt:** Assoc Prof Med, NY Med Coll

Keltz, Theodore MD (Cv) - **Spec Exp:** Echocardiography; Nuclear Cardiology; **Hospital:** Sound Shore Med Ctr - Westchester (page 711), NY-Presby Hosp (page 100); **Address:** 150 Lockwood Ave, Ste 28, New Rochelle, NY 10801-4913; **Phone:** 914-633-7870; **Board Cert:** Internal Medicine 1983; Cardiovascular Disease 1985; Critical Care Medicine 1989; **Med School:** Albany Med Coll 1980; **Resid:** Internal Medicine, Mount Sinai 1983; **Fellow:** Cardiovascular Disease, Montefiore Hosp Med Ctr 1985; **Fac Appt:** Assoc Clin Prof Med, Albert Einstein Coll Med

Levine, Evan MD (Cv) - **Spec Exp:** Cardiac Stress Testing; Weight Reduction; **Hospital:** Montefiore Med Ctr, St John's Riverside Hosp; **Address:** Riverside Cardiology, 955 Yonkers Ave, Ste 200, Yonkers, NY 10704; **Phone:** 914-237-1332; **Board Cert:** Internal Medicine 1988; Cardiovascular Disease 2000; **Med School:** Mount Sinai Sch Med 1985; **Resid:** Internal Medicine, Montefiore Med Ctr 1988; **Fellow:** Cardiovascular Disease, Montefiore Med Ctr 1990; **Fac Appt:** Asst Clin Prof Med, Albert Einstein Coll Med

Matos, Marshall MD (Cv) - **Spec Exp:** Coronary Artery Disease; Preventive Cardiology; Arrhythmias; Cholesterol/Lipid Disorders; **Hospital:** Sound Shore Med Ctr - Westchester (page 711), NYU Med Ctr (page 102); **Address:** 140 Lockwood Ave, Ste 310, New Rochelle, NY 10801-4909; **Phone:** 914-576-7171; **Board Cert:** Internal Medicine 1983; Cardiovascular Disease 1985; **Med School:** Albert Einstein Coll Med 1977; **Resid:** Internal Medicine, Bronx Muni Hosp 1981; **Fellow:** Cardiovascular Disease, Albert Einstein Coll Med 1983; **Fac Appt:** Asst Prof Med, NYU Sch Med

McClung, John A MD (Cv) - **Spec Exp:** Echocardiography; **Hospital:** Westchester Med Ctr (page 713); **Address:** 19 Bradhurst Ave, Ste 700, Hawthorne, NY 10532; **Phone:** 914-593-7800; **Board Cert:** Internal Medicine 1980; Cardiovascular Disease 1983; **Med School:** NY Med Coll 1975; **Resid:** Internal Medicine, Lincoln Med Ctr 1979; Internal Medicine, Our Lady of Mercy Hosp 1979; **Fellow:** Cardiovascular Disease, Westchester Med Ctr 1982; **Fac Appt:** Assoc Prof Med, NY Med Coll

Medina, Emma MD (Cv) - **Spec Exp:** Non-Invasive Cardiology; **Hospital:** Sound Shore Med Ctr - Westchester (page 711), Montefiore Med Ctr - Weiler-Einstein Div; **Address:** 140 Lockwood Ave, Ste 310, New Rochelle, NY 10801-4909; **Phone:** 914-632-1600; **Board Cert:** Internal Medicine 1982; Cardiovascular Disease 1985; **Med School:** NYU Sch Med 1979; **Resid:** Internal Medicine, Jacobi Med Ctr 1982; **Fellow:** Cardiovascular Disease, Jacobi Med Ctr 1984; **Fac Appt:** Asst Clin Prof Med, Albert Einstein Coll Med

Mercando, Anthony MD (Cv) - **Spec Exp:** Cholesterol/Lipid Disorders; Pacemakers/Defibrillators; Preventive Cardiology; **Hospital:** Lawrence Hosp Ctr, NY-Presby Hosp (page 100); **Address:** 688 White Plains Rd, Ste 201, Scarsdale, NY 10583; **Phone:** 914-722-6300; **Board Cert:** Internal Medicine 1983; Cardiovascular Disease 1987; **Med School:** Harvard Med Sch 1980; **Resid:** Internal Medicine, Montefiore Hosp Med Ctr 1984; **Fellow:** Cardiovascular Disease, Montefiore Hosp Med Ctr 1986; **Fac Appt:** Assoc Clin Prof Med, Columbia P&S

Mercurio, Peter MD (Cv) - **Spec Exp:** Echocardiography; Stress Echocardiography; Nuclear Cardiology; **Hospital:** Northern Westchester Hosp, Westchester Med Ctr (page 713); **Address:** 1888 Commerce St, Yorktown Heights, NY 10598-4431; **Phone:** 914-962-4000; **Board Cert:** Internal Medicine 1978; Cardiovascular Disease 1983; **Med School:** NYU Sch Med 1975; **Resid:** Internal Medicine, Bellevue Hosp 1979; **Fellow:** Cardiovascular Disease, Bellevue Hosp 1981; **Fac Appt:** Asst Clin Prof Med, NYU Sch Med

Monteferrante, Judith MD (Cv) - **Spec Exp:** Nuclear Cardiology; Heart Disease in Women; Preventive Cardiology; **Hospital:** White Plains Hosp Ctr (page 714), Westchester Med Ctr (page 713); **Address:** Primary Care & Cardiovascular Assocs, 15 N Broadway Fl 2, White Plains, NY 10601; **Phone:** 914-428-6000; **Board Cert:** Internal Medicine 1981; Cardiovascular Disease 1985; **Med School:** Mount Sinai Sch Med 1978; **Resid:** Internal Medicine, St Vincent's Hosp 1981; **Fellow:** Cardiovascular Disease, Westchester Med Ctr 1983; **Fac Appt:** Asst Clin Prof Med, NY Med Coll

Ozick, Hershel MD (Cv) - **Spec Exp:** Preventive Cardiology; Hypertension; Heart Failure; **Hospital:** Sound Shore Med Ctr - Westchester (page 711), NY-Presby Hosp (page 100); **Address:** 175 Memorial Hwy, Ste 1-1, New Rochelle, NY 10801; **Phone:** 914-235-3535; **Board Cert:** Internal Medicine 1980; Cardiovascular Disease 1983; Critical Care Medicine 1999; **Med School:** NYU Sch Med 1977; **Resid:** Internal Medicine, Downstate Med Ctr 1980; **Fellow:** Cardiovascular Disease, Maimonides Medical Ctr 1983; **Fac Appt:** Asst Clin Prof Med, NY Med Coll

Perry-Bottinger, Lynne MD (Cv) - **Spec Exp:** Cardiac Catheterization; Coronary Angioplasty/Stents; Heart Disease in Women; **Hospital:** NY-Presby Hosp (page 100), Sound Shore Med Ctr - Westchester (page 711); **Address:** Clinical & Interventional Cardiology, 140A Lockwood Ave, New Rochelle, NY 10801; **Phone:** 914-576-7577; **Board Cert:** Cardiovascular Disease 1997; **Med School:** Yale Univ 1986; **Resid:** Internal Medicine, Yale-New Haven Hosp 1990; **Fellow:** Cardiovascular Disease, Johns Hopkins Hosp 1993; Interventional Cardiology, Johns Hopkins Hosp 1994; **Fac Appt:** Asst Clin Prof Med, Columbia P&S

Price Jr, Thomas J MD (Cv) - **Hospital:** Mount Vernon Hosp (page 712), Sound Shore Med Ctr - Westchester (page 711); **Address:** 105 Stevens Ave, Ste 603, Mt Vernon, NY 10550; **Phone:** 914-664-4052; **Board Cert:** Internal Medicine 1984; Cardiovascular Disease 1987; **Med School:** Univ Cincinnati 1975; **Resid:** Internal Medicine, Harlem Hosp 1979; **Fellow:** Cardiovascular Disease, Harlem Hosp 1983; **Fac Appt:** Asst Clin Prof Med, Columbia P&S

Pucillo, Anthony MD (Cv) - **Spec Exp:** Coronary Angioplasty/Stents; Peripheral Vascular Disease; **Hospital:** Westchester Med Ctr (page 713); **Address:** 19 Bradhurst Ave, Ste 700, Hawthorne, NY 10532; **Phone:** 914-593-7800; **Board Cert:** Internal Medicine 1981; Cardiovascular Disease 1983; Interventional Cardiology 2000; **Med School:** Mount Sinai Sch Med 1978; **Resid:** Internal Medicine, Columbia-Presby Med Ctr 1981; **Fellow:** Cardiovascular Disease, Columbia-Presby Med Ctr 1984; **Fac Appt:** Assoc Prof Med, NY Med Coll

Sheikh, Shahid MD (Cv) - **Hospital:** St John's Riverside Hosp; **Address:** 970 N Broadway, Ste 210, Yonkers, NY 10701-1311; **Phone:** 914-963-0111; **Board Cert:** Internal Medicine 1977; Cardiovascular Disease 1979; **Med School:** Pakistan 1971; **Resid:** Internal Medicine, Lady of Mercy Med Ctr 1976

Silver, Michael MD (Cv) - **Spec Exp:** Hypertension; Cholesterol/Lipid Disorders; Coronary Artery Disease; **Hospital:** White Plains Hosp Ctr (page 714); **Address:** Mid-Westchester Medical Associates, 33 Davis Ave, White Plains, NY 10605-1015; **Phone:** 914-948-3630; **Board Cert:** Internal Medicine 1980; Cardiovascular Disease 1983; **Med School:** SUNY Downstate 1977; **Resid:** Internal Medicine, Thomas Jefferson Univ Hosp 1980; **Fellow:** Cardiovascular Disease, Presby-Hosp Univ Penn 1982

Tartaglia, Joseph J MD (Cv) - **Spec Exp:** Angina; Congestive Heart Failure; Arrhythmias; **Hospital:** White Plains Hosp Ctr (page 714), Greenwich Hosp; **Address:** 311 North St, Ste 301, White Plains, NY 10605-2232; **Phone:** 914-946-3388; **Board Cert:** Internal Medicine 1988; Cardiovascular Disease 2001; Geriatric Medicine 2004; **Med School:** Italy 1984; **Resid:** Internal Medicine, Our Lady of Mercy Med Ctr 1988; **Fellow:** Cardiovascular Disease, N Shore Univ Hosp 1990; **Fac Appt:** Asst Clin Prof Med, NY Med Coll

Weiss, Melvin MD (Cv) - **Spec Exp:** Angioplasty; Congestive Heart Failure; Diabetes; Coronary Artery Disease; **Hospital:** Westchester Med Ctr (page 713); **Address:** 19 Bradhurst Ave, Ste 700, Hawthorne, NY 10532-2140; **Phone:** 914-593-7800; **Board Cert:** Internal Medicine 1972; Cardiovascular Disease 1975; Interventional Cardiology 1999; **Med School:** SUNY Hlth Sci Ctr 1967; **Resid:** Internal Medicine, New York Hosp 1971; **Fellow:** Cardiovascular Disease, Columbia P&S 1972; **Fac Appt:** Prof Med, NY Med Coll

Weissman, Ronald MD (Cv) - **Spec Exp:** Coronary Artery Disease; Congestive Heart Failure; Arrhythmias; **Hospital:** White Plains Hosp Ctr (page 714), Westchester Med Ctr (page 713); **Address:** 15 N Broadway Fl 2, White Plains, NY 10601; **Phone:** 914-428-6000; **Board Cert:** Internal Medicine 1980; Cardiovascular Disease 1983; **Med School:** NY Med Coll 1977; **Resid:** Internal Medicine, LI Jewish Hosp 1980; **Fellow:** Cardiovascular Disease, LI Jewish Hosp 1982; **Fac Appt:** Assoc Clin Prof Med, NY Med Coll

Zimmerman, Franklin (Bud) MD (Cv) - **Spec Exp:** Preventive Cardiology; Sports Medicine-Cardiology; Cholesterol/Lipid Disorders; **Hospital:** Phelps Meml Hosp Ctr, Westchester Med Ctr (page 713); **Address:** 465 N State Rd, Briarcliff Manor, NY 10510-1468; **Phone:** 914-762-5810; **Board Cert:** Internal Medicine 1983; Cardiovascular Disease 1987; Critical Care Medicine 1989; **Med School:** Brown Univ 1980; **Resid:** Internal Medicine, St Luke's-Roosevelt Hosp Ctr 1983; **Fellow:** Cardiovascular Disease, St Luke's-Roosevelt Hosp Ctr 1988; **Fac Appt:** Asst Prof Med, Columbia P&S

CHILD & ADOLESCENT PSYCHIATRY

Cohen, Lee MD (ChAP) - **Spec Exp:** Anxiety & Mood Disorders; Psychopharmacology; ADD/ADHD; **Hospital:** NY-Presby Hosp (page 100), St Luke's - Roosevelt Hosp Ctr - Roosevelt Div (page 90); **Address:** 623 Warburton Ave, Hastings On Hudson, NY 10706-1523; **Phone:** 914-478-1330; **Board Cert:** Psychiatry 1987; Child & Adolescent Psychiatry 1988; **Med School:** SUNY Stony Brook 1982; **Resid:** Pediatrics, Mount Sinai 1983; Psychiatry, Mount Sinai 1985; **Fellow:** Child & Adolescent Psychiatry, Columbia-Presby 1987; **Fac Appt:** Asst Clin Prof Psyc, Columbia P&S

Hajal, Fady MD (ChAP) - **Spec Exp:** ADD/ADHD; Anxiety Disorders; Mood Disorders; **Hospital:** Stony Lodge Hosp; **Address:** Stony Lodge Hospital, 40 Croton Dam Rd, Ossining, NY 10562; **Phone:** 914-941-7400; **Board Cert:** Psychiatry 1976; Child & Adolescent Psychiatry 1979; **Med School:** Lebanon 1968; **Resid:** Psychiatry, Boston City Hosp 1972; **Fellow:** Child & Adolescent Psychiatry, Univ Mich Med Ctr 1974

Hyler, Irene MD (ChAP) - **Spec Exp:** Psychotherapy; Psychoanalysis; **Hospital:** NY-Presby Hosp (page 100); **Address:** 2A Berkeley Rd, Scarsdale, NY 10583-1102; **Phone:** 914-472-8447; **Board Cert:** Psychiatry 1984; Child & Adolescent Psychiatry 1986; **Med School:** Albert Einstein Coll Med 1979; **Resid:** Psychiatry, Albert Einstein 1982; **Fellow:** Child & Adolescent Psychiatry, Albert Einstein 1984; **Fac Appt:** Asst Clin Prof Psyc, Cornell Univ-Weill Med Coll

Pincus, Emile MD (ChAP) - **Spec Exp:** Substance Abuse; Suicide; **Hospital:** Stony Lodge Hosp; **Address:** 40 Croton Dam Rd, Ossining, NY 10562; **Phone:** 914-941-7400; **Board Cert:** Psychiatry 1986; **Med School:** Mount Sinai Sch Med 1978; **Resid:** Psychiatry, St Lukes Hosp Ctr 1979; Psychiatry, Mt Sinai Med Ctr 1982; **Fellow:** Child & Adolescent Psychiatry, NY Hosp-Cornell Med Ctr 1984

Rubinstein, Boris MD (ChAP) - **Spec Exp:** Psychopharmacology; Neuro-Psychiatry; Mood Disorders; **Hospital:** NY-Presby Hosp (page 100); **Address:** 623 Warburton Ave, Hastings On Hudson, NY 10706; **Phone:** 914-478-1330; **Board Cert:** Pediatrics 1976; Psychiatry 1979; Child & Adolescent Psychiatry 1981; **Med School:** Mexico 1970; **Resid:** Pediatrics, Chldns Hosp 1974; Psychiatry, Bronx Muni Hosp-Albert Einstein 1976; **Fellow:** Child & Adolescent Psychiatry, Bronx Muni Hosp-Albert Einstein 1978; Public Health & Genl Preventive Med, Harvard-Sch Pub Hlth 1974; **Fac Appt:** Assoc Clin Prof Psyc, Columbia P&S

Schreiber, Klaus MD (ChAP) - **Spec Exp:** Developmental Disorders; **Address:** 11 Neperan Rd, Tarrytown, NY 10591; **Phone:** 914-332-0270; **Board Cert:** Psychiatry 1976; Child & Adolescent Psychiatry 1986; **Med School:** Germany 1966; **Resid:** Psychiatry, Elmhurst City Hosp Ctr 1971; Psychiatry, Westchester Med Ctr; **Fellow:** Child & Adolescent Psychiatry, Westchester Med Ctr 1973; Child & Adolescent Psychiatry, Albert Einstein Coll Med 1982; **Fac Appt:** Asst Prof Psyc, NY Med Coll

Seaver, Robert MD (ChAP) - **Spec Exp:** Forensic Psychiatry; Art & Creativity; **Address:** 83 S Bedford Ave Fl 2nd, Mt Kisco, NY 10549; **Phone:** 914-241-8979; **Board Cert:** Pediatrics 1978; Psychiatry 1984; Child & Adolescent Psychiatry 1986; **Med School:** Mount Sinai Sch Med 1973; **Resid:** Pediatrics, Mt Sinai Hosp 1975; Psychiatry, NY Hosp-Westchester Div; **Fellow:** Pediatrics, St Luke's-Roosevelt Hosp Ctr 1976; Child & Adolescent Psychiatry, Jacobi Med Ctr 1985

Slater, Jonathan MD (ChAP) - **Spec Exp:** Psychopharmacology; Medical Illness in Psychiatry; **Hospital:** NY-Presby Hosp (page 100); **Address:** 1 Bridge St, Ste 24, Irvington, NY 10533; **Phone:** 914-591-4135; **Board Cert:** Psychiatry 1991; Child & Adolescent Psychiatry 1993; **Med School:** Columbia P&S 1985; **Resid:** Psychiatry, Columbia-Presby Med Ctr 1990; **Fellow:** Research, NY State Psychiatric Inst 1986; Child & Adolescent Psychiatry, Columbia-Presby Med Ctr 1992; **Fac Appt:** Assoc Clin Prof Psyc, Columbia P&S

Child Neurology

Jacobson, Ronald MD (ChiN) - **Spec Exp:** Epilepsy; Headache; ADD/ADHD; **Hospital:** Westchester Med Ctr (page 713), White Plains Hosp Ctr (page 714); **Address:** 125 S Broadway, White Plains, NY 10605; **Phone:** 914-997-1692; **Board Cert:** Pediatrics 1981; Child Neurology 1984; **Med School:** Albert Einstein Coll Med 1975; **Resid:** Pediatrics, Yale-New Haven Hosp 1979; **Fellow:** Pediatric Neurology, Univ Minn Med Ctr 1982; **Fac Appt:** Assoc Clin Prof N, NY Med Coll

Kang, Harriet MD (ChiN) - **Spec Exp:** Epilepsy/Seizure Disorders; **Hospital:** Beth Israel Med Ctr- Kings Hwy Div (page 90); **Address:** 141 S Central Park Ave, Hartsdale, NY 10530; **Phone:** 914-428-0529; **Board Cert:** Pediatrics 1979; Child Neurology 1981; Clinical Neurophysiology 1996; **Med School:** Johns Hopkins Univ 1974; **Resid:** Pediatrics, Johns Hopkins Hosp 1976; Child Neurology, Univ Minn Med Ctr 1979; **Fellow:** Clinical Neurophysiology, Univ Minn Med Ctr 1980; **Fac Appt:** Assoc Prof Ped, Albert Einstein Coll Med

Kutscher, Martin MD (ChiN) - **Spec Exp:** ADD/ADHD; Seizure Disorders; Asperger's Syndrome; **Hospital:** Westchester Med Ctr (page 713), White Plains Hosp Ctr (page 714); **Address:** 125 S Broadway, White Plains, NY 10605-1405; **Phone:** 914-997-1692; **Board Cert:** Pediatrics 1986; Child Neurology 1989; **Med School:** Columbia P&S 1981; **Resid:** Pediatrics, St Christopher's Hosp 1984; Neurology, Albert Einstein Med Ctr 1987; **Fellow:** Child Neurology, Albert Einstein Med Coll 1989; **Fac Appt:** Assoc Clin Prof Ped, NY Med Coll

CLINICAL GENETICS

Brenholz, Pauline MD (CG) - **Spec Exp:** Genetic Disorders; Amniocentesis; **Hospital:** Phelps Meml Hosp Ctr; **Address:** 280 Mamaroneck Ave, Ste 205, White Plains, NY 10605-1456; **Phone:** 914-997-6535; **Board Cert:** Clinical Genetics 1982; Pediatrics 1982; Clinical Cytogenetics 1982; **Med School:** Albert Einstein Coll Med 1973; **Resid:** Pediatrics, Montefiore Hosp Med Ctr 1976; **Fellow:** Clinical Genetics, Albert Einstein 1979

Shapiro, Lawrence R MD (CG) - **Spec Exp:** Dysmorphology; Prenatal Diagnosis; Hereditary Cancer; Developmental Disorders; **Hospital:** Westchester Med Ctr (page 713); **Address:** Regional Med Genetics Ctr, 19 Bradhurst Ave, Ste 1600, Hawthorne, NY 10532-2140; **Phone:** 914-593-8900; **Board Cert:** Pediatrics 1967; Clinical Genetics 1982; Clinical Cytogenetics 1982; **Med School:** NYU Sch Med 1962; **Resid:** Pediatrics, Chldns Hosp 1964; Pediatrics, Bellevue Hosp 1965; **Fellow:** Clinical Genetics, NYU Med Ctr 1965; Clinical Genetics, Mount Sinai Med Ctr 1968; **Fac Appt:** Prof Ped, NY Med Coll

COLON & RECTAL SURGERY

Bruce, Christopher J MD (CRS) - **Spec Exp:** Colon & Rectal Cancer; **Hospital:** White Plains Hosp Ctr (page 714); **Address:** 15 N Broadway, Ste J, White Plains, NY 10601; **Phone:** 914-997-1599; **Board Cert:** Surgery 1996; Colon & Rectal Surgery 1997; **Med School:** UMDNJ-NJ Med Sch, Newark 1989; **Resid:** Surgery, UMDNJ Univ Hosp 1995

Burg, Richard MD (CRS) - **Spec Exp:** Colonoscopy; **Hospital:** White Plains Hosp Ctr (page 714), Sound Shore Med Ctr - Westchester (page 711); **Address:** 12 Greenridge Ave, Ste 201, White Plains, NY 10605; **Phone:** 914-949-0760; **Board Cert:** Surgery 1971; Colon & Rectal Surgery 1994; **Med School:** Tulane Univ 1965; **Resid:** Surgery, Univ Wisconsin Hosp 1970; **Fellow:** Colon & Rectal Surgery, St Vincent's Hosp 1977; **Fac Appt:** Asst Clin Prof S, NY Med Coll

Cohen, Martin A MD (CRS) - **Spec Exp:** Colon & Rectal Cancer; Hemorrhoids; Laparoscopic Surgery; **Hospital:** Northern Westchester Hosp, Comm Hosp - Dobbs Ferry; **Address:** 666 Lexington Ave, Ste 101, Mt Kisco, NY 10549; **Phone:** 914-666-2778; **Board Cert:** Surgery 1995; Colon & Rectal Surgery 1986; **Med School:** Hahnemann Univ 1979; **Resid:** Surgery, LI Jewish-Hillside Hosp 1984; **Fellow:** Colon & Rectal Surgery, Allentown Affil Hosps 1985

DERMATOLOGY

Bank, David MD (D) - **Spec Exp:** Liposuction; Skin Laser Surgery; Botox Therapy; **Hospital:** NY-Presby Hosp (page 100), Northern Westchester Hosp; **Address:** 359 E Main St, Ste 4G, Mt Kisco, NY 10549-3035; **Phone:** 914-241-3003; **Board Cert:** Dermatology 1989; **Med School:** Columbia P&S 1985; **Resid:** Internal Medicine, Montefiore Hosp Med Ctr 1986; Dermatology, Columbia-Presby Med Ctr 1989; **Fac Appt:** Assoc Clin Prof D, Columbia P&S

Berkowitz, Rhonda MD (D) - **Hospital:** Phelps Meml Hosp Ctr; **Address:** 325 S Highland Ave, Briarcliff Manor, NY 10510-2031; **Phone:** 914-941-5769; **Board Cert:** Dermatology 1986; **Med School:** NYU Sch Med 1982; **Resid:** Internal Medicine, N Shore Univ Hosp 1983; Dermatology, Columbia-Presby Med Ctr 1986

Bronin, Andrew MD (D) - **Spec Exp:** Skin Cancer; Melanoma; **Hospital:** Greenwich Hosp, Yale - New Haven Hosp (page 984); **Address:** 4 Rye Ridge Plaza, Rye Brook, NY 10573-2820; **Phone:** 914-253-8080; **Board Cert:** Dermatology 1981; **Med School:** NY Med Coll 1975; **Resid:** Dermatology, New York Hosp 1979; **Fac Appt:** Assoc Clin Prof D, Yale Univ

Davis, Ira C MD (D) - **Spec Exp:** Mohs' Surgery; Cosmetic Dermatology; Dermatologic Surgery; Skin Cancer; **Hospital:** Westchester Med Ctr (page 713), St Vincent Cath Med Ctr - Staten Island (page 375); **Address:** 280 N Central Park Ave, Ste 114, Hartsdale, NY 10530; **Phone:** 914-288-0500; **Board Cert:** Dermatology 1990; **Med School:** NYU Sch Med 1986; **Resid:** Dermatology, Duke Univ Med Ctr 1990; **Fellow:** Dermatologic Pharmacology, NYU Med Ctr 1991; Mohs Surgery, Wake Forest Univ Med Ctr 1993; **Fac Appt:** Asst Clin Prof D, NY Med Coll

Eisert, Jack MD (D) - **Spec Exp:** Psoriasis; Contact Dermatitis; Acne; **Hospital:** Phelps Meml Hosp Ctr, NY-Presby Hosp (page 100); **Address:** 200 S Broadway, Ste 208, Tarrytown, NY 10591; **Phone:** 914-631-4666; **Board Cert:** Dermatology 1961; **Med School:** SUNY Hlth Sci Ctr 1956; **Resid:** Dermatology, Columbia-Presby Med Ctr 1960; **Fac Appt:** Assoc Clin Prof D, Columbia P&S

Felsenstein, Jerome M MD (D) - **Hospital:** Phelps Meml Hosp Ctr, NYU Med Ctr (page 102); **Address:** 100 S Highland Ave, Ossining, NY 10562; **Phone:** 914-941-5770; **Board Cert:** Dermatology 1976; **Med School:** NYU Sch Med 1971; **Resid:** Dermatology, Kings County Hosp 1975

Goldberg, Neil S MD (D) - **Spec Exp:** Skin Cancer; Pediatric Dermatology; Acne; **Hospital:** White Plains Hosp Ctr (page 714), Lawrence Hosp Ctr; **Address:** 222 Westchester Ave, Ste 203, White Plains, NY 10604-2926; **Phone:** 914-761-8140; **Board Cert:** Dermatology 1986; **Med School:** Northwestern Univ 1982; **Resid:** Dermatology, Northwestern Meml Hosp 1986

Grossman, Marc E MD (D) - **Spec Exp:** Skin Diseases in Transplants/Cancer; Psoriasis; Rare Skin Disorders; **Hospital:** NY-Presby Hosp (page 100), White Plains Hosp Ctr (page 714); **Address:** 12 Greenridge Ave, White Plains, NY 10605-1238; **Phone:** 914-946-1101; **Board Cert:** Internal Medicine 1977; Dermatology 1978; **Med School:** Univ Pennsylvania 1974; **Resid:** Internal Medicine, Hosp Univ Penn 1976; **Fellow:** Dermatology, Columbia-Presby Med Ctr 1979; **Fac Appt:** Prof D, Columbia P&S

Halperin, Alan MD (D) - **Spec Exp:** Dermatopathology; **Hospital:** Montefiore Med Ctr - Weiler-Einstein Div, Montefiore Med Ctr; **Address:** 100 Midland Ave, Port Chester, NY 10573; **Phone:** 914-636-0136; **Board Cert:** Dermatology 1975; Dermatopathology 1977; **Med School:** NYU Sch Med 1970; **Resid:** Dermatology, Albert Einstein Coll Med 1974; **Fac Appt:** Assoc Clin Prof Med, Albert Einstein Coll Med

Kaplan, Sherri MD (D) - **Hospital:** Comm Hosp - Dobbs Ferry; **Address:** 1055 Saw Mill River Rd, Ste 208, Ardsley, NY 10502; **Phone:** 914-693-7191; **Board Cert:** Dermatology 1987; **Med School:** NY Med Coll 1983; **Resid:** Dermatology, NY Med Coll 1987; **Fac Appt:** Asst Clin Prof D, NY Med Coll

Klar, Tobi MD (D) - **Hospital:** Sound Shore Med Ctr - Westchester (page 711), Montefiore Med Ctr - Weiler-Einstein Div; **Address:** 150 Lockwood Ave, Ste 20, New Rochelle, NY 10801; **Phone:** 914-636-2039; **Board Cert:** Dermatology 1989; **Med School:** SUNY Downstate 1981; **Resid:** Dermatology, Downstate Med Ctr 1986

Lerman, Jay S MD (D) - **Spec Exp:** Acne; Eczema; Warts; **Hospital:** White Plains Hosp Ctr (page 714); **Address:** 280 Dobbs Ferry Rd, Ste 205, White Plains, NY 10607-1912; **Phone:** 914-949-9196; **Board Cert:** Dermatology 1974; **Med School:** SUNY Downstate 1969; **Resid:** Dermatology, Jacobi Med Ctr 1973; **Fac Appt:** Asst Clin Prof D, Albert Einstein Coll Med

Levy, Ross MD (D) - **Spec Exp:** Skin Laser Surgery; Dermatologic Surgery; Skin Cancer; **Hospital:** Northern Westchester Hosp, Montefiore Med Ctr; **Address:** Mt Kisco Med Grp, 110 S Bedford Rd, Mt Kisco, NY 10549; **Phone:** 914-242-1355; **Board Cert:** Dermatology 1981; **Med School:** Albert Einstein Coll Med 1976; **Resid:** Internal Medicine, Montefiore Hosp Med Ctr 1978; **Fellow:** Dermatology, Albert Einstein Coll Med 1981; **Fac Appt:** Assoc Clin Prof Med, Albert Einstein Coll Med

Lukash, Barbara MD (D) - **Spec Exp:** Skin Cancer; Acne; Psoriasis; **Hospital:** NY-Presby Hosp (page 100); **Address:** 14 Lawton St, New Rochelle, NY 10801; **Phone:** 914-712-2800; **Board Cert:** Dermatology 1980; **Med School:** Tulane Univ 1976; **Resid:** Dermatology, Univ Chicago Hosps 1980; **Fac Appt:** Assoc Clin Prof D, Columbia P&S

Mackler, Karen MD (D) - **Spec Exp:** Pediatric Dermatology; Skin Cancer; **Hospital:** Sound Shore Med Ctr - Westchester (page 711); **Address:** 150 Lockwood Ave, Ste 34, New Rochelle, NY 10801-4914; **Phone:** 914-576-7070; **Board Cert:** Pediatrics 1978; Dermatology 1983; **Med School:** NYU Sch Med 1973; **Resid:** Pediatrics, NY Hosp 1976; Dermatology, Montefiore Hosp Med Ctr 1983; **Fac Appt:** Asst Prof D, Albert Einstein Coll Med

Mattison, Timothy MD (D) - **Hospital:** Northern Westchester Hosp; **Address:** 90 S Bedford Rd, Mt Kisco, NY 10549-3412; **Phone:** 914-242-1355; **Board Cert:** Dermatology 1980; **Med School:** Dartmouth Med Sch 1976; **Resid:** Dermatology, New York Univ Med Ctr 1980

Mermelstein, Harold MD (D) - **Spec Exp:** Cosmetic Dermatology; Aging Skin; **Hospital:** NYU Med Ctr (page 102), Lawrence Hosp Ctr; **Address:** 559 Gramatan Ave, Mt Vernon, NY 10552-3234; **Phone:** 914-667-2242; **Board Cert:** Dermatology 1979; **Med School:** NY Med Coll 1975; **Resid:** Dermatology, NYU Med Ctr 1979; **Fellow:** Dermatologic Surgery, NYU Med Ctr 1980; **Fac Appt:** Assoc Clin Prof D, NYU Sch Med

Narins, Rhoda MD (D) - **Spec Exp:** Liposuction; Cosmetic Dermatology; Botox Therapy; **Hospital:** NYU Med Ctr (page 102), White Plains Hosp Ctr (page 714); **Address:** 222 Westchester Ave, Ste 300, White Plains, NY 10604-2925; **Phone:** 914-684-1000; **Board Cert:** Dermatology 1970; **Med School:** NYU Sch Med 1965; **Resid:** Dermatology, NYU Med Ctr 1969; **Fac Appt:** Clin Prof D, NYU Sch Med

Newburger, Amy MD (D) - **Spec Exp:** Contact Dermatitis; Cosmetic Dermatology; **Hospital:** White Plains Hosp Ctr (page 714); **Address:** 2 Overhill Rd, Ste 330, Scarsdale, NY 10583; **Phone:** 914-725-1800; **Board Cert:** Dermatology 1979; **Med School:** NYU Sch Med 1974; **Resid:** Dermatology, Univ Miami Hosps 1978

Rosenthal, Elizabeth MD (D) - **Hospital:** Jacobi Med Ctr; **Address:** 1600 Harrison Ave, Ste 303, Mamaroneck, NY 10543-3151; **Phone:** 914-698-2190; **Board Cert:** Dermatology 1975; **Med School:** NYU Sch Med 1967; **Resid:** Dermatology, Henry Ford Hosp 1969; Dermatology, Roosevelt Hosp 1970; **Fellow:** Dermatology, Boston Univ Med Ctr 1974; **Fac Appt:** Asst Clin Prof D, Albert Einstein Coll Med

Schliftman, Alan MD (D) - **Spec Exp:** Laser Surgery; **Hospital:** White Plains Hosp Ctr (page 714); **Address:** 244 Westchester Ave, Ste 211, White Plains, NY 10604-2926; **Phone:** 914-761-1400; **Board Cert:** Dermatology 1981; **Med School:** Geo Wash Univ 1977; **Resid:** Dermatology, Albert Einstein 1980

Stillman, Michael MD (D) - **Spec Exp:** Skin Cancer; Acne; Eczema; **Hospital:** Northern Westchester Hosp; **Address:** 39 Smith Ave, Mt Kisco, NY 10549-2838; **Phone:** 914-241-3330; **Board Cert:** Dermatology 1973; **Med School:** SUNY Downstate 1967; **Resid:** Dermatology, NYU Med Ctr 1973; **Fellow:** Dermatology, Letterman Army Inst Rsch 1970

Sturza, Jeffrey MD (D) - **Spec Exp:** Psoriasis; Laser Surgery; Cosmetic Dermatology; **Hospital:** Phelps Meml Hosp Ctr; **Address:** 200 S Broadway, Ste 208, Tarrytown, NY 10591; **Phone:** 914-631-4666; **Board Cert:** Dermatology 1988; **Med School:** SUNY Hlth Sci Ctr 1984; **Resid:** Dermatology, Cook Co Hosp 1988

Treiber, Ruth Kaplan MD (D) - **Spec Exp:** Acne; Botox Therapy; **Hospital:** NY-Presby Hosp (page 100); **Address:** 175 Purchase St, Rye, NY 10580; **Phone:** 914-967-2153; **Board Cert:** Dermatology 1983; **Med School:** Cornell Univ-Weill Med Coll 1978; **Resid:** Internal Medicine, New York Hosp 1980; Dermatology, Columbia-Presby Med Ctr 1983; **Fac Appt:** Assoc Clin Prof D, Columbia P&S

Zweibel, Stuart M MD/PhD (D) - **Spec Exp:** Mohs' Surgery; Laser Surgery; **Hospital:** Northern Westchester Hosp; **Address:** 185 Kisco Ave, Ste 3, Mt Kisco, NY 10549; **Phone:** 914-242-2020; **Board Cert:** Dermatology 1989; **Med School:** Mount Sinai Sch Med 1985; **Resid:** Dermatology, Rhode Island Hosp 1989; **Fellow:** Mohs Surgery, Univ of Wisconsin Hosp 1991

DIAGNOSTIC RADIOLOGY

Botet, Jose MD (DR) - **Spec Exp:** Interventional Radiology; **Hospital:** White Plains Hosp Ctr (page 714); **Address:** White Plains Hosp Ctr, Dept Rad, Davis Ave at East Post Rd, White Plains, NY 10605; **Phone:** 914-681-1260; **Board Cert:** Diagnostic Radiology 1982; **Med School:** Mexico 1973; **Resid:** Radiology, St Luke's-Roosevelt Hosp Ctr 1978; **Fellow:** Interventional Radiology, Meml Sloan Kettering Cancer Ctr 1979

Chisolm, Alvin MD (DR) - **Spec Exp:** Women's Imaging; Ultrasound; CT Scan; **Hospital:** Sound Shore Med Ctr - Westchester (page 711); **Address:** 16 Guion Pl, New Rochelle, NY 10801-5503; **Phone:** 914-632-5000 x3790; **Board Cert:** Radiology 1973; **Med School:** NY Med Coll 1968; **Resid:** Radiology, Montefiore Hosp Med Ctr 1972

Kelly, Anna MD (DR) - **Spec Exp:** Neuroradiology; **Hospital:** Lawrence Hosp Ctr; **Address:** Lawrence Hospital,Dept Radiology, 55 Palmer Ave Fl 2, Bronxville, NY 10708; **Phone:** 914-787-3058; **Board Cert:** Diagnostic Radiology 1986; Neuroradiology 1995; **Med School:** Univ Cincinnati 1982; **Resid:** Diagnostic Radiology, NY Hosp-Cornell Med Ctr 1986; **Fellow:** Neurological Radiology, NY Hosp-Cornell Med Ctr 1999

Khoury, Paul MD (DR) - **Hospital:** White Plains Hosp Ctr (page 714); **Address:** White Plains Hospital, Dept Radiology, Davis Ave @ East Post Rd, White Plains, NY 10601; **Phone:** 914-681-1219; **Board Cert:** Diagnostic Radiology 1979; Nuclear Radiology 1980; **Med School:** Lebanon 1973; **Resid:** Radiology, Hotel Dieu de France Hosp 1975; Diagnostic Radiology, St Luke's-Roosevelt Hosp Ctr 1978

Klein, Robert M MD (DR) - **Spec Exp:** Musculoskeletal Imaging; Bone Densitometry; **Hospital:** Westchester Med Ctr (page 713); **Address:** Westchester Med Center, Dept Rad, Valhalla, NY 10595; **Phone:** 914-493-7355; **Board Cert:** Radiology 1971; Nuclear Medicine 1975; **Med School:** SUNY Upstate Med Univ 1963; **Resid:** Radiology, Kings County Hosp 1969; **Fac Appt:** Prof Rad, NY Med Coll

Kutcher, Rosalyn MD (DR) - **Spec Exp:** Mammography; Ultrasound; Women's Imaging; **Hospital:** White Plains Hosp Ctr (page 714); **Address:** 90 S Rich St, Rye Brook, NY 10573; **Phone:** 914-935-0011; **Board Cert:** Diagnostic Radiology 1975; **Med School:** SUNY Hlth Sci Ctr 1970; **Resid:** Diagnostic Radiology, Montefiore Hosp Med Ctr 1974; **Fac Appt:** Prof Rad, Albert Einstein Coll Med

Leslie, Denise MD (DR) - **Spec Exp:** Neuroradiology; **Address:** East Westchester Radiology, 503 Grasslands Rd, Ste 100, Valhalla, NY 10595; **Phone:** 914-345-0376; **Board Cert:** Diagnostic Radiology 1985; Neuroradiology 1995; **Med School:** SUNY Buffalo 1981; **Resid:** Diagnostic Radiology, Westchester Co Med Ctr 1985; **Fellow:** Neuroradiology, Westchester Co Med Ctr 1987; **Fac Appt:** Asst Prof Rad, NY Med Coll

LoRusso, Diane MD (DR) - **Spec Exp:** Breast Imaging; Women's Health; Ultrasound; MRI; **Address:** Rye Radiology Assoc, 30 Rye Ridge Plaza, Rye Brook, NY 10573-2830; **Phone:** 914-253-9200; **Board Cert:** Diagnostic Radiology 1974; **Med School:** SUNY Upstate Med Univ 1969; **Resid:** Diagnostic Radiology, Montefiore Med Ctr 1974

Miller, Karen L MD (DR) - **Spec Exp:** Mammography; CT Scan; **Hospital:** Phelps Meml Hosp Ctr; **Address:** Phelps Meml Hosp, Dept Radiology, 701 N Broadway, Sleepy Hollow, NY 10591-1020; **Phone:** 914-366-3450; **Board Cert:** Diagnostic Radiology 1990; **Med School:** NY Med Coll 1981; **Resid:** Diagnostic Radiology, Westchester Co Med Ctr 1990; **Fellow:** Diagnostic Radiology, Westchester Co Med Ctr 1991

Novich, Ira MD (DR) - **Spec Exp:** Nuclear Medicine; **Hospital:** Sound Shore Med Ctr - Westchester (page 711); **Address:** New Rochelle Radiology, 175 Memorial Hwy, Ste 14, New Rochelle, NY 10801-5637; **Phone:** 914-633-7700; **Board Cert:** Diagnostic Radiology 1974; Nuclear Medicine 1974; **Med School:** Albert Einstein Coll Med 1969; **Resid:** Diagnostic Radiology, Maimonides Medical Ctr 1970; **Fellow:** Diagnostic Radiology, Albert Einstein 1974; **Fac Appt:** Asst Clin Prof Rad, Albert Einstein Coll Med

ENDOCRINOLOGY, DIABETES & METABOLISM

Albin, Joan MD (EDM) - **Spec Exp:** Diabetes; Thyroid Disorders; Polycystic Ovarian Syndrome; **Hospital:** Sound Shore Med Ctr - Westchester (page 711); **Address:** 140 Lockwood Ave, Ste 212, New Rochelle, NY 10801-4908; **Phone:** 914-235-8503; **Board Cert:** Internal Medicine 1972; Endocrinology, Diabetes & Metabolism 1973; **Med School:** NY Med Coll 1967; **Resid:** Internal Medicine, Metropolitan Hosp 1969; Internal Medicine, Montefiore Hosp Med Ctr 1970; **Fellow:** Endocrinology, Diabetes & Metabolism, Mount Sinai Hosp 1971; Endocrinology, Diabetes & Metabolism, New York Med Coll 1972; **Fac Appt:** Assoc Clin Prof Med, Albert Einstein Coll Med

Bloomgarden, David K MD (EDM) - **Spec Exp:** Diabetes; Osteoporosis; Thyroid Disorders; **Hospital:** White Plains Hosp Ctr (page 714); **Address:** Endocrinology & Diabetes Associates, 222 Westchester Ave, Ste 306, White Plains, NY 10604-2906; **Phone:** 914-684-0202; **Board Cert:** Internal Medicine 1980; Endocrinology, Diabetes & Metabolism 1983; **Med School:** NYU Sch Med 1977; **Resid:** Internal Medicine, Jacobi Med Ctr 1980; **Fellow:** Endocrinology, Diabetes & Metabolism, Albert Einstein 1982

Blum, David MD (EDM) - **Spec Exp:** Diabetes; Osteoporosis; Thyroid Disorders; **Hospital:** Sound Shore Med Ctr - Westchester (page 711); **Address:** 175 Memorial Hwy, Ste 1-7, New Rochelle, NY 10801; **Phone:** 914-633-8680; **Board Cert:** Internal Medicine 1977; Endocrinology, Diabetes & Metabolism 1979; **Med School:** Northwestern Univ 1974; **Resid:** Internal Medicine, Mount Sinai Hosp 1977; **Fellow:** Endocrinology, Mount Sinai Hosp 1979; **Fac Appt:** Asst Clin Prof Med, NY Med Coll

Eufemio, Michael MD (EDM) - **Spec Exp:** Osteoporosis; Diabetes; Thyroid Disorders; **Hospital:** Sound Shore Med Ctr - Westchester (page 711); **Address:** 140 Lockwood Ave, Ste 308, New Rochelle, NY 10801-4909; **Phone:** 914-636-5700; **Board Cert:** Internal Medicine 1977; Endocrinology, Diabetes & Metabolism 1972; **Med School:** Geo Wash Univ 1960; **Resid:** Internal Medicine, DC Genl Hosp 1962; Internal Medicine, VA Med Ctr 1966; **Fellow:** Endocrinology, Diabetes & Metabolism, VA Med Ctr 1967; **Fac Appt:** Assoc Clin Prof Med, NY Med Coll

Gitler, Ellen MD (EDM) - **Spec Exp:** Cardiac Rehabilitation; **Hospital:** Burke Rehab Hosp (page 105); **Address:** 785 Mamaroneck Ave, White Plains, NY 10605-2523; **Phone:** 914-597-2409; **Board Cert:** Internal Medicine 1980; Endocrinology, Diabetes & Metabolism 1983; **Med School:** Cornell Univ-Weill Med Coll 1977; **Resid:** Internal Medicine, Bronx Municipal Hosp 1980; **Fellow:** Endocrinology, Diabetes & Metabolism, Mt Sinai Hosp 1982

Hellerman, James MD (EDM) - **Spec Exp:** Thyroid Disorders; Diabetes; Calcium Disorders; **Hospital:** Phelps Meml Hosp Ctr, St Barnabas Hosp - Bronx; **Address:** 200 S Broadway, Ste 100, Tarrytown, NY 10591-4504; **Phone:** 914-631-9300; **Board Cert:** Internal Medicine 1979; Endocrinology 1983; **Med School:** Univ Rochester 1976; **Resid:** Internal Medicine, Montefiore Med Ctr 1980; **Fellow:** Endocrinology, Diabetes & Metabolism, Mass Genl Hosp 1984

Kantor, Alan MD (EDM) - **Spec Exp:** Thyroid Disorders; Osteoporosis; Diabetes; Endocrine Tumors; **Hospital:** Northern Westchester Hosp; **Address:** 1940 Commerce St, Ste 310, Yorktown Heights, NY 10598; **Phone:** 914-245-1111; **Board Cert:** Internal Medicine 1981; Endocrinology, Diabetes & Metabolism 1983; **Med School:** South Africa 1975; **Resid:** Internal Medicine, La Guardia Hosp 1980; Internal Medicine, LI Jewish-Hillside Med Ctr 1981; **Fellow:** Endocrinology, Diabetes & Metabolism, Meml Sloan Kettering Cancer Ctr 1983; **Fac Appt:** Asst Clin Prof Med, NY Med Coll

Kleinbaum, Jerry MD (EDM) - **Spec Exp:** Diabetes; **Hospital:** Hudson Valley Hosp Ctr, Putnam Hosp Ctr; **Address:** 48 Route 6, Mahapoc Ave, Ste 103, Yorktown Heights, NY 10598; **Phone:** 914-248-4000; **Board Cert:** Internal Medicine 1979; Endocrinology 1985; **Med School:** Tufts Univ 1976; **Resid:** Internal Medicine, Bronx Municipal Hosp 1980; **Fellow:** Endocrinology, Diabetes & Metabolism, Albert Einstein 1982

Marshall, Merville MD (EDM) - **Spec Exp:** Thyroid Disorders; Diabetes; Pituitary & Adrenal Disorders; **Hospital:** Westchester Med Ctr (page 713); **Address:** Endocrine Institute, 21 Seymour Pl, White Plains, NY 10605; **Phone:** 914-949-8650; **Board Cert:** Internal Medicine 1977; Endocrinology, Diabetes & Metabolism 1981; **Med School:** Columbia P&S 1974; **Resid:** Internal Medicine, St Luke's-Roosevelt Hosp Ctr 1976; **Fellow:** Endocrinology, Diabetes & Metabolism, Nat Inst Health 1979

Powell, Jeffrey S MD (EDM) - **Hospital:** Northern Westchester Hosp; **Address:** 90 S Bedford Rd, Mount Kisco, NY 10549; **Phone:** 914-241-1050; **Board Cert:** Internal Medicine 1998; Endocrinology, Diabetes & Metabolism 2000; **Med School:** Albert Einstein Coll Med 1995; **Resid:** Internal Medicine, Columbia-Presby Med Ctr 1998; **Fellow:** Endocrinology, Diabetes & Metabolism, Columbia-Presby Med Ctr 1999

Pretto, Zorayda MD (EDM) - **Hospital:** White Plains Hosp Ctr (page 714); **Address:** Mid-Westchester Medical Assocs, 33 Davis Ave, Lower Level, White Plains, NY 10605; **Phone:** 914-948-3630; **Board Cert:** Internal Medicine 1993; Endocrinology, Diabetes & Metabolism 1995; **Med School:** Panama 1986; **Resid:** Internal Medicine, St John's Episcopal Hosp 1991; **Fellow:** Endocrinology, Diabetes & Metabolism, Beth Israel Hosp 1993

Ross, Herbert MD (EDM) - **Spec Exp:** Diabetes; Thyroid Disorders; Osteoporosis; **Hospital:** White Plains Hosp Ctr (page 714); **Address:** 33 Davis Ave, White Plains, NY 10605-1030; **Phone:** 914-946-5354; **Board Cert:** Internal Medicine 1964; Endocrinology, Diabetes & Metabolism 1972; **Med School:** Switzerland 1955; **Resid:** Internal Medicine, VA Hosp 1959; Internal Medicine, Montefiore Hosp Med Ctr 1962; **Fellow:** Endocrinology, Diabetes & Metabolism, Flower Fifth Ave Hosp 1963

FAMILY MEDICINE

Annabi, Iyad N MD (FMed) **PCP** - **Hospital:** St John's Riverside Hosp; **Address:** 472 Palmer Rd, Yonkers, NY 10701; **Phone:** 914-375-2300; **Board Cert:** Family Medicine 2001; **Med School:** Mexico 1988; **Resid:** Family Medicine, St Joseph Med Ctr 1993

Apuzzo, Thomas MD (FMed) **PCP** - **Hospital:** Saint Joseph's Med Ctr - Yonkers, St John's Riverside Hosp; **Address:** 955 Yonkers Ave, Yonkers, NY 10704; **Phone:** 914-237-0994; **Board Cert:** Family Medicine 2002; **Med School:** Italy 1985; **Resid:** Family Medicine, St Joseph's Med Ctr 1989

Coloka-Kump, Rodika DO (FMed) **PCP** - **Spec Exp:** Preventive Medicine; **Hospital:** Saint Joseph's Med Ctr - Yonkers, St John's Riverside Hosp; **Address:** 461 Riverdale Ave, Yonkers, NY 10705-2970; **Phone:** 914-965-0117; **Board Cert:** Family Medicine 1998; **Med School:** NY Coll Osteo Med 1988; **Resid:** Family Medicine, NY Methodist Hosp 1989St Joseph's Med Ctr 1991

Gottesfeld, Peter MD (FMed) **PCP** - **Spec Exp:** Preventive Medicine; Headache; Pain Management; ADD/ADHD; **Hospital:** Northern Westchester Hosp, Hudson Valley Hosp Ctr; **Address:** 101 S Bedford Rd Ste 412 Bldg, Mt Kisco, NY 10549-3455; **Phone:** 914-241-7800; **Board Cert:** Family Medicine 2003; **Med School:** UMDNJ-RW Johnson Med Sch 1985; **Resid:** Family Medicine, Thomas Jefferson U Hosp 1988; **Fac Appt:** Assoc Clin Prof FMed, NY Med Coll

Heinegg, Philip MD (FMed) **PCP** - **Spec Exp:** Complementary Medicine; **Hospital:** Sound Shore Med Ctr - Westchester (page 711); **Address:** 1890 Palmer Ave, Ste 305, Larchmont, NY 10538-3031; **Phone:** 914-834-9606; **Board Cert:** Family Medicine 2003; **Med School:** France 1980; **Resid:** Family Medicine, S Nassau Comm Hosp 1983

Kelly, Stephen P MD (FMed) **PCP** - **Spec Exp:** Tropical Medicine; **Hospital:** Comm Hosp - Dobbs Ferry, St John's Riverside Hosp; **Address:** 18 Ashford Ave, Ste MW, Dobbs Ferry, NY 10522-1800; **Phone:** 914-693-1660; **Board Cert:** Family Medicine 2003; **Med School:** Univ Cincinnati 1975; **Resid:** Family Medicine, John F Kennedy Hosp 1978; **Fac Appt:** Asst Clin Prof FMed, NY Med Coll

Merker, Edward MD (FMed) **PCP** - **Spec Exp:** Geriatrics; **Hospital:** Phelps Meml Hosp Ctr; **Address:** 180 Marble Ave, Pleasantville, NY 10570; **Phone:** 914-769-7300 x202; **Board Cert:** Family Medicine 1998; **Med School:** Albert Einstein Coll Med 1981; **Resid:** Family Medicine, Overlook Hosp 1984; **Fac Appt:** Asst Clin Prof FMed, Albert Einstein Coll Med

Miller, Daniel MD (FMed) **PCP** - **Hospital:** Saint Joseph's Med Ctr - Yonkers; **Address:** St Josephs Family Hlth Ctr, 81 S Broadway, Yonkers, NY 10701; **Phone:** 914-375-3200; **Board Cert:** Family Medicine 2000; **Med School:** Univ Cincinnati 1984; **Resid:** Family Medicine, Montefiore Hosp Med Ctr 1987; **Fac Appt:** Asst Prof FMed, NY Med Coll

Miller, Ellen G MD (FMed) **PCP** - **Spec Exp:** Women's Health; **Hospital:** Saint Joseph's Med Ctr - Yonkers; **Address:** Family Hlth Ctr, 81 S Broadway, Yonkers, NY 10701; **Phone:** 914-375-3200; **Board Cert:** Family Medicine 1980; **Med School:** Univ Rochester 1977; **Resid:** Family Medicine, Montefiore Hosp Med Ctr 1980; **Fac Appt:** Prof FMed, NY Med Coll

Piccirilli, Dora MD (FMed) **PCP** - **Hospital:** Phelps Meml Hosp Ctr; **Address:** Family Medical Care, 180 Marble Ave, Pleasantville, NY 10570; **Phone:** 914-769-7300; **Board Cert:** Family Medicine 1991; **Med School:** SUNY Hlth Sci Ctr 1988; **Resid:** Overlook Hosp 1991

Strongwater, Richard F MD (FMed) **PCP** - **Spec Exp:** Parenting Issues; Travel Medicine; **Hospital:** Phelps Meml Hosp Ctr; **Address:** Family Medical Care, 180 Marble Ave, Pleasantville, NY 10570; **Phone:** 914-769-7300; **Board Cert:** Family Medicine 1998; **Med School:** SUNY Upstate Med Univ 1981; **Resid:** Family Medicine, Overlook Hosp 1984

Sutton, Ira MD (FMed) **PCP** - **Spec Exp:** Preventive Medicine; Skin Diseases; **Hospital:** Sound Shore Med Ctr - Westchester (page 711); **Address:** 77 Quaker Ridge Rd, Ste 101, New Rochelle, NY 10804; **Phone:** 914-636-0077; **Board Cert:** Family Medicine 1983; **Med School:** Albert Einstein Coll Med 1980; **Resid:** Family Medicine, Rhode Island Med Ctr 1983

Yudin, Howard MD (FMed) **PCP** - **Hospital:** Greenwich Hosp, Sound Shore Med Ctr - Westchester (page 711); **Address:** 18 Rye Ridge Plaza, Rye Brook, NY 10573-2820; **Phone:** 914-251-1261; **Board Cert:** Family Medicine 2002; **Med School:** Univ Montreal 1974; **Resid:** Family Medicine, Jewish Genl Hosp 1976

GASTROENTEROLOGY

Abemayor, Elie M MD (Ge) - **Spec Exp:** Inflammatory Bowel Disease; Endoscopy; Peptic Ulcer Disease; **Hospital:** Northern Westchester Hosp, NYU Med Ctr (page 102); **Address:** 91 Smith Ave, Mt Kisco, NY 10549-2810; **Phone:** 914-241-9026; **Board Cert:** Internal Medicine 1988; Gastroenterology 2005; **Med School:** SUNY Stony Brook 1985; **Resid:** Internal Medicine, NYU-Bellevue Med Ctr 1988; **Fellow:** Gastroenterology, NYU/Manhattan VA Med Ctr 1990; **Fac Appt:** Asst Clin Prof Med, NYU Sch Med

Antonelle, Robert MD (Ge) - **Spec Exp:** Gastroesophageal Reflux Disease (GERD); Liver & Biliary Disease; Colonoscopy; **Hospital:** White Plains Hosp Ctr (page 714); **Address:** 311 North St, rm 302, White Plains, NY 10605-2232; **Phone:** 914-949-7171; **Board Cert:** Internal Medicine 1992; Gastroenterology 1995; **Med School:** NY Med Coll 1989; **Resid:** Internal Medicine, Westchester Med Ctr 1990; **Fellow:** Gastroenterology, Westchester Med Ctr 1994; **Fac Appt:** Asst Clin Prof Med, NY Med Coll

Auerbach, Mitchell E MD (Ge) - **Spec Exp:** Colonoscopy; Crohn's Disease; Ulcerative Colitis; **Hospital:** Saint Joseph's Med Ctr - Yonkers, St John's Riverside Hosp; **Address:** 469 N Broadway, Yonkers, NY 10701-1923; **Phone:** 914-969-1115; **Board Cert:** Internal Medicine 1994; Gastroenterology 1997; **Med School:** Tufts Univ 1991; **Resid:** Internal Medicine, Mt Sinai Hosp 1994; **Fellow:** Gastroenterology, Mt Sinai Hosp 1996

Chinitz, Marvin MD (Ge) - **Spec Exp:** Colonoscopy; Inflammatory Bowel Disease; Liver Disease; **Hospital:** Northern Westchester Hosp; **Address:** Mt Kisco Medical Group, 90 S Bedford Rd, Mt Kisco, NY 10549-3422; **Phone:** 914-241-1050; **Board Cert:** Internal Medicine 1982; Gastroenterology 1985; **Med School:** Boston Univ 1978; **Resid:** Internal Medicine, Boston Med Ctr 1981; **Fellow:** Gastroenterology, Montefiore Med Ctr 1984; **Fac Appt:** Asst Prof Med, Albert Einstein Coll Med

Dworkin, Brad MD (Ge) - **Spec Exp:** Motility Disorders; Endoscopic Ultrasound; Endoscopy; **Hospital:** Westchester Med Ctr (page 713); **Address:** NY Medical College, Munger Pavilion, Ste 206, Valhalla, NY 10595; **Phone:** 914-493-7337; **Board Cert:** Internal Medicine 1979; Gastroenterology 1981; **Med School:** Jefferson Med Coll 1976; **Resid:** Internal Medicine, New York Hosp 1979; **Fellow:** Gastroenterology, Meml Sloan Kettering Cancer Ctr 1981; **Fac Appt:** Prof Med, NY Med Coll

Ehrlich, James B MD (Ge) - **Spec Exp:** Ulcerative Colitis; Colonoscopy; **Hospital:** Lawrence Hosp Ctr; **Address:** 1 Pondfield Rd, Ste 301, Bronxville, NY 10708-3706; **Phone:** 914-779-3333; **Board Cert:** Internal Medicine 1983; Gastroenterology 1985; **Med School:** Univ Hlth Sci/Chicago Med Sch 1980; **Resid:** Internal Medicine, Univ Illinois 1983; **Fellow:** Gastroenterology, Michael Reese Med Ctr 1985

Field, Barry E MD (Ge) - **Spec Exp:** Ulcerative Colitis; Crohn's Disease; **Hospital:** Phelps Meml Hosp Ctr; **Address:** 777 N Broadway, Ste 305, Sleepy Hollow, NY 10591-1040; **Phone:** 914-366-6120; **Board Cert:** Internal Medicine 1976; Gastroenterology 1979; **Med School:** Albert Einstein Coll Med 1972; **Resid:** Internal Medicine, Metropolitan Hosp Ctr 1976; **Fellow:** Gastroenterology, Harbor Genl Hosp 1978

Geders, Jane MD/PhD (Ge) - **Spec Exp:** Hepatitis C; Nutrition; Colon Cancer Screening; **Hospital:** Northern Westchester Hosp, Putnam Hosp Ctr; **Address:** 90 S Bedford Rd, Mt Kisco, NY 10549; **Phone:** 914-242-1307; **Board Cert:** Internal Medicine 2001; Gastroenterology 2003; **Med School:** Univ S Fla Coll Med 1987; **Resid:** Internal Medicine, Meml Sloan Kettering Cancer Ctr 1988; Internal Medicine, N Shore Univ Hosp 1990; **Fellow:** Gastroenterology, Mt Sinai Med Ctr 1992; Hepatology, Mt Sinai Med Ctr 1993; **Fac Appt:** Asst Prof Med, NYU Sch Med

Gendler, Seth MD (Ge) - **Spec Exp:** Pancreatic/Biliary Endoscopy (ERCP); Biliary Disease; Pancreatic Disease; **Hospital:** Sound Shore Med Ctr - Westchester (page 711); **Address:** 140 Lockwood Ave, Ste 104, New Rochelle, NY 10801-4907; **Phone:** 914-235-9333; **Board Cert:** Internal Medicine 1986; Gastroenterology 2001; **Med School:** Rush Med Coll 1983; **Resid:** Internal Medicine, St Lukes Hosp 1986; **Fellow:** Gastroenterology, St Lukes Hosp 1988; Endoscopy, Univ Hosp 1989; **Fac Appt:** Assoc Prof Med, NY Med Coll

Genn, David A MD (Ge) - **Spec Exp:** Liver Disease; Colon Cancer; Gastroesophageal Reflux Disease (GERD); Barrett's Esophagus; **Hospital:** Hudson Valley Hosp Ctr; **Address:** 1985 Crompond Rd, Cortlandt Manor, NY 10567-4146; **Phone:** 914-739-2400; **Board Cert:** Internal Medicine 1992; Gastroenterology 2003; **Med School:** Boston Univ 1988; **Resid:** Internal Medicine, Montefiore Med Ctr 1991; **Fellow:** Gastroenterology, Westchester Med Ctr 1993

Goldblatt, Robert MD (Ge) - **Spec Exp:** Liver Disease; Biliary Disease; Endoscopy; **Hospital:** NY-Presby Hosp (page 100), Greenwich Hosp; **Address:** 18 Rye Ridge Plaza, Rye Brook, NY 10573; **Phone:** 914-253-9252; **Board Cert:** Internal Medicine 1978; Gastroenterology 1979; **Med School:** Geo Wash Univ 1974; **Resid:** Internal Medicine, Univ FL-Shands Hosp 1977; **Fellow:** Gastroenterology, Yale-New Haven Hosp 1979; **Fac Appt:** Asst Prof Med, Cornell Univ-Weill Med Coll

Gould, Richard MD (Ge) - **Spec Exp:** Colonoscopy; Gastroscopy; **Hospital:** Lawrence Hosp Ctr; **Address:** 1 Pondfield Rd W, Ste 1R, Bronxville, NY 10708; **Phone:** 914-779-6200; **Board Cert:** Internal Medicine 1975; Gastroenterology 1977; **Med School:** SUNY Upstate Med Univ 1972; **Resid:** Internal Medicine, Montefiore Hosp Med Ctr 1975; **Fellow:** Gastroenterology, Montefiore Hosp Med Ctr 1977; **Fac Appt:** Assoc Clin Prof Med, Columbia P&S

Heier, Stephen MD (Ge) - **Spec Exp:** Colonoscopy/Polypectomy; Gastric & Esophageal Disorders; Pancreatic/Biliary Endoscopy (ERCP); **Hospital:** Westchester Med Ctr (page 713); **Address:** New York Medical College, Munger Pavilion, rm 408, Valhalla, NY 10595; **Phone:** 914-493-8699; **Board Cert:** Internal Medicine 1979; Gastroenterology 1981; **Med School:** Albany Med Coll 1976; **Resid:** Internal Medicine, Flower Fifth Ave/Metro Hosps 1979; **Fellow:** Gastroenterology, Tufts Univ 1981; **Fac Appt:** Clin Prof Med, NY Med Coll

Kahn, Oren MD (Ge) - **Spec Exp:** Colon Cancer; Inflammatory Bowel Disease; Peptic Ulcer Disease; **Hospital:** Northern Westchester Hosp; **Address:** 90 S Bedford Rd, Mount Kisco, NY 10549; **Phone:** 914-241-1050; **Board Cert:** Internal Medicine 2004; Gastroenterology 1997; **Med School:** Albert Einstein Coll Med 1990; **Resid:** Internal Medicine, Mt Sinai Med Ctr 1994; **Fellow:** Gastroenterology, Mt Sinai Med Ctr 1996; **Fac Appt:** Assoc Clin Prof Med, Mount Sinai Sch Med

Katz, Henry J MD (Ge) - **Hospital:** Montefiore Med Ctr, Comm Hosp - Dobbs Ferry; **Address:** 1234 Central Park Ave, Yonkers, NY 10704-1068; **Phone:** 914-793-1600; **Board Cert:** Internal Medicine 1983; Gastroenterology 1985; **Med School:** Albany Med Coll 1980; **Resid:** Internal Medicine, Bellevue Hosp 1983; **Fellow:** Gastroenterology, Montefiore Med Ctr 1985

Kozicky, Orest MD (Ge) - **Spec Exp:** Colitis; Peptic Ulcer Disease; Gastroesophageal Reflux Disease (GERD); **Hospital:** St John's Riverside Hosp, Saint Joseph's Med Ctr - Yonkers; **Address:** 469 N Broadway, Yonkers, NY 10701-1923; **Phone:** 914-969-1115; **Board Cert:** Internal Medicine 1985; Gastroenterology 1987; **Med School:** NY Med Coll 1981; **Resid:** Internal Medicine, Jacobi Med Ctr 1985; **Fellow:** Gastroenterology, Montefiore Hosp Med Ctr 1987; **Fac Appt:** Asst Clin Prof Med, Albert Einstein Coll Med

Kressner, Michael MD (Ge) - **Spec Exp:** Colon Cancer; Inflammatory Bowel Disease; Biliary Disease; **Hospital:** Sound Shore Med Ctr - Westchester (page 711), Mount Vernon Hosp (page 712); **Address:** 140 Lockwood Ave, Ste 110, New Rochelle, NY 10801-4907; **Phone:** 914-636-5222; **Board Cert:** Internal Medicine 1980; Gastroenterology 1983; **Med School:** SUNY Buffalo 1977; **Resid:** Internal Medicine, Albert Einstein 1980; **Fellow:** Gastroenterology, Albert Einstein 1982; **Fac Appt:** Asst Clin Prof Med, NY Med Coll

Landau, Steven MD (Ge) - **Spec Exp:** Inflammatory Bowel Disease; Colon Cancer; **Hospital:** White Plains Hosp Ctr (page 714); **Address:** 30 Greenridge Ave, White Plains, NY 10605; **Phone:** 914-328-8555; **Board Cert:** Internal Medicine 1984; Gastroenterology 1987; **Med School:** NYU Sch Med 1981; **Resid:** Internal Medicine, Jacobi Med Ctr 1982; Internal Medicine, Albert Einstein Coll Med 1984; **Fellow:** Gastroenterology, Mount Sinai Hosp 1986; **Fac Appt:** Asst Prof Med, Albert Einstein Coll Med

Lebovics, Edward MD (Ge) - **Spec Exp:** Hepatitis B & C; Pancreatic/Biliary Endoscopy (ERCP); Crohn's Disease; Liver Disease; **Hospital:** Westchester Med Ctr (page 713); **Address:** NY Med College-Div Gastroenterology, Munger Pavilion, Ste 206, Valhalla, NY 10595; **Phone:** 914-493-7337; **Board Cert:** Internal Medicine 1983; Gastroenterology 1985; **Med School:** NYU Sch Med 1980; **Resid:** Internal Medicine, Jewish Hosp 1983; **Fellow:** Hepatology, Mount Sinai Hosp 1984; Gastroenterology, NY Med Coll 1986; **Fac Appt:** Prof Med, NY Med Coll

Liss, Mark MD (Ge) - **Spec Exp:** Endoscopy; Peptic Acid Disorders; Inflammatory Bowel Disease; **Hospital:** Sound Shore Med Ctr - Westchester (page 711), Montefiore Med Ctr; **Address:** 140 Lockwood Ave, Ste 318, New Rochelle, NY 10801; **Phone:** 914-633-0888; **Board Cert:** Internal Medicine 1980; Gastroenterology 1983; **Med School:** Mount Sinai Sch Med 1977; **Resid:** Internal Medicine, Mt Sinai Hosp 1980; **Fellow:** Gastroenterology, Montefiore Hosp Med Ctr 1982; **Fac Appt:** Asst Clin Prof Med, Albert Einstein Coll Med

Rosemarin, Jack MD (Ge) - **Spec Exp:** Colon Cancer; Peptic Acid Disorders; Nutrition; **Hospital:** White Plains Hosp Ctr (page 714), NY United Hosp Med Ctr; **Address:** 222 Westchester Ave, Ste 308, White Plains, NY 10604-2925; **Phone:** 914-683-1555; **Board Cert:** Internal Medicine 1982; Gastroenterology 1983; **Med School:** NY Med Coll 1978; **Resid:** Internal Medicine, NY Med Coll 1981; **Fellow:** Gastroenterology, Yale Affil Hosps 1983

Roston, Alfred MD (Ge) - **Spec Exp:** Pancreatic/Biliary Endoscopy (ERCP); **Hospital:** White Plains Hosp Ctr (page 714); **Address:** 222 Westchester Ave, Ste 308, White Plains, NY 10604; **Phone:** 914-683-1555; **Board Cert:** Gastroenterology 1995; **Med School:** NYU Sch Med 1989; **Resid:** Internal Medicine, Mt Sinai Hosp 1992; **Fellow:** Gastroenterology, NY Hosp-Cornell Univ Med 1994

Salama, Meir MD (Ge) - **Spec Exp:** Colonoscopy; Endoscopy; **Hospital:** Montefiore Med Ctr; **Address:** Intercounty Medical Bldg, 955 Yonkers Ave, rm 200, Yonkers, NY 10704; **Phone:** 914-237-0011; **Board Cert:** Internal Medicine 2000; Gastroenterology 1993; **Med School:** NY Med Coll 1987; **Resid:** Internal Medicine, Montefiore Hosp Med Ctr 1990; **Fellow:** Gastroenterology, NY Med Ctr 1992

Shapiro, Neil MD (Ge) - **Spec Exp:** Endoscopy; Liver Disease; Inflammatory Bowel Disease; **Hospital:** White Plains Hosp Ctr (page 714), Greenwich Hosp; **Address:** 18 Rye Ridge Plaza, Rye Brook, NY 10573; **Phone:** 914-253-9252; **Board Cert:** Internal Medicine 1978; Gastroenterology 1981; **Med School:** Wayne State Univ 1975; **Resid:** Internal Medicine, Beth Israel Hosp 1978; **Fellow:** Gastroenterology, Montefiore Hosp Med Ctr 1980; **Fac Appt:** Asst Clin Prof Med, Cornell Univ-Weill Med Coll

Taffet, Sanford MD (Ge) - **Spec Exp:** Inflammatory Bowel Disease; Colon Cancer; Liver Disease; **Hospital:** Sound Shore Med Ctr - Westchester (page 711), Mount Vernon Hosp (page 712); **Address:** 140 Lockwood Ave, Ste 110, New Rochelle, NY 10801-4907; **Phone:** 914-636-5222; **Board Cert:** Internal Medicine 1980; Gastroenterology 1981; **Med School:** NY Med Coll 1976; **Resid:** Internal Medicine, Maimonides Med Ctr 1979; **Fellow:** Gastroenterology, Albert Einstein Med Ctr 1981; **Fac Appt:** Assoc Clin Prof Med, NY Med Coll

Torman, Julie MD (Ge) - **Spec Exp:** Colon Cancer Screening; Swallowing Disorders; **Hospital:** Phelps Meml Hosp Ctr; **Address:** 2005 Albany Post Rd, Ste 15, Croton-on-Hudson, NY 10520; **Phone:** 914-271-4212; **Board Cert:** Internal Medicine 1983; Gastroenterology 1989; **Med School:** Univ Nevada 1980; **Resid:** Internal Medicine, Brigham & Womens Hosp 1983; **Fellow:** Gastroenterology, Stanford Univ Med Ctr 1985

Wayne, Peter MD (Ge) - **Spec Exp:** Hepatitis; Pancreatic/Biliary Endoscopy (ERCP); **Hospital:** Saint Joseph's Med Ctr - Yonkers, St John's Riverside Hosp; **Address:** 469 N Broadway, Yonkers, NY 10701-1923; **Phone:** 914-969-1115; **Board Cert:** Internal Medicine 1979; Gastroenterology 1981; **Med School:** Albert Einstein Coll Med 1976; **Resid:** Internal Medicine, Montefiore Hosp Med Ctr 1979; **Fellow:** Gastroenterology, Mount Sinai Hosp 1981

Wolf, David C MD (Ge) - **Spec Exp:** Liver Failure; Transplant Medicine-Liver; Liver Disease; **Hospital:** Westchester Med Ctr (page 713); **Address:** NY Med Coll, Div GI, Munger Pavilion, Rm 206, Valhalla, NY 10595; **Phone:** 914-493-7337; **Board Cert:** Internal Medicine 1988; Gastroenterology 2001; **Med School:** Columbia P&S 1985; **Resid:** Internal Medicine, NY Presby Hosp 1988; **Fellow:** Gastroenterology, Albert Einstein Coll Med 1991; **Fac Appt:** Assoc Clin Prof Med, NY Med Coll

GERIATRIC MEDICINE

Kalchthaler, Thomas DO (Ger) **PCP** - **Hospital:** Saint Joseph's Med Ctr - Yonkers, Sound Shore Med Ctr - Westchester (page 711); **Address:** 69 S Broadway, Yonkers, NY 10701-4004; **Phone:** 914-376-5555; **Board Cert:** Internal Medicine 1976; Geriatric Medicine 1992; **Med School:** Chicago Coll Osteo Med 1971; **Resid:** Internal Medicine, Elmhurst Hosp 1975; **Fellow:** Geriatric Medicine, Elmhurst Hosp 1974; **Fac Appt:** Asst Prof Med, NY Med Coll

GYNECOLOGIC ONCOLOGY

Kwon, Tae MD (GO) - **Spec Exp:** Uterine Cancer; Cervical Cancer; Ovarian Cancer; **Hospital:** Our Lady of Mercy Med Ctr, Phelps Meml Hosp Ctr; **Address:** 33 W Main St, Ste 304, Elmsford, NY 10523; **Phone:** 914-592-3811; **Board Cert:** Obstetrics & Gynecology 1978; Gynecologic Oncology 1981; **Med School:** South Korea 1965; **Resid:** Obstetrics & Gynecology, Lenox Hill Hosp 1974; Gynecologic Oncology, Lenox Hill Hosp 1976; **Fellow:** Gynecologic Oncology, Univ Mississippi Hosp 1978; **Fac Appt:** Assoc Prof ObG, NY Med Coll

HEMATOLOGY

Caron, Philip C MD/PhD (Hem) - **Hospital:** Phelps Meml Hosp Ctr; **Address:** 777 N Broadway, Ste 102, Sleepy Hollow, NY 10591; **Phone:** 914-366-0664; **Board Cert:** Internal Medicine 1989; Medical Oncology 2003; Hematology 1997; **Med School:** NY Med Coll 1986; **Resid:** Internal Medicine, Mt Sinai Hosp 1989; **Fellow:** Hematology & Oncology, Meml Sloan Kettering Cancer Ctr 1992

Lester, Thomas J MD (Hem) - **Hospital:** Northern Westchester Hosp; **Address:** Katonah Medical Group, 111 Bedford Rd, Katonah, NY 10536-2190; **Phone:** 914-232-3135; **Board Cert:** Internal Medicine 1982; Hematology 1984; Medical Oncology 1987; **Med School:** Rutgers Univ 1979; **Resid:** Internal Medicine, Mt Sinai Hosp 1982; **Fellow:** Hematology, Mt Sinai Hosp 1984; Medical Oncology, Meml Sloan Kettering Cancer Ctr 1986

Nelson, John C MD (Hem) - **Hospital:** Westchester Med Ctr (page 713); **Address:** Westchester Hem/Onc Grp, 19 Bradhurst Ave, Ste 2100, Hawthorne, NY 10532; **Phone:** 914-493-8353; **Board Cert:** Internal Medicine 1974; Hematology 1976; **Med School:** Harvard Med Sch 1971; **Resid:** Internal Medicine, Mount Sinai Med Ctr 1974; **Fellow:** Hematology, Westchester Med Ctr 1976; **Fac Appt:** Assoc Prof Med, NY Med Coll

INFECTIOUS DISEASE

Berkey, Peter MD (Inf) - **Spec Exp:** Immune Deficiency; Tick-borne Diseases; Travel Medicine; **Hospital:** St John's Riverside Hosp, Saint Joseph's Med Ctr - Yonkers; **Address:** 970 N Broadway, Ste 212, Yonkers, NY 10701-1311; **Phone:** 914-376-1543; **Board Cert:** Internal Medicine 1985; Infectious Disease 1988; **Med School:** Univ Puerto Rico 1980; **Resid:** Internal Medicine, Westchester Med Ctr 1984; **Fellow:** Infectious Disease, MD Anderson Hosp 1988

Horowitz, Harold MD (Inf) - **Spec Exp:** AIDS/HIV; Tick-borne Diseases; Travel Medicine; **Hospital:** Westchester Med Ctr (page 713); **Address:** NY Med Coll, Div Inf Disease, Munger Pavilion, Ste 245, Valhalla, NY 10595; **Phone:** 914-493-8865; **Board Cert:** Internal Medicine 1983; Infectious Disease 1988; **Med School:** NYU Sch Med 1979; **Resid:** Internal Medicine, Univ Wisconsin Hosp 1983; **Fellow:** Infectious Disease, New England Med Ctr 1986; **Fac Appt:** Prof Med, NY Med Coll

Lederman, Jeffrey A MD (Inf) - **Hospital:** Sound Shore Med Ctr - Westchester (page 711); **Address:** Sound Shore Medical Ctr, 16 Guion Pl Fl 2, New Rochelle, NY 10802; **Phone:** 914-637-1657; **Board Cert:** Internal Medicine 2000; Infectious Disease 2000; **Med School:** Jefferson Med Coll 1988; **Resid:** Internal Medicine, Mt Sinai Hosp 1991; **Fellow:** Infectious Disease, Montefiore Med Ctr 1995

Nadelman, Robert MD (Inf) - **Spec Exp:** Tick-borne Diseases; Lyme Disease; **Hospital:** Westchester Med Ctr (page 713); **Address:** NY Med Coll, Div Inf Dis, Munger Pavillion, rm 245, Valhalla, NY 10595; **Phone:** 914-493-8865; **Board Cert:** Internal Medicine 1983; Infectious Disease 1988; **Med School:** Albert Einstein Coll Med 1980; **Resid:** Internal Medicine, Beth Israel Hosp 1983; **Fellow:** Infectious Disease, Beth Israel Hosp 1985; **Fac Appt:** Prof Med, NY Med Coll

Rush, Thomas MD (Inf) - **Spec Exp:** AIDS/HIV; Lyme Disease; Travel Medicine; **Hospital:** Phelps Meml Hosp Ctr, Putnam Hosp Ctr; **Address:** 540 N State Rd, Briarcliff Manor, NY 10510; **Phone:** 914-762-2276; **Board Cert:** Internal Medicine 1981; Infectious Disease 1984; **Med School:** Rush Med Coll 1978; **Resid:** Internal Medicine, Genesee Hosp 1981; **Fellow:** Infectious Disease, Strong Meml Hosp 1983; **Fac Appt:** Asst Clin Prof Med, NY Med Coll

Wormser, Gary MD (Inf) - **Spec Exp:** Lyme Disease; AIDS/HIV; Diagnostic Problems; **Hospital:** Westchester Med Ctr (page 713); **Address:** New York Medical College, Munger Pavilion, rm 245, Valhalla, NY 10595; **Phone:** 914-493-8865; **Board Cert:** Internal Medicine 1978; Infectious Disease 1982; **Med School:** Johns Hopkins Univ 1972; **Resid:** Internal Medicine, Mount Sinai Hosp 1975; **Fellow:** Infectious Disease, Mount Sinai Hosp 1977; **Fac Appt:** Prof Med, NY Med Coll

INTERNAL MEDICINE

Abenavoli, Tancredi J MD (IM) `PCP` - **Hospital:** White Plains Hosp Ctr (page 714); **Address:** 446 Westchester Ave, Port Chester, NY 10573; **Phone:** 914-939-1573; **Board Cert:** Internal Medicine 1979; Cardiovascular Disease 1981; **Med School:** NYU Sch Med 1976; **Resid:** Internal Medicine, VA Hosp/NYU Med Ctr 1979; **Fellow:** Cardiovascular Disease, VA Hosp/NYU Med Ctr 1981

Alpert, Barbara MD (IM) `PCP` - **Spec Exp:** Osteoporosis; Lyme Disease; **Hospital:** Northern Westchester Hosp; **Address:** 90 S Bedford Rd, Mt Kisco, NY 10549; **Phone:** 914-241-1050; **Board Cert:** Internal Medicine 1987; **Med School:** Univ Pennsylvania 1984; **Resid:** Internal Medicine, NY-Cornell Hosp 1987

Alter, Sheldon MD (IM) `PCP` - **Spec Exp:** Kidney Disease; **Hospital:** White Plains Hosp Ctr (page 714); **Address:** 33 Davis Ave, White Plains, NY 10605-1030; **Phone:** 914-946-5354; **Board Cert:** Internal Medicine 1980; Nephrology 1972; **Med School:** Univ Hlth Sci/Chicago Med Sch 1961; **Resid:** Internal Medicine, Montefiore Hosp Med Ctr 1964; **Fellow:** Nephrology, St Luke's Hosp 1966

Altholz, Jeffrey MD (IM) `PCP` - **Spec Exp:** Occupational Medicine; Addiction Medicine; **Hospital:** Phelps Meml Hosp Ctr, Comm Hosp - Dobbs Ferry; **Address:** 160 S Central Ave, Elmsford, NY 10523; **Phone:** 914-345-3135; **Board Cert:** Internal Medicine 2003; **Med School:** Albert Einstein Coll Med 1986; **Resid:** Internal Medicine, St Vincents Hosp 1989; **Fellow:** Internal Medicine, St Vincents Hosp 1990

Bagg, Jennifer G MD (IM) - **Hospital:** Sound Shore Med Ctr - Westchester (page 711); **Address:** 1255 North Ave, New Rochelle, NY 10804; **Phone:** 914-576-2010; **Board Cert:** Internal Medicine 2005; **Med School:** NY Med Coll 1988; **Resid:** Internal Medicine, Cabrini Med Ctr 1991

Berman, Daniel MD (IM) `PCP` - **Spec Exp:** Infectious Disease; **Hospital:** White Plains Hosp Ctr (page 714), NY Westchester Sq Med Ctr; **Address:** 56 Doyer Ave, Ste 1E, White Plains, NY 10605; **Phone:** 914-948-0500; **Board Cert:** Internal Medicine 1985; Infectious Disease 1988; **Med School:** NYU Sch Med 1982; **Resid:** Internal Medicine, NYU Med Ctr 1985; **Fellow:** Infectious Disease, NYU Med Ctr 1989

Colangelo, Daniel MD (IM) `PCP` - **Hospital:** White Plains Hosp Ctr (page 714); **Address:** 1600 Harrison Ave, Ste G 105, Mamaroneck, NY 10543-3149; **Phone:** 914-698-4466; **Board Cert:** Internal Medicine 2004; **Med School:** NYU Sch Med 1980; **Resid:** Internal Medicine, Lenox Hill Hosp 1983

Croen, Kenneth MD (IM) `PCP` - **Spec Exp:** Infectious Disease; Herpes Simplex; **Hospital:** White Plains Hosp Ctr (page 714); **Address:** 259 Heathcote Rd, Scarsdale, NY 10583-4523; **Phone:** 914-723-8100; **Board Cert:** Internal Medicine 1984; Infectious Disease 1988; **Med School:** Albert Einstein Coll Med 1980; **Resid:** Internal Medicine, Columbia-Presby Hosp 1984; **Fellow:** Infectious Disease, Natl Inst Hlth 1989

De Angelis, Arthur MD (IM) `PCP` - **Spec Exp:** Cholesterol/Lipid Disorders; Heart Disease; **Hospital:** Greenwich Hosp; **Address:** 3020 Westchester Ave Fl 2, Purchase, NY 10577; **Phone:** 914-253-6464; **Board Cert:** Internal Medicine 1975; Cardiovascular Disease 1977; **Med School:** SUNY Buffalo 1969; **Resid:** Internal Medicine, Montefiore Hosp Med Ctr 1971; **Fellow:** Cardiovascular Disease, Mt Sinai Hosp 1975; **Fac Appt:** Asst Clin Prof Med, Cornell Univ-Weill Med Coll

Dennett, Ronald MD (IM) `PCP` - **Hospital:** Lawrence Hosp Ctr, Montefiore Med Ctr; **Address:** 1254 Central Park Ave, Yonkers, NY 10704-1059; **Phone:** 914-965-1771; **Board Cert:** Internal Medicine 1980; **Med School:** Univ VT Coll Med 1977; **Resid:** Internal Medicine, Univ Colorado Hosp 1980; **Fac Appt:** Asst Clin Prof Med, Albert Einstein Coll Med

Elkind, Arthur H MD (IM) - **Spec Exp:** Headache; **Hospital:** Mount Vernon Hosp (page 712); **Address:** 12 N 7th Ave, Mount Vernon, ny 10550; **Phone:** 914-667-2230; **Board Cert:** Internal Medicine 1964; **Med School:** SUNY Downstate 1957; **Resid:** Internal Medicine, Maimonides Hosp 1961; **Fellow:** Metabolism, Montefiore Med Ctr 1962; **Fac Appt:** Asst Clin Prof Med, NY Med Coll

Fazio, Nelson M MD (IM) `PCP` - **Spec Exp:** Skin Diseases; Hypertension; Obesity; **Hospital:** Lawrence Hosp Ctr; **Address:** 133 Montgomery Ave Fl Ground, Scarsdale, NY 10583; **Phone:** 914-713-8517; **Board Cert:** Internal Medicine 1986; **Med School:** NY Med Coll 1981; **Resid:** Internal Medicine, Westchester Med Ctr 1984; **Fellow:** Infectious Disease, Montefiore Hosp Med Ctr 1994

Federman, Harold MD (IM) `PCP` - **Spec Exp:** Hospice-Palliative Care; **Hospital:** Northern Westchester Hosp; **Address:** 336 Route 202 Bailey Bldg, Somers, NY 10589; **Phone:** 914-277-0843; **Board Cert:** Internal Medicine 1972; **Med School:** NYU Sch Med 1964; **Resid:** Internal Medicine, Bellevue Hosp/NYU Med Ctr 1971; **Fac Appt:** Asst Prof Med, NYU Sch Med

Finkelstein, Michael MD (IM) - **Spec Exp:** Complementary Medicine; **Hospital:** Northern Westchester Hosp; **Address:** Center for Health & Healing, 39 Smith Ave, Mt Kisko, NY 10549; **Phone:** 914-244-9393; **Board Cert:** Internal Medicine 1989; **Med School:** Univ Pennsylvania 1986; **Resid:** Internal Medicine, Lenox Hill Hosp 1989

Fiorentino, Thomas MD (IM) - **Spec Exp:** Palliative Care; **Hospital:** St John's Riverside Hosp; **Address:** 984 North Broadway, Ste 303, Yonkers, NY 10701; **Phone:** 914-969-0770; **Board Cert:** Internal Medicine 1975; **Med School:** NY Med Coll 1972; **Resid:** Internal Medicine, Metropolitan Hosp 1976

Goldman, Jack S MD (IM) `PCP` - **Spec Exp:** Colonoscopy/Polypectomy; Liver Disease; Endoscopy; **Hospital:** Saint Joseph's Med Ctr - Yonkers, Montefiore Med Ctr; **Address:** 750 McLean Ave, Yonkers, NY 10704; **Phone:** 914-237-8686; **Board Cert:** Internal Medicine 1975; Gastroenterology 1979; **Med School:** Albert Einstein Coll Med 1961; **Resid:** Internal Medicine, Bronx Lebanon Hosp 1963; Internal Medicine, VA Med Ctr 1966; **Fellow:** Gastroenterology, VA Med Ctr 1965

Herzog, David A MD (IM) **PCP** - **Spec Exp:** Cholesterol/Lipid Disorders; Preventive Medicine; **Hospital:** Sound Shore Med Ctr - Westchester (page 711); **Address:** 1380 Boston Post Rd, Larchmont, NY 10538; **Phone:** 914-833-1080; **Board Cert:** Internal Medicine 1984; **Med School:** Mount Sinai Sch Med 1981; **Resid:** Internal Medicine, St Luke's Hosp 1984; **Fac Appt:** Asst Clin Prof Med, NY Med Coll

Higgins, William MD (IM) **PCP** - **Spec Exp:** Alzheimer's Disease; **Hospital:** Hudson Valley Hosp Ctr; **Address:** 1985 Crompond Rd, Cortlandt Manor, NY 10566-4146; **Phone:** 914-739-3597; **Board Cert:** Internal Medicine 2002; **Med School:** Geo Wash Univ 1986; **Resid:** Internal Medicine, Lenox Hill Hosp 1989; **Fellow:** Pulmonary Disease, Lenox Hill Hosp 1991; **Fac Appt:** Assoc Clin Prof Med, NY Med Coll

Hopkins, Arthur MD (IM) **PCP** - **Hospital:** Montefiore Med Ctr; **Address:** 1010 Central Park Ave, Yonkers, NY 10704; **Phone:** 914-964-4183; **Board Cert:** Internal Medicine 1986; **Med School:** Univ Pennsylvania 1983; **Resid:** Internal Medicine, Hosp Univ Penn 1986; **Fac Appt:** Asst Prof Med, Albert Einstein Coll Med

Isaacs, Ellen MD (IM) - **Spec Exp:** Hypertension; Heart Disease; **Hospital:** Saint Joseph's Med Ctr - Yonkers, St John's Riverside Hosp; **Address:** 1019 Yonkers Ave, Yonkers, NY 10704; **Phone:** 914-963-9493; **Board Cert:** Internal Medicine 1972; Cardiovascular Disease 1981; **Med School:** NYU Sch Med 1969; **Resid:** Internal Medicine, Bellevue Hosp 1972; **Fellow:** Cardiovascular Disease, St Vincent's Hosp Med Ctr 1974; **Fac Appt:** Asst Prof Med, NY Med Coll

Kaplan, Kenneth C MD (IM) **PCP** - **Spec Exp:** Cardiology; Vascular Ultrasound; **Hospital:** Phelps Meml Hosp Ctr; **Address:** 160 N State Rd, Briarcliff Manor, NY 10510; **Phone:** 914-762-3821; **Board Cert:** Internal Medicine 1970; Cardiovascular Disease 1975; **Med School:** NYU Sch Med 1962; **Resid:** Internal Medicine, Bellevue Hosp 1966; **Fellow:** Cardiovascular Disease, Bellevue Hosp/NYU 1969

Kapoor, Satish MD (IM) **PCP** - **Spec Exp:** Asthma; Emphysema; Preventive Medicine; **Hospital:** Phelps Meml Hosp Ctr, Comm Hosp - Dobbs Ferry; **Address:** 362 N Broadway Fl 2, North Tarrytown, NY 10591-1040; **Phone:** 914-631-2070; **Board Cert:** Internal Medicine 1979; **Med School:** India 1972; **Resid:** Internal Medicine, Kingsbrook Jewish MC 1979; **Fellow:** Pulmonary Disease, Queens Hosp 1981

Karmen, Carol MD (IM) **PCP** - **Spec Exp:** Cancer Screening; Preventive Medicine; **Hospital:** Westchester Med Ctr (page 713); **Address:** 311 North St, Ste 207, White Plains, NY 10605; **Phone:** 914-681-0926; **Board Cert:** Internal Medicine 1996; **Med School:** Albert Einstein Coll Med 1986; **Resid:** Internal Medicine, Westchester Med Ctr 1990; **Fac Appt:** Asst Prof Med, NY Med Coll

Lans, David DO (IM) **PCP** - **Spec Exp:** Rheumatoid Arthritis; Lupus/SLE; Asthma; Osteoporosis; **Hospital:** Sound Shore Med Ctr - Westchester (page 711), Lawrence Hosp Ctr; **Address:** 838 Pelhamdale Ave, New Rochelle, NY 10801-1032; **Phone:** 914-235-5577; **Board Cert:** Internal Medicine 1984; Allergy & Immunology 1987; Rheumatology 1988; **Med School:** Univ Osteo Med & Hlth Sci, Des Moines 1981; **Resid:** Internal Medicine, Downstate Univ Hosp 1985; **Fellow:** Allergy & Immunology, New Eng Med Ctr 1987; Rheumatology, Hosp For Special Surgery 1989; **Fac Appt:** Asst Clin Prof Med, NY. Med Coll

Lebofsky, Martin MD (IM) - **Spec Exp:** Kidney Disease; Hypertension; Dialysis Care; **Hospital:** Lawrence Hosp Ctr, Saint Joseph's Med Ctr - Yonkers; **Address:** 1 Stone Pl, Bronxville, NY 10708-3406; **Phone:** 914-337-9004; **Board Cert:** Internal Medicine 1975; Nephrology 1978; **Med School:** Albert Einstein Coll Med 1972; **Resid:** Internal Medicine, Harlem Hosp 1975; **Fellow:** Nephrology, Montefiore Hosp Med Ctr 1978

Lechner, Michael MD (IM) **PCP** - **Spec Exp:** Geriatric Medicine; Rehabilitation-Geriatric; **Hospital:** Phelps Meml Hosp Ctr; **Address:** 14 Church St, Ste 208, Ossining, NY 10562-4831; **Phone:** 914-762-0722; **Board Cert:** Internal Medicine 1980; Geriatric Medicine 1992; **Med School:** Albert Einstein Coll Med 1961; **Resid:** Internal Medicine, Westchester Med Ctr 1963; **Fellow:** Hematology, LI Jewish Med Ctr 1965

Melman, Martin MD (IM) **PCP** - **Spec Exp:** Hypertension; Asthma; Geriatric Medicine; **Hospital:** Phelps Meml Hosp Ctr; **Address:** 87 Grand St, Croton On Hudson, NY 10520-2518; **Phone:** 914-271-4845; **Board Cert:** Internal Medicine 1977; **Med School:** NY Med Coll 1974; **Resid:** Internal Medicine, Metropolitan Hosp Ctr 1977; Internal Medicine, Westchester Med Ctr 1978; **Fac Appt:** Asst Clin Prof Med, NY Med Coll

Pappas, Steven MD (IM) **PCP** - **Spec Exp:** Occupational Medicine; Preventive Medicine; **Hospital:** Sound Shore Med Ctr - Westchester (page 711), St John's Riverside Hosp; **Address:** 266 White Plains Rd, Eastchester, NY 10709; **Phone:** 914-793-1115; **Board Cert:** Internal Medicine 1982; Emergency Medicine 2000; **Med School:** Albert Einstein Coll Med 1978; **Resid:** Internal Medicine, St Luke's Roosevelt Hosp Ctr 1981

Peterson, Stephen J MD (IM) **PCP** - **Spec Exp:** Forensic Medicine; **Hospital:** Westchester Med Ctr (page 713); **Address:** Westchester Med Ctr, Munger Pavilion 256, Valhalla, NY 10595; **Phone:** 914-493-8370; **Board Cert:** Internal Medicine 1985; **Med School:** Philippines 1982; **Resid:** Internal Medicine, Metropolitan Hosp Ctr 1986; **Fac Appt:** Clin Prof Med, NY Med Coll

Plesset, Maxwell MD (IM) **PCP** - **Spec Exp:** Infectious Disease; **Hospital:** Northern Westchester Hosp; **Address:** 1825 Commerce St, Yorktown Hts, NY 10598-4432; **Phone:** 914-962-5060; **Board Cert:** Internal Medicine 1976; **Med School:** Univ Pittsburgh 1968; **Resid:** Internal Medicine, North Shore Univ Hosp 1976

Ridge, Gerald MD (IM) **PCP** - **Spec Exp:** Geriatric Medicine; **Hospital:** Lawrence Hosp Ctr, NY-Presby Hosp (page 100); **Address:** 14 Studio Arcade, Bronxville, NY 10708; **Phone:** 914-779-9066; **Board Cert:** Internal Medicine 1998; Geriatric Medicine 1997; **Med School:** UCSF 1979; **Resid:** Internal Medicine, Einstein-Bronx Muni Hosp Ctr 1981; Neurology, Columbia-Presby Med Ctr 1982; **Fellow:** Internal Medicine, NY-Cornell Hosp 1983; **Fac Appt:** Clin Prof Med, Columbia P&S

Rosch, Elliott MD (IM) **PCP** - **Spec Exp:** Preventive Medicine; Cholesterol/Lipid Disorders; Hypertension; **Hospital:** St John's Riverside Hosp; **Address:** 1010 N Broadway, Yonkers, NY 10701-1303; **Phone:** 914-965-4424; **Board Cert:** Internal Medicine 1981; **Med School:** Univ Pennsylvania 1978; **Resid:** Internal Medicine, Pennsylvania Hosp 1981

Saltzman-Gabelman, Lori MD (IM) **PCP** - **Hospital:** White Plains Hosp Ctr (page 714), Greenwich Hosp; **Address:** 210 Westchester Ave, White Plains, NY 10604-2914; **Phone:** 914-682-0700; **Board Cert:** Internal Medicine 1989; **Med School:** NY Med Coll 1986; **Resid:** Internal Medicine, Westchester Med Ctr 1989; **Fac Appt:** , NY Med Coll

Seicol, Noel MD (IM) **PCP** - **Spec Exp:** Asthma & Allergy; Menopause Problems; Osteoporosis; **Hospital:** Greenwich Hosp, Sound Shore Med Ctr - Westchester (page 711); **Address:** 33 Cedar St, Rye, NY 10580-2031; **Phone:** 914-967-3483; **Board Cert:** Internal Medicine 1984; Allergy & Immunology 1984; **Med School:** SUNY Hlth Sci Ctr 1950; **Resid:** Internal Medicine, Montefiore Hosp Med Ctr 1952; Internal Medicine, Beth Israel Hosp 1953; **Fellow:** Internal Medicine, VA Med Ctr 1954

Sheehy, Albert MD (IM) `PCP` - **Hospital:** Phelps Meml Hosp Ctr; **Address:** 362 N Broadway Fl 2, Sleepy Hollow, NY 10591; **Phone:** 914-631-2070; **Board Cert:** Internal Medicine 1982; **Med School:** Univ Rochester 1963; **Resid:** St Vincent's Hosp & Med Ctr 1967Kings County Hosp 1968; **Fellow:** Pulmonary Disease, Kings County Hosp 1969

Soltren, Rafael MD (IM) `PCP` - **Spec Exp:** Diabetes; Hypertension; **Hospital:** Phelps Meml Hosp Ctr; **Address:** 100 S Highland Ave, Ossining, NY 10562; **Phone:** 914-941-1277; **Board Cert:** Internal Medicine 1985; **Med School:** Cornell Univ-Weill Med Coll 1981; **Resid:** Internal Medicine, Montefiore Hosp Med Ctr 1984

Starke, Charles MD (IM) `PCP` - **Hospital:** Phelps Meml Hosp Ctr, Westchester Med Ctr (page 713); **Address:** 516 N State Rd, Briarcliff Manor, NY 10510-1526; **Phone:** 914-762-4460; **Board Cert:** Internal Medicine 1978; **Med School:** Albert Einstein Coll Med 1975; **Resid:** Internal Medicine, Georgetown Univ Hosp 1978

Welch, Peter MD (IM) - **Spec Exp:** Lyme Disease; Tick-borne Diseases; **Hospital:** Northern Westchester Hosp; **Address:** 16 Orchard Drive, Armonk, NY 10504; **Phone:** 914-273-3404; **Board Cert:** Internal Medicine 1977; Infectious Disease 1980; **Med School:** SUNY Buffalo 1974; **Resid:** Internal Medicine, New York Hosp 1977; **Fellow:** Infectious Disease, New York Hosp 1979

Wolfe, Mary J MD (IM) `PCP` - **Spec Exp:** Women's Health; **Hospital:** Phelps Meml Hosp Ctr; **Address:** 14 Church St, Ossining, NY 10562; **Phone:** 914-941-1334; **Board Cert:** Internal Medicine 1980; Emergency Medicine 1996; **Med School:** Penn State Univ-Hershey Med Ctr 1976; **Resid:** Internal Medicine, Westchester Med Ctr 1979

Zarowitz, William MD (IM) `PCP` - **Spec Exp:** Occupational Medicine; Preventive Medicine; **Hospital:** White Plains Hosp Ctr (page 714); **Address:** 143 Maple Ave, White Plains, NY 10601; **Phone:** 914-683-8610; **Board Cert:** Internal Medicine 1981; **Med School:** NY Med Coll 1978; **Resid:** Internal Medicine, Montefiore Hosp Med Ctr 1981

Maternal & Fetal Medicine

Hsu, Chaur Dong MD (MF) - **Spec Exp:** Pregnancy-High Risk; Prenatal Diagnosis; Pregnancy Loss; Hypertension in Pregnancy; **Hospital:** Westchester Med Ctr (page 713); **Address:** NY Medical College, Dept OB/GYN, Munger Pavilion, rm 617, Valhalla, NY 10595; **Phone:** 914-593-8950; **Board Cert:** Obstetrics & Gynecology 2005; Maternal & Fetal Medicine 2005; **Med School:** Taiwan 1982; **Resid:** Obstetrics & Gynecology, Veterans Genl Hosp 1985; Obstetrics & Gynecology, Beth Israel Med Ctr 1990; **Fellow:** Maternal & Fetal Medicine, Johns Hopkins Hosp 1993; **Fac Appt:** Prof ObG, NY Med Coll

Leikin, Enid MD (MF) - **Spec Exp:** Infectious Disease; Genetic Disorders; **Hospital:** White Plains Hosp Ctr (page 714), Westchester Med Ctr (page 713); **Address:** 15 N Broadway, White Plains, NY 10601; **Phone:** 914-328-8444; **Board Cert:** Obstetrics & Gynecology 1997; Maternal & Fetal Medicine 1997; **Med School:** Cornell Univ-Weill Med Coll 1980; **Resid:** Surgery, Mt Sinai Med Ctr 1981; Obstetrics & Gynecology, New York Hosp 1984; **Fellow:** Maternal & Fetal Medicine, Grady Meml Hosp-Emory Univ 1986

Lescale, Keith B MD (MF) - **Spec Exp:** Pregnancy-High Risk; **Hospital:** White Plains Hosp Ctr (page 714); **Address:** White Plains Hospital, Div Perinatology, Davis Ave at E Post Rd Fl 5, White Plains, NY 10601; **Phone:** 914-681-2164; **Board Cert:** Obstetrics & Gynecology 2006; Maternal & Fetal Medicine 2005; **Med School:** Louisiana State Univ 1987; **Resid:** Obstetrics & Gynecology, New Orleans/LSU Med Ctr 1991; Maternal & Fetal Medicine, NY Hosp-Cornell Med Ctr 1993; **Fac Appt:** Asst Clin Prof ObG, Cornell Univ-Weill Med Coll

Mootabar, Hamid MD (MF) - **Spec Exp:** Pregnancy-High Risk; **Hospital:** Lawrence Hosp Ctr, NY-Presby Hosp (page 100); **Address:** Amniocentesis & Genetics Ctr, 77 Pondfield Rd, Bronxville, NY 10708; **Phone:** 914-337-2102; **Board Cert:** Obstetrics & Gynecology 1975; Maternal & Fetal Medicine 1983; **Med School:** Iran 1966; **Resid:** Obstetrics & Gynecology, Roosevelt Hosp 1973; **Fellow:** Maternal & Fetal Medicine, Roosevelt Hosp 1979; **Fac Appt:** Assoc Clin Prof ObG, Columbia P&S

Sullivan, Christopher A MD (MF) - **Hospital:** Northern Westchester Hosp; **Address:** No Westchester Hosp Perinatal Group, 400 E Main St Fl 5, Mount Kisco, NY 10549; **Phone:** 914-666-1010; **Board Cert:** Obstetrics & Gynecology 2004; Maternal & Fetal Medicine 2004; **Med School:** Albany Med Coll 1989; **Resid:** Obstetrics & Gynecology, St Barnabas Med Ctr 1993; **Fellow:** Maternal & Fetal Medicine, Univ of Miss Med Ctr 1995; **Fac Appt:** Asst Clin Prof ObG, Columbia P&S

Tejani, Nergesh MD (MF) - **Hospital:** Jacobi Med Ctr; **Address:** 5 Shady Lane, Ossining, NY 10562; **Phone:** 718-918-6300; **Board Cert:** Obstetrics & Gynecology 1975; Maternal & Fetal Medicine 1979; **Med School:** India 1956; **Resid:** Obstetrics & Gynecology, New York Methodist Hosp 1973

Medical Oncology

Ahmed, Tauseef MD (Onc) - **Spec Exp:** Bone Marrow Transplant; Lymphoma; Brain Tumors; Genitourinary Cancer; **Hospital:** Westchester Med Ctr (page 713); **Address:** NY Medical Coll, Medical Oncology, Munger Pavillon, rm 250, Valhalla, NY 10595; **Phone:** 914-493-8374; **Board Cert:** Internal Medicine 1980; Hematology 1982; Medical Oncology 1983; **Med School:** Pakistan 1976; **Resid:** Internal Medicine, Sinai Hosp 1980; **Fellow:** Medical Oncology, Meml Sloan Kettering Cancer Ctr 1983; **Fac Appt:** Prof Med, NY Med Coll

Bernhardt, Bernard MD (Onc) - **Spec Exp:** Lung Cancer; Prostate Cancer; Breast Cancer; **Hospital:** Sound Shore Med Ctr - Westchester (page 711); **Address:** 50 Guion Pl, New Rochelle, NY 10801-5512; **Phone:** 914-632-5397; **Board Cert:** Internal Medicine 1968; Hematology 1972; Medical Oncology 1973; **Med School:** Northwestern Univ 1961; **Resid:** Internal Medicine, DC Genl Hosp 1963; Internal Medicine, NY Med Coll 1966; **Fellow:** Hematology, Montefiore Hosp Med Ctr 1968; **Fac Appt:** Clin Prof Med, NY Med Coll

Chia, Gloria MD (Onc) - **Spec Exp:** Lung Cancer; Breast Cancer; Solid Tumors; **Hospital:** Phelps Meml Hosp Ctr, Meml Sloan Kettering Cancer Ctr (page 109); **Address:** 777 N Broadway, Ste 201, Sleepy Hollow, NY 10591; **Phone:** 914-366-0664; **Board Cert:** Internal Medicine 1996; Medical Oncology 1997; **Med School:** Philippines 1965; **Resid:** Internal Medicine, VA Med Ctr 1969; Hematology, LI Coll Hosp 1971; **Fellow:** Medical Oncology, Albert Einstein Coll Med 1974

Feldman, Stuart MD (Onc) - **Spec Exp:** Breast Cancer; Lymphoma; **Hospital:** White Plains Hosp Ctr (page 714), NY-Presby Hosp (page 100); **Address:** 210 Westchester Ave, White Plains, NY 10604; **Phone:** 914-681-5200; **Board Cert:** Internal Medicine 1980; Hematology 1982; Medical Oncology 1985; **Med School:** Geo Wash Univ 1977; **Resid:** Internal Medicine, New York Hosp-Cornell 1980; **Fellow:** Hematology & Oncology, Mem Sloan Kettering Cancer Ctr 1983; **Fac Appt:** Asst Clin Prof Med, Cornell Univ-Weill Med Coll

Fialk, Mark A MD (Onc) - **Hospital:** White Plains Hosp Ctr (page 714); **Address:** 259 Heathcote Rd, Scarsdale, NY 10583; **Phone:** 914-723-8100; **Board Cert:** Internal Medicine 1976; Medical Oncology 1977; Hematology 1978; **Med School:** Tufts Univ 1973; **Resid:** Internal Medicine, NY Hosp-Cornell Med Ctr 1975; Internal Medicine, Meml Sloan-Kettering Cancer Ctr 1976; **Fellow:** Hematology & Oncology, NY Hosp-Cornell Med Ctr 1978; Infectious Disease, Meml Sloan-Kettering Cancer Ctr 1979; **Fac Appt:** Asst Clin Prof Med, NY Med Coll

Mills, Nancy Ellyn MD (Onc) - **Spec Exp:** Breast Cancer; Gynecologic Cancer; **Hospital:** Phelps Meml Hosp Ctr, Meml Sloan Kettering Cancer Ctr (page 109); **Address:** Meml Sloan Kettering @ Phelps, 777 N Broadway, Ste 102, Sleepy Hollow, NY 10591; **Phone:** 914-366-0664; **Board Cert:** Internal Medicine 2000; Medical Oncology 2003; Hematology 2004; **Med School:** Mount Sinai Sch Med 1987; **Resid:** Internal Medicine, Mt Sinai Med Ctr 1990; **Fellow:** Hematology & Oncology, NYU Med Ctr 1993; **Fac Appt:** Asst Clin Prof Med, Cornell Univ-Weill Med Coll

Mittelman, Abraham MD (Onc) - **Spec Exp:** Breast Cancer; Melanoma; Prostate Cancer; **Hospital:** Westchester Med Ctr (page 713), Northern Westchester Hosp; **Address:** 311 North St, Ste 305, White Plains, NY 10605; **Phone:** 914-681-0025; **Med School:** Mexico 1977; **Resid:** Internal Medicine, Kings Co Hosp 1980; **Fellow:** Medical Oncology, Meml Sloan Kettering Canc Ctr 1981; **Fac Appt:** Assoc Prof Med, NY Med Coll

Phillips, Elizabeth MD (Onc) - **Spec Exp:** Breast Cancer; Lymphoma; Colon Cancer; **Hospital:** Sound Shore Med Ctr - Westchester (page 711); **Address:** Advanced Oncology Assocs, 50 Guion Pl, Ste 32, New Rochelle, NY 10801-4914; **Phone:** 914-632-5397; **Board Cert:** Internal Medicine 1974; Hematology 1976; Medical Oncology 1977; **Med School:** Univ Wash 1969; **Resid:** Internal Medicine, Harlem Hosp 1972; Hematology, Montefiore Hosp Med Ctr 1973; **Fellow:** Hematology & Oncology, Mem Sloan Kettering Canc Ctr 1976; **Fac Appt:** Assoc Clin Prof Med, NY Med Coll

Provenzano, Anthony MD (Onc) - **Spec Exp:** Lung Cancer; **Hospital:** Lawrence Hosp Ctr, Mount Vernon Hosp (page 712); **Address:** 1 Pondfield Rd W, Ste 1, Bronxville, NY 10708-2635; **Phone:** 914-961-3421; **Board Cert:** Internal Medicine 1979; Medical Oncology 1981; **Med School:** Cornell Univ-Weill Med Coll 1976; **Resid:** Internal Medicine, Lenox Hill Hosp 1978; **Fellow:** Medical Oncology, St Vincents Hosp 1979; **Fac Appt:** Asst Clin Prof Med, NY Med Coll

Puccio, Carmelo MD (Onc) - **Spec Exp:** Breast Cancer; Lung Cancer; Solid Tumors; Gynecologic Cancer; **Hospital:** Westchester Med Ctr (page 713), Sound Shore Med Ctr - Westchester (page 711); **Address:** NY Med Coll, Munger Pavillion, rm 250, Valhalla, NY 10595; **Phone:** 914-493-8374; **Board Cert:** Internal Medicine 1984; Medical Oncology 1989; **Med School:** Mexico 1979; **Resid:** Internal Medicine, Maimonides Med Ctr 1984; **Fellow:** Medical Oncology, Westchesr Co Med Ctr 1985; **Fac Appt:** Asst Prof Med, NY Med Coll

Rosen, Norman MD (Onc) - **Hospital:** St John's Riverside Hosp, Montefiore Med Ctr; **Address:** 984 N Broadway, Ste 311, Yonkers, NY 10701-1308; **Phone:** 914-965-2060; **Board Cert:** Internal Medicine 1975; Medical Oncology 1977; **Med School:** Tufts Univ 1972; **Resid:** Internal Medicine, Montefiore Hosp Med Ctr 1975; **Fellow:** Hematology & Oncology, Montefiore Hosp Med Ctr 1977; **Fac Appt:** Asst Clin Prof Med, Albert Einstein Coll Med

Sadan, Sara MD (Onc) - **Spec Exp:** Hematology; **Hospital:** White Plains Hosp Ctr (page 714); **Address:** 244 Westchester Ave, Ste 411, White Plains, NY 10604; **Phone:** 914-684-8100; **Board Cert:** Internal Medicine 1992; Medical Oncology 1995; **Med School:** Israel 1984; **Resid:** Internal Medicine, St Luke's-Roosevelt Hosp Ctr 1991; **Fellow:** Hematology & Oncology, Meml Sloan Kettering Cancer Ctr 1994

Saponara, Eduardo M MD (Onc) - **Spec Exp:** Breast Cancer; Gastrointestinal Cancer; Lymphoma; Lung Cancer; **Hospital:** Lawrence Hosp Ctr, Mount Sinai Med Ctr (page 98); **Address:** 77 Pondfield Rd, Bronxville, NY 10708-3809; **Phone:** 914-793-1500; **Board Cert:** Internal Medicine 1977; Hematology 1978; Medical Oncology 1979; Geriatric Medicine 1994; **Med School:** Peru 1973; **Resid:** Internal Medicine, Westchester Med Ctr 1976; **Fellow:** Hematology & Oncology, Flower Fifth Ave Hospital/NY Med Coll 1978; Oncology, Mount Sinai Hosp 1979; **Fac Appt:** Asst Clin Prof Med, NY Med Coll

Schneider, Robert MD (Onc) - **Spec Exp:** Breast Cancer; Genitourinary Cancer; **Hospital:** Northern Westchester Hosp, Westchester Med Ctr (page 713); **Address:** 101 S Bedford, Ste 202A, Mt Kisco, NY 10549-3456; **Phone:** 914-666-8976; **Board Cert:** Internal Medicine 1979; Medical Oncology 1985; **Med School:** Albert Einstein Coll Med 1975; **Resid:** Internal Medicine, Jacobi Med Ctr 1978; **Fellow:** Medical Oncology, Meml Sloan Kettering Cancer Ctr 1980

Schwartz, Simeon MD (Onc) - **Spec Exp:** Breast Cancer; **Hospital:** White Plains Hosp Ctr (page 714), NY-Presby Hosp (page 100); **Address:** 210 Westchester Ave, White Plains, NY 10604-2901; **Phone:** 914-681-5200; **Board Cert:** Internal Medicine 1980; Medical Oncology 1983; Hematology 1984; **Med School:** Yale Univ 1977; **Resid:** Internal Medicine, NY Hosp 1980; **Fellow:** Hematology & Oncology, Meml Sloan Kettering Cancer Ctr 1983; **Fac Appt:** Assoc Clin Prof Med, Cornell Univ-Weill Med Coll

Seiter, Karen MD (Onc) - **Spec Exp:** Hematologic Disorders; Leukemia; Myelodysplastic Syndromes; **Hospital:** Westchester Med Ctr (page 713); **Address:** NY Med College, Munger Pavillion, rm 250, Valhalla, NY 10595; **Phone:** 914-493-8374; **Board Cert:** Internal Medicine 1988; Medical Oncology 2001; Hematology 2002; **Med School:** NY Med Coll 1985; **Resid:** Internal Medicine, Albert Einstein Hosp 1988; **Fellow:** Hematology & Oncology, Memorial Sloan Kettering Med Ctr 1991; **Fac Appt:** Prof Med, NY Med Coll

Neonatal-Perinatal Medicine

Jaile-Marti, Jesus MD (NP) - **Spec Exp:** Lung Disease of Prematurity; Neonatal Nutrition; **Hospital:** White Plains Hosp Ctr (page 714), NY-Presby Hosp (page 100); **Address:** White Plains Hospital Ctr, Div of Neonatology, Davis Ave at East Post Rd, White Plains, NY 10601; **Phone:** 914-681-2282; **Board Cert:** Pediatrics 2005; Neonatal-Perinatal Medicine 2003; **Med School:** Columbia P&S 1987; **Resid:** Pediatrics, Columbia-Presby Med Ctr 1990; **Fellow:** Neonatology, Columbia-Presby Med Ctr 1993

La Gamma, Edmund F MD (NP) - **Spec Exp:** Neonatal Infections; Prematurity/Low Birth Weight Infants; Necrotizing Enterocolitis; **Hospital:** Westchester Med Ctr (page 713); **Address:** Maria Fareri Chldns Hosp, Grasslands Rd Fl 2, Valhalla, NY 10595-0001; **Phone:** 914-493-8558; **Board Cert:** Pediatrics 1981; Neonatal-Perinatal Medicine 1981; **Med School:** NY Med Coll 1976; **Resid:** Pediatrics, New York Hosp-Cornell Med Ctr 1978; **Fellow:** Neonatal-Perinatal Medicine, New York Hosp-Cornell 1980; Cardiovascular Disease, UCSF Med Ctr 1981; **Fac Appt:** Prof Ped, NY Med Coll

NEPHROLOGY

Adler, Stephen MD (Nep) - **Spec Exp:** Kidney Failure; Glomerulonephritis; Hypertension; **Hospital:** Westchester Med Ctr (page 713), White Plains Hosp Ctr (page 714); **Address:** 19 Bradhurst Ave, Ste 100, Hawthorne, NY 10532-2169; **Phone:** 914-493-7701; **Board Cert:** Internal Medicine 1979; Nephrology 1982; **Med School:** NYU Sch Med 1976; **Resid:** Internal Medicine, Mt. Sinai Hosp 1979; **Fellow:** Nephrology, Boston Univ Med Ctr 1982; **Fac Appt:** Prof Med, NY Med Coll

Buzzeo, Louis MD (Nep) - **Spec Exp:** Hypertension; **Hospital:** Phelps Meml Hosp Ctr; **Address:** 777 N Broadway St, Ste 203, Sleepy Hollow, NY 10591-1019; **Phone:** 914-332-9100; **Board Cert:** Internal Medicine 1975; Nephrology 1978; **Med School:** Tufts Univ 1972; **Resid:** Internal Medicine, St Vincent's Hosp & Med Ctr 1975; **Fellow:** Nephrology, NYU Med Ctr 1977

Das Gupta, Manash K MD (Nep) - **Spec Exp:** Hypertension; Kidney Disease; Dialysis Care; **Hospital:** Montefiore Med Ctr, Comm Hosp - Dobbs Ferry; **Address:** 9A Central Park Ave, Yonkers, NY 10705-4746; **Phone:** 914-376-3330; **Board Cert:** Internal Medicine 1980; Nephrology 2002; **Med School:** India 1966; **Resid:** Internal Medicine, Methodist Hosp 1972; **Fellow:** Nephrology, Montefiore Hosp Med Ctr 1974; **Fac Appt:** Assoc Clin Prof Med, Albert Einstein Coll Med

Garrick, Renee MD (Nep) - **Spec Exp:** Hypertension; Dialysis Care; **Hospital:** Westchester Med Ctr (page 713); **Address:** Nephrology Assocs of Westechester, 19 Bradhurst Ave, Ste 100, Hawthorn, NY 10532; **Phone:** 914-493-7701; **Board Cert:** Internal Medicine 1981; Nephrology 1984; **Med School:** Rush Med Coll 1978; **Resid:** Internal Medicine, Jacobi Med Ctr 1981; **Fellow:** Nephrology, Hosp Univ Penn 1984; **Fac Appt:** Clin Prof Med, NY Med Coll

Joshi, Anil MD (Nep) - **Hospital:** St John's Riverside Hosp, Saint Joseph's Med Ctr - Yonkers; **Address:** 970 N Broadway, Ste 311, Yonkers, NY 10701-1311; **Phone:** 914-969-3635; **Board Cert:** Internal Medicine 1973; Nephrology 1976; **Med School:** India 1964; **Resid:** Internal Medicine, Bergen Pines Co Hosp 1970; **Fellow:** Nephrology, Holy Name Hosp 1973; Renal Disease, Bronx VA Hosp 1973

Reda, Dominick MD (Nep) - **Spec Exp:** Hypertension; Kidney Disease; **Hospital:** Saint Joseph's Med Ctr - Yonkers; **Address:** 136 S Broadway, Yonkers, NY 10705-2970; **Phone:** 914-965-0621; **Board Cert:** Internal Medicine 1987; Nephrology 1990; **Med School:** Italy 1983; **Resid:** Internal Medicine, Our Lady of Mercy 1987; **Fellow:** Nephrology, Lincoln Med Ctr 1989

Rie, Jonathan MD (Nep) - **Spec Exp:** Hypertension; Kidney Stones; **Hospital:** White Plains Hosp Ctr (page 714); **Address:** 33 Davis Ave, White Plains, NY 10605; **Phone:** 914-948-3630; **Board Cert:** Internal Medicine 1988; Nephrology 2000; **Med School:** NY Med Coll 1985; **Resid:** Internal Medicine, Montefiore Hosp Med Ctr 1988; **Fellow:** Nephrology, Montefiore Hosp Med Ctr 1990

Saltzman, Martin MD (Nep) - **Spec Exp:** Kidney Disease; Hypertension; **Hospital:** Northern Westchester Hosp, Putnam Hosp Ctr; **Address:** 41 S Bedford Rd, Mt Kisco, NY 10549; **Phone:** 914-666-5588; **Board Cert:** Internal Medicine 1977; Nephrology 1978; **Med School:** SUNY Downstate 1972; **Resid:** Internal Medicine, Kings County Hosp 1973; Internal Medicine, Harlem Hosp 1974; **Fellow:** Nephrology, Univ Hosp 1976

NEUROLOGICAL SURGERY

Duffy, Kent R MD (NS) - **Spec Exp:** Pituitary Tumors; Brain Surgery; Spinal Surgery; **Hospital:** White Plains Hosp Ctr (page 714), Northern Westchester Hosp; **Address:** 244 Westchester Ave, Ste 310, White Plains, NY 10604-2926; **Phone:** 914-948-2288; **Board Cert:** Neurological Surgery 1993; **Med School:** Temple Univ 1980; **Resid:** Surgery, UCLA Med Ctr 1982; Neurological Surgery, UCLA Med Ctr 1988; **Fac Appt:** Asst Clin Prof NS, NY Med Coll

Kornel, Ezriel MD (NS) - **Spec Exp:** Spinal Surgery-Minimally Invasive; Brain Tumors; Aneurysm-Cerebral; **Hospital:** Northern Westchester Hosp, Lawrence Hosp Ctr; **Address:** 244 Westchester Ave, Ste 310, White Plains, NY 10604; **Phone:** 914-948-0444; **Board Cert:** Neurological Surgery 1987; **Med School:** Rush Med Coll 1978; **Resid:** Surgery, Washington Hosp Ctr 1979; Neurological Surgery, Geo Wash Univ Hosp 1984; **Fac Appt:** Asst Clin Prof NS, Columbia P&S

Lansen, Thomas A MD (NS) - **Spec Exp:** Stereotactic Radiosurgery; Hydrocephalus; Brain Tumors; **Hospital:** Northern Westchester Hosp, Lawrence Hosp Ctr; **Address:** 244 Westchester Ave, Ste 310, White Plains, NY 10604; **Phone:** 914-948-8448; **Board Cert:** Neurological Surgery 1983; **Med School:** Med Coll Wisc 1973; **Resid:** Surgery, NYU Med Ctr 1974; Neurological Surgery, Univ Fla-Shands Hosp 1980; **Fac Appt:** Assoc Prof NS, NY Med Coll

Murali, Raj MD (NS) - **Spec Exp:** Trigeminal Neuralgia; Skull Base Surgery; Aneurysm-Cerebral; Pituitary Tumors; **Hospital:** Westchester Med Ctr (page 713), St Vincent Cath Med Ctrs - Manhattan (page 375); **Address:** Westchester Med Ctr, Dept Neurosurgery, Munger Pavilion, Ste 329, Valhalla, NY 10595; **Phone:** 914-493-8392; **Board Cert:** Neurological Surgery 1982; **Med School:** India 1968; **Resid:** Neurological Surgery, Royal Infirm-Univ Edinburgh 1974; Neurological Surgery, NYU Med Ctr 1979; **Fac Appt:** Prof NS, NY Med Coll

Robbins, John MD (NS) - **Spec Exp:** Spinal Surgery; Brain Tumors; **Hospital:** Phelps Meml Hosp Ctr, Northern Westchester Hosp; **Address:** 245 Saw Mill River Rd, Ste 106, Hawthorne, NY 10532; **Phone:** 914-375-6222; **Board Cert:** Neurological Surgery 1991; **Med School:** Brown Univ 1978; **Resid:** Surgery, Montefiore Hosp Med Ctr 1982; Neurological Surgery, NY Hosp 1988

Rosner, Saran MD (NS) - **Spec Exp:** Spinal Surgery; Brain & Spinal Cord Tumors; **Hospital:** Phelps Meml Hosp Ctr, Hudson Valley Hosp Ctr; **Address:** 245 Saw Mill River Rd, Hawthorne, NY 10532; **Phone:** 914-741-2666; **Board Cert:** Neurological Surgery 1986; **Med School:** Columbia P&S 1976; **Resid:** Surgery, Johns Hopkins Hosp 1978; Neurological Surgery, Columbia-Presby Med Ctr 1983

Stern, Jack MD/PhD (NS) - **Spec Exp:** Spinal Reconstructive Surgery; Brain Tumors; Trigeminal Neuralgia; **Hospital:** White Plains Hosp Ctr (page 714), Northern Westchester Hosp; **Address:** 244 Westchester Ave, Ste 310, White Plains, NY 10604; **Phone:** 914-948-6688; **Board Cert:** Neurological Surgery 1982; **Med School:** Albert Einstein Coll Med 1971; **Resid:** Surgery, Bellevue Hosp 1976; Neurological Surgery, Columbia-Presby Med Ctr 1980; **Fac Appt:** Clin Prof NS, Yale Univ

Neurology

Ahluwalia, Brij M Singh MD (N) - **Spec Exp:** Dementia; Cerebrovascular Disease; Multiple Sclerosis; **Hospital:** Westchester Med Ctr (page 713); **Address:** 19 Bradhurst St, Ste 2800, Hawthorne, NY 10532; **Phone:** 914-345-1313; **Board Cert:** Neurology 1974; **Med School:** India 1961; **Resid:** Internal Medicine, Beekman Downtown Hosp 1969; Neurology, Metropolitan Hosp 1972; **Fac Appt:** Prof N, NY Med Coll

Dickoff, David MD (N) - **Spec Exp:** Epilepsy/Seizure Disorders; Neuromuscular Disorders; Parkinson's Disease; **Hospital:** St John's Riverside Hosp, Mount Sinai Med Ctr (page 98); **Address:** 984 N Broadway, rm 509, Yonkers, NY 10701; **Phone:** 914-968-0620; **Board Cert:** Neurology 1987; **Med School:** Albany Med Coll 1982; **Resid:** Neurology, Mt Sinai Hosp 1986; **Fellow:** Neurological Muscular Disease, Columbia-Presby Med Ctr 1987; **Fac Appt:** Asst Clin Prof N, Mount Sinai Sch Med

Gross, Elliott MD (N) - **Spec Exp:** Alzheimer's Disease; Parkinson's Disease; Headache; **Hospital:** Montefiore Med Ctr; **Address:** 10 Rye Ridge Plaza, Ste 203, Rye Brook, NY 10573-2828; **Phone:** 914-251-1010; **Board Cert:** Neurology 1969; **Med School:** Albert Einstein Coll Med 1962; **Resid:** Neurology, Albert Einstein 1966; **Fellow:** Neurology, Albert Einstein 1970; **Fac Appt:** Asst Clin Prof N, Albert Einstein Coll Med

Jordan, Barry D MD (N) - **Spec Exp:** Brain Injury-Traumatic; Sports Neurology; Alzheimer's Disease; Memory Disorders; **Hospital:** Burke Rehab Hosp (page 105); **Address:** Burke Rehabilitation Hosp, 785 Mamaroneck Ave, White Plains, NY 10605; **Phone:** 914-597-2332; **Board Cert:** Neurology 1989; **Med School:** Harvard Med Sch 1981; **Resid:** Neurology, New York Hosp 1986; **Fellow:** Hosp Spec Surgery 1987UCLA Med Ctr 1998; **Fac Appt:** Assoc Prof N, Cornell Univ-Weill Med Coll

Kranzler, L Stephan MD (N) - **Hospital:** White Plains Hosp Ctr (page 714); **Address:** 244 Westchester Ave, White Plains, NY 10604; **Phone:** 914-946-9444; **Board Cert:** Neurology 1990; **Med School:** Univ Pennsylvania 1985; **Resid:** Neurology, Neuro Inst/Columbia-Presby Med Ctr 1989

Marks, Stephen MD (N) - **Spec Exp:** Stroke; Alzheimer's Disease; Dementia; **Hospital:** Westchester Med Ctr (page 713); **Address:** NY Medical College, Dept Neuro, Munger Pavilion, Valhalla, NY 10595; **Phone:** 914-345-1313; **Board Cert:** Neurology 1985; **Med School:** NY Med Coll 1980; **Resid:** Neurology, Mount Sinai Hosp 1984; **Fellow:** Stroke, Duke Univ Med Ctr 1985; **Fac Appt:** Assoc Clin Prof N, NY Med Coll

Reding, Michael MD (N) - **Spec Exp:** Neuro-Rehabilitation; **Hospital:** Burke Rehab Hosp (page 105); **Address:** 785 Mamaroneck Ave, White Plains, NY 10605-2523; **Phone:** 914-597-2470; **Board Cert:** Internal Medicine 1976; Neurology 1981; **Med School:** Univ Kans 1973; **Resid:** Internal Medicine, Univ Nebraska Med Ctr 1976; Neurology, Univ Nebraska Med Ctr 1979; **Fellow:** Neurology, NY Hosp/Cornell 1980; **Fac Appt:** Assoc Prof N, Cornell Univ-Weill Med Coll

Selman, Jay E MD (N) - **Spec Exp:** Epilepsy/Seizure Disorders; Headache; Tourette's Syndrome; Pediatric Neurology; **Hospital:** Northern Westchester Hosp; **Address:** 117 Smith Ave, Mt Kisco, NY 10549-2815; **Phone:** 914-666-8080; **Board Cert:** Pediatrics 1978; Child Neurology 1980; Clinical Neurophysiology 1997; Neurodevelopmental Disabilities 2002; **Med School:** Univ Tex SW, Dallas 1973; **Resid:** Pediatrics, Jacobi Med Ctr 1975; Neurology, Jacobi Med Ctr 1978; **Fellow:** Child Neurology, Jacobi Med Ctr 1977; **Fac Appt:** Assoc Clin Prof N, Columbia P&S

Singh, Avtar MD (N) - **Spec Exp:** Stroke; Epilepsy; Headache; **Hospital:** White Plains Hosp Ctr (page 714); **Address:** 244 Westchester Ave, Ste 315, White Plains, NY 10604; **Phone:** 914-946-2552; **Board Cert:** Neurology 1978; **Med School:** India 1967; **Resid:** Neurology, Metropolitan Hosp Ctr 1976; **Fac Appt:** Assoc Clin Prof N, NY Med Coll

Weintraub, Michael MD (N) - **Spec Exp:** Carpal Tunnel Syndrome; Peripheral Nerve Disorders; Pain-Back & Neck; Diabetic Neuropathy; **Hospital:** Phelps Meml Hosp Ctr, Putnam Hosp Ctr; **Address:** 325 S Highland Ave, Briarcliff Manor, NY 10510-2093; **Phone:** 914-941-0788; **Board Cert:** Neurology 1972; **Med School:** SUNY Buffalo 1966; **Resid:** Neurology, EJ Meyer Meml Hosp 1968; **Fellow:** Neurology, Yale-New Haven Hosp 1970; **Fac Appt:** Clin Prof N, NY Med Coll

NEURORADIOLOGY

Tenner, Michael MD (NRad) - **Spec Exp:** Stroke; Aneurysm-Cerebral; Arteriovenous Malformations; Carotid Artery Stents; **Hospital:** Westchester Med Ctr (page 713); **Address:** NY Med Coll, Dept Radiology, Route 100, Valhalla, NY 10595; **Phone:** 914-493-8158; **Board Cert:** Radiology 1967; Neuroradiology 1995; **Med School:** Univ MD Sch Med 1960; **Resid:** Radiology, Univ Maryland Hosp 1962; Radiology, Univ Maryland Hosp 1966; **Fellow:** Neuroradiology, Neurological Inst-Columbia Presby 1968; **Fac Appt:** Prof Rad, NY Med Coll

OBSTETRICS & GYNECOLOGY

Armbruster, Robert MD (ObG) - **Spec Exp:** Laparoscopy; Colposcopy; Pregnancy-High Risk; **Hospital:** Lawrence Hosp Ctr, Westchester Med Ctr (page 713); **Address:** 77 Pondfield Rd, Bronxville, NY 10708-3809; **Phone:** 914-337-3229; **Board Cert:** Obstetrics & Gynecology 1984; **Med School:** Washington Univ, St Louis 1977; **Resid:** Obstetrics & Gynecology, UCLA Med Ctr 1979; Obstetrics & Gynecology, NY-Cornell Hosp 1981

Burns, Elisa MD (ObG) PCP - **Spec Exp:** Minimally Invasive Surgery; Colposcopy; Pregnancy-High Risk; **Hospital:** Northern Westchester Hosp; **Address:** 90 S Bedford Rd, Mt Kisco, NY 10549-3433; **Phone:** 914-241-1050; **Board Cert:** Obstetrics & Gynecology 1997; **Med School:** Columbia P&S 1982; **Resid:** Obstetrics & Gynecology, Columbia-Presby Hosp 1986

Carolan, Stephen MD (ObG) PCP - **Spec Exp:** Laparoscopic Surgery; Uterine Fibroids; **Hospital:** Greenwich Hosp; **Address:** 14 Rye Ridge Plaza, Ste 244, Rye Brook, NY 10573; **Phone:** 914-253-4912; **Board Cert:** Obstetrics & Gynecology 1990; **Med School:** NY Med Coll 1984; **Resid:** Obstetrics & Gynecology, Univ Conn Hlth Ctr 1988

Eilen, Bonnie MD (ObG) PCP - **Hospital:** White Plains Hosp Ctr (page 714); **Address:** 30 Davis Ave, White Plains, NY 10605; **Phone:** 914-946-7274; **Board Cert:** Obstetrics & Gynecology 2004; **Med School:** Albert Einstein Coll Med 1977; **Resid:** Obstetrics & Gynecology, Bronx Municipal Hosp 1981; **Fac Appt:** Asst Clin Prof ObG, Albert Einstein Coll Med

Florio, Philip MD (ObG) PCP - **Spec Exp:** Pregnancy-High Risk; Laparoscopic Surgery; Osteoporosis; Gynecologic Cancer; **Hospital:** St John's Riverside Hosp; **Address:** 1022 N Broadway, Yonkers, NY 10701-1303; **Phone:** 914-963-0284; **Board Cert:** Obstetrics & Gynecology 1981; **Med School:** SUNY Upstate Med Univ 1974; **Resid:** Obstetrics & Gynecology, St Barnabas 1978

Giuffrida, Regina MD (ObG) PCP - **Spec Exp:** Menopause Problems; **Hospital:** Northern Westchester Hosp; **Address:** 90 S Bedford Rd, Mt Kisco, NY 10549; **Phone:** 914-241-1050; **Board Cert:** Obstetrics & Gynecology 1996; **Med School:** NY Med Coll 1980; **Resid:** Obstetrics & Gynecology, UCSD Med Ctr 1984

Grano, Vanessa MD (ObG) - **Spec Exp:** Laparoscopic Surgery; Pap Smear Abnormalities; **Hospital:** Greenwich Hosp; **Address:** Westchester Medical Group, 14 Rye Ridge Plaza, Ste 244, Rye Brook, NY 10573-2858; **Phone:** 914-253-4912; **Board Cert:** Obstetrics & Gynecology 2003; **Med School:** SUNY Downstate 1988; **Resid:** Obstetrics & Gynecology, Columbia-Presby Hosp 1993

Greenlee, Robert MD (ObG) - **Spec Exp:** Vulvar Disease; Colposcopy; Sexual Dysfunction; Menopause Problems; **Hospital:** Lawrence Hosp Ctr, Sound Shore Med Ctr - Westchester (page 711); **Address:** 838 Pelhamdale Ave, New Rochelle, NY 10801-1032; **Phone:** 914-235-2900; **Board Cert:** Obstetrics & Gynecology 1982; **Med School:** Mexico 1975; **Resid:** Obstetrics & Gynecology, St Luke's Roosevelt Hosp 1980

Hayworth, Scott MD (ObG) PCP - **Spec Exp:** Minimally Invasive & Laser Surgery; Pregnancy-High Risk; Menopause Problems; **Hospital:** Northern Westchester Hosp; **Address:** 90 S Bedford Rd, Mt Kisco, NY 10549-3412; **Phone:** 914-241-1050; **Board Cert:** Obstetrics & Gynecology 2005; **Med School:** Cornell Univ-Weill Med Coll 1984; **Resid:** Obstetrics & Gynecology, Mount Sinai Med Ctr 1988; **Fac Appt:** Asst Clin Prof ObG, Mount Sinai Sch Med

Kalinsky, Jay MD (ObG) - **Spec Exp:** Pregnancy-High Risk; **Hospital:** Hudson Valley Hosp Ctr; **Address:** 1985 Crompond Rd, Ste B, Cortlandt Manor, NY 10567-4146; **Phone:** 914-739-1697 x224; **Board Cert:** Obstetrics & Gynecology 1980; **Med School:** Univ Miami Sch Med 1973; **Resid:** Obstetrics & Gynecology, Bronx Municipal Hosp 1977

Kirshenbaum, Nancy MD (ObG) - **Spec Exp:** Pregnancy-High Risk; Ultrasound; **Hospital:** Montefiore Med Ctr - Weiler-Einstein Div; **Address:** 700 White Plains Rd, Ste 270, Scarsdale, NY 10583; **Phone:** 914-423-4111; **Board Cert:** Obstetrics & Gynecology 1997; Maternal & Fetal Medicine 1997; **Med School:** Mount Sinai Sch Med 1980; **Resid:** Obstetrics & Gynecology, NYU Med Ctr 1984; **Fellow:** Maternal & Fetal Medicine, NYU Med Ctr 1986; **Fac Appt:** Assoc Clin Prof ObG, Albert Einstein Coll Med

Klugman, Susan MD (ObG) PCP - **Spec Exp:** Pregnancy-High Risk; Adolescent Gynecology; Reproductive Genetics; **Hospital:** Montefiore Med Ctr - Weiler-Einstein Div; **Address:** 2345 Boston Post Rd, Larchmont, NY 10538-3556; **Phone:** 914-833-0444; **Board Cert:** Obstetrics & Gynecology 1995; **Med School:** NYU Sch Med 1988; **Resid:** Obstetrics & Gynecology, Albert Einstein 1992; **Fellow:** Genetics, Albert Einstein 2004; **Fac Appt:** Asst Prof ObG, Albert Einstein Coll Med

Loiacono, Anthony F MD (ObG) - **Spec Exp:** Hysteroscopic Surgery; Laparoscopic Surgery; **Hospital:** White Plains Hosp Ctr (page 714); **Address:** 280 Mamaroneck Ave, White Plains, NY 10605-1438; **Phone:** 914-949-0108; **Board Cert:** Obstetrics & Gynecology 1966; **Med School:** SUNY Downstate 1959; **Resid:** Obstetrics & Gynecology, St John's Episcopal Hosp 1963; **Fac Appt:** Asst Clin Prof, NY Med Coll

Meacham, Kevin MD (ObG) - **Spec Exp:** Pregnancy-High Risk; Laparoscopic Surgery; Gynecologic Surgery; **Hospital:** Sound Shore Med Ctr - Westchester (page 711); **Address:** 2071 Boston Post Rd, Larchmont, NY 10538-3701; **Phone:** 914-833-1000; **Board Cert:** Obstetrics & Gynecology 1993; **Med School:** NY Med Coll 1986; **Resid:** Obstetrics & Gynecology, Long Island Jewish Med Ctr 1990

Mendelowitz, Lawrence MD (ObG) - **Spec Exp:** Pelvic Reconstruction; Laparoscopic Hysterectomy; Gynecologic Surgery-Benign; Pregnancy-High Risk; **Hospital:** Phelps Meml Hosp Ctr, Westchester Med Ctr (page 713); **Address:** 325 S Highland Ave, Briarcliff Manor, NY 10510; **Phone:** 914-941-5656; **Board Cert:** Obstetrics & Gynecology 1996; **Med School:** NYU Sch Med 1976; **Resid:** Obstetrics & Gynecology, Bellevue Hosp-NYU 1980

Nelson, William S MD (ObG) - **Spec Exp:** Menopause Problems; **Hospital:** Greenwich Hosp; **Address:** Rye Brook Ob/Gyn, 14 Rye Ridge Plz, Ste 244, Rye Brook, NY 10573-2802; **Phone:** 914-253-4912; **Board Cert:** Obstetrics & Gynecology 1981; **Med School:** Albert Einstein Coll Med 1960; **Resid:** Obstetrics & Gynecology, Maimonides Med Ctr 1965; **Fac Appt:** Asst Clin Prof ObG, Albert Einstein Coll Med

Pawl, Nancy MD (ObG) - **Spec Exp:** Women's Health; Menopause Problems; **Hospital:** Montefiore Med Ctr - Weiler-Einstein Div, Sound Shore Med Ctr - Westchester (page 711); **Address:** Larchmont Women's Center, 2345 Boston Post Rd, Larchmont, NY 10538; **Phone:** 914-833-0444; **Board Cert:** Obstetrics & Gynecology 2004; **Med School:** Harvard Med Sch 1980; **Resid:** Obstetrics & Gynecology, Columbia-Presby Med Ctr 1984; **Fac Appt:** Asst Prof ObG, Albert Einstein Coll Med

Razmzan, Shahram MD (ObG) - **Spec Exp:** Laparoscopic Surgery; Pregnancy-High Risk; **Hospital:** St John's Riverside Hosp, Saint Joseph's Med Ctr - Yonkers; **Address:** 656 Yonkers Ave, Southern Westchester OB/GYN Associates, LLP, Yonkers, NY 10704-2641; **Phone:** 914-963-3366; **Board Cert:** Obstetrics & Gynecology 2005; **Med School:** Grenada 1982; **Resid:** Obstetrics & Gynecology, Westchester Co Med Ctr 1987

Reilly, Kevin B MD (ObG) **PCP** - **Spec Exp:** Ultrasound; Prenatal Diagnosis; **Hospital:** Northern Westchester Hosp, NY-Presby Hosp (page 100); **Address:** 90 S Bedford Rd, Mt Kisco, NY 10549-3412; **Phone:** 914-242-1380; **Board Cert:** Obstetrics & Gynecology 2005; **Med School:** SUNY Hlth Sci Ctr 1970; **Resid:** Obstetrics & Gynecology, Columbia-Presby Hosp 1977; **Fac Appt:** Asst Clin Prof ObG, Columbia P&S

Schneider, Ronald MD (ObG) - **Spec Exp:** Laparoscopic Surgery; Hysteroscopic Surgery; **Hospital:** Sound Shore Med Ctr - Westchester (page 711); **Address:** 110 Lockwood Ave, Ste 300, New Rochelle, NY 10801; **Phone:** 914-632-8164; **Board Cert:** Obstetrics & Gynecology 1981; **Med School:** NY Med Coll 1975; **Resid:** Obstetrics & Gynecology, LI Jewish Med Ctr 1979

Silverman, Barney MD (ObG) **PCP** - **Spec Exp:** Menopause Problems; Complementary Medicine; **Hospital:** White Plains Hosp Ctr (page 714); **Address:** 170 Maple Ave, Ste 309, White Plains, NY 10601-4782; **Phone:** 914-949-8338; **Board Cert:** Obstetrics & Gynecology 1993; **Med School:** Univ Louisville Sch Med 1964; **Resid:** Obstetrics & Gynecology, Hosp U Penn 1971; **Fac Appt:** Assoc Clin Prof ObG, Yale Univ

Suvannavejh, Chaisurat MD (ObG) **PCP** - **Hospital:** Lawrence Hosp Ctr, Mount Vernon Hosp (page 712); **Address:** 559 Gramatan Ave, Mt Vernon, NY 10552; **Phone:** 914-668-8601; **Board Cert:** Obstetrics & Gynecology 1976; **Med School:** Thailand 1968; **Resid:** Obstetrics & Gynecology, Mount Vernon Hosp 1973

Ullman, Joel MD (ObG) - **Spec Exp:** Laparoscopic Surgery-Complex; Uro-Gynecology; Vulvar Disease; Vaginal Surgery; **Hospital:** Sound Shore Med Ctr - Westchester (page 711); **Address:** 2071 Boston Post Rd, Larchmont, NY 10538-3701; **Phone:** 914-833-1000; **Board Cert:** Obstetrics & Gynecology 1978; **Med School:** NY Med Coll 1963; **Resid:** Obstetrics & Gynecology, Beth Israel Med Ctr 1969; **Fac Appt:** Asst Clin Prof ObG, Albert Einstein Coll Med

Westchester

Young, Constance MD (ObG) - **Spec Exp:** Pelvic Surgery; Menopause Problems; **Hospital:** Phelps Meml Hosp Ctr, White Plains Hosp Ctr (page 714); **Address:** 358 N Broadway, Ste 202, Sleepy Hollow, NY 10591; **Phone:** 914-524-9612; **Board Cert:** Obstetrics & Gynecology 2000; **Med School:** Cornell Univ-Weill Med Coll 1983; **Resid:** Obstetrics & Gynecology, North Shore Univ Hosp 1987

OPHTHALMOLOGY

Bansal, Rajendra K MD (Oph) - **Spec Exp:** Glaucoma; **Hospital:** Mount Vernon Hosp (page 712); **Address:** 105 Stevens Ave, Ste 306, Mt Vernon, NY 10550-2686; **Phone:** 914-664-3168; **Board Cert:** Ophthalmology 1977; **Med School:** India 1967; **Resid:** Ophthalmology, Univ Delhi Hosp 1973; **Fellow:** Glaucoma, Columbia Presby Med Ctr 1979; **Fac Appt:** Asst Clin Prof Oph, Columbia P&S

Brustein, Harris MD (Oph) - **Hospital:** Sound Shore Med Ctr - Westchester (page 711); **Address:** 77 Quaker Ridge Rd, Ste 203, New Rochelle, NY 10804-2821; **Phone:** 914-235-0022; **Board Cert:** Ophthalmology 1976; **Med School:** Albert Einstein Coll Med 1970; **Resid:** Ophthalmology, Montefiore Med Ctr 1974; **Fellow:** Pediatric Ophthalmology, Chldns Hosp 1975

Dieck, William MD (Oph) - **Spec Exp:** Cataract Surgery; Glaucoma; **Hospital:** Northern Westchester Hosp; **Address:** 185 Kisco Ave, Mt Kisco, NY 10549; **Phone:** 914-666-4939; **Board Cert:** Ophthalmology 1990; **Med School:** NY Med Coll 1983; **Resid:** Internal Medicine, Westchester Co Med Ctr 1985; Ophthalmology, NY Med Coll 1988

Fleischman, Jay MD (Oph) - **Spec Exp:** Diabetic Eye Disease/Retinopathy; Macular Degeneration; **Hospital:** Montefiore Med Ctr; **Address:** 600 Mamaroneck Ave, Ste 103, Harrison, NY 10528; **Phone:** 914-315-5111; **Board Cert:** Ophthalmology 1980; **Med School:** Columbia P&S 1975; **Resid:** Ophthalmology, Johns Hopkins Hosp 1979; **Fac Appt:** Assoc Prof Oph, Albert Einstein Coll Med

Forman, Scott MD (Oph) - **Spec Exp:** Botox Therapy; Eye Muscle Disorders; Neuro-Ophthalmology; **Hospital:** Westchester Med Ctr (page 713); **Address:** Westchester Med Ctr, Dept Ophth, Macy Pavilion, Valhalla, NY 10595; **Phone:** 914-493-7666; **Board Cert:** Ophthalmology 1989; **Med School:** UMDNJ-RW Johnson Med Sch 1981; **Resid:** Ophthalmology, New York Med Coll 1986; **Fellow:** Neurological Ophthalmology, Columbia-Presby Med Ctr 1987; **Fac Appt:** Assoc Prof Oph, NY Med Coll

Glassman, Morris MD (Oph) - **Spec Exp:** Cataract Surgery; Glaucoma; **Hospital:** Northern Westchester Hosp, Westchester Med Ctr (page 713); **Address:** 1940 Commerce St, Ste 101, Yorktown Heights, NY 10598; **Phone:** 914-962-5506; **Board Cert:** Ophthalmology 1975; **Med School:** NYU Sch Med 1968; **Resid:** Ophthalmology, Montefiore Med Ctr 1974; **Fac Appt:** Assoc Clin Prof Oph, Albert Einstein Coll Med

Greenbaum, Allen MD (Oph) - **Spec Exp:** Laser Refractive Surgery; **Hospital:** White Plains Hosp Ctr (page 714); **Address:** 170 Maple Ave, Ste 402, White Plains, NY 10601; **Phone:** 914-949-9200; **Board Cert:** Ophthalmology 1985; **Med School:** Mount Sinai Sch Med 1979; **Resid:** Ophthalmology, Mount Sinai Hosp 1983

Greenberg, Steven C MD (Oph) - **Spec Exp:** Pediatric Ophthalmology; **Address:** 2 Rye Ridge Plaza, Rye Brook, NY 10573; **Phone:** 914-253-6502; **Board Cert:** Ophthalmology 1987; **Med School:** Univ Conn 1982; **Resid:** Ophthalmology, NYU Med Ctr 1986; **Fellow:** Pediatric Ophthalmology, Manhattan EET Hosp 1987

Horowitz, Marc MD (Oph) - **Spec Exp:** Retinopathy of Prematurity; Strabismus; **Hospital:** Westchester Med Ctr (page 713), White Plains Hosp Ctr (page 714); **Address:** 14 Harwood Ct, Ste 209, Scarsdale, NY 10583; **Phone:** 914-723-5511; **Board Cert:** Ophthalmology 1983; **Med School:** Mount Sinai Sch Med 1978; **Resid:** Ophthalmology, St Luke's Roosevelt Hosp Ctr 1982; **Fellow:** Pediatric Ophthalmology, Chldns Hosp 1983; **Fac Appt:** Clin Prof Oph, NY Med Coll

Lederman, Martin E MD (Oph) - **Spec Exp:** Pediatric Ophthalmology; Eye Muscle Disorders; Diagnostic Problems; **Hospital:** White Plains Hosp Ctr (page 714), NY-Presby Hosp (page 100); **Address:** 3020 Westchester Ave, Ste 402, Purchase, NY 10577; **Phone:** 914-417-6441; **Board Cert:** Ophthalmology 2005; **Med School:** Albert Einstein Coll Med 1964; **Resid:** Ophthalmology, Albert Einstein Coll of Med 1968; **Fellow:** Pediatric Ophthalmology, Chldns Hosp 1970; **Fac Appt:** Assoc Clin Prof Oph, Columbia P&S

Lippman, Jay MD (Oph) - **Spec Exp:** Cataract Surgery; LASIK-Refractive Surgery; Cornea Transplant; **Hospital:** New York Eye & Ear Infirm (page 110); **Address:** 828 Pelhamdale Ave, New Rochelle, NY 10801; **Phone:** 914-636-3600; **Board Cert:** Ophthalmology 1972; **Med School:** Univ Hlth Sci/Chicago Med Sch 1964; **Resid:** Ophthalmology, Montefiore Med Ctr 1970; **Fac Appt:** Clin Prof Oph, NY Med Coll

Magaro, Joseph MD (Oph) - **Spec Exp:** Cataract Surgery; **Hospital:** Lawrence Hosp Ctr, Manhattan Eye, Ear & Throat Hosp; **Address:** 77 Pondfield Rd, Bronxville, NY 10708-3809; **Phone:** 914-337-8844; **Board Cert:** Ophthalmology 1967; **Med School:** Boston Univ 1961; **Resid:** Ophthalmology, Manhattan Eye, Ear & Throat Hosp 1965

Markowitz, Allan MD (Oph) - ; **Address:** 3505 Hill Blvd, Ste K, Yorktown Heights, NY 10598-1283; **Phone:** 914-245-3303; **Board Cert:** Ophthalmology 1979; **Med School:** Albert Einstein Coll Med 1974; **Resid:** Ophthalmology, Albert Einstein 1978; **Fac Appt:** Asst Clin Prof Oph, Albert Einstein Coll Med

McKee, Heather MD (Oph) - **Spec Exp:** Cataract Surgery; Glaucoma; **Hospital:** Comm Hosp - Dobbs Ferry, Westchester Med Ctr (page 713); **Address:** 200 S Broadway, Ste 202, Tarrytown, NY 10591-4504; **Phone:** 914-631-7300; **Board Cert:** Ophthalmology 1981; **Med School:** Duke Univ 1976; **Resid:** Ophthalmology, Strong Meml Hosp 1980; **Fac Appt:** Asst Clin Prof Oph, NY Med Coll

Mignone, Biagio MD (Oph) - **Spec Exp:** Cataract Surgery; Glaucoma; **Hospital:** Mount Vernon Hosp (page 712), Our Lady of Mercy Med Ctr; **Address:** 202 Stevens Ave, Mt Vernon, NY 10550-2534; **Phone:** 914-664-6001; **Board Cert:** Ophthalmology 1980; **Med School:** NY Med Coll 1975; **Resid:** Ophthalmology, UMDNJ med Ctr 1979; **Fac Appt:** Asst Clin Prof Oph, NY Med Coll

Miller, Brian MD (Oph) - **Spec Exp:** Cataract Surgery; Glaucoma; **Hospital:** Sound Shore Med Ctr - Westchester (page 711), Montefiore Med Ctr - Weiler-Einstein Div; **Address:** 1600 Harrison Ave, Ste 203, Mamaroneck, NY 10543-3145; **Phone:** 914-698-0670; **Board Cert:** Ophthalmology 1975; **Med School:** Temple Univ 1971; **Resid:** Ophthalmology, Temple U Hosp 1975; **Fac Appt:** Asst Clin Prof Oph, Albert Einstein Coll Med

Mooney, Robert M MD (Oph) - **Spec Exp:** Glaucoma; Contact lenses; **Hospital:** Northern Westchester Hosp; **Address:** 185 Kisco Ave, Ste 5, Mt Kisco, NY 10549-1409; **Phone:** 914-666-4939; **Board Cert:** Ophthalmology 1982; **Med School:** Italy 1972; **Resid:** Ophthalmology, Westchester Co Med Ctr 1977; **Fac Appt:** Asst Clin Prof Oph, NY Med Coll

Morello, Robert MD (Oph) - **Spec Exp:** Geriatric Ophthalmology; **Hospital:** Sound Shore Med Ctr - Westchester (page 711); **Address:** 120 Warren St, New Rochelle, NY 10801; **Phone:** 914-633-7214; **Board Cert:** Ophthalmology 1985; **Med School:** Mexico 1976; **Resid:** Internal Medicine, Bronx Lebanon Hosp 1978; Ophthalmology, Bronx Lebanon Hosp 1981

Most, Richard W MD (Oph) - **Spec Exp:** Pediatric Ophthalmology; Strabismus; Tear Duct Disorders; Amblyopia; **Hospital:** Northern Westchester Hosp, Mount Sinai Med Ctr (page 98); **Address:** 101 S Bedford Rd, Ste 401, Mt Kisco, NY 10549; **Phone:** 914-241-2206; **Board Cert:** Ophthalmology 1977; **Med School:** Italy 1971; **Resid:** Pathology, Maimonides Med Ctr 1973; Ophthalmology, Lenox Hill Hosp 1976; **Fellow:** Pediatric Ophthalmology, Bellevue Hosp/NYU 1977; Pediatric Ophthalmology, Childrens Hosp Natl Med Ctr 1978; **Fac Appt:** Assoc Prof Oph, Mount Sinai Sch Med

Phillips, Howard MD (Oph) - **Spec Exp:** LASIK-Refractive Surgery; Corneal Disease; **Hospital:** Phelps Meml Hosp Ctr; **Address:** 24 Saw Mill River Rd, Hawthorne, NY 10532; **Phone:** 914-345-3937; **Board Cert:** Ophthalmology 1982; **Med School:** NYU Sch Med 1977; **Resid:** Ophthalmology, New York Univ Med Ctr 1981; **Fellow:** Retina, New York Univ Med Ctr 1982

Ray, Audell MD (Oph) - **Spec Exp:** Cataract Surgery; **Hospital:** Lawrence Hosp Ctr; **Address:** Bronxville Eye Associates, 77 Pondfield Rd, Bronxville, NY 10708-3809; **Phone:** 914-337-8844; **Board Cert:** Ophthalmology 1979; **Med School:** Columbia P&S 1974; **Resid:** Ophthalmology, Manhattan EET 1978

Salzman, Jacqueline MD (Oph) - **Spec Exp:** Cataract Surgery; Diabetic Eye Disease; Glaucoma; **Hospital:** Phelps Meml Hosp Ctr; **Address:** 200 S Broadway, Ste 211, Tarrytown, NY 10591-4504; **Phone:** 914-332-5394; **Board Cert:** Ophthalmology 1985; **Med School:** NYU Sch Med 1979; **Resid:** Ophthalmology, Bellevue Hosp 1983; **Fellow:** Retina, Bellevue Hosp 1984

Solomon, Ira MD (Oph) - **Spec Exp:** Glaucoma; **Hospital:** Lawrence Hosp Ctr, Lenox Hill Hosp (page 94); **Address:** 700 White Plains Rd, Ste 343, Scarsdale, NY 10583; **Phone:** 914-725-5400; **Board Cert:** Ophthalmology 1989; **Med School:** Jefferson Med Coll 1982; **Resid:** Ophthalmology, Montefiore Hosp Med Ctr 1986; **Fellow:** Glaucoma, New York Eye & Ear Infirmary 1987; **Fac Appt:** Asst Clin Prof Oph, Albert Einstein Coll Med

Solomon, Sherry MD (Oph) - **Spec Exp:** Diabetic Eye Disease/Retinopathy; Macular Degeneration; Retinitis Pigmentosa; Retinal Detachment; **Hospital:** Lawrence Hosp Ctr, Sound Shore Med Ctr - Westchester (page 711); **Address:** 700 White Plains Rd, Ste 343, Scarsdale, NY 10583; **Phone:** 914-725-5400; **Board Cert:** Ophthalmology 1991; **Med School:** Albert Einstein Coll Med 1986; **Resid:** Ophthalmology, Montefiore Hosp Med Ctr 1990; **Fellow:** Retina, NYU Med Ctr 1991; **Fac Appt:** Asst Clin Prof Oph, Albert Einstein Coll Med

Stein, Mitchell MD (Oph) - **Spec Exp:** Cataract Surgery; Cornea & External Eye Disease; **Hospital:** Northern Westchester Hosp; **Address:** 69 S Moger Ave, Mount Kisco, NY 10549-2217; **Phone:** 914-666-2961; **Board Cert:** Internal Medicine 1982; Ophthalmology 1987; **Med School:** Albert Einstein Coll Med 1979; **Resid:** Internal Medicine, Bronx Muni Hosp 1982; Ophthalmology, SUNY-Downstate Med Ctr 1986; **Fellow:** Cornea, Mount Sinai Hosp/Beth Israel Hosp 1987; **Fac Appt:** Asst Clin Prof Med, Albert Einstein Coll Med

Sussman, John MD (Oph) - **Spec Exp:** Glaucoma; Cataract Surgery; **Hospital:** Phelps Meml Hosp Ctr; **Address:** 24 Saw Mill River Rd, Ste 202, Hawthorne, NY 10532; **Phone:** 914-631-9191; **Board Cert:** Ophthalmology 1965; **Med School:** NYU Sch Med 1959; **Resid:** Ophthalmology, Montefiore Hosp Med Ctr 1963

Zaidman, Gerald MD (Oph) - **Spec Exp:** Laser Vision Surgery; Cornea Transplant; Cataract Surgery; **Hospital:** Westchester Med Ctr (page 713), Our Lady of Mercy Med Ctr; **Address:** Westchester Med Ctr, Macy Pavilion, Dept Opth, rm 1100, Valhalla, NY 10595; **Phone:** 914-493-1599; **Board Cert:** Ophthalmology 1981; **Med School:** Albert Einstein Coll Med 1975; **Resid:** Ophthalmology, Beth Abraham Hosp 1977; Ophthalmology, Lenox Hill Hosp 1980; **Fellow:** Cornea & Ext Eye Disease, Univ Pittsburgh 1982; **Fac Appt:** Prof Oph, NY Med Coll

ORTHOPAEDIC SURGERY

Brown, Charles B MD (OrS) - **Spec Exp:** Arthroscopic Surgery; Joint Replacement; Knee Surgery; **Hospital:** Northern Westchester Hosp; **Address:** 90 S Bedford Rd Fl 1, Mt Kisco, NY 10549-3422; **Phone:** 914-241-1050; **Board Cert:** Orthopaedic Surgery 1977; **Med School:** Columbia P&S 1969; **Resid:** Surgery, Columbia Presby Med Ctr 1972; Orthopaedic Surgery, Columbia Presby Med Ctr 1975; **Fellow:** Orthopaedic Surgery, Columbia Presby Med Ctr 1976

Burak, George MD (OrS) - **Spec Exp:** Sports Injuries; Arthritis; **Hospital:** Phelps Meml Hosp Ctr; **Address:** 24 Saw Mill River Rd, Ste 206, Hawthorne, NY 10532; **Phone:** 914-631-7777; **Board Cert:** Orthopaedic Surgery 1971; **Med School:** SUNY Upstate Med Univ 1964; **Resid:** Orthopaedic Surgery, Kings County Hosp 1969; **Fac Appt:** Asst Prof OrS, SUNY Downstate

Cristofaro, Robert MD (OrS) - **Spec Exp:** Pediatric Orthopaedic Surgery; Pediatric Sports Medicine; Foot & Hip Disorders-Complex Pediatric; **Hospital:** Westchester Med Ctr (page 713), Greenwich Hosp; **Address:** Blind Brook Ln & Purchase St, Rye, NY 10580; **Phone:** 914-967-8708; **Board Cert:** Orthopaedic Surgery 1978; **Med School:** SUNY Downstate 1971; **Resid:** Surgery, Montefiore Hosp 1972; Orthopaedic Surgery, Montefiore Hosp 1976; **Fellow:** Pediatric Orthopaedic Surgery, Rancho Los Amigos Med Ctr 1977; **Fac Appt:** Assoc Clin Prof OrS, NY Med Coll

Delbello, Damon MD (OrS) - **Spec Exp:** Pediatric Orthopaedic Surgery; Spinal Surgery; Scoliosis; **Hospital:** Westchester Med Ctr (page 713), Northern Westchester Hosp; **Address:** Blind Brook Ln, Rye, NY 10580; **Phone:** 914-967-8708; **Board Cert:** Orthopaedic Surgery 1996; **Med School:** NY Med Coll 1988; **Resid:** Surgery, Westchester Med Ctr 1989; Orthopaedic Surgery, Westchester Med CTr 1993; **Fellow:** Pediatric Orthopaedic Surgery, Shriners Hosp 1994; **Fac Appt:** Asst Prof OrS, NY Med Coll

Edelson, Charles MD (OrS) - **Spec Exp:** Reconstructive Surgery; Sports Medicine; Joint Replacement; **Hospital:** St John's Riverside Hosp, Saint Joseph's Med Ctr - Yonkers; **Address:** 970 N Broadway, Ste 204, Yonkers, NY 10701-1310; **Phone:** 914-476-4343; **Board Cert:** Orthopaedic Surgery 1979; **Med School:** NY Med Coll 1973; **Resid:** Surgery, Montefiore Med Ctr 1975; Orthopaedic Surgery, Montefiore Med Ctr 1978

Galeno, John MD (OrS) - **Spec Exp:** Spinal Surgery; Sports Medicine; **Hospital:** Westchester Med Ctr (page 713); **Address:** 222 Westchester Ave, Ste 204, White Plains, NY 10604; **Phone:** 914-288-0036; **Board Cert:** Orthopaedic Surgery 1998; **Med School:** Italy 1979; **Resid:** Orthopaedic Surgery, Westchester Med Ctr 1984; **Fellow:** Spinal Surgery, Toronto Genl Hosp 1985

Gundy, Edward MD (OrS) - **Spec Exp:** Geriatric Orthopaedic Surgery; Sports Medicine; **Hospital:** White Plains Hosp Ctr (page 714), Greenwich Hosp; **Address:** 210 Westchester Ave, White Plains, NY 10604; **Phone:** 914-682-6540; **Board Cert:** Orthopaedic Surgery 1983; **Med School:** Cornell Univ-Weill Med Coll 1976; **Resid:** Surgery, Roosevelt Hosp 1978; Orthopaedic Surgery, Hosp Special Surg 1981

Habermann, Edward MD (OrS) - **Spec Exp:** Hip & Knee Replacement; Bone Tumors; Arthritis; **Hospital:** Montefiore Med Ctr, Montefiore Med Ctr - Weiler-Einstein Div; **Address:** 335 Whippoorwill Road Rd, Chappaqua, NY 10514-2312; **Phone:** 914-238-1791; **Board Cert:** Orthopaedic Surgery 1994; **Med School:** SUNY Upstate Med Univ 1959; **Resid:** Surgery, Hosp Joint Dis 1963; Orthopaedic Surgery, Hosp Joint Dis 1966; **Fellow:** Hip Surgery, Wrighton Hosp 1967; **Fac Appt:** Prof OrS, Albert Einstein Coll Med

Holder, Jonathan L MD (OrS) - **Spec Exp:** Sports Medicine; Foot & Ankle Surgery; **Hospital:** White Plains Hosp Ctr (page 714), Westchester Med Ctr (page 713); **Address:** 170 Maple Ave, Ste 109, White Plains, NY 10601; **Phone:** 914-421-0600; **Board Cert:** Orthopaedic Surgery 2003; **Med School:** NY Med Coll 1985; **Resid:** Orthopaedic Surgery, Metropolitan Hosp Ctr 1990; **Fac Appt:** Asst Clin Prof OrS, NY Med Coll

Karas, Evan MD (OrS) - **Spec Exp:** Shoulder Surgery; **Hospital:** Northern Westchester Hosp; **Address:** 90 S Bedford Rd, Mt Kisco, NY 10549; **Phone:** 914-241-1050; **Board Cert:** Orthopaedic Surgery 1999; **Med School:** NYU Sch Med 1991; **Resid:** Orthopaedic Surgery, Mt Sinai Hosp 1996; **Fellow:** Sports Medicine, Univ Penn 1997

Levin, Howard MD (OrS) - **Spec Exp:** Knee Surgery; Shoulder Surgery; **Hospital:** Northern Westchester Hosp; **Address:** 1888 Commerce St, Yorktown Heights, NY 10598; **Phone:** 914-962-7712; **Board Cert:** Orthopaedic Surgery 1979; **Med School:** SUNY Hlth Sci Ctr 1973; **Resid:** Orthopaedic Surgery, Hosp for Joint Diseases 1978

Maddalo, Anthony MD (OrS) - **Spec Exp:** Sports Medicine; Shoulder & Knee Injuries; **Hospital:** Phelps Meml Hosp Ctr; **Address:** 24 Saw Mill River Rd, Ste 206, Hawthorne, NY 10532; **Phone:** 914-631-7777; **Board Cert:** Orthopaedic Surgery 1999; **Med School:** NY Med Coll 1981; **Resid:** Orthopaedic Surgery, Lenox Hill Hosp 1986

Mann, Ronald L MD (OrS) - **Spec Exp:** Pediatric Orthopaedic Surgery; Joint Replacement; Sports Medicine; **Hospital:** Northern Westchester Hosp; **Address:** 1888 Commerce St, Yorktown Heights, NY 10598-4431; **Phone:** 914-962-7712; **Board Cert:** Orthopaedic Surgery 1999; **Med School:** Univ Pennsylvania 1980; **Resid:** Surgery, Mount Sinai Hosp 1982; Orthopaedic Surgery, Mount Sinai Hosp 1985; **Fellow:** Pediatric Orthopaedic Surgery, Hosp for Special Surgery 1986

Nelson Jr, John M MD (OrS) - **Spec Exp:** Pediatric Orthopaedic Surgery; Joint Replacement; Sports Medicine; **Hospital:** Sound Shore Med Ctr - Westchester (page 711), Westchester Med Ctr (page 713); **Address:** Blind Brook Lane on Purchase St, Rye, NY 10580; **Phone:** 914-967-8708; **Board Cert:** Orthopaedic Surgery 1998; **Med School:** Mount Sinai Sch Med 1979; **Resid:** Orthopaedic Surgery, Hosp for Joint Diseases 1984; **Fellow:** Pediatric Orthopaedic Surgery, Scottish Rite Chldns Hosp 1985

Peress, Richard MD (OrS) - **Spec Exp:** Spinal Reconstructive Surgery; **Hospital:** Phelps Meml Hosp Ctr; **Address:** 100 S Highland Ave, Park Profl Bldg, Ste 1, Ossining, NY 10562-5634; **Phone:** 914-762-9300; **Board Cert:** Orthopaedic Surgery 1989; **Med School:** Columbia P&S 1981; **Resid:** Surgery, St Luke's-Roosevelt Hosp Ctr 1983; Orthopaedic Surgery, Columbia-Presby Med Ctr 1986; **Fellow:** Spinal Surgery, Leatherman Spine Ctr/Univ Louisville 1987

Purcell, Ralph MD (OrS) - **Spec Exp:** Hand Surgery; **Hospital:** Phelps Meml Hosp Ctr, White Plains Hosp Ctr (page 714); **Address:** 200 S Broadway, Ste 104, Tarrytown, NY 10591; **Phone:** 914-631-1142; **Board Cert:** Orthopaedic Surgery 2000; **Med School:** Columbia P&S 1979; **Resid:** Surgery, Beth Israel-Harvard Univ 1982; Orthopaedic Surgery, NY Orth Hosp-Columbia Univ 1985; **Fellow:** Hand Surgery, NYU Med Ctr 1986

Seebacher, J Robert MD (OrS) - **Spec Exp:** Hip Replacement; Knee Replacement; Joint Replacement; **Hospital:** Phelps Meml Hosp Ctr; **Address:** Hudson Valley Bone & Joint Surgeons, 239 N Broadway, Sleepy Hollow, NY 10591-2674; **Phone:** 914-631-7777; **Board Cert:** Orthopaedic Surgery 1984; **Med School:** Georgetown Univ 1976; **Resid:** Surgery, Mount Sinai Hosp 1978; Orthopaedic Surgery, Hosp for Special Surgery 1981; **Fellow:** Pediatric Orthopaedic Surgery, Hosp for Sick Children 1982

Small, Steven MD (OrS) - **Spec Exp:** Sports Medicine; **Hospital:** Hudson Valley Hosp Ctr; **Address:** 1985 Crompond Rd, Bldg E, Cortland Manor, NY 10567; **Phone:** 914-739-2121; **Board Cert:** Orthopaedic Surgery 1997; **Med School:** NY Med Coll 1979; **Resid:** Orthopaedic Surgery, Westchester Med Ctr 1984

Taddonio, Rudolph MD (OrS) - **Spec Exp:** Scoliosis; Spinal Surgery; **Hospital:** Stamford Hosp, Northern Westchester Hosp; **Address:** Scoliosis & Spinal Surgery, 244 Westchester Ave, Ste 316, White Plains, NY 10604; **Phone:** 914-288-0045; **Board Cert:** Orthopaedic Surgery 1977; **Med School:** NY Med Coll 1971; **Resid:** Surgery, Metropolitian Hosp Ctr 1975; **Fellow:** Spinal Surgery, Rush Presbyterian-St Luke's Med Ctr 1976; **Fac Appt:** Clin Prof OrS, NY Med Coll

Walsh, William MD (OrS) - **Spec Exp:** Running Injuries; Arthroscopic Surgery; Joint Replacement; **Hospital:** Westchester Med Ctr (page 713), White Plains Hosp Ctr (page 714); **Address:** University Orthopaedics, 19 Bradhurst Ave, Ste 1300 N, Hawthorn, NY 10532; **Phone:** 914-789-2725; **Board Cert:** Orthopaedic Surgery 1972; **Med School:** NY Med Coll 1964; **Resid:** Surgery, St Vincent's Hosp & Med Ctr 1966; Orthopaedic Surgery, Bellevue Hosp 1971; **Fac Appt:** Assoc Prof S, NY Med Coll

Zelicof, Steven B MD (OrS) - **Spec Exp:** Joint Reconstruction; Arthritis; Sports Medicine; **Hospital:** Sound Shore Med Ctr - Westchester (page 711), Westchester Med Ctr (page 713); **Address:** 311 North St, Ste 206, White Plains, NY 10605-2232; **Phone:** 914-686-0111; **Board Cert:** Orthopaedic Surgery 2003; **Med School:** Univ Pennsylvania 1983; **Resid:** Surgery, Lenox Hill Hosp 1985; Orthopaedic Surgery, Hosp Special Surg 1989; **Fellow:** Orthopaedic Surgery, Brigham & Women's Hosp 1990; **Fac Appt:** Assoc Clin Prof OrS, NY Med Coll

OTOLARYNGOLOGY

Fox, Mark MD (Oto) - **Spec Exp:** Head & Neck Cancer; Sinus Surgery; **Hospital:** Lawrence Hosp Ctr, Sound Shore Med Ctr - Westchester (page 711); **Address:** 700 White Plains Rd, Ste 30, Scarsdale, NY 10583-5013; **Phone:** 914-725-4266; **Board Cert:** Otolaryngology 1979; **Med School:** NY Med Coll 1973; **Resid:** Surgery, Metropolitan Hosp Ctr 1974; Otolaryngology, Manhattan EET Hosp 1979; **Fac Appt:** Asst Clin Prof Oto, Columbia P&S

Jamal, Habib MD (Oto) - **Hospital:** Greenwich Hosp; **Address:** 14 Rye Ridge Plz, Ste 231, Rye Brook, NY 10573; **Phone:** 914-253-4985; **Board Cert:** Otolaryngology 1979; **Med School:** Pakistan 1974; **Resid:** Surgery, Baylor Coll Med 1976; Otolaryngology, Albert Einstein 1979

Jay, Judith MD (Oto) - **Spec Exp:** Endoscopic Sinus Surgery; Pediatric Otolaryngology; **Hospital:** Phelps Meml Hosp Ctr; **Address:** 425 N State Rd, Briarcliff Manor, NY 10510-1469; **Phone:** 914-945-0505; **Board Cert:** Otolaryngology 1984; **Med School:** Hahnemann Univ 1979; **Resid:** Surgery, Abington Meml Hosp 1980; Otolaryngology, Mount Sinai Hosp 1984

Kase, Steven B MD (Oto) - **Spec Exp:** Sinus Disorders; Pediatric Otolaryngology; **Hospital:** White Plains Hosp Ctr (page 714), Westchester Med Ctr (page 713); **Address:** 75 S Broadway Fl 3, White Plains, NY 10601; **Phone:** 914-681-0300; **Board Cert:** Otolaryngology 1981; **Med School:** Loyola Univ-Stritch Sch Med 1976; **Resid:** Surgery, St Francis Hosp 1977; Otolaryngology, NY EE Infirm 1980

Kates, Matthew MD (Oto) - **Spec Exp:** Sinus Disorders/Surgery; Thyroid Surgery; Balance Disorders; **Hospital:** Sound Shore Med Ctr - Westchester (page 711), Lawrence Hosp Ctr; **Address:** 26 Burling Ln, New Rochelle, NY 10801-4914; **Phone:** 914-636-0104; **Board Cert:** Otolaryngology 1992; **Med School:** Cornell Univ-Weill Med Coll 1986; **Resid:** Surgery, St Vincent's Hosp 1988; Otolaryngology, Manhattan EET Hosp 1991

Lawrence, David MD (Oto) - **Spec Exp:** Pediatric Otolaryngology; **Hospital:** Greenwich Hosp; **Address:** 3000 Westchester Ave, Purchase, NY 10577; **Phone:** 914-253-0868; **Board Cert:** Otolaryngology 1974; **Med School:** Albany Med Coll 1969; **Resid:** Surgery, Lenox Hill Hosp 1971; Otolaryngology, NY EE Infirm 1974

Lewis, Lawrence MD (Oto) - **Spec Exp:** Sinus Surgery; **Hospital:** Northern Westchester Hosp; **Address:** 344 Main St, Ste 004, Mt Kisco, NY 10549; **Phone:** 914-241-0516; **Board Cert:** Otolaryngology 1976; **Med School:** SUNY Buffalo 1969; **Resid:** Surgery, Montefiore Hosp Med Ctr 1971; **Fellow:** Otolaryngology, U Conn Hlth Ctr 1976

Merer, David M MD (Oto) - **Spec Exp:** Pediatric Otolaryngology; **Hospital:** Westchester Med Ctr (page 713); **Address:** 1056 Saw Mill River Rd, Ste 101, Ardsley, NY 10502; **Phone:** 914-693-7636; **Board Cert:** Otolaryngology 1996; **Med School:** Albert Einstein Coll Med 1990; **Resid:** Otolaryngology, Montefiore Med Ctr 1995; **Fellow:** Pediatric Otolaryngology, Montefiore Med Ctr 1996; **Fac Appt:** Assoc Prof Oto, NY Med Coll

Moscatello, Augustine L MD (Oto) - **Spec Exp:** Nasal & Sinus Disorders; Head & Neck Surgery; **Hospital:** Westchester Med Ctr (page 713); **Address:** 1055 Sawmill River Rd, Ste 101, Ardsley, NY 10502; **Phone:** 914-693-7636; **Board Cert:** Otolaryngology 1987; **Med School:** Mount Sinai Sch Med 1982; **Resid:** Surgery, Mount Sinai Hosp 1987; Otolaryngology, Mount Sinai Hosp 1987; **Fac Appt:** Assoc Prof Oto, NY Med Coll

Nevins, Stuart MD (Oto) - **Spec Exp:** Snoring/Sleep Apnea; **Hospital:** White Plains Hosp Ctr (page 714); **Address:** Ear, Nose, & Throat Assocs, 75 S Broadway, Fl 3rd, White Plains, NY 10601; **Phone:** 914-949-3888; **Board Cert:** Otolaryngology 1968; **Med School:** Albany Med Coll 1960; **Resid:** Surgery, Albany Med Ctr 1964; Otolaryngology, Manhattan EE&T 1967

Ryback, Hyman MD (Oto) - **Spec Exp:** Endoscopic Sinus Surgery; Laryngeal Surgery; Snoring/Sleep Apnea; Reconstructive Surgery; **Hospital:** White Plains Hosp Ctr (page 714); **Address:** 75 S Broadway Fl 3, White Plains, NY 10601; **Phone:** 914-949-3888; **Board Cert:** Otolaryngology 1977; **Med School:** McGill Univ 1970; **Resid:** Surgery, Jewish Genl Hosp 1973; Otolaryngology, Mount Sinai Hosp 1977

Schaffer, Dean MD (Oto) - **Spec Exp:** Nasal & Sinus Disorders; Ear Disorders; **Hospital:** Northern Westchester Hosp; **Address:** Box 710, Goldens Bridge, NY 10526-0710; **Phone:** 914-232-3112; **Board Cert:** Otolaryngology 1980; **Med School:** Albert Einstein Coll Med 1976; **Resid:** Surgery, Montefiore Hosp Med Ctr 1977; Otolaryngology, Johns Hopkins Hosp 1980

Shapiro, Barry M MD (Oto) - **Spec Exp:** Endoscopic Sinus Surgery; Sleep Disorders/Apnea; **Hospital:** Phelps Meml Hosp Ctr; **Address:** 425 N State Rd, Briarcliff Manor, NY 10510-1469; **Phone:** 914-945-0505; **Board Cert:** Otolaryngology 1983; **Med School:** Mount Sinai Sch Med 1978; **Resid:** Surgery, Mount Sinai 1979; Otolaryngology, Mount Sinai 1982; **Fac Appt:** Asst Clin Prof Oto, Mount Sinai Sch Med

Siglock, Timothy MD (Oto) - **Spec Exp:** Ear Disorders/Surgery; Sinus Surgery; Voice Disorders; **Hospital:** Hudson Valley Hosp Ctr; **Address:** 3630 Hill Blvd, Ste 202, Jefferson Valley, NY 10535-1502; **Phone:** 914-245-7700; **Board Cert:** Otolaryngology 1986; **Med School:** Belgium 1981; **Resid:** Otolaryngology, New York Eye and Ear Infirmary 1986; **Fellow:** Research, House Ear Institute 1987

Vecchiotti, Arthur MD (Oto) - **Spec Exp:** Asthma & Allergy; Nasal & Sinus Surgery; Pediatric Otolaryngology; **Hospital:** Phelps Meml Hosp Ctr, Westchester Med Ctr (page 713); **Address:** 245 N Broadway, Ste 101, Sleepy Hollow, NY 10591-2647; **Phone:** 914-631-6161; **Board Cert:** Otolaryngology 1978; **Med School:** Italy 1971; **Resid:** Surgery, Metropolitan Hosp Ctr 1976; Otolaryngology, Manhattan EET Hosp 1978; **Fac Appt:** Asst Prof Oto, NY Med Coll

PAIN MEDICINE

Epstein, Lawrence J MD (PM) - **Hospital:** St John's Riverside Hosp; **Address:** Pain Medicine Wellness Ctr of New York, 220 Westchester Ave, White Plains, NY 10604; **Phone:** 914-289-1507; **Board Cert:** Anesthesiology 1987; Pain Medicine 2004; **Med School:** Israel 1983; **Resid:** Anesthesiology, SUNY Brooklyn Med Ctr 1986; **Fellow:** Obstetrics & Anesthesiology, SUNY Brooklyn Med Ctr 1987

Gevirtz, Clifford MD (PM) - **Spec Exp:** Opiate Addiction; Palliative Care; Herpetic Neuralgia (Shingles); **Hospital:** N Shore Univ Hosp at Forest Hills; **Address:** Somnia, 627 West St, Harrison, NY 10528; **Phone:** 914-636-6210; **Board Cert:** Anesthesiology 1997; Pain Medicine 2004; **Med School:** Tulane Univ 1981; **Resid:** Surgery, Montefiore Hosp Med Ctr 1982; Anesthesiology, Jacobi Med Ctr 1985; **Fellow:** Pain Medicine, Mass Genl Hosp 1986

Kestenbaum, Alan MD (PM) - **Spec Exp:** Pain-Back; Pain-Cancer; **Hospital:** Lawrence Hosp Ctr; **Address:** 1 Pondfield Rd, Ste 201, Bronxville, NY 10708-2670; **Phone:** 914-337-0434; **Board Cert:** Anesthesiology 1990; Pain Medicine 1996; **Med School:** Boston Univ 1985; **Resid:** Anesthesiology, LI Jewish Med Ctr 1988; **Fellow:** Pain Medicine, Meml Sloan Kettering Cancer Ctr 1989

Kizelshteyn, Grigory MD (PM) - **Hospital:** St John's Riverside Hosp; **Address:** Pain Medicine Wellness Ctr of New York, 220 Westchester Ave, White Plains, NY 10604; **Phone:** 914-289-1507; **Board Cert:** Anesthesiology 1991; Pain Medicine 2004; **Med School:** Russia 1975; **Resid:** Anesthesiology, Westchester Med Ctr 1986

Lu, Gabriel MD (PM) - **Spec Exp:** Pain-Back & Neck; Acupuncture; **Hospital:** Montefiore Med Ctr; **Address:** 112 Penn Rd, Scarsdale, NY 10583-7558; **Phone:** 914-725-4240; **Board Cert:** Anesthesiology 1984; Pain Medicine 1997; **Med School:** China 1968; **Resid:** Surgery, St Lukes Hospital 1976; Anesthesiology, Albert Einstein 1978; **Fellow:** Anesthesiology, Albert Einstein 1979; **Fac Appt:** Prof Anes, Albert Einstein Coll Med

PEDIATRIC CARDIOLOGY

Fish, Bernard MD (PCd) - **Spec Exp:** Cardiac Imaging; Fetal Echocardiography; **Hospital:** Westchester Med Ctr (page 713), St John's Riverside Hosp; **Address:** NY Med Coll, Ped Cardiology, Munger Pavillion, Ste 618, Valhalla, NY 10595; **Phone:** 914-594-4370; **Board Cert:** Pediatrics 1974; Pediatric Cardiology 1975; **Med School:** Univ Chicago-Pritzker Sch Med 1969; **Resid:** Pediatrics, Montefiore Hosp Med Ctr 1971; Pediatric Cardiology, Montefiore Hosp Med Ctr 1973; **Fellow:** Pediatric Cardiology, Yale-New Haven Hosp 1975; **Fac Appt:** Assoc Prof Ped, NY Med Coll

Gewitz, Michael MD (PCd) - **Spec Exp:** Neonatal Cardiology; Kawasaki Disease; Echocardiography; **Hospital:** Westchester Med Ctr (page 713), Vassar Bros Med Ctr; **Address:** Maria Fareri Chldns Hosp, Rte 100, Munger Pavillion, Ste 618, Valhalla, NY 10595; **Phone:** 914-594-4370; **Board Cert:** Pediatrics 1979; Pediatric Cardiology 1981; **Med School:** Hahnemann Univ 1974; **Resid:** Pediatrics, Chldns Hosp 1976; Pediatrics, Hosp Sick Chldn 1977; **Fellow:** Pediatric Cardiology, Yale-New Haven Hosp 1979; **Fac Appt:** Prof Ped, NY Med Coll

Issenberg, Henry MD (PCd) - **Spec Exp:** Cardiac Catheterization; Fetal Echocardiography; Congenital Heart Disease-Adult & Child; **Hospital:** Westchester Med Ctr (page 713), Our Lady of Mercy Med Ctr; **Address:** New York Med College, Dept Ped Cardiology, Munger Pavilion, rm 618, Valhalla, NY 10595; **Phone:** 914-594-4370; **Board Cert:** Pediatrics 1979; Pediatric Cardiology 1979; **Med School:** Emory Univ 1974; **Resid:** Pediatrics, Jacobi Med Ctr 1977; **Fellow:** Pediatric Cardiology, Childrens Med Ctr 1980; **Fac Appt:** Assoc Prof Ped, NY Med Coll

Levin, Aaron MD (PCd) - **Spec Exp:** Cardiac Catheterization; Heart Disease-Congenital; Kawasaki Disease; **Hospital:** Westchester Med Ctr (page 713); **Address:** Munger Pavilion, Ste 618, Valhalla, NY 10595; **Phone:** 914-594-4370; **Board Cert:** Pediatrics 1965; Pediatric Cardiology 1967; **Med School:** South Africa 1953; **Resid:** Pediatrics, Coronation Hosp 1960; Pediatrics, Charing Cross Hosp 1963; **Fellow:** Pediatric Cardiology, Duke Univ Med Ctr 1966; **Fac Appt:** Prof Ped, NY Med Coll

Woolf, Paul MD (PCd) - **Spec Exp:** Arrhythmias; **Hospital:** Westchester Med Ctr (page 713); **Address:** New York Medical College, Munger Pavillion, rm 618, Valhalla, NY 10595; **Phone:** 914-594-4370; **Board Cert:** Pediatrics 1982; Pediatric Cardiology 1983; **Med School:** Columbia P&S 1977; **Resid:** Pediatrics, Children's Hosp 1980; **Fellow:** Pediatric Cardiology, Children's Hosp 1983; **Fac Appt:** Assoc Prof Ped, NY Med Coll

PEDIATRIC CRITICAL CARE MEDICINE

Goltzman, Carey MD (PCCM) - **Spec Exp:** Respiratory Failure; Sepsis & Septic Shock; **Hospital:** Westchester Med Ctr (page 713); **Address:** NY Med Coll, Chldns Physicians of Westchester, Maria Fareri Chlds Hosp, PCCM, rm 2237, Valhalla, NY 10595; **Phone:** 914-493-7513; **Board Cert:** Pediatrics 2000; Pediatric Critical Care Medicine 2000; **Med School:** Mexico 1981; **Resid:** Pediatrics, Westchester Med Ctr 1987; **Fellow:** Pediatric Critical Care Medicine, Henry Ford Hosp 1989; **Fac Appt:** Asst Prof Ped, NY Med Coll

PEDIATRIC ENDOCRINOLOGY

Handelsman, Dan MD (PEn) - **Hospital:** Phelps Meml Hosp Ctr, Westchester Med Ctr (page 713); **Address:** 325 S Highland Ave, Briarcliff Manor, NY 10510; **Phone:** 914-762-0015; **Board Cert:** Pediatrics 1973; **Med School:** Albert Einstein Coll Med 1968; **Resid:** Pediatrics, Babies Hosp 1969; Pediatrics, Montefiore Hosp 1971; **Fellow:** Genetics and Metabolism, Albert Einstein 1973; **Fac Appt:** Assoc Clin Prof Ped, NY Med Coll

Lebinger, Tessa MD (PEn) - **Spec Exp:** Diabetes; Growth Disorders; Thyroid Disorders; **Hospital:** Nyack Hosp, White Plains Hosp Ctr (page 714); **Address:** 121 Bon Air Ave, New Rochelle, NY 10804; **Phone:** 914-633-4446; **Board Cert:** Pediatrics 1982; Pediatric Endocrinology 1983; **Med School:** Albert Einstein Coll Med 1976; **Resid:** Pediatrics, Jacobi Med Ctr 1978; **Fellow:** Pediatric Endocrinology, Montefiore Hosp Med Ctr 1981; **Fac Appt:** Asst Clin Prof Ped, NY Med Coll

Noto, Richard MD (PEn) - **Spec Exp:** Growth/Development Disorders; Diabetes; Lead Poisoning; **Hospital:** Westchester Med Ctr (page 713), St Vincent Cath Med Ctrs - Westchester (page 375); **Address:** 701 N Broadway, Sleepy Hollow, NY 10591; **Phone:** 914-366-3400; **Board Cert:** Pediatrics 1981; Pediatric Endocrinology 1983; **Med School:** Mount Sinai Sch Med 1976; **Resid:** Pediatrics, Beth Israel Med Ctr 1978; **Fellow:** Pediatric Endocrinology, NY Hosp 1979; Pediatric Endocrinology, N Shore Univ Hosp 1981; **Fac Appt:** Asst Prof Ped, NY Med Coll

Romano, Alicia MD (PEn) - **Spec Exp:** Growth/Development Disorders; Diabetes; **Hospital:** Westchester Med Ctr (page 713), Our Lady of Mercy Med Ctr; **Address:** 701 N Broadway, Diabetes & Endocrine Ctr, Sleepy Hollow, NY 10591; **Phone:** 914-366-3400; **Board Cert:** Pediatric Endocrinology 1999; **Med School:** SUNY Stony Brook 1985; **Resid:** Pediatrics, Schneider Chldns Hosp 1988; **Fellow:** Pediatric Endocrinology, Schneider Chldns Hosp 1991; **Fac Appt:** Asst Prof Ped, NY Med Coll

Saenger, Paul MD (PEn) - **Spec Exp:** Short Stature in Children; Turner's Syndrome; Sexual Differentiation Disorders; **Hospital:** Montefiore Med Ctr; **Address:** 150 Lockwood Ave, New Rochelle, NY 10801; **Phone:** 914-636-5924; **Board Cert:** Pediatrics 1973; Pediatric Endocrinology 1978; **Med School:** Germany 1969; **Resid:** Pediatrics, Montefiore Hosp Med Ctr 1970; Pediatrics, Albert Einstein Coll Med 1971; **Fellow:** Pediatric Endocrinology, Cornell Univ Med Ctr 1975; **Fac Appt:** Prof Ped, Albert Einstein Coll Med

PEDIATRIC GASTROENTEROLOGY

Berezin, Stuart MD (PGe) - **Hospital:** Westchester Med Ctr (page 713); **Address:** NY Med College, Div Ped Gastroenterology, Munger Pavillion, rm 101, Valhalla, NY 10595; **Phone:** 914-594-4610; **Board Cert:** Pediatrics 1980; Pediatric Gastroenterology 1990; **Med School:** Hahnemann Univ 1976; **Resid:** Pediatrics, Metrohealth Med Ctr 1979; Gastroenterology, Chldns Hosp; **Fac Appt:** Assoc Prof Ped, NY Med Coll

Birnbaum, Audrey MD (PGe) - **Spec Exp:** Food Allergy; Inflammatory Bowel Disease/Crohn's; **Hospital:** Northern Westchester Hosp; **Address:** 110 S Bedford Rd, Mount Kisco, NY 10549; **Phone:** 914-241-1050; **Board Cert:** Pediatrics 2000; Pediatric Gastroenterology 2000; **Med School:** NYU Sch Med 1986; **Resid:** Pediatrics, Mt Sinai Hosp 1989; **Fellow:** Pediatric Gastroenterology, Mt Sinai Hosp 1991

Halata, Michael MD (PGe) - **Spec Exp:** Inflammatory Bowel Disease; Functional Bowel Disorders; Gastroesophageal Reflux Disease (GERD); **Hospital:** Westchester Med Ctr (page 713); **Address:** Munger Pavilion, Rm 101, Div Ped Gastroenterology, Valhalla, NY 10595; **Phone:** 914-594-4610; **Board Cert:** Pediatrics 1980; Pediatric Gastroenterology 2004; **Med School:** UMDNJ-NJ Med Sch, Newark 1974; **Resid:** Pediatrics, NY Med Coll 1977; **Fellow:** Pediatric Gastroenterology, NY Med Coll 1979; **Fac Appt:** Assoc Clin Prof Ped, NY Med Coll

Newman, Leonard MD (PGe) - **Spec Exp:** Inflammatory Bowel Disease; Celiac Disease; **Hospital:** Westchester Med Ctr (page 713), Our Lady of Mercy Med Ctr; **Address:** NY Med College, Dept Ped, Munger Pavillion - rm 123, Valhalla, NY 10595; **Phone:** 914-594-4610; **Board Cert:** Pediatrics 1975; Pediatric Gastroenterology 1990; **Med School:** NY Med Coll 1970; **Resid:** Pediatrics, UCSD Med Ctr 1972; Pediatrics, NY Med Coll 1973; **Fellow:** Gastroenterology, Bronx Lebanon Hosp/Einstein 1974; **Fac Appt:** Prof Ped, NY Med Coll

PEDIATRIC HEMATOLOGY-ONCOLOGY

Jayabose, Somasundaram MD (PHO) - **Spec Exp:** Sickle Cell Disease; Leukemia; Lymphoma; **Hospital:** Westchester Med Ctr (page 713), Good Samaritan Hosp - Suffern; **Address:** NY Med Coll, Dept Pediatrics, Munger Pavilion, rm 110, Valhalla, NY 10595; **Phone:** 914-493-7997; **Board Cert:** Pediatrics 1975; Pediatric Hematology-Oncology 1976; **Med School:** India 1969; **Resid:** Pediatrics, Metropolitan Hosp Ctr 1974; **Fellow:** Pediatric Hematology-Oncology, LI Jewish Med Ctr 1976; **Fac Appt:** Prof Ped, NY Med Coll

Marcus, Judith R MD (PHO) - **Spec Exp:** Leukemia; Lymphoma; Bleeding Disorders; Wilms' Tumor; **Hospital:** NY-Presby Hosp (page 100), White Plains Hosp Ctr (page 714); **Address:** 147 Underhill Ave, White Plains, NY 10604-2539; **Phone:** 914-684-0220; **Board Cert:** Pediatrics 1997; Pediatric Hematology-Oncology 1997; **Med School:** NYU Sch Med 1971; **Resid:** Pediatrics, Bronx Muni Hosp-Albert Einstein 1974; **Fellow:** Pediatric Hematology-Oncology, Mem Sloan Kettering Cancer Ctr 1979; **Fac Appt:** Clin Prof Ped, Columbia P&S

Sandoval, Claudio MD (PHO) - **Hospital:** Westchester Med Ctr (page 713), Metropolitan Hosp Ctr - NY; **Address:** NY Med Coll, Munger Pavillion, rm 110, Valhalla, NY 10595; **Phone:** 914-493-7997; **Board Cert:** Pediatrics 1990; Pediatric Hematology-Oncology 1994; **Med School:** NY Med Coll 1987; **Resid:** Pediatrics, Schneider Chldns Hosp 1990; **Fellow:** Pediatric Hematology-Oncology, St Jude Chldns Rsch Hosp

Tugal, Oya MD (PHO) - **Spec Exp:** Leukemia & Lymphoma; Brain Tumors; Langerhans Cell Histiocytoma; **Hospital:** Westchester Med Ctr (page 713), Good Samaritan Hosp - Suffern; **Address:** NY Med Coll, Dept Peds, Munger Pavillion, rm 110, Valhalla, NY 10595; **Phone:** 914-493-7997; **Board Cert:** Pediatrics 1986; Pediatric Hematology-Oncology 1987; **Med School:** Turkey 1974; **Resid:** Pediatrics, Hacettepe Med Ctr 1977; Pediatrics, Westchester Med Ctr 1985; **Fellow:** Allergy & Immunology, Hacettepe Med Ctr 1978; Pediatric Hematology-Oncology, Mount Sinai Hosp 1987; **Fac Appt:** Assoc Clin Prof Ped, NY Med Coll

PEDIATRIC INFECTIOUS DISEASE

Munoz, Jose Luis MD (PInf) - **Spec Exp:** Lyme Disease; Immune Deficiency; AIDS/HIV; **Hospital:** Westchester Med Ctr (page 713); **Address:** Ped Infectious Disease, 19 Bradhurst Ave, Hawthorne, NY 10532; **Phone:** 914-493-8333; **Board Cert:** Pediatrics 1989; Pediatric Infectious Disease 2002; **Med School:** Yale Univ 1978; **Resid:** Pediatrics, Yale New Haven Hosp 1981; **Fellow:** Pediatric Infectious Disease, Univ Rochester 1984; **Fac Appt:** Assoc Prof Ped, NY Med Coll

PEDIATRIC NEPHROLOGY

Weiss, Robert A MD (PNep) - **Spec Exp:** Kidney Failure; Nephrotic Syndrome; **Hospital:** Westchester Med Ctr (page 713); **Address:** Pediatric Nephrology, NY Med Coll, Munger Pavilion, rm 116, Valhalla, NY 10595; **Phone:** 914-493-7583; **Board Cert:** Pediatrics 1976; Pediatric Nephrology 1979; **Med School:** Georgetown Univ 1971; **Resid:** Pediatrics, Bellevue Hosp Ctr 1974; **Fellow:** Pediatric Nephrology, Westchester Med Ctr 1977; **Fac Appt:** Prof Ped, NY Med Coll

PEDIATRIC OTOLARYNGOLOGY

Keller, Jeffrey MD (PO) - **Spec Exp:** Sleep Disorders/Apnea; Ear Infections; Sinusitis; Otitis Media; **Hospital:** Northern Westchester Hosp, Mount Sinai Med Ctr (page 98); **Address:** 90 S Bedford Rd, Mount Kisco, NY 10549; **Phone:** 914-242-1355; **Board Cert:** Otolaryngology 1996; **Med School:** Stanford Univ 1990; **Resid:** Otolaryngology, Mt Sinai Hosp 1995; **Fellow:** Pediatric Otolaryngology, Children's Hosp 1996; **Fac Appt:** Asst Prof Oto, Mount Sinai Sch Med

PEDIATRIC PULMONOLOGY

Dozor, Allen J MD (PPul) - **Spec Exp:** Asthma; Cystic Fibrosis; **Hospital:** Westchester Med Ctr (page 713); **Address:** NY Med College, Munger Pavilion, Pediatric Pulmonology, Ste 106, Valhalla, NY 10595-1600; **Phone:** 914-493-7585; **Board Cert:** Pediatrics 1981; Pediatric Pulmonology 2003; **Med School:** Penn State Univ-Hershey Med Ctr 1977; **Resid:** Pediatrics, St Vincent's Hosp & Med Ctr 1980; **Fellow:** Pediatric Pulmonology, Chldns Hosp 1982; **Fac Appt:** Prof Ped, NY Med Coll

Lowenthal, Diana MD (PPul) - **Spec Exp:** Asthma; Cystic Fibrosis; Cough; **Hospital:** Westchester Med Ctr (page 713); **Address:** NY Med Coll, Munger Pavilion, rm 106, Valhalla, NY 10595; **Phone:** 914-493-7585; **Board Cert:** Pediatrics 2000; Pediatric Pulmonology 2000; **Med School:** Albert Einstein Coll Med 1986; **Resid:** Pediatrics, Albert Einstein Coll Med 1989; **Fellow:** Pulmonary Disease, Mount Sinai Hosp 1992; **Fac Appt:** Asst Prof Ped, NY Med Coll

PEDIATRIC SURGERY

Holgersen, Leif MD (PS) - **Spec Exp:** Congenital Anomalies; Tumor Surgery; Endoscopy; **Hospital:** St Luke's - Roosevelt Hosp Ctr - Roosevelt Div (page 90), Lawrence Hosp Ctr; **Address:** PO Box 667, Purchase, NY 10577; **Phone:** 914-337-2455; **Board Cert:** Surgery 1971; Pediatric Surgery 1995; **Med School:** UMDNJ-NJ Med Sch, Newark 1965; **Resid:** Surgery, St Luke's-Roosevelt Hosp Ctr 1970; Pediatric Surgery, Chldns Hosp 1974; **Fac Appt:** Asst Prof S, Columbia P&S

Liebert, Peter MD (PS) - **Spec Exp:** Chest Deformities; Intestinal Surgery; Hernia; **Hospital:** White Plains Hosp Ctr (page 714), Northern Westchester Hosp; **Address:** 222 Westchester Ave, Ste 403, White Plains, NY 10604; **Phone:** 914-428-3533; **Board Cert:** Surgery 1968; Pediatric Surgery 1995; **Med School:** Harvard Med Sch 1961; **Resid:** Surgery, Peter Bent Brigham Hosp 1964; Surgery, Montefiore Hosp 1966; **Fellow:** Pediatric Surgery, Childrens Hosp 1968; **Fac Appt:** Assoc Clin Prof S, Columbia P&S

San Filippo, J Anthony MD (PS) - **Spec Exp:** Newborn Surgery; Tumor Surgery; Hernia; **Hospital:** Westchester Med Ctr (page 713), Northern Westchester Hosp; **Address:** 303 North St, Ste 102, White Plains, NY 10605; **Phone:** 914-761-5437; **Board Cert:** Surgery 1973; Pediatric Surgery 1975; **Med School:** Georgetown Univ 1965; **Resid:** Surgery, Bellevue Hosp 1967; Surgery, N Shore Univ Hosp 1970; **Fellow:** Pediatric Surgery, Children's Hosp 1972; **Fac Appt:** Prof S, NY Med Coll

Stringel, Gustavo MD (PS) - **Spec Exp:** Minimally Invasive Surgery; Cancer Surgery; Neonatal Surgery; **Hospital:** Westchester Med Ctr (page 713); **Address:** New York Med College, Div Ped Surgery, Munger Pavilion, rm 321, Valhalla, NY 10595; **Phone:** 914-493-7620; **Board Cert:** Surgery 1997; Pediatric Surgery 1995; Surgical Critical Care 1997; **Med School:** Mexico 1971; **Resid:** Surgery, U Toronto 1977; **Fellow:** Pediatric Surgery, Hosp Sick Chldn 1979; **Fac Appt:** Prof S, NY Med Coll

Zitsman, Jeffrey MD (PS) - **Spec Exp:** Minimally Invasive Surgery; Chest Wall Deformities; Obesity/Bariatric Surgery; **Hospital:** White Plains Hosp Ctr (page 714), NY-Presby Hosp (page 100); **Address:** 688 White Plains Rd, Ste 223, Scarsdale, NY 10583-5015; **Phone:** 914-722-6737; **Board Cert:** Surgery 2001; Pediatric Surgery 1995; Surgical Critical Care 1994; **Med School:** Tufts Univ 1976; **Resid:** Surgery, New England Med Ctr 1981; **Fellow:** Pediatric Surgery, Babies Hosp/Columbia Presby Med Ctr 1985; **Fac Appt:** Assoc Clin Prof S, Columbia P&S

PEDIATRICS

Acker, Peter J MD (Ped) PCP - **Hospital:** Greenwich Hosp, Westchester Med Ctr (page 713); **Address:** 12 Rye Ridge Plz, Rye Brook, NY 10573; **Phone:** 914-251-1100; **Board Cert:** Pediatrics 1988; **Med School:** Israel 1982; **Resid:** Pediatrics, NYU-Bellevue Hosp 1985; **Fellow:** Ambulatory Pediatrics, NYU-Bellevue Hosp 1987

Altman, Robin MD (Ped) PCP - **Spec Exp:** Sudden Infant Death Syndrome (SIDS); Weight Gain-Inadequate; **Hospital:** Westchester Med Ctr (page 713); **Address:** General Pediatrics, 19 Bradhurst Ave, Ste 800, Hawthorne, NY 10532; **Phone:** 914-593-8850; **Board Cert:** Pediatrics 1987; **Med School:** Robert W Johnson Med Sch 1983; **Resid:** Pediatrics, Colum-Presby Med Ctr 1986; **Fac Appt:** Asst Prof Ped, NY Med Coll

Amler, David MD (Ped) PCP - **Spec Exp:** Adolescent Medicine; **Hospital:** White Plains Hosp Ctr (page 714); **Address:** 15 N Broadway, White Plains, NY 10601; **Phone:** 914-948-4422; **Board Cert:** Pediatrics 1982; **Med School:** SUNY Buffalo 1969; **Resid:** Pediatrics, NYU Med Ctr 1972

Bailey, Michele L MD (Ped) PCP - **Spec Exp:** Adolescent Medicine; Asthma; **Hospital:** Our Lady of Mercy Med Ctr; **Address:** 16 North Broadway, Ste LMG, White Plains, NY 10601; **Phone:** 914-686-1848; **Board Cert:** Pediatrics 2002; **Med School:** West Indies 1989; **Resid:** Pediatrics, Lincoln Med Ctr 1994; **Fac Appt:** Asst Clin Prof Ped, NY Med Coll

Baskind, Larry MD (Ped) PCP - **Hospital:** Hudson Valley Hosp Ctr; **Address:** 35 S Riverside Ave, Ste 101, Croton-On-Hudson, NY 10520; **Phone:** 914-271-2424; **Board Cert:** Pediatrics 2003; **Med School:** UMDNJ-NJ Med Sch, Newark 1983; **Resid:** Pediatrics, Chldns Hosp 1987

Berkowitz, Norman MD (Ped) PCP - **Hospital:** Greenwich Hosp, Westchester Med Ctr (page 713); **Address:** 12 Rye Ridge Plaza, Rye Brook, NY 10573-2820; **Phone:** 914-251-1100; **Board Cert:** Pediatrics 1972; **Med School:** SUNY Buffalo 1967; **Resid:** Pediatrics, Mount Sinai 1970; **Fellow:** Pediatrics, St Christopher Hosp Chldn 1973

Berman, Morton MD (Ped) PCP - **Spec Exp:** Developmental Disorders; **Hospital:** White Plains Hosp Ctr (page 714), NYU Med Ctr (page 102); **Address:** 244 Westchester Ave, Ste 210, White Plains, NY 10604; **Phone:** 914-948-7016; **Board Cert:** Pediatrics 1972; **Med School:** NYU Sch Med 1966; **Resid:** Pediatrics, Bellevue Hosp 1970; **Fac Appt:** Asst Clin Prof Ped, NYU Sch Med

Bomback, Fredric MD (Ped) PCP - **Spec Exp:** Infectious Disease; Complex Diagnosis; **Hospital:** White Plains Hosp Ctr (page 714), NY-Presby Hosp (page 100); **Address:** 99 Fieldstone Drive, Hartsdale, NY 10530; **Phone:** 914-428-2120; **Board Cert:** Pediatrics 1984; **Med School:** NYU Sch Med 1969; **Resid:** Pediatrics, Albert Einstein Med Ctr 1972; **Fellow:** Genetics and Metabolism, Albert Einstein Med Ctr 1976; **Fac Appt:** Clin Prof Ped, Columbia P&S

Boyer, Joseph MD (Ped) **PCP** - **Hospital:** Westchester Med Ctr (page 713); **Address:** New York Med Coll, Pediatric Pulmonology, Munger Pavilion, rm 106, Valhalla, NY 10595; **Phone:** 914-493-7585; **Board Cert:** Pediatrics 2000; Pediatric Pulmonology 1998; **Med School:** SUNY Downstate 1988; **Resid:** Pediatrics, Westchester Co Med Ctr 1991; **Fellow:** Pediatric Pulmonology, Westchester Co Med Ctr 1995

Brittis, Robert J MD (Ped) **PCP** - **Hospital:** St John's Riverside Hosp; **Address:** 984 N Broadway, Ste 506, Yonkers, NY 10701; **Phone:** 914-963-7668; **Board Cert:** Pediatrics 1968; **Med School:** Italy 1963; **Resid:** Pediatrics, Hackensack Univ Med Ctr 1965; Pediatrics, Kings County Hosp 1966

Brown, Jeffrey MD (Ped) **PCP** - **Spec Exp:** Diagnostic Problems; Behavioral Disorders; Learning Disorders; **Hospital:** Greenwich Hosp, Westchester Med Ctr (page 713); **Address:** 12 Rye Ridge Plaza, Rye Brook, NY 10573-2855; **Phone:** 914-251-1100; **Board Cert:** Pediatrics 1972; **Med School:** Univ MD Sch Med 1965; **Resid:** Pediatrics, Mount Sinai Hosp 1970; **Fellow:** Neonatal-Perinatal Medicine, NY Hosp-Cornell Med Ctr 1971; **Fac Appt:** Assoc Clin Prof Ped, Cornell Univ-Weill Med Coll

Coven, Barbara MD (Ped) **PCP** - **Spec Exp:** Adolescent Medicine; **Hospital:** Greenwich Hosp, White Plains Hosp Ctr (page 714); **Address:** Westchester Med Group, Dept Pediatrics, 210 Westchester Ave Fl 2, White Plains, NY 10604; **Phone:** 914-682-0731; **Board Cert:** Pediatrics 1986; **Med School:** Boston Univ 1980; **Resid:** Pediatrics, Boston City Hosp 1983; **Fellow:** Psychosomatic Medicine, Chldns Hosp Med Ctr 1983

Edis, Gloria MD (Ped) **PCP** - **Hospital:** Lawrence Hosp Ctr, White Plains Hosp Ctr (page 714); **Address:** 2 Overhill Rd, Ste 220, Scarsdale, NY 10583-5316; **Phone:** 914-725-0800; **Board Cert:** Pediatrics 1970; **Med School:** NYU Sch Med 1963; **Resid:** Pediatrics, Montefiore Hosp Med Ctr 1964; Pediatrics, Columbia-Presby 1968; **Fac Appt:** Assoc Clin Prof Ped, Cornell Univ-Weill Med Coll

Glassman, Ben MD (Ped) **PCP** - **Spec Exp:** Adolescent Medicine; Sexually Transmitted Diseases; Eating Disorders; **Hospital:** Greenwich Hosp, Westchester Med Ctr (page 713); **Address:** 1600 Harrison Ave, Ste 307, Mamaroneck, NY 10543; **Phone:** 914-698-0564; **Board Cert:** Pediatrics 1974; **Med School:** Israel 1969; **Resid:** Pediatrics, Mt Sinai Hosp 1973; **Fellow:** Adolescent Medicine, Mt Sinai Hosp 1976; Ambulatory Pediatrics, Mt Sinai Hosp 1976; **Fac Appt:** Asst Clin Prof Ped, NY Med Coll

Hartz, Cindi MD (Ped) **PCP** - **Spec Exp:** Adolescent Medicine; **Hospital:** Sound Shore Med Ctr - Westchester (page 711); **Address:** 1415 Boston Post Rd, Larchmont, NY 10538; **Phone:** 914-833-1502; **Board Cert:** Pediatrics 2003; **Med School:** Mount Sinai Sch Med 1983; **Resid:** Pediatrics, Mt Sinai Hosp 1986; **Fellow:** Hematology & Oncology, Mt Sinai Hosp 1987

Katz, Kenneth MD (Ped) **PCP** - **Spec Exp:** Prematurity/Low Birth Weight Infants; Infectious Disease; **Hospital:** White Plains Hosp Ctr (page 714), NY-Presby Hosp (page 100); **Address:** 99 Fieldstone Dr, Hartsdale, NY 10530-1564; **Phone:** 914-428-2120; **Board Cert:** Pediatrics 1978; **Med School:** NY Med Coll 1973; **Resid:** Pediatrics, Bronx Muni Hosp 1976; **Fellow:** Developmental-Behavioral Pediatrics, Albert Einstein Coll Med 1978; **Fac Appt:** Clin Prof Ped, Columbia P&S

Levitt, Miriam MD (Ped) **PCP** - **Spec Exp:** Travel Medicine; **Hospital:** Lawrence Hosp Ctr, Montefiore Med Ctr; **Address:** 1 Pondfield Rd, Bronxville, NY 10708-3706; **Phone:** 914-961-3604; **Board Cert:** Pediatrics 1975; **Med School:** Albert Einstein Coll Med 1971; **Resid:** Pediatrics, Montefiore Hosp Med Ctr 1973; **Fac Appt:** Asst Clin Prof Ped, Albert Einstein Coll Med

Lubell, Harry R MD (Ped) `PCP` - **Hospital:** Phelps Meml Hosp Ctr, Westchester Med Ctr (page 713); **Address:** 245 N Broadway, Ste 201, Sleepy Hollow, NY 10591-2657; **Phone:** 914-332-4141; **Board Cert:** Pediatrics 1969; **Med School:** Univ Hlth Sci/Chicago Med Sch 1964; **Resid:** Pediatrics, Montefiore Hosp Med Ctr 1967; **Fellow:** Pediatric Hematology-Oncology, Babies Hosp-Columbia Preby 1970; **Fac Appt:** Asst Clin Prof Ped, NY Med Coll

Richel, Peter MD (Ped) `PCP` - **Spec Exp:** Ambulatory Care; **Hospital:** Northern Westchester Hosp; **Address:** 36 Smith Ave, Mt Kisco, NY 10549; **Phone:** 914-666-6655; **Board Cert:** Pediatrics 2001; **Med School:** Dominican Republic 1983; **Resid:** Pediatrics, Albany Med Ctr 1987; **Fellow:** Ambulatory Pediatrics, St Luke's-Roosevelt Hosp Ctr 1988; **Fac Appt:** Asst Clin Prof Ped, Albert Einstein Coll Med

Versfelt, Mary MD (Ped) `PCP` - **Spec Exp:** Adolescent Medicine; Chronic Disease; Newborn Care; **Hospital:** Greenwich Hosp; **Address:** 12 Rye Ridge Plaza, Rye Brook, NY 10573-2820; **Phone:** 914-251-1100; **Board Cert:** Pediatrics 1983; **Med School:** Columbia P&S 1978; **Resid:** Pediatrics, Columbia Presy Med Ctr 1981; **Fac Appt:** Assoc Clin Prof Ped, Columbia P&S

Wager, Marc MD (Ped) `PCP` - **Spec Exp:** Adolescent Medicine; **Hospital:** Sound Shore Med Ctr - Westchester (page 711); **Address:** 140 Lockwood Ave, Ste 115, New Rochelle, NY 10801-4907; **Phone:** 914-235-3800; **Board Cert:** Pediatrics 1986; **Med School:** Albert Einstein Coll Med 1981; **Resid:** Pediatrics, Jacobi Med Ctr 1984; **Fellow:** Adolescent Medicine, Montefiore Med Ctr 1986; **Fac Appt:** Asst Clin Prof Ped, Albert Einstein Coll Med

Wasserman, Eugene MD (Ped) `PCP` - **Spec Exp:** ADD/ADHD; **Hospital:** Greenwich Hosp; **Address:** 1600 Harrison Ave, Ste 307, Mamaroneck, NY 10543-3151; **Phone:** 914-698-0564; **Board Cert:** Pediatrics 1961; **Med School:** Univ Hlth Sci/Chicago Med Sch 1956; **Resid:** Pediatrics, Mount Sinai Hosp Med Ctr 1959; **Fac Appt:** Clin Prof Ped, NY Med Coll

PHYSICAL MEDICINE & REHABILITATION

Nelson, Mario MD (PMR) - **Spec Exp:** Spinal Cord Injury; Electrodiagnosis; Pain Management; **Hospital:** Westchester Med Ctr (page 713), Our Lady of Mercy Med Ctr; **Address:** 311 North St, Ste 202, White Plains, NY 10605; **Phone:** 914-428-6838; **Board Cert:** Physical Medicine & Rehabilitation 1986; **Med School:** Haiti 1978; **Resid:** Surgery, State Univ Hosp 1981; Physical Medicine & Rehabilitation, Westchester Medical Ctr 1985; **Fellow:** Spinal Cord Injury Medicine, Westchester Medical Ctr 1986; **Fac Appt:** Assoc Clin Prof PMR, NY Med Coll

Pechman, Karen M MD (PMR) - **Spec Exp:** Electrodiagnosis; Musculoskeletal Disorders; Amputee Rehabilitation; **Hospital:** Burke Rehab Hosp (page 105), White Plains Hosp Ctr (page 714); **Address:** 170 Maple Ave, Ste 510, White Plains, NY 10601; **Phone:** 914-683-0020; **Board Cert:** Physical Medicine & Rehabilitation 1987; **Med School:** Boston Univ 1980; **Resid:** Physical Medicine & Rehabilitation, Montefiore-Weiler Einstein Div 1986; **Fellow:** Research, NYU Sch Med 1982; **Fac Appt:** Asst Clin Prof PMR, Cornell Univ-Weill Med Coll

Pici, Ralph A MD (PMR) - **Hospital:** Lawrence Hosp Ctr; **Address:** Lawrence Hospital, Physical Med & Rehab, 55 Palmer Ave Fl 2, Bronxville, NY 10708; **Phone:** 914-787-3370; **Board Cert:** Physical Medicine & Rehabilitation 1974; **Med School:** Italy 1965; **Resid:** Pediatrics, Grasslands Hosp 1967; Physical Medicine & Rehabilitation, Montefiore-Weiler Einstein Div 1972

Randolph, Audrey MD (PMR) - **Spec Exp:** Musculoskeletal Disorders; Gait Disorders; Sports Medicine; **Hospital:** Westchester Med Ctr (page 713), Our Lady of Mercy Med Ctr; **Address:** 311 North St, Ste 202, White Plains, NY 10605-2232; **Phone:** 914-428-6838; **Board Cert:** Physical Medicine & Rehabilitation 1970; **Med School:** Med Coll PA Hahnemann 1964; **Resid:** Physical Medicine & Rehabilitation, NYU Med Ctr 1968; **Fac Appt:** Prof PMR, NY Med Coll

PLASTIC SURGERY

Bernard, Robert W MD (PlS) - **Spec Exp:** Cosmetic Surgery-Face; Cosmetic Surgery-Body; Breast Reconstruction; **Hospital:** White Plains Hosp Ctr (page 714), Northern Westchester Hosp; **Address:** 10 Chester Ave Fl 3, White Plains, NY 10601-5112; **Phone:** 914-761-8667; **Board Cert:** Surgery 1973; Plastic Surgery 1975; **Med School:** Univ VT Coll Med 1967; **Resid:** Surgery, NYU Med Ctr 1972; Plastic Surgery, NYU Med Ctr 1974

Khoury, F Frederic MD (PlS) - **Spec Exp:** Cosmetic Surgery-Liposuction; Cosmetic Surgery-Breast; Cosmetic Surgery-Face; **Hospital:** White Plains Hosp Ctr (page 714), Greenwich Hosp; **Address:** 22 Rye Ridge Plz, Rye Brook, NY 10573-2820; **Phone:** 914-253-9300; **Board Cert:** Plastic Surgery 2004; **Med School:** Lebanon 1971; **Resid:** Surgery, St Luke's-Roosevelt Hosp Ctr 1976; Plastic Surgery, St Luke's-Roosevelt Hosp Ctr 1979; **Fellow:** Surgery, St Louis Hosp 1977

Kleinman, Andrew MD (PlS) - **Spec Exp:** Cosmetic Surgery; Breast Reconstruction; **Hospital:** Sound Shore Med Ctr - Westchester (page 711); **Address:** 175 Memorial Hwy, LL17, New Rochelle, NY 10801-5635; **Phone:** 914-632-8500; **Board Cert:** Plastic Surgery 1989; **Med School:** Univ Rochester 1979; **Resid:** Surgery, Geo Wash Univ Hosp 1981; Surgery, Harvard Surg Svcs 1982; **Fellow:** Plastic Surgery, Baylor Coll Med 1985

Miclat Jr, Marciano MD (PlS) - **Spec Exp:** Cosmetic Surgery; Breast Reconstruction; Hand Surgery; **Hospital:** Sound Shore Med Ctr - Westchester (page 711); **Address:** 175 Memorial Hwy, Ste 2-4, New Rochelle, NY 10801; **Phone:** 914-636-8657; **Board Cert:** Plastic Surgery 1978; **Med School:** Philippines 1969; **Resid:** Surgery, Albert Einstein 1974; Plastic Surgery, Albert Einstein 1977

Newman, Scott E MD (PlS) - **Spec Exp:** Breast Augmentation; **Hospital:** St John's Riverside Hosp, Sound Shore Med Ctr - Westchester (page 711); **Address:** 1 Odell Plaza, Yonkers, NY 10701; **Phone:** 914-423-9000; **Board Cert:** Plastic Surgery 1996; **Med School:** NY Med Coll 1985; **Resid:** Surgery, Westchester Med Ctr 1990; Plastic Surgery, Mt Sinai Hosp 1993

Petro, Jane MD (PlS) - **Spec Exp:** Breast Surgery; Reconstructive Surgery-Pediatric; Abdominal Wall Reconstruction; **Hospital:** Northern Westchester Hosp; **Address:** 303 North St, Ste 207, White Plains, NY 10605; **Phone:** 914-428-8881; **Board Cert:** Plastic Surgery 1982; **Med School:** Penn State Univ-Hershey Med Ctr 1972; **Resid:** Surgery, Harrisburg Hosp 1976; Plastic Surgery, MS Hershey Med Ctr 1978; **Fellow:** Burn Surgery, Montefiore Hosp Med Ctr 1979; **Fac Appt:** Prof PlS, NY Med Coll

Reiffel, Robert S MD (PlS) - **Spec Exp:** Cosmetic & Reconstructive Surgery; Hand Surgery; **Hospital:** White Plains Hosp Ctr (page 714); **Address:** 12 Greenridge Ave, Ste 203, White Plains, NY 10605-1238; **Phone:** 914-683-1400; **Board Cert:** Plastic Surgery 1981; Hand Surgery 1990; **Med School:** Columbia P&S 1972; **Resid:** Surgery, Roosevelt Hosp 1977; Plastic Surgery, NYU Med Ctr 1979; **Fellow:** Hand Surgery, NYU Med Ctr 1980

Salisbury, Roger E MD (PlS) - **Spec Exp:** Burn Care; Hand Reconstruction; Body Contouring; **Hospital:** Westchester Med Ctr (page 713); **Address:** Westchester Med Ctr, Burn Ctr, Macy Pavillion, Valhalla, NY 10595; **Phone:** 914-493-8660; **Board Cert:** Surgery 1972; Plastic Surgery 1978; **Med School:** Albert Einstein Coll Med 1966; **Resid:** Surgery, T Jefferson Univ Hosp 1971; Plastic Surgery, Temple Univ Hosp 1976; **Fellow:** Hand Surgery, T Jefferson Univ Hosp 1969; **Fac Appt:** Prof S, NY Med Coll

Salzberg, C Andrew MD (PlS) - **Spec Exp:** Breast Surgery; Cosmetic Surgery-Face; Laser Surgery; Wound Healing/Care; **Hospital:** Westchester Med Ctr (page 713), Comm Hosp - Dobbs Ferry; **Address:** 155 White Plains Rd, Ste 109, Tarrytown, NY 10591; **Phone:** 914-366-6139; **Board Cert:** Plastic Surgery 1989; **Med School:** Univ Fla Coll Med 1981; **Resid:** Surgery, Mount Sinai 1987; **Fellow:** Plastic Surgery, Mount Sinai 1987; **Fac Appt:** Assoc Prof PlS, NY Med Coll

Smith, Aloysius G MD (PlS) - **Spec Exp:** Cosmetic Surgery-Breast; Breast Reconstruction; Hand Surgery; **Hospital:** Saint Joseph's Med Ctr - Yonkers, Our Lady of Mercy Med Ctr; **Address:** Intercounty Medical Plaza, 955 Yonkers Ave, Ste 17, Yonkers, NY 10704; **Phone:** 914-237-6002; **Board Cert:** Plastic Surgery 1985; **Med School:** Jamaica 1973; **Resid:** Surgery, Metropolitan Hosp 1979; Plastic Surgery, Mayo Clinic 1982; **Fellow:** Hand Surgery, Metropolitan Hosp 1980; **Fac Appt:** Asst Clin Prof S, NY Med Coll

PREVENTIVE MEDICINE

Cimino, Joseph MD (PrM) - **Spec Exp:** Nutrition; Environmental Medicine; **Hospital:** Westchester Med Ctr (page 713), Calvary Hosp (page 106); **Address:** NY Med Coll, Community & Preventive Med, Munger Pavilion, Valhalla, NY 10595; **Phone:** 914-594-4253; **Board Cert:** Occupational Medicine 1969; **Med School:** SUNY Buffalo 1962; **Resid:** Preventive Medicine, Harvard Sch Public Health 1965; Preventive Medicine, NYC Health Dept 1966; **Fac Appt:** Prof PrM, NY Med Coll

Mamtani, Ravinder MD (PrM) - **Spec Exp:** Complementary Medicine; Preventive Medicine; Acupuncture; Nutrition; **Hospital:** Westchester Med Ctr (page 713), Calvary Hosp (page 106); **Address:** NY Med Coll, Community & Preventive Med, Munger Pavilion, Valhalla, NY 10595; **Phone:** 914-594-4253; **Board Cert:** Public Health & Genl Preventive Med 1989; Occupational Medicine 1994; **Med School:** India 1975; **Resid:** Internal Medicine, Bryntirion Hosp 1979; Preventive Medicine, Derbyshire Health Authority 1981; **Fellow:** Preventive Medicine, NY Medical Coll 1987; **Fac Appt:** Clin Prof PrM, NY Med Coll

PSYCHIATRY

Addonizio, Gerard C MD (Psyc) - **Spec Exp:** Psychotherapy; Psychopharmacology; Depression; Anxiety Disorders; **Hospital:** NY-Presby Hosp (page 100); **Address:** 21 Bloomingdale Rd, White Plains, NY 10605-1504; **Phone:** 914-997-5864; **Board Cert:** Psychiatry 1983; Geriatric Psychiatry 1994; **Med School:** Columbia P&S 1978; **Resid:** Psychiatry, Yale-New Haven Hosp 1982; **Fac Appt:** Prof Psyc, Cornell Univ-Weill Med Coll

Alexopoulos, George MD (Psyc) - **Spec Exp:** Geriatric Psychiatry; Depression; Psychopharmacology; **Hospital:** NY-Presby Hosp (page 100); **Address:** 21 Bloomingdale Rd, White Plains, NY 10605; **Phone:** 914-997-5767; **Board Cert:** Psychiatry 1978; Geriatric Psychiatry 2001; **Med School:** Greece 1970; **Resid:** Psychiatry, UMDNJ Univ Hosp 1976; Psychiatry, NY Presby Hosp-Westch Div 1977; **Fellow:** Biological Psychiatry, NY Hosp-Cornell Med Ctr 1978; **Fac Appt:** Prof Psyc, Cornell Univ-Weill Med Coll

Badikian, Arthur MD (Psyc) - **Spec Exp:** Mood Disorders; Geriatric Psychiatry; Psychiatry in Physical Illness; Women's Health-Mental Health; **Hospital:** St Vincent Cath Med Ctrs - Westchester (page 375); **Address:** 303 North St, rm 204, White Plains, NY 10605; **Phone:** 914-948-4277; **Board Cert:** Psychiatry 1981; Geriatric Psychiatry 1996; **Med School:** Univ Fla Coll Med 1976; **Resid:** Psychiatry, Westchester Med Ctr 1980; **Fac Appt:** Assoc Prof Psyc, NY Med Coll

Bauman, Jonathan MD (Psyc) - **Spec Exp:** Mood Disorders; Anxiety Disorders; Personality Disorders; **Hospital:** Four Winds Hosp; **Address:** 800 Cross River Rd, Katonah, NY 10536-3549; **Phone:** 914-763-8151; **Board Cert:** Psychiatry 1978; **Med School:** Georgetown Univ 1974; **Resid:** Psychiatry, Univ Va Med Ctr 1975; Psychiatry, Georgetown Univ Med Ctr 1977; **Fac Appt:** Asst Prof Psyc, Albert Einstein Coll Med

Bemporad, Jules MD (Psyc) - **Spec Exp:** Child & Adolescent Psychiatry; Psychotherapy; ADD/ADHD; **Hospital:** Westchester Med Ctr (page 713); **Address:** Two Brambach Ave, Scarsdale, NY 10583-5236; **Phone:** 914-723-3882; **Board Cert:** Psychiatry 1969; Child & Adolescent Psychiatry 1969; **Med School:** Univ Fla Coll Med 1962; **Resid:** Psychiatry, NY Med Coll 1966; Child & Adolescent Psychiatry, Colum-Presby Hosp 1968; **Fac Appt:** Clin Prof Psyc, NY Med Coll

Blumenfield, Michael MD (Psyc) - **Spec Exp:** Psychotherapy; Psychopharmacology; Post Traumatic Stress Disorder; **Hospital:** Westchester Med Ctr (page 713), White Plains Hosp Ctr (page 714); **Address:** 16 Donellan Rd, Scarsdale, NY 10583-2008; **Phone:** 914-472-5035; **Board Cert:** Psychiatry 1970; Psychosomatic Medicine 2005; **Med School:** SUNY Downstate 1964; **Resid:** Psychiatry, Kings County Hosp 1968; **Fellow:** Psychosomatic Medicine, Kings County Hosp 1971; **Fac Appt:** Prof Psyc, NY Med Coll

Dolan, Anna MD (Psyc) - **Spec Exp:** Anxiety & Depression; Phobias; Geriatric Psychiatry; **Hospital:** St John's Riverside Hosp, Pk Care Pavillion; **Address:** 984 N Broadway, Yonkers, NY 10705; **Phone:** 914-476-1208; **Board Cert:** Psychiatry 1976; **Med School:** St Louis Univ 1960; **Resid:** Surgery, St Louis Univ-Chldns Hosp 1963; Psychiatry, Inst Penn Hosp 1968

Dulit, Rebecca A MD (Psyc) - **Spec Exp:** Personality Disorders-Borderline; Suicide; Post Traumatic Stress Disorder; Disaster Psychiatry; **Hospital:** NY-Presby Hosp (page 100), NY-Presby Hosp (page 100); **Address:** 45 Popham Rd, Ste D, Scarsdale, NY 10583; **Phone:** 914-722-0608; **Board Cert:** Psychiatry 1991; **Med School:** Mount Sinai Sch Med 1985; **Resid:** Psychiatry, Payne Whitney Clinic-Cornell 1989; **Fellow:** Research, Payne Whitney Clinic-Cornell 1992; **Fac Appt:** Assoc Clin Prof Psyc, Cornell Univ-Weill Med Coll

Gabel, Richard MD (Psyc) - **Spec Exp:** Psychopharmacology; Psychotherapy; **Hospital:** White Plains Hosp Ctr (page 714), St Vincent Cath Med Ctrs - Westchester (page 375); **Address:** 12 Greenridge Ave, White Plains, NY 10605; **Phone:** 914-681-0202; **Board Cert:** Psychiatry 1982; **Med School:** NYU Sch Med 1976; **Resid:** Psychiatry, Mass Genl Hosp 1980

Halmi, Katherine MD (Psyc) - **Spec Exp:** Eating Disorders; **Hospital:** NY-Presby Hosp (page 100); **Address:** NY Presby Hosp - Westchester Div, 21 Bloomingdale Rd, White Plains, NY 10605; **Phone:** 914-997-5875; **Board Cert:** Pediatrics 1970; Psychiatry 1977; **Med School:** Univ Iowa Coll Med 1965; **Resid:** Pediatrics, Univ Iowa Hosp 1968; Psychiatry, Univ Iowa Hosp 1972; **Fellow:** Child Development, Univ Iowa Hosp 1969; **Fac Appt:** Prof Psyc, Cornell Univ-Weill Med Coll

Harlam, Dean MD (Psyc) - **Spec Exp:** Depression; Bipolar/Mood Disorders; Psychopharmacology; **Hospital:** St Vincent Cath Med Ctrs - Westchester (page 375); **Address:** St Vincent's Hospital, 275 North St, Harrison, NY 10528; **Phone:** 914-925-5490; **Board Cert:** Psychiatry 1979; **Med School:** Albert Einstein Coll Med 1972; **Resid:** Psychiatry, Bronx Municipal Hosp/Einstein 1976; **Fellow:** Psychiatry, NY Hosp-Cornell Med Ctr 1977; **Fac Appt:** Assoc Prof Psyc, NY Med Coll

Kernberg, Otto MD (Psyc) - **Spec Exp:** Psychoanalysis; Personality Disorders; **Hospital:** NY-Presby Hosp (page 100); **Address:** 21 Bloomingdale Rd, White Plains, NY 10605; **Phone:** 914-997-5714; **Board Cert:** Psychiatry 1970; **Med School:** Chile 1953; **Resid:** Psychoanalysis, Psychoanalytic Inst 1958; Psychiatry, Menninger Meml Hosp 1968; **Fellow:** Psychiatry, Johns Hopkins Hosp 1960; **Fac Appt:** Prof Psyc, Cornell Univ-Weill Med Coll

Klagsbrun, Samuel C MD (Psyc) - **Spec Exp:** Psychiatry in Cancer; Psychiatry in Terminal Illness; **Hospital:** Four Winds Hosp; **Address:** Four Winds Hospital, 800 Cross River Rd, Katonah, NY 10536; **Phone:** 914-763-8151; **Board Cert:** Psychiatry 1977; **Med School:** Univ Hlth Sci/Chicago Med Sch 1962; **Resid:** Psychiatry, Yale-New Haven Hosp 1966; **Fac Appt:** Clin Prof Psyc, Albert Einstein Coll Med

Levin, Andrew Paul MD (Psyc) - **Spec Exp:** Psychiatry in Trauma; Forensic Psychiatry; Psychopharmacology; **Address:** 141 N Central Ave, Hartsdale, NY 10530-1912; **Phone:** 914-949-7699; **Board Cert:** Psychiatry 1985; Forensic Psychiatry 1996; **Med School:** Univ Pennsylvania 1980; **Resid:** Psychiatry, NYS Psych Inst 1984; **Fellow:** Anxiety Disorder, NYS Psych Inst 1986; **Fac Appt:** Asst Clin Prof Psyc, Columbia P&S

Lew, Arthur MD (Psyc) - **Spec Exp:** Psychoanalysis; Psychotherapy; Child & Adolescent Psychiatry; **Address:** 225 Lyncroft Rd, New Rochelle, NY 10804-4120; **Phone:** 914-632-9679; **Board Cert:** Psychiatry 1974; Child & Adolescent Psychiatry 1979; **Med School:** SUNY Downstate 1968; **Resid:** Psychiatry, SUNY Downstate Med Ctr 1972; **Fellow:** Child & Adolescent Psychiatry, SUNY Downstate Med Ctr 1975; **Fac Appt:** Clin Prof Psyc, NYU Sch Med

Loeb, Laurence MD (Psyc) - **Spec Exp:** Forensic Psychiatry; Child & Adolescent Psychiatry; **Hospital:** NY-Presby Hosp (page 100); **Address:** 180 E Hartsdale Ave, Ste 1C, Hartsdale, NY 10530; **Phone:** 914-723-1446; **Board Cert:** Psychiatry 1959; Forensic Psychiatry 1981; **Med School:** SUNY Downstate 1953; **Resid:** Psychiatry, NY Hosp 1955; Child & Adolescent Psychiatry, NY Hosp 1959; **Fellow:** Child & Adolescent Psychiatry, Albert Einstein 1960; **Fac Appt:** Assoc Clin Prof Psyc, Cornell Univ-Weill Med Coll

Meyers, Barnett MD (Psyc) - **Spec Exp:** Depression; Geriatric Psychiatry; Psychopharmacology; **Hospital:** NY-Presby Hosp (page 100); **Address:** 21 Bloomingdale Rd, White Plains, NY 10605-1504; **Phone:** 914-997-5721; **Board Cert:** Psychiatry 1975; Geriatric Psychiatry 2001; **Med School:** NYU Sch Med 1966; **Resid:** Psychiatry, Bronx Muni Hosp 1972; **Fac Appt:** Prof Psyc, Cornell Univ-Weill Med Coll

Milone, Richard MD (Psyc) - **Spec Exp:** Depression; Psychopharmacology; **Hospital:** St Vincent Cath Med Ctrs - Westchester (page 375); **Address:** 275 North St, Harrison, NY 10528; **Phone:** 914-925-5311; **Board Cert:** Psychiatry 1970; **Med School:** Creighton Univ 1963; **Resid:** Psychiatry, St Vincent's Hosp & Med Ctr 1967; **Fac Appt:** Assoc Clin Prof Psyc, NY Med Coll

Neschis, Ronald MD (Psyc) - **Spec Exp:** Geriatric Psychiatry; **Hospital:** Saint Joseph's Med Ctr - Yonkers; **Address:** 18 Linden Ave, Larchmont, NY 10538-4139; **Phone:** 914-834-3470; **Board Cert:** Psychiatry 1972; Geriatric Psychiatry 1994; **Med School:** SUNY Downstate 1963; **Resid:** Psychiatry, Montefiore Hosp Med Ctr 1969

Opler, Lewis MD (Psyc) - **Spec Exp:** Psychopharmacology; Psychotherapy; **Hospital:** NY-Presby Hosp (page 100); **Address:** 765 Gramatan Ave, Mount Vernon, NY 10552; **Phone:** 914-668-4799; **Board Cert:** Psychiatry 1983; **Med School:** Albert Einstein Coll Med 1976; **Resid:** Psychiatry, Jacobi Med Ctr 1979

Perlman, Barry B MD (Psyc) - **Hospital:** Saint Joseph's Med Ctr - Yonkers; **Address:** St Joseph's Med Ctr-Dept of Psychiatry, 127 S Broadway, Yonkers, NY 10701-4006; **Phone:** 914-378-7342; **Board Cert:** Psychiatry 1977; **Med School:** Yale Univ 1971; **Resid:** Psychiatry, Mount Sinai Hosp 1975; **Fac Appt:** Assoc Clin Prof Psyc, NY Med Coll

Perry, Bradford MD (Psyc) - **Spec Exp:** Anxiety & Mood Disorders; Psychopharmacology; **Hospital:** NY-Presby Hosp (page 100), White Plains Hosp Ctr (page 714); **Address:** 455 Central Park Ave, Ste 214, Scarsdale, NY 10583-1034; **Phone:** 914-472-2167; **Board Cert:** Psychiatry 1989; **Med School:** Univ Miami Sch Med 1984; **Resid:** Psychiatry, NY Hosp 1988; **Fellow:** Psychiatry, Columbia-Presby Ned Ctr 1989; **Fac Appt:** Assoc Clin Prof Psyc, Cornell Univ-Weill Med Coll

Russakoff, L Mark MD (Psyc) - **Spec Exp:** Mood Disorders; Anxiety Disorders; **Hospital:** Phelps Meml Hosp Ctr; **Address:** Phelps Memorial Hospital, 701 N Broadway, Sleepy Hollow, NY 10591-1020; **Phone:** 914-366-3600; **Board Cert:** Psychiatry 1976; **Med School:** SUNY Downstate 1971; **Resid:** Psychiatry, Yale-New Haven Hosp 1975

Scharfman, Edward L MD (Psyc) - **Spec Exp:** Anxiety & Mood Disorders; Panic Disorder; ADD/ADHD; Phobias; **Address:** 111 N Central Ave, Ste 421, Hartsdale, NY 10530-1914; **Phone:** 914-632-6646; **Board Cert:** Psychiatry 1983; **Med School:** SUNY Downstate 1978; **Resid:** Psychiatry, Univ Hosp/Kings Co Hosp Ctr-SUNY Downstate 1982; **Fellow:** Psychopharmacology, New England Med Ctr-Tufts 1984; **Fac Appt:** Asst Clin Prof Psyc, Columbia P&S

Seaman, Cheryl MD (Psyc) - **Spec Exp:** Anxiety Disorders; Depression; Addiction Psychiatry; **Address:** 427 Manville Rd, Pleasantville, NY 10570; **Phone:** 917-741-0071; **Board Cert:** Psychiatry 1986; Geriatric Psychiatry 2001; **Med School:** Columbia P&S 1979; **Resid:** Psychiatry, NY Hosp-Westchester Div 1983

Singer, Elliot MD (Psyc) - **Hospital:** Rye Hosp Ctr; **Address:** Rye Hospital Ctr, 754 Boston Post Rd, Rye, NY 10580-2724; **Phone:** 914-967-4567; **Board Cert:** Psychiatry 1977; **Med School:** Univ VT Coll Med 1965; **Resid:** Psychiatry, NY Hosp 1971; **Fellow:** Psychiatry, Cornell Med Ctr 1971; **Fac Appt:** Asst Clin Prof Psyc, NY Med Coll

Stabinsky, Susan MD (Psyc) - **Spec Exp:** Psychotherapy; Psychopharmacology; Addiction Psychiatry; **Hospital:** VA Hudson Valley-FDR/Montrose; **Address:** 15 Boulder Trail, Armonk, NY 10504-1008; **Phone:** 914-273-6637; **Board Cert:** Psychiatry 1986; Addiction Psychiatry 2004; Geriatric Psychiatry 2000; **Med School:** Mexico 1978; **Resid:** Psychiatry, Montefiore Hosp Med Ctr 1984; **Fellow:** Psychiatry, Montefiore Hosp Med Ctr 1985; **Fac Appt:** Asst Clin Prof Psyc, NY Med Coll

Sullivan, Timothy B MD (Psyc) - **Spec Exp:** Bipolar/Mood Disorders; Psychotherapy & Psychopharmacology; Schizophrenia; **Hospital:** St Vincent Cath Med Ctrs - Westchester (page 375); **Address:** 275 North St, Harrison, NY 10528-1524; **Phone:** 914-925-5485; **Board Cert:** Internal Medicine 1981; Psychiatry 1986; **Med School:** Dartmouth Med Sch 1977; **Resid:** Internal Medicine, St Vincent's Hosp & Med Ctr 1980; Psychiatry, NY Presby Hosp-Westch Div 1985; **Fac Appt:** Asst Prof Psyc, NY Med Coll

Sussman, Robert B MD (Psyc) - **Spec Exp:** Substance Abuse; Psychopharmacology; Anxiety & Depression; **Address:** 167 Purchase St, Rye, NY 10580-2137; **Phone:** 914-967-1363; **Board Cert:** Psychiatry 1964; Addiction Psychiatry 1993; **Med School:** SUNY Buffalo 1957; **Resid:** Psychiatry, Stanford Univ Med Ctr 1960; Addiction Psychiatry, Hillside Hosp 1963; **Fac Appt:** Asst Clin Prof Psyc, Cornell Univ-Weill Med Coll

Turato, Mariann MD (Psyc) - **Spec Exp:** Anxiety Disorders; Depression; Women's Health-Mental Health; **Hospital:** St Vincent Cath Med Ctrs - Westchester (page 375), NY-Presby Hosp (page 100); **Address:** 1 Elm St, Ste 0B, Tuckahoe, NY 10707; **Phone:** 914-395-3135; **Board Cert:** Psychiatry 1992; **Med School:** Albert Einstein Coll Med 1986; **Resid:** Psychiatry, NY Hosp 1990

Zolkind, Neil MD (Psyc) - **Spec Exp:** Depression; Anxiety Disorders; **Hospital:** Westchester Med Ctr (page 713); **Address:** Westchester Med Ctr - Behavioral Hlth Ctr, Valhalla, NY 10595; **Phone:** 914-493-1818; **Board Cert:** Psychiatry 1981; **Med School:** Geo Wash Univ 1976; **Resid:** Psychiatry, UCLA Neuropsyc Hosp 1980; **Fac Appt:** Asst Prof Psyc, NY Med Coll

PULMONARY DISEASE

Binder, Ralph E MD (Pul) - **Spec Exp:** Asthma; Chronic Obstructive Lung Disease (COPD); **Hospital:** Lawrence Hosp Ctr; **Address:** 1 Pondfield Rd, Bronxville, NY 10708; **Phone:** 914-337-1610; **Board Cert:** Internal Medicine 1978; Pulmonary Disease 1980; **Med School:** Yale Univ 1975; **Resid:** Internal Medicine, Bronx Municipal Hosp 1978; **Fellow:** Pulmonary Disease, Boston Med Ctr 1980; **Fac Appt:** Asst Prof Med, Columbia P&S

Brill, Joseph MD (Pul) - **Spec Exp:** Sarcoidosis; Chronic Obstructive Lung Disease (COPD); Asthma; **Hospital:** St John's Riverside Hosp, Saint Joseph's Med Ctr - Yonkers; **Address:** 102 Park Ave, Yonkers, NY 10703; **Phone:** 914-968-1611; **Board Cert:** Internal Medicine 1988; Pulmonary Disease 2002; **Med School:** Mexico 1981; **Resid:** Internal Medicine, Mt Sinai/Elmhurst City Hosp 1986; **Fellow:** Pulmonary Disease, Mt Sinai/Elmhurst City Hosp 1988

Casino, Joseph MD (Pul) - **Spec Exp:** Asthma; Sleep Disorders; **Hospital:** Sound Shore Med Ctr - Westchester (page 711); **Address:** 2365 Boston Post Rd, Ste 103, Larchmont, NY 10538; **Phone:** 914-833-2020; **Board Cert:** Internal Medicine 1989; Pulmonary Disease 2000; Critical Care Medicine 2001; **Med School:** Italy 1984; **Resid:** Internal Medicine, New Rochelle Med Ctr 1988; **Fellow:** Pulmonary Critical Care Medicine, RW Johnson Univ Hosp 1991; **Fac Appt:** Asst Clin Prof Med, NY Med Coll

Chodosh, Ronald MD (Pul) - **Spec Exp:** Chronic Obstructive Lung Disease (COPD); Asthma; Pulmonary Infections; **Hospital:** Phelps Meml Hosp Ctr, Hudson Valley Hosp Ctr; **Address:** 310 N Highland Ave, Ste 2, Ossining, NY 10562; **Phone:** 914-762-4144; **Board Cert:** Internal Medicine 1971; Pulmonary Disease 1978; Critical Care Medicine 1997; **Med School:** Switzerland 1965; **Resid:** Internal Medicine, Maimonides Med Ctr 1970; Pulmonary Disease, Montefiore Med Ctr 1971; **Fac Appt:** Asst Prof Med, Albert Einstein Coll Med

De Matteo, Robert MD (Pul) - **Spec Exp:** Asthma; Emphysema; Lung Cancer-Early Detection; **Hospital:** St John's Riverside Hosp, Saint Joseph's Med Ctr - Yonkers; **Address:** 970 N Broadway, Ste 209, Yonkers, NY 10701; **Phone:** 914-965-3366; **Board Cert:** Internal Medicine 1988; Pulmonary Disease 1998; **Med School:** Mexico 1982; **Resid:** Internal Medicine, Mount Sinai/Bronx VA Hosp 1985; **Fellow:** Pulmonary Disease, Westchester Med Ctr 1988

Delorenzo, Lawrence MD (Pul) - **Spec Exp:** Asthma; Emphysema; **Hospital:** Westchester Med Ctr (page 713); **Address:** Westchester Med Ctr, Pulmonary Lab - Macy Pavillion, Valhalla, NY 10595; **Phone:** 914-493-7518; **Board Cert:** Internal Medicine 1979; Pulmonary Disease 1982; Critical Care Medicine 1999; **Med School:** NY Med Coll 1976; **Resid:** Internal Medicine, Metropolitan Hosp Ctr 1979; **Fellow:** Pulmonary Disease, Metropolitan Hosp Ctr 1981; **Fac Appt:** Assoc Clin Prof Med, NY Med Coll

DiCosmo, Bruno F MD (Pul) - **Spec Exp:** Chronic Obstructive Lung Disease (COPD); Asthma; **Hospital:** White Plains Hosp Ctr (page 714), Greenwich Hosp; **Address:** 745 E Boston Post Rd, Mamaroneck, NY 10543-4140; **Phone:** 914-698-6900; **Board Cert:** Internal Medicine 2001; Pulmonary Disease 2004; Critical Care Medicine 1995; **Med School:** Univ Conn 1988; **Resid:** Internal Medicine, Univ Conn Hlth Ctr 1991; **Fellow:** Pulmonary Disease, Yale-New Haven Hosp 1994; Critical Care Medicine, Yale-New Haven Hosp 1994; **Fac Appt:** Asst Clin Prof Med, Cornell Univ-Weill Med Coll

Frimer, Richard MD (Pul) - **Hospital:** White Plains Hosp Ctr (page 714); **Address:** 170 Maple Ave, Ste G1, White Plains, NY 10601-4710; **Phone:** 914-328-0932; **Board Cert:** Internal Medicine 1983; Pulmonary Disease 1986; Critical Care Medicine 1998; **Med School:** SUNY Buffalo 1980; **Resid:** Internal Medicine, Montefiore Med Ctr 1983; **Fellow:** Pulmonary Disease, NYU Med Ctr 1985

Jacobowitz, Marilyn MD (Pul) - **Spec Exp:** Asthma; **Hospital:** Northern Westchester Hosp; **Address:** 90 S Bedford Rd, Mt Kisco, NY 10549-3412; **Phone:** 914-241-1050; **Board Cert:** Internal Medicine 2002; Pulmonary Disease 2004; Critical Care Medicine 2005; **Med School:** NYU Sch Med 1989; **Resid:** Internal Medicine, Mt Sinai Hosp 1992; **Fellow:** Pulmonary Disease, Mt Sinai Hosp 1995

Lehrman, Gary R MD (Pul) - **Hospital:** Phelps Meml Hosp Ctr, Comm Hosp - Dobbs Ferry; **Address:** 160 N State Rd, Briarcliff Manor, NY 10510-1443; **Phone:** 914-762-8383; **Board Cert:** Internal Medicine 1982; Pulmonary Disease 1986; Critical Care Medicine 1999; **Med School:** NYU Sch Med 1979; **Resid:** Pulmonary Disease, LI Jewish Med Ctr 1984

Lehrman, Stuart MD (Pul) - **Spec Exp:** Lung Cancer; Asthma; **Hospital:** Westchester Med Ctr (page 713); **Address:** Pulmonary Lab, Macy Pavilion, Valhalla, NY 10595; **Phone:** 914-493-7518; **Board Cert:** Internal Medicine 1981; Pulmonary Disease 1984; Critical Care Medicine 1996; **Med School:** SUNY Hlth Sci Ctr 1978; **Resid:** Internal Medicine, Cedars-Sinai Med Ctr 1981; **Fellow:** Pulmonary Disease, Cedars-Sinai Med Ctr 1983; **Fac Appt:** Assoc Clin Prof Med, NY Med Coll

Mandel, Michael MD (Pul) - **Spec Exp:** Sleep Disorders/Apnea; Chronic Obstructive Lung Disease (COPD); Asthma; **Hospital:** Sound Shore Med Ctr - Westchester (page 711); **Address:** 2365 Boston Post Rd, Larchmont, NY 10538; **Phone:** 914-833-2020; **Board Cert:** Internal Medicine 1986; Pulmonary Disease 1999; Critical Care Medicine 2001; **Med School:** Columbia P&S 1983; **Resid:** Internal Medicine, St Lukes Roosevelt Hosp 1987; **Fellow:** Pulmonary Critical Care Medicine, UMDNJ Med Ctr 1989; **Fac Appt:** Asst Prof Med, NY Med Coll

Meixler, Steven MD (Pul) - **Spec Exp:** Asthma; Emphysema; Cough-Chronic; **Hospital:** White Plains Hosp Ctr (page 714); **Address:** 210 Westchester Ave, White Plains, NY 10604; **Phone:** 914-682-0700; **Board Cert:** Internal Medicine 1987; Pulmonary Disease 2000; Critical Care Medicine 2000; **Med School:** Boston Univ 1984; **Resid:** Internal Medicine, VA Med Ctr 1988; **Fellow:** Pulmonary Disease, Bellevue Hosp/NYU 1990

Novitch, Richard MD (Pul) - **Spec Exp:** Pulmonary Rehabilitation; **Hospital:** Burke Rehab Hosp (page 105), NY-Presby Hosp (page 100); **Address:** 785 Mamaroneck Ave, White Plains, NY 10605; **Phone:** 914-597-2226; **Board Cert:** Internal Medicine 1987; Pulmonary Disease 1990; **Med School:** Mexico 1983; **Resid:** Internal Medicine, UMDNJ Med Ctr 1987; Pulmonary Disease, UMDNJ Med Ctr 1989; **Fac Appt:** Asst Clin Prof Med, Cornell Univ-Weill Med Coll

Schreiber, Michael MD (Pul) - **Spec Exp:** Asthma; Emphysema; **Hospital:** St John's Riverside Hosp, Saint Joseph's Med Ctr - Yonkers; **Address:** 970 N Broadway, Ste 304, Yonkers, NY 10701; **Phone:** 914-423-8517; **Board Cert:** Internal Medicine 1976; Pulmonary Disease 1978; **Med School:** Univ Ariz Coll Med 1973; **Resid:** Internal Medicine, Montefiore Hosp Med Ctr 1976; **Fellow:** Pulmonary Disease, NYU Med Ctr 1978; **Fac Appt:** Asst Clin Prof Med, NY Med Coll

Sherling, Bruce E MD (Pul) - **Hospital:** White Plains Hosp Ctr (page 714), Greenwich Hosp; **Address:** Westchester Medical Group, 745 E Boston Post Rd, Mamaroneck, NY 10543; **Phone:** 914-698-6900; **Board Cert:** Internal Medicine 1976; Pulmonary Disease 1978; **Med School:** NY Med Coll 1973; **Resid:** Internal Medicine, Metropolitan Hosp Ctr 1974; **Fellow:** Pulmonary Disease, Metropolitan Hosp Ctr 1977; Pulmonary Disease, Lenox Hill Hosp 1978

Weinberg, Harlan MD (Pul) - **Spec Exp:** Asthma; Critical Care Medicine; **Hospital:** Northern Westchester Hosp; **Address:** 83 S Bedford Rd, Mt. Kisco, NY 10549; **Phone:** 914-241-8356; **Board Cert:** Internal Medicine 1984; Pulmonary Disease 1986; Critical Care Medicine 2002; **Med School:** Univ Conn 1981; **Resid:** Internal Medicine, McGaw Med Ctr-Northwestern 1984; **Fellow:** Pulmonary Disease, Cedars-Sinai Med Ctr 1986

RADIATION ONCOLOGY

Lehrman, David B MD (RadRO) - **Spec Exp:** Breast Cancer; Prostate Cancer; **Hospital:** Sound Shore Med Ctr - Westchester (page 711); **Address:** 175 Memorial Hwy, New Rochelle, NY 10801-5642; **Phone:** 914-633-3525; **Board Cert:** Therapeutic Radiology 1980; **Med School:** Dalhousie Univ 1974; **Resid:** Surgery, SUNY Downstate Med Ctr 1977; Radiation Oncology, NYU Med Ctr 1980

Moorthy, Chitti MD (RadRO) - **Spec Exp:** Prostate Cancer; Breast Cancer; **Hospital:** Westchester Med Ctr (page 713); **Address:** NY Med College-Dept Radiation Med, Macy Pavilion rm 1297, Valhalla, NY 10595; **Phone:** 914-493-8561; **Board Cert:** Radiation Oncology 1979; **Med School:** India 1974; **Resid:** Surgery, Michael Reese Hosp 1976; Radiation Oncology, Michael Reese Hosp 1979; **Fellow:** Brachytherapy, Meml Sloan Kettering Cancer Ctr 1980; **Fac Appt:** Prof RadRO, NY Med Coll

Tinger, Alfred MD (RadRO) - **Spec Exp:** Prostate Cancer; Brachytherapy; Brain Tumors; **Hospital:** Northern Westchester Hosp, St John's Riverside Hosp; **Address:** 970 N Broadway, Yonkers, NY 10701; **Phone:** 914-969-1600; **Board Cert:** Radiation Oncology 1997; **Med School:** SUNY Downstate 1992; **Resid:** Radiology, Washington Univ Med Ctr 1997

REPRODUCTIVE ENDOCRINOLOGY

Santoro, Nanette MD (RE) - **Spec Exp:** Menopause Problems; Menstrual Disorders; Infertility; **Hospital:** Montefiore Med Ctr; **Address:** 141 S Central Ave, Ste 201, Hartsdale, NY 10530-2319; **Phone:** 914-997-1060; **Board Cert:** Obstetrics & Gynecology 1998; Reproductive Endocrinology 1998; **Med School:** Albany Med Coll 1979; **Resid:** Obstetrics & Gynecology, Beth Israel Med Ctr 1983; **Fellow:** Reproductive Endocrinology, Mass Genl Hosp 1986; **Fac Appt:** Prof ObG, Albert Einstein Coll Med

Stangel, John MD (RE) - **Spec Exp:** Infertility-IVF; Endometriosis; Pregnancy Loss; **Hospital:** Northern Westchester Hosp, Phelps Meml Hosp Ctr; **Address:** 70 Maple Ave, Rye, NY 10580-1568; **Phone:** 914-967-6800; **Board Cert:** Obstetrics & Gynecology 1976; Reproductive Endocrinology 1981; **Med School:** NY Med Coll 1969; **Resid:** Obstetrics & Gynecology, Mount Sinai Med Ctr 1974; **Fellow:** Reproductive Endocrinology, Metropolitan Hosp Ctr 1976

RHEUMATOLOGY

Ash, Julia Y MD (Rhu) - **Spec Exp:** Lupus/SLE; Rheumatoid Arthritis; Psoriatic Arthritis; Scleroderma; **Hospital:** Westchester Med Ctr (page 713); **Address:** NY Med Coll, Div Rheumatology, Munger Pavilion - rm G73, Valhalla, NY 10595; **Phone:** 914-594-4444; **Board Cert:** Internal Medicine 1991; Rheumatology 1994; **Med School:** SUNY Stony Brook 1987; **Resid:** Internal Medicine, Winthrop Univ Hosp 1990; **Fellow:** Rheumatology, Mass Genl Hosp 1992; Rheumatology, Hosp Joint Diseases 1993; **Fac Appt:** Asst Prof Med, NY Med Coll

Barone, Richard P MD (Rhu) - **Spec Exp:** Rheumatoid Arthritis; Lupus/SLE; Psoriatic Arthritis; **Hospital:** Sound Shore Med Ctr - Westchester (page 711); **Address:** 421 Huguenot St Fl 4 - Ste 44, New Rochelle, NY 10801-7004; **Phone:** 914-235-3065; **Med School:** Italy 1971; **Resid:** Internal Medicine, Brooklyn Jewish Hosp & Med Ctr 1974; **Fellow:** Rheumatology, Brooklyn Jewish Hosp & Med Ctr 1976; **Fac Appt:** Assoc Clin Prof Med, NY Med Coll

Berger, Jack MD (Rhu) - **Spec Exp:** Rheumatoid Arthritis; **Hospital:** White Plains Hosp Ctr (page 714); **Address:** 210 Westchester Ave, White Plains, NY 10604; **Phone:** 914-682-6532; **Board Cert:** Internal Medicine 1979; Rheumatology 1982; **Med School:** Albert Einstein Coll Med 1976; **Resid:** Rheumatology, Bellevue Hosp 1979; **Fellow:** Rheumatology, Bellevue Hosp 1981

Burns, Mark MD (Rhu) - **Spec Exp:** Lupus Nephritis; Rheumatoid Arthritis; **Hospital:** Sound Shore Med Ctr - Westchester (page 711), Montefiore Med Ctr; **Address:** 421 Huguenot St, Ste 44, New Rochelle, NY 10801-7021; **Phone:** 914-235-3065; **Board Cert:** Internal Medicine 1980; Rheumatology 1984; **Med School:** UCSF 1977; **Resid:** Internal Medicine, Montefiore Hosp Med Ctr 1980; **Fellow:** Rheumatology, Montefiore Hosp Med Ctr 1983; **Fac Appt:** Asst Clin Prof Med, Albert Einstein Coll Med

Futran-Sheinberg, Jacobo MD (Rhu) - **Spec Exp:** Arthritis; Lupus/SLE; Lupus Nephritis; **Hospital:** St John's Riverside Hosp, Hosp For Special Surgery (page 108); **Address:** 970 N Broadway, Ste 312, Yonkers, NY 10701-1311; **Phone:** 914-968-4695; **Board Cert:** Internal Medicine 1995; Rheumatology 1996; **Med School:** Mexico 1980; **Resid:** Internal Medicine, Natl Med Ctr 1984; **Fellow:** Rheumatology, Univ Toronto Med Ctr 1986; Immunology, Univ IA Hosp 1988; **Fac Appt:** Assoc Prof Med, Cornell Univ-Weill Med Coll

Mascarenhas, Bento MD (Rhu) - **Spec Exp:** Arthritis; Lupus/SLE; Osteoporosis; **Hospital:** Burke Rehab Hosp (page 105), Hosp For Special Surgery (page 108); **Address:** 785 Mammaroneck Ave, White Plains, NY 10605; **Phone:** 914-948-6405; **Board Cert:** Internal Medicine 1972; Rheumatology 1974; **Med School:** India 1961; **Resid:** Internal Medicine, Westchester Med Ctr 1967; **Fellow:** Internal Medicine, Cornell Univ Med Ctr 1970; Rheumatology, Hosp for Special Surg 1970; **Fac Appt:** Clin Prof Med, NY Med Coll

Reinitz, Elizabeth MD (Rhu) - **Spec Exp:** Rheumatoid Arthritis; Lupus/SLE; Osteoarthritis; Gout; **Hospital:** White Plains Hosp Ctr (page 714); **Address:** 259 Heathcote Rd, Scarsdale, NY 10583; **Phone:** 914-723-8100; **Board Cert:** Internal Medicine 1979; Rheumatology 1982; **Med School:** Albert Einstein Coll Med 1976; **Resid:** Internal Medicine, Boston City Hosp 1979; **Fellow:** Rheumatology, Montefiore Hosp Med Ctr 1981; **Fac Appt:** Assoc Prof Med, Albert Einstein Coll Med

Sloane, Lori MD (Rhu) - **Spec Exp:** Rheumatoid Arthritis; **Hospital:** Northern Westchester Hosp; **Address:** Westchester Medical Associates, 322 Underhill Ave, Yorktown Heights, NY 10598; **Phone:** 914-962-5501; **Board Cert:** Internal Medicine 1989; Rheumatology 1992; **Med School:** SUNY Downstate 1986; **Resid:** Internal Medicine, Jacobi Med Ctr 1989; **Fellow:** Rheumatology, Montefiore Hosp Med Ctr 1991; **Fac Appt:** Asst Clin Prof Med, Albert Einstein Coll Med

SPORTS MEDICINE

Cavaliere, Gregg MD (SM) - **Spec Exp:** Rotator Cuff Surgery; Knee Injuries/Ligament Surgery; Shoulder Instability; **Hospital:** Phelps Meml Hosp Ctr, St John's Riverside Hosp; **Address:** 24 Saw Mill River Rd, Ste 2, Hawthorne, NY 10532; **Phone:** 914-631-7777; **Board Cert:** Orthopaedic Surgery 2004; **Med School:** NY Med Coll 1987; **Resid:** Orthopaedic Surgery, Lenox Hill Hosp 1992; **Fellow:** Sports Medicine, NYU Med Ctr 1993

Luks, Howard J MD (SM) - **Hospital:** Westchester Med Ctr (page 713); **Address:** 19 Bradhurst Ave, Hawthorne, NY 10532; **Phone:** 914-789-2735; **Board Cert:** Orthopaedic Surgery 1999; **Med School:** NY Med Coll 1991; **Resid:** Orthopaedic Surgery, LI Jewish Med Ctr 1996

SURGERY

Ashikari, Andrew Y MD (S) - **Spec Exp:** Breast Cancer; **Hospital:** Comm Hosp - Dobbs Ferry, Westchester Med Ctr (page 713); **Address:** Ashikari Comprehensive Breast Ctr, Community Hospital, 128 Ashford Ave, Dobbs Ferry, NY 10522; **Phone:** 914-693-5025; **Board Cert:** Surgery 1997; **Med School:** Univ Pittsburgh 1991; **Resid:** Surgery, Montefiore Med Ctr 1996; **Fellow:** Surgical Oncology, Univ Chicago Hosps 1997

Butt, Khalid M H MD (S) - **Spec Exp:** Transplant-Kidney; Vascular Surgery; Vascular Access; Thyroid & Parathyroid Surgery; **Hospital:** Westchester Med Ctr (page 713); **Address:** 19 Bradhurst Ave, Ste 3150, Hawthorne, NY 10532-2140; **Phone:** 914-493-1990; **Board Cert:** Surgery 1972; Thoracic Surgery 1972; **Med School:** Pakistan 1962; **Resid:** Surgery, Queens Hosp 1965; Surgery, Kings Co Hosp 1970; **Fellow:** Thoracic Surgery, Kings Co Hosp 1971; **Fac Appt:** Prof S, NY Med Coll

Cahan, Anthony MD (S) - **Spec Exp:** Breast Surgery; **Hospital:** Northern Westchester Hosp, Beth Israel Med Ctr - Petrie Division (page 90); **Address:** 311 North St, Ste 308, White Plains, NY 10605; **Phone:** 914-681-9481; **Board Cert:** Surgery 1998; **Med School:** Cornell Univ-Weill Med Coll 1982, **Resid:** Surgery, New York Hosp 1987

Cehelsky, John Ihor MD (S) - **Spec Exp:** Laparoscopic Surgery; Breast Surgery; **Hospital:** Northern Westchester Hosp; **Address:** Mt Kisco Med Grp, 110 S Bedford Rd, Mt Kisco, NY 10549; **Phone:** 914-242-1360; **Board Cert:** Surgery 1994; **Med School:** Ohio State Univ 1977; **Resid:** Surgery, St Lukes Hosp 1982

Elwyn, Katherine E MD (S) - **Spec Exp:** Breast Cancer; Breast Disease; **Hospital:** Northern Westchester Hosp; **Address:** 344 E Main St, Ste 403, Mount Kisco, NY 10549-3036; **Phone:** 914-244-9058; **Board Cert:** Surgery 2001; **Med School:** SUNY Hlth Sci Ctr 1976; **Resid:** Surgery, SUNY Brooklyn Med Ctr 1981; **Fellow:** Surgical Oncology, MD Anderson Cancer Ctr 1983

Finkelstein, Jacob MD (S) - **Spec Exp:** Breast Surgery; **Hospital:** White Plains Hosp Ctr (page 714), Sound Shore Med Ctr - Westchester (page 711); **Address:** 33 Cedar St, Rye, NY 10580; **Phone:** 914-967-7979; **Board Cert:** Surgery 1970; **Med School:** NYU Sch Med 1963; **Resid:** Surgery, Mount Sinai Med Ctr 1969

Gandhi, Govindan MD (S) - **Spec Exp:** Gallbladder Surgery-Laparoscopic; Breast Disease; Carotid Artery Surgery; **Hospital:** St John's Riverside Hosp, Saint Joseph's Med Ctr - Yonkers; **Address:** 970 N Broadway, Ste 309, Yonkers, NY 10701; **Phone:** 914-965-0625; **Board Cert:** Surgery 1980; **Med School:** India 1973; **Resid:** Surgery, Cabrini Med Ctr 1977; Surgery, New Rochelle Hosp Med Ctr 1979

Gordon, Mark S MD (S) - **Spec Exp:** Breast Surgery; Melanoma; Pancreatic Surgery; **Hospital:** White Plains Hosp Ctr (page 714); **Address:** 2 Longview Ave, Ste 302, White Plains, NY 10601; **Phone:** 914-684-5884; **Board Cert:** Surgery 1997; **Med School:** Northwestern Univ 1982; **Resid:** Surgery, NY Hosp/Cornell Med Ctr 1987; **Fellow:** Surgical Oncology, Meml Sloan Kettering Cancer Ctr 1989; **Fac Appt:** Asst Clin Prof S, NY Med Coll

Homan, William P MD/PhD (S) - **Spec Exp:** Obesity/Bariatric Surgery; **Hospital:** White Plains Hosp Ctr (page 714); **Address:** 170 Maple Ave, Ste 502, White Plains, NY 10601; **Phone:** 914-948-1000; **Board Cert:** Surgery 1997; **Med School:** Cornell Univ-Weill Med Coll 1973; **Resid:** Surgery, New York Hosp-Cornell Med Ctr 1978; **Fellow:** Surgery, Radcliffe Infirmary 1980

Josephson, Lynn MD (S) - **Spec Exp:** Breast Surgery; Gallbladder Surgery-Laparoscopic; **Hospital:** White Plains Hosp Ctr (page 714); **Address:** 170 Maple Ave, Ste 502, White Plains, NY 10601; **Phone:** 914-949-4609; **Board Cert:** Surgery 2002; **Med School:** Mount Sinai Sch Med 1977; **Resid:** Surgery, Columbia-Presby Med Ctr 1981

Kassel, Barry MD (S) - **Spec Exp:** Breast Surgery; Laparoscopic Surgery; **Hospital:** Northern Westchester Hosp; **Address:** 90 S Bedford Rd, Mount Kisco, NY 10549; **Phone:** 914-241-1050; **Board Cert:** Surgery 1998; **Med School:** SUNY Buffalo 1973; **Resid:** Surgery, Albert Einstein 1977; Surgery, NYU Med Ctr 1979

Kim, Zung Wan MD (S) - **Spec Exp:** Varicose Veins; Carotid & Leg Arterial Bypass Surg; **Hospital:** White Plains Hosp Ctr (page 714); **Address:** 265 Purchase St, Rye, NY 10580; **Phone:** 914-967-2588; **Board Cert:** Surgery 1973; **Med School:** South Korea 1964; **Resid:** Surgery, Hosp for Joint Diseases 1967; Surgery, New York Methodist Hosp 1970

Krakovitz, Evan MD (S) - **Spec Exp:** Colon & Rectal Cancer & Surgery; Hemorrhoids; Laparoscopic Surgery; **Hospital:** White Plains Hosp Ctr (page 714), Greenwich Hosp; **Address:** Surgical Specialties, 210 Westchester Ave, White Plains, NY 10604; **Phone:** 914-682-6557; **Board Cert:** Surgery 2006; Colon & Rectal Surgery 1997; **Med School:** Hahnemann Univ 1989; **Resid:** Surgery, Graduate Hospital 1994; **Fellow:** Colon & Rectal Surgery, RWJ Univ Hosp 1995

Pass, Helen MD (S) - **Spec Exp:** Breast Cancer; Breast Disease; Breast Surgery; **Hospital:** Lawrence Hosp Ctr; **Address:** Breast Care Ctr - Lawrence Hosp, 55 W Palmer Ave, Fl 5, Bronxville, NY 10708; **Phone:** 914-787-4000; **Board Cert:** Surgery 2003; **Med School:** Univ Mich Med Sch 1987; **Resid:** Surgery, Univ Tex Hlth Sci Ctr/MD Anderson Cancer Ctr 1989; Surgery, Georgetown Univ Hosp 1994; **Fellow:** Surgical Oncology, NCI/NIH 1992; **Fac Appt:** Asst Prof S, Columbia P&S

Policastro, Anthony MD (S) - **Spec Exp:** Breast Surgery; Hernia; **Hospital:** Westchester Med Ctr (page 713); **Address:** 19 Bradhurst Ave, Ste 1700, Hawthorne, NY 10532; **Phone:** 914-347-0162; **Board Cert:** Surgery 2000; Surgical Critical Care 1992; **Med School:** Creighton Univ 1985; **Resid:** Surgery, Westchester Co Med Ctr 1990; **Fellow:** Surgical Critical Care, Westchester Co Med Ctr 1991; **Fac Appt:** Asst Prof S, NY Med Coll

Rajdeo, Heena MD (S) - **Spec Exp:** Dialysis Access Surgery; Thyroid & Parathyroid Surgery; Laparoscopic Surgery; **Hospital:** Westchester Med Ctr (page 713); **Address:** Munger Pavilion, Ste 551, Northeast Surgical Group, Valhalla, NY 10595; **Phone:** 914-493-7378; **Board Cert:** Surgery 2002; **Med School:** India 1969; **Resid:** Surgery, KEM Hosp 1972; Surgery, Westchester Med Ctr 1982; **Fac Appt:** Asst Prof S, NY Med Coll

Raniolo, Robert MD (S) - **Spec Exp:** Breast Surgery; Abdominal Surgery; Hernia; **Hospital:** Phelps Meml Hosp Ctr; **Address:** 777 N Broadway, Ste 204, Sleepy Hollow, NY 10591-1019; **Phone:** 914-631-3660; **Board Cert:** Surgery 1998; **Med School:** Mexico 1981; **Resid:** Surgery, Lincoln Hosp 1988

Savino, John MD (S) - **Spec Exp:** Critical Care; Trauma; Pancreatic Surgery; **Hospital:** Westchester Med Ctr (page 713); **Address:** NY Med Coll, Dept Surg, Munger Pavillion, Valhalla, NY 10595; **Phone:** 914-594-4352; **Board Cert:** Surgery 1975; Surgical Critical Care 1995; **Med School:** Italy 1968; **Resid:** Surgery, Metropolitan Hosp Ctr 1974; **Fac Appt:** Prof S, NY Med Coll

Walsh, Bruce MD (S) - **Spec Exp:** Critical Care; Trauma; Laparoscopic Abdominal Surgery; **Hospital:** Sound Shore Med Ctr - Westchester (page 711); **Address:** 140 Lockwood Ave, Ste 103, New Rochelle, NY 10801; **Phone:** 914-636-3373; **Board Cert:** Surgery 1996; Surgical Critical Care 2001; **Med School:** Mexico 1979; **Resid:** Surgery, New Rochelle Med Ctr 1986; **Fellow:** Surgical Critical Care, Westchester Med Ctr 1987

Wertkin, Martin MD (S) - **Spec Exp:** Breast Cancer; Breast Surgery; **Hospital:** St John's Riverside Hosp, Phelps Meml Hosp Ctr; **Address:** 1034 N Broadway, Yonkers, NY 10701; **Phone:** 914-965-2026; **Board Cert:** Surgery 1999; **Med School:** SUNY Hlth Sci Ctr 1972; **Resid:** Surgery, Mount Sinai Med Ctr 1978; **Fac Appt:** Asst Clin Prof S, Mount Sinai Sch Med

THORACIC SURGERY

Lafaro, Rocco J MD (TS) - **Spec Exp:** Minimally Invasive Cardiac Surgery; **Hospital:** Westchester Med Ctr (page 713); **Address:** Westchester Med Ctr, Div Cardiothor Surg, Macy Weiss Pavillion, rm 128, Valhalla, NY 10595; **Phone:** 914-493-7676; **Board Cert:** Thoracic Surgery 1991; **Med School:** NY Med Coll 1982; **Resid:** Surgery, Metropolitan Hosp Ctr 1984; Surgery, Westchester Med Ctr 1986; **Fellow:** Thoracic Surgery, Bronx Muni Hosp Ctr 1991; Thoracic Surgery, Montefiore Med Ctr 1993

Lansman, Steven MD/PhD (TS) - **Spec Exp:** Coronary Artery Surgery; Heart Valve Surgery; Ventricular Assist Device (LVAD); Transplant-Heart; **Hospital:** Westchester Med Ctr (page 713); **Address:** Westchester Medical Ctr, Macy Pavilion, rm 114, Valhalla, NY 10595; **Phone:** 914-493-8793; **Board Cert:** Thoracic Surgery 1986; **Med School:** SUNY Hlth Sci Ctr 1977; **Resid:** Surgery, Montefiore Hosp Med Ctr 1982; **Fellow:** Thoracic Surgery, Univ Hosp 1984; **Fac Appt:** Prof S, NY Med Coll

Spielvogel, David MD (TS) - **Spec Exp:** Aneurysm-Aortic; Transplant-Heart; Coronary Artery Surgery; Heart Valve Surgery; **Hospital:** Westchester Med Ctr (page 713); **Address:** Westchester Medical Ctr, Macey Pavilion, rm 114, Valhalla, NY 10595; **Phone:** 914-493-8793; **Board Cert:** Surgery 1996; Thoracic Surgery 2000; **Med School:** SUNY Downstate 1990; **Resid:** Surgery, SUNY Health Sci Ctr 1995; Thoracic Surgery, Mount Sinai Med Ctr 1998; **Fellow:** Cardiac Surgery, Harefield Hosp 1999; **Fac Appt:** Assoc Prof S, NY Med Coll

Streisand, Robert MD (TS) - **Spec Exp:** Video Assisted Thoracic Surgery (VATS); **Hospital:** White Plains Hosp Ctr (page 714), St John's Riverside Hosp; **Address:** 10 Chester Ave, White Plains, NY 10601-5112; **Phone:** 914-948-6633; **Board Cert:** Surgery 1973; Thoracic Surgery 1975; **Med School:** SUNY Downstate 1966; **Resid:** Surgery, Kings County Hosp 1973; Thoracic Surgery, Baylor Coll Med 1968

Urology

Bromberg, Warren MD (U) - **Spec Exp:** Prostate Cancer; Bladder Cancer; Incontinence-Female; **Hospital:** Northern Westchester Hosp; **Address:** Mount Kisco Medical Group, 110 S Bedford Rd, Mt Kisco, NY 10549-3408; **Phone:** 914-242-1520; **Board Cert:** Urology 1993; **Med School:** Johns Hopkins Univ 1985; **Resid:** Urology, Northwestern Meml Hosp 1991

Choudhury, Muhammad MD (U) - **Spec Exp:** Urologic Cancer; Prostate Cancer; Bladder Cancer; **Hospital:** Westchester Med Ctr (page 713); **Address:** 19 Bradhurst Ave, Ste 1900, Hawthorne, NY 10532-2144; **Phone:** 914-347-1900; **Board Cert:** Urology 1982; **Med School:** Bangladesh 1972; **Resid:** Urology, Columbia-Presby Med Ctr 1978; Urology, NY Med Coll 1980; **Fellow:** Urologic Oncology, Roswell Park Cancer Inst 1981; **Fac Appt:** Prof U, NY Med Coll

Eshghi, A Majid MD (U) - **Spec Exp:** Kidney Stones; Laparoscopic Surgery; **Hospital:** Westchester Med Ctr (page 713); **Address:** 19 Bradhurst Ave, Ste 1900, Hawthorne, NY 10532; **Phone:** 914-347-1900; **Board Cert:** Urology 1997; **Med School:** Iran 1976; **Resid:** Surgery, St Barnabas Med Ctr 1981; Urology, LI Jewish Med Ctr 1985; **Fac Appt:** Prof U, NY Med Coll

Fagin, Bernard H MD (U) - **Spec Exp:** Prostate Disease; Urologic Cancer; Kidney Stones; **Hospital:** Hudson Valley Hosp Ctr, Putnam Hosp Ctr; **Address:** 1985 Crompond Rd, Bldg D, Cortland Manor, NY 10567-4146; **Phone:** 914-739-1219; **Board Cert:** Urology 1977; **Med School:** NY Med Coll 1967; **Resid:** Surgery, Brookdale Hosp Ctr 1969; Urology, Albert Einstein Coll Med 1973

Glassman, Charles N MD (U) - **Spec Exp:** Prostate Cancer; Incontinence; Pediatric Urology; Sexual Dysfunction; **Hospital:** White Plains Hosp Ctr (page 714); **Address:** 170 Maple Ave, Ste 104, White Plains, NY 10601-4707; **Phone:** 914-949-7556; **Board Cert:** Urology 1980; **Med School:** Tufts Univ 1973; **Resid:** Surgery, UCSF Med Ctr 1975; Urology, UCSF Med Ctr 1978; **Fellow:** Pediatric Urology, Mayo Clinic 1979

Hershman, Jack MD (U) - **Spec Exp:** Prostate Cancer; Kidney Stones; Incontinence; **Hospital:** Phelps Meml Hosp Ctr, Northern Westchester Hosp; **Address:** 777 N Broadway, Ste 309, Sleepy Hollow, NY 10591; **Phone:** 914-631-3331; **Board Cert:** Urology 1998; **Med School:** Mount Sinai Sch Med 1981; **Resid:** Surgery, Lenox Hill Hosp 1983; Urology, Montefiore Hosp Med Ctr 1986

Housman, Arno MD (U) - **Spec Exp:** Kidney Stones; Urologic Cancer; Incontinence; **Hospital:** Phelps Meml Hosp Ctr, Westchester Med Ctr (page 713); **Address:** 325 S Highland Ave, Briarcliff Manor, NY 10510-2093; **Phone:** 914-941-0617; **Board Cert:** Urology 1999; **Med School:** SUNY Downstate 1980; **Resid:** Surgery, SUNY-Kings Co Hosp Ctr 1983; Urology, Yale-New Haven Hosp 1986

Kogan, Stanley J MD (U) - **Spec Exp:** Pediatric Urology; Genital Surgery-Pediatric; **Hospital:** Westchester Med Ctr (page 713), NY-Presby Hosp (page 100); **Address:** 19 Bradhurst Ave, Ste 2575, Hawthorne, NY 10532; **Phone:** 914-493-8628; **Board Cert:** Urology 1976; **Med School:** SUNY Hlth Sci Ctr 1966; **Resid:** Surgery, Montefiore Med Ctr 1968; Urology, Montefiore Med Ctr 1973; **Fellow:** Pediatric Urology, Alder Hay Hosp Sick Chldn 1974; **Fac Appt:** Prof U, NY Med Coll

Lerner, Seth E MD (U) - **Spec Exp:** Prostate Cancer; **Hospital:** White Plains Hosp Ctr (page 714); **Address:** 170 Maple Ave, Ste 104, White Plains, NY 10601; **Phone:** 914-949-7556; **Board Cert:** Urology 1997; **Med School:** SUNY Downstate 1988; **Resid:** Surgery, Montefiore-Weiler Einstein Div 1990; Urology, Montefiore-Weler Einstein Div 1994; **Fellow:** Urologic Oncology, Mayo Clinic 1995; **Fac Appt:** Asst Prof U, Albert Einstein Coll Med

Matthews, Gerald J MD (U) - **Spec Exp:** Infertility-Male; Impotence; **Hospital:** Westchester Med Ctr (page 713), Our Lady of Mercy Med Ctr; **Address:** Medical Arts Atrium, 19 Bradhurst Ave, Ste 1900, Hawthorne, NY 10532-2144; **Phone:** 914-347-1900; **Board Cert:** Urology 1998; **Med School:** NY Med Coll 1986; **Resid:** Urology, Lenox Hill Hosp 1993; Surgery, St Francis Hosp Med Ctr 1989; **Fellow:** Urology, NY Hosp-Cornell Med Ctr 1995; Urology, Rockefeller Univ Hosp 1995; **Fac Appt:** Assoc Prof U, NY Med Coll

Owens, George MD (U) - **Spec Exp:** Erectile Dysfunction; Prostate Disease; Minimally Invasive Surgery; **Hospital:** White Plains Hosp Ctr (page 714), Westchester Med Ctr (page 713); **Address:** 311 North St, Ste 201, White Plains, NY 10605-2232; **Phone:** 914-946-1406; **Board Cert:** Urology 1996; **Med School:** NY Med Coll 1979; **Resid:** Surgery, Montefiore Hosp Med Ctr 1981; Urology, Montefiore Hosp Med Ctr 1984; **Fellow:** Urology, NY Med Coll 1985; **Fac Appt:** Assoc Clin Prof U, NY Med Coll

Putignano, Joseph MD (U) - **Spec Exp:** Bladder Surgery; Laser Surgery; Kidney Stones; Prostate Surgery; **Hospital:** Lawrence Hosp Ctr, Westchester Med Ctr (page 713); **Address:** 26 Pondfield Rd W, Bronxville, NY 10708; **Phone:** 914-793-1200; **Board Cert:** Urology 1975; **Med School:** Canada 1965; **Resid:** Urology, St Luke's-Roosevelt Hosp Ctr 1971; **Fac Appt:** Assoc Prof U, NY Med Coll

Riechers, Roger MD (U) - **Spec Exp:** Incontinence-Female; Prostate Cancer; **Hospital:** Northern Westchester Hosp; **Address:** 90 S Bedford Rd, Mt Kisco, NY 10549; **Phone:** 914-242-1520; **Board Cert:** Urology 1976; **Med School:** NYU Sch Med 1968; **Resid:** Urology, Mount Sinai 1973

Roberts, Larry P MD (U) - **Spec Exp:** Infertility-Male; Erectile Dysfunction; Incontinence; **Hospital:** Sound Shore Med Ctr - Westchester (page 711); **Address:** 175 Memorial Hwy, Ste 32, New Rochelle, NY 10801-5641; **Phone:** 914-235-2929; **Board Cert:** Urology 1981; **Med School:** Univ Miami Sch Med 1974; **Resid:** Urology, Albert Einstein Med Coll 1979; Surgery, Univ Miami Hosps 1976; **Fac Appt:** Asst Clin Prof U, Albert Einstein Coll Med

Schrager, Alan MD (U) - **Spec Exp:** Voiding Dysfunction; Erectile Dysfunction; Urologic Cancer; **Hospital:** Greenwich Hosp, Sound Shore Med Ctr - Westchester (page 711); **Address:** 1600 Harrison Ave, Ste G102, Mamaroneck, NY 10543-3124; **Phone:** 914-698-8106; **Board Cert:** Urology 1975; **Med School:** Univ Hlth Sci/Chicago Med Sch 1966; **Resid:** Surgery, Maimonides Med Ctr 1970; Urology, SUNY Downstate 1973

Shalit, Shimon MD (U) - **Spec Exp:** Prostate Disease; Incontinence-Female; Prostate Cancer; **Hospital:** White Plains Hosp Ctr (page 714); **Address:** 12 Greenridge Ave, White Plains, NY 10605; **Phone:** 914-948-3128; **Board Cert:** Urology 1979; **Med School:** Israel 1957; **Resid:** Surgery, Beilinson 1962; Urology, New York Univ. Med. Center 1965; **Fellow:** Neurology, New York Univ. Center 1966; **Fac Appt:** Asst Clin Prof U, NYU Sch Med

Siegel, Judy F MD (U) - **Spec Exp:** Voiding Dysfunction-Female; Voiding Dysfunction-Pediatric; **Hospital:** St John's Riverside Hosp, Phelps Meml Hosp Ctr; **Address:** 623 Walburn Ave, Hastings-on-Hudson, NY 10706; **Phone:** 914-478-3001; **Board Cert:** Urology 1999; **Med School:** Univ VT Coll Med 1988; **Resid:** Surgery, LI Jewish Med Ctr 1990; Urology, LI Jewish Med Ctr 1994; **Fellow:** Pediatric Urology, Schneider Chldns Hosp 1996

VASCULAR SURGERY

Babu, Sateesh MD (VascS) - **Spec Exp:** Carotid Artery Surgery; Aneurysm-Aortic; Lower Limb Arterial Disease; **Hospital:** Westchester Med Ctr (page 713), Northern Westchester Hosp; **Address:** 19 Bradhurst Ave, Medical Arts Atrium/Westchester Med Ctr, Hawthorne, NY 10532-2140; **Phone:** 914-593-1200; **Board Cert:** Surgery 1995; Vascular Surgery 2001; **Med School:** India 1969; **Resid:** Surgery, Jewish Memorial Hosp 1972; Surgery, Metropolitan Hosp 1975; **Fellow:** Vascular Surgery, Metropolitan Hosp 1977; **Fac Appt:** Prof S, NY Med Coll

Karanfilian, Richard MD (VascS) - **Spec Exp:** Varicose Veins; Carotid Artery Surgery; Endovascular Surgery; **Hospital:** Sound Shore Med Ctr - Westchester (page 711), Mount Vernon Hosp (page 712); **Address:** 150 Lockwood Ave, Ste 14, New Rochelle, NY 10801-4912; **Phone:** 914-636-1700; **Board Cert:** Surgery 2002; Vascular Surgery 1996; **Med School:** Italy 1977; **Resid:** Surgery, UMDNJ-NJ Med Sch 1983; **Fellow:** Vascular Surgery, UMDNJ-NJ Med Sch 1985; **Fac Appt:** Assoc Clin Prof S, NY Med Coll

Schwartz, Kenneth S MD (VascS) - **Spec Exp:** Arterial Disease; Vein Disorders; Dialysis Access Surgery; **Hospital:** White Plains Hosp Ctr (page 714), Greenwich Hosp; **Address:** 14 Harwood Ct, Ste 326, Scarsdale, NY 10583-4122; **Phone:** 914-723-7737; **Board Cert:** Surgery 2002; **Med School:** Albert Einstein Coll Med 1977; **Resid:** Surgery, Montefiore Hosp Med Ctr 1981; **Fellow:** Peripheral Vascular Surgery, USC Med Ctr 1982; **Fac Appt:** Asst Clin Prof S, NY Med Coll

Tannenbaum, Gary MD (VascS) - **Spec Exp:** Diabetic Leg/Foot; Wound Healing/Care; Arterial Bypass Surgery; **Hospital:** St John's Riverside Hosp; **Address:** 984 N Broadway, Ste 501, Yonkers, NY 10701-1308; **Phone:** 914-965-2606; **Board Cert:** Surgery 2000; Vascular Surgery 2002; **Med School:** Columbia P&S 1983; **Resid:** Surgery, Columbia-Presby Med Ctr 1989; Vascular Surgery, New England Deaconness 1992; **Fellow:** Transplant Surgery, Columbia-Presby Med Ctr 1987; Surgical Critical Care, Columbia-Presby Med Ctr 1990

Weintraub, Neil MD (VascS) - **Spec Exp:** Carotid Artery Surgery; Aneurysm-Aortic; Dialysis Access Surgery; **Hospital:** White Plains Hosp Ctr (page 714), Saint Joseph's Med Ctr - Yonkers; **Address:** 14 Harwood Ct, Ste 326, Scarsdale, NY 10583-4120; **Phone:** 914-723-7737; **Board Cert:** Surgery 1985; Vascular Surgery 1998; **Med School:** Univ Chicago-Pritzker Sch Med 1979; **Resid:** Surgery, NYU Med Ctr 1984; **Fellow:** Vascular Surgery, NYU Med Ctr 1985; **Fac Appt:** Asst Clin Prof S, NY Med Coll

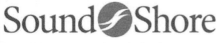

MEDICAL CENTER OF WESTCHESTER

16 Guion Place   New Rochelle, NY 10802
914-632-5000
Physician Referral Service: 914-MDs-LINE

Sponsorship: Private, Not-for-profit, Teaching
Beds: 471: 321 Acute, 50 Short-term Rehabilitation and 100 Long-term Care
Accreditation: Joint Commission on Accreditation of Healthcare Organizations (JCAHO)

Sound Shore Medical Center(SSMC) is a 471-bed, private, not-for-profit hospital and one of the largest private teaching hospitals between New York City and Albany. Sound Shore Medical Center provides comprehensive primary, acute, emergency and short-term rehabilitation and long-term healthcare. Residents of southern Westchester, the Sound Shore region, the northern Bronx and beyond benefit from their century-long commitment to quality patient care.

SSMC's slogan, *Care. For Life.*, exemplifies their healthcare expertise that spans the life cycle – from prenatal through extended care.

Emergency Services
New York State-designated:
- Level II - Area Trauma Center
- Stroke Center

Maternal and Child Health Services
New York State-designated:
- Perinatal Hospital
  - o Antepartum Testing Laboratory, 1st Trimester Screening Center of Excellence
  - o Level 3 Neonatal Intensive Care Nursery

Medical Services
Cancer Program designated Commission on Cancer of the American College of Surgeons, with commendation:
- o Gladys and Murray Goldstein Cancer Center
- o Solomon Katz Breast Center
- o Mobile Mammography Service
- Travel Health Center
- Sleep Center
- Center for Arthritis and Total Joint Surgery
- The Spine Center
- Diabetes Education Center
- Kirschenbaum Mental Health Clinic

Surgical Services
Center of Excellence by the American Society for Bariatric Surgery
- o Bariatric Surgical Weight Loss Program
- Orthopaedic and Neurological Spine Center
- Gastro-Reflux Center
- GI Endoscopy Suite
- The Spine Center

Cardiology Services
- Chest Pain Center
- Harriet and Bernard Miller Adult Cardiac Catheterization Laboratory
- Cardiac Rehabilitation Center

Geriatrics Services
- Center for Sound Aging
- Physician Home Visit Program
- Ludington Adult Day Services Program
- Health Access – information and referral service for seniors
- Schaffer Extended Care Center (Beds: 50 short-term rehabilitation and 100 long-term)

Care. For Life.
www.ssmc.org
Member of Sound Shore Health System and Pinnacle Healthcare

744

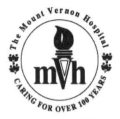

The Mount Vernon Hospital

12 North Seventh Avenue
Mount Vernon, NY 10550
914-664-8000
Physician Referral Service: 914-664-8000 x3050

Sponsorship: Private, Not-for-profit, Teaching
Beds: 228
Accreditation: Joint Commission on Accreditation of Healthcare Organizations (JCAHO)

The Mount Vernon Hospital (MVH) is a private, not-for-profit, teaching hospital providing inpatient, critical care and ambulatory services using the latest technology. Mount Vernon Hospital is a New York State-designated Stroke Center and home to one of the largest and most advanced Chronic Wound Treatment and Hyperbaric Centers in the northeast and one of only two hyperbaric centers in Westchester County. These notable distinctions complement their other outstanding services:

- Pain Management Center
  - o Low Back Pain Management Center
- Center for Foot & Ankle Care
- Family Health and Wellness Center
- Behavioral Health Services
  - o Assertive Community Treatment
    - A multidisciplinary team takes services directly to individuals in their own environment
  - o Intensive Case Management
    - With Assertive Community Treatment, team coordinates necessary outpatient medical and mental healthcare and life needs
  - o Kirschenbaum Mental Health Clinic
- In-patient Psychiatric Unit

Recognizing the need to address the full-spectrum of healthcare needs within their service area and beyond, Mount Vernon Hospital is also a New York State-designated HIV/AIDS Center.

Mount Vernon Hospital is one of only five hospitals selected by the New York State to take part in a statewide Transitional Care Unit demonstration project. It will explore continued hospital care for individuals whose condition warrants discharge but for whom prior living arrangements or nursing home placement is not yet suitable. When this three-year study ends, MVH will have contributed immeasurably to the State's assessment of this growing healthcare issue.

Educating healthcare professionals has been central to MVH's mission for more than a century. Mount Vernon is home to The Dorothea Hopfer School of Nursing and the only Podiatry residency in Westchester. The hospital is also home to the County's only, freestanding internal medicine residency program. From an application pool of thousands, Mount Vernon Hospital selects 24 graduating medical students for this highly regarded program.

Mount Vernon Hospital's educational mission ensures that it remains at the forefront of healthcare.

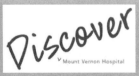

Mount Vernon Hospital
www.mtvernonhospital.org
Sound Shore Health System and Pinnacle Healthcare Member

745

Sponsored Page

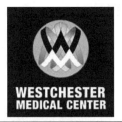

WESTCHESTER MEDICAL CENTER

Valhalla Campus
Valhalla, NY 10595
Tel. 1-877-WMC-DOCS
http://www.worldclassmedicine.com

Sponsorship:	Public Benefit Corporation
Beds:	900 beds
Accreditation:	Joint Commission on Accreditation of Healthcare Organizations (JCAHO); American College of Surgeons Verification for Level 1 Trauma Center with Pediatric Commitment; American College of Surgeons Verification for Burn Center

REGIONAL MEDICAL CENTER

As an academic medical center and the region's advanced care and Level 1 Trauma Center, Westchester Medical Center is on the leading edge of medical research and advances in clinical care. Over 3.5 million people in the Hudson Valley region, northern New Jersey and lower Connecticut rely on our services.

FOUR MAJOR FACILITIES

With four major facilities—our University Hospital, Maria Fareri Children's Hospital, Behavioral Health Center and Taylor Care Center (for skilled nursing and sub-acute)—Westchester Medical Center's renowned specialty services have made us the referral hospital of choice for physicians and patients seeking the highest level and quality of care.

CENTERS OF EXCELLENCE

The academic affiliate of New York Medical College, Westchester Medical Center is home to one of New York State's largest kidney transplant programs and one of only four liver transplant programs in the state. Maria Fareri Children's Hospital at Westchester Medical Center is the only all-specialty children's hospital in the region. Our renowned pediatric specialists treat over 20,000 children each year. The Children's Hospital is also home to the only Level IV regional neonatal intensive care unit and pediatric intensive care unit, as well as a specialized high-risk obstetrics center.

The Heart Center at Westchester Medical Center boasts one of the most highly regarded cardiology and cardiac surgery programs on the East Coast. With fully equipped medevac helicopters, our STAT Flight team responds in minutes to accidents and other emergencies, and carries critical inter-hospital patient transfers from throughout the region and beyond.

Westchester Medical Center's Trauma and Burn Center features the only burn center between New York City and the Canadian border; our Arlin Cancer Institute offers the latest cancer therapies, including bone marrow and stem cell transplants; and our Neuroscience Center offers neurosurgical and neurological care, including "knifeless" brain surgery, specialized stroke (brain attack) service, a cerebrovascular center and an epilepsy program.

QUALITY HEALTHCARE

Westchester Medical Center is recognized throughout New York's Hudson Valley region as a leader in quality healthcare. Westchester Medical Center is recognized as a "Distinguished Hospital for Clinical Excellence" by HealthGrades, the industry's quality experts, and number one in the region for cardiac services, heart surgery and angioplasty/stents. In addition, Westchester Medical Center was recognized as the top hospital in Westchester County for an unprecedented fifth year in a row, receiving National Research Corporation's "Consumers Choice Award for Best Overall Quality and Image."

Physician Referral: For information on Westchester Medical Center's physicians and surgeons, visit us at www.worldclassmedicine.com or call 1-877-WMC-DOCS.

779

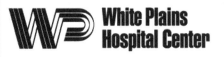

White Plains Hospital Center

Davis Avenue at East Post Road
White Plains, New York 10601
914-681-0600
www.wphospital.org

Beds: 292
Sponsorship: Private, Not-for-Profit
Accreditation: Joint Commission on Accreditation of Healthcare Organizations, Commission on Cancer of the American College of Surgeons, College of American Pathologists, American Registry of Radiological Technology, American Society of Radiological Technology, American Society for Bariatric Surgery

A LEADING COMMUNITY HOSPITAL

White Plains Hospital Center (WPHC) is a 292-bed community hospital that has been serving the Westchester area and its environs since 1893. In addition to a wide range of general acute care services, the Hospital offers highly sophisticated specialty programs in Oncology, Orthopedics, Obstetrics, Radiology, and Stroke Care. Although classified as a community hospital, WPHC offers some levels of service normally found in large academic medical centers.

HealthGrades™, the nation's leading independent health care ratings organization, recently ranked WPHC in the top 5% in the nation for overall outcomes in 26 different medical procedures and diagnoses.

The Hospital is a member of the New York-Presbyterian Healthcare System and the Stellaris Health Network.

MEDICAL STAFF

With nearly 700 members on its medical and dental staff, WPHC is well-positioned to deliver both general and subspecialty care. Many of these physicians have trained at well-known academic medical centers, and approximately 90% are board-certified.

CENTERS OF EXCELLENCE

The Hospital's Centers of Excellence include:

The Ruth and Jerome A. Siegel Stroke Center: The Hospital was the first in Westchester County to receive Stroke Center designation from the New York State Department of Health. The Stroke Center has been also cited by HealthGrades™ as being among the top 10% in the nation for stroke care.

The Westchester Orthopaedic Institute: The care delivered by this partnership between the Hospital and many of its orthopedic surgeons is renowned for the scope of its services that range from pre-op education to follow-up care after surgery for a wide array of bone, joint, and spine conditions. More hip and knee replacement surgeries have been performed at WPHC than at any other hospital in Westchester.

The William & Sylvia Silberstein Neonatal & Maternity Center: A redesigned and refurbished Labor & Delivery unit, backed up by a Level III Neonatal Intensive Care Unit – the highest designation available to a community hospital – is part of the reason why this program leads Westchester County in number of deliveries, year after year. The maternity program recently received a five-star rating from HealthGrades™.

The Dickstein Cancer Treatment Center: The only freestanding outpatient oncology treatment program in the County anchors a wide range of services that include a linear accelerator for radiation therapy, as well as a state-of-the-art infusion center for chemotherapy and other intravenous treatments. In addition, the Dickstein Center's Complementary Care Program provides various support groups, and classes in yoga, mental imagery, art therapy, and meditation.

Bariatric Surgery Center: The hospital's accredited Bariatric Surgery Center offers a comprehensive program for surgical weight loss. Procedures include laparoscopic Roux-en-Y bypass and Vertical Banded Gastroplasty.

GROWING FOR THE FUTURE

A major capital campaign raised more than $39 million for numerous clinical services, including expansion of the Emergency Department.

Physician Referral: To choose a White Plains Hospital Center doctor, call the 24-hour Physician Referral Service at (914) 681-1010.

769

Sponsored Page

The State of New Jersey

Bergen

Bergen

Allergy & Immunology

Falk, Theodore MD (A&I) - **Spec Exp:** Asthma; Immune Deficiency; Chronic Fatigue Syndrome; **Hospital:** Holy Name Hosp (page 761), Englewood Hosp & Med Ctr (page 760); **Address:** 63 Grand Ave, River Edge, NJ 07661-1930; **Phone:** 201-487-2900; **Board Cert:** Pediatrics 1982; **Med School:** Belgium 1977; **Resid:** Pediatrics, Long Island Jewish Med Ctr 1980; **Fellow:** Allergy & Immunology, Nassau Co Med Ctr 1982

Goodstein, Carolyn E MD (A&I) - **Spec Exp:** Asthma; Rhinitis; Urticaria; **Hospital:** Englewood Hosp & Med Ctr (page 760), Hackensack Univ Med Ctr (page 92); **Address:** 180 N Dean St, Ste 18, Englewood, NJ 07631-2534; **Phone:** 201-871-4755; **Board Cert:** Internal Medicine 1974; Allergy & Immunology 1980; **Med School:** SUNY Downstate 1964; **Resid:** Internal Medicine, Montefiore Med Ctr 1967; Allergy & Immunology, Roosevelt Hosp 1971

Harish, Ziv MD (A&I) - **Spec Exp:** Asthma & Sinusitis; Hay Fever; Urticaria; Eczema; **Hospital:** Englewood Hosp & Med Ctr (page 760), Holy Name Hosp (page 761); **Address:** 200 Engle St, Ste 18, Englewood, NJ 07631; **Phone:** 201-871-7475; **Board Cert:** Pediatrics 1989; Allergy & Immunology 2001; **Med School:** Israel 1983; **Resid:** Pediatrics, Albert Einstein Med Ctr 1989; **Fellow:** Allergy & Immunology, Albert Einstein Med Ctr 1991; **Fac Appt:** Asst Clin Prof Med, Albert Einstein Coll Med

Lo Galbo, Peter MD (A&I) - **Spec Exp:** Asthma; Food Allergy; **Hospital:** Pascack Valley Hosp, Good Samaritan Hosp - Suffern; **Address:** 177 N Dean St, South Penthouse, Englewood, NJ 07631; **Phone:** 201-722-9850; **Board Cert:** Pediatrics 1983; Allergy & Immunology 1983; Pediatric Rheumatology 2001; Clinical & Laboratory Immunology 1994; **Med School:** SUNY Stony Brook 1978; **Resid:** Pediatrics, Mount Sinai Med Ctr 1980; **Fellow:** Allergy & Immunology, Duke Univ Med Ctr 1982; **Fac Appt:** Asst Clin Prof Ped, Albert Einstein Coll Med

Michelis, Mary Ann MD (A&I) - **Spec Exp:** Asthma; Immune Deficiency; **Hospital:** Hackensack Univ Med Ctr (page 92), Valley Hosp (page 762); **Address:** Hackensack Univ Medical Ctr, 30 Prospect Ave, rm 3674, Hackensack, NJ 07601-1915; **Phone:** 201-996-2065; **Board Cert:** Internal Medicine 1978; Allergy & Immunology 1981; **Med School:** Univ Pittsburgh 1975; **Resid:** Internal Medicine, Lenox Hill Hosp 1978; **Fellow:** Allergy & Immunology, NY Hosp-Cornell Med Ctr 1978; **Fac Appt:** Assoc Clin Prof Med, UMDNJ-NJ Med Sch, Newark

Minikes, Neil MD (A&I) - **Spec Exp:** Asthma; Food Allergy; Hay Fever; Sinus Disorders; **Hospital:** Englewood Hosp & Med Ctr (page 760), NY-Presby Hosp (page 100); **Address:** 570 Peirmont Rd, 17 Closter Commons, Closter, NJ 07624; **Phone:** 201-768-8811; **Board Cert:** Pediatrics 1986; Allergy & Immunology 1991; **Med School:** Columbia P&S 1980; **Resid:** Pediatrics, Columbia Presby Med Ctr 1983; **Fellow:** Allergy & Immunology, LI Jewish Med Ctr 1990; **Fac Appt:** Asst Clin Prof Ped, Columbia P&S

Cardiovascular Disease

Berkowitz, Walter MD (Cv) - **Spec Exp:** Arrhythmias; Coronary Artery Disease; Hypertension; **Hospital:** Englewood Hosp & Med Ctr (page 760), NY-Presby Hosp (page 100); **Address:** 2200 Fletcher Ave, Fort Lee, NJ 07024-5005; **Phone:** 201-461-6200; **Board Cert:** Internal Medicine 1969; Cardiovascular Disease 1972; **Med School:** SUNY Downstate 1962; **Resid:** Internal Medicine, Mt Sinai Hosp 1965; **Fellow:** Cardiovascular Disease, Montefiore Med Ctr 1967

Blood, David K MD (Cv) - **Spec Exp:** Nuclear Cardiology; Transplant Medicine-Heart; **Hospital:** Englewood Hosp & Med Ctr (page 760), NY-Presby Hosp (page 100); **Address:** 163 Engle St, 1C Bldg, Englewood, NJ 07631; **Phone:** 201-569-3313; **Board Cert:** Internal Medicine 1972; Cardiovascular Disease 1975; **Med School:** Columbia P&S 1966; **Resid:** Internal Medicine, Bellevue Hosp 1970; Internal Medicine, Harlem Hosp 1972; **Fellow:** Cardiovascular Disease, Columbia-Presby Med Ctr 1974; **Fac Appt:** Assoc Clin Prof Med, Columbia P&S

Conroy Jr, Daniel P MD (Cv) - **Hospital:** PBI Regional- Passaic, St Mary's Hosp - Passaic; **Address:** 358 Valley Brook Ave, Lyndhurst, NJ 07071; **Phone:** 201-460-0142; **Board Cert:** Internal Medicine 1979; Cardiovascular Disease 1981; **Med School:** Mexico 1975; **Resid:** Internal Medicine, St Michael's Med Ctr 1978; **Fellow:** Cardiovascular Disease, St Michael's Med Ctr 1980

Eisenberg, Sheldon MD (Cv) - **Spec Exp:** Nuclear Cardiology; Preventive Cardiology; Coronary Artery Disease; **Hospital:** Pascack Valley Hosp, Hackensack Univ Med Ctr (page 92); **Address:** 333 Old Hook Rd, Ste 200, Westwood, NJ 07675-3200; **Phone:** 201-664-0201; **Board Cert:** Internal Medicine 1979; Cardiovascular Disease 1981; Critical Care Medicine 1997; **Med School:** Cornell Univ-Weill Med Coll 1976; **Resid:** Internal Medicine, N Shore Univ Hosp 1979; **Fellow:** Cardiovascular Disease, N Shore Univ Hosp 1981

Erlebacher, Jay A MD (Cv) - **Spec Exp:** Pacemakers; Congestive Heart Failure; Cardiac Stress Testing; **Hospital:** Englewood Hosp & Med Ctr (page 760); **Address:** 200 Grand Ave, Ste 202, Englewood, NJ 07631-4363; **Phone:** 201-569-4901; **Board Cert:** Internal Medicine 1978; Cardiovascular Disease 1981; **Med School:** SUNY Upstate Med Univ 1975; **Resid:** Internal Medicine, Einstein-Bronx Muni Hosp Ctr 1978; **Fellow:** Cardiovascular Disease, Johns Hopkins Hosp 1980; **Fac Appt:** Asst Clin Prof Med, Cornell Univ-Weill Med Coll

Goldfischer, Jerome D MD (Cv) - **Spec Exp:** Heart Valve Disease; Preventive Cardiology; Ischemic Heart Disease; **Hospital:** Englewood Hosp & Med Ctr (page 760), Montefiore Med Ctr; **Address:** 1555 Center Ave, Fort Lee, NJ 07024-4612; **Phone:** 201-945-1144; **Board Cert:** Internal Medicine 1962; Cardiovascular Disease 1975; **Med School:** NYU Sch Med 1955; **Resid:** Internal Medicine, Montefiore Hosp Med Ctr 1960; **Fellow:** Cardiovascular Disease, Montefiore Hosp Med Ctr 1963; **Fac Appt:** Asst Clin Prof Med, Albert Einstein Coll Med

Goldweit, Richard MD (Cv) - **Spec Exp:** Interventional Cardiology; Sleep Disorders/Cardiac Risk; Peripheral Vascular Disease; Cardiac Catheterization; **Hospital:** Englewood Hosp & Med Ctr (page 760); **Address:** 200 Grand Ave, Ste 202, Englewood, NJ 07631-4363; **Phone:** 201-569-4901; **Board Cert:** Internal Medicine 1985; Cardiovascular Disease 1987; Interventional Cardiology 1999; **Med School:** Cornell Univ-Weill Med Coll 1982; **Resid:** Internal Medicine, New York Hosp 1985; **Fellow:** Cardiovascular Disease, New York Hosp-Cornell Med Ctr 1987

Haft, Jacob I MD (Cv) - **Spec Exp:** Coronary Artery Disease; Arrhythmias; Heart Failure; **Hospital:** Saint Michael's Med Ctr, Hackensack Univ Med Ctr (page 92); **Address:** 20 Prospect Ave, Hackensack, NJ 07601; **Phone:** 201-343-8505; **Board Cert:** Internal Medicine 1968; Cardiovascular Disease 1973; Cardiac Electrophysiology 1994; **Med School:** Columbia P&S 1962; **Resid:** Internal Medicine, Beth Israel Hosp 1964; Internal Medicine, Bellevue-Columbia P&S 1968; **Fellow:** Cardiovascular Disease, Mt Sinai Hosp 1965; Cardiovascular Disease, Peter Bent Brigham Hosp 1969; **Fac Appt:** Prof Med, Seton Hall Univ Sch Grad Med Ed

Krakoff, Lawrence MD (Cv) - **Spec Exp:** Hypertension; **Hospital:** Englewood Hosp & Med Ctr (page 760), Mount Sinai Med Ctr (page 98); **Address:** 350 Engle St, Dept of Medicine, Englewood, NJ 07631; **Phone:** 201-894-3510; **Board Cert:** Internal Medicine 1971; **Med School:** Columbia P&S 1963; **Resid:** Internal Medicine, Columbia Presby Med Ctr 1968; **Fellow:** Cardiovascular Disease, Columbia Presby Med Ctr 1970; **Fac Appt:** Prof Med, Mount Sinai Sch Med

Landers, David B MD (Cv) - **Spec Exp:** Cardiac Catheterization; Coronary Angioplasty/Stents; **Hospital:** Hackensack Univ Med Ctr (page 92), Holy Name Hosp (page 761); **Address:** 222 Cedar Ln, Ste 208, Teaneck, NJ 07666-4312; **Phone:** 201-907-0442; **Board Cert:** Internal Medicine 1983; Cardiovascular Disease 1987; Interventional Cardiology 1999; **Med School:** Georgetown Univ 1979; **Resid:** Internal Medicine, St Vincents Hosp 1982; **Fellow:** Cardiovascular Disease, Westchester Co Med Ctr 1985; **Fac Appt:** Asst Clin Prof Med, UMDNJ-NJ Med Sch, Newark

Landzberg, Joel MD (Cv) - **Spec Exp:** Preventive Cardiology; Coronary Angioplasty/Stents; Heart Valve Disease; **Hospital:** Pascack Valley Hosp, Hackensack Univ Med Ctr (page 92); **Address:** 333 Old Hook Rd, Ste 200, Westwood, NJ 07675-3200; **Phone:** 201-664-0201; **Board Cert:** Internal Medicine 1986; Cardiovascular Disease 1989; Interventional Cardiology 2003; **Med School:** Columbia P&S 1983; **Resid:** Internal Medicine, Vanderbilt Univ Hosp 1986; **Fellow:** Cardiology Research, Moffit Hosp-UCSF 1987; Cardiovascular Disease, Brigham & Womens Hosp 1991; **Fac Appt:** Asst Clin Prof Med, UMDNJ-NJ Med Sch, Newark

Lau, Henry MD (Cv) - **Hospital:** Hackensack Univ Med Ctr (page 92); **Address:** 211 Essex St, Ste 403, Hackensack, NJ 07601; **Phone:** 201-646-0044; **Board Cert:** Internal Medicine 1977; Cardiovascular Disease 1981; **Med School:** Taiwan 1973; **Resid:** Internal Medicine, Hackensack Univ Med Ctr 1977; **Fellow:** Cardiovascular Disease, Hackensack Univ Med Ctr 1980

Lauricella, Joseph MD (Cv) - **Spec Exp:** Coronary Artery Disease; **Hospital:** Holy Name Hosp (page 761), Hackensack Univ Med Ctr (page 92); **Address:** 292 Columbia Ave, Fort Lee, NJ 07024-4124; **Phone:** 201-224-0050; **Board Cert:** Internal Medicine 1985; **Med School:** Mexico 1978; **Resid:** Internal Medicine, Rutgers Univ Med Ctr 1985

Pumill, Rick MD (Cv) - **Spec Exp:** Coronary Artery Disease; Hypertension; Congestive Heart Failure; **Hospital:** Hackensack Univ Med Ctr (page 92), Meadowlands Hosp Med Ctr; **Address:** 103 River Rd Fl 2, Edgewater, NJ 07020-1002; **Phone:** 201-941-8100; **Board Cert:** Internal Medicine 1988; Cardiovascular Disease 2001; **Med School:** Dominica 1984; **Resid:** Internal Medicine, Jersey City Med Ctr 1988; **Fellow:** Cardiovascular Disease, Jersey City Med Ctr 1990

Rossakis, Constantine MD (Cv) - **Spec Exp:** Interventional Cardiology; **Hospital:** Hackensack Univ Med Ctr (page 92); **Address:** 357 Prospect Ave, Hackensack, NJ 07601-2505; **Phone:** 201-489-3440; **Board Cert:** Internal Medicine 1986; Cardiovascular Disease 1989; **Med School:** NYU Sch Med 1983; **Resid:** Internal Medicine, New York Hosp-Cornell Med Ctr 1986; **Fellow:** Cardiovascular Disease, New York Hosp-Cornell Med Ctr 1989; **Fac Appt:** Asst Clin Prof Med, Cornell Univ-Weill Med Coll

Rothman, Howard MD (Cv) - **Spec Exp:** Cholesterol/Lipid Disorders; Angina; Women's Health; **Hospital:** Englewood Hosp & Med Ctr (page 760), NY-Presby Hosp (page 100); **Address:** 2200 Fletcher Ave, Fort Lee, NJ 07024-5005; **Phone:** 201-461-6200; **Board Cert:** Internal Medicine 1975; Cardiovascular Disease 1979; **Med School:** Univ Cincinnati 1970; **Resid:** Internal Medicine, New York Hosp-Cornell Med Ctr 1975; **Fellow:** Cardiovascular Disease, New York Hosp-Cornell Med Ctr 1976; **Fac Appt:** Asst Clin Prof Med, Columbia P&S

Salerno, William MD (Cv) - **Hospital:** Hackensack Univ Med Ctr (page 92); **Address:** 38 Mayhill St, Heartcare Center, Saddle Brook, NJ 07663-5307; **Phone:** 201-843-1019; **Board Cert:** Internal Medicine 1987; Cardiovascular Disease 1989; Critical Care Medicine 2001; **Med School:** Mexico 1982; **Resid:** Internal Medicine, Hackensack Med Ctr 1986; Critical Care Medicine, Norwalk Hosp 1987; **Fellow:** Cardiovascular Disease, Hackensack Med Ctr 1989; Interventional Cardiology, Hackensack Med Ctr 1990; **Fac Appt:** Assoc Clin Prof Med, UMDNJ-NJ Med Sch, Newark

Sotsky, Gerald MD (Cv) - **Hospital:** Valley Hosp (page 762); **Address:** 1200 E Ridgewood Ave, Ridgewood, NJ 07450; **Phone:** 201-670-8660; **Board Cert:** Internal Medicine 1984; Cardiovascular Disease 1987; Critical Care Medicine 1989; **Med School:** Mount Sinai Sch Med 1981; **Resid:** Internal Medicine, Mt Sinai Med Ctr 1984; **Fellow:** Cardiovascular Disease, Mt Sinai Med Ctr 1986

Teichholz, Louis MD (Cv) - **Spec Exp:** Mitral Valve Disease; Complementary Medicine; Echocardiography; **Hospital:** Hackensack Univ Med Ctr (page 92); **Address:** Hackensack Univ Med Ctr, 30 Prospect Ave, Ste 4655, Hackensack, NJ 07601; **Phone:** 201-996-2314; **Board Cert:** Internal Medicine 1972; Cardiovascular Disease 1975; **Med School:** Harvard Med Sch 1966; **Resid:** Internal Medicine, Peter Bent Brigham Hosp 1968; **Fellow:** Cardiovascular Disease, Peter Bent Brigham Hosp 1972; **Fac Appt:** Prof Med, UMDNJ-NJ Med Sch, Newark

Weinstock, Murray MD (Cv) - **Spec Exp:** Cholesterol/Lipid Disorders; Angina; Hypertension; **Hospital:** Hackensack Univ Med Ctr (page 92); **Address:** 150 Overlook Ave, Hackensack, NJ 07601; **Phone:** 201-489-5999; **Board Cert:** Cardiovascular Disease 1975; Internal Medicine 1972; **Med School:** Boston Univ 1965; **Resid:** Internal Medicine, Albert Einstein Med Ctr 1968; Cardiovascular Disease, VA Hospital 1970; **Fellow:** Cardiovascular Disease, Mt Sinai Med Ctr 1969; **Fac Appt:** Asst Prof Med, UMDNJ-NJ Med Sch, Newark

CHILD & ADOLESCENT PSYCHIATRY

Levine, Allwyn MD (ChAP) - **Spec Exp:** Forensic Psychiatry; ADD/ADHD; Anxiety & Depression; **Address:** 179 S Maple Ave, Ridgewood, NJ 07450-4541; **Phone:** 201-652-4335; **Board Cert:** Psychiatry 1977; Child & Adolescent Psychiatry 1981; **Med School:** SUNY Buffalo 1967; **Resid:** Psychiatry, Univ Mich Med 1973; **Fellow:** Child & Adolescent Psychiatry, Univ Mich Med 1975

CLINICAL GENETICS

Wallerstein, Robert MD (CG) - **Spec Exp:** Connective Tissue Disorders; Chromosome Disorders; Genetic Disorders; **Hospital:** Hackensack Univ Med Ctr (page 92); **Address:** Hackensack Univ Med Ctr, 30 Prospect Ave, Ste 258, Hackensack, NJ 07601; **Phone:** 201-996-5264; **Board Cert:** Pediatrics 2002; Clinical Genetics 1996; Clinical Cytogenetics 1996; **Med School:** UMDNJ-RW Johnson Med Sch 1991; **Resid:** Pediatrics, RW Johnson Med Sch 1994; **Fellow:** Clinical Genetics, Jefferson Med Coll 1996; **Fac Appt:** Assoc Prof Ped, UMDNJ-NJ Med Sch, Newark

COLON & RECTAL SURGERY

Helbraun, Mark MD (CRS) - **Spec Exp:** Colonoscopy; Rectal Cancer; **Hospital:** Hackensack Univ Med Ctr (page 92), Pascack Valley Hosp; **Address:** 20 Prospect Ave, Ste 811, Hackensack, NJ 07601; **Phone:** 201-525-1660; **Board Cert:** Colon & Rectal Surgery 1978; **Med School:** Wayne State Univ 1972; **Resid:** Surgery, New York Hosp-Cornell 1977; **Fellow:** Colon & Rectal Surgery, Lahey Clinic 1978

McConnell, John MD (CRS) - **Spec Exp:** Colonoscopy; Ultrasound; Inflammatory Bowel Disease; **Hospital:** Valley Hosp (page 762), Chilton Meml Hosp; **Address:** 414 Saddle River Rd, Fair Lawn, NJ 07410-5624; **Phone:** 201-791-4002; **Board Cert:** Surgery 1999; Colon & Rectal Surgery 1980; **Med School:** Columbia P&S 1974; **Resid:** Surgery, St Luke's Hosp 1979; **Fellow:** Colon & Rectal Surgery, Lehigh Valley Hosp 1980

Nizin, Joel MD (CRS) - **Spec Exp:** Colon Cancer; Inflammatory Bowel Disease; **Hospital:** Valley Hosp (page 762), Chilton Meml Hosp; **Address:** 414 Saddle River Rd, Fair Lawn, NJ 07410-5624; **Phone:** 201-791-4002; **Board Cert:** Surgery 1997; Colon & Rectal Surgery 1987; **Med School:** Howard Univ 1978; **Resid:** Surgery, St Luke's Hosp 1983; **Fellow:** Colon & Rectal Surgery, Univ Minn Med Ctr 1984

Waxenbaum, Steven MD (CRS) - **Spec Exp:** Laparoscopic Surgery; Hemorrhoids; Colon Cancer; **Hospital:** Valley Hosp (page 762), Englewood Hosp & Med Ctr (page 760); **Address:** 216 Engle St, Englewood, NJ 07631; **Phone:** 201-567-7615; **Board Cert:** Surgery 2003; Colon & Rectal Surgery 2004; **Med School:** UMDNJ-RW Johnson Med Sch 1988; **Resid:** Surgery, Westchester Med Ctr 1993; **Fellow:** Colon & Rectal Surgery, Lehigh Valley Hosp 1994

White, Ronald A MD (CRS) - **Spec Exp:** Hemorrhoids; Colon & Rectal Cancer; Colonoscopy; **Hospital:** Englewood Hosp & Med Ctr (page 760), Valley Hosp (page 762); **Address:** 216 Engle St, Ste 203, Englewood, NJ 07631-2428; **Phone:** 201-567-7615; **Board Cert:** Surgery 1996; Colon & Rectal Surgery 1988; **Med School:** Boston Univ 1981; **Resid:** Surgery, Montefiore Hosp 1986; **Fellow:** Colon & Rectal Surgery, RW Johnson Med Sch 1987

CRITICAL CARE MEDICINE

Cornell, James MD/PhD (CCM) - **Spec Exp:** Respiratory Distress Syndrome; Lung Cancer; Chronic Obstructive Lung Disease (COPD); **Hospital:** Valley Hosp (page 762); **Address:** 31-00 Broadway, Fair Lawn, NJ 07410-2305; **Phone:** 201-796-2255; **Board Cert:** Internal Medicine 2002; Pulmonary Disease 1999; **Med School:** Cornell Univ-Weill Med Coll 1988; **Resid:** Internal Medicine, New York Hosp-Cornell 1991; Pulmonary Disease, Meml Sloan Kettering Cancer Ctr 1991; **Fellow:** Pulmonary Critical Care Medicine, New York Hosp-Cornell 1994

Melamed, Marc S MD (CCM) - **Spec Exp:** Asthma; Respiratory Failure; Sepsis; **Hospital:** Valley Hosp (page 762); **Address:** 44 Godwin Ave, Ste 201, Midland Park, NJ 07432-1969; **Phone:** 201-689-7755; **Board Cert:** Internal Medicine 1980; Critical Care Medicine 1997; **Med School:** NYU Sch Med 1977; **Resid:** Internal Medicine, Montefiore Med Ctr 1980; **Fellow:** Critical Care Medicine, Montefiore Med Ctr 1981

DERMATOLOGY

Ashinoff, Robin MD (D) - **Spec Exp:** Mohs' Surgery; Laser Surgery; Cosmetic Dermatology; **Hospital:** Hackensack Univ Med Ctr (page 92), NYU Med Ctr (page 102); **Address:** 360 Essex St, Ste 201, Hackensack, NJ 07601; **Phone:** 201-336-6880; **Board Cert:** Dermatology 1989; **Med School:** NYU Sch Med 1985; **Resid:** Dermatology, NYU Med Ctr 1989; **Fellow:** Mohs Surgery, NYU Med Ctr 1991; **Fac Appt:** Assoc Clin Prof D, NYU Sch Med

Brauner, Gary MD (D) - **Spec Exp:** Skin Laser Surgery; Black/Asian Skin Care; Cosmetic Dermatology; Laser Hair Removal; **Hospital:** Englewood Hosp & Med Ctr (page 760), Mount Sinai Med Ctr (page 98); **Address:** 1625 Anderson Ave, Fort Lee, NJ 07024; **Phone:** 201-461-5522; **Board Cert:** Dermatology 1972; Dermatopathology 1978; **Med School:** Harvard Med Sch 1967; **Resid:** Dermatology, Jewish Hosp 1968; Dermatology, Mass Genl Hosp 1971; **Fac Appt:** Assoc Clin Prof D, Mount Sinai Sch Med

Corey, Timothy MD (D) - **Spec Exp:** Psoriasis; Skin Cancer; **Hospital:** Valley Hosp (page 762), NY-Presby Hosp (page 100); **Address:** 400 Rt 17 S, Ridgewood, NJ 07450; **Phone:** 201-652-4536; **Board Cert:** Dermatology 1979; **Med School:** Columbia P&S 1975; **Resid:** Dermatology, Columbia Presby Med Ctr 1979; **Fac Appt:** Asst Clin Prof D, Columbia P&S

Fine, Herbert MD (D) - **Spec Exp:** Acne; **Hospital:** Pascack Valley Hosp; **Address:** 390 Old Hook Rd, Westwood, NJ 07675-2616; **Phone:** 201-666-9550; **Board Cert:** Dermatology 1969; **Med School:** Univ Hlth Sci/Chicago Med Sch 1961; **Resid:** Dermatology, Bellevue Hosp 1967; **Fac Appt:** Asst Clin Prof D, NYU Sch Med

Fishman, Miriam MD (D) - **Spec Exp:** Pediatric Dermatology; Skin Cancer; **Hospital:** Englewood Hosp & Med Ctr (page 760); **Address:** 216 Engle St, Ste 104, Englewood, NJ 07631-2428; **Phone:** 201-569-5678; **Board Cert:** Dermatology 1984; **Med School:** NYU Sch Med 1978; **Resid:** Pediatrics, Montefiore Med Ctr 1981; Dermatology, Albert Einstein Med Ctr 1984

Fried, Sharon MD (D) - **Spec Exp:** Skin Cancer; Acne; Psoriasis; **Hospital:** Englewood Hosp & Med Ctr (page 760); **Address:** 180 N Dean St, Englewood, NJ 07631-2534; **Phone:** 201-569-9800; **Board Cert:** Internal Medicine 1983; Dermatology 1987; **Med School:** NYU Sch Med 1980; **Resid:** Internal Medicine, NYU Med Ctr 1983; Dermatology, SUNY Downstate HSC 1985

Grodberg, Michele MD (D) - **Spec Exp:** Cosmetic Dermatology; Hair Removal-Laser; Botox Therapy; **Hospital:** Englewood Hosp & Med Ctr (page 760); **Address:** 106 Grand Ave Fl 3, Englewood, NJ 07631-3574; **Phone:** 201-567-8884; **Board Cert:** Dermatology 2001; **Med School:** NYU Sch Med 1987; **Resid:** Dermatology, NYU Med Ctr 1991

Heldman, Jay MD (D) - **Spec Exp:** Dermatologic Surgery; **Hospital:** Valley Hosp (page 762); **Address:** 2300 Route 208 S, Fair Lawn, NJ 07410-1559; **Phone:** 201-797-7770; **Board Cert:** Dermatology 1981; **Med School:** Columbia P&S 1977; **Resid:** Internal Medicine, Columbia-Presby Med Ctr 1978; Dermatology, Mt Sinai Med Ctr 1981

Possick, Paul MD (D) - **Spec Exp:** Skin Cancer; **Hospital:** Pascack Valley Hosp; **Address:** 390 Old Hook Rd Fl 2, Westwood, NJ 07675-2616; **Phone:** 201-666-9550; **Board Cert:** Dermatology 1969; **Med School:** Tufts Univ 1964; **Resid:** Internal Medicine, Montefiore Hosp 1966; Dermatology, Univ Hosp 1968; **Fac Appt:** Asst Prof D, NYU Sch Med

Rapaport, Jeffrey A MD (D) - **Spec Exp:** Cosmetic Dermatology; Scar Revision; Skin Laser Surgery; **Hospital:** Englewood Hosp & Med Ctr (page 760), Holy Name Hosp (page 761); **Address:** 333 Sylvan Ave, Ste 207, Englewood Cliffs, NJ 07632; **Phone:** 201-227-1555; **Board Cert:** Dermatology 1983; **Med School:** Emory Univ 1979; **Resid:** Dermatology, Jefferson Univ Hosp 1982

Scherl, Sharon MD (D) - **Spec Exp:** Skin Cancer; Psoriasis; Cosmetic Dermatology; **Hospital:** Englewood Hosp & Med Ctr (page 760); **Address:** 45 Central Ave, Tenafly, NJ 07670; **Phone:** 201-568-8400; **Board Cert:** Dermatology 1999; **Med School:** NY Med Coll 1988; **Resid:** Dermatology, Metropolitian Hosp Ctr 1992

Sweeney, Eugene MD (D) - **Spec Exp:** Skin Cancer; Pediatric Dermatology; Acne; **Hospital:** Holy Name Hosp (page 761), Englewood Hosp & Med Ctr (page 760); **Address:** 757 Teaneck Rd, Teaneck, NJ 07666-4846; **Phone:** 201-837-3939; **Board Cert:** Dermatology 1967; **Med School:** NY Med Coll 1960; **Resid:** Dermatology, Columbia-Presby Med Ctr 1966; **Fac Appt:** Assoc Prof D, Columbia P&S

DIAGNOSTIC RADIOLOGY

Baldasar, Jack L MD (DR) - **Spec Exp:** MRI; **Hospital:** NY Westchester Sq Med Ctr; **Address:** 177 N Dean St Fl P2, Englewood, NJ 07631; **Phone:** 201-871-1950; **Board Cert:** Diagnostic Radiology 1979; **Med School:** SUNY Hlth Sci Ctr 1974; **Resid:** Diagnostic Radiology, Bronx Muni Hosp 1979

Budin, Joel A MD (DR) - **Spec Exp:** Neuroradiology; **Hospital:** Hackensack Univ Med Ctr (page 92); **Address:** 130 Kinderkamack Rd, Riveredge, NJ 07661; **Phone:** 201-488-1188; **Board Cert:** Diagnostic Radiology 1975; **Med School:** Columbia P&S 1969; **Resid:** Diagnostic Radiology, Columbia-Presby Med Ctr 1975

Calem-Grunat, Jaclyn A MD (DR) - **Spec Exp:** Breast Imaging; **Hospital:** Valley Hosp (page 762); **Address:** Radiology Assocs of Ridgewood, 20 Franklin Tpke, Waldwick, NJ 07463; **Phone:** 201-445-8822; **Board Cert:** Diagnostic Radiology 1994; **Med School:** Mount Sinai Sch Med 1988; **Resid:** Internal Medicine, Beeth Israel Med Ctr 1990; Diagnostic Radiology, Harbor-UCLA Med Ctr 1994; **Fellow:** Breast Imaging, UCLA Med Ctr 1995

Krinsky, Glenn MD (DR) - **Spec Exp:** MRI; Musculoskeletal Imaging; **Hospital:** Valley Hosp (page 762); **Address:** Radiology Assocs of Ridgewood, 20 Franklin Tpke, Waldwick, NJ 07463; **Phone:** 201-445-8822; **Board Cert:** Diagnostic Radiology 1994; **Med School:** NYU Sch Med 1988; **Resid:** Surgical Pathology, Bellevue Hosp 1990; Diagnostic Radiology, Bellevue Hosp 1993; **Fellow:** Magnetic Resonance Imaging, NYU/Bellevue Hosp 1994

Levy, Lauren S MD (DR) - **Spec Exp:** Breast Imaging; **Hospital:** Valley Hosp (page 762); **Address:** Radiology Assocs of Ridgewood, 20 Franklin Tpke, Waldwick, NJ 07463; **Phone:** 201-445-8822; **Board Cert:** Diagnostic Radiology 1996; **Med School:** SUNY Downstate 1991; **Resid:** Diagnostic Radiology, NYU-Bellevue Hosp 1996; **Fellow:** Mammography, NYU-Bellevue Hosp 1997

Lubat, Edward MD (DR) - **Spec Exp:** Abdominal Imaging; Thoracic Radiology; Musculoskeletal Imaging; Nuclear Medicine; **Hospital:** Valley Hosp (page 762); **Address:** 20 Franklin Tpke, Waldwick, NJ 07463-1749; **Phone:** 201-445-8822; **Board Cert:** Diagnostic Radiology 1989; Nuclear Medicine 1989; **Med School:** Jefferson Med Coll 1982; **Resid:** Radiology, NYU Med Ctr 1988; **Fellow:** Nuclear Medicine, NYU Med Ctr 1985

Rambler, Louis MD (DR) - **Spec Exp:** Ultrasound; **Hospital:** Valley Hosp (page 762); **Address:** 20 Franklin Tpke, Waldwick, NJ 07463-1749; **Phone:** 201-445-8822; **Board Cert:** Diagnostic Radiology 1977; **Med School:** Cornell Univ-Weill Med Coll 1971; **Resid:** Diagnostic Radiology, Columbia-Presby Med Ctr 1977

Sorabella, Philip MD (DR) - **Spec Exp:** Nuclear Medicine; Breast Imaging; **Hospital:** Valley Hosp (page 762); **Address:** 20 Franklin Tpke, Waldwick, NJ 07463-1749; **Phone:** 201-445-8822; **Board Cert:** Diagnostic Radiology 1974; Nuclear Medicine 1974; **Med School:** Columbia P&S 1968; **Resid:** Diagnostic Radiology, Columbia-Presby 1974

ENDOCRINOLOGY, DIABETES & METABOLISM

Cobin, Rhoda MD (EDM) - **Spec Exp:** Thyroid Disorders; Diabetes; Pituitary Disorders; **Hospital:** Valley Hosp (page 762), Mount Sinai Med Ctr (page 98); **Address:** 75 N Maple Ave, Ridgewood, NJ 07450; **Phone:** 201-444-5552; **Board Cert:** Internal Medicine 1972; Endocrinology, Diabetes & Metabolism 1975; **Med School:** Univ Puerto Rico 1969; **Resid:** Internal Medicine, Beth Israel Med Ctr 1972; **Fellow:** Endocrinology, Diabetes & Metabolism, Mt Sinai Hosp 1974; **Fac Appt:** Clin Prof Med, Mount Sinai Sch Med

Goldman, Michael MD (EDM) - **Spec Exp:** Thyroid Disorders; Diabetes; Pituitary Disorders; Cholesterol/Lipid Disorders; **Hospital:** Englewood Hosp & Med Ctr (page 760); **Address:** 600 E Palisade Ave, Englewood Cliffs, NJ 07632-1826; **Phone:** 201-568-1108; **Board Cert:** Internal Medicine 1980; Endocrinology, Diabetes & Metabolism 1981; **Med School:** NY Med Coll 1973; **Resid:** Internal Medicine, Englewood Hosp 1978; **Fellow:** Endocrinology, Diabetes & Metabolism, Columbia-Presby Med Ctr 1980; **Fac Appt:** Asst Prof Med, Mount Sinai Sch Med

Hochstein, Martin MD (EDM) - **Spec Exp:** Thyroid Disorders; Diabetes; Osteoporosis; **Hospital:** Valley Hosp (page 762), Hackensack Univ Med Ctr (page 92); **Address:** 1 Sears Drive, Paramus, NJ 07652; **Phone:** 201-261-2560; **Board Cert:** Internal Medicine 1973; Endocrinology, Diabetes & Metabolism 1975; **Med School:** Univ Louisville Sch Med 1969; **Resid:** Internal Medicine, Maimoides Med Ctr 1971; Internal Medicine, Jacobi Med Ctr 1972; **Fellow:** Endocrinology, Diabetes & Metabolism, Johns Hopkins Med Ctr 1975; **Fac Appt:** Assoc Clin Prof Med, UMDNJ-RW Johnson Med Sch

Tohme, Jack MD (EDM) - **Spec Exp:** Osteoporosis; Thyroid Disorders; **Hospital:** Valley Hosp (page 762), NY-Presby Hosp (page 100); **Address:** 265 Ackerman Ave, Ste 101, Ridgewood, NJ 07450-4203; **Phone:** 201-444-4363; **Board Cert:** Internal Medicine 1978; Endocrinology, Diabetes & Metabolism 1979; **Med School:** Lebanon 1974; **Resid:** Internal Medicine, American Univ Hosp 1976; **Fellow:** Endocrinology, Diabetes & Metabolism, Columbia-Presby Med Ctr 1977; Endocrinology, Diabetes & Metabolism, Barnes Hosp/Wash Univ 1979; **Fac Appt:** Asst Clin Prof Med, Columbia P&S

Wehmann, Robert MD/PhD (EDM) - **Spec Exp:** Diabetes; Thyroid Disorders; Pituitary Disorders; **Hospital:** Pascack Valley Hosp, Hackensack Univ Med Ctr (page 92); **Address:** 400 Old Hook Rd, Ste 1-4, Westwood, NJ 07675-2720; **Phone:** 201-666-1400; **Board Cert:** Internal Medicine 1977; Endocrinology 1979; **Med School:** Albany Med Coll 1974; **Resid:** Internal Medicine, VA Med Ctr 1976; **Fellow:** Endocrinology, Nat Inst Hlth 1979

Wiesen, Mark MD (EDM) - **Spec Exp:** Diabetes; Thyroid Disorders; Osteoporosis; **Hospital:** Hackensack Univ Med Ctr (page 92), Holy Name Hosp (page 761); **Address:** 870 Palisade Ave, Ste 203, Teaneck, NJ 07666; **Phone:** 201-836-5655; **Board Cert:** Internal Medicine 1978; Endocrinology, Diabetes & Metabolism 1981; **Med School:** Columbia P&S 1975; **Resid:** Internal Medicine, Brookdale Hosp 1978; **Fellow:** Endocrinology, Diabetes & Metabolism, Mt Sinai Hosp 1981; **Fac Appt:** Asst Clin Prof Med, UMDNJ-NJ Med Sch, Newark

FAMILY MEDICINE

Bello, Mary MD (FMed) `PCP` - **Spec Exp:** Adolescent Medicine; Geriatric Care; **Hospital:** Valley Hosp (page 762); **Address:** 400 Franklin Tpke, Ste 106, Mahwah, NJ 07430-3517; **Phone:** 201-327-3333; **Board Cert:** Family Medicine 2002; **Med School:** West Indies 1984; **Resid:** Family Medicine, St Joseph's Hosp 1987; **Fac Appt:** Asst Clin Prof FMed, UMDNJ-NJ Med Sch, Newark

Gross, Harvey MD (FMed) `PCP` - **Spec Exp:** Geriatrics; Dementia; Myasthenia Gravis; **Hospital:** Englewood Hosp & Med Ctr (page 760), Holy Name Hosp (page 761); **Address:** 370 Grand Ave, Englewood, NJ 07631; **Phone:** 201-567-3370; **Board Cert:** Family Medicine 1999; Geriatric Medicine 2000; **Med School:** Boston Univ 1970; **Resid:** Family Medicine, Southside Hosp 1974; **Fac Appt:** Asst Clin Prof Med, Mount Sinai Sch Med

Karatoprak, Ohan MD (FMed) - **Spec Exp:** Asthma; Nutrition; **Hospital:** Holy Name Hosp (page 761), Hackensack Univ Med Ctr (page 92); **Address:** 420 Deerwood Rd, Fort Lee, NJ 07024-1643; **Phone:** 201-886-8877; **Board Cert:** Family Medicine 1998; Geriatric Medicine 2003; **Med School:** Turkey 1977; **Resid:** Surgery, Brookdale Univ Hosp 1983; Family Medicine, Southside Hosp 1986; **Fac Appt:** Asst Clin Prof FMed, UMDNJ-NJ Med Sch, Newark

GASTROENTEROLOGY

Chessler, Richard MD (Ge) - **Spec Exp:** Gallbladder Disease; Colonoscopy; **Hospital:** Englewood Hosp & Med Ctr (page 760), Holy Name Hosp (page 761); **Address:** 1555 Center Ave, Fort Lee, NJ 07024-4612; **Phone:** 201-945-6564 x320; **Board Cert:** Internal Medicine 1972; Gastroenterology 1975; **Med School:** Univ Hlth Sci/Chicago Med Sch 1969; **Resid:** Internal Medicine, NY Med Coll/Flower-Fifth Ave Hosp 1972; **Fellow:** Gastroenterology, NY Med Coll/Flower-Fifth Ave Hosp 1974; **Fac Appt:** Asst Clin Prof Med, Mount Sinai Sch Med

Feit, David MD (Ge) - **Spec Exp:** Hepatitis; **Hospital:** Hackensack Univ Med Ctr (page 92); **Address:** 385 Prospect Ave, Hackensack, NJ 07601; **Phone:** 201-488-3003; **Board Cert:** Internal Medicine 1984; Gastroenterology 1989; **Med School:** Columbia P&S 1981; **Resid:** Internal Medicine, Columbia-Presby Med Ctr 1984; **Fellow:** Gastroenterology, Columbia-Presby Med Ctr 1987

Friedrich, Ivan MD (Ge) - **Spec Exp:** Colonoscopy; Pancreatic/Biliary Endoscopy (ERCP); Gallbladder Disease; **Hospital:** Englewood Hosp & Med Ctr (page 760), Holy Name Hosp (page 761); **Address:** 420 Grand Ave, Englewood, NJ 07631-4152; **Phone:** 201-569-7044; **Board Cert:** Internal Medicine 1979; Gastroenterology 1981; **Med School:** Albany Med Coll 1976; **Resid:** Internal Medicine, Montefiore Med Ctr 1979; **Fellow:** Gastroenterology, Mt Sinai Med Ctr 1982; **Fac Appt:** Asst Clin Prof Med, Mount Sinai Sch Med

Goldfarb, Joel MD (Ge) - **Spec Exp:** Hepatitis; Colonoscopy/Polypectomy; Colon Cancer; **Hospital:** Holy Name Hosp (page 761), Englewood Hosp & Med Ctr (page 760); **Address:** 1600 Parker Ave, Fort Lee, NJ 07024-7050; **Phone:** 201-461-2507; **Board Cert:** Internal Medicine 1978; Gastroenterology 1981; **Med School:** NYU Sch Med 1975; **Resid:** Internal Medicine, NYU Med Ctr 1978; **Fellow:** Hepatology, Yale-New Haven Hosp 1979; Gastroenterology, Columbia-Presby Med Ctr 1981; **Fac Appt:** Asst Clin Prof Med, Mount Sinai Sch Med

Klein, Walter A MD (Ge) - **Spec Exp:** Esophageal Disorders; Gastroesophageal Reflux Disease (GERD); Colon Polyps & Cancer; **Hospital:** Englewood Hosp & Med Ctr (page 760), Pascack Valley Hosp; **Address:** 274 County Rd, Ste A, Tenafly, NJ 07670; **Phone:** 201-568-0493; **Board Cert:** Internal Medicine 2000; Gastroenterology 2000; **Med School:** Cornell Univ-Weill Med Coll 1987; **Resid:** Internal Medicine, NY Hosp-Cornell Med Ctr 1990; **Fellow:** Gastroenterology, Temple Univ Hosp 1992; **Fac Appt:** Asst Clin Prof Med, Mount Sinai Sch Med

Margulis, Stephen MD (Ge) - **Spec Exp:** Hepatitis; Colonoscopy/Polypectomy; Peptic Ulcer Disease; **Hospital:** Pascack Valley Hosp, Valley Hosp (page 762); **Address:** 466 Old Hook Rd, Ste 1, Emerson, NJ 07630-1368; **Phone:** 201-967-8221; **Board Cert:** Internal Medicine 1984; Gastroenterology 1987; **Med School:** Brown Univ 1981; **Resid:** Internal Medicine, New York Hosp-Cornell 1984; **Fellow:** Gastroenterology, New York Hosp-Cornell 1987

Nikias, George A MD (Ge) - **Spec Exp:** Hepatitis; **Hospital:** Hackensack Univ Med Ctr (page 92); **Address:** 130 Kinderkamack Rd, Ste 301, River Edge, NJ 07661; **Phone:** 201-489-7772; **Board Cert:** Internal Medicine 2002; Gastroenterology 1995; **Med School:** NY Med Coll 1989; **Resid:** Internal Medicine, North Shore Univ Hosp 1992; **Fellow:** Gastroenterology, Meml Sloan Kettering Cancer Ctr 1993

Panella, Vincent S MD (Ge) - **Spec Exp:** Colon Cancer; Hepatitis C; Inflammatory Bowel Disease; Endoscopy; **Hospital:** Englewood Hosp & Med Ctr (page 760), Holy Name Hosp (page 761); **Address:** 420 Grand Ave, Englewood, NJ 07631-4141; **Phone:** 201-569-7044; **Board Cert:** Internal Medicine 1985; Gastroenterology 1987; **Med School:** NY Med Coll 1982; **Resid:** Internal Medicine, North Shore Univ Hosp 1985; **Fellow:** Gastroenterology, Mem Sloan-Kettering Cancer Cntr 1987; **Fac Appt:** Asst Clin Prof Med, Mount Sinai Sch Med

Rahmin, Michael G MD (Ge) - **Spec Exp:** Endoscopy; **Hospital:** Valley Hosp (page 762); **Address:** 140 Chestnut St, Ste 300, Ridgewood, NJ 07452; **Phone:** 201-444-2600; **Board Cert:** Internal Medicine 2002; Gastroenterology 2005; **Med School:** NYU Sch Med 1989; **Resid:** Internal Medicine, Mt Sinai Hosp 1992; **Fellow:** Gastroenterology, New York Hosp 1995

Roth, Joseph MD (Ge) - **Spec Exp:** Endoscopy; Inflammatory Bowel Disease; **Hospital:** PBI Regional- Passaic, PBI Regional- Passaic; **Address:** 71 Union Ave, Rutherford, NJ 07070-1272; **Phone:** 201-842-0020; **Board Cert:** Internal Medicine 1984; Gastroenterology 1987; **Med School:** Univ Pittsburgh 1981; **Resid:** Internal Medicine, Lenox Hill Hosp 1984; **Fellow:** Gastroenterology, Univ Conn Hlth Ctr 1986

Rubin, Kenneth MD (Ge) - **Spec Exp:** Colon Cancer; Inflammatory Bowel Disease; Gastroesophageal Reflux Disease (GERD); Endoscopy; **Hospital:** Englewood Hosp & Med Ctr (page 760), Mount Sinai Med Ctr (page 98); **Address:** 420 Grand Ave, Englewood, NJ 07631-4152; **Phone:** 201-569-7044; **Board Cert:** Internal Medicine 1978; Gastroenterology 1981; **Med School:** UMDNJ-NJ Med Sch, Newark 1975; **Resid:** Internal Medicine, Bronx Municipal Hosp 1979; **Fellow:** Gastroenterology, Mount Sinai Hosp 1981; **Fac Appt:** Asst Clin Prof Med, Mount Sinai Sch Med

Rubinoff, Mitchell MD (Ge) - **Spec Exp:** Hepatitis; Gastroesophageal Reflux Disease (GERD); **Hospital:** Valley Hosp (page 762); **Address:** 140 Chestnut St, Ste 300, Ridgewood, NJ 07450-2536; **Phone:** 201-444-2600; **Board Cert:** Internal Medicine 1982; Gastroenterology 1985; **Med School:** Mount Sinai Sch Med 1979; **Resid:** Internal Medicine, Columbia-Presby Med Ctr 1982; **Fellow:** Gastroenterology, Columbia-Presby Med Ctr 1985

Zingler, Barry MD (Ge) - **Spec Exp:** Colon Cancer; Hepatitis; Gastroesophageal Reflux Disease (GERD); **Hospital:** Englewood Hosp & Med Ctr (page 760), Holy Name Hosp (page 761); **Address:** 1555 Center Ave, Fort Lee, NJ 07024-4612; **Phone:** 201-945-6564; **Board Cert:** Internal Medicine 1988; Gastroenterology 1991; **Med School:** Rutgers Univ 1985; **Resid:** Internal Medicine, NYU Med Ctr 1988; **Fellow:** Gastroenterology, NYU Med Ctr 1990

Zucker, Ira MD (Ge) - **Spec Exp:** Colon Cancer; Gastroesophageal Reflux Disease (GERD); Ulcerative Colitis/Crohn's; **Hospital:** Pascack Valley Hosp, Hackensack Univ Med Ctr (page 92); **Address:** 452 Old Hook Rd, Emerson, NJ 07630; **Phone:** 201-666-3900; **Board Cert:** Internal Medicine 1984; Gastroenterology 1987; **Med School:** Univ Hlth Sci/Chicago Med Sch 1981; **Resid:** Internal Medicine, St Vincents Hosp 1984; **Fellow:** Gastroenterology, St Vincents Hosp 1986

GERIATRIC MEDICINE

Leifer, Bennett MD (Ger) **PCP** - **Spec Exp:** Dementia; Alzheimer's Disease; **Hospital:** Valley Hosp (page 762); **Address:** 301 Godwin Ave, Midland Park, NJ 07432-1544; **Phone:** 201-444-4526; **Board Cert:** Internal Medicine 2000; Geriatric Medicine 2000; **Med School:** SUNY Upstate Med Univ 1986; **Resid:** Internal Medicine, Hartford Hosp 1989; **Fellow:** Geriatric Medicine, Mt Sinai Hosp 1991

GYNECOLOGIC ONCOLOGY

Gafori, Iraj MD (GO) - **Hospital:** Hackensack Univ Med Ctr (page 92), Newark Beth Israel Med Ctr; **Address:** 20 Prospect Ave, Ste 801, Hackensack, NJ 07601-1963; **Phone:** 201-489-1808; **Board Cert:** Obstetrics & Gynecology 1979; **Med School:** Iran 1969; **Resid:** Surgery, Montefiore Med Ctr 1974; Obstetrics & Gynecology, W Virginia Med Ctr 1977; **Fellow:** Gynecologic Oncology, Hahnemann Univ Hosp 1981; **Fac Appt:** Assoc Clin Prof ObG, UMDNJ-NJ Med Sch, Newark

HAND SURGERY

Fakharzadeh, Frederick MD (HS) - **Hospital:** Hackensack Univ Med Ctr (page 92), Valley Hosp (page 762); **Address:** 22 Madison Ave, FL 3, Paramus, NJ 07652-2721; **Phone:** 201-587-7767; **Board Cert:** Orthopaedic Surgery 1999; Hand Surgery 1999; **Med School:** Columbia P&S 1980; **Resid:** Surgery, Roosevelt Hosp 1982; Orthopaedic Surgery, Columbia-Presby Med Ctr 1985; **Fellow:** Hand Surgery, Thomas Jefferson Univ Hosp 1986

Gurland, Mark MD (HS) - **Spec Exp:** Carpal Tunnel Syndrome; Wrist/Hand Injuries; Arthritis Hand Surgery; **Hospital:** Hackensack Univ Med Ctr (page 92), Englewood Hosp & Med Ctr (page 760); **Address:** 216 Engle St, Englewood, NJ 07631-2448; **Phone:** 201-568-4066; **Board Cert:** Orthopaedic Surgery 1999; Hand Surgery 1999; **Med School:** NYU Sch Med 1979; **Resid:** Surgery, Hosp U Penn 1980; Orthopaedic Surgery, Hosp For Joint Disease 1984; **Fellow:** Hand Surgery, Thos Jefferson U Hosp

Miller-Breslow, Anne MD (HS) - **Spec Exp:** Rheumatoid Arthritis; Wrist/Hand Injuries; Arthroscopic Surgery; **Hospital:** Englewood Hosp & Med Ctr (page 760), Holy Name Hosp (page 761); **Address:** 401 S Van Brunt St Fl 3, Englewood, NJ 07631-2904; **Phone:** 201-569-2770; **Board Cert:** Orthopaedic Surgery 2002; Hand Surgery 2002; **Med School:** Harvard Med Sch 1983; **Resid:** Orthopaedic Surgery, Montefiore Med Ctr 1988; **Fellow:** Hand Surgery, New England Med Ctr 1989

Rosenstein, Roger G MD (HS) - **Spec Exp:** Arthritis Hand Surgery; Nerve Compression; Carpal Tunnel Syndrome; **Hospital:** Hackensack Univ Med Ctr (page 92), Valley Hosp (page 762); **Address:** 22 Madison Ave, Ste 3-1, Paramus, NJ 07652-5474; **Phone:** 201-587-7767; **Board Cert:** Orthopaedic Surgery 1984; Hand Surgery 2000; **Med School:** Columbia P&S 1975; **Resid:** Surgery, St Luke's Roosevelt Hosp Ctr 1977; Orthopaedic Surgery, Columbia-Presby Med Ctr 1980; **Fellow:** Hand Surgery, Thomas Jefferson Univ Hosp 1981; **Fac Appt:** Assoc Clin Prof OrS, UMDNJ-NJ Med Sch, Newark

HEMATOLOGY

Fernbach, Barry R MD (Hem) - **Hospital:** Valley Hosp (page 762); **Address:** 1 Valley Health Plaza, Paramus, NJ 07652; **Phone:** 201-634-5353; **Board Cert:** Internal Medicine 1974; Medical Oncology 1977; Hematology 1982; **Med School:** Harvard Med Sch 1971; **Resid:** Internal Medicine, Mt Sinai Hosp 1973; Hematology, Mt Sinai Hosp 1976; **Fellow:** Neoplastic Diseases, Mt Sinai Hosp 1977

Harper, Harry MD (Hem) - **Spec Exp:** Lung Cancer; **Hospital:** Hackensack Univ Med Ctr (page 92), Holy Name Hosp (page 761); **Address:** 20 Prospect Ave, Ste 400, Hackensack, NJ 07601-1271; **Phone:** 201-996-5900; **Board Cert:** Internal Medicine 1980; Hematology 1982; Medical Oncology 1983; **Med School:** Baylor Coll Med 1977; **Resid:** Internal Medicine, New York Hosp-Cornell 1983; **Fellow:** Hematology & Oncology, Meml Sloan Kettering Cancer Ctr 1983

Israel, Alan MD (Hem) - **Hospital:** Pascack Valley Hosp, Valley Hosp (page 762); **Address:** 270 Old Hook Rd, Westwood, NJ 07675-3102; **Phone:** 201-666-4949; **Board Cert:** Internal Medicine 1982; Medical Oncology 1985; Hematology 1986; **Med School:** NYU Sch Med 1979; **Resid:** Internal Medicine, Mt Sinai Hosp 1982; **Fellow:** Hematology & Oncology, Meml Sloan Kettering Cancer Ctr 1984; Hematology, LI Jewish Hosp 1985

Pecora, Andrew L MD (Hem) - **Spec Exp:** Stem Cell Transplant; Myelodysplastic Syndromes; Melanoma; Immunotherapy; **Hospital:** Hackensack Univ Med Ctr (page 92); **Address:** The Cancer Ctr at Hackensack Univ Med Ctr, 20 Prospect Ave, Ste 400, Hackensack, NJ 07601; **Phone:** 201-996-5900; **Board Cert:** Internal Medicine 1986; Hematology 1988; Medical Oncology 1989; **Med School:** UMDNJ-NJ Med Sch, Newark 1983; **Resid:** Internal Medicine, New York Hosp-Cornell Med Ctr 1986; **Fellow:** Hematology & Oncology, Meml Sloan Kettering Cancer Ctr 1988; **Fac Appt:** Prof Med, UMDNJ-NJ Med Sch, Newark

INFECTIOUS DISEASE

Birch, Thomas MD (Inf) - **Spec Exp:** AIDS/HIV; Lyme Disease; Travel Medicine; **Hospital:** Holy Name Hosp (page 761), Englewood Hosp & Med Ctr (page 760); **Address:** 185 Cedar Ln, Ste 8, Teaneck, NJ 07666; **Phone:** 201-287-0051; **Board Cert:** Internal Medicine 1986; Infectious Disease 2004; **Med School:** Univ Wisc 1983; **Resid:** Internal Medicine, Montefiore Med Ctr 1986; **Fellow:** Infectious Disease, Montefiore Med Ctr 1993

Cicogna, Cristina E MD (Inf) - **Spec Exp:** Infections in Immunocompromised Patients; **Hospital:** Hackensack Univ Med Ctr (page 92); **Address:** 20 Prospect Ave, Ste 507, Hackensack, NJ 07601; **Phone:** 201-487-4088; **Board Cert:** Internal Medicine 2002; Infectious Disease 2002; **Med School:** Switzerland 1986; **Resid:** Internal Medicine, St Luke's Roosevelt Hosp 1989; **Fellow:** Infectious Disease, Meml Sloan Kettering Cancer Ctr 1991; **Fac Appt:** Asst Prof Med, UMDNJ-RW Johnson Med Sch

Greenman, James L MD (Inf) - **Spec Exp:** AIDS/HIV; Lyme Disease; **Hospital:** Overlook Hosp (page 88); **Address:** Medical Diagnostic Assocs, 525 Central Ave, Westfield, NJ 07675; **Phone:** 908-233-0895; **Board Cert:** Internal Medicine 1985; Infectious Disease 1988; **Med School:** Albert Einstein Coll Med 1982; **Resid:** Internal Medicine, Columbia-Presby Med Ctr 1985; **Fellow:** Infectious Disease, Montefiore Med Ctr 1988

Gross, Peter A MD (Inf) - **Spec Exp:** Viral Infections; Travel Medicine; **Hospital:** Hackensack Univ Med Ctr (page 92); **Address:** 20 Prospect Ave, Ste 507, Hackensack, NJ 07601-1962; **Phone:** 201-487-4088; **Board Cert:** Internal Medicine 1971; Infectious Disease 1976; **Med School:** Yale Univ 1964; **Resid:** Internal Medicine, Yale-New Haven Hosp 1966; Internal Medicine, Peter Bent Brigham Hosp 1969; **Fellow:** Virology, Yale-New Haven Hosp 1971; **Fac Appt:** Prof PrM, UMDNJ-NJ Med Sch, Newark

Kocher, Jeffrey MD (Inf) - **Spec Exp:** Hepatitis B & C; AIDS/HIV; Fungal Infections; Lyme Disease; **Hospital:** Englewood Hosp & Med Ctr (page 760), Holy Name Hosp (page 761); **Address:** 25 Rockwood Pl, Englewood, NJ 07631-4957; **Phone:** 201-568-3335; **Board Cert:** Internal Medicine 1983; Infectious Disease 1986; **Med School:** Cornell Univ-Weill Med Coll 1980; **Resid:** Internal Medicine, New York Hosp 1983; Internal Medicine, St Barnabas Hosp 1984; **Fellow:** Infectious Disease, New York Hosp 1986; **Fac Appt:** Assoc Clin Prof Med, Mount Sinai Sch Med

Levine, Jerome F MD (Inf) - **Spec Exp:** AIDS/HIV; Hospital Acquired Infections; Bone Infections; **Hospital:** Hackensack Univ Med Ctr (page 92); **Address:** 20 Prospect Ave, Ste 507, Hackensack, NJ 07601; **Phone:** 201-487-4088; **Board Cert:** Internal Medicine 1979; Infectious Disease 1982; **Med School:** NYU Sch Med 1976; **Resid:** Internal Medicine, NYU/Manhattan VA Hosp 1980; **Fellow:** Infectious Disease, Manhattan VA Hosp 1982; **Fac Appt:** Assoc Clin Prof Med, UMDNJ-NJ Med Sch, Newark

Weisholtz, Steven MD (Inf) - **Spec Exp:** AIDS/HIV; Antibiotic Resistance; Travel Medicine; **Hospital:** Englewood Hosp & Med Ctr (page 760), Holy Name Hosp (page 761); **Address:** 25 Rockwood Pl, Englewood, NJ 07631-4957; **Phone:** 201-568-3335; **Board Cert:** Internal Medicine 1981; Infectious Disease 1984; **Med School:** Univ Pennsylvania 1978; **Resid:** Internal Medicine, New York Hosp 1981; **Fellow:** Infectious Disease, New York Hosp 1983; **Fac Appt:** Asst Clin Prof Med, Mount Sinai Sch Med

INTERNAL MEDICINE

Bromberg, Assia MD (IM) **PCP** - **Spec Exp:** Asthma; Emphysema; Women's Health; **Hospital:** Valley Hosp (page 762); **Address:** 19-20 Fair Lawn Ave, Fairlawn, NJ 07410; **Phone:** 201-794-1963; **Board Cert:** Internal Medicine 1989; Pulmonary Disease 2004; **Med School:** Israel 1974; **Resid:** Anesthesiology, Chaim Sheba Med Ctr 1981; Internal Medicine, Englewood Hosp 1989; **Fellow:** Pulmonary Disease, Bellevue-NYU Med Ctr 1992

Brunnquell, Stephen MD (IM) **PCP** - **Hospital:** Englewood Hosp & Med Ctr (page 760), Pascack Valley Hosp; **Address:** 24 Elm St, Harrington Park, NJ 07640-1902; **Phone:** 201-784-0123; **Board Cert:** Internal Medicine 2002; **Med School:** UMDNJ-NJ Med Sch, Newark 1989; **Resid:** Internal Medicine, Montefiore Hosp Med Ctr 1992; **Fac Appt:** Asst Clin Prof Med, Mount Sinai Sch Med

Fields, Sheila MD (IM) `PCP` - **Spec Exp:** Anemia; Hypertension; **Hospital:** Pascack Valley Hosp, Valley Hosp (page 762); **Address:** 270 Old Hook Rd, Westwood, NJ 07675; **Phone:** 201-666-4949; **Board Cert:** Internal Medicine 1973; **Med School:** SUNY Hlth Sci Ctr 1968; **Resid:** Internal Medicine, Mount Sinai Hosp 1972; **Fellow:** Hematology, Mount Sinai Hosp 1974

Lan, Vivian E MD (IM) `PCP` - **Spec Exp:** Women's Health; Eating Disorders; **Hospital:** Valley Hosp (page 762), Pascack Valley Hosp; **Address:** 466 Old Hook Rd, Ste 1, Emerson, NJ 07630; **Phone:** 201-967-8221; **Board Cert:** Internal Medicine 1997; **Med School:** Mount Sinai Sch Med 1994; **Resid:** Internal Medicine, Mt Sinai Med Ctr 1997

Miguel, Eduardo MD (IM) `PCP` - **Spec Exp:** Rheumatoid Arthritis; **Hospital:** Englewood Hosp & Med Ctr (page 760); **Address:** 12 E Pallisade Ave, Englewood, NJ 07631; **Phone:** 201-871-3280; **Board Cert:** Internal Medicine 1982; **Med School:** Paraguay 1966; **Resid:** Internal Medicine, VA Med Ctr 1969; Internal Medicine, NY Polyclinic Hosp 1972; **Fellow:** Rheumatology, Albert Einstein Med Ctr 1973

Pelavin, Martin MD (IM) `PCP` - **Hospital:** Pascack Valley Hosp; **Address:** 215 Old Tappan Rd, Old Tappan, NJ 07675-7428; **Phone:** 201-666-1000; **Board Cert:** Internal Medicine 1976; **Med School:** NYU Sch Med 1973; **Resid:** Internal Medicine, Montefiore Hosp Med Ctr 1976; **Fac Appt:** Asst Clin Prof Med, NY Med Coll

Scibetta, Maria MD (IM) `PCP` - **Hospital:** Valley Hosp (page 762); **Address:** 42 N Franklin Tpke, Ramsey, NJ 07446-2034; **Phone:** 201-327-8765; **Board Cert:** Internal Medicine 2003; **Med School:** UMDNJ-RW Johnson Med Sch 1990; **Resid:** Internal Medicine, Mount Sinai Hosp 1993

Shapiro, Jonathan MD (IM) `PCP` - **Hospital:** Englewood Hosp & Med Ctr (page 760); **Address:** 25 Rockwood Pl, Engelwood, NJ 07631; **Phone:** 201-568-3335; **Board Cert:** Internal Medicine 1995; **Med School:** NYU Sch Med 1993; **Resid:** Internal Medicine, Bellevue Med Ctr 1996

Volpe, Anthony Peter MD (IM) `PCP` - **Spec Exp:** Hypertension; **Hospital:** Pascack Valley Hosp; **Address:** 466 Old Hook Rd, Ste 14, Emerson, NJ 07630-1368; **Phone:** 201-262-6485; **Board Cert:** Internal Medicine 1995; **Med School:** Mexico 1981; **Resid:** Internal Medicine, Texas Tech Hlth Scis Ctr 1986

Wasserman, Kenneth MD (IM) `PCP` - **Hospital:** Englewood Hosp & Med Ctr (page 760), Holy Name Hosp (page 761); **Address:** 401 S Van Brunt St, Ste 402, Englewood, NJ 07631-4200; **Phone:** 201-567-1140 x10; **Board Cert:** Internal Medicine 1982; **Med School:** Albert Einstein Coll Med 1979; **Resid:** Internal Medicine, Lenox Hill Hosp 1982

MATERNAL & FETAL MEDICINE

Frieden, Faith MD (MF) - **Spec Exp:** Prenatal Ultrasound; Prenatal Diagnosis; **Hospital:** Englewood Hosp & Med Ctr (page 760); **Address:** 350 Engle St, Englewood, NJ 07631-1808; **Phone:** 201-894-3669; **Board Cert:** Obstetrics & Gynecology 2005; Maternal & Fetal Medicine 2005; **Med School:** Mount Sinai Sch Med 1984; **Resid:** Obstetrics & Gynecology, Beth Israel Med Ctr 1988; **Fellow:** Maternal & Fetal Medicine, Bellevue Hosp 1990; **Fac Appt:** Asst Clin Prof ObG, Mount Sinai Sch Med

MEDICAL ONCOLOGY

Attas, Lewis MD (Onc) - **Spec Exp:** Breast Cancer; Lymphoma; **Hospital:** Englewood Hosp & Med Ctr (page 760), Holy Name Hosp (page 761); **Address:** 25 Rockwood Pl Fl 1, Englewood, NJ 07631-4957; **Phone:** 201-568-5250; **Board Cert:** Internal Medicine 1985; Medical Oncology 1987; Hematology 1988; **Med School:** Mount Sinai Sch Med 1982; **Resid:** Internal Medicine, Montefiore Hosp Med Ctr 1985; **Fellow:** Medical Oncology, North Shore Univ Hosp 1988; **Fac Appt:** Assoc Clin Prof Med, Mount Sinai Sch Med

Forte, Francis A MD (Onc) - **Spec Exp:** Breast Cancer; Bleeding Disorders; **Hospital:** Englewood Hosp & Med Ctr (page 760), Holy Name Hosp (page 761); **Address:** 25 Rockwood Pl, Englewood, NJ 07631; **Phone:** 201-568-5250; **Board Cert:** Internal Medicine 1971; Hematology 1972; Medical Oncology 1973; **Med School:** Albert Einstein Coll Med 1964; **Resid:** Internal Medicine, Mount Sinai Hosp 1968; **Fellow:** Hematology, Mount Sinai Hosp 1969; **Fac Appt:** Asst Prof Med, Mount Sinai Sch Med

Hesdorffer, Charles MD (Onc) - **Spec Exp:** Stem Cell Transplant; Immunotherapy; Melanoma; Sarcoma; **Hospital:** Hackensack Univ Med Ctr (page 92); **Address:** Hackensack Univ Medical Ctr, 20 Prospect Ave, Ste 400, Hackensack, NJ 07601; **Phone:** 201-996-5900; **Board Cert:** Internal Medicine 1995; Medical Oncology 1997; **Med School:** South Africa 1978; **Resid:** Internal Medicine, Univ Wittwatersrand Hosp 1984; **Fellow:** Hematology & Oncology, Columbia-Presby Hosp 1988; **Fac Appt:** Prof Med, UMDNJ-NJ Med Sch, Newark

Krutchik, Allan MD (Onc) - **Spec Exp:** Breast Cancer; **Hospital:** Wayne Hosp, Chilton Meml Hosp; **Address:** 795 Franklin Ave, Ste 106, Franklin Lakes, NJ 07417; **Phone:** 201-848-8791; **Board Cert:** Internal Medicine 1976; Medical Oncology 2001; **Med School:** Univ Hlth Sci/Chicago Med Sch 1973; **Resid:** Internal Medicine, Beth Israel Hosp 1976; **Fellow:** Medical Oncology, MD Anderson Cancer Ctr 1978; **Fac Appt:** Asst Clin Prof Med, UMDNJ-NJ Med Sch, Newark

Pascal, Mark MD (Onc) - **Spec Exp:** Lung Cancer; Breast Cancer; Neuro-Oncology; **Hospital:** Hackensack Univ Med Ctr (page 92), Holy Name Hosp (page 761); **Address:** 20 Prospect Ave, Fl 4 - Ste 400, Hackensack, NJ 07601-1997; **Phone:** 201-996-5900; **Board Cert:** Internal Medicine 1977; Medical Oncology 1979; **Med School:** Jefferson Med Coll 1973; **Resid:** Internal Medicine, NY Hosp 1977; Pathology, Cornell U Med Ctr 1976; **Fellow:** Hematology & Oncology, Meml Sloan Kettering Cancer Ctr 1979

Rakowski, Thomas MD (Onc) - **Hospital:** Valley Hosp (page 762); **Address:** 301 Godwin Ave, Midland Park, NJ 07432-4426; **Phone:** 201-444-4526; **Board Cert:** Internal Medicine 1979; Medical Oncology 1981; **Med School:** SUNY Upstate Med Univ 1976; **Resid:** Internal Medicine, SUNY Hlth Sci Ctr 1979; Hematology, NY Presby Hosp-Columbia Campus 1981

Schleider, Michael MD (Onc) - **Spec Exp:** Breast Cancer; Colon Cancer; Bleeding/Coagulation Disorders; **Hospital:** Englewood Hosp & Med Ctr (page 760); **Address:** 25 Rockwood Pl, Englewood, NJ 07631; **Phone:** 201-568-5250; **Board Cert:** Internal Medicine 1974; Hematology 1976; Medical Oncology 1977; **Med School:** Univ Pennsylvania 1969; **Resid:** Internal Medicine, New York Hosp 1974; **Fellow:** Hematology & Oncology, New York Hosp 1977

Waintraub, Stanley MD (Onc) - **Spec Exp:** Breast Cancer; Gynecologic Cancer; Bleeding/Coagulation Disorders; **Hospital:** Hackensack Univ Med Ctr (page 92), Holy Name Hosp (page 761); **Address:** Northern NJ Cancer Associates, 20 Prospect Ave, Fl 4, Hackensack, NJ 07601-1271; **Phone:** 201-996-5900; **Board Cert:** Internal Medicine 1980; Hematology 1982; Medical Oncology 1983; **Med School:** NY Med Coll 1977; **Resid:** Internal Medicine, Metropolitan Hosp Ctr 1980; **Fellow:** Hematology, Montefiore Hosp Med Ctr 1982; Medical Oncology, Meml Sloan Kettering Cancer Ctr 1983; **Fac Appt:** Asst Clin Prof Med, UMDNJ-NJ Med Sch, Newark

NEONATAL-PERINATAL MEDICINE

Carlin, Elizabeth MD (NP) - **Hospital:** Englewood Hosp & Med Ctr (page 760), Mount Sinai Med Ctr (page 98); **Address:** 350 Engle St, Englewood Hosp & Med Ctr, Englewood, NJ 07631-1808; **Phone:** 201-894-3021; **Board Cert:** Pediatrics 1994; Neonatal-Perinatal Medicine 1997; **Med School:** Boston Univ 1990; **Resid:** Pediatrics, Boston City Hosp 1993; **Fellow:** Neonatal-Perinatal Medicine, Mount Sinai 1996; **Fac Appt:** Asst Clin Prof Ped, Mount Sinai Sch Med

Manginello, Frank MD (NP) - **Hospital:** Valley Hosp (page 762), Chilton Meml Hosp; **Address:** The Valley Hosp, 223 N Van Dien Ave, Ridgewood, NJ 07450-2736; **Phone:** 201-447-8388; **Board Cert:** Pediatrics 1978; Neonatal-Perinatal Medicine 1979; **Med School:** Georgetown Univ 1973; **Resid:** Pediatrics, Georgetown Univ Hosp 1974; Pediatrics, Georgetown Univ Hosp 1975; **Fellow:** Perinatal Medicine, NY Hosp-Cornell Med Ctr 1977; **Fac Appt:** Asst Prof Ped, UMDNJ-NJ Med Sch, Newark

Pane, Carmela MD (NP) - **Spec Exp:** Prematurity/Low Birth Weight Infants; Neonatal Chronic Lung Disease; **Hospital:** Valley Hosp (page 762); **Address:** 223 N Van Dien Ave, Ridgewood, NJ 07450-2726; **Phone:** 201-447-8288; **Board Cert:** Neonatal-Perinatal Medicine 2004; **Med School:** Geo Wash Univ 1984; **Resid:** Pediatrics, Chldns Hosp 1987; **Fellow:** Neonatal-Perinatal Medicine, Chldns Hosp 1989

Perl, Harold MD (NP) - **Spec Exp:** Pulmonary Disease; Jaundice & Bilirubin Metabolism; Sudden Infant Death Syndrome (SIDS); **Hospital:** Hackensack Univ Med Ctr (page 92); **Address:** Hackensack Univ Med Ctr, Dept Pediatrics, 30 Prospect Ave Bldg Imus - rm 217, Hackensack, NJ 07601-1914; **Phone:** 201-996-5362; **Board Cert:** Pediatrics 1980; Neonatal-Perinatal Medicine 1983; **Med School:** Albert Einstein Coll Med 1975; **Resid:** Pediatrics, Montefiore Hosp Med Ctr 1978; **Fellow:** Neonatal-Perinatal Medicine, Albert Einstein 1980; **Fac Appt:** Asst Clin Prof Ped, UMDNJ-NJ Med Sch, Newark

Sison, Joseph MD (NP) - **Hospital:** Englewood Hosp & Med Ctr (page 760); **Address:** 350 Engle St, Englewood, NJ 07631-1808; **Phone:** 201-894-3321; **Board Cert:** Pediatrics 2000; Neonatal-Perinatal Medicine 1997; **Med School:** Philippines 1984; **Resid:** Pediatrics, Jersey Shore Med Ctr 1992; Neonatal-Perinatal Medicine, Vanderbilt Univ Hosp 1993; **Fellow:** Neonatal-Perinatal Medicine, New York Hosp 1995; **Fac Appt:** Clin Prof Ped, Mount Sinai Sch Med

NEPHROLOGY

Fein, Deborah A MD (Nep) - **Spec Exp:** Hypertension; Kidney Disease; **Hospital:** Englewood Hosp & Med Ctr (page 760), Holy Name Hosp (page 761); **Address:** 177 N Dean St, Ste 207, Englewood, NJ 07631-2501; **Phone:** 201-567-0446; **Board Cert:** Internal Medicine 1983; Nephrology 2004; **Med School:** Tufts Univ 1980; **Resid:** Internal Medicine, Roosevelt Hosp 1982; **Fellow:** Nephrology, NY Hosp 1985

Grodstein, Gerald MD (Nep) - **Spec Exp:** Hypertension; Dialysis Care; **Hospital:** Englewood Hosp & Med Ctr (page 760); **Address:** 177 N Dean St, Ste 205, Englewood, NJ 07631-2527; **Phone:** 201-567-0446; **Board Cert:** Internal Medicine 1977; Nephrology 1980; **Med School:** SUNY Downstate 1974; **Resid:** Internal Medicine, Kings County Hosp 1977; **Fellow:** Nephrology, UCLA Med Ctr 1978

Kozlowski, Jeffrey MD (Nep) - **Spec Exp:** Hypertension; Dialysis Care; Diabetic Kidney Disease; **Hospital:** Valley Hosp (page 762), Hackensack Univ Med Ctr (page 92); **Address:** 44 Godwin Ave, Midland Park, NJ 07432; **Phone:** 201-447-0013; **Board Cert:** Internal Medicine 1981; Nephrology 1984; **Med School:** NYU Sch Med 1978; **Resid:** Internal Medicine, VA Med Ctr 1981; **Fellow:** Nephrology, NYU Med Ctr 1984

Levin, David N MD (Nep) - **Spec Exp:** Hypertension; Dialysis Care; **Hospital:** Holy Name Hosp (page 761), Hackensack Univ Med Ctr (page 92); **Address:** 870 Palisade Ave, Ste 202, Teaneck, NJ 07666-3419; **Phone:** 201-836-0897; **Board Cert:** Internal Medicine 1979; Nephrology 1981; **Med School:** UMDNJ-NJ Med Sch, Newark 1976; **Resid:** Internal Medicine, Jacobi Medical Center 1979; **Fellow:** Nephrology, Albert Einstein 1981

Nathin, Donald MD (Nep) - **Spec Exp:** Hypertension; Dialysis Care; Kidney Disease; **Hospital:** Pascack Valley Hosp, Hackensack Univ Med Ctr (page 92); **Address:** 150 Washington Ave, Dumont, NJ 07628-2305; **Phone:** 201-387-2040; **Board Cert:** Internal Medicine 1980; Nephrology 1996; **Med School:** Univ Hlth Sci/Chicago Med Sch 1961; **Resid:** Internal Medicine, Brookdale Hospital 1963; Nephrology, Montefiore Hospital 1967; **Fac Appt:** Assoc Clin Prof Med, NY Med Coll

Pattner, Austin MD (Nep) - **Spec Exp:** Hypertension; Dialysis Care; Kidney Disease; **Hospital:** Englewood Hosp & Med Ctr (page 760), Hackensack Univ Med Ctr (page 92); **Address:** 177 N Dean St, Ste 207, Englewood, NJ 07631-2527; **Phone:** 201-567-0445; **Board Cert:** Internal Medicine 1974; Nephrology 1976; **Med School:** SUNY Upstate Med Univ 1966; **Resid:** Internal Medicine, Roosevelt Hosp 1969; Internal Medicine, Columbia-Presby Med Ctr 1970; **Fellow:** Nephrology, Columbia-Presby Med Ctr 1972; **Fac Appt:** Asst Prof Med, Mount Sinai Sch Med

Rigolosi, Robert S MD (Nep) - **Spec Exp:** Kidney Disease; Hypertension; Dialysis Care; **Hospital:** Holy Name Hosp (page 761), Valley Hosp (page 762); **Address:** Holy Name Hospital, 718 Teaneck Rd, Teaneck, NJ 07666-4281; **Phone:** 201-833-3223; **Med School:** Italy 1963; **Resid:** Internal Medicine, Bronx VA Hosp 1967; **Fellow:** Renal Disease, Georgetown Univ Hosp 1969

Tartini, Albert MD (Nep) - **Spec Exp:** Dialysis Care; Hypertension; Anemia; Osteoporosis; **Hospital:** Valley Hosp (page 762), Holy Name Hosp (page 761); **Address:** Holy Name Hospital, 718 Teaneck Rd, Teaneck, NJ 07666; **Phone:** 201-833-3223; **Board Cert:** Internal Medicine 1988; Nephrology 2000; **Med School:** Grenada 1984; **Resid:** Internal Medicine, St Joseph Hosp Med Ctr 1988; **Fellow:** Nephrology, Univ Vermont Med Ctr 1990

Weizman, Howard MD (Nep) - **Spec Exp:** Dialysis Care; Hypertension; **Hospital:** Hackensack Univ Med Ctr (page 92), Valley Hosp (page 762); **Address:** 44 Godwin Ave, Midland Park, NJ 07432-1976; **Phone:** 201-447-0013; **Board Cert:** Internal Medicine 1985; Nephrology 2002; **Med School:** Albert Einstein Coll Med 1982; **Resid:** Internal Medicine, Bronx Muni Hosp 1985; **Fellow:** Nephrology, Mount Sinai Med Ctr 1987

NEUROLOGICAL SURGERY

Carpenter, Duncan MD (NS) - **Spec Exp:** Spinal Surgery; Spinal Reconstructive Surgery; **Hospital:** Valley Hosp (page 762); **Address:** 225 Dayton St, Ridgewood, NJ 07450-4407; **Phone:** 201-612-0020; **Board Cert:** Neurological Surgery 1987; **Med School:** Columbia P&S 1978; **Resid:** Surgery, St Lukes Hosp 1980; Neurological Surgery, NY Neuro Inst-Columbia 1985

Goulart, Hamilton MD (NS) - **Spec Exp:** Spinal Disc Replacement; Spinal Reconstructive Surgery; Spinal Surgery; **Hospital:** Valley Hosp (page 762); **Address:** 225 Dayton St, Ridgewood, NJ 07450-4407; **Phone:** 201-612-0020; **Board Cert:** Neurological Surgery 1985; **Med School:** Brazil 1975; **Resid:** Neurological Surgery, Mount Sinai Med Ctr 1982

Roth, Patrick A MD (NS) - **Spec Exp:** Spinal Surgery; Brain Tumors; **Hospital:** Hackensack Univ Med Ctr (page 92), Holy Name Hosp (page 761); **Address:** 20 Prospect Ave, Ste 907, Hackensack, NJ 07601; **Phone:** 201-342-2550; **Board Cert:** Neurological Surgery 1997; **Med School:** Albert Einstein Coll Med 1987; **Resid:** Neurological Surgery, New England Med Ctr 1994

Vingan, Roy D MD (NS) - **Spec Exp:** Brain Surgery; Spinal Surgery; **Hospital:** Hackensack Univ Med Ctr (page 92); **Address:** 20 Prospect Ave, Ste 907, Hackensack, NJ 07601; **Phone:** 201-342-2550; **Board Cert:** Neurological Surgery 1995; **Med School:** SUNY Downstate 1985; **Resid:** Neurological Surgery, Univ Hosp 1992; **Fac Appt:** Asst Clin Prof NS, UMDNJ-NJ Med Sch, Newark

NEUROLOGY

Alweiss, Gary MD (N) - **Spec Exp:** Electromyography; Carpal Tunnel Syndrome; Headache; **Hospital:** Englewood Hosp & Med Ctr (page 760), Hackensack Univ Med Ctr (page 92); **Address:** 200 Grand Ave, Ste 101, Englewood, NJ 07631; **Phone:** 201-894-5805; **Board Cert:** Neurology 1993; **Med School:** Mount Sinai Sch Med 1988; **Resid:** Neurology, Mount Sinai Med Ctr 1992; **Fellow:** Nuclear Medicine, Columbia-Presby Med Ctr 1993

Effron, Charles MD (N) - **Spec Exp:** Peripheral Neuropathy; **Hospital:** Mount Sinai Med Ctr (page 98); **Address:** 365 W Passaic St, Rochelle Park, NJ 07662; **Phone:** 212-987-6110; **Board Cert:** Neurology 1989; **Med School:** Brown Univ 1983; **Resid:** Neurology, Mt Sinai Hosp 1987

Klein, Patricia MD (N) - **Spec Exp:** Headache; Dizziness; Stroke; **Hospital:** Pascack Valley Hosp, Hackensack Univ Med Ctr (page 92); **Address:** 10 Fairview Ave, Westwood, NJ 07675; **Phone:** 201-263-0101; **Board Cert:** Neurology 1980; **Med School:** UMDNJ-NJ Med Sch, Newark 1976; **Resid:** Neurology, UMDNJ 1979; **Fac Appt:** Asst Clin Prof N, UMDNJ-NJ Med Sch, Newark

Perron, Reed C MD (N) - **Hospital:** Valley Hosp (page 762); **Address:** 1200 E Ridgewood Ave, Ridgewood, NJ 07450; **Phone:** 201-444-0868; **Board Cert:** Neurology 1974; **Med School:** Univ Rochester 1966; **Resid:** Internal Medicine, Cleveland Clinic 1970; Neurology, Albert Einstein Coll Med 1973

Rabin, Aaron MD/PhD (N) - **Spec Exp:** Parkinson's Disease; Dementia; Peripheral Neuropathy; **Hospital:** Englewood Hosp & Med Ctr (page 760); **Address:** 177 N Dean St, Englewood, NJ 07631-2533; **Phone:** 201-568-3412; **Board Cert:** Neurology 1981; **Med School:** Albert Einstein Coll Med 1976; **Resid:** Neurology, Albert Einstein Coll Med 1980; **Fellow:** Neuroelectrophysiology, Neuro Inst-Columbia Presby Hosp 1981; **Fac Appt:** Asst Clin Prof Med, Mount Sinai Sch Med

Van Engel, Daniel MD (N) - **Spec Exp:** Electromyography; **Hospital:** Valley Hosp (page 762); **Address:** 1200 E Ridgewood Ave, East Wing Fl 2, Ridgewood, NJ 07450-3957; **Phone:** 201-444-0868; **Board Cert:** Neurology 1980; **Med School:** SUNY Upstate Med Univ 1973; **Resid:** Internal Medicine, North Shore Univ Hosp-Cornell 1975; Neurology, Alebert Einstein 1978

Van Slooten, David MD (N) - **Spec Exp:** Electromyography; Headache; Dementia; **Hospital:** Pascack Valley Hosp, Valley Hosp (page 762); **Address:** 550 Kinderkamack Rd, Oradell, NJ 07649; **Phone:** 201-261-6222; **Board Cert:** Neurology 1989; Clinical Neurophysiology 2004; **Med School:** UMDNJ-NJ Med Sch, Newark 1984; **Resid:** Neurology, UMDNJ Univ Hosp 1988; **Fellow:** Clinical Neurophysiology, VA Med Ctr 1989

Willner, Joseph H MD (N) - **Spec Exp:** Multiple Sclerosis; Myasthenia Gravis; Peripheral Neuropathy; **Hospital:** Englewood Hosp & Med Ctr (page 760), Hackensack Univ Med Ctr (page 92); **Address:** 200 Grand Ave, Ste 101, Englewood, NJ 07631-4363; **Phone:** 201-894-5805; **Board Cert:** Neurology 1978; **Med School:** NYU Sch Med 1970; **Resid:** Neurology, Columbia-Presby Hosp 1977; **Fac Appt:** Assoc Clin Prof N, Columbia P&S

NEURORADIOLOGY

Lerner, Elliot MD (NRad) - **Hospital:** Valley Hosp (page 762); **Address:** Radiology Assocs of Ridgewood, 20 Franklin Tpke, Waldwick, NJ 07463-1749; **Phone:** 201-445-8822; **Board Cert:** Radiology 1990; Neuroradiology 2004; **Med School:** Brown Univ 1985; **Resid:** Diagnostic Radiology, Hosp Univ Penn 1989; **Fellow:** Neuroradiology, Hosp Univ Penn 1991

NUCLEAR MEDICINE

Brunetti, Jacqueline MD (NuM) - **Spec Exp:** PET Imaging; Tumor Imaging; **Hospital:** Holy Name Hosp (page 761); **Address:** Holy Name Hosp, Dept Radiology, 718 Teaneck Rd, Teaneck, NJ 07666-4281; **Phone:** 201-833-3280; **Board Cert:** Diagnostic Radiology 1979; Nuclear Medicine 1980; **Med School:** SUNY Downstate 1975; **Resid:** Diagnostic Radiology, St Vincents Hosp Med Ctr 1979; Nuclear Radiology, St Vincents Hosp Med Ctr 1980; **Fellow:** Nuclear Medicine, St Vincents Hosp Med Ctr 1980; **Fac Appt:** Assoc Clin Prof Rad, Columbia P&S

OBSTETRICS & GYNECOLOGY

Butler, David MD (ObG) **PCP** - **Spec Exp:** Gynecologic Surgery; Menopause Problems; **Hospital:** Holy Name Hosp (page 761), Englewood Hosp & Med Ctr (page 760); **Address:** 420 Grand Ave, Ste 201, Englewood, NJ 07631-4152; **Phone:** 201-871-4040; **Board Cert:** Obstetrics & Gynecology 1972; **Med School:** SUNY Hlth Sci Ctr 1965; **Resid:** Obstetrics & Gynecology, St Vincent's Hosp 1970

Faust, Michael MD (ObG) - **Spec Exp:** Pregnancy-High Risk; Menopause Problems; Gynecologic Surgery; **Hospital:** Valley Hosp (page 762); **Address:** 581 N Franklin Tpke, Ramsey, NJ 07446; **Phone:** 201-236-2100; **Board Cert:** Obstetrics & Gynecology 1998; **Med School:** Univ Pittsburgh 1983; **Resid:** Obstetrics & Gynecology, Thomas Jefferson Univ Hosp 1987

Hurst, Wendy MD (ObG) - **Spec Exp:** Pregnancy-High Risk; Laparoscopic Surgery; Preconception Planning; **Hospital:** Englewood Hosp & Med Ctr (page 760); **Address:** 370 Grand Ave, Ste 202, Englewood, NJ 07631-4109; **Phone:** 201-894-9599; **Board Cert:** Obstetrics & Gynecology 2004; **Med School:** Tufts Univ 1986; **Resid:** Obstetrics & Gynecology, Hosp Univ Penn 1990

McCormack, Barbara MD (ObG) **`PCP`** - **Spec Exp:** Menopause Problems; Pediatric Gynecology; **Hospital:** Englewood Hosp & Med Ctr (page 760); **Address:** 473 Sylvan Ave, Englewood Cliffs, NJ 07632; **Phone:** 201-569-5151; **Board Cert:** Obstetrics & Gynecology 1989; **Med School:** Albert Einstein Coll Med 1971; **Resid:** Obstetrics & Gynecology, Bronx Municipal Hosp 1975

Schulze, Ruth MD (ObG) - **Spec Exp:** Vulvar Disease; Gynecology Only; **Hospital:** Valley Hosp (page 762); **Address:** 550 N Maple Ave, Ridgewood, NJ 07450; **Phone:** 201-445-5500; **Board Cert:** Obstetrics & Gynecology 2004; **Med School:** SUNY Stony Brook 1983; **Resid:** Obstetrics & Gynecology, Baystate Med Ctr 1987

OPHTHALMOLOGY

Burke, Patricia MD (Oph) - **Spec Exp:** Corneal Disease; Cataract Surgery; **Hospital:** Holy Name Hosp (page 761); **Address:** One Sears Drive, Paramus, NJ 07652; **Phone:** 201-599-0123; **Board Cert:** Ophthalmology 1991; **Med School:** UMDNJ-NJ Med Sch, Newark 1986; **Resid:** Ophthalmology, Columbia-Presby Med Ctr 1990; **Fellow:** Cornea, Manhattan EET Hosp 1991

DeLuca, Joseph A MD (Oph) - **Spec Exp:** Anterior Segment Surgery; Laser Refractive Surgery; Trauma; Cataract Surgery; **Hospital:** Clara Maass Med Ctr; **Address:** 20 Park Ave Fl 1, Lyndhurst, NJ 07071; **Phone:** 201-896-0096; **Board Cert:** Ophthalmology 1991; **Med School:** Rutgers Univ 1985; **Resid:** Ophthalmology, United Hosp Med Ctr 1990; **Fac Appt:** Asst Clin Prof Oph, UMDNJ-NJ Med Sch, Newark

Hersh, Peter MD (Oph) - **Spec Exp:** LASIK-Refractive Surgery; Cornea Transplant; **Hospital:** UMDNJ-Univ Hosp-Newark; **Address:** 300 Frank W Burr Blvd, Teaneck, NJ 07666-6704; **Phone:** 201-883-0505; **Board Cert:** Ophthalmology 1987; **Med School:** Johns Hopkins Univ 1982; **Resid:** Internal Medicine, Lenox Hill Hosp 1983; Ophthalmology, Mass Eye & Ear Infirm 1986; **Fellow:** Cornea & Ext Eye Disease, Mass Eye & Ear Infirm 1987; **Fac Appt:** Prof Oph, UMDNJ-NJ Med Sch, Newark

Kaiden, Jeffrey MD (Oph) - **Spec Exp:** Glaucoma; Cataract Surgery; Laser Refractive Surgery; **Hospital:** Pascack Valley Hosp, Hackensack Univ Med Ctr (page 92); **Address:** 300 Fairview Ave, Westwood, NJ 07675-1703; **Phone:** 201-666-4014; **Board Cert:** Ophthalmology 1978; **Med School:** Univ Fla Coll Med 1973; **Resid:** Ophthalmology, Mount Sinai Hosp 1977

Liva, Douglas MD (Oph) - **Spec Exp:** LASIK-Refractive Surgery; Cataract Surgery; Glaucoma; **Hospital:** Valley Hosp (page 762); **Address:** 1 W Ridgewood Ave, Ste 101, Paramus, NJ 07652-2350; **Phone:** 201-444-7770; **Board Cert:** Ophthalmology 1987; **Med School:** Univ Miami Sch Med 1981; **Resid:** Ophthalmology, UMDNJ Affil Hosps 1986

Norden, Richard MD (Oph) - **Spec Exp:** LASIK-Refractive Surgery; **Hospital:** Valley Hosp (page 762); **Address:** 1144 E Ridgewood Ave, Ridgewood, NJ 07450-3915; **Phone:** 201-444-2442; **Board Cert:** Ophthalmology 1985; **Med School:** Southern IL Univ 1980; **Resid:** Ophthalmology, UMDNJ Med Ctr 1984; **Fellow:** Cornea & Refractive Surgery, NY Eye & Ear Infirm 1986; **Fac Appt:** Asst Clin Prof Oph, NY Med Coll

Seidenberg, Boyd MD (Oph) - **Spec Exp:** Cataract Surgery; Glaucoma; **Hospital:** Valley Hosp (page 762); **Address:** 85 S Maple Ave, Ste 4, Ridgewood, NJ 07450-4500; **Phone:** 201-447-2700; **Board Cert:** Ophthalmology 1970; **Med School:** Columbia P&S 1962; **Resid:** Internal Medicine, Columbia-Bellvue 1963; Ophthalmology, NYU Medical Ctr 1968; **Fellow:** Ophthalmology, NYU Medical Ctr 1969

Silbert, Glenn MD (Oph) - **Spec Exp:** Cataract Surgery; Lens Implants; **Hospital:** Hackensack Univ Med Ctr (page 92), New York Eye & Ear Infirm (page 110); **Address:** 316 State St, Hackensack, NJ 07601-5529; **Phone:** 201-342-8115; **Board Cert:** Ophthalmology 1985; **Med School:** Columbia P&S 1979; **Resid:** Ophthalmology, NYU Med Ctr 1983; **Fac Appt:** Asst Prof Oph, NY Med Coll

Solomon, Edward MD (Oph) - **Spec Exp:** Cataract Surgery; Laser Surgery; **Hospital:** Valley Hosp (page 762); **Address:** 85 S Maple Ave, Ridgewood, NJ 07450-4500; **Phone:** 201-444-3010; **Board Cert:** Ophthalmology 1976; **Med School:** Tufts Univ 1968; **Resid:** Ophthalmology, NYU Med Ctr 1974

Stabile, John MD (Oph) - **Spec Exp:** Cataract Surgery; Oculoplastic Surgery; LASIK-Refractive Surgery; **Hospital:** Englewood Hosp & Med Ctr (page 760), Holy Name Hosp (page 761); **Address:** 111 Dean Drive, Tenafly, NJ 07670-2764; **Phone:** 201-567-5995; **Board Cert:** Ophthalmology 1981; **Med School:** NY Med Coll 1976; **Resid:** Internal Medicine, Lincoln Med Ctr 1977; Ophthalmology, St Luke's-Roosevelt Hosp Ctr 1980; **Fellow:** Oculoplastic Surgery, Columbia-Presby 1981; **Fac Appt:** Clin Prof Oph, Columbia P&S

Weinberg, Martin MD (Oph) - **Spec Exp:** Neuro-Ophthalmology; Glaucoma; **Hospital:** Englewood Hosp & Med Ctr (page 760), Hackensack Univ Med Ctr (page 92); **Address:** 405 Cedar Ln, Ste 5, Teaneck, NJ 07666-1715; **Phone:** 201-836-8333; **Board Cert:** Ophthalmology 1989; **Med School:** Eastern VA Med Sch 1979; **Resid:** Ophthalmology, Kings County Hosp 1986; **Fellow:** Ocular Pathology, Scheie Eye Inst-Univ Penn 1983; Ocular Oncology, Manhattan EET Hosp 1987

ORTHOPAEDIC SURGERY

Altman, Wayne MD (OrS) - **Spec Exp:** Carpal Tunnel Syndrome; Knee Injuries; Hand & Wrist Injuries; **Hospital:** Meadowlands Hosp Med Ctr, Mountainside Hosp (page 88); **Address:** 85 Orient Way, FL 1, Rutherford, NJ 07070-2045; **Phone:** 201-438-5888; **Board Cert:** Orthopaedic Surgery 1999; Hand Surgery 1992; **Med School:** UMDNJ-NJ Med Sch, Newark 1978; **Resid:** Orthopaedic Surgery, UMDNJ- Newark 1983; **Fellow:** Hand Surgery, Thomas Jefferson Univ Hosp 1984

Berman, Mark MD (OrS) - **Spec Exp:** Knee Surgery; Shoulder Surgery; Sports Medicine; **Hospital:** Hackensack Univ Med Ctr (page 92), Holy Name Hosp (page 761); **Address:** 211 Essex St, Ste 402, Hackensack, NJ 07601-3246; **Phone:** 201-489-8250; **Board Cert:** Orthopaedic Surgery 2000; **Med School:** Mount Sinai Sch Med 1981; **Resid:** Surgery, Mount Sinai Hosp 1983; Orthopaedic Surgery, Univ Hosp 1986; **Fellow:** Sports Medicine, Lenox Hill Hosp 1987

Doidge, Robert DO (OrS) - **Spec Exp:** Knee Surgery; Shoulder Surgery; Sports Medicine; **Hospital:** Englewood Hosp & Med Ctr (page 760), Pascack Valley Hosp; **Address:** 370 Grand Ave, Ste 100, Englewood, NJ 07631-4109; **Phone:** 201-567-5700; **Board Cert:** Orthopaedic Surgery 2005; **Med School:** Philadelphia Coll Osteo Med 1986; **Resid:** Orthopaedic Surgery, Oakland Genl Hosp 1991; **Fellow:** Sports Medicine, Michigan State Univ 1992

Esformes, Ira MD (OrS) - **Spec Exp:** Sports Medicine; Arthroscopic Surgery; Joint Replacement; **Hospital:** Pascack Valley Hosp, Hackensack Univ Med Ctr (page 92); **Address:** 440 Old Hook Rd Fl 2, Emerson, NJ 07630-1325; **Phone:** 201-261-3333; **Board Cert:** Orthopaedic Surgery 1985; **Med School:** Albany Med Coll 1977; **Resid:** Surgery, North Shore Univ Hosp 1979; Orthopaedic Surgery, Hosp For Joint Diseases 1983

Feldman, David N MD (OrS) - **Spec Exp:** Joint Replacement; **Hospital:** Englewood Hosp & Med Ctr (page 760), Holy Name Hosp (page 761); **Address:** 309 Engle St, Englewood, NJ 07631; **Phone:** 201-503-0447; **Board Cert:** Orthopaedic Surgery 2003; **Med School:** SUNY Hlth Sci Ctr 1986; **Resid:** Ophthalmology, Maimonides Med Ctr 1991

Gennace, Ronald MD (OrS) - **Hospital:** Clara Maass Med Ctr, Saint Michael's Med Ctr; **Address:** 312 Belleville Tpke, Ste 2A, North Arlington, NJ 07031; **Phone:** 201-997-8777; **Board Cert:** Orthopaedic Surgery 1982; **Med School:** UMDNJ-NJ Med Sch, Newark 1976; **Resid:** Orthopaedic Surgery, St Joseph's Hosp & Med Ctr 1980

Hartzband, Mark A MD (OrS) - **Spec Exp:** Knee Replacement; Hip Replacement; **Hospital:** Hackensack Univ Med Ctr (page 92), Lenox Hill Hosp (page 94); **Address:** 10 Forest Ave, Paramus, NJ 07652; **Phone:** 201-291-4040; **Board Cert:** Orthopaedic Surgery 1997; **Med School:** McGill Univ 1978; **Resid:** Surgery, Montefiore Hosp Med Ctr 1981; Orthopaedic Surgery, Montefiore Hosp Med Ctr 1984

Livingston, Lawrence MD (OrS) - **Spec Exp:** Sports Medicine; Shoulder & Knee Injuries; Hip & Knee Replacement; Arthroscopic Surgery; **Hospital:** Pascack Valley Hosp; **Address:** 21 Phillips Pkwy, Montvale, NJ 07645; **Phone:** 201-573-1202; **Board Cert:** Orthopaedic Surgery 1981; **Med School:** Med Coll Wisc 1975; **Resid:** Orthopaedic Surgery, Hosp Joint Diseases 1980

Lloyd, J Mervyn MD (OrS) - **Spec Exp:** Joint Replacement; Sports Medicine; **Hospital:** Pascack Valley Hosp, Valley Hosp (page 762); **Address:** 221 Old Hook Rd, Westwood, NJ 07675; **Phone:** 201-666-0013; **Board Cert:** Orthopaedic Surgery 2006; **Med School:** England 1971; **Resid:** Orthopaedic Surgery, St George's Hosp 1981; Orthopaedic Surgery, Mt Carmel Mercy Hosp 1983

McIlveen, Stephen J MD (OrS) - **Spec Exp:** Shoulder & Knee Surgery; Hip & Knee Replacement; Sports Medicine; **Hospital:** Valley Hosp (page 762), Hackensack Univ Med Ctr (page 92); **Address:** 1 W Ridgewood Ave, Paramus, NJ 07652; **Phone:** 201-670-6702; **Board Cert:** Orthopaedic Surgery 1983; **Med School:** NYU Sch Med 1973; **Resid:** Surgery, Columbia Presby Med Ctr 1975; Orthopaedic Surgery, Columbia Presby Med Ctr 1978; **Fellow:** Joint Replacement Surgery, Columbia Presby Med Ctr 1979; **Fac Appt:** Asst Prof OrS, Columbia P&S

Pizzurro, Joseph MD (OrS) - **Spec Exp:** Hip & Knee Replacement; **Hospital:** Valley Hosp (page 762); **Address:** 85 S Maple Ave, Ridgewood, NJ 07450-4561; **Phone:** 201-445-2830; **Board Cert:** Orthopaedic Surgery 1972; **Med School:** St Louis Univ 1963; **Resid:** Surgery, Bronx VA Hosp 1968; Orthopaedic Surgery, Bellevue Hosp Ctr/NYU 1971; **Fellow:** Orthopaedic Surgery, Amer Acad Ortho Surg 1975

Pollock, Roger G MD (OrS) - **Spec Exp:** Rotator Cuff Surgery; Shoulder Arthroscopic Surgery; Shoulder Injuries; **Hospital:** NY-Presby Hosp (page 100), Valley Hosp (page 762); **Address:** 1 W Ridgewood Ave, Ste 202, Paramus, NJ 07652; **Phone:** 201-612-9774; **Board Cert:** Orthopaedic Surgery 2004; **Med School:** Columbia P&S 1985; **Resid:** Surgery, St Luke's-Roosevelt 1987; Orthopaedic Surgery, Columbia-Presby Med Ctr 1991; **Fellow:** Shoulder Surgery, Columbia-Presby Med Ctr 1992; **Fac Appt:** Asst Prof OrS, Columbia P&S

Salzer Jr, Richard L MD (OrS) - **Spec Exp:** Knee Injuries; Joint Replacement; Pediatric Orthopaedic Surgery; **Hospital:** Englewood Hosp & Med Ctr (page 760), Holy Name Hosp (page 761); **Address:** 401 S Van Brunt St Fl 3rd, Englewood, NJ 07631-4625; **Phone:** 201-569-2770; **Board Cert:** Orthopaedic Surgery 1979; **Med School:** Tufts Univ 1973; **Resid:** Surgery, St Paul's Hosp 1975; Orthopaedic Surgery, Hosp Special Surgery 1978

Self, Edward MD (OrS) - **Spec Exp:** Shoulder Surgery; Shoulder Injuries; **Hospital:** Valley Hosp (page 762); **Address:** 385 S Maple Ave, Ste 101, Ridgewood, NJ 07452-1545; **Phone:** 201-447-1188; **Board Cert:** Orthopaedic Surgery 1980; **Med School:** Columbia P&S 1970; **Resid:** Surgery, St Luke's-Roosevelt Hosp Ctr 1972; Orthopaedic Surgery, Columbia-Presby Med Ctr 1977; **Fellow:** Shoulder Surgery, Columbia-Presby Med Ctr; **Fac Appt:** Asst Clin Prof OrS, Columbia P&S

OTOLARYNGOLOGY

Eisenberg, Lee MD (Oto) - **Spec Exp:** Pediatric Otolaryngology; Thyroid Surgery; Ear Surgery; **Hospital:** Englewood Hosp & Med Ctr (page 760), Hackensack Univ Med Ctr (page 92); **Address:** 177 N Dean St, South Penthouse, Englewood, NJ 07631-2527; **Phone:** 201-567-2771; **Board Cert:** Otolaryngology 1977; **Med School:** SUNY Hlth Sci Ctr 1971; **Resid:** Surgery, Valley Med Ctr 1974; Otolaryngology, UCSF Med Ctr 1977; **Fac Appt:** Assoc Clin Prof Oto, Columbia P&S

Garay, Kenneth MD (Oto) - **Spec Exp:** Nasal & Sinus Disorders; **Hospital:** Meadowlands Hosp Med Ctr; **Address:** 475 Grand Ave, Englewood, NJ 07631-4956; **Phone:** 201-871-4545; **Board Cert:** Otolaryngology 1982; **Med School:** Temple Univ 1978; **Resid:** Surgery, Abington Meml Hosp 1979; Otolaryngology, Columbia-Presby 1982

Henick, David H MD (Oto) - **Spec Exp:** Nasal & Sinus Surgery; Endoscopic Sinus Surgery; Head & Neck Surgery; **Hospital:** Hackensack Univ Med Ctr (page 92), Englewood Hosp & Med Ctr (page 760); **Address:** 301 Bridge Plz N Fl 3, Fort Lee, NJ 07024-5059; **Phone:** 201-592-8200; **Board Cert:** Otolaryngology 1993; **Med School:** SUNY Buffalo 1987; **Resid:** Otolaryngology, Montefiore Med Ctr 1992; **Fellow:** Head and Neck Surgery, Montefiore Med Ctr 1993; Rhinoplasty & Sinus Surgery, Hosp Univ Penn 1994; **Fac Appt:** Asst Clin Prof Oto, UMDNJ-NJ Med Sch, Newark

Ho, Bryan MD (Oto) - **Spec Exp:** Pediatric Otolaryngology; Sinus Surgery; Thyroid Surgery; **Hospital:** Englewood Hosp & Med Ctr (page 760), Holy Name Hosp (page 761); **Address:** 216 Engle St, Ste 101, Englewood, NJ 07631-2428; **Phone:** 201-816-9800; **Board Cert:** Otolaryngology 1995; **Med School:** Mount Sinai Sch Med 1989; **Resid:** Surgery, Mt Sinai Med Ctr 1990; **Fellow:** Otolaryngology, Mt Sinai Med Ctr 1994

Katz, Harry MD (Oto) - **Spec Exp:** Sinus Disorders; **Hospital:** Valley Hosp (page 762), Holy Name Hosp (page 761); **Address:** 44 Godwin Ave, Midland Park, NJ 07432-1959; **Phone:** 201-445-2900; **Board Cert:** Otolaryngology 1982; **Med School:** NYU Sch Med 1977; **Resid:** Otolaryngology, NYU Med Ctr-Bellevue 1981

Lehrer, Joel MD (Oto) - **Spec Exp:** Dizziness; Balance Disorders; Ear Infections; Hearing Loss; **Hospital:** Holy Name Hosp (page 761), Valley Hosp (page 762); **Address:** 315 Cedar Lane, Teaneck, NJ 07666-3442; **Phone:** 201-837-2174; **Board Cert:** Otolaryngology 1964; **Med School:** SUNY Upstate Med Univ 1956; **Resid:** Surgery, Kings County Hosp 1960; Otolaryngology, Mount Sinai 1963; **Fellow:** Otolaryngology, Mount Sinai 1964; **Fac Appt:** Assoc Clin Prof Oto, UMDNJ-NJ Med Sch, Newark

Low, Ronald B MD (Oto) - **Spec Exp:** Head & Neck Surgery; Rhinoplasty; Sinus Surgery; **Hospital:** Hackensack Univ Med Ctr (page 92), Pascack Valley Hosp; **Address:** 20 Prospect Ave, Ste 909, Hackensack, NJ 07601-5013; **Phone:** 201-489-6520; **Board Cert:** Otolaryngology 1974; **Med School:** UMDNJ-NJ Med Sch, Newark 1969; **Resid:** Surgery, Montefiore Hosp 1971; Otolaryngology, NYU-Bellevue Hosp Ctr 1974; **Fac Appt:** Asst Clin Prof Oto

Rosen, Arie MD (Oto) - **Spec Exp:** Head & Neck Tumors; Sinus Disorders; Facial Plastic Surgery; Ear Surgery; **Hospital:** Hackensack Univ Med Ctr (page 92), Englewood Hosp & Med Ctr (page 760); **Address:** 2 S Summit Ave, Hackensack, NJ 07601-1117; **Phone:** 201-996-9200; **Board Cert:** Otolaryngology 1995; **Med School:** Israel 1982; **Resid:** Otolaryngology, Univ of Chicago-Pritzker Sch of Medicine 1994; **Fellow:** Otolaryngology, Lenox Hill Hosp 1989; **Fac Appt:** Asst Prof Oto

Scherl, Michael MD (Oto) - **Spec Exp:** Hearing Loss/Tinnitus; Nasal & Sinus Disorders; **Hospital:** Englewood Hosp & Med Ctr (page 760), Pascack Valley Hosp; **Address:** 219 Old Hook Rd, Westwood, NJ 07675; **Phone:** 201-666-8787; **Board Cert:** Otolaryngology 1987; **Med School:** Albany Med Coll 1982; **Resid:** Surgery, Mount Sinai 1984; Otolaryngology, Mount Sinai 1987; **Fac Appt:** , Mount Sinai Sch Med

Steckowych, Jayde MD (Oto) - **Spec Exp:** Sinus Disorders; Voice Disorders; **Hospital:** Valley Hosp (page 762), NY-Presby Hosp (page 100); **Address:** 400 Franklin Tpke, Ste 200, Mahwah, NJ 07430-3516; **Phone:** 201-825-6163; **Board Cert:** Otolaryngology 1993; **Med School:** Philippines 1981; **Resid:** Surgery, Harlem Hosp 1983; Internal Medicine, Harlem Hosp 1988; **Fellow:** Otolaryngology, Columbia-Presby 1992

Surow, Jason MD (Oto) - **Spec Exp:** Pediatric Otolaryngology; Sinus Disorders; Voice Disorders; **Hospital:** Valley Hosp (page 762), Holy Name Hosp (page 761); **Address:** 44 Godwin Ave, Midland Park, NJ 07432-1959; **Phone:** 201-445-2900; **Board Cert:** Otolaryngology 1987; **Med School:** Univ Pennsylvania 1982; **Resid:** Surgery, Hosp Univ Penn 1984; Otolaryngology, Hosp Univ Penn 1987

Tobias, Geoffrey MD (Oto) - **Spec Exp:** Rhinoplasty Revision; Nasal Reconstruction; Cosmetic Surgery-Face; **Hospital:** Englewood Hosp & Med Ctr (page 760), Mount Sinai Med Ctr (page 98); **Address:** 214 Engle St, Englewood, NJ 07631; **Phone:** 201-567-6770; **Board Cert:** Otolaryngology 1978; **Med School:** Tufts Univ 1973; **Resid:** Otolaryngology, Mount Sinai Med Ctr 1978

PATHOLOGY

Sanchez, Miguel A MD (Path) - **Spec Exp:** Breast Cancer; Thyroid Cancer; **Hospital:** Englewood Hosp & Med Ctr (page 760); **Address:** Englewood Hosp & Med Ctr, Dept Pathology, 350 Engle St, Englewood, NJ 07631-1898; **Phone:** 201-894-3423; **Board Cert:** Anatomic Pathology 1975; Clinical Pathology 1979; Cytopathology 1991; **Med School:** Spain 1969; **Resid:** Pathology, Englewood Hosp 1972; Pathology, Temple Univ 1973; **Fellow:** Pathology, Meml Sloan Kettering Cancer Ctr 1974; **Fac Appt:** Assoc Prof Path, Mount Sinai Sch Med

PEDIATRIC ALLERGY & IMMUNOLOGY

Colenda, Maryann MD (PA&I) - **Spec Exp:** Asthma-Adult & Pediatric; Allergy; **Hospital:** Englewood Hosp & Med Ctr (page 760), Meadowlands Hosp Med Ctr; **Address:** 811 Abbott Blvd, Fort Lee, NJ 07024-4116; **Phone:** 201-224-2256; **Board Cert:** Pediatrics 1976; Allergy & Immunology 1979; **Med School:** NY Med Coll 1971; **Resid:** Pediatrics, Columbia Presby Med Ctr 1974; **Fellow:** Allergy & Immunology, Columbia Presby Med Ctr 1978; **Fac Appt:** Assoc Clin Prof Ped, Columbia P&S

Hicks, Patricia MD (PA&I) - **Spec Exp:** Asthma & Sinusitis; Asthma in Pregnancy; **Hospital:** Valley Hosp (page 762); **Address:** 119 1st St, Hohokus, NJ 07423-1575; **Phone:** 201-444-5277; **Board Cert:** Pediatrics 1978; Allergy & Immunology 2001; **Med School:** Penn State Univ-Hershey Med Ctr 1973; **Resid:** Pediatrics, Columbia-Presby Med Ctr 1976; **Fellow:** Allergy & Immunology, Columbia-Presby Med Ctr 1981

PEDIATRIC CARDIOLOGY

Messina, John MD (PCd) - **Spec Exp:** Critical Care; Interventional Cardiology; Congenital Heart Disease; **Hospital:** St Joseph's Regl Med Ctr - Paterson, Valley Hosp (page 762); **Address:** 1 Broadway, Ste 203, Elmwood Park, NJ 07407; **Phone:** 973-569-6250; **Board Cert:** Pediatrics 1989; Pediatric Cardiology 2002; **Med School:** West Indies 1986; **Resid:** Pediatrics, St Joseph's Hosp & Med Ctr 1988; **Fellow:** Pediatric Cardiology, New York Hosp 1992; **Fac Appt:** Asst Prof Ped, Columbia P&S

Tozzi, Robert MD (PCd) - **Spec Exp:** Fetal Echocardiography; Sports Medicine; **Hospital:** Hackensack Univ Med Ctr (page 92); **Address:** 155 Polifly Rd Fl 1 - Ste 106, Hackensack, NJ 07601; **Phone:** 201-487-7617; **Board Cert:** Pediatrics 1987; Pediatric Cardiology 1999; **Med School:** UMDNJ-NJ Med Sch, Newark 1983; **Resid:** Pediatrics, UMDNJ Univ Hosp 1987; **Fellow:** Pediatric Cardiology, NYU Med Ctr 1991

PEDIATRIC ENDOCRINOLOGY

Novogroder, Michael MD (PEn) - **Spec Exp:** Growth/Development Disorders; Pubertal Disorders; Thyroid Disorders; **Hospital:** Englewood Hosp & Med Ctr (page 760); **Address:** 704 Palisade Ave, Teaneck, NJ 07666; **Phone:** 201-836-4301; **Board Cert:** Pediatrics 1974; Pediatric Endocrinology 1980; **Med School:** SUNY Hlth Sci Ctr 1969; **Resid:** Pediatrics, Jacobi Med Ctr 1973; **Fellow:** Pediatric Endocrinology, New York Hosp 1976; **Fac Appt:** Clin Prof Ped, Columbia P&S

PEDIATRIC HEMATOLOGY-ONCOLOGY

Diamond, Steven MD (PHO) - **Spec Exp:** Pediatric Cancers; Sickle Cell Disease; Hemophilia; **Hospital:** Hackensack Univ Med Ctr (page 92); **Address:** 30 Prospect Ave, Hackensack, NJ 07601-1914; **Phone:** 201-996-5437; **Board Cert:** Pediatrics 1979; Pediatric Hematology-Oncology 1980; **Med School:** Univ Pennsylvania 1974; **Resid:** Pediatrics, Mount Sinai Hosp 1977; **Fellow:** Pediatric Hematology-Oncology, Beth Israel Hosp 1979; **Fac Appt:** Asst Clin Prof Ped, UMDNJ-NJ Med Sch, Newark

Flug, Frances MD (PHO) - **Spec Exp:** Bleeding/Coagulation Disorders; Sickle Cell Disease; Pediatric Cancers; **Hospital:** Hackensack Univ Med Ctr (page 92); **Address:** 30 Prospect Ave, FL 1, Hackensack, NJ 07601-2129; **Phone:** 201-996-5437; **Board Cert:** Pediatrics 1984; Pediatric Hematology-Oncology 1984; **Med School:** SUNY Downstate 1979; **Resid:** Pediatrics, Bellevue/NYU Med Ctr 1982; **Fellow:** Pediatric Hematology-Oncology, Bellevue/NYU Med Ctr 1984; **Fac Appt:** Assoc Prof Ped, UMDNJ-NJ Med Sch, Newark

Halpern, Steven MD (PHO) - **Spec Exp:** Leukemia; Brain Tumors; Hemophilia; **Hospital:** Hackensack Univ Med Ctr (page 92), Overlook Hosp (page 88); **Address:** 30 Prospect Ave Fl 1-WFAN, Hackensack, NJ 07601; **Phone:** 201-996-5437; **Board Cert:** Pediatrics 1981; Pediatric Hematology-Oncology 1982; **Med School:** Univ Hlth Sci/Chicago Med Sch 1976; **Resid:** Pediatrics, St Christopher's Hosp for Children 1979; **Fellow:** Pediatric Hematology-Oncology, Childrens Hosp 1982; **Fac Appt:** Asst Prof Ped, UMDNJ-NJ Med Sch, Newark

Harris, Michael B MD (PHO) - **Spec Exp:** Leukemia & Lymphoma; Bone Tumors; Sarcoma-Soft Tissue; **Hospital:** Hackensack Univ Med Ctr (page 92); **Address:** Tomorrows Chldns Inst, JM Sanzari Chldns Hosp, 30 Prospect Ave, Imus 1-TCI, rm PC116, Hackensack, NJ 07601; **Phone:** 201-996-5437; **Board Cert:** Pediatrics 1974; Pediatric Hematology-Oncology 1974; **Med School:** Albert Einstein Coll Med 1969; **Resid:** Pediatrics, Chldns Hosp 1971; **Fellow:** Pediatric Hematology-Oncology, Chldns Hosp 1974; **Fac Appt:** Prof Ped, UMDNJ-NJ Med Sch, Newark

PEDIATRIC INFECTIOUS DISEASE

Boscamp, Jeffrey R MD (PInf) - **Spec Exp:** Fevers of Unknown Origin; Lyme Disease; **Hospital:** Hackensack Univ Med Ctr (page 92); **Address:** 30 Prospect Ave, WFAN Bldg Fl 3, Hackensack, NJ 07601; **Phone:** 201-996-5308; **Board Cert:** Pediatrics 1986; Pediatric Infectious Disease 2002; **Med School:** NY Med Coll 1981; **Resid:** Pediatrics, Columbia-Presby Med Ctr 1984; Internal Medicine, Greenwich Hosp 1985; **Fellow:** Infectious Disease, Montefiore Med Ctr 1987; **Fac Appt:** Assoc Prof Ped, UMDNJ-Univ Med Dent NJ

PEDIATRIC NEPHROLOGY

Lieberman, Kenneth MD (PNep) - **Spec Exp:** Nephrotic Syndrome; Glomerulonephritis; Kidney Failure-Chronic; Hypertension; **Hospital:** Hackensack Univ Med Ctr (page 92), Lenox Hill Hosp (page 94); **Address:** The Joseph M Sanzari Chlds Hosp, 30 Prospect Ave, Hackensack, NJ 07601; **Phone:** 201-336-8228; **Board Cert:** Pediatrics 1981; Pediatric Nephrology 1982; **Med School:** Albert Einstein Coll Med 1977; **Resid:** Pediatrics, Mount Sinai Hosp 1979; **Fellow:** Nephrology, New York Hosp-Cornell 1981; **Fac Appt:** Prof Ped, UMDNJ-NJ Med Sch, Newark

PEDIATRIC OTOLARYNGOLOGY

Respler, Don MD (PO) - **Spec Exp:** Airway Disorders; Sinus Disorders; Head & Neck Tumors; Sleep Disorders/Apnea; **Hospital:** Hackensack Univ Med Ctr (page 92), Valley Hosp (page 762); **Address:** 2 South Summit Ave, Hackensack, NJ 07601-1117; **Phone:** 201-996-9200; **Board Cert:** Otolaryngology 1986; **Med School:** Mount Sinai Sch Med 1981; **Resid:** Surgery, Beth Israel Hosp 1983; Otolaryngology, UMDNJ-NJ Med Sch 1986; **Fellow:** Pediatric Otolaryngology, Chldns Hosp 1988; **Fac Appt:** Asst Clin Prof S, UMDNJ-NJ Med Sch, Newark

PEDIATRIC PULMONOLOGY

Kanengiser, Steven MD (PPul) - **Spec Exp:** Asthma; Cough-Chronic; Sleep Disorders; **Hospital:** Valley Hosp (page 762), St Joseph's Regl Med Ctr - Paterson; **Address:** 505 Goffle Rd, Ridgewood, NJ 07450; **Phone:** 201-447-8026; **Board Cert:** Pediatrics 2003; Pediatric Pulmonology 2002; **Med School:** UCSF 1984; **Resid:** Pediatrics, Children's Hosp 1987; **Fellow:** Pediatric Pulmonology, Westchester Med Ctr 1994; **Fac Appt:** Asst Clin Prof Ped, Columbia P&S

PEDIATRIC RHEUMATOLOGY

Haines, Kathleen A MD (PRhu) - **Spec Exp:** Juvenile Arthritis; Lupus/SLE; Immune Deficiency; **Hospital:** Hackensack Univ Med Ctr (page 92), NYU Med Ctr (page 102); **Address:** Hackensack Univ Med Ctr, Don Imus Ped Ctr, 30 Prospect Ave Fl 3, Hackensack, NJ 07601; **Phone:** 201-996-5306; **Board Cert:** Pediatrics 1980; Allergy & Immunology 1981; Pediatric Rheumatology 2000; Clinical & Laboratory Immunology 1994; **Med School:** Albert Einstein Coll Med 1975; **Resid:** Pediatrics, New York Hosp 1977; **Fellow:** Allergy & Immunology, New York Hosp 1980; Rheumatology, NYU Med Sch 1982; **Fac Appt:** Assoc Prof Ped, UMDNJ-NJ Med Sch, Newark

Kimura, Yukiko MD (PRhu) - **Spec Exp:** Juvenile Arthritis; Lupus/SLE; Dermatomyositis; Vasculitis; **Hospital:** Hackensack Univ Med Ctr (page 92); **Address:** Hackensack Univ Med Ctr, 30 Prospect Ave, Hackensack, NJ 07601-1915; **Phone:** 201-996-5306; **Board Cert:** Pediatrics 1987; Pediatric Rheumatology 2000; **Med School:** Albert Einstein Coll Med 1982; **Resid:** Pediatrics, Babies Hosp/Columbia Presby 1985; **Fellow:** Pediatric Rheumatology, Babies Hosp/Columbia Presby 1990; **Fac Appt:** Assoc Prof Ped, UMDNJ-NJ Med Sch, Newark

PEDIATRIC SURGERY

Friedman, David L MD (PS) - **Spec Exp:** Neonatal Surgery; Gastroesophageal Reflux Disease (GERD); Laparoscopic Surgery; **Hospital:** Valley Hosp (page 762), Hackensack Univ Med Ctr (page 92); **Address:** 30 W Century Rd, Ste 235, Paramus, NJ 07652-1433; **Phone:** 201-225-9440; **Board Cert:** Surgery 1977; Pediatric Surgery 1999; **Med School:** SUNY Downstate 1971; **Resid:** Surgery, Univ Hosp 1976; **Fellow:** Pediatric Surgery, Univ Hosp 1977; **Fac Appt:** Asst Prof S, Columbia P&S

Gandhi, Rajinder MD (PS) - **Spec Exp:** Gastrointestinal Surgery; Laparoscopic Surgery; Chest Wall Deformities; **Hospital:** Valley Hosp (page 762); **Address:** 30 W Century Rd, Ste 235, Paramus, NJ 07652; **Phone:** 201-225-9440; **Board Cert:** Surgery 1975; Pediatric Surgery 1997; **Med School:** Burma 1966; **Resid:** Surgery, Montefiore Med Ctr-Einstein Div 1974; Pediatric Surgery, Columbia-Presby Med Ctr 1977; **Fellow:** Gastroenterology, Columbia-Presby Med Ctr 1975; **Fac Appt:** Assoc Clin Prof S, Columbia P&S

Valda, Victor MD (PS) - **Spec Exp:** Congenital Anomalies; Cancer Surgery; **Hospital:** Hackensack Univ Med Ctr (page 92), Valley Hosp (page 762); **Address:** 5 Summit Ave, Ste 6, Hackensack, NJ 07601-1271; **Phone:** 201-343-6885; **Board Cert:** Surgery 1974; Pediatric Surgery 1995; **Med School:** Bolivia 1962; **Resid:** Surgery, Mt Zion Hosp; Surgery, Maricopa Med Ctr 1972; **Fellow:** Pediatric Surgery, St Christopher's Hosp 1974

PEDIATRICS

Asnes, Russell MD (Ped) `PCP` - **Spec Exp:** Diagnostic Problems; **Hospital:** Englewood Hosp & Med Ctr (page 760), Hackensack Univ Med Ctr (page 92); **Address:** 32 Franklin St, Tenafly, NJ 07670-2005; **Phone:** 201-569-2400; **Board Cert:** Pediatrics 1969; **Med School:** Tufts Univ 1963; **Resid:** Pediatrics, Johns Hopkins Hosp 1966; **Fellow:** Neonatology, Babies Hosp/Columbia 1968; **Fac Appt:** Clin Prof Ped, Columbia P&S

Bases, Hugh MD (Ped) - **Spec Exp:** Developmental & Behavioral Disorders; Autism; ADD/ADHD; **Hospital:** Hackensack Univ Med Ctr (page 92); **Address:** Hackensack Univ, Institute Child Dvlpt, 60 Prospect Ave, Hackensack, NJ 07601; **Phone:** 201-996-5353; **Board Cert:** Pediatrics 1997; Developmental-Behavioral Pediatrics 2002; **Med School:** Yale Univ 1994; **Resid:** Pediatrics, Yale-New Haven Hosp 1997; **Fellow:** Developmental-Behavioral Pediatrics, Yale-New Haven Hosp 2000; **Fac Appt:** Assoc Prof Ped, UMDNJ-NJ Med Sch, Newark

Buchalter, Maury MD (Ped) `PCP` - **Spec Exp:** Asthma; Infectious Disease; ADD/ADHD; **Hospital:** Hackensack Univ Med Ctr (page 92), Englewood Hosp & Med Ctr (page 760); **Address:** 301 Bridge Plaza N, Fort Lee, NJ 07670; **Phone:** 201-592-8787; **Board Cert:** Pediatrics 1988; **Med School:** Mount Sinai Sch Med 1984; **Resid:** Pediatrics, Mount Sinai Hosp 1987; **Fellow:** Infectious Disease, Chldns Hosp 1988

Hages, Harry MD (Ped) `PCP` - **Hospital:** Pascack Valley Hosp; **Address:** 215 Old Tappan Rd, Old Tappan, NJ 07675-7000; **Phone:** 201-666-1000; **Board Cert:** Pediatrics 1973; **Med School:** Univ Pittsburgh 1966; **Resid:** Pediatrics, Chldns Hosp 1968; Pediatrics, NY Hosp 1969

Harlow, Paul MD (Ped) - **Spec Exp:** Anemia; Bleeding Disorders; **Hospital:** Hackensack Univ Med Ctr (page 92), Valley Hosp (page 762); **Address:** 90 Prospect Ave, Hackensack, NJ 07601; **Phone:** 201-342-4001; **Board Cert:** Pediatrics 1979; Pediatric Hematology-Oncology 1980; **Med School:** SUNY Hlth Sci Ctr 1974; **Resid:** Pediatrics, Jacobi Med Ctr 1977; **Fellow:** Pediatric Hematology-Oncology, Children's Hosp 1977

Hyatt, Alexander C MD (Ped) `PCP` - **Hospital:** Englewood Hosp & Med Ctr (page 760), Mount Sinai Med Ctr (page 98); **Address:** Englewood Hospital, Dept Pediatrics, 350 Engle St, Englewood, NJ 07631; **Phone:** 201-894-3158; **Board Cert:** Pediatrics 1980; Infectious Disease 2002; **Med School:** Mount Sinai Sch Med 1975; **Resid:** Pediatrics, Johns Hopkins Hosp 1978; **Fellow:** Infectious Disease, Mount Sinai Med Ctr 1979; **Fac Appt:** Assoc Prof Ped, Mount Sinai Sch Med

Kanter, Alan MD (Ped) `PCP` - **Spec Exp:** ADD/ADHD; Autism; **Hospital:** Englewood Hosp & Med Ctr (page 760), NY-Presby Hosp (page 100); **Address:** 704 Palisade Ave, Teaneck, NJ 07666-3198; **Phone:** 201-836-4301; **Board Cert:** Pediatrics 1977; **Med School:** Albert Einstein Coll Med 1970; **Resid:** Pediatrics, St Christopher's Hosp 1971; Pediatrics, Montefiore Hosp Med Ctr 1975; **Fac Appt:** Assoc Clin Prof Ped, Columbia P&S

Kolsky, Neil MD (Ped) `PCP` - **Hospital:** Holy Name Hosp (page 761), Hackensack Univ Med Ctr (page 92); **Address:** 870 Palisade Ave, Teaneck, NJ 07666-3419; **Phone:** 201-692-1661; **Board Cert:** Pediatrics 1972; **Med School:** UMDNJ-NJ Med Sch, Newark 1966; **Resid:** Pediatrics, Johns Hopkins Hosp 1969

Kushner, Susan MD (Ped) `PCP` - **Spec Exp:** Atopic Dermatitis; Allergic Rhinitis; Asthma; Otitis Media; **Hospital:** Hackensack Univ Med Ctr (page 92), Valley Hosp (page 762); **Address:** 90 Prospect Ave, Hackensack, NJ 07601-1909; **Phone:** 201-342-4001; **Board Cert:** Pediatrics 1997; **Med School:** SUNY Upstate Med Univ 1986; **Resid:** Pediatrics, LI Jewish Med Ctr 1989

Namerow, David MD (Ped) `PCP` - **Spec Exp:** Adolescent Medicine; Behavioral Disorders; **Hospital:** Valley Hosp (page 762), St Joseph's Regl Med Ctr - Paterson; **Address:** 2020 Fair Lawn Ave, Fair Lawn, NJ 07410-2319; **Phone:** 201-791-4545; **Board Cert:** Pediatrics 1977; **Med School:** Univ Louisville Sch Med 1972; **Resid:** Pediatrics, Children's Hosp 1975; **Fellow:** Adolescent Medicine, Univ MD Hosp 1977; **Fac Appt:** Asst Clin Prof Ped, NY Med Coll

O'Brien, Daryl H MD (Ped) - **Hospital:** Pascack Valley Hosp; **Address:** Broadway Pediatric Assocs, 336 Center Ave, Westwood, NJ 07675; **Phone:** 201-664-7444; **Board Cert:** Pediatrics 1986; **Med School:** Dartmouth Med Sch 1979; **Resid:** Pediatrics, Duke Univ Med Ctr 1982

Schuss, Steven A MD (Ped) `PCP` - **Hospital:** Englewood Hosp & Med Ctr (page 760), Hackensack Univ Med Ctr (page 92); **Address:** 197 Cedar Ln, Teaneck, NJ 07666-4301; **Phone:** 201-836-7171; **Board Cert:** Pediatrics 1986; **Med School:** Albert Einstein Coll Med 1979; **Resid:** Pediatrics, Montefiore Hosp Med Ctr 1983; **Fac Appt:** Asst Clin Prof Ped, Albert Einstein Coll Med

Sugarman, Lynn B MD (Ped) PCP - **Hospital:** Englewood Hosp & Med Ctr (page 760), Hackensack Univ Med Ctr (page 92); **Address:** 32 Franklin St, Tenafly, NJ 07670-2005; **Phone:** 201-569-2400; **Board Cert:** Pediatrics 1981; **Med School:** Harvard Med Sch 1977; **Resid:** Pediatrics, Bronx Muni Hosp Ctr 1981; **Fellow:** Pediatric Critical Care Medicine, Bronx Muni Hosp Ctr 1983; **Fac Appt:** Assoc Clin Prof Ped, Columbia P&S

PHYSICAL MEDICINE & REHABILITATION

Liss, Donald MD (PMR) - **Spec Exp:** Pain-Back; Sports Medicine; Osteoarthritis; **Hospital:** Englewood Hosp & Med Ctr (page 760), Palisades Med Ctr; **Address:** 15 Engle St, rm 205, Englewood, NJ 07631-2920; **Phone:** 201-567-2277; **Board Cert:** Physical Medicine & Rehabilitation 1984; **Med School:** Wayne State Univ 1979; **Resid:** Physical Medicine & Rehabilitation, Columbia-Presby Med Ctr 1982; **Fac Appt:** Assoc Clin Prof PMR, Columbia P&S

Zimmerman, Jerald R MD (PMR) - **Spec Exp:** Polio Rehabilitation; Musculoskeletal Disorders; Pain Management; **Hospital:** Englewood Hosp & Med Ctr (page 760); **Address:** 370 Grand Ave, Ste 102, Englewood, NJ 07631; **Phone:** 201-567-3370; **Board Cert:** Physical Medicine & Rehabilitation 1989; **Med School:** Univ IL Coll Med 1982; **Resid:** Orthopaedic Surgery, Univ Minn Med Ctr 1985; **Fellow:** Physical Medicine & Rehabilitation, Columbia-Presby Med Ctr 1988; **Fac Appt:** Asst Prof PMR, UMDNJ-RW Johnson Med Sch

PLASTIC SURGERY

Bloomenstein, Richard MD (PlS) - **Spec Exp:** Cosmetic Surgery; Reconstructive Surgery; Wound Healing/Care; **Hospital:** Englewood Hosp & Med Ctr (page 760), Valley Hosp (page 762); **Address:** 177 N Dean St, Englewood, NJ 07631; **Phone:** 201-569-2244; **Board Cert:** Plastic Surgery 1970; **Med School:** SUNY Downstate 1959; **Resid:** Surgery, Kings Co Hosp 1965; Plastic Surgery, Montefiore Hosp Med Ctr 1967

D'Amico, Richard MD (PlS) - **Spec Exp:** Cosmetic Surgery-Face; Cosmetic Surgery-Liposuction; Breast Augmentation; **Hospital:** Englewood Hosp & Med Ctr (page 760), Holy Name Hosp (page 761); **Address:** 180 N Dean St, Ste 3NE, Englewood, NJ 07631-2534; **Phone:** 201-567-9595; **Board Cert:** Plastic Surgery 1986; **Med School:** NYU Sch Med 1976; **Resid:** Surgery, Tulsa Med Ctr 1979; Surgery, Strong Meml Hosp 1981; **Fellow:** Plastic Reconstructive Surgery, Columbia-Presby Med Ctr 1983; **Fac Appt:** Asst Clin Prof PlS, Mount Sinai Sch Med

Hall, Craig D MD (PlS) - **Spec Exp:** Cosmetic Surgery; Craniofacial Surgery; Breast Surgery; **Hospital:** Hackensack Univ Med Ctr (page 92), Englewood Hosp & Med Ctr (page 760); **Address:** 146 Rt 17 N, Hackensack, NJ 07601-2261; **Phone:** 201-488-2101; **Board Cert:** Plastic Surgery 1990; **Med School:** Univ Chicago-Pritzker Sch Med 1981; **Resid:** Surgery, Montefiore Hosp Med Ctr 1985; Plastic Surgery, Montefiore Hosp Med Ctr 1987; **Fellow:** Craniofacial Surgery, Humana Intl Craniofacial Inst 1988; **Fac Appt:** Assoc Prof PlS, UMDNJ-NJ Med Sch, Newark

Lipson, David E MD (PlS) - **Spec Exp:** Breast Augmentation; Body Contouring; Facial Rejuvenation; **Hospital:** Valley Hosp (page 762); **Address:** 2300 Route 208 South, Fair Lawn, NJ 07410; **Phone:** 201-797-7770; **Board Cert:** Plastic Surgery 1981; **Med School:** Albert Einstein Coll Med 1971; **Resid:** Surgery, Bellevue/NYU Med Ctr 1976; Plastic Surgery, Bellevue/NYU Med Ctr 1978

Ponamgi, Suri MD (PlS) - **Spec Exp:** Cosmetic & Reconstructive Surgery; **Hospital:** Trinitas Hosp, Palisades Med Ctr; **Address:** 1101 Palisades Ave, Fort Lee, NJ 07024-6329; **Phone:** 201-224-8831; **Board Cert:** Plastic Surgery 1984; **Med School:** India 1970; **Resid:** Surgery, Bronx Lebonon Hosp 1979; Plastic Surgery, NY Methodist Hosp 1982; **Fellow:** Bronx Lebonon Hosp 1980

Rauscher, Gregory MD (PlS) - **Spec Exp:** Cosmetic Surgery-Face & Breast; Liposuction; Hand Surgery; **Hospital:** Hackensack Univ Med Ctr (page 92), Englewood Hosp & Med Ctr (page 760); **Address:** 20 Prospect Ave, Ste 600, Hackensack, NJ 07601-1962; **Phone:** 201-488-1916; **Board Cert:** Plastic Surgery 1979; **Med School:** SUNY Downstate 1972; **Resid:** Surgery, Kings County Hosp 1976; Plastic Surgery, Kings County Hosp 1978; **Fellow:** Hand & Microvascular Surgery, Kings County Hosp 1975; **Fac Appt:** Prof PlS, UMDNJ-NJ Med Sch, Newark

Rothenberg, Bennett C MD (PlS) - **Spec Exp:** Reconstructive Surgery; Cosmetic Surgery-Face; Cosmetic Surgery-Breast; **Hospital:** St Barnabas Med Ctr; **Address:** 219 Paterson Ave, Fair Lawn, NJ 07410; **Phone:** 201-812-7400; **Board Cert:** Plastic Surgery 1998; **Med School:** Howard Univ 1986; **Resid:** Surgery, St Barnabas Med Ctr 1991; Plastic Surgery, Univ Okla Hlth Sci Ctr 1993

Sternschein, Michael MD (PlS) - **Spec Exp:** Cosmetic Surgery-Face & Breast; Cosmetic Surgery-Liposuction; Laser Surgery; **Hospital:** Pascack Valley Hosp, Valley Hosp (page 762); **Address:** 1200 E Ridgewood Ave Fl 2 West Wing, Ridgewood, NJ 07450; **Phone:** 201-444-1188; **Board Cert:** Plastic Surgery 1985; **Med School:** Columbia P&S 1976; **Resid:** Surgery, Columbia-Presby Med Ctr 1980; Plastic Surgery, Columbia-Presby Med Ctr 1982; **Fellow:** Microsurgery, Columbia-Presby Med Ctr 1982

Zubowski, Robert MD (PlS) - **Spec Exp:** Rhinoplasty; Liposuction & Body Contouring; Eyelid Cosmetic & Reconstructive Surgery; **Hospital:** Valley Hosp (page 762); **Address:** 1 Sears Drive Fl 1, Paramus, NJ 07652; **Phone:** 201-261-7550; **Board Cert:** Plastic Surgery 2003; **Med School:** Mexico 1983; **Resid:** Surgery, Westchester County Med Ctr 1991; **Fellow:** Plastic Surgery, Cleveland Clinic 1994; **Fac Appt:** Asst Clin Prof S, NY Med Coll

PSYCHIATRY

Chertoff, Harvey MD (Psyc) - **Spec Exp:** Anxiety & Mood Disorders; Psychoanalysis; **Hospital:** Englewood Hosp & Med Ctr (page 760), NY-Presby Hosp (page 100); **Address:** 205 Engle St, Englewood, NJ 07631-2409; **Phone:** 201-567-4970; **Board Cert:** Psychiatry 1978; Geriatric Psychiatry 1996; Addiction Psychiatry 1998; Forensic Psychiatry 1999; **Med School:** Albert Einstein Coll Med 1966; **Resid:** Psychiatry, Columbia-Presby Med Ctr 1970; **Fac Appt:** Asst Clin Prof Psyc, Columbia P&S

Farkas, Edward MD (Psyc) - **Spec Exp:** Depression in the Elderly; Psychotherapy-Men's Issues; **Hospital:** Holy Name Hosp (page 761); **Address:** 175 Cedar Ln, Ste A, Teaneck, NJ 07666-4315; **Phone:** 201-692-8354; **Board Cert:** Psychiatry 1988; **Med School:** Italy 1979; **Resid:** Psychiatry, Bronx Lebanon Hosp 1981; Psychiatry, St Luke's-Roosevelt Hosp Ctr 1983; **Fellow:** Psychiatry, William Allison White Inst 1983

Gurland, Frances E MD (Psyc) - **Spec Exp:** Eating Disorders; ADD/ADHD; **Address:** 216 Engle St, Englewood, NJ 07631-2444; **Phone:** 201-568-4066; **Board Cert:** Psychiatry 1991; **Med School:** SUNY Hlth Sci Ctr 1989; **Resid:** Psychiatry, St Luke's-Roosevelt Hosp Ctr 1991; **Fellow:** Child & Adolescent Psychiatry, Mount Sinai Hosp 1994; **Fac Appt:** Asst Clin Prof Psyc, Mount Sinai Sch Med

Napoli, Joseph C MD (Psyc) - **Spec Exp:** Post Traumatic Stress Disorder; Trauma Psychiatry; **Hospital:** Englewood Hosp & Med Ctr (page 760); **Address:** 2185 Lemoine Ave, Fort Lee, NJ 07024-6030; **Phone:** 201-461-0212; **Board Cert:** Psychiatry 1978; **Med School:** Georgetown Univ 1972; **Resid:** Psychiatry, Presby Hosp/NY State Psych Inst 1976; Psychoanalysis, Columbia Univ Psychoanalysis Ctr 1985; **Fac Appt:** Asst Clin Prof Psyc, Columbia P&S

Narula, Amarjot S MD (Psyc) - **Spec Exp:** Geriatric Psychiatry; Mood Disorders; **Hospital:** Valley Hosp (page 762), Barnert Hosp; **Address:** 65 N Maple Ave, Ridgewood, NJ 07450-1600; **Phone:** 201-670-4423; **Board Cert:** Psychiatry 1992; Geriatric Psychiatry 1996; **Med School:** India 1979; **Resid:** Psychiatry, Middletown Psychiatric Ctr 1988; **Fellow:** Psychiatry, Metropolitan Hosp 1989

Rosenfeld, David N MD (Psyc) - **Spec Exp:** Mood Disorders; Anxiety Disorders; Personality Disorders; Geriatric Psychiatry; **Hospital:** Valley Hosp (page 762); **Address:** 265 Ackerman Ave, Ste 202, Ridgewood, NJ 07450-4200; **Phone:** 201-447-5630; **Board Cert:** Psychiatry 1995; **Med School:** UMDNJ-RW Johnson Med Sch 1988; **Resid:** Psychiatry, Mount Sinai Sch Med 1990; Psychiatry, Bergen Pines Co 1994

Samuels, Steven MD (Psyc) - **Spec Exp:** Dementia; Depression; Geriatric Psychiatry; **Hospital:** Englewood Hosp & Med Ctr (page 760); **Address:** Englewood Hosp, Behavioral Health Unit, 350 Engel St, Englewood, NJ 07631; **Phone:** 201-681-2915; **Board Cert:** Psychiatry 1994; Geriatric Psychiatry 1996; **Med School:** SUNY Buffalo 1989; **Resid:** Psychiatry, St Vincent's Hosp & Med Ctr 1993; **Fellow:** Geriatric Psychiatry, Hosp Univ Penn 1995; **Fac Appt:** Asst Prof Psyc, Mount Sinai Sch Med

Videtti, Nicholas F MD (Psyc) - **Spec Exp:** Psychopharmacology; Electroconvulsive Therapy (ECT); **Hospital:** Valley Hosp (page 762); **Address:** 127 Union St, Ridgewood, NJ 07450; **Phone:** 201-444-4103; **Board Cert:** Psychiatry 1979; **Med School:** Italy 1961; **Resid:** Psychiatry, VA Hosp 1966

Wagle, Sharad MD (Psyc) - **Spec Exp:** Depression; Anxiety Disorders; **Hospital:** Holy Name Hosp (page 761), Pascack Valley Hosp; **Address:** 718 Teaneck Rd, Teaneck, NJ 07666; **Phone:** 201-833-3291; **Board Cert:** Psychiatry 1996; Child & Adolescent Psychiatry 1997; **Med School:** India 1971; **Resid:** Psychiatry, Hackensack Univ Med Ctr 1976; Psychiatry, Psychoanalytic Inst 1978; **Fellow:** Child & Adolescent Psychiatry, Albert Einstein 1978

PULMONARY DISEASE

Birns, Robert MD (Pul) - **Spec Exp:** Asthma; Emphysema; **Hospital:** Holy Name Hosp (page 761), Englewood Hosp & Med Ctr (page 760); **Address:** 200 Grand Ave, Ste 102, Englewood, NJ 07631-4363; **Phone:** 201-871-3636; **Board Cert:** Internal Medicine 1974; Pulmonary Disease 1976; **Med School:** Washington Univ, St Louis 1970; **Resid:** Internal Medicine, Boston City Hosp 1972; **Fellow:** Pulmonary Disease, Boston City Hosp 1973

Brauntuch, Glenn R MD (Pul) - **Hospital:** Englewood Hosp & Med Ctr (page 760); **Address:** 180 Engle St, Englewood, NJ 07631-2507; **Phone:** 201-567-2050; **Board Cert:** Internal Medicine 1981; Pulmonary Disease 1984; **Med School:** Columbia P&S 1978; **Resid:** Internal Medicine, St Lukes-Roosevelt Hosp 1981; **Fellow:** Pulmonary Disease, NYU Med Ctr 1984

Di Pasquale, Laurene MD (Pul) - **Spec Exp:** Asthma; Sleep Disorders; **Hospital:** Pascack Valley Hosp; **Address:** 400 Old Hook Rd, Westwood, NJ 07675-2732; **Phone:** 201-664-8663; **Board Cert:** Internal Medicine 2003; **Med School:** Dominican Republic 1982; **Resid:** Internal Medicine, Mountainside Hosp 1988; **Fellow:** Pulmonary Disease, Bronx Lebanon 1990

Engler, Mitchell MD (Pul) - **Spec Exp:** Pulmonary Disease; Critical Care; Sleep Disorders; **Hospital:** Holy Name Hosp (page 761), Englewood Hosp & Med Ctr (page 760); **Address:** 180 Engle St, Englewood, NJ 07631-2541; **Phone:** 201-568-8010; **Board Cert:** Internal Medicine 1981; Pulmonary Disease 1988; **Med School:** Boston Univ 1978; **Resid:** Internal Medicine, St Lukes Hosp 1981; **Fellow:** Pulmonary Disease, St Lukes Hosp 1983

Levine, Selwyn MD (Pul) - **Spec Exp:** Chronic Obstructive Lung Disease(COPD); Asthma; **Hospital:** Holy Name Hosp (page 761), Englewood Hosp & Med Ctr (page 760); **Address:** Pulmonary Assocs of Northern NJ, 200 Grand Ave, Ste 102, Englewood, NJ 07631; **Phone:** 201-871-3636; **Board Cert:** Internal Medicine 1985; Pulmonary Disease 1988; **Med School:** NYU Sch Med 1982; **Resid:** Internal Medicine, Bellevue Hosp/NYU Med Ctr 1985; **Fellow:** Pulmonary Disease, Albert Einstein 1987

Malovany, Robert MD (Pul) - **Spec Exp:** Exercise Physiology; **Hospital:** Englewood Hosp & Med Ctr (page 760), Holy Name Hosp (page 761); **Address:** 180 Engle St, Englewood, NJ 07631-2507; **Phone:** 201-568-8010; **Board Cert:** Internal Medicine 1973; Pulmonary Disease 1976; **Med School:** Jefferson Med Coll 1970; **Resid:** Internal Medicine, Montefiore Hosp Med Ctr 1973; **Fellow:** Pulmonary Disease, Montefiore Hosp Med Ctr 1975; **Fac Appt:** Asst Clin Prof Med, Mount Sinai Sch Med

Polkow, Melvin MD (Pul) - **Spec Exp:** Asthma; Sarcoidosis; Pulmonary Fibrosis; **Hospital:** Hackensack Univ Med Ctr (page 92); **Address:** 211 Essex St, Ste 302, Hackensack, NJ 07601; **Phone:** 201-498-1311; **Board Cert:** Internal Medicine 1980; Pulmonary Disease 1982; Critical Care Medicine 1996; **Med School:** SUNY Downstate 1977; **Resid:** Internal Medicine, Lenox Hill Hosp 1980; **Fellow:** Pulmonary Critical Care Medicine, Univ Hosp 1982; **Fac Appt:** Asst Clin Prof Med, UMDNJ-NJ Med Sch, Newark

Rose, Henry J MD (Pul) - **Spec Exp:** Asthma; Emphysema; Sleep Disorders; Lung Cancer; **Hospital:** PBI Regional- Passaic, Clara Maass Med Ctr; **Address:** 639 Ridge Rd, Lyndhurst, NJ 07071-3219; **Phone:** 201-939-8741; **Board Cert:** Internal Medicine 1982; Pulmonary Disease 1984; Critical Care Medicine 1991; **Med School:** UMDNJ-NJ Med Sch, Newark 1979; **Resid:** Internal Medicine, Univ of Medicine & Dentistry 1982; **Fellow:** Pulmonary Disease, Bronx Municipal Hosp 1984

Simon, Clifford J MD (Pul) - **Spec Exp:** Asthma; Lung Cancer; **Hospital:** Englewood Hosp & Med Ctr (page 760), Holy Name Hosp (page 761); **Address:** 180 Engle St, Englewood, NJ 07631; **Phone:** 201-567-2050; **Board Cert:** Internal Medicine 1976; Pulmonary Disease 1980; **Med School:** Cornell Univ-Weill Med Coll 1973; **Resid:** Internal Medicine, Dartmouth 1975; **Fellow:** Pulmonary Disease, Bellevue Hosp 1977

RADIATION ONCOLOGY

Dubin, David MD (RadRO) - **Spec Exp:** Breast Cancer; Brachytherapy; Prostate Cancer; **Hospital:** Englewood Hosp & Med Ctr (page 760); **Address:** Englewood Hosp, Dept Radiation Oncology, 350 Engle St, Englewood, NJ 07631-1808; **Phone:** 201-894-3125; **Board Cert:** Radiation Oncology 1991; **Med School:** Albert Einstein Coll Med 1986; **Resid:** Radiation Oncology, St Barnabas Hosp 1990

Gejerman, Glen MD (RadRO) - **Spec Exp:** Prostate Cancer; Intensity Modulated Radiotherapy (IMRT); **Hospital:** Hackensack Univ Med Ctr (page 92); **Address:** Hackensack Univ Med Ctr, Radiation Oncology, 30 Prospect Ave, St John Basement, Hackensack, NJ 07601; **Phone:** 201-996-2210; **Board Cert:** Radiation Oncology 1996; **Med School:** UMDNJ-NJ Med Sch, Newark 1990; **Resid:** Radiation Oncology, Montefiore Med Ctr/Albert Einstein 1995; **Fac Appt:** Asst Clin Prof RadRO, Albert Einstein Coll Med

Wesson, Michael MD (RadRO) - **Spec Exp:** Breast Cancer; Prostate Cancer; Brachytherapy; **Hospital:** Valley Hosp (page 762); **Address:** 223 N Van Dien Ave, Ridgewood, NJ 07450-2726; **Phone:** 201-634-5403; **Board Cert:** Radiation Oncology 1987; **Med School:** Univ VA Sch Med 1983; **Resid:** Radiation Oncology, Meml Sloan Kettering Cancer Ctr 1987

REPRODUCTIVE ENDOCRINOLOGY

Lesorgen, Philip MD (RE) - **Spec Exp:** Infertility; Infertility-IVF; Polycystic Ovarian Syndrome; **Hospital:** Englewood Hosp & Med Ctr (page 760), Hackensack Univ Med Ctr (page 92); **Address:** 106 Grand Ave Fl 4, Englewood, NJ 07631-3570; **Phone:** 201-569-6979; **Board Cert:** Obstetrics & Gynecology 1984; **Med School:** Boston Univ 1977; **Resid:** Obstetrics & Gynecology, LI Jewish Med Ctr 1981; **Fellow:** Reproductive Endocrinology, Thomas Jefferson Univ Hosp 1983; **Fac Appt:** Asst Clin Prof ObG, Seton Hall Univ Sch Grad Med Ed

Navot, Daniel MD (RE) - **Spec Exp:** Infertility-IVF; **Hospital:** Pascack Valley Hosp, Valley Hosp (page 762); **Address:** 400 Old Hook Rd, Westwood, NJ 07675-2732; **Phone:** 201-666-4200; **Board Cert:** Obstetrics & Gynecology 2002; Reproductive Endocrinology 2002; **Med School:** Israel 1978; **Resid:** Obstetrics & Gynecology, Hassadah Hosp 1983; **Fellow:** Reproductive Endocrinology, Jones Inst 1987; **Fac Appt:** Prof ObG, NY Med Coll

Slowey, Michael J MD (RE) - **Spec Exp:** Infertility-IVF; Infertility-Male & Female; Minimally Invasive Surgery; **Hospital:** Englewood Hosp & Med Ctr (page 760), Holy Name Hosp (page 761); **Address:** 25 Rockwood Pl, Englewood, NJ 07631-4957; **Phone:** 201-569-7773; **Board Cert:** Obstetrics & Gynecology 2004; Reproductive Endocrinology 2004; **Med School:** Univ Tenn Coll Med, Memphis 1987; **Resid:** Obstetrics & Gynecology, Naval Med Ctr 1991; **Fellow:** Reproductive Endocrinology, Michael Reese/Univ Illinois 1993

Weiss, Gerson MD (RE) - **Spec Exp:** Infertility; Menopause Problems; **Hospital:** Hackensack Univ Med Ctr (page 92), UMDNJ-Univ Hosp-Newark; **Address:** 214 Terrace Ave, Hasbrouck Heights, NJ 07604-1815; **Phone:** 201-288-6330; **Board Cert:** Obstetrics & Gynecology 1993; Reproductive Endocrinology 1974; **Med School:** NYU Sch Med 1964; **Resid:** Obstetrics & Gynecology, Bellevue Hosp Ctr 1969; **Fellow:** Reproductive Endocrinology, Univ Pittsburgh 1973; **Fac Appt:** Prof ObG, UMDNJ-NJ Med Sch, Newark

RHEUMATOLOGY

Kopelman, Rima G MD (Rhu) - **Spec Exp:** Rheumatoid Arthritis; Lupus/SLE; Vasculitis; **Hospital:** Valley Hosp (page 762), NY-Presby Hosp (page 100); **Address:** 301 Godwin Ave, Midland Park, NJ 07432-1544; **Phone:** 201-444-4526; **Board Cert:** Internal Medicine 1980; Rheumatology 1984; **Med School:** Columbia P&S 1977; **Resid:** Internal Medicine, Columbia-Presby 1981; **Fellow:** Rheumatology, Columbia-Presby 1983; **Fac Appt:** Asst Prof Med, Columbia P&S

Marcus, Ralph MD (Rhu) - **Spec Exp:** Rheumatoid Arthritis; Osteoporosis; Lupus/SLE; **Hospital:** Holy Name Hosp (page 761), Hackensack Univ Med Ctr (page 92); **Address:** 1415 Queen Anne Rd, Ste 102, Teaneck, NJ 07666-3521; **Phone:** 201-837-7788; **Board Cert:** Internal Medicine 1975; Rheumatology 1976; **Med School:** Albert Einstein Coll Med 1969; **Resid:** Internal Medicine, Mount Sinai Hosp 1974; **Fellow:** Rheumatology, Nat Inst Hlth 1972; Rheumatology, Hosp Special Surg 1976; **Fac Appt:** Assoc Clin Prof Med, UMDNJ-NJ Med Sch, Newark

Rosner, Steven MD (Rhu) - **Spec Exp:** Rheumatoid Arthritis; Fibromyalgia; Lupus/SLE; **Hospital:** Pascack Valley Hosp, Valley Hosp (page 762); **Address:** 452 Old Hook Rd, Emerson, NJ 07630; **Phone:** 201-666-3900; **Board Cert:** Internal Medicine 1979; Rheumatology 2004; **Med School:** NY Med Coll 1976; **Resid:** Internal Medicine, Metropolitan Hosp 1979; **Fellow:** Rheumatology, SUNY Downstate Med Ctr 1981; **Fac Appt:** Asst Clin Prof Med, UMDNJ-NJ Med Sch, Newark

Salem, Noel MD (Rhu) - **Hospital:** Englewood Hosp & Med Ctr (page 760); **Address:** 285 Engle St, Englewood, NJ 07631-2406; **Phone:** 201-871-0223; **Board Cert:** Internal Medicine 1976; Rheumatology 1998; Geriatric Medicine 2004; **Med School:** SUNY Buffalo 1972; **Resid:** Internal Medicine, USPHS Hosp-Staten Island, NY & USPHS Hosp 1974; **Fellow:** Rheumatology, Columbia-Presby 1976; **Fac Appt:** Asst Prof Med, Mount Sinai Sch Med

Zalkowitz, Alan MD (Rhu) - **Spec Exp:** Lupus/SLE; Rheumatoid Arthritis; Polymyositis; **Hospital:** Valley Hosp (page 762); **Address:** 31-00 Broadway, Fair Lawn, NJ 07410-2331; **Phone:** 201-796-2255; **Board Cert:** Internal Medicine 1977; Rheumatology 1982; **Med School:** Belgium 1970; **Resid:** Internal Medicine, Stamford Hosp 1972; **Fellow:** Rheumatology, Mount Sinai Hosp 1974

Sports Medicine

Gross, Michael L MD (SM) - **Hospital:** Hackensack Univ Med Ctr (page 92); **Address:** 25 Prospect Ave, Hackensack, NJ 07601; **Phone:** 201-343-2277; **Board Cert:** Orthopaedic Surgery 2002; **Med School:** NYU Sch Med 1983; **Resid:** Orthopaedic Surgery, Montefiore Med Ctr 1988; **Fellow:** Sports Medicine, UCLA Med Ctr 1989

Kelly, Michael A MD (SM) - **Spec Exp:** Knee Surgery; **Hospital:** Hackensack Univ Med Ctr (page 92), Lenox Hill Hosp (page 94); **Address:** 360 Essex St, Ste 303, Hackensack, NJ 07601; **Phone:** 201-336-8861; **Board Cert:** Orthopaedic Surgery 1999; **Med School:** Georgetown Univ 1979; **Resid:** Surgery, St Vincents Hosp 1981; Orthopaedic Surgery, Columbia-Presby Hosp 1984; **Fellow:** Knee Surgery, Hosp for Special Surgery 1985

Savatsky, Gary MD (SM) - **Spec Exp:** Shoulder & Knee Injuries; **Hospital:** Hackensack Univ Med Ctr (page 92); **Address:** 2 Forest Ave, Paramus, NJ 07652; **Phone:** 201-587-1111; **Board Cert:** Orthopaedic Surgery 1997; **Med School:** Columbia P&S 1975; **Resid:** Surgery, St Luke's-Roosevelt Hosp Ctr 1978; Orthopaedic Surgery, Hosp for Special Surgery 1983; **Fellow:** Orthopaedic Surgery, Hosp for Special Surgery 1979

Surgery

Ahlborn, Thomas N MD (S) - **Spec Exp:** Breast Surgery; Gastrointestinal Surgery; Hernia; **Hospital:** Valley Hosp (page 762); **Address:** 385 S Maple Ave, Glen Rock, NJ 07452; **Phone:** 201-444-5757; **Board Cert:** Surgery 2005; **Med School:** Columbia P&S 1980; **Resid:** Surgery, Columbia-Presby Hosp 1985; **Fellow:** Vascular Surgery, Columbia-Presby Hosp 1986

Ballantyne, Garth MD (S) - **Spec Exp:** Laparoscopic Surgery; Gastroesophageal Reflux Disease (GERD); Colon Cancer; **Hospital:** Hackensack Univ Med Ctr (page 92); **Address:** 20 Prospect Ave, Ste 901, Hackensack, NJ 07601-1974; **Phone:** 201-996-2959; **Board Cert:** Surgery 1984; Colon & Rectal Surgery 1985; **Med School:** Columbia P&S 1977; **Resid:** Surgery, UCLA Med Ctr 1980; Surgery, Northwestern Univ 1982; **Fellow:** Colon & Rectal Surgery, Mayo Clinic 1984; **Fac Appt:** Prof S, UMDNJ-NJ Med Sch, Newark

Benson, Douglas MD (S) - **Spec Exp:** Trauma; Critical Care; **Hospital:** Hackensack Univ Med Ctr (page 92), Holy Name Hosp (page 761); **Address:** 83 Summit Ave, Hackensack, NJ 07601-1262; **Phone:** 201-646-0010; **Board Cert:** Surgery 1995; Surgical Critical Care 1995; **Med School:** UMDNJ-NJ Med Sch, Newark 1971; **Resid:** Surgery, UMDNJ 1975; **Fac Appt:** Asst Clin Prof S, UMDNJ-NJ Med Sch, Newark

Bruck, Harold M MD (S) - **Spec Exp:** Breast Surgery; Cancer Surgery; Vein Disorders; **Hospital:** Valley Hosp (page 762); **Address:** 385 S Maple Ave, Ste 204, Ridgewood, NJ 07452-1545; **Phone:** 201-652-2800; **Board Cert:** Surgery 1969; **Med School:** Columbia P&S 1962; **Resid:** Surgery, Bellevue Hosp 1967; Surgery, Columbia-Presby Hosp 1968

Bufalini, Bruno MD (S) - **Spec Exp:** Laparoscopic Surgery; **Hospital:** Englewood Hosp & Med Ctr (page 760); **Address:** 200 Grand Ave, Englewood, NJ 07631-4371; **Phone:** 201-871-0303; **Med School:** Italy 1971; **Resid:** Surgery, Englewood Hosp 1976

Christoudias, George MD (S) - **Spec Exp:** Laparoscopic Hernia Repair; Laparoscopic Cholecystectomy; Cancer Surgery; **Hospital:** Holy Name Hosp (page 761); **Address:** 741 Teaneck Rd, Teaneck, NJ 07666; **Phone:** 201-833-2888; **Med School:** Greece 1969; **Resid:** Surgery, Downstate-Kings Co Med Ctr 1975; **Fellow:** Surgical Oncology, Downstate-Kings Co Med Ctr 1976

Davies, Richard MD (S) - **Spec Exp:** Cancer Surgery; Breast Cancer; Colon & Rectal Cancer; **Hospital:** Hackensack Univ Med Ctr (page 92); **Address:** Hackensack Univ Med Ctr, Dept Surgery, 30 Prospect Ave, Hackensack, NJ 07601-1914; **Phone:** 201-996-2625; **Board Cert:** Surgery 2003; **Med School:** England 1973; **Resid:** Surgery, Tulane Univ Med Ctr 1980; Research, Yale Univ Sch Med 1981; **Fellow:** Surgical Oncology, Meml Sloan-Kettering Cancer Ctr 1983; **Fac Appt:** Prof S, UMDNJ-NJ Med Sch, Newark

Fan, Peter MD (S) - **Spec Exp:** Laparoscopic Abdominal Surgery; Laparoscopic Hernia Repair; **Hospital:** Hackensack Univ Med Ctr (page 92); **Address:** 110 Summit Ave, Hackensack, NJ 07601-2205; **Phone:** 201-646-0066; **Board Cert:** Surgery 1974; **Med School:** England 1961; **Resid:** Surgery, Whittington Hosp 1964; Surgery, Hammersmith Hosp 1966; **Fac Appt:** Clin Prof S, UMDNJ-NJ Med Sch, Newark

Fried, Kenneth MD (S) - **Spec Exp:** Carotid Artery Surgery; Laparoscopic Surgery; **Hospital:** Englewood Hosp & Med Ctr (page 760), Holy Name Hosp (page 761); **Address:** 180 N Dean St, Ste 2 South, Englewood, NJ 07631-2541; **Phone:** 201-568-8666; **Board Cert:** Surgery 1994; **Med School:** NYU Sch Med 1978; **Resid:** Surgery, NYU Med Ctr 1983; **Fellow:** Vascular Surgery, NYU Med Ctr 1984; **Fac Appt:** Asst Clin Prof S, Mount Sinai Sch Med

Ganepola, G.A.P. MD (S) - **Spec Exp:** Cancer Surgery; **Hospital:** Valley Hosp (page 762); **Address:** 400 Franklin Tpke, Ste 110, Mahwah, NJ 07430-3517; **Phone:** 201-236-0400; **Board Cert:** Surgery 1975; **Med School:** Japan 1967; **Resid:** Surgery, Harlem Hosp-Columbia P&S 1974; **Fac Appt:** Assoc Clin Prof S, Columbia P&S

Ibrahim, Ibrahim M MD (S) - **Spec Exp:** Laparoscopic Surgery; Obesity/Bariatric Surgery; **Hospital:** Englewood Hosp & Med Ctr (page 760), Holy Name Hosp (page 761); **Address:** Bariatric Ctr, 350 Engle St, Englewood, NJ 07631; **Phone:** 201-227-5533; **Board Cert:** Surgery 1974; Vascular Surgery 1992; **Med School:** NYU Sch Med 1966; **Resid:** Surgery, NYU Med Ctr 1973; **Fellow:** Vascular Surgery, NYU Med Ctr 1974; **Fac Appt:** Assoc Prof S, Mount Sinai Sch Med

Joseph, Patricia MD (S) - **Spec Exp:** Breast Cancer; **Hospital:** Holy Name Hosp (page 761), Englewood Hosp & Med Ctr (page 760); **Address:** 610 E Palisade Ave, Englewood Cliffs, NJ 07632-1808; **Phone:** 201-567-5111; **Board Cert:** Surgery 1994; **Med School:** Univ Fla Coll Med 1979; **Resid:** Surgery, Montefiore Hosp Med Ctr 1984

Licata Jr, Joseph J MD (S) - **Spec Exp:** Laparoscopic Surgery; Breast Surgery; **Hospital:** Valley Hosp (page 762), Pascack Valley Hosp; **Address:** 245 E Main St, Ramsey, NJ 07446; **Phone:** 201-327-0220; **Board Cert:** Surgery 2002; **Med School:** Mexico 1984; **Resid:** Surgery, New York Med Coll 1991

Pereira, Stephen MD (S) - **Spec Exp:** Laparoscopic Abdominal Surgery; **Hospital:** Hackensack Univ Med Ctr (page 92); **Address:** 90 Prospect Ave, Ste 1D, Hackensack, NJ 07601-1918; **Phone:** 201-343-3433; **Board Cert:** Surgery 1997; **Med School:** UMDNJ-RW Johnson Med Sch 1991; **Resid:** Surgery, Northwestern Univ 1996; **Fellow:** Laparoscopic Surgery, Hackensack Univ Med Ctr; **Fac Appt:** Asst Clin Prof S, UMDNJ-NJ Med Sch, Newark

Schmidt, Hans J MD (S) - **Spec Exp:** Obesity/Bariatric Surgery; Abdominal Surgery-Laparoscopic; **Hospital:** Hackensack Univ Med Ctr (page 92); **Address:** 385 Prospect Ave, Hackensack, NJ 07601-2205; **Phone:** 201-646-1121; **Board Cert:** Surgery 1998; **Med School:** UMDNJ-NJ Med Sch, Newark 1991; **Resid:** Surgery, UMDNJ Univ Hosp 1997

Shapiro, Michael E MD (S) - **Spec Exp:** Transplant Surgery; Parathyroid Surgery; Dialysis Access Surgery; **Hospital:** Hackensack Univ Med Ctr (page 92); **Address:** 30 Prospect Ave, Hackensack, NJ 07601-1914; **Phone:** 201-996-2608; **Board Cert:** Surgery 1995; **Med School:** Univ Rochester 1977; **Resid:** Surgery, Beth Israel Med Ctr 1983; **Fac Appt:** Assoc Prof S, UMDNJ-NJ Med Sch, Newark

Silvestri, Fred MD (S) - **Spec Exp:** Laparoscopic Surgery; Hyperbaric Medicine; **Hospital:** Englewood Hosp & Med Ctr (page 760); **Address:** 375 Engle St, Englewood, NJ 07631; **Phone:** 201-894-0400; **Board Cert:** Surgery 2000; Surgical Critical Care 2002; **Med School:** SUNY Downstate 1983; **Resid:** Surgery, Staten Island Hosp 1988; **Fellow:** Vascular Surgery, Englewood Hosp 1989; Surgical Critical Care, North Shore Hosp 1990

Sussman, Barry MD (S) - **Spec Exp:** Breast Surgery; Laparoscopic Surgery; **Hospital:** Englewood Hosp & Med Ctr (page 760), Holy Name Hosp (page 761); **Address:** 375 Engle St, Englewood, NJ 07631-1823; **Phone:** 201-894-0400; **Board Cert:** Surgery 1998; Vascular Surgery 1995; **Med School:** NYU Sch Med 1973; **Resid:** Surgery, NYU Med Ctr 1978; **Fellow:** Vascular Surgery, Englewood Hosp 1979; **Fac Appt:** Asst Clin Prof S, Mount Sinai Sch Med

Walsky, Robert MD (S) - **Spec Exp:** Breast Surgery; **Hospital:** Pascack Valley Hosp, Valley Hosp (page 762); **Address:** 452 Old Hook Rd, Ste 302, Emerson, NJ 07630-1368; **Phone:** 201-967-1105; **Board Cert:** Surgery 1996; **Med School:** Univ Louisville Sch Med 1969; **Resid:** Surgery, Mount Sinai Hosp 1975; **Fac Appt:** Asst Clin Prof S, NY Med Coll

Yiengpruksawan, Anusak MD (S) - **Spec Exp:** Liver & Biliary Surgery; Endoscopic Ultrasound; Robotic Surgery; Minimally Invasive Surgery; **Hospital:** Valley Hosp (page 762), Pascack Valley Hosp; **Address:** 1200 E Ridgewood Ave, Ridgewood, NJ 07450; **Phone:** 201-493-1005; **Board Cert:** Surgery 2001; **Med School:** Japan 1978; **Resid:** Surgery, Harlem Hosp 1989; **Fellow:** Surgical Oncology, Meml Sloan Kettering Cancer Ctr 1991

THORACIC SURGERY

Elmann, Elie MD (TS) - **Spec Exp:** Robotic Heart Surgery; Minimally Invasive Cardiac Surgery; Heart Valve Surgery; **Hospital:** Hackensack Univ Med Ctr (page 92), Pascack Valley Hosp; **Address:** 20 Prospect Ave, Ste 900, Hackensack, NJ 07601; **Phone:** 201-996-2261; **Board Cert:** Surgery 2004; Thoracic Surgery 1996; **Med School:** NY Med Coll 1987; **Resid:** Surgery, Cabrini Med Ctr/NY Med Coll 1992; **Fellow:** Thoracic Surgery, SUNY Downstate 1995; **Fac Appt:** Asst Prof S, UMDNJ-NJ Med Sch, Newark

Ergin, M Arisan MD (TS) - **Spec Exp:** Cardiac Surgery; Transfusion Free Surgery; Aneurysm; **Hospital:** Englewood Hosp & Med Ctr (page 760); **Address:** 350 Engle St, Ste 1000, Englewood, NJ 07631-1808; **Phone:** 201-894-3636; **Board Cert:** Thoracic Surgery 1997; **Med School:** Turkey 1968; **Resid:** Surgery, Kings Co Hosp 1973; **Fellow:** Thoracic Surgery, Kings Co Hosp-SUNY 1976; **Fac Appt:** Prof S, Mount Sinai Sch Med

Lee, Youngick MD (TS) - **Spec Exp:** Lung Cancer; Esophageal Cancer; Video Assisted Thoracic Surgery (VATS); Esophageal Disorders; **Hospital:** Valley Hosp (page 762), Englewood Hosp & Med Ctr (page 760); **Address:** 145 Prospect St, Ridgewood, NJ 07450-4493; **Phone:** 201-652-3641; **Board Cert:** Thoracic Surgery 2005; Surgery 1974; **Med School:** South Korea 1963; **Resid:** Surgery, St Clare's Hosp 1968; Thoracic Surgery, Metro Hosp-NY Med Coll 1970; **Fellow:** Cardiothoracic Surgery, Univ Oregon 1982; **Fac Appt:** Asst Clin Prof S, NY Med Coll

Zairis, Ignatios MD (TS) - **Hospital:** Englewood Hosp & Med Ctr (page 760), Holy Name Hosp (page 761); **Address:** 741 Teaneck Rd, Teaneck, NJ 07666-4243; **Phone:** 201-837-8282; **Board Cert:** Surgery 2000; **Med School:** Greece 1973; **Resid:** Surgery, Downstate Med Ctr 1984; Cardiothoracic Surgery, Downstate Med Ctr 1984

UROLOGY

Basralian, Kevin R MD (U) - **Spec Exp:** Infertility-Male; Prostate Benign Disease; **Hospital:** Hackensack Univ Med Ctr (page 92), Holy Name Hosp (page 761); **Address:** 20 Prospect Ave, Ste 719, Hackensack, NJ 07601; **Phone:** 201-343-0082; **Board Cert:** Urology 2000; **Med School:** Mexico 1979; **Resid:** Surgery, Lenox Hill Hosp 1982; Urology, Lenox Hill Hosp 1985; **Fellow:** Pediatric Urology, Westchester Co Med Ctr 1985

Berdini, Jeffrey L MD (U) - **Spec Exp:** Kidney Stones; Prostate Cancer; Vasectomy Reversal; **Hospital:** Pascack Valley Hosp, Valley Hosp (page 762); **Address:** 92 Kinderkamack Rd, Woodcliff Lake, NJ 07677-8050; **Phone:** 201-391-1515; **Board Cert:** Urology 1980; **Med School:** UMDNJ-NJ Med Sch, Newark 1973; **Resid:** Urology, UNDMJ Affil Hosps 1978

Esposito, Michael P MD (U) - **Spec Exp:** Laparoscopic Kidney Surgery; Prostate Cancer/Robotic Surgery; Minimally Invasive Urologic Surgery; Adrenal Surgery; **Hospital:** Hackensack Univ Med Ctr (page 92), Valley Hosp (page 762); **Address:** 5 Summit Ave Fl 2, Hackensack, NJ 07601; **Phone:** 201-487-8866; **Board Cert:** Urology 2003; **Med School:** UMDNJ-NJ Med Sch, Newark 1994; **Resid:** Urology, UMDNJ Med Ctr 2000; **Fellow:** Urologic Laparoscopic Surgery-Endourology, Royal Infirmary/Western Genl Hosp 2001; **Fac Appt:** Asst Clin Prof S, UMDNJ-NJ Med Sch, Newark

Frey, Howard MD (U) - **Spec Exp:** Prostate Cancer; Bladder Cancer; Kidney Cancer; **Hospital:** Valley Hosp (page 762); **Address:** 4 Godwin Ave, Midland Park, NJ 07432-1980; **Phone:** 201-444-7070; **Board Cert:** Urology 2003; **Med School:** Johns Hopkins Univ 1977; **Resid:** Surgery, Johns Hopkins Hosp 1979; Urology, UCLA Med Ctr 1983

Hajjar, John H MD (U) - **Spec Exp:** Laparoscopic Surgery; Prostate Surgery; **Hospital:** Valley Hosp (page 762); **Address:** 1501 Broadway, Ste 1, Fair Lawn, NJ 07410-6001; **Phone:** 201-791-4544; **Board Cert:** Urology 2001; **Med School:** Georgetown Univ 1981; **Resid:** Surgery, NYU Med Ctr 1983; Urology, NYU-Bellevue/Sloan Ketterin 1987; **Fellow:** Research, NYU Med Ctr 1988

Katz, Steven A MD (U) - **Spec Exp:** Transfusion Free Cancer Surgery; Prostate Cancer; Prostate Surgery; **Hospital:** Englewood Hosp & Med Ctr (page 760), Holy Name Hosp (page 761); **Address:** 75 S Dean St, Englewood, NJ 07631-3512; **Phone:** 201-816-1900; **Board Cert:** Urology 1978; **Med School:** SUNY Buffalo 1969; **Resid:** Urology, Metropolitan Hosp Ctr 1976

Lanteri, Vincent J MD (U) - **Spec Exp:** Prostate Cancer/Robotic Surgery; Urologic Cancer; Minimally Invasive Urologic Surgery; **Hospital:** Hackensack Univ Med Ctr (page 92), Valley Hosp (page 762); **Address:** 5 Summit Ave Fl 2, Hackensack, NJ 07601; **Phone:** 201-487-8866; **Board Cert:** Urology 1982; **Med School:** Mexico 1974; **Resid:** Surgery, UMDNJ Med Ctr 1977; Urology, UMDNJ Med Ctr 1980; **Fellow:** Urologic Oncology, Roswell Park Cancer Inst 1981

Munver, Ravi MD (U) - **Spec Exp:** Prostate Cancer/Robotic Surgery; Minimally Invasive Urologic Surgery; Endourology; **Hospital:** Hackensack Univ Med Ctr (page 92); **Address:** 360 Essex St, Ste 403, Hackensack, NJ 07601; **Phone:** 201-336-8090; **Board Cert:** Urology 2005; **Med School:** Cornell Univ-Weill Med Coll 1996; **Resid:** Urology, Duke Univ Med Ctr 2002; **Fellow:** Endourology, New York Hosp-Cornell Med Ctr 2003; **Fac Appt:** Asst Prof U, UMDNJ-NJ Med Sch, Newark

Rosen, Jay S MD (U) - **Spec Exp:** Prostate Cancer/Robotic Surgery; Robotic Urologic Surgery; Kidney Stones; Genitourinary Cancer; **Hospital:** Hackensack Univ Med Ctr (page 92), Valley Hosp (page 762); **Address:** 1200 E Ridgewood Ave Bldg West Fl 2, Ridgewood, NJ 07450; **Phone:** 201-444-5988; **Board Cert:** Urology 2004; **Med School:** Mexico 1978; **Resid:** Urology, Mayo Clinic 1984; **Fac Appt:** Asst Clin Prof U, UMDNJ-NJ Med Sch, Newark

Sadeghi-Nejad, Hossein MD (U) - **Spec Exp:** Infertility-Male; Erectile Dysfunction; Microsurgery; Peyronie's Disease; **Hospital:** Hackensack Univ Med Ctr (page 92), UMDNJ-Univ Hosp-Newark; **Address:** 20 Prospect Ave, rm 711, Hackensack, NJ 07601; **Phone:** 201-342-7977; **Board Cert:** Urology 2000; **Med School:** McGill Univ 1989; **Resid:** Surgery, UCSF Med Ctr 1991; Urology, Boston Univ Med Ctr 1996; **Fellow:** Microsurgery, Boston Univ Med Ctr 1997; **Fac Appt:** Assoc Prof U, UMDNJ-NJ Med Sch, Newark

Sawczuk, Ihor S MD (U) - **Spec Exp:** Kidney Cancer; Bladder Cancer; Prostate Cancer/Robotic Surgery; **Hospital:** Hackensack Univ Med Ctr (page 92), NY-Presby Hosp (page 100); **Address:** Hackensack Univ Med Ctr, 360 Essex St, Hackensack, NJ 07601; **Phone:** 201-336-8090; **Board Cert:** Urology 1996; **Med School:** Med Coll PA Hahnemann 1979; **Resid:** Surgery, St Vincent's Hosp & Med Ctr 1981; Urology, Columbia-Presby Med Ctr 1984; **Fellow:** Urologic Oncology, Columbia-Presby Med Ctr 1986; **Fac Appt:** Prof U, Columbia P&S

Vitenson, Jack MD (U) - **Spec Exp:** Prostate Cancer; Bladder Cancer; Erectile Dysfunction; **Hospital:** Hackensack Univ Med Ctr (page 92); **Address:** 277 Forest Ave, Paramus, NJ 07652; **Phone:** 201-489-8900; **Board Cert:** Urology 1974; **Med School:** NY Med Coll 1965; **Resid:** Surgery, VA Med Ctr 1967; Urology, Metropolitan Hosp Ctr 1970; **Fac Appt:** Assoc Clin Prof U, UMDNJ-NJ Med Sch, Newark

Wasserman, Gary D MD (U) - **Spec Exp:** Laparoscopic Kidney Surgery; Prostate Surgery; Incontinence; **Hospital:** Englewood Hosp & Med Ctr (page 760), Holy Name Hosp (page 761); **Address:** 106 Grand Ave, Englewood, NJ 07631-3506; **Phone:** 201-569-7777; **Board Cert:** Urology 2001; **Med School:** Tulane Univ 1985; **Resid:** Surgery, Geo Wash Univ Med Ctr 1987; Urology, Tulane Univ Med Ctr 1991

VASCULAR SURGERY

Dardik, Herbert MD (VascS) - **Spec Exp:** Limb Salvage; Carotid Artery Surgery; Aneurysm-Aortic; **Hospital:** Englewood Hosp & Med Ctr (page 760); **Address:** Englewood Hosp, Dept Surgery, 350 Engle St, Englewood, NJ 07631-1823; **Phone:** 201-894-3689; **Board Cert:** Surgery 1966; Vascular Surgery 2001; **Med School:** NYU Sch Med 1960; **Resid:** Surgery, Montefiore Hosp Med Ctr 1965; **Fac Appt:** Clin Prof S, Mount Sinai Sch Med

De Groote, Robert MD (VascS) - **Spec Exp:** Stroke; Carotid Artery Surgery; **Hospital:** Hackensack Univ Med Ctr (page 92), Holy Name Hosp (page 761); **Address:** 83 Summit Ave, Hackensack, NJ 07601; **Phone:** 201-646-0010; **Board Cert:** Surgery 2004; Vascular Surgery 1997; Surgical Critical Care 1990; **Med School:** Mexico 1978; **Resid:** Surgery, UMDNJ Univ Hosp 1984; **Fellow:** Critical Care Medicine, UMDNJ Univ Hosp 1982; Vascular Surgery, UMDNJ Univ Hosp 1986; **Fac Appt:** Asst Clin Prof S, UMDNJ-NJ Med Sch, Newark

Elias, Steven MD (VascS) - **Spec Exp:** Vein Disorders; Wound Healing/Care; Endovascular Surgery; Varicose Veins; **Hospital:** Englewood Hosp & Med Ctr (page 760), Mount Sinai Med Ctr (page 98); **Address:** 350 Engle St, Englewood, NJ 07631-2541; **Phone:** 201-894-3252; **Board Cert:** Surgery 1997; **Med School:** SUNY Buffalo 1979; **Resid:** Surgery, Millard Filmore Hosp 1981; **Fellow:** Peripheral Vascular Surgery, Englewood Hosp 1985; **Fac Appt:** Asst Prof S, Mount Sinai Sch Med

Geuder, James MD (VascS) - **Spec Exp:** Carotid Artery Surgery; Aneurysm-Aortic; Endovascular Surgery; Peripheral Vascular Disease; **Hospital:** Hackensack Univ Med Ctr (page 92), Pascack Valley Hosp; **Address:** 20 Prospect Ave, Ste 707, Hackensack, NJ 07601-1963; **Phone:** 201-488-2220; **Board Cert:** Surgery 1997; Vascular Surgery 1999; **Med School:** Med Coll Wisc 1981; **Resid:** Surgery, UMDNJ Med Ctr 1986; **Fellow:** Vascular Surgery, NYU Med Ctr 1988

Manno, Joseph MD (VascS) - **Spec Exp:** Arterial Disease; Angioplasty; **Hospital:** Holy Name Hosp (page 761), Hackensack Univ Med Ctr (page 92); **Address:** 83 Summit Ave, Hackensack, NJ 07601-1262; **Phone:** 201-646-0010; **Board Cert:** Surgery 1999; Vascular Surgery 1993; **Med School:** Oral Roberts Sch Med 1982; **Resid:** Surgery, Univ of Med & Dentistry 1987; **Fellow:** Vascular Surgery, Univ of Med & Dentistry 1989

Moss, Charles M MD (VascS) - **Spec Exp:** Wound Healing/Care; **Hospital:** Hackensack Univ Med Ctr (page 92); **Address:** 20 Prospect Ave, Ste 707, Hackensack, NJ 07601; **Phone:** 201-488-2220; **Board Cert:** Surgery 1973; Vascular Surgery 2003; Undersea & Hyperbaric Medicine 2006; **Med School:** Tulane Univ 1967; **Resid:** Surgery, Montefiore Med Ctr 1972

Wolodiger, Fred MD (VascS) - **Spec Exp:** Arterial Bypass Surgery-Leg; Carotid Artery Surgery; Laparoscopic Surgery; **Hospital:** Englewood Hosp & Med Ctr (page 760), Holy Name Hosp (page 761); **Address:** 375 Engle St, Englewood, NJ 07631; **Phone:** 201-894-0400; **Board Cert:** Surgery 2004; Vascular Surgery 1997; **Med School:** SUNY Hlth Sci Ctr 1980; **Resid:** Surgery, North Shore Univ Hosp 1985; **Fellow:** Vascular Surgery, Englewood Hosp 1987

Regional Medical Centers
New Jersey (Bergen)

ENGLEWOOD HOSPITAL AND MEDICAL CENTER

E N G L E W O O D
HOSPITAL AND MEDICAL CENTER
AN AFFILIATE OF MOUNT SINAI SCHOOL OF MEDICINE

350 Engle Stree[t]
Englewood, New Jersey 0763[1]
(201) 894-300[0]
www.englewoodhospital.com

GENERAL DESCRIPTION

Englewood Hospital and Medical Center provides primary, secondary and tertiary care. We are a leader in innovative services and state-of-the-art clinical programs, and are among two percent of U.S. hospitals to achieve Magnet status for nursing. For seven consecutive years, we are home to more top-rated doctors than any other hospital in New Jersey.

AFFILIATIONS AND TEACHING PROGRAMS

Englewood Hospital and Medical Center is affiliated with The Mount Sinai School of Medicine. Through our affiliation, residents in surgery, pediatrics and pathology, as well as critical care medicine fellows, rotate through our Medical Center. Our institution also maintains a free-standing residency program in medicine and a fellowship in vascular surgery.

SPECIAL PROGRAMS AND SERVICES

Bloodless Medicine and Surgery - The New Jersey Institute for the Advancement of Bloodless Medicine and Surgery is a national and international research, education and referral center founded in 1994. Today, 95% of all our surgeries are performed transfusion-free. Englewood recently completed a demonstration project to help establish transfusion-free care as the standard for the nation.

Breast Care Center Our Cytodiagnosis and Breast Care Center offers rapid, highly accurate and frequently conclusive diagnoses in a matter of hours, usually without surgery. Designated by Congress in 1994 as a national model for breast cancer diagnosis and management, and recently acknowledged by the American College of Pathology for detecting tumors at least one-half the size of those detected at 95% of all other institutions in the U.S., this facility offers the most comprehensive and reliable means for the early diagnosis and treatment of breast cancer.

The Family Birth Place - Our newly renovated Family Birth Place is located in a dedicated wing that offers a family-centered birthing experience, including state-of-the-art equipment and exceptional services to help the entire family welcome their baby into a warm and reassuring environment. Our team of award-winning physicians and nurses provide the ultimate in expertise, skill and personal attention. We are the only hospital in New Jersey to have specialists in both maternal-fetal and neonatal medicine named among "Best Doctors" by *New York* and *NJ Monthly* magazines.

Heart & Vascular Institute of New Jersey - At the Heart & Vascular Institute of New Jersey, our patients have access to world-renowned experts in all areas of cardiology services, including interventional cardiology, cardiac surgery and vascular surgery. The Institute provides cross-specialty access to advanced medical treatment, diagnostic procedures, surgical modalities and rehabilitative services, resulting in a superior level of continuity of care. We employ the latest in diagnostic technology, including a new 64-Slice CT Scanner and an upgraded Cardiac Catheterization Lab. The New Jersey Department of Health and Senior Services has recognized Englewood Hospital as one of the top New Jersey hospitals for isolated coronary bypass surgery since the program's inception.

Radiology and Imaging - Committed to providing the most advanced and comprehensive services, we offer three Spiral CT Scanners, one 64 slice multi-detector CT, three 1.5 Tesla high-field MRI machines, a dedicated breast coil for detailed breast imaging, and 4-D ultrasound imaging in our antepartum testing unit. Additionally, Englewood recently added the latest generation PET/CT scanner for the most advanced diagnostic imaging in cancer care.

For a referral to one of our physicians, call 201-894-3456.

Sponsored Page

Holy Name Hospital

Member
NewYork-Presbyterian Healthcare System
Affiliate: Columbia University College of Physicians & Surgeons

718 Teaneck Road
Teaneck, NJ 07666
(201) 833-3000
www.holyname.org

GENERAL OVERVIEW

Founded and sponsored in 1925 by the Sisters of St. Joseph of Peace, Holy Name Hospital is a comprehensive 361-bed acute care medical center that has stayed true to its community roots. Centers of excellence in cardiovascular services, cancer care, orthopedic services, dialysis treatment, women's health care and neurology services, and other state-of-the-art diagnostic, treatment and health management services, provide high-quality health care from prevention through treatment to recovery and wellness.

WORLD-CLASS MEDICAL CARE

Holy Name Hospital is distinguished by its long history of innovation and record of achievements. It was the first hospital in New Jersey and the third in the world to use respiratory gating technology to treat lung cancer. It is the first hospital in the nation to receive three J.D. Power and Associates Distinguished Hospital Awards for Inpatient, Outpatient and Emergency Service Excellence. For two consecutive years (2005 and 2006) Holy Name received the HealthGrades® Distinguished Hospital Award for Clinical Excellence™. It is among a select group of hospitals in the state to receive Primary Stroke Center designation from the Joint Commission on Accreditation of Healthcare Organizations. Its Institute for Clinical Research exceeds the highest standards for carrying out today's most promising clinical trials. The new Interventional Institute is using revolutionary technology to treat chronic and inoperable conditions without surgery. And the PET/CT Center joins a handful of prestigious medical institutions in the United States to perform Cardiac PET stress testing.

SERVICE-DRIVEN

Each year, the hospital serves more than 25,000 inpatients and 44,000 Emergency Department patients. There are more than 600 board-certified physicians within all specialties and sub-specialties on the medical staff. The hospital is a member of the NewYork-Presbyterian Healthcare System and academically affiliated with the Columbia University College of Physicians and Surgeons.

Holy Name Hospital Centers of Excellence include:

- Cardiovascular Services

- Regional Cancer Center

- Bone & Joint Center

- The Institute for Clinical Research

- Primary Stroke Center

- The BirthPlace

- The Interventional Institute

- Regional Dialysis Center

- Emergency Services

- Multiple Sclerosis Center

- Northern NJ Center for Sleep Medicine

- PET/CT Center

For more information about our Centers of Excellence or any service, call (201) 833-3000

778

THE VALLEY HOSPITAL

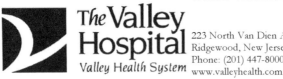

The Valley Hospital
Valley Health System

223 North Van Dien Avenue
Ridgewood, New Jersey 07450
Phone: (201) 447-8000
www.valleyhealth.com

Sponsorship:	Voluntary Not-for Profit
Beds:	431 Acute Care Beds
Accreditation:	Accredited by the Joint Commission on Accreditation of Healthcare Organizations

PROFILE
Serving more than 440,000 people in Bergen County and adjoining communities, and affiliated with The New York Presbyterian Healthcare System, Valley has received the J.D. Power & Associates Distinguished Hospital Award for Service Excellence and the Magnet Award for Nursing Excellence.

MEDICAL STAFF
The Valley Hospital has more than 700 physicians on its Active Medical Staff and 91 percent of the Active Staff is Board Certified.

CARDIOLOGY
Known throughout northern New Jersey for its medical and technical excellence, Valley is a leader in the field of cardiology services. The service includes a full range of diagnostic and interventional cardiac treatment services, including cardiac surgery, coronary angioplasty and electrophysiology studies. A leader in cardiac care research, Valley offers medical and procedural clinical trials that are at the forefront of coronary care. Valley has also established a relationship with NewYork-Presbyterian Healthcare System to offer the services of *The Valley Columbia Heart Center.*

ONCOLOGY
Certified by the American College of Surgeons as a Community Hospital Comprehensive Cancer Program, Valley is widely known for its prostate seed implant program which it played a leading role in pioneering. Additional innovative treatments include Intensity Modulated Radiation Therapy. The hospital recently opened a free-standing, full-service Cancer Center, designed to bring clinical and support services to patients and their families in an easily-accessible off-site location.

OBSTETRICS
The hospital offers a full range of maternity services, including Maternal-Fetal Medicine, a newly renovated and enhanced Neonatal Intensive Care Unit directed by 4 neonatologists, a Maternal & Child Health home care program, and a full-service Center for Child Development. The hospital also offers a Center for Fertility including a new, state-of-the-art embryology laboratory.

SURGERY
The Valley Hospital is also known for its comprehensive Surgical Program, including pioneering advances in surgical oncology and a full-service Center for Minimally Invasive and Robotic Surgery.

Physician Referral	*Valley Connection* 1-800-VALLEY 1
	A free, seven-day telephone referral service providing callers with information on programs the hospital offers, registration for community programs, and information on the more than 700 Active Medical Staff physicians affiliated with The Valley Hospital.

797

Essex

Essex

ADOLESCENT MEDICINE

Johnson, Robert L MD (AM) - **Spec Exp:** AIDS/HIV; Abuse/Neglect; **Hospital:** UMDNJ-Univ Hosp-Newark; **Address:** 185 S Orange Ave, rm C677, Newark, NJ 07103-2714; **Phone:** 973-972-5277; **Board Cert:** Pediatrics 1977; **Med School:** UMDNJ-NJ Med Sch, Newark 1972; **Resid:** Pediatrics, Martland Hosp 1974; **Fellow:** Adolescent Medicine, NYU Med Ctr 1976

Stanford, Paulette D MD (AM) - **Spec Exp:** AIDS/HIV in Adolescents; Adolescent Gynecology; Adolescent Behavior-High Risk; **Hospital:** UMDNJ-Univ Hosp-Newark; **Address:** UMDNJ - Dept Pediatrics, Adolescent Med, 90 Bergen St, Ste 4300, Newark, NJ 07103; **Phone:** 973-972-2100; **Board Cert:** Pediatrics 1984; Adolescent Medicine 2002; **Med School:** UMDNJ-NJ Med Sch, Newark 1975; **Resid:** Pediatrics, UMDNJ-Univ Hosp 1977; **Fellow:** Adolescent Medicine, UMDNJ-Univ Hosp 1979; **Fac Appt:** Prof Ped, UMDNJ-NJ Med Sch, Newark

ALLERGY & IMMUNOLOGY

Bielory, Leonard MD (A&I) - **Spec Exp:** Complementary Medicine; Asthma; Eye Allergy; **Hospital:** UMDNJ-Univ Hosp-Newark, St Barnabas Med Ctr; **Address:** 90 Bergen St, Ste 4700, Newark, NJ 07103-2499; **Phone:** 973-972-2762; **Board Cert:** Internal Medicine 1984; Allergy & Immunology 1985; Clinical & Laboratory Immunology 1986; **Med School:** UMDNJ-NJ Med Sch, Newark 1980; **Resid:** Internal Medicine, Univ Md Hosp 1982; Hematology, Natl Inst Hlth 1983; **Fellow:** Allergy & Immunology, Natl Inst Hlth 1985; **Fac Appt:** Prof Med, UMDNJ-NJ Med Sch, Newark

Perlman, Donald B MD (A&I) - **Spec Exp:** Asthma; Food Allergy; **Hospital:** St Barnabas Med Ctr; **Address:** 101 Old Short Hills Rd, Ste 407, West Orange, NJ 07052-1023; **Phone:** 973-736-7722; **Board Cert:** Pediatrics 1978; Allergy & Immunology 1979; **Med School:** Mount Sinai Sch Med 1973; **Resid:** Pediatrics, Mt Sinai Hosp 1976; **Fellow:** Allergy & Immunology, Duke Univ Med Ctr 1978; **Fac Appt:** Asst Clin Prof Ped, UMDNJ-NJ Med Sch, Newark

Weiss, Steven J MD (A&I) - **Spec Exp:** Asthma; Sinus Disorders; **Hospital:** St Barnabas Med Ctr; **Address:** 209 S Livingston Ave, Ste 6, Livingston, NJ 07039-4042; **Phone:** 973-992-4171; **Board Cert:** Internal Medicine 1985; Allergy & Immunology 1987; **Med School:** Univ Hlth Sci/Chicago Med Sch 1982; **Resid:** Internal Medicine, St Luke's Roosevelt Hosp Ctr 1985; **Fellow:** Allergy & Immunology, St Luke's Roosevelt Hosp Ctr 1987; **Fac Appt:** Asst Clin Prof Med, Mount Sinai Sch Med

CARDIAC ELECTROPHYSIOLOGY

Correia, Joaquim MD (CE) - **Spec Exp:** Arrhythmias; Pacemakers; Defibrillators; **Hospital:** UMDNJ-Univ Hosp-Newark, Trinitas Hosp; **Address:** 243 Chestnut St, Ste 2L, Newark, NJ 07105; **Phone:** 973-589-8668; **Board Cert:** Internal Medicine 1989; Cardiovascular Disease 2001; Cardiac Electrophysiology 2004; **Med School:** NYU Sch Med 1986; **Resid:** Internal Medicine, Columbia-Presby Med Ctr 1989; **Fellow:** Cardiovascular Disease, Columbia-Presby Med Ctr 1992; Cardiac Electrophysiology, Columbia-Presby Med Ctr 1993; **Fac Appt:** Asst Prof Med, UMDNJ-NJ Med Sch, Newark

Costeas, Constantinos A MD (CE) - **Spec Exp:** Arrhythmias; Radiofrequency Ablation; Pacemakers; **Hospital:** Saint Michael's Med Ctr, St Barnabas Med Ctr; **Address:** 101 Old Short Hills Rd, Ste 120, West Orange, NJ 07052; **Phone:** 973-731-9598; **Board Cert:** Cardiovascular Disease 1997; Cardiac Electrophysiology 1998; **Med School:** SUNY Stony Brook 1989; **Resid:** Internal Medicine, Univ Hosp 1992; **Fellow:** Cardiovascular Disease, St Vincent's Hosp 1996; Cardiac Electrophysiology, Columbia-Presby Med Ctr 1998

Rothbart, Stephen MD (CE) - **Spec Exp:** Cardiac Catheterization; Pacemakers; Defibrillators; **Hospital:** Newark Beth Israel Med Ctr, St Barnabas Med Ctr; **Address:** 201 Lyons Ave, Fl G4, Newark, NJ 07112-2027; **Phone:** 973-926-8590; **Board Cert:** Internal Medicine 1981; Cardiovascular Disease 1983; Cardiac Electrophysiology 1992; **Med School:** UMDNJ-NJ Med Sch, Newark 1977; **Resid:** Internal Medicine, Univ Hosp 1978; **Fellow:** Cardiovascular Disease, Newark Beth Israel Med Ctr 1983; **Fac Appt:** Asst Clin Prof Med, UMDNJ-NJ Med Sch, Newark

CARDIOVASCULAR DISEASE

Bahler, Alan MD (Cv) - **Hospital:** St Barnabas Med Ctr; **Address:** 201 S Livingston Ave 2F Bldg, Livingston, NJ 07039-4040; **Phone:** 973-535-9292; **Board Cert:** Internal Medicine 1974; **Med School:** Cornell Univ-Weill Med Coll 1971; **Resid:** Internal Medicine, Peter B Brigham Hosp 1973; **Fellow:** Cardiovascular Disease, Peter B Brigham Hosp 1973; Cardiovascular Disease, Mt Sinai Hosp 1975

Ciccone, John MD (Cv) - **Spec Exp:** Interventional Cardiology; Complementary Medicine; **Hospital:** St Barnabas Med Ctr, Morristown Mem Hosp (page 88); **Address:** 741 Northfield Ave, Ste 205, West Orange, NJ 07052; **Phone:** 973-467-1544; **Board Cert:** Internal Medicine 1982; Cardiovascular Disease 1985; **Med School:** UMDNJ-NJ Med Sch, Newark 1979; **Resid:** Internal Medicine, UMDNJ-Univ Hosp 1982; **Fellow:** Cardiovascular Disease, UMDNJ-Newark Beth Israel Hosp 1984; **Fac Appt:** Asst Clin Prof Med, UMDNJ-NJ Med Sch, Newark

Goldstein, Jonathan E MD (Cv) - **Spec Exp:** Interventional Cardiology; Cardiac Catheterization; **Hospital:** Saint Michael's Med Ctr, St Barnabas Med Ctr; **Address:** Saint Michael's Med Ctr, Dept Medicine, 111 Central Ave, Newark, NJ 07102; **Phone:** 973-877-5430; **Board Cert:** Internal Medicine 1978; Cardiovascular Disease 1981; Interventional Cardiology 1999; **Med School:** UMDNJ-NJ Med Sch, Newark 1973; **Resid:** Internal Medicine, Univ Miami Hosps 1976; **Fellow:** Cardiovascular Disease, Boston Med Ctr 1978; **Fac Appt:** Assoc Prof Med, Seton Hall Univ Sch Grad Med Ed

Klapholz, Marc MD (Cv) - **Spec Exp:** Congestive Heart Failure; Angioplasty; **Hospital:** UMDNJ-Univ Hosp-Newark; **Address:** 185 S Orange Ave Med Sci Bldg, I-536, Newark, NJ 07103; **Phone:** 973-972-4731; **Board Cert:** Internal Medicine 1989; Cardiovascular Disease 2002; Interventional Cardiology 1999; **Med School:** Albert Einstein Coll Med 1986; **Resid:** Internal Medicine, Bronx Muni Hosp 1989; **Fellow:** Cardiovascular Disease, Montefiore Med Ctr 1992

Miller, Kenneth Paul MD (Cv) - **Spec Exp:** Interventional Cardiology; **Hospital:** Mountainside Hosp (page 88), St Barnabas Med Ctr; **Address:** 62 S Fullerton Ave, Montclair, NJ 07042-2629; **Phone:** 973-746-8585; **Board Cert:** Internal Medicine 1981; Cardiovascular Disease 1989; Interventional Cardiology 2002; **Med School:** NYU Sch Med 1982; **Resid:** Internal Medicine, Bronx Muni Hosp 1986; **Fellow:** Cardiovascular Disease, Columbia Presby Med Ctr 1989

Rogal, Gary J MD (Cv) - **Spec Exp:** Echocardiography; Coronary Artery Disease; **Hospital:** St Barnabas Med Ctr, Newark Beth Israel Med Ctr; **Address:** 769 Northfield Ave, Ste 220, W Orange, NJ 07052; **Phone:** 973-731-9442; **Board Cert:** Internal Medicine 1981; Cardiovascular Disease 1983; **Med School:** Geo Wash Univ 1978; **Resid:** Internal Medicine, LI Jewish Med Ctr 1981; **Fellow:** Cardiovascular Disease, Strong Meml Hosp 1984

Saroff, Alan MD (Cv) - **Spec Exp:** Heart Valve Disease; Cholesterol/Lipid Disorders; Arrhythmias; Preventive Cardiology; **Hospital:** Mountainside Hosp (page 88); **Address:** Montclair Cardiology Group, 123 Highland Ave, Ste 302, Glen Ridge, NJ 07028-1522; **Phone:** 973-748-9555; **Board Cert:** Internal Medicine 1972; Cardiovascular Disease 1975; **Med School:** SUNY Upstate Med Univ 1965; **Resid:** Internal Medicine, SUNY-Syracuse Med Ctr 1967; Internal Medicine, New York Hosp 1970; **Fellow:** Cardiovascular Disease, Columbia Presby Med Ctr 1972; Cardiac Electrophysiology, Columbia Presby Med Ctr 1973; **Fac Appt:** Assoc Clin Prof Med, Columbia P&S

Shamoon, Fayez E MD (Cv) - **Spec Exp:** Interventional Cardiology; Coronary Artery Disease; Nuclear Cardiology; **Hospital:** Saint Michael's Med Ctr, Clara Maass Med Ctr; **Address:** Saint Michael's Med Ctr, Dept Cardiology, 268 Martin Lutherr King Jr Blvd, Newark, NJ 07102; **Phone:** 973-877-5160; **Board Cert:** Internal Medicine 1991; Cardiovascular Disease 1995; Interventional Cardiology 1999; **Med School:** Jordan 1981; **Resid:** Internal Medicine, Jordan Univ Hosp 1985; Internal Medicine, Saint Michael's Med Ctr 1992; **Fellow:** Cardiovascular Disease, Saint Michael's Med Ctr 1995; Interventional Cardiology, Saint Michael's Med Ctr 1996; **Fac Appt:** Assoc Prof Med, Seton Hall Univ Sch Grad Med Ed

Wangenheim, Paul MD (Cv) - **Spec Exp:** Interventional Cardiology; Complementary Medicine; Echocardiography; **Hospital:** St Barnabas Med Ctr, Morristown Mem Hosp (page 88); **Address:** 741 Northfield Ave, Ste 205, West Orange, NJ 07052; **Phone:** 973-467-1544; **Board Cert:** Internal Medicine 1985; Cardiovascular Disease 1987; **Med School:** UMDNJ-NJ Med Sch, Newark 1982; **Resid:** Internal Medicine, VA Med Ctr 1985; Internal Medicine, Univ Hosp/Newark Beth Israel Med Ctr 1985; **Fellow:** Cardiovascular Disease, Newark Beth Israel Med Ctr 1987

Werres, Roland MD (Cv) - **Spec Exp:** Angioplasty; Pacemakers; Congestive Heart Failure; **Hospital:** Newark Beth Israel Med Ctr, St Barnabas Med Ctr; **Address:** 2130 Millburn Ave, Ste A4, Maplewood, NJ 07040; **Phone:** 973-275-9300; **Board Cert:** Internal Medicine 1974; Cardiovascular Disease 1977; **Med School:** Germany 1967; **Resid:** Internal Medicine, Newark Beth Israel Med Ctr 1974; **Fellow:** Cardiovascular Disease, Newark Beth Israel Med Ctr 1976

Wu, Chia F MD (Cv) - **Hospital:** St Barnabas Med Ctr; **Address:** 35 Park Ave, W Orange, NJ 07052-5526; **Phone:** 973-325-3445; **Board Cert:** Internal Medicine 1972; Cardiovascular Disease 1975; **Med School:** Taiwan 1969; **Resid:** Internal Medicine, Martland Hosp 1972; **Fellow:** Cardiovascular Disease, Martland Hosp 1974; **Fac Appt:** Asst Clin Prof Med, UMDNJ-NJ Med Sch, Newark

Zucker, Mark Jay MD (Cv) - **Spec Exp:** Transplant Medicine-Heart; Heart Failure; Pulmonary Hypertension; **Hospital:** Newark Beth Israel Med Ctr, St Barnabas Med Ctr; **Address:** Heart Failure Trmt & Transplant Program, 201 Lyons Ave, Ste L4, Newark, NJ 07112; **Phone:** 973-926-7205; **Board Cert:** Internal Medicine 1984; Cardiovascular Disease 1987; **Med School:** Northwestern Univ 1981; **Resid:** Internal Medicine, Northwestern Meml Hosp 1984; **Fellow:** Cardiovascular Disease, Northwestern Meml Hosp 1987; **Fac Appt:** Assoc Clin Prof Med, Mount Sinai Sch Med

CHILD & ADOLESCENT PSYCHIATRY

Bartlett, Jacqueline MD (ChAP) - **Spec Exp:** Stress Management; ADD/ADHD; Mood Disorders; **Hospital:** UMDNJ-Univ Hosp-Newark; **Address:** 183 S Orange Ave, BHSB - rmF1534, Newark, NJ 07103; **Phone:** 973-972-2977; **Board Cert:** Psychiatry 1983; **Med School:** Univ Cincinnati 1971; **Resid:** Pediatrics, Montefiore Hospital 1976; Psychiatry, Columbia-Presby Med Ctr 1981; **Fellow:** Child & Adolescent Psychiatry, Columbia-Presby Med Ctr 1979; **Fac Appt:** Assoc Prof Ped, UMDNJ-NJ Med Sch, Newark

CHILD NEUROLOGY

Pak, Jayoung MD (ChiN) - **Spec Exp:** Epilepsy/Seizure Disorders; Brain Mapping; **Hospital:** UMDNJ-Univ Hosp-Newark; **Address:** UMDNJ Doctor's Office Ctr, 90 Bergen St , rm 8100, Newark, NJ 07103-2406; **Phone:** 973-972-5204; **Board Cert:** Child Neurology 1993; Clinical Neurophysiology 1993; **Med School:** South Korea 1978; **Resid:** Pediatrics, Ewha Women's Univ 1983; Pediatrics, UMDNJ-Univ Hosp 1988; **Fellow:** Child Neurology, UMDNJ-Univ Hosp 1991; Epilepsy, Columbia-Presby Med Ctr 1993; **Fac Appt:** Assoc Prof N, UMDNJ-NJ Med Sch, Newark

CLINICAL GENETICS

Desposito, Franklin MD (CG) - **Spec Exp:** Birth Defects; Genetic Disorders; **Hospital:** UMDNJ-Univ Hosp-Newark; **Address:** 90 Bergen St, Ste 5400, Newark, NJ 07103; **Phone:** 973-972-3300; **Board Cert:** Pediatrics 1986; Clinical Genetics 1982; Clinical Cytogenetics 1990; Clinical Molecular Genetics 2004; **Med School:** Univ Hlth Sci/Chicago Med Sch 1957; **Resid:** Pediatrics, Long Island Jewish Hosp 1961; **Fellow:** Hematology, Univ Wisc Sch Med 1963; **Fac Appt:** Prof Ped, UMDNJ-NJ Med Sch, Newark

COLON & RECTAL SURGERY

Holmes, Nathaniel J MD (CRS) - **Spec Exp:** Colon & Rectal Cancer; Laparoscopic Surgery; **Hospital:** Mountainside Hosp (page 88), Overlook Hosp (page 88); **Address:** 1 Bay Ave, Montclair, NJ 07042; **Phone:** 973-429-6689; **Board Cert:** Surgery 1996; Colon & Rectal Surgery 1999; **Med School:** Univ Pittsburgh 1987; **Resid:** Surgery, RW Johnson Univ Hosp 1993; **Fellow:** Colon & Rectal Surgery, St Vincent Health Ctr 1994

Rothberg, Robert MD (CRS) - **Spec Exp:** Colon & Rectal Cancer; Colonoscopy; Inflammatory Bowel Disease; **Hospital:** Mountainside Hosp (page 88), Clara Maass Med Ctr; **Address:** 39 S Fullerton Ave, Montclair, NJ 07042-6303; **Phone:** 973-744-0550; **Board Cert:** Surgery 1990; Colon & Rectal Surgery 1978; **Med School:** NYU Sch Med 1972; **Resid:** Surgery, Hackensack Hosp 1977; Colon & Rectal Surgery, Muhlenberg Hosp 1978

CRITICAL CARE MEDICINE

Shah, Smita MD (CCM) - **Hospital:** St Barnabas Med Ctr, Newark Beth Israel Med Ctr; **Address:** 96 Millburn Ave, Ste 200-A, Millburn, NJ 07040; **Phone:** 973-763-6800; **Board Cert:** Internal Medicine 1986; Pulmonary Disease 2000; Critical Care Medicine 2001; **Med School:** India 1980; **Resid:** Internal Medicine, St Mary's Hosp 1986; **Fellow:** Pulmonary Disease, Temple Univ Hosp 1988

DERMATOLOGY

Brodkin, Roger MD (D) - **Spec Exp:** Skin Allergies; Skin Cancer; Melanoma; **Hospital:** St Barnabas Med Ctr, UMDNJ-Univ Hosp-Newark; **Address:** Center for Dermatology, 101 Old Short Hills Rd, Ste 401, W Orange, NJ 07052-1023; **Phone:** 973-736-9535; **Board Cert:** Dermatology 1964; **Med School:** Jefferson Med Coll 1958; **Resid:** Dermatology, Bellevue Hosp 1962; Dermatology, NYU 1961; **Fac Appt:** Clin Prof D, UMDNJ-NJ Med Sch, Newark

Connolly, Adrian L MD (D) - **Spec Exp:** Mohs' Surgery; Skin Cancer; **Hospital:** St Barnabas Med Ctr; **Address:** 101 Old Short Hills Rd, Ste 503, West Orange, NJ 07052-1023; **Phone:** 973-731-9131; **Board Cert:** Dermatology 1999; **Med School:** UMDNJ-NJ Med Sch, Newark 1975; **Resid:** Dermatology, NYU Med Ctr 1979; **Fellow:** Mohs Surgery, NYU Med Ctr 1980; **Fac Appt:** Asst Clin Prof D, UMDNJ-NJ Med Sch, Newark

Downie, Jeanine B MD (D) - **Spec Exp:** Cosmetic Dermatology; Botox Therapy; Black/Asian Skin Care; Skin Laser Surgery; **Hospital:** Overlook Hosp (page 88), Mountainside Hosp (page 88); **Address:** 51 Park St, Montclair, NJ 07042; **Phone:** 973-509-6900; **Board Cert:** Dermatology 1998; **Med School:** SUNY Hlth Sci Ctr 1992; **Resid:** Pediatrics, NY Hosp-Cornell Med Ctr 1994; Dermatology, Mt Sinai Med Ctr 1997

Liftin, Alan MD (D) - **Spec Exp:** Cosmetic Dermatology; **Hospital:** St Barnabas Med Ctr; **Address:** 22 Old Short Hills Rd, Ste 103, Livingston, NJ 07039-5605; **Phone:** 973-535-5800; **Board Cert:** Dermatology 1990; Dermatopathology 1989; **Med School:** Mount Sinai Sch Med 1987; **Resid:** Pathology, Mt Sinai Hosp 1985; Dermatology, Mt Sinai Hosp 1990; **Fellow:** Dermatopathology, Hosp U Penn 1986

Machler, Brian MD (D) - **Hospital:** St Barnabas Med Ctr; **Address:** 101 Old Short Hills Rd, West Orange, NJ 07052; **Phone:** 973-736-9535; **Board Cert:** Dermatology 2004; **Med School:** Univ Ala 1991; **Resid:** Dermatology, Jackson Meml Hosp 1995

Rozanski, Reuben MD (D) - **Spec Exp:** Cosmetic Dermatology; Acne; Rosacea; **Hospital:** Mountainside Hosp (page 88); **Address:** 200 Highland Ave, Glen Ridge, NJ 07028-1528; **Phone:** 973-748-9474; **Board Cert:** Internal Medicine 1974; Dermatology 1979; **Med School:** Boston Univ 1970; **Resid:** Internal Medicine, Montefiore Med Ctr 1974; Dermatology, Albert Einstein Coll Med 1976

Schwartz, Robert A MD (D) - **Spec Exp:** Skin Cancer; Atopic Dermatitis; Rosacea; **Hospital:** UMDNJ-Univ Hosp-Newark; **Address:** 185 S Orange Ave, Bldg MSB - rm H 576, Newark, NJ 07103; **Phone:** 973-972-2505; **Board Cert:** Dermatology 1978; Clinical & Laboratory Dematologic Immunology 1985; **Med School:** NY Med Coll 1974; **Resid:** Dermatology, Univ Hosp 1977; Dermatology, Roswell Park Meml Inst 1978; **Fellow:** Dermatopathology, NJ Med Sch Affil Hosps 1990; **Fac Appt:** Prof D, UMDNJ-NJ Med Sch, Newark

Seibt, R Stephen MD (D) - **Spec Exp:** Skin Cancer; Aging Skin; **Hospital:** St Luke's - Roosevelt Hosp Ctr - Roosevelt Div (page 90), NY-Presby Hosp (page 100); **Address:** 92 Old Northfield Rd, W Orange, NJ 07052-5337; **Phone:** 973-736-0885; **Med School:** Univ Minn 1976; **Resid:** Dermatology, USPHS Hosp-Staten Island NY & USPHS Hosp 1980; **Fac Appt:** Assoc Prof D, Columbia P&S

DIAGNOSTIC RADIOLOGY

Jewel, Kenneth MD (DR) - **Spec Exp:** MRI; CT Scan; **Address:** 116 Park St, Montclair, NJ 07042-2930; **Phone:** 973-746-2525; **Board Cert:** Diagnostic Radiology 1973; **Med School:** SUNY Buffalo 1968; **Resid:** Radiology, Staten Island USPHS Hosp 1971; **Fellow:** Diagnostic Radiology, Columbia-Presby Hosp 1972

Lee, Huey-jen MD (DR) - **Spec Exp:** Brain Imaging; Head & Neck Imaging; Spine Neuroradiologic Diagnosis; Brain Tumors; **Hospital:** UMDNJ-Univ Hosp-Newark; **Address:** 150 Bergen St, Ste C320, Newark, NJ 07103; **Phone:** 973-972-4202; **Board Cert:** Radiology 1990; Neuroradiology 2004; **Med School:** Taiwan 1976; **Resid:** Pediatrics, Taipei Jen-Ai Hosp 1979; Radiology, Beth Israel Med Ctr 1988; **Fellow:** Neuroradiology, NY Med Coll 1989; **Fac Appt:** Prof Rad, UMDNJ-NJ Med Sch, Newark

Lutzker, Letty G MD (DR) - **Hospital:** St Barnabas Med Ctr; **Address:** St Barnabas Med Ctr, Dept Nuclear Med, 94 Old Short Hills Rd, Livingston, NJ 07039-5672; **Phone:** 973-322-5814; **Board Cert:** Diagnostic Radiology 1973; Nuclear Medicine 1974; Nuclear Radiology 1977; **Med School:** Albert Einstein Coll Med 1968; **Resid:** Diagnostic Radiology, Montefiore Med Ctr 1972; **Fac Appt:** Assoc Clin Prof NuM, Albert Einstein Coll Med

Norton, Karen MD (DR) - **Spec Exp:** Pediatric Radiology; **Hospital:** Newark Beth Israel Med Ctr; **Address:** 201 Lyons Ave, Newark, NJ 07112; **Phone:** 973-926-7689; **Board Cert:** Diagnostic Radiology 1984; Pediatric Radiology 2005; **Med School:** Mount Sinai Sch Med 1980; **Resid:** Pediatrics, NYU Med Ctr 1981; Radiology, Mount Sinai Hosp 1984; **Fellow:** Pediatric Radiology, Mount Sinai Hosp 1985; **Fac Appt:** Prof Rad, Mount Sinai Sch Med

Reese, Ronald MD (DR) - **Spec Exp:** MRI; CT Scan; **Hospital:** Chilton Meml Hosp; **Address:** 116 Park St, Montclair, NJ 07042-2930; **Phone:** 973-746-2525; **Board Cert:** Diagnostic Radiology 1988; **Med School:** Penn State Univ-Hershey Med Ctr 1983; **Resid:** Internal Medicine, Nassau County Med Ctr 1984; Diagnostic Radiology, NYU Med Ctr 1988; **Fellow:** Magnetic Resonance Imaging, NYU Med Ctr 1988

Sanders, Linda MD (DR) - **Spec Exp:** Breast Imaging; **Hospital:** St Barnabas Med Ctr; **Address:** St Barnabas Med Ctr, Dept Radiology, 94 Old Short Hills Rd, Livingston, NJ 07039; **Phone:** 973-322-7850; **Board Cert:** Diagnostic Radiology 1986; **Med School:** Univ Pennsylvania 1982; **Resid:** Diagnostic Radiology, Columbia-Presby Med Ctr 1986; **Fellow:** Mammography, Meml Sloan-Kettering Cancer Ctr 1987

Whelan, Charles MD (DR) - **Spec Exp:** Ultrasound; PET Imaging; **Address:** 116 Park St, Montclair, NJ 07042-2930; **Phone:** 973-746-2525; **Board Cert:** Radiology 1973; Nuclear Medicine 1975; **Med School:** Univ VA Sch Med 1967; **Resid:** Surgery, Boston City Hosp 1969; Radiology, Columbia-Presby Med Ctr 1972; **Fellow:** Nuclear Medicine, NYU Med Ctr 1973; **Fac Appt:** Assoc Clin Prof Rad, NYU Sch Med

ENDOCRINOLOGY, DIABETES & METABOLISM

Baranetsky, Nicholas G MD (EDM) - **Hospital:** Saint Michael's Med Ctr; **Address:** 111 Central Ave, Saint Michael's Medical Ctr, Newark, NJ 07102-2011; **Phone:** 973-877-5185; **Board Cert:** Internal Medicine 1977; Endocrinology, Diabetes & Metabolism 1981; **Med School:** NY Med Coll 1974; **Resid:** Internal Medicine, Stamford Hosp 1977; **Fellow:** Endocrinology, Diabetes & Metabolism, VA Med Ctr-Wadsworth 1979; **Fac Appt:** Prof Med, Seton Hall Univ Sch Grad Med Ed

Dower, Samuel MD (EDM) - **Hospital:** St Barnabas Med Ctr; **Address:** 200 S Orange Ave, Livingston, NJ 07039; **Phone:** 973-322-7200; **Board Cert:** Internal Medicine 1984; Endocrinology 1987; **Med School:** NYU Sch Med 1981; **Resid:** Internal Medicine, Bronx Muni Hosp 1984; **Fellow:** Endocrinology, Mount Sinai Hosp 1985

Gewirtz, George MD (EDM) - **Hospital:** St Barnabas Med Ctr; **Address:** 200 S Orange Ave, Livingston, NJ 07039; **Phone:** 973-322-7200; **Board Cert:** Internal Medicine 1972; Endocrinology 1975; **Med School:** Harvard Med Sch 1965; **Resid:** Internal Medicine, Bellevue Hosp Ctr-NYU 1967; Internal Medicine, Columbia-Presby Med Ctr 1971; **Fellow:** Endocrinology, Diabetes & Metabolism, Mt Sinai Hosp 1973

Schneider, George MD (EDM) - **Spec Exp:** Diabetes; Thyroid Disorders; Cholesterol/Lipid Disorders; **Hospital:** Newark Beth Israel Med Ctr, St Barnabas Med Ctr; **Address:** 204 Eagle Rock Ave, Roseland, NJ 07068-1723; **Phone:** 973-228-2047; **Board Cert:** Internal Medicine 1971; Endocrinology, Diabetes & Metabolism 1973; **Med School:** Tufts Univ 1965; **Resid:** Internal Medicine, Bellevue Hosp 1967; Internal Medicine, Strong Meml Hosp 1970; **Fellow:** Endocrinology, Diabetes & Metabolism, Yale-New Haven Hosp 1972; **Fac Appt:** Assoc Clin Prof Med, UMDNJ-NJ Med Sch, Newark

Sherry, Stephen MD (EDM) - **Spec Exp:** Thyroid Disorders; Diabetes; Osteoporosis; **Hospital:** Mountainside Hosp (page 88); **Address:** 119 Grove St, Montclair, NJ 07042-2629; **Phone:** 973-744-3733; **Board Cert:** Internal Medicine 1979; Endocrinology, Diabetes & Metabolism 1981; **Med School:** Univ Conn 1976; **Resid:** Internal Medicine, New Eng Deaconess 1979; **Fellow:** Endocrinology, Diabetes & Metabolism, New Eng Deaconess 1981; **Fac Appt:** Asst Clin Prof Med, UMDNJ-NJ Med Sch, Newark

FAMILY MEDICINE

Cirello, Richard MD (FMed) PCP - **Hospital:** Mountainside Hosp (page 88); **Address:** 271 Grove Ave, Verona, NJ 07044; **Phone:** 973-239-2600; **Board Cert:** Family Medicine 2004; **Med School:** Mexico 1975; **Resid:** Family Medicine, Mountainside Hosp 1979; **Fac Appt:** Asst Clin Prof FMed, Rutgers Univ

Johnson, Mark S MD (FMed) PCP - **Spec Exp:** Hypertension; Cardiology; **Hospital:** UMDNJ-Univ Hosp-Newark; **Address:** New Jersey Family Practice Ctr, 90 Bergen St, Ste LL 0300, Newark, NJ 07103-2425; **Phone:** 973-972-2112; **Board Cert:** Family Medicine 2002; **Med School:** UMDNJ-NJ Med Sch, Newark 1979; **Resid:** Family Medicine, Univ S Alabama Med Ctr 1982; **Fellow:** Family Medicine, Univ NC Hosps 1984; **Fac Appt:** Prof FMed, UMDNJ-NJ Med Sch, Newark

McCampbell, Edwin MD (FMed) PCP - **Spec Exp:** Hypertension; **Hospital:** Columbus Hosp, East Orange Gen Hosp; **Address:** 85 S Harrison St, Ste 201, E Orange, NJ 07018; **Phone:** 973-672-3829; **Board Cert:** Family Medicine 2001; **Med School:** Howard Univ 1968; **Resid:** Internal Medicine, Kaiser Hosp 1971; Cardiovascular Disease, Howard Univ Hosp 1982; **Fellow:** Family Medicine, Howard Univ Hosp 1972; **Fac Appt:** Assoc Prof FMed, UMDNJ-NJ Med Sch, Newark

GASTROENTEROLOGY

De Pasquale, Joseph MD (Ge) - **Spec Exp:** Liver & Biliary Disease; Crohn's Disease; Gastroesophageal Reflux Disease (GERD); **Hospital:** Clara Maass Med Ctr, Saint Michael's Med Ctr; **Address:** 5 Franklin Ave, Ste 109, Belleville, NJ 07109; **Phone:** 973-759-7240; **Board Cert:** Internal Medicine 1986; Gastroenterology 1989; **Med School:** Italy 1983; **Resid:** Internal Medicine, St Michael's Med Ctr 1986; **Fellow:** Gastroenterology, St Michael's Med Ctr 1988; **Fac Appt:** Assoc Prof Med, Seton Hall Univ Sch Grad Med Ed

Finkelstein, Warren MD (Ge) - **Spec Exp:** Ulcerative Colitis; Crohn's Disease; Inflammatory Bowel Disease; **Hospital:** Mountainside Hosp (page 88); **Address:** 123 Highland Ave, Ste 103, Glen Ridge, NJ 07028-1522; **Phone:** 973-429-8800; **Board Cert:** Internal Medicine 1975; Gastroenterology 1983; **Med School:** Med Coll VA 1972; **Resid:** Internal Medicine, Boston City Hosp 1974; Internal Medicine, Boston VA Med Ctr 1975; **Fellow:** Gastroenterology, Mass Genl Hosp 1977; **Fac Appt:** Assoc Clin Prof Med, UMDNJ-NJ Med Sch, Newark

Fiske, Steven MD (Ge) - **Spec Exp:** Inflammatory Bowel Disease/Crohn's; Colonoscopy; Peptic Acid Disorders; **Hospital:** St Barnabas Med Ctr, Clara Maass Med Ctr; **Address:** 741 Northfield Ave, Ste 101, W Orange, NJ 07052; **Phone:** 973-325-5775; **Board Cert:** Internal Medicine 1977; Gastroenterology 1979; **Med School:** NYU Sch Med 1974; **Resid:** Internal Medicine, Bellevue Hosp/NYU Med Ctr 1976; **Fellow:** Gastroenterology, Brigham & Women's Hosp 1978; **Fac Appt:** Assoc Prof Med, Seton Hall Univ Sch Grad Med Ed

Groisser, Victor MD (Ge) - **Spec Exp:** Colon & Rectal Cancer Detection; Crohn's Disease; Barrett's Esophagus; Gastroesophageal Reflux Disease (GERD); **Hospital:** Mountainside Hosp (page 88), Clara Maass Med Ctr; **Address:** 21 Plymouth St, Montclair, NJ 07042-2698; **Phone:** 973-746-5166; **Board Cert:** Internal Medicine 1966; Gastroenterology 1972; **Med School:** SUNY Downstate 1952; **Resid:** Internal Medicine, Montefiore Med Ctr 1957; Gastroenterology, Manhattan VA Hosp 1958; **Fellow:** Gastroenterology, Manhattan VA Hosp/Cornell 1959; **Fac Appt:** Clin Prof Med, UMDNJ-NJ Med Sch, Newark

Kenny, Raymond MD (Ge) - **Spec Exp:** Liver Disease; Hepatitis C; Inflammatory Bowel Disease/Crohn's; **Hospital:** Mountainside Hosp (page 88), St Barnabas Med Ctr; **Address:** 123 Highland Ave, Ste 103, Glen Ridge, NJ 07028; **Phone:** 973-429-8800; **Board Cert:** Internal Medicine 1984; Gastroenterology 1987; **Med School:** SUNY Stony Brook 1981; **Resid:** Internal Medicine, Mayo Clinic 1984; **Fellow:** Gastroenterology, Univ Penn Med Ctr 1986; **Fac Appt:** Asst Clin Prof Med, UMDNJ-NJ Med Sch, Newark

Mogan, Glen MD (Ge) - **Spec Exp:** Inflammatory Bowel Disease; Peptic Ulcer Disease; Gastroesophageal Reflux Disease (GERD); **Hospital:** St Barnabas Med Ctr; **Address:** 741 N Field Ave, Ste 204, West Orange, NJ 07052-1104; **Phone:** 973-731-8686; **Board Cert:** Internal Medicine 1978; Gastroenterology 1981; **Med School:** SUNY Upstate Med Univ 1975; **Resid:** Internal Medicine, Mount Sinai Hosp 1978; **Fellow:** Gastroenterology, Mount Sinai Hosp 1980; **Fac Appt:** Assoc Clin Prof Med, UMDNJ-RW Johnson Med Sch

Schrader, Zalman MD (Ge) - **Spec Exp:** Endoscopy; Colonoscopy; Inflammatory Bowel Disease; **Hospital:** St Barnabas Med Ctr, Morristown Mem Hosp (page 88); **Address:** 101 Old Short Hills Rd, Ste 217, W Orange, NJ 07052-1023; **Phone:** 973-731-4600; **Board Cert:** Internal Medicine 1968; Gastroenterology 1972; **Med School:** Albert Einstein Coll Med 1961; **Resid:** Internal Medicine, Bronx Municipal Hosp 1967; **Fellow:** Gastroenterology, New York Hosp-Cornell Med Ctr 1969

Sloan, William MD (Ge) - **Spec Exp:** Liver Disease; Inflammatory Bowel Disease; Endoscopy; **Hospital:** St Barnabas Med Ctr, Morristown Mem Hosp (page 88); **Address:** 101 Old Short Hills Rd, Ste 217, West Orange, NJ 07052-1023; **Phone:** 973-731-4600; **Board Cert:** Internal Medicine 1972; Gastroenterology 1972; **Med School:** Univ Pennsylvania 1965; **Resid:** Internal Medicine, Mt Sinai Hosp 1970; **Fellow:** Gastroenterology, Mt Sinai Hosp 1972

GYNECOLOGIC ONCOLOGY

Denehy, Thad MD (GO) - **Spec Exp:** Uterine Cancer; Ovarian Cancer; Pelvic Reconstruction; **Hospital:** St Barnabas Med Ctr; **Address:** Gynecologic Cancer & Pelvic Surgery, 101 Old Short Hills Rd, Ste 400, West Orange, NJ 07052; **Phone:** 973-243-9300; **Board Cert:** Obstetrics & Gynecology 2004; Gynecologic Oncology 2004; **Med School:** Wake Forest Univ 1984; **Resid:** Obstetrics & Gynecology, St Barnabas Med Ctr 1988; **Fellow:** Gynecologic Oncology, Strong Meml Hosp 1990

HEMATOLOGY

Cohen, Alice MD (Hem) - **Spec Exp:** Bleeding/Coagulation Disorders; **Hospital:** Newark Beth Israel Med Ctr, St Barnabas Med Ctr; **Address:** Newark Beth Israel Med Ctr, Div Hem, 201 Lyons Ave at Osborne Terrace, Newark, NJ 07112; **Phone:** 973-926-7230; **Board Cert:** Internal Medicine 1984; Hematology 1986; Medical Oncology 2001; **Med School:** Univ Hlth Sci/Chicago Med Sch 1981; **Resid:** Internal Medicine, NYU-Man VA Med Ctr 1984; **Fellow:** Hematology & Oncology, Geo Wash Univ Med Ctr 1986; Hematology & Oncology, Columbia Presby Med Ctr 1987; **Fac Appt:** Assoc Clin Prof Med, Columbia P&S

Zager, Robert MD (Hem) - **Hospital:** Mountainside Hosp (page 88); **Address:** Richard F Harries Ambulatory Care Pav, 1 Bay Ave, Ste 1, Montclair, NJ 07042; **Phone:** 973-259-3555; **Board Cert:** Internal Medicine 1973; Hematology 1974; Medical Oncology 1975; **Med School:** Cornell Univ-Weill Med Coll 1968; **Resid:** Internal Medicine, New York Hosp 1970; Medical Oncology, Natl Cancer Inst-NIH 1972; **Fellow:** Hematology & Oncology, New York Hosp 1974; **Fac Appt:** Asst Clin Prof Med, UMDNJ-NJ Med Sch, Newark

Zauber, N Peter MD (Hem) - **Hospital:** St Barnabas Med Ctr; **Address:** 22 Old Short Hills Rd, Ste 108, Livingston, NJ 07039; **Phone:** 973-533-9299; **Board Cert:** Internal Medicine 1976; Hematology 1978; **Med School:** Johns Hopkins Univ 1971; **Resid:** Internal Medicine, NY-Meml Hosps 1973; Internal Medicine, Baltimore City Hosp 1976; **Fellow:** Hematology & Oncology, Presby Hosp 1978

INFECTIOUS DISEASE

Ellner, Jerrold Jay MD (Inf) - **Spec Exp:** AIDS/HIV; Tuberculosis; Infections-Neurologic; **Hospital:** UMDNJ-Univ Hosp-Newark; **Address:** UMDNJ-New Jersey Med Sch, Dept Medicine, 185 S Orange Ave, MSB, rm I 506, Newark, NJ 07103; **Phone:** 973-972-4595; **Board Cert:** Internal Medicine 1973; Infectious Disease 1978; **Med School:** Johns Hopkins Univ 1970; **Resid:** Internal Medicine, Johns Hopkins Hosp 1972; Infectious Disease, National Inst of Allergy & Infectious Disease 1975; **Fac Appt:** Prof Med, UMDNJ-NJ Med Sch, Newark

Slim, Jihad MD (Inf) - **Spec Exp:** AIDS/HIV; Hepatitis C; Hospital Acquired Infections; **Hospital:** Saint Michael's Med Ctr, Clara Maass Med Ctr - West Hudson Div; **Address:** Saint Michael's Medical Ctr, 268 Dr Martin Luther King Jr Blvd, Newark, NJ 07102; **Phone:** 973-877-5482; **Board Cert:** Internal Medicine 1986; Infectious Disease 1988; **Med School:** Lebanon 1980; **Resid:** Internal Medicine, Broussais Hosp 1983; Internal Medicine, Saint Michael's Med Ctr 1986; **Fellow:** Infectious Disease, Saint Michaels Med Ctr 1988; **Fac Appt:** Asst Prof Med, Seton Hall Univ Sch Grad Med Ed

Smith, Leon G MD (Inf) - **Spec Exp:** Fevers of Unknown Origin; Bone/Joint Infections; Hepatitis; **Hospital:** Saint Michael's Med Ctr, St Barnabas Med Ctr; **Address:** 111 Central Ave C Bldg Fl 6, Newark, NJ 07102-2011; **Phone:** 973-877-5481; **Board Cert:** Internal Medicine 1963; Infectious Disease 1974; **Med School:** Georgetown Univ 1956; **Resid:** Infectious Disease, Nat Inst Hlth 1959; Internal Medicine, Yale-New Haven Hosp 1962; **Fellow:** Infectious Disease, Yale-New Haven Hosp 1960; **Fac Appt:** Prof Med, UMDNJ-NJ Med Sch, Newark

Smith, Stephen M MD (Inf) - **Spec Exp:** AIDS/HIV; **Hospital:** Saint Michael's Med Ctr, St Barnabas Med Ctr; **Address:** 268 Dr Martin Luther King Blvd, Saint Michael's Med Ctr, Newark, NJ 07102; **Phone:** 973-877-2711; **Board Cert:** Internal Medicine 1992; Infectious Disease 1994; **Med School:** Yale Univ 1989; **Resid:** Internal Medicine, Univ VA 1991; **Fellow:** Infectious Disease, Natl Inst Allergy & Inf Dis 1993; **Fac Appt:** Asst Prof Med, Seton Hall Univ Sch Grad Med Ed

Soroko, Theresa MD (Inf) - **Spec Exp:** AIDS/HIV; Lyme Disease; Skin/Soft Tissue Infection; **Hospital:** Mountainside Hosp (page 88), Clara Maass Med Ctr; **Address:** 199 Broad St, Ste 2A, Bloomfield, NJ 07003-2635; **Phone:** 973-748-4583; **Board Cert:** Internal Medicine 1988; Infectious Disease 1992; **Med School:** Grenada 1985; **Resid:** Internal Medicine, St Michael's Med Ctr 1988; **Fellow:** Infectious Disease, St Michael's Med Ctr 1990; **Fac Appt:** Asst Clin Prof Med, UMDNJ-NJ Med Sch, Newark

INTERNAL MEDICINE

Atkin, Suzanne MD (IM) - **Hospital:** UMDNJ-Univ Hosp-Newark; **Address:** University Hospital, D217, 150 Bergen St, rm D217, Newark, NJ 07103; **Phone:** 973-972-0440; **Board Cert:** Internal Medicine 1982; Emergency Medicine 2000; **Med School:** UMDNJ-NJ Med Sch, Newark 1979; **Resid:** Internal Medicine, UMDNJ-NJ Med Sch 1982; **Fac Appt:** Assoc Prof Med, UMDNJ-NJ Med Sch, Newark

Bains, Yatinder MD (IM) `PCP` - **Spec Exp:** Liver Disease; Inflammatory Bowel Disease; Gastroesophageal Reflux Disease (GERD); **Hospital:** Columbus Hosp, Jersey City Med Ctr; **Address:** 116 Millburn Ave, Ste 214, Millburn, NJ 07104; **Phone:** 201-376-2121; **Board Cert:** Internal Medicine 1991; Gastroenterology 1993; **Med School:** UMDNJ-NJ Med Sch, Newark 1987; **Resid:** Internal Medicine, UMDNJ 1990; **Fellow:** Gastroenterology, UMDNJ 1992; **Fac Appt:** Med, UMDNJ-RW Johnson Med Sch

Chrisanderson, Donna MD (IM) - **Hospital:** St Barnabas Med Ctr; **Address:** 2040 Millburn Ave, Ste 402, Maplewood, NJ 07040; **Phone:** 973-378-9070; **Board Cert:** Internal Medicine 1994; **Med School:** Med Coll GA 1988; **Resid:** Internal Medicine, Greenwich Hosp 1991; **Fellow:** Internal Medicine, Univ Alabama Hosp 1993

DeCosimo, Diana R MD (IM) `PCP` - **Spec Exp:** Women's Health; Geriatric Care; Preventive Medicine; **Hospital:** UMDNJ-Univ Hosp-Newark, Hackensack Univ Med Ctr (page 92); **Address:** Doctors Office Ctr, 90 Bergen St, Ste 4500, Newark, NJ 07103-2425; **Phone:** 973-972-2500; **Board Cert:** Internal Medicine 1977; Cardiovascular Disease 1979; **Med School:** Boston Univ 1974; **Resid:** Internal Medicine, Worcester City Hosp 1977; **Fellow:** Cardiovascular Disease, Univ Mass Med Ctr 1979; **Fac Appt:** Assoc Prof Med, UMDNJ-NJ Med Sch, Newark

Di Giacomo, William A MD (IM) `PCP` - **Hospital:** Saint Michael's Med Ctr, Overlook Hosp (page 88); **Address:** 1072 S Orange Ave, Newark, NJ 07106; **Phone:** 973-623-5309; **Board Cert:** Internal Medicine 1978; **Med School:** Mexico 1974; **Resid:** Internal Medicine, St Michaels Med Ctr 1978; **Fac Appt:** Assoc Prof Med, Seton Hall Univ Sch Grad Med Ed

Fortunato, Dana MD (IM) `PCP` - **Spec Exp:** Asthma; Obesity; **Hospital:** Mountainside Hosp (page 88); **Address:** 127 Pine St, Montclair, NJ 07042-4835; **Phone:** 973-744-4075; **Board Cert:** Internal Medicine 1978; Pulmonary Disease 1980; **Med School:** UMDNJ-NJ Med Sch, Newark 1975; **Resid:** Internal Medicine, St Michael's Med Ctr 1977; **Fellow:** Pulmonary Disease, St Michael's Med Ctr 1979

Gribbon, John MD (IM) `PCP` - **Spec Exp:** Hypertension; Diabetes; **Hospital:** Mountainside Hosp (page 88); **Address:** 62 S Fullerton Ave, Montclair, NJ 07042-2686; **Phone:** 973-744-3382; **Board Cert:** Internal Medicine 1980; **Med School:** UMDNJ-NJ Med Sch, Newark 1977; **Resid:** Internal Medicine, UMDNJ-NJ Med Schl 1980; **Fac Appt:** Asst Clin Prof Med, UMDNJ-NJ Med Sch, Newark

Haggerty, Mary A MD (IM) `PCP` - **Spec Exp:** Preventive Medicine; Hypertension; **Hospital:** Newark Beth Israel Med Ctr; **Address:** 2115 Millburn Ave, Maplewood, NJ 07040-3724; **Phone:** 973-275-1322; **Board Cert:** Internal Medicine 2000; Geriatric Medicine 2000; **Med School:** UMDNJ-NJ Med Sch, Newark 1979; **Resid:** Internal Medicine, UMDNJ-Univ Hosp 1982; **Fac Appt:** Assoc Clin Prof Med, UMDNJ-NJ Med Sch, Newark

Peyser, Donald MD (IM) - **Spec Exp:** Cardiology; **Hospital:** St Barnabas Med Ctr; **Address:** 225 Millburn Ave, Ste 104A, Millburn, NJ 07041; **Phone:** 973-467-5800; **Board Cert:** Internal Medicine 1974; **Med School:** Univ Rochester 1958; **Resid:** Internal Medicine, Boston VA Hosp 1963; **Fellow:** Cardiovascular Disease, Peter Bent Brigham Hosp 1964

Rommer, James A MD (IM) `PCP` - **Hospital:** St Barnabas Med Ctr; **Address:** 349 E Northfield Rd, Ste 110, Livingston, NJ 07039; **Phone:** 973-992-2227; **Board Cert:** Internal Medicine 1981; **Med School:** Cornell Univ-Weill Med Coll 1978; **Resid:** Internal Medicine, NY Hosp-Cornell Med Ctr 1981; **Fellow:** Internal Medicine, Johns Hopkins Med Sch 1982; **Fac Appt:** Asst Clin Prof Med, Mount Sinai Sch Med

Russo, John A MD (IM) `PCP` - **Hospital:** St Barnabas Med Ctr; **Address:** 1500 Pleasant Valley Way Ave, Ste 201, West Orange, NJ 07052; **Phone:** 973-736-8119; **Board Cert:** Internal Medicine 1988; **Med School:** Mexico 1981; **Resid:** Internal Medicine, UMDNJ Med Ctr 1987

INTERVENTIONAL CARDIOLOGY

Cohen, Marc MD (IC) - **Hospital:** Newark Beth Israel Med Ctr; **Address:** Newark Beth Israel Med Ctr, Cath Lab Admin, 201 Lyons Ave, Newark, NJ 07112; **Phone:** 973-926-7852; **Board Cert:** Internal Medicine 1980; Cardiovascular Disease 1983; Interventional Cardiology 1999; **Med School:** NYU Sch Med 1977; **Resid:** Internal Medicine, Mt Sinai Hosp 1980; **Fellow:** Cardiovascular Disease, Mt Sinai Hosp 1982; **Fac Appt:** Prof Med, Mount Sinai Sch Med

MATERNAL & FETAL MEDICINE

Bardeguez, Arlene D MD (MF) - **Spec Exp:** AIDS/HIV in Pregnancy; Pregnancy-High Risk; **Hospital:** UMDNJ-Univ Hosp-Newark, Columbus Hosp; **Address:** 90 Bergen St, Ste 5100, Newark, NJ 07103; **Phone:** 973-972-2700; **Board Cert:** Obstetrics & Gynecology 1998; Maternal & Fetal Medicine 1998; **Med School:** Univ Puerto Rico 1981; **Resid:** Obstetrics & Gynecology, Catholic Med Ctr 1985; **Fellow:** Maternal & Fetal Medicine, Nassau Co Med Ctr 1987; Maternal & Fetal Medicine, Columbia Univ 2001; **Fac Appt:** Prof ObG, UMDNJ-NJ Med Sch, Newark

Smith Jr, Leon G MD (MF) - **Spec Exp:** Ultrasound; Prenatal Diagnosis; Perinatal Infections; Amniocentesis; **Hospital:** St Barnabas Med Ctr; **Address:** New Jersey Perinatal Assocs, 94 Old Short Hills Rd, East Wing, Ste 402, Livingston, NJ 07039-5672; **Phone:** 973-322-5287; **Board Cert:** Obstetrics & Gynecology 2004; Maternal & Fetal Medicine 2004; **Med School:** Georgetown Univ 1985; **Resid:** Obstetrics & Gynecology, Tulane Univ Hosp 1989; **Fellow:** Maternal & Fetal Medicine, Baylor Univ Hosp 1991

MEDICAL ONCOLOGY

Botti, Anthony Charles MD (Onc) - **Spec Exp:** Lymphoma; Multiple Myeloma; **Hospital:** St Barnabas Med Ctr; **Address:** 349 E Northfield Rd, Ste 200, Livingston, NJ 07039-4806; **Phone:** 973-597-0900; **Board Cert:** Internal Medicine 1985; Medical Oncology 1987; Hematology 1988; **Med School:** Spain 1982; **Resid:** Internal Medicine, Interfaith Med Ctr 1985; **Fellow:** Hematology & Oncology, LI Coll Hosp 1988

Kane, Michael J MD (Onc) - **Spec Exp:** Breast Cancer; Colon Cancer; **Hospital:** Mountainside Hosp (page 88); **Address:** Mountainside Cancer Ctr, 1 Bay Ave, Montclair, NJ 07042; **Phone:** 973-429-6746; **Board Cert:** Internal Medicine 1986; Medical Oncology 1989; **Med School:** UMDNJ-NJ Med Sch, Newark 1983; **Resid:** Internal Medicine, Thomas Jefferson Univ Hosp 1986; **Fellow:** Medical Oncology, Mount Sinai Hosp 1988

Lippman, Alan MD (Onc) - **Hospital:** Clara Maass Med Ctr, St Barnabas Med Ctr; **Address:** 36 Newark Ave, Belleville, NJ 07109; **Phone:** 973-751-8880; **Board Cert:** Internal Medicine 1973; Medical Oncology 1975; **Med School:** Hahnemann Univ 1965; **Resid:** Internal Medicine, Newark Beth Israel Med Ctr 1970; **Fellow:** Medical Oncology, Meml Sloan Kettering Canc Hosp 1972; **Fac Appt:** Assoc Clin Prof Med, UMDNJ-NJ Med Sch, Newark

Michaelson, Richard MD (Onc) - **Spec Exp:** Breast Cancer; **Hospital:** St Barnabas Med Ctr; **Address:** St Barnabas Med Ctr-East Wing Fl 2, 94 Old Short Hills Rd, Livingston, NJ 07039; **Phone:** 973-322-5362; **Board Cert:** Internal Medicine 1979; Medical Oncology 1981; **Med School:** Univ Pennsylvania 1976; **Resid:** Internal Medicine, Hosp Univ Penn 1979; **Fellow:** Medical Oncology, Meml Sloan Kettering Canc Ctr 1981

Sagorin, Charles MD (Onc) - **Hospital:** Mountainside Hosp (page 88); **Address:** 127 Pine St, Ste 6, Montclair, NJ 07042-4868; **Phone:** 973-783-3300; **Board Cert:** Internal Medicine 1981; Medical Oncology 1983; Hematology 1986; **Med School:** SUNY Downstate 1971; **Resid:** Internal Medicine, Bronx Municipal Hosp 1973; **Fellow:** Hematology, Montefiore Med Ctr 1974; Medical Oncology, Montefiore Med Ctr 1978

NEPHROLOGY

Byrd, Lawrence H MD (Nep) - **Spec Exp:** Hypertension; Kidney Disease; **Hospital:** St Barnabas Med Ctr, Bayonne Med Ctr; **Address:** 22 Old Short Hills Rd, Ste 212, Livingston, NJ 07039-5605; **Phone:** 973-994-4550; **Board Cert:** Internal Medicine 1977; Nephrology 1978; **Med School:** Med Coll PA 1973; **Resid:** Internal Medicine, UMDNJ-Univ Hosp 1976; **Fellow:** Nephrology, NY Hosp-Cornell Med Ctr 1978; **Fac Appt:** Asst Clin Prof Med, UMDNJ-NJ Med Sch, Newark

Grasso, Michael MD (Nep) - **Spec Exp:** Kidney Disease; **Hospital:** Newark Beth Israel Med Ctr; **Address:** 111 Northfield Ave, Ste 311, West Orange, NJ 07052-4703; **Phone:** 973-325-2103; **Board Cert:** Internal Medicine 1974; Nephrology 1976; **Med School:** Univ MD Sch Med 1970; **Resid:** Internal Medicine, Univ MD Hosp 1974; **Fellow:** Nephrology, Newark Beth Israel Hosp 1976

Lyman, Neil MD (Nep) - **Spec Exp:** Dialysis Care; Kidney Failure; **Hospital:** St Barnabas Med Ctr, Clara Maass Med Ctr; **Address:** 769 Northfield Ave, Ste 200, West Orange, NJ 07052-1106; **Phone:** 973-736-2212; **Board Cert:** Internal Medicine 1976; Nephrology 1980; **Med School:** Albert Einstein Coll Med 1973; **Resid:** Internal Medicine, Mt Sinai Hosp 1976; Nephrology, Mt Sinai Hosp 1979; **Fellow:** Nephrology, Boston Med Ctr 1977; **Fac Appt:** Asst Prof Med, UMDNJ-NJ Med Sch, Newark

Mulgaonkar, Shamkant MD (Nep) - **Spec Exp:** Transplant Medicine-Kidney; **Hospital:** St Barnabas Med Ctr, Newark Beth Israel Med Ctr; **Address:** St Barnabas Med Ctr, 94 Old Short Hills Rd, Ste 306, Livingston, NJ 07039; **Phone:** 973-322-8216; **Board Cert:** Internal Medicine 1981; Nephrology 1982; **Med School:** India 1975; **Resid:** Internal Medicine, Morristown Meml Hosp 1980; **Fellow:** Nephrology, St Barnabas Med Ctr 1982

Sipzner, Robert MD (Nep) - **Hospital:** Bayonne Med Ctr, St Barnabas Med Ctr; **Address:** 22 Old Short Hills Rd, Ste 212, Livingston, NJ 07039; **Phone:** 973-994-4550; **Board Cert:** Internal Medicine 1985; Nephrology 1988; **Med School:** NYU Sch Med 1982; **Resid:** Internal Medicine, SUNY Downstate 1985; **Fellow:** Nephrology, Univ Tenn Hlth Sci Ctr 1987

Thomsen, Stephen MD (Nep) - **Spec Exp:** Diabetes; Hypertension; **Hospital:** Christ Hosp, Mountainside Hosp (page 88); **Address:** 123 Highland Ave, Ste G2, Glen Ridge, NJ 07028; **Phone:** 973-429-1881; **Board Cert:** Internal Medicine 1981; Nephrology 1996; **Med School:** Italy 1977; **Resid:** Internal Medicine, Mountainside Hosp 1980; **Fellow:** Nephrology, UMDNJ-Univ Hosp 1982

NEUROLOGICAL SURGERY

Carmel, Peter MD (NS) - **Spec Exp:** Brain Tumors-Pediatric; Skull Base Surgery; Pediatric Neurosurgery; **Hospital:** UMDNJ-Univ Hosp-Newark; **Address:** 90 Bergen St, Ste 8100, Newark, NJ 07101; **Phone:** 973-972-2323; **Board Cert:** Neurological Surgery 1969; Pediatric Neurological Surgery 1996; **Med School:** NYU Sch Med 1960; **Resid:** Neurological Surgery, Neuro Inst/Columbia Presby Med Ctr 1967; **Fac Appt:** Prof NS, UMDNJ-NJ Med Sch, Newark

Frank, Donald MD (NS) - **Spec Exp:** Spinal Surgery; Carpal Tunnel Syndrome; Trigeminal Neuralgia; **Hospital:** Clara Maass Med Ctr; **Address:** 96 Gates Ave, Montclair, NJ 07042; **Phone:** 973-744-7111; **Board Cert:** Neurological Surgery 1972; **Med School:** Duke Univ 1962; **Resid:** Neurological Surgery, NYU Med Ctr 1966; Neurological Surgery, Albert Einstein 1969; **Fellow:** Neurological Surgery, NYU Med Ctr 1970; **Fac Appt:** Asst Clin Prof NS, NYU Sch Med

Heary, Robert F MD (NS) - **Spec Exp:** Spinal Surgery; Spinal Cord Injury; Spinal Deformity; **Hospital:** UMDNJ-Univ Hosp-Newark, Hackensack Univ Med Ctr (page 92); **Address:** UMDNJ-NJ Med Sch, Div Neurosurg, 90 Bergen St, Ste 8100, Newark, NJ 07103-2499; **Phone:** 973-972-2334; **Board Cert:** Neurological Surgery 1999; **Med School:** Univ Pittsburgh 1986; **Resid:** Surgery, UMDNJ Univ Hosp 1989; Neurological Surgery, UMDNJ Univ Hosp 1994; **Fellow:** Orthopaedic Surgery, Thomas Jefferson Univ Hosp 1995; **Fac Appt:** Assoc Prof NS, UMDNJ-NJ Med Sch, Newark

Hubschmann, Otakar R MD (NS) - **Spec Exp:** Spinal Surgery; Cerebrovascular Neurosurgery; Brain Surgery; **Hospital:** St Barnabas Med Ctr, Newark Beth Israel Med Ctr; **Address:** 101 Old Short Hills Rd, Ste 409, W Orange, NJ 07052-1023; **Phone:** 973-322-6732; **Board Cert:** Neurological Surgery 1978; **Med School:** Czech Republic 1967; **Resid:** Surgery, Montefiore Med Ctr 1970; Neurological Surgery, Montefiore Med Ctr 1976

Schulder, Michael MD (NS) - **Spec Exp:** Brain Tumors; Movement Disorders; Skull Base Surgery; **Hospital:** UMDNJ-Univ Hosp-Newark, Overlook Hosp (page 88); **Address:** New Jersey Med Sch, 90 Bergen St Fl 8, Newark, NJ 07103-2425; **Phone:** 973-972-2907; **Board Cert:** Neurological Surgery 1991; **Med School:** Columbia P&S 1982; **Resid:** Neurological Surgery, Montefiore Hosp Med Ctr/Albert Einstein 1988; **Fac Appt:** Assoc Prof NS, UMDNJ-NJ Med Sch, Newark

NEUROLOGY

Blady, David MD (N) - **Spec Exp:** Parkinson's Disease; Dementia; Multiple Sclerosis; **Hospital:** Mountainside Hosp (page 88), Clara Maass Med Ctr; **Address:** 230 Sherman Ave, Ste#K, Glen Ridge, NJ 07028-1520; **Phone:** 973-743-9555; **Board Cert:** Neurology 1990; **Med School:** SUNY Downstate 1983; **Resid:** Neurology, Bellevue Hosp/NYU Med Ctr 1987

Cook, Stuart MD (N) - **Spec Exp:** Multiple Sclerosis; Infectious & Demyelinating Diseases; **Hospital:** UMDNJ-Univ Hosp-Newark; **Address:** 65 Bergen St, rm 1435, Newark, NJ 07101; **Phone:** 973-972-9181; **Board Cert:** Neurology 1970; **Med School:** Univ VT Coll Med 1962; **Resid:** Neurology, Albert Einstein Coll Med 1968; **Fac Appt:** Prof N, UMDNJ-NJ Med Sch, Newark

Fellus, Jonathan L MD (N) - **Spec Exp:** Brain Injury; Neuro-Rehabilitation; Stroke; Dementia; **Hospital:** Kessler Inst for Rehab - East Orange; **Address:** Kessler Inst Rehab, 240 Central Ave, East Orange, NJ 07018; **Phone:** 973-414-4768; **Board Cert:** Neurology 1998; **Med School:** UMDNJ-RW Johnson Med Sch 1992; **Resid:** Neurology, Penn Hosp 1996; **Fellow:** Neurological Rehabilitation, Kernan Hosp-Univ Md Med Ctr 1997; **Fac Appt:** Asst Clin Prof N, UMDNJ-NJ Med Sch, Newark

Geller, Eric B MD (N) - **Spec Exp:** Epilepsy; **Hospital:** St Barnabas Med Ctr; **Address:** St Barnabas Inst Neurolgy & Neurosurg, 101 Old Short Hills Rd, Ste 415, West Orange, NJ 07052; **Phone:** 973-322-6600; **Board Cert:** Neurology 1995; Clinical Neurophysiology 1996; **Med School:** Brown Univ 1989; **Resid:** Neurology, Harvard Med Sch Prog 1993; **Fellow:** Clinical Neurophysiology, Cleveland Clinic 1995

Marks, David A MD (N) - **Spec Exp:** Epilepsy/Seizure Disorders; Headache; Migraine; **Hospital:** UMDNJ-Univ Hosp-Newark; **Address:** 90 Bergen St, Ste 8100, Newark, NJ 07103; **Phone:** 973-972-2550; **Board Cert:** Neurology 1989; **Med School:** South Africa 1983; **Resid:** Neurology, Boston Med Ctr 1988; **Fellow:** Neurological Physiology, New England Med Ctr 1989; Epilepsy, Yale-New Haven Hosp 1991; **Fac Appt:** Assoc Prof Med, UMDNJ-NJ Med Sch, Newark

Ruderman, Marvin MD (N) - **Spec Exp:** Neuromuscular Disorders; Peripheral Neuropathy; Myasthenia Gravis; **Hospital:** St Barnabas Med Ctr, Mountainside Hosp (page 88); **Address:** 1099 Bloomfield Ave, West Caldwell, NJ 07006-7129; **Phone:** 973-439-7000; **Board Cert:** Neurology 1981; **Med School:** Columbia P&S 1976; **Resid:** Neurology, Barnes Hosp 1980; **Fellow:** Neuromuscular Disease, Columbia-Presby Med Ctr 1981; **Fac Appt:** Asst Clin Prof N, UMDNJ-NJ Med Sch, Newark

OBSTETRICS & GYNECOLOGY

Apuzzio, Joseph MD (ObG) - **Spec Exp:** Prenatal Diagnosis; Pregnancy-High Risk; Infectious Disease; **Hospital:** UMDNJ-Univ Hosp-Newark, Columbus Hosp; **Address:** UMDNJ Med Sch, Dept OB/GYN & Women's Hlth, 185 S Orange Ave, MSB-rm E506, Newark, NJ 07103-2714; **Phone:** 973-972-5557; **Board Cert:** Obstetrics & Gynecology 2004; Maternal & Fetal Medicine 2004; **Med School:** UMDNJ-NJ Med Sch, Newark 1973; **Resid:** Obstetrics & Gynecology, UMDNJ-Univ Hosp 1976; **Fellow:** Maternal & Fetal Medicine, UMDNJ-Univ Hosp 1982; **Fac Appt:** Prof ObG, UMDNJ-NJ Med Sch, Newark

Cooperman, Alan S MD (ObG) - **Spec Exp:** Laparoscopic Surgery; Pelvic Surgery; Colposcopy; **Hospital:** Overlook Hosp (page 88), St Barnabas Med Ctr; **Address:** 235 Millburn Ave, Millburn, NJ 07041-1738; **Phone:** 973-467-9440; **Board Cert:** Obstetrics & Gynecology 1979; **Med School:** Italy 1968; **Resid:** Obstetrics & Gynecology, Newark Beth Israel Med Ctr 1973

Luciani, Richard L MD (ObG) - **Spec Exp:** Laparoscopic Surgery; Pregnancy-High Risk; Endometriosis; **Hospital:** Overlook Hosp (page 88), St Barnabas Med Ctr; **Address:** 235 Millburn Ave, Millburn, NJ 07041; **Phone:** 973-467-9440; **Board Cert:** Obstetrics & Gynecology 1982; **Med School:** UMDNJ-NJ Med Sch, Newark 1976; **Resid:** Obstetrics & Gynecology, St Barnabas Hosp 1980

Quartell, Anthony C MD (ObG) - **Spec Exp:** Laparoscopic Surgery-Complex; Pelvic Reconstruction; **Hospital:** St Barnabas Med Ctr; **Address:** 316 Eisenhower Pkwy, Ste 202, Livingston, NJ 07039-1718; **Phone:** 973-716-9600; **Board Cert:** Obstetrics & Gynecology 1978; **Med School:** UMDNJ-NJ Med Sch, Newark 1969; **Resid:** Surgery, New Jersey Coll 1971; Obstetrics & Gynecology, St Barnabas Med Ctr 1976; **Fac Appt:** Asst Clin Prof ObG, Mount Sinai Sch Med

Sladowski, Catherine MD (ObG) - **Hospital:** St Barnabas Med Ctr; **Address:** 207 Pompton Ave, Verona, NJ 07044-3018; **Phone:** 973-239-0052; **Board Cert:** Obstetrics & Gynecology 1976; **Med School:** Med Coll PA Hahnemann 1970; **Resid:** Obstetrics & Gynecology, St Barnabas Hosp 1974

OPHTHALMOLOGY

Cangemi, Francis E MD (Oph) - **Spec Exp:** Diabetic Eye Disease/Retinopathy; Macular Degeneration; Retinal Detachment; **Hospital:** Clara Maass Med Ctr, Valley Hosp (page 762); **Address:** 36 Newark Ave, Ste 212, Belleville, NJ 07109-3504; **Phone:** 973-751-8808; **Board Cert:** Ophthalmology 1976; **Med School:** NY Med Coll 1969; **Resid:** Internal Medicine, Mayo Clinic 1971; Ophthalmology, New York Eye & Ear 1975; **Fellow:** Vitreoretinal Surgery, Mass EE Infirm 1976; **Fac Appt:** Assoc Clin Prof Oph, UMDNJ-NJ Med Sch, Newark

Caputo, Anthony R MD (Oph) - **Spec Exp:** Pediatric Ophthalmology; Strabismus; **Hospital:** Columbus Hosp; **Address:** 556 Eagle Rock Ave, Ste 203, Roseland, NJ 07068-1500; **Phone:** 973-228-3111; **Board Cert:** Ophthalmology 1976; **Med School:** Italy 1969; **Resid:** Ophthalmology, UMDNJ-Univ Hosp 1974; **Fellow:** Ophthalmology, Wills Eye Hosp 1975; **Fac Appt:** Prof Oph, UMDNJ-NJ Med Sch, Newark

Cohen, Steven MD (Oph) - **Spec Exp:** Retinal/Vitreous Surgery; Diabetic Eye Disease; Macular Degeneration; **Hospital:** St Barnabas Med Ctr, Overlook Hosp (page 88); **Address:** 349 E Northfield Rd, Ste 100, Livingston, NJ 07039-4807; **Phone:** 973-716-0123; **Board Cert:** Ophthalmology 1984; **Med School:** NYU Sch Med 1978; **Resid:** Ophthalmology, LI Jewish Med Ctr 1982; **Fellow:** Vitreoretinal Surgery, Univ Chicago Hosps 1985

Davidson, Lawrence MD (Oph) - **Spec Exp:** LASIK-Refractive Surgery; Cataract Surgery; Glaucoma; **Hospital:** Mountainside Hosp (page 88), St Barnabas Med Ctr; **Address:** 825 Bloomfield Ave Fl 1, Verona, NJ 07044-1300; **Phone:** 973-239-4000; **Board Cert:** Ophthalmology 1975; **Med School:** SUNY Downstate 1969, **Resid:** Ophthalmology, Manhattan EE&T Hosp 1973

Frohman, Larry P MD (Oph) - **Spec Exp:** Neuro-Ophthalmology; Sarcoidosis; Vision Loss-Unexplained Loss; **Hospital:** UMDNJ-Univ Hosp-Newark; **Address:** 90 Bergen St, Ste 6174, Newark, NJ 07103-2425; **Phone:** 973-972-2065; **Board Cert:** Ophthalmology 1985; **Med School:** Univ Pennsylvania 1980; **Resid:** Ophthalmology, Bellevue Hosp 1984; **Fellow:** Neurological Ophthalmology, Bellevue Hosp/NYU 1985; **Fac Appt:** Assoc Prof Oph, UMDNJ-NJ Med Sch, Newark

Glatt, Herbert MD (Oph) - **Spec Exp:** Cataract Surgery-Lens Implant; LASIK-Refractive Surgery; **Hospital:** Mountainside Hosp (page 88), Clara Maass Med Ctr; **Address:** 1025 Broad St, Bloomfield, NJ 07003-2844; **Phone:** 973-338-1001; **Board Cert:** Ophthalmology 1991; **Med School:** Mexico 1979; **Resid:** Ophthalmology, UMDNJ-NJ Med Sch 1983; **Fac Appt:** Asst Clin Prof Oph, UMDNJ-NJ Med Sch, Newark

Langer, Paul MD (Oph) - **Spec Exp:** Oculoplastic Surgery; Orbital Surgery; Thyroid Eye Disease; **Hospital:** UMDNJ-Univ Hosp-Newark; **Address:** 90 Bergen St Fl 6 - Ste 6100, Newark, NJ 07101; **Phone:** 973-972-2065; **Board Cert:** Ophthalmology 1994; **Med School:** Johns Hopkins Univ 1989; **Resid:** Ophthalmology, UCSF Med Ctr 1993; **Fellow:** Ophthalmic Plastic Surgery, Univ Utah 1995; Orbital Surgery, Moorfields Eye Hosp 1995; **Fac Appt:** Asst Prof Oph, UMDNJ-NJ Med Sch, Newark

Miller, Philip MD (Oph) - **Spec Exp:** Laser Refractive Surgery; Cataract Surgery; Glaucoma; **Hospital:** St Barnabas Med Ctr; **Address:** 211 Irvington Ave, South Orange, NJ 07079; **Phone:** 973-763-2324; **Board Cert:** Ophthalmology 1967; **Med School:** Northwestern Univ 1961; **Resid:** Ophthalmology, Downstate Univ Med Ctr 1965

Turbin, Roger E MD (Oph) - **Spec Exp:** Neuro-Ophthalmology; Orbital Tumors/Cancer; **Hospital:** UMDNJ-Univ Hosp-Newark; **Address:** UMDNJ Dept Ophthalmology, DOC-Ste 6100, PO Box 1709, Newark, NJ 07101-1709; **Phone:** 973-972-2065; **Board Cert:** Ophthalmology 1999; **Med School:** Washington Univ, St Louis 1993; **Resid:** Ophthalmology, NYU Med Ctr 1997; **Fellow:** Neurological Ophthalmology, NYU/NY Eye & Ear/Beth Israel 1998; Oculoplastic Surgery, Allegheny Genl Hosp 1999

Wagner, Rudolph MD (Oph) - **Spec Exp:** Strabismus; Eye Disorders-Congenital; Botox Therapy; Pediatric Ophthalmology; **Hospital:** St Barnabas Med Ctr, UMDNJ-Univ Hosp-Newark; **Address:** Childrens Eye Care Ctr New Jersey, 495 N 13th St, Newark, NJ 07107-1317; **Phone:** 973-485-3186; **Board Cert:** Ophthalmology 1983; **Med School:** UMDNJ-NJ Med Sch, Newark 1978; **Resid:** Ophthalmology, NJ Med Sch Affil Hosp 1982; **Fellow:** Pediatric Ophthalmology, Wills Eye Hosp 1983; **Fac Appt:** Assoc Clin Prof Oph, UMDNJ-NJ Med Sch, Newark

Zarbin, Marco MD/PhD (Oph) - **Spec Exp:** Macular Degeneration; Diabetic Eye Disease/Retinopathy; Eye Trauma; **Hospital:** UMDNJ-Univ Hosp-Newark, Columbus Hosp; **Address:** 90 Bergen St, Bldg DOC - Ste 6156, Newark, NJ 07103-2499; **Phone:** 973-972-2065; **Board Cert:** Ophthalmology 1989; **Med School:** Johns Hopkins Univ 1984; **Resid:** Ophthalmology, Johns Hopkins Hosp 1988; **Fellow:** Vitreoretinal Surgery, Johns Hopkins Hosp 1990; **Fac Appt:** Prof Oph, UMDNJ-NJ Med Sch, Newark

ORTHOPAEDIC SURGERY

Benevenia, Joseph MD (OrS) - **Spec Exp:** Limb Salvage; Bone Cancer; Sarcoma-Soft Tissue; **Hospital:** UMDNJ-Univ Hosp-Newark; **Address:** 90 Bergen St, Ste 1200, Newark, NJ 07103; **Phone:** 973-972-2150; **Board Cert:** Orthopaedic Surgery 2003; **Med School:** UMDNJ-NJ Med Sch, Newark 1984; **Resid:** Orthopaedic Surgery, UMDNJ-NJ Med Sch Hosp 1988; **Fellow:** Orthopaedic Oncology, Case Western Reserve Univ 1991; **Fac Appt:** Assoc Prof OrS, UMDNJ-NJ Med Sch, Newark

Chase, Mark MD (OrS) - **Spec Exp:** Sports Medicine; **Hospital:** Mountainside Hosp (page 88); **Address:** 200 Highland Ave, Glen Ridge, NJ 07028-1521; **Phone:** 973-746-2200; **Board Cert:** Orthopaedic Surgery 2002; **Med School:** Boston Univ 1983; **Resid:** Orthopaedic Surgery, Boston Univ Affil Hosps 1988

Decter, Edward MD (OrS) - **Spec Exp:** Knee Reconstruction; Shoulder Reconstruction; **Hospital:** St Barnabas Med Ctr; **Address:** 1500 Pleasant Valley Way, West Orange, NJ 07052; **Phone:** 973-669-5600; **Board Cert:** Orthopaedic Surgery 1982; **Med School:** Creighton Univ 1975; **Resid:** Orthopaedic Surgery, Hosp Joint Dis 1980

Mendes, John MD (OrS) - **Spec Exp:** Hip & Knee Replacement; Foot & Ankle Surgery; Spinal Disorders; **Hospital:** Mountainside Hosp (page 88); **Address:** 200 Highland Ave, Glen Ridge, NJ 07028-1521; **Phone:** 973-746-2200; **Board Cert:** Orthopaedic Surgery 1984; **Med School:** Cornell Univ-Weill Med Coll 1976; **Resid:** Surgery, Bryn Mawr Hosp 1978; Orthopaedic Surgery, Hosp Special Surg 1981; **Fellow:** Penn Hosp 1982

Schob, Clifford MD (OrS) - **Spec Exp:** Sports Medicine; Shoulder & Knee Surgery; **Hospital:** Overlook Hosp (page 88), St Barnabas Med Ctr; **Address:** 235 Millburn Ave, Millburn, NJ 07041; **Phone:** 973-258-1177; **Board Cert:** Orthopaedic Surgery 2003; **Med School:** UMDNJ-RW Johnson Med Sch 1982; **Resid:** Surgery, Long Island Jewish Med Ctr 1984; Orthopaedic Surgery, Long Island Jewish Med Ctr 1988; **Fellow:** Sports Medicine, Am Sports Med Inst

Seidenstein, Michael MD (OrS) - **Spec Exp:** Arthroscopic Surgery; Joint Replacement; **Hospital:** Newark Beth Israel Med Ctr; **Address:** 81 Northfield Ave, Ste 304, West Orange, NJ 07052-5338; **Phone:** 973-736-8080; **Board Cert:** Orthopaedic Surgery 1977; **Med School:** NY Med Coll 1970; **Resid:** Orthopaedic Surgery, Hosp for Joint Diseases 1975; **Fellow:** Hip Surgery, Wrightington Hosp Ctr 1975A-O Fellowship 1978; **Fac Appt:** Asst Prof OrS, UMDNJ-NJ Med Sch, Newark

OTOLARYNGOLOGY

Baredes, Soly MD (Oto) - **Spec Exp:** Head & Neck Cancer; Skull Base Surgery; Voice Disorders; Swallowing Disorders; **Hospital:** UMDNJ-Univ Hosp-Newark; **Address:** 90 Bergen St, Ste 8100, Newark, NJ 07103-2425; **Phone:** 973-226-3444; **Board Cert:** Otolaryngology 1981; **Med School:** Columbia P&S 1976; **Resid:** Otolaryngology, Columbia-Presby Med Ctr 1980; **Fellow:** Head and Neck Surgery, Beth Israel Hosp 1981; **Fac Appt:** Assoc Prof Oto, UMDNJ-NJ Med Sch, Newark

Fieldman, Robert MD (Oto) - **Spec Exp:** Chronic Sinusitis; Pediatric Otolaryngology; **Hospital:** St Barnabas Med Ctr, Newark Beth Israel Med Ctr; **Address:** 741 Northfield Ave, Ste 104, W Orange, NJ 07052-1104; **Phone:** 973-243-0600; **Board Cert:** Otolaryngology 1986; **Med School:** Tulane Univ 1981; **Resid:** Otolaryngology, NY Hosp-Cornell Med Ctr 1983; **Fac Appt:** Asst Clin Prof S, UMDNJ-NJ Med Sch, Newark

Jahn, Anthony MD (Oto) - **Spec Exp:** Voice Disorders/Professional Voice Care; Hearing Loss; **Hospital:** St Barnabas Med Ctr, St Luke's - Roosevelt Hosp Ctr - Roosevelt Div (page 90); **Address:** 556 Eagle Rock Ave, Roseland, NJ 07068; **Phone:** 973-226-2262; **Board Cert:** Otolaryngology 1979; **Med School:** Canada 1974; **Resid:** Otolaryngology, Toronto Genl Hosp 1979; **Fac Appt:** Prof Oto, Columbia P&S

Morrow, Todd MD (Oto) - **Spec Exp:** Cosmetic Surgery-Face; Rhinoplasty; **Hospital:** St Barnabas Med Ctr, Newark Beth Israel Med Ctr; **Address:** 741 Northfield Ave, Ste 104, West Orange, NJ 07052; **Phone:** 973-243-0600; **Board Cert:** Otolaryngology 1992; Facial Plastic & Reconstructive Surgery 1995; **Med School:** Jefferson Med Coll 1986; **Resid:** Otolaryngology, UMDNJ-Univ Hosp 1991; **Fellow:** Facial Plastic & Reconstructive Surgery, Univ Toronto 1992; **Fac Appt:** Asst Clin Prof Oto, UMDNJ-NJ Med Sch, Newark

Zbar, Lloyd MD (Oto) - **Spec Exp:** Hearing & Balance Disorders; Nasal & Sinus Disorders; Voice Disorders; **Hospital:** Mountainside Hosp (page 88); **Address:** 200 Highland Ave, Glen Ridge, NJ 07028-1528; **Phone:** 973-744-2424; **Board Cert:** Otolaryngology 1970; **Med School:** Canada 1964; **Resid:** Surgery, French Hosp 1966; Otolaryngology, NYU-Bellevue Hosp Ctr 1969; **Fellow:** Otolaryngology, NYU-Bellevue Hosp Ctr 1970; **Fac Appt:** Assoc Clin Prof Oto, NYU Sch Med

PATHOLOGY

Heller, Debra MD (Path) - **Spec Exp:** Gynecologic Pathology; **Hospital:** UMDNJ-Univ Hosp-Newark; **Address:** UMDNJ-NJ Med Sch Dept Pathology, 185 S Orange Ave, Newark, NJ 07101; **Phone:** 973-972-0751; **Board Cert:** Anatomic Pathology 1988; Obstetrics & Gynecology 2005; Pediatric Pathology 1999; **Med School:** NY Med Coll 1977; **Resid:** Obstetrics & Gynecology, Beth Israel Med Ctr 1981; Anatomic Pathology, Mt Sinai Med Ctr 1988; **Fellow:** Pediatric Pathology, Mt Sinai Med Ctr 1987; Gynecologic Pathology, Mt Sinai Med Ctr 1989; **Fac Appt:** Prof Path, UMDNJ-NJ Med Sch, Newark

Lara, Jonathan F MD (Path) - **Spec Exp:** Breast Cancer; **Hospital:** St Barnabas Med Ctr; **Address:** St Barnabas Medical Ctr, Dept Pathology, 94 Old Short Hills Rd, Livingston, NJ 07039-5672; **Phone:** 973-322-5762; **Board Cert:** Anatomic & Clinical Pathology 1988; Cytopathology 1997; **Med School:** Philippines 1984; **Resid:** Pathology, St Barnabas Med Ctr 1988; **Fellow:** Surgical Pathology, Meml Sloan Kettering Cancer Ctr 1989; **Fac Appt:** Asst Clin Prof Path, UMDNJ-NJ Med Sch, Newark

PEDIATRIC ALLERGY & IMMUNOLOGY

Fost, Arthur MD (PA&I) - **Spec Exp:** Asthma; Sinusitis; Urticaria; **Hospital:** Clara Maass Med Ctr, Mountainside Hosp (page 88); **Address:** 197 Bloomfield Ave, Verona, NJ 07044-2702; **Phone:** 973-857-0330; **Board Cert:** Pediatrics 1968; Allergy & Immunology 1972; **Med School:** Jefferson Med Coll 1963; **Resid:** Pediatrics, Chldns Hosp 1965; Pediatrics, Hosp Univ Penn 1966; **Fellow:** Allergy & Immunology, St Vincents Hosp 1968; **Fac Appt:** Assoc Clin Prof Ped, UMDNJ-NJ Med Sch, Newark

Morrison, Susan MD (PA&I) - **Spec Exp:** Allergy & Immunology; Infectious Disease; Travel Medicine; **Hospital:** Clara Maass Med Ctr; **Address:** 36 Newark Ave, Ste 322, Belleville, NJ 07109; **Phone:** 973-450-0100; **Board Cert:** Pediatrics 1986; Allergy & Immunology 1999; Pediatric Infectious Disease 2002; **Med School:** UMDNJ-NJ Med Sch, Newark 1981; **Resid:** Pediatrics, UMDNJ-Univ Hosp 1985; **Fellow:** Pediatric Allergy & Immunology, UMDNJ-Univ Hosp 1988; Pediatric Infectious Disease, UMDNJ-Univ Hosp 1988; **Fac Appt:** Prof Ped, UMDNJ-NJ Med Sch, Newark

Torre, Arthur MD (PA&I) - **Spec Exp:** Asthma; Diving Medicine; **Hospital:** St Joseph's Regl Med Ctr - Paterson; **Address:** 25 Hollywood Ave, Fairfield, NJ 07004-1113; **Phone:** 973-882-0880; **Board Cert:** Pediatrics 1975; **Med School:** UMDNJ-NJ Med Sch, Newark 1970; **Resid:** Pediatrics, Martland Hosp 1972; **Fellow:** Pediatric Allergy & Immunology, Martland Hosp 1973; **Fac Appt:** Assoc Clin Prof Ped, UMDNJ-NJ Med Sch, Newark

PEDIATRIC CARDIOLOGY

Connor, Thomas M MD (PCd) - **Hospital:** St Barnabas Med Ctr, NY-Presby Hosp (page 100); **Address:** 101 Old Short Hills Rd, Ste 104, W Orange, NJ 07052; **Phone:** 973-731-5550; **Board Cert:** Pediatrics 1973; Pediatric Cardiology 1977; **Med School:** Italy 1966; **Resid:** Pediatrics, Grasslands Hosp 1970; **Fellow:** Pediatric Cardiology, Yale-New Haven Hosp 1972; **Fac Appt:** Assoc Prof Ped, Columbia P&S

Fernandes, John MD (PCd) - **Spec Exp:** Heart Disease-Congenital; Fetal Cardiology; **Hospital:** NY-Presby Hosp (page 100), St Barnabas Med Ctr; **Address:** 349 E Northfield Rd, Ste 201, Livingston, NJ 07039-4086; **Phone:** 973-533-1031; **Board Cert:** Pediatrics 1989; Pediatric Cardiology 1999; **Med School:** India 1983; **Resid:** Pediatrics, Hahnemann Univ 1988; **Fellow:** Pediatric Cardiology, NYU Med Ctr 1991; Pediatric Cardiology, Johns Hopkins Hosp 1990; **Fac Appt:** Assoc Clin Prof Ped, Columbia P&S

Friedman, Deborah MD (PCd) - **Spec Exp:** Fetal Cardiology; Echocardiography; Fetal Echocardiography; **Hospital:** St Barnabas Med Ctr; **Address:** St Barnabas Med Ctr, Dept Pediatrics, 94 Old Short Hills Rd, Livingston, NJ 07039; **Phone:** 973-322-5690; **Board Cert:** Pediatrics 1982; Pediatric Cardiology 1983; Pediatric Critical Care Medicine 2000; **Med School:** Univ Chicago-Pritzker Sch Med 1977; **Resid:** Pediatrics, Bronx Muni Hosp Ctr 1980; **Fellow:** Pediatric Cardiology, NYU Med Ctr 1983; **Fac Appt:** Prof Ped, Mount Sinai Sch Med

Langsner, Alan MD (PCd) - **Spec Exp:** Fetal Echocardiography; Congenital Heart Disease-Adult & Child; Preventive Cardiology; **Hospital:** St Barnabas Med Ctr, NYU Med Ctr (page 102); **Address:** 405 Northfield Ave, Ste 204, West Orange, NJ 07052-3023; **Phone:** 973-736-9997; **Board Cert:** Pediatrics 1983; Pediatric Cardiology 2002; **Med School:** Mexico 1977; **Resid:** Pediatrics, Metropolitan Hosp Ctr 1980; **Fellow:** Pediatric Cardiology, NYU Med Ctr 1983; **Fac Appt:** Asst Prof Ped, NYU Sch Med

PEDIATRIC CRITICAL CARE MEDICINE

Davis, Alan MD (PCCM) - **Spec Exp:** Sepsis & Septic Shock; Respiratory Failure; Pain Management; **Hospital:** St Barnabas Med Ctr; **Address:** 94 Old Short Hills Rd, 4rth Fl, West Wing/PICU, Livingston, NJ 07039; **Phone:** 973-322-8264; **Board Cert:** Pediatrics 1986; Pediatric Critical Care Medicine 2002; **Med School:** Univ Louisville Sch Med 1982; **Resid:** Pediatrics, Chldns Meml Hosp 1985; **Fellow:** Pediatric Critical Care Medicine, Chldns Hosp Natl Med Ctr 1987; **Fac Appt:** Assoc Clin Prof Ped, UMDNJ-NJ Med Sch, Newark

PEDIATRIC ENDOCRINOLOGY

Anhalt, Henry DO (PEn) - **Spec Exp:** Diabetes; Obesity; Growth Disorders; **Hospital:** St Barnabas Med Ctr, Newark Beth Israel Med Ctr; **Address:** 200 S Orange Ave, Livingston, NJ 07039; **Phone:** 973-322-7223; **Board Cert:** Pediatrics 2002; Pediatric Endocrinology 1997; **Med School:** NY Coll Osteo Med 1988; **Resid:** Pediatrics, Winthrop Univ Hosp 1992; **Fellow:** Pediatric Endocrinology, Stanford Univ Med Ctr 1995; **Fac Appt:** Assoc Prof Ped, SUNY Hlth Sci Ctr

PEDIATRIC GASTROENTEROLOGY

Sunaryo, Francis MD (PGe) - **Spec Exp:** Inflammatory Bowel Disease, Gastroesophageal Reflux Disease (GERD); **Hospital:** Newark Beth Israel Med Ctr, St Barnabas Med Ctr; **Address:** 400 Osborne Terrace, L-5, Newark, NJ 07112; **Phone:** 973-926-7280; **Board Cert:** Pediatrics 1982; Pediatric Gastroenterology 1998; **Med School:** Indonesia 1973; **Resid:** Pediatrics, North Shore Univ Hosp 1979; **Fellow:** Pediatric Gastroenterology, Chldns Hosp 1982; **Fac Appt:** Asst Prof Ped, UMDNJ-Univ Med Dent NJ

PEDIATRIC HEMATOLOGY-ONCOLOGY

Kamalakar, Peri MD (PHO) - **Spec Exp:** Sickle Cell Disease; Thalassemia; Leukemia; Solid Tumors; **Hospital:** Newark Beth Israel Med Ctr, Monmouth Med Ctr; **Address:** Childrens Hosp NJ, Fund Childrens Ctr, 201 Lyons Ave, Newark, NJ 07112-2027; **Phone:** 973-926-7161; **Board Cert:** Pediatrics 1975; Pediatric Hematology-Oncology 1997; **Med School:** India 1967; **Resid:** Pediatrics, Beth Israel Med Ctr 1973; **Fellow:** Pediatric Hematology-Oncology, Childrens Hosp 1976; **Fac Appt:** Asst Clin Prof Ped, UMDNJ-NJ Med Sch, Newark

PEDIATRIC INFECTIOUS DISEASE

Oleske, James MD (PInf) - **Spec Exp:** AIDS/HIV; Pediatric Allergy & Immunology; Palliative Care; **Hospital:** UMDNJ-Univ Hosp-Newark; **Address:** UMDNJ Dept Ped, MSB-F 572, 185 S Orange Ave, Newark, NJ 07103; **Phone:** 973-972-5066; **Board Cert:** Pediatrics 1976; Allergy & Immunology 1977; Pediatric Infectious Disease 2002; Diagnostic Lab Immunology 1986; **Med School:** UMDNJ-NJ Med Sch, Newark 1971; **Resid:** Pediatrics, Martland Hosp 1973; **Fellow:** Public Health, Columbia-Presby 1974; Pediatric Infectious Disease, Grady Meml Hosp/Emory Univ 1976; **Fac Appt:** Prof Ped, UMDNJ-NJ Med Sch, Newark

PEDIATRIC NEPHROLOGY

Roberti, M Isabel MD (PNep) - **Spec Exp:** Transplant Medicine-Kidney; Kidney Failure; **Hospital:** St Barnabas Med Ctr; **Address:** 94 Old Short Hills Rd, Ste 304, Livingston, NJ 07039; **Phone:** 973-322-5264; **Board Cert:** Pediatrics 2003; Pediatric Nephrology 1997; **Med School:** Brazil 1983; **Resid:** Pediatrics, Hosp Sao Paulo 1986; **Fellow:** Pediatric Nephrology, Hosp Sao Paulo 1989; Pediatric Nephrology, Mount Sinai Hosp 1995; **Fac Appt:** Assoc Clin Prof Ped, Mount Sinai Sch Med

PEDIATRIC PULMONOLOGY

Aguila, Helen MD (PPul) - **Spec Exp:** Asthma; Tuberculosis; **Hospital:** UMDNJ-Univ Hosp-Newark, Columbus Hosp; **Address:** 90 Bergen St, Ste 4100, Newark, NJ 07103; **Phone:** 973-972-5773; **Board Cert:** Pediatrics 1983; Pediatric Pulmonology 2004; **Med School:** Philippines 1974; **Resid:** Pediatrics, Staten Island Hosp 1979; Pediatrics, Kings Co Hosp/Downstate Med Ctr 1980; **Fellow:** Pediatric Pulmonology, Chldns Hosp Michigan 1983; **Fac Appt:** Asst Prof Ped, UMDNJ-NJ Med Sch, Newark

Bisberg, Dorothy Stein MD (PPul) - **Spec Exp:** Asthma; Cystic Fibrosis; **Hospital:** St Barnabas Med Ctr; **Address:** 200 South Orange Ave, Livingston, NJ 07039; **Phone:** 973-322-7600; **Board Cert:** Pediatrics 1977; Pediatric Pulmonology 2000; **Med School:** Cornell Univ-Weill Med Coll 1972; **Resid:** Pediatrics, Montefiore Hosp Med Ctr 1974; Pediatrics, Bronx Lebanon Hosp 1975; **Fac Appt:** Asst Prof Ped, UMDNJ-NJ Med Sch, Newark

Kottler, William MD (PPul) - **Spec Exp:** Asthma; Cystic Fibrosis; **Hospital:** St Barnabas Med Ctr, Overlook Hosp (page 88); **Address:** 48 Essex St, Millburn, NJ 07041; **Phone:** 973-218-0900; **Board Cert:** Pediatrics 1990; Pediatric Pulmonology 1994; **Med School:** France 1987; **Resid:** Pediatrics, Overlook Hosp 1990; **Fellow:** Pulmonary Disease, Shands Hosp 1993; **Fac Appt:** Asst Prof Ped, UMDNJ-NJ Med Sch, Newark

Lee, Haesoon MD (PPul) - **Spec Exp:** Asthma; Bronchitis; Sleep Apnea; **Hospital:** UMDNJ-Univ Hosp-Newark; **Address:** New Jersey Med Sch - Dept Pediatrics, 185 S Orange Ave, MSB-F540, Newark, NJ 07103; **Phone:** 973-972-5773; **Board Cert:** Pediatrics 1979; Pediatric Pulmonology 2004; **Med School:** South Korea 1972; **Resid:** Pediatrics, St Francis Hosp 1975; **Fellow:** Pediatric Pulmonology, Albert Einstein Coll Med 1977; **Fac Appt:** Assoc Prof Ped, UMDNJ-NJ Med Sch, Newark

PEDIATRIC SURGERY

Bethel, Colin MD (PS) - **Spec Exp:** Minimally Invasive Surgery; **Hospital:** UMDNJ-Univ Hosp-Newark, St Barnabas Med Ctr; **Address:** 90 Bergen St, Ste 7100, Newark, NJ 07103; **Phone:** 973-972-0212; **Board Cert:** Surgery 1996; Pediatric Surgery 2000; **Med School:** Columbia P&S 1987; **Resid:** Surgery, Yale-New Haven Hosp 1995; **Fellow:** Pediatric Surgery, Chldns Hosp 1997; **Fac Appt:** Asst Prof S, UMDNJ-NJ Med Sch, Newark

PEDIATRICS

Boodish, Wesley MD (Ped) `PCP` - **Hospital:** St Barnabas Med Ctr, Overlook Hosp (page 88); **Address:** 159 Millburn Ave, Millburn, NJ 07041-1849; **Phone:** 913-912-0155; **Board Cert:** Pediatrics 1965; **Med School:** Scotland 1960; **Resid:** Pediatrics, US Naval Hosp 1964

Gruenwald, Laurence D MD (Ped) `PCP` - **Spec Exp:** Asthma; Behavioral Disorders; **Hospital:** St Barnabas Med Ctr, Overlook Hosp (page 88); **Address:** 90 Millburn Ave, Ste 101, Millburn, NJ 07041-1933; **Phone:** 973-378-7990; **Board Cert:** Pediatrics 1981; **Med School:** UMDNJ-NJ Med Sch, Newark 1975; **Resid:** Pediatrics, Chldns Hosp Natl Med Ctr 1978; **Fac Appt:** Asst Clin Prof Ped, UMDNJ-RW Johnson Med Sch

Marcus, Richard MD (Ped) `PCP` - **Spec Exp:** ADD/ADHD; **Hospital:** Clara Maass Med Ctr; **Address:** 242 Washington Ave, Ste A, Nutley, NJ 07110-1994; **Phone:** 973-667-6676; **Board Cert:** Pediatrics 1988; **Med School:** UMDNJ-NJ Med Sch, Newark 1982; **Resid:** Pediatrics, UMDNJ-Univ Hosp 1985; **Fac Appt:** Asst Prof Ped, UMDNJ-NJ Med Sch, Newark

Prystowsky, Barry MD (Ped) - **Hospital:** Clara Maass Med Ctr, St Barnabas Med Ctr; **Address:** 562 Kingsland St, Nutley, NJ 07110-1069; **Phone:** 973-235-0101; **Board Cert:** Pediatrics 1986; **Med School:** UMDNJ-NJ Med Sch, Newark 1981; **Resid:** Pediatrics, UMDNJ Univ Hosp 1984

Rigtrup, Edward MD (Ped) `PCP` - **Hospital:** Mountainside Hosp (page 88), St Barnabas Med Ctr; **Address:** 73 Park St, Montclair, NJ 07042-2903; **Phone:** 973-746-7375; **Board Cert:** Pediatrics 1980; **Med School:** NY Med Coll 1975; **Resid:** Pediatrics, Chldns Natl Med Ctr 1978; **Fac Appt:** Assoc Clin Prof Ped, NY Med Coll

PHYSICAL MEDICINE & REHABILITATION

Bach, John MD (PMR) - **Spec Exp:** Mechanical Ventilation; Spinal Cord Injury; Neuromuscular Disorders; **Hospital:** UMDNJ-Univ Hosp-Newark; **Address:** 150 Bergen St, Ste B403, Newark, NJ 07103-2425; **Phone:** 973-972-7195; **Board Cert:** Physical Medicine & Rehabilitation 1986; **Med School:** UMDNJ-NJ Med Sch, Newark 1976; **Resid:** Physical Medicine & Rehabilitation, NYU Med Ctr 1980; **Fellow:** Neurological Muscular Disease, Univ Hosp 1983; **Fac Appt:** Prof PMR, UMDNJ-NJ Med Sch, Newark

Cole, Jeffrey L MD (PMR) - **Spec Exp:** Pain Management; Neuromuscular Disorders; Electromyography; **Hospital:** Kessler Inst for Rehab - W Orange; **Address:** Kessler Inst for Rehabilitation, 1199 Pleasant Valley Way, West Orange, NJ 07052; **Phone:** 973-243-6943; **Board Cert:** Physical Medicine & Rehabilitation 1983; Pain Medicine 2003; **Med School:** Mexico 1977; **Resid:** Internal Medicine, NY Hosp-Queens Med Ctr 1979; Physical Medicine & Rehabilitation, Montefiore Med Ctr 1982

Francis, Kathleen MD (PMR) - **Spec Exp:** Lymphedema; Amyotrophic Lateral Sclerosis (ALS); Neurodegenerative Disorders; **Address:** 200 S Orange Ave, Livingston, NJ 07039; **Phone:** 973-322-7366; **Board Cert:** Physical Medicine & Rehabilitation 2004; **Med School:** UMDNJ-NJ Med Sch, Newark 1989; **Resid:** Physical Medicine & Rehabilitation, UMDNJ-Kessler Inst Rehab 1993; **Fac Appt:** Asst Clin Prof PMR, UMDNJ-NJ Med Sch, Newark

Kirshblum, Steven C MD (PMR) - **Spec Exp:** Spinal Cord Injury; **Hospital:** Kessler Inst for Rehab - W Orange, St Barnabas Hosp - Bronx; **Address:** 1199 Pleasant Valley Way, West Orange, NJ 07052-1424; **Phone:** 973-731-3600; **Board Cert:** Physical Medicine & Rehabilitation 1991; Spinal Cord Injury Medicine 1998; **Med School:** Univ Hlth Sci/Chicago Med Sch 1986; **Resid:** Physical Medicine & Rehabilitation, Mount Sinai Med Ctr 1990; **Fac Appt:** Prof PMR, UMDNJ-NJ Med Sch, Newark

PLASTIC SURGERY

Berlet, Anthony C MD (PlS) - **Hospital:** Hackensack Univ Med Ctr (page 92), Chilton Meml Hosp; **Address:** 908 Pompton Ave, Ste A-1, Cedar Grove, NJ 07009; **Phone:** 973-857-7757; **Board Cert:** Plastic Surgery 1996; **Med School:** UMDNJ-NJ Med Sch, Newark 1986; **Resid:** Surgery, Albert Einstein Med Ctr 1991; Plastic Surgery, UMDNJ-NJ Med Ctr 1993; **Fac Appt:** Asst Clin Prof PlS, UMDNJ-NJ Med Sch, Newark

DiBernardo, Barry E MD (PlS) - **Spec Exp:** Laser Cosmetic Surgery; Hair Restoration/Transplant; Cosmetic Surgery-Face & Body; **Hospital:** Mountainside Hosp (page 88), Clara Maass Med Ctr; **Address:** 29 Park St, Montclair, NJ 07042; **Phone:** 973-509-2000; **Board Cert:** Plastic Surgery 1994; **Med School:** Cornell Univ-Weill Med Coll 1984; **Resid:** Surgery, Mt Sinai Hosp 1989; Plastic Surgery, Montefiore Med Ctr 1991; **Fac Appt:** Assoc Clin Prof PlS, UMDNJ-NJ Med Sch, Newark

Friedlander, Beverly MD (PlS) - **Spec Exp:** Breast Augmentation; Cosmetic Surgery-Face & Body; Cosmetic Surgery-Liposuction; **Hospital:** Overlook Hosp (page 88), St Barnabas Med Ctr; **Address:** 636 Morris Tpke, Ste 2G, Short Hills, NJ 07078-2608; **Phone:** 973-912-9120; **Board Cert:** Plastic Surgery 1990; **Med School:** SUNY Downstate 1980; **Resid:** Surgery, Kings Co Hosp 1984; Plastic Surgery, Montefiore Med Ctr 1987

Granick, Mark S MD (PlS) - **Spec Exp:** Rhinoplasty; Cosmetic Surgery; **Hospital:** UMDNJ-Univ Hosp-Newark; **Address:** NJ Medical School Plastic Surgery, 90 Bergen St, Ste 7200, Newark, NJ 07103; **Phone:** 973-972-8092; **Board Cert:** Otolaryngology 1982; Plastic Surgery 1985; **Med School:** UMDNJ-NJ Med Sch, Newark 1977; **Resid:** Otolaryngology, Mass E&E Hosp 1982; Plastic Surgery, U Pittsburgh Med Ctr 1984; **Fac Appt:** Prof PlS, Hahnemann Univ

LoVerme, Paul J MD (PlS) - **Spec Exp:** Cosmetic Surgery-Face; Liposuction & Body Contouring; Breast Reconstruction & Augmentation; **Hospital:** Mountainside Hosp (page 88), St Barnabas Med Ctr; **Address:** 825 Bloomfield Ave, Ste 205, Verona, NJ 07044; **Phone:** 973-857-9499; **Board Cert:** Plastic Surgery 1987; **Med School:** UMDNJ-NJ Med Sch, Newark 1978; **Resid:** Surgery, UMDNJ Univ Hosp 1983; Plastic Surgery, Med Coll Hosp 1985; **Fellow:** Surgical Oncology, UMDNJ Univ Hosp 1982; **Fac Appt:** Assoc Clin Prof PlS, UMDNJ-NJ Med Sch, Newark

Rosen, Allen D MD (PlS) - **Spec Exp:** Breast Reconstruction; Cosmetic Surgery-Face; Body Contouring; **Hospital:** Mountainside Hosp (page 88), PBI Regional- Passaic; **Address:** 37 N Fullerton Ave, Montclair, NJ 07042; **Phone:** 973-233-1933; **Board Cert:** Plastic Surgery 1991; **Med School:** SUNY Buffalo 1983; **Resid:** Surgery, Columbia Presby Med Ctr 1986; Plastic Surgery, Columbia Presby Med Ctr 1988; **Fellow:** Hand Surgery, Columbia Presby Med Ctr 1987; **Fac Appt:** Asst Clin Prof PlS, UMDNJ-NJ Med Sch, Newark

PREVENTIVE MEDICINE

Weiss, Stanley H MD (PrM) - **Spec Exp:** Cancer Epidemiology & Control; AIDS Related Infections; Bioterrorism Preparedness; Infections in Cancer Patients; **Hospital:** UMDNJ-Univ Hosp-Newark; **Address:** NJ Medical School, 30 Bergen St, ADMC, Ste 1614, Newark, NJ 07107-3000; **Phone:** 973-972-7716; **Board Cert:** Internal Medicine 1981; Medical Oncology 1985; **Med School:** Harvard Med Sch 1978; **Resid:** Internal Medicine, Montefiore Med Ctr 1981; **Fellow:** Medical Oncology, National Cancer Inst 1985; Epidemiology, National Cancer Inst 1987; **Fac Appt:** Prof PrM, UMDNJ-NJ Med Sch, Newark

PSYCHIATRY

Caracci, Giovanni MD (Psyc) - **Spec Exp:** Geriatric Psychiatry; Psychopharmacology; Psychotherapy; **Hospital:** UMDNJ-Univ Hosp-Newark; **Address:** 183 S Orange Ave, rm E1453, Box 1709, Newark, NJ 07101; **Phone:** 973-972-9712; **Board Cert:** Psychiatry 1990; Geriatric Psychiatry 2001; **Med School:** Italy 1977; **Resid:** Psychiatry, Metropolitan Hosp 1983; **Fellow:** Psychiatry, Metropolitan Hosp 1984; **Fac Appt:** Assoc Prof Psyc, Mount Sinai Sch Med

Faber, Mark MD (Psyc) - **Spec Exp:** Anxiety Disorders; Depression; ADD/ADHD; **Hospital:** St Barnabas Med Ctr; **Address:** 594 Valley Rd, Upper Montclair, NJ 07043-1882; **Phone:** 973-746-6711; **Board Cert:** Psychiatry 1993; Child & Adolescent Psychiatry 1995; **Med School:** Dominica 1988; **Resid:** Psychiatry, CT Valley Hosp-Yale 1991; **Fellow:** Child & Adolescent Psychiatry, UMDNJ-RW Johnson Sch Med 1993; Sleep Medicine, UMDNJ-RW Johnson Sch Med 1996

Nucci, Annamaria MD (Psyc) - **Spec Exp:** Psychopharmacology; Relationship Problems; Depression; **Address:** 5 Westview Ct, Cedar Grove, NJ 07009-1937; **Phone:** 973-857-2609; **Board Cert:** Psychiatry 1978; **Med School:** Italy 1971; **Resid:** Psychiatry, Payne Whitney Clinic 1976; **Fellow:** Child & Adolescent Psychiatry, New York Hosp-Cornell 1976; **Fac Appt:** Asst Clin Prof Psyc, NY Med Coll

Schleifer, Steven MD (Psyc) - **Spec Exp:** Depression; Psychoneuroimmunology; Anxiety Disorders; **Hospital:** UMDNJ-Univ Hosp-Newark; **Address:** 183 S Orange Ave Bldg BHSB F1430, Newark, NJ 07103; **Phone:** 973-972-5023; **Board Cert:** Psychiatry 1980; **Med School:** Mount Sinai Sch Med 1975; **Resid:** Psychiatry, USC Med Ctr 1976; Psychiatry, Mount Sinai Med Ctr 1979; **Fac Appt:** Prof Psyc, UMDNJ-NJ Med Sch, Newark

Zornitzer, Michael MD (Psyc) - **Spec Exp:** Psychotherapy; Mood Disorders; Obsessive Compulsive Disorder; **Hospital:** St Barnabas Med Ctr; **Address:** 2 W Northfield Rd, Ste 305, Livingston, NJ 07039-3789; **Phone:** 973-992-6090; **Board Cert:** Psychiatry 1976; **Med School:** SUNY Downstate 1971; **Resid:** Psychiatry, Albert Einstein Coll Med 1975; **Fac Appt:** Asst Clin Prof Psyc, NY Coll Osteo Med

PULMONARY DISEASE

Dadaian, Jack MD (Pul) - **Spec Exp:** Sleep Disorders; Bronchoscopy; Laryngoscopy; Pulmonary Rehabilitation; **Hospital:** Mountainside Hosp (page 88), St Barnabas Med Ctr; **Address:** 123 Highland Ave, Ste 301, Glen Ridge, NJ 07028-1522; **Phone:** 973-746-7474; **Board Cert:** Internal Medicine 1968; Pulmonary Disease 1969; **Med School:** UMDNJ-NJ Med Sch, Newark 1962; **Resid:** Internal Medicine, Jersey City Med Ctr 1966; Pulmonary Disease, Bronx Muni Hosp 1967; **Fellow:** Pulmonary Disease, UMDNJ-NJ Coll Med 1968

Greenberg, Martin J MD (Pul) - **Spec Exp:** Asthma; Emphysema; **Hospital:** St Barnabas Med Ctr; **Address:** 124 East Mt Pleasant Ave, Livingston, NJ 07039; **Phone:** 973-994-4130; **Board Cert:** Internal Medicine 1987; Pulmonary Disease 1992; **Med School:** Dominica 1983; **Resid:** Internal Medicine, Univ Hosp UMDNJ 1986; **Fellow:** Pulmonary Disease, Newark Beth Israel 1989

Karetzky, Monroe MD (Pul) - **Spec Exp:** Asthma; Sleep Disorders; **Hospital:** Newark Beth Israel Med Ctr; **Address:** 201 Lyons Ave, Newark, NJ 07112; **Phone:** 973-926-7597; **Board Cert:** Pain Medicine 1974; Critical Care Medicine 1999; Geriatric Medicine 2002; **Med School:** Cornell Univ-Weill Med Coll 1963; **Resid:** Internal Medicine, Mary I Bassett Hosp 1966; **Fellow:** Cardiopulmonary Disease, Mary I Bassett Hosp 1967; **Fac Appt:** Assoc Clin Prof Med, UMDNJ-NJ Med Sch, Newark

Labissiere, Jean-Claude MD (Pul) - **Spec Exp:** Asthma; **Hospital:** St Barnabas Med Ctr; **Address:** 92 Old Northfield Rd, West Orange, NJ 07052; **Phone:** 973-736-5552; **Board Cert:** Internal Medicine 1988; Pulmonary Disease 1994; **Med School:** Haiti 1977; **Resid:** Internal Medicine, Lincoln Med Ctr 1984; **Fellow:** Pulmonary Disease, UMDNJ/E Orange VA Hosp 1986

Reichman, Lee B MD (Pul) - **Spec Exp:** Tuberculosis; Mycobacterial Infections; **Hospital:** UMDNJ-Univ Hosp-Newark; **Address:** 225 Warren St, Box 1709, Newark, NJ 07101-1709; **Phone:** 973-972-3270; **Board Cert:** Internal Medicine 1972; Pulmonary Disease 1972; **Med School:** NYU Sch Med 1964; **Resid:** Internal Medicine, Bellevue Hosp 1965; Internal Medicine, Harlem Hosp 1969; **Fellow:** Pulmonary Disease, Harlem Hosp-Columbia P&S 1970; **Fac Appt:** Prof Med, UMDNJ-NJ Med Sch, Newark

Safirstein, Benjamin MD (Pul) - **Spec Exp:** Asthma; Sarcoidosis; **Hospital:** Mount Sinai Med Ctr (page 98), Saint Michael's Med Ctr; **Address:** 62 South Fullerton Ave, Montclair, NJ 07042; **Phone:** 973-744-9125; **Board Cert:** Internal Medicine 1970; Pulmonary Disease 1974; **Med School:** Univ Hlth Sci/Chicago Med Sch 1965; **Resid:** Internal Medicine, Mount Sinai Hosp 1969; **Fellow:** Pulmonary Disease, Inst Dis Chest 1972

RADIATION ONCOLOGY

Goodman, Robert L MD (RadRO) - **Spec Exp:** Breast Cancer; Lymphoma; **Hospital:** St Barnabas Med Ctr; **Address:** St Barnabas Med Ctr, Dept Rad Oncology, 94 Old Short Hills Rd, Livingston, NJ 07039; **Phone:** 973-322-5133; **Board Cert:** Internal Medicine 1971; Therapeutic Radiology 1974; Medical Oncology 1975; **Med School:** Columbia P&S 1966; **Resid:** Internal Medicine, Beth Israel Hosp 1970; Radiation Therapy, Harvard Joint Ctr Rad Therapy 1974; **Fellow:** Hematology, Presby Hosp 1969

Stabile, Richard MD (RadRO) - **Spec Exp:** Brachytherapy; **Hospital:** Mountainside Hosp (page 88); **Address:** Mountainside Hosp, Dept Rad Onc, 1 Bay Ave, Montclair, NJ 07042; **Phone:** 973-429-6096; **Board Cert:** Therapeutic Radiology 1975; **Med School:** NY Med Coll 1971; **Resid:** Radiation Oncology, Mount Sinai Hosp 1974

Zablow, Andrew MD (RadRO) - **Spec Exp:** Prostate Cancer; Head & Neck Cancer; Gynecologic Cancer; **Hospital:** St Barnabas Med Ctr; **Address:** St Barnabas Med Ctr, Dept Radiation Onc, 94 Old Short Hills Rd, Livingston, NJ 07039-5672; **Phone:** 973-322-5630 x5632; **Board Cert:** Radiation Oncology 1987; **Med School:** Mexico 1981; **Resid:** Radiation Oncology, St Barnabas Med Ctr 1986

REPRODUCTIVE ENDOCRINOLOGY

Annos, Thomas MD (RE) - **Spec Exp:** Infertility-IVF; Endometriosis; Polycystic Ovarian Syndrome; **Hospital:** St Barnabas Med Ctr, Overlook Hosp (page 88); **Address:** Short Hills Fertility Ctr, 40 Farley Pl, Short Hills, NJ 07078-3319; **Phone:** 973-467-0099; **Board Cert:** Obstetrics & Gynecology 1978; Reproductive Endocrinology 1982; **Med School:** Geo Wash Univ 1972; **Resid:** Obstetrics & Gynecology, Thomas Jefferson Univ Hosp 1976; **Fellow:** Reproductive Endocrinology, Beth Israel Deaconess/Harvard 1980

RHEUMATOLOGY

Cannarozzi, Nicholas MD (Rhu) - **Spec Exp:** Rheumatoid Arthritis; Lupus Nephritis; Osteoporosis; **Hospital:** Mountainside Hosp (page 88); **Address:** 127 Pine St, Montclair, NJ 07042-4835; **Phone:** 973-783-6000; **Board Cert:** Internal Medicine 1980; Rheumatology 1972; **Med School:** Hahnemann Univ 1965; **Resid:** Internal Medicine, Philadelphia Genl Hosp 1967; Internal Medicine, St Michaels Med Ctr 1968; **Fellow:** Rheumatology, Yale Univ Sch Med 1969; Rheumatology, Yale Univ Sch Med 1972

Kramer, Neil MD (Rhu) - **Spec Exp:** Rheumatoid Arthritis; **Hospital:** St Barnabas Med Ctr; **Address:** 200 S Orange Ave, Livingston, NJ 07039-5817; **Phone:** 973-322-7400; **Board Cert:** Internal Medicine 1977; Rheumatology 1980; **Med School:** Univ Pennsylvania 1974; **Resid:** Internal Medicine, Manhattan VA Hosp/NYU Med Ctr 1978; **Fellow:** Rheumatology, NYU Med Ctr 1980; **Fac Appt:** Asst Clin Prof Med, Mount Sinai Sch Med

Panush, Richard MD (Rhu) - **Spec Exp:** Arthritis; **Hospital:** St Barnabas Med Ctr; **Address:** 101 Old Short Hills Rd, Ste 106, Livingston, NJ 07052; **Phone:** 973-322-6256; **Board Cert:** Internal Medicine 1972; Rheumatology 1972; **Med School:** Univ Mich Med Sch 1967; **Resid:** Internal Medicine, Duke Univ Hosp 1969; **Fellow:** Rheumatology, Peter Bent Brigham Hosp 1971; **Fac Appt:** Prof Med, Mount Sinai Sch Med

Rosenstein, Elliot D MD (Rhu) - **Spec Exp:** Rheumatoid Arthritis; Lupus/SLE; Sjogren's Syndrome; **Hospital:** St Barnabas Med Ctr; **Address:** 200 S Orange Ave, Livingston, NJ 07039-5817; **Phone:** 973-322-7400; **Board Cert:** Internal Medicine 1981; Rheumatology 1984; **Med School:** Mount Sinai Sch Med 1978; **Resid:** Internal Medicine, NYU/Bellevue Hosp 1982; **Fellow:** Rheumatology, NYU/Bellevue Hosp 1984; **Fac Appt:** Assoc Clin Prof Med, Mount Sinai Sch Med

Simon, Jonathan MD (Rhu) - **Hospital:** Mountainside Hosp (page 88); **Address:** 1018 Broad St, Bloomfield, NJ 07003-2807; **Phone:** 973-338-3383; **Board Cert:** Internal Medicine 1981; Rheumatology 1984; **Med School:** NYU Sch Med 1978; **Resid:** Internal Medicine, UMDNJ Univ Hosp 1981; **Fellow:** Rheumatology, UMDNJ Univ Hosp 1983

SURGERY

Blackwood, M Michele MD (S) - **Spec Exp:** Breast Cancer; Breast Surgery; Sentinel Node Surgery; Breast Cancer - Young Women; **Hospital:** Saint Michael's Med Ctr; **Address:** St Michaels Med Ctr - The Breast Center, 111 Central Ave, Newark, NJ 07102; **Phone:** 973-877-5189; **Board Cert:** Surgery 2003; **Med School:** Med Univ SC 1988; **Resid:** Surgery, Stamford Hosp 1993; **Fellow:** Surgical Oncology, Meml Sloan Kettering Cancer Ctr 1994; **Fac Appt:** Asst Clin Prof S, Columbia P&S

Brief, Donald MD (S) - **Spec Exp:** Breast Cancer & Surgery; Cancer Surgery; Endocrine Surgery; **Hospital:** Newark Beth Israel Med Ctr; **Address:** 225 Millburn Ave, Ste 104B, Millburn, NJ 07041-1712; **Phone:** 973-379-5888; **Board Cert:** Surgery 1980; **Med School:** Harvard Med Sch 1957; **Resid:** Surgery, Peter Bent Brigham Hosp 1964; **Fac Appt:** Clin Prof S, UMDNJ-NJ Med Sch, Newark

Chamberlain, Ronald S MD (S) - **Spec Exp:** Liver & Biliary Surgery; Cancer Surgery; Laparoscopic Surgery; Pancreatic Cancer; **Hospital:** St Barnabas Med Ctr; **Address:** St Barnabas Med Ctr, Dept Surgery, 94 Old Short Hills Rd, Livingston, NJ 07039; **Phone:** 973-322-8976; **Board Cert:** Surgery 1999; **Med School:** Geo Wash Univ 1991; **Resid:** Surgery, Geo Wash Univ Med Ctr 1997; **Fellow:** Surgical Oncology, Natl Cancer Inst-NIH 1996; Surgical Oncology, Meml Sloan-Kettering Canc Ctr 1999

Chang, Patrick KS MD (S) - **Spec Exp:** Melanoma; Thyroid & Parathyroid Surgery; Hernia; **Hospital:** St Barnabas Med Ctr; **Address:** 101 Old Short Hills Rd, Ste 206, West Orange, NJ 07052; **Phone:** 973-731-5005; **Board Cert:** Surgery 1997; **Med School:** Australia 1970; **Resid:** Surgery, St Barnabas Hosp 1976; **Fellow:** Surgical Oncology, Meml Sloan Kettering Cancer Ctr 1980; **Fac Appt:** Assoc Clin Prof S, UMDNJ-NJ Med Sch, Newark

Deitch, Edwin MD (S) - **Spec Exp:** Critical Care; Trauma; Burn Care; **Hospital:** UMDNJ-Univ Hosp-Newark; **Address:** 185 S Orange Ave, MSB, rm G506, Newark, NJ 07103; **Phone:** 973-972-5045; **Board Cert:** Surgery 1997; Surgical Critical Care 1995; **Med School:** Univ MD Sch Med 1973; **Resid:** Surgery, US Public Hlth Svc Hosp 1976; Surgery, US Public Hlth Svc Hosp 1978; **Fac Appt:** Prof S, UMDNJ-NJ Med Sch, Newark

Fletcher, H Stephen MD (S) - **Spec Exp:** Vascular Surgery; Breast Surgery; **Hospital:** St Barnabas Med Ctr, Overlook Hosp (page 88); **Address:** 1500 Pleasant Valley Way, Ste 302, West Orange, NJ 07052-2956; **Phone:** 973-325-9779; **Board Cert:** Surgery 1973; **Med School:** Geo Wash Univ 1967; **Resid:** Surgery, Geo Wash U Med Ctr 1972; **Fac Appt:** Assoc Clin Prof S, UMDNJ-NJ Med Sch, Newark

Mansour, E Hani MD (S) - **Spec Exp:** Burn Care; **Hospital:** St Barnabas Med Ctr; **Address:** St Barnabas Med Ctr, Dept Surgery, 94 Old Short Hills Rd, Livingston, NJ 07039; **Phone:** 973-322-5924; **Board Cert:** Surgery 1999; Surgical Critical Care 1999; **Med School:** Lebanon 1973; **Resid:** Surgery, Union Meml Hosp 1979; **Fellow:** Burn Surgery, Brooke Army Med Ctr

Munoz, Eric MD (S) - **Hospital:** UMDNJ-Univ Hosp-Newark, Overlook Hosp (page 88); **Address:** 150 Bergen St, Mezz North, rm 237-A, Newark, NJ 07103; **Phone:** 973-972-3665; **Board Cert:** Surgery 1995; **Med School:** Albert Einstein Coll Med 1974; **Resid:** Surgery, Yale-New Haven Hosp 1978; **Fac Appt:** Asst Prof S, SUNY Upstate Med Univ

Petrone, Sylvia MD (S) - **Spec Exp:** Burn Care; Critical Care; **Hospital:** St Barnabas Med Ctr; **Address:** St Barnabas Med Ctr, Dept Surgery, 94 Old Short Hills Rd, Livingston, NJ 07039-5672; **Phone:** 973-322-5924; **Board Cert:** Surgery 2001; Surgical Critical Care 1998; **Med School:** Loyola Univ-Stritch Sch Med 1977; **Resid:** Surgery, Boston Univ Med Ctr 1982; **Fellow:** Burn Surgery, NY Hosp-Cornell Univ 1983

Raina, Suresh MD (S) - **Spec Exp:** Endocrine Surgery; **Hospital:** UMDNJ-Univ Hosp-Newark; **Address:** UMDNJ School - Surgery, 185 S Orange Ave, Ste D215, MS H/578, Newark, NJ 07103; **Phone:** 973-972-6294; **Board Cert:** Surgery 1998; **Med School:** India 1971; **Resid:** Surgery, UMDNJ-NJ Med Sch 1977; **Fellow:** Surgical Oncology, UMDNJ-NJ Med Sch 1978; Surgical Oncology, Roswell Park Cancer Inst 1979; **Fac Appt:** Assoc Prof S, UMDNJ-NJ Med Sch, Newark

Santoro, Elissa J MD (S) - **Spec Exp:** Breast Cancer; Cancer Surgery; **Hospital:** St Barnabas Med Ctr; **Address:** 200 S Orange Ave, Livingston, NJ 07039-5817; **Phone:** 973-533-0222; **Board Cert:** Surgery 1971; **Med School:** Med Coll PA Hahnemann 1965; **Resid:** Surgery, Womens Med Coll Hosp 1967; Surgery, St Vincent's Hosp 1970; **Fellow:** Surgical Oncology, St Vincent's Hosp 1969; Surgical Oncology, New York Med Coll 1971

Seltzer, Murray H MD (S) - **Spec Exp:** Breast Cancer; Breast Surgery; **Hospital:** St Barnabas Med Ctr; **Address:** 200 S Orange Ave, Livingston, NJ 07039-5817; **Phone:** 973-992-8484; **Board Cert:** Surgery 1972; **Med School:** Univ Pennsylvania 1965; **Resid:** Surgery, Hosp Univ Penn 1971; **Fellow:** Research, Hosp Univ Penn 1970; **Fac Appt:** Clin Prof S, UMDNJ-NJ Med Sch, Newark

THORACIC SURGERY

Connolly, Mark W MD (TS) - **Spec Exp:** Minimally Invasive Cardiac Surgery; **Hospital:** Saint Michael's Med Ctr; **Address:** St Michael's Med Ctr, Cathedral Cardiothoracic Surgeons, 268 Dr Martin Luther King Jr Blvd, Newark, NJ 07102; **Phone:** 973-877-5300; **Board Cert:** Thoracic Surgery 2001; **Med School:** Northwestern Univ 1982; **Resid:** Surgery, Bellevue/NYU Med Ctr 1988; Cardiothoracic Surgery, Emory Univ Hosps 1991; **Fellow:** Surgical Research, Maimonides Med Ctr 1986

Forman, Mark MD (TS) - **Spec Exp:** Lung Cancer; Thoracic Surgery; Vascular Surgery; **Hospital:** St Barnabas Med Ctr, Columbus Hosp; **Address:** 1500 Pleasant Valley Way, Ste 302, West Orange, NJ 07052; **Phone:** 973-324-0988; **Board Cert:** Surgery 1983; Thoracic Surgery 1997; **Med School:** Tulane Univ 1976; **Resid:** Surgery, LI Jewish Med Ctr 1981; Thoracic Surgery, Montefiore Hosp Med Ctr 1982; **Fellow:** Thoracic Surgery, Montefiore Hosp Med Ctr 1984

Saunders, Craig R MD (TS) - **Spec Exp:** Cardiac Surgery; Minimally Invasive Surgery; **Hospital:** Newark Beth Israel Med Ctr, St Barnabas Med Ctr; **Address:** 201 Lyons Ave, Ste G5, Newark, NJ 07112; **Phone:** 973-926-6938; **Board Cert:** Thoracic Surgery 2000; **Med School:** Univ Iowa Coll Med 1970; **Resid:** Surgery, Univ Iowa Hosps 1978; Thoracic Surgery, Cleveland Clinic 1980

Starr, Joanne P MD (TS) - **Spec Exp:** Pediatric Cardiothoracic Surgery; Congenital Heart Surgery; **Hospital:** Chldns Hosp NJ at Newark, Newark Beth Israel Med Ctr; **Address:** Childrens Heart Center, 201 Lyons Ave, Newark, NJ 07112; **Phone:** 973-926-4900; **Board Cert:** Surgery 1997; Thoracic Surgery 2000; **Med School:** NY Med Coll ; **Resid:** Surgery, NY Presbyterian Hosp 1996; Cardiothoracic Surgery, NY Presbyterian Hosp 1998; **Fellow:** Pediatric Cardiac Surgery, Childrens Hosp 1999

Syracuse, Donald MD (TS) - **Spec Exp:** Pacemakers; Lung Cancer; Carotid Artery Surgery; **Hospital:** Mountainside Hosp (page 88); **Address:** 5 Franklin Ave, Ste 310, Belleville, NJ 07109-3522; **Phone:** 973-759-9000; **Board Cert:** Thoracic Surgery 2002; **Med School:** Columbia P&S 1973; **Resid:** Surgery, Columbia Presby Hosp 1979; Thoracic Surgery, Columbia Presby Hosp 1981; **Fellow:** Cardiovascular Surgery, Nat Inst Health 1977; **Fac Appt:** Clin Prof S, UMDNJ-NJ Med Sch, Newark

UROLOGY

Boorjian, Peter MD (U) - **Spec Exp:** Kidney Stones; Prostate Benign Disease; Urinary Tract Infections; Urologic Cancer; **Hospital:** Mountainside Hosp (page 88); **Address:** 777 Bloomfield Ave, Glen Ridge, NJ 07028; **Phone:** 973-746-3322; **Board Cert:** Urology 1978; **Med School:** SUNY Downstate 1971; **Resid:** Surgery, Med Coll VA 1973; Urology, SUNY Downstate 1976

Ciccone, Patrick MD (U) - **Spec Exp:** Prostate Cancer; **Hospital:** Clara Maass Med Ctr, St Barnabas Med Ctr; **Address:** 36 Newark Ave, Ste 200, Belleville, NJ 07109; **Phone:** 973-759-6180; **Board Cert:** Urology 1975; **Med School:** Georgetown Univ 1967; **Resid:** Surgery, VA Med Ctr 1969; Urology, VA Med Ctr 1972

Katz, Jeffrey I MD (U) - **Spec Exp:** Prostate Disease; Kidney Stones; Urologic Cancer; **Hospital:** St Barnabas Med Ctr; **Address:** 741 Northfield Ave, Ste 206, W Orange, NJ 07052; **Phone:** 973-325-6100; **Board Cert:** Urology 1978; **Med School:** Italy 1970; **Resid:** Surgery, Mt Sinai Hosp 1973; Urology, Albert Einstein 1976

Linsenmeyer, Todd MD (U) - **Spec Exp:** Infertility-Male in Spinal Cord Injury; Voiding Dysfunction/Spinal Cord Injury; Urodynamins in Spinal Cord Injury; **Hospital:** Kessler Inst for Rehab - W Orange; **Address:** Kessler Inst Rehab, 1199 Pleasant Valley Way, West Orange, NJ 07052; **Phone:** 973-731-3900 x2274; **Board Cert:** Urology 1996; Physical Medicine & Rehabilitation 1990; **Med School:** Univ Hawaii JA Burns Sch Med 1979; **Resid:** Urology, Tripler AMC 1984; **Fellow:** Physical Medicine & Rehabilitation, Stanford Hosp 1989; **Fac Appt:** Assoc Prof S, UMDNJ-NJ Med Sch, Newark

Seidman, Barry MD (U) - **Spec Exp:** Sexual Dysfunction; Incontinence; Genitourinary Cancer; **Hospital:** Overlook Hosp (page 88); **Address:** Atlantic Coast Urologic Implant Center, 107 Millburn Ave, Millburn, NJ 07041; **Phone:** 973-379-1523; **Board Cert:** Urology 2004; **Med School:** Mount Sinai Sch Med 1978; **Resid:** Urology, Mt Sinai 1983

Stock, Jeffrey A MD (U) - **Spec Exp:** Pediatric Urology; Robotic Surgery-Pediatric; Minimally Invasive Surgery-Pediatric; **Hospital:** Newark Beth Israel Med Ctr, Chldns Hosp NJ at Newark; **Address:** 101 Old Short Hills Rd, Ste 203, West Orange, NJ 07052-1023; **Phone:** 973-325-7188; **Board Cert:** Urology 1996; **Med School:** Mount Sinai Sch Med 1988; **Resid:** Surgery, UMDNJ- Univ Hosp 1990; Urology, UMDNJ - Univ Hosp 1993; **Fellow:** Pediatric Urology, UCSD Med Ctr 1994; **Fac Appt:** Assoc Clin Prof U, UMDNJ-NJ Med Sch, Newark

Strauss, Bernard MD (U) - **Spec Exp:** Kidney Stones; Prostate Disease; Sexual Dysfunction; **Hospital:** St Barnabas Med Ctr; **Address:** 741 Northfield Ave, Ste 206, W Orange, NJ 07052; **Phone:** 973-325-6100; **Board Cert:** Urology 1973; **Med School:** Albert Einstein Coll Med 1964; **Resid:** Surgery, Marquette Univ Affil Hosp 1966; **Fellow:** Urology, Bronx Municipal Hosp 1969; **Fac Appt:** Asst Clin Prof S, UMDNJ-NJ Med Sch, Newark

VASCULAR & INTERVENTIONAL RADIOLOGY

Bakal, Curtis MD (VIR) - **Hospital:** UMDNJ-Univ Hosp-Newark; **Address:** 150 Bergen, Ste C-318, Newark, NJ 07103; **Phone:** 973-972-5188; **Board Cert:** Public Health & Genl Preventive Med 1980; Diagnostic Radiology 1984; Vascular & Interventional Radiology 2003; **Med School:** Harvard Med Sch 1976; **Resid:** Public Health & Genl Preventive Med, NY Hlth Dept 1980; Radiology, Mass Genl Hosp 1984; **Fellow:** Vascular & Interventional Radiology, NY Med Coll 1985; **Fac Appt:** Prof Rad, Albert Einstein Coll Med

VASCULAR SURGERY

Brener, Bruce J MD (VascS) - **Spec Exp:** Endovascular Surgery; Minimally Invasive Vascular Surgery; Carotid Artery Surgery; **Hospital:** Newark Beth Israel Med Ctr, St Barnabas Med Ctr; **Address:** 200 South Orange Ave, Livingston, NJ 07039; **Phone:** 973-322-7233; **Board Cert:** Surgery 1972; Vascular Surgery 1993; **Med School:** Harvard Med Sch 1966; **Resid:** Surgery, Chldns Hosp Med Ctr 1968; Surgery, Peter Bent Brigham Hosp 1972; **Fellow:** Vascular Surgery, Mass Genl Hosp 1973; **Fac Appt:** Assoc Clin Prof S, Columbia P&S

Hobson II, Robert Wayne MD (VascS) - **Spec Exp:** Carotid Artery Surgery; **Hospital:** UMDNJ-Univ Hosp-Newark, St Clare's Hosp - Denville; **Address:** UMDNJ-New Jersey Med Sch, 30 Bergen St, Bldg 6, rm 620, Newark, NJ 07101; **Phone:** 973-972-6633; **Board Cert:** Surgery 1972; Vascular Surgery 2003; **Med School:** Geo Wash Univ 1963; **Resid:** Surgery, Walter Reed AMC 1971; **Fellow:** Vascular Surgery, Walter Reed AMC 1973; **Fac Appt:** Prof S, UMDNJ-NJ Med Sch, Newark

Jamil, Zafar MD (VascS) - **Spec Exp:** Endovascular Surgery; **Hospital:** Saint Michael's Med Ctr, St Clare's Hosp - Denville; **Address:** 306 Martin Luther King Jr Blvd, Newark, NJ 07102; **Phone:** 973-877-5059; **Board Cert:** Surgery 1998; Vascular Surgery 2001; **Med School:** Pakistan 1971; **Resid:** Surgery, UMDNJ Univ Hosp 1977; **Fellow:** Vascular Surgery, UMDNJ-NJ Med Sch 1978; **Fac Appt:** Clin Prof S, UMDNJ-NJ Med Sch, Newark

Padberg, Frank MD (VascS) - **Spec Exp:** Vein Disorders; Aneurysm-Abdominal Aortic; Carotid Artery Surgery; **Hospital:** UMDNJ-Univ Hosp-Newark, Saint Michael's Med Ctr; **Address:** 90 Bergen St, Ste 7200, Newark, NJ 07103-2425; **Phone:** 973-972-9371; **Board Cert:** Surgery 2000; Vascular Surgery 2005; **Med School:** Univ Ark 1973; **Resid:** Surgery, New England-Deaconess Hosp 1976; Vascular Surgery, Aberdeen Royal Infirm 1977; **Fellow:** Surgery, New England-Deaconess Hosp 1979; Peripheral Vascular Surgery, Lahey Clinic 1981; **Fac Appt:** Prof S, UMDNJ-NJ Med Sch, Newark

Hudson

Hudson

CARDIOVASCULAR DISEASE

Cruz, Merle Correa MD (Cv) - **Spec Exp:** Heart Disease; **Hospital:** Christ Hosp; **Address:** 201 St Paul Ave, Unit 1-D, Jersey City, NJ 07306; **Phone:** 201-653-7533; **Board Cert:** Internal Medicine 1983; Cardiovascular Disease 1985; **Med School:** Philippines 1976; **Resid:** Internal Medicine, Jersey City Med Ctr 1982; **Fellow:** Cardiovascular Disease, Brookdale Hosp Med Ctr 1984

Elkind, Barry M MD (Cv) - **Spec Exp:** Cardiac Catheterization; Cardiac Stress Testing; Preventive Cardiology; **Hospital:** Bayonne Med Ctr, Newark Beth Israel Med Ctr; **Address:** 654 Broadway, Bayonne, NJ 07002-4726; **Phone:** 201-243-9999; **Board Cert:** Internal Medicine 1979; Cardiovascular Disease 1981; **Med School:** UMDNJ-NJ Med Sch, Newark 1976; **Resid:** Internal Medicine, Boston City Hosp 1979; **Fellow:** Cardiovascular Disease, New England Med Ctr 1982

Moussa, Ghias MD (Cv) - **Spec Exp:** Heart Valve Disease; Congestive Heart Failure; **Hospital:** Greenville Hosp, Christ Hosp; **Address:** 1815 Kennedy Blvd, Jersey City, NJ 07305; **Phone:** 201-333-3311; **Board Cert:** Internal Medicine 1989; Cardiovascular Disease 1991; **Med School:** Syria 1979; **Resid:** Internal Medicine, Jersey City Med Ctr 1989; **Fellow:** Cardiovascular Disease, Jersey City Med Ctr 1991; **Fac Appt:** Assoc Prof Med, UMDNJ-NJ Med Sch, Newark

DERMATOLOGY

Beckett, MarieAnne G MD (D) - **Spec Exp:** Skin Diseases; **Hospital:** Meadowlands Hosp Med Ctr, St Mary's Hosp - Passaic; **Address:** 1 Harmon Plaza, Secaucus, NJ 07094-2925; **Phone:** 201-348-8911; **Board Cert:** Dermatology 1990; **Med School:** NY Med Coll 1986; **Resid:** Dermatology, NY Med Coll 1990

Blank, Ellen MD (D) - **Spec Exp:** Acne; **Hospital:** Mount Sinai Med Ctr (page 98), Bayonne Med Ctr; **Address:** 333 Avenue C, Bayonne, NJ 07002; **Phone:** 201-858-4800; **Board Cert:** Dermatology 1979; **Med School:** Mount Sinai Sch Med 1975; **Resid:** Dermatology, Mount Sinai Hosp 1979

Kopec, Anna V MD (D) - **Spec Exp:** Cosmetic Dermatology; Hair & Nail Disorders; **Hospital:** Bayonne Med Ctr; **Address:** 730 Kennedy Blvd, Bayonne, NJ 07002-1838; **Phone:** 201-858-4300; **Board Cert:** Dermatology 1980; **Med School:** UMDNJ-NJ Med Sch, Newark 1975; **Resid:** Dermatology, Albert Einstein 1979; **Fac Appt:** Assoc Clin Prof D, Albert Einstein Coll Med

DIAGNOSTIC RADIOLOGY

Byk, Cheryl MD (DR) - **Spec Exp:** Mammography; Nuclear Medicine; **Address:** 550 Summit Ave, Jersey City, NJ 07306; **Phone:** 201-656-5050; **Board Cert:** Diagnostic Radiology 1976; Nuclear Radiology 1977; **Med School:** UMDNJ-NJ Med Sch, Newark 1972; **Resid:** Diagnostic Radiology, St Vincent's Hosp 1976; **Fellow:** Nuclear Medicine, St Vincent's Hosp 1977; **Fac Appt:** Asst Clin Prof Rad, Mount Sinai Sch Med

ENDOCRINOLOGY, DIABETES & METABOLISM

Cam, Jenny Rose MD (EDM) - **Spec Exp:** Diabetes; Osteoporosis; Obesity; Adrenal Disorders; **Hospital:** Meadowlands Hosp Med Ctr, Christ Hosp; **Address:** 10 Huron Ave, Ste 1P, Jersey City, NJ 07306; **Phone:** 201-656-6003; **Board Cert:** Internal Medicine 1988; Endocrinology, Diabetes & Metabolism 1989; **Med School:** Philippines 1979; **Resid:** Internal Medicine, Interfaith Med Ctr 1987; **Fellow:** Endocrinology, Diabetes & Metabolism, UMDNJ-Univ Hosp 1989

FAMILY MEDICINE

Levine, Martin S DO (FMed) **PCP** - **Spec Exp:** Sports Medicine; Hypertension; Diabetes; **Hospital:** Christ Hosp, Bayonne Med Ctr; **Address:** 789 Avenue C, Bayonne, NJ 07002; **Phone:** 201-339-2620; **Board Cert:** Family Medicine 2005; **Med School:** Kirksville Coll Osteo Med 1980; **Resid:** Family Medicine, Kennedy Meml Hosp 1983; **Fac Appt:** Asst Clin Prof FMed, UMDNJ Sch Osteo Med

Sklower, Jay A DO (FMed) **PCP** - **Spec Exp:** Geriatric Medicine; Diabetes; Cholesterol/Lipid Disorders; **Hospital:** Christ Hosp, Jersey City Med Ctr; **Address:** 600 Pavonia Ave, 2nd Fl, Ste AB, Jersey City, NJ 07306-2929; **Phone:** 201-216-3040; **Board Cert:** Family Medicine 1998; **Med School:** Univ Hlth Sci, Coll Osteo Med 1971; **Resid:** Family Medicine, Union Meml Hosp

GASTROENTEROLOGY

Hahn, John C MD (Ge) - **Spec Exp:** Colonoscopy; Peptic Acid Disorders; **Hospital:** Bayonne Med Ctr; **Address:** 534 Avenue E, Ste 1C, Bayonne, NJ 07002; **Phone:** 201-823-0450; **Board Cert:** Internal Medicine 1988; Gastroenterology 2000; **Med School:** UMDNJ-NJ Med Sch, Newark 1985; **Resid:** Internal Medicine, Univ Hosp 1988; **Fellow:** Gastroenterology, Univ Hosp 1990

Prakash, Anaka MD (Ge) - **Spec Exp:** Gallbladder Disease; Colonoscopy; Peptic Ulcer Disease; Pancreatic/Biliary Endoscopy (ERCP); **Hospital:** Bayonne Med Ctr, Greenville Hosp; **Address:** 534 Ave E, Ste 1A, Bayonne, NJ 07002; **Phone:** 201-858-8444; **Board Cert:** Internal Medicine 1976; Gastroenterology 1977; **Med School:** India 1973; **Resid:** Internal Medicine, St Josephs Hosp 1975; **Fellow:** Gastroenterology, CMDNJ-Newark 1977

Spira, Robert S MD (Ge) - **Spec Exp:** Liver Disease; Inflammatory Bowel Disease; **Hospital:** Saint Michael's Med Ctr, Clara Maass Med Ctr; **Address:** 655 Kearny Ave, Ste 103, Kearny, NJ 07032; **Phone:** 201-955-6290; **Board Cert:** Internal Medicine 1978; Gastroenterology 1981; **Med School:** NYU Sch Med 1975; **Resid:** Internal Medicine, Bellevue Hosp/NYU Med Ctr 1978; **Fellow:** Gastroenterology, VA Med Ctr 1981

GERIATRIC MEDICINE

Brown, Mitchell Lee MD (Ger) **PCP** - **Spec Exp:** Alzheimer's Disease; **Hospital:** Bayonne Med Ctr; **Address:** 2 Joan Ree Terrace, Bayonne, NJ 07002; **Phone:** 201-339-2220; **Board Cert:** Internal Medicine 2000; Geriatric Medicine 2002; **Med School:** West Indies 1987; **Resid:** Internal Medicine, St Elizabeth Hosp 1990; **Fellow:** Geriatric Medicine, St Vincent's Hosp & Med Ctr 1992

Condo, Dominick MD (Ger) - **Hospital:** Bayonne Med Ctr; **Address:** 622 Broadway, Bayonne, NJ 07002; **Phone:** 201-436-2800; **Board Cert:** Internal Medicine 1984; Geriatric Medicine 1994; **Med School:** Mexico 1980; **Resid:** Internal Medicine, St Michael's Med Ctr 1984

Reisner, Michelle MD (Ger) **PCP** - **Hospital:** Jersey City Med Ctr; **Address:** 196 Jewitt Ave, Jersey City, NJ 07304; **Phone:** 201-332-3354; **Board Cert:** Internal Medicine 1989; Geriatric Medicine 1994; **Med School:** South Africa 1983; **Resid:** Internal Medicine, Jersey City Med Ctr 1989

GYNECOLOGIC ONCOLOGY

Sommers, Gara M MD (GO) - **Spec Exp:** Gynecologic Cancer; **Hospital:** St Mary Hosp - Hoboken, Christ Hosp; **Address:** 129 Washington St, Ste 100, Hoboken, NJ 07030; **Phone:** 201-792-9011; **Board Cert:** Obstetrics & Gynecology 2004; Gynecologic Oncology 2004; **Med School:** NYU Sch Med 1981; **Resid:** Obstetrics & Gynecology, NYU Med Ctr 1985; **Fellow:** Gynecologic Oncology, Barnes Jewish Hosp 1988; Research, Beckman Inst-City of Hope; **Fac Appt:** Asst Clin Prof ObG, Albert Einstein Coll Med

INTERNAL MEDICINE

Cardiello, Gary P MD (IM) PCP - **Spec Exp:** Diabetes; Hypertension; Hemochromatosis; **Hospital:** Clara Maass Med Ctr - West Hudson Div, Saint Michael's Med Ctr; **Address:** 744 Broadway, Bayonne, NJ 07002; **Phone:** 201-436-8888; **Board Cert:** Internal Medicine 1983; **Med School:** Italy 1983; **Resid:** Internal Medicine, St Michael's Med Ctr 1986

Mutterperl, Mitchell MD (IM) PCP - **Spec Exp:** Hypertension; Cholesterol/Lipid Disorders; Cardiovascular Disease; **Hospital:** Bayonne Med Ctr; **Address:** 19 W 33rd St, rm B2, Bayonne, NJ 07002-3916; **Phone:** 201-858-0090; **Board Cert:** Internal Medicine 1985; **Med School:** Italy 1981; **Resid:** Internal Medicine, UMDNJ-NJ Med Sch 1985

Wozniak, Deborah MD (IM) PCP - **Spec Exp:** Heart Failure; Diabetes; Osteoporosis; **Hospital:** Bayonne Med Ctr, St Mary Hosp - Hoboken; **Address:** 19 E 27th St, Bayonne, NJ 07002; **Phone:** 201-823-1066; **Board Cert:** Internal Medicine 1979; **Med School:** UMDNJ-NJ Med Sch, Newark 1976; **Resid:** Internal Medicine, St Joseph's Hosp & Med Ctr 1979

MEDICAL ONCOLOGY

Iyengar, Devarajan P MD (Onc) - **Spec Exp:** Breast Cancer; Colon & Rectal Cancer; **Hospital:** Bayonne Med Ctr; **Address:** 27 E 29th St, Bayonne, NJ 07002; **Phone:** 201-858-1211; **Board Cert:** Internal Medicine 1982; Medical Oncology 1985; **Med School:** India 1977; **Resid:** Internal Medicine, St Clare's Hosp 1980; **Fellow:** Medical Oncology, Univ Medicine & Dentistry 1982; Medical Oncology, Newark Beth Israel 1983

NEONATAL-PERINATAL MEDICINE

Aly, Sayed MD (NP) - **Hospital:** Bayonne Med Ctr; **Address:** 770 Kennedy Blvd, Bayonne, NJ 07002-2859; **Phone:** 201-823-3769; **Board Cert:** Pediatrics 1985; **Med School:** Egypt 1977; **Resid:** Pediatrics, Hahnemann; **Fellow:** Neonatal-Perinatal Medicine, Babies Hosp/Columbia Presby Med Ctr; **Fac Appt:** Asst Clin Prof Ped, Columbia P&S

NEUROLOGY

Anselmi, Gregory MD (N) - **Spec Exp:** Migraine; Multiple Sclerosis; **Hospital:** Bayonne Med Ctr, St Mary Hosp - Hoboken; **Address:** 1222 Kennedy Blvd, Bayonne, NJ 07002-3822; **Phone:** 201-339-6531; **Board Cert:** Neurology 2002; **Med School:** Italy 1988; **Resid:** Internal Medicine, SUNY/Univ Hosp 1989; **Fellow:** Neurology, St Vincent's Hosp & Med Ctr 1992

Sadeghi, Hooshang MD (N) - **Spec Exp:** Parkinson's Disease; Seizure Disorders; Botox for Facial Spasms/Dystonia; **Hospital:** Bayonne Med Ctr, Christ Hosp; **Address:** 631 Broadway, FL 3, Bayonne, NJ 07002-3846; **Phone:** 201-823-2888; **Board Cert:** Neurology 1977; **Med School:** Iran 1967; **Resid:** Neurology, UMDNJ Med Ctr 1975; **Fac Appt:** Asst Clin Prof N, UMDNJ-NJ Med Sch, Newark

OBSTETRICS & GYNECOLOGY

Banzon, Manuel MD (ObG) - **Spec Exp:** Laparoscopic Surgery; Vaginal Surgery; **Hospital:** Meadowlands Hosp Med Ctr, Hackensack Univ Med Ctr (page 92); **Address:** 714 10th St, Secaucus, NJ 07094; **Phone:** 201-864-4442; **Board Cert:** Obstetrics & Gynecology 1979; **Med School:** Philippines 1962; **Resid:** Obstetrics & Gynecology, Jersey City Med Ctr 1969

Kitzis, Hugo D MD (ObG) - **Spec Exp:** Gynecologic Surgery; Menopause Problems; **Hospital:** Hackensack Univ Med Ctr (page 92), Palisades Med Ctr; **Address:** 7400 Bergenline Ave, North Bergen, NJ 07047-5449; **Phone:** 201-869-5488; **Board Cert:** Obstetrics & Gynecology 1975; **Med School:** Argentina 1967; **Resid:** Surgery, St Francis Hosp 1971; Obstetrics & Gynecology, St Francis Hosp 1974

Masson, Lalitha MD (ObG) - **Hospital:** Christ Hosp; **Address:** 506 Washington St, Hoboken, NJ 07030; **Phone:** 201-963-8554; **Board Cert:** Obstetrics & Gynecology 1973; **Med School:** India 1964; **Resid:** Margaret Hogue Hosp 1969St Clares Hosp 1970; **Fellow:** Infertility, UMDNJ-NJ Sch Med 1971

Uy, Vena MD (ObG) `PCP` - **Hospital:** Christ Hosp, Meadowlands Hosp Med Ctr; **Address:** 142 Palisade Ave, Ste 102, Jersey City, NJ 07306; **Phone:** 201-653-0506; **Board Cert:** Obstetrics & Gynecology 1977; **Med School:** Philippines 1968; **Resid:** Obstetrics & Gynecology, UMDNJ-NJ Hosp 1973; **Fellow:** Gynecologic Pathology, Magee Woman's Hosp 1974

OPHTHALMOLOGY

Constad, William H MD (Oph) - **Spec Exp:** Cornea Transplant; Cataract Surgery; Refractive Surgery; **Hospital:** Jersey City Med Ctr, UMDNJ-Univ Hosp-Newark; **Address:** 600 Pavonia Ave Fl 6, Jersey City, NJ 07306; **Phone:** 201-963-3937; **Board Cert:** Ophthalmology 1985; **Med School:** Med Coll PA Hahnemann 1980; **Resid:** Ophthalmology, UMDNJ Univ Hosp 1984; **Fellow:** Cornea, NY Eye & Ear Infirm 1985; **Fac Appt:** Clin Prof Oph, UMDNJ-NJ Med Sch, Newark

Tchorbajian, Kirk MD (Oph) - **Spec Exp:** Cataract Surgery; **Hospital:** St Mary Hosp - Hoboken, Union Hosp - NJ; **Address:** 1 McWilliams Pl, Jersey City, NJ 07302-1609; **Phone:** 201-795-0808; **Board Cert:** Ophthalmology 1991; **Med School:** France 1981; **Resid:** Ophthalmology, UMDNJ 1985; Surgery, St Clares 1992; **Fellow:** Ophthalmology, UMDNJ 1986

ORTHOPAEDIC SURGERY

Granatir, Charles MD (OrS) - **Hospital:** Clara Maass Med Ctr - West Hudson Div; **Address:** 586 Kearny Ave, Kearny, NJ 07032; **Phone:** 201-997-7667; **Board Cert:** Orthopaedic Surgery 1989; **Med School:** Hahnemann Univ 1979; **Resid:** Orthopaedic Surgery, Montefiore Hosp Med Ctr 1984

Irving III, Henry C MD (OrS) - **Spec Exp:** Joint Replacement; Sports Medicine; **Hospital:** Jersey City Med Ctr, Christ Hosp; **Address:** 600 Pavonia Ave Fl 7, Jersey City, NJ 07306-2929; **Phone:** 201-216-9300; **Board Cert:** Orthopaedic Surgery 1980; **Med School:** Meharry Med Coll 1972; **Resid:** Orthopaedic Surgery, UMDNJ-Univ Hosp 1977

OTOLARYNGOLOGY

Laskey, Richard S MD (Oto) - **Spec Exp:** Liposuction; **Hospital:** St Mary Hosp - Hoboken, Christ Hosp; **Address:** 331 Grand St Fl Ground, Hoboken, NJ 07030; **Phone:** 201-795-5103; **Board Cert:** Otolaryngology 1984; **Med School:** Albert Einstein Coll Med 1979; **Resid:** Otolaryngology, NYU Med Ctr 1983; Plastic Surgery, Boston Univ Med Ctr 1986

PEDIATRICS

Bonforte, Richard J MD (Ped) - **Spec Exp:** Cystic Fibrosis; Asthma; Infections-Respiratory; **Hospital:** Jersey City Med Ctr, Mount Sinai Med Ctr (page 98); **Address:** Chldns Hosp of Hudson Co @ Jersey City Med Ctr, 355 Grand St, Jersey City, NJ 07032; **Phone:** 201-915-2456; **Board Cert:** Pediatrics 1970; **Med School:** Georgetown Univ 1965; **Resid:** Pediatrics, Mt Sinai Hosp 1968; **Fellow:** Infectious Disease, Mt Sinai Hosp 1972; **Fac Appt:** Prof Ped, Mount Sinai Sch Med

Skripkus, Aldona MD (Ped) **PCP** - **Hospital:** Clara Maass Med Ctr; **Address:** 381 Kearny Ave, Kearny, NJ 07032; **Phone:** 201-991-4824; **Board Cert:** Pediatrics 1971; **Med School:** Med Coll PA Hahnemann 1966; **Resid:** Pediatrics, Childrens Hosp 1969

PHYSICAL MEDICINE & REHABILITATION

Filippone, Mark A MD (PMR) - **Spec Exp:** Electrodiagnosis; **Hospital:** Christ Hosp, St Mary Hosp - Hoboken; **Address:** 2012 John F Kennedy Blvd, Jersey City, NJ 07305-1526; **Phone:** 201-332-6855; **Board Cert:** Physical Medicine & Rehabilitation 1980; **Med School:** Georgetown Univ 1974; **Resid:** Pediatrics, St Vincent's Hosp & Med Ctr 1976; Physical Medicine & Rehabilitation, Bronx Muni Hosp-Einstein 1978; **Fac Appt:** Asst Clin Prof PMR, Albert Einstein Coll Med

PSYCHIATRY

Gewolb, Eric B MD (Psyc) - **Spec Exp:** Anxiety Disorders; Dementia; Bipolar/Mood Disorders; **Hospital:** Bayonne Med Ctr; **Address:** 830 Kennedy Blvd, Bayonne, NJ 07002-2872; **Phone:** 201-339-0200; **Board Cert:** Psychiatry 1979; **Med School:** Tulane Univ 1974; **Resid:** Psychiatry, Mount Sinai Hosp 1978

Jacoby, Jacob H MD/PhD (Psyc) - **Spec Exp:** Psychopharmacology; Mood Disorders; Addiction Psychiatry; **Hospital:** Bayonne Med Ctr, St Barnabas Med Ctr; **Address:** 654 Avenue C, Ste 201, Bayonne, NJ 07002-3899; **Phone:** 201-339-0323; **Board Cert:** Psychiatry 1993; Addiction Psychiatry 1993; **Med School:** SUNY Buffalo 1980; **Resid:** Psychiatry, U of Pittsburgh 1981; Psychiatry, Western Psychiatric Institute 1983; **Fellow:** Addiction Psychiatry, Albert Einstein; **Fac Appt:** Assoc Clin Prof Psyc, UMDNJ-NJ Med Sch, Newark

Kurani, Devendra MD (Psyc) - **Spec Exp:** Depression; Anxiety Disorders; Panic Disorder; **Hospital:** St Barnabas Med Ctr, Christ Hosp; **Address:** 221 Palisade Ave, FL 2, Jersey City, NJ 07306-1110; **Phone:** 201-656-3116; **Board Cert:** Psychiatry 1986; **Med School:** Burma 1976; **Resid:** Psychiatry, Warley Hosp 1982; Psychiatry, Harlem Hosp 1983

Moraille, Pascale MD (Psyc) - **Spec Exp:** Autism; Developmental Disorders; ADD/ADHD; **Hospital:** St Mary Hosp - Hoboken; **Address:** 506 3rd St, Hoboken, NJ 07030; **Phone:** 201-792-8200; **Board Cert:** Psychiatry 1993; Child & Adolescent Psychiatry 1995; **Med School:** Ponce Med Sch 1988; **Resid:** Psychiatry, UMDNJ-NJ Med Sch 1991; **Fellow:** Child & Adolescent Psychiatry, UMDNJ-NJ Med Sch 1993

PULMONARY DISEASE

Elamir, Mazhar MD (Pul) - **Spec Exp:** Sleep Disorders; Allergy; Asthma; **Hospital:** Christ Hosp, Greenville Hosp; **Address:** 192 Harrison Ave, Jersey City, NJ 07304; **Phone:** 201-333-5363; **Board Cert:** Internal Medicine 1987; Pulmonary Disease 1994; **Med School:** Egypt 1981; **Resid:** Internal Medicine, Jersey City Med Ctr 1987; **Fellow:** Pulmonary Disease, Interfaith Med Ctr 1991

RHEUMATOLOGY

Lahita, Robert G MD (Rhu) - **Spec Exp:** Lupus/SLE; Endocrinology & Joint Disorders; Immunodeficiency Disorders; **Hospital:** Jersey City Med Ctr, St Vincent Cath Med Ctrs - Manhattan (page 375); **Address:** 610 Washington Blvd, Jersey City, NJ 07310; **Phone:** 201-222-1266; **Board Cert:** Internal Medicine 2004; Rheumatology 1997; **Med School:** Jefferson Med Coll 1973; **Resid:** Internal Medicine, New York Hosp-Cornell 1976; **Fellow:** Rheumatology, Rockefeller Hosp 1978; **Fac Appt:** Prof Med, Mount Sinai Sch Med

Scarpa, Nicholas P MD (Rhu) - **Spec Exp:** Lupus/SLE; Rheumatoid Arthritis; Osteoporosis; **Hospital:** Christ Hosp, NY-Presby Hosp (page 100); **Address:** 600 Pavonia Ave Fl 5 - Ste 1, Jersey City, NJ 07306-2923; **Phone:** 201-216-3050; **Board Cert:** Internal Medicine 1983; Rheumatology 1986; **Med School:** UMDNJ-NJ Med Sch, Newark 1980; **Resid:** Internal Medicine, Hackensack Univ Med Ctr 1983; **Fellow:** Rheumatology, New York Hosp-Cornell Med Ctr 1985; **Fac Appt:** Asst Clin Prof Med, UMDNJ-NJ Med Sch, Newark

SURGERY

Di Giacomo, Jody C MD (S) - **Spec Exp:** Trauma; Critical Care; Wound Healing/Care; **Hospital:** Jersey City Med Ctr; **Address:** Jersey City Med Ctr, Dept Surgery/Trauma, 355 Grand St, Jersey City, NJ 07302; **Phone:** 201-915-2197; **Board Cert:** Surgery 2004; Surgical Critical Care 1996; Undersea & Hyperbaric Medicine 2004; **Med School:** Temple Univ 1986; **Resid:** Surgery, St Francis Med Ctr 1992; **Fellow:** Surgical Critical Care, Hosp U Penn 1994

Gildengers, Jaime MD (S) - **Spec Exp:** Gallbladder Surgery; Colon Surgery; Breast Surgery; **Hospital:** Palisades Med Ctr, Christ Hosp; **Address:** 313 60th St, West New York, NJ 07093; **Phone:** 201-854-0406; **Board Cert:** Surgery 1995; **Med School:** Argentina 1965; **Resid:** Surgery, Mt Sinai Med Ctr 1970; Surgery, St Clares Hosp 1973; **Fellow:** Surgical Research, St Clares Hosp 1974; **Fac Appt:** Asst Clin Prof S, UMDNJ-NJ Med Sch, Newark

McGovern Jr, Patrick Joseph MD (S) - **Spec Exp:** Vascular Surgery; Gallbladder Surgery; Carotid Artery Surgery; **Hospital:** Bayonne Med Ctr, Christ Hosp; **Address:** 631 Broadway, Bayonne, NJ 07002; **Phone:** 201-858-5705; **Board Cert:** Surgery 1993; Vascular Surgery 1998; **Med School:** UMDNJ-NJ Med Sch, Newark 1978; **Resid:** Surgery, UMDNJ-Univ Hosp 1983; **Fellow:** Vascular Surgery, UMDNJ-RWJ Univ Hosp 1984

Popovich, Joseph F MD (S) - **Spec Exp:** Vascular Surgery; **Hospital:** Christ Hosp, Meadowlands Hosp Med Ctr; **Address:** 679 Montgomery St, Jersey City, NJ 07304; **Phone:** 201-209-9110; **Board Cert:** Surgery 1994; **Med School:** UMDNJ-RW Johnson Med Sch 1987; **Resid:** Med Ctr Hosp 1993Univ of Medicine & Dentistry 1991; **Fellow:** St Francis Hosp 1988

Sultan, Ronald H MD (S) - **Spec Exp:** Hernia; **Hospital:** Christ Hosp; **Address:** 2255 John F Kennedy Blvd, Jersey City, NJ 07304-1428; **Phone:** 201-434-3305; **Board Cert:** Surgery 1999; **Med School:** NYU Sch Med 1973; **Resid:** Surgery, Bronx Muni Hosps 1977; Surgery, Albert Einstein Med Ctr 1980

UROLOGY

Di Bella Jr, Louis J MD (U) - **Spec Exp:** Prostate Surgery; Kidney Stones; Laparoscopic Surgery; **Hospital:** Meadowlands Hosp Med Ctr, Palisades Med Ctr; **Address:** 110B Meadowlands Pkwy, Ste 302, Secaucus, NJ 07094; **Phone:** 201-867-1297; **Board Cert:** Urology 1980; **Med School:** UMDNJ-NJ Med Sch, Newark 1972; **Resid:** Urology, Martland Med Ctr 1976

Katz, Herbert I MD (U) - **Spec Exp:** Urologic Cancer; Erectile Dysfunction; Kidney Stones; **Hospital:** Bayonne Med Ctr; **Address:** 534 Ave E, Ste 2A, Bayonne, NJ 07002; **Phone:** 201-823-1303; **Board Cert:** Urology 1981; **Med School:** Temple Univ 1974; **Resid:** Surgery, Abington Meml Hosp 1976; Urology, Monterfiore-Weiler Einstein Med Ctr 1979

Lehrhoff, Bernard MD (U) - **Spec Exp:** Prostate Cancer; Kidney Stones; Sexual Dysfunction; **Hospital:** Overlook Hosp (page 88), St Barnabas Med Ctr; **Address:** 659 Kearny Ave, Kearny, NJ 07032; **Phone:** 908-654-5100; **Board Cert:** Urology 1984; **Med School:** UMDNJ-NJ Med Sch, Newark 1976; **Resid:** Urology, Bellevue Hosp 1982; **Fac Appt:** Asst Clin Prof U, Columbia P&S

Shulman, Yale MD (U) - **Spec Exp:** Urologic Cancer; Kidney Stones; Sexual Dysfunction; **Hospital:** Christ Hosp, Bayonne Med Ctr; **Address:** 2255 Kennedy Blvd, Jersey City, NJ 07304-1428; **Phone:** 201-433-1057; **Board Cert:** Urology 1984; **Med School:** Albert Einstein Coll Med 1976; **Resid:** Surgery, Montefiore Hosp Med Ctr 1978; Urology, NYU Med Ctr 1982; **Fac Appt:** Assoc Clin Prof U, NYU Sch Med

Steigman, Elliott G MD (U) - **Spec Exp:** Kidney Stones; Prostate Benign Disease; **Hospital:** Christ Hosp; **Address:** 142 Palisade Ave, Ste 211, Jersey City, NJ 07306-1108; **Phone:** 201-435-2244; **Board Cert:** Urology 1982; **Med School:** SUNY Downstate 1975; **Resid:** Surgery, Brookdale Hosp Med Ctr 1977; Urology, SUNY Downstate Med Ctr 1980

Mercer

Mercer

ALLERGY & IMMUNOLOGY

Ricketti, Anthony J MD (A&I) - **Spec Exp:** Asthma in Pregnancy; Allergic Aspergillosis; Eosinophilic Lung Disorders; **Hospital:** St Francis Med Ctr - Trenton, Robert Wood Johnson Univ Hosp Hamilton (page 853); **Address:** Allergy & Pulmonary Assoc, 1542 Kuser Rd, Ste B7, Trenton, NJ 08619-3829; **Phone:** 609-581-1400; **Board Cert:** Internal Medicine 1981; Allergy & Immunology 1983; Pulmonary Disease 1986; Critical Care Medicine 1999; **Med School:** Hahnemann Univ 1978; **Resid:** Internal Medicine, Cleveland Clin Fdn 1981; Allergy & Immunology, Northwestern Univ 1983; **Fellow:** Pulmonary Disease, Northwestern Univ 1984; **Fac Appt:** Asst Clin Prof Med, UMDNJ-RW Johnson Med Sch

Winant, John MD (A&I) - **Spec Exp:** Asthma; **Hospital:** Univ Med Ctr - Princeton, Capital Hlth Sys - Mercer Campus; **Address:** 8 Quakerbridge Plaza, Mercerville, NJ 08619-1255; **Phone:** 609-890-8782; **Board Cert:** Pediatrics 1980; Allergy & Immunology 1987; **Med School:** Univ Cincinnati 1975; **Resid:** Pediatrics, Chldns Hosp Med Ctr 1978; **Fellow:** Allergy & Immunology, Chldns Hosp Med Ctr 1980

CARDIOVASCULAR DISEASE

Costin, Andrew MD (Cv) - **Hospital:** Univ Med Ctr - Princeton; **Address:** 419 N Harrison St, Princeton, NJ 08540; **Phone:** 609-924-9300; **Board Cert:** Internal Medicine 1989; Cardiovascular Disease 2003; **Med School:** Yale Univ 1986; **Resid:** Internal Medicine, New York Hosp 1989; **Fellow:** Cardiovascular Disease, Hosp Univ Penn 1993

George, Abraham MD (Cv) - **Hospital:** Capital Hlth Sys - Mercer Campus; **Address:** 416 Bellevue Ave, Ste 301, Trenton, NJ 08618; **Phone:** 609-394-9699; **Board Cert:** Internal Medicine 1981; Cardiovascular Disease 1983; **Med School:** India 1973; **Resid:** Surgery, French Hosp 1977; Internal Medicine, St Francis Med Ctr 1980; **Fellow:** Cardiovascular Disease, Univ Louisville Sch Med 1982

Hagaman, John MD (Cv) - **Spec Exp:** Heart Failure; **Hospital:** Univ Med Ctr - Princeton; **Address:** 281 Witherspoon St, Ste 210, Princeton, NJ 08540-3210; **Phone:** 609-921-7456; **Board Cert:** Internal Medicine 1977; Cardiovascular Disease 1981; **Med School:** Columbia P&S 1974; **Resid:** Internal Medicine, Univ Mich Hosp 1977; **Fellow:** Cardiovascular Disease, NC Meml Hosp 1980; **Fac Appt:** Asst Clin Prof Med, Robert W Johnson Med Sch

Samuel, Steven MD (Cv) - **Spec Exp:** Congestive Heart Failure; Heart Disease in Women; **Hospital:** St Francis Med Ctr - Trenton, Robert Wood Johnson Univ Hosp Hamilton (page 853); **Address:** Trenton Cardiology Consultants, 1235 Whitehorse Mercerville Rd C Bldg - Ste 317, Mercerville, NJ 08619-3826; **Phone:** 609-585-2040; **Board Cert:** Internal Medicine 1982; Cardiovascular Disease 1985; **Med School:** Albert Einstein Coll Med 1978; **Resid:** Family Medicine, Southside Hosp 1979; Internal Medicine, Univ Hosp SUNY 1982; **Fellow:** Cardiovascular Disease, Univ Hosp SUNY 1984

COLON & RECTAL SURGERY

Hardy III, Howard MD (CRS) - **Hospital:** St Francis Med Ctr - Trenton, Capital Hlth Sys - Mercer Campus; **Address:** 3131 Princeton Pike 3C Bldg - Ste 201, Lawrenceville, NJ 08648-2201; **Phone:** 609-896-1700; **Board Cert:** Colon & Rectal Surgery 1991; **Med School:** Columbia P&S 1980; **Resid:** Surgery, St Luke's Roosevelt Hosp Ctr 1985; **Fellow:** Colon & Rectal Surgery, Univ Tex Med Ctr 1986

DERMATOLOGY

Bagel, Jerry MD (D) - **Spec Exp:** Psoriasis; Atopic Dermatitis; **Hospital:** Univ Med Ctr - Princeton; **Address:** 59 One Mile Rd, Ste G, East Windsor, NJ 08520-2505; **Phone:** 609-443-4500; **Board Cert:** Dermatology 1985; **Med School:** Mount Sinai Sch Med 1981; **Resid:** Dermatology, Columbia-Presby Med Ctr 1985; **Fac Appt:** Asst Clin Prof D, Columbia P&S

Kazenoff, Steven MD (D) - **Spec Exp:** Skin Cancer; Hair & Nail Disorders; Skin Diseases; Hair Restoration/Transplant; **Hospital:** Univ Med Ctr - Princeton; **Address:** 419 N Harrison St, Princeton, NJ 08540-3594; **Phone:** 609-924-9300; **Board Cert:** Internal Medicine 1982; Dermatology 1985; **Med School:** Jefferson Med Coll 1979; **Resid:** Internal Medicine, SUNY Stony Brook Hosp 1982; Dermatology, CWRU Univ Hosp 1985; **Fac Appt:** Asst Clin Prof D, UMDNJ-RW Johnson Med Sch

Notterman, Robyn MD (D) - **Hospital:** Univ Med Ctr - Princeton; **Address:** 601 Ewing St, Ste 13, Princeton, NJ 08540; **Phone:** 609-924-1033; **Board Cert:** Dermatology 1994; **Med School:** Cornell Univ-Weill Med Coll 1983; **Resid:** Dermatology, NYU Med Ctr 1992

Vine, John MD (D) - **Spec Exp:** Mohs' Surgery; Cosmetic Dermatology; Hypohidrosis/Axillary Liposuction; **Hospital:** Univ Med Ctr - Princeton; **Address:** 253 Witherspoon St, Ste L, Princeton, NJ 08540; **Phone:** 609-683-0101; **Board Cert:** Dermatology 1996; **Med School:** Brown Univ 1992; **Resid:** Dermatology, Univ Tex MD Anderson Cancer Ctr 1996; **Fellow:** Mohs Surgery, Scripps Clinic 1997

DIAGNOSTIC RADIOLOGY

Compito, Gerard MD (DR) - **Hospital:** Univ Med Ctr - Princeton; **Address:** 419 N Harrison St, Ste G, Princeton, NJ 08540-3521; **Phone:** 609-921-3345; **Board Cert:** Diagnostic Radiology 1990; Neuroradiology 1995; **Med School:** SUNY Upstate Med Univ 1985; **Resid:** Diagnostic Radiology, NY Hosp-Cornell 1990; **Fellow:** Neuroradiology, NY Hosp-Cornell 1992

Ford, Robert R MD (DR) - **Spec Exp:** CT Scan; MRI; Nuclear Medicine; Ultrasound; **Hospital:** Univ Med Ctr - Princeton; **Address:** Radpharm, 103 Carnegie Center, Ste 200, Princeton, NJ 08540; **Phone:** 609-936-2604; **Board Cert:** Diagnostic Radiology 1988; Neuroradiology 1996; **Med School:** Rutgers Univ 1983; **Resid:** Internal Medicine, R W Johnson Univ Hosp 1985; Diagnostic Radiology, NY Hosp-Cornell 1988

Namm, Joel MD (DR) - **Hospital:** St Francis Med Ctr - Trenton, St Mary Med Ctr; **Address:** 1255 Whitehorse Mercerville Rd, Radiology Affiliates of Central NJ, Hamilton Township, NJ 08619-3813; **Phone:** 609-585-8800; **Board Cert:** Radiology 1971; **Med School:** SUNY Downstate 1966; **Resid:** Radiology, Downstate Med Ctr 1970; **Fellow:** Radiology, Yale-New Haven Hosp 1971; **Fac Appt:** Asst Prof Rad, Yale Univ

ENDOCRINOLOGY, DIABETES & METABOLISM

Kennedy, John W MD (EDM) - **Spec Exp:** Diabetes; Thyroid Disorders; Osteoporosis; **Hospital:** Robert Wood Johnson Univ Hosp Hamilton (page 853), Univ Med Ctr - Princeton; **Address:** Diabetes & Endocrinology Assoc, 1235 Whitehorse Mercerville Rd, Ste 301, Hamilton, NJ 08619; **Phone:** 609-581-7725; **Board Cert:** Internal Medicine 1995; Endocrinology, Diabetes & Metabolism 1997; **Med School:** Jefferson Med Coll 1992; **Resid:** Internal Medicine, Thomas Jefferson Univ Hosp 1995; **Fellow:** Endocrinology, Deaconess Hosp/Joslin Diabetes Ctr 1996; **Fac Appt:** Asst Clin Prof Med, UMDNJ-RW Johnson Med Sch

FAMILY MEDICINE

Rednor, Jeffrey DO (FMed) `PCP` - **Spec Exp:** Diabetes; Pain-Back; Cardiology; **Hospital:** Robert Wood Johnson Univ Hosp Hamilton (page 853); **Address:** 1 Washington Blvd, Ste A, Robbinsville, NJ 08691-3119; **Phone:** 609-448-4353; **Board Cert:** Family Medicine 1992; **Med School:** UMDNJ Sch Osteo Med 1989; **Resid:** Family Medicine, Kennedy Mem Hosp 1992

GASTROENTEROLOGY

Afridi, Shariq MD (Ge) - **Spec Exp:** Liver Disease; **Hospital:** Robert Wood Johnson Univ Hosp Hamilton (page 853), St Francis Med Ctr - Trenton; **Address:** 2107 Klockner Rd Bldg 6, Trenton, NJ 08690-3403; **Phone:** 609-586-1319; **Board Cert:** Internal Medicine 2002; Gastroenterology 2003; **Med School:** Pakistan 1986; **Resid:** Internal Medicine, Bridgeport Hosp 1991; **Fellow:** Gastroenterology, Bridgeport Hosp 1993

De Antonio, Joseph MD (Ge) - **Spec Exp:** Liver Disease; **Hospital:** Capital Health Sys - Fuld Campus; **Address:** 2999 Princeton Pike, Lawrenceville, NJ 08648; **Phone:** 609-882-2185; **Board Cert:** Internal Medicine 1989; Gastroenterology 2004; **Med School:** St Louis Univ 1982; **Resid:** Internal Medicine, Vet Affairs Med Ctr 1989; **Fellow:** Gastroenterology, Bellevue Hosp Ctr 1991

Fidanzato, Michael MD (Ge) - **Spec Exp:** Colon Cancer Screening; Gastroesophageal Reflux Disease (GERD); Irritable Bowel Syndrome; Hepatitis; **Hospital:** Univ Med Ctr - Princeton; **Address:** 601 Ewing St, Ste C-7, Princeton, NJ 08540; **Phone:** 609-921-7620; **Board Cert:** Internal Medicine 1985; Gastroenterology 1991; **Med School:** NY Med Coll 1982; **Resid:** Internal Medicine, St Vincent's Hosp & Med Ctr 1985; **Fellow:** Gastroenterology, St Vincent's Hosp & Med Ctr 1987

Iqbal, Riaz MD (Ge) - **Hospital:** Robert Wood Johnson Univ Hosp Hamilton (page 853); **Address:** 2105 Klockner Rd Bldg 6, Hamilton, NJ 08690-3403; **Phone:** 609-586-1319; **Board Cert:** Internal Medicine 1977; Gastroenterology 1979; **Med School:** Pakistan 1966; **Resid:** Internal Medicine, NJ Med Sch 1971; **Fellow:** Gastroenterology, NJ Med Sch 1973; **Fac Appt:** Asst Clin Prof FMed, UMDNJ-NJ Med Sch, Newark

Marin, Geobel MD (Ge) - **Spec Exp:** Peptic Ulcer Disease; Colonoscopy; Inflammatory Bowel Disease; **Hospital:** Capital Hlth Sys - Mercer Campus; **Address:** 416 Bellevue Ave, Ste 101, Trenton, NJ 08618; **Phone:** 609-394-8844; **Board Cert:** Internal Medicine 1969; Gastroenterology 1972; **Med School:** Columbia P&S 1962; **Resid:** Internal Medicine, Philadelphia Genl Hosp 1966; **Fellow:** Gastroenterology, Philadelphia Genl Hosp 1968

Meirowitz, Robert MD (Ge) - **Spec Exp:** Inflammatory Bowel Disease; Colon Polyps & Cancer; Colonoscopy; **Hospital:** Univ Med Ctr - Princeton; **Address:** 281 Witherspoon St, Ste 230, Princeton, NJ 08540-3210; **Phone:** 609-924-1422; **Board Cert:** Internal Medicine 1987; Gastroenterology 2001; **Med School:** NY Med Coll 1984; **Resid:** Internal Medicine, UMDNJ-RW Johnson Univ Hosp 1988; **Fellow:** Gastroenterology, Univ Maryland 1990; **Fac Appt:** Asst Clin Prof Med, Robert W Johnson Med Sch

Rosner, Bruce MD (Ge) - **Spec Exp:** Liver Disease; Gastroesophageal Reflux Disease (GERD); Colon Cancer; **Hospital:** St Francis Med Ctr - Trenton; **Address:** 2275 Whitehorse Mercerville Rd Bldg 2, Trenton, NJ 08619-2643; **Phone:** 609-890-0200; **Board Cert:** Internal Medicine 1979; Gastroenterology 1983; **Med School:** Univ Pennsylvania 1976; **Resid:** Internal Medicine, Penn Hosp 1979; **Fellow:** Gastroenterology, Hahnemann Univ 1981

Rubin, Marc R MD (Ge) - **Hospital:** St Francis Med Ctr - Trenton; **Address:** Gastroenterology Associates, 2275 Whitehorse Mercerville Rd, Ste 2, Trenton, NJ 08619-2643; **Phone:** 609-890-0200; **Board Cert:** Internal Medicine 1977; Gastroenterology 1979; **Med School:** Albert Einstein Coll Med 1974; **Resid:** Internal Medicine, Penn Hosp 1977; **Fellow:** Gastroenterology, Univ Hosp 1979

Sachs, Jonathan R MD (Ge) - **Spec Exp:** Colon Cancer Screening; Gastroesophageal Reflux Disease (GERD); Inflammatory Bowel Disease; **Hospital:** Univ Med Ctr - Princeton; **Address:** 281 Witherspoon St, Ste 230, Princeton, NJ 08542-3210; **Phone:** 609-924-1422; **Board Cert:** Internal Medicine 1987; Gastroenterology 1989; **Med School:** Med Coll PA Hahnemann 1984; **Resid:** Internal Medicine, Temple Univ Hosp 1987; **Fellow:** Gastroenterology, Graduate Hosp 1987

HAND SURGERY

Ark, Jon Wong Tze-Jen MD (HS) - **Spec Exp:** Hand Surgery; Carpal Tunnel Syndrome; Foot & Ankle Surgery; Arthritis Hand Surgery; **Hospital:** Univ Med Ctr - Princeton; **Address:** 325 Princeton Ave, Princeton, NJ 08540-1617; **Phone:** 609-924-8131; **Board Cert:** Orthopaedic Surgery 1996; Hand Surgery 1997; **Med School:** UMDNJ-RW Johnson Med Sch 1987; **Resid:** Orthopaedic Surgery, Columbia-Presby Med Ctr 1992; **Fellow:** Hand Surgery, Mass Genl Hosp 1993; Foot/Ankle Surgery, Jefferson Hosp 1995

INFECTIOUS DISEASE

Aufiero, Patrick MD (Inf) - **Hospital:** Robert Wood Johnson Univ Hosp Hamilton (page 853), Capital Hlth Sys - Mercer Campus; **Address:** 2085 Klockner Rd, Hamilton, NJ 08690; **Phone:** 609-587-4122; **Board Cert:** Internal Medicine 1995; Infectious Disease 1996; **Med School:** West Indies 1984; **Resid:** Internal Medicine, St Michael's Med Ctr 1989; **Fellow:** Infectious Disease, St Michael's Med Ctr 1991

Gekowski, Kathleen MD (Inf) - **Spec Exp:** Travel Medicine; AIDS/HIV; Lyme Disease; **Hospital:** Capital Hlth Sys - Mercer Campus, Robert Wood Johnson Univ Hosp Hamilton (page 853); **Address:** 408 Bellevue Ave, Trenton, NJ 08618-4502; **Phone:** 609-392-1988; **Board Cert:** Internal Medicine 1979; Infectious Disease 1984; **Med School:** Hahnemann Univ 1976; **Resid:** Internal Medicine, Univ Illinois Hosp 1979; **Fellow:** Infectious Disease, Yale Univ 1982; **Fac Appt:** Assoc Clin Prof Med, UMDNJ-RW Johnson Med Sch

Nahass, Ronald MD (Inf) - **Spec Exp:** Hepatitis; **Hospital:** Robert Wood Johnson Univ Hosp - New Brunswick (page 853), Univ Med Ctr - Princeton; **Address:** 411 Courtyard Drive, Hillsborough, NJ 08844; **Phone:** 908-725-2522; **Board Cert:** Internal Medicine 1985; Infectious Disease 1988; **Med School:** UMDNJ-RW Johnson Med Sch 1982; **Resid:** Internal Medicine, RWJ Univ Hosp 1985; **Fellow:** Infectious Disease, RWJ Univ Hosp 1988; **Fac Appt:** Clin Prof Med, UMDNJ-RW Johnson Med Sch

Porwancher, Richard MD (Inf) - **Spec Exp:** Lyme Disease; AIDS/HIV; Bioterrorism Preparedness; **Hospital:** St Francis Med Ctr - Trenton, Robert Wood Johnson Univ Hosp Hamilton (page 853); **Address:** 1245 Whitehorse-Mercerville Rd, Ste 411, Mercerville, NJ 08619-3831; **Phone:** 609-581-2000; **Board Cert:** Internal Medicine 1980; Infectious Disease 1982; **Med School:** Northwestern Univ 1977; **Resid:** Internal Medicine, Med Coll Wisconsin Affil Hosps 1980; **Fellow:** Infectious Disease, VA Med Ctr 1982; **Fac Appt:** Assoc Clin Prof Med, Robert W Johnson Med Sch

INTERNAL MEDICINE

Lancefield, Margaret MD (IM) PCP - **Hospital:** Univ Med Ctr - Princeton; **Address:** Princeton Healthcare Med Assocs, 253 Witherspoon St, Lambert House FL 2, Princeton, NJ 08540-3211; **Phone:** 609-497-4301; **Board Cert:** Internal Medicine 1987; **Med School:** Yale Univ 1984; **Resid:** Internal Medicine, Hosp Univ Penn 1987; **Fac Appt:** Assoc Clin Prof Med, UMDNJ-RW Johnson Med Sch

Levenberg, Steven MD (IM) - **Hospital:** St Francis Med Ctr - Trenton; **Address:** 667 Chambers St, Trenton, NJ 08611-3701; **Phone:** 609-393-4656; **Board Cert:** Internal Medicine 1982; **Med School:** Jefferson Med Coll 1979; **Resid:** Internal Medicine, Thomas Jefferson Univ Hosp 1982; **Fac Appt:** Asst Clin Prof Med, UMDNJ-RW Johnson Med Sch

Schaeffer, Mark A MD (IM) - **Hospital:** Univ Med Ctr - Princeton; **Address:** 281 Witherspoon St, Ste 220, Princeton, NJ 08542; **Phone:** 609-921-3362; **Board Cert:** Internal Medicine 1989; **Med School:** NY Med Coll 1984; **Resid:** Internal Medicine, RW Johnson Univ Hosp 1989

Shelmet, John J MD (IM) - **Spec Exp:** Diabetes; **Hospital:** Univ Med Ctr - Princeton; **Address:** 3131 Princeton Pike, Bldg 2B, Ste 104, Lawrenceville, NJ 08648-2526; **Phone:** 609-896-8050; **Board Cert:** Internal Medicine 1984; **Med School:** UMDNJ-RW Johnson Med Sch 1981; **Resid:** Internal Medicine, Middlesex Genl Hosp/Univ Hosp 1984; **Fellow:** Diabetes, Temple Univ 1986; **Fac Appt:** Clin Prof Med, Robert W Johnson Med Sch

Warren, Ronald MD (IM) - **Spec Exp:** Pulmonary Disease; **Hospital:** Capital Health Sys - Fuld Campus; **Address:** Pulmonary & Internal Medicine, 40 Fuld St, Ste 201, Trenton, NJ 08638-5247; **Phone:** 609-695-4422; **Board Cert:** Internal Medicine 1972; **Med School:** Univ Pennsylvania 1968; **Resid:** Internal Medicine, Presbyterian Hosp 1970; Internal Medicine, Grady Meml Hosp 1971; **Fellow:** Pulmonary Disease, Emory Hosps 1972

Yamane, Michael MD (IM) PCP - **Spec Exp:** Geriatrics; **Hospital:** Capital Hlth Sys - Mercer Campus; **Address:** 2480 Pennington Rd, Ste 108, Pennington, NJ 08534-5227; **Phone:** 609-737-6700; **Board Cert:** Internal Medicine 1984; **Med School:** UCSF 1981; **Resid:** Internal Medicine, Univ Hawaii 1984

INTERVENTIONAL CARDIOLOGY

Shanahan, Andrew MD (IC) - **Spec Exp:** Angioplasty; **Hospital:** Univ Med Ctr - Princeton, Robert Wood Johnson Univ Hosp - New Brunswick (page 853); **Address:** Cardiology Assocs of Princeton, 281 Witherspoon St, Ste 210, Princeton, NJ 08542; **Phone:** 609-921-7456; **Board Cert:** Internal Medicine 2005; Cardiovascular Disease 2005; Interventional Cardiology 2001; **Med School:** Med Coll Wisc 1989; **Resid:** Internal Medicine, St Lukes-Roosevelt Hosp 1992; **Fellow:** Cardiovascular Disease, St Lukes-Roosevelt Hosp 1995

MEDICAL ONCOLOGY

Grossman, Bernard MD (Onc) - **Hospital:** Capital Hlth Sys - Mercer Campus, Robert Wood Johnson Univ Hosp Hamilton (page 853); **Address:** 408 Bellevue Ave, Trenton, NJ 08618; **Phone:** 609-396-5800; **Board Cert:** Internal Medicine 1977; Medical Oncology 1979; Hematology 1980; **Med School:** Temple Univ 1974; **Resid:** Internal Medicine, Albany Med 1977; **Fellow:** Hematology & Oncology, George Wash Univ Hosp 1979; Oncology, Fox Chase Cancer Ctr 1980

Pennacchi, John MD (Onc) - **Hospital:** Robert Wood Johnson Univ Hosp Hamilton (page 853); **Address:** Cancer Inst of NJ-Hamilton, 2575 Klockner Rd, Hamilton, NJ 08690; **Phone:** 609-631-6960; **Board Cert:** Internal Medicine 1987; Medical Oncology 1997; **Med School:** UMDNJ-RW Johnson Med Sch 1987; **Resid:** Internal Medicine, Robert Wood Johnson Univ Hosp 1990; **Fellow:** Hematology & Oncology, Fox Chase Cancer Ctr 1993; Hematology & Oncology, Temple Univ Hosp 1993; **Fac Appt:** Assoc Prof Med, UMDNJ-RW Johnson Med Sch

Schaebler, David MD (Onc) - **Hospital:** Capital Hlth Sys - Mercer Campus, Robert Wood Johnson Univ Hosp Hamilton (page 853); **Address:** Mercer Medical Center, 408 Bellevue Ave, Trenton, NJ 08618; **Phone:** 609-396-5800; **Board Cert:** Internal Medicine 2002; Medical Oncology 2003; **Med School:** Jefferson Med Coll 1988; **Resid:** Internal Medicine, Cooper Univ Med Ctr 1991; **Fellow:** Medical Oncology, Fox Chase 1994

Sierocki, John MD (Onc) - **Spec Exp:** Breast Cancer; Lung Cancer; Lymphoma; **Hospital:** Univ Med Ctr - Princeton; **Address:** Princeton Med Grp, 419 N Harrison St, Ste 101, Princeton, NJ 08540-3521; **Phone:** 609-924-9300; **Board Cert:** Internal Medicine 1976; Medical Oncology 1979; **Med School:** Hahnemann Univ 1973; **Resid:** Internal Medicine, Hahnemann Univ Hosp 1976; **Fellow:** Medical Oncology, Meml Sloan-Kettering Cancer Ctr 1978; **Fac Appt:** Assoc Clin Prof Med, UMDNJ-RW Johnson Med Sch

Yi, Peter MD (Onc) - **Spec Exp:** Breast Cancer; Lymphoma; Prostate Cancer; **Hospital:** Univ Med Ctr - Princeton; **Address:** 419 N Harrison St, Princeton, NJ 08540; **Phone:** 609-924-9300; **Board Cert:** Internal Medicine 1987; Medical Oncology 1989; Hematology 1999; **Med School:** Cornell Univ-Weill Med Coll 1984; **Resid:** Internal Medicine, Brigham & Women's Hosp 1987; **Fellow:** Hematology & Oncology, New York Hosp-Cornell Med Ctr 1990; **Fac Appt:** Asst Clin Prof Med, Robert W Johnson Med Sch

NEONATAL-PERINATAL MEDICINE

Axelrod, Randi MD (NP) - **Hospital:** Capital Hlth Sys - Mercer Campus; **Address:** 446 Bellevue Ave, Trenton, NJ 08618; **Phone:** 609-393-2236; **Board Cert:** Pediatrics 2001; Neonatal-Perinatal Medicine 2001; **Med School:** Mount Sinai Sch Med 1987; **Resid:** Pediatrics, St Christopher's Hosp 1990; **Fellow:** Neonatal-Perinatal Medicine, St Christopher's Hosp Chldn-Temple 1993

NEPHROLOGY

Cohen, Barry H MD (Nep) - **Hospital:** Capital Hlth Sys - Mercer Campus; **Address:** 40 Fuld St, Ste 401, Trenton, NJ 08638-5247; **Phone:** 609-599-1004; **Board Cert:** Internal Medicine 1971; Nephrology 1974; **Med School:** Hahnemann Univ 1965; **Resid:** Internal Medicine, Hahnemann Univ Hosp 1968; **Fellow:** Nephrology, Hahnemann Univ 1969

Ruddy, Michael MD (Nep) - **Spec Exp:** Hypertension; Renovascular Disease; Diabetic Kidney Disease; **Hospital:** Univ Med Ctr - Princeton, Robert Wood Johnson Univ Hosp - New Brunswick (page 853); **Address:** 88 Princeton-Hightstown Rd, Princeton Junction, NJ 08550-1100; **Phone:** 609-750-7330; **Board Cert:** Internal Medicine 1977; Nephrology 1980; **Med School:** UMDNJ-NJ Med Sch, Newark 1974; **Resid:** Internal Medicine, Rutgers Affil Hosps 1977; **Fellow:** Nephrology, NY Hosp-Cornell Med Ctr 1980; **Fac Appt:** Assoc Clin Prof Med, Robert W Johnson Med Sch

Somerstein, Michael MD (Nep) - **Spec Exp:** Hypertension; Diabetes; **Hospital:** Capital Health Sys - Fuld Campus, St Francis Med Ctr - Trenton; **Address:** 40 Fuld St, Ste 401, Trenton, NJ 08638-5293; **Phone:** 609-599-1004; **Board Cert:** Internal Medicine 1977; **Med School:** Univ Cincinnati 1966; **Resid:** Internal Medicine, Hahnemann Hosp 1969; **Fellow:** Nephrology, Hahnemann Hosp 1970

Sudhakar, Telechery MD (Nep) - **Spec Exp:** Kidney Disease; **Hospital:** Capital Hlth Sys - Mercer Campus, Capital Health Sys - Fuld Campus; **Address:** 40 Fuld St, Ste 401, Trenton, NJ 08638; **Phone:** 609-599-1004; **Board Cert:** Internal Medicine 1977; Nephrology 1978; **Med School:** India 1971; **Resid:** Internal Medicine, Helene Fuld Med Ctr 1976; **Fellow:** Nephrology, Washington VA Hosp 1978

Wei, Fong MD (Nep) - **Spec Exp:** Hypertension; Kidney Stones; **Hospital:** Univ Med Ctr - Princeton; **Address:** 419 N Harrison St, Princeton, NJ 08540-3594; **Phone:** 609-924-9300; **Board Cert:** Internal Medicine 1976; Nephrology 1976; **Med School:** Tufts Univ 1967; **Resid:** Internal Medicine, Boston City Hosp 1969; Internal Medicine, Bronx Municipal Hosp 1970; **Fellow:** Nephrology, Univ NC Hosp 1972; **Fac Appt:** Assoc Clin Prof Med, Robert W Johnson Med Sch

NEUROLOGICAL SURGERY

Abud, Ariel MD (NS) - **Spec Exp:** Neck & Back Surgery; Carpal Tunnel Syndrome; Brain Surgery; **Hospital:** Capital Health Sys - Fuld Campus, Robert Wood Johnson Univ Hosp Hamilton (page 853); **Address:** 3100 Princeton Pike, Bldg 1 - Ste A, Lawrenceville, NJ 08648; **Phone:** 609-219-0280; **Board Cert:** Neurological Surgery 1976; **Med School:** Mexico 1966; **Resid:** Surgery, Hackensack Hosp 1968; Neurological Surgery, Univ Hosp 1972; **Fellow:** Neurological Surgery, Hosp Sick Children

Chiurco, Anthony MD (NS) - **Spec Exp:** Aneurysm-Cerebral; Brain Tumors; Spinal Disc Replacement; **Hospital:** Univ Med Ctr - Princeton, Capital Hlth Sys - Mercer Campus; **Address:** 3131 Princeton Pike Bldg 4 - Ste 201, Lawrenceville, NJ 08648; **Phone:** 609-895-8898; **Board Cert:** Neurological Surgery 1977; **Med School:** Jefferson Med Coll 1967; **Resid:** Surgery, Univ Iowa Coll Med 1971; Neurological Surgery, Univ Iowa 1975; **Fellow:** Neurological Surgery, Penn Hosp 1976; **Fac Appt:** Asst Clin Prof NS, Robert W Johnson Med Sch

Pizzi, Francis MD (NS) - **Spec Exp:** Pain-Back & Neck; Spinal Disc Replacement; **Hospital:** St Francis Med Ctr - Trenton, Hunterdon Med Ctr; **Address:** 3131 Princeton Pike Bldg 4 - Ste 201, Lawrenceville, NJ 08648-2526; **Phone:** 609-895-8898; **Board Cert:** Neurological Surgery 1977; **Med School:** NY Med Coll 1969; **Resid:** Neurological Surgery, Hosp Univ Penn 1975

NEUROLOGY

Kaiser, Paul MD (N) - **Hospital:** Robert Wood Johnson Univ Hosp Hamilton (page 853); **Address:** 3131 Princeton Pike 3C Bldg - Ste 202, Lawrenceville, NJ 08648-2526; **Phone:** 609-896-1701; **Board Cert:** Neurology 1993; Clinical Neurophysiology 1999; **Med School:** Jefferson Med Coll 1988; **Resid:** Neurology, Temple Univ Hosp 1992; **Fellow:** Neurology, Temple Univ Hosp 1993

Kososky, Charles MD (N) - **Hospital:** St Francis Med Ctr - Trenton; **Address:** St Francis Med Ctr, Neurosci Inst, 601 Hamilton Ave, Trenton, NJ 08629; **Phone:** 609-599-5792; **Board Cert:** Neurology 1981; Clinical Neurophysiology 1997; **Med School:** UMDNJ-NJ Med Sch, Newark 1975; **Resid:** Internal Medicine, Kings Co Hosp; Neurology, UMDNJ-Univ Hosp

Vester, John MD (N) - **Spec Exp:** Parkinson's Disease; Stroke; Peripheral Neuropathy; **Hospital:** Univ Med Ctr - Princeton; **Address:** 1000 Herrontown Rd, Princeton, NJ 08540; **Phone:** 609-497-0100; **Board Cert:** Neurology 1979; **Med School:** Georgetown Univ 1973; **Resid:** Internal Medicine, Hartford Hosp 1975; Neurology, Georgetown Univ Hosp 1978

Witte, Arnold S MD (N) - **Spec Exp:** Neuromuscular Disorders; Parkinson's Disease; Electromyography; **Hospital:** Capital Hlth Sys - Mercer Campus, Capital Health Sys - Fuld Campus; **Address:** 2 Princess Rd, Lawrenceville, NJ 08648; **Phone:** 609-895-9000; **Board Cert:** Internal Medicine 1981; Neurology 1983; **Med School:** Tufts Univ 1977; **Resid:** Internal Medicine, Hosp Univ Penn 1979; Neurology, Hosp Univ Penn 1982; **Fellow:** Neurology, Hosp Univ Penn 1983

OBSTETRICS & GYNECOLOGY

Brickner, Gary R MD (ObG) PCP - **Spec Exp:** Menopause Problems; Gynecology Only; Menstrual Disorders; **Hospital:** Capital Hlth Sys - Mercer Campus, Robert Wood Johnson Univ Hosp Hamilton (page 853); **Address:** Quakerbridge Pl, Bldg 1A, Hamilton, NJ 08619-1241; **Phone:** 609-689-9991; **Board Cert:** Obstetrics & Gynecology 1981; **Med School:** Univ Pittsburgh 1975; **Resid:** Obstetrics & Gynecology, Pennsylvania Hosp 1979

Friedman, Alan MD (ObG) - **Spec Exp:** Pregnancy-High Risk; Infertility; **Hospital:** Univ Med Ctr - Princeton; **Address:** 253 Witherspoon St, Ste R, Princeton, NJ 08540; **Phone:** 609-683-9292; **Board Cert:** Obstetrics & Gynecology 2004; **Med School:** Univ Chicago-Pritzker Sch Med 1982; **Resid:** Obstetrics & Gynecology, NYU Medical Ctr 1986

Lemmerling, L J MD (ObG) - **Spec Exp:** Laparoscopic Surgery; Infertility; Incontinence; **Hospital:** Univ Med Ctr - Princeton; **Address:** 601 Ewing St, Ste A4, Princeton, NJ 08540-2754; **Phone:** 609-921-1500; **Board Cert:** Obstetrics & Gynecology 1980; **Med School:** Belgium 1970; **Resid:** Obstetrics & Gynecology, Womens Hosp-Columbia Univ 1975

OPHTHALMOLOGY

Matossian, Cynthia MD (Oph) - **Spec Exp:** Cataract Surgery; Glaucoma; **Hospital:** Capital Health Sys - Fuld Campus, Doylestown Hosp; **Address:** 1230 Parkway Ave, Ste 103, Ewing, NJ 08628; **Phone:** 609-882-8833; **Board Cert:** Ophthalmology 1987; **Med School:** Penn State Univ-Hershey Med Ctr 1981; **Resid:** Ophthalmology, Geo Wash U Med Ctr 1985

Safran, Steven MD (Oph) - **Spec Exp:** Cataract Surgery; Laser Vision Surgery; Glaucoma; **Hospital:** Capital Hlth Sys - Mercer Campus, Robert Wood Johnson Univ Hosp Hamilton (page 853); **Address:** 132 Franklin Corner Rd, Ste A-1, Lawrenceville, NJ 08648; **Phone:** 609-896-3931; **Board Cert:** Ophthalmology 1992; **Med School:** SUNY Downstate 1987; **Resid:** Internal Medicine, Beth Israel Med Ctr 1988; Ophthalmology, NYU Med Ctr 1991; **Fellow:** Cornea & Ext Eye Disease, Duke Univ Med Ctr 1992

Wong, Michael Y MD (Oph) - **Spec Exp:** LASIK-Refractive Surgery; Cataract Surgery-Lens Implant; Glaucoma; **Hospital:** Univ Med Ctr - Princeton, Wills Eye Hosp; **Address:** 419 N Harrison St, Ste 104, Princeton, NJ 08540-3521; **Phone:** 609-921-9437; **Board Cert:** Ophthalmology 1983; **Med School:** Albany Med Coll 1978; **Resid:** Ophthalmology, Wills Eye Hosp 1982

Wong, Richard H MD (Oph) - **Spec Exp:** Cataract Surgery-Lens Implant; LASIK-Refractive Surgery; **Hospital:** Univ Med Ctr - Princeton; **Address:** 419 N Harrison St, Ste 104, Princeton, NJ 08540-3521; **Phone:** 609-921-9437; **Board Cert:** Internal Medicine 1982; Ophthalmology 1987; **Med School:** UMDNJ-NJ Med Sch, Newark 1979; **Resid:** Internal Medicine, T Jefferson Univ Hosp 1982; Ophthalmology, Wills Eye Hosp 1985

ORTHOPAEDIC SURGERY

Abrams, Jeffrey MD (OrS) - **Spec Exp:** Shoulder Surgery; Sports Medicine; Arthroscopic Surgery; **Hospital:** Univ Med Ctr - Princeton; **Address:** 325 Princeton Ave, Princeton, NJ 08540-1617; **Phone:** 609-924-8131; **Board Cert:** Orthopaedic Surgery 1999; **Med School:** SUNY Upstate Med Univ 1980; **Resid:** Orthopaedic Surgery, Thomas Jefferson Univ Hosp 1985; Sports Medicine, Fell-Aspen Valley Hosp 1986; **Fellow:** Shoulder Surgery, Univ Western Ontario 1986; Sports Medicine, Hughston Sports Med Hosp 1986

Costa, Leon N MD (OrS) - **Spec Exp:** Arthroscopic Surgery; Joint Replacement; **Hospital:** Univ Med Ctr - Princeton, Capital Hlth Sys - Mercer Campus; **Address:** 256 Bunn Dr, Ste 2, Princeton, NJ 08540-2859; **Phone:** 609-924-9229; **Board Cert:** Orthopaedic Surgery 1999; **Med School:** Geo Wash Univ 1980; **Resid:** Surgery, Hosp Univ Penn 1982; Orthopaedic Surgery, NY Ortho Hosp/Colum-Presby 1984; **Fellow:** Sports Medicine, NY Ortho Hosp/Colum-Presby 1985

Eingorn, David MD (OrS) - **Hospital:** Capital Hlth Sys - Mercer Campus, St Mary Med Ctr; **Address:** 3120 Princeton Pike, Lawrenceville, NJ 08648; **Phone:** 609-896-0444; **Board Cert:** Orthopaedic Surgery 1997; **Med School:** Temple Univ 1979; **Resid:** Orthopaedic Surgery, Thomas Jefferson Univ Hosp 1984; Hand Surgery, Thomas Jefferson Univ Hosp 1984

Glick, Ronald MD (OrS) - **Hospital:** Capital Health Sys - Fuld Campus, Robert Wood Johnson Univ Hosp Hamilton (page 853); **Address:** 4065 Quakerbridge Rd, Princeton Junction, NJ 08550; **Phone:** 609-394-3804; **Board Cert:** Orthopaedic Surgery 1977; **Med School:** Univ MD Sch Med 1968; **Resid:** Orthopaedic Surgery, Albert Einstein

Gomez, William MD (OrS) - **Spec Exp:** Sports Medicine; Arthroscopic Surgery; **Hospital:** St Francis Med Ctr - Trenton, Robert Wood Johnson Univ Hosp Hamilton (page 853); **Address:** Trenton Orthopaedic Group, 1225 Whitehorse Mercerville Rd, Bldg D, Ste 220, Trenton, NJ 08619-3876; **Phone:** 609-581-2200; **Board Cert:** Orthopaedic Surgery 2001; **Med School:** Columbia P&S 1982; **Resid:** Surgery, St Vincent's Hosp 1984; Orthopaedic Surgery, Columbia-Presby Med Ctr 1987; **Fellow:** Sports Medicine, Univ Pittsburgh Hosp 1988

Grenis, Michael S MD (OrS) - **Spec Exp:** Carpal Tunnel Syndrome; Hand & Wrist Injuries; **Hospital:** Univ Med Ctr - Princeton, Capital Hlth Sys - Mercer Campus; **Address:** 256 Bunn, Ste 2, Princeton, NJ 08540; **Phone:** 609-924-9229; **Board Cert:** Orthopaedic Surgery 2000; **Med School:** NY Med Coll 1984; **Resid:** Surgery, NYU-Bellevue Hosp 1985; Orthopaedic Surgery, NYU-Bellevue Hosp 1989; **Fellow:** Hand Surgery, NYU-Bellevue Hosp 1990

Gutowski, W Thomas MD (OrS) - **Spec Exp:** Hip Replacement; Knee Replacement; Arthroscopic Surgery; **Hospital:** Univ Med Ctr - Princeton; **Address:** Princeton Orthopaedic Assocs, 325 Princeton Ave, Princeton, NJ 08540; **Phone:** 609-924-8131; **Board Cert:** Orthopaedic Surgery 1998; **Med School:** Cornell Univ-Weill Med Coll 1980; **Resid:** Orthopaedic Surgery, Yale-New Haven Hosp 1985

Taitsman, James MD (OrS) - **Spec Exp:** Sports Medicine; **Hospital:** Capital Hlth Sys - Mercer Campus, Robert Wood Johnson Univ Hosp Hamilton (page 853); **Address:** 123 Franklin Corner Rd, Ste 114, Lawrenceville, NJ 08648-2526; **Phone:** 609-896-0707; **Board Cert:** Orthopaedic Surgery 1977; **Med School:** Univ Rochester 1971; **Resid:** Surgery, Yale-New Haven Hosp 1973; Orthopaedic Surgery, Yale-New Haven Hosp 1976

OTOLARYNGOLOGY

Davidson, William D MD (Oto) - **Hospital:** Capital Hlth Sys - Mercer Campus; **Address:** 3131 Princeton Pike Bldg 6 - Ste 100, Lawrenceville, NJ 08648; **Phone:** 609-912-1000; **Board Cert:** Otolaryngology 1987; **Med School:** Univ VA Sch Med 1982; **Resid:** Surgery, Presby Hosp 1984; Otolaryngology, Univ Texas 1987

Farmer, Howard S MD (Oto) - **Spec Exp:** Endoscopic Sinus Surgery; Hearing Disorders; Snoring/Sleep Apnea; **Hospital:** Univ Med Ctr - Princeton; **Address:** 3100 Princeton Pike Bldg 4 - Ste 2G, Lawrenceville, NJ 08648; **Phone:** 609-895-6655; **Board Cert:** Otolaryngology 1966; **Med School:** Washington Univ, St Louis 1959; **Resid:** Surgery, Mt Sinai Hosp 1961; Otolaryngology, Barnes Hosp-Wash Univ 1966; **Fac Appt:** Assoc Clin Prof S, UMDNJ-RW Johnson Med Sch

Haroldson, Olaf MD (Oto) - **Spec Exp:** Hearing Disorders; Voice Disorders; **Hospital:** Univ Med Ctr - Princeton; **Address:** Nassau Ear Nose & Throat, 812 Executive Dr, Princeton, NJ 08540-1530; **Phone:** 609-655-3000; **Board Cert:** Otolaryngology 1965; **Med School:** Univ Mich Med Sch 1959; **Resid:** Otolaryngology, Columbia-Presby Med Ctr 1963; Surgery, Columbia-Presby Med Ctr 1964

Kay, Scott MD (Oto) - **Spec Exp:** Facial Paralysis; Otology; Hearing Loss; Sinus Surgery; **Hospital:** Univ Med Ctr - Princeton; **Address:** 457 N Harrison St, Ste 101, Princeton, NJ 08540-3522; **Phone:** 609-924-0518; **Board Cert:** Otolaryngology 1993; **Med School:** Univ Pennsylvania 1986; **Resid:** Surgery, Mt Sinai Hosp 1988; Otolaryngology, Columbia-Presby Med Ctr 1992; **Fellow:** Facial Plastic Surgery, Shadyside Hosp 1993; **Fac Appt:** Prof S, Robert W Johnson Med Sch

Li, Ronald MD (Oto) - **Spec Exp:** Cosmetic Surgery-Face; Sinus Disorders; Voice Disorders; **Hospital:** Univ Med Ctr - Princeton; **Address:** 812 Executive Drive Bldg 8, Princeton, NJ 08540; **Phone:** 609-921-1000; **Board Cert:** Otolaryngology 1990; **Med School:** Mount Sinai Sch Med 1984; **Resid:** Otolaryngology, Montefiore Med Ctr 1989; **Fac Appt:** Asst Prof Oto, Robert W Johnson Med Sch

Moses, Brett MD (Oto) - **Hospital:** St Francis Med Ctr - Trenton; **Address:** 8 Quakerbridge Plaza, Hamilton, NJ 08619-1255; **Phone:** 609-890-7800; **Board Cert:** Otolaryngology 1994; **Med School:** Jefferson Med Coll 1982; **Resid:** Otolaryngology, Johns Hopkins Univ Hosp 1992; **Fellow:** Otolaryngology, Johns Hopkins Univ Hosp 1993

PAIN MEDICINE

Loren, Gary M MD (PM) - **Spec Exp:** Pain-Back; Reflex Sympathetic Dystrophy (RSD); **Hospital:** St Francis Med Ctr - Trenton; **Address:** 1666 Hamilton Ave, Hamilton Township, NJ 08629; **Phone:** 609-584-9080; **Board Cert:** Anesthesiology 1988; Pain Medicine 2002; **Med School:** Univ Pittsburgh 1984; **Resid:** Anesthesiology, LI Jewish Med Ctr 1987; **Fellow:** Pediatrics, LI Jewish Med Ctr 1988

PEDIATRIC ENDOCRINOLOGY

Boim, Marilynn MD (PEn) - **Hospital:** Capital Hlth Sys - Mercer Campus, Robert Wood Johnson Univ Hosp Hamilton (page 853); **Address:** 1255 Whitehorse Mercerville Rd, B Bldg - Ste 510, Mercerville, NJ 08619-3800; **Phone:** 609-581-4480; **Board Cert:** Pediatrics 1987; Pediatric Endocrinology 2002; **Med School:** Emory Univ 1982; **Resid:** Pediatrics, Mt Sinai Hosp; **Fellow:** Pediatric Endocrinology, Mt Sinai Hosp

PEDIATRICS

Baiser, Dennis MD (Ped) `PCP` - **Spec Exp:** Developmental Disorders; Asthma; **Hospital:** Capital Hlth Sys - Mercer Campus, Robert Wood Johnson Univ Hosp Hamilton (page 853); **Address:** 1255 Whitehorse Mercerville Rd, B Bldg - Ste 510, Mercerville, NJ 08619-3800; **Phone:** 609-581-4480; **Board Cert:** Pediatrics 1983; **Med School:** NY Med Coll 1978; **Resid:** Pediatrics, Children's Hosp 1981; **Fac Appt:** Ped, Univ Pennsylvania

Palsky, Glenn MD (Ped) - **Spec Exp:** Adolescent Medicine; **Hospital:** Capital Hlth Sys - Mercer Campus, Univ Med Ctr - Princeton; **Address:** 132 Franklin Corner Rd, Lawrenceville, NJ 08648-2526; **Phone:** 609-896-4141; **Board Cert:** Pediatrics 1978; **Med School:** Penn State Univ-Hershey Med Ctr 1973; **Resid:** Pediatrics, Albany Med Ctr 1977

Raymond, Gerald M MD (Ped) `PCP` - **Hospital:** Univ Med Ctr - Princeton; **Address:** 196 Princeton Heights Town Rd, West Windsor, NJ 08550; **Phone:** 609-799-5335; **Board Cert:** Pediatrics 1987; **Med School:** Penn State Univ-Hershey Med Ctr 1983; **Resid:** Pediatrics, Columbus Chldns Hosp 1986

Saltstein, Elliott MD (Ped) - **Hospital:** Capital Hlth Sys - Mercer Campus, Robert Wood Johnson Univ Hosp Hamilton (page 853); **Address:** 1225 Whitehorse-Mercerville Rd, D Bldg - Ste 203, Mercerville, NJ 08619-3882; **Phone:** 609-581-5100; **Board Cert:** Pediatrics 1975; **Med School:** SUNY Downstate 1969; **Resid:** Pediatrics, Kings County Hosp

PHYSICAL MEDICINE & REHABILITATION

Agri, Robyn MD (PMR) - **Spec Exp:** Acupuncture; **Hospital:** St Lawrence Rehab Ctr; **Address:** 2381 Lawrenceville Rd, St Lawrence Rehabilitation Ctr, Lawrenceville, NJ 08648-2024; **Phone:** 609-896-9500; **Board Cert:** Physical Medicine & Rehabilitation 1990; Pain Medicine 1994; **Med School:** SUNY Upstate Med Univ 1985; **Resid:** Physical Medicine & Rehabilitation, Hosp of Univ Penn 1989

Gribbin, Dorota MD (PMR) - **Spec Exp:** Industrial Injuries; Sports Injuries; Pain Management; **Hospital:** Robert Wood Johnson Univ Hosp Hamilton (page 853), Univ Med Ctr - Princeton; **Address:** 2333 Whitehorse Mercerville Rd, Ste 8, Mercerville, NJ 06819; **Phone:** 609-588-0540; **Board Cert:** Physical Medicine & Rehabilitation 2003; **Med School:** Poland 1984; **Resid:** Internal Medicine, Beth Israel Med Ctr 1989; Physical Medicine & Rehabilitation, New York Hosp-Cornell Med Ctr 1992; **Fellow:** Pain Medicine, Univ P&M Hosp 1985; **Fac Appt:** Asst Clin Prof PMR, Columbia P&S

PLASTIC SURGERY

Cimino, Ernest MD (PlS) - **Spec Exp:** Cosmetic Surgery; Trauma Reconstruction; **Hospital:** Capital Hlth Sys - Mercer Campus; **Address:** Yardley Plastic Surgery, 416 Bellevue Ave, Ste 404, Trenton, NJ 08618-4513; **Phone:** 609-396-5509; **Board Cert:** Plastic Surgery 1991; **Med School:** NYU Sch Med 1982; **Resid:** Surgery, St Vincents Hosp 1986; Plastic Surgery, Indiana Univ Med Ctr 1989

Mercer

Drimmer, Marc A MD (PIS) - **Spec Exp:** Cosmetic Surgery; **Hospital:** Univ Med Ctr - Princeton; **Address:** 842 State Rd, Princeton, NJ 08540-1439; **Phone:** 609-924-1026; **Board Cert:** Plastic Surgery 1981; **Med School:** Belgium 1974; **Resid:** Surgery, Beth Israel Med Ctr 1977; Plastic Surgery, Univ Hosp 1979

Leach, Thomas A MD (PIS) - **Spec Exp:** Cosmetic Surgery-Face; Cosmetic Surgery-Breast; Liposuction; **Hospital:** Univ Med Ctr - Princeton, Robert Wood Johnson Univ Hosp - New Brunswick (page 853); **Address:** 932 State Rd, Princeton, NJ 08540; **Phone:** 609-921-7161; **Board Cert:** Plastic Surgery 1994; **Med School:** UMDNJ-NJ Med Sch, Newark 1985; **Resid:** Surgery, UMDNJ Med Ctr 1990; **Fellow:** Plastic Surgery, UMDNJ Med Ctr 1992

Malik, Parvaiz MD (PIS) - **Spec Exp:** Cosmetic Surgery; Reconstructive Surgery; Hand Surgery; **Hospital:** Robert Wood Johnson Univ Hosp Hamilton (page 853), Capital Health Sys - Fuld Campus; **Address:** 1542 Kuser Rd, Ste B2, Hamilton, NJ 08619-3829; **Phone:** 609-585-0044; **Board Cert:** Plastic Surgery 1983; **Med School:** Pakistan 1972; **Resid:** Surgery, Flushing Hosp 1980; **Fellow:** Plastic Surgery, St Louis Univ Hosp 1982

Smotrich, Gary MD (PIS) - **Hospital:** Capital Hlth Sys - Mercer Campus; **Address:** Lawrenceville Plastic Surgery, 3131 Princeton Pike Bldg 5 - Ste 205, Lawrenceville, NJ 08648-2300; **Phone:** 609-896-2525; **Board Cert:** Plastic Surgery 1991; **Med School:** Univ Conn 1982; **Resid:** Surgery, Boston Univ Med Ctr 1987; Plastic Surgery, U Louisville 1989

PSYCHIATRY

Khouri, Philippe J MD (Psyc) - **Spec Exp:** Neuro-Psychiatry; Bipolar/Mood Disorders; Geriatric Psychiatry; **Hospital:** Univ Med Ctr - Princeton; **Address:** Princetown House, 905 Herrontown Rd, Princeton, NJ 08540; **Phone:** 609-497-3300; **Board Cert:** Psychiatry 1977; Geriatric Psychiatry 1994; **Med School:** Lebanon 1972; **Resid:** Psychiatry, Strong Meml Hosp 1973; Psychiatry, Univ Tenn Med Ctr 1975; **Fellow:** Genetics and Metabolism, Nat Inst Mntl Hlth 1977; **Fac Appt:** Prof Psyc, Robert W Johnson Med Sch

Leifer, Marvin W MD (Psyc) - **Spec Exp:** Psychopharmacology; Anxiety & Mood Disorders; **Hospital:** Univ Med Ctr - Princeton, Capital Hlth Sys - Mercer Campus; **Address:** 42 North Tulane St, Princeton, NJ 08542; **Phone:** 609-497-1810; **Board Cert:** Psychiatry 1972; **Med School:** SUNY Downstate 1970; **Resid:** Psychiatry, Albert Einstein 1974; **Fellow:** Psychopharmacology, Albert Einstein 1976

Schneider, Samuel MD (Psyc) - **Spec Exp:** Mood Disorders; Personality Disorders; Addiction/Substance Abuse; **Hospital:** Univ Med Ctr - Princeton; **Address:** 33 N State Rd, Ste H, Princeton, NJ 08540-1304; **Phone:** 609-924-3980; **Board Cert:** Psychiatry 1982; Internal Medicine 1978; **Med School:** Penn State Univ-Hershey Med Ctr 1975; **Resid:** Internal Medicine, MS Hershey Med Ctr 1977; Psychiatry, Coll Med NJ 1983

PULMONARY DISEASE

Deitz, Joel MD (Pul) - **Spec Exp:** Respiratory Failure; Chronic Obstructive Lung Disease (COPD); **Hospital:** Univ Med Ctr - Princeton; **Address:** Princeton Healthcare Med Assocs, 253 Witherspoon St, 2nd Fl-Lambert House, Princeton, NJ 08540-3211; **Phone:** 609-497-4301; **Board Cert:** Internal Medicine 1980; Pulmonary Disease 1984; Critical Care Medicine 1997; **Med School:** Tufts Univ 1977; **Resid:** Internal Medicine, Med Coll Va Med Ctr 1980; **Fellow:** Pulmonary Disease, Duke Univ Med Ctr 1984

Goldblatt, Kenneth MD (Pul) - **Spec Exp:** Asthma; Emphysema; **Hospital:** Univ Med Ctr - Princeton; **Address:** Princeton Hosp Med Assoc, 253 Witherspoon St, Fl 2, Princeton, NJ 08540-3211; **Phone:** 609-497-4301; **Board Cert:** Internal Medicine 1975; Pulmonary Disease 1978; **Med School:** NY Med Coll 1972; **Resid:** Internal Medicine, CMDNJ-Rutgers 1975; **Fellow:** Pulmonary Disease, CMDNJ-Rutgers 1977; **Fac Appt:** Assoc Prof Med, UMDNJ-RW Johnson Med Sch

Harman, John MD (Pul) - **Hospital:** Capital Hlth Sys - Mercer Campus; **Address:** 2480 Pennington Rd, Ste 104, Pennington, NJ 08534; **Phone:** 609-737-7544; **Board Cert:** Internal Medicine 1972; **Med School:** Univ Pennsylvania 1969; **Resid:** Internal Medicine, Presby Hosp 1972

Seelagy, Marc MD (Pul) - **Spec Exp:** Sleep Disorders; Lung Disease; Critical Care Medicine; **Hospital:** St Francis Med Ctr - Trenton, Robert Wood Johnson Univ Hosp Hamilton (page 853); **Address:** Allergy & Pulmonary Assoc, 1542 Kuser Rd, Ste B7, Trenton, NJ 08619-3829; **Phone:** 609-581-1400; **Board Cert:** Internal Medicine 1989; Pulmonary Disease 2002; Critical Care Medicine 2003; **Med School:** Univ Chicago-Pritzker Sch Med 1986; **Resid:** Internal Medicine, Univ Colorado Hosp 1989; **Fellow:** Pulmonary Disease, Johns Hopkins Hosp 1993; Critical Care Medicine, Johns Hopkins Hosp 1993

RADIATION ONCOLOGY

Baumann, John MD (RadRO) - **Spec Exp:** Breast Cancer; Cervical Cancer; Prostate Cancer; **Hospital:** Univ Med Ctr - Princeton, CentraState Med Ctr; **Address:** University Med Ctr - Radiation Oncology, 253 Witherspoon St, Princeton, NJ 08540; **Phone:** 609-497-4304; **Board Cert:** Radiation Oncology 1981; **Med School:** Harvard Med Sch 1977; **Resid:** Internal Medicine, Walter Reed AMC 1978; Radiation Oncology, Harvard Joint Program 1981; **Fellow:** Radiation Oncology, Harvard Joint Program

Fram, Daniel K MD (RadRO) - **Spec Exp:** Prostate Cancer; **Hospital:** Capital Hlth Sys - Mercer Campus; **Address:** Capital Hlth Sys at Mercer, Rad Onc, 446 Bellevue Ave, Trenton, NJ 08618-4502; **Phone:** 609-394-4244; **Board Cert:** Radiation Oncology 1991; **Med School:** Univ VT Coll Med 1985; **Resid:** Radiation Oncology, Univ California 1990; **Fac Appt:** Asst Clin Prof RadRO, Univ Pennsylvania

Soffen, Edward MD (RadRO) - **Spec Exp:** Prostate Cancer; Breast Cancer; Intravascular Brachytherapy (IVB); **Hospital:** Univ Med Ctr - Princeton, CentraState Med Ctr; **Address:** Med Ctr at Princeton, Dept Rad Onc, 253 Witherspoon St, Princeton, NJ 08540-3298; **Phone:** 609-497-4304; **Board Cert:** Radiation Oncology 1991; **Med School:** Temple Univ 1986; **Resid:** Radiation Oncology, Hosp Univ Penn 1990; **Fac Appt:** Asst Clin Prof Rad, UMDNJ-RW Johnson Med Sch

RHEUMATOLOGY

Carney, Alexander MD (Rhu) - **Hospital:** Univ Med Ctr - Princeton; **Address:** 8 Quakerbridge Plaza, Ste H, Mercerville, NJ 08619; **Phone:** 609-588-9044; **Board Cert:** Internal Medicine 1972; **Med School:** Cornell Univ-Weill Med Coll 1966; **Resid:** Internal Medicine, Univ Iowa Hosp 1972; **Fellow:** Rheumatology, Univ Iowa Hosp 1974

Gordon, Richard D MD (Rhu) - **Hospital:** St Francis Med Ctr - Trenton, Capital Health Sys - Fuld Campus; **Address:** 2275 Whitehorse Mercerville Rd, Ste 8, Mercerville, NJ 08619; **Phone:** 609-587-9898; **Board Cert:** Internal Medicine 1978; Rheumatology 1980; **Med School:** Jefferson Med Coll 1975; **Resid:** Internal Medicine, Geo Wash Hosp/VA Hosp 1978; **Fellow:** Rheumatology, Georgetown Univ 1979; Rheumatology, St Vincents Hosp 1980

SURGERY

Abouchedid, Claude MD (S) - **Spec Exp:** Breast Surgery; **Hospital:** Robert Wood Johnson Univ Hosp Hamilton (page 853); **Address:** 1542 Kuser Rd, Ste B3, Trenton, NJ 08619-3829; **Phone:** 609-585-2323; **Board Cert:** Surgery 1968; **Med School:** Lebanon 1963; **Resid:** Surgery, Meml Sloan Kettering Cancer Ctr; Surgery, St Francis Hosp 1967; **Fellow:** Surgery, St Francis Hosp

Davidson, J Thomas MD (S) - **Spec Exp:** Vascular Surgery; **Hospital:** Univ Med Ctr - Princeton; **Address:** Princeton Surgery Associates, 281 Witherspoon St, Ste 120, Princeton, NJ 08540-3210; **Phone:** 609-921-7223; **Board Cert:** Surgery 1974; **Med School:** Cornell Univ-Weill Med Coll 1966; **Resid:** Surgery, NYU Hosp-Bellevue Hosp 1973; **Fellow:** Vascular Surgery, NYU Hosp-Bellevue Hosp 1974; **Fac Appt:** Assoc Clin Prof S, UMDNJ-RW Johnson Med Sch

Davison Jr, Henry MD (S) - **Spec Exp:** Cancer Surgery; Laparoscopic Surgery; **Hospital:** Univ Med Ctr - Princeton; **Address:** 281 Witherspoon St, Ste 120, Princeton, NJ 08540-3210; **Phone:** 609-921-7223; **Board Cert:** Surgery 1993; **Med School:** Columbia P&S 1987; **Resid:** Surgery, Columbia-Presby Med Ctr 1992

Dultz, Rachel MD (S) - **Spec Exp:** Breast Surgery; Breast Cancer; **Hospital:** Univ Med Ctr - Princeton; **Address:** Princeton Surgical Assocs, 281 Witherspoon St, Ste 120, Princeton, NJ 08540; **Phone:** 609-921-7223; **Board Cert:** Surgery 1998; **Med School:** SUNY Downstate 1991; **Resid:** Surgery, Robert Wood Johnson Univ Hosp 1997; **Fellow:** Breast Surgery, Baylor Univ Med Ctr 1998

Jordan, Lawrence MD (S) - **Spec Exp:** Laparoscopic Surgery; Biliary Surgery; **Hospital:** Univ Med Ctr - Princeton; **Address:** 281 Witherspoon St, Ste 120, Princeton, NJ 08540; **Phone:** 609-921-7223; **Board Cert:** Surgery 1998; **Med School:** Cornell Univ-Weill Med Coll 1983; **Resid:** Surgery, Columbia-Presby Med Ctr 1988

Kahn, Steven P MD (S) - **Hospital:** Univ Med Ctr - Princeton; **Address:** 281 Witherspoon St, Ste 120, Princeton, NJ 08540; **Phone:** 609-921-7223; **Board Cert:** Surgery 1975; **Med School:** NY Med Coll 1967; **Resid:** Surgery, Univ Mich Med Ctr 1973; **Fac Appt:** Assoc Clin Prof S, UMDNJ-RW Johnson Med Sch

Schell, Harold S MD (S) - **Spec Exp:** Breast Cancer; Thyroid & Parathyroid Surgery; Gastrointestinal Surgery; **Hospital:** Capital Hlth Sys - Mercer Campus, Capital Health Sys - Fuld Campus; **Address:** 416 Bellevue Ave, Ste 406, Trenton, NJ 08618; **Phone:** 609-392-8100; **Board Cert:** Surgery 2002; **Med School:** Boston Univ 1970; **Resid:** Surgery, St Vincent's Hosp & Med Ctr 1975

THORACIC SURGERY

Laub, Glenn W MD (TS) - **Spec Exp:** Cardiac Surgery; Minimally Invasive Surgery; **Hospital:** St Francis Med Ctr - Trenton, Robert Wood Johnson Univ Hosp Hamilton (page 853); **Address:** St Francis Med Ctr Heart Hosp, 601 Hamilton Ave, rm 109, Trenton, NJ 08629-1986; **Phone:** 609-599-5307; **Board Cert:** Thoracic Surgery 1997; **Med School:** Dartmouth Med Sch 1981; **Resid:** Surgery, NYU-Bellevue Med Ctr 1986; Cardiothoracic Surgery, Allegheny Genl Hosp 1988; **Fac Appt:** Assoc Prof S, UMDNJ-RW Johnson Med Sch

UROLOGY

Orland, Steven MD (U) - **Spec Exp:** Prostate Disease; Incontinence; Erectile Dysfunction; **Hospital:** Capital Health Sys - Fuld Campus, Capital Hlth Sys - Mercer Campus; **Address:** 6 Colonial Lake Drive, Ste D, Lawrenceville, NJ 08648-4126; **Phone:** 609-882-5564; **Board Cert:** Urology 1999; **Med School:** Columbia P&S 1981; **Resid:** Surgery, Hosp Univ Penn 1983; Urology, Hosp Univ Penn 1987

Rezvan, Masoud MD (U) - **Spec Exp:** Prostate Disease; Kidney Stones; **Hospital:** St Francis Med Ctr - Trenton; **Address:** 3131 Princeton Pike Bldg 5 - Ste 109, Lawrenceville, NJ 08648; **Phone:** 609-912-1145; **Board Cert:** Urology 1980; **Med School:** Iran 1969; **Resid:** Surgery, St Francis Med Ctr 1972; Urology, Columbia Univ-Delafield Div 1975

Rosenberg, Stanley MD (U) - **Spec Exp:** Prostate Cancer; Urinary Tract Infections; Impotence; **Hospital:** Univ Med Ctr - Princeton, Robert Wood Johnson Univ Hosp - New Brunswick (page 853); **Address:** 281 Witherspoon St, Ste 100, Princeton, NJ 08540-3210; **Phone:** 609-924-6487; **Board Cert:** Urology 1968; **Med School:** Columbia P&S 1957; **Resid:** Surgery, Bellevue Hosp 1959; Urology, Columbia-Presby Med Ctr 1964; **Fac Appt:** Clin Prof U, Robert W Johnson Med Sch

Rossman, Barry R MD (U) - **Spec Exp:** Incontinence; Prostate Cancer; Vasectomy-Scalpelless; **Hospital:** Univ Med Ctr - Princeton, Robert Wood Johnson Univ Hosp - New Brunswick (page 853); **Address:** 281 Witherspoon St, Ste 100, Princeton, NJ 08542-3210; **Phone:** 609-924-6487; **Board Cert:** Urology 2000; **Med School:** Boston Univ 1983; **Resid:** Surgery, Montefiore Med Ctr 1985; Urology, Montefiore Med Ctr 1989; **Fac Appt:** Assoc Clin Prof U, UMDNJ-RW Johnson Med Sch

Vukasin, Alexander P MD (U) - **Spec Exp:** Laparoscopic Surgery; Urologic Cancer; Urology-Female; **Hospital:** Univ Med Ctr - Princeton, Robert Wood Johnson Univ Hosp - New Brunswick (page 853); **Address:** 281 Witherspoon St, Ste 100, Princeton, NJ 08542; **Phone:** 609-924-6487; **Board Cert:** Urology 1997; **Med School:** Yale Univ 1989; **Resid:** Urology, New York Hosp 1995; **Fac Appt:** Asst Clin Prof U, UMDNJ-RW Johnson Med Sch

VASCULAR SURGERY

Abud, Alfredo MD (VascS) - **Hospital:** Capital Health Sys - Fuld Campus, St Francis Med Ctr - Trenton; **Address:** 40 Fuld St, Ste 403, Trenton, NJ 08638; **Phone:** 609-656-8622; **Med School:** Mexico 1970; **Resid:** Surgery, St Francis Hosp 1979; **Fellow:** Cardiovascular Surgery, Cleveland Clinic 1980

Goldman, Kenneth Alan MD (VascS) - **Spec Exp:** Carotid Artery Surgery; Aneurysm-Aortic; Varicose Veins; **Hospital:** Univ Med Ctr - Princeton; **Address:** 281 Witherspoon St, Ste 120, Princeton, NJ 08540-3210; **Phone:** 609-921-7223; **Board Cert:** Surgery 1994; Vascular Surgery 1996; **Med School:** NYU Sch Med 1988; **Resid:** Surgery, Bellevue Hosp 1993; **Fellow:** Vascular Surgery, NYU Med Ctr 1994

Middlesex

Castle Connolly Top Doctors: New York Metro Area 10th Edition

ADDICTION PSYCHIATRY

Ziedonis, Douglas M MD (AdP) - **Spec Exp:** Nicotine Dependence; **Hospital:** UMDNJ-Univ Behavioral HealthCare, Robert Wood Johnson Univ Hosp - New Brunswick (page 853); **Address:** Univ Behavioral Healthcare Ctr, 671 Hoes Ln, rm D349, Piscataway, NJ 08854; **Phone:** 732-235-4341; **Board Cert:** Psychiatry 1994; Addiction Psychiatry 1996; **Med School:** Penn State Univ-Hershey Med Ctr 1985; **Resid:** Psychiatry, UCLA Med Ctr 1989; **Fellow:** Addiction Psychiatry, UCLA Med Ctr 1990; **Fac Appt:** Prof Psyc, Robert W Johnson Med Sch

ADOLESCENT MEDICINE

Picciano, Anne MD (AM) **PCP** - **Spec Exp:** Adolescent Medicine; **Hospital:** JFK Med Ctr - Edison; **Address:** 65 James St, Edison, NJ 08818; **Phone:** 732-321-7493; **Board Cert:** Family Medicine 2002; Adolescent Medicine 2003; **Med School:** Univ Pennsylvania 1987; **Resid:** Family Medicine, W Jersey Health Sys 1990; **Fac Appt:** Asst Clin Prof FMed, UMDNJ-RW Johnson Med Sch

Snyder, Barbara K MD (AM) - **Spec Exp:** Eating Disorders; Pediatric Gynecology; **Hospital:** Robert Wood Johnson Univ Hosp - New Brunswick (page 853); **Address:** Childrens Health Inst New Jersey, 89 French St, Ste 2230, New Brunswick, NJ 08901; **Phone:** 732-235-6230; **Board Cert:** Pediatrics 1985; Adolescent Medicine 2002; **Med School:** Geo Wash Univ 1979; **Resid:** Pediatrics, Chldns National Med Ctr 1981; Pediatrics, Upstate Med Ctr 1982; **Fellow:** Adolescent Medicine, Univ Rochester 1988; **Fac Appt:** Assoc Prof Ped, Robert W Johnson Med Sch

ALLERGY & IMMUNOLOGY

Blum, Jay MD (A&I) - **Spec Exp:** Rhinitis; Asthma; Hives; **Hospital:** St Peter's Univ Hosp, Robert Wood Johnson Univ Hosp - New Brunswick (page 853); **Address:** 85 Raritan Ave, Highland Park, NJ 08904-2439; **Phone:** 732-846-7861; **Board Cert:** Internal Medicine 1978; Allergy & Immunology 1979; **Med School:** Univ Pennsylvania 1974; **Resid:** Internal Medicine, Beth Israel Hosp 1977; **Fellow:** Allergy & Immunology, New York Hosp 1979

Kesarwala, Hemant MD (A&I) - **Spec Exp:** Food Allergy; Asthma; **Hospital:** St Peter's Univ Hosp, Robert Wood Johnson Univ Hosp - New Brunswick (page 853); **Address:** 3084 State Route 27, Ste 6, Kendall Park, NJ 08824-1657; **Phone:** 732-821-0595; **Board Cert:** Pediatrics 1979; Allergy & Immunology 1979; Pediatric Infectious Disease 2002; **Med School:** India 1971; **Resid:** Pediatrics, Lincoln Hosp 1976; **Fellow:** Infectious Disease, UMDNJ-Rutgers Med Sch 1978; Allergy & Immunology, Children's Hosp 1979; **Fac Appt:** Clin Prof Ped, Drexel Univ Coll Med

Leibner, Donald MD (A&I) - **Spec Exp:** Asthma & Allergy; Cough-Chronic; Insect Allergies; **Hospital:** Robert Wood Johnson Univ Hosp - New Brunswick (page 853), St Peter's Univ Hosp; **Address:** 579-A Cranbury Rd, Ste 103, East Brunswick, NJ 08816-5426; **Phone:** 732-390-4900; **Board Cert:** Pediatrics 2003; Allergy & Immunology 2005; **Med School:** SUNY Downstate 1981; **Resid:** Pediatrics, UMDNJ-Rutgers 1984; **Fellow:** Allergy & Immunology, Long Island Coll Hosp 1986

CARDIOVASCULAR DISEASE

Kostis, John B MD (Cv) - **Spec Exp:** Hypertension; Coronary Artery Disease; Cholesterol/Lipid Disorders; **Hospital:** Robert Wood Johnson Univ Hosp - New Brunswick (page 853), St Peter's Univ Hosp; **Address:** 125 Paterson St, Ste 5200, New Brunswick, NJ 08903-0019; **Phone:** 732-235-7685; **Board Cert:** Internal Medicine 1973; Cardiovascular Disease 1973; **Med School:** Greece 1960; **Resid:** Internal Medicine, Evanglismos Hosp 1964; Internal Medicine, Cumberland Med Ctr 1967; **Fellow:** Cardiovascular Disease, Philadelphia Genl Hosp 1969; **Fac Appt:** Prof Med, UMDNJ-RW Johnson Med Sch

Lauer, Robert MD (Cv) - **Spec Exp:** Nuclear Cardiology; **Hospital:** Muhlenberg Regional Med Ctr, Overlook Hosp (page 88); **Address:** Central Jersey Cardiology, 1511 Park Ave, Ste 2, South Plainfield, NJ 07080-5516; **Phone:** 908-756-4438; **Board Cert:** Internal Medicine 1981; Cardiovascular Disease 1985; **Med School:** Columbia P&S 1978; **Resid:** Internal Medicine, Presbyterian Hosp 1981; **Fellow:** Cardiovascular Disease, Presbyterian Hosp 1983

Mermelstein, Erwin MD (Cv) - **Spec Exp:** Cholesterol/Lipid Disorders; Cardiac Catheterization; Coronary Angioplasty/Stents; Congestive Heart Failure; **Hospital:** Robert Wood Johnson Univ Hosp - New Brunswick (page 853), St Peter's Univ Hosp; **Address:** 593 Cranbury Rd, East Brunswick, NJ 08816; **Phone:** 732-390-3333; **Board Cert:** Cardiovascular Disease 1983; Interventional Cardiology 1999; **Med School:** Cornell Univ-Weill Med Coll 1978; **Resid:** Internal Medicine, New York Hosp 1981; **Fellow:** Cardiovascular Disease, Hosp Univ Penn 1983; **Fac Appt:** Assoc Clin Prof Med, Robert W Johnson Med Sch

Mondrow, Daniel MD (Cv) - **Spec Exp:** Cardiac Catheterization; Nuclear Stress Testing; Critical Care Medicine; **Hospital:** JFK Med Ctr - Edison, Robert Wood Johnson Univ Hosp - New Brunswick (page 853); **Address:** 280 Main St, Metuchen, NJ 08840-2429; **Phone:** 732-494-3177; **Board Cert:** Internal Medicine 1979; Cardiovascular Disease 1985; **Med School:** SUNY Downstate 1976; **Resid:** Internal Medicine, Brookdale Hosp Med Ctr 1979; **Fellow:** Cardiovascular Disease, St Vincents Hosp 1981

Shell, Roger MD (Cv) - **Spec Exp:** Coronary Artery Disease; Heart Valve Disease; Cholesterol/Lipid Disorders; **Hospital:** Robert Wood Johnson Univ Hosp - New Brunswick (page 853), St Peter's Univ Hosp; **Address:** 593 Cranberry Rd, East Brunswick, NJ 08816; **Phone:** 732-390-3333; **Board Cert:** Internal Medicine 1980; Cardiovascular Disease 1983; **Med School:** Rutgers Univ 1977; **Resid:** Internal Medicine, Rutgers Med Sch 1980; **Fellow:** Cardiovascular Disease, Presby Hosp-Univ Penn 1982; **Fac Appt:** Asst Clin Prof Med, Robert W Johnson Med Sch

Shindler, Daniel MD (Cv) - **Spec Exp:** Echocardiography; **Hospital:** Robert Wood Johnson Univ Hosp - New Brunswick (page 853); **Address:** Univ Med Grp, 125 Paterson St, Ste 5200, New Brunswick, NJ 08901; **Phone:** 732-235-7854; **Board Cert:** Internal Medicine 1987; Cardiovascular Disease 2002; **Med School:** Spain 1979; **Resid:** Internal Medicine, US Public 1981; Internal Medicine, Robert Wood Johnson Hosp 1984; **Fellow:** Cardiovascular Disease, Robert Wood Johnson Hosp 1983; **Fac Appt:** Assoc Prof Med, UMDNJ-RW Johnson Med Sch

CHILD NEUROLOGY

Wollack, Jan B MD (ChiN) - **Spec Exp:** Epilepsy; Neurodevelopmental Disabilities; **Hospital:** Robert Wood Johnson Univ Hosp - New Brunswick (page 853); **Address:** RW Johnson Professional Ctr, 97 Patterson St, New Brunswick, NJ 08901; **Phone:** 732-235-6230; **Board Cert:** Pediatrics 1988; Child Neurology 1987; Neurodevelopmental Disabilities 2001; **Med School:** Columbia P&S 1981; **Resid:** Pediatrics, Colum-Presby Med Ctr 1983; Neurology, Colum-Presby Med Ctr 1986; **Fac Appt:** Assoc Prof Ped, UMDNJ-RW Johnson Med Sch

CLINICAL GENETICS

Sklower Brooks, Susan MD (CG) - **Spec Exp:** Birth Defects; Inborn Errors of Metabolism; Developmental Disorders; **Hospital:** Robert Wood Johnson Univ Hosp - New Brunswick (page 853); **Address:** Dept of Pediatrics, Div of Med Genetics, 97 Paterson St Fl 4 - rm 445, New Brunswick, NJ 08903; **Phone:** 732-235-6350; **Board Cert:** Pediatrics 1979; Clinical Genetics 1982; Clinical Biochemical Genetics 1984; **Med School:** Mount Sinai Sch Med 1975; **Resid:** Pediatrics, Mount Sinai Hosp 1977; **Fellow:** Clinical Genetics, Mount Sinai Hosp 1979; **Fac Appt:** Assoc Prof Ped, UMDNJ-RW Johnson Med Sch

COLON & RECTAL SURGERY

Eisenstat, Theodore E MD (CRS) - **Spec Exp:** Colon & Rectal Cancer; Inflammatory Bowel Disease; **Hospital:** Robert Wood Johnson Univ Hosp - New Brunswick (page 853), JFK Med Ctr - Edison; **Address:** 3900 Park Ave, Ste 101, Edison, NJ 08820-3032; **Phone:** 732-494-6640; **Board Cert:** Surgery 1974; Colon & Rectal Surgery 1994; **Med School:** NY Med Coll 1968; **Resid:** Surgery, Thomas Jefferson Univ Hosp 1971; Surgery, Pennsylvania Hosp 1973; **Fellow:** Colon & Rectal Surgery, Muhlenberg Med Ctr 1978; **Fac Appt:** Clin Prof S, UMDNJ-RW Johnson Med Sch

Oliver, Gregory C MD (CRS) - **Spec Exp:** Colon & Rectal Cancer; Incontinence-Fecal; Ulcerative Colitis; Crohn's Disease; **Hospital:** JFK Med Ctr - Edison, Muhlenberg Regional Med Ctr; **Address:** 3900 Park Ave, Ste 101, Edison, NJ 08820; **Phone:** 732-494-6640; **Board Cert:** Colon & Rectal Surgery 1986; **Med School:** Geo Wash Univ 1976; **Resid:** Surgery, Geo Wash Univ Med Ctr 1983; Surgery, UMDNJ-Rutgers 1985; **Fac Appt:** Assoc Clin Prof S, UMDNJ-RW Johnson Med Sch

Zinkin, Lewis MD (CRS) - **Spec Exp:** Colon Cancer; Inflammatory Bowel Disease; **Hospital:** Robert Wood Johnson Univ Hosp - New Brunswick (page 853), St Peter's Univ Hosp; **Address:** 620 Cranbury Rd, Ste 111, East Brunswick, NJ 08816; **Phone:** 732-238-2662; **Board Cert:** Colon & Rectal Surgery 1978; Surgery 1986; **Med School:** UMDNJ-NJ Med Sch, Newark 1970; **Resid:** Surgery, St Vincent's Hosp & Med Ctr 1977; Colon & Rectal Surgery, Greater Baltimore Med Ctr 1978; **Fac Appt:** Assoc Clin Prof S, Robert W Johnson Med Sch

DERMATOLOGY

Milgraum, Sandy MD (D) - **Spec Exp:** Skin Laser Surgery; Tattoo Removal; Cosmetic Dermatology; **Hospital:** Robert Wood Johnson Univ Hosp - New Brunswick (page 853); **Address:** Academic Dermatology Ctr, 81 Brunswick Woods Drive, East Brunswick, NJ 08816-5601; **Phone:** 732-613-0300; **Board Cert:** Dermatology 1986; **Med School:** Australia 1983; **Resid:** Dermatology, Univ Mich Hosp 1986; **Fac Appt:** Asst Clin Prof D, Robert W Johnson Med Sch

Pappert, Amy S MD (D) - **Hospital:** Robert Wood Johnson Univ Hosp - New Brunswick (page 853); **Address:** Robert Wood Johnson Univ Hosp, Dermatology, 125 Paterson St, Clin Acad Bldg, Ste 5100B, New Brunswick, NJ 08901; **Phone:** 732-235-7993; **Board Cert:** Dermatology 2001; **Med School:** UMDNJ-RW Johnson Med Sch 1989; **Resid:** Dermatology, Columbia Presby Med Ctr 1994; **Fellow:** Research, Columbia Presby Med Ctr 1991; **Fac Appt:** Asst Prof D, UMDNJ-RW Johnson Med Sch

DIAGNOSTIC RADIOLOGY

Epstein, Robert MD (DR) - **Spec Exp:** MRI; Musculoskeletal Disorders; **Hospital:** Robert Wood Johnson Univ Hosp - New Brunswick (page 853), St Peter's Univ Hosp; **Address:** University Radiology Group, 579A Cranbury Rd Fl 3rd, East Brunswick, NJ 08816; **Phone:** 732-390-0040; **Board Cert:** Diagnostic Radiology 1995; **Med School:** Duke Univ 1990; **Resid:** Diagnostic Radiology, Thomas Jefferson Univ Hosp 1995; **Fellow:** Musculoskeletal Imaging, Hosp Univ Penn 1996

Rosenfeld, David MD (DR) - **Spec Exp:** Pediatric Radiology; **Hospital:** Robert Wood Johnson Univ Hosp - New Brunswick (page 853), St Peter's Univ Hosp; **Address:** Univ Radiology Group, 579A Cranbury Rd Fl 3, East Brunswick, NJ 08816; **Phone:** 732-390-0030; **Board Cert:** Radiology 1972; Pediatric Radiology 1995; **Med School:** Univ Pittsburgh 1967; **Resid:** Radiology, Montefiore Hosp 1971; **Fac Appt:** Clin Prof Rad, UMDNJ-RW Johnson Med Sch

Underberg-Davis, Sharon MD (DR) - **Spec Exp:** Pediatric Radiology; **Hospital:** St Peter's Univ Hosp, Robert Wood Johnson Univ Hosp Hamilton (page 853); **Address:** Univ Radiology Group, 579A Cranbury Rd Fl 3, East Brunswick, NJ 08816; **Phone:** 732-390-0030; **Board Cert:** Diagnostic Radiology 1993; Pediatric Radiology 2004; **Med School:** Harvard Med Sch 1988; **Resid:** Diagnostic Radiology, Hosp Univ Penn 1993; **Fellow:** Pediatric Radiology, Childrens Hosp 1995

ENDOCRINOLOGY, DIABETES & METABOLISM

Agrin, Richard MD (EDM) - **Spec Exp:** Thyroid Disorders; Parathyroid Disease; Diabetes; **Hospital:** Robert Wood Johnson Univ Hosp - New Brunswick (page 853), Somerset Med Ctr; **Address:** 137 Louis St, New Brunswick, NJ 08901; **Phone:** 732-545-1065; **Board Cert:** Internal Medicine 1974; Endocrinology 1977; **Med School:** Univ Pennsylvania 1971; **Resid:** Internal Medicine, USPHS Hosp 1975; **Fellow:** Endocrinology, Boston Univ Hosp 1977; **Fac Appt:** Assoc Clin Prof Med, UMDNJ-RW Johnson Med Sch

Amorosa, Louis MD (EDM) - **Spec Exp:** Diabetes; Endocrine Tumors; Thyroid Disorders; **Hospital:** Robert Wood Johnson Univ Hosp - New Brunswick (page 853); **Address:** Clinic Academic Bldg, 125 Paterson St, New Brunswick, NJ 08901; **Phone:** 732-235-7219; **Board Cert:** Endocrinology, Diabetes & Metabolism 1975; Internal Medicine 1972; **Med School:** UMDNJ-NJ Med Sch, Newark 1969; **Resid:** Internal Medicine, Bronx Municipal Hosps 1972; Internal Medicine, Kings County Hosp 1973; **Fellow:** Endocrinology, Diabetes & Metabolism, Mount Sinai Hosp 1975; **Fac Appt:** Prof Med, UMDNJ-RW Johnson Med Sch

Bucholtz, Harvey K MD (EDM) - **Spec Exp:** Diabetes; Thyroid Disorders; Osteoporosis; **Hospital:** JFK Med Ctr - Edison, Newark Beth Israel Med Ctr; **Address:** 2 Lincoln Hwy, Ste 501, Edison, NJ 08820; **Phone:** 732-549-7470; **Board Cert:** Internal Medicine 1973; Endocrinology 1975; **Med School:** SUNY Hlth Sci Ctr 1968; **Resid:** Internal Medicine, Univ Michigan Med Ctr 1971; **Fellow:** Endocrinology, Duke Univ Med Ctr 1975; **Fac Appt:** Asst Clin Prof Med, UMDNJ-NJ Med Sch, Newark

Maman, Arie MD (EDM) - **Spec Exp:** Thyroid Disorders; Diabetes; Pituitary Disorders; **Hospital:** Robert Wood Johnson Univ Hosp - New Brunswick (page 853), St Peter's Univ Hosp; **Address:** D3 Brier Hill Ct, East Brunswick, NJ 08816-3335; **Phone:** 732-613-0707; **Board Cert:** Internal Medicine 1977; Endocrinology, Diabetes & Metabolism 1979; **Med School:** France 1974; **Resid:** Internal Medicine, Jewish Hosp 1975; Internal Medicine, Jewish Hosp 1977; **Fellow:** Endocrinology, Diabetes & Metabolism, Univ Colorado Med Ctr 1979; **Fac Appt:** Assoc Clin Prof Med, UMDNJ-RW Johnson Med Sch

Spiler, Ira MD (EDM) - **Spec Exp:** Pituitary Disorders; Thyroid Disorders; Calcium Disorders; **Hospital:** Raritan Bay Med Ctr - Perth Amboy, Robert Wood Johnson Univ Hosp - New Brunswick (page 853); **Address:** 3 Hospital Plz, Ste 307, Old Bridge, NJ 08857-3095; **Phone:** 732-360-1122; **Board Cert:** Internal Medicine 1976; Endocrinology, Diabetes & Metabolism 1979; **Med School:** Albert Einstein Coll Med 1971; **Resid:** Internal Medicine, Bronx Municipal Hosp 1973; Internal Medicine, Boston City Hosp 1976; **Fellow:** Endocrinology, Tufts-New England Med Ctr 1978; **Fac Appt:** Assoc Clin Prof Med, UMDNJ-RW Johnson Med Sch

Family Medicine

Lansing, Martha MD (FMed) `PCP` - **Spec Exp:** Psychosomatic Disorders; Women's Health; **Hospital:** Capital Health Sys - Fuld Campus; **Address:** 666 Plainsboro Rd, Ste 640, Plainsboro, NJ 08536; **Phone:** 609-275-0487; **Board Cert:** Family Medicine 1998; **Med School:** Univ Okla Coll Med 1982; **Resid:** Family Medicine, Univ Tenn 1984; Family Medicine, Williamsport Hosp/Univ Penn 1985; **Fac Appt:** Assoc Prof FMed, UMDNJ-RW Johnson Med Sch

Swee, David MD (FMed) `PCP` - **Hospital:** Robert Wood Johnson Univ Hosp - New Brunswick (page 853), St Peter's Univ Hosp; **Address:** 317 George St, New Brunswick, NJ 08901-1977; **Phone:** 732-235-8993; **Board Cert:** Family Medicine 2001; **Med School:** Canada 1974; **Resid:** Family Medicine, Somerset Med Ctr 1977; **Fac Appt:** Prof FMed, UMDNJ-RW Johnson Med Sch

Tierney, Peter MD (FMed) `PCP` - **Hospital:** Univ Med Ctr - Princeton; **Address:** 666 Plainsboro Rd, Ste 1316, Plainsboro, NJ 08536; **Phone:** 609-275-8100; **Board Cert:** Family Medicine 1999; **Med School:** Univ VA Sch Med 1983; **Resid:** Family Medicine, Hunterdon Med Ctr 1986

Winter, Robin Okner MD (FMed) `PCP` - **Spec Exp:** Geriatric Medicine; **Hospital:** JFK Med Ctr - Edison; **Address:** JFK Med Ctr - Family Practice Ctr, 65 James St, Edison, NJ 08818; **Phone:** 732-321-7487; **Board Cert:** Family Medicine 2005; Geriatric Medicine 1997; **Med School:** Albert Einstein Coll Med 1978; **Resid:** Family Medicine, Hunterdon Med Ctr 1981; **Fac Appt:** Assoc Clin Prof FMed, UMDNJ-RW Johnson Med Sch

Gastroenterology

Hodes, Steven MD (Ge) - **Hospital:** Raritan Bay Med Ctr - Perth Amboy, JFK Med Ctr - Edison; **Address:** 205 May St, Ste 201, Edison, NJ 08837; **Phone:** 732-661-9225; **Board Cert:** Internal Medicine 1977; Gastroenterology 1979; **Med School:** Albert Einstein Coll Med 1974; **Resid:** Internal Medicine, Montefiore Hosp Med Ctr 1976; **Fellow:** Gastroenterology, Mount Sinai -Bronx VA Hosps 1977

Lenger, Ellis S MD (Ge) - **Spec Exp:** Biliary Disease; Peptic Ulcer Disease; **Hospital:** Robert Wood Johnson Univ Hosp - New Brunswick (page 853), St Peter's Univ Hosp; **Address:** Gastroenterology, 465 Cranbury Rd, Ste 102, East Brunswick, NJ 08816-5405; **Phone:** 732-390-1995; **Board Cert:** Internal Medicine 1982; Gastroenterology 1987; **Med School:** SUNY Downstate 1979; **Resid:** Internal Medicine, NY Hosp 1982; Gastroenterology, Beth Israel 1984; **Fac Appt:** Asst Clin Prof Med, UMDNJ-RW Johnson Med Sch

Pitchumoni, Capecomorin S MD (Ge) - **Spec Exp:** Pancreatic Disease; Gastroesophageal Reflux Disease (GERD); **Hospital:** St Peter's Univ Hosp; **Address:** St Peters Univ Hosp, 254 Easton Ave CARES Bldg Fl 4 - Ste 4013, New Brunswick, NJ 08903; **Phone:** 732-745-7939; **Board Cert:** Internal Medicine 1977; Gastroenterology 1971; **Med School:** India 1960; **Resid:** Internal Medicine, Norwalk Hosp 1968; **Fellow:** Gastroenterology, Yale New Haven Hosp 1969Metropolitan Hosp Ctr 1971; **Fac Appt:** Clin Prof Med, Robert W Johnson Med Sch

Plumser, Allan MD (Ge) - **Spec Exp:** Endoscopy; Pancreatic/Biliary Endoscopy (ERCP); Liver Disease; **Hospital:** Robert Wood Johnson Univ Hosp - New Brunswick (page 853), St Peter's Univ Hosp; **Address:** 265 Cranbury Rd, Ste 102, East Brunswick, NJ 08816; **Phone:** 732-390-1995; **Board Cert:** Internal Medicine 1981; Gastroenterology 1983; **Med School:** NY Med Coll 1978; **Resid:** Internal Medicine, SUNY Stonybrook Med Ctr 1981; **Fellow:** Gastroenterology, SUNY Stonybrook Med Ctr 1983; **Fac Appt:** Asst Prof Med, UMDNJ-RW Johnson Med Sch

Rosenheck, David MD (Ge) - **Hospital:** JFK Med Ctr - Edison, Raritan Bay Med Ctr - Old Bridge Div; **Address:** 205 May St, Ste 201, Edison, NJ 08837; **Phone:** 732-661-9225; **Board Cert:** Internal Medicine 1986; Gastroenterology 1989; **Med School:** UMDNJ-NJ Med Sch, Newark 1983; **Resid:** Internal Medicine, UMDNJ Med Ctr 1986; **Fellow:** Gastroenterology, UMDNJ Med Ctr 1988

GERIATRIC MEDICINE

Bullock, Richard B MD (Ger) `PCP` - **Spec Exp:** Hypertension; Cholesterol/Lipid Disorders; Dementia; **Hospital:** JFK Med Ctr - Edison, Muhlenberg Regional Med Ctr; **Address:** 224 May St, Ste E, Edison, NJ 08837-3266; **Phone:** 732-661-2020; **Board Cert:** Internal Medicine 1984; Geriatric Medicine 2000; **Med School:** Mount Sinai Sch Med 1981; **Resid:** Internal Medicine, Mt Sinai Hosp 1984; **Fac Appt:** Asst Clin Prof Med, Robert W Johnson Med Sch

Leventhal, Elaine MD/PhD (Ger) - **Spec Exp:** Behavioral Disorders; Women's Health; **Hospital:** Robert Wood Johnson Univ Hosp - New Brunswick (page 853); **Address:** 125 Paterson St, Ste 2300, New Brunswick, NJ 08901-1962; **Phone:** 732-235-6968; **Board Cert:** Internal Medicine 1979; Geriatric Medicine 2000; **Med School:** Univ Wisc 1974; **Resid:** Internal Medicine, Univ Wisconsin Hosp 1977; **Fellow:** Geriatric Medicine, William S Middleton/VA Meml Hosp 1981; **Fac Appt:** Prof Med, UMDNJ-RW Johnson Med Sch

GYNECOLOGIC ONCOLOGY

Carlson, John MD (GO) - **Spec Exp:** Gynecologic Cancer; Ovarian Cancer; Gynecologic Surgery-Complex; **Hospital:** St Peter's Univ Hosp; **Address:** St Peter's University Hosp, 254 Easton Ave, New Brunswick, NJ 08901; **Phone:** 732-937-6003; **Board Cert:** Obstetrics & Gynecology 1981; Gynecologic Oncology 1982; **Med School:** Georgetown Univ 1974; **Resid:** Obstetrics & Gynecology, Hartford Hosp 1975; Obstetrics & Gynecology, Hosp Univ Penn 1978; **Fellow:** Gynecologic Oncology, MD Anderson Hosp 1980; **Fac Appt:** Prof ObG, UMDNJ-RW Johnson Med Sch

Goldberg, Michael I MD (GO) - **Spec Exp:** Ovarian Cancer; Uterine Cancer; **Hospital:** St Peter's Univ Hosp, Robert Wood Johnson Univ Hosp - New Brunswick (page 853); **Address:** 78 Easton Ave, New Brunswick, NJ 08901-1865; **Phone:** 732-828-3300; **Board Cert:** Obstetrics & Gynecology 1977; Gynecologic Oncology 1980; **Med School:** Italy 1970; **Resid:** Obstetrics & Gynecology, Maimonides Med Ctr 1975; **Fellow:** Gynecologic Oncology, Jackson Meml Hosp 1977; **Fac Appt:** Clin Prof ObG, UMDNJ-RW Johnson Med Sch

Rodriguez, Lorna MD/PhD (GO) - **Spec Exp:** Ovarian Cancer; Cervical Cancer; **Hospital:** Robert Wood Johnson Univ Hosp - New Brunswick (page 853); **Address:** Cancer Institute of New Jersey, 195 Little Albany St, rm 2001, New Brunswick, NJ 08903; **Phone:** 732-235-6777; **Board Cert:** Obstetrics & Gynecology 1997; Gynecologic Oncology 1997; **Med School:** Puerto Rico 1979; **Resid:** Obstetrics & Gynecology, Cooper Med CtrHo 1983; **Fellow:** Gynecologic Oncology, Univ Michigan 1985

HAND SURGERY

Coyle, Michael P MD (HS) - **Spec Exp:** Arthritis Hand Surgery; Nerve Compression; Dupuytren's Contracture; **Hospital:** Robert Wood Johnson Univ Hosp - New Brunswick (page 853), St Peter's Univ Hosp; **Address:** 215 Easton Ave, New Brunswick, NJ 08901-1722; **Phone:** 732-545-0400; **Board Cert:** Orthopaedic Surgery 2005; Hand Surgery 2000; **Med School:** Columbia P&S 1968; **Resid:** Surgery, UCSF-Moffitt Hosp 1970; Orthopaedic Surgery, NY Orth Hosp 1976; **Fellow:** NY Orth Hosp 1973; Hand Surgery, NY Orth Hosp 1977; **Fac Appt:** Clin Prof OrS, UMDNJ-RW Johnson Med Sch

HEMATOLOGY

Karp, George MD (Hem) - **Spec Exp:** Coagulation Disorders; Anemia; Breast Cancer; **Hospital:** Robert Wood Johnson Univ Hosp - New Brunswick (page 853), St Peter's Univ Hosp; **Address:** 205 Easton Ave, New Brunswick, NJ 08901; **Phone:** 732-828-9570; **Board Cert:** Internal Medicine 1979; Medical Oncology 1981; Hematology 1982; **Med School:** Columbia P&S 1976; **Resid:** Internal Medicine, Univ Chicago Hosps 1978; **Fellow:** Medical Oncology, Natl Cancer Inst 1979; Hematology, Dana Farber Cancer Inst 1982; **Fac Appt:** Clin Prof Med, Robert W Johnson Med Sch

Saidi, Parvin MD (Hem) - **Spec Exp:** Bleeding/Coagulation Disorders; **Hospital:** Robert Wood Johnson Univ Hosp - New Brunswick (page 853); **Address:** One Robert Wood Johnson Pl Fl 3, Box 19, New Brunswick, NJ 08901-1928; **Phone:** 732-235-7679; **Board Cert:** Internal Medicine 1974; Hematology 1974; Medical Oncology 1979; **Med School:** Harvard Med Sch 1956; **Resid:** Internal Medicine, UCSF Med Ctr 1961; **Fellow:** Hematology, UCSF Med Ctr 1964; **Fac Appt:** Prof Med, Robert W Johnson Med Sch

Strair, Roger MD/PhD (Hem) - **Spec Exp:** Leukemia; Lymphoma; Bone Marrow Transplant; **Hospital:** Robert Wood Johnson Univ Hosp - New Brunswick (page 853), St Peter's Univ Hosp; **Address:** Cancer Inst of NJ, 195 Little Albany St, New Brunswick, NJ 08901; **Phone:** 732-235-6044; **Board Cert:** Internal Medicine 1984; Hematology 1986; Medical Oncology 1987; **Med School:** Albert Einstein Coll Med 1981; **Resid:** Internal Medicine, Brigham & Women's Hosp 1984; **Fellow:** Hematology & Oncology, Brigham & Women's Hosp 1988; **Fac Appt:** Assoc Prof Med, UMDNJ-RW Johnson Med Sch

INFECTIOUS DISEASE

Middleton, John R MD (Inf) - **Spec Exp:** AIDS/HIV; Osteomyelitis; **Hospital:** Raritan Bay Med Ctr - Perth Amboy; **Address:** Raritan Bay Infectious Disease, 1 Hospital Plaza, Ste 208, Old Bridge, NJ 08857-3093; **Phone:** 732-360-2700; **Board Cert:** Internal Medicine 1973; Infectious Disease 1980; **Med School:** UMDNJ-NJ Med Sch, Newark 1970; **Resid:** Internal Medicine, NY Hosp-Cornell Med Ctr 1973; **Fellow:** Infectious Disease, RWJ Univ Hosp 1977; **Fac Appt:** Assoc Clin Prof Med, Rutgers Univ

Sensakovic, John W MD/PhD (Inf) - **Spec Exp:** Lyme Disease; Fevers of Unknown Origin; Bone Infections; **Hospital:** Saint Michael's Med Ctr, JFK Med Ctr - Edison; **Address:** 113 James St, Edison, NJ 08820; **Phone:** 732-549-3449; **Board Cert:** Internal Medicine 1982; Infectious Disease 1984; **Med School:** UMDNJ-NJ Med Sch, Newark 1977; **Resid:** Internal Medicine, St Michael's Med Ctr 1980; **Fellow:** Infectious Disease, St Michael's Med Ctr 1982; **Fac Appt:** Prof Med, Seton Hall Univ Sch Grad Med Ed

Weinstein, Melvin P MD (Inf) - **Spec Exp:** Bone/Joint Infections; Infective Endocarditis; **Hospital:** Robert Wood Johnson Univ Hosp - New Brunswick (page 853); **Address:** 1 Robert Wood Johnson Pl, New Brunswick, NJ 08901-1928; **Phone:** 732-235-7713; **Board Cert:** Internal Medicine 1975; Infectious Disease 1978; Medical Microbiology 1983; **Med School:** Geo Wash Univ 1970; **Resid:** Internal Medicine, Hartford Hosp 1975; **Fellow:** Infectious Disease, Univ Colo Hosp 1977; **Fac Appt:** Prof Med, UMDNJ-RW Johnson Med Sch

INTERNAL MEDICINE

Carson, Jeffrey MD (IM) `PCP` - **Hospital:** Robert Wood Johnson Univ Hosp - New Brunswick (page 853); **Address:** 125 Paterson St, Ste 5, New Brunswick, NJ 08901; **Phone:** 732-235-6968; **Board Cert:** Internal Medicine 1980; **Med School:** Hahnemann Univ 1977; **Resid:** Internal Medicine, Hahnemann Univ Hosp 1980; **Fellow:** Internal Medicine, Hosp Univ Penn 1982; **Fac Appt:** Prof Med, UMDNJ-RW Johnson Med Sch

Cassidy, Brian MD (IM) `PCP` - **Hospital:** Muhlenberg Regional Med Ctr; **Address:** 3910 Park Ave, Ste 8, Edison, NJ 08820; **Phone:** 732-767-3130; **Board Cert:** Internal Medicine 1988; **Med School:** Grenada 1985; **Resid:** Internal Medicine, Muhlenberg Med Ctr 1988

DeSilva Jr, Derrick M MD (IM) - **Spec Exp:** Complementary Medicine; Preventive Cardiology; **Hospital:** Raritan Bay Med Ctr - Perth Amboy; **Address:** 629 Amboy Ave Fl 2, Edison, NJ 08837; **Phone:** 732-738-8801; **Med School:** Dominican Republic 1982; **Resid:** Internal Medicine, Raritan Bay Med Ctr-Perth Amboy Div 1988

Gil, Constante MD (IM) `PCP` - **Spec Exp:** Hypertension; Diabetes; Heart Failure; **Hospital:** Raritan Bay Med Ctr - Perth Amboy; **Address:** 220 Market St, Ste 2, Perth Amboy, NJ 08861; **Phone:** 732-826-1609; **Board Cert:** Internal Medicine 2000; **Med School:** Dominican Republic 1981; **Resid:** Internal Medicine, Raritan Bay Med Ctr-Perth Amboy Div 1989; **Fac Appt:** Assoc Clin Prof Med, UMDNJ-RW Johnson Med Sch

Guillen, Gregorio MD (IM) `PCP` - **Spec Exp:** Geriatric Medicine; **Hospital:** Raritan Bay Med Ctr - Perth Amboy, JFK Med Ctr - Edison; **Address:** 796 Amboy Ave, Peth Amboy, NJ 08861; **Phone:** 732-442-6020; **Board Cert:** Internal Medicine 1998; **Med School:** Dominican Republic 1982; **Resid:** Internal Medicine, Raritan Bay Med Ctr 1990; **Fellow:** Geriatric Medicine, Univ Florida 1992

INTERVENTIONAL CARDIOLOGY

Altmann, Dory B MD (IC) - **Hospital:** Robert Wood Johnson Univ Hosp - New Brunswick (page 853); **Address:** Cardiology Assocs of New Brunswick, 593 Cranbury Rd, East Brunswick, NJ 08816; **Phone:** 732-390-3333; **Board Cert:** Internal Medicine 1989; Cardiovascular Disease 2000; Interventional Cardiology 1999; **Med School:** Yale Univ 1986; **Resid:** Internal Medicine, New England Med Ctr 1989; **Fellow:** Cardiovascular Disease, Mt Sinai Hosp 1992; Interventional Cardiology, Washington Hosp Ctr 1993; **Fac Appt:** Asst Clin Prof Med, UMDNJ-RW Johnson Med Sch

MATERNAL & FETAL MEDICINE

Benito, Carlos W MD (MF) - **Spec Exp:** Pregnancy Loss; Prenatal Diagnosis; **Hospital:** St Peter's Univ Hosp; **Address:** St Peters Univ Hosp, Dept Maternal-Fetal Med, 254 Easton Ave, MOB 4, New Brunswick, NJ 08903; **Phone:** 732-745-8549; **Board Cert:** Obstetrics & Gynecology 1997; Maternal & Fetal Medicine 1999; **Med School:** UMDNJ-RW Johnson Med Sch 1993; **Resid:** Obstetrics & Gynecology, UMDNJ-RWJ Med Ctr 1997; **Fellow:** Maternal & Fetal Medicine, UMDNJ-RWJ Med Ctr 1999

Thornton, Yvonne S MD (MF) - **Spec Exp:** Ultrasound; Chorionic Villus Sampling; Prenatal Diagnosis; **Hospital:** St Peter's Univ Hosp; **Address:** St Peter's Univ Hosp, Maternal/Fetal Medicine, 254 Easton Ave, New Brunswick, NJ 08901; **Phone:** 732-745-8549; **Board Cert:** Obstetrics & Gynecology 1998; Maternal & Fetal Medicine 1998; **Med School:** Columbia P&S 1973; **Resid:** Obstetrics & Gynecology, St Luke's-Roosevelt Hosp Ctr 1977; **Fellow:** Maternal & Fetal Medicine, Sloane Hosp/Columbia Presby Med Ctr 1979

Vintzileos, Anthony M MD (MF) - **Spec Exp:** Ultrasound; Fetal Therapy; **Hospital:** Robert Wood Johnson Univ Hosp - New Brunswick (page 853); **Address:** RW Johnson Med Sch, Dept Ob/Gyn, 125 Paterson St, Clin Acad Bldg, rm 2150, New Brunswick, NJ 08901; **Phone:** 732-235-6600; **Board Cert:** Obstetrics & Gynecology 1999; Maternal & Fetal Medicine 1999; **Med School:** Greece 1975; **Resid:** Obstetrics & Gynecology, St Josephs Hosp Med Ctr 1981; **Fellow:** Maternal & Fetal Medicine, Univ Conn Hlth Ctr 1983; **Fac Appt:** Prof ObG, UMDNJ-RW Johnson Med Sch

MEDICAL ONCOLOGY

Aisner, Joseph MD (Onc) - **Spec Exp:** Lung Cancer; Solid Tumors; **Hospital:** Robert Wood Johnson Univ Hosp - New Brunswick (page 853); **Address:** Cancer Inst of New Jersey, 195 Little Albany St, rm 2012, New Brunswick, NJ 08903-2681; **Phone:** 732-235-6777; **Board Cert:** Internal Medicine 1973; Medical Oncology 1975; **Med School:** Wayne State Univ 1970; **Resid:** Internal Medicine, Georgetown Univ Hosp 1972; **Fellow:** Medical Oncology, Natl Cancer Inst 1975

Hait, William MD/PhD (Onc) - **Spec Exp:** Breast Cancer; **Hospital:** Robert Wood Johnson Univ Hosp - New Brunswick (page 853); **Address:** Cancer Inst of NJ, 195 Little Albany St, New Brunswick, NJ 08901-1914; **Phone:** 732-235-8064; **Board Cert:** Internal Medicine 1982; Medical Oncology 1987; **Med School:** Med Coll PA 1978; **Resid:** Internal Medicine, Yale-New Haven Hosp 1982; **Fellow:** Medical Oncology, Yale Univ Sch Med 1983; **Fac Appt:** Prof Med, UMDNJ-RW Johnson Med Sch

Miskoff, A Richard DO (Onc) - **Spec Exp:** Breast Cancer; Lung Cancer; **Hospital:** JFK Med Ctr - Edison, Raritan Bay Med Ctr - Old Bridge Div; **Address:** 3 Hospital Plaza, Fl 2 - Ste 203, Old Bridge, NJ 08857-3093; **Phone:** 732-360-2280; **Board Cert:** Internal Medicine 1974; Hematology 1982; Medical Oncology 1975; **Med School:** Univ Hlth Sci, Coll Osteo Med 1968; **Resid:** Internal Medicine, Detroit Osteopathic Hosp 1970; Internal Medicine, Brooke Army Med Ctr 1972; **Fellow:** Hematology & Oncology, Walter Reed Hosp 1974; **Fac Appt:** Asst Clin Prof Med, UMDNJ-RW Johnson Med Sch

Nissenblatt, Michael MD (Onc) - **Spec Exp:** Breast Cancer; Colon Cancer; Hereditary Cancer; Familial Cancer; **Hospital:** Robert Wood Johnson Univ Hosp - New Brunswick (page 853), St Peter's Univ Hosp; **Address:** 205 Easton Ave, New Brunswick, NJ 08901-1722; **Phone:** 732-828-9570; **Board Cert:** Internal Medicine 1976; Medical Oncology 1979; **Med School:** Columbia P&S 1973; **Resid:** Internal Medicine, Johns Hopkins Hosp 1976; **Fellow:** Medical Oncology, Johns Hopkins Hosp 1978; **Fac Appt:** Clin Prof Med, Robert W Johnson Med Sch

Salwitz, James MD (Onc) - **Hospital:** St Peter's Univ Hosp, Robert Wood Johnson Univ Hosp Hamilton (page 853); **Address:** Central Jersey Oncology Ctr, Brierhill Ct, J2 Bldg, East Brunswick, NJ 08816; **Phone:** 732-828-9570; **Board Cert:** Internal Medicine 1984; Medical Oncology 1987; **Med School:** Rutgers Univ 1981; **Resid:** Internal Medicine, Northwestern Univ/ McGaw Med Ctr 1984; **Fellow:** Medical Oncology, NIH-Natl Canc Inst 1987

Shypula, Gregory MD (Onc) - **Spec Exp:** Hematology; **Hospital:** Raritan Bay Med Ctr - Perth Amboy, JFK Med Ctr - Edison; **Address:** 1030 St Georges Ave, Ste 307, Avenel, NJ 07001-1330; **Phone:** 732-750-1200; **Board Cert:** Internal Medicine 1989; Medical Oncology 2001; Hematology 1997; **Med School:** Poland 1981; **Resid:** Internal Medicine, T Marciniak Univ 1984; Internal Medicine, Raritan Bay Med Ctr-Perth Amboy Div 1988; **Fellow:** Hematology & Oncology, St Luke's-Roosevelt Hosp Ctr 1992; **Fac Appt:** Assoc Clin Prof Med, Columbia P&S

Toppmeyer, Deborah MD (Onc) - **Spec Exp:** Breast Cancer; Hereditary Cancer; **Hospital:** Robert Wood Johnson Univ Hosp - New Brunswick (page 853), St Peter's Univ Hosp; **Address:** Cancer Inst of New Jersey, 195 Little Albany St, New Brunswick, NJ 08901-1914; **Phone:** 732-235-6777; **Board Cert:** Internal Medicine 1988; Medical Oncology 1993; **Med School:** Albany Med Coll 1985; **Resid:** Internal Medicine, Univ Pittsburgh Hlth Ctr Hosp 1988; **Fellow:** Oncology, Dana Farber Cancer Inst 1993

NEONATAL-PERINATAL MEDICINE

Hiatt, I Mark MD (NP) - **Spec Exp:** Respiratory Failure; Prematurity/Low Birth Weight Infants; Ethics; **Hospital:** St Peter's Univ Hosp, Robert Wood Johnson Univ Hosp - New Brunswick (page 853); **Address:** St Peter's Univ Hosp, Div Neonatal Med, 254 Easton Ave, New Brunswick, NJ 08903; **Phone:** 732-745-8523; **Board Cert:** Pediatrics 1978; Neonatal-Perinatal Medicine 1979; **Med School:** Cornell Univ-Weill Med Coll 1972; **Resid:** Pediatrics, New York Hosp 1975; **Fellow:** Neonatal-Perinatal Medicine, Babies Hosp-Columbia Univ 1977; **Fac Appt:** Prof Ped, UMDNJ-RW Johnson Med Sch

Lambert, George MD (NP) - **Spec Exp:** Environmental Toxicology-Autism; Neonatal Critical Care; **Hospital:** Robert Wood Johnson Univ Hosp - New Brunswick (page 853); **Address:** 170 Frelinghuysen Rd, Piscataway, NJ 08854; **Phone:** 732-235-7900; **Board Cert:** Pediatrics 1979; Neonatal-Perinatal Medicine 1979; **Med School:** Univ IL Coll Med 1972; **Resid:** Pediatrics, Johns Hopkins Hosp 1974; **Fellow:** Pharmacology, Natl Inst Hlth 1976; Neonatal-Perinatal Medicine, Chldns Hosp 1978; **Fac Appt:** Assoc Prof Ped, UMDNJ-RW Johnson Med Sch

Mehta, Rajeev MD (NP) - **Spec Exp:** Neonatal Critical Care; **Hospital:** Robert Wood Johnson Univ Hosp - New Brunswick (page 853); **Address:** RW Johnson Med Sch-UMDNJ, 1 RW Johnson Pl, MEB 348, New Brunswick, NJ 08903-1766; **Phone:** 732-235-7036; **Board Cert:** Pediatrics 2001; Neonatal-Perinatal Medicine 2001; **Med School:** India 1979; **Resid:** Pediatrics, Queens Park/St Mary's/Dudley Rd Hosps 1985; Pediatrics, Univ Hosp 1990; **Fellow:** Neonatology, Bradford Royal Infirmary 1989; Neonatology, North Shore Univ Hosp 1993; **Fac Appt:** Assoc Prof Ped, UMDNJ-RW Johnson Med Sch

NEPHROLOGY

Covit, Andrew MD (Nep) - **Spec Exp:** Hypertension; Kidney Failure; Renovascular Disease; **Hospital:** Robert Wood Johnson Univ Hosp - New Brunswick (page 853), St Peter's Univ Hosp; **Address:** 8 Old Bridge Tpke, South River, NJ 08882; **Phone:** 732-390-4888; **Board Cert:** Internal Medicine 1982; Nephrology 1986; **Med School:** SUNY Downstate 1979; **Resid:** Internal Medicine, NY Hosp 1982; **Fellow:** Nephrology, NY Hosp 1984; **Fac Appt:** Assoc Clin Prof Med, UMDNJ-RW Johnson Med Sch

Sherman, Richard A MD (Nep) - **Spec Exp:** Dialysis Care; Fluid & Electrolyte Disorders; **Hospital:** Robert Wood Johnson Univ Hosp - New Brunswick (page 853); **Address:** 1 RJ Johnson Pl, Box 19, Dept Med-Nephrology, New Brunswick, NJ 08903-0019; **Phone:** 732-235-6512; **Board Cert:** Internal Medicine 1978; Nephrology 1980; **Med School:** Albert Einstein Coll Med 1975; **Resid:** Internal Medicine, Metropolitan Hosp 1977; **Fellow:** Nephrology, Albert Einstein 1979; **Fac Appt:** Prof Med, Robert W Johnson Med Sch

NEUROLOGICAL SURGERY

Nosko, Michael MD/PhD (NS) - **Spec Exp:** Aneurysm-Cerebral; Brain Tumors; Pituitary Tumors; Cerebrovascular Neurosurgery; **Hospital:** Robert Wood Johnson Univ Hosp - New Brunswick (page 853), Univ Med Ctr - Princeton; **Address:** 125 Paterson St, CAB - Ste 2100, New Brunswick, NJ 08903; **Phone:** 732-235-7757; **Board Cert:** Neurological Surgery 1993; **Med School:** Univ Toronto 1982; **Resid:** Neurological Surgery, Toronto Genl Hosp 1986; Neurological Surgery, Walter Mackenzie Ctr 1991; **Fellow:** Research, Alberta Heritage Fdn Med Rsch 1986; **Fac Appt:** Assoc Prof NS, UMDNJ-RW Johnson Med Sch

Ruzicka, Petr MD (NS) - **Spec Exp:** Craniofacial Surgery; Spinal Cord Surgery-Pediatric; Pediatric Neurosurgery; **Hospital:** Robert Wood Johnson Univ Hosp - New Brunswick (page 853); **Address:** 125 Paterson St, Ste 2100, Clinical Academic Bldg - Ped Neurosurgery, New Brunswick, NJ 08901; **Phone:** 732-235-7756; **Board Cert:** Neurological Surgery 1990; Pediatric Neurological Surgery 1998; **Med School:** Univ Minn 1974; **Resid:** Surgery, Univ Hawaii Hosp 1978; Neurological Surgery, Fairview Univ Med Ctr 1983; **Fellow:** Pediatric Neurological Surgery, Univ Minnesota Hosp 1983; **Fac Appt:** Assoc Prof NS, UMDNJ-RW Johnson Med Sch

NEUROLOGY

Gizzi, Martin MD/PhD (N) - **Spec Exp:** Neuro-Ophthalmology; Balance Disorders; Progressive Supranuclear Palsy (PSP); **Hospital:** JFK Med Ctr - Edison, Muhlenberg Regional Med Ctr; **Address:** NJ Neuroscience Insitute, 65 James St, Edison, NJ 08820-3947; **Phone:** 732-321-7010; **Board Cert:** Neurology 1990; **Med School:** Univ Miami Sch Med 1985; **Resid:** Neurology, Mount Sinai Hosp 1989; **Fellow:** Neurological Ophthalmology, Mount Sinai Hosp 1991; **Fac Appt:** Prof N, Seton Hall Univ Sch Grad Med Ed

Golbe, Lawrence MD (N) - **Spec Exp:** Parkinson's Disease; Progressive Supranuclear Palsy (PSP); Movement Disorders; **Hospital:** Robert Wood Johnson Univ Hosp - New Brunswick (page 853); **Address:** 97 Paterson St, rm 208, New Brunswick, NJ 08901-2160; **Phone:** 732 235-7733; **Board Cert:** Neurology 1984; **Med School:** NYU Sch Med 1978; **Resid:** Internal Medicine, Hahnemann Univ Hosp 1980; Neurology, Bellevue Hosp 1983; **Fac Appt:** Prof N, UMDNJ-RW Johnson Med Sch

Lazar, Mark H MD (N) - **Spec Exp:** Headache; Pain Management; Acupuncture; **Hospital:** Robert Wood Johnson Univ Hosp - New Brunswick (page 853); **Address:** 573 Cranbury Rd, Ste A5, East Brunswick, NJ 08816-4026; **Phone:** 732-254-5101; **Board Cert:** Neurology 1982; **Med School:** NYU Sch Med 1977; **Resid:** Neurology, NYU Med Ctr 1981; **Fellow:** Neurology, NY-Cornell Med Ctr 1982; Clinical Neurophysiology, Columbia-Presby Med Ctr 1983; **Fac Appt:** Asst Prof N, UMDNJ-RW Johnson Med Sch

Lepore, Frederick MD (N) - **Spec Exp:** Neuro-Ophthalmology; Botox Therapy for Blepharospasm; Migraine; Epilepsy; **Hospital:** Robert Wood Johnson Univ Hosp - New Brunswick (page 853); **Address:** Dept Neurology, 97 Paterson St, rm 225, New Brunswick, NJ 08901-2160; **Phone:** 732-235-7731; **Board Cert:** Neurology 1981; **Med School:** Univ Rochester 1975; **Resid:** Internal Medicine, Univ Michigan Med Ctr 1976; Neurology, Univ Virginia Hlth Sci Ctr 1979; **Fellow:** Neurological Ophthalmology, Bascom Palmer Eye Inst 1980; **Fac Appt:** Prof N, Robert W Johnson Med Sch

Oh, Youn MD (N) - **Spec Exp:** Headache; Stroke; **Hospital:** JFK Med Ctr - Edison, Robert Wood Johnson Univ Hosp at Rahway (page 853); **Address:** 34-36 Progress St, Ste B3, Edison, NJ 08820; **Phone:** 908-757-6633; **Board Cert:** Neurology 1979; Psychiatry 1981; **Med School:** South Korea 1964; **Resid:** Neurology, UMDNJ-NJ Med Sch 1975; Psychiatry, Harvard Psy Svc/Boston City Hosp 1973; **Fac Appt:** Assoc Clin Prof N, UMDNJ-RW Johnson Med Sch

Rosenberg, Michael MD (N) - **Spec Exp:** Neuro-Ophthalmology; Neuro-Otology; Balance Disorders; **Hospital:** JFK Med Ctr - Edison; **Address:** New Jersey Neuroscience Inst, 65 James St, Edison, NJ 08818; **Phone:** 732-321-7010; **Board Cert:** Neurology 1983; **Med School:** Baylor Coll Med 1976; **Resid:** Neurology, Letterman AMC 1981; **Fellow:** Neurological Ophthalmology, Bascom-Palmer Eye Inst 1981; **Fac Appt:** Prof N, Seton Hall Univ Sch Grad Med Ed

Sage, Jacob MD (N) - **Spec Exp:** Parkinson's Disease; **Hospital:** Robert Wood Johnson Univ Hosp - New Brunswick (page 853); **Address:** UMDNJ, Dept Neurology, 97 Paterson St, New Brunswick, NJ 08901; **Phone:** 732-235-7733; **Board Cert:** Neurology 1979; **Med School:** Univ Pittsburgh 1972; **Resid:** Neurology, Univ Pittsburgh Hosps 1978; **Fellow:** Neurological Chemistry, NY Hosp-Cornell Univ 1980; **Fac Appt:** Prof N, UMDNJ-RW Johnson Med Sch

NEURORADIOLOGY

Keller, Irwin MD (NRad) - **Spec Exp:** Brain & Spine Imaging; Interventional Neuroradiology; Aneurysm-Cerebral; **Hospital:** Robert Wood Johnson Univ Hosp - New Brunswick (page 853), St Peter's Univ Hosp; **Address:** 579A Cranbury Rd, East Brunswick, NJ 08816-5405; **Phone:** 732-390-0040; **Board Cert:** Diagnostic Radiology 1984; Neuroradiology 1995; **Med School:** NY Med Coll 1980; **Resid:** Diagnostic Radiology, Montefiore Hosp Med Ctr 1984; **Fellow:** Neuroradiology, NYU Med Ctr 1986; **Fac Appt:** Assoc Clin Prof Rad, UMDNJ-RW Johnson Med Sch

Roychowdhury, Sudipta MD (NRad) - **Spec Exp:** Interventional Neuroradiology; **Hospital:** Robert Wood Johnson Univ Hosp - New Brunswick (page 853); **Address:** University Radiology Group, 579A Cranbury Rd, East Brunswick, NJ 08816; **Phone:** 732-390-0040; **Board Cert:** Diagnostic Radiology 1997; Neuroradiology 1999; **Med School:** Northwestern Univ 1992; **Resid:** Diagnostic Radiology, Northwestern Univ 1997; **Fellow:** Neuroradiology, Univ Penn 1999

Schonfeld, Steven MD (NRad) - **Spec Exp:** Spine Imaging & Intervention; Interventional Neuroradiology; **Hospital:** St Peter's Univ Hosp, Robert Wood Johnson Univ Hosp - New Brunswick (page 853); **Address:** University Radiology Group, 579A Cranbury Rd Fl 3, East Brunswick, NJ 08816; **Phone:** 732-390-0040; **Board Cert:** Diagnostic Radiology 1982; Neuroradiology 1995; **Med School:** Mount Sinai Sch Med 1978; **Resid:** Diagnostic Radiology, Montefiore Hosp Med Ctr 1982; **Fellow:** Neuroradiology, NYU Med Ctr 1984; **Fac Appt:** Assoc Clin Prof Rad, UMDNJ-RW Johnson Med Sch

NUCLEAR MEDICINE

Stahl, Theodore MD (NuM) - **Hospital:** Robert Wood Johnson Univ Hosp - New Brunswick (page 853), St Peter's Univ Hosp; **Address:** 303 George St, New Brunswick, NJ 08901; **Phone:** 732-249-4410; **Board Cert:** Nuclear Medicine 1972; **Med School:** Hahnemann Univ 1957; **Resid:** Internal Medicine, Albert Einstein Med Ctr 1959; Internal Medicine, Bronx VA Hosp 1961; **Fellow:** Endocrinology, Columbia-Presby Hosp 1963; Nuclear Medicine, Albert Einstein Med Ctr 1972; **Fac Appt:** Clin Prof Med, UMDNJ-RW Johnson Med Sch

OBSTETRICS & GYNECOLOGY

Bachmann, Gloria MD (ObG) - **Spec Exp:** Menopause Problems; Sexual Dysfunction; Pelvic Surgery; **Hospital:** Robert Wood Johnson Univ Hosp - New Brunswick (page 853); **Address:** Women's Hlth Inst, Clinical Academic Bldg, 125 Paterson St, Ste 2104, New Brunswick, NJ 08901; **Phone:** 732-235-7633; **Board Cert:** Obstetrics & Gynecology 1981; **Med School:** Univ Pennsylvania 1974; **Resid:** Obstetrics & Gynecology, Hosp Univ Penn 1978; **Fac Appt:** Prof ObG, UMDNJ-RW Johnson Med Sch

Bochner, Ronnie MD (ObG) - **Spec Exp:** Gynecologic Surgery-Laparoscopic; Uterine Fibroids; Menopause Problems; **Hospital:** Robert Wood Johnson Univ Hosp - New Brunswick (page 853); **Address:** 3270 Rt 27, Ste 2200, Kendall Park, NJ 08824-1458; **Phone:** 732-422-8989; **Board Cert:** Obstetrics & Gynecology 2005; **Med School:** Mount Sinai Sch Med 1981; **Resid:** Obstetrics & Gynecology, LI Jewish Med Ctr 1985; **Fac Appt:** Asst Clin Prof ObG, Robert W Johnson Med Sch

Rathauser, Robert MD (ObG) - **Spec Exp:** Gynecology Only; **Hospital:** Robert Wood Johnson Univ Hosp - New Brunswick (page 853); **Address:** 3270 Route 27, Ste 2200, Kendall Park, NJ 08824; **Phone:** 732-422-8989; **Board Cert:** Obstetrics & Gynecology 2005; **Med School:** NY Med Coll 1979; **Resid:** Obstetrics & Gynecology, LI Jewish Med Ctr 1983; **Fac Appt:** Assoc Prof ObG, UMDNJ-RW Johnson Med Sch

OCCUPATIONAL MEDICINE

Gochfeld, Michael MD/PhD (OM) - **Spec Exp:** Environmental Medicine; Chemical Exposure; Mercury Toxic Exposure; **Hospital:** Robert Wood Johnson Univ Hosp - New Brunswick (page 853); **Address:** Enviro & Occupational Health - EOHSI, 170 Frelinghuysen Rd, Ste 200, Piscataway, NJ 08854; **Phone:** 732-445-0123 x627; **Board Cert:** Occupational Medicine 1983; **Med School:** Albert Einstein Coll Med 1965; **Resid:** Behavioral Medicine, Rockefeller Univ 1977; **Fac Appt:** Prof OM, UMDNJ-RW Johnson Med Sch

Kipen, Howard MD (OM) - **Spec Exp:** Environmental Medicine; Occupational Disease; Lung Disease; **Hospital:** Robert Wood Johnson Univ Hosp - New Brunswick (page 853); **Address:** UMDNJ-RWJ Med Sch, EOHSI, 170 Frelinghuysen Rd, Piscataway, NJ 08854; **Phone:** 732-445-0123 x629; **Board Cert:** Internal Medicine 1982; Occupational Medicine 1986; **Med School:** UCSF 1979; **Resid:** Internal Medicine, Columbia Presby Med Ctr 1982; Occupational Medicine, Mt Sinai Hosp 1984; **Fac Appt:** Prof Med, UMDNJ-RW Johnson Med Sch

OPHTHALMOLOGY

Engel, J Mark MD (Oph) - **Spec Exp:** Pediatric Ophthalmology; **Hospital:** Robert Wood Johnson Univ Hosp - New Brunswick (page 853), St Peter's Univ Hosp; **Address:** University Childrens Eye Ctr, 4 Cornwall Ct, East Brunswick, NJ 08816; **Phone:** 732-613-9191; **Board Cert:** Ophthalmology 2003; **Med School:** Loyola Univ-Stritch Sch Med 1986; **Resid:** Internal Medicine, Evanston Hosp 1988; Ophthalmology, Interfaith Med Ctr 1991; **Fellow:** Pediatric Ophthalmology, Children's Meml Hosp 1992; **Fac Appt:** , UMDNJ-NJ Med Sch, Newark

Grabowski, Wayne MD (Oph) - **Spec Exp:** Diabetic Eye Disease; Laser Vision Surgery; **Hospital:** Univ Med Ctr - Princeton; **Address:** 5 Centre Drive, Ste 1B, Monroe, NJ 08831; **Phone:** 609-409-2777; **Board Cert:** Ophthalmology 1982; **Med School:** Albany Med Coll 1977; **Resid:** Ophthalmology, Albany Med Ctr 1981; **Fellow:** Vitreoretinal Surgery, Wills Eye Hosp 1983

Santamaria II, Jaime MD (Oph) - **Spec Exp:** Cataract Surgery; Corneal Surgery; LASIK-Refractive Surgery; Intraocular Lenses; **Hospital:** Raritan Bay Med Ctr - Perth Amboy, NY-Presby Hosp (page 100); **Address:** Santamaria Eye Center, 104 Market St, Perth Amboy, NJ 08861-4412; **Phone:** 732-826-5159 x200; **Board Cert:** Ophthalmology 1979; **Med School:** Columbia P&S 1973; **Resid:** Ophthalmology, Columbia-Presby Med Ctr 1978; **Fac Appt:** Asst Clin Prof Oph, Columbia P&S

ORTHOPAEDIC SURGERY

Butler, Mark S MD (OrS) - **Spec Exp:** Trauma; **Hospital:** Robert Wood Johnson Univ Hosp - New Brunswick (page 853), St Peter's Univ Hosp; **Address:** 215 Easton Ave, New Brunswick, NJ 08901; **Phone:** 732-545-0400; **Board Cert:** Orthopaedic Surgery 1993; **Med School:** UMDNJ-RW Johnson Med Sch 1984; **Resid:** Orthopaedic Surgery, RWJ Med Sch 1989

Garfinkel, Matthew J MD (OrS) - **Spec Exp:** Shoulder & Knee Surgery; Arthroscopic Surgery; Sports Medicine; **Hospital:** JFK Med Ctr - Edison; **Address:** 10 Parsonage Rd, Ste 500, Edison, NJ 08837-2429; **Phone:** 732-494-6226; **Board Cert:** Orthopaedic Surgery 2002; **Med School:** Cornell Univ-Weill Med Coll 1986; **Resid:** Orthopaedic Surgery, Montefiore/Weiler Einsten Med Ctr 1991; **Fellow:** Sports Medicine, Lankenau Hosp 1992

Leddy, Joseph MD (OrS) - **Spec Exp:** Hand Surgery; Shoulder Surgery; **Hospital:** Robert Wood Johnson Univ Hosp - New Brunswick (page 853), St Peter's Univ Hosp; **Address:** University Orthopaedic Group, 215 Easton Ave, New Brunswick, NJ 08901; **Phone:** 732-545-0400; **Board Cert:** Orthopaedic Surgery 1995; Hand Surgery 1995; **Med School:** Jefferson Med Coll 1965; **Resid:** Surgery, NY Hosp 1967; Orthopaedic Surgery, Columbia-Presby Hosp 1970; **Fellow:** Hand Surgery, Boyes-Stark Ashworth 1971; **Fac Appt:** Prof OrS, Robert W Johnson Med Sch

Lombardi, Joseph MD (OrS) - **Spec Exp:** Spinal Surgery; Spinal Disc Replacement; **Hospital:** JFK Med Ctr - Edison; **Address:** 10 Parsonage Rd, Ste 500, Edison, NJ 08837-2475; **Phone:** 732-494-6226; **Board Cert:** Orthopaedic Surgery 1987; **Med School:** UMDNJ-RW Johnson Med Sch 1978; **Resid:** Internal Medicine, St Vincent's Hosp & Med Ctr 1979; Orthopaedic Surgery, Univ of Medicine & Dentistry 1983; **Fellow:** Spinal Surgery, Long Beach Mem Med Ctr 1984

Piskun, Andrew MD (OrS) - **Spec Exp:** Trauma; Sports Injuries; Arthroscopic Surgery; **Hospital:** Robert Wood Johnson Univ Hosp - New Brunswick (page 853), St Peter's Univ Hosp; **Address:** 1132 S Washington Ave, Piscataway, NJ 08854-3335; **Phone:** 732-752-8484; **Board Cert:** Orthopaedic Surgery 1984; **Med School:** UMDNJ-RW Johnson Med Sch 1977; **Resid:** Orthopaedic Surgery, UMDNJ-RW Johnson Univ Hosp 1982; **Fac Appt:** Asst Clin Prof OrS, UMDNJ-RW Johnson Med Sch

Reich, Steven MD (OrS) - **Spec Exp:** Spinal Surgery; Spinal Injury; **Hospital:** Robert Wood Johnson Univ Hosp - New Brunswick (page 853), St Peter's Univ Hosp; **Address:** Orthopaedic Assocs, 2186 Rte 27 Ste 1A, New Brunswick, NJ 08902; **Phone:** 732-422-1222; **Board Cert:** Orthopaedic Surgery 2005; **Med School:** Albert Einstein Coll Med 1986; **Resid:** Orthopaedic Surgery, Hosp for Joint Dis 1991; **Fellow:** Spinal Surgery, Pennsylvania Hosp 1992; Spinal Surgery, Thomas Jefferson Univ Hosp 1992

OTOLARYNGOLOGY

Edelman, Bruce MD (Oto) - **Spec Exp:** Ear Disorders; Sinusitis; **Hospital:** St Peter's Univ Hosp; **Address:** B3 Cornwall Drive, East Brunswick, NJ 08816-3390; **Phone:** 732-238-0300; **Board Cert:** Otolaryngology 1990; **Med School:** NYU Sch Med 1984; **Resid:** Surgery, Albert Einstein 1986; Otolaryngology, NYU Med Ctr 1990; **Fellow:** Pediatric Otolaryngology, Children's Hosp 1991

Glasgold, Alvin MD (Oto) - **Spec Exp:** Cosmetic Surgery-Face; Rhinoplasty; Rhinoplasty Revision; **Hospital:** Robert Wood Johnson Univ Hosp - New Brunswick (page 853), Manhattan Eye, Ear & Throat Hosp; **Address:** 31 River Rd, Highland Park, NJ 08904; **Phone:** 732-846-6540; **Board Cert:** Otolaryngology 1967; Facial Plastic & Reconstructive Surgery 2002; **Med School:** NY Med Coll 1961; **Resid:** Surgery, Bronx VA Hosp 1963; Otolaryngology, Bronx VA Hosp/ Columbia Coll of P&S 1966; **Fac Appt:** Clin Prof S, UMDNJ-RW Johnson Med Sch

Miller, Andrew J MD (Oto) - **Spec Exp:** Facial Plastic Surgery; **Hospital:** JFK Med Ctr - Edison; **Address:** Assocs in Plastic Surg, 1150 Amboy Ave, Edison, NJ 08837; **Phone:** 732-548-3200; **Board Cert:** Otolaryngology 2000; Facial Plastic & Reconstructive Surgery 2002; **Med School:** Baylor Coll Med 1994; **Resid:** Otolaryngology, Tulane Univ Med Ctr 1999

Rosenbaum, Jeffrey MD (Oto) - **Spec Exp:** Head & Neck Surgery; Cosmetic Surgery-Face; **Hospital:** St Peter's Univ Hosp, Robert Wood Johnson Univ Hosp - New Brunswick (page 853); **Address:** B3 Cornwall Drive, East Brunswick, NJ 08816-3352; **Phone:** 732-238-0300; **Board Cert:** Otolaryngology 1978; **Med School:** Albany Med Coll 1973; **Resid:** Surgery, Hartford Hosp 1975; Otolaryngology, NYU Med Ctr 1978; **Fellow:** Plastic Surgery, Wayne Co Genl Hosp 1979; **Fac Appt:** Assoc Prof Oto, NYU Sch Med

PAIN MEDICINE

Grubb, William R MD (PM) - **Hospital:** Robert Wood Johnson Univ Hosp - New Brunswick (page 853); **Address:** New Jersey Pain Institute, 125 Patterson St, Ste 3100, New Brunswick, NJ 08901; **Phone:** 732-937-8841; **Board Cert:** Anesthesiology 1990; Pain Medicine 1996; **Med School:** Geo Wash Univ 1985; **Resid:** Anesthesiology, George Washington Univ Med Ctr 1989; **Fellow:** Cardiac Anesthesiology, Univ S Florida 1994; **Fac Appt:** Asst Prof Anes, Robert W Johnson Med Sch

Levin, Alexander MD (PM) - **Spec Exp:** Pain-Chronic; **Address:** Pain Control Ctr of New Jersey, 561 Cranbury Rd, East Brunswick, NJ 08816-5400; **Phone:** 732-651-1300; **Board Cert:** Anesthesiology 1990; Pain Medicine 1996; **Med School:** Russia 1979; **Resid:** Anesthesiology, Westch Med Ctr 1986; **Fellow:** Pain Medicine, U of Cinciinatti Med Ctr

PATHOLOGY

Barnard, Nicola MD (Path) - **Spec Exp:** Gynecologic Pathology; Breast Pathology; Surgical Pathology; **Hospital:** Robert Wood Johnson Univ Hosp - New Brunswick (page 853); **Address:** 1 Robert Wood Johnson Pl, Dept Surgical Pathology, New Brunswick, NJ 08903; **Phone:** 732-937-8590; **Board Cert:** Anatomic Pathology 1981; **Med School:** England 1975; **Resid:** Anatomic Pathology, Yale-New Haven Hosp 1980; Anatomic Pathology, Beth Israel Deaconess Hosp 1982; **Fellow:** Clinical Pathology, Harvard Univ 1982; **Fac Appt:** Assoc Prof Path, Robert W Johnson Med Sch

PEDIATRIC CARDIOLOGY

Agarwal, Kishan MD (PCd) - **Spec Exp:** Echocardiography; Chest Pain; Heart Disease in Newborns; Arrhythmias; **Hospital:** JFK Med Ctr - Edison, Deborah Hrt & Lung Ctr; **Address:** 450 Plainfield Rd, Edison, NJ 08820-2628; **Phone:** 732-494-9500; **Board Cert:** Pediatrics 1990; Pediatric Cardiology 1990; **Med School:** India 1969; **Resid:** Pediatrics, St John's Episcopal Hosp 1977; Pediatrics, SUNY Downstate Med Ctr 1979; **Fellow:** Pediatric Cardiology, Mayo Clinic 1981; **Fac Appt:** Clin Prof Ped, UMDNJ-RW Johnson Med Sch

Gaffney, Joseph W MD (PCd) - **Spec Exp:** Echocardiography; Fetal Echocardiography; Critical Care; **Hospital:** Robert Wood Johnson Univ Hosp - New Brunswick (page 853), NY-Presby Hosp (page 100); **Address:** RWJ Univ Hosp, Ambulatory Care Bldg, 1 RWJ Plaza Fl 1 - Ste C, New Brunswick, NJ 08903; **Phone:** 732-235-7905; **Board Cert:** Pediatrics 1999; Pediatric Cardiology 2006; **Med School:** NY Med Coll 1981; **Resid:** Pediatrics, Brookdale Hosp Med Ctr 1984; **Fellow:** Pediatric Cardiology, Babies Hosp/Columbia-Presby 1987; **Fac Appt:** Assoc Prof Ped, UMDNJ-RW Johnson Med Sch

Kurer, Cheryl C MD (PCd) - **Spec Exp:** Arrhythmias; Heart Disease-Congenital & Acquired; **Hospital:** St Peter's Univ Hosp, Chldns Hosp of Philadelphia, The; **Address:** CHOP Cardiac Ctr at St Peter's Univ Hosp, 254 Easton Ave, New Brunswick, NJ 08901; **Phone:** 732-846-2855; **Board Cert:** Pediatrics 1987; Pediatric Cardiology 2005; **Med School:** Mount Sinai Sch Med 1983; **Resid:** Pediatrics, Mt Sinai Hosp 1986; **Fellow:** Pediatric Cardiology, Chldns Hosp 1989; **Fac Appt:** Assoc Clin Prof Ped, Robert W Johnson Med Sch

PEDIATRIC CRITICAL CARE MEDICINE

Bojko, Thomas MD (PCCM) - **Spec Exp:** Asthma; Sepsis & Septic Shock; Pneumonia; **Hospital:** Robert Wood Johnson Univ Hosp - New Brunswick (page 853), Staten Island Univ Hosp-North Site; **Address:** 89 French St, rm 2232, New Brunswick, NJ 08901; **Phone:** 732-235-7887; **Board Cert:** Pediatrics 1999; Pediatric Critical Care Medicine 2002; **Med School:** Italy 1985; **Resid:** Pediatrics, Newark-Beth Israel Med Ctr 1991; **Fellow:** Pediatric Critical Care Medicine, NY Hosp-Cornell Med Ctr 1994; **Fac Appt:** Assoc Prof Ped, UMDNJ-RW Johnson Med Sch

Notterman, Daniel A MD (PCCM) - **Spec Exp:** Critical Care; **Hospital:** Robert Wood Johnson Univ Hosp - New Brunswick (page 853); **Address:** RW Johnson Univ Hosp, Dept Pediatrics, 1 Robert Wood Johnson Pl, New Brunswick, NJ 08903; **Phone:** 732-235-7900; **Board Cert:** Pediatrics 1983; Pediatric Critical Care Medicine 2003; **Med School:** NYU Sch Med 1978; **Resid:** Pediatrics, Bellevue Hosp-NYU Med Ctr 1981; **Fellow:** Pharmacology, New York Hosp-Cornell 1983; Molecular Biology, Princeton Univ 1997; **Fac Appt:** Prof Ped, Robert W Johnson Med Sch

PEDIATRIC ENDOCRINOLOGY

Salas, Max MD (PEn) - **Spec Exp:** Growth Disorders; Pubertal Disorders; Diabetes; **Hospital:** St Peter's Univ Hosp; **Address:** 254 Easton Ave Fl 3rd, New Brunswick, NJ 08901-1766; **Phone:** 732-745-8574; **Board Cert:** Pediatrics 1969; Pediatric Endocrinology 1986; **Med School:** Mexico 1964; **Resid:** Pediatrics, Children's Hosp 1967; Pediatrics, Children's Hosp 1968; **Fellow:** Pediatric Endocrinology, Children's Hosp 1979; Pediatric Endocrinology, N Shore Univ Hosp 1980; **Fac Appt:** Assoc Prof Ped, UMDNJ-RW Johnson Med Sch

Skuza, Kathryn MD (PEn) - **Spec Exp:** Diabetes; Thyroid Disorders; **Hospital:** St Peter's Univ Hosp; **Address:** St Peter's Univ Hosp, 254 Eastern Ave, New Brunswick, NJ 08901; **Phone:** 732-745-8574; **Board Cert:** Pediatrics 1987; Pediatric Endocrinology 2004; **Med School:** Poland 1982; **Resid:** Pediatrics, UMDNJ-Chldns Hosp 1985; **Fellow:** Endocrinology, Diabetes & Metabolism, UMDNJ-Chldns Hosp 1988; **Fac Appt:** Asst Prof Ped, UMDNJ-NJ Med Sch, Newark

PEDIATRIC GASTROENTEROLOGY

Koniaris, Soula MD (PGe) - **Spec Exp:** Nutrition; **Hospital:** Robert Wood Johnson Univ Hosp - New Brunswick (page 853); **Address:** 89 French St Fl 2, New Brunswick, NJ 08901-1928; **Phone:** 732-235-7885; **Board Cert:** Pediatrics 1991; Pediatric Gastroenterology 1997; **Med School:** Univ Tenn Coll Med, Memphis 1988; **Resid:** Pediatrics, Montefiore Hosp Med Ctr 1991; **Fellow:** Pediatric Gastroenterology, North Shore Univ Hosp 1994; **Fac Appt:** Asst Prof Ped, UMDNJ-RW Johnson Med Sch

PEDIATRIC HEMATOLOGY-ONCOLOGY

Drachtman, Richard MD (PHO) - **Spec Exp:** Pediatric Cancers; Sickle Cell Disease; **Hospital:** Robert Wood Johnson Univ Hosp - New Brunswick (page 853), Jersey Shore Univ Med Ctr; **Address:** Cancer Inst of New Jersey, 195 Little Albany St, New Brunswick, NJ 08903-2681; **Phone:** 732-235-5437; **Board Cert:** Pediatrics 2000; Pediatric Hematology-Oncology 2000; **Med School:** Univ Hlth Sci/Chicago Med Sch 1984; **Resid:** Pediatrics, N Shore Univ Hosp 1988; **Fellow:** Pediatric Hematology-Oncology, Mount Sinai Hosp 1991; **Fac Appt:** Assoc Prof Ped, UMDNJ-RW Johnson Med Sch

Ettinger, Lawrence MD (PHO) - **Spec Exp:** Leukemia; Thalassemia; Sickle Cell Disease; **Hospital:** St Peter's Univ Hosp; **Address:** 254 Easton Ave, New Brunswick, NJ 08901-1766; **Phone:** 732-745-6674; **Board Cert:** Pediatrics 1978; Pediatric Hematology-Oncology 1978; **Med School:** Case West Res Univ 1973; **Resid:** Pediatrics, Univ Maryland Hosp 1975; Pediatrics, Chldns Hosp 1976; **Fellow:** Pediatric Hematology-Oncology, Roswell Park Cancer Inst 1978; **Fac Appt:** Prof Ped, Drexel Univ Coll Med

Kamen, Barton A MD/PhD (PHO) - **Spec Exp:** Drug Development; Leukemia; **Hospital:** Robert Wood Johnson Univ Hosp - New Brunswick (page 853); **Address:** Cancer Inst of New Jersey, 195 Little Albany St, rm 3507, New Brunswick, NJ 08903; **Phone:** 732-235-8131; **Board Cert:** Pediatrics 1981; Pediatric Hematology-Oncology 1987; **Med School:** Case West Res Univ 1976; **Resid:** Pediatrics, Yale-New Haven Hosp 1978; **Fellow:** Pediatric Hematology-Oncology, Yale-New Haven Hosp 1980; **Fac Appt:** Prof Ped, UMDNJ-RW Johnson Med Sch

PEDIATRIC INFECTIOUS DISEASE

Whitley-Williams, Patricia MD (PInf) - **Hospital:** Robert Wood Johnson Univ Hosp - New Brunswick (page 853); **Address:** RWJ Med Sch, Dept Peds, One Robert Wood Johnson Pl, MEB, rm 322, New Brunswick, NJ 08901; **Phone:** 732-235-7894; **Board Cert:** Pediatrics 1980; Pediatric Infectious Disease 1997; **Med School:** Johns Hopkins Univ 1975; **Resid:** Pediatrics, Chldns Hosp Med Ctr 1978; **Fellow:** Pediatric Infectious Disease, Boston City Hosp 1980; **Fac Appt:** Assoc Prof Ped, UMDNJ-RW Johnson Med Sch

PEDIATRIC NEPHROLOGY

Singh, Anup MD (PNep) - **Hospital:** St Peter's Univ Hosp; **Address:** St Peter's Univ Hospital, MOB-3, 254 Easton Ave, New Brunswick, NJ 08901; **Phone:** 732-745-8600 x5489; **Board Cert:** Pediatrics 2000; Pediatric Nephrology 2003; **Med School:** Philippines 1985; **Resid:** Pediatrics, SUNY-Downstate Med Ctr 1991; **Fellow:** Pediatric Nephrology, SUNY-Downstate Med Ctr 1994

Weiss, Lynne MD (PNep) - **Spec Exp:** Hypertension; Kidney Disease; Kidney Failure-Chronic; **Hospital:** Robert Wood Johnson Univ Hosp - New Brunswick (page 853); **Address:** RW Johnson Med Sch, 1 RW Johnson Pl, New Brunswick, NJ 08903-0019; **Phone:** 732-235-6230; **Board Cert:** Pediatrics 1979; Pediatric Nephrology 1982; **Med School:** Hahnemann Univ 1974; **Resid:** Pediatrics, Michael Reese Hosp 1977; **Fellow:** Pediatric Nephrology, Michael Reese Hosp 1979; **Fac Appt:** Prof Ped, UMDNJ-RW Johnson Med Sch

PEDIATRIC OTOLARYNGOLOGY

Traquina, Diana N MD (PO) - **Spec Exp:** Airway Disorders; Ear Disorders; Sinus Disorders; **Hospital:** Robert Wood Johnson Univ Hosp - New Brunswick (page 853); **Address:** 181 Somerset St Fl 2, New Brunswick, NJ 08901; **Phone:** 732-247-2401; **Board Cert:** Otolaryngology 1989; **Med School:** Yale Univ 1984; **Resid:** Surgery, Yale-New Haven Hosp 1986; Otolaryngology, Yale-New Haven Hosp 1989; **Fellow:** Pediatric Otolaryngology, Montefiore-Weiler Enstein Hosp 1990; **Fac Appt:** Assoc Prof Ped, UMDNJ-RW Johnson Med Sch

PEDIATRIC PULMONOLOGY

Turcios, Nelson MD (PPul) - **Spec Exp:** Cystic Fibrosis; Breathing Disorders; **Hospital:** St Peter's Univ Hosp, Somerset Med Ctr; **Address:** 254 Easton Ave, MOB , Ste 3160, New Brunswick, NJ 08901; **Phone:** 732-565-5467; **Board Cert:** Pediatrics 1982; Pediatric Pulmonology 2000; **Med School:** El Salvador 1973; **Resid:** Pediatrics, Univ Mississippi Med Ctr 1978; Pediatrics, Univ Maryland Hosp 1980; **Fellow:** Pediatric Pulmonology, Childrens Hosp 1982; **Fac Appt:** Assoc Prof Ped, UMDNJ-NJ Med Sch, Newark

PEDIATRIC SURGERY

Price, Mitchell MD (PS) - **Spec Exp:** Laparoscopic/Minimally Invasive Surgery; Cancer Surgery; Congenital Anomalies; **Hospital:** Robert Wood Johnson Univ Hosp - New Brunswick (page 853); **Address:** UMDNJ RWJ Med Sch, One Robert Wood Johnson Pl, CN-19, New Brunswick, NJ 08903-0019; **Phone:** 732-235-7821; **Board Cert:** Surgery 1996; Pediatric Surgery 1998; **Med School:** Univ Chicago-Pritzker Sch Med 1986; **Resid:** Surgery, NYU Med Ctr 1988; Surgery, NYU Med Ctr 1994; **Fellow:** Pediatric Surgery-ECMO, Babies Hosp/Columbia 1991; Pediatric Surgery, Univ Colo/Denver Chldn's Hosp 1996; **Fac Appt:** Asst Prof S, UMDNJ-RW Johnson Med Sch

PEDIATRICS

Blackman, Edward MD (Ped) PCP - **Spec Exp:** Allergy; Asthma; Adolescent Medicine; **Hospital:** St Peter's Univ Hosp, Robert Wood Johnson Univ Hosp - New Brunswick (page 853); **Address:** 1950 Highway 27, North Brunswick, NJ 08902-1300; **Phone:** 732-940-5511; **Board Cert:** Pediatrics 1972; **Med School:** Temple Univ 1967; **Resid:** Pediatrics, US Naval Hosp 1970; **Fac Appt:** Asst Clin Prof Ped, UMDNJ-RW Johnson Med Sch

Brennan, George MD (Ped) PCP - **Spec Exp:** Learning Disorders; Developmental Disorders; **Hospital:** St Peter's Univ Hosp, Robert Wood Johnson Univ Hosp - New Brunswick (page 853); **Address:** 100 Perrine Rd, Old Bridge, NJ 08857; **Phone:** 732-316-0900; **Board Cert:** Pediatrics 1965; **Med School:** Loyola Univ-Stritch Sch Med 1957; **Resid:** Pediatrics, St Vincent's Hosp & Med Ctr 1960; **Fac Appt:** Assoc Clin Prof Ped, UMDNJ-RW Johnson Med Sch

Cohen, Richard MD (Ped) PCP - **Hospital:** St Peter's Univ Hosp, Robert Wood Johnson Univ Hosp - New Brunswick (page 853); **Address:** 1598 US Highway 130, North Brunswick, NJ 08902-3040; **Phone:** 732-297-0603; **Board Cert:** Pediatrics 1974; **Med School:** Jefferson Med Coll 1968; **Resid:** Pediatrics, St Luke's Hosp 1970; **Fellow:** Pediatrics, Thomas Jeffferson Hosp 1972; **Fac Appt:** Asst Clin Prof Ped, UMDNJ-RW Johnson Med Sch

Rhoads, Frances MD (Ped) PCP - **Spec Exp:** Breast Feeding Problems; Child Development; **Hospital:** St Peter's Univ Hosp; **Address:** 123 How Lane, New Brunswick, NJ 08901-3639; **Phone:** 732-745-8519; **Board Cert:** Pediatrics 1981; **Med School:** England 1965; **Resid:** Pediatrics, Philadelphia Genl Hosp 1968; Pediatrics, Kapiolani Chldns Med Ctr; **Fellow:** Child Development, Kapiolani Chldns Med Ctr 1975; **Fac Appt:** Clin Prof Ped, UMDNJ-RW Johnson Med Sch

PLASTIC SURGERY

Borah, Gregory MD (PlS) - **Spec Exp:** Cosmetic Surgery-Face; Cosmetic Surgery-Breast; Hand Surgery; **Hospital:** Robert Wood Johnson Univ Hosp - New Brunswick (page 853); **Address:** UMDNJ Medical Center - Div Plastic Surgery, 1 Robert Wood Johnson MEB 506, New Brunswick, NJ 08901-1928; **Phone:** 732-235-7865; **Board Cert:** Plastic Surgery 1986; Hand Surgery 1996; **Med School:** Harvard Med Sch 1978; **Resid:** Surgery, Mass Genl Hosp 1983; Plastic Surgery, Yale-New Haven Hosp 1985; **Fac Appt:** Prof PlS, UMDNJ-RW Johnson Med Sch

Middlesex

Herbstman, Robert A MD (PlS) - **Spec Exp:** Cosmetic Surgery-Face; Cosmetic Surgery-Body; Breast Reconstruction; **Hospital:** Robert Wood Johnson Univ Hosp - New Brunswick (page 853), St Peter's Univ Hosp; **Address:** 579A Cranbury Rd, Ste 202, East Brunswick, NJ 08816; **Phone:** 732-254-1919; **Board Cert:** Plastic Surgery 1992; **Med School:** Univ Rochester 1982; **Resid:** Surgery, RWJohnson Univ Med Ctr 1987; Plastic Surgery, RWJohnson Univ Med Ctr 1989

Nini, Kevin MD (PlS) - **Spec Exp:** Facial Plastic Surgery; Breast Surgery; Liposuction & Body Contouring; **Hospital:** St Peter's Univ Hosp, Robert Wood Johnson Univ Hosp - New Brunswick (page 853); **Address:** 78 Easton Ave, Fl 2nd, New Brunswick, NJ 08901-5400; **Phone:** 732-418-0709; **Board Cert:** Plastic Surgery 1994; **Med School:** UMDNJ-RW Johnson Med Sch 1984; **Resid:** Surgery, Pennsylvania Hosp 1989; Plastic Surgery, Shands Hosp-Univ Fla 1991; **Fellow:** Plastic Surgery, Univ Miami Hosps 1992

Olson, Robert MD (PlS) - **Spec Exp:** Cleft Palate/Lip; Head & Neck Surgery; Wound Healing/Care; **Hospital:** St Peter's Univ Hosp, Robert Wood Johnson Univ Hosp - New Brunswick (page 853); **Address:** 78 Easton Ave, New Brunswick, NJ 08901-1838; **Phone:** 732-418-0709; **Board Cert:** Plastic Surgery 1982; **Med School:** Univ Pennsylvania 1974; **Resid:** Surgery, Peter Bent Brigham Hosp 1979; Plastic Surgery, Mayo Clinic 1981; **Fac Appt:** Assoc Prof S, UMDNJ-RW Johnson Med Sch

Wey, Philip D MD (PlS) - **Spec Exp:** Cosmetic Surgery-Face; Breast Cosmetic & Reconstructive Surgery; Liposuction & Body Contouring; **Hospital:** Robert Wood Johnson Univ Hosp - New Brunswick (page 853), St Peter's Univ Hosp; **Address:** 78 Easton Ave Fl 2, New Brunswick, NJ 08901-1838; **Phone:** 732-418-0709; **Board Cert:** Plastic Surgery 1996; **Med School:** Brown Univ 1986; **Resid:** Surgery, Northwestern Univ /McGaw Med Ctr 1990; Plastic Surgery, NY Cornell Med Ctr 1992; **Fellow:** Breast Surgery, NYU/Meml Sloan-Kettering Cancer Ctr 1993; **Fac Appt:** Assoc Clin Prof S, UMDNJ-RW Johnson Med Sch

PSYCHIATRY

Jones Jr, Frank A MD (Psyc) - **Spec Exp:** Depression; Anxiety Disorders; Mood Disorders; **Address:** 2186 Route 27, Ste 2A, North Brunswick, NJ 08902; **Phone:** 732-422-0800; **Board Cert:** Psychiatry 1977; **Med School:** Case West Res Univ 1972; **Resid:** Psychiatry, Boston State Hosp 1973; Psychiatry, Worcester State Hosp 1975; **Fac Appt:** Clin Prof Psyc, UMDNJ-RW Johnson Med Sch

Menza, Matthew MD (Psyc) - **Spec Exp:** Psychopharmacology; Depression; Anxiety Disorders; **Hospital:** Robert Wood Johnson Univ Hosp - New Brunswick (page 853); **Address:** RW Johnson Med Sch, Dept Psychiatry, 671 Hoes Ln, Piscataway, NJ 08854; **Phone:** 732-235-7647; **Board Cert:** Psychiatry 1985; **Med School:** Temple Univ 1980; **Resid:** Psychiatry, NYU -Bellevue Hospital 1984; **Fellow:** Psychiatry, Harvard Med Sch 1985; **Fac Appt:** Prof Psyc, UMDNJ-RW Johnson Med Sch

Zykorie, David MD (Psyc) - **Spec Exp:** Depression; Anxiety Disorders; ADD/ADHD; **Address:** 25 Brunswick Woods Dr, East Brunswick, NJ 08816-5601; **Phone:** 732-257-9599; **Board Cert:** Psychiatry 1975; **Med School:** NYU Sch Med 1969; **Resid:** Psychiatry, Yale U Sch Med 1973; **Fac Appt:** Asst Clin Prof Psyc, Robert W Johnson Med Sch

PULMONARY DISEASE

Goldberg, Jory MD (Pul) - **Spec Exp:** Lung Disease; Asthma; **Hospital:** Univ Med Ctr - Princeton; **Address:** 9 Centre Dr, Ste 100A, Monroetownship, NJ 08831-1564; **Phone:** 609-655-1700; **Board Cert:** Internal Medicine 1981; Pulmonary Disease 1984; Critical Care Medicine 1995; **Med School:** Mexico 1976; **Resid:** Internal Medicine, City Hosp Ctr Elmhurst 1979; Internal Medicine, Monmouth Hosp 1980; **Fellow:** Pulmonary Disease, Bergen County Hosp 1982

Harangozo, Andrea MD (Pul) - **Hospital:** Robert Wood Johnson Univ Hosp - New Brunswick (page 853), St Peter's Univ Hosp; **Address:** 593 Cranbury Rd, Ste 1-A, East Brunswick, NJ 08816; **Phone:** 732-613-8880; **Board Cert:** Internal Medicine 1989; Pulmonary Disease 1994; Critical Care Medicine 1995; **Med School:** NYU Sch Med 1984; **Resid:** Internal Medicine, UMDNJ-RWJ Univ Hosp 1987; **Fellow:** Pulmonary Disease, UMDNJ-RWJ Univ Hosp 1990; **Fac Appt:** Asst Clin Prof Med, UMDNJ-RW Johnson Med Sch

Melillo, Nicholas MD (Pul) - **Spec Exp:** Chronic Obstructive Lung Disease (COPD); Lung Cancer; Asthma; **Hospital:** JFK Med Ctr - Edison; **Address:** Middlesex Pulmonary Assocs, 106 James St, Edison, NJ 08820-3945; **Phone:** 732-906-0091; **Board Cert:** Internal Medicine 1983; Pulmonary Disease 1986; Critical Care Medicine 1996; **Med School:** UMDNJ-NJ Med Sch, Newark 1979; **Resid:** Internal Medicine, St Michael's Med Ctr 1983; **Fellow:** Pulmonary Disease, St Michael's Med Ctr 1985; Critical Care Medicine, St Michael's Med Ctr 1986; **Fac Appt:** Assoc Clin Prof Med, Seton Hall Univ Sch Grad Med Ed

Paz, Harold L MD (Pul) - **Spec Exp:** Sarcoidosis; **Hospital:** Robert Wood Johnson Univ Hosp - New Brunswick (page 853); **Address:** UMDNJ RW Johnson Medical School, 125 Paterson St, Ste 1400, New Brunswick, NJ 08901; **Phone:** 732-235-6300; **Board Cert:** Internal Medicine 1985; Pulmonary Disease 1988; **Med School:** Univ Rochester 1982; **Resid:** Internal Medicine, Northwestern Meml Med Ctr 1986; **Fellow:** Pulmonary Disease, Johns Hopkins Hosp 1988; **Fac Appt:** Prof Med, Robert W Johnson Med Sch

Riley, David MD (Pul) - **Spec Exp:** Pulmonary Fibrosis; Interstitial Lung Disease; **Hospital:** Robert Wood Johnson Univ Hosp - New Brunswick (page 853); **Address:** RWJ Univ Hosp, Med Education Bldg 572, 1 Robert Wood Johnson Pl, New Brunswick, NJ 08903-0019; **Phone:** 732-235-7840; **Board Cert:** Internal Medicine 1980; Pulmonary Disease 1974; **Med School:** Univ MD Sch Med 1968; **Resid:** Internal Medicine, Baltimore City Hosps 1970; Internal Medicine, Johns Hopkins Hosp 1973; **Fellow:** Pulmonary Disease, Hosp Univ Penn 1972; **Fac Appt:** Prof Med, UMDNJ-RW Johnson Med Sch

Schiffman, Philip MD (Pul) - **Spec Exp:** Occupational Lung Disease; Sarcoidosis; Asthma; **Hospital:** Robert Wood Johnson Univ Hosp - New Brunswick (page 853), St Peter's Univ Hosp; **Address:** 593 Cranbury Road, Ste B, East Brunswick, NJ 08816; **Phone:** 732-613-8880; **Board Cert:** Internal Medicine 1975; Pulmonary Disease 1978; Critical Care Medicine 1996; **Med School:** SUNY Downstate 1972; **Resid:** Internal Medicine, LI Jewish Med Ctr 1975; Pulmonary Disease, LAC/ Harbor-UCLA Med Ctr 1977; **Fac Appt:** Clin Prof Med, UMDNJ-RW Johnson Med Sch

Wolf, Barry MD (Pul) - **Spec Exp:** Asthma; Critical Care; **Hospital:** JFK Med Ctr - Edison, Robert Wood Johnson Univ Hosp - New Brunswick (page 853); **Address:** 2 Lincoln Hwy, Ste 301, Edison, NJ 08820; **Phone:** 732-549-7380; **Board Cert:** Internal Medicine 1985; Pulmonary Disease 1988; Critical Care Medicine 2001; **Med School:** NYU Sch Med 1982; **Resid:** Internal Medicine, Bellevue Hosp/VA Hosp 1986; **Fellow:** Pulmonary Critical Care Medicine, Bellevue Hosp-NYU 1988

RADIATION ONCOLOGY

Haas, Alexander MD (RadRO) - **Spec Exp:** Breast Cancer; Prostate Cancer; **Hospital:** St Peter's Univ Hosp, Robert Wood Johnson Univ Hosp - New Brunswick (page 853); **Address:** St Peter's Univ Hosp, Dept Rad Oncology, 254 Easton Ave, New Brunswick, NJ 08901-1766; **Phone:** 732-745-8590; **Board Cert:** Radiation Oncology 1972; **Med School:** Yugoslavia 1962; **Resid:** Diagnostic Radiology, Univ WA Med Ctr 1968; Radiation Oncology, Univ WA Med Ctr 1972; **Fellow:** Neoplastic Diseases, Thomas Jefferson Univ Hosp 1973; **Fac Appt:** Assoc Clin Prof Rad, UMDNJ-RW Johnson Med Sch

Haffty, Bruce MD (RadRO) - **Spec Exp:** Breast Cancer; Head & Neck Cancer; Lung Cancer; **Hospital:** Robert Wood Johnson Univ Hosp - New Brunswick (page 853), Robert Wood Johnson Univ Hosp Hamilton (page 853); **Address:** The Cancer Institute of New Jersey, 195 Little Albany St, New Brunswick, NJ 08903; **Phone:** 732-253-3939; **Board Cert:** Radiation Oncology 1988; **Med School:** Yale Univ 1984; **Resid:** Radiation Oncology, Yale-New Haven Hosp 1988; **Fac Appt:** Prof RadRO, Robert W Johnson Med Sch

Knee, Robert MD (RadRO) - **Spec Exp:** Brachytherapy; Pediatric Cancers; **Hospital:** St Peter's Univ Hosp; **Address:** St Peter's Medical Ctr, 254 Easton Ave, New Brunswick, NJ 08901; **Phone:** 732-745-8590; **Board Cert:** Therapeutic Radiology 1983; **Med School:** SUNY Downstate 1978; **Resid:** Radiology, SUNY Downstate 1983; **Fellow:** Radiology, Univ Texas/MD Anderson Hosp 1984; **Fac Appt:** Asst Clin Prof Rad, UMDNJ-RW Johnson Med Sch

Macher, Mark MD (RadRO) - **Hospital:** JFK Med Ctr - Edison; **Address:** JFK Med Ctr, MidState Rad Oncology, 65 James St, Edison, NJ 08820-3948; **Phone:** 732-321-7167; **Board Cert:** Radiation Oncology 1986; **Med School:** Howard Univ 1982; **Resid:** Radiology, New York Univ Med Ctr 1985; **Fellow:** Radiology, Univ Hosp 1986

REPRODUCTIVE ENDOCRINOLOGY

Kemmann, Ekkehard MD (RE) - **Spec Exp:** Infertility-IVF; Endometriosis; Polycystic Ovarian Syndrome; **Hospital:** Robert Wood Johnson Univ Hosp - New Brunswick (page 853), St Peter's Univ Hosp; **Address:** 303 George St, Ste 250, New Brunswick, NJ 08901; **Phone:** 732-235-7301; **Board Cert:** Obstetrics & Gynecology 2003; Reproductive Endocrinology 2003; **Med School:** Germany 1967; **Resid:** Obstetrics & Gynecology, Kings County Hosp 1973; **Fellow:** Reproductive Endocrinology, SUNY Downstate Med Ctr 1976; **Fac Appt:** Prof ObG, UMDNJ-RW Johnson Med Sch

RHEUMATOLOGY

Lichtbroun, Alan MD (Rhu) - **Spec Exp:** Rheumatoid Arthritis; Sjogren's Syndrome; Fibromyalgia; **Hospital:** Robert Wood Johnson Univ Hosp - New Brunswick (page 853), JFK Med Ctr - Edison; **Address:** 63 Brunswick Woods Dr, East Brunswick, NJ 08816-5601; **Phone:** 732-613-1900; **Board Cert:** Internal Medicine 1980; Rheumatology 1984; **Med School:** SUNY Downstate 1977; **Resid:** Internal Medicine, LI Jewish-Hillside Med Ctr 1980; **Fellow:** Rheumatology, Mt Sinai Hosp 1982; **Fac Appt:** Asst Clin Prof Med, UMDNJ-RW Johnson Med Sch

SURGERY

August, David MD (S) - **Spec Exp:** Cancer Surgery; Gastrointestinal Cancer; Breast Cancer; Sarcoma-Soft Tissue; **Hospital:** Robert Wood Johnson Univ Hosp - New Brunswick (page 853); **Address:** Canc Inst NJ, 195 Little Albany St, New Brunswick, NJ 08903-1914; **Phone:** 732-235-7701; **Board Cert:** Surgery 1995; **Med School:** Yale Univ 1980; **Resid:** Surgery, Yale-New Haven Hosp 1986; **Fellow:** Surgical Oncology, Natl Cancer Inst 1984; **Fac Appt:** Prof S, UMDNJ-RW Johnson Med Sch

Boyarsky, Andrew MD (S) - **Spec Exp:** Endocrine Surgery; Laparoscopic Surgery-Complex; Trauma; **Hospital:** Robert Wood Johnson Univ Hosp - New Brunswick (page 853); **Address:** UMDNJ-RW Johnson Med Sch, Dept Surgery, New Brunswick, NJ 08903; **Phone:** 732-235-7920; **Board Cert:** Surgery 1994; Surgical Critical Care 1998; **Med School:** Rutgers Univ 1980; **Resid:** Surgery, RWJ Univ Hosp 1985; **Fellow:** Vascular Surgery, Maimonides Medical Ctr 1986; **Fac Appt:** Assoc Prof S, UMDNJ-RW Johnson Med Sch

Brolin, Robert E MD (S) - **Spec Exp:** Obesity/Bariatric Surgery; Gastrointestinal Surgery; **Hospital:** Univ Med Ctr - Princeton; **Address:** 4250 US Highway Rte 1 N, Ste 1, Monmouth Junction, NJ 08852; **Phone:** 732-274-3434; **Board Cert:** Surgery 2001; **Med School:** Univ Mich Med Sch 1974; **Resid:** Surgery, Univ Pittsburgh Med Ctr 1980

Chung-Loy, Harold MD (S) - **Spec Exp:** Transplant-Kidney; **Hospital:** JFK Med Ctr - Edison, Robert Wood Johnson Univ Hosp at Rahway (page 853); **Address:** 98 James St, Ste 202, Edison, NJ 08820; **Phone:** 732-548-1000; **Board Cert:** Surgery 1995; **Med School:** Howard Univ 1980; **Resid:** Surgery, Mount Sinai 1985; **Fellow:** Transplant Surgery, Mount Sinai 1983

Dasmahapatra, Kumar MD (S) - **Spec Exp:** Cancer Surgery; Breast Surgery; Laparoscopic Surgery; **Hospital:** Raritan Bay Med Ctr - Perth Amboy, JFK Med Ctr - Edison; **Address:** 225 May St, Ste A, Edison, NJ 08837; **Phone:** 732-346-5400; **Board Cert:** Surgery 1998; **Med School:** India 1973; **Resid:** Surgery, Grace Hosp 1979; **Fellow:** Surgical Oncology, Roswell Park Meml Inst 1982; **Fac Appt:** Assoc Clin Prof S, UMDNJ-NJ Med Sch, Newark

Goydos, James S MD (S) - **Spec Exp:** Cancer Surgery; Melanoma; **Hospital:** Robert Wood Johnson Univ Hosp - New Brunswick (page 853), St Peter's Univ Hosp; **Address:** Cancer Inst of NJ, 195 Little Albany St, New Brunswick, NJ 08901; **Phone:** 732-235-7563; **Board Cert:** Surgery 2004; **Med School:** UMDNJ-RW Johnson Med Sch 1988; **Resid:** Surgery, New Britain Gen Hosp 1993; **Fellow:** Surgical Oncology, Univ Pittsburgh Sch Med 1995; **Fac Appt:** Assoc Prof S, Robert W Johnson Med Sch

Kearney, Thomas MD (S) - **Spec Exp:** Breast Cancer; **Hospital:** Robert Wood Johnson Univ Hosp - New Brunswick (page 853); **Address:** Cancer Institute New Jersey, 195 Little Albany St, New Brunswick, NJ 08901; **Phone:** 732-235-6777; **Board Cert:** Surgery 2000; **Med School:** Georgetown Univ 1984; **Resid:** Surgery, Cedars Sinai Med Ctr 1992; **Fellow:** Surgical Oncology, Univ Chicago-Pritzker Sch Med 1995; **Fac Appt:** Assoc Prof S, UMDNJ-RW Johnson Med Sch

Lowry, Stephen MD (S) - **Spec Exp:** Cancer Surgery; **Hospital:** Robert Wood Johnson Univ Hosp - New Brunswick (page 853); **Address:** 125 Patterson St, Ste 7300, New Brunswick, NJ 08901; **Phone:** 732-235-6096; **Board Cert:** Surgery 1982; **Med School:** Univ Mich Med Sch 1971; **Resid:** Surgery, U Utah Med Ctr 1975; Surgery, NCI-NIH 1978; **Fellow:** Surgical Oncology, Memorial-Sloan Kettering Cancer Ctr 1982

Middlesex

Swaminathan, A P MD (S) - **Spec Exp:** Breast Surgery; Laparoscopic Surgery; **Hospital:** Raritan Bay Med Ctr - Perth Amboy, JFK Med Ctr - Edison; **Address:** 225 May St, Ste A, Edison, NJ 08837; **Phone:** 732-346-5400; **Board Cert:** Surgery 1974; **Med School:** India 1965; **Resid:** Surgery, Queens Genl Hosp 1972Martland Hosp 1973; **Fac Appt:** Prof S, UMDNJ-NJ Med Sch, Newark

THORACIC SURGERY

Spotnitz, Alan J MD (TS) - **Spec Exp:** Coronary Artery Surgery; Heart Valve Surgery; **Hospital:** Robert Wood Johnson Univ Hosp - New Brunswick (page 853); **Address:** 125 Paterson St, rm 7319-A, New Brunswick, NJ 08901; **Phone:** 732-235-7805; **Board Cert:** Thoracic Surgery 2000; **Med School:** Columbia P&S 1970; **Resid:** Surgery, Beth Israel Hosp 1975; Cardiothoracic Surgery, Presbyterian Hosp 1979; **Fac Appt:** Clin Prof TS, UMDNJ-RW Johnson Med Sch

UROLOGY

Fleisher, Michael MD (U) - **Spec Exp:** Pediatric Urology; Transplant-Kidney; **Hospital:** St Peter's Univ Hosp, Monmouth Med Ctr; **Address:** Pediatric Urology Assocs, 557 Cranbury Rd, East Brunswick, NJ 08816-5400; **Phone:** 732-613-9144; **Board Cert:** Urology 1984; **Med School:** SUNY Downstate 1977; **Resid:** Urology, SUNY Downstate Med Ctr 1982; **Fellow:** Transplant Medicine, Montefiore Hosp Med Ctr 1979; Pediatric Urology, Hosp Sick Chldn 1983; **Fac Appt:** Assoc Clin Prof U, Robert W Johnson Med Sch

Grubman, Jerold MD (U) - **Spec Exp:** Prostate Cancer; Incontinence; Prostate Disease; **Hospital:** JFK Med Ctr - Edison, Raritan Bay Med Ctr - Perth Amboy; **Address:** 10 Parsonage Rd, Ste 118, Edison, NJ 08837-2429; **Phone:** 732-494-9400; **Board Cert:** Urology 1976; **Med School:** Albert Einstein Coll Med 1966; **Resid:** Urology, Bronx Municipal Hosp 1973; **Fac Appt:** Asst Clin Prof U, Rutgers Univ

Solomon, Michael J MD (U) - **Spec Exp:** Pediatric & Adult Urology; **Hospital:** St Peter's Univ Hosp, Robert Wood Johnson Univ Hosp - New Brunswick (page 853); **Address:** 579A Cranbury Rd, Ste 105, East Brunswick, NJ 08816-4026; **Phone:** 732-390-8700; **Board Cert:** Urology 1981; **Med School:** Univ Pennsylvania 1973; **Resid:** Surgery, New England Med Ctr/Harvard 1976; Urology, Lahey Clinic 1979; **Fellow:** Pediatric Urology, Mass Genl Hosp 1981; **Fac Appt:** Assoc Clin Prof U, UMDNJ-RW Johnson Med Sch

Weiss, Robert E MD (U) - **Spec Exp:** Bladder Cancer; Kidney Cancer; Testicular Cancer; **Hospital:** Robert Wood Johnson Univ Hosp - New Brunswick (page 853), Univ Med Ctr - Princeton; **Address:** 1 Robert Wood Johnson Pl Ste MB588, New Brunswick, NJ 08901-1928; **Phone:** 732-235-7775; **Board Cert:** Urology 2003; **Med School:** NYU Sch Med 1985; **Resid:** Surgery, Mount Sinai Med Ctr 1987; Urology, Mount Sinai Med Ctr 1991; **Fellow:** Urologic Oncology, Meml Sloan Kettering Cancer Ctr 1994; **Fac Appt:** Assoc Prof U, UMDNJ-RW Johnson Med Sch

VASCULAR & INTERVENTIONAL RADIOLOGY

Denny, Donald F MD (VIR) - **Hospital:** Univ Med Ctr - Princeton; **Address:** Princeton Radiology, 3674 Route 27, Kendall Park, NJ 08824; **Phone:** 732-821-5563; **Board Cert:** Diagnostic Radiology 1982; Vascular & Interventional Radiology 2005; **Med School:** Hahnemann Univ 1978; **Resid:** Diagnostic Radiology, Yale-New Haven Hosp 1982; **Fellow:** Diagnostic Radiology, Brigham & Woomens Hosp 1983

Nosher, John MD (VIR) - **Spec Exp:** Endovascular Surgery; Uterine Fibroid Embolization; Radiofrequency Ablation; **Hospital:** Robert Wood Johnson Univ Hosp - New Brunswick (page 853); **Address:** UMDNJ-RW Johnson Med Sch-Dept Radiology, MEB 404, Box 19, New Brunswick, NJ 08903-0019; **Phone:** 732-235-7721; **Board Cert:** Diagnostic Radiology 1975; Vascular & Interventional Radiology 1995; **Med School:** Jefferson Med Coll 1970; **Resid:** Radiology, Columbia Presby Med Ctr 1975; **Fac Appt:** Clin Prof Rad, UMDNJ-RW Johnson Med Sch

Siegel, Randall MD (VIR) - **Spec Exp:** Endovascular Surgery; Vascular Access; Pediatric Interventional Radiology; **Hospital:** Robert Wood Johnson Univ Hosp - New Brunswick (page 853), St Peter's Univ Hosp; **Address:** University Radiology Group, 579A Cranbury Rd, East Brunswick, NJ 08816; **Phone:** 732-937-8617; **Board Cert:** Diagnostic Radiology 1991; Vascular & Interventional Radiology 2005; **Med School:** Univ Pennsylvania 1986; **Resid:** Diagnostic Radiology, RWJ Univ Hosp 1991; **Fellow:** Vascular & Interventional Radiology, RWJ Univ Hosp 1992; **Fac Appt:** Asst Clin Prof Rad, UMDNJ-RW Johnson Med Sch

Vascular Surgery

Graham, Alan M MD (VascS) - **Spec Exp:** Endovascular Surgery; Aneurysm-Abdominal Aortic; Carotid Artery Surgery; **Hospital:** Robert Wood Johnson Univ Hosp - New Brunswick (page 853); **Address:** 1 Robert Wood Johnson Pl, MEB Bldg - rm 541, Box 19, New Brunswick, NJ 08901; **Phone:** 732-235-8770; **Board Cert:** Surgery 1994; Vascular Surgery 1996; **Med School:** Canada 1979; **Resid:** Surgery, McGill Univ Med Ctr 1984; **Fellow:** Vascular Surgery, Univ Chicago Hosps 1986; **Fac Appt:** Prof S, UMDNJ-RW Johnson Med Sch

Konigsberg, Stephen MD (VascS) - **Spec Exp:** Carotid Artery Surgery; Thyroid & Parathyroid Surgery; Hernia; **Hospital:** Robert Wood Johnson Univ Hosp - New Brunswick (page 853), St Peter's Univ Hosp; **Address:** 31 River Rd, Highland Park, NJ 08904-1731; **Phone:** 732-846-9500; **Board Cert:** Surgery 1970; Vascular Surgery 1998; **Med School:** Harvard Med Sch 1962; **Resid:** Surgery, Peter Bent Brigham Hosp 1966; Surgery, Albert Einstein 1968; **Fac Appt:** Assoc Clin Prof S, UMDNJ-RW Johnson Med Sch

Shindelman, Larry MD (VascS) - **Spec Exp:** Endovascular Surgery; Vascular Access; Carotid Artery Surgery; Lower Limb Arterial Disease; **Hospital:** Robert Wood Johnson Univ Hosp - New Brunswick (page 853), CentraState Med Ctr; **Address:** 465 Cranbury Rd, Ste 204, New Brunswick, NJ 08816; **Phone:** 732-698-0606; **Board Cert:** Surgery 2002; Vascular Surgery 1999; **Med School:** SUNY Downstate 1977; **Resid:** Surgery, Mt Sinai Hosp 1982; **Fellow:** Vascular Surgery, Mt Sinai Hosp 1983; **Fac Appt:** Assoc Clin Prof S, UMDNJ-RW Johnson Med Sch

Simpson, Alec MD (VascS) - **Spec Exp:** Stroke Prevention; Diabetic Leg/Foot; **Hospital:** Muhlenberg Regional Med Ctr, JFK Med Ctr - Edison; **Address:** 1511 Park Ave, S Plainfield, NJ 07080; **Phone:** 908-561-9500; **Board Cert:** Surgery 1997; Vascular Surgery 1995; **Med School:** Panama 1970; **Resid:** Surgery, Beth Israel Med Ctr 1977; **Fellow:** Vascular Surgery, Middlesex Genl Hosp 1978; **Fac Appt:** Asst Clin Prof S, UMDNJ-RW Johnson Med Sch

ROBERT WOOD JOHNSON
UNIVERSITY HOSPITAL

One Robert Wood Johnson Place
New Brunswick, NJ 08903-2601
General Information (732) 828-3000
Physician Referral 888-44-RWJUH
www.rwjuh.edu

OVERVIEW

One of the nation's leading academic health centers, the 584-bed Robert Wood Johnson University Hospital is the principal teaching hospital of UMDNJ-Robert Wood Johnson Medical School and the hub of a clinically-integrated medical campus that includes The Cardiovascular Institute of New Jersey, The Cancer Institute of New Jersey, The Child Health Institute of New Jersey and The Bristol-Myers Squibb Children's Hospital.

CENTERS OF EXCELLENCE

The Heart Center of New Jersey offers complete diagnostic capabilities and treatment options for heart disease, including the latest minimally invasive and robotic techniques. Home to one of the busiest cardiac catheterization programs in the region, the Heart Center performs more than 11,000 cardiac interventional procedures annually. The Advanced Heart Failure and Transplant Program offers specialized care for patients with heart failure, including medical management, surgically implanted assist devices, and a Medicare-certified heart transplantation program.

The Cancer Hospital of New Jersey is the flagship hospital of The Cancer Institute of New Jersey, the state's only National Cancer Institute-designated Comprehensive Cancer Center. This 123-bed hospital offers outpatient chemotherapy, a bone marrow transplant unit, medical oncology, surgical oncology, radiation oncology and an urgent-care center.

The Bristol-Myers Squibb Children's Hospital (www.bmsch.org) is a state-designated acute care children's hospital providing pediatric specialties and subspecialties including cardiac surgery, hematology-oncology, orthopaedics and neurosurgery.

Regional Perinatal Center offers the latest technology to treat high-risk pregnancies, as well as the most critically ill newborns. The Center's renowned maternal-fetal medicine and neonatology specialists provide a full array of services and surgical support for babies and families.

The Center for Kidney and Pancreas Transplantation is one of a select few programs in the state to offer kidney and pancreas transplantation. A team of physicians, surgeons, nurses and health professionals offer adult and pediatric patients the full spectrum of care.

The Level I Trauma Center provides a skilled shock/trauma team composed of general surgeons, orthopaedic surgeons, neurosurgeons and anesthesiologists. The Center provides care for adults and children.

The Thoracic Center of New Jersey treats patients with a variety of medical problems affecting the lungs, esophagus and mediastinum. It is a major referral center for surgery on lung and esophageal cancers.

LEADERSHIP

Ranked among the nation's top five hospitals for patient safety initiatives in 2005 by *Consumers Digest Magazine*. Most top-rated physicians of all New Jersey hospitals listed in Castle Connolly *Top Doctors NY-Metro (9th Edition)*. Winner of the prestigious Magnet Award for Nursing Excellence for nine consecutive years. Ranked sixth in the nation in hospital quality analysis commissioned by The Commonwealth Fund.

Flagship hospital of the Robert Wood Johnson Health System & Network.

539

Monmouth

Monmouth

ALLERGY & IMMUNOLOGY

Gross, Gary L MD (A&I) - **Spec Exp:** Asthma; Cough-Chronic; Sinus Disorders; **Hospital:** Jersey Shore Univ Med Ctr, Monmouth Med Ctr; **Address:** 802 W Park Ave, Ste 213, Ocean Township, NJ 07712-4556; **Phone:** 732-695-2555; **Board Cert:** Allergy & Immunology 1987; Pediatrics 1986; **Med School:** NYU Sch Med 1981; **Resid:** Pediatrics, Children's Hosp 1984; **Fellow:** Allergy & Immunology, Children's Hosp 1986; **Fac Appt:** Assoc Clin Prof Ped, Robert W Johnson Med Sch

Hirsch, Andrew MD (A&I) - **Spec Exp:** Asthma; Sinusitis; Allergic Rhinitis; **Hospital:** Riverview Med Ctr, Monmouth Med Ctr; **Address:** Allergy & Asthma Assocs, 258 Broad St, Red Bank, NJ 07701-5623; **Phone:** 732-741-8900; **Board Cert:** Pediatrics 1991; Allergy & Immunology 2005; **Med School:** Temple Univ 1988; **Resid:** Pediatrics, New York Hosp 1991; **Fellow:** Allergy & Immunology, Thomas Jefferson Univ Hosp 1993

Picone, Frank J MD (A&I) - **Spec Exp:** Asthma; Sinus Disorders; Allergy; **Hospital:** Riverview Med Ctr, Monmouth Med Ctr; **Address:** 709 Sycamore Ave, Tinton Falls, Red Bank, NJ 07701; **Phone:** 732-747-8188; **Board Cert:** Pediatrics 1973; Allergy & Immunology 1975; **Med School:** UMDNJ-NJ Med Sch, Newark 1967; **Resid:** Pediatrics, Jackson Meml Hosp 1970; **Fellow:** Allergy & Immunology, Chldns Hosp Med Ctr 1974; **Fac Appt:** Asst Clin Prof Ped, Drexel Univ Coll Med

Sher, Ellen R MD (A&I) - **Spec Exp:** Asthma & Sinusitis; Nasal Allergies; Insect Allergies; **Hospital:** Monmouth Med Ctr, Riverview Med Ctr; **Address:** 802 W Park Ave, Ste 213, Ocean Township, NJ 07712; **Phone:** 732-695-2555; **Board Cert:** Internal Medicine 1989; Allergy & Immunology 2003; **Med School:** Georgetown Univ 1986; **Resid:** Internal Medicine, Thomas Jefferson Univ Hosp 1989; **Fellow:** Pulmonary Disease, Thomas Jefferson Univ Hosp 1990; Allergy & Immunology, Natl Jewish Ctr Resp Dis 1992; **Fac Appt:** Asst Clin Prof Med, UMDNJ-NJ Med Sch, Newark

CARDIOVASCULAR DISEASE

Adelson, Richard MD (Cv) - **Hospital:** Jersey Shore Univ Med Ctr; **Address:** 1820 Corlies Ave, Ste 4B, Neptune, NJ 07753-4860; **Phone:** 732-776-8500; **Board Cert:** Internal Medicine 1986; Cardiovascular Disease 1989; Interventional Cardiology 2001; **Med School:** Albert Einstein Coll Med 1983; **Resid:** Internal Medicine, Montefiore Hosp-Albert Einstein 1986; Cardiovascular Disease, Loma Linda Univ Med Ctr 1989; **Fellow:** Cardiovascular Disease, Montefiore Hosp-Albert Einstein 1988; Interventional Cardiology, Newark Beth Israel Hosp 1990

Beauregard, Lou-Anne M MD (Cv) - **Spec Exp:** Arrhythmias; Heart Disease in Women; **Hospital:** Robert Wood Johnson Univ Hosp - New Brunswick (page 853), CentraState Med Ctr; **Address:** Heart Specialists of Central Jersey, 100 Craig Rd Fl 2, Manalapan, NJ 07726; **Phone:** 732-866-0800; **Board Cert:** Internal Medicine 1983; Cardiovascular Disease 1985; Cardiac Electrophysiology 2002; **Med School:** Med Coll PA 1980; **Resid:** Internal Medicine, Temple Univ Hosp 1983; **Fellow:** Cardiovascular Disease, Med Coll Penn 1985; Cardiac Electrophysiology, Cooper Hosp 1986; **Fac Appt:** Assoc Clin Prof Med, Robert W Johnson Med Sch

Daniels, Jeffrey MD (Cv) - **Hospital:** Monmouth Med Ctr, Jersey Shore Univ Med Ctr; **Address:** 215 Brighton Ave, Long Branch, NJ 07740; **Phone:** 732-222-5143; **Board Cert:** Internal Medicine 1983; Cardiovascular Disease 1985; **Med School:** Albany Med Coll 1980; **Resid:** Internal Medicine, Mount Sinai Hosp 1983; **Fellow:** Cardiovascular Disease, Mount Sinai Hosp 1985; **Fac Appt:** Asst Clin Prof Med, Drexel Univ Coll Med

Watson, Rita MD (Cv) - **Spec Exp:** Cardiac Catheterization; Peripheral Vascular Disease; Heart Valve Disease; **Hospital:** Jersey Shore Univ Med Ctr, Monmouth Med Ctr; **Address:** 215 Brighton Ave, Long Branch, NJ 07740; **Phone:** 732-222-5143; **Board Cert:** Internal Medicine 1979; Cardiovascular Disease 1983; Interventional Cardiology 1999; **Med School:** Harvard Med Sch 1976; **Resid:** Internal Medicine, Hosp Univ Penn 1979; **Fellow:** Cardiovascular Disease, NHLBI-Natl Inst Hlth 1981

COLON & RECTAL SURGERY

Arvanitis, Michael MD (CRS) - **Spec Exp:** Laparoscopic Surgery; Colon & Rectal Cancer; Ulcerative Colitis; **Hospital:** Monmouth Med Ctr; **Address:** 1131 Broad St, Ste 105, Shrewsbury, NJ 07702-4329; **Phone:** 732-389-1331; **Board Cert:** Colon & Rectal Surgery 2001; **Med School:** Hahnemann Univ 1982; **Resid:** Surgery, St Vincent's Hosp 1987; **Fellow:** Colon & Rectal Surgery, Cleveland Clinic 1988; **Fac Appt:** Assoc Prof S, Hahnemann Univ

DERMATOLOGY

Grossman, Kenneth MD (D) - **Spec Exp:** Melanoma; Psoriasis; Skin Cancer; **Hospital:** Riverview Med Ctr; **Address:** 180 White Rd, Ste 103, Little Silver, NJ 07739-1166; **Phone:** 732-842-5222; **Board Cert:** Internal Medicine 1980; Dermatology 1983; **Med School:** SUNY Hlth Sci Ctr 1977; **Resid:** Internal Medicine, Nassau County Med Ctr 1980; Dermatology, Albert Einstein Coll Med 1983

Hametz, Irwin MD (D) - **Hospital:** CentraState Med Ctr; **Address:** 77-55 Schanck Rd, Ste B-3, Freehold, NJ 07728; **Phone:** 732-462-9800; **Board Cert:** Dermatology 1978; **Med School:** NY Med Coll 1973; **Resid:** Pediatrics, Long Island Jewish-Hillside Med Ctr 1975; Dermatology, Brown Univ Affil Hosps 1978; **Fac Appt:** Asst Clin Prof Med, UMDNJ-RW Johnson Med Sch

DIAGNOSTIC RADIOLOGY

Chalal, Jeffrey MD (DR) - **Hospital:** CentraState Med Ctr; **Address:** 901 W Main St, Ground Fl, Freehold, NJ 07728; **Phone:** 732-462-4844; **Board Cert:** Diagnostic Radiology 1982; **Med School:** Univ Pennsylvania 1977; **Resid:** Diagnostic Radiology, Columbia-Presby Med Ctr 1981; **Fellow:** Cross Sectional Imaging, Columbia-Presby Med Ctr 1982

ENDOCRINOLOGY, DIABETES & METABOLISM

Luria, Martin MD (EDM) - **Spec Exp:** Thyroid Disorders; Diabetes; **Hospital:** Monmouth Med Ctr, Riverview Med Ctr; **Address:** 170 Morris Ave, Ste F, Long Branch, NJ 07740-6660; **Phone:** 732-222-8874; **Board Cert:** Internal Medicine 1976; Endocrinology, Diabetes & Metabolism 1977; **Med School:** NYU Sch Med 1971; **Resid:** Internal Medicine, Kings County Hosp 1974; **Fellow:** Endocrinology, Diabetes & Metabolism, Mt Sinai Hosp 1976

Nassberg, Barton MD (EDM) - **Spec Exp:** Thyroid Disorders; Diabetes; **Hospital:** Bayshore Community Hosp, Riverview Med Ctr; **Address:** 723 N Beers St, Ste 2G, Holmdel, NJ 07733-1512; **Phone:** 732-739-0200; **Board Cert:** Internal Medicine 1982; Endocrinology, Diabetes & Metabolism 1984; **Med School:** Belgium 1979; **Resid:** Internal Medicine, Mountainside Hosp 1982; **Fellow:** Endocrinology, Diabetes & Metabolism, MS Hershey Med Ctr 1984

FAMILY MEDICINE

Catanese, Vincent J MD (FMed) PCP - **Spec Exp:** Hypertension; Diabetes; Functional Bowel Disorders; **Hospital:** Bayshore Community Hosp, Riverview Med Ctr; **Address:** 733 N Beers St, Ste U3, Holmdel, NJ 07733; **Phone:** 732-264-8484; **Board Cert:** Family Medicine 1999; **Med School:** Penn State Univ-Hershey Med Ctr 1978; **Resid:** Family Medicine, Conemaugh Valley Meml Hosp 1981

Liquori, Frances DO (FMed) PCP - **Hospital:** CentraState Med Ctr, Kimball Med Ctr; **Address:** Howell Family Medical Ctr, 3701 Rte 9 N, Howell, NJ 07731-3396; **Phone:** 732-364-4555; **Board Cert:** Family Medicine 2001; **Med School:** Univ Osteo Med & Hlth Sci, Des Moines 1984; **Resid:** Family Medicine, Mountainside Hosp 1988

GASTROENTEROLOGY

Binns, Joseph MD (Ge) - **Spec Exp:** Colonoscopy; **Hospital:** Riverview Med Ctr; **Address:** Red Bank Gastroenterology Assocs, 365 Broad St, Ste 1-E, Red Bank, NJ 07701; **Phone:** 732-842-4294; **Board Cert:** Internal Medicine 2000; Gastroenterology 2003; **Med School:** UMDNJ-RW Johnson Med Sch 1987; **Resid:** Internal Medicine, Pennsylvania Hosp 1990; **Fellow:** Gastroenterology, Graduate Hosp 1992

Fiest, Thomas DO (Ge) - **Spec Exp:** Colitis; Liver Disease; **Hospital:** Monmouth Med Ctr, Jersey Shore Univ Med Ctr; **Address:** 142 Route 35, Eatontown, NJ 07724; **Phone:** 732-389-5004; **Board Cert:** Internal Medicine 1989; Gastroenterology 1995; **Med School:** Philadelphia Coll Osteo Med 1985; **Resid:** Internal Medicine, Monmouth Med Ctr 1990; **Fellow:** Gastroenterology, Jersey City Med Ctr 1993

Ludwig, Shelly MD (Ge) - **Spec Exp:** Inflammatory Bowel Disease; Hepatitis B & C; Gastroesophageal Reflux Disease (GERD); **Hospital:** CentraState Med Ctr, Robert Wood Johnson Univ Hosp - New Brunswick (page 853); **Address:** 535 Iron Bridge Rd, Ste 12, Freehold, NJ 07728-5301; **Phone:** 732-780-4224; **Board Cert:** Internal Medicine 1977; Gastroenterology 1979; **Med School:** Albert Einstein Coll Med 1974; **Resid:** Internal Medicine, LAC-Harbor UCLA Med Ctr 1977; **Fellow:** Gastroenterology, Wadsworth VA Hosp/UCLA 1979; **Fac Appt:** Assoc Clin Prof Med, Robert W Johnson Med Sch

Schwartz, Mitchell S MD (Ge) - **Spec Exp:** Colitis; Gallbladder Disease; Liver Disease; **Hospital:** Monmouth Med Ctr, Jersey Shore Univ Med Ctr; **Address:** 1907 Highway 35, Ste 1, Oakhurst, NJ 07755; **Phone:** 732-517-0060; **Board Cert:** Internal Medicine 1986; Gastroenterology 1989; **Med School:** Albert Einstein Coll Med 1983; **Resid:** Internal Medicine, Bronx Municipal Hosp 1987; **Fellow:** Gastroenterology, Montefiore Hosp Med Ctr/Albert Einstein 1989

Tendler, Michael MD (Ge) - **Spec Exp:** Colon Cancer; Gastroesophageal Reflux Disease (GERD); Hepatitis C; **Hospital:** CentraState Med Ctr; **Address:** 50 Franklin Ln, Ste 201, Manalapan, NJ 07726; **Phone:** 732-972-6996; **Board Cert:** Internal Medicine 2001; Gastroenterology 2003; **Med School:** UMDNJ-RW Johnson Med Sch 1986; **Resid:** Internal Medicine, New York Hospital 1990; **Fellow:** Gastroenterology, UMDNJ 1992

Turtel, Penny MD (Ge) - **Spec Exp:** Inflammatory Bowel Disease; Celiac Disease; Colon Polyps & Cancer; **Hospital:** Monmouth Med Ctr, Jersey Shore Univ Med Ctr; **Address:** 1907 Highway 35, Ste 1, Oakhurst, NJ 07755-2760; **Phone:** 732-517-0060; **Board Cert:** Internal Medicine 1989; Gastroenterology 1991; **Med School:** Cornell Univ-Weill Med Coll 1986; **Resid:** Internal Medicine, Mount Sinai Hosp 1989; **Fellow:** Gastroenterology, Mount Sinai Hosp 1991

HEMATOLOGY

Lerner, William MD (Hem) - **Spec Exp:** Palliative Care; **Hospital:** Jersey Shore Univ Med Ctr, Ocean Med Ctr; **Address:** 1707 Atlantic Ave, Manasquan, NJ 08736-1147; **Phone:** 732-528-0760; **Board Cert:** Internal Medicine 1980; Hematology 1982; Medical Oncology 1983; **Med School:** Belgium 1977; **Resid:** Internal Medicine, Albert Einstein Med Ctr 1980; **Fellow:** Hematology, NYU Med Ctr 1981; Oncology, NYU Med Ctr 1983

Topilow, Arthur MD (Hem) - **Spec Exp:** Lymphoma; Multiple Myeloma; **Hospital:** Jersey Shore Univ Med Ctr, Ocean Med Ctr; **Address:** 1707 Atlantic Ave, Manasquan, NJ 08736-1147; **Phone:** 732-528-0760; **Board Cert:** Internal Medicine 1971; Hematology 1972; Medical Oncology 1981; **Med School:** NY Med Coll 1967; **Resid:** Internal Medicine, Flower/NY Metro Hosp 1970; **Fellow:** Hematology, Flower/NY Metro Hosp 1972; **Fac Appt:** Assoc Clin Prof Med, UMDNJ-NJ Med Sch, Newark

INTERNAL MEDICINE

Burkett, Eric N MD (IM) `PCP` - **Spec Exp:** Hypertension; Diabetes; Geriatric Medicine; **Hospital:** Monmouth Med Ctr; **Address:** 223 Monmouth Rd, Ste 1A, West Long Branch, NJ 07764-1029; **Phone:** 732-229-3838; **Board Cert:** Internal Medicine 1976; Geriatric Medicine 1992; **Med School:** Hahnemann Univ 1971; **Resid:** Internal Medicine, Monmouth Med Ctr 1976

Courtney, Barbara MD (IM) `PCP` - **Spec Exp:** Geriatrics; **Hospital:** Monmouth Med Ctr; **Address:** Monmouth Medical Group, 565 Highway 35, Red Bank, NJ 07701; **Phone:** 732-842-0290; **Board Cert:** Internal Medicine 1980; Geriatric Medicine 2002; **Med School:** Hahnemann Univ 1977; **Resid:** Internal Medicine, Monmouth Med Ctr 1980; **Fac Appt:** Med

Glowacki, Jan S MD (IM) `PCP` - **Spec Exp:** Preventive Medicine; Diagnostic Problems; **Hospital:** Riverview Med Ctr, Monmouth Med Ctr; **Address:** 569 River Rd, Fair Haven, NJ 07704-3262; **Phone:** 732-530-0100; **Board Cert:** Internal Medicine 1980; **Med School:** Jefferson Med Coll 1977; **Resid:** Internal Medicine, Monmouth Med Ctr 1980

Granet, Kenneth M MD (IM) `PCP` - **Hospital:** Monmouth Med Ctr; **Address:** 615 Hope Rd, Bldg 4 - Ste 3, Eatontown, NJ 07724-1273; **Phone:** 732-542-3030; **Board Cert:** Internal Medicine 1987; **Med School:** SUNY Downstate 1984; **Resid:** Internal Medicine, N Shore Univ Hosp 1987; **Fac Appt:** Asst Clin Prof Med, Hahnemann Univ

Masterson, Raymond M MD (IM) `PCP` - **Spec Exp:** Hypertension; Diabetes; Cholesterol/Lipid Disorders; **Hospital:** Jersey Shore Univ Med Ctr; **Address:** 700 Crescent Pl, Sea Girt, NJ 08750-2804; **Phone:** 732-974-0340; **Board Cert:** Internal Medicine 1986; **Med School:** Philippines 1978; **Resid:** Internal Medicine, St Michaels Med Ctr 1982

MEDICAL ONCOLOGY

Fitzgerald, Denis MD (Onc) - **Spec Exp:** Breast Cancer; Lung Cancer; Hemochromatosis; **Hospital:** Riverview Med Ctr; **Address:** 180 White Rd, Ste 101, Little Silver, NJ 07739; **Phone:** 732-530-8666; **Board Cert:** Internal Medicine 1981; Medical Oncology 1985; Hematology 1986; **Med School:** SUNY Hlth Sci Ctr 1978; **Resid:** Internal Medicine, St Vincent's Hosp Med Ctr 1982; **Fellow:** Hematology & Oncology, Strong Meml Hosp 1985

Greenberg, Susan MD (Onc) - **Spec Exp:** Breast Cancer; Lymphoma; Lung Cancer; **Hospital:** Jersey Shore Univ Med Ctr, Monmouth Med Ctr; **Address:** 39 Sycamore Ave, Little Silver, NJ 07739-1208; **Phone:** 732-576-8610; **Board Cert:** Internal Medicine 1981; Medical Oncology 1983; **Med School:** Med Coll PA Hahnemann 1978; **Resid:** Internal Medicine, Hosp Med Coll Penn 1981; **Fellow:** Medical Oncology, Columbia-Presby Med Ctr 1983

Sharon, David MD (Onc) - **Spec Exp:** Breast Cancer; Lung Cancer; Gastrointestinal Cancer; **Hospital:** Monmouth Med Ctr; **Address:** The Cancer Ctr - Monmouth Med Ctr, 100 State Highway 36, Ste 1B, West Long Branch, NJ 07764-6205; **Phone:** 732-222-1711; **Board Cert:** Internal Medicine 1980; Medical Oncology 1983; **Med School:** NY Med Coll 1977; **Resid:** Internal Medicine, Beth Israel Med Ctr 1980; **Fellow:** Medical Oncology, Mount Sinai Med Ctr 1982

Walsh, Christina MD (Onc) - **Spec Exp:** Cancer Genetics; Breast Cancer; **Hospital:** Riverview Med Ctr; **Address:** 180 White Rd, Ste 101, Little Silver, NJ 07739; **Phone:** 732-530-8666; **Board Cert:** Internal Medicine 1980; Hematology 1982; Medical Oncology 1985; **Med School:** Georgetown Univ 1977; **Resid:** Internal Medicine, Georgetown Univ Hosp 1980; **Fellow:** Hematology, Georgetown Univ Hosp 1981; Hematology & Oncology, NYU Medical Ctr 1984

NEPHROLOGY

Flis, Raymond S DO (Nep) - **Spec Exp:** Hypertension; Kidney Disease; **Hospital:** Monmouth Med Ctr, Riverview Med Ctr; **Address:** 6 Industrial Way W, Ste B, Eatontown, NJ 07724-2268; **Phone:** 732-460-1200; **Board Cert:** Internal Medicine 1974; Nephrology 1976; **Med School:** Kirksville Coll Osteo Med 1971; **Resid:** Internal Medicine, Cooper Hosp 1974; **Fellow:** Nephrology, Thomas Jefferson Univ Hosp 1975; Nephrology, Temple Univ Hosp 1976; **Fac Appt:** Assoc Clin Prof Med, Drexel Univ Coll Med

Manning, Eric MD (Nep) - **Spec Exp:** Hypertension; **Hospital:** Robert Wood Johnson Univ Hosp - New Brunswick (page 853), Somerset Med Ctr; **Address:** 719 Route 206, Ste 100, Hillsborough, NJ 08844; **Phone:** 908-904-9055; **Board Cert:** Internal Medicine 1989; Nephrology 2002; **Med School:** UC Davis 1985; **Resid:** Internal Medicine, Boston Univ Hosp 1988; **Fellow:** Nephrology, Boston Univ Hosp 1992

NEUROLOGICAL SURGERY

Rosenblum, Bruce MD (NS) - **Spec Exp:** Spinal Surgery; Brain Tumors; Stereotactic Radiosurgery; **Hospital:** Riverview Med Ctr, Bayshore Community Hosp; **Address:** 160 Ave at the Commons, Shrewsbury, NJ 07702; **Phone:** 732-460-1522; **Board Cert:** Neurological Surgery 1991; **Med School:** Mount Sinai Sch Med 1982; **Resid:** Neurological Surgery, Mount Sinai Med Ctr 1986; **Fellow:** Stroke, Natl Inst Health 1988

NEUROLOGY

Gilson, Noah MD (N) - **Spec Exp:** Multiple Sclerosis; Headache; Parkinson's Disease; **Hospital:** Monmouth Med Ctr, Riverview Med Ctr; **Address:** 107 Monmouth Rd, Ste 110, West Long Branch, NJ 07764; **Phone:** 732-935-1850; **Board Cert:** Neurology 1987; **Med School:** Loyola Univ-Stritch Sch Med 1982; **Resid:** Neurology, Mount Sinai Hosp 1986

Herman, Martin MD (N) - **Spec Exp:** Multiple Sclerosis; Epilepsy; Migraine; **Hospital:** Monmouth Med Ctr, Riverview Med Ctr; **Address:** 107 Monmouth Rd, Ste 110, West Long Branch, NJ 07764-1000; **Phone:** 732-935-1850; **Board Cert:** Neurology 1973; **Med School:** Northwestern Univ 1964; **Resid:** Neurology, Univ VA Hlth Sci Ctr 1970; **Fellow:** Clinical Neurophysiology, Columbia-Presby Hosp 1971; **Fac Appt:** Assoc Clin Prof N, Drexel Univ Coll Med

Holland, Neil R MD (N) - **Spec Exp:** Neuromuscular Disorders; Peripheral Neuropathy; Electrodiagnosis; **Hospital:** Monmouth Med Ctr, Riverview Med Ctr; **Address:** 107 Monmouth Rd, Ste 110, West Long Branch, NJ 07764; **Phone:** 732-935-1850; **Board Cert:** Neurology 2000; Clinical Neurophysiology 2001; **Med School:** England 1991; **Resid:** Neurology, Johns Hopkins Univ Hosp 1996; **Fellow:** Clinical Neurophysiology, Johns Hopkins Univ Hosp 1997

Silbert, Paul MD (N) - **Spec Exp:** Parkinson's Disease; Migraine; Carpal Tunnel Syndrome; **Hospital:** Jersey Shore Univ Med Ctr; **Address:** 2100 Corlies Ave, Ste 10, Neptune, NJ 07753-6116; **Phone:** 732-776-8866; **Board Cert:** Neurology 1980; **Med School:** Jefferson Med Coll 1971; **Resid:** Neurology, Columbia-Presbyterian 1975; **Fellow:** Neurology, Columbia-Presbyterian 1975; **Fac Appt:** Asst Clin Prof N, Robert W Johnson Med Sch

OBSTETRICS & GYNECOLOGY

Goldstein, Steven MD (ObG) - **Spec Exp:** Laparoscopic Hysterectomy; Ultrasound; Menopause Problems; Minimally Invasive Surgery; **Hospital:** CentraState Med Ctr; **Address:** 501 Iron Bridge Rd, Ste 4, Freehold, NJ 07728; **Phone:** 732-431-1807; **Board Cert:** Obstetrics & Gynecology 2004; **Med School:** SUNY Downstate 1985; **Resid:** Obstetrics & Gynecology, RWJ Univ Hosp 1989

Seigel, Mark J MD (ObG) - **Spec Exp:** Adolescent Gynecology; Minimally Invasive Surgery; **Hospital:** CentraState Med Ctr, Monmouth Med Ctr; **Address:** 501 Iron Bridge Rd, Ste 4, Freehold, NJ 07728-5305; **Phone:** 732-431-1807; **Board Cert:** Obstetrics & Gynecology 1997; **Med School:** Geo Wash Univ 1980; **Resid:** Obstetrics & Gynecology, Columbia-Presby Med Ctr 1984

OPHTHALMOLOGY

Engel, Mark MD (Oph) - **Spec Exp:** Cataract Surgery; Glaucoma; **Hospital:** Bayshore Community Hosp, Riverview Med Ctr; **Address:** 733 N Beers St, Ste U4, Holmdel, NJ 07733-1528; **Phone:** 732-739-0707; **Board Cert:** Ophthalmology 1977; **Med School:** SUNY Downstate 1971; **Resid:** Ophthalmology, SUNY Downstate 1975

Goldberg, Daniel MD (Oph) - **Spec Exp:** LASIK-Refractive Surgery; Corneal Disease; Cataract Surgery; **Hospital:** Monmouth Med Ctr; **Address:** 180 White Rd, Ste 202, Little Silver, NJ 07739-1166; **Phone:** 732-219-9220; **Board Cert:** Ophthalmology 1979; **Med School:** SUNY Downstate 1974; **Resid:** Ophthalmology, SUNY Downstate 1978; **Fellow:** Cornea, Eye & Ear Hosp 1979; **Fac Appt:** Assoc Clin Prof Oph, Drexel Univ Coll Med

Talansky, Marvin MD (Oph) - **Spec Exp:** Cataract Surgery; Diabetic Eye Disease; LASIK-Refractive Surgery; **Hospital:** Jersey Shore Univ Med Ctr, Monmouth Med Ctr; **Address:** 3333 Fairmont Ave, Asbury Park, NJ 07712-4010; **Phone:** 732-988-4000; **Board Cert:** Ophthalmology 1978; **Med School:** Med Univ SC 1973; **Resid:** Ophthalmology, Storm Eye Inst 1978; **Fellow:** Retina, Storm Eye Inst 1986

ORTHOPAEDIC SURGERY

Bade III, Harry A MD (OrS) - **Spec Exp:** Joint Replacement; Shoulder Arthroscopic Surgery; Hand Surgery; **Hospital:** Riverview Med Ctr, Monmouth Med Ctr; **Address:** Professional Orthopedics Assoc, 776 Shrewsbury Ave, Ste 201, Tinton Falls, NJ 07724-3006; **Phone:** 732-530-4949 x218; **Board Cert:** Orthopaedic Surgery 1984; **Med School:** Jefferson Med Coll 1976; **Resid:** Surgery, Roosevelt Hosp 1978; Orthopaedic Surgery, Hosp for Special Surg 1981; **Fellow:** Shoulder Surgery, Hosp for Special Surg 1982; Hand Surgery, Roosevelt Hosp 1982

Grossman, Robert B MD (OrS) - **Spec Exp:** Knee Surgery; **Hospital:** Monmouth Med Ctr, Riverview Med Ctr; **Address:** 35 Gilbert St S, Tinton Falls, NJ 07701-4917; **Phone:** 732-530-1515; **Board Cert:** Orthopaedic Surgery 1978; **Med School:** Univ MD Sch Med 1972; **Resid:** Orthopaedic Surgery, Univ Vermont Med Ctr 1976; **Fellow:** Sports Medicine, Lenox Hill Hosp 1977; **Fac Appt:** Assoc Prof OrS, Hahnemann Univ

OTOLARYNGOLOGY

Rossos, Paul MD (Oto) - **Spec Exp:** Pediatric Otolaryngology; Sinus Disorders; **Hospital:** CentraState Med Ctr, Robert Wood Johnson Univ Hosp Hamilton (page 853); **Address:** 501 Iron Bridge Rd, Ste 11, Freehold, NJ 07728-5305; **Phone:** 732-409-2500; **Board Cert:** Otolaryngology 1988; **Med School:** Grenada 1981; **Resid:** Surgery, UMDNJ Hosps 1983; Otolaryngology, UMDNJ Hosps 1986

Scaccia, Frank J MD (Oto) - **Spec Exp:** Cosmetic Surgery-Face; Rhinoplasty; **Hospital:** Riverview Med Ctr; **Address:** Riverside Plastic Surgery & Sinus Ctr, 70 E Front St Fl 3, Red Bank, NJ 07701; **Phone:** 732-747-5300; **Board Cert:** Otolaryngology 1993; Facial Plastic & Reconstructive Surgery 1995; **Med School:** Wake Forest Univ 1985; **Resid:** Surgery, Monmouth Med Ctr 1988; Otolaryngology, Univ Hosp Cleveland 1992

Shah, Darsit K MD (Oto) - **Spec Exp:** Head & Neck Cancer; Thyroid & Parathyroid Surgery; Parotid Surgery; **Hospital:** Monmouth Med Ctr; **Address:** Central Jersey Otolaryngology, 1131 Broad St, Shrewsbury, NJ 07702; **Phone:** 732-389-3388; **Board Cert:** Otolaryngology 1997; **Med School:** Med Coll PA 1991; **Resid:** Surgery, Mt Sinai Hosp 1992; Otolaryngology, Mt Sinai Hosp 1996; **Fellow:** Neurotology, Michigan Ear Inst

PAIN MEDICINE

Bram, Harris MD (PM) - **Spec Exp:** Pain-Back & Neck; **Hospital:** Monmouth Med Ctr, St Peter's Univ Hosp; **Address:** 200 White Rd, Ste 205, Little Silver, NJ 07739; **Phone:** 732-345-1180; **Board Cert:** Anesthesiology 1993; Pain Medicine 1993; **Med School:** Univ Ark 1988; **Resid:** Anesthesiology, Hahnemann Unin Hosp 1992; **Fellow:** Pain Medicine, TJefferson Univ Hosp 1993

Haber, Daran MD (PM) - **Spec Exp:** Pain-Back & Neck; Reflex Sympathetic Dystrophy (RSD); Pain-Muscle & Nerve; **Hospital:** Riverview Med Ctr; **Address:** One River View Plaza, Red Bank, NJ 07701-1864; **Phone:** 732-530-2295; **Board Cert:** Anesthesiology 1992; Pain Medicine 1996; **Med School:** Puerto Rico 1986; **Resid:** Anesthesiology, New Jersey Hosp 1989; Anesthesiology, Albert Einstein 1989; **Fellow:** Anesthesiology, Albert Einstein 1990; Pain Medicine, Yale University 1991

Staats, Peter MD (PM) - **Spec Exp:** Pain-Cancer; Pain-Back; **Hospital:** Riverview Med Ctr, CentraState Med Ctr; **Address:** Metzger Pain Management, 160 Avenue at the Commons, Ste 1, Shrewsbury, NJ 07702; **Phone:** 732-380-0200; **Board Cert:** Anesthesiology 1994; Pain Medicine 2005; **Med School:** Univ Mich Med Sch 1989; **Resid:** Anesthesiology, Johns Hopkins Hosp 1993; **Fellow:** Pain Medicine, Johns Hopkins Hosp 1994

PEDIATRIC OTOLARYNGOLOGY

Tavill, Michael A MD (PO) - **Hospital:** Monmouth Med Ctr, Jersey Shore Univ Med Ctr; **Address:** Central Jersey Otolaryngology, 1131 Broad Street, Shrewsbury, NJ 07702; **Phone:** 732-389-3388; **Board Cert:** Otolaryngology 1997; **Med School:** Case West Res Univ 1991; **Resid:** Otolaryngology, Hosp Univ Penn 1996; **Fellow:** Pediatric Otolaryngology, Childrens Hosp 1997

PEDIATRIC SURGERY

Saad, Saad A MD (PS) - **Spec Exp:** Neonatal Surgery; Thoracic Surgery; Laparoscopic Surgery; **Hospital:** Monmouth Med Ctr; **Address:** Childrens Surgery & Pediatric Laparoscopy, 615 Hope Rd, Victoria Plaza - Bldg 1A, Eatontown, NJ 07724; **Phone:** 732-935-0407; **Board Cert:** Surgery 2001; Pediatric Surgery 2003; **Med School:** Egypt 1971; **Resid:** Surgery, Martland Hosp 1977; **Fellow:** Pediatric Surgery, Med Univ South Carolina 1979

PEDIATRICS

Murphy, Robert MD (Ped) **PCP** - **Spec Exp:** ADD/ADHD; Asthma; Vaccines; **Hospital:** Monmouth Med Ctr; **Address:** 223 Monmouth Rd, Ste 1, West Long Branch, NJ 07764-1029; **Phone:** 732-229-4540; **Board Cert:** Pediatrics 1982; **Med School:** Vanderbilt Univ 1977; **Resid:** Pediatrics, Yale-New Haven Hosp 1980

PHYSICAL MEDICINE & REHABILITATION

Braddom, Randall L MD (PMR) - **Spec Exp:** Electromyography; Stroke Rehabilitation; Spinal Cord Injury; Musculoskeletal Disorders; **Hospital:** Riverview Med Ctr; **Address:** Orthopaedic, Sports Medicine & Rehab Ctr, 80 Oak Hill Rd, rm 368, Red Bank, NJ 07701; **Phone:** 732-741-2313; **Board Cert:** Physical Medicine & Rehabilitation 1974; **Med School:** Ohio State Univ 1968; **Resid:** Physical Medicine & Rehabilitation, Ohio State Univ Hosp 1973; **Fac Appt:** Clin Prof PMR, UMDNJ-NJ Med Sch, Newark

PLASTIC SURGERY

Dudick, Stephen T MD (PlS) - **Spec Exp:** Breast Reconstruction & Augmentation; Cosmetic Surgery; Cleft Palate/Lip; Body Contouring after Weight Loss; **Hospital:** Jersey Shore Univ Med Ctr, Monmouth Med Ctr; **Address:** 252 Broad St, Red Bank, NJ 07701; **Phone:** 732-741-1303; **Board Cert:** Plastic Surgery 1993; **Med School:** Mexico 1975; **Resid:** Surgery, St Vincents Hosp 1981; Plastic Surgery, Indiana Univ Med Ctr 1983

Elkwood, Andrew I MD (PlS) - **Spec Exp:** Cosmetic Surgery-Face; Peripheral Nerve Surgery; Reconstructive Surgery; **Hospital:** Monmouth Med Ctr, Riverview Med Ctr; **Address:** Plastic Surgery Ctr, 535 Sycamore Ave, Shrewsbury, NJ 07702; **Phone:** 732-741-0970; **Board Cert:** Surgery 1995; Plastic Surgery 1998; **Med School:** Albany Med Coll 1988; **Resid:** Surgery, NYU Med Ctr 1994; **Fellow:** Plastic Reconstructive Surgery, NYU Med Ctr 1996

Glicksman, Caroline MD (PlS) - **Spec Exp:** Breast Reconstruction & Augmentation; Cosmetic Surgery-Breast; **Hospital:** Jersey Shore Univ Med Ctr; **Address:** 2164 Hwy 35, Bldg A, Sea Girt, NJ 08750; **Phone:** 732-974-2424; **Board Cert:** Plastic Surgery 1994; **Med School:** SUNY Downstate 1985; **Resid:** Surgery, Mt Sinai Hosp 1988; Plastic Surgery, New York Hosp-Cornell Med Ctr 1991; **Fellow:** Cosmetic Plastic Surgery, Mass Genl Hosp-Newton Wellesley Hosp 1992

Hetzler, Peter MD (PlS) - **Spec Exp:** Breast Cosmetic & Reconstructive Surgery; Cosmetic Surgery; Melanoma; **Hospital:** Riverview Med Ctr, Monmouth Med Ctr; **Address:** 200 White Rd, Ste 211, Little Silver, NJ 07739-1162; **Phone:** 732-219-0447; **Board Cert:** Plastic Surgery 1991; **Med School:** Univ Mich Med Sch 1981; **Resid:** Surgery, MS Hershey Med Ctr 1986; Plastic Reconstructive Surgery, MS Hershey Med Ctr 1988; **Fellow:** Microsurgery, York Hosp Trauma Ctr 1988; Cosmetic Plastic Surgery, Manhattan Eye & Ear Hosp 1989

Rose, Michael I MD (PlS) - **Spec Exp:** Body Contouring after Weight Loss; Cosmetic Surgery-Face; Eyelid Cosmetic & Reconstructive Surgery; Cosmetic Surgery-Breast; **Hospital:** Jersey Shore Univ Med Ctr, Monmouth Med Ctr; **Address:** Plastic Surgery Center, 535 Sycamore Ave, Shrewsbury, NJ 07702; **Phone:** 732-741-0970; **Board Cert:** Surgery 2001; Plastic Surgery 2003; **Med School:** NYU Sch Med 1994; **Resid:** Surgery, NYU/Bellevue Med Ctr 2000; **Fellow:** Plastic Surgery, Emory Univ Med Ctr 2002

Samra, Said MD (PlS) - **Spec Exp:** Reconstructive Surgery; Hand Surgery; Cosmetic Surgery; **Hospital:** Bayshore Community Hosp, Raritan Bay Med Ctr - Perth Amboy; **Address:** 733 N Beers St, Ste U1, Holmdel, NJ 07733-1528; **Phone:** 732-739-2100; **Board Cert:** Plastic Surgery 1988; **Med School:** Syria 1973; **Resid:** Surgery, CMDNJ-NJ Med Sch 1980; **Fellow:** Plastic Surgery, St Barnabas Hosp 1982

PSYCHIATRY

Rubin, Kenneth MD (Psyc) - **Spec Exp:** Mood Disorders; Anxiety Disorders; Dementia; **Hospital:** Monmouth Med Ctr; **Address:** 170 Morris Ave, Ste D, Long Branch, NJ 07740-6660; **Phone:** 732-870-3535; **Board Cert:** Psychiatry 1979; Geriatric Psychiatry 1995; **Med School:** SUNY Downstate 1974; **Resid:** Psychiatry, Kings County Hosp 1977; **Fac Appt:** Assoc Clin Prof Psyc, Drexel Univ Coll Med

PULMONARY DISEASE

Davis, George MD (Pul) - **Spec Exp:** Critical Care; Chronic Obstructive Lung Disease (COPD); Sepsis; **Hospital:** Monmouth Med Ctr; **Address:** 279 3rd Ave, Ste 510, Long Branch, NJ 07740; **Phone:** 732-870-0650; **Board Cert:** Internal Medicine 1976; Pulmonary Disease 1980; Critical Care Medicine 1987; **Med School:** Hahnemann Univ 1972; **Resid:** Internal Medicine, Monmouth Med Ctr 1977; **Fellow:** Pulmonary Disease, Monmouth Med Ctr 1979

Markowitz, Daniel MD (Pul) - **Spec Exp:** Critical Care; **Hospital:** Jersey Shore Univ Med Ctr; **Address:** 2640 Rte 70 Bldg 6A, Manasquan, NJ 08736-2610; **Phone:** 732-528-5900; **Board Cert:** Internal Medicine 1974; Pulmonary Disease 1976; Critical Care Medicine 2001; **Med School:** Albert Einstein Coll Med 1971; **Resid:** Internal Medicine, Univ Mich Med Ctr 1974; **Fellow:** Pulmonary Critical Care Medicine, Univ Mich Med Ctr 1976

REPRODUCTIVE ENDOCRINOLOGY

Damien, Miguel MD (RE) - **Hospital:** Riverview Med Ctr; **Address:** East Coast Infertility & Ivf, 200 White Rd, Ste 214, Little Silver, NJ 07739-1162; **Phone:** 732-758-6511 x111; **Board Cert:** Obstetrics & Gynecology 1998; Reproductive Endocrinology 1998; **Med School:** Dartmouth Med Sch 1982; **Resid:** Obstetrics & Gynecology, Beth Israel Deconess Hosp 1986; **Fellow:** Reproductive Endocrinology, Beth Israel Deconess Hosp 1988; Reproductive Endocrinology, Univ Conn Hosp 1989

RHEUMATOLOGY

Schwartzberg, Mori MD (Rhu) - **Spec Exp:** Rheumatoid Arthritis; Spondylitis; Osteoarthritis; **Hospital:** Jersey Shore Univ Med Ctr; **Address:** 10 Neptune Blvd, Ste 106, Neptune, NJ 07753-4848; **Phone:** 732-988-5030; **Board Cert:** Internal Medicine 1976; Rheumatology 1978; **Med School:** SUNY Upstate Med Univ 1973; **Resid:** Internal Medicine, Nassau County Med Ctr 1976; **Fellow:** Rheumatology, Albert Einstein Med Ctr 1978; **Fac Appt:** Asst Clin Prof Med, UMDNJ-RW Johnson Med Sch

Wasser, Kenneth MD (Rhu) - **Spec Exp:** Rheumatoid Arthritis; Lupus Nephritis; Psoriatic Arthritis; **Hospital:** Riverview Med Ctr, Monmouth Med Ctr; **Address:** 43 Gilbert St N, Tinton Falls, NJ 07701; **Phone:** 732-530-7999; **Board Cert:** Internal Medicine 1981; Rheumatology 1982; **Med School:** Case West Res Univ 1977; **Resid:** Internal Medicine, Univ Hosps 1980; Rheumatology, Univ Hosps 1982; **Fac Appt:** Asst Clin Prof Med, Drexel Univ Coll Med

SPORTS MEDICINE

Halpern, Brian MD (SM) - **Spec Exp:** Primary Care Sports Medicine; Knee Injuries; Shoulder Injuries; **Hospital:** Hosp For Special Surgery (page 108); **Address:** 475 County Road 520, Marlboro, NJ 07746-1059; **Phone:** 732-946-2100; **Board Cert:** Family Medicine 2002; Sports Medicine 1995; **Med School:** Cornell Univ-Weill Med Coll 1981; **Resid:** Family Medicine, Univ Md Med Ctr 1984; **Fellow:** Sports Medicine, Hughston Ortho Clinic 1985; **Fac Appt:** Asst Clin Prof Med, Cornell Univ-Weill Med Coll

Rice, Stephen G MD/PhD (SM) - **Spec Exp:** Primary Care Sports Medicine; Musculoskeletal Injuries; **Hospital:** Jersey Shore Univ Med Ctr; **Address:** Jersey Shore Sports Med Ctr, 1944 Route 33, Ste 204, Neptune, NJ 07753; **Phone:** 732-776-2433; **Board Cert:** Pediatrics 1981; Sports Medicine 2004; **Med School:** NYU Sch Med 1974; **Resid:** Pediatrics, Chldn's Hosp Med Ctr 1977; **Fac Appt:** Assoc Clin Prof Ped, UMDNJ-RW Johnson Med Sch

Sclafani, Michael MD (SM) - **Spec Exp:** Knee Injuries/Ligament Surgery; Shoulder Instability; **Hospital:** Jersey Shore Univ Med Ctr; **Address:** Orthopedic Institute, 2164 Route 35, Sea Girt, NJ 08750; **Phone:** 732-974-0404; **Board Cert:** Orthopaedic Surgery 1996; **Med School:** NYU Sch Med 1988; **Resid:** Orthopaedic Surgery, NYU Med Ctr 1993; **Fellow:** Sports Medicine, American Sports Med Inst 1994

SURGERY

Arbour, Robert MD (S) - **Spec Exp:** Vascular Surgery; **Hospital:** Bayshore Community Hosp, Riverview Med Ctr; **Address:** 213 Main St, Matawan, NJ 07747-3285; **Phone:** 732-566-2363; **Board Cert:** Surgery 1972; **Med School:** UMDNJ-NJ Med Sch, Newark 1965; **Resid:** Surgery, Georgetown Univ Hosp 1971

Borao, Frank J MD (S) - **Spec Exp:** Laparoscopic Abdominal Surgery; Obesity/Bariatric Surgery; Gastroesophageal Reflux Disease (GERD); Critical Care; **Hospital:** Monmouth Med Ctr; **Address:** 1131 Broad St, Ste 105, Shrewsbury, NJ 07702; **Phone:** 732-389-1331; **Board Cert:** Surgery 2000; **Med School:** UMDNJ-NJ Med Sch, Newark 1994; **Resid:** Surgery, Monmouth Med Ctr 1999; **Fellow:** Laparoscopic Surgery, White Plains Hosp 2000; **Fac Appt:** Asst Clin Prof S, Hahnemann Univ

Goldfarb, Michael A MD (S) - **Spec Exp:** Breast Surgery; Laparoscopic Surgery; **Hospital:** Monmouth Med Ctr; **Address:** 279 Third Ave, Ste 103, Long Branch, NJ 07740-6413; **Phone:** 732-870-6060; **Board Cert:** Surgery 1973; **Med School:** NYU Sch Med 1967; **Resid:** Surgery, Beth Israel Med Ctr 1972; **Fac Appt:** Assoc Prof S, Seton Hall Univ Sch Grad Med Ed

Schreiber, Martha MD (S) - **Spec Exp:** Breast Disease; Breast Cancer; **Hospital:** Ocean Med Ctr, Jersey Shore Univ Med Ctr; **Address:** 1540 Hwy 138 W, Ste 201, Wall, NJ 07719-3765; **Phone:** 732-280-0020; **Board Cert:** Surgery 2000; **Med School:** UMDNJ-RW Johnson Med Sch 1977; **Resid:** Surgery, Monmouth Med Ctr 1982

THORACIC SURGERY

Neibart, Richard MD (TS) - **Spec Exp:** Coronary Artery Surgery; **Hospital:** Jersey Shore Univ Med Ctr; **Address:** 1944 Route 33, Ste 201, Neptune, NJ 07753-4463; **Phone:** 732-776-4618; **Board Cert:** Surgery 1997; Thoracic Surgery 1999; **Med School:** Mount Sinai Sch Med 1982; **Resid:** Surgery, St Vincents Med Ctr 1987; **Fellow:** Thoracic Surgery, Univ Miami-Jackson Meml Hosp 1989

UROLOGY

Ebani, Jack MD (U) - **Spec Exp:** Prostate Cancer; Incontinence; **Hospital:** Jersey Shore Univ Med Ctr, Ocean Med Ctr; **Address:** 1820 Corlies Ave, Neptune, NJ 07753-4860; **Phone:** 732-774-4551; **Board Cert:** Urology 2005; **Med School:** SUNY Hlth Sci Ctr 1979; **Resid:** Surgery, N Shore Univ Hosp 1981; Urology, NYU Med Ctr 1985

Geltzeiler, Jules MD (U) - **Spec Exp:** Prostate Cancer; Incontinence; **Hospital:** Monmouth Med Ctr, Jersey Shore Univ Med Ctr; **Address:** Shore Urology, 279 3rd Ave, Ste 101, Long Branch, NJ 07740-6205; **Phone:** 732-222-2111; **Board Cert:** Urology 2004; **Med School:** Hahnemann Univ 1979; **Resid:** Surgery, Monmouth Med Ctr 1981; Urology, Geo Wash Univ Med Ctr 1984; **Fac Appt:** Asst Clin Prof S, Drexel Univ Coll Med

Grebler, Arnold MD (U) - **Spec Exp:** Urologic Cancer; Kidney Stones; Incontinence; Impotence; **Hospital:** Monmouth Med Ctr, Jersey Shore Univ Med Ctr; **Address:** Shore Urology, 279 3rd Ave, Ste 101, Long Branch, NJ 07740; **Phone:** 732-222-2111; **Board Cert:** Urology 1982; **Med School:** Italy 1974; **Resid:** Surgery, Maimonides Med Ctr 1976; Urology, Maimonides Med Ctr 1979; **Fac Appt:** Assoc Clin Prof U, Hahnemann Univ

Litvin, Y Samuel MD (U) - **Spec Exp:** Infertility; Prostate Disease; **Hospital:** Monmouth Med Ctr, Riverview Med Ctr; **Address:** Shore Urology, 279 3rd Ave, Ste 101, Long Branch, NJ 07740-6205; **Phone:** 732-222-2111; **Board Cert:** Urology 1994; **Med School:** UCLA 1986; **Resid:** Surgery, Beth Israel Med Ctr 1988; Urology, Beth Israel Med Ctr 1991

Rose, John MD (U) - **Hospital:** Riverview Med Ctr, Bayshore Community Hosp; **Address:** 70 E Front St, Red Bank, NJ 07701-1851; **Phone:** 732-741-5923; **Board Cert:** Urology 1977; **Med School:** Cornell Univ-Weill Med Coll 1968; **Resid:** Surgery, Cornell Univ/NY Hosp 1970; Urology, Univ Virginia 1974

Rotolo, James MD (U) - **Spec Exp:** Prostate Disease; Urologic Cancer; Kidney Stones; **Hospital:** Ocean Med Ctr, Jersey Shore Univ Med Ctr; **Address:** 2401 Hwy 35, Manasquan, NJ 08736; **Phone:** 732-223-7877; **Board Cert:** Urology 2000; **Med School:** Georgetown Univ 1984; **Resid:** Surgery, Georgetown Univ Hosp 1986; Urology, Georgetown Univ Hosp 1990

Morris

Morris

Specialty & Subspecialty	Page
Allergy & Immunology	873
Cardiac Electrophysiology	873
Cardiovascular Disease	873
Child Neurology	874
Colon & Rectal Surgery	874
Dermatology	874
Diagnostic Radiology	875
Family Medicine	875
Gastroenterology	875
Geriatric Medicine	876
Gynecologic Oncology	876
Hand Surgery	876
Hematology	876
Infectious Disease	876
Internal Medicine	877
Medical Oncology	877
Neonatal-Perinatal Medicine	878
Nephrology	878
Neurological Surgery	878
Neurology	878
Obstetrics & Gynecology	879
Ophthalmology	879
Orthopaedic Surgery	880
Otolaryngology	881
Pain Medicine	881
Pediatric Cardiology	881
Pediatric Endocrinology	881
Pediatric Gastroenterology	882
Pediatric Pulmonology	882
Pediatrics	882
Physical Medicine & Rehabilitation	883
Plastic Surgery	883
Psychiatry	884
Pulmonary Disease	884
Radiation Oncology	884
Reproductive Endocrinology	884
Rheumatology	885
Surgery	885
Thoracic Surgery	885
Urology	885

ALLERGY & IMMUNOLOGY

Applebaum, Eric MD (A&I) - **Spec Exp:** Asthma; Food Allergy; Sinus Disorders; Rhinitis; **Hospital:** Morristown Mem Hosp (page 88), St Clare's Hosp - Denville; **Address:** 50 Cherry Hill Rd, Ste 301, Parsippany, NJ 07054-1101; **Phone:** 973-335-1700; **Board Cert:** Allergy & Immunology 2003; **Med School:** Albert Einstein Coll Med 1987; **Resid:** Internal Medicine, LI Jewish Med Ctr 1990; **Fellow:** Allergy & Immunology, LI Jewish Med Ctr 1992

Chernack, William J MD (A&I) - **Spec Exp:** Asthma; Sinus Disorders; Insect Allergies; **Hospital:** Morristown Mem Hosp (page 88), NY-Presby Hosp (page 100); **Address:** 28 Franklin Pl, Morristown, NJ 07960-5305; **Phone:** 973-538-7271; **Board Cert:** Pediatrics 1975; Allergy & Immunology 1977; **Med School:** NY Med Coll 1970; **Resid:** Pediatrics, Columbia-Presby Med Ctr 1972; **Fellow:** Allergy & Immunology, Columbia-Presby Med Ctr 1974; **Fac Appt:** Asst Clin Prof Ped, Columbia P&S

CARDIAC ELECTROPHYSIOLOGY

Winters, Stephen Leslie MD (CE) - **Spec Exp:** Arrhythmias; Catheter Ablation; Pacemakers/Defibrillators; **Hospital:** Morristown Mem Hosp (page 88), Overlook Hosp (page 88); **Address:** Morristown Meml Hosp, 100 Madison Ave, Morristown, NJ 07962; **Phone:** 973-971-4261; **Board Cert:** Internal Medicine 1982; Cardiovascular Disease 1985; Cardiac Electrophysiology 2002; **Med School:** Mount Sinai Sch Med 1979; **Resid:** Internal Medicine, Mt Sinai Med Ctr 1981; **Fellow:** Cardiovascular Disease, Mt Sinai Med Ctr 1985; Cardiac Electrophysiology, Mt Sinai Med Ctr 1986; **Fac Appt:** Assoc Prof Med, UMDNJ-NJ Med Sch, Newark

CARDIOVASCULAR DISEASE

Blum, Mark A MD (Cv) - **Spec Exp:** Interventional Cardiology; Cholesterol/Lipid Disorders; **Hospital:** Morristown Mem Hosp (page 88), St Barnabas Med Ctr; **Address:** 95 Madison Ave, Ste A-10, Morristown, NJ 07960; **Phone:** 973-889-9001; **Board Cert:** Internal Medicine 1986; Cardiovascular Disease 1989; Interventional Cardiology 1999; **Med School:** Mount Sinai Sch Med 1983; **Resid:** Internal Medicine, Montefiore Hosp Med Ctr 1985; Internal Medicine, Mt Sinai Hosp 1986; **Fellow:** Cardiovascular Disease, Mt Sinai Hosp 1988; Cardiovascular Disease, Newark Beth Israel Hosp 1989; **Fac Appt:** Asst Clin Prof Med, UMDNJ-NJ Med Sch, Newark

Fisch, Arthur MD (Cv) - **Spec Exp:** Echocardiography; Coronary Artery Disease; Heart Valve Disease; **Hospital:** Morristown Mem Hosp (page 88); **Address:** 182 South St, Ste 5, Morristown, NJ 07960-5350; **Phone:** 973-267-3944; **Board Cert:** Internal Medicine 1972; Cardiovascular Disease 1975; **Med School:** Boston Univ 1969; **Resid:** Internal Medicine, UCLA Med Ctr 1972; **Fellow:** Cardiovascular Disease, Hosp Univ Penn 1974

Raska, Karel MD (Cv) - **Spec Exp:** Preventive Cardiology; Hypertension; Echocardiography; **Hospital:** Morristown Mem Hosp (page 88); **Address:** 182 South St, Ste 5, Morristown, NJ 07960-5350; **Phone:** 973-267-3944; **Board Cert:** Internal Medicine 1992; Cardiovascular Disease 1995; **Med School:** Harvard Med Sch 1989; **Resid:** Internal Medicine, Mass Genl Hosp 1992; **Fellow:** Cardiovascular Disease, Johns Hopkins Hosp 1995

Smart, Frank W MD (Cv) - **Spec Exp:** Congestive Heart Failure; Transplant Medicine-Heart; Ventricular Assist Device(LVAD); **Hospital:** Morristown Mem Hosp (page 88); **Address:** Morristown Meml Hosp, Dept Cardio Med, 100 Madison Ave, Morristown, NJ 07962; **Phone:** 973-971-5597; **Board Cert:** Internal Medicine 1988; Cardiovascular Disease 2001; **Med School:** Louisiana State Univ 1985; **Resid:** Internal Medicine, Ochsner Fdn Hosp 1988; **Fellow:** Cardiovascular Disease, Baylor Coll Med 1991

CHILD NEUROLOGY

Bennett, Harvey S MD (ChiN) - **Spec Exp:** Cerebral Palsy; Tourette's Syndrome; **Hospital:** Morristown Mem Hosp (page 88), Overlook Hosp (page 88); **Address:** Goryeb Children's Hosp, 100 Madison Ave, Morristown, NJ 07962; **Phone:** 973-971-5700; **Board Cert:** Pediatrics 1979; Child Neurology 1991; **Med School:** Albert Einstein Coll Med 1976; **Resid:** Pediatrics, St Christopher's Hosp Chldn 1978; Child Neurology, Albert Einstein Med Ctr 1981; **Fac Appt:** Clin Prof N, SUNY Downstate

Grossman, Elliot MD (ChiN) - **Spec Exp:** Migraine; ADD/ADHD; Tourette's Syndrome; **Hospital:** St Barnabas Med Ctr, Morristown Mem Hosp (page 88); **Address:** 205 Ridgedale Ave, Florham Park, NJ 07932; **Phone:** 973-966-6333; **Board Cert:** Pediatrics 1987; Child Neurology 1990; **Med School:** Meharry Med Coll 1980; **Resid:** Pediatrics, Bellevue Hosp 1982; Pediatrics, Boston Med Ctr 1983; **Fellow:** Pediatric Neurology, Boston Med Ctr 1986; **Fac Appt:** Asst Prof N, UMDNJ-NJ Med Sch, Newark

COLON & RECTAL SURGERY

Moskowitz, Richard L MD (CRS) - **Spec Exp:** Colon & Rectal Cancer; Anorectal Disorders; Inflammatory Bowel Disease; **Hospital:** Morristown Mem Hosp (page 88), St Clare's Hosp - Dover; **Address:** 111 Madison Ave, Ste 312, Morristown, NJ 07960-6083; **Phone:** 973-267-1225; **Board Cert:** Surgery 1991; Colon & Rectal Surgery 1985; **Med School:** Penn State Univ-Hershey Med Ctr 1978; **Resid:** Surgery, LI Jewish-Hillside Med Ctr 1983; Colon & Rectal Surgery, Greater Baltimore Med Ctr 1984; **Fellow:** Colon & Rectal Surgery, St Marks Hosp 1985

DERMATOLOGY

Almeida, Laila MD (D) - **Spec Exp:** Psoriasis; Acne; Skin Cancer; **Hospital:** St Clare's Hosp - Denville, NY-Presby Hosp (page 100); **Address:** 199 Baldwin Rd, Ste 230, Parsippany, NJ 07054-2043; **Phone:** 973-335-2560; **Board Cert:** Internal Medicine 1986; Dermatology 1989; **Med School:** Univ Mich Med Sch 1983; **Resid:** Internal Medicine, Columbia-Presby 1986; Dermatology, Columbia-Presby 1989

Bisaccia, Emil MD (D) - **Spec Exp:** Skin Cancer; Cosmetic Dermatology; **Hospital:** Morristown Mem Hosp (page 88), NY-Presby Hosp (page 100); **Address:** 182 South St, Ste 1, Morristown, NJ 07960; **Phone:** 973-267-0300; **Board Cert:** Dermatology 1984; Facial Plastic & Reconstructive Surgery 1989; **Med School:** Med Coll OH 1979; **Resid:** Dermatology, Ohio State Univ Hosps 1982; Dermatology, Columbia Presby Hosp 1983; **Fac Appt:** Clin Prof D, Columbia P&S

Marinaro, Robert MD (D) - **Spec Exp:** Cosmetic Dermatology; **Hospital:** Morristown Mem Hosp (page 88); **Address:** 20 Community Pl, Morristown, NJ 07960-7501; **Phone:** 973-538-4544; **Board Cert:** Dermatology 1986; **Med School:** Univ Rochester 1981; **Resid:** Internal Medicine, Strong Meml Hosp 1983; Dermatology, Case Western Res U Hosps 1986; **Fac Appt:** Asst Clin Prof D, Columbia P&S

DIAGNOSTIC RADIOLOGY

Claps, Richard J MD (DR) - **Spec Exp:** Nuclear Medicine; Ultrasound; Mammography; **Hospital:** St Clare's Hosp - Denville; **Address:** 25 Pocono Rd, Denville, NJ 07834; **Phone:** 973-625-6000; **Board Cert:** Diagnostic Radiology 1973; Nuclear Medicine 1975; Nuclear Radiology 1978; **Med School:** NY Med Coll 1968; **Resid:** Radiology, Metropolitan Hosp 1972

FAMILY MEDICINE

Holland Jr, Elbridge MD (FMed) **PCP** - **Hospital:** Overlook Hosp (page 88); **Address:** 492 Main St, Chatham, NJ 07928; **Phone:** 973-635-2432; **Board Cert:** Family Medicine 2002; Geriatric Medicine 1997; **Med School:** Univ Chicago-Pritzker Sch Med 1975; **Resid:** Family Medicine, Overlook Hosp 1978; **Fac Appt:** Asst Clin Prof FMed, UMDNJ-NJ Med Sch, Newark

GASTROENTEROLOGY

Dalena, John M MD (Ge) - **Spec Exp:** Endoscopy; Irritable Bowel Syndrome; Cancer Prevention; **Hospital:** Morristown Mem Hosp (page 88); **Address:** 65 Ridgedale Ave, Cedar Knolls, NJ 07927; **Phone:** 973-401-0500; **Board Cert:** Internal Medicine 1988; Gastroenterology 2001; **Med School:** UMDNJ-NJ Med Sch, Newark 1985; **Resid:** Internal Medicine, Mount Sinai Hosp 1988; **Fellow:** Gastroenterology, UMDNJ-Univ Hosp 1990; **Fac Appt:** Asst Prof Med, UMDNJ-NJ Med Sch, Newark

Freedman, Pamela MD (Ge) - **Spec Exp:** Peptic Acid Disorders; Colon Cancer; Irritable Bowel Syndrome; **Hospital:** St Clare's Hosp - Denville, St Clare's Hosp - Dover; **Address:** 369 W Blackwell St, Dover, NJ 07801-2560; **Phone:** 973-361-7660; **Board Cert:** Internal Medicine 1983; Gastroenterology 1985; **Med School:** Albert Einstein Coll Med 1980; **Resid:** Internal Medicine, Montefiore Hosp Med Ctr 1983; **Fellow:** Gastroenterology, Bellevue Hosp/NYU 1985

Samach, Michael MD (Ge) - **Spec Exp:** Colonoscopy; Gastroesophageal Reflux Disease (GERD); Hepatitis C; **Hospital:** Morristown Mem Hosp (page 88); **Address:** 101 Madison Ave, Ste 100, Morristown, NJ 07960; **Phone:** 973-455-0404; **Board Cert:** Internal Medicine 1974; Gastroenterology 1979; **Med School:** NYU Sch Med 1971; **Resid:** Internal Medicine, Montefiore Hosp Med Ctr 1974; **Fellow:** Gastroenterology, Montefiore Hosp Med Ctr 1978

Soriano, John MD (Ge) - **Hospital:** St Clare's Hosp - Denville, Morristown Mem Hosp (page 88); **Address:** 16 Pocono Rd, Ste 310, Denville, NJ 07834; **Phone:** 973-627-4430; **Board Cert:** Internal Medicine 1986; Gastroenterology 2003; **Med School:** Mexico 1981; **Resid:** Internal Medicine, Morristown Meml Hosp 1987; **Fellow:** Gastroenterology, Long Island Coll Hosp 1989

Stein, Lawrence B MD (Ge) - **Spec Exp:** Hepatitis; Gastroesophageal Reflux Disease (GERD); Endoscopy; **Hospital:** Morristown Mem Hosp (page 88), St Barnabas Med Ctr; **Address:** 195 Columbia Tpke, Florham Park, NJ 07932; **Phone:** 973-410-0960; **Board Cert:** Internal Medicine 1972; Gastroenterology 1973; **Med School:** Univ Minn 1965; **Resid:** Internal Medicine, Albert Einstein 1967; Internal Medicine, Albert Einstein 1970; **Fellow:** Gastroenterology, Albert Einstein 1972

GERIATRIC MEDICINE

Ryan, Joseph MD (Ger) - **Spec Exp:** Dementia; **Hospital:** Morristown Mem Hosp (page 88), **Address:** 95 Madison Ave, Ste 411, Morristown, NJ 07962; **Phone:** 973-971-7022; **Board Cert:** Internal Medicine 1974; Gastroenterology 1981; Geriatric Medicine 1988; **Med School:** SUNY Downstate 1970; **Resid:** Internal Medicine, Univ Hosp 1973; **Fellow:** Gastroenterology, St Vincent's Hosp & Med Ctr 1975; **Fac Appt:** Asst Prof Med, Columbia P&S

GYNECOLOGIC ONCOLOGY

Heller, Paul B MD (GO) - **Spec Exp:** Gynecologic Cancer; **Hospital:** Morristown Mem Hosp (page 88), Overlook Hosp (page 88); **Address:** Morristown Meml Hosp, Women's Cancer Ctr, 100 Madison Ave, Morristown, NJ 07960; **Phone:** 973-971-5900; **Board Cert:** Obstetrics & Gynecology 1975; Gynecologic Oncology 1982; **Med School:** NY Med Coll 1968; **Resid:** Obstetrics & Gynecology, Metroplitan Hosp 1971; Obstetrics & Gynecology, Beth Israel Med Ctr 1973; **Fellow:** Gynecologic Oncology, Metropolitan Hosp 1977; **Fac Appt:** Clin Prof ObG, Temple Univ

HAND SURGERY

Ende, Leigh MD (HS) - **Spec Exp:** Arthritis; Carpal Tunnel Syndrome; Hand & Upper Extremity Surgery; **Hospital:** St Clare's Hosp - Dover, Newton Meml Hosp; **Address:** 715 Rte 10 E, Randolph, NJ 07869; **Phone:** 973-366-5565; **Board Cert:** Orthopaedic Surgery 2000; Hand Surgery 2000; **Med School:** Tulane Univ 1978; **Resid:** Orthopaedic Surgery, UMDNJ-Univ Hosp 1983; **Fellow:** Hand Surgery, Columbia Presby Med Ctr 1984

Miller, Jeffrey K MD (HS) - **Spec Exp:** Carpal Tunnel Syndrome; Dupuytren's Contracture; **Hospital:** Morristown Mem Hosp (page 88), St Barnabas Med Ctr; **Address:** 301 E Hanover Ave, Morristown, NJ 07960; **Phone:** 973-538-5200; **Board Cert:** Orthopaedic Surgery 2000; Hand Surgery 2000; **Med School:** Univ Pittsburgh 1981; **Resid:** Surgery, Geo Wash Univ Med Ctr; Orthopaedic Surgery, Boston Univ Med Ctr 1986; **Fellow:** Hand Surgery, Thomas Jefferson Med Ctr 1987

HEMATOLOGY

Frank, Martin MD (Hem) - **Hospital:** Chilton Meml Hosp; **Address:** Collins Pavilion, 97 West Pkwy, Pompton Plains, NJ 07444; **Phone:** 973-831-5451; **Board Cert:** Hematology 1990; Medical Oncology 1989; Internal Medicine 1985; **Med School:** Geo Wash Univ 1982; **Resid:** Hematology, Montefiore Hosp Med Ctr 1986

INFECTIOUS DISEASE

Allegra, Donald MD (Inf) - **Spec Exp:** Tropical Diseases; AIDS/HIV; International Health; **Hospital:** St Clare's Hosp - Denville, Morristown Mem Hosp (page 88); **Address:** 765 Rte 10 E, Randolph, NJ 07869; **Phone:** 973-989-0068; **Board Cert:** Infectious Disease 1982; Internal Medicine 1978; **Med School:** Harvard Med Sch 1974; **Resid:** Internal Medicine, Univ Colorado Affil Hosps 1978; **Fellow:** Infectious Disease, Emory Univ Hosp 1981

McManus, Edward MD (Inf) - **Hospital:** St Clare's Hosp - Denville, Morristown Mem Hosp (page 88); **Address:** 765 Route 10 E, Randolph, NJ 07869; **Phone:** 973-989-0068; **Board Cert:** Internal Medicine 1985; Infectious Disease 1988; **Med School:** UMDNJ-NJ Med Sch, Newark 1982; **Resid:** Internal Medicine, Univ Wisconsin Hosp 1986; **Fellow:** Infectious Disease, Nat Inst Health 1989

INTERNAL MEDICINE

Najarian, James MD (IM) - **Hospital:** Morristown Mem Hosp (page 88); **Address:** 121 Center Grove Rd, Ste 13-14, Randolph, NJ 07869; **Phone:** 973-361-3737; **Board Cert:** Nephrology 1996; Internal Medicine 1975; **Med School:** Univ Wisc 1972; **Resid:** Internal Medicine, Beth Israel Hosp 1975; **Fellow:** Nephrology, Montefiore Hosp Med Ctr 1978

Randazzo, Jean MD (IM) **PCP** - **Hospital:** Morristown Mem Hosp (page 88); **Address:** Internal Medicine of Morristown, 95 Madison Ave, Ste A-00, Morristown, NJ 07960; **Phone:** 973-538-1388; **Board Cert:** Internal Medicine 2003; **Med School:** Tufts Univ 1990; **Resid:** Internal Medicine, Morristown Meml Hosp 1994; **Fac Appt:** Asst Clin Prof Med, UMDNJ-NJ Med Sch, Newark

Scaduto, Philip MD (IM) **PCP** - **Spec Exp:** Hypertension; Diabetes; Geriatrics; Preventive Medicine; **Hospital:** St Clare's Hosp - Denville; **Address:** 223 W Main St, Boonton, NJ 07005-1166; **Phone:** 973-335-8656; **Board Cert:** Internal Medicine 1986; Geriatric Medicine 1990; **Med School:** UMDNJ-NJ Med Sch, Newark 1983; **Resid:** Internal Medicine, UMDNJ-Univ Hosp 1986

Silva, Waldemar MD (IM) - **Hospital:** Chilton Meml Hosp; **Address:** 488 Newark Pompton Tpke, Pompton Plains, NJ 07444; **Phone:** 973-835-9100; **Board Cert:** Internal Medicine 1987; **Med School:** Harvard Med Sch 1982

Storch, Kenneth J MD/PhD (IM) - **Spec Exp:** Nutrition; Diabetes; Cholesterol/Lipid Disorders; **Hospital:** Morristown Mem Hosp (page 88), Overlook Hosp (page 88); **Address:** Medical Nutrition Clinic, 7 Columbia Tpke, Florham Park, NJ 07932; **Phone:** 973-765-9355; **Board Cert:** Internal Medicine 1982; **Med School:** SUNY Downstate 1979; **Resid:** Internal Medicine, Staten Island Hosp 1982; **Fellow:** Nutrition & Metabolism, MIT 1986; Nutrition & Metabolism, New England Deaconess 1988; **Fac Appt:** Asst Clin Prof Med, UMDNJ-NJ Med Sch, Newark

Weine, Gary MD (IM) **PCP** - **Spec Exp:** Hypertension; Cholesterol/Lipid Disorders; **Hospital:** Morristown Mem Hosp (page 88); **Address:** 95 Madison Ave, Ste 405, Morristown, NJ 07960-7336; **Phone:** 973-829-9998; **Board Cert:** Internal Medicine 1979; **Med School:** Cornell Univ-Weill Med Coll 1976; **Resid:** Internal Medicine, New York Hosp 1979; **Fac Appt:** Asst Clin Prof Med, UMDNJ-NJ Med Sch, Newark

MEDICAL ONCOLOGY

Adler, Kenneth MD (Onc) - **Spec Exp:** Lymphoma; Breast Cancer; **Hospital:** Morristown Mem Hosp (page 88); **Address:** 100 Madison Ave, Box 1089, Morristown, NJ 07962; **Phone:** 973-538-5210; **Board Cert:** Internal Medicine 1976; Hematology 1978; **Med School:** Albany Med Coll 1973; **Resid:** Internal Medicine, Albany Med Ctr 1976; **Fellow:** Hematology & Oncology, Albany Med Ctr 1978; **Fac Appt:** Asst Clin Prof Med, UMDNJ-NJ Med Sch, Newark

Casper, Ephraim MD (Onc) - **Spec Exp:** Gastrointestinal Cancer; Sarcoma; Pancreatic Cancer; **Hospital:** St Clare's Hosp - Denville, Meml Sloan Kettering Cancer Ctr (page 109); **Address:** Meml Sloan-Kettering Cancer Ctr at Saint Clare's, 23 Pocono Rd, Denville, NJ 07834; **Phone:** 973-983-7330; **Board Cert:** Internal Medicine 1977; Medical Oncology 1979; **Med School:** Rush Med Coll 1974; **Resid:** Internal Medicine, Rush Presbyterian-St Lukes Hosp 1977; **Fellow:** Medical Oncology, Meml Sloan Kettering Cancer Ctr 1979; **Fac Appt:** Prof Med, Cornell Univ-Weill Med Coll

Farber, Charles MD/PhD (Onc) - **Spec Exp:** Lymphoma; Leukemia; **Hospital:** Morristown Mem Hosp (page 88); **Address:** Carol G. Simon Cancer Center, 100 Madison Ave, Box 1089, Morristown, NJ 07962; **Phone:** 973-538-5210; **Board Cert:** Hematology 1996; Medical Oncology 1991; Internal Medicine 1990; **Med School:** NYU Sch Med 1986; **Resid:** Internal Medicine, NY Hosp 1988; **Fellow:** Medical Oncology, NY Hosp; **Fac Appt:** Asst Clin Prof Med, UMDNJ-NJ Med Sch, Newark

Papish, Steven MD (Onc) - **Spec Exp:** Breast Cancer; Lymphoma; Gynecologic Cancer; **Hospital:** Morristown Mem Hosp (page 88); **Address:** Carol Simon Cancer Ctr, 100 Madison Ave, Box 1089, Morristown, NJ 07962-1089; **Phone:** 973-538-5210; **Board Cert:** Internal Medicine 1977; Hematology 1980; Medical Oncology 1981; **Med School:** Univ Pennsylvania 1974; **Resid:** Internal Medicine, Geo Wash Univ Med Ctr 1978; **Fellow:** Hematology, New England Med Ctr 1979; Medical Oncology, Dana Farber Canc Inst 1981; **Fac Appt:** Asst Prof Med, UMDNJ-RW Johnson Med Sch

NEONATAL-PERINATAL MEDICINE

Skolnick, Lawrence MD (NP) - **Spec Exp:** Neonatal Care; **Hospital:** Morristown Mem Hosp (page 88), Overlook Hosp (page 88); **Address:** 100 Madison Ave, Morristown, NJ 07960-6136; **Phone:** 973-971-5488; **Board Cert:** Pediatrics 1975; Neonatal-Perinatal Medicine 1977; **Med School:** NYU Sch Med 1972; **Resid:** Pediatrics, Albert Einstein 1975; **Fellow:** Neonatal-Perinatal Medicine, Duke Univ Med Ctr 1977; **Fac Appt:** Assoc Clin Prof Ped, UMDNJ-NJ Med Sch, Newark

NEPHROLOGY

Fine, Paul MD (Nep) - **Spec Exp:** Hypertension; Kidney Failure; Dialysis Care; **Hospital:** Morristown Mem Hosp (page 88), St Clare's Hosp - Denville; **Address:** 2 Franklin Pl, Morristown, NJ 07960-5305; **Phone:** 973-267-7673; **Board Cert:** Internal Medicine 1982; Nephrology 1984; **Med School:** Yale Univ 1979; **Resid:** Internal Medicine, New York Hosp 1982; **Fellow:** Nephrology, Kidney Ctr-Cornell Univ Med Ctr 1984

NEUROLOGICAL SURGERY

Beyerl, Brian D MD (NS) - **Spec Exp:** Brain Tumors; Stereotactic Radiosurgery; Arteriovenous Malformations; **Hospital:** Morristown Mem Hosp (page 88), Overlook Hosp (page 88); **Address:** 310 Madison Ave, Morristown, NJ 07960; **Phone:** 973-285-7800; **Board Cert:** Neurological Surgery 1990; **Med School:** Johns Hopkins Univ 1980; **Resid:** Surgery, Johns Hopkins Univ Hosp 1981; Neurological Surgery, Mass General Hosp 1986; **Fac Appt:** Asst Clin Prof NS, UMDNJ-NJ Med Sch, Newark

Zampella, Edward J MD (NS) - **Spec Exp:** Stereotactic Radiosurgery; Pediatric Neurosurgery; Pain Management; Brain Tumors; **Hospital:** Overlook Hosp (page 88), Morristown Mem Hosp (page 88); **Address:** Atlantic Neurosurgical Specialists, 310 Madison Ave Fl 2, Morristown, NJ 07960; **Phone:** 973-285-7800; **Board Cert:** Neurological Surgery 1991; Pain Medicine 1997; **Med School:** Univ Ala 1982; **Resid:** Neurological Surgery, Univ Alabama Hosp 1988; **Fellow:** Neurology, Natl Hosp Nervous Disorders-Queen Square 1985; **Fac Appt:** Assoc Prof NS, UMDNJ-NJ Med Sch, Newark

NEUROLOGY

Cerny, Kenneth MD (N) - **Hospital:** Morristown Mem Hosp (page 88); **Address:** 310 Madison Ave, Morristown, NJ 07960; **Phone:** 973-285-1446; **Board Cert:** Neurology 1983; **Med School:** Columbia P&S 1976; **Resid:** Neurology, Barnes Hosp 1978; Neurology, Albert Einstein Med Ctr 1981

Fox, Stuart MD (N) - **Spec Exp:** Neuromuscular Disorders; Headache; **Hospital:** Morristown Mem Hosp (page 88); **Address:** 310 Madison Ave, Ste 120, Morristown, NJ 07960-6092; **Phone:** 973-285-1446; **Board Cert:** Internal Medicine 1978; Neurology 1982; **Med School:** Cornell Univ-Weill Med Coll 1975; **Resid:** Internal Medicine, Univ Mich Med Ctr 1978; Neurology, Albert Einstein 1981; **Fellow:** Clinical Neurophysiology, LI Jewish-Hillside Hosp 1982; **Fac Appt:** Asst Clin Prof Med, Columbia P&S

OBSTETRICS & GYNECOLOGY

Dreyfuss, Patricia MD (ObG) - **Hospital:** St Clare's Hosp - Denville; **Address:** 115 Route 46 West, Bldg D - Ste 27, Mountain Lakes, NJ 07046; **Phone:** 973-334-3345; **Board Cert:** Obstetrics & Gynecology 1985; **Med School:** Rutgers Univ 1979; **Resid:** Obstetrics & Gynecology, St Barnabas Hosp 1983

Gluck, Ian MD (ObG) **PCP** - **Hospital:** Morristown Mem Hosp (page 88); **Address:** 261 James St, Ste 3-C, Morristown, NJ 07960; **Phone:** 973-538-1515; **Board Cert:** Obstetrics & Gynecology 1985; **Med School:** NY Med Coll 1979; **Resid:** Obstetrics & Gynecology, Emory Univ/Grady Meml Hosp 1983; **Fac Appt:** Asst Clin Prof ObG, UMDNJ-NJ Med Sch, Newark

Iammatteo, Matthew MD (ObG) - **Spec Exp:** Pregnancy-High Risk; Hysteroscopic Surgery; Laparoscopic Surgery; **Hospital:** Morristown Mem Hosp (page 88); **Address:** 111 Madison Ave, Ste 311, Morristown, NJ 07960; **Phone:** 973-971-9950; **Board Cert:** Obstetrics & Gynecology 1991; **Med School:** Dominica 1985; **Resid:** Obstetrics & Gynecology, St Michael's Med Ctr 1989

Mohr, Robert F MD (ObG) **PCP** - **Spec Exp:** Gynecology Only; Gynecologic Surgery; **Hospital:** Morristown Mem Hosp (page 88); **Address:** 390 Route 10, Randolph, NJ 07869; **Phone:** 973-328-1262; **Board Cert:** Obstetrics & Gynecology 1983; **Med School:** Hahnemann Univ 1977; **Resid:** Obstetrics & Gynecology, Northwestern Meml Hosp 1981

Steer, Robert MD (ObG) - **Spec Exp:** Pregnancy-High Risk; **Hospital:** Morristown Mem Hosp (page 88); **Address:** 32 Maple Ave, Morristown, NJ 07960-5217; **Phone:** 973-993-1919; **Board Cert:** Obstetrics & Gynecology 2003; **Med School:** Cornell Univ-Weill Med Coll 1986; **Resid:** Obstetrics & Gynecology, New York Hosp 1990

Wallis, Joseph J DO (ObG) - **Spec Exp:** Laparoscopic Surgery; Endoscopy; Infertility; **Hospital:** St Clare's Hosp - Denville, St Clare's Hosp - Dover; **Address:** 600 Mt Pleasant Ave, Dover, NJ 07801-1629; **Phone:** 973-989-9000; **Board Cert:** Obstetrics & Gynecology 1977; **Med School:** Philadelphia Coll Osteo Med 1970; **Resid:** Obstetrics & Gynecology, St Michael's Med Ctr 1975

OPHTHALMOLOGY

Kazam, Ezra MD (Oph) - **Spec Exp:** Glaucoma; Cataract Surgery; Refractive Surgery; **Hospital:** Morristown Mem Hosp (page 88); **Address:** 2 Washington Pl, Morristown, NJ 07960-4220; **Phone:** 973-267-8755; **Board Cert:** Ophthalmology 1978; **Med School:** SUNY Downstate 1973; **Resid:** Ophthalmology, Montefiore Hosp 1977; **Fac Appt:** Asst Clin Prof Oph, Albert Einstein Coll Med

Pinke, Robert S MD (Oph) - **Spec Exp:** Cataract Surgery; Glaucoma; Laser Refractive Surgery; **Hospital:** St Clare's Hosp - Dover; **Address:** 66 Sunset Strip, Ste 107, Succasunna, NJ 07876; **Phone:** 973-584-4451; **Board Cert:** Ophthalmology 1989; **Med School:** Mount Sinai Sch Med 1984; **Resid:** Ophthalmology, Methodist Hosp-Baylor Coll Med 1988

Sachs, Ronald MD (Oph) - **Spec Exp:** Macular Degeneration; Diabetic Eye Disease/Retinopathy; Retinal Disorders; **Hospital:** Morristown Mem Hosp (page 88), St Clare's Hosp - Denville; **Address:** 8 Saddle Rd, Ste 201, Cedar Knolls, NJ 07927; **Phone:** 973-539-3600; **Board Cert:** Ophthalmology 2003; **Med School:** NYU Sch Med 1988; **Resid:** Ophthalmology, Montefiore Med Ctr 1992; **Fellow:** Retina, Albert Einstein Med Ctr 1993

Silverman, Cary MD (Oph) - **Spec Exp:** LASIK-Refractive Surgery; Cataract Surgery; **Hospital:** St Barnabas Med Ctr; **Address:** 46 Eagle Rock Ave, East Hanover, NJ 07936; **Phone:** 973-560-1500; **Board Cert:** Ophthalmology 1987; **Med School:** UMDNJ-NJ Med Sch, Newark 1982; **Resid:** Ophthalmology, Hahnemann Univ Hosp 1986; **Fac Appt:** Clin Prof Oph, UMDNJ-RW Johnson Med Sch

ORTHOPAEDIC SURGERY

Baydin, Jeffrey MD (OrS) - **Hospital:** Morristown Mem Hosp (page 88); **Address:** 50 Cherry Hill Rd, Ste 203, Parsippany, NJ 07054; **Phone:** 973-263-2828; **Board Cert:** Orthopaedic Surgery 1976; **Med School:** Tufts Univ 1969; **Resid:** Surgery, Boston City Hosp-Harvard 1971; Orthopaedic Surgery, Tufts-New England Med Ctr 1975

Cubelli, Ken MD (OrS) - **Hospital:** St Clare's Hosp - Denville; **Address:** 109 US Highway 46, Denville, NJ 07834; **Phone:** 973-625-1221; **Board Cert:** Orthopaedic Surgery 1997; **Med School:** NYU Sch Med 1979; **Resid:** Orthopaedic Surgery, UMDNJ-NJ Med Sch 1984

Dowling, William MD (OrS) - **Spec Exp:** Joint Replacement; **Hospital:** Morristown Mem Hosp (page 88), Overlook Hosp (page 88); **Address:** 131 Madison Ave, Ste 130, Morristown, NJ 07960; **Phone:** 973-998-5990; **Board Cert:** Orthopaedic Surgery 1978; **Med School:** UMDNJ-NJ Med Sch, Newark 1971; **Resid:** Orthopaedic Surgery, UMDNJ-Newark 1976

Feldman, David J MD (OrS) - **Spec Exp:** Pediatric Orthopaedic Surgery; **Hospital:** St Clare's Hosp - Denville; **Address:** 16 Pocono Rd, Ste 100, Denville, NJ 07834; **Phone:** 973-625-5700; **Board Cert:** Orthopaedic Surgery 1979; **Med School:** Boston Univ 1972; **Resid:** Surgery, Mt Sinai Med Ctr 1974; Orthopaedic Surgery, Mt Sinai Med Ctr 1977; **Fellow:** Pediatric Orthopaedic Surgery, Stanford Univ Med Ctr 1978

Hurley, John A MD (OrS) - **Spec Exp:** Sports Medicine; Knee Surgery; Shoulder Surgery; **Hospital:** Morristown Mem Hosp (page 88); **Address:** 111 Madison Ave, Morristown, NJ 07962-1446; **Phone:** 973-971-6898; **Board Cert:** Orthopaedic Surgery 1999; **Med School:** NYU Sch Med 1980; **Resid:** Orthopaedic Surgery, UMDNJ 1985; **Fellow:** Sports Medicine, Cleveland Clinic 1986; **Fac Appt:** Asst Clin Prof S, UMDNJ-NJ Med Sch, Newark

Rieger, Mark MD (OrS) - **Spec Exp:** Pediatric Orthopaedic Surgery; Scoliosis; Hip Disorders-Pediatric; **Hospital:** Morristown Mem Hosp (page 88), St Barnabas Med Ctr; **Address:** 218 Ridgedale Ave, Ste 104, Cedar Knolls, NJ 07927-2109; **Phone:** 973-538-7700; **Board Cert:** Orthopaedic Surgery 2002; **Med School:** Univ Conn 1983; **Resid:** Orthopaedic Surgery, LI Jewish Hosp 1988; **Fellow:** Pediatric Orthopaedic Surgery, DuPont Inst 1989

Taffet, Berton MD (OrS) - **Hospital:** Morristown Mem Hosp (page 88); **Address:** 95 Madison Ave, Ste A07, Morristown, NJ 07960; **Phone:** 973-984-0404; **Board Cert:** Orthopaedic Surgery 2001; **Med School:** Albert Einstein Coll Med 1978; **Resid:** Orthopaedic Surgery, Mt Sinai Med Ctr 1983; **Fellow:** Joint Replacement Surgery, Univ Colorado Hosp 1984

OTOLARYNGOLOGY

Fleming, Gregory MD (Oto) - **Spec Exp:** Endoscopic Sinus Surgery; Sleep Disorders/Apnea; **Hospital:** Morristown Mem Hosp (page 88), Overlook Hosp (page 88); **Address:** 26 Madison Ave, Morristown, NJ 07960; **Phone:** 973-267-1850; **Board Cert:** Otolaryngology 1988; **Med School:** Univ Mass Sch Med 1982; **Resid:** Surgery, Univ Mass Med Ctr 1984; Otolaryngology, Mass EE Infirm 1988

Lachman, Reid MD (Oto) - **Hospital:** Morristown Mem Hosp (page 88); **Address:** 95 Madison Ave, Ste 105, Morristown, NJ 07960; **Phone:** 973-644-0808; **Board Cert:** Otolaryngology 1986; **Med School:** NY Med Coll 1981; **Resid:** Otolaryngology, Montefiore Hosp Med Ctr 1986

Taylor, Howard MD (Oto) - **Spec Exp:** Hearing Loss; Sinus Surgery; Throat Disorders; Voice Disorders; **Hospital:** Chilton Meml Hosp; **Address:** 51 State Highway 23 S, Riverdale, NJ 07457-1625; **Phone:** 973-831-1220; **Board Cert:** Otolaryngology 1980; **Med School:** Columbia P&S 1976; **Resid:** Otolaryngology, Univ Chicago Hosps 1980; **Fellow:** Facial Plastic Surgery, Hosp Med Coll Penn 1981; **Fac Appt:** Asst Clin Prof Oto, UMDNJ-NJ Med Sch, Newark

PAIN MEDICINE

Rudman, Michael E MD (PM) - **Hospital:** Morristown Mem Hosp (page 88); **Address:** Morristown Meml Hosp, Pain Mgmt Ctr, 95 Madison Ave, Ste 402, Morristown, NJ 07960; **Phone:** 973-971-6824; **Board Cert:** Pain Medicine 1996; Anesthesiology 1993; **Med School:** Penn State Univ-Hershey Med Ctr 1988; **Resid:** Anesthesiology, Hosp Univ Penn 1992

PEDIATRIC CARDIOLOGY

Donnelly, Christine MD (PCd) - **Spec Exp:** Fetal Echocardiography; Heart Disease-Congenital; Cardiac Catheterization; **Hospital:** Morristown Mem Hosp (page 88), NY-Presby Hosp (page 100); **Address:** 100 Madison Ave, Morristown, NJ 07960-6136; **Phone:** 973-971-5996; **Board Cert:** Pediatrics 1985; Pediatric Cardiology 1985; **Med School:** Columbia P&S 1978; **Resid:** Pediatrics, Columbia-Presby Med Ctr 1981; **Fellow:** Pediatric Cardiology, Columbia-Presby Med Ctr 1984; **Fac Appt:** Assoc Clin Prof Ped, Columbia P&S

PEDIATRIC ENDOCRINOLOGY

Chin, Daisy MD (PEn) - **Spec Exp:** Thyroid Disorders; Growth Disorders; Pubertal Disorders; **Hospital:** Morristown Mem Hosp (page 88); **Address:** Morristown Mem Hosp, 100 Madison Ave, Box 53, Morristown, NJ 07962; **Phone:** 973-971-4340; **Board Cert:** Pediatrics 2003; Pediatric Endocrinology 1999; **Med School:** SUNY Downstate 1992; **Resid:** Pediatrics, Columbia Presby Med Ctr 1995; **Fellow:** Pediatric Endocrinology, NYU Med Ctr 1998; **Fac Appt:** Asst Prof Ped, Columbia P&S

Starkman, Harold MD (PEn) - **Spec Exp:** Diabetes; Growth Disorders; **Hospital:** Morristown Mem Hosp (page 88), Overlook Hosp (page 88); **Address:** 100 Madison Ave, Morristown, NJ 07962-6136; **Phone:** 973-971-4340; **Board Cert:** Pediatrics 1980; Pediatric Endocrinology 1983; **Med School:** Albert Einstein Coll Med 1976; **Resid:** Pediatrics, Mount Sinai Hosp 1978; Pediatrics, New York Hosp 1979; **Fellow:** Pediatric Endocrinology, New York Hosp 1980; Pediatric Endocrinology, Joslin Diabetes Center 1983; **Fac Appt:** Assoc Prof Ped, UMDNJ-NJ Med Sch, Newark

PEDIATRIC GASTROENTEROLOGY

Mones, Richard MD (PGe) - **Spec Exp:** Inflammatory Bowel Disease/Crohn's; Nutrition; **Hospital:** Morristown Mem Hosp (page 88), Overlook Hosp (page 88); **Address:** Morristown Meml Hosp, Ped Gastroenterology, 100 Madison Ave, Box 82, Morristown, NJ 07962; **Phone:** 973-971-5676; **Board Cert:** Pediatrics 1976; Pediatric Gastroenterology 2005; **Med School:** NY Med Coll 1971; **Resid:** Pediatrics, Babies/Columbia-Presby Hosps 1973; **Fellow:** Pediatric Gastroenterology, Babies/Columbia-Presby Hosps 1977; **Fac Appt:** Assoc Clin Prof Ped, Columbia P&S

Rosh, Joel MD (PGe) - **Spec Exp:** Inflammatory Bowel Disease; Celiac Disease; Liver Disease; **Hospital:** Morristown Mem Hosp (page 88), Overlook Hosp (page 88); **Address:** Dept Peds Gastroenterology & Nutrition, 100 Madison Ave, Morristown, NJ 07960-6136; **Phone:** 973-971-5676; **Board Cert:** Pediatrics 1989; Pediatric Gastroenterology 2000; **Med School:** Albert Einstein Coll Med 1986; **Resid:** Pediatrics, Babies Hosp/Columbia-Presby Med Ctr 1989; **Fellow:** Pediatric Gastroenterology, Mount Sinai Med Ctr 1991; **Fac Appt:** Assoc Prof Ped, UMDNJ-NJ Med Sch, Newark

PEDIATRIC PULMONOLOGY

Atlas, Arthur B MD (PPul) - **Spec Exp:** Asthma; Cystic Fibrosis; Lung Disease; **Hospital:** Morristown Mem Hosp (page 88), Overlook Hosp (page 88); **Address:** Morristown Meml Hosp, Resp Ctr for Chldn, 100 Madison Ave, Morristown, NJ 07962; **Phone:** 973-971-4142; **Board Cert:** Pediatrics 2001; Pediatric Pulmonology 2000; **Med School:** Mexico 1982; **Resid:** Pediatrics, St Louis Chldns Hosp 1986; **Fellow:** Allergy & Immunology, St Louis Chldns Hosp 1989; Pediatric Pulmonology, Chldns Hosp/Univ Pittsburgh 1991; **Fac Appt:** Asst Clin Prof Ped, UMDNJ-NJ Med Sch, Newark

PEDIATRICS

Cohen, Martin MD (Ped) `PCP` - **Spec Exp:** Growth Disorders; Asthma; Allergy; **Hospital:** Morristown Mem Hosp (page 88); **Address:** 261 James St, Ste 1G, Morristown, NJ 07960-6331; **Phone:** 973-540-9393; **Board Cert:** Pediatrics 1972; **Med School:** SUNY Hlth Sci Ctr 1967; **Resid:** Pediatrics, Children's Hosp 1970; **Fac Appt:** Asst Clin Prof Ped, Columbia P&S

Gotfried, Fern MD (Ped) - **Hospital:** Morristown Mem Hosp (page 88); **Address:** Franklin Pediatrics, 91 S Jefferson Rd Fl 2, Whippany, NJ 07981; **Phone:** 973-538-6116; **Board Cert:** Pediatrics 1986; Adolescent Medicine 2002; **Med School:** Rutgers Univ 1980; **Resid:** Pediatrics, Strong Memorial Hosp 1983; **Fellow:** Adolescent Medicine, Strong Memorial Hosp 1985

Handler, Robert MD (Ped) `PCP` - **Spec Exp:** Asthma; Allergy; Behavioral Disorders; **Hospital:** Morristown Mem Hosp (page 88), St Clare's Hosp - Denville; **Address:** 1140 Parsippany Blvd, Ste 102, Parsippany, NJ 07054; **Phone:** 973-263-0066; **Board Cert:** Pediatrics 1980; **Med School:** UMDNJ-NJ Med Sch, Newark 1975; **Resid:** Pediatrics, Chldns Hosp 1978; **Fac Appt:** Asst Clin Prof Ped, UMDNJ-NJ Med Sch, Newark

Suda, Anjuli MD (Ped) - **Spec Exp:** Pulmonary Disease; **Hospital:** Chilton Meml Hosp; **Address:** 170 Kinnelon Rd, Ste 28, Kinnelon, NJ 07405; **Phone:** 973-838-0001; **Board Cert:** Pediatrics 1988; **Med School:** India 1976; **Resid:** Pediatrics, St Joseph's Hosp & Med Ctr 1985

PHYSICAL MEDICINE & REHABILITATION

Malanga, Gerard MD (PMR) - **Spec Exp:** Pain-Back & Neck; Sports Medicine; Electrodiagnosis; **Hospital:** Overlook Hosp (page 88); **Address:** 95 Mt Kemble Ave, Bldg T-4, Morristown, NJ 07960; **Phone:** 973-267-2293; **Board Cert:** Physical Medicine & Rehabilitation 2003; Pain Medicine 2002; **Med School:** UMDNJ-NJ Med Sch, Newark 1982; **Resid:** Physical Medicine & Rehabilitation, UMDNJ Affil Hosp 1992; **Fellow:** Sports Medicine, Mayo Clinic 1993; **Fac Appt:** Assoc Clin Prof PMR, UMDNJ-NJ Med Sch, Newark

Mulford, Gregory MD (PMR) - **Spec Exp:** Sports Medicine; Electrodiagnosis; **Hospital:** Morristown Mem Hosp (page 88), Overlook Hosp (page 88); **Address:** Associates in Rehab Medicine, 95 Mt Kemble Ave Thebaud Bldg Fl 4, Morristown, NJ 07960; **Phone:** 973-267-2293; **Board Cert:** Physical Medicine & Rehabilitation 1990; **Med School:** UMDNJ-RW Johnson Med Sch 1985; **Resid:** Physical Medicine & Rehabilitation, Columbia-Presby Hosp 1989; **Fac Appt:** Asst Clin Prof PMR, Columbia P&S

PLASTIC SURGERY

Colon, Francisco G MD (PlS) - **Spec Exp:** Cosmetic Surgery-Face & Body; Reconstructive Plastic Surgery; **Hospital:** St Barnabas Med Ctr, Morristown Mem Hosp (page 88); **Address:** PeerGroup Plastic Surgery Ctr, 124 Columbia Tpke, Florham Park, NJ 07932; **Phone:** 973-822-3000; **Board Cert:** Plastic Surgery 1997; **Med School:** Columbia P&S 1987; **Resid:** Surgery, St Lukes Roosevelt Hosp 1992; Plastic Surgery, Beth Israel Deaconess Hosp 1992

Hawrylo, Richard MD (PlS) - **Spec Exp:** Cosmetic Surgery-Breast; Cosmetic Surgery-Face & Eyelid; Abdominoplasty; Liposuction; **Hospital:** St Barnabas Med Ctr, Morristown Mem Hosp (page 88); **Address:** 124 Columbia Tpke, Florham Park, NJ 07932-2106; **Phone:** 973-822-3000; **Board Cert:** Plastic Surgery 1980; **Med School:** Wake Forest Univ 1972; **Resid:** Surgery, Bellevue/NYU Med Ctr 1977; Plastic Surgery, Bellevue/NYU Med Ctr 1979

Lange, David J MD (PlS) - **Spec Exp:** Cosmetic Surgery-Breast; Liposuction & Body Contouring; Craniofacial Surgery/Reconstruction; **Hospital:** St Barnabas Med Ctr, Morristown Mem Hosp (page 88); **Address:** 124 Columbia Tpke, Florham Park, NJ 07932-2183; **Phone:** 973-822-3000; **Board Cert:** Plastic Surgery 1990; **Med School:** Mexico 1979; **Resid:** Surgery, St Banabas Med Ctr 1985; **Fellow:** Plastic Surgery, St Louis Univ 1987

Rafizadeh, Farhad MD (PlS) - **Spec Exp:** Breast Reconstruction; Cosmetic Surgery-Face; **Hospital:** Morristown Mem Hosp (page 88), St Barnabas Med Ctr; **Address:** 101 Madison Ave, Ste 105, Morristown, NJ 07960; **Phone:** 973-267-0928; **Board Cert:** Plastic Surgery 1986; **Med School:** Switzerland 1975; **Resid:** Surgery, St Barnabas Med Ctr 1981; Surgery, Morristown Meml Hosp 1982; **Fellow:** Plastic Surgery, New York Hosp-Cornell Med Ctr 1984

Starker, Isaac MD (PlS) - **Spec Exp:** Cosmetic Surgery-Face; Cosmetic Surgery-Body; Breast Reconstruction; **Hospital:** Morristown Mem Hosp (page 88), St Barnabas Med Ctr; **Address:** 124 Columbia Tpke, Florham Park, NJ 07932; **Phone:** 973-822-3000; **Board Cert:** Plastic Surgery 1992; **Med School:** NYU Sch Med 1981; **Resid:** Surgery, St Luke's-Roosevelt Hosp Ctr 1986; Plastic Surgery, Montefiore Med Ctr 1988; **Fellow:** Hand Surgery, St Luke's-Roosevelt Hosp Ctr 1989

Weinstein, Larry MD (PlS) - **Spec Exp:** Breast Cosmetic & Reconstructive Surgery; Cosmetic Surgery-Face; Liposuction & Body Contouring; **Hospital:** Morristown Mem Hosp (page 88), Overlook Hosp (page 88); **Address:** 385 State Rte 24, Ste 3K, Chester, NJ 07930-2910; **Phone:** 908-879-2222; **Board Cert:** Plastic Surgery 1993; **Med School:** Mexico 1979; **Resid:** Surgery, Univ Hosp/Morristown Meml Hosp 1984; Surgical Oncology, Meml Sloan-Kettering Cancer Ctr 1985; **Fellow:** Plastic Surgery, Univ Pittsburgh 1986; Plastic Surgery, SUNY-Brooklyn Med Ctr 1988

PSYCHIATRY

Sofair, Jane MD (Psyc) - **Spec Exp:** Anxiety & Depression; Women's Health; **Hospital:** Morristown Mem Hosp (page 88); **Address:** 35 Airport Rd, Ste 350, Morristown, NJ 07960; **Phone:** 973-292-0960; **Board Cert:** Psychiatry 1986; **Med School:** NYU Sch Med 1980; **Resid:** Psychiatry, NYU Med Ctr 1984; **Fac Appt:** , Columbia P&S

PULMONARY DISEASE

Benton, Marc MD (Pul) - **Spec Exp:** Asthma; Sleep Disorders/Apnea; Emphysema; **Hospital:** Morristown Mem Hosp (page 88), Overlook Hosp (page 88); **Address:** 8 Saddle Rd, Cedar Knolls, NJ 07927; **Phone:** 973-267-9393; **Board Cert:** Internal Medicine 1985; Pulmonary Disease 1988; Critical Care Medicine 2005; Sleep Medicine 1995; **Med School:** Mount Sinai Sch Med 1982; **Resid:** Internal Medicine, Mt Sinai Sch Med 1985; **Fellow:** Pulmonary Disease, NYU Med Ctr 1988

RADIATION ONCOLOGY

Wong, James R MD (RadRO) - **Spec Exp:** Stereotactic Radiosurgery; Prostate Cancer; Lung Cancer; **Hospital:** Morristown Mem Hosp (page 88); **Address:** Morristown Meml Hosp, Dept Rad Oncology, 100 Madison Ave, Box 9, Morristown, NJ 07960; **Phone:** 973-971-5329; **Board Cert:** Radiation Oncology 1993; **Med School:** Harvard Med Sch 1986; **Resid:** Radiation Oncology, Harvard Jt Ctr for Rad Therapy 1992; **Fac Appt:** Assoc Clin Prof RadRO, Columbia P&S

REPRODUCTIVE ENDOCRINOLOGY

Bergh, Paul A MD (RE) - **Spec Exp:** Infertility-IVF; **Hospital:** Morristown Mem Hosp (page 88), St Barnabas Med Ctr; **Address:** 111 Madison Ave, Ste 100, Morristown, NJ 07962; **Phone:** 973-971-4600; **Board Cert:** Obstetrics & Gynecology 2004; Reproductive Endocrinology 2004; **Med School:** UMDNJ-RW Johnson Med Sch 1983; **Resid:** Obstetrics & Gynecology, St Banabas Hosp 1989; **Fellow:** Reproductive Endocrinology, Mount Sinai Med Ctr 1991

Scott, Richard T MD (RE) - **Spec Exp:** Infertility; Infertility-IVF; Fertility Preservation in Cancer; **Hospital:** Morristown Mem Hosp (page 88), St Barnabas Med Ctr; **Address:** Reproductive Medicine Assocs, 111 Madison Ave, Ste 100, Morristown, NJ 07962; **Phone:** 973-971-4600; **Board Cert:** Obstetrics & Gynecology 2004; Reproductive Endocrinology 2004; **Med School:** Univ VA Sch Med 1983; **Resid:** Obstetrics & Gynecology, Wilford Hall USAF Med Ctr 1987; **Fellow:** Reproductive Endocrinology, Jones Inst Reproductive Med 1989

RHEUMATOLOGY

Pasik, Deborah MD (Rhu) - **Spec Exp:** Rheumatoid Arthritis; **Hospital:** Morristown Mem Hosp (page 88); **Address:** Atlantic Rheumatology, 8 Saddle Rd, Ste 102, Cedar Knolls, NJ 07927; **Phone:** 973-984-9796; **Board Cert:** Internal Medicine 1985; Rheumatology 1988; **Med School:** Mount Sinai Sch Med 1982; **Resid:** Internal Medicine, Beth Israel Hosp 1985; **Fellow:** Rheumatology, NYU Med Ctr 1988

SURGERY

Rolandelli, Rolando MD (S) - **Spec Exp:** Crohn's Disease; Inflammatory Bowel Disease; **Hospital:** Morristown Mem Hosp (page 88), Overlook Hosp (page 88); **Address:** 100 Madison Ave, rm 78, Morristown, NJ 07962; **Phone:** 973-971-7200; **Board Cert:** Surgery 1999; **Med School:** Argentina 1977; **Resid:** Surgery, Buenos Aires 1982; Surgery, Grad Hosp 1990; **Fellow:** Metabolism, Univ Penn 1984

THORACIC SURGERY

Brown III, John MD (TS) - **Spec Exp:** Cardiac Surgery-Adult; Thoracic Cancers; Heart Valve Surgery; **Hospital:** Morristown Mem Hosp (page 88); **Address:** 100 Madison Ave, Morristown, NJ 07960-1956; **Phone:** 973-971-7300; **Board Cert:** Surgery 2001; Thoracic Surgery 2004; **Med School:** Cornell Univ-Weill Med Coll 1986; **Resid:** Surgery, NY Hosp-Cornell Univ Med Ctr 1991; **Fellow:** Thoracic Surgery, NY Hosp-Meml Sloan Kettering 1993

Parr, Grant MD (TS) - **Spec Exp:** Cardiac Surgery; Heart Valve Disease; **Hospital:** Morristown Mem Hosp (page 88), Overlook Hosp (page 88); **Address:** MidAtlantic Surg Assocs, 100 Madison Ave, Morristown, NJ 07962; **Phone:** 973-971-7300; **Board Cert:** Thoracic Surgery 1997; **Med School:** Cornell Univ-Weill Med Coll 1969; **Resid:** Surgery, Univ Hosps 1971; Surgery, Univ Alabama Hosp 1977; **Fellow:** Cardiothoracic Surgery, Univ Alabama Hosp 1977; **Fac Appt:** Asst Clin Prof S, Columbia P&S

Widmann, Mark D MD (TS) - **Spec Exp:** Minimally Invasive Thoracic Surgery; Video Assisted Thoracic Surgery (VATS); **Hospital:** Morristown Mem Hosp (page 88); **Address:** PO Box 1348, Morristown, NJ 07962-1348; **Phone:** 973-644-4844; **Board Cert:** Surgery 1996; Thoracic Surgery 1999; **Med School:** Yale Univ 1987; **Resid:** Surgery, Yale-New Haven Hosp 1995; **Fellow:** Thoracic Surgery, Univ Iowa Hosps & Clinics 1998

UROLOGY

Atlas, Ian MD (U) - **Spec Exp:** Prostate Cancer; Bladder Cancer; Urologic Cancer; **Hospital:** Morristown Mem Hosp (page 88); **Address:** Adult & Pediatric Urology Group, 261 James St, Ste 3-A, Morristown, NJ 07960-6348; **Phone:** 973-539-0333; **Board Cert:** Urology 2002; **Med School:** Mount Sinai Sch Med 1984; **Resid:** Urology, Mount Sinai Med Ctr 1989; **Fellow:** Urologic Oncology, Meml Sloan Kettering Cancer Ctr 1992

Chaikin, David C MD (U) - **Spec Exp:** Voiding Dysfunction; Urology-Female; **Hospital:** Morristown Mem Hosp (page 88); **Address:** Morristown Urology, 261 James St, Ste 1A, Morristown, NJ 07960; **Phone:** 973-539-1050; **Board Cert:** Urology 1999; **Med School:** Albert Einstein Coll Med 1992; **Resid:** Urology, Hosp Univ Penn 1997; **Fellow:** Female Urology, New York Hosp-Cornell Med Ctr 1999; **Fac Appt:** Asst Clin Prof U, Cornell Univ-Weill Med Coll

Colton, Marc D MD (U) - **Spec Exp:** Prostate Cancer; Urologic Cancer; Kidney Stones; Robotic Surgery; **Hospital:** St Clare's Hosp - Denville, Morristown Mem Hosp (page 88); **Address:** 16 Pocono Rd, Ste 205, Denville, NJ 07869; **Phone:** 973-627-0060; **Board Cert:** Urology 2005; **Med School:** Med Coll PA Hahnemann 1989; **Resid:** Surgery, Temple Univ Hosp 1991; Urology, Temple Univ Hosp 1995

Passaic

Passaic

ADDICTION PSYCHIATRY

Hindin, Lee MD (AdP) - **Hospital:** St Barnabas Med Ctr; **Address:** 1149 Bloomfield Ave, Clifton, NJ 07012; **Phone:** 973-365-2300; **Board Cert:** Psychiatry 1984; **Med School:** UMDNJ-NJ Med Sch, Newark 1977; **Resid:** Psychiatry, UCLA-Neuropsyc Inst 1982

ALLERGY & IMMUNOLOGY

Klein, Robert MD (A&I) - **Spec Exp:** Asthma; Sinusitis; Urticaria; **Hospital:** NY-Presby Hosp (page 100), PBI Regional- Passaic; **Address:** 1005 Clifton Ave, Clifton, NJ 07013-3597; **Phone:** 973-773-7400; **Board Cert:** Pediatrics 1981; **Med School:** NY Med Coll 1976; **Resid:** Pediatrics, Beth Israel Hosp 1979; **Fellow:** Allergy & Immunology, Columbia-Presby Med Ctr 1984; **Fac Appt:** Asst Clin Prof Med, Columbia P&S

CARDIOVASCULAR DISEASE

Salimi, Mostafa MD (Cv) - **Hospital:** Wayne Hosp, St Joseph's Regl Med Ctr - Paterson; **Address:** 510 Hamburg Tpke, Ste 201, Wayne, NJ 07470; **Phone:** 973-942-1141; **Board Cert:** Internal Medicine 1973; Cardiovascular Disease 1977; **Med School:** Iran 1964; **Resid:** Internal Medicine, VA Hospital 1970; **Fellow:** Cardiovascular Disease, George Washington Univ Hosp 1972

Schwarz, Michael MD (Cv) - **Hospital:** PBI Regional- Passaic; **Address:** 1198 Clifton Ave, Clifton, NJ 07013; **Phone:** 973-779-0019; **Board Cert:** Cardiovascular Disease 1995; **Med School:** UMDNJ-NJ Med Sch, Newark 1988; **Resid:** Internal Medicine, Bronx Muni Hosp Ctr 1991; Cardiovascular Disease, Montefiore Med Ctr 1994

Siepser, Stuart MD (Cv) - **Spec Exp:** Coronary Artery Disease; Hypertension; Nuclear Stress Testing; Cholesterol/Lipid Disorders; **Hospital:** Chilton Meml Hosp, Morristown Mem Hosp (page 88); **Address:** 1777 Hamburg Tpke, Ste 302, Wayne, NJ 07470-5243; **Phone:** 973-831-9222; **Board Cert:** Internal Medicine 1972; Cardiovascular Disease 1975; **Med School:** NYU Sch Med 1968; **Resid:** Internal Medicine, NYU Med Ctr 1970; Cardiovascular Disease, NYU Med Ctr 1972; **Fac Appt:** Asst Clin Prof Med, UMDNJ-NJ Med Sch, Newark

Strobeck, John E MD/PhD (Cv) - **Spec Exp:** Congestive Heart Failure; Nuclear Cardiology; Cardiac Imaging; **Hospital:** Valley Hosp (page 762); **Address:** 297 Lafayette Ave, Hawthorne, NJ 07506; **Phone:** 973-423-9388; **Board Cert:** Internal Medicine 1979; Cardiovascular Disease 1983; **Med School:** Univ Cincinnati 1974; **Resid:** Internal Medicine, Peter Bent Brigham Hospital 1976; **Fellow:** Cardiovascular Disease, Albert Einstein Coll Med 1978

Weiss, E Michael MD (Cv) - **Spec Exp:** Preventive Cardiology; **Hospital:** PBI Regional- Passaic; **Address:** Cardiac Care Ctr, 842 Clifton Ave, Clifton, NJ 07013-1881; **Phone:** 973-777-2418; **Board Cert:** Internal Medicine 1984; Cardiovascular Disease 1995; **Med School:** Romania 1980; **Resid:** Internal Medicine, Hackensack Med Ctr 1983; **Fellow:** Cardiovascular Disease, Hackensack Med Ctr 1985; **Fac Appt:** Asst Clin Prof Med, UMDNJ-NJ Med Sch, Newark

DERMATOLOGY

Maier, Herbert MD (D) - **Spec Exp:** Acne; Connective Tissue Disorders; Rosacea; **Hospital:** St Joseph's Wayne Hosp; **Address:** 220 Hamburg Tpke Fl 2 - Ste 22, Wayne, NJ 07470-2132; **Phone:** 973-595-6338; **Board Cert:** Dermatology 1975; **Med School:** Geo Wash Univ 1967; **Resid:** Dermatology, Mount Sinai 1973

ENDOCRINOLOGY, DIABETES & METABOLISM

Berkowitz, Richard H MD (EDM) - **Spec Exp:** Diabetes; Cholesterol/Lipid Disorders; Thyroid Disorders; **Hospital:** Chilton Meml Hosp; **Address:** 2025 Hamburg Tpke, Ste D, Wayne, NJ 07470-6250; **Phone:** 973-839-5070; **Board Cert:** Internal Medicine 1975; Endocrinology 1977; **Med School:** SUNY Hlth Sci Ctr 1972; **Resid:** Internal Medicine, Montefiore Med Ctr 1974; Internal Medicine, UMDNJ-Univ Hospital 1975; **Fellow:** Endocrinology, Beth Israel Med Ctr 1977

GASTROENTEROLOGY

Baum, Howard B MD (Ge) - **Spec Exp:** Endoscopy; **Hospital:** PBI Regional- Passaic; **Address:** 540 Broadway, Passaic, NJ 07055; **Phone:** 973-472-2100; **Board Cert:** Internal Medicine 1980; Gastroenterology 1983; **Med School:** Cornell Univ-Weill Med Coll 1977; **Resid:** Internal Medicine, Dartmouth-Hitchcock Med Ctr 1980; **Fellow:** Gastroenterology, NY Presby-Cornell Med Ctr

Bleicher, Robert MD (Ge) - **Spec Exp:** Inflammatory Bowel Disease; Irritable Bowel Syndrome; Liver Disease; **Hospital:** Chilton Meml Hosp; **Address:** 1825 Route 23 South, Wayne, NJ 07470; **Phone:** 973-633-1484; **Board Cert:** Internal Medicine 1981; Gastroenterology 1983; **Med School:** Columbia P&S 1978; **Resid:** Internal Medicine, Northwestern Meml Hosp 1981; **Fellow:** Gastroenterology, Northwestern Meml Hosp 1983

Farkas, John J MD (Ge) - **Hospital:** St Joseph's Regl Med Ctr - Paterson, Wayne Hosp; **Address:** 716 Broad St, FL 1, Clifton, NJ 07013; **Phone:** 973-777-5717; **Board Cert:** Internal Medicine 1989; **Med School:** West Indies 1983; **Resid:** Internal Medicine, St Joseph's Hosp&Med Ctr 1986; **Fellow:** Gastroenterology, St Joseph's Hosp&Med Ctr 1988

GERIATRIC MEDICINE

Lewko, Michael MD (Ger) - **Hospital:** St Joseph's Regl Med Ctr - Paterson; **Address:** 871 Allwood Rd, Clifton, NJ 07012; **Phone:** 973-754-4152; **Board Cert:** Internal Medicine 1988; Geriatric Medicine 2004; Rheumatology 2002; **Med School:** Rutgers Univ 1985; **Resid:** Internal Medicine, RW Johnson Univ Hosp 1988; **Fellow:** Geriatric Medicine, Roger Williams Med Ctr 1989; Rheumatology, Hosp Univ Penn 1991

INFECTIOUS DISEASE

Krieger, Richard MD (Inf) - **Spec Exp:** Lyme Disease; Endocarditis; **Hospital:** Chilton Meml Hosp, St Joseph's Wayne Hosp; **Address:** 2035 Hamburg Tpke, Ste F, Wayne, NJ 07470-6251; **Phone:** 973-831-9228; **Board Cert:** Internal Medicine 1981; Infectious Disease 1984; **Med School:** UMDNJ-NJ Med Sch, Newark 1978; **Resid:** Internal Medicine, Med Coll Penn Hosp 1981; **Fellow:** Infectious Disease, Med Coll Penn 1983

Weiss, Gabriella A MD (Inf) - **Hospital:** PBI Regional- Passaic; **Address:** 842 Clifton Avenue, Clifton, NJ 07013-1800; **Phone:** 973-777-2418; **Board Cert:** Internal Medicine 1985; **Med School:** Romania 1979; **Resid:** Internal Medicine, Hackensack Med Ctr 1984; **Fellow:** Infectious Disease, Hackensack Med Ctr 1985

INTERNAL MEDICINE

De Giacomo, Frank MD (IM) **PCP** - **Hospital:** PBI Regional- Passaic; **Address:** 540 Broadway, Passaic, NJ 07055-1956; **Phone:** 973-472-2100; **Board Cert:** Internal Medicine 1972; **Med School:** Harvard Med Sch 1965; **Resid:** Internal Medicine, Bellevue Hosp 1968; **Fellow:** Cardiovascular Disease, W Roxbury 1969

Gajdos, Robert MD (IM) `PCP` - **Hospital:** Mountainside Hosp (page 88), St Mary's Hosp - Passaic; **Address:** 1005 Clifton Ave, Clifton, NJ 07013-3520; **Phone:** 973-777-2005; **Board Cert:** Internal Medicine 1989; **Med School:** Grenada 1985; **Resid:** Internal Medicine, Mountainside Hosp 1989

Galton, Barry MD (IM) `PCP` - **Spec Exp:** Cardiology; Hypertension; **Hospital:** Chilton Meml Hosp; **Address:** 1777 Hamburg Tpke, Ste 302, Wayne, NJ 07470-5243; **Phone:** 973-831-9222; **Board Cert:** Internal Medicine 1980; **Med School:** Columbia P&S 1958; **Resid:** Internal Medicine, Bronx Muni Hosp Ctr 1962; **Fellow:** Cardiovascular Disease, NY Heart Assn 1961; Internal Medicine, Bronx Muni Hosp Ctr 1962

Gold, Jeffrey L MD (IM) `PCP` - **Hospital:** St Joseph's Regl Med Ctr - Paterson, PBI Regional- Passaic; **Address:** 1135 Broad St, Ste 205, Clifton, NJ 07013-3346; **Phone:** 973-471-8850; **Board Cert:** Internal Medicine 1983; **Med School:** Mexico 1977; **Resid:** Internal Medicine, St Josephs Hosp 1981; **Fac Appt:** Asst Clin Prof Med, UMDNJ-NJ Med Sch, Newark

Jawetz, Harold MD (IM) - **Spec Exp:** Chronic Obstructive Lung Disease (COPD); Pulmonary Disease; Asthma; **Hospital:** PBI Regional- Passaic; **Address:** 540 Broadway, Passaic, NJ 07055-1956; **Phone:** 973-472-2100; **Board Cert:** Internal Medicine 1974; **Med School:** Albert Einstein Coll Med 1971; **Resid:** Internal Medicine, Montefiore Hosp Med Ctr 1974; **Fellow:** Pulmonary Disease, Montefiore Hosp Med Ctr 1978

MEDICAL ONCOLOGY

Uhm, Kyudong MD (Onc) - **Hospital:** PBI Regional- Passaic; **Address:** 1117 Route 46 East, Ste 205, Clifton, NJ 07013; **Phone:** 973-471-0981; **Board Cert:** Internal Medicine 1978; Hematology 1980; **Med School:** South Korea 1969; **Resid:** Internal Medicine, Englewood 1977; Hematology, Montefiore Hosp Med Ctr 1978; **Fellow:** Medical Oncology, Montefiore Hosp Med Ctr 1980

NEPHROLOGY

Vitting, Kevin E MD (Nep) - **Spec Exp:** Hypertension; Kidney Failure; **Hospital:** St Joseph's Regl Med Ctr - Paterson, Wayne Hosp; **Address:** 510 Hamburg Tpke, Ste 108, Wayne, NJ 07470; **Phone:** 973-389-1119; **Board Cert:** Internal Medicine 1985; Nephrology 1988; **Med School:** UMDNJ-RW Johnson Med Sch 1982; **Resid:** Internal Medicine, Lenox Hill Hosp 1985; **Fellow:** Nephrology, Lenox Hill Hosp 1987; **Fac Appt:** Asst Clin Prof Med, Mount Sinai Sch Med

NEUROLOGY

Chodosh, Eliot MD (N) - **Spec Exp:** Stroke; Multiple Sclerosis; **Hospital:** Wayne Hosp, Chilton Meml Hosp; **Address:** 220 Hamburg Tpke, Ste 16, Wayne, NJ 07470-2193; **Phone:** 973-942-4778; **Board Cert:** Neurology 1987; **Med School:** Mexico 1981; **Resid:** Neurology, Boston Univ Med Ctr 1986; **Fellow:** Cerebrovascular Disease, Boston Univ Med Ctr 1987

Knep, Stanley MD (N) - **Spec Exp:** Electromyography; Parkinson's Disease; Headache; **Hospital:** St Joseph's Regl Med Ctr - Paterson, PBI Regional- Passaic; **Address:** 50 Mt Prospect Ave, Clifton, NJ 07013; **Phone:** 973-471-3680; **Board Cert:** Neurology 1977; Internal Medicine 1970; **Med School:** South Africa 1965; **Resid:** Internal Medicine, Johannesburg Hosp 1970; Neurology, Albert Einstein 1975; **Fac Appt:** Asst Clin Prof N, Seton Hall Univ Sch Grad Med Ed

OBSTETRICS & GYNECOLOGY

Burns, Les A MD (ObG) **PCP** - **Spec Exp:** Menopause Problems; Pap Smear Abnormalities; Hysterectomy Alternatives; **Hospital:** Chilton Meml Hosp, St Joseph's Regl Med Ctr - Paterson; **Address:** 1784 Hamburg Tpke, Wayne, NJ 07470-4023; **Phone:** 973-831-9925; **Board Cert:** Obstetrics & Gynecology 1998; **Med School:** Hahnemann Univ 1981; **Resid:** Obstetrics & Gynecology, Danbury Hosp 1985

Kierce, Roger MD (ObG) - **Hospital:** St Joseph's Regl Med Ctr - Paterson; **Address:** Willowbrook Obstetrics & Gynecology, 57 Willowbrook Blvd, Wayne, NJ 07470-7045; **Phone:** 973-754-4075; **Board Cert:** Obstetrics & Gynecology 2001; **Med School:** UMDNJ-NJ Med Sch, Newark 1986; **Resid:** Obstetrics & Gynecology, St Josephs Hosp 1990

OPHTHALMOLOGY

Giliberti, Orazio MD (Oph) - **Spec Exp:** Laser-Refractive Surgery; Cataract Surgery; Corneal Surgery; **Hospital:** UMDNJ-Univ Hosp-Newark, Clara Maass Med Ctr; **Address:** Giliberti Eye and Laser Center, 415 Totowa Rd, Totowa, NJ 07512-2081; **Phone:** 973-595-0011; **Board Cert:** Ophthalmology 1989; **Med School:** Grenada 1982; **Resid:** Ophthalmology, UMDNJ Affil Hosps 1987; **Fellow:** Ophthalmology, Pennsylvania Hosp 1984; Refractive Surgery, Vision Sculpting; **Fac Appt:** Asst Prof Oph, UMDNJ-NJ Med Sch, Newark

Vogel, Mitchell MD (Oph) - **Spec Exp:** Corneal Disease; Refractive Surgery; Uveitis; **Hospital:** St Mary's Hosp - Passaic, Overlook Hosp (page 88); **Address:** 124 Gregory Ave, Ste 104, Passaic, NJ 07055-4856; **Phone:** 973-779-0808; **Board Cert:** Ophthalmology 1999; **Med School:** Temple Univ 1991; **Resid:** Ophthalmology, Nassau Co Med Ctr 1995; **Fellow:** Cornea, Univ Tex SW Med Ctr 1996

ORTHOPAEDIC SURGERY

Drillings, Gary MD (OrS) - **Spec Exp:** Knee Injuries; Shoulder Injuries; Sports Medicine; **Hospital:** Chilton Meml Hosp; **Address:** 1777 Hamburg Tpke, Ste 305, Wayne, NJ 07470; **Phone:** 973-831-6666; **Board Cert:** Orthopaedic Surgery 2004; **Med School:** SUNY Upstate Med Univ 1985; **Resid:** Orthopaedic Surgery, Northwestern Med Ctr 1990; **Fellow:** Sports Medicine, Lenox Hill Hosp 1991

Reicher, Oscar MD (OrS) - **Spec Exp:** Reconstructive Surgery; Sports Medicine; **Hospital:** Chilton Meml Hosp, Wayne Hosp; **Address:** 2035 Hamburg Tpke, Ste D, Wayne, NJ 07470; **Phone:** 973-616-0200; **Board Cert:** Orthopaedic Surgery 1997; **Med School:** Univ Pittsburgh 1979; **Resid:** Orthopaedic Surgery, Vanderbilt Univ Hosp 1984

OTOLARYNGOLOGY

Cece, John MD (Oto) - **Spec Exp:** Sinus Surgery; Cosmetic Surgery-Face; Rhinoplasty; **Hospital:** PBI Regional-Passaic, Clara Maass Med Ctr; **Address:** 1001 Clifton Ave, Clifton, NJ 07013; **Phone:** 973-777-5151; **Board Cert:** Otolaryngology 1986; Facial Plastic & Reconstructive Surgery 1986; **Med School:** UMDNJ-RW Johnson Med Sch 1981; **Resid:** Otolaryngology, Mt Sinai Med Ctr 1986

La Bagnara Jr, James MD (Oto) - **Spec Exp:** Thyroid & Parathyroid Surgery; Pediatric Otolaryngology; **Hospital:** St Joseph's Regl Med Ctr - Paterson, St Joseph's Wayne Hosp; **Address:** 311 Lexington Ave, Paterson, NJ 07502-1010; **Phone:** 973-942-1300; **Board Cert:** Otolaryngology 1978; **Med School:** UMDNJ-NJ Med Sch, Newark 1974; **Resid:** Otolaryngology, UMDNJ Affil Hosp 1978; Otolaryngology, Newark EE Hosp 1981; **Fac Appt:** Assoc Clin Prof Oto, UMDNJ-NJ Med Sch, Newark

Mattel, Stephen MD (Oto) - **Spec Exp:** Sinus Surgery; Thyroid Surgery; **Hospital:** PBI Regional- Passaic; **Address:** 1070 Clifton Ave, Clifton, NJ 07013-3619; **Phone:** 973-773-9880; **Board Cert:** Otolaryngology 1981; **Med School:** NYU Sch Med 1977; **Resid:** Surgery, Mount Sinai Hosp 1978; Otolaryngology, Bellevue Hosp 1981

PEDIATRIC HEMATOLOGY-ONCOLOGY

Bonilla, Mary Ann MD (PHO) - **Hospital:** St Joseph's Regl Med Ctr - Paterson; **Address:** St Joseph's Children's Hospital, 703 Main St, Paterson, NJ 07503; **Phone:** 973-754-3230; **Board Cert:** Pediatrics 1986; Pediatric Hematology-Oncology 2004; **Med School:** Loyola Univ-Stritch Sch Med 1981; **Resid:** Pediatrics, Brookdale Hosp 1984; **Fellow:** Pediatric Hematology-Oncology, Meml Sloan Kettering Canc Ctr 1988; **Fac Appt:** Asst Prof Ped, Columbia P&S

PEDIATRIC NEPHROLOGY

Salcedo, Jose MD (PNep) - **Spec Exp:** Hypertension; Dialysis Care; Kidney Failure; **Hospital:** St Joseph's Regl Med Ctr - Paterson, Morristown Mem Hosp (page 88); **Address:** 703 Main St, Paterson, NJ 07053-2621; **Phone:** 973-754-2570; **Board Cert:** Pediatrics 1976; Pediatric Nephrology 1976; **Med School:** Mexico 1970; **Resid:** Pediatrics, UMDNJ-Martland Hosp 1974; **Fellow:** Pediatric Nephrology, Chldns Hosp Natl Med Ctr 1976; Nephrology, Armed Forces Inst Path 1977; **Fac Appt:** Assoc Clin Prof Ped, UMDNJ-NJ Med Sch, Newark

PEDIATRIC PULMONOLOGY

Nachajon, Roberto MD (PPul) - **Spec Exp:** Asthma; Cystic Fibrosis; Sleep Disorders; Bronchoscopy; **Hospital:** St Joseph's Regl Med Ctr - Paterson; **Address:** St Josephs Chldns Hosp - Div Pediatric Pulmonology, 703 Main St, Paterson, NJ 07503; **Phone:** 973-754-2550; **Board Cert:** Pediatrics 2001; Pediatric Pulmonology 2004; **Med School:** Uruguay 1985; **Resid:** Pediatrics, Chldns Hosp Uruguay 1990; Pediatrics, Beth Israel Med Ctr 1993; **Fellow:** Pediatric Pulmonology, Childrens Hosp 1996

PEDIATRICS

Scofield, Lisa MD (Ped) `PCP` - **Hospital:** St Joseph's Regl Med Ctr - Paterson, Chilton Meml Hosp; **Address:** 57 Willowbrook Blvd, Ste 421, Wayne, NJ 07470; **Phone:** 973-754-4025; **Board Cert:** Pediatrics 2002; **Med School:** UMDNJ-NJ Med Sch, Newark 1990; **Resid:** Pediatrics, New York Hosp-Cornell 1994

PLASTIC SURGERY

Ganchi, Parham A MD/PhD (PlS) - **Spec Exp:** Cosmetic Surgery-Face & Body; Liposuction & Body Contouring; **Hospital:** Wayne Hosp; **Address:** 342 Hamburg Tpke, Ste 202, Wayne, NJ 07470; **Phone:** 973-942-6600; **Board Cert:** Surgery 2000; Plastic Surgery 2003; **Med School:** Duke Univ 1994; **Resid:** Surgery, Brigham & Women's Hosp 1999; Plastic Surgery, Brigham & Women's Hosp 2002; **Fac Appt:** Asst Prof PlS, UMDNJ-NJ Med Sch, Newark

PULMONARY DISEASE

Amoruso, Robert MD (Pul) - **Spec Exp:** Asthma; Critical Care; **Hospital:** St Joseph's Regl Med Ctr - Paterson, Wayne Hosp; **Address:** 999 McBride Ave, Ste 201C, West Patterson, NJ 07424; **Phone:** 973-256-0287; **Board Cert:** Internal Medicine 1979; Pulmonary Disease 1982; Critical Care Medicine 1997; **Med School:** Italy 1975; **Resid:** Internal Medicine, St Joseph's Hosp Med Ctr 1979; **Fellow:** Pulmonary Disease, College Hosp-UMDNJ 1981

Passaic

Grizzanti, Joseph DO (Pul) - **Spec Exp:** Lung Cancer; Asthma; Allergy; Immunologic Lung Disease; **Hospital:** Valley Hosp (page 762); **Address:** 297 Lafayette Ave, Hawthorne, NJ 07506; **Phone:** 973-790-4111; **Board Cert:** Internal Medicine 1979; Pulmonary Disease 1982; Allergy & Immunology 1985; **Med School:** Philadelphia Coll Osteo Med 1979; **Resid:** Internal Medicine, Univ Hosp 1979; Allergy & Immunology, Montefiore-Albert Einstein 1984; **Fellow:** Pulmonary Disease, Montefiore-Albert Einstein 1981; **Fac Appt:** Assoc Clin Prof Med, Albert Einstein Coll Med

O'Donnell, Timothy DO (Pul) - **Spec Exp:** Asthma; Lung Cancer; Interstitial Lung Disease; **Hospital:** Chilton Meml Hosp, Morristown Mem Hosp (page 88); **Address:** 525 Wanaque Ave, Pompton Lakes, NJ 07442-1833; **Phone:** 973-616-6166; **Board Cert:** Internal Medicine 1989; Pulmonary Disease 2002; Critical Care Medicine 2003; **Med School:** UMDNJ Sch Osteo Med 1985; **Resid:** Internal Medicine, NJ Med Sch/Univ Hosp 1989; **Fellow:** Pulmonary Critical Care Medicine, UMDNJ/Newark Beth Israel Med Ctr 1992

REPRODUCTIVE ENDOCRINOLOGY

Ransom, Mark MD (RE) - **Spec Exp:** Infertility; **Hospital:** St Joseph's Wayne Hosp, Hackensack Univ Med Ctr (page 92); **Address:** 57 Willowbrook Blvd, Wayne, NJ 07470; **Phone:** 973-754-4055; **Board Cert:** Obstetrics & Gynecology 2004; Reproductive Endocrinology 2004; **Med School:** UMDNJ-RW Johnson Med Sch 1987; **Resid:** Obstetrics & Gynecology, RWJ Univ Hosp 1991; **Fellow:** Reproductive Endocrinology, RWJ Univ Hosp 1992

RHEUMATOLOGY

Goldberg, Marc A MD (Rhu) - **Spec Exp:** Rheumatoid Arthritis; Osteoporosis; Osteoarthritis; **Hospital:** PBI Regional- Passaic, PBI Regional- Passaic; **Address:** 200 Gregory Ave, Passaic, NJ 07055-3802; **Phone:** 973-473-2597; **Board Cert:** Internal Medicine 1972; Rheumatology 1976; **Med School:** Med Coll VA 1969; **Resid:** Internal Medicine, Univ Maryland Hosp 1972; Rheumatology, Johns Hopkins Hosp 1973; **Fellow:** Rheumatology, Hosp Univ Penn 1976

SURGERY

Buckley, Michael Kevin MD (S) - **Spec Exp:** Anal Disorders & Reconstruction; Colon & Rectal Cancer; **Hospital:** PBI Regional- Passaic, PBI Regional- Passaic; **Address:** 1100 Clifton Ave Fl 1, Clifton, NJ 07013-3631; **Phone:** 973-778-0100; **Board Cert:** Surgery 1996; Colon & Rectal Surgery 1989; **Med School:** Ireland 1979; **Resid:** Surgery, RWJ Univ Hosp 1987; **Fellow:** Colon & Rectal Surgery, Cook Co Hosp 1988

Budd, Daniel MD (S) - **Spec Exp:** Breast Cancer; Endocrine Surgery; Gastrointestinal Surgery; **Hospital:** Barnert Hosp, Valley Hosp (page 762); **Address:** 707 Broadway, Paterson, NJ 07514; **Phone:** 973-742-3371; **Board Cert:** Surgery 1975; **Med School:** Duke Univ 1969; **Resid:** Surgery, Columbia-Presby Hosp 1974; **Fac Appt:** Assoc Clin Prof S, UMDNJ-NJ Med Sch, Newark

Feigenbaum, Howard MD (S) - **Spec Exp:** Gastrointestinal Surgery; Colon Surgery; **Hospital:** Chilton Meml Hosp; **Address:** 227 Hamburg Tpke, Pompton Lakes, NJ 07442-1838; **Phone:** 973-839-7999; **Board Cert:** Surgery 1988; **Med School:** NYU Sch Med 1971; **Resid:** Surgery, Bellevue Hosp 1977

THORACIC SURGERY

Christakos, Manny MD (TS) - **Spec Exp:** Cardiovascular Surgery; **Hospital:** St Joseph's Wayne Hosp, PBI Regional- Passaic; **Address:** 871 Allwood Rd, Clifton, NJ 07012-1922; **Phone:** 973-779-2270; **Board Cert:** Thoracic Surgery 1997; Surgery 1978; **Med School:** SUNY Buffalo 1971; **Resid:** Surgery, EJ Meyer Meml Hosp 1976; Thoracic Surgery, Univ of Calif 1980; **Fellow:** Thoracic Surgery, Univ of Calif 1980

Ciocon, Hermogenes MD (TS) - **Spec Exp:** Cardiovascular Surgery; **Hospital:** Chilton Meml Hosp, Wayne Hosp; **Address:** 871 Allwood Rd Fl 2, Clifton, NJ 07013; **Phone:** 973-779-2270; **Board Cert:** Thoracic Surgery 1974; Surgery 1969; **Med School:** Philippines 1961; **Resid:** Thoracic Surgery, Flower Fifth Ave Hosp 1969; Thoracic Surgery, Metro Hosp Ctr 1969

Goldenberg, Bruce MD (TS) - **Spec Exp:** Coronary Artery Surgery; Heart Valve Surgery; Minimally Invasive Cardiac Surgery; **Hospital:** PBI Regional- Passaic, Mountainside Hosp (page 88); **Address:** PBI Regional Medical Ctr, 350 Boulevard, Passaic, NJ 07055; **Phone:** 973-365-4722; **Board Cert:** Thoracic Surgery 2003; Surgery 1983; **Med School:** Northwestern Univ 1976; **Resid:** Surgery, NYU Med Ctr 1981; Thoracic Surgery, NYU Med Ctr 1983

Kaushik, Raj R MD (TS) - **Spec Exp:** Cardiac Surgery; **Hospital:** PBI Regional- Passaic, Mountainside Hosp (page 88); **Address:** PBI Regional Med Ctr, Div Cardiac Surgery, 350 Boulevard, Passaic, NJ 07055; **Phone:** 973-365-4567; **Board Cert:** Thoracic Surgery 1999; **Med School:** India 1979; **Resid:** Surgery, Bridgeport Hosp 1985; Cardiothoracic Surgery, Newark Beth Israel Med Ctr 1988; **Fellow:** Cardiac Surgery, Baylor Univ 1989; Cardiac Surgery, Univ W Ontario Med Ctr 1990

UROLOGY

Levine, Seth MD (U) - **Spec Exp:** Prostate Cancer; **Hospital:** Chilton Meml Hosp, Valley Hosp (page 762); **Address:** 1777 Hamburg Tpke, Ste 304, Wayne, NJ 07470; **Phone:** 973-616-8400; **Board Cert:** Urology 1980; **Med School:** Tufts Univ 1971; **Resid:** Surgery, Mount Sinai Hosp 1973; Urology, Mount Sinai Hosp 1978

Schlecker, Burton A MD (U) - **Spec Exp:** Incontinence-Female; **Hospital:** PBI Regional- Passaic, Chilton Meml Hosp; **Address:** 1033 Clifton Ave, Clifton, NJ 07013-3631; **Phone:** 973-473-5700; **Board Cert:** Urology 1998; **Med School:** NYU Sch Med 1981; **Resid:** Surgery, Lennox Hill Hosp 1983; Urology, Hosp U Penn 1986

Somerset

Somerset

ALLERGY & IMMUNOLOGY

Caucino, Julie DO (A&I) - **Spec Exp:** Asthma & Allergy; Food Allergy; Urticaria; **Hospital:** Univ Med Ctr - Princeton, Somerset Med Ctr; **Address:** 24 Vreeland Drive, Skillnan, NJ 08558-2621; **Phone:** 609-921-2202; **Board Cert:** Internal Medicine 2001; Allergy & Immunology 2003; **Med School:** Kirksville Coll Osteo Med 1987; **Resid:** Internal Medicine, RWJ Univ Hosp 1991; **Fellow:** Allergy & Immunology, Albert Einstein 1991

Fox, James MD (A&I) - **Spec Exp:** Asthma; Urticaria; Food Allergy; **Hospital:** Somerset Med Ctr, Hunterdon Med Ctr; **Address:** 3461 US Highway 22, Somerville, NJ 08876-6021; **Phone:** 908-725-4777; **Board Cert:** Pediatrics 1981; Allergy & Immunology 1983; **Med School:** Yale Univ 1977; **Resid:** Pediatrics, Bronx Municipal Hosp Ctr 1980; **Fellow:** Allergy & Immunology, Columbia-Presby Med Ctr 1982

Krol, Kristine MD (A&I) - **Spec Exp:** Insect Allergies; Drug Sensitivity; **Hospital:** Staten Island Univ Hosp - South Site, Somerset Med Ctr; **Address:** 177 W High St, Somerville, NJ 08876; **Phone:** 908-725-8666; **Board Cert:** Internal Medicine 1987; **Med School:** SUNY Downstate 1981; **Resid:** Internal Medicine, Staten Island Hosp 1985; **Fellow:** Allergy & Immunology, Mass Genl Hosp 1987; **Fac Appt:** Asst Clin Prof Med, SUNY Downstate

Pedinoff, Andrew MD (A&I) - **Spec Exp:** Allergy; Asthma; Hay Fever; **Hospital:** Univ Med Ctr - Princeton; **Address:** Princeton Allergy & Asthma Assoc, 24 Vreeland Drive, Skilman, NJ 08558; **Phone:** 609-921-2202; **Board Cert:** Pediatrics 1998; Allergy & Immunology 2003; **Med School:** Dominican Republic 1984; **Resid:** Pediatrics, Georgetown Univ Hosp 1987; **Fellow:** Allergy & Immunology, Georgetown Univ Hosp 1989; **Fac Appt:** Asst Clin Prof Ped, UMDNJ-RW Johnson Med Sch

Schulhafer, Edwin MD (A&I) - **Spec Exp:** Asthma; Sinus Disorders; **Hospital:** Somerset Med Ctr, Hunterdon Med Ctr; **Address:** 712 Courtyard Drive, Hillsborough, NJ 08844; **Phone:** 908-526-0200; **Board Cert:** Allergy & Immunology 1997; Internal Medicine 1988; **Med School:** UMDNJ-NJ Med Sch, Newark 1983; **Resid:** Internal Medicine, Overlook Hosp 1986; **Fellow:** Allergy & Immunology, Long Island Hosp 1988

Southern, D Loren MD (A&I) - **Spec Exp:** Asthma; Allergy; Hives; **Hospital:** Univ Med Ctr - Princeton; **Address:** 24 Vreeland Drive, Skillman, NJ 08558; **Phone:** 609-921-2202; **Board Cert:** Pediatrics 1976; **Med School:** Columbia P&S 1971; **Resid:** Pediatrics, Columbia-Presby Med Ctr 1974; **Fellow:** Allergy & Immunology, Columbia-Presby Med Ctr 1976

CARDIOVASCULAR DISEASE

Leeds, Richard MD (Cv) - **Spec Exp:** Cardiac Catheterization; Invasive Cardiology; **Hospital:** Somerset Med Ctr, Robert Wood Johnson Univ Hosp - New Brunswick (page 853); **Address:** 225 Jackson St, Bridgewater, NJ 08807; **Phone:** 908-526-8668; **Board Cert:** Cardiovascular Disease 1987; Internal Medicine 1984; **Med School:** NY Med Coll 1981; **Resid:** Internal Medicine, Beth Israel 1985; **Fellow:** Cardiovascular Disease, St Vincent's Hosp & Med Ctr 1986

Saulino, Patrick MD (Cv) - **Spec Exp:** Cardiac Catheterization; Heart Failure; **Hospital:** Somerset Med Ctr, Robert Wood Johnson Univ Hosp - New Brunswick (page 853); **Address:** 225 Jackson Street, Bridgewater, NJ 08807; **Phone:** 908-526-8668; **Board Cert:** Internal Medicine 1984; Cardiovascular Disease 1987; **Med School:** Georgetown Univ 1981; **Resid:** Internal Medicine, Georgetown Univ Hosp 1984; Cardiovascular Disease, Georgetown Univ Hosp 1985; **Fellow:** Cardiovascular Disease, UMDNJ-RW Johnson Sch Med 1987; Cardiovascular Disease, Georgetown Univ Hosp 1988

Stroh, Jack MD (Cv) - **Spec Exp:** Angioplasty & Stent Placement; Hypertension; Cholesterol/Lipid Disorders; **Hospital:** Robert Wood Johnson Univ Hosp - New Brunswick (page 853), St Peter's Univ Hosp; **Address:** 75 Veronica Ave, Somerset, NJ 08873-5002; **Phone:** 732-247-7444; **Board Cert:** Internal Medicine 1987; Cardiovascular Disease 1989; Interventional Cardiology 1999; **Med School:** Albert Einstein Coll Med 1984; **Resid:** Internal Medicine, Boston Univ Med Ctr 1987; **Fellow:** Cardiovascular Disease, New York Univ Med Ctr 1990

COLON & RECTAL SURGERY

Sadler, Daniel MD (CRS) - **Hospital:** Somerset Med Ctr; **Address:** 704 Route 202 S, Bridgewater, NJ 08807-2552; **Phone:** 908-526-5600; **Board Cert:** Surgery 2003; Colon & Rectal Surgery 2006; **Med School:** W VA Univ 1987; **Resid:** Surgery, Charleston Area Med Ctr 1993; **Fellow:** Colon & Rectal Surgery, UMDNJ-RW Johnson Univ Hosp 1994

DERMATOLOGY

Fox, Alissa MD (D) - **Spec Exp:** Acne; Psoriasis; **Hospital:** Somerset Med Ctr, Hunterdon Med Ctr; **Address:** 3461 US Highway 22, Somerville, NJ 08876-6021; **Phone:** 908-725-4777; **Board Cert:** Dermatology 1984; **Med School:** NYU Sch Med 1980; **Resid:** Dermatology, New York Hosp 1984

Wrone, David A MD (D) - **Spec Exp:** Skin Laser Surgery; Cosmetic Dermatology; Mohs' Surgery; Skin Cancer; **Hospital:** Robert Wood Johnson Univ Hosp - New Brunswick (page 853); **Address:** 1543 Highway 27, Somerset, NJ 08873; **Phone:** 732-579-1290; **Board Cert:** Dermatology 2001; **Med School:** Stanford Univ 1996; **Resid:** Dermatology, Univ Wisconsin Med Ctr 1998; Dermatology, Mass Genl Hosp 2001; **Fellow:** Mohs Surgery, UCLA Med Ctr 2002

DIAGNOSTIC RADIOLOGY

Melville, Gordon MD (DR) - **Spec Exp:** Neuroradiology; MRI; **Hospital:** Somerset Med Ctr; **Address:** 16 Mountain Blvd, Warren, NJ 07059-6331; **Phone:** 908-769-7200; **Board Cert:** Diagnostic Radiology 1984; Neuroradiology 2006; **Med School:** Univ NC Sch Med 1979; **Resid:** Diagnostic Radiology, George Washington Univ Hosp 1984; **Fellow:** Neuroradiology, Mass Genl Hosp 1985; **Fac Appt:** Asst Clin Prof Rad, Robert W Johnson Med Sch

Yang, Roger MD (DR) - **Spec Exp:** Breast Imaging; Women's Imaging; **Hospital:** Somerset Med Ctr; **Address:** Somerset Med Ctr, Dept Radiology, 110 Rehill Ave, Somerville, NJ 08876; **Phone:** 908-685-2930; **Board Cert:** Diagnostic Radiology 1997; **Med School:** Northwestern Univ 1992; **Resid:** Diagnostic Radiology, Univ Hosp 1997; **Fellow:** Women''s Imaging, Univ Hosp 1998; **Fac Appt:** Asst Clin Prof Rad, SUNY Downstate

FAMILY MEDICINE

Corson, Richard L MD (FMed) **PCP** - **Hospital:** Somerset Med Ctr; **Address:** 211 Courtyard Drive, Hillsborough, NJ 08844; **Phone:** 908-722-9962; **Board Cert:** Family Medicine 2004; **Med School:** Rutgers Univ 1983

Frisoli, Anthony MD (FMed) **PCP** - **Spec Exp:** Sports Medicine; Geriatrics; **Hospital:** Somerset Med Ctr; **Address:** 1973 Washington Valley Rd, Martinsville, NJ 08836; **Phone:** 732-560-9225; **Board Cert:** Family Medicine 2005; **Med School:** Rutgers Univ 1983; **Resid:** Family Medicine, Somerset Med Ctr 1986

Jobanputra, Kishor MD (FMed) PCP - **Spec Exp:** Geriatric Medicine; Preventive Medicine; **Hospital:** Hunterdon Med Ctr; **Address:** 2143 S Branch Rd, Branchburg, NJ 08876; **Phone:** 908-369-8871; **Board Cert:** Family Medicine 2000; Geriatric Medicine 1996; **Med School:** India 1969; **Resid:** Family Medicine, Somerset Med Ctr 1976; **Fac Appt:** Asst Clin Prof FMed, UMDNJ-RW Johnson Med Sch

Ziering, Thomas MD (FMed) PCP - **Spec Exp:** Anxiety & Depression; Skin Diseases; Gay/Lesbian/Transgender Health; **Hospital:** Morristown Mem Hosp (page 88); **Address:** 39 Olcott Fl 2, Bernardsville, NJ 07924-2317; **Phone:** 908-221-1919; **Board Cert:** Family Medicine 2003; **Med School:** UMDNJ-NJ Med Sch, Newark 1987; **Resid:** Family Medicine, Somerset Med Ctr 1990; **Fac Appt:** Assoc Clin Prof FMed, Robert W Johnson Med Sch

GASTROENTEROLOGY

Accurso, Charles MD (Ge) - **Spec Exp:** Endoscopy; Peptic Acid Disorders; Gastroesophageal Reflux Disease (GERD); **Hospital:** Somerset Med Ctr; **Address:** 511 Courtyard Dr, Bldg 500, Hillsborough, NJ 08844-2017; **Phone:** 908-218-9222; **Board Cert:** Internal Medicine 1987; Gastroenterology 1989; **Med School:** UMDNJ-NJ Med Sch, Newark 1984; **Resid:** Internal Medicine, UMDNJ/NJ Med Sch-Univ Hosp 1987; **Fellow:** Gastroenterology, Univ Hosp/NJ Med Sch 1989; **Fac Appt:** Asst Clin Prof Med, UMDNJ-NJ Med Sch, Newark

Ferges, Mitchell MD (Ge) - **Spec Exp:** Liver Disease; **Hospital:** St Peter's Univ Hosp, Robert Wood Johnson Univ Hosp - New Brunswick (page 853); **Address:** 33 Clyde Rd, Ste 102, Somerset, NJ 08873; **Phone:** 732-873-9200; **Board Cert:** Internal Medicine 1978; Gastroenterology 1981; **Med School:** UMDNJ-RW Johnson Med Sch 1975; **Resid:** Internal Medicine, UMDNJ Rutgers Affil Hosps 1978; **Fellow:** Gastroenterology, UMDNJ Univ Hosp 1980; **Fac Appt:** Asst Clin Prof Med, UMDNJ-RW Johnson Med Sch

HEMATOLOGY

Toomey, Kathleen C MD (Hem) - **Spec Exp:** Breast Cancer; **Hospital:** Somerset Med Ctr, Robert Wood Johnson Univ Hosp - New Brunswick (page 853); **Address:** 107 Cedar Grove Ln, Ste 101, Somerset, NJ 08873; **Phone:** 732-356-8300; **Board Cert:** Internal Medicine 1982; Medical Oncology 1987; Hematology 2003; **Med School:** Italy 1979; **Resid:** Internal Medicine, St Peters Med Ctr 1982; **Fellow:** Hematology & Oncology, UMDNJ-Rutgers Med Sch 1985

INFECTIOUS DISEASE

Herman, David J MD (Inf) - **Spec Exp:** Lyme Disease; AIDS/HIV; Travel Medicine; **Hospital:** Somerset Med Ctr, Robert Wood Johnson Univ Hosp - New Brunswick (page 853); **Address:** 411 Courtyard Drive, Hillsborough, NJ 08844; **Phone:** 908-725-2522; **Board Cert:** Internal Medicine 1988; Infectious Disease 2000; **Med School:** Univ MO-Columbia Sch Med 1985; **Resid:** Internal Medicine, Northwestern Univ 1988; **Fellow:** Infectious Disease, Univ Minn 1991; **Fac Appt:** Asst Clin Prof Med, Robert W Johnson Med Sch

Martinez, Homar MD (Inf) - **Spec Exp:** Travel Medicine; **Hospital:** Somerset Med Ctr, Ocean Med Ctr; **Address:** 3461 US Highway 22E Ave E Bldg, Branchburg, NJ 08876; **Phone:** 732-764-9392; **Board Cert:** Internal Medicine 1994; Infectious Disease 1997; **Med School:** Mexico 1985; **Resid:** Internal Medicine, St Vincents Hosp 1990; **Fellow:** Infectious Disease, Long Island Coll Hosp 1992

INTERNAL MEDICINE

Bell, Kevin MD (IM) **PCP** - **Spec Exp:** Lyme Disease; Hypertension; **Hospital:** Overlook Hosp (page 88); **Address:** 10 Mountain Blvd, Warren, NJ 07059; **Phone:** 908-226-9000; **Board Cert:** Internal Medicine 1978; **Med School:** Columbia P&S 1975; **Resid:** Internal Medicine, Univ Wisconsin Med Ctr 1979; **Fac Appt:** Asst Clin Prof Med, Columbia P&S

MEDICAL ONCOLOGY

Wu, Hen-vai MD (Onc) - **Hospital:** Somerset Med Ctr; **Address:** 107 Cedar Grove Ln, Somerset, NJ 08873; **Phone:** 732-356-8300; **Board Cert:** Internal Medicine 1977; Hematology 1978; Medical Oncology 1981; **Med School:** Taiwan 1972; **Resid:** Internal Medicine, Mount Vernon Hosp 1974; Internal Medicine, Helene Fuld Med Ctr 1975; **Fellow:** Hematology, Robert W Johnson Univ Hosp 1977; Medical Oncology, Robert W Johnson Univ Hosp 1980; **Fac Appt:** Asst Clin Prof Med, UMDNJ-NJ Med Sch, Newark

NEONATAL-PERINATAL MEDICINE

Chavez, Alberto MD (NP) - **Hospital:** Somerset Med Ctr; **Address:** Somerset Med Ctr, Maternal Child Health, 110 Rehill Ave, Somerville, NJ 08876; **Phone:** 908-685-2868; **Board Cert:** Neonatal-Perinatal Medicine 1997; Pediatrics 1985; **Med School:** Peru 1972; **Resid:** Pediatrics, Univ San Marco 1976; Pediatrics, UMDNJ 1982; **Fellow:** Neonatology, UMDNJ 1985

NEPHROLOGY

Kabis, Suzanne MD (Nep) - **Spec Exp:** Lupus Nephritis; Hypertension; Glomerulonephritis; **Hospital:** Robert Wood Johnson Univ Hosp - New Brunswick (page 853), St Peter's Univ Hosp; **Address:** 1350 Hamilton St, Somerset, NJ 08873; **Phone:** 732-246-2626; **Board Cert:** Internal Medicine 1982; Nephrology 1988; **Med School:** Rutgers Univ 1979; **Resid:** Internal Medicine, NC Meml Hosp 1982; **Fellow:** Nephrology, NC Meml Hosp 1985; **Fac Appt:** Asst Clin Prof Med, Robert W Johnson Med Sch

NEUROLOGY

Friedlander, Devin MD (N) - **Spec Exp:** Headache; Botox Therapy; **Hospital:** Robert Wood Johnson Univ Hosp - New Brunswick (page 853), St Peter's Univ Hosp; **Address:** Princeton & Rutgers Neurology, 75 Veronica Ave, Ste 202, Somerset, NJ 08873; **Phone:** 732-246-1311; **Board Cert:** Neurology 2003; **Med School:** UMDNJ-RW Johnson Med Sch 1989; **Resid:** Neurology, Albert Einstein Med Ctr 1993; **Fellow:** Neurological Physiology, Lyons VA Med Ctr 1994

OBSTETRICS & GYNECOLOGY

Sanderson, Rhonda MD (ObG) - **Spec Exp:** Gynecology Only; **Hospital:** Overlook Hosp (page 88); **Address:** 8 Mountain Blvd, Warren, NJ 07059; **Phone:** 908-754-5775; **Board Cert:** Obstetrics & Gynecology 1996; **Med School:** Hahnemann Univ 1980; **Resid:** Obstetrics & Gynecology, Womens/Infants Hosp 1984

OPHTHALMOLOGY

Salz, Alan MD (Oph) - **Hospital:** Somerset Med Ctr; **Address:** 201 Union Ave Bldg 2 - Ste F, Bridgewater, NJ 08807; **Phone:** 908-231-1110; **Board Cert:** Ophthalmology 1987; **Med School:** Boston Univ 1981; **Resid:** Ophthalmology, Wills Eye Hosp 1985

Wachtel, Daniel MD (Oph) - **Spec Exp:** Cataract Surgery; **Hospital:** Somerset Med Ctr; **Address:** 515 Church St, Bound Brook, NJ 08805; **Phone:** 732-356-7283; **Board Cert:** Ophthalmology 1968; **Med School:** NYU Sch Med 1962; **Resid:** Ophthalmology, NYU-Bellevue Hosp 1966; **Fellow:** Ophthalmology, NYU-Bellevue Hosp 1967

ORTHOPAEDIC SURGERY

D'Agostini, Robert MD (OrS) - **Spec Exp:** Joint Replacement; **Hospital:** Morristown Mem Hosp (page 88); **Address:** 1590 Route 206 N, Bedminster, NJ 07921; **Phone:** 908-234-2002; **Board Cert:** Orthopaedic Surgery 1998; **Med School:** UMDNJ-RW Johnson Med Sch 1980; **Resid:** Orthopaedic Surgery, Georgetown Univ Hosp 1985

Johnson, Albert MD (OrS) - **Spec Exp:** Hand Surgery; Hip & Knee Replacement; **Hospital:** Somerset Med Ctr; **Address:** 1081 Route 22 W, Bridgewater, NJ 08807; **Phone:** 908-722-0822; **Board Cert:** Orthopaedic Surgery 1977; **Med School:** India 1967; **Resid:** Surgery, New England Med Ctr; Orthopaedic Surgery, New England Med Ctr 1975; **Fellow:** Hand Surgery, St Luke's-Roosevelt Hosp Ctr

Schneider, Stephen MD (OrS) - **Spec Exp:** Sports Medicine; Trauma; Joint Replacement; **Hospital:** Somerset Med Ctr, Robert Wood Johnson Univ Hosp - New Brunswick (page 853); **Address:** 515 Church St, Bound Brook, NJ 08805-1743; **Phone:** 732-469-6160; **Board Cert:** Orthopaedic Surgery 1985; **Med School:** Mexico 1972; **Resid:** Orthopaedic Surgery, NYU Hosp 1978; **Fac Appt:** Assoc Clin Prof OrS, UMDNJ-RW Johnson Med Sch

OTOLARYNGOLOGY

Bortniker, David MD (Oto) - **Spec Exp:** Sinus Disorders/Surgery; Hearing Disorders-Pediatric; Head & Neck Surgery; **Hospital:** Somerset Med Ctr, Overlook Hosp (page 88); **Address:** 242 E Main St, Somerville, NJ 08876; **Phone:** 908-704-9696; **Board Cert:** Otolaryngology 1985; **Med School:** Albert Einstein Coll Med 1980; **Resid:** Otolaryngology, Montefiore Hosp Med Ctr 1984; **Fellow:** Head and Neck Surgery, Beth Israel Med Ctr 1985; **Fac Appt:** Asst Prof S, UMDNJ-RW Johnson Med Sch

Kunzman, Kenneth MD (Oto) - **Hospital:** Somerset Med Ctr; **Address:** 56 Union Ave, Somerville, NJ 08876; **Phone:** 908-722-1022; **Board Cert:** Otolaryngology 1973; **Med School:** UMDNJ-NJ Med Sch, Newark 1964; **Resid:** Surgery, Hartford Hosp 1966; Otolaryngology, Hosp Univ Penn 1969

PEDIATRICS

Katz, Andrea G MD (Ped) **PCP** - **Spec Exp:** Developmental & Behavioral Disorders; Chronic Illness; Obesity; **Hospital:** Overlook Hosp (page 88), St Barnabas Med Ctr; **Address:** 76 Stirling Rd, Ste 201, Warren, NJ 07059; **Phone:** 908-755-5437; **Board Cert:** Pediatrics 1999; **Med School:** NY Med Coll 1988; **Resid:** Pediatrics, NY Hosp-Cornell Med Ctr 1991

PLASTIC SURGERY

Perry, Arthur MD (PlS) - **Spec Exp:** Cosmetic Surgery-Face; Liposuction; Rhinoplasty; **Hospital:** Robert Wood Johnson Univ Hosp - New Brunswick (page 853), Somerset Med Ctr; **Address:** 3055 Route 27, Franklin Park, NJ 08823-1315; **Phone:** 732-422-9600; **Board Cert:** Plastic Surgery 1989; **Med School:** Albany Med Coll 1981; **Resid:** Surgery, Beth Israel Deaconess Med Ctr 1984; Plastic Surgery, Univ Chicago Med Ctr 1987; **Fellow:** Burn Surgery, New York Hosp-Cornell 1985; Cosmetic Plastic Surgery, Univ Miami/Baker-Gordon Assoc; **Fac Appt:** Assoc Clin Prof PlS, Robert W Johnson Med Sch

PSYCHIATRY

Donnellan, Joseph MD (Psyc) - **Spec Exp:** Eating Disorders; **Hospital:** Somerset Med Ctr; **Address:** 422 Courtyard Drive, Hillsborough, NJ 08844; **Phone:** 908-725-5595; **Board Cert:** Psychiatry 1991; **Med School:** UMDNJ-NJ Med Sch, Newark 1986; **Resid:** Psychiatry, UMDNJ/Newark 1990

Nadel, William MD (Psyc) - **Spec Exp:** Mood Disorders; **Hospital:** Muhlenberg Regional Med Ctr; **Address:** Behav Med Consultants, 65 Mountain Blvd, Ste 210, Warren, NJ 07059; **Phone:** 732-356-5665; **Board Cert:** Psychiatry 1975; **Med School:** Case West Res Univ 1968; **Resid:** Psychiatry, Albert Einstein 1972; **Fellow:** Social Psychiatry, Albert Einstein 1973

Rochford, Joseph MD (Psyc) - **Spec Exp:** Depression; Anxiety Disorders; Eating Disorders; **Hospital:** Somerset Med Ctr; **Address:** 407 Omni Drive, Hillsborough, NJ 08844; **Phone:** 908-359-2312; **Board Cert:** Psychiatry 1975; **Med School:** Yale Univ 1969; **Resid:** Psychiatry, Penn Univ Med Ctr 1973; **Fac Appt:** Assoc Clin Prof Psyc, UMDNJ-RW Johnson Med Sch

PULMONARY DISEASE

Arno, Louis MD (Pul) - **Hospital:** Somerset Med Ctr, St Peter's Univ Hosp; **Address:** 489 Union Ave, Bridge Water, NJ 08807; **Phone:** 732-356-9950; **Board Cert:** Pulmonary Disease 1994; Internal Medicine 2002; Critical Care Medicine 1997; **Med School:** Grenada 1986; **Resid:** Internal Medicine, Seton Hall Univ Hosp 1990; **Fellow:** Pulmonary Disease, Seton Hall Univ Hosp 1992; Critical Care Medicine, Seton Hall Univ Hosp 1993

REPRODUCTIVE ENDOCRINOLOGY

Dlugi, Alexander M MD (RE) - **Spec Exp:** Infertility; Infertility-IVF; **Hospital:** Somerset Med Ctr, Morristown Mem Hosp (page 88); **Address:** Sher Inst for Reproductive Medicine - NJ, One Robertson Drive, Ste 24, Bedminster, NJ 07921; **Phone:** 908-781-0666; **Board Cert:** Obstetrics & Gynecology 1985; Reproductive Endocrinology 1987; **Med School:** Univ Pennsylvania 1977; **Resid:** Obstetrics & Gynecology, Johns Hopkins Hosp 1981; **Fellow:** Reproductive Endocrinology, Yale-New Haven Hosp 1983

Treiser, Susan L MD/PhD (RE) - **Spec Exp:** Infertility; Infertility-IVF; **Hospital:** St Peter's Univ Hosp; **Address:** IVF NJ Fertility & Gynecology Ctr, 81 Veronica Ave, Somerset, NJ 08873; **Phone:** 732-220-9060; **Board Cert:** Obstetrics & Gynecology 2004; Reproductive Endocrinology 2004; **Med School:** Georgetown Univ 1983; **Resid:** Obstetrics & Gynecology, UMDNJ Med Ctr 1988; **Fellow:** Reproductive Endocrinology, Columbia Presby Med Ctr 1990

RHEUMATOLOGY

McWhorter, John MD (Rhu) - **Spec Exp:** Arthritis; Osteoporosis; Lupus/SLE; Scleroderma; **Hospital:** Somerset Med Ctr, Robert Wood Johnson Univ Hosp - New Brunswick (page 853); **Address:** 201 Union Ave, Ste 2D, Bridgewater, NJ 08807-3002; **Phone:** 908-722-5380; **Board Cert:** Internal Medicine 1973; Rheumatology 1974; **Med School:** UMDNJ-NJ Med Sch, Newark 1968; **Resid:** Internal Medicine, Thomas Jefferson Univ Hosp 1971; Internal Medicine, Harlem Hosp 1972; **Fellow:** Rheumatology, Columbia-Presby Med Ctr 1975; **Fac Appt:** Asst Prof Med, UMDNJ-NJ Med Sch, Newark

Whitman III, Hendricks MD (Rhu) - **Spec Exp:** Rheumatoid Arthritis; Scleroderma; **Hospital:** Overlook Hosp (page 88), Morristown Mem Hosp (page 88); **Address:** 34 Mountain Blvd, B Bldg, Warren, NJ 07059; **Phone:** 908-769-0100; **Board Cert:** Internal Medicine 1978; Rheumatology 1980; **Med School:** Univ NC Sch Med 1975; **Resid:** Internal Medicine, NY Hosp-Cornell 1978; **Fellow:** Rheumatology, NY Hosp-Cornell 1980; **Fac Appt:** Asst Clin Prof Med, Cornell Univ-Weill Med Coll

SURGERY

Buch, Edward MD (S) - **Spec Exp:** Endovascular Surgery; Vein Disorders; Hernia; Laparoscopic Surgery; **Hospital:** Somerset Med Ctr; **Address:** 611 Courtyard Drive Bldg 600, Hillsborough, NJ 08844; **Phone:** 908-722-0030; **Board Cert:** Vascular Surgery 2000; Surgery 1996; **Med School:** SUNY Downstate 1981; **Resid:** Surgery, Downstate 1981; Surgery, Downstate 1985; **Fellow:** Vascular Surgery, Medical Coll of Virginia 1986

Drascher, Gary MD (S) - **Spec Exp:** Laparoscopic Surgery-Complex; Aneurysm; Carotid Artery Surgery; **Hospital:** Somerset Med Ctr, Robert Wood Johnson Univ Hosp - New Brunswick (page 853); **Address:** 515 Church St, Ste 1, Bound Brook, NJ 08805-1743; **Phone:** 732-356-0770; **Board Cert:** Surgery 1996; **Med School:** Mount Sinai Sch Med 1981; **Resid:** Internal Medicine, St Luke's-Roosevelt Hosp Ctr 1982; Surgery, St Luke's-Roosevelt Hosp Ctr 1987; **Fellow:** Vascular Surgery, Englewood Hosp 1989

McManus, Susan MD (S) - **Spec Exp:** Breast Surgery; **Hospital:** St Peter's Univ Hosp, Hunterdon Med Ctr; **Address:** 1553 Route 27, Ste 3100, Somerset, NJ 08873; **Phone:** 732-846-3300; **Board Cert:** Surgery 1995; **Med School:** Mexico 1979; **Resid:** Surgery, Beth Israel Med Ctr 1985; **Fac Appt:** Asst Clin Prof S, UMDNJ-RW Johnson Med Sch

THORACIC SURGERY

Caccavale, Robert J MD (TS) - **Spec Exp:** Video Assisted Thoracic Surgery (VATS); **Hospital:** St Peter's Univ Hosp, Robert Wood Johnson Univ Hosp - New Brunswick (page 853); **Address:** 35 Clyde Rd, Ste 104, Somerset, NJ 08873; **Phone:** 732-247-3002; **Board Cert:** Thoracic Surgery 1997; **Med School:** SUNY Buffalo 1981; **Resid:** Surgery, NYU Med Ctr 1984; Surgery, Booth Meml Med Ctr 1986; **Fellow:** Thoracic Surgery, Downstate Med Ctr 1988; **Fac Appt:** Assoc Prof S, Robert W Johnson Med Sch

UROLOGY

Lifland, John MD (U) - **Spec Exp:** Urologic Cancer; Infertility-Male; Sexual Dysfunction; **Hospital:** Somerset Med Ctr; **Address:** 72 West End Ave, Somerville, NJ 08876; **Phone:** 908-725-3535; **Board Cert:** Urology 1975; **Med School:** Univ VA Sch Med 1965; **Resid:** Surgery, Penn Hosp 1967; Urology, Penn Hosp 1972

Union

Union

ALLERGY & IMMUNOLOGY

Brown, David K MD (A&I) - **Spec Exp:** Asthma; Sinus Disorders; Headache; **Hospital:** Overlook Hosp (page 88); **Address:** 33 Overlook Rd, Ste 307, Summit, NJ 07901-3563; **Phone:** 908-522-9696; **Board Cert:** Internal Medicine 1984; Allergy & Immunology 1987; **Med School:** Med Coll OH 1981; **Resid:** Internal Medicine, Overlook Hosp 1984; **Fellow:** Allergy & Immunology, St Luke's-Roosevelt Hosp Ctr 1986

Bukosky, Richard MD (A&I) - **Spec Exp:** Asthma; Hives; **Hospital:** Trinitas Hosp, Union Hosp - NJ; **Address:** 926 N Wood Ave, Linden, NJ 07036-4040; **Phone:** 908-925-3318; **Board Cert:** Allergy & Immunology 1977; **Med School:** Med Coll Wisc 1960; **Resid:** Internal Medicine, VA Hosp 1966; **Fellow:** Allergy & Immunology, Milwaukee Co Genl Hosp 1968

Goodman, Alan MD (A&I) - **Spec Exp:** Rhinitis; Sinus Disorders; **Hospital:** St Barnabas Med Ctr, Union Hosp - NJ; **Address:** 381 Chestnut St, Union, NJ 07083; **Phone:** 908-688-6200; **Board Cert:** Internal Medicine 1985; Allergy & Immunology 1999; **Med School:** SUNY Upstate Med Univ 1982; **Resid:** Internal Medicine, Washington Hosp Ctr 1985; **Fellow:** Allergy & Immunology, St Luke's-Roosevelt Hosp Ctr 1988

Le Benger, Kerry S MD (A&I) - **Spec Exp:** Asthma; Allergy; **Hospital:** Overlook Hosp (page 88), St Barnabas Med Ctr; **Address:** 120 Summit Ave, Summit, NJ 07901-2885; **Phone:** 908-277-8681; **Board Cert:** Internal Medicine 1983; Allergy & Immunology 1985; **Med School:** NY Med Coll 1980; **Resid:** Internal Medicine, Lenox Hill Hosp 1983; **Fellow:** Allergy & Immunology, New York Hosp 1985; **Fac Appt:** Asst Clin Prof Med, UMDNJ-NJ Med Sch, Newark

Maccia, Clement MD (A&I) - **Spec Exp:** Rhinitis; Asthma; Urticaria; Eczema; **Hospital:** Muhlenberg Regional Med Ctr; **Address:** 19 Holly St, Cranford, NJ 07016; **Phone:** 908-276-0666; **Board Cert:** Pediatrics 1980; Allergy & Immunology 1985; **Med School:** Italy 1971; **Resid:** Pediatrics, Muhlenberg Med Ctr 1974; **Fellow:** Allergy & Immunology, Univ Hosp 1976; **Fac Appt:** Clin Prof A&I, Robert W Johnson Med Sch

Mendelson, Joel S MD (A&I) - **Spec Exp:** Infectious Disease; Food Allergy; **Hospital:** St Barnabas Med Ctr; **Address:** 1124 Springfield Ave, Mountainside, NJ 07092; **Phone:** 908-233-4477; **Board Cert:** Pediatrics 1987; Allergy & Immunology 1999; Pediatric Infectious Disease 2005; **Med School:** Dominican Republic 1982; **Resid:** Pediatrics, St Luke's-Roosevelt Hosp 1985; **Fellow:** Allergy & Immunology, UMDNJ Med Ctr 1987; Infectious Disease, UMDNJ Med Ctr 1987

CARDIOVASCULAR DISEASE

Brodyn, Nicholas DO (Cv) - **Spec Exp:** Transesophageal Echocardiography; Cardiac Catheterization; **Hospital:** Union Hosp - NJ, Saint Michael's Med Ctr; **Address:** 1216 Rt 22 W, Mountainside, NJ 07092; **Phone:** 908-654-1200; **Board Cert:** Internal Medicine 1987; Cardiovascular Disease 1991; **Med School:** Univ Osteo Med & Hlth Sci, Des Moines 1983; **Resid:** Internal Medicine, St Michael's Med Ctr 1987; **Fellow:** Cardiovascular Disease, St Michael's Med Ctr 1989

Kalischer, Alan MD (Cv) - **Spec Exp:** Echocardiography; Cardiac Stress Testing; Arrhythmias & Pacemakers; Heart Valve Disease; **Hospital:** Muhlenberg Regional Med Ctr, Overlook Hosp (page 88); **Address:** 2253 South Ave, Scotch Plains, NJ 07076-4688; **Phone:** 908-654-3080; **Board Cert:** Internal Medicine 1982; Cardiovascular Disease 1985; **Med School:** NY Med Coll 1977; **Resid:** Internal Medicine, Kings County Hosp 1980; **Fellow:** Cardiovascular Disease, Columbia-Presby Med Ctr 1984; **Fac Appt:** Asst Clin Prof Med, UMDNJ-RW Johnson Med Sch

Sachs, R Gregory MD (Cv) - **Spec Exp:** Heart Disease; Heart Valve Disease; Congenital Heart Disease-Adult; **Hospital:** Overlook Hosp (page 88), Morristown Mem Hosp (page 88); **Address:** 120 Summit Ave, Summit, NJ 07901; **Phone:** 908-273-4300; **Board Cert:** Internal Medicine 1972; Cardiovascular Disease 1976; **Med School:** Georgetown Univ 1966; **Resid:** Internal Medicine, Georgetown Univ Hosp 1968; **Fellow:** Cardiovascular Disease, Emory Hosp 1970; Cardiovascular Disease, National Heart Hosp 1971; **Fac Appt:** Asst Clin Prof Med, Columbia P&S

Slama, Robert MD (Cv) - **Spec Exp:** Echocardiography; Preventive Cardiology; **Hospital:** Overlook Hosp (page 88), Morristown Mem Hosp (page 88); **Address:** 129 Summit Ave, Summit, NJ 07901; **Phone:** 908-273-4300 x8714; **Board Cert:** Internal Medicine 1974; Cardiovascular Disease 1977; **Med School:** Temple Univ 1971; **Resid:** Internal Medicine, Boston Med Ctr 1973; Internal Medicine, Georgetown Univ Hosp 1974; **Fellow:** Cardiovascular Disease, Boston Univ Med Ctr 1976

Stein, Elliott MD (Cv) - **Hospital:** Overlook Hosp (page 88); **Address:** 211 Mountain Ave, Springfield, NJ 07081; **Phone:** 973-467-0005; **Board Cert:** Internal Medicine 1974; Cardiovascular Disease 1974; **Med School:** Jefferson Med Coll 1964; **Resid:** Internal Medicine, Mount Sinai Hosp 1969; Cardiovascular Disease, Mount Sinai Hosp 1971

Williams, Edward MD (Cv) - **Hospital:** Trinitas Hosp, Robert Wood Johnson Univ Hosp at Rahway (page 853); **Address:** 1317 Morris Ave, Union, NJ 07083; **Phone:** 908-964-9370; **Board Cert:** Internal Medicine 1971; Cardiovascular Disease 1974; **Med School:** Columbia P&S 1964; **Resid:** Internal Medicine, St Luke's Hosp 1969; **Fellow:** Cardiovascular Disease, St Luke's Hosp 1971

CHILD & ADOLESCENT PSYCHIATRY

Greenberg, Rosalie MD (ChAP) - **Spec Exp:** Bipolar/Mood Disorders; ADD/ADHD; **Hospital:** Overlook Hosp (page 88), NY-Presby Hosp (page 100); **Address:** 33 Overlook Rd, Ste 406, Summit, NJ 07901; **Phone:** 908-598-0200; **Board Cert:** Psychiatry 1982; Child & Adolescent Psychiatry 1983; **Med School:** Columbia P&S 1976; **Resid:** Psychiatry, Columbia-Presby Hosp 1979; **Fellow:** Child & Adolescent Psychiatry, Columbia-Presby Hosp 1981; **Fac Appt:** Asst Clin Prof Psyc, Columbia P&S

CHILD NEUROLOGY

Traeger, Eveline MD (ChiN) - **Spec Exp:** Autism; ADD/ADHD; Learning Disorders; **Hospital:** Children's Specialized Hosp; **Address:** 150 New Providence Rd, Mountainside, NJ 07092; **Phone:** 908-233-3720 x5491; **Board Cert:** Pediatrics 1999; Child Neurology 1995; Clinical Genetics 1990; **Med School:** SUNY Buffalo 1984; **Resid:** Child Neurology, Yeshiva Univ 1986; Pediatrics, Jacobi Med Ctr 1988

COLON & RECTAL SURGERY

Groff, Walter MD (CRS) - **Spec Exp:** Colonoscopy; Rectal Cancer/Sphincter Preservation; Laparoscopic Surgery; **Hospital:** Overlook Hosp (page 88); **Address:** 33 Overlook Rd, Ste 412, Summit, NJ 07901-3564; **Phone:** 908-598-0220; **Board Cert:** Colon & Rectal Surgery 1980; **Med School:** Albany Med Coll 1970; **Resid:** Surgery, St Vincent's Hosp 1979; Colon & Rectal Surgery, Muhlenberg Med Ctr 1980; **Fac Appt:** Assoc Prof S, Columbia P&S

DERMATOLOGY

Eisenberg, Richard R MD (D) - **Spec Exp:** Skin Cancer; Melanoma; **Hospital:** Overlook Hosp (page 88); **Address:** 40 Sterling Rd, Ste 203, Watchung, NJ 07069; **Phone:** 908-753-4144; **Board Cert:** Internal Medicine 1985; Dermatology 1989; **Med School:** Cornell Univ-Weill Med Coll 1982; **Resid:** Internal Medicine, NY Hosp-Cornell Med Ctr 1985; Dermatology, NY Hosp-Cornell/Meml Sloan Kettering Cancer Ctr 1989

Gruber, Gabriel MD (D) - **Spec Exp:** Psoriasis; Phototherapy; **Hospital:** Overlook Hosp (page 88), St Barnabas Med Ctr; **Address:** Summit Medical Group, 1 Diamond Hill Rd, Berkeley Heights, NJ 07922; **Phone:** 908-273-4300; **Board Cert:** Internal Medicine 1976; Dermatology 1977; **Med School:** Harvard Med Sch 1972; **Resid:** Internal Medicine, Boston Med Ctr 1974; Dermatology, Mass General Hosp 1977

Weinberger, George I MD (D) - **Spec Exp:** Skin Cancer; **Hospital:** Muhlenberg Regional Med Ctr; **Address:** 190 Greenbrook Rd, N Plainfield, NJ 07060-3903; **Phone:** 908-561-8070; **Board Cert:** Dermatology 1977; **Med School:** UMDNJ-NJ Med Sch, Newark 1973; **Resid:** Dermatology, Henry Ford Hosp 1977

DIAGNOSTIC RADIOLOGY

Donnelly, Brian MD (DR) - **Spec Exp:** Bone Disorders; MRI; Chest Radiology; **Hospital:** Overlook Hosp (page 88); **Address:** Westfield Imaging Center, 118 Elm St, Westfield, NJ 07090; **Phone:** 908-232-0290; **Board Cert:** Diagnostic Radiology 1975; **Med School:** Jefferson Med Coll 1971; **Resid:** Diagnostic Radiology, Columbia Presby Med Ctr 1975

ENDOCRINOLOGY, DIABETES & METABOLISM

Fuhrman, Robert MD (EDM) - **Spec Exp:** Diabetes; Thyroid Disorders; Osteoporosis; **Hospital:** Overlook Hosp (page 88); **Address:** 552 Westfield Ave, Westfield, NJ 07090-3312; **Phone:** 908-654-3377; **Board Cert:** Internal Medicine 1971; Endocrinology, Diabetes & Metabolism 1972; **Med School:** Univ Hlth Sci/Chicago Med Sch 1966; **Resid:** Internal Medicine, Mount Sinai Hosp 1970; Nuclear Medicine, VA Hospital 1970; **Fellow:** Endocrinology, Diabetes & Metabolism, Mount Sinai Hosp 1970; **Fac Appt:** Asst Clin Prof Med, UMDNJ-NJ Med Sch, Newark

Rosenbaum, Robert MD (EDM) - **Spec Exp:** Thyroid Disorders; Diabetes; Osteoporosis; **Hospital:** Overlook Hosp (page 88); **Address:** 120 Summit Ave, Summit, NJ 07901-2804; **Phone:** 908-273-4300; **Board Cert:** Internal Medicine 1978; Endocrinology, Diabetes & Metabolism 1981; **Med School:** Columbia P&S 1975; **Resid:** Internal Medicine, Montefiore Hosp Med Ctr 1978; **Fellow:** Endocrinology, Diabetes & Metabolism, Montefiore Hosp Med Ctr 1980; **Fac Appt:** Asst Clin Prof Med, UMDNJ-NJ Med Sch, Newark

Silverman, Mitchell MD (EDM) - **Spec Exp:** Diabetes; Thyroid Disorders; Adrenal Disorders; **Hospital:** St Barnabas Med Ctr, Newark Beth Israel Med Ctr; **Address:** 2333 Morris Ave, Ste B-9, Union, NJ 07083; **Phone:** 908-964-5511; **Board Cert:** Internal Medicine 1983; Endocrinology 1988; **Med School:** Duke Univ 1980; **Resid:** Internal Medicine, Emory Univ Hosp 1983; **Fellow:** Endocrinology, Diabetes & Metabolism, NY Hosp-Meml Sloan-Kettering 1988

FAMILY MEDICINE

Eisenstat, Steven DO (FMed) `PCP` - **Spec Exp:** Osteoporosis; Hypertension; Alzheimer's Disease; **Hospital:** Union Hosp - NJ, Overlook Hosp (page 88); **Address:** 1050 Galloping Hill Rd, Ste 202, Union, NJ 07083-7980; **Phone:** 908-688-4845; **Board Cert:** Family Medicine 1993; Geriatric Medicine 1991; **Med School:** Ohio State Univ 1984; **Resid:** Family Medicine, Union Hosp 1987; **Fac Appt:** Asst Clin Prof FMed, NY Coll Osteo Med

Kaye, Susan MD (FMed) `PCP` - **Spec Exp:** Women's Health; **Hospital:** Overlook Hosp (page 88); **Address:** 33 Overlook Rd, Ste L-01, Summit, NJ 07901-3561; **Phone:** 908-522-5700; **Board Cert:** Family Medicine 2001; **Med School:** NYU Sch Med 1979; **Resid:** Family Medicine, Overlook Hosp 1982; **Fellow:** Family Medicine, Faculty Develop Ctr 1983; **Fac Appt:** Assoc Clin Prof FMed, UMDNJ-NJ Med Sch, Newark

Rosenberg, Amy MD (FMed) `PCP` - **Hospital:** Overlook Hosp (page 88); **Address:** 563 Westfield Ave, Westfield, NJ 07090-3125; **Phone:** 908-232-5858; **Board Cert:** Family Medicine 1998; **Med School:** Univ Pennsylvania 1982; **Resid:** Family Medicine, Overlook Hosp 1985

Tabachnick, John F MD (FMed) `PCP` - **Hospital:** Overlook Hosp (page 88); **Address:** 417 W Broad St, Westfield, NJ 07090; **Phone:** 908-232-5858; **Board Cert:** Family Medicine 1994; **Med School:** Mount Sinai Sch Med 1979; **Resid:** Family Medicine, Overlook Hosp 1982; **Fac Appt:** Asst Clin Prof FMed, UMDNJ Sch Osteo Med

GASTROENTEROLOGY

Goldenberg, David MD (Ge) - **Spec Exp:** Inflammatory Bowel Disease/Crohn's; Biliary Disease; Gastroesophageal Reflux Disease (GERD); **Hospital:** Muhlenberg Regional Med Ctr, JFK Med Ctr - Edison; **Address:** 1165 Park Ave, Plainfield, NJ 07060; **Phone:** 908-754-2992; **Board Cert:** Gastroenterology 1981; Internal Medicine 1977; **Med School:** NY Med Coll 1974; **Resid:** Internal Medicine, Metropolitan Hosp 1977; **Fellow:** Gastroenterology, Emory Univ Hosp 1980; **Fac Appt:** Asst Clin Prof Med, UMDNJ-RW Johnson Med Sch

Kerner, Michael MD (Ge) - **Spec Exp:** Colonoscopy; Biliary Disease; Gastroesophageal Reflux Disease (GERD); Inflammatory Bowel Disease; **Hospital:** Overlook Hosp (page 88); **Address:** 25 Morris Ave, Springfield, NJ 07081-1406; **Phone:** 973-467-1313; **Board Cert:** Internal Medicine 1975; Gastroenterology 1977; **Med School:** Wake Forest Univ 1971; **Resid:** Internal Medicine, NYU Med Ctr 1974; **Fellow:** Gastroenterology, Manhattan VA-Bellevue Hosp 1976; **Fac Appt:** Asst Clin Prof Med, UMDNJ-NJ Med Sch, Newark

Levinson, Joel MD (Ge) - **Spec Exp:** Inflammatory Bowel Disease; Gastroesophageal Reflux Disease (GERD); Liver Disease; **Hospital:** Overlook Hosp (page 88); **Address:** 25 Morris Ave, Springfield, NJ 07081; **Phone:** 973-467-1313; **Board Cert:** Internal Medicine 1970; Gastroenterology 1972; **Med School:** Georgetown Univ 1963; **Resid:** Internal Medicine, Georgetown Univ Hosp 1965; Internal Medicine, Vanderbilt Univ Hosp 1968; **Fellow:** Gastroenterology, Univ Chicago Hosp 1970; **Fac Appt:** Asst Clin Prof Med, UMDNJ-NJ Med Sch, Newark

Mahal, Pradeep MD (Ge) - **Spec Exp:** Gastrointestinal Cancer; **Hospital:** Union Hosp - NJ, Trinitas Hosp; **Address:** 1308 Morris Ave, Ste 202, Union, NJ 07083; **Phone:** 908-851-6767; **Board Cert:** Gastroenterology 1981; Internal Medicine 1978; Geriatric Medicine 2002; Medical Oncology 1983; **Med School:** India 1975; **Resid:** Internal Medicine, UMDNJ Univ Hosp 1978; **Fellow:** Medical Oncology, MD Anderson Tumor Inst 1980; Gastroenterology, MD Anderson Tumor Inst 1980

Tempera, Patrick MD (Ge) - **Spec Exp:** Biliary Disease; Pancreatic Disease; Gastroesophageal Reflux Disease (GERD); **Hospital:** Union Hosp - NJ, Trinitas Hosp; **Address:** 2333 Morris Ave, Ste C-1, Union, NJ 07083; **Phone:** 908-851-2771; **Board Cert:** Internal Medicine 1990; Gastroenterology 2004; **Med School:** Grenada 1986; **Resid:** Surgery, Brooklyn Hosp 1987; Internal Medicine, Seton Hall Univ Hosp 1990; **Fellow:** Gastroenterology, Seton Hall Univ Hosp 1992; **Fac Appt:** Assoc Prof Med, Seton Hall Univ Sch Grad Med Ed

GERIATRIC MEDICINE

Solomon, Robert B MD (Ger) `PCP` - **Spec Exp:** Alzheimer's Disease; Osteoporosis; **Hospital:** Trinitas Hosp, Overlook Hosp (page 88); **Address:** 744 Galloping Hill Rd, Roselle Park, NJ 07204-1758; **Phone:** 908-241-0044; **Board Cert:** Internal Medicine 1980; Geriatric Medicine 1988; **Med School:** SUNY Hlth Sci Ctr 1977; **Resid:** Internal Medicine, Westchester Med Ctr 1980; **Fellow:** Geriatric Medicine, New York Hosp 1981

HEMATOLOGY

Kessler, William MD (Hem) - **Hospital:** Trinitas Hosp; **Address:** Medical Offices, 225 Williamson St, Elizabeth, NJ 07207; **Phone:** 908-994-8773; **Board Cert:** Internal Medicine 1978; Hematology 1980; **Med School:** Albert Einstein Coll Med 1975; **Resid:** Internal Medicine, UMDNJ-Newark 1978; **Fellow:** Hematology, VA Hosp 1979

INFECTIOUS DISEASE

Farrer, William MD (Inf) - **Spec Exp:** AIDS/HIV; Diabetic Leg/Foot Infections; Travel Medicine; **Hospital:** Trinitas Hosp; **Address:** 240 Williamson St, Ste 502, Elizabeth, NJ 07207-3625; **Phone:** 908-994-5300; **Board Cert:** Internal Medicine 1978; Infectious Disease 1980; **Med School:** Harvard Med Sch 1975; **Resid:** Internal Medicine, Montefiore Hosp Med Ctr 1978; **Fellow:** Infectious Disease, Montefiore-Weiler Einstein Med Ctr 1980; **Fac Appt:** Assoc Prof Med, Seton Hall Univ Sch Grad Med Ed

Roland, Robert DO (Inf) - **Spec Exp:** AIDS/HIV; Travel Medicine; Hepatitis C; **Hospital:** Union Hosp - NJ, Trinitas Hosp; **Address:** 1308 Morris Ave, Ste 204, Union, NJ 07083; **Phone:** 908-810-9200; **Board Cert:** Internal Medicine 1990; Infectious Disease 1992; **Med School:** Kirksville Coll Osteo Med 1985; **Resid:** Internal Medicine, Union Hosp 1989; **Fellow:** Infectious Disease, Kennedy Meml Hosp 1991; **Fac Appt:** Asst Clin Prof Med, NY Coll Osteo Med

INTERNAL MEDICINE

Feldman, Jeffrey MD (IM) `PCP` - **Spec Exp:** Hypertension; Cholesterol/Lipid Disorders; Diabetes; **Hospital:** Overlook Hosp (page 88), Muhlenberg Regional Med Ctr; **Address:** 440 Chestnut St Fl 1, Union, NJ 07083-9306; **Phone:** 908-686-9330; **Board Cert:** Nephrology 1982; Internal Medicine 1979; **Med School:** Hahnemann Univ 1976; **Resid:** Internal Medicine, Bronx Municipal Hosp 1979; **Fellow:** Nephrology, SUNY Hlth Sci Ctr 1981

Goodgold, Abraham MD (IM) `PCP` - **Hospital:** Trinitas Hosp, Union Hosp - NJ; **Address:** 310 W Jersey St, Elizabeth Medical Group, Elizabeth, NJ 07202-1832; **Phone:** 908-351-2222; **Board Cert:** Internal Medicine 1977; **Med School:** NYU Sch Med 1973; **Resid:** Infectious Disease, Montefiore Med Ctr 1976; **Fellow:** Endocrinology, Mt Sinai Med Ctr 1978

Hwang, Cheng-hong DO (IM) `PCP` - **Spec Exp:** Pulmonary Disease; **Hospital:** Union Hosp - NJ, Robert Wood Johnson Univ Hosp at Rahway (page 853); **Address:** 1457 Raritan Rd, Ste 201, Clark, NJ 07066; **Phone:** 908-272-2270; **Board Cert:** Internal Medicine 1983; Pulmonary Disease 1984; **Med School:** Coll Osteo Med 1978; **Resid:** Internal Medicine, USPHS Hosp-Staten Island NY & USPHS Hosp 1981; **Fellow:** Pulmonary Disease, UMDNJ-Univ Hosp 1983

Khimani, Karim MD (IM) `PCP` - **Spec Exp:** Geriatric Medicine; **Hospital:** Trinitas Hosp, Union Hosp - NJ; **Address:** 240 Williamson St, Ste 306, Elizabeth, NJ 07202; **Phone:** 908-352-5071; **Board Cert:** Internal Medicine 1986; Geriatric Medicine 1990; **Med School:** Dominican Republic 1982; **Resid:** Internal Medicine, St Elizabeth Hosp 1985

Maglaras, Nicholas MD (IM) - **Hospital:** Trinitas Hosp, Union Hosp - NJ; **Address:** 236 E Westfield Ave, Roselle Park, NJ 07204; **Phone:** 908-245-8222; **Board Cert:** Internal Medicine 1991; Internal Medicine 1996; **Med School:** Grenada 1987; **Resid:** Internal Medicine, Elmhurst Hosp 1990; **Fellow:** Pulmonary Disease, Elmhurst Hosp 1992

INTERVENTIONAL CARDIOLOGY

Lux, Michael MD (IC) - **Hospital:** Overlook Hosp (page 88), Morristown Mem Hosp (page 88); **Address:** Assocs in Cardiovascular Disease, 211 Mountain Ave, Springfield, NJ 07081-1581; **Phone:** 973-467-0005; **Board Cert:** Internal Medicine 1980; Cardiovascular Disease 1985; Interventional Cardiology 2002; **Med School:** NYU Sch Med 1977; **Resid:** Internal Medicine, Johns Hopkins Hosp 1980; **Fellow:** Cardiovascular Disease, Johns Hopkins Hosp 1983

Mich, Robert MD (IC) - **Hospital:** Morristown Mem Hosp (page 88); **Address:** 29 South St, FL 2, New Providence, NJ 07974-1996; **Phone:** 908-464-4200; **Board Cert:** Internal Medicine 1984; Cardiovascular Disease 1985; Interventional Cardiology 2002; **Med School:** Johns Hopkins Univ 1979; **Resid:** Internal Medicine, Johns Hopkins Hosp 1982; **Fellow:** Cardiovascular Disease, Vanderbilt Univ Hosp 1984; Cardiovascular Disease, Mass Genl Hosp 1986

MEDICAL ONCOLOGY

Leff, Charles MD (Onc) - **Spec Exp:** Breast Cancer; Lung Cancer; Colon Cancer; **Hospital:** Muhlenberg Regional Med Ctr, Somerset Med Ctr; **Address:** 1314 Park Ave, Plainfield, NJ 07060; **Phone:** 908-754-0400; **Board Cert:** Internal Medicine 1972; Hematology 1974; Medical Oncology 1975; **Med School:** SUNY Upstate Med Univ 1968; **Resid:** Internal Medicine, Mt Sinai Hosp 1971; **Fellow:** Hematology & Oncology, Mt Sinai Hosp 1975

Lowenthal, Dennis MD (Onc) - **Spec Exp:** Lung Cancer; Lymphoma; Prostate Cancer; **Hospital:** Overlook Hosp (page 88); **Address:** The Cancer Center at Overlook Hospital, 99 Beauvoir Ave, Summit, NJ 07902; **Phone:** 908-608-0078; **Board Cert:** Internal Medicine 1982; Medical Oncology 1985; Hematology 1986; **Med School:** Boston Univ 1979; **Resid:** Internal Medicine, Montefiore Med Ctr 1982; **Fellow:** Hematology, Montefiore Med Ctr 1983; Medical Oncology, Mem Sloan Kettering Cancer Ctr 1986; **Fac Appt:** Asst Clin Prof Med, UMDNJ-NJ Med Sch, Newark

Wax, Michael MD (Onc) - **Hospital:** Overlook Hosp (page 88); **Address:** 120 Summit Ave, Summit, NJ 07901-2804; **Phone:** 908-219-3080; **Board Cert:** Internal Medicine 1980; Medical Oncology 1983; **Med School:** Med Coll PA Hahnemann 1977; **Resid:** Internal Medicine, Hosp Med Coll Penn 1980; **Fellow:** Hematology & Oncology, Univ Wash Med Ctr 1980; **Fac Appt:** Asst Clin Prof Med, UMDNJ-NJ Med Sch, Newark

NEPHROLOGY

Alterman, Lloyd MD (Nep) - **Spec Exp:** Hypertension; Chronic Kidney Disease; **Hospital:** Overlook Hosp (page 88), St Barnabas Med Ctr; **Address:** 120 Summit Ave, Summit, NJ 07901-2885; **Phone:** 908-273-4300; **Board Cert:** Internal Medicine 1980; Nephrology 1982; **Med School:** Wayne State Univ 1977; **Resid:** Internal Medicine, Overlook Hosp 1980; **Fellow:** Nephrology, Montefiore Med Ctr 1982

Goldstein, Carl MD (Nep) - **Spec Exp:** Hypertension; Glomerulonephritis; Kidney Failure; **Hospital:** Overlook Hosp (page 88); **Address:** 215 North Ave W, Westfield, NJ 07090-1428; **Phone:** 908-232-4321; **Board Cert:** Internal Medicine 1981; Nephrology 1984; **Med School:** Washington Univ, St Louis 1978; **Resid:** Internal Medicine, Univ Minn Med Ctr 1981; **Fellow:** Nephrology, Hosp Univ Penn 1984; **Fac Appt:** Assoc Clin Prof Med, UMDNJ-RW Johnson Med Sch

McAnally, James MD (Nep) - **Spec Exp:** Kidney Disease; Hypertension; Diabetes; **Hospital:** Trinitas Hosp, Union Hosp - NJ; **Address:** 240 Williamson St, Ste 307, Elizabeth, NJ 07202-3672; **Phone:** 908-994-9200; **Board Cert:** Internal Medicine 1978; Nephrology 1980; **Med School:** UMDNJ-NJ Med Sch, Newark 1975; **Resid:** Internal Medicine, CMDNJ-Newark Affil Hosp 1978; Internal Medicine, Georgetown Univ Hosp 1980; **Fellow:** Nephrology, Georgetown Univ Hosp 1980; **Fac Appt:** Assoc Clin Prof Med, Seton Hall Univ Sch Grad Med Ed

NEUROLOGICAL SURGERY

Fineman, Sanford MD (NS) - **Spec Exp:** Brain Tumors; Pain Management; Spinal Surgery; **Hospital:** Union Hosp - NJ, Robert Wood Johnson Univ Hosp at Rahway (page 853); **Address:** 2333 Morris Ave, Ste B-8, Union, NJ 07083-5737; **Phone:** 908-688-8800; **Board Cert:** Neurological Surgery 1985; **Med School:** Temple Univ 1976; **Resid:** Neurological Surgery, Thomas Jefferson Univ Hosp 1981; **Fellow:** Neurological Surgery, Presbyterian Hosp 1982

Friedlander, Marvin E MD (NS) - **Spec Exp:** Spinal Diseases; **Hospital:** Union Hosp - NJ, Overlook Hosp (page 88); **Address:** 700 Rahway Ave, Union, NJ 07083; **Phone:** 908-688-1999; **Board Cert:** Neurological Surgery 1994; **Med School:** SUNY Downstate 1982; **Resid:** Neurological Surgery, Kings Co Hosp 1989; **Fellow:** Metabolism, SUNY Downstate Med Ctr 1984

Hodosh, Richard M MD (NS) - **Spec Exp:** Acoustic Neuroma; Neurovascular Surgery; Spinal Surgery; **Hospital:** Overlook Hosp (page 88), Morristown Mem Hosp (page 88); **Address:** Atlantic Brain & Spine Inst, 99 Beavoir Ave Fl 7, Summit, NJ 07902; **Phone:** 908-522-4979; **Board Cert:** Neurological Surgery 1980; **Med School:** Univ Cincinnati 1972; **Resid:** Neurological Surgery, Univ Tex Hlth Scis Ctr 1978; **Fellow:** Neuroradiology, Natl Hosp Neur Dis 1975; Neurological Surgery, Kanto Hosp 1976; **Fac Appt:** Clin Prof NS, UMDNJ-NJ Med Sch, Newark

NEUROLOGY

Halperin, John MD (N) - **Spec Exp:** Lyme Disease; Neuromuscular Disorders; Multiple Sclerosis; **Hospital:** Overlook Hosp (page 88), N Shore Univ Hosp at Manhasset; **Address:** Dept Neurosciences, Overlook Hospital, Summit, NJ 07902; **Phone:** 908-522-3501; **Board Cert:** Internal Medicine 1978; Neurology 1982; Clinical Neurophysiology 1996; **Med School:** Harvard Med Sch 1975; **Resid:** Internal Medicine, Univ Chicago Hosps 1977; Neurology, Mass Genl Hosp 1980; **Fellow:** Neurology, Mass Genl Hosp 1983; **Fac Appt:** Prof N, NYU Sch Med

Pollock, Jeffrey MD (N) - **Hospital:** Overlook Hosp (page 88); **Address:** 47 Maple St, Ste 104, Summit, NJ 07901; **Phone:** 908-277-2722; **Board Cert:** Neurology 1987; **Med School:** Med Coll GA 1982; **Resid:** Internal Medicine, Rutgers Univ 1983; Neurology, UMDNJ Med Ctr 1986; **Fellow:** VA Med Ctr 1986

Sachs, Stephen MD (N) - **Hospital:** Union Hosp - NJ, Robert Wood Johnson Univ Hosp at Rahway (page 853); **Address:** 700 N Broad St, Ste 201, Elizabeth, NJ 07208; **Phone:** 908-354-3994; **Board Cert:** Neurology 1977; **Med School:** Univ Pennsylvania 1971; **Resid:** Internal Medicine, Bellevue Hosp 1973; Neurology, Columbia-Presby Med Ctr 1976; **Fac Appt:** Asst Clin Prof N, UMDNJ-NJ Med Sch, Newark

Schanzer, Bernard MD (N) - **Spec Exp:** Stroke; Headache; Multiple Sclerosis; **Hospital:** Trinitas Hosp, Robert Wood Johnson Univ Hosp at Rahway (page 853); **Address:** 700 N Broad St, Ste 201, Elizabeth, NJ 07208-2310; **Phone:** 908-354-3994; **Board Cert:** Neurology 1972; **Med School:** Belgium 1962; **Resid:** Internal Medicine, Maimonides Med Ctr 1965; Neurology, Bronx Municipal Med Ctr 1970; **Fac Appt:** Assoc Clin Prof N, UMDNJ-NJ Med Sch, Newark

NEURORADIOLOGY

Horner, Neil MD (NRad) - **Spec Exp:** MRI of the Nervous System; MRI of Brain Tumors; Spine Imaging & Intervention; **Hospital:** Overlook Hosp (page 88); **Address:** Overlook Hosp, Dept Radiology, 99 Beauvoir Ave, Summit, NJ 07901; **Phone:** 908-522-2066; **Board Cert:** Diagnostic Radiology 1988; Nuclear Radiology 1989; Neuroradiology 1995; **Med School:** Rutgers Univ 1983; **Resid:** Diagnostic Radiology, NYU Med Ctr 1988; **Fellow:** Neuroradiology, NYU Med Ctr 1989; Nuclear Radiology, NYU Med Ctr 1989; **Fac Appt:** Asst Clin Prof Rad, Columbia P&S

OBSTETRICS & GYNECOLOGY

Soffer, Jeffrey MD (ObG) - **Hospital:** Overlook Hosp (page 88); **Address:** 522 E Broad St, Westfield, NJ 07090; **Phone:** 908-561-8444; **Board Cert:** Obstetrics & Gynecology 1983; **Med School:** Howard Univ 1975; **Resid:** Obstetrics & Gynecology, Hosp Univ Penn 1978

OPHTHALMOLOGY

Confino, Joel MD (Oph) - **Spec Exp:** Laser Vision Surgery; Cataract Surgery; Corneal Disease & Transplant; **Hospital:** Overlook Hosp (page 88), Muhlenberg Regional Med Ctr; **Address:** 592 Springfield Ave, Westfield, NJ 07090-1002; **Phone:** 908-789-8999; **Board Cert:** Ophthalmology 1985; **Med School:** Albert Einstein Coll Med 1980; **Resid:** Ophthalmology, Mt Sinai 1984; **Fellow:** Cornea & Ext Eye Disease, Univ California 1985

Natale, Benjamin DO (Oph) - **Spec Exp:** LASIK-Refractive Surgery; Cataract Surgery; **Hospital:** Union Hosp - NJ, St Mary Hosp - Hoboken; **Address:** 1050 Galloping Hill Rd, Union, NJ 07083-7983; **Phone:** 908-964-7878; **Board Cert:** Ophthalmology 1991; **Med School:** Coll Osteo Med 1980; **Resid:** Family Medicine, Union Hosp 1982; Ophthalmology, Univ of Medicine & Dentistry 1985; **Fellow:** Refractive Surgery, Newark Eye & Ear Infirmary 1986

Tchorbajian, Kourkin MD (Oph) - **Spec Exp:** Cataract Surgery; Glaucoma; **Hospital:** Union Hosp - NJ; **Address:** 1050 Galloping Hill Rd, Union, NJ 07083; **Phone:** 908-964-7878; **Board Cert:** Ophthalmology 1991; **Med School:** France 1981; **Resid:** Ophthalmology, UMDNJ-Univ Hosp 1985; Surgery, St Clares Hosp 1992; **Fellow:** Ophthalmology, UMDNJ-Univ Hosp 1986

ORTHOPAEDIC SURGERY

Barmakian, Joseph MD (OrS) - **Spec Exp:** Carpal Tunnel Syndrome; Nerve & Tendon Reconstruction; Shoulder Reconstruction; **Hospital:** Overlook Hosp (page 88), JFK Med Ctr - Edison; **Address:** 523 Westfield Ave, Westfield, NJ 07090-3300; **Phone:** 908-654-1100; **Board Cert:** Orthopaedic Surgery 2003; Hand Surgery 2003; **Med School:** UMDNJ-RW Johnson Med Sch 1984; **Resid:** Surgery, Geo Wash Univ Med Ctr 1986; Orthopaedic Surgery, Columbia-Presby Med Ctr 1989; **Fellow:** Hand Surgery, Hosp for Joint Diseases 1990

Botwin, Clifford DO (OrS) - **Spec Exp:** Arthroscopic Surgery; Hip Surgery; Knee Surgery; **Hospital:** Union Hosp - NJ, Bayonne Med Ctr; **Address:** 900 Stuyvesant Ave, Union, NJ 07083-6936; **Phone:** 908-964-6600; **Resid:** Orthopaedic Surgery, Delaware Valley Hosp 1976

Gallick, Gregory MD (OrS) - **Spec Exp:** Sports Medicine; Knee Reconstruction; Shoulder Reconstruction; **Hospital:** Overlook Hosp (page 88); **Address:** 2780 Morris Ave, Ste 2-C, Union, NJ 07083; **Phone:** 908-686-6665; **Board Cert:** Orthopaedic Surgery 1999; **Med School:** Rutgers Univ 1980; **Resid:** Surgery, Univ of Medicine & Dentistry 1981; Orthopaedic Surgery, Univ of Medicine & Dentistry 1985; **Fellow:** Interventional Cardiology, Southern California Sports Medicine 1986

Innella, Robin DO (OrS) - **Spec Exp:** Sports Medicine; Hip & Knee Replacement; Fractures; **Hospital:** Union Hosp - NJ, Bayonne Med Ctr; **Address:** 900 Stuyvesant Ave, Union, NJ 07083-6936; **Phone:** 908-964-6600; **Board Cert:** Orthopaedic Surgery 1989; **Med School:** Philadelphia Coll Osteo Med 1982; **Resid:** Orthopaedic Surgery, UMDNJ 1987; **Fac Appt:** Asst Clin Prof S, UMDNJ-NJ Med Sch, Newark

Mackessy, Richard P MD (OrS) - **Spec Exp:** Hand Surgery; **Hospital:** Trinitas Hosp, Robert Wood Johnson Univ Hosp at Rahway (page 853); **Address:** 210 W St George Ave, Linden, NJ 07036; **Phone:** 908-486-1111; **Board Cert:** Orthopaedic Surgery 1997; Hand Surgery 1994; **Med School:** UMDNJ-NJ Med Sch, Newark 1978; **Resid:** Surgery, St Vincents Hosp 1980; Orthopaedic Surgery, St Lukes Hosp 1983; **Fellow:** Hand Surgery, Thomas Jefferson Univ Hosp 1984

Nuzzo, Roy MD (OrS) - **Spec Exp:** Pediatric Orthopaedic Surgery; Cerebral Palsy; **Hospital:** Overlook Hosp (page 88); **Address:** Overlook Hosp, 99 Beauvoir Ave, Ste 750, Summit, NJ 07901; **Phone:** 908-522-5801; **Board Cert:** Orthopaedic Surgery 1977; **Med School:** Cornell Univ-Weill Med Coll 1970; **Resid:** Surgery, Yale-New Haven Hosp 1972; Orthopaedic Surgery, Mass Genl Hosp 1975; **Fellow:** Research, Chldns Hosp Med Ctr 1974

Sarokhan, Alan MD (OrS) - **Spec Exp:** Hip Replacement; Knee Replacement; Hand Surgery; **Hospital:** Overlook Hosp (page 88), St Barnabas Med Ctr; **Address:** Medical Arts Bldg, 33 Overlook Rd, Ste 201, Summit, NJ 07901-3562; **Phone:** 908-522-4555; **Board Cert:** Orthopaedic Surgery 1994; **Med School:** Harvard Med Sch 1977; **Resid:** Surgery, Peter Bent Brigham Hosp 1979; Orthopaedic Surgery, Harvard Affil Hosps 1982; **Fellow:** Hand Surgery, Roosevelt Hosp 1984

OTOLARYNGOLOGY

Carniol, Paul MD (Oto) - **Spec Exp:** Laser Surgery; Facial Rejuvenation; Cosmetic Surgery; **Hospital:** Overlook Hosp (page 88); **Address:** Medical Arts Bldg, 33c Overlook Rd, Ste 401, Summit, NJ 07901; **Phone:** 908-598-1400; **Board Cert:** Otolaryngology 1981; Facial Plastic & Reconstructive Surgery 1991; **Med School:** Univ Pennsylvania 1976; **Resid:** Surgery, Hosp Univ Penn 1977; Surgery, North Shore Univ Hosp 1978; **Fellow:** Otolaryngology, Mass Eye & Ear Infirm 1981; Plastic Surgery, Hosp Univ Penn 1983; **Fac Appt:** Assoc Clin Prof S, UMDNJ-NJ Med Sch, Newark

Drake III, William MD (Oto) - **Spec Exp:** Endoscopic Sinus Surgery; Head & Neck Surgery; Thyroid & Parathyroid Surgery; Pediatric Otolaryngology; **Hospital:** Overlook Hosp (page 88); **Address:** Westfield Ear Nose & Throat, 189 Elm St, Westfield, NJ 07090; **Phone:** 908-233-5500; **Board Cert:** Otolaryngology 1995; **Med School:** UMDNJ-NJ Med Sch, Newark 1989; **Resid:** Otolaryngology, Mt Sinai Med Ctr 1994

Eden, Avrim MD (Oto) - **Spec Exp:** Meniere's Disease; Hearing Loss; **Hospital:** UMDNJ-Univ Hosp-Newark; **Address:** 1 Diamond Hill Rd, Berkeley Heights, NJ 07922; **Phone:** 908-273-4300; **Board Cert:** Otolaryngology 1974; **Med School:** South Africa 1968; **Resid:** Otolaryngology, Univ Toronto Hosps 1974; **Fellow:** Otolaryngology, Univ Hosp Zurich 1975; **Fac Appt:** Clin Prof Oto, UMDNJ-NJ Med Sch, Newark

Kwartler, Jed A MD (Oto) - **Spec Exp:** Acoustic Neuroma; Balance Disorders; Cochlear Implants; Otology; **Hospital:** Overlook Hosp (page 88), Hackensack Univ Med Ctr (page 92); **Address:** 1 Diamond Hill Rd, Berkeley Heights, NJ 07922; **Phone:** 908-273-4300; **Board Cert:** Otolaryngology 1988; **Med School:** UMDNJ-NJ Med Sch, Newark 1983; **Resid:** Surgery, UMDNJ/Univ Hosp 1985; Otolaryngology, UMDNJ/Univ Hosp 1988; **Fellow:** Otology & Neurotology, St Vincent's Hosp & Med Ctr 1990; **Fac Appt:** Assoc Clin Prof Oto, UMDNJ-NJ Med Sch, Newark

Scharf, Richard DO (Oto) - **Spec Exp:** Sinus Disorders/Surgery; Cosmetic Surgery-Face; **Hospital:** Union Hosp - NJ, Bayonne Med Ctr; **Address:** 505 Chestnut St, Roselle Park, NJ 07204; **Phone:** 908-241-0200; **Board Cert:** Otolaryngology 1998; **Med School:** Univ Hlth Sci, Coll Osteo Med 1982; **Resid:** Otolaryngology, Flint Hosp 1990; **Fac Appt:** Assoc Clin Prof Oto, NY Coll Osteo Med

PAIN MEDICINE

Ashendorf, Douglas MD (PM) - **Spec Exp:** Headache; Fibromyalgia; Reflex Sympathetic Dystrophy (RSD); Pain-Neuropathic; **Hospital:** St Barnabas Med Ctr; **Address:** 67 Walnut Ave, Ste 105, Clark, NJ 07066-1640; **Phone:** 732-382-1700; **Board Cert:** Physical Medicine & Rehabilitation 1987; Pain Medicine 2000; **Med School:** Mexico 1978; **Resid:** Orthopaedic Surgery, Harlem Hosp Ctr 1983; Physical Medicine & Rehabilitation, Mt. Sinai Med Ctr 1985; **Fac Appt:** Asst Clin Prof Med, Seton Hall Univ Sch Grad Med Ed

Choi, Young K MD (PM) - **Spec Exp:** Pain-Back; Reflex Sympathetic Dystrophy (RSD); Spinal Epiduroscopy; **Hospital:** Robert Wood Johnson Univ Hosp at Rahway (page 853); **Address:** RW Johnson U Hosp at Rahway, Pain Ctr, 865 Stone St, Rahway, NJ 07065; **Phone:** 732-815-7605; **Board Cert:** Anesthesiology 1990; Pain Medicine 2005; **Med School:** South Korea 1973; **Resid:** Anesthesiology, Yale-New Haven Hosp 1983; **Fellow:** Pain Medicine, RWJohnson Univ Hosp 1991; **Fac Appt:** Assoc Prof Anes, UMDNJ-RW Johnson Med Sch

PEDIATRIC CARDIOLOGY

Leichter, Donald MD (PCd) - **Spec Exp:** Heart Disease-Congenital; Fetal Echocardiography; Echocardiography; **Hospital:** Overlook Hosp (page 88), NY-Presby Hosp (page 100); **Address:** 47 Maple St, Ste 206, Summit, NJ 07901; **Phone:** 908-522-5566; **Board Cert:** Pediatrics 1988; Pediatric Cardiology 2003; **Med School:** Cornell Univ-Weill Med Coll 1980; **Resid:** Pediatrics, Chldns Hosp Natl Med Ctr 1983; **Fellow:** Pediatric Cardiology, Columbia Presby Med Ctr 1985; **Fac Appt:** Assoc Clin Prof Ped, Columbia P&S

PEDIATRIC GASTROENTEROLOGY

Tyshkov, Michael MD (PGe) - **Spec Exp:** Nutrition; Crohn's Disease; Colitis; **Hospital:** Staten Island Univ Hosp-North Site, Overlook Hosp (page 88); **Address:** 33 Overlook Rd, Ste 207, Summit, NJ 07901; **Phone:** 908-273-2300; **Board Cert:** Pediatrics 1999; Pediatric Gastroenterology 1995; **Med School:** Russia 1977; **Resid:** Pediatrics, Flushing Hosp 1989; **Fellow:** Pediatric Gastroenterology, NY Med Coll 1991; **Fac Appt:** Asst Clin Prof Ped, Columbia P&S

PEDIATRICS

Ayyanathan, K MD (Ped) PCP - **Hospital:** Trinitas Hosp, JFK Med Ctr - Edison; **Address:** Linden Pediatric Group, 517 Rahway Ave, Elizabeth, NJ 07202-2308; **Phone:** 908-527-1247; **Board Cert:** Pediatrics 1983; **Med School:** India 1975; **Resid:** Pediatrics, St Elizabeth Hosp 1977; Pediatrics, Rahway Hosp 1979

Corbo, Emanuel MD (Ped) PCP - **Spec Exp:** Vaccines; Asthma; Otitis Media; Pneumonia; **Hospital:** Overlook Hosp (page 88), Trinitas Hosp; **Address:** 443 E Westfield Ave, Roselle Park, NJ 07204; **Phone:** 908-245-2442; **Board Cert:** Pediatrics 1992; **Med School:** Grenada 1985; **Resid:** Pediatrics, Newark Beth Israel Med Ctr 1990; **Fellow:** Pediatrics, Newark Beth Israel Med Ctr 1991

Davis, Kenneth J MD (Ped) PCP - **Hospital:** Overlook Hosp (page 88), Trinitas Hosp; **Address:** 701 Newark Ave, Elizabeth, NJ 07208; **Phone:** 908-354-9500; **Board Cert:** Pediatrics 1985; **Med School:** Albert Einstein Coll Med 1980; **Resid:** Pediatrics, Bellevue Hosp 1983

Mehta, Uday MD (Ped) - **Spec Exp:** Autism; ADD/ADHD; Neurodevelopmental Disabilities; **Hospital:** Children's Specialized Hosp; **Address:** 150 New Providence Rd, Mountainside, NJ 07092; **Phone:** 908-233-3720; **Board Cert:** Pediatrics 1983; Developmental-Behavioral Pediatrics 2004; **Med School:** India 1971; **Resid:** Pediatrics, Overlook Hosp 1980; **Fellow:** Child Development, Chldns Hosp 1981; **Fac Appt:** Asst Clin Prof Ped, Robert W Johnson Med Sch

Oxman, David MD (Ped) **PCP** - **Hospital:** St Barnabas Med Ctr; **Address:** 1050 Galloping Hill Rd, Ste 200, Union, NJ 07083; **Phone:** 908-688-9900; **Board Cert:** Pediatrics 1980; **Med School:** Univ Hlth Sci/Chicago Med Sch 1974; **Resid:** Pediatrics, LI Jewish Med Ctr 1977

Panza, Robert MD (Ped) - **Hospital:** Overlook Hosp (page 88); **Address:** 566 Westfield Ave, Westfield, NJ 07090; **Phone:** 908-233-7171; **Board Cert:** Pediatrics 1997; **Med School:** Italy 1985; **Resid:** Pediatrics, Overlook Hosp 1989

Panzner, Elizabeth MD (Ped) **PCP** - **Spec Exp:** Acne; Allergy; Asthma; **Hospital:** St Barnabas Med Ctr, Overlook Hosp (page 88); **Address:** 1050 Galloping Hill Rd, Ste 200, Union, NJ 07083-9417; **Phone:** 908-688-9900; **Board Cert:** Pediatrics 2004; **Med School:** Mexico 1984; **Resid:** Pediatrics, UMDNJ-Univ Hosp 1988

Saraiya, Narendra MD (Ped) **PCP** - **Spec Exp:** Asthma; Anemia; Sickle Cell Disease; **Hospital:** Trinitas Hosp; **Address:** 817 Rahway Ave, Elizabeth, NJ 07202; **Phone:** 908-353-5750; **Board Cert:** Pediatrics 1988; Pediatric Hematology-Oncology 2002; **Med School:** India 1971; **Resid:** Pediatrics, New York Methodist Hosp 1980; **Fellow:** Pediatric Hematology-Oncology, Maimonides Medical Ctr 1982; Pediatric Hematology-Oncology, Children's Hosp Buffalo 1984

Vigorita, John MD (Ped) **PCP** - **Spec Exp:** Learning Disorders; Sports Medicine; **Hospital:** Overlook Hosp (page 88); **Address:** 33 Overlook Rd, Ste 101, Summit, NJ 07901; **Phone:** 908-273-1112; **Board Cert:** Pediatrics 2002; **Med School:** Mexico 1974; **Resid:** Pediatrics, Overlook Hosp 1978

Yalamanchi, Krishan MD (Ped) - **Spec Exp:** Neurodevelopmental Disabilities; Brain Injury; **Hospital:** Children's Specialized Hosp, Newark Beth Israel Med Ctr; **Address:** 150 New Providence Rd, Mountainside, NJ 07092; **Phone:** 908-301-5461; **Board Cert:** Pediatrics 2004; Neurodevelopmental Disabilities 2004; **Med School:** India 1981

Zanger, Norman MD (Ped) **PCP** - **Hospital:** St Barnabas Med Ctr, Overlook Hosp (page 88); **Address:** 1050 Galloping Hill Rd, Pediatric Medical Group, Union, NJ 07083-9417; **Phone:** 908-688-9900; **Board Cert:** Pediatrics 1972; **Med School:** Belgium 1966; **Resid:** Pediatrics, Newark Beth Israel 1972; **Fac Appt:** Asst Clin Prof Ped, UMDNJ-Univ Med Dent NJ

PHYSICAL MEDICINE & REHABILITATION

Armento, Michael J MD (PMR) - **Spec Exp:** Cerebral Palsy; Spina Bifida; Spinal Cord Injury-Pediatric; **Hospital:** Children's Specialized Hosp; **Address:** Children's Specialized Hospital, 150 New Providence Rd, Mountainside, NJ 07092; **Phone:** 908-301-5416; **Board Cert:** Physical Medicine & Rehabilitation 2003; Spinal Cord Injury Medicine 2002; Pediatric Rehabilitation Medicine 2004; **Med School:** UMDNJ-NJ Med Sch, Newark 1988; **Resid:** Physical Medicine & Rehabilitation, UMDNJ Med Ctr 1992; **Fellow:** Pediatric Rehabilitation Medicine, Chldns Specialty Hosp 1994; **Fac Appt:** Asst Clin Prof Ped, UMDNJ-NJ Med Sch, Newark

Diamond, Martin MD (PMR) - **Spec Exp:** Cerebral Palsy; Neuromuscular Disorders; Electrodiagnosis; **Hospital:** Children's Specialized Hosp, Newark Beth Israel Med Ctr; **Address:** 150 New Providence Rd, Mountainside, NJ 07092; **Phone:** 908-301-5416; **Board Cert:** Pediatrics 1983; Physical Medicine & Rehabilitation 1982; Pediatric Rehabilitation Medicine 2003; **Med School:** Univ Pittsburgh 1975; **Resid:** Pediatrics, Chldns Hosp Natl Med Ctr 1978; Physical Medicine & Rehabilitation, Sinai Hosp 1980; **Fac Appt:** Assoc Clin Prof PMR, UMDNJ-NJ Med Sch, Newark

Novick, Ellen MD (PMR) - **Spec Exp:** Electrodiagnosis; Pain-Back & Neck; Sports Medicine; **Address:** 210 W St Georges Ave, Linden, NJ 07036; **Phone:** 908-486-1111; **Board Cert:** Physical Medicine & Rehabilitation 1986; **Med School:** Mount Sinai Sch Med 1982; **Resid:** Physical Medicine & Rehabilitation, Albert Einstein 1985; **Fac Appt:** Asst Clin Prof Med, UMDNJ-NJ Med Sch, Newark

PLASTIC SURGERY

Jeffries III, James M MD (PlS) - **Spec Exp:** Cosmetic Surgery-Face; Breast Reconstruction; **Hospital:** Muhlenberg Regional Med Ctr, JFK Med Ctr - Edison; **Address:** 1024 Park Ave, Ste 4, Plainfield, NJ 07060; **Phone:** 908-755-0009; **Board Cert:** Plastic Surgery 1997; **Med School:** UMDNJ-NJ Med Sch, Newark 1983; **Resid:** Surgery, UMDNJ Med Ctr 1991; Plastic Surgery, UMDNJ Med Ctr 1994

Tepper, Howard MD (PlS) - **Spec Exp:** Cosmetic Surgery; Breast Surgery; Hand Surgery; **Hospital:** Overlook Hosp (page 88), Union Hosp - NJ; **Address:** 522 E Broad St, Westfield, NJ 07090-2116; **Phone:** 908-654-6540; **Board Cert:** Plastic Surgery 1983; **Med School:** Albert Einstein Coll Med 1975; **Resid:** Surgery, Montefiore Hosp Med Ctr 1979; Plastic Surgery, Montefiore Hosp Med Ctr 1981; **Fellow:** Hand Surgery, St Luke's-Roosevelt Hosp Ctr 1979

Zeitels, Jerrold R MD (PlS) - **Spec Exp:** Cosmetic Surgery-Face; Liposuction & Body Contouring; **Hospital:** Overlook Hosp (page 88), Robert Wood Johnson Univ Hosp at Rahway (page 853); **Address:** 522 E Broad St Fl 2, Westfield, NJ 07090; **Phone:** 908-654-6540; **Board Cert:** Plastic Surgery 1989; Hand Surgery 1999; **Med School:** Univ Chicago-Pritzker Sch Med 1980; **Resid:** Surgery, U Michigan Med Ctr 1985; Plastic Surgery, Hosp U Penn 1987

PSYCHIATRY

Kaplan, Gabriel MD (Psyc) - **Spec Exp:** Psychopharmacology; ADD/ADHD; Depression; **Hospital:** St Mary Hosp - Hoboken; **Address:** 535 Morris Ave, Springfield, NJ 07081-1426; **Phone:** 201-659-6060; **Board Cert:** Psychiatry 1987; Child & Adolescent Psychiatry 1989; **Med School:** Argentina 1980; **Resid:** Psychiatry, NY Hosp-Cornell 1986; Child & Adolescent Psychiatry, NY Hosp-Cornell 1988; **Fac Appt:** Asst Clin Prof Psyc, UMDNJ-NJ Med Sch, Newark

Miller, David G MD (Psyc) - **Spec Exp:** Psychopharmacology; Major Depression; ADD/ADHD; Bipolar/Mood Disorders; **Hospital:** St Barnabas Med Ctr; **Address:** 28 Milburn Ave, Ste 5, Springfield, NJ 07081; **Phone:** 973-218-1770; **Board Cert:** Psychiatry 1985; **Med School:** Univ Rochester 1980; **Resid:** Psychiatry, Strong Meml Hosp-Univ Rochester 1984

Richardson, William T MD (Psyc) - **Spec Exp:** Adolescent Psychiatry; Family Therapy; Psychopharmacology; **Hospital:** Overlook Hosp (page 88), Morristown Mem Hosp (page 88); **Address:** 33 Overlook Rd, Ste 210, Summit, NJ 07901-3570; **Phone:** 908-598-0008; **Board Cert:** Psychiatry 1980; **Med School:** McGill Univ 1967; **Resid:** Psychiatry, Jewish Genl Hosp 1971; Psychiatry, Payne Whitney Psych Clinic 1974

Silver, Bennett MD (Psyc) - **Spec Exp:** Child & Adolescent Psychiatry; ADD/ADHD; Anxiety Disorders; **Hospital:** St Mary Hosp - Hoboken; **Address:** 535 Morris Ave, Springfield, NJ 07081; **Phone:** 973-376-1020; **Board Cert:** Psychiatry 1979; **Med School:** SUNY Downstate 1974; **Resid:** Psychiatry, Mount Sinai Hosp 1978; **Fellow:** Child & Adolescent Psychiatry, Mount Sinai Hosp 1980

Villafranca, Manuel MD (Psyc) - **Spec Exp:** Psychopharmacology; Depression; Anxiety Disorders; **Hospital:** Summit Oaks Hosp; **Address:** 220 Lenox Ave, Westfield, NJ 07090; **Phone:** 908-232-9369; **Board Cert:** Psychiatry 1982; **Med School:** Philippines 1971; **Resid:** Psychiatry, St Vincent's Hosp & Med Ctr 1978; **Fellow:** Child & Adolescent Psychiatry, St Vincent's Hosp & Med Ctr 1980; **Fac Appt:** Asst Clin Prof Psyc, Robert W Johnson Med Sch

PULMONARY DISEASE

Cerrone, Federico MD (Pul) - **Spec Exp:** Asthma; Sleep Disorders/Apnea; Chronic Obstructive Lung Disease (COPD); **Hospital:** Overlook Hosp (page 88), Morristown Mem Hosp (page 88); **Address:** 1 Springfield Ave, Summit, NJ 07901; **Phone:** 908-934-0555; **Board Cert:** Internal Medicine 1989; Pulmonary Disease 2002; Critical Care Medicine 2003; Sleep Medicine 1998; **Med School:** Georgetown Univ 1986; **Resid:** Internal Medicine, Bronx Municipal Hosp 1989; **Fellow:** Pulmonary Critical Care Medicine, Georgetown Univ Hosp 1992; **Fac Appt:** Asst Clin Prof Med, UMDNJ-NJ Med Sch, Newark

Sussman, Robert MD (Pul) - **Spec Exp:** Asthma; Emphysema; **Hospital:** Overlook Hosp (page 88), Morristown Mem Hosp (page 88); **Address:** 1 Springfield Ave, Summit, NJ 07901; **Phone:** 908-934-0555; **Board Cert:** Internal Medicine 1984; Pulmonary Disease 1987; Critical Care Medicine 1999; **Med School:** Albert Einstein Coll Med 1981; **Resid:** Internal Medicine, Montefiore Hosp Med Ctr 1984; **Fellow:** Pulmonary Disease, NYU/Bellevue Hosp 1987; **Fac Appt:** Asst Clin Prof Med, Columbia P&S

RADIATION ONCOLOGY

Schwartz, Louis MD (RadRO) - **Spec Exp:** Stereotactic Radiosurgery; **Hospital:** Overlook Hosp (page 88); **Address:** Overlook Hosp, Dept Rad Oncology, 33 Overlook Rd, Ste L5, Summit, NJ 07901-3561; **Phone:** 908-522-2871; **Board Cert:** Therapeutic Radiology 1979; Pediatrics 1981; **Med School:** SUNY Hlth Sci Ctr 1974; **Resid:** Pediatrics, NY Methodist Hosp 1976; Pediatrics, Chldns Hosp Med Ctr 1977; **Fellow:** Therapeutic Radiology, Columbia-Presby Hosp 1979

RHEUMATOLOGY

Brodman, Richard R MD (Rhu) - **Spec Exp:** Lupus/SLE; Arthritis; Osteoporosis; **Hospital:** Muhlenberg Regional Med Ctr; **Address:** 345 Somerset St, Ste 107, North Plainfield, NJ 07060; **Phone:** 908-561-7440; **Board Cert:** Internal Medicine 1976; Rheumatology 1982; **Med School:** SUNY Downstate 1973; **Resid:** Internal Medicine, Rhode Island Hosp 1976; **Fellow:** Rheumatology, Brigham & Women's Hosp 1978; **Fac Appt:** Assoc Clin Prof Med, UMDNJ-RW Johnson Med Sch

Worth, David MD (Rhu) - **Spec Exp:** Rheumatoid Arthritis; Osteoporosis; **Hospital:** Overlook Hosp (page 88), Union Hosp - NJ; **Address:** 2376 Morris Ave, Union, NJ 07083-5707; **Phone:** 908-686-6616; **Board Cert:** Internal Medicine 1974; Rheumatology 1978; **Med School:** Univ Rochester 1971; **Resid:** Internal Medicine, Montefiore Med Ctr 1974; **Fellow:** Rheumatology, Montefiore Med Ctr 1975; Rheumatology, Montefiore Med Ctr 1978; **Fac Appt:** Asst Clin Prof Med, UMDNJ-NJ Med Sch, Newark

SPORTS MEDICINE

Levy, Andrew S MD (SM) - **Spec Exp:** Cartilage Damage & Transplant; Ligament Reconstruction; Shoulder Surgery; **Hospital:** St Barnabas Med Ctr, Morristown Mem Hosp (page 88); **Address:** 33 Overlook Rd, Ste 409, Summit, NJ 07901-3564; **Phone:** 908-598-9199; **Board Cert:** Orthopaedic Surgery 1994; **Med School:** Temple Univ 1987; **Resid:** Orthopaedic Surgery, Albert Einstein Med Ctr 1994; **Fellow:** Sports Medicine, Duke Univ Med Ctr 1995; Shoulder Surgery, Duke Univ Med Ctr 1995; **Fac Appt:** Assoc Clin Prof OrS, UMDNJ-NJ Med Sch, Newark

SURGERY

Befeler, David MD (S) - **Spec Exp:** Breast Disease; Laparoscopic Surgery; **Hospital:** Overlook Hosp (page 88); **Address:** 555 Westfield Ave, Westfield, NJ 07090; **Phone:** 908-232-6000; **Board Cert:** Surgery 1966; **Med School:** Columbia P&S 1959; **Resid:** Surgery, St Vincent's Hosp 1964; **Fac Appt:** Assoc Clin Prof S, Columbia P&S

Colaco, Rodolfo MD (S) - **Spec Exp:** Hernia; Gallbladder Surgery; Laparoscopic Surgery; **Hospital:** Trinitas Hosp, Union Hosp - NJ; **Address:** 431 Elmora Ave, Elizabeth, NJ 07208; **Phone:** 908-353-4177; **Board Cert:** Surgery 1992; **Med School:** India 1974; **Resid:** Surgery, St Vincent Hosp 1980; Surgery, St Elizabeth Hosp 1983

Digioia, Julia MD (S) - **Hospital:** Overlook Hosp (page 88), Bayonne Med Ctr; **Address:** Medical Arts Ctr, 33 Overlook Rd, Ste 205, Summit, NJ 07901; **Phone:** 908-522-3200; **Board Cert:** Surgery 1994; **Med School:** Italy 1979; **Resid:** Surgery, Jersey City Med Ctr 1984

Frost, James H MD (S) - **Spec Exp:** Breast Cancer; Colon Cancer; Laparoscopic Surgery; **Hospital:** Union Hosp - NJ, Trinitas Hosp; **Address:** 700 N Broad St, Ste 301, Elizabeth, NJ 07208-2310; **Phone:** 908-354-3779; **Board Cert:** Surgery 1997; **Med School:** Mexico 1982; **Resid:** Surgery, Univ Illinois Med Ctr 1988

Huston, Jan A MD (S) - **Spec Exp:** Breast Surgery; **Hospital:** St Barnabas Med Ctr, Overlook Hosp (page 88); **Address:** 47 Maple St, Ste 406, Summit, NJ 07901; **Phone:** 908-918-0001; **Board Cert:** Surgery 1998; **Med School:** Mich State Univ 1982; **Resid:** Surgery, St Barnabas Hosp 1987; Vascular Surgery, Lehigh Valley Hosp 1988; **Fac Appt:** Asst Prof S, UMDNJ-RW Johnson Med Sch

Nitzberg, Richard MD (S) - **Spec Exp:** Laparoscopic Surgery; Vein Disorders; **Hospital:** Overlook Hosp (page 88); **Address:** 33 Overlook Rd, Medical Arts , Ste 103, Summit, NJ 07901; **Phone:** 908-219-3030; **Board Cert:** Surgery 1989; Vascular Surgery 1992; **Med School:** Harvard Med Sch 1983; **Resid:** Surgery, Columbia-Presby Med Ctr 1988; **Fellow:** Vascular Surgery, New England Med Ctr 1990

Starker, Paul MD (S) - **Spec Exp:** Laparoscopic Surgery; Minimally Invasive Surgery; **Hospital:** Overlook Hosp (page 88); **Address:** 33 Overlook Rd, Ste 405, Summit, NJ 07901-3564; **Phone:** 908-608-9001; **Board Cert:** Surgery 1995; **Med School:** Columbia P&S 1980; **Resid:** Surgery, Columbia-Presby Med Ctr 1986; **Fellow:** Metabolism, Columbia-Presby Med Ctr 1982; **Fac Appt:** Asst Prof S, Columbia P&S

Wegryn, Robert MD (S) - **Spec Exp:** Laparoscopic Colon Surgery; Vascular Surgery; Laparoscopic Surgery-GERD; **Hospital:** Trinitas Hosp, St Barnabas Med Ctr; **Address:** 700 N Broad St, Ste 301, Elizabeth, NJ 07208-2310; **Phone:** 908-354-3779; **Board Cert:** Surgery 1969; **Med School:** Cornell Univ-Weill Med Coll 1963; **Resid:** Surgery, Strong Meml Hosp 1968; **Fac Appt:** Asst Clin Prof S, UMDNJ-NJ Med Sch, Newark

THORACIC SURGERY

Bolanowski, Paul J P MD (TS) - **Spec Exp:** Tracheal Stenosis; Thymus Surgery; Lung Cancer; **Hospital:** UMDNJ-Univ Hosp-Newark, Trinitas Hosp; **Address:** 219 S Broad St, Fl 1, Elizabeth, NJ 07202; **Phone:** 908-352-8110; **Board Cert:** Surgery 1972; Thoracic Surgery 1974; **Med School:** UMDNJ-NJ Med Sch, Newark 1965; **Resid:** Surgery, Yale-New Haven Hosp 1968; Surgery, UMDNJ-Univ Hosp 1970; **Fellow:** Cardiothoracic Surgery, UMDNJ-Univ Hosp 1972; **Fac Appt:** Assoc Prof S, UMDNJ-NJ Med Sch, Newark

Lozner, Jerrold MD (TS) - **Spec Exp:** Lung Cancer; Breast Cancer; **Hospital:** Overlook Hosp (page 88); **Address:** 33 Overlook Rd, Ste 103 - rm 107, Summit, NJ 07901; **Phone:** 908-219-3030; **Board Cert:** Surgery 1999; Thoracic Surgery 2001; **Med School:** Univ Louisville Sch Med 1971; **Resid:** Surgery, Univ Cincinnati Med Ctr 1976; **Fellow:** Cardiothoracic Surgery, Univ Cincinnati Med Ctr 1978; **Fac Appt:** Assoc Clin Prof S, Columbia P&S

UROLOGY

Ring, Kenneth S MD (U) - **Spec Exp:** Pediatric Urology; Urologic Cancer; Kidney Stones; **Hospital:** Overlook Hosp (page 88), Union Hosp - NJ; **Address:** 275 Orchard St, Westfield, NJ 07090-3133; **Phone:** 908-654-5100; **Board Cert:** Urology 2001; **Med School:** Mount Sinai Sch Med 1985; **Resid:** Surgery, Mount Sinai Hosp 1987; Urology, Columbia-Presby Med Ctr 1991

Ritter, Joseph MD (U) - **Hospital:** Overlook Hosp (page 88); **Address:** Dept Urology, 120 Summit Ave Fl 3, Summit, NJ 07901; **Phone:** 908-277-8679; **Board Cert:** Urology 1971; **Med School:** UMDNJ-NJ Med Sch, Newark 1963; **Resid:** Urology, Albert Einstein 1968

VASCULAR SURGERY

Sales, Clifford MD (VascS) - **Spec Exp:** Varicose Veins; Aneurysm-Abdominal Aortic; Peripheral Vascular Disease; **Hospital:** Overlook Hosp (page 88), St Barnabas Med Ctr; **Address:** 1801 E 2nd St, Scotch Plains, NJ 07076-1749; **Phone:** 908-490-1699; **Board Cert:** Surgery 1992; Vascular Surgery 2002; **Med School:** Mount Sinai Sch Med 1986; **Resid:** Surgery, Montefiore Hosp Med Ctr 1991; **Fellow:** Vascular Surgery, Montefiore Hosp Med Ctr 1993; **Fac Appt:** Asst Clin Prof S, Mount Sinai Sch Med

The State of Connecticut

Fairfield

Fairfield

ADOLESCENT MEDICINE

Schneider, Marcie MD (AM) - **Spec Exp:** Eating Disorders; Obesity; Menstrual Disorders; **Hospital:** Greenwich Hosp; **Address:** 1011 High Ridge Rd, Stamford, CT 06905; **Phone:** 203-329-9666; **Board Cert:** Pediatrics 1987; Adolescent Medicine 2002; **Med School:** Albert Einstein Coll Med 1983; **Resid:** Pediatrics, Montefiore Med Ctr 1986; **Fellow:** Adolescent Medicine, N Shore Univ Hosp 1988; **Fac Appt:** Asst Clin Prof Ped, Yale Univ

ALLERGY & IMMUNOLOGY

Bell, Jonathan MD (A&I) - **Spec Exp:** Asthma; Insect Allergies; Sinusitis; **Hospital:** Danbury Hosp; **Address:** 107 Newtown Rd, Ste 1B, Danbury, CT 06810-4156; **Phone:** 203-748-7433; **Board Cert:** Pediatrics 1986; Allergy & Immunology 1987; **Med School:** Georgetown Univ 1980; **Resid:** Pediatrics, St Christopher's Hosp Chldn 1983; **Fellow:** Pediatric Allergy & Immunology, Chldns Hosp 1987; **Fac Appt:** Asst Clin Prof A&I, NY Med Coll

Lindner, Paul S MD (A&I) - **Spec Exp:** Asthma; Hay Fever; Food Allergy; **Hospital:** Stamford Hosp; **Address:** 22 Fifth St, Stamford, CT 06905-5030; **Phone:** 203-978-0072; **Board Cert:** Internal Medicine 1989; Allergy & Immunology 2001; **Med School:** SUNY Buffalo 1985; **Resid:** Internal Medicine, Stamford Hosp 1989; **Fellow:** Allergy & Immunology, Nassau Co Med Ctr 1991

Litchman, Mark MD (A&I) - **Spec Exp:** Asthma; Immune Deficiency; Lupus/SLE; **Hospital:** Greenwich Hosp, Yale - New Haven Hosp (page 984); **Address:** 21 Dearfield Drive, Greenwich, CT 06831-5335; **Phone:** 203-869-2080; **Board Cert:** Internal Medicine 1987; Allergy & Immunology 1999; Rheumatology 1988; **Med School:** Rush Med Coll 1984; **Resid:** Internal Medicine, Greenwich Hosp 1987; **Fellow:** Allergy & Immunology, Yale-New Haven Hosp 1989; Rheumatology, Yale-New Haven Hosp 1989; **Fac Appt:** Assoc Clin Prof Med, Yale Univ

Rockwell, William MD (A&I) - **Hospital:** Bridgeport Hosp, St Vincent's Med Ctr - Bridgeport; **Address:** 4675 Main St, Bridgeport, CT 06606-1834; **Phone:** 203-374-6103; **Board Cert:** Pediatrics 1979; Allergy & Immunology 1981; **Med School:** Albany Med Coll 1973; **Resid:** Pediatrics, Bridgeport Hosp 1976; **Fellow:** Allergy & Immunology, Long Island Coll Hosp 1981

Santilli, John MD (A&I) - **Spec Exp:** Allergy; Sinusitis; **Hospital:** St Vincent's Med Ctr - Bridgeport; **Address:** 4675 Main St, Bridgeport, CT 06606-1834; **Phone:** 203-374-6103; **Board Cert:** Pediatrics 1973; Allergy & Immunology 1983; **Med School:** Georgetown Univ 1968; **Resid:** Pediatrics, Georgetown Univ Hosp 1971; **Fellow:** Allergy & Immunology, Georgetown Univ Hosp 1973

CARDIOVASCULAR DISEASE

Casale, Linda MD (Cv) - **Spec Exp:** Non-Invasive Cardiology; Women's Health; Echocardiography; **Hospital:** Bridgeport Hosp; **Address:** 1305 Post Rd, Fairfield, CT 06824; **Phone:** 203-292-2000; **Board Cert:** Cardiovascular Disease 2003; **Med School:** NY Med Coll 1986; **Resid:** Internal Medicine, Montefiore Med Ctr 1989; **Fellow:** Cardiovascular Disease, UC San Diego 1992

Copen, David MD (Cv) - **Spec Exp:** Cardiac Catheterization; Coronary Artery Disease; Congestive Heart Failure; **Hospital:** Danbury Hosp; **Address:** 24 Hospital Ave, 6th fl Tower, Danbury, CT 06810-6099; **Phone:** 203-797-7155; **Board Cert:** Internal Medicine 1972; Cardiovascular Disease 1975; **Med School:** SUNY Downstate 1969; **Resid:** Internal Medicine, Yale-New Haven Hosp 1972; **Fellow:** Cardiovascular Disease, Mass Genl Hosp 1974; **Fac Appt:** Assoc Clin Prof Med, Yale Univ

Fisher, Lawrence MD (Cv) - **Spec Exp:** Cardiac Catheterization; Pacemakers; Heart Valve Disease; **Hospital:** Danbury Hosp, Bridgeport Hosp; **Address:** 25 Germantown Rd, Ste 2B, Danbury, CT 06810-6035; **Phone:** 203-794-0090; **Board Cert:** Internal Medicine 1988; Cardiovascular Disease 2001; **Med School:** SUNY Buffalo 1985; **Resid:** Internal Medicine, Bronx Muni Hosp 1988; **Fellow:** Cardiovascular Disease, Albert Einstein Coll Med 1990

Horowitz, Steven MD (Cv) - **Spec Exp:** Nuclear Cardiology; PET Imaging; Preventive Cardiology; **Hospital:** Stamford Hosp; **Address:** 30 Shelburne Rd, Stamford, CT 06904-9317; **Phone:** 203-325-7480; **Board Cert:** Internal Medicine 1975; Cardiovascular Disease 1979; **Med School:** NY Med Coll 1972; **Resid:** Internal Medicine, Beth Israel Hosp 1976; **Fellow:** Cardiovascular Disease, Mt Sinai Hosp 1978; Cardiology Research, Mt Sinai Hosp 1979

Keller, Andrew M MD (Cv) - **Spec Exp:** Echocardiography; Cardiac Imaging; **Hospital:** Danbury Hosp; **Address:** Danbury Hospital, Div Cardiology, 24 Hospital Ave Fl 6, Danbury, CT 06810-6099; **Phone:** 203-797-7219; **Board Cert:** Internal Medicine 1982; Cardiovascular Disease 1985; **Med School:** Ohio State Univ 1979; **Resid:** Internal Medicine, Duke Univ Med Ctr Hosps 1982; **Fellow:** Cardiovascular Disease, Univ Texas-SW Med Ctr 1985; **Fac Appt:** Assoc Clin Prof Med, Columbia P&S

Kosinski, Edward MD (Cv) - **Spec Exp:** Angioplasty; **Hospital:** St Vincent's Med Ctr - Bridgeport; **Address:** 4675 Main St, Bridgeport, CT 06606-4201; **Phone:** 203-683-5100; **Board Cert:** Internal Medicine 1976; Cardiovascular Disease 1979; **Med School:** Wake Forest Univ 1973; **Resid:** Internal Medicine, Columbia-Presby Med Ctr 1976; **Fellow:** Cardiovascular Disease, Peter Bent Brigham Hosp 1978; **Fac Appt:** Assoc Clin Prof Med, Columbia P&S

Krauthamer, Martin MD (Cv) - **Spec Exp:** Cholesterol/Lipid Disorders; Pacemakers; **Hospital:** Norwalk Hosp, Stamford Hosp; **Address:** 40 Cross St, Ste 202, Norwalk, CT 06851-4647; **Phone:** 203-845-2160; **Board Cert:** Internal Medicine 1970; Cardiovascular Disease 1971; **Med School:** SUNY Downstate 1962; **Resid:** Internal Medicine, Montefiore Hosp 1965; Cardiovascular Disease, Montefiore Hosp 1966; **Fellow:** Cardiovascular Disease, Montefiore Hosp 1967; **Fac Appt:** Assoc Clin Prof Med, Yale Univ

Landesman, Richard Howard MD (Cv) - **Hospital:** Stamford Hosp; **Address:** 80 Mill River St, Ste 1300, Stamford, CT 06902-3733; **Phone:** 203-348-7410; **Board Cert:** Internal Medicine 1971; Cardiovascular Disease 1973; **Med School:** Univ VT Coll Med 1966; **Resid:** Internal Medicine, St Luke's Hosp 1969; **Fellow:** Cardiovascular Disease, St Luke's Hosp 1971; **Fac Appt:** Assoc Clin Prof Med, NY Med Coll

Meizlish, Jay Lewis MD (Cv) - **Spec Exp:** Interventional Cardiology; Nuclear Cardiology; **Hospital:** Bridgeport Hosp; **Address:** 1305 Post Rd, Fairfield, CT 06824; **Phone:** 203-292-2000; **Board Cert:** Internal Medicine 1980; Cardiovascular Disease 1983; Nuclear Medicine 1984; Interventional Cardiology 2000; **Med School:** NYU Sch Med 1977; **Resid:** Internal Medicine, Harbor-UCLA Med Ctr 1980; **Fellow:** Cardiovascular Disease, Yale Univ Sch Med 1983; Nuclear Medicine, Yale Univ Sch Med

Neeson, Francis MD (Cv) - **Hospital:** Greenwich Hosp; **Address:** 75 Holly Hill Ln, Greenwich, CT 06830; **Phone:** 203-869-6960; **Board Cert:** Internal Medicine 1988; Cardiovascular Disease 2001; **Med School:** NYU Sch Med 1985; **Resid:** Internal Medicine, Bronx Muni Hosp 1988; **Fellow:** Cardiovascular Disease, Albert Einstein Coll Med 1991

Zarich, Stuart MD (Cv) - **Spec Exp:** Echocardiography; Diabetes & Heart Disease; Cholesterol/Lipid Disorders; **Hospital:** Bridgeport Hosp; **Address:** Bridgeport Hosp, Cardiology Div, 267 Grant St Fl 10, Bridgeport, CT 06610; **Phone:** 203-384-3844; **Board Cert:** Internal Medicine 1984; Cardiovascular Disease 1989; **Med School:** SUNY Upstate Med Univ 1981; **Resid:** Internal Medicine, Beth Israel Deaconess Hosp; **Fellow:** Cardiovascular Disease, Beth Israel Deaconess Hosp/Harvard; **Fac Appt:** Asst Clin Prof Med, Yale Univ

COLON & RECTAL SURGERY

Guthrie, James MD (CRS) - **Hospital:** Norwalk Hosp; **Address:** 148 East Ave, Ste 3B, Norwalk, CT 06851; **Phone:** 203-853-1705; **Board Cert:** Surgery 1972; Colon & Rectal Surgery 1972; **Med School:** NYU Sch Med 1961; **Resid:** Surgery, NYU Med Ctr 1966; **Fellow:** Colon & Rectal Surgery, St Marks Hosp 1974; **Fac Appt:** Asst Prof S, Yale Univ

Hirshorn, Steven MD (CRS) - **Spec Exp:** Colonoscopy; **Hospital:** St Vincent's Med Ctr - Bridgeport, Bridgeport Hosp; **Address:** 2660 Main St, Ste 302, Bridgeport, CT 06606-4237; **Phone:** 203-331-8700; **Board Cert:** Surgery 1991; Colon & Rectal Surgery 1993; **Med School:** Cornell Univ-Weill Med Coll 1977; **Resid:** Surgery, North Shore Univ Hosp 1982; **Fellow:** Colon & Rectal Surgery, Greater Baltimore Med Ctr 1983

Littlejohn, Charles E MD (CRS) - **Spec Exp:** Colon & Rectal Cancer; **Hospital:** Stamford Hosp, Norwalk Hosp; **Address:** 70 Mill River St, Stamford, CT 06902; **Phone:** 203-323-8989; **Board Cert:** Colon & Rectal Surgery 1985; **Med School:** Dartmouth Med Sch 1978; **Resid:** Surgery, Univ Rochester Affil Hosps 1980; Surgery, UMDNJ Med Ctr 1983; **Fellow:** Colon & Rectal Surgery, UMDNJ Med Ctr 1984; **Fac Appt:** Asst Clin Prof S, Columbia P&S

Thornton, Scott MD (CRS) - **Spec Exp:** Laparoscopic Surgery; Colon & Rectal Cancer; **Hospital:** Bridgeport Hosp; **Address:** 2660 Main St, Ste 302, Bridgeport, CT 06606-4237; **Phone:** 203-331-8700; **Board Cert:** Colon & Rectal Surgery 2003; Surgery 2005; **Med School:** Univ Pittsburgh 1986; **Resid:** Surgery, Univ Conn Sch Med 1991; Colon & Rectal Surgery, UMDNJ-NJ Med Sch 1992; **Fac Appt:** Clin Prof S, Yale Univ

DERMATOLOGY

Cohen, Ivan S MD (D) - **Spec Exp:** Hair Restoration/Transplant; **Hospital:** St Vincent's Med Ctr - Bridgeport; **Address:** Center for Hair Transplantation, 1305 Post Rd, Fairfield, CT 06824; **Phone:** 203-259-7709; **Board Cert:** Dermatology 1974; **Med School:** SUNY Downstate 1967; **Resid:** Dermatology, Yale Univ 1973; **Fac Appt:** Assoc Clin Prof D, Yale Univ

Connors, Richard MD (D) - **Spec Exp:** Skin Cancer; **Hospital:** Greenwich Hosp; **Address:** 1 Perryridge Rd, Greenwich, CT 06830-4607; **Phone:** 203-622-0808; **Board Cert:** Dermatology 1974; Dermatopathology 1976; **Med School:** Cornell Univ-Weill Med Coll 1967; **Resid:** Dermatology, New York Hosp 1974; **Fellow:** Dermatopathology, NYU Med Ctr 1975; **Fac Appt:** Assoc Clin Prof D, NYU Sch Med

Fairfield

Maiocco, Kenneth MD (D) - **Spec Exp:** Skin Cancer; Botox Therapy; Aging Skin; **Hospital:** St Vincent's Med Ctr - Bridgeport, Bridgeport Hosp; **Address:** 4639 Main St, Bridgeport, CT 06606-1873; **Phone:** 203-374-5546; **Board Cert:** Dermatology 1976; **Med School:** Univ Rochester 1967; **Resid:** Surgery, St Vincents Med Ctr 1971; Dermatology, Geisinger Med Ctr 1975

Mayer, Fern MD (D) - **Hospital:** Stamford Hosp; **Address:** 132 Morgan St, Stamford, CT 06905; **Phone:** 203-969-0123; **Board Cert:** Dermatology 1990; **Med School:** NYU Sch Med 1986; **Resid:** Dermatology, Downstate Med Ctr 1990

Pesce, Joseph MD (D) - **Hospital:** St Vincent's Med Ctr - Bridgeport, Bridgeport Hosp; **Address:** 4699 Main St, CPPC, Ste 212, Bridgeport, CT 06606-1830; **Phone:** 203-372-8949; **Board Cert:** Dermatology 1972; **Med School:** Belgium 1967; **Resid:** Internal Medicine, Hosp of St Raphael 1968; Dermatology, Dartmouth/Hitchcock Med Ctr 1971

Pruzan, Debra L MD (D) - **Hospital:** Stamford Hosp; **Address:** 1290 Summer St, Ste 3600, Stamford, CT 06905; **Phone:** 203-325-3576; **Board Cert:** Dermatology 1990; **Med School:** Univ Pennsylvania 1986; **Resid:** Dermatology, SUNY Health Sci Ctr. 1990; **Fac Appt:** Asst Prof D, Albert Einstein Coll Med

Sibrack, Laurence MD (D) - **Spec Exp:** Skin Cancer; Cosmetic Dermatology; **Hospital:** Danbury Hosp, Yale - New Haven Hosp (page 984); **Address:** 73 Sand Pit Rd, Ste 207, Danbury, CT 06810; **Phone:** 203-792-4151; **Board Cert:** Dermatology 1978; **Med School:** Univ Mich Med Sch 1974; **Resid:** Dermatology, Yale-New Haven Hosp 1978; **Fac Appt:** Asst Prof D, Yale Univ

DIAGNOSTIC RADIOLOGY

Bauman, James S MD (DR) - **Spec Exp:** Mammography; **Hospital:** Norwalk Hosp; **Address:** 148 East Ave, Norwalk, CT 06851; **Phone:** 203-838-4886; **Board Cert:** Diagnostic Radiology 1984; **Med School:** Cornell Univ-Weill Med Coll 1980; **Resid:** Radiology, NY Hosp-Cornell 1984; **Fellow:** Ultrasound, NYU Med Ctr 1985

Cohen, Steven M MD (DR) - **Spec Exp:** Ultrasound; Breast Imaging; CT Scan; MRI; **Hospital:** Bridgeport Hosp; **Address:** Bridgeport Hospital, Dept Radiology, 267 Grant St, Bridgeport, CT 06610; **Phone:** 203-384-3170; **Board Cert:** Diagnostic Radiology 1987; **Med School:** NY Med Coll 1983; **Resid:** Internal Medicine, Stamford Hosp 1984; Diagnostic Radiology, Montefiore Hosp 1987; **Fellow:** Ultrasound/CT/MRI, Thomas Jefferson Univ Hosp 1989; **Fac Appt:** Asst Prof Rad, Columbia P&S

Lee, Ronald MD (DR) - **Spec Exp:** MRI; CT Scan; **Hospital:** Norwalk Hosp; **Address:** Norwalk Radiology, 148 East Ave, Ste 1R, Norwalk, CT 06851; **Phone:** 203-851-5645; **Board Cert:** Diagnostic Radiology 1991; **Med School:** NYU Sch Med 1986; **Resid:** Diagnostic Radiology, Bellevue/NYU Med Ctr 1991; **Fellow:** Magnetic Resonance Imaging, Johns Hopkins Hosp 1992

Mullen, David MD (DR) - **Hospital:** Greenwich Hosp; **Address:** 49 Lake Ave, Greenwich, CT 06830-4502; **Phone:** 203-869-6220; **Board Cert:** Diagnostic Radiology 1987; **Med School:** Albert Einstein Coll Med 1983; **Resid:** Diagnostic Radiology, Columbia-Presby Med Ctr 1985; **Fellow:** Abdominal Imaging, Columbia-Presby Med Ctr 1986; **Fac Appt:** Asst Clin Prof Rad, Columbia P&S

Russo, Robert MD (DR) - **Spec Exp:** MRI; **Address:** 2660 Main St, Bridgeport, CT 06606; **Phone:** 203-331-4500; **Board Cert:** Diagnostic Radiology 1977; **Med School:** Tulane Univ 1973; **Resid:** Diagnostic Radiology, Yale-New Haven Hosp 1977

Strauss, Edward MD (DR) - **Spec Exp:** Nuclear Medicine; Interventional Radiology; **Hospital:** Norwalk Hosp; **Address:** Norwalk Hosp, Radiology, 24 Stevens St, Norwalk, CT 06856-3894; **Phone:** 203-852-2715; **Board Cert:** Diagnostic Radiology 1983; Nuclear Medicine 1984; Vascular & Interventional Radiology 2005; **Med School:** Yale Univ 1979; **Resid:** Radiology, Yale-New Haven Hosp 1983; **Fellow:** Nuclear Medicine, Yale-New Haven Hosp 1984

ENDOCRINOLOGY, DIABETES & METABOLISM

Goldberg-Berman, Judith C MD/PhD (EDM) - **Spec Exp:** Diabetes; Thyroid Disorders; Osteoporosis; **Hospital:** Greenwich Hosp; **Address:** 4 Dearfield Drive, Ste 102, Greenwich, CT 06831; **Phone:** 203-622-9160; **Board Cert:** Internal Medicine 2000; Endocrinology, Diabetes & Metabolism 2000; **Med School:** Cornell Univ-Weill Med Coll 1987; **Resid:** Internal Medicine, NYU Med Ctr-Bellevue Hosp 1990; **Fellow:** Endocrinology, Cornell-NY Hosp-Meml Sloan Kettering 1993

Padilla, Alfred MD (EDM) - **Spec Exp:** Diabetes; **Hospital:** Greenwich Hosp, Montefiore Med Ctr; **Address:** 4 Dearfield Dr, Ste 102, Greenwich, CT 06831-5351; **Phone:** 203-622-9160; **Board Cert:** Internal Medicine 1975; Endocrinology, Diabetes & Metabolism 1977; **Med School:** Northwestern Univ 1972; **Resid:** Internal Medicine, Univ Chicago Hosp 1975; **Fellow:** Endocrinology, Diabetes & Metabolism, Columbia Presby Hosp 1977; **Fac Appt:** Asst Clin Prof Med, Albert Einstein Coll Med

FAMILY MEDICINE

Acosta, Rod MD (FMed) PCP - **Spec Exp:** Geriatric Care; **Hospital:** Stamford Hosp; **Address:** Stamford Family Practice, 32 Strawberry Hill Ct, Stamford, CT 06905; **Phone:** 203-977-2566; **Board Cert:** Family Medicine 1987; Geriatric Medicine 1992; **Med School:** Univ Tex SW, Dallas 1984; **Resid:** Family Medicine, St Josephs Med Ctr 1987

Farrell, Matthew MD (FMed) PCP - **Spec Exp:** Sports Medicine; Sports Medicine-Aging Athlete; Adolescent Medicine; **Hospital:** Danbury Hosp; **Address:** 60 Old New Milford Rd, Ste 2A, Brookfield, CT 06804-2430; **Phone:** 203-775-6365; **Board Cert:** Geriatric Medicine 1996; Family Medicine 2001; Sports Medicine 2003; Adolescent Medicine 2002; **Med School:** Columbia P&S 1980; **Resid:** Family Medicine, Somerset Med Ctr 1983; **Fac Appt:** Asst Clin Prof FMed, Univ Conn

Filiberto, Cosmo MD (FMed) PCP - **Spec Exp:** Geriatric Care; Cholesterol/Lipid Disorders; Cardiology; Geriatrics; **Hospital:** St Vincent's Med Ctr - Bridgeport, Bridgeport Hosp; **Address:** 3715 Main St, Ste 200, Bridgeport, CT 06606-3615; **Phone:** 203-372-4065; **Board Cert:** Family Medicine 1999; Geriatric Medicine 2000; **Med School:** Italy 1976; **Resid:** Family Medicine, Lutheran Med Ctr 1980; **Fac Appt:** Asst Clin Prof FMed, Univ Conn

Mallozzi, Angelo MD (FMed) PCP - **Hospital:** Stamford Hosp; **Address:** 32 Strawberry Hill Court, Tully Health Ctr, Ste 41096, Stamford, CT 06902; **Phone:** 203-977-2566; **Board Cert:** Family Medicine 2001; **Med School:** Italy 1978; **Resid:** Family Medicine, St Josephs Hosp 1982

GASTROENTEROLOGY

Bonheim, Nelson MD (Ge) - **Spec Exp:** Inflammatory Bowel Disease; Hepatitis C; Colon Cancer; **Hospital:** Greenwich Hosp; **Address:** 500 W Putnam Ave, Ste 100, Greenwich, CT 06830; **Phone:** 203-863-2900; **Board Cert:** Internal Medicine 1973; Gastroenterology 1975; **Med School:** Univ Hlth Sci/Chicago Med Sch 1970; **Resid:** Internal Medicine, Bronx Muni Hosp 1973; **Fellow:** Gastroenterology, NY Hosp-Cornell Med Ctr 1975; **Fac Appt:** Assoc Prof Med, Yale Univ

Gardner, Peter MD (Ge) - **Spec Exp:** Liver Disease; **Hospital:** Stamford Hosp; **Address:** 166 W Broad St, Ste 303, Stamford, CT 06902; **Phone:** 203-967-2100; **Board Cert:** Internal Medicine 1982; Gastroenterology 1987; **Med School:** Georgetown Univ 1979; **Resid:** Internal Medicine, St Vincents Med Ctr 1982; **Fellow:** Gastroenterology, Univ Conn Hlth Ctr 1984; **Fac Appt:** Asst Clin Prof Med, Columbia P&S

Grossman, Edward MD (Ge) - **Spec Exp:** Inflammatory Bowel Disease; Malabsorption; **Hospital:** St Vincent's Med Ctr - Bridgeport, Bridgeport Hosp; **Address:** 425 Post Rd, Fairfield, CT 06430-6059; **Phone:** 203-292-9000; **Board Cert:** Internal Medicine 1970; Gastroenterology 1973; **Med School:** Albert Einstein Coll Med 1963; **Resid:** Internal Medicine, Bronx Muni Hosp Ctr 1968; **Fellow:** Gastroenterology, NY Hosp-Cornell Med Ctr 1970; **Fac Appt:** Assoc Clin Prof Med, Yale Univ

Gruss, Claudia MD (Ge) - **Spec Exp:** Colonoscopy; Gastroesophageal Reflux Disease (GERD); Inflammatory Bowel Disease; **Hospital:** Norwalk Hosp; **Address:** 73 Redding Rd, Box 270, Georgetown, CT 06829; **Phone:** 203-544-9517; **Board Cert:** Internal Medicine 1980; Gastroenterology 1983; **Med School:** Brown Univ 1977; **Resid:** Internal Medicine, Rhode Island Hosp 1980; **Fellow:** Gastroenterology, Rhode Island Hosp 1982

Mauer, Kenneth MD (Ge) - **Spec Exp:** Endoscopy; Inflammatory Bowel Disease/Crohn's; Capsule Endoscopy; **Hospital:** St Vincent's Med Ctr - Bridgeport, Bridgeport Hosp; **Address:** 425 Post Rd, Fairfield, CT 06824; **Phone:** 203-292-9000; **Board Cert:** Internal Medicine 1986; Gastroenterology 1989; **Med School:** NYU Sch Med 1983; **Resid:** Internal Medicine, Bronx Muni Hosp Ctr 1987; **Fellow:** Gastroenterology, Mount Sinai Hosp 1989

Sheinbaum, Richard MD (Ge) - **Hospital:** Stamford Hosp; **Address:** 32 Strawberry Hill Ct Fl 4 - Ste 1, Stamford, CT 06902; **Phone:** 203-348-5355; **Board Cert:** Internal Medicine 1983; Gastroenterology 1987; **Med School:** Temple Univ 1979; **Resid:** Surgery, Mt. Sinai Medical Hospital 1981; Internal Medicine, Stamford Hospital 1983; **Fellow:** Gastroenterology, Cedars-Sinai Medical Ctr 1985; **Fac Appt:** Asst Clin Prof Med, NY Med Coll

Taubin, Howard L MD (Ge) - **Spec Exp:** Colon Cancer Screening; Gastroesophagael Reflux Disease (GERD); Inflammatory Bowel Disease; **Hospital:** Bridgeport Hosp; **Address:** 2890 Main St, Stratford, CT 06614; **Phone:** 203-375-1200; **Board Cert:** Internal Medicine 1972; Gastroenterology 1973; **Med School:** Univ VA Sch Med 1965; **Resid:** Internal Medicine, Montefiore Hosp 1967; Internal Medicine, Yale-New Haven Hosp 1970; **Fellow:** Gastroenterology, Yale-New Haven Hosp 1973; **Fac Appt:** Assoc Clin Prof Med, Yale Univ

Waldstreicher, Stuart MD (Ge) - **Spec Exp:** Celiac Disease; Inflammatory Bowel Disease/Crohn's; **Hospital:** Stamford Hosp; **Address:** 166 W Broad St, Ste 303, Stamford, CT 06902-3661; **Phone:** 203-967-2100; **Board Cert:** Internal Medicine 1985; Gastroenterology 1987; **Med School:** NY Med Coll 1982; **Resid:** Internal Medicine, Overlook Hosp 1985; **Fellow:** Gastroenterology, Westchester Co Med Ctr 1987; **Fac Appt:** Asst Clin Prof Med, Columbia P&S

GERIATRIC MEDICINE

Spivack, Barney MD (Ger) - **Spec Exp:** Musculoskeletal Disorders; Dementia; Memory Disorders; **Hospital:** Stamford Hosp; **Address:** 3 Farm Rd, New Canaan, CT 06840; **Phone:** 203-594-5311; **Board Cert:** Internal Medicine 1981; Rheumatology 1984; Geriatric Medicine 1999; **Med School:** Mount Sinai Sch Med 1978; **Resid:** Internal Medicine, Bellevue Hosp 1981; **Fellow:** Rheumatology, Rhode Island Hosp 1983; **Fac Appt:** Assoc Prof Med, Columbia P&S

HAND SURGERY

Brown, Lionel MD (HS) - **Spec Exp:** Hand Reconstruction; Carpal Tunnel Syndrome; **Hospital:** Danbury Hosp; **Address:** 35 Tamarack Ave, Danbury, CT 06811; **Phone:** 203-792-4263; **Board Cert:** Surgery 1990; Hand Surgery 1989; **Med School:** UCSF 1968; **Resid:** Surgery, UCSF Med Ctr 1975; **Fellow:** Hand Surgery, UCSF Med Ctr

Rago, Thomas MD (HS) - **Hospital:** Bridgeport Hosp, St Vincent's Med Ctr - Bridgeport; **Address:** 3101 Main St, Bridgeport, CT 06606; **Phone:** 203-374-5892; **Board Cert:** Orthopaedic Surgery 1997; Hand Surgery 1997; **Med School:** Columbia P&S 1977; **Resid:** Surgery, Roosevelt Hosp 1979; Orthopaedic Surgery, Presby Hosp 1982; **Fellow:** Hand Surgery, Columbia-Presby Med Ctr 1983

HEMATOLOGY

Bar, Michael MD (Hem) - **Spec Exp:** Bone Marrow Transplant; Bleeding/Coagulation Disorders; Lymphoma; Multiple Myeloma; **Hospital:** Stamford Hosp; **Address:** 34 Shelburne Rd, Bennett Cancer Ctr, Stamford, CT 06902-3658; **Phone:** 203-325-2695; **Board Cert:** Internal Medicine 1986; Hematology 2000; Medical Oncology 1989; **Med School:** Columbia P&S 1983; **Resid:** Internal Medicine, Columbia-Presby Med Ctr 1986; **Fellow:** Hematology & Oncology, UCSF Med Ctr 1990; **Fac Appt:** Asst Clin Prof Med, Columbia P&S

INFECTIOUS DISEASE

McLeod, Gavin MD (Inf) - **Spec Exp:** AIDS/HIV; Travel Medicine; Hospital Acquired Infections; **Hospital:** Stamford Hosp; **Address:** 166 W Broad St, Ste 202, Stamford, CT 06902; **Phone:** 203-353-1427; **Board Cert:** Internal Medicine 1988; Infectious Disease 2002; **Med School:** Univ Conn 1985; **Resid:** Internal Medicine, North Shore Univ Hosp 1988; **Fellow:** Infectious Disease, New England Deaconess 1992; **Fac Appt:** Asst Clin Prof Med, Columbia P&S

Parry, Michael MD (Inf) - **Spec Exp:** AIDS/HIV; Antibiotic Resistance; Lyme Disease; Pneumonia; **Hospital:** Stamford Hosp; **Address:** 166 W Broad St, Ste 202, Stamford, CT 06902; **Phone:** 203-353-1427; **Board Cert:** Internal Medicine 1974; Infectious Disease 1978; **Med School:** Columbia P&S 1970; **Resid:** Internal Medicine, Columbia-Presby Med Ctr 1974; Internal Medicine, UCSF Med Ctr 1973; **Fellow:** Infectious Disease, Columbia-Presby Med Ctr 1976; **Fac Appt:** Clin Prof Med, Columbia P&S

Sabetta, James MD (Inf) - **Spec Exp:** Travel Medicine; Tropical Diseases; **Hospital:** Greenwich Hosp; **Address:** 5 Perryridge Rd, Ste 108, Greenwich, CT 06830; **Phone:** 203-869-8838; **Board Cert:** Internal Medicine 1981; Infectious Disease 1984; **Med School:** Brown Univ 1978; **Resid:** Internal Medicine, Rhode Island Hosp 1981; **Fellow:** Infectious Disease, Yale-New Haven Hosp 1984; **Fac Appt:** Assoc Clin Prof Med, Yale Univ

Saul, Zane MD (Inf) - **Spec Exp:** Lyme Disease; AIDS/HIV; **Hospital:** Bridgeport Hosp; **Address:** 2890 Main St, Ste D, Stratford, CT 06614; **Phone:** 203-259-8087; **Board Cert:** Internal Medicine 2000; Infectious Disease 2000; **Med School:** Grenada 1985; **Resid:** Internal Medicine, Brooklyn Hosp 1988; **Fellow:** Infectious Disease, Hackensack Univ Med Ctr 1990

Yee, Arthur MD (Inf) - **Spec Exp:** Lyme Disease; Infections-Respiratory; **Hospital:** Norwalk Hosp; **Address:** 40 Cross St, Norwalk, CT 06851; **Phone:** 203-845-4838; **Board Cert:** Internal Medicine 1986; Infectious Disease 1988; **Med School:** Univ Conn 1982; **Resid:** Internal Medicine, Columbia-Presby Med Ctr 1985; **Fellow:** Infectious Disease, Hosp Univ Penn 1988; **Fac Appt:** Asst Clin Prof Med, Yale Univ

INTERNAL MEDICINE

Altbaum, Robert MD (IM) **PCP** - **Spec Exp:** Hypertension; Asthma; Osteoporosis; **Hospital:** Norwalk Hosp; **Address:** 162 Kings Hwy N, Westport, CT 06880-2425; **Phone:** 203-226-0731; **Board Cert:** Internal Medicine 1978; **Med School:** Harvard Med Sch 1975; **Resid:** Internal Medicine, Mass Genl Hosp 1977; Internal Medicine, Yale-New Haven Hosp 1979

Andrews Jr, Joseph MD (IM) **PCP** - **Hospital:** Norwalk Hosp; **Address:** 83 East Ave, Ste 212, Norwalk, CT 06851; **Phone:** 203-853-2707; **Board Cert:** Internal Medicine 1974; **Med School:** Yale Univ 1968; **Resid:** Internal Medicine, St Francis Hosp 1973; **Fellow:** Infectious Disease, St Francis Hosp 1974; **Fac Appt:** Asst Clin Prof Med, Yale Univ

Bivona, James J MD (IM) **PCP** - **Hospital:** Stamford Hosp; **Address:** Stamford Primary Care, 1275 Summer St, Stamford, CT 06905; **Phone:** 203-325-2667; **Board Cert:** Internal Medicine 2000; **Med School:** Dominica 1997; **Resid:** Internal Medicine, Stamford Hosp 2000

Blumberg, Joel M MD (IM) **PCP** - **Spec Exp:** Preventive Cardiology; Hypertension; Echocardiography; **Hospital:** Greenwich Hosp; **Address:** 2 1/2 Dearfield Dr, Greenwich, CT 06831-5329; **Phone:** 203-661-4242; **Board Cert:** Internal Medicine 1972; Cardiovascular Disease 1974; **Med School:** NYU Sch Med 1966; **Resid:** Internal Medicine, Bellevue Hosp 1971; **Fellow:** Cardiovascular Disease, New York Hosp 1973; **Fac Appt:** Asst Clin Prof Med, Yale Univ

Costanzo, Joseph MD (IM) **PCP** - **Hospital:** Stamford Hosp; **Address:** 80 Mill River St, Ste 2400, Stamford, CT 06902; **Phone:** 203-348-9455; **Board Cert:** Internal Medicine 2000; **Med School:** Harvard Med Sch 1987; **Resid:** Internal Medicine, Bronx Muni Hosp 1990

Do Rosario, Arnold MD (IM) **PCP** - **Spec Exp:** Preventive Medicine; Geriatric Care; **Hospital:** St Vincent's Med Ctr - Bridgeport; **Address:** 4699 Main St, Ste 105, Bridgeport, CT 06606; **Phone:** 203-374-6162; **Board Cert:** Internal Medicine 1978; Geriatric Medicine 1988; **Med School:** Spain 1975; **Resid:** Internal Medicine, St Vincent's Med Ctr 1978

Dreyer, Neil P MD (IM) **PCP** - **Spec Exp:** Hypertension; Kidney Disease; Preventive Medicine; **Hospital:** Stamford Hosp; **Address:** 51 Schuyler Ave, Stamford, CT 06902; **Phone:** 203-327-1187; **Board Cert:** Internal Medicine 1980; Nephrology 1974; **Med School:** NYU Sch Med 1967; **Resid:** Internal Medicine, Bronx Municipal Hosp Ctr 1972; **Fellow:** Nephrology, Albert Einstein Med Ctr 1973; **Fac Appt:** Asst Clin Prof Med, Columbia P&S

Finnerty, James MD (IM) `PCP` - **Hospital:** Danbury Hosp; **Address:** 2 Elizabeth St, Ste 111, Bethel, CT 06801-2100; **Phone:** 203-791-2221; **Board Cert:** Internal Medicine 1983; **Med School:** Georgetown Univ 1979; **Resid:** Internal Medicine, Naval Hosp 1983

Herbin, Joseph MD (IM) `PCP` - **Spec Exp:** Lyme Disease; Infectious Disease in Elderly; **Hospital:** St Vincent's Med Ctr - Bridgeport; **Address:** 2150 Black Rock Tpke, Ste 201, Fairfield, CT 06825; **Phone:** 203-384-0451; **Board Cert:** Internal Medicine 1972; **Med School:** Switzerland 1965; **Resid:** Internal Medicine, St Vincent's Hosp & Med Ctr 1970; **Fellow:** Infectious Disease, Med Ctr Hosp 1971; **Fac Appt:** Asst Clin Prof Med, Columbia P&S

Hoffman, Pamela MD (IM) `PCP` - **Spec Exp:** Geriatrics; **Hospital:** St Vincent's Med Ctr - Bridgeport; **Address:** 2800 Main St, Bridgeport, CT 06606-4201; **Phone:** 203-576-5710; **Board Cert:** Internal Medicine 1983; Geriatric Medicine 1998; **Med School:** Univ VA Sch Med 1978; **Resid:** Internal Medicine, St Vincent's Hosp & Med Ctr 1981; **Fellow:** Geriatric Medicine, Jewish Inst Geriatric Care 1983

Klein, Neil MD (IM) - **Spec Exp:** Inflammatory Bowel Disease/Crohn's; Ulcerative Colitis; **Hospital:** Stamford Hosp; **Address:** 1450 Washington Blvd, Stamford, CT 06902-2451; **Phone:** 203-327-9321; **Board Cert:** Internal Medicine 1974; Gastroenterology 1975; **Med School:** Cornell Univ-Weill Med Coll 1960; **Resid:** Internal Medicine, NY Hosp; Internal Medicine, NY Hosp 1965; **Fellow:** Gastroenterology, NY Hosp 1967; **Fac Appt:** Clin Prof Med, Columbia P&S

Mickley, Diane W MD (IM) - **Spec Exp:** Eating Disorders; **Hospital:** Greenwich Hosp; **Address:** 7 Riversville Rd Fl 3, Greenwich, CT 06831; **Phone:** 203-531-1909; **Board Cert:** Internal Medicine 1974; **Med School:** Tufts Univ 1971; **Resid:** Internal Medicine, Barnes Jewish Hosp 1973; Internal Medicine, Montefiore Med Ctr 1974; **Fac Appt:** Assoc Clin Prof Med, Yale Univ

Mickley, Steven P MD (IM) `PCP` - **Hospital:** Greenwich Hosp; **Address:** 7 Riversville Rd, FL 1, Glenville Medical Assoc, Greenwich, CT 06831-3697; **Phone:** 203-531-1808; **Board Cert:** Internal Medicine 1974; **Med School:** Harvard Med Sch 1971; **Resid:** Internal Medicine, Barnes Hospital 1973; Internal Medicine, USPHS 1974; **Fac Appt:** Asst Clin Prof Med, Yale Univ

Molloy, Edward Michael MD (IM) `PCP` - **Spec Exp:** Hypertension; Diabetes; Preventive Medicine; **Hospital:** St Vincent's Med Ctr - Bridgeport; **Address:** 134 Round Hill Rd, Fl 2, Fairfield, CT 06824; **Phone:** 203-255-0695; **Board Cert:** Internal Medicine 1974; **Med School:** UMDNJ-NJ Med Sch, Newark 1966; **Resid:** Internal Medicine, St Vincent's Hosp & Med Ctr 1972

Olin, Craig H MD (IM) `PCP` - **Hospital:** Stamford Hosp; **Address:** 51 Schuyler Ave, Stamford, CT 06902-3730; **Phone:** 203-327-1187; **Board Cert:** Internal Medicine 1996; **Med School:** NYU Sch Med 1993; **Resid:** Internal Medicine, New York Hosp-Cornell 1996

Osnoss, Kenneth MD (IM) `PCP` - **Spec Exp:** Asthma; Lung Disease; **Hospital:** Danbury Hosp; **Address:** 24 Hospital Ave, Medical Associates, Danbury, CT 06810-6099; **Phone:** 203-797-7173; **Board Cert:** Internal Medicine 1978; Pulmonary Disease 1980; **Med School:** Tufts Univ 1975; **Resid:** Internal Medicine, Hosp Univ Penn 1978; **Fellow:** Pulmonary Disease, Hosp Univ Penn 1980

Rosa, Joseph MD (IM) `PCP` - **Spec Exp:** Endocrinology; **Hospital:** St Vincent's Med Ctr - Bridgeport; **Address:** 4699 Main St, Ste 105, Bridgeport, CT 06606; **Phone:** 203-374-6162; **Board Cert:** Internal Medicine 1987; Endocrinology 1989; **Med School:** Mexico 1982; **Resid:** Internal Medicine, St Vincents Med Ctr 1986; **Fellow:** Endocrinology, Diabetes & Metabolism, Univ Conn Med Ctr 1988; **Fac Appt:** Assoc Prof Med, Columbia P&S

Sennett, Margaret A MD (IM) `PCP` - **Spec Exp:** Women's Health; Geriatrics; **Hospital:** Greenwich Hosp; **Address:** 75 Holly Hill Ln, Greenwich, CT 06830; **Phone:** 203-869-6960; **Board Cert:** Internal Medicine 1979; Geriatric Medicine 1994; **Med School:** SUNY Upstate Med Univ 1976; **Resid:** Internal Medicine, Greenwich Hosp 1979

Skluth, Myra MD (IM) `PCP` - **Spec Exp:** Women's Health; Diabetes; Cardiovascular Disease; **Hospital:** Norwalk Hosp; **Address:** 87 East Ave, Norwalk, CT 06851-4908; **Phone:** 203-866-4455; **Board Cert:** Internal Medicine 1989; Geriatric Medicine 1994; **Med School:** Albert Einstein Coll Med 1986; **Resid:** Internal Medicine, Montefiore Hosp Med Ctr 1989; **Fac Appt:** Asst Clin Prof Med, Yale Univ

Slogoff, Frederick B MD (IM) `PCP` - **Hospital:** Stamford Hosp; **Address:** 51 Schuyler Ave, Stamford, CT 06902; **Phone:** 203-327-1187; **Board Cert:** Internal Medicine 1999; **Med School:** Mount Sinai Sch Med 1996; **Resid:** Internal Medicine, New York Hosp 1999

Tepper, Deborah E MD (IM) `PCP` - **Spec Exp:** Women's Health; Headache; **Hospital:** Stamford Hosp; **Address:** Medical Assocs of Stamford, 1100 Bedford St, Stamford, CT 06905; **Phone:** 203-323-4458; **Board Cert:** Internal Medicine 1998; **Med School:** Univ Wash 1995; **Resid:** Internal Medicine, Univ Washington Med Ctr 1998

Thomas, Bryon S MD (IM) `PCP` - **Spec Exp:** Rehabilitation-Geriatric; **Hospital:** Danbury Hosp; **Address:** 24 Hospital Ave, Danbury, CT 06810; **Phone:** 203-797-7173; **Board Cert:** Internal Medicine 1978; Geriatric Medicine 2002; **Med School:** Univ Pittsburgh 1975; **Resid:** Internal Medicine, Mt Sinai Hosp 1978; **Fac Appt:** Asst Clin Prof Med, Yale Univ

Turetsky, Arthur MD (IM) - **Hospital:** Bridgeport Hosp; **Address:** 15 Corporate Dr, Trumbull, CT 06611; **Phone:** 203-261-3980; **Board Cert:** Internal Medicine 1977; Pulmonary Disease 1980; **Med School:** Albert Einstein Coll Med 1974; **Resid:** Internal Medicine, Einstein Bronx Muncipal Hosp Ctr 1977; Pulmonary Disease, Bronx Municipal Hosp 1979; **Fac Appt:** Asst Clin Prof Med, Albert Einstein Coll Med

Walsh, Francis X MD (IM) `PCP` - **Spec Exp:** Kidney Disease; Hypertension; Dialysis Care; **Hospital:** Greenwich Hosp, Stamford Hosp; **Address:** 31 River Rd, Ste 200, Cos Cob, CT 06830-5694; **Phone:** 203-661-9433; **Board Cert:** Internal Medicine 1972; Nephrology 1974; **Med School:** NY Med Coll 1967; **Resid:** Internal Medicine, Greenwich Hosp 1970; **Fellow:** Nephrology, Duke Univ Med Ctr 1972; **Fac Appt:** Asst Clin Prof Med, Yale Univ

Weiner, Jay MD (IM) `PCP` - **Hospital:** Danbury Hosp; **Address:** Danbury Internal Med Assoc, 7 Germantown Rd, Danbury, CT 06810-6035; **Phone:** 203-744-4511; **Board Cert:** Internal Medicine 1967; Geriatric Medicine 1994; **Med School:** Univ Pennsylvania 1959; **Resid:** Internal Medicine, Montefiore Hosp 1962; Hematology, Montefiore Hosp 1963; **Fac Appt:** Asst Clin Prof Med, Yale Univ

Zucker, Michael MD (IM) **PCP** - **Hospital:** Stamford Hosp; **Address:** 555 Newfield Ave, Stamford, CT 06905-3330; **Phone:** 203-359-4444; **Board Cert:** Internal Medicine 1988; **Med School:** NYU Sch Med 1985; **Resid:** Internal Medicine, Stamford Hospital 1988

INTERVENTIONAL CARDIOLOGY

Driesman, Mitchell MD (IC) - **Spec Exp:** Cardiac Catheterization; **Hospital:** Bridgeport Hosp; **Address:** 1305 Post Rd, Fairfield, CT 06430-6016; **Phone:** 203-292-2000; **Board Cert:** Internal Medicine 1980; Cardiovascular Disease 1983; Interventional Cardiology 1999; **Med School:** Brown Univ 1977; **Resid:** Internal Medicine, Tufts-New Eng Med Ctr 1980; **Fellow:** Cardiovascular Disease, Mt Sinai Hosp 1982; **Fac Appt:** Asst Clin Prof Med, Yale Univ

Wasserman, Hal S MD (IC) - **Spec Exp:** Mitral Valve Prolapse; **Hospital:** Danbury Hosp; **Address:** 24 Hospital Ave, 7 Tower, Danbury, CT 06810; **Phone:** 203-739-7600; **Board Cert:** Internal Medicine 1985; Cardiovascular Disease 1987; Interventional Cardiology 1999; **Med School:** Columbia P&S 1982; **Resid:** Internal Medicine, Columbia-Presby Med Ctr 1985; **Fellow:** Cardiovascular Disease, Columbia-Presby Med Ctr 1988

MATERNAL & FETAL MEDICINE

Bond, Annette L MD (MF) - **Spec Exp:** Pregnancy-High Risk; Multiple Gestation; Prenatal Diagnosis; Hypertension in Pregnancy; **Hospital:** Greenwich Hosp; **Address:** Greenwich Hosp, 5 Perryridge Rd, rm 1-251, Greenwich, CT 06830; **Phone:** 203-863-3674; **Board Cert:** Obstetrics & Gynecology 2002; Maternal & Fetal Medicine 2002; **Med School:** Harvard Med Sch 1984; **Resid:** Obstetrics & Gynecology, NY Hosp-Cornell Med Ctr 1987; **Fellow:** Perinatal Medicine, NY Hosp-Cornell Med Ctr 1990

Laifer, Steven A MD (MF) - **Spec Exp:** Prenatal Diagnosis; Obesity in Pregnancy; **Hospital:** Bridgeport Hosp, St Vincent's Med Ctr - Bridgeport; **Address:** 267 Grant St Fl 5, Bridgeport, CT 06610-2805; **Phone:** 203-384-3544; **Board Cert:** Obstetrics & Gynecology 2002; Maternal & Fetal Medicine 2002; **Med School:** SUNY Downstate 1982; **Resid:** Obstetrics & Gynecology, Johns Hopkins Hosp 1987; **Fellow:** Maternal & Fetal Medicine, Magee Womens Hosp 1989; **Fac Appt:** Asst Clin Prof ObG, Yale Univ

Stiller, Robert J MD (MF) - **Hospital:** Bridgeport Hosp; **Address:** Bridgeport Hospital, Ante Natal Testing, 267 Grant St, Bridgeport, CT 06610; **Phone:** 203-384-3544; **Board Cert:** Obstetrics & Gynecology 1996; Maternal & Fetal Medicine 1996; **Med School:** UMDNJ-RW Johnson Med Sch 1979; **Resid:** Obstetrics & Gynecology, Univ Conn Med Ctr 1983; **Fellow:** Maternal & Fetal Medicine, Hosp U Penn 1985; **Fac Appt:** Assoc Clin Prof ObG, Yale Univ

MEDICAL ONCOLOGY

Boyd, D Barry MD (Onc) - **Spec Exp:** Complementary Medicine; Acupuncture; Breast Cancer; **Hospital:** Greenwich Hosp; **Address:** 15 Valley Drive, Greenwich, CT 06831; **Phone:** 203-869-2111; **Board Cert:** Internal Medicine 1982; Medical Oncology 1987; **Med School:** Cornell Univ-Weill Med Coll 1979; **Resid:** Internal Medicine, NY Hosp-Cornell Med Ctr 1982; **Fellow:** Hematology & Oncology, NY Hosp-Cornell Med Ctr 1986; **Fac Appt:** Asst Clin Prof Med, Yale Univ

Fairfield

Burd, Robert MD (Onc) - **Spec Exp:** Non-Hodgkin's Lymphoma; Breast Cancer; Bleeding/Coagulation Disorders; **Hospital:** St Vincent's Med Ctr - Bridgeport, Bridgeport Hosp; **Address:** 425 Post Rd, Fairfield, CT 06430-6232; **Phone:** 203-255-4545; **Board Cert:** Internal Medicine 1980; Medical Oncology 1975; Hematology 1972; **Med School:** Columbia P&S 1963; **Resid:** Internal Medicine, Bronx Municipal Hosp 1966; **Fellow:** Hematology, Montefiore Hosp Med Ctr 1967; **Fac Appt:** Assoc Clin Prof Med, Yale Univ

Cooper, Robert MD (Onc) - **Spec Exp:** Breast Cancer; Lymphoma; Colon & Rectal Cancer; **Hospital:** Danbury Hosp; **Address:** Praxair Cancer Center, 24 Hospital Ave, Danbury, CT 06810; **Phone:** 203-792-5303; **Board Cert:** Internal Medicine 1974; Medical Oncology 1981; **Med School:** Univ Pittsburgh 1971; **Resid:** Internal Medicine, Pennsylvania Hosp 1974; **Fellow:** Hematology & Oncology, Unic Colorado Med Ctr 1978; **Fac Appt:** Asst Clin Prof Med, Yale Univ

Folman, Robert S MD (Onc) - **Spec Exp:** Breast Cancer; Lung Cancer; Colon & Rectal Cancer; **Hospital:** Bridgeport Hosp, St Vincent's Med Ctr - Bridgeport; **Address:** 15 Corporate Dr, Ste 210, Trumbull, CT 06611-1351; **Phone:** 203-459-0262; **Board Cert:** Medical Oncology 1977; Internal Medicine 1975; **Med School:** SUNY Buffalo 1972; **Resid:** Internal Medicine, Buffalo Gen Hosp 1975; Internal Medicine, Meml Sloan Kettering Cancer Ctr 1976; **Fellow:** Medical Oncology, Meml Sloan Kettering Cancer Ctr 1977; **Fac Appt:** Asst Prof Med, Yale Univ

Hollister Jr, Dickerman MD (Onc) - **Spec Exp:** Breast Cancer; Lung Cancer; Colon Cancer; Leukemia & Lymphoma; **Hospital:** Greenwich Hosp; **Address:** 77 Lafayette Pl, Greenwich, CT 06830; **Phone:** 203-863-3737; **Board Cert:** Internal Medicine 1978; Hematology 1980; Medical Oncology 1981; **Med School:** Univ VA Sch Med 1975; **Resid:** Internal Medicine, New York Hosp-Cornell Med Ctr 1978; **Fellow:** Hematology & Oncology, New York Hosp-Cornell Med Ctr 1981; **Fac Appt:** Asst Clin Prof Med, Yale Univ

Kloss, Robert MD (Onc) - **Spec Exp:** Breast Cancer; Colon Cancer; Lung Cancer; **Hospital:** Danbury Hosp; **Address:** 95 Locust Ave Fl 1, Danbury, CT 06810-6010; **Phone:** 203-797-7029; **Board Cert:** Internal Medicine 1979; Medical Oncology 1981; **Med School:** Jefferson Med Coll 1976; **Resid:** Internal Medicine, Univ Hosp 1979; **Fellow:** Hematology & Oncology, Columbia-Presby Med Ctr 1981

Lo, K M Steve MD (Onc) - **Spec Exp:** Breast Cancer; Lymphoma; Multiple Myeloma; **Hospital:** Stamford Hosp; **Address:** 34 Shelburne Rd, Stamford, CT 06902-3658; **Phone:** 203-325-2695; **Board Cert:** Internal Medicine 1989; Medical Oncology 1991; Hematology 1992; **Med School:** Harvard Med Sch 1985; **Resid:** Internal Medicine, Brigham & Women's Hosp 1988; **Fellow:** Hematology & Oncology, Dana Farber Cancer Inst 1991; Hematology, Dana Farber Cancer Inst 1992; **Fac Appt:** Asst Clin Prof Med, Columbia P&S

Weinstein, Paul MD (Onc) - **Spec Exp:** Breast Cancer; Lung Cancer; Colon Cancer; **Hospital:** Stamford Hosp; **Address:** 34 Shelburne Rd, Bennett Cancer Ctr, Hematology-Oncology, Stamford, CT 06902-3658; **Phone:** 203-325-2695; **Board Cert:** Internal Medicine 1973; Medical Oncology 1977; Hematology 1978; **Med School:** Univ Hlth Sci/Chicago Med Sch 1970; **Resid:** Internal Medicine, Montefiore Med Ctr 1973; **Fellow:** Hematology & Oncology, Montefiore Med Ctr 1975; **Fac Appt:** Assoc Clin Prof Med, Columbia P&S

Zelkowitz, Richard S MD (Onc) - **Spec Exp:** Breast Cancer; Hematology; **Hospital:** Norwalk Hosp; **Address:** 40 Cross St, Norwalk, CT 06851; **Phone:** 203-845-4890; **Board Cert:** Internal Medicine 1986; Hematology 1988; Medical Oncology 1989; **Med School:** NY Med Coll 1983; **Resid:** Internal Medicine, Westchester Co Med Ctr 1986; **Fellow:** Hematology & Oncology, Brown Univ Hosps 1989

Neonatal-Perinatal Medicine

Herzlinger, Robert A MD (NP) - **Spec Exp:** Neonatology; **Hospital:** Bridgeport Hosp, Yale - New Haven Hosp (page 984); **Address:** Bridgeport Hosp, 267 Grant St, Bridgeport, CT 06610-2870; **Phone:** 203-384-3486; **Board Cert:** Pediatrics 1973; Neonatal-Perinatal Medicine 1977; **Med School:** NY Med Coll 1969; **Resid:** Pediatrics, NY Med Coll 1971; Pediatrics, Columbia-Presby Med Ctr 1972; **Fellow:** Neonatal-Perinatal Medicine, Columbia-Presby Med Ctr 1973; Neonatal-Perinatal Medicine, Albert Einstein Coll Med 1976

Theofanidis, Stylianos MD (NP) - **Hospital:** Greenwich Hosp, Yale - New Haven Hosp (page 984); **Address:** 5 Perryridge Rd, Greenwich, CT 06830-4608; **Phone:** 203-863-3515; **Board Cert:** Pediatrics 1989; Neonatal-Perinatal Medicine 1997; **Med School:** Greece 1980; **Resid:** Pediatrics, St Lukes Hosp 1985; **Fellow:** Neonatal-Perinatal Medicine, New York Hosp-Cornell 1987; **Fac Appt:** Asst Clin Prof Ped, Yale Univ

Nephrology

Brown, Eric MD (Nep) - **Spec Exp:** Kidney Disease; Hypertension; Glomerulonephritis; **Hospital:** Stamford Hosp, Greenwich Hosp; **Address:** 30 Commerce Rd, Stamford, CT 06902-4550; **Phone:** 203-324-7666; **Board Cert:** Internal Medicine 1988; Nephrology 2001; **Med School:** Emory Univ 1985; **Resid:** Internal Medicine, Johns Hopkins Hosp 1988; **Fellow:** Nephrology, Yale-New Haven Hosp 1990; **Fac Appt:** Asst Clin Prof Med, Yale Univ

Chan, Brenda MD (Nep) - **Spec Exp:** Dialysis Care; Kidney Failure-Chronic; Lupus Nephritis; Glomerulonephritis; **Hospital:** Stamford Hosp; **Address:** Stamford Nephrology, 30 Commerce Rd, Stamford, CT 06902; **Phone:** 203-324-7666; **Board Cert:** Internal Medicine 1994; Nephrology 1996; **Med School:** Mount Sinai Sch Med 1990; **Resid:** Internal Medicine, Montefiore Med Ctr 1993; **Fellow:** Nephrology, Albert Einstein 1996

Feintzeig, Irwin MD (Nep) - **Spec Exp:** Kidney Disease; Hypertension; Dialysis Care; **Hospital:** Bridgeport Hosp, St Vincent's Med Ctr - Bridgeport; **Address:** 900 Madison Ave, Ste 209, Bridgeport, CT 06606-5534; **Phone:** 203-335-0195; **Board Cert:** Nephrology 1984; Internal Medicine 1982; **Med School:** Univ Chicago-Pritzker Sch Med 1979; **Resid:** Internal Medicine, Temple Univ Hosp 1982; **Fellow:** Nephrology, Boston Univ Med Ctr 1985; **Fac Appt:** Asst Clin Prof Med, Yale Univ

Fogel, Mitchell A MD (Nep) - **Spec Exp:** Lupus Nephritis; Glomerulonephritis; Kidney Disease; **Hospital:** St Vincent's Med Ctr - Bridgeport, Bridgeport Hosp; **Address:** 900 Madison Ave, Ste 209, Bridgeport, CT 06606-5534; **Phone:** 203-335-0195; **Board Cert:** Internal Medicine 1986; Nephrology 1988; **Med School:** Univ Pennsylvania 1982; **Resid:** Internal Medicine, Boston Univ Med Ctr 1985; **Fellow:** Nephrology, Boston Univ Med Ctr 1988

Garfinkel, Howard B MD (Nep) - **Spec Exp:** Hypertension; Kidney Disease; Kidney Stones; **Hospital:** Danbury Hosp; **Address:** 24 Hospital Ave, Danbury, CT 06810-6099; **Phone:** 203-797-7104; **Board Cert:** Internal Medicine 1972; Nephrology 1972; **Med School:** Tufts Univ 1965; **Resid:** Internal Medicine, Cleveland Metro Genl Hosp 1970; **Fellow:** Renal Disease, Tufts-New Eng Med Ctr 1972; **Fac Appt:** Assoc Clin Prof Med, Yale Univ

Hines, William H MD (Nep) - **Spec Exp:** Dialysis Care; Hypertension; Kidney Disease; **Hospital:** Stamford Hosp, Greenwich Hosp; **Address:** 30 Commerce Rd, Stamford, CT 06902-4550; **Phone:** 203-324-7666; **Board Cert:** Internal Medicine 1984; Nephrology 1986; **Med School:** Cornell Univ-Weill Med Coll 1981; **Resid:** Internal Medicine, Hosp Univ Penn 1984; **Fellow:** Nephrology, Hosp Univ Penn 1988; **Fac Appt:** Asst Clin Prof Med, Columbia P&S

NEUROLOGICAL SURGERY

Camel, Mark MD (NS) - **Spec Exp:** Brain Tumors; Spinal Surgery; **Hospital:** Greenwich Hosp; **Address:** 6 Greenwich Office Park, Greenwich, CT 06831-5151; **Phone:** 203-869-1145 x616; **Board Cert:** Neurological Surgery 1990; **Med School:** Washington Univ, St Louis 1981; **Resid:** Neurological Surgery, Barnes Jewish Hosp 1986; **Fellow:** Neurological Surgery, Barnes Jewish Hosp 1987; **Fac Appt:** Asst Clin Prof S, Columbia P&S

Dila, Carl MD (NS) - **Spec Exp:** Spinal Surgery; Brain Tumors; **Hospital:** Stamford Hosp, Greenwich Hosp; **Address:** 70 Mill River St, Ste LL3, Stamford, CT 06902; **Phone:** 203-324-3504; **Board Cert:** Neurological Surgery 1973; **Med School:** Wayne State Univ 1962; **Resid:** Neurological Surgery, Montreal Genl Hosp 1971; Neurological Surgery, Montreal Neur Inst 1971; **Fellow:** Neurological Pathology, Montreal Neur Inst 1970

Lipow, Kenneth MD (NS) - **Spec Exp:** Spinal Surgery; Brain Surgery; **Hospital:** Bridgeport Hosp; **Address:** CT Neurosurgical Specialists, 267 Grant St Fl 8, Bridgeport, CT 06610-2870; **Phone:** 203-384-4500; **Board Cert:** Neurological Surgery 1989; **Med School:** Albert Einstein Coll Med 1978; **Resid:** Neurological Surgery, Albert Einstein Coll Med 1984; **Fac Appt:** Asst Clin Prof NS, NYU Sch Med

Mintz, Abraham MD (NS) - **Spec Exp:** Spinal Diseases; **Hospital:** St Vincent's Med Ctr - Bridgeport, Bridgeport Hosp; **Address:** 5520 Park Ave, Ste 210, Trumbull, CT 06611; **Phone:** 203-372-6460; **Board Cert:** Neurological Surgery 1992; **Med School:** Mexico 1982; **Resid:** Neurological Surgery, Jackson Meml Hosp/Univ Miami 1989

Nijensohn, Daniel MD (NS) - **Spec Exp:** Spinal Surgery; Brain Tumors; Gamma Knife Radiosurgery; Aneurysm-Cerebral; **Hospital:** St Vincent's Med Ctr - Bridgeport, Bridgeport Hosp; **Address:** 340 Capitol Ave, Bridgeport, CT 06606-5445; **Phone:** 203-336-3303; **Board Cert:** Neurological Surgery 1979; **Med School:** Argentina 1970; **Resid:** Surgery, Baylor Coll Med 1971; Surgery, Mayo Clinic 1972; **Fellow:** Neurological Surgery, Mayo Clinic 1976; **Fac Appt:** Assoc Clin Prof NS, Yale Univ

Rosenstein, C Cory MD (NS) - **Spec Exp:** Cerebrovascular Neurosurgery; Brain Tumors; Spinal Surgery; **Hospital:** Stamford Hosp, Greenwich Hosp; **Address:** 70 Mill River St, Ste LL3, Stamford, CT 06902-3275; **Phone:** 203-324-3504; **Board Cert:** Neurological Surgery 1994; **Med School:** Case West Res Univ 1985; **Resid:** Neurological Surgery, Univ Hosp 1991; **Fellow:** Neurological Surgery, Univ Hosp 1990

Shahid, Syed Javed MD (NS) - **Spec Exp:** Brain Tumors; Neck & Back Surgery; **Hospital:** Danbury Hosp, Norwalk Hosp; **Address:** 148 East Ave, Ste 3D, Norwalk, CT 06851; **Phone:** 203-853-0003; **Board Cert:** Neurological Surgery 1983; **Med School:** Pakistan 1972; **Resid:** Surgery, Kings County Hosp 1977; Neurological Surgery, Kings County Hosp 1980

NEUROLOGY

Camp, Walter A MD (N) - **Spec Exp:** Headache; Multiple Sclerosis; **Hospital:** Greenwich Hosp; **Address:** 49 Lake Ave, Greenwich, CT 06830; **Phone:** 203-869-6446; **Board Cert:** Neurology 1965; **Med School:** Emory Univ 1957; **Resid:** Internal Medicine, Univ Okla Med Ctr 1959; Neurology, NY Hosp-Cornell Med Ctr 1961; **Fellow:** Neurology, Natl Inst Neur Disease 1962; **Fac Appt:** Asst Clin Prof N, Yale Univ

Engel, Murray MD (N) - **Hospital:** Greenwich Hosp, Stamford Hosp; **Address:** 1290 Summer St, Ste 3300, Stamford, CT 06905; **Phone:** 203-359-1790; **Board Cert:** Pediatrics 1979; Neurology 1980; Neurodevelopmental Disabilities 2001; **Med School:** Univ Chicago-Pritzker Sch Med 1972; **Resid:** Neurology, Yale-New Haven Hosp 1976; Neurology, Columbia Presby Med Ctr 1977

Gross, Jeffrey MD (N) - **Spec Exp:** Multiple Sclerosis; **Hospital:** St Vincent's Med Ctr - Bridgeport, Milford Hosp; **Address:** 75 Kings Highway Cutoff, Fairfield, CT 06824; **Phone:** 203-333-1133; **Board Cert:** Neurology 1985; **Med School:** Case West Res Univ 1978; **Resid:** Internal Medicine, Hosp Univ Penn 1980; Neurology, Hosp Univ Penn 1983; **Fellow:** Neurological Muscular Disease, Hosp Univ Penn 1984

Murphy, John MD (N) - **Spec Exp:** Parkinson's Disease; Multiple Sclerosis; Stroke; **Hospital:** Danbury Hosp; **Address:** 69 Sand Pit Rd, Ste 300, Danbury, CT 06810-4088; **Phone:** 203-748-2551; **Board Cert:** Neurology 1991; **Med School:** Rutgers Univ 1985; **Resid:** Neurology, Univ Hosp 1989; **Fac Appt:** Asst Clin Prof N, NY Med Coll

Resor, Louise MD (N) - **Hospital:** Stamford Hosp; **Address:** 1290 Summer St, Ste 3200, Stamford, CT 06905; **Phone:** 203-978-0283; **Board Cert:** Neurology 1980; **Med School:** Washington Univ, St Louis 1974; **Resid:** Neurology, Columbia-Presby 1978; **Fellow:** Babies Hosp 1979

Sena, Kanaga N MD (N) - **Spec Exp:** Stroke; Neuro-Rehabilitation; **Hospital:** Bridgeport Hosp, Griffin Hosp; **Address:** 2590 Main St, Stratford, CT 06615-5838; **Phone:** 203-377-5988; **Board Cert:** Neurology 1979; **Med School:** Sri Lanka 1968; **Resid:** Internal Medicine, Bridgeport Hosp 1973; Neurology, Yale-New Haven Med Ctr 1976; **Fac Appt:** Assoc Clin Prof N, Yale Univ

Siegel, Kenneth C MD (N) - **Spec Exp:** Parkinson's Disease; Headache; **Hospital:** St Vincent's Med Ctr - Bridgeport, Milford Hosp; **Address:** 75 King's Highway Cutoff, Fairfield, CT 06824; **Phone:** 203-333-1133; **Board Cert:** Neurology 1975; **Med School:** Meharry Med Coll 1969; **Resid:** Neurology, Bellevue Med Ctr/NYU 1973; **Fac Appt:** Assoc Clin Prof N, Yale Univ

NUCLEAR MEDICINE

Gupta, Shiv MD (NuM) - **Spec Exp:** Osteoporosis; **Hospital:** Danbury Hosp; **Address:** 24 Hospital Ave, Danbury, CT 06810; **Phone:** 203-797-7222; **Board Cert:** Nuclear Medicine 1981; **Med School:** India 1966; **Resid:** Nuclear Medicine, Univ Conn Hlth Ctr 1980; Internal Medicine, Danbury Hosp 1981; **Fellow:** Nuclear Medicine, Auckland Hosp 1978; **Fac Appt:** Clin Prof NuM, Univ Conn

Johns, William MD (NuM) - **Hospital:** Danbury Hosp; **Address:** 24 Hospital Ave, Danbury, CT 06810; **Phone:** 203-797-7222; **Board Cert:** Internal Medicine 1986; Nuclear Medicine 1988; **Med School:** Univ Conn 1983; **Resid:** Internal Medicine, Danbury Hosp 1986; Nuclear Medicine, Brigham & Women's Hosp 1988

OBSTETRICS & GYNECOLOGY

Ayoub, Thomas MD (ObG) - **Spec Exp:** Menopause Problems; **Hospital:** Norwalk Hosp; **Address:** 30 Stevens St, Ste B, Norwalk, CT 06851; **Phone:** 203-644-1100; **Board Cert:** Obstetrics & Gynecology 2003; **Med School:** NYU Sch Med 1980; **Resid:** Obstetrics & Gynecology, Bellevue Hosp Ctr 1984

Besser, Gary MD (ObG) - **Spec Exp:** Laparoscopic Surgery-Complex; Uro-Gynecology; Pelvic Surgery; **Hospital:** Stamford Hosp; **Address:** Whittingham Pavilion, 190 W Broad St, Ste G-401, Stamford, CT 06902-3661; **Phone:** 203-325-4321; **Board Cert:** Obstetrics & Gynecology 2004; **Med School:** SUNY Downstate 1982; **Resid:** Obstetrics & Gynecology, Stamford Hosp 1986; **Fac Appt:** Asst Prof ObG, NY Med Coll

Rosenman, Stephen MD (ObG) - **Spec Exp:** Pelvic Reconstruction; Gynecologic Surgery; Vaginal Surgery; **Hospital:** Bridgeport Hosp, St Vincent's Med Ctr - Bridgeport; **Address:** 267 Grant St, Bridgeport, CT 06610-2805; **Phone:** 203-384-3990; **Board Cert:** Obstetrics & Gynecology 1991; **Med School:** Belgium 1972; **Resid:** Obstetrics & Gynecology, Bridgeport Hosp 1976; **Fac Appt:** Asst Clin Prof ObG, Yale Univ

Weinstein Jr, David B MD (ObG) - **Spec Exp:** Pregnancy-High Risk; **Hospital:** Stamford Hosp; **Address:** Stamford Hospital, Whittingham Pavilion, 190 W Broad St, Ste G-401, Stamford, CT 06902; **Phone:** 203-325-4321; **Board Cert:** Obstetrics & Gynecology 2003; **Med School:** Univ Chicago-Pritzker Sch Med 1969; **Resid:** Obstetrics & Gynecology, NY Hosp-Cornell 1974; **Fac Appt:** Asst Clin Prof ObG, Cornell Univ-Weill Med Coll

OPHTHALMOLOGY

Eisner, Leslie MD (Oph) - **Spec Exp:** Cataract Surgery-Lens Implant; Contact lenses; LASIK-Refractive Surgery; **Hospital:** Stamford Hosp; **Address:** 70 Mill River St, Stamford, CT 06902; **Phone:** 203-359-2020; **Board Cert:** Ophthalmology 1985; **Med School:** Canada 1978; **Resid:** Ophthalmology, Georgetown Univ Hosp 1983

Manjoney, Delia MD (Oph) - **Spec Exp:** Cataract Surgery; Glaucoma; Laser-Refractive Surgery; **Hospital:** St Vincent's Med Ctr - Bridgeport, Bridgeport Hosp; **Address:** 2720 Main St, Bridgeport, CT 06606; **Phone:** 203-576-6500; **Board Cert:** Pediatrics 1982; Ophthalmology 1988; **Med School:** Univ VT Coll Med 1977; **Resid:** Pediatrics, Parkland Hosp/Chldns Med Ctr 1980; Ophthalmology, Colum Presby Med Ctr/Harkness 1986

Musto, Anthony MD (Oph) - **Spec Exp:** Cataract Surgery; Oculoplastic Surgery; Eyelid Surgery; **Hospital:** Bridgeport Hosp; **Address:** 3060 Main St, Stratford, CT 06614-4945; **Phone:** 203-375-5819; **Board Cert:** Ophthalmology 1975; **Med School:** Georgetown Univ 1968; **Resid:** Ophthalmology, USPHS 1971; Ophthalmology, Manhattan Eye & Ear 1973; **Fac Appt:** Asst Clin Prof Oph, Yale Univ

Robbins, Kim P MD (Oph) - **Spec Exp:** Cataract Surgery; LASIK-Refractive Surgery; **Hospital:** Bridgeport Hosp; **Address:** 4695 Main St, Bridgeport, CT 06606; **Phone:** 203-371-5800; **Board Cert:** Ophthalmology 1985; **Med School:** NY Med Coll 1978; **Resid:** Internal Medicine, Stamford Hosp 1980; Ophthalmology, St Vincents Hosp 1983

Siderides, Elizabeth MD (Oph) - **Spec Exp:** Cataract Surgery; **Hospital:** Stamford Hosp; **Address:** 1275 Summer St, Stamford Ophthalmology, Stamford, CT 06905-3725; **Phone:** 203-327-5808; **Board Cert:** Ophthalmology 1991; **Med School:** Columbia P&S 1985; **Resid:** Ophthalmology, NYU Med Ctr 1989

Spector, Scott MD (Oph) - **Spec Exp:** Retinal Disorders; **Hospital:** Norwalk Hosp, Bridgeport Hosp; **Address:** 605 West Ave, Norwalk, CT 06850; **Phone:** 203-853-9900; **Board Cert:** Ophthalmology 1987; **Med School:** NY Med Coll 1982; **Resid:** Ophthalmology, NY Ear & Ear Infirm 1985; **Fellow:** Retina, Scheie Eye Inst- Univ Penn 1986

Wasserman, Eric MD (Oph) - **Spec Exp:** Cataract Surgery; Glaucoma; **Hospital:** Stamford Hosp; **Address:** 1275 Summer St, Ste 200, Stamford, CT 06905-5315; **Phone:** 203-978-0800; **Board Cert:** Ophthalmology 1988; **Med School:** NY Med Coll 1979; **Resid:** Ophthalmology, NY Med Coll 1983; **Fellow:** Anterior Segment - External Disease, John H Sheets Eye Fdn 1984

ORTHOPAEDIC SURGERY

Bindelglass, David MD (OrS) - **Spec Exp:** Arthritis; Minimally Invasive Surgery; Hip Replacement; Knee Replacement; **Hospital:** Bridgeport Hosp, St Vincent's Med Ctr - Bridgeport; **Address:** 75 Kings Highway Cutoff, Fairfield, CT 06824; **Phone:** 203-337-2600; **Board Cert:** Orthopaedic Surgery 1994; **Med School:** Columbia P&S 1985; **Resid:** Surgery, Beth Israel Hosp 1987; Orthopaedic Surgery, Columbia-Presby 1990; **Fellow:** Orthopaedic Surgery, Kerlan-Jobe Orthopaedic Clinic 1991

Carolan, Patrick J MD (OrS) - **Spec Exp:** Joint Replacement; Arthroscopic Surgery; **Hospital:** St Vincent's Med Ctr - Bridgeport, Griffin Hosp; **Address:** 3909 Main St, Bridgeport, CT 06606-2815; **Phone:** 203-372-4565; **Board Cert:** Orthopaedic Surgery 1972; **Med School:** UMDNJ-NJ Med Sch, Newark 1963; **Resid:** Orthopaedic Surgery, Letterman AMC 1970; Orthopaedic Surgery, Martin AMC 1966

Crowe, John F MD (OrS) - **Spec Exp:** Hip & Knee Replacement; Upper Extremity Surgery; Sports Medicine; **Hospital:** Greenwich Hosp, Hosp For Special Surgery (page 108); **Address:** 6 Greenwich Office Park, Greenwich, CT 06831-6086; **Phone:** 203-869-1145 x263; **Board Cert:** Orthopaedic Surgery 1977; **Med School:** Cornell Univ-Weill Med Coll 1971; **Resid:** Surgery, Roosevelt Hosp 1973; Orthopaedic Surgery, Hosp Special Surgery 1976

Hermele, Herbert MD (OrS) - **Spec Exp:** Trauma; **Hospital:** Bridgeport Hosp; **Address:** 75 Kings Hwy Cutoff, Fairfield, CT 06824; **Phone:** 203-337-2600; **Board Cert:** Orthopaedic Surgery 1975; **Med School:** Albert Einstein Coll Med 1969; **Resid:** Orthopaedic Surgery, Albert Einstein 1974

Hughes, Peter MD (OrS) - **Spec Exp:** Hip Replacement; Knee Replacement; Sports Medicine; **Hospital:** Stamford Hosp; **Address:** 90 Morgan St, Ste 207, Stamford, CT 06905; **Phone:** 203-325-4087; **Board Cert:** Orthopaedic Surgery 1978; **Med School:** NY Med Coll 1972; **Resid:** Orthopaedic Surgery, Metropolitan Hosp Ctr 1976; **Fellow:** Surgery, Hosp for Special Surg 1977; **Fac Appt:** Asst Clin Prof OrS, Columbia P&S

Spak, James I MD (OrS) - **Spec Exp:** Sports Medicine; **Hospital:** St Vincent's Med Ctr - Bridgeport; **Address:** Orthopaedic & Sports Med Ctr, 888 White Plains Rd, Trumbull, CT 06611; **Phone:** 203-268-2882; **Board Cert:** Orthopaedic Surgery 2000; **Med School:** Harvard Med Sch 1992; **Resid:** Orthopaedic Surgery, Brigham & Womens Hosp 1997; **Fellow:** Sports Medicine, Tahoe Fracture & Ortho Cl 1998; Trauma, Lake Tahoe Fracture & Ortho Cl 1998

Stovell, Peter MD (OrS) - **Spec Exp:** Joint Replacement; Sports Medicine; **Hospital:** Norwalk Hosp; **Address:** 40 Cross St, Ste 300, Norwalk, CT 06851-5726; **Phone:** 203-853-1811; **Board Cert:** Orthopaedic Surgery 1976; **Med School:** Columbia P&S 1968; **Resid:** Surgery, St Luke's-Roosevelt Hosp Ctr 1970; Orthopaedic Surgery, Hosp for Special Surgery 1975

Fairfield

Troy, Allen MD (OrS) - **Spec Exp:** Foot & Ankle Surgery; Sports Medicine; **Hospital:** Stamford Hosp; **Address:** 61 4th St, Stamford, CT 06905-5010; **Phone:** 203-324-0307; **Board Cert:** Orthopaedic Surgery 2000; **Med School:** SUNY Downstate 1979; **Resid:** Orthopaedic Surgery, NYU Med Ctr 1984; **Fellow:** Foot/Ankle Surgery, Hosp Joint Disease 1985; **Fac Appt:** Asst Clin Prof OrS, Columbia P&S

Wilchinsky, Mark MD (OrS) - **Spec Exp:** Arthroscopic Surgery; Joint Replacement; **Hospital:** St Vincent's Med Ctr - Bridgeport, Griffin Hosp; **Address:** 3909 Main St, Bridgeport, CT 06606-2815; **Phone:** 203-372-4565; **Board Cert:** Orthopaedic Surgery 1997; **Med School:** Tulane Univ 1979; **Resid:** Surgery, Univ Mass Med Ctr 1980; Orthopaedic Surgery, Univ Mass Med Ctr 1984; **Fac Appt:** Asst Prof OrS, Univ Mass Sch Med

OTOLARYNGOLOGY

Coffey, Tom MD (Oto) - **Spec Exp:** Snoring/Sleep Apnea; Hearing Disorders; **Hospital:** Bridgeport Hosp, St Vincent's Med Ctr - Bridgeport; **Address:** 15 Corporate Drive, Trumbull, CT 06611; **Phone:** 203-452-7081; **Board Cert:** Otolaryngology 1992; **Med School:** Columbia P&S 1986; **Resid:** Surgery, Yale-New Haven Hosp 1988; Otolaryngology, Yale-New Haven Hosp 1991

Gordon, Neil A MD (Oto) - **Spec Exp:** Cosmetic Surgery-Face; **Hospital:** Bridgeport Hosp; **Address:** 539 Danbury Rd, Wilton, CT 06897; **Phone:** 203-661-1715; **Board Cert:** Otolaryngology 1996; Facial Plastic & Reconstructive Surgery 1998; **Med School:** Albert Einstein Coll Med 1990; **Resid:** Otolaryngology, Yale-New Haven Hosp 1995; **Fellow:** Facial Plastic Surgery, Tulane Univ Med Ctr 1996

Klarsfeld, Jay MD (Oto) - **Spec Exp:** Sinus Disorders; Thyroid & Parathyroid Surgery; **Hospital:** Danbury Hosp; **Address:** 107 Newtown Rd, Ste 2A, Danbury, CT 06810-4151; **Phone:** 203-830-4700; **Board Cert:** Otolaryngology 1986; **Med School:** Mount Sinai Sch Med 1981; **Resid:** Surgery, Mt Sinai Hosp 1983; Otolaryngology, Mt Sinai Hosp 1986

Klenoff, Bruce MD (Oto) - **Spec Exp:** Ear Disorders/Surgery; Sinus Disorders/Surgery; Pediatric Otolaryngology; **Hospital:** Stamford Hosp; **Address:** Ear, Nose & Throat Ctr - Tully Hlth Ctr, 32 Strawberry Hill Ct, Fl 4 - Ste 4, Stamford, CT 06902; **Phone:** 203-324-4123; **Board Cert:** Otolaryngology 1976; **Med School:** Tufts Univ 1969; **Resid:** Surgery, St Elizabeth Hosp 1973; Otolaryngology, Mass Eye & Ear Infirm 1976; **Fac Appt:** Asst Clin Prof S, Columbia P&S

Levin, Richard MD (Oto) - **Spec Exp:** Sinus Disorders; Ear Infections; Facial Plastic/Reconstructive Surgery; **Hospital:** St Vincent's Med Ctr - Bridgeport, Bridgeport Hosp; **Address:** 1305 Post Rd, Fairfield, CT 06824; **Phone:** 203-259-4700; **Board Cert:** Otolaryngology 1993; **Med School:** Tufts Univ 1987; **Resid:** Otolaryngology, Mount Sinai 1993; **Fac Appt:** Asst Prof S, Yale Univ

Levine, Steven B MD (Oto) - **Spec Exp:** Snoring/Sleep Apnea; Sinus Disorders; Facial Plastic Surgery; **Hospital:** Bridgeport Hosp; **Address:** 160 Hawley Ln, Ste 202, Trumbull, CT 06611; **Phone:** 203-380-3707; **Board Cert:** Otolaryngology 1986; **Med School:** Univ Rochester 1981; **Resid:** Surgery, Penn Hosp 1983; Otolaryngology, Hosp Univ Penn 1986; **Fellow:** Otolaryngology, NY Hosp; **Fac Appt:** Asst Clin Prof S, Yale Univ

Lipton, Richard J MD (Oto) - **Spec Exp:** Head & Neck Surgery; **Hospital:** Danbury Hosp; **Address:** 107 Newtown Rd, Ste 2A, Danbury, CT 06810-4545; **Phone:** 203-830-4700; **Board Cert:** Otolaryngology 1990; **Med School:** Mayo Med Sch 1985; **Resid:** Surgery, Mayo Clinic 1986; Otolaryngology, Mayo Clinic 1990

Miles, Richard J MD/DDS (Oto) - **Spec Exp:** Nasal & Sinus Disorders; Snoring/Sleep Apnea; Ear Disorders; Facial Plastic Surgery; **Hospital:** Stamford Hosp; **Address:** 32 Strawberry Hill Ct Fl 4, Stamford, CT 06902; **Phone:** 203-353-0000; **Board Cert:** Otolaryngology 1995; **Med School:** Med Coll VA 1987; **Resid:** Otolaryngology, NYU Med Ctr 1993; **Fellow:** Plastic Surgery, Deaconess Hosp 1994

Salzer, Stephen MD (Oto) - **Spec Exp:** Thyroid & Parathyroid Surgery; Pediatric Otolaryngology; Sinus Disorders/Surgery; **Hospital:** Greenwich Hosp, Stamford Hosp; **Address:** 49 Lake Ave Fl 1, Greenwich, CT 06830-4519; **Phone:** 203-869-2030; **Board Cert:** Otolaryngology 1995; **Med School:** Johns Hopkins Univ 1989; **Resid:** Otolaryngology, Yale-New Haven Hosp 1994; **Fellow:** Otolaryngology, Laennel Hosp; **Fac Appt:** Assoc Clin Prof Oto, Yale Univ

PAIN MEDICINE

Kloth, David S MD (PM) - **Spec Exp:** Pain-Back; Pain-Cancer; **Hospital:** Danbury Hosp, St Mary's Hosp - Waterbury; **Address:** Connecticut Pain Care, 109 Newtown Rd, Danbury, CT 06810; **Phone:** 203-792-7246; **Board Cert:** Anesthesiology 1992; Pain Medicine 1996; **Med School:** NYU Sch Med 1987; **Resid:** Anesthesiology, Hosp U Penn 1991

PEDIATRIC CARDIOLOGY

Berkwits, Kieve MD (PCd) - **Spec Exp:** Congenital Heart Disease; **Hospital:** Bridgeport Hosp; **Address:** Bridgeport Hosp, Dept Peds, 267 Grant St, Box 5000, Bridgeport, CT 06610; **Phone:** 203-384-3783; **Board Cert:** Pediatrics 1986; Pediatric Cardiology 2003; **Med School:** Mexico 1979; **Resid:** Pediatrics, Beth Israel Med Ctr 1983; **Fellow:** Pediatric Cardiology, NY Hosp/Cornell Univ 1985; **Fac Appt:** Asst Clin Prof Ped, Yale Univ

Snyder, Michael MD (PCd) - **Spec Exp:** Heart Murmurs; Echocardiography; Fetal Echocardiography; **Hospital:** Stamford Hosp, NY-Presby Hosp (page 100); **Address:** Darien Med Ctr, 1500 Boston Post Rd Fl 1, Darien, CT 06820-5936; **Phone:** 203-662-0313; **Board Cert:** Pediatrics 1984; Pediatric Cardiology 1985; **Med School:** Cornell Univ-Weill Med Coll 1979; **Resid:** Pediatrics, New York Hosp 1982; **Fellow:** Pediatric Cardiology, New York Hosp 1984; **Fac Appt:** Assoc Prof Ped, Columbia P&S

PEDIATRIC GASTROENTEROLOGY

Glassman, Mark MD (PGe) - **Spec Exp:** Inflammatory Bowel Disease/Crohn's; Gastroesophageal Reflux Disease (GERD); Diarrheal Diseases; Food Allergy; **Hospital:** Sound Shore Med Ctr - Westchester (page 711), Stamford Hosp; **Address:** 149 East Ave, Ste 39, Norwalk, CT 06851-5711; **Phone:** 203-853-7170; **Board Cert:** Pediatrics 1983; Pediatric Gastroenterology 1998; **Med School:** SUNY Buffalo 1978; **Resid:** Pediatrics, Yale-New Haven Hosp 1981; **Fellow:** Gastroenterology, Chldns Hosp 1983; **Fac Appt:** Prof Ped, NY Med Coll

PEDIATRIC HEMATOLOGY-ONCOLOGY

Ertl, John MD (PHO) - **Hospital:** Danbury Hosp; **Address:** 41 Germantown Rd, Ste 201, Danbury, CT 06810-4000; **Phone:** 203-744-1680; **Board Cert:** Pediatrics 1977; Pediatric Hematology-Oncology 1978; **Med School:** SUNY Downstate 1970; **Resid:** Pediatrics, Rhode Island Hosp 1973; **Fellow:** Pediatric Hematology-Oncology, UC Davis Medical Center 1977

PEDIATRIC NEPHROLOGY

Kennedy, Thomas MD (PNep) - **Spec Exp:** Hypertension; Fluid & Electrolyte Disorders; **Hospital:** Bridgeport Hosp, Yale - New Haven Hosp (page 984); **Address:** 267 Grant St, Bridgeport, CT 06610-2805; **Phone:** 203-384-3712; **Board Cert:** Pediatrics 1977; Pediatric Nephrology 1979; **Med School:** Cornell Univ-Weill Med Coll 1972; **Resid:** Pediatrics, Childrens Hosp 1975; **Fellow:** Nephrology, Childrens Hosp 1979; **Fac Appt:** Clin Prof Ped, Yale Univ

PEDIATRIC PULMONOLOGY

Dworkin, Gregory MD (PPul) - **Spec Exp:** Asthma; Chronic Lung Disease; **Hospital:** Danbury Hosp; **Address:** 24 Hospital Ave, Danbury, CT 06810; **Phone:** 203-797-7027; **Board Cert:** Pediatrics 1987; Pediatric Pulmonology 1998; **Med School:** Albany Med Coll 1982; **Resid:** Pediatrics, Mount Sinai 1985; Pediatrics, Mount Sinai 1986; **Fellow:** Pediatric Pulmonology, Mount Sinai 1989; **Fac Appt:** Asst Clin Prof Ped, NY Med Coll

Hen Jr, Jacob MD (PPul) - **Spec Exp:** Asthma; **Hospital:** Bridgeport Hosp, CT Chldns Med Ctr; **Address:** Bridgeport Hosp, Dept Peds, 267 Grant St, Box 5000, Bridgeport, CT 06610-2870; **Phone:** 203-384-3711; **Board Cert:** Pediatrics 1980; Pediatric Pulmonology 2006; Pediatric Critical Care Medicine 2003; **Med School:** UMDNJ-NJ Med Sch, Newark 1975; **Resid:** Pediatrics, UMDNJ-Univ Hosp 1977; **Fellow:** Pediatric Pulmonology, Yale-New Haven Hosp 1981; **Fac Appt:** Assoc Clin Prof Ped, Yale Univ

Sadeghi, Hossein MD (PPul) - **Spec Exp:** Asthma; Neonatal Chronic Lung Disease; Cystic Fibrosis; **Hospital:** Stamford Hosp, NY-Presby Hosp (page 100); **Address:** 32 Strawberry Hill Ct, Stamford, CT 06902; **Phone:** 203-967-5949; **Board Cert:** Pediatrics 1995; Pediatric Pulmonology 1998; **Med School:** Australia 1990; **Resid:** Pediatrics, Royal Chldns Hosp 1992; Pediatrics, Med Coll Va Hosp 1995; **Fellow:** Pediatric Pulmonology, NY Med Coll 1998; **Fac Appt:** Asst Clin Prof Ped, Columbia P&S

PEDIATRICS

Chessin, Robert MD (Ped) `PCP` - **Spec Exp:** Child Development; Developmental Disorders; **Hospital:** Bridgeport Hosp, St Vincent's Med Ctr - Bridgeport; **Address:** 4699 Main St, Ste 215, Bridgeport, CT 06606-1830; **Phone:** 203-452-8322; **Board Cert:** Pediatrics 1978; Developmental-Behavioral Pediatrics 2004; **Med School:** Johns Hopkins Univ 1973; **Resid:** Pediatrics, Duke Univ Med Ctr 1976; **Fac Appt:** Assoc Clin Prof Ped, Yale Univ

Freedman, Richard MD (Ped) `PCP` - **Spec Exp:** Neonatology; **Hospital:** Bridgeport Hosp; **Address:** 4699 Main St, Ste 215, Bridgeport, CT 06606-1830; **Phone:** 203-452-8322; **Board Cert:** Pediatrics 1979; Neonatal-Perinatal Medicine 1981; **Med School:** Boston Univ 1975; **Resid:** Pediatrics, Yale-New Haven Hosp 1978; **Fellow:** Neonatology, Yale-New Haven Hosp 1980; **Fac Appt:** Assoc Clin Prof Ped, Yale Univ

Gundy, John MD (Ped) `PCP` - **Spec Exp:** Developmental Disorders; Child Abuse; **Hospital:** Danbury Hosp; **Address:** 300 Federal Rd, Brookfield, CT 06804-2412; **Phone:** 203-775-1118; **Board Cert:** Pediatrics 1981; **Med School:** Cornell Univ-Weill Med Coll 1962; **Resid:** Pediatrics, Chldns Hosp 1966; **Fac Appt:** Assoc Clin Prof Ped, Yale Univ

Hochstadt, Judith MD (Ped) `PCP` - **Spec Exp:** Diabetes; Pubertal Disorders; **Hospital:** Bridgeport Hosp, St Vincent's Med Ctr - Bridgeport; **Address:** 15 Corporate Dr, Trumbull, CT 06611-1351; **Phone:** 203-452-8322; **Board Cert:** Pediatrics 1983; **Med School:** SUNY Downstate 1978; **Resid:** Pediatrics, Yale-New Haven Hosp 1981; **Fellow:** Pediatric Endocrinology, Yale-New Haven Hosp 1982; **Fac Appt:** Assoc Clin Prof Ped, Yale Univ

Keller, Barry MD (Ped) `PCP` - **Spec Exp:** Growth/Development Disorders; **Hospital:** Danbury Hosp; **Address:** 16 Hospital Ave, Ste 304, Danbury, CT 06810; **Phone:** 203-743-1201; **Board Cert:** Pediatrics 1971; **Med School:** SUNY Downstate 1965; **Resid:** Pediatrics, Jewish Hospital 1967; Pediatrics, Montefiore Hosp Med Ctr 1968; **Fellow:** Pediatric Endocrinology, Bronx Muni Hosp 1971

Kenefick, Timothy MD (Ped) `PCP` - **Spec Exp:** ADD/ADHD; **Hospital:** Stamford Hosp; **Address:** 126 Morgan St, Stamford, CT 06905-5431; **Phone:** 203-327-1055; **Board Cert:** Pediatrics 2003; **Med School:** Cornell Univ-Weill Med Coll 1984; **Resid:** Pediatrics, NY Hosp-Cornell Med Ctr 1987; Pediatrics, NY Hosp-Cornell Med Ctr 1988

Klenk, Rosemary MD (Ped) `PCP` - **Spec Exp:** ADD/ADHD; **Hospital:** Stamford Hosp; **Address:** 183 Cherry St, New Canaan, CT 06840; **Phone:** 203-972-5232; **Board Cert:** Pediatrics 1987; **Med School:** Cornell Univ-Weill Med Coll 1980; **Resid:** Pediatrics, Columbia-Presby Med Ctr 1983

Korval, Arnold MD (Ped) `PCP` - **Spec Exp:** Adolescent Medicine; **Hospital:** Greenwich Hosp, Stamford Hosp; **Address:** 8 West End Ave, Old Greenwich, CT 06870-1642; **Phone:** 203-637-0186; **Board Cert:** Pediatrics 1979; **Med School:** St Louis Univ 1974; **Resid:** Pediatrics, Children's Hosp-Univ Penn 1977

Levine, Dorothy MD (Ped) `PCP` - **Spec Exp:** Pediatrics; **Hospital:** Stamford Hosp; **Address:** 166 W Broad St,, Ste 103, Stamford, CT 06902; **Phone:** 203-323-1770; **Board Cert:** Pediatrics 1985; **Med School:** Albert Einstein Coll Med 1980; **Resid:** Pediatrics, Columbia-Presby Med Ctr 1983; **Fac Appt:** Asst Clin Prof Ped, Columbia P&S

Mongillo, Nicholas MD (Ped) `PCP` - **Spec Exp:** AIDS/HIV; Sports Medicine; ADD/ADHD; **Hospital:** Bridgeport Hosp, Yale - New Haven Hosp (page 984); **Address:** 7365 Main St, Stratford, CT 06614; **Phone:** 203-381-9990; **Board Cert:** Pediatrics 2003; **Med School:** Grenada 1987; **Resid:** Pediatrics, Bridgeport Hosp 1990

Morelli, Alan MD (Ped) `PCP` - **Hospital:** Stamford Hosp; **Address:** 166 W Broad St, Ste 103, Stamford, CT 06902; **Phone:** 203-323-1770; **Board Cert:** Pediatrics 1987; **Med School:** NY Med Coll 1982; **Resid:** Pediatrics, Yale-New Haven Hosp 1985

Schutzengel, Roy MD (Ped) `PCP` - **Spec Exp:** Growth Disorders; Developmental Disorders; **Hospital:** Bridgeport Hosp, St Vincent's Med Ctr - Bridgeport; **Address:** 3180 Main St, Ste G1, Bridgeport, CT 06606; **Phone:** 203-371-7111; **Board Cert:** Pediatrics 1996; **Med School:** Univ Pennsylvania 1984; **Resid:** Pediatrics, UC Davis Medical Center 1988; **Fellow:** Pediatric Endocrinology, Nat Inst Health 1986; Pediatric Hematology-Oncology, Yale-New Haven Hosp 1989

Smith, Marilyn MD (Ped) `PCP` - **Hospital:** St Vincent's Med Ctr - Bridgeport, Bridgeport Hosp; **Address:** 401 Monroe Tpke, Monroe, CT 06468; **Phone:** 203-452-1063; **Board Cert:** Pediatrics 1998; **Med School:** Univ Cincinnati 1987; **Resid:** Pediatrics, Yale-New Haven Hosp 1990

Swidler, Sanford MD (Ped) `PCP` - **Hospital:** Stamford Hosp; **Address:** 126 Morgan St, Stamford, CT 06905-5431; **Phone:** 203-327-1055; **Board Cert:** Pediatrics 1987; **Med School:** NYU Sch Med 1980; **Resid:** Pediatrics, Bellevue Hosp 1984; **Fac Appt:** Asst Clin Prof Ped, Columbia P&S

PHYSICAL MEDICINE & REHABILITATION

Grant, Linda MD (PMR) - **Hospital:** Greenwich Hosp; **Address:** 5 Perryridge Rd, Greenwich, CT 06830; **Phone:** 203-863-3290; **Board Cert:** Physical Medicine & Rehabilitation 1990; **Med School:** Rutgers Univ 1985; **Resid:** Physical Medicine & Rehabilitation, NYU Med Ctr 1989

Petrillo, Claudio R MD (PMR) - **Spec Exp:** Spinal Cord Injury; Stroke Rehabilitation; Amputee Rehabilitation; **Hospital:** Norwalk Hosp; **Address:** 698 West Ave, Norwalk, CT 06850-3816; **Phone:** 203-523-0100; **Board Cert:** Physical Medicine & Rehabilitation 1977; **Med School:** Brazil 1972; **Resid:** Physical Medicine & Rehabilitation, NYU-Rusk Inst 1976; **Fellow:** Spinal Cord Injury Medicine, NYU-Rusk Inst 1979; **Fac Appt:** Assoc Prof PMR, Mount Sinai Sch Med

PLASTIC SURGERY

Gewirtz, Harold MD (PlS) - **Spec Exp:** Cosmetic Surgery-Face; Breast Cosmetic & Reconstructive Surgery; Craniofacial Surgery/Reconstruction; **Hospital:** Stamford Hosp, Greenwich Hosp; **Address:** 70 Mill River St, Stamford, CT 06902-3725; **Phone:** 203-325-1381; **Board Cert:** Plastic Surgery 1984; Hand Surgery 1998; **Med School:** Johns Hopkins Univ 1975; **Resid:** Surgery, UCLA Med Ctr 1980; Plastic Surgery, NYU Med Ctr 1982; **Fac Appt:** Assoc Clin Prof PlS, Columbia P&S

Goldenberg, David MD (PlS) - **Spec Exp:** Cosmetic Surgery; Breast Reconstruction; Wound Healing/Care; **Hospital:** Danbury Hosp; **Address:** 107 Newtown Rd, Ste 2C, Danbury, CT 06810-4151; **Phone:** 203-791-9661; **Board Cert:** Plastic Surgery 1990; **Med School:** NY Med Coll 1982; **Resid:** Surgery, Montefiore Med Ctr-Einstein Div 1986; **Fellow:** Plastic Surgery, Montefiore Med Ctr-Einstein Div 1988

Newman, Fredric A MD (PlS) - **Spec Exp:** Cosmetic Surgery-Face; Liposuction & Body Contouring; Breast Reconstruction; **Hospital:** Greenwich Hosp; **Address:** 722 Post Rd, Ste 200, Darien, CT 06820; **Phone:** 203-656-9999; **Board Cert:** Plastic Surgery 1985; **Med School:** SUNY Downstate 1974; **Resid:** Surgery, Beth Israel Med Ctr 1977; Surgery, SUNY Downstate 1979; **Fellow:** Plastic Reconstructive Surgery, NYU Med Ctr 1981; Plastic Surgery, Jackson Meml Hosp 1982

Nolan, William MD (PlS) - **Spec Exp:** Cosmetic Surgery-Face; Hand Surgery; **Hospital:** Stamford Hosp; **Address:** 39 Pine St, New Canaan, CT 06840; **Phone:** 203-966-2717; **Board Cert:** Plastic Surgery 1987; **Med School:** UCLA 1976; **Resid:** Plastic Surgery, Stanford Univ Med Ctr 1984; **Fellow:** Hand Surgery, St Lukes Roosevelt Hosp 1981; **Fac Appt:** Asst Clin Prof S, Cornell Univ-Weill Med Coll

O'Connell, Joseph B MD (PlS) - **Spec Exp:** Cosmetic Surgery-Liposuction; Cosmetic Surgery-Face; Cosmetic Surgery-Breast; **Hospital:** Bridgeport Hosp; **Address:** 208 Post Rd W, Westport, CT 06880; **Phone:** 203-454-0044; **Board Cert:** Plastic Surgery 1992; **Med School:** Cornell Univ-Weill Med Coll 1981; **Resid:** Surgery, St Vincents Med Ctr 1986; **Fellow:** Plastic Surgery, New York Hosp 1988

Rein, Joel MD (PlS) - **Spec Exp:** Liposuction & Body Contouring; Cosmetic Surgery-Breast; Cosmetic Surgery-Face; Rhinoplasty; **Hospital:** Greenwich Hosp, Stamford Hosp; **Address:** 2 1/2 Deerfield Drive, Greenwich, CT 06830; **Phone:** 203-869-9850; **Board Cert:** Plastic Surgery 1973; Surgery 1971; **Med School:** Columbia P&S 1963; **Resid:** Surgery, Columbia-Presby 1970; Plastic Surgery, Columbia-Presby 1972; **Fellow:** Hand Surgery, St Luke's-Roosevelt Hosp Ctr

Rosenstock, Arthur MD (PlS) - **Spec Exp:** Cosmetic Surgery-Face; Eyelid Surgery; Cosmetic Surgery-Breast; **Hospital:** Stamford Hosp; **Address:** 1290 Summer St, Ste 3100, Stamford, CT 06905-5326; **Phone:** 203-359-1959; **Board Cert:** Plastic Surgery 1985; **Med School:** Belgium 1976; **Resid:** Surgery, Westchester Co Med Ctr 1981; **Fellow:** Plastic Reconstructive Surgery, Med Coll Virginia 1983; **Fac Appt:** Asst Clin Prof S, Columbia P&S

PSYCHIATRY

Caraccio, Babette MD (Psyc) - **Spec Exp:** Anxiety Disorders; Depression; **Hospital:** Greenwich Hosp; **Address:** 23 Mianus View Ter, Cos Cob, CT 06807-2219; **Phone:** 203-622-7428; **Board Cert:** Psychiatry 1988; Child & Adolescent Psychiatry 1989; **Med School:** NYU Sch Med 1982; **Resid:** Psychiatry, NYU Med Ctr 1984; **Fellow:** Child & Adolescent Psychiatry, NY Hosp-Westchester Div 1985

Hart, Sidney MD (Psyc) - **Spec Exp:** Anxiety Disorders; Mood Disorders; Psychotherapy; **Hospital:** Greenwich Hosp; **Address:** 282 Railroad Ave Fl 2, Greenwich, CT 06830; **Phone:** 203-622-1722; **Board Cert:** Psychiatry 1973; **Med School:** Albert Einstein Coll Med 1964; **Resid:** Psychiatry, Bronx Municipal Hosp 1971; **Fellow:** Liason Psychiatry, Montefiore Hosp Med Ctr 1973

Lorefice, Laurence MD (Psyc) - **Spec Exp:** Depression; Panic Disorder; Obsessive-Compulsive Disorder; Bipolar/Mood Disorders; **Address:** 404 Sound Beach Ave, Old Greenwich, CT 06870-2222; **Phone:** 203-637-4006; **Board Cert:** Psychiatry 1979; **Med School:** Univ Pennsylvania 1975; **Resid:** Psychiatry, Mass General Hosp 1979

Mueller, F Carl MD (Psyc) - **Spec Exp:** Anxiety & Depression; Obsessive-Compulsive Disorder; Psychopharmacology; **Hospital:** Stamford Hosp; **Address:** 999 Summer St, Ste 200, Stamford, CT 06905; **Phone:** 203-357-7773; **Board Cert:** Psychiatry 1987; Geriatric Psychiatry 2000; **Med School:** Univ Conn 1982; **Resid:** Psychiatry, Yale-New Haven Hosp 1983; **Fellow:** Psychiatry, Yale-New Haven Hosp 1986; **Fac Appt:** Asst Clin Prof Psyc, Yale Univ

Schechter, Justin MD (Psyc) - **Spec Exp:** Anxiety Disorders; Mood Disorders; Eating Disorders; Forensic Psychiatry; **Hospital:** Stamford Hosp; **Address:** 22 Fifth St, Stamford, CT 06905-5030; **Phone:** 203-323-7760; **Board Cert:** Psychiatry 1986; Forensic Psychiatry 1998; **Med School:** SUNY Stony Brook 1981; **Resid:** Psychiatry, Yale-New Haven 1985; **Fac Appt:** Asst Clin Prof Psyc, Yale Univ

Shapiro, Bruce MD (Psyc) - **Spec Exp:** Forensic Psychiatry; Psychopharmacology; Anxiety & Depression; Bipolar/Mood Disorders; **Address:** 666 W Glenbrook Rd, River Suite, Stamford, CT 06906; **Phone:** 203-327-4144; **Board Cert:** Psychiatry 1976; Geriatric Psychiatry 1996; Forensic Psychiatry 1996; **Med School:** NY Med Coll 1972; **Resid:** Psychiatry, Metropolitan Hosp Ctr 1975; **Fac Appt:** Clin Prof Psyc, Columbia P&S

Sheftell, Fred MD (Psyc) - **Spec Exp:** Headache; **Hospital:** Greenwich Hosp; **Address:** 778 Long Ridge Rd, Stamford, CT 06902; **Phone:** 203-968-1799; **Board Cert:** Psychiatry 1972; **Med School:** NY Med Coll 1966; **Resid:** Psychiatry, Metropolitan Hosp Ctr 1970; **Fac Appt:** Asst Clin Prof Psyc, NY Med Coll

Smith, Jo Ann MD (Psyc) - **Spec Exp:** Mood Disorders; Anxiety Disorders; Women's Health-Mental Health; **Hospital:** St Vincent's Med Ctr - Bridgeport; **Address:** 160 Hawley Ln, Ste 001, Trumbull, CT 06611-5300; **Phone:** 203-377-0111; **Board Cert:** Psychiatry 1980; **Med School:** SUNY Hlth Sci Ctr 1974; **Resid:** Psychiatry, Georgetown Univ Hosp 1979

Tamerin, John MD (Psyc) - **Spec Exp:** Psychotherapy; Bipolar/Mood Disorders; Substance Abuse; Alcohol Abuse; **Hospital:** NY-Presby Hosp (page 100), Greenwich Hosp; **Address:** 27 Stag Ln, Greenwich, CT 06831-3137; **Phone:** 203-661-8282; **Board Cert:** Psychiatry 1970; Addiction Psychiatry 1993; **Med School:** NYU Sch Med 1963; **Resid:** Psychiatry, Yale-New Haven Hosp 1965; Psychiatry, Mt Sinai Med Ctr 1967; **Fellow:** Child Psychiatry, Mt Sinai Med Ctr 1967; **Fac Appt:** Assoc Clin Prof Psyc, Cornell Univ-Weill Med Coll

PULMONARY DISEASE

Brown, Robert B MD (Pul) - **Spec Exp:** Critical Care; **Hospital:** St Vincent's Med Ctr - Bridgeport; **Address:** 2800 Main St, Bridgeport, CT 06606; **Phone:** 203-576-5711; **Board Cert:** Internal Medicine 1981; Pulmonary Disease 1984; Critical Care Medicine 1996; **Med School:** SUNY Downstate 1978; **Resid:** Internal Medicine, Westchester Med Ctr 1981; **Fellow:** Pulmonary Disease, NY Med Coll 1984; **Fac Appt:** Asst Prof Med, NY Med Coll

Krasnogor, Lester MD (Pul) - **Spec Exp:** Asthma; Emphysema; Cough-Chronic; Sleep Apnea; **Hospital:** Stamford Hosp; **Address:** 190 W Broad St, Stamford, CT 06902; **Phone:** 203-348-2437; **Board Cert:** Internal Medicine 1970; Pulmonary Disease 1972; Critical Care Medicine 1997; **Med School:** NYU Sch Med 1963; **Resid:** Internal Medicine, Duke Univ Med Ctr 1965; Internal Medicine, Univ Pittsburgh 1969; **Fellow:** Pulmonary Disease, Yale-New Haven Hosp 1968; **Fac Appt:** Assoc Clin Prof Med, Columbia P&S

Krinsley, James MD (Pul) - **Spec Exp:** Asthma; Emphysema; Critical Care; **Hospital:** Stamford Hosp; **Address:** 190 W Broad St, Pulmonary Associates, Stamford, CT 06902; **Phone:** 203-348-2437; **Board Cert:** Internal Medicine 1983; Pulmonary Disease 1986; Critical Care Medicine 1999; **Med School:** Cornell Univ-Weill Med Coll 1980; **Resid:** Internal Medicine, NYU/VA Med Ctr 1983; **Fellow:** Pulmonary Disease, Yale-New Haven Hosp 1986; **Fac Appt:** Assoc Clin Prof Med, Columbia P&S

Kurtz, Caroline MD (Pul) - **Spec Exp:** Asthma; Emphysema; **Hospital:** Norwalk Hosp; **Address:** 30 Stevens St, Ste C, Norwalk, CT 06850; **Phone:** 203-855-3888; **Board Cert:** Internal Medicine 1988; Pulmonary Disease 2000; Critical Care Medicine 2000; **Med School:** NYU Sch Med 1984; **Resid:** Internal Medicine, Mt Sinai Hosp 1987; **Fellow:** Pulmonary Critical Care Medicine, Mt Sinai Hosp 1990

Marino, A Michael MD (Pul) - **Spec Exp:** Asthma; Bronchitis; Emphysema; **Hospital:** Greenwich Hosp; **Address:** 5 Perryridge Rd, Greenwich, CT 06830; **Phone:** 203-661-5379; **Board Cert:** Internal Medicine 1970; Pulmonary Disease 1972; **Med School:** Georgetown Univ 1964; **Resid:** Internal Medicine, VA Med Ctr 1967; **Fellow:** Pulmonary Disease, VA Med Ctr 1969; **Fac Appt:** Assoc Prof Med, Yale Univ

McCalley, Stuart MD (Pul) - **Spec Exp:** Sleep Disorders; Chronic Obstructive Lung Disease (COPD); Asthma; **Hospital:** Greenwich Hosp; **Address:** 75 Holly Hill Ln, Greenwich, CT 06830; **Phone:** 203-869-6960; **Board Cert:** Internal Medicine 1972; Pulmonary Disease 1974; **Med School:** Case West Res Univ 1969; **Resid:** Internal Medicine, Univ Conn Hlth Ctr 1971; Internal Medicine, Univ Vermont Med Ctr 1972; **Fellow:** Pulmonary Disease, Albert Einstein/Bronx Muni Hosp 1974; **Fac Appt:** Asst Clin Prof Med, Yale Univ

Sachs, Paul MD (Pul) - **Spec Exp:** Pulmonary Rehabilitation; Asthma; **Hospital:** Stamford Hosp; **Address:** 190 W Broad St, Stamford, CT 06902-3633; **Phone:** 203-348-2437; **Board Cert:** Internal Medicine 1985; Pulmonary Disease 1988; Critical Care Medicine 1999; **Med School:** NYU Sch Med 1982; **Resid:** Internal Medicine, NY Hosp 1985; **Fellow:** Pulmonary Disease, Montefior Med Ctr 1987

Winter, Stephen MD (Pul) - **Spec Exp:** Respiratory Failure; Sepsis; Critical Care; **Hospital:** Norwalk Hosp, VA Conn Hlthcre Sys; **Address:** Norwalk Hosp, Sect Pulm & Crit Care Med, Maple St, Norwalk, CT 06856; **Phone:** 203-852-2392; **Board Cert:** Internal Medicine 1984; Pulmonary Disease 1986; Critical Care Medicine 1997; **Med School:** Cornell Univ-Weill Med Coll 1981; **Resid:** Internal Medicine, NY Hosp 1984; **Fellow:** Pulmonary Disease, Yale-New Haven Hosp 1987; **Fac Appt:** Clin Prof Med, Yale Univ

RADIATION ONCOLOGY

Dowling, Sean MD (RadRO) - **Spec Exp:** Breast Cancer; Gynecologic Cancer; **Hospital:** Stamford Hosp; **Address:** Dept Radiation Oncology, 34 Shelburne Rd, Stamford, CT 06902; **Phone:** 203-325-7886; **Board Cert:** Internal Medicine 1986; Radiation Oncology 1990; **Med School:** Yale Univ 1983; **Resid:** Internal Medicine, Yale-New Haven Hosp 1986; Radiation Oncology, Yale-New Haven Hosp 1989

Fass, Daniel E MD (RadRO) - **Spec Exp:** Prostate Cancer; Breast Cancer; Head & Neck Cancer; **Hospital:** Greenwich Hosp; **Address:** 77 Lafayette Pl, Ste 290, Greenwich, CT 06830; **Phone:** 203-863-3773; **Board Cert:** Radiation Oncology 1987; **Med School:** Howard Univ 1983; **Resid:** Radiation Oncology, NYU Med Ctr 1986; **Fellow:** Brachytherapy, Meml Sloan Kettering Cancer Ctr 1987; **Fac Appt:** Asst Prof Med, Cornell Univ-Weill Med Coll

Masino, Frank A MD (RadRO) - **Spec Exp:** Breast Cancer; Prostate Cancer; Brachytherapy; **Hospital:** Stamford Hosp; **Address:** 34 Shelburne Rd, Stamford, CT 06902-3628; **Phone:** 203-276-7886; **Board Cert:** Therapeutic Radiology 1982; **Med School:** Albert Einstein Coll Med 1978; **Resid:** Therapeutic Radiology, Yale-New Haven Hosp 1982

Spera, John A MD (RadRO) - **Spec Exp:** Breast Cancer; Prostate Cancer; Intensity Modulated Radiotherapy (IMRT); **Hospital:** Danbury Hosp; **Address:** Dept Rad Onc, 24 Hospital Ave, Danbury, CT 06810-6099; **Phone:** 203-797-7190; **Board Cert:** Radiation Oncology 1987; **Med School:** Georgetown Univ 1979; **Resid:** Surgery, Hosp Univ Penn 1981; Urology, Hosp Univ Penn 1983; **Fellow:** Radiation Oncology, Hosp Univ Penn 1987

REPRODUCTIVE ENDOCRINOLOGY

Doyle, Michael MD (RE) - **Spec Exp:** Infertility-IVF; Endometriosis; **Hospital:** Norwalk Hosp; **Address:** 4920 Main St, Ste 301, Bridgeport, CT 06606-1813; **Phone:** 203-373-1200; **Board Cert:** Obstetrics & Gynecology 2001; **Med School:** Georgetown Univ 1990; **Resid:** Obstetrics & Gynecology, Hosp U Penn 1993; **Fellow:** Reproductive Endocrinology, Yale New Haven Hosp 1995

Ginsburg, Frances MD (RE) - **Spec Exp:** Infertility; Menopause Problems; Endometriosis; **Hospital:** Stamford Hosp; **Address:** Stamford Hospital, Box 9317, Stamford, CT 06904-9317; **Phone:** 203-276-7559; **Board Cert:** Obstetrics & Gynecology 1996; Reproductive Endocrinology 1996; **Med School:** NYU Sch Med 1980; **Resid:** Obstetrics & Gynecology, Bellevue Hosp Ctr-NYU 1984; **Fellow:** Reproductive Endocrinology, Bellevue Hosp Ctr-NYU 1986; **Fac Appt:** Asst Clin Prof ObG, Columbia P&S

Fairfield

Witt, Barry R MD (RE) - **Spec Exp:** Infertility-IVF; **Hospital:** Greenwich Hosp, NYU Med Ctr (page 102); **Address:** 55 Holly Hill Ln, Ste 270, Greenwich, CT 06830; **Phone:** 203-863-2990; **Board Cert:** Obstetrics & Gynecology 2003; Reproductive Endocrinology 2003; **Med School:** NY Med Coll 1984; **Resid:** Obstetrics & Gynecology, Montefiore-Weiler/Einstein Med Ctr 1988; **Fellow:** Reproductive Endocrinology, Tulane Univ Med Ctr 1990; **Fac Appt:** Assoc Prof ObG, NYU Sch Med

RHEUMATOLOGY

Danehower, Richard L MD (Rhu) - **Spec Exp:** Rheumatoid Arthritis; Temporal Arteritis; Psoriatic Arthritis; Osteoarthritis; **Hospital:** Greenwich Hosp; **Address:** 49 Lake Ave, Greenwich, CT 06830-4501; **Phone:** 203-869-5715; **Board Cert:** Internal Medicine 1971; Rheumatology 1974; **Med School:** Univ Pennsylvania 1965; **Resid:** Internal Medicine, Univ Michigan Med Ctr 1969; **Fellow:** Rheumatology, Univ Michigan Med Ctr 1970; **Fac Appt:** Asst Clin Prof Med, Yale Univ

Miller, Kenneth Alan MD (Rhu) - **Spec Exp:** Rheumatoid Arthritis; Osteoporosis; Lyme Disease; **Hospital:** Danbury Hosp, New Milford Hosp; **Address:** 27 Hospital Ave, Ste 205, Danbury, CT 06810-5954; **Phone:** 203-794-0599; **Board Cert:** Internal Medicine 1978; Rheumatology 1980; **Med School:** Rush Med Coll 1975; **Resid:** Internal Medicine, GW Univ Hosp 1978; **Fellow:** Rheumatology, Worcester City Hosp-Univ Mass 1980

Nascimento, Joao M A MD (Rhu) - **Spec Exp:** Rheumatoid Arthritis; Lupus/SLE; Psoriatic Arthritis; **Hospital:** St Vincent's Med Ctr - Bridgeport, Bridgeport Hosp; **Address:** 3203 Main St, Bridgeport, CT 06606-4225; **Phone:** 203-371-6969; **Board Cert:** Internal Medicine 1989; Rheumatology 2002; **Med School:** Portugal 1984; **Resid:** Internal Medicine, Bridgeport Hosp 1989; **Fellow:** Rheumatology, Brown Univ Med Ctr 1991; **Fac Appt:** Asst Clin Prof Med, Columbia P&S

SURGERY

Bull, Sherman MD (S) - **Spec Exp:** Breast Surgery; Cancer Surgery; Laparoscopic Cholecystectomy; Hernia; **Hospital:** Stamford Hosp; **Address:** 22 Long Ridge Rd, Ste 2, Stamford, CT 06905-3803; **Phone:** 203-327-2777; **Board Cert:** Surgery 1969; **Med School:** Columbia P&S 1962; **Resid:** Surgery, Columbia-Presby Med Ctr 1967; **Fellow:** Pediatric Surgery, Babies Hosp 1969; **Fac Appt:** Asst Clin Prof S, Columbia P&S

McWhorter, Philip MD (S) - **Hospital:** Greenwich Hosp; **Address:** 77 Lafayette Pl, Ste 301, Greenwich, CT 06830; **Phone:** 203-863-4300; **Board Cert:** Surgery 1997; **Med School:** Cornell Univ-Weill Med Coll 1973; **Resid:** Surgery, NY Hosp 1977

Passeri, Daniel J MD (S) - **Spec Exp:** Cancer Surgery; Laparoscopic Surgery; **Hospital:** St Vincent's Med Ctr - Bridgeport, Bridgeport Hosp; **Address:** 888 White Plains Rd Fl 2 - Ste 206, Trumbull, CT 06611-4552; **Phone:** 203-459-2666; **Board Cert:** Surgery 2000; **Med School:** Yale Univ 1975; **Resid:** Yale-New Haven Hosp 1980; **Fac Appt:** Assoc Clin Prof S, NY Med Coll

Ward, Barbara MD (S) - **Spec Exp:** Breast Cancer; Breast Disease; **Hospital:** Greenwich Hosp; **Address:** 77 Lafayette Pl, Ste 301, Greenwich, CT 06830-5426; **Phone:** 203-863-4250; **Board Cert:** Surgery 2002; **Med School:** Temple Univ 1983; **Resid:** Surgery, Yale-New Haven Hosp 1990; **Fellow:** Surgical Oncology, Natl Cancer Inst 1987; **Fac Appt:** Assoc Clin Prof S, Yale Univ

Wasson, Dennis MD (S) - **Spec Exp:** Breast Surgery; **Hospital:** Bridgeport Hosp; **Address:** 2900 Main St, Ste 1F, Stratford, CT 06614; **Phone:** 203-378-4500; **Board Cert:** Surgery 1968; **Med School:** Ireland 1957; **Resid:** Surgery, Soston Univ Med Ctr 1966; Surgery, Royal Victoria Hosp 1963; **Fellow:** Surgery, Harvard Surgery Svcs 1964

THORACIC SURGERY

De France, John MD (TS) - **Spec Exp:** Lung Cancer; Aneurysm-Aortic; Peripheral Vascular Disease; **Hospital:** Danbury Hosp; **Address:** 27 Hospital Ave, Ste 405, Danbury, CT 06810-5907; **Phone:** 203-797-1811; **Board Cert:** Surgery 1975; Thoracic Surgery 1995; **Med School:** Jefferson Med Coll 1969; **Resid:** Surgery, Polyclinic Hosp 1974; Thoracic Surgery, VA Med Ctr 1976

Frymus, Michael MD (TS) - **Spec Exp:** Minimally Invasive Cardiac Surgery; Heart Valve Surgery; Coronary Revascularization; **Hospital:** Danbury Hosp; **Address:** Danbury Hosp, Dept Cardiothoracic Surg, 24 Hospital Ave, Danbury, CT 06810; **Phone:** 203-739-6950; **Board Cert:** Thoracic Surgery 2001; Surgery 1997; **Med School:** Georgetown Univ 1981; **Resid:** Surgery, Waterbury Hosp 1986; Cardiothoracic Surgery, Montefiore Med Ctr 1989

Lettera, James V MD (TS) - **Spec Exp:** Lung Cancer; Minimally Invasive Thoracic Surgery; **Hospital:** St Vincent's Med Ctr - Bridgeport, Bridgeport Hosp; **Address:** 52 Beach Rd, Ste 207, Fairfield, CT 06824; **Phone:** 203-255-2003; **Board Cert:** Thoracic Surgery 2003; **Med School:** Georgetown Univ 1977; **Resid:** Surgery, St Vincent's Hosp Med Ctr 1982; Thoracic Surgery, Jackson Meml Hosp 1984; **Fac Appt:** Asst Clin Prof S, NY Med Coll

Rose, Daniel MD (TS) - **Spec Exp:** Minimally Invasive Surgery; Cardiothoracic Surgery; **Hospital:** St Vincent's Med Ctr - Bridgeport, Bridgeport Hosp; **Address:** 2800 Main St, Bridgeport, CT 06606; **Phone:** 203-576-5708; **Board Cert:** Thoracic Surgery 2001; **Med School:** Univ Colorado 1974; **Resid:** Surgery, Bellevue Hosp-NYU 1979; Cardiovascular Surgery, Natl Heart & Lung Inst 1980; **Fellow:** Cardiothoracic Surgery, Bellevue Hosp-NYU 1982; **Fac Appt:** Asst Prof S, SUNY Downstate

Sanchez, Juan A MD (TS) - **Spec Exp:** Mitral Valve Surgery; Coronary Artery Surgery; Esophageal Surgery; Lung Surgery; **Hospital:** Bridgeport Hosp, St Vincent's Med Ctr - Bridgeport; **Address:** Box 860, Monroe, CT 06468; **Phone:** 203-375-0658; **Board Cert:** Thoracic Surgery 2004; **Med School:** Univ Fla Coll Med 1984; **Resid:** Surgery, Georgetown Univ 1989; Thoracic Surgery, Yale-New Haven Hosp 1993; **Fellow:** Research, Columbia-Presby Med Ctr 1990; Transplant Surgery, Yale-New Haven Hosp 1991

Walker, Michael J MD (TS) - **Spec Exp:** Lung Cancer; Minimally Invasive Surgery; Clinical Trials; **Hospital:** Danbury Hosp; **Address:** Danbury Hosp, 27 Hospital Ave, Ste 405, Danbury, CT 06810; **Phone:** 203-797-1811; **Board Cert:** Thoracic Surgery 2004; **Med School:** Jefferson Med Coll 1988; **Resid:** Surgery, Jefferson Hosp 1993; **Fellow:** Cardiothoracic Surgery, U Washington Med Ctr 1995; **Fac Appt:** Asst Clin Prof S, NY Med Coll

UROLOGY

Andriani, Rudy MD (U) - **Spec Exp:** Urologic Cancer; Kidney Stones; Incontinence; **Hospital:** Stamford Hosp, Greenwich Hosp; **Address:** 166 W Broad St, Ste 404, Stamford, CT 06902-3661; **Phone:** 203-356-9692; **Board Cert:** Urology 1999; **Med School:** NY Med Coll 1981; **Resid:** Surgery, St Vincent's Hosp & Med Ctr 1983; Urology, Duke U Med Ctr 1987; **Fac Appt:** Asst Clin Prof S, Columbia P&S

Burbige, Kevin MD (U) - **Spec Exp:** Hypospadias; Birth Defects; Urinary Reconstruction-Pediatric; **Hospital:** NY-Presby Hosp (page 100), Lenox Hill Hosp (page 94); **Address:** The Tully Health Center, 32 Strawberry Hill Ct, Stamford, CT 06902; **Phone:** 877-359-4211; **Board Cert:** Urology 1984; **Med School:** Wayne State Univ 1976; **Resid:** Surgery, Boston Univ Med Ctr 1978; Urology, Boston Univ Med Ctr 1981; **Fellow:** Pediatric Urology, Childrens Hosp 1982; **Fac Appt:** Assoc Prof U, Columbia P&S

Ranta, Jeffrey A MD (U) - **Spec Exp:** Prostate Cancer; Bladder Cancer; Kidney Stones; **Hospital:** Greenwich Hosp, Stamford Hosp; **Address:** 49 Lake Ave, Greenwich, CT 06830-4520; **Phone:** 203-869-1285; **Board Cert:** Urology 2004; **Med School:** Georgetown Univ 1979; **Resid:** Surgery, Georgetown Univ Hosp 1981; Urology, Lahey Clinic 1984

Viner, Nicholas MD (U) - **Spec Exp:** Prostate Cancer; Kidney Stones; Bladder Cancer; **Hospital:** Bridgeport Hosp, St Vincent's Med Ctr - Bridgeport; **Address:** 160 Hawley Ln, Trumbull, CT 06611-6058; **Phone:** 203-375-3456; **Board Cert:** Urology 1977; **Med School:** Vanderbilt Univ 1968; **Resid:** Surgery, Greenwich Hosp 1970; Urology, Vanderbilt Univ Hosp 1974

Waxberg, Jonathan MD (U) - **Spec Exp:** Prostate Cancer; Minimally Invasive Surgery; Erectile Dysfunction; **Hospital:** Stamford Hosp, Greenwich Hosp; **Address:** 35 Hoyt St, Stamford, CT 06905-5602; **Phone:** 203-324-2268; **Board Cert:** Urology 1999; **Med School:** Univ Cincinnati 1980; **Resid:** Urology, Maimonides Med Ctr 1986

Zuckerman, Howard L MD (U) - **Spec Exp:** Incontinence; Prostate Cancer; Pediatric Urology; **Hospital:** Bridgeport Hosp, St Vincent's Med Ctr - Bridgeport; **Address:** 160 Hawley Ln Ste 002 Bldg, Trumbull, CT 06611-5300; **Phone:** 203-375-3456; **Board Cert:** Urology 1977; **Med School:** St Louis Univ 1967; **Resid:** Surgery, Med Coll Virginia Hosp 1969; Urology, Albert Einstein Coll Med 1975

VASCULAR & INTERVENTIONAL RADIOLOGY

Hamet, Marc R MD (VIR) - **Spec Exp:** Osteoporosis Spine-Vertebroplasty; Uterine Fibroid Embolization; Endovascular Surgery; Carotid Artery Stents; **Hospital:** Stamford Hosp; **Address:** Stamford Radiological Assoc, PO Box 1092, Stamford, CT 06904-1092; **Phone:** 203-276-7860; **Board Cert:** Diagnostic Radiology 1995; Vascular & Interventional Radiology 1998; Neuroradiology 1999; **Med School:** Univ MD Sch Med 1991; **Resid:** Diagnostic Radiology, Univ Maryland Med Sys 1995; **Fellow:** Neuroradiology, Univ Maryland Med Sys 1996; Interventional Radiology, Johns Hopkins Univ Hosp 1998

VASCULAR SURGERY

Dietzek, Alan M MD (VascS) - **Spec Exp:** Aneurysm-Aortic; Minimally Invasive Vascular Surgery; Arterial Bypass Surgery-Leg; Carotid Artery Surgery; **Hospital:** Danbury Hosp; **Address:** 69 Sandpit Rd, Ste 204, Danbury, CT 06810; **Phone:** 203-798-6986; **Board Cert:** Surgery 1999; Vascular Surgery 2001; **Med School:** Loyola Univ-Stritch Sch Med 1983; **Resid:** Surgery, LI Jewish Med Ctr 1988; **Fellow:** Vascular Surgery, Montefiore Med Ctr 1990; **Fac Appt:** Asst Clin Prof VascS, NYU Sch Med

New Haven

New Haven

ADDICTION PSYCHIATRY

Schottenfeld, Richard MD (AdP) - **Spec Exp:** Drug Abuse; Alcohol Abuse; **Hospital:** Yale - New Haven Hosp (page 984); **Address:** Connecticut Mental Health Ctr, 34 Park St, rm S-204, New Haven, CT 06519; **Phone:** 203-974-7349; **Board Cert:** Psychiatry 1984; Addiction Psychiatry 1994; **Med School:** Yale Univ 1976; **Resid:** Psychiatry, Yale Psych Inst 1982; **Fellow:** Epidemiology, Yale Univ 1984; **Fac Appt:** Assoc Prof Psyc, Yale Univ

ALLERGY & IMMUNOLOGY

Askenase, Philip MD (A&I) - **Spec Exp:** Asthma; Urticaria; Sinusitis; **Hospital:** Yale - New Haven Hosp (page 984); **Address:** PO Box 208013, New Haven, CT 06520-8013; **Phone:** 203-785-4143; **Board Cert:** Internal Medicine 1973; Allergy & Immunology 1974; **Med School:** Yale Univ 1965; **Resid:** Internal Medicine, Boston City Hosp 1967; **Fellow:** Allergy & Immunology, Yale Univ 1971; **Fac Appt:** Prof Med, Yale Univ

Kaufman, Richard E MD (A&I) - **Spec Exp:** Asthma; Urticaria; Allergy; **Hospital:** Yale - New Haven Hosp (page 984), Hosp of St Raphael; **Address:** 960 Main St, Branford, CT 06405; **Phone:** 203-488-6358; **Board Cert:** Internal Medicine 1976; Allergy & Immunology 1979; **Med School:** Yale Univ 1971; **Resid:** Internal Medicine, Yale-New Haven Hosp 1976; **Fellow:** Immunology, Yale-New Haven Hosp 1978; **Fac Appt:** Assoc Clin Prof Med, Yale Univ

CARDIAC ELECTROPHYSIOLOGY

Batsford, William P MD (CE) - **Spec Exp:** Arrhythmias; **Hospital:** Yale - New Haven Hosp (page 984); **Address:** Yale Univ Sch Med, Section Cardiovascular Med, 333 Cedar St, 3 FMP, Box 208017, New Haven, CT 06520-8017; **Phone:** 203-785-4126; **Board Cert:** Internal Medicine 1972; Cardiovascular Disease 1977; **Med School:** Albany Med Coll 1969; **Resid:** Internal Medicine, Hosp Univ Penn 1972; **Fac Appt:** Prof Med, Yale Univ

CARDIOVASCULAR DISEASE

Cabin, Henry S MD (Cv) - **Spec Exp:** Interventional Cardiology; Cardiac Catheterization; **Hospital:** Yale - New Haven Hosp (page 984); **Address:** PO Box 208017, New Haven, CT 06520-8017; **Phone:** 203-785-4129; **Board Cert:** Internal Medicine 1978; Cardiovascular Disease 1983; Interventional Cardiology 2000; **Med School:** Yale Univ 1975; **Resid:** Internal Medicine, Yale-New Haven Hosp 1978; **Fellow:** Internal Medicine, Natl Heart Lung and Blood Inst 1981; Cardiovascular Disease, Yale New Haven Hosp 1982; **Fac Appt:** Prof Med, Yale Univ

Cleman, Michael W MD (Cv) - **Spec Exp:** Interventional Cardiology; Angioplasty; Cardiac Catheterization; **Hospital:** Yale - New Haven Hosp (page 984), Hosp of St Raphael; **Address:** 333 Cedar St, Fitkin Fl 3, Box 208017, New Haven, CT 06520-8017; **Phone:** 203-785-4129; **Board Cert:** Internal Medicine 1980; Cardiovascular Disease 1985; Interventional Cardiology 2000; **Med School:** Johns Hopkins Univ 1977; **Resid:** Internal Medicine, Univ Fla-Shands Hosp 1980; **Fellow:** Cardiovascular Disease, Yale-New Haven Hosp 1981; **Fac Appt:** Prof Med, Yale Univ

Cohen, Lawrence S MD (Cv) - **Spec Exp:** Coronary Artery Disease; Heart Valve Disease; Geriatric Cardiology; **Hospital:** Yale - New Haven Hosp (page 984); **Address:** Yale Univ Sch Med - Cardiology, 333 Cedar St, Ste FMP 313, Box 208017, New Haven, CT 06520-8017; **Phone:** 203-785-4128; **Board Cert:** Internal Medicine 1966; Cardiovascular Disease 1967; **Med School:** NYU Sch Med 1958; **Resid:** Internal Medicine, Yale-New Haven Hosp 1960; Internal Medicine, Yale-New Haven Hosp 1965; **Fellow:** Research, Peter Bent Brigham Hosp 1964; **Fac Appt:** Prof Med, Yale Univ

Freed, Lisa A MD (Cv) - **Spec Exp:** Heart Disease in Women; Mitral Valve Prolapse; **Hospital:** Yale - New Haven Hosp (page 984); **Address:** The Cardiology Group, 60 Temple St, Ste 6C, New Haven, CT 06510; **Phone:** 203-773-3055; **Board Cert:** Internal Medicine 1995; Cardiovascular Disease 1999; **Med School:** Johns Hopkins Univ 1992; **Resid:** Internal Medicine, New York Hosp-Cornell Med Ctr 1995; **Fellow:** Cardiovascular Disease, Mass Genl Hosp 1998; Cardiovascular Disease, Framingham Heart Study 1999

Zaret, Barry L MD (Cv) - **Spec Exp:** Nuclear Cardiology; Heart Failure; Coronary Artery Disease; **Hospital:** Yale - New Haven Hosp (page 984); **Address:** 333 Cedar St, 3-FMP, New Haven, CT 06520-8017; **Phone:** 203-785-4127; **Board Cert:** Internal Medicine 1973; Cardiovascular Disease 1973; **Med School:** NYU Sch Med 1966; **Resid:** Internal Medicine, Bellevue Hosp Ctr 1969; **Fellow:** Cardiovascular Disease, Johns Hopkins Hosp 1971; **Fac Appt:** Prof Med, Yale Univ

CHILD & ADOLESCENT PSYCHIATRY

Gammon, G Davis MD (ChAP) - **Hospital:** Yale - New Haven Hosp (page 984); **Address:** 33 Edgehill Terr, Hamden, CT 06517; **Phone:** 203-865-6540; **Board Cert:** Psychiatry 1981; Child & Adolescent Psychiatry 1992; **Med School:** Temple Univ 1976; **Resid:** Psychiatry, Yale-New Haven Hosp 1980; Child & Adolescent Psychiatry, Yale-New Haven Hosp 1982; **Fellow:** Epidemiology, Yale-New Haven Hosp 1984

King, Robert A MD (ChAP) - **Spec Exp:** Tourette's Syndrome; Obsessive-Compulsive Disorder; Psychoanalysis; **Hospital:** Yale - New Haven Hosp (page 984); **Address:** 230 S Frontage Rd, Box 207900, New Haven, CT 06519-1124; **Phone:** 203-785-5880; **Board Cert:** Psychiatry 1974; Child & Adolescent Psychiatry 1981; **Med School:** Harvard Med Sch 1968; **Resid:** Pediatrics, Chldns Hosp 1969; Psychiatry, Mass Mental Hlth Ctr 1971; **Fellow:** Child Psychiatry, Chldns Hosp 1972; Child Psychiatry, Chldns Hosp Natl Med Ctr 1974; **Fac Appt:** Prof Psyc, Yale Univ

Leckman, James F MD (ChAP) - **Spec Exp:** Tourette's Syndrome; Obsessive-Compulsive Disorder; Autism; **Hospital:** Yale - New Haven Hosp (page 984); **Address:** Yale Child Study Ctr, 230 S Frontage Rd, Box 207900, New Haven, CT 06520; **Phone:** 203-785-7971; **Board Cert:** Psychiatry 1980; Child & Adolescent Psychiatry 1982; **Med School:** Univ New Mexico 1973; **Resid:** Psychiatry, Yale Univ 1979; Child & Adolescent Psychiatry, Yale Chld Stdy Ctr 1980; **Fellow:** Psychiatry, Natl Inst Mental Hlth 1976; **Fac Appt:** Prof Psyc, Yale Univ

Lewis, Dorothy Otnow MD (ChAP) - **Spec Exp:** Dissociative Disorders; Aggression Disorders; **Hospital:** Yale - New Haven Hosp (page 984); **Address:** 100 York St, New Haven, CT 06511; **Phone:** 203-624-3933; **Board Cert:** Psychiatry 1972; **Med School:** Yale Univ 1963; **Resid:** Psychiatry, Yale-New Haven Hosp 1967; **Fellow:** Child & Adolescent Psychiatry, Yale-New Haven Hosp 1969; **Fac Appt:** Asst Prof Psyc, Yale Univ

Madigan, Janet MD (ChAP) - **Spec Exp:** Developmental Disorders; Psychotherapy; Psychoanalysis; **Hospital:** Yale - New Haven Hosp (page 984); **Address:** 240 Bradley St, New Haven, CT 06510-1103; **Phone:** 203-787-5420; **Board Cert:** Psychiatry 1982; Child & Adolescent Psychiatry 1986; **Med School:** NY Med Coll 1977; **Resid:** Psychiatry, Yale-New Haven Hosp 1981; **Fellow:** Child & Adolescent Psychiatry, Yale-New Haven Hosp 1983; **Fac Appt:** Asst Clin Prof Psyc, Yale Univ

Volkmar, Fred R MD (ChAP) - **Spec Exp:** Autism; Asperger's Syndrome; Developmental Disorders; Mental Retardation; **Hospital:** Yale - New Haven Hosp (page 984); **Address:** Yale Child Study Ctr, 230 S Frontage Rd, Box 207900, New Haven, CT 06519-1124; **Phone:** 203-785-2510; **Board Cert:** Psychiatry 1981; Child & Adolescent Psychiatry 1988; **Med School:** Stanford Univ 1976; **Resid:** Psychiatry, Stanford Univ 1980; Child & Adolescent Psychiatry, Yale Univ Child Study Ctr 1982; **Fac Appt:** Prof Psyc, Yale Univ

CHILD NEUROLOGY

Shaywitz, Bennett A MD (ChiN) - **Spec Exp:** Learning Disorders; Dyslexia; Headache; **Hospital:** Yale - New Haven Hosp (page 984); **Address:** Yale Univ Sch Med, Dept Peds, 333 Cedar St, LMP-3089, New Haven, CT 06520; **Phone:** 203-785-4641; **Board Cert:** Pediatrics 1968; Child Neurology 1973; **Med School:** Washington Univ, St Louis 1963; **Resid:** Pediatrics, Bronx Muni Hosp Ctr 1967; **Fellow:** Child Neurology, Albert Einstein Coll Med 1970; **Fac Appt:** Prof Ped, Yale Univ

CLINICAL GENETICS

Mahoney, Maurice J MD (CG) - **Spec Exp:** Fetal Therapy; Prenatal Diagnosis; **Hospital:** Yale - New Haven Hosp (page 984); **Address:** Yale Genetics Consultation Serv, 333 Cedar St, rm WWW330, New Haven, CT 06520-8005; **Phone:** 203-785-2661; **Board Cert:** Pediatrics 1967; Clinical Genetics 1982; Clinical Biochemical Genetics 1982; **Med School:** Univ Pittsburgh 1962; **Resid:** Pediatrics, Johns Hopkins Hosp 1965; Pediatrics, Childrens Hosp 1966; **Fellow:** Clinical Genetics, Yale Univ Sch Med 1970; **Fac Appt:** Prof CG, Yale Univ

Seashore, Margretta MD (CG) - **Spec Exp:** Inherited Metabolic Disorders; **Hospital:** Yale - New Haven Hosp (page 984); **Address:** Yale Univ Sch Med, Dept Genetics, 333 Cedar St, rm 305, Box 208005, New Haven, CT 06520-8005; **Phone:** 203-785-2660; **Board Cert:** Pediatrics 1970; Clinical Biochemical Genetics 1982; Clinical Genetics 1982; **Med School:** Yale Univ 1965; **Resid:** Pediatrics, Yale-New Haven Hosp 1968; **Fellow:** Clinical Genetics, Yale-New Haven Hosp 1970; **Fac Appt:** Prof CG, Yale Univ

COLON & RECTAL SURGERY

Longo, Walter E MD (CRS) - **Spec Exp:** Colon & Rectal Cancer; Gastrointestinal Surgery; Inflammatory Bowel Disease; **Hospital:** Yale - New Haven Hosp (page 984); **Address:** Yale Univ Sch Med, Dept Surg, Box 208062, New Haven, CT 06520-8062; **Phone:** 203-785-2616; **Board Cert:** Surgery 2001; Colon & Rectal Surgery 2006; **Med School:** NY Med Coll 1984; **Resid:** Surgery, Yale-New Haven Hosp 1990; **Fellow:** Research, Yale-New Haven Hosp 1988; Colon & Rectal Surgery, Cleveland Clinic 1991; **Fac Appt:** Prof S, Yale Univ

DERMATOLOGY

Bolognia, Jean MD (D) - **Spec Exp:** Melanoma; Skin Cancer; **Hospital:** Yale - New Haven Hosp (page 984); **Address:** 2 Church St S, Ste 305, New Haven, CT 06519; **Phone:** 203-789-1249; **Board Cert:** Dermatology 1985; **Med School:** Yale Univ 1980; **Resid:** Internal Medicine, Yale-New Haven Hosp 1982; Dermatology, Yale-New Haven Hosp 1985; **Fellow:** Dermatology, Yale Univ 1987; **Fac Appt:** Prof D, Yale Univ

Braverman, Irwin MD (D) - **Spec Exp:** Psoriasis; Lupus/SLE; Cutaneous Lymphoma; **Hospital:** Yale - New Haven Hosp (page 984); **Address:** Yale Dermatology, 2 Church St S, Ste 305, New Haven, CT 06519; **Phone:** 203-789-1249; **Board Cert:** Dermatology 1963; Dermatopathology 1982; **Med School:** Yale Univ 1955; **Resid:** Internal Medicine, Yale-New Haven Hosp 1956; Internal Medicine, Yale-New Haven Hosp 1959; **Fellow:** Dermatology, Yale-New Haven Hosp 1962; **Fac Appt:** Prof D, Yale Univ

Edelson, Richard MD (D) - **Spec Exp:** Cutaneous Lymphoma; Immune Deficiency-Skin Disorders; **Hospital:** Yale - New Haven Hosp (page 984); **Address:** 800 Howard Ave, New Haven, CT 06519-1369; **Phone:** 203-789-1249; **Board Cert:** Dermatology 1977; **Med School:** Yale Univ 1970; **Resid:** Dermatology, Mass Genl Hosp 1972; Dermatology, Natl Inst Hlth 1975; **Fac Appt:** Prof D, Yale Univ

Heald, Peter MD (D) - **Spec Exp:** Cutaneous Lymphoma; **Hospital:** Yale - New Haven Hosp (page 984); **Address:** 2 Church St S, Ste 305, New Haven, CT 06519; **Phone:** 203-789-1249; **Board Cert:** Internal Medicine 1982; Dermatology 1984; Clinical & Laboratory Dematologic Immunology 1987; **Med School:** Duke Univ 1979; **Resid:** Internal Medicine, Duke Univ Med Ctr; **Fellow:** Dermatology, Hosp Univ Penn

Leffell, David J MD (D) - **Spec Exp:** Mohs' Surgery; Melanoma; Skin Cancer; Skin Laser Surgery; **Hospital:** Yale - New Haven Hosp (page 984), Hosp of St Raphael; **Address:** 40 Temple St, Ste 5A, New Haven, CT 06510; **Phone:** 203-785-3466; **Board Cert:** Internal Medicine 1984; Dermatology 1987; **Med School:** McGill Univ 1981; **Resid:** Internal Medicine, New York Hosp 1984; Dermatology, Yale-New Haven Hosp 1986; **Fellow:** Dermatology, Yale Univ 1987; Dermatologic Surgery, Univ Michigan Med Ctr 1988; **Fac Appt:** Prof D, Yale Univ

Savin, Ronald MD (D) - **Spec Exp:** Hair Loss; Skin Tumors; Psoriasis; **Hospital:** Yale - New Haven Hosp (page 984), Hosp of St Raphael; **Address:** 134 Park St, New Haven, CT 06511-5416; **Phone:** 203-865-6143; **Board Cert:** Dermatology 1968; **Med School:** Univ Fla Coll Med 1961; **Resid:** Dermatology, Yale-New Haven Hosp 1965; **Fac Appt:** Clin Prof D, Yale Univ

DIAGNOSTIC RADIOLOGY

McCarthy, Shirley M MD/PhD (DR) - **Spec Exp:** Gynecologic Cancer; Pelvic Imaging; Uterine Fibroids; **Hospital:** Yale - New Haven Hosp (page 984); **Address:** Yale-New Haven Hosp, Tompkins East-2, 789 Howard Ave, New Haven, CT 06519; **Phone:** 203-785-5251; **Board Cert:** Diagnostic Radiology 1983; **Med School:** Yale Univ 1979; **Resid:** Radiology, Yale-New Haven Hosp 1983; **Fellow:** Cross Sectional Imaging, UCSF Med Ctr 1984; **Fac Appt:** Prof Rad, Yale Univ

McClennan, Bruce MD (DR) - **Spec Exp:** Genitourinary Imaging; Abdominal Imaging; **Hospital:** Yale - New Haven Hosp (page 984); **Address:** Yale-New Haven Hosp, Dept Radiology, 333 Cedar St, TE-2, New Haven, CT 06520; **Phone:** 203-785-2384; **Board Cert:** Diagnostic Radiology 1972; **Med School:** SUNY Upstate Med Univ 1967; **Resid:** Radiology, Mary Imogene Bassett Hosp 1968; **Fellow:** Radiology, Columbia-Presby Med Ctr 1971; **Fac Appt:** Prof Rad, Yale Univ

Weinreb, Jeffrey C MD (DR) - **Spec Exp:** MRI; Breast Cancer; Abdominal Imaging; **Hospital:** Yale - New Haven Hosp (page 984); **Address:** Yale Univ Sch Medicine, Dept Radiology, 333 Cedar St, rm MRC147, Box 208042, New Haven, CT 06520-8042; **Phone:** 203-785-5913; **Board Cert:** Diagnostic Radiology 1983; **Med School:** Mount Sinai Sch Med 1978; **Resid:** Diagnostic Radiology, LI Jewish Med Ctr 1982; **Fellow:** Ultrasound/CT, Hosp Univ Penn 1983; **Fac Appt:** Prof Rad, Yale Univ

ENDOCRINOLOGY, DIABETES & METABOLISM

Inzucchi, Sylvio MD (EDM) - **Spec Exp:** Diabetes; Pituitary Disorders; Growth Hormone Therapy-Adult; **Hospital:** Yale - New Haven Hosp (page 984); **Address:** Yale Univ Sch Med, Div Endocrinology, Box 208020, New Haven, CT 06520-8020; **Phone:** 203-737-1932; **Board Cert:** Internal Medicine 1988; Endocrinology, Diabetes & Metabolism 1995; **Med School:** Harvard Med Sch 1985; **Resid:** Internal Medicine, Yale New-Haven Hosp 1988; **Fellow:** Endocrinology, Diabetes & Metabolism, Yale Univ Sch Med 1994; **Fac Appt:** Prof Med, Yale Univ

Sherwin, Robert MD (EDM) - **Spec Exp:** Diabetes; **Hospital:** Yale - New Haven Hosp (page 984); **Address:** Yale Univ Sch Med, Sect Endocrinology, 333 Cedar St, Box 208020, New Haven, CT 06520-8020; **Phone:** 203-785-4183; **Board Cert:** Internal Medicine 1972; **Med School:** Albert Einstein Coll Med 1967; **Resid:** Internal Medicine, Mt Sinai Hosp 1969; Internal Medicine, Mt Sinai Hosp 1972; **Fellow:** Metabolism, Yale-New Haven Hosp 1973; **Fac Appt:** Prof Med, Yale Univ

Wysolmerski, John J MD (EDM) - **Spec Exp:** Metabolic Bone Disease; Osteoporosis; Parathyroid Disorders; **Hospital:** Yale - New Haven Hosp (page 984); **Address:** Yale Sch Med - Div Endocrinology, Box 208020, New Haven, CT 06520-8020; **Phone:** 203-737-1932; **Board Cert:** Internal Medicine 1989; Endocrinology, Diabetes & Metabolism 1993; **Med School:** Yale Univ 1986; **Resid:** Internal Medicine, New England Med Ctr 1989; **Fellow:** Endocrinology, Yale Univ Sch Med 1993; **Fac Appt:** Assoc Prof Med, Yale Univ

GERIATRIC MEDICINE

Cooney Jr, Leo M MD (Ger) - **Spec Exp:** Rheumatology; **Hospital:** Yale - New Haven Hosp (page 984); **Address:** 20 York St, Tompkins 17, New Haven, CT 06520; **Phone:** 203-688-2204; **Board Cert:** Internal Medicine 1974; Rheumatology 1978; Geriatric Medicine 2000; **Med School:** Yale Univ 1969; **Resid:** Internal Medicine, Boston City Hosp 1971; Internal Medicine, Boston City Hosp 1974; **Fellow:** Rheumatology, Boston Med Ctr 1975; **Fac Appt:** Prof Med, Yale Univ

Tinetti, Mary E MD (Ger) - **Spec Exp:** Falls in the Elderly; Geriatric Functional Assessment; **Hospital:** Yale - New Haven Hosp (page 984); **Address:** Yale-New Haven Hosp, Adler Geriatric Ctr, 789 Howard Ave, Tompkins Basement, Box 208057, New Haven, CT 06510; **Phone:** 203-688-6361; **Board Cert:** Internal Medicine 1981; Geriatric Medicine 1988; **Med School:** Univ Mich Med Sch 1978; **Resid:** Internal Medicine, Univ Minnesota 1981; **Fellow:** Geriatric Medicine, Univ Rochester 1984; **Fac Appt:** Prof Med, Yale Univ

GERIATRIC PSYCHIATRY

van Dyck, Christopher H MD (GerPsy) - **Spec Exp:** Alzheimer's Disease; Neuroimaging; **Hospital:** Yale - New Haven Hosp (page 984); **Address:** One Church St, Ste 600, New Haven, CT 06510-3330; **Phone:** 203-764-8100; **Board Cert:** Psychiatry 1991; Geriatric Psychiatry 2005; **Med School:** Northwestern Univ 1984; **Resid:** Psychiatry, Yale-New Haven Hosp 1988; **Fellow:** Geriatric Psychiatry, Yale-New Haven Hosp 1990; **Fac Appt:** Assoc Prof Psyc, Yale Univ

GYNECOLOGIC ONCOLOGY

Rutherford, Thomas MD (GO) - **Spec Exp:** Ovarian Cancer; Uterine Cancer; **Hospital:** Yale - New Haven Hosp (page 984); **Address:** Yale Univ Sch Med Dept Ob-Gyn, 333 Cedar St, Box 208063, New Haven, CT 06520; **Phone:** 203-785-6301; **Board Cert:** Obstetrics & Gynecology 1997; Gynecologic Oncology 2000; **Med School:** Med Coll OH 1989; **Resid:** Obstetrics & Gynecology, Cooper Hosp MC-UMDNJ 1993; **Fellow:** Gynecologic Oncology, Yale Univ Sch Med 1995; **Fac Appt:** Assoc Prof ObG, Yale Univ

Schwartz, Peter E MD (GO) - **Spec Exp:** Ovarian Cancer; Uterine Cancer; Gynecologic Surgery-Complex; **Hospital:** Yale - New Haven Hosp (page 984), Hosp of St Raphael; **Address:** Yale Univ Sch Med, Dept Ob/Gyn, 333 Cedar St, rm FMB-316, New Haven, CT 06510-3289; **Phone:** 203-785-4014; **Board Cert:** Obstetrics & Gynecology 1973; Gynecologic Oncology 1979; **Med School:** Albert Einstein Coll Med 1966; **Resid:** Obstetrics & Gynecology, Yale-New Haven Hosp 1970; **Fellow:** Gynecologic Oncology, MD Anderson Cancer Ctr 1975; **Fac Appt:** Prof ObG, Yale Univ

HAND SURGERY

Thomson, J Grant MD (HS) - **Spec Exp:** Carpal Tunnel Syndrome; Hand Reconstruction; Microsurgery; **Hospital:** Yale - New Haven Hosp (page 984), Hosp of St Raphael; **Address:** Yale Plastic Surgery, 333 Cedar St, Box 208041, New Haven, CT 06520-8041; **Phone:** 203-737-5130; **Board Cert:** Hand Surgery 2004; Plastic Surgery 2004; **Med School:** McGill Univ 1983; **Resid:** Surgery, Montreal Genl Hosp 1988; Plastic Surgery, Montreal Genl Hosp 1990; **Fellow:** Hand Surgery, Barnes Jewish Hosp 1991; **Fac Appt:** Assoc Prof PlS, Yale Univ

HEMATOLOGY

Berliner, Nancy MD (Hem) - **Spec Exp:** Leukemia; Multiple Myeloma; Hodgkin's Disease; **Hospital:** Yale - New Haven Hosp (page 984); **Address:** Sect of Hematology, Dpt of Internal Med, 333 Cedar St, Box 208021, New Haven, CT 06520-8021; **Phone:** 203-785-4144; **Board Cert:** Internal Medicine 1982; Hematology 1984; **Med School:** Yale Univ 1979; **Resid:** Internal Medicine, Brigham Womens Hosp 1982; **Fellow:** Hematology, Brigham Womens Hosp 1985; **Fac Appt:** Prof Med, Yale Univ

Duffy, Thomas P MD (Hem) - **Spec Exp:** Mast Cell Diseases; Leukemia; Lymphoma; **Hospital:** Yale - New Haven Hosp (page 984); **Address:** Yale Univ, Sect Hematology, 333 Cedar St, rm 403-WWW, Box 208021, New Haven, CT 06520-8021; **Phone:** 203-785-4744; **Board Cert:** Internal Medicine 1972; Hematology 1974; **Med School:** Johns Hopkins Univ 1962; **Resid:** Internal Medicine, Johns Hopkins Hosp 1965; **Fellow:** Hematology, Johns Hopkins Hosp 1970; **Fac Appt:** Prof Med, Yale Univ

Forget, Bernard MD (Hem) - **Spec Exp:** Thalassemia; Hemolytic Anemia; **Hospital:** Yale - New Haven Hosp (page 984); **Address:** Yale Univ Sch Med, Hematology Sect, PO Box 208021, New Haven, CT 06520-8021; **Phone:** 203-785-4144; **Board Cert:** Internal Medicine 1971; Hematology 1973; **Med School:** McGill Univ 1963; **Resid:** Internal Medicine, Mass Genl Hosp 1965; Clinical Pathology, Mass Genl Hosp 1968; **Fellow:** Hematology, Peter Bent Brigham Hosp 1971; **Fac Appt:** Prof Med, Yale Univ

INFECTIOUS DISEASE

Andriole, Vincent MD (Inf) - **Spec Exp:** Infective Endocarditis; Urinary Tract Infections; Fungal Infections; **Hospital:** Yale - New Haven Hosp (page 984); **Address:** Yale Univ Dept Internal Medicine, 333 Cedar St, Box 208022, New Haven, CT 06520-8022; **Phone:** 203-785-4141; **Board Cert:** Internal Medicine 1964; Infectious Disease 1976; **Med School:** Yale Univ 1957; **Resid:** Internal Medicine, NC Meml Hosp-UNC 1959; **Fellow:** Infectious Disease, Natl Inst A&I 1961; Infectious Disease, Yale Univ Sch Med 1963; **Fac Appt:** Prof Med, Yale Univ

Quagliarello, Vincent MD (Inf) - **Spec Exp:** Meningitis; Pneumonia; Endocarditis; **Hospital:** Yale - New Haven Hosp (page 984); **Address:** Yale Univ Sch Med, TAC 169A, 300 Cedar St, New Haven, CT 06520-8022; **Phone:** 203-785-7570; **Board Cert:** Internal Medicine 1985; Infectious Disease 1989; **Med School:** Washington Univ, St Louis 1980; **Resid:** Internal Medicine, Yale-New Haven Hosp 1984; **Fellow:** Infectious Disease, Univ VA Hlth Sci Ctr 1987; **Fac Appt:** Prof Med, Yale Univ

INTERNAL MEDICINE

Barry, Michele MD (IM) - **Spec Exp:** Travel Medicine; Tropical Diseases; **Hospital:** Yale - New Haven Hosp (page 984); **Address:** 333 Cedar St, PO BOX 208025, New Haven, CT 06520-8025; **Phone:** 203-688-2476; **Board Cert:** Internal Medicine 1980; **Med School:** Albert Einstein Coll Med 1977; **Resid:** Internal Medicine, Yale-New Haven Hosp 1981; **Fellow:** Rheumatology, Yale-New Haven Hosp 1981; Tropical Medicine, Walter Reed AMC 1981; **Fac Appt:** Prof Med, Yale Univ

Eilbott, David J MD (IM) **PCP** - **Hospital:** Yale - New Haven Hosp (page 984), Hosp of St Raphael; **Address:** 500 E Main St, Ste 212, Branford, Ct 06405-2937; **Phone:** 203-481-5665; **Board Cert:** Internal Medicine 1986; **Med School:** Univ Rochester 1981; **Resid:** Internal Medicine, Waterbury Hosp 1985; **Fellow:** Infectious Disease, SUNY 1988; **Fac Appt:** Asst Clin Prof Med, Yale Univ

Kernan, Walter MD (IM) **PCP** - **Spec Exp:** Stroke; **Hospital:** Yale - New Haven Hosp (page 984); **Address:** 20 York St, New Haven, CT 06520-1744; **Phone:** 203-688-2984; **Board Cert:** Internal Medicine 1987; **Med School:** Dartmouth Med Sch 1984; **Resid:** Internal Medicine, Johns Hopkins Hosp 1987; **Fellow:** Internal Medicine, Yale New Haven Hosp 1989; **Fac Appt:** Prof Med, Yale Univ

O'Connor, Patrick MD (IM) **PCP** - **Spec Exp:** Substance Abuse; **Hospital:** Yale - New Haven Hosp (page 984); **Address:** Yale Univ Sch Med, PO Box 208025, New Haven, CT 06520-8025; **Phone:** 203-688-6532; **Board Cert:** Internal Medicine 1986; **Med School:** Albany Med Coll 1982; **Resid:** Internal Medicine, Univ Rochester 1985; **Fellow:** Internal Medicine, Yale-New Haven Hosp 1988; **Fac Appt:** Prof Med, Yale Univ

Wilson, Madeline S MD (IM) - **Hospital:** Yale - New Haven Hosp (page 984); **Address:** 789 Howard Ave, Ste Dana 3, New Haven, CT 06510; **Phone:** 203-785-7411; **Board Cert:** Internal Medicine 2002; **Med School:** Harvard Med Sch 1988; **Resid:** Internal Medicine, Yale-New Haven Hosp

INTERVENTIONAL CARDIOLOGY

Schoenfeld, Mark MD (IC) - **Spec Exp:** Arrhythmias; **Hospital:** Hosp of St Raphael; **Address:** 330 Orchard St, Ste 210, New Haven, CT 06511; **Phone:** 203-867-5400; **Board Cert:** Internal Medicine 1982; Cardiovascular Disease 1985; Cardiac Electrophysiology 2002; **Med School:** Harvard Med Sch 1979; **Resid:** Internal Medicine, Mass Genl Hosp 1982; **Fellow:** Cardiovascular Disease, Mass Genl Hosp 1985; Cardiac Electrophysiology, Mass Genl Hosp 1986; **Fac Appt:** Clin Prof Med, Yale Univ

MATERNAL & FETAL MEDICINE

Copel, Joshua MD (MF) - **Spec Exp:** Prenatal Diagnosis; Fetal Echocardiography; Pregnancy-High Risk; **Hospital:** Yale - New Haven Hosp (page 984); **Address:** Yale Univ Sch Med, Dept OB/GYN, 333 Cedar St, Box 208063, New Haven, CT 06520-8063; **Phone:** 203-785-2671; **Board Cert:** Obstetrics & Gynecology 1995; Maternal & Fetal Medicine 1995; **Med School:** Tufts Univ 1979; **Resid:** Obstetrics & Gynecology, Pennsylvania Hosp 1983; **Fellow:** Maternal & Fetal Medicine, Yale-New Haven Hosp 1985; **Fac Appt:** Prof ObG, Yale Univ

Lockwood, Charles MD (MF) - **Spec Exp:** Prematurity Prevention; Miscarriage-Recurrent; Multiple Gestation; **Hospital:** Yale - New Haven Hosp (page 984); **Address:** Yale Univ Sch Med, Dept Ob-Gyn, 333 Cedar St, rm FMB 335, New Haven, CT 06520-8063; **Phone:** 203-737-2970; **Board Cert:** Obstetrics & Gynecology 1997; Maternal & Fetal Medicine 1997; **Med School:** Univ Pennsylvania 1981; **Resid:** Obstetrics & Gynecology, Pennsylvania Hosp 1985; **Fellow:** Maternal & Fetal Medicine, Yale-New Haven Hosp 1987; Thrombosis, Mt Sinai Med Ctr 1991; **Fac Appt:** Prof ObG, Yale Univ

Magriples, Urania MD (MF) - **Spec Exp:** Pregnancy-High Risk; **Hospital:** Yale - New Haven Hosp (page 984); **Address:** Yale Univ Sch Med - Dept Ob/Gyn, 333 Cedar St, PO Box 208063, New Haven, CT 06520-8063; **Phone:** 203-785-3463; **Board Cert:** Obstetrics & Gynecology 1995; Maternal & Fetal Medicine 1999; **Med School:** Mount Sinai Sch Med 1987; **Resid:** Obstetrics & Gynecology, Yale-New Haven Hosp 1991; **Fellow:** Perinatal Medicine, Yale-New Haven Hosp 1994; **Fac Appt:** Assoc Prof ObG, Yale Univ

MEDICAL ONCOLOGY

Chu, Edward MD (Onc) - **Spec Exp:** Colon & Rectal Cancer; Gastrointestinal Cancer; Clinical Trials; **Hospital:** Yale - New Haven Hosp (page 984), VA Conn Hlthcre Sys; **Address:** Yale Cancer Ctr, 333 Cedar St, PO Box 208032, New Haven, CT 06520-8032; **Phone:** 203-785-6879; **Board Cert:** Internal Medicine 1986; Medical Oncology 1989; **Med School:** Brown Univ 1983; **Resid:** Internal Medicine, Roger Williams Hosp 1987; **Fellow:** Hematology & Oncology, Natl Cancer Inst 1990; Internal Medicine, Natl Cancer Inst 1992; **Fac Appt:** Prof Med, Yale Univ

Cooper, Dennis MD (Onc) - **Spec Exp:** Lymphoma; Stem Cell Transplant; Leukemia; **Hospital:** Yale - New Haven Hosp (page 984); **Address:** Yale Univ Sch Med, 333 Cedar St, WWW 211, New Haven, CT 06520; **Phone:** 203-737-5751; **Board Cert:** Internal Medicine 1983; Medical Oncology 1985; **Med School:** Rush Med Coll 1979; **Resid:** Internal Medicine, Yale-New Haven Hosp 1982; Internal Medicine, Presby-Univ Hosp 1983; **Fellow:** Medical Oncology, Yale-New Haven Hosp 1985; **Fac Appt:** Assoc Prof Med, Yale Univ

De Vita Jr, Vincent T MD (Onc) - **Spec Exp:** Lymphoma; Hodgkin's Disease; **Hospital:** Yale - New Haven Hosp (page 984); **Address:** 333 Cedar St, rm WWW-205, Box 208028, New Haven, CT 06520-8028; **Phone:** 203-737-1010; **Board Cert:** Internal Medicine 1974; Hematology 1972; Medical Oncology 1973; **Med School:** Geo Wash Univ 1961; **Resid:** Internal Medicine, Geo Wash Hosp 1963; Internal Medicine, Yale-New Haven Hosp 1966; **Fellow:** Medical Oncology, Natl Cancer Inst 1965; **Fac Appt:** Prof Med, Yale Univ

Lacy, Jill MD (Onc) - **Spec Exp:** Colon & Rectal Cancer; Brain Tumors; Gastrointestinal Cancer; **Hospital:** Yale - New Haven Hosp (page 984); **Address:** Yale Univ Sch Med - Div Medical Oncology, 333 Cedar St, PO Box 208032, New Haven, CT 06520-8032; **Phone:** 203-688-4191; **Board Cert:** Internal Medicine 1982; Medical Oncology 2005; **Med School:** Yale Univ 1978; **Resid:** Internal Medicine, Yale-New Haven Hosp 1981; **Fellow:** Medical Oncology, Yale-New Haven Hosp 1985; **Fac Appt:** Assoc Prof Med, Yale Univ

Lundberg, Walter B MD (Onc) - **Spec Exp:** Lymphoma; Colon Cancer; Lung Cancer; **Hospital:** Hosp of St Raphael; **Address:** 1450 Chapel St, New Haven, CT 06511; **Phone:** 203-867-5420; **Board Cert:** Internal Medicine 1973; Hematology 1974; Blood Banking Transfusion Medicine 1974; Medical Oncology 1975; **Med School:** Columbia P&S 1970; **Resid:** Internal Medicine, Columbia Presby Hosp 1972; Medical Oncology, Yale-New Haven Hosp 1976; **Fellow:** Internal Medicine, Harvard Med Sch 1971; **Fac Appt:** Assoc Clin Prof Med, Yale Univ

NEONATAL-PERINATAL MEDICINE

Ehrenkranz, Richard MD (NP) - **Spec Exp:** Critical Care; Nutrition; **Hospital:** Yale - New Haven Hosp (page 984); **Address:** Yale Univ-Dept Ped, PO Box 208064, New Haven, CT 06520-8064; **Phone:** 203-688-2320; **Board Cert:** Neonatal-Perinatal Medicine 1979; Pediatrics 1977; **Med School:** SUNY Downstate 1972; **Resid:** Pediatrics, Yale-New Haven Hosp 1974; **Fellow:** Neonatal-Perinatal Medicine, Yale Univ 1978; **Fac Appt:** Prof Ped, Yale Univ

Gross, Ian MD (NP) - **Spec Exp:** Breathing Disorders; Critical Care; **Hospital:** Yale - New Haven Hosp (page 984); **Address:** Yale Sch Med, Dept Peds, 333 Cedar St, PO Box 208064, New Haven, CT 06520-8064; **Phone:** 203-688-2320; **Board Cert:** Pediatrics 1974; Neonatal-Perinatal Medicine 1977; **Med School:** South Africa 1967; **Resid:** Pediatrics, Univ Witwatersrand Affil Hosps 1971; Pediatrics, Chldns Hosp Med Ctr 1972; **Fellow:** Pediatrics, Harvard Med Sch 1973; Neonatal-Perinatal Medicine, Yale Univ Sch Med 1974; **Fac Appt:** Prof Ped, Yale Univ

NEPHROLOGY

Aronson, Peter S MD (Nep) - **Spec Exp:** Acid-Base Disorders; Electrolyte Disorders; **Hospital:** Yale - New Haven Hosp (page 984), VA Conn Hlthcre Sys; **Address:** Yale Sch Med, Dept Medicine, PO Box 208029, New Haven, CT 06520-8029; **Phone:** 203-785-4186; **Board Cert:** Internal Medicine 1973; Nephrology 1976; **Med School:** NYU Sch Med 1970; **Resid:** Internal Medicine, NC Meml Hosp 1972; **Fellow:** Nephrology, Yale Univ Sch Med 1977; **Fac Appt:** Prof Med, Yale Univ

Kliger, Alan MD (Nep) - **Spec Exp:** Kidney Disease; Kidney Disease-Metabolic; **Hospital:** Hosp of St Raphael; **Address:** 136 Sherman Ave, New Haven, CT 06511-5238; **Phone:** 203-787-0117; **Board Cert:** Internal Medicine 1973; Nephrology 1976; **Med School:** SUNY Upstate Med Univ 1970; **Resid:** Internal Medicine, SUNY Upstate Med Ctr 1973; **Fellow:** Nephrology, Georgetown Univ Hosp 1975; **Fac Appt:** Clin Prof Med, Yale Univ

Rastegar, Asghar MD (Nep) - **Spec Exp:** Glomerulonephritis; Amyloidosis; Acid-Base Disorders; **Hospital:** Yale - New Haven Hosp (page 984); **Address:** Yale Sch Med - Div Nephrology, 333 Cedar St, Box 208056, New Haven, CT 06520-8056; **Phone:** 203-785-4184; **Board Cert:** Internal Medicine 1972; Nephrology 1978; **Med School:** Univ Wisc 1968; **Resid:** Internal Medicine, Hosp Univ Penn 1973; **Fellow:** Nephrology, Hosp Univ Penn 1972; **Fac Appt:** Prof Med, Yale Univ

NEUROLOGICAL SURGERY

de Lotbiniere, Alain MD (NS) - **Spec Exp:** Movement Disorders; Pain Management; Brain Tumors; Pituitary Tumors; **Hospital:** Yale - New Haven Hosp (page 984), Northern Westchester Hosp; **Address:** Yale Univ Sch Med, Dept Neurosurgery, 333 Cedar St, Box 208082, New Haven, CT 06520-8082; **Phone:** 203-785-2808; **Board Cert:** Neurological Surgery 1994; **Med School:** McGill Univ 1981; **Resid:** Surgery, Royal Victoria Hosp 1983; Neurological Surgery, Royal Victoria Hosp 1988; **Fellow:** Neurological Surgery, Univ of Cambridge 1989; **Fac Appt:** Assoc Prof NS, Yale Univ

Duncan, Charles C MD (NS) - **Spec Exp:** Pediatric Neurosurgery; **Hospital:** Yale - New Haven Hosp (page 984); **Address:** Yale Univ Sch Med, PO Box 208082, New Haven, CT 06520-8082; **Phone:** 203-785-2809; **Board Cert:** Neurological Surgery 1979; Pediatric Neurological Surgery 1996; **Med School:** Duke Univ 1971; **Resid:** Neurological Surgery, Duke Univ Med Ctr 1977; **Fac Appt:** Prof NS, Yale Univ

Piepmeier, Joseph MD (NS) - **Spec Exp:** Neuro-Oncology; Brain & Spinal Cord Tumors; **Hospital:** Yale - New Haven Hosp (page 984); **Address:** Yale Sch Med, Dept Neurosurgery, 333 Cedar St, TMP-410, New Haven, CT 06520; **Phone:** 203-785-2791; **Board Cert:** Neurological Surgery 1984; **Med School:** Univ Tenn Coll Med, Memphis 1975; **Resid:** Neurological Surgery, Yale-New Haven Hosp 1982; **Fac Appt:** Prof NS, Yale Univ

Spencer, Dennis D MD (NS) - **Spec Exp:** Epilepsy/Seizure Disorders; Brain Tumors; **Hospital:** Yale - New Haven Hosp (page 984), Hosp of St Raphael; **Address:** Yale Univ Sch Med, Dept Neurosurgery, 333 Cedar St, TMP-4, New Haven, CT 06520; **Phone:** 203-785-4891; **Board Cert:** Neurological Surgery 1980; **Med School:** Washington Univ, St Louis 1971; **Resid:** Surgery, Barnes Hosp 1972; Neurological Surgery, Yale-New Haven Hosp 1976; **Fac Appt:** Prof NS, Yale Univ

NEUROLOGY

Goldstein, Jonathan M MD (N) - **Spec Exp:** Myasthenia Gravis; Peripheral Neuropathy; **Hospital:** Yale - New Haven Hosp (page 984); **Address:** Yale Univ, Dept Neurology, PO Box 208018, New Haven, CT 06520-8018; **Phone:** 203-785-4085; **Board Cert:** Clinical Neurophysiology 1994; Neurology 1991; **Med School:** Brown Univ 1986; **Resid:** Neurology, Yale-New Haven Hosp 1990; **Fellow:** Clinical Neurophysiology, Yale-New Haven Hosp 1991; Neurological Immunology, Yale-New Haven Hosp 1992; **Fac Appt:** Assoc Prof N, Yale Univ

Katz, Amiram MD (N) - **Spec Exp:** Seizure Disorders; Lyme Disease; Diving Medicine; **Hospital:** Norwalk Hosp; **Address:** 291 S Lambert Rd, Ste 5, Orange, CT 06477; **Phone:** 203-795-5425; **Board Cert:** Neurology 1993; **Med School:** Israel 1976; **Resid:** Neurology, Sheba Hospital 1980; Neurology, Tel Aviv Med Ctr 1984; **Fellow:** Clinical Neurophysiology, Cleveland Clinic 1988; Epilepsy, Yale Univ 1991; **Fac Appt:** Asst Clin Prof N, Yale Univ

Spencer, Susan S MD (N) - **Spec Exp:** Epilepsy/Seizure Disorders; **Hospital:** Yale - New Haven Hosp (page 984); **Address:** Yale Univ Sch Med, Dept Neurology, 333 Cedar St, Box 208018, New Haven, CT 06520-8018; **Phone:** 203-785-3865; **Board Cert:** Neurology 1980; Clinical Neurophysiology 1988; **Med School:** Univ Rochester 1974; **Resid:** Neurology, Yale-New Haven Hosp 1978; **Fellow:** Epilepsy, Yale New Haven Hosp-Yale Univ 1980; **Fac Appt:** Prof N, Yale Univ

OBSTETRICS & GYNECOLOGY

Fine, Emily A MD (ObG) - **Spec Exp:** Menopause Problems; Vulvar Disease; **Hospital:** Yale - New Haven Hosp (page 984); **Address:** 60 Washington Ave, Ste 201, Hamden, CT 06518; **Phone:** 203-230-2939; **Board Cert:** Obstetrics & Gynecology 1984; **Med School:** Yale Univ 1978; **Resid:** Obstetrics & Gynecology, Yale-New Haven Hosp 1982; **Fac Appt:** Asst Clin Prof ObG, Yale Univ

Lynch, Vincent J MD (ObG) - **Spec Exp:** Laparoscopic Surgery; Menopause Problems; Heart Disease in Pregnancy; **Hospital:** Yale - New Haven Hosp (page 984); **Address:** 2 Church St S, Ste 209, New Haven, CT 06519; **Phone:** 203-787-2264; **Board Cert:** Obstetrics & Gynecology 1986; **Med School:** NY Med Coll 1967; **Resid:** Obstetrics & Gynecology, Yale-New Haven Hosp 1972; **Fac Appt:** Clin Prof ObG, Yale Univ

Richman, Susan M MD (ObG) - **Spec Exp:** Menopause Problems; Pap Smear Abnormalities; Vulvar Disease; **Hospital:** Yale - New Haven Hosp (page 984); **Address:** Yale Sch Med-Dept Ob/Gyn, 333 Cedar St, Box 208063, New Haven, CT 06520; **Phone:** 203-785-4176; **Board Cert:** Obstetrics & Gynecology 1985; **Med School:** Albert Einstein Coll Med 1979; **Resid:** Obstetrics & Gynecology, Yale-New Haven Hosp 1983; **Fac Appt:** Asst Prof ObG, Yale Univ

OCCUPATIONAL MEDICINE

Cullen, Mark R MD (OM) - **Spec Exp:** Mesothelioma; **Hospital:** Yale - New Haven Hosp (page 984); **Address:** 135 College St, Ste 392, New Haven, CT 06510; **Phone:** 203-785-6434; **Board Cert:** Internal Medicine 1979; Occupational Medicine 1986; **Med School:** Yale Univ 1976; **Resid:** Internal Medicine, Yale-New Haven Hosp 1980; **Fac Appt:** Prof Med, Yale Univ

ORTHOPAEDIC SURGERY

Friedlaender, Gary E MD (OrS) - **Spec Exp:** Bone & Soft Tissue Tumors; Limb Surgery/Reconstruction; Fractures-Non Union; **Hospital:** Yale - New Haven Hosp (page 984); **Address:** Yale Univ Sch Med, Dept Orthopedic Surg, 800 Howard Ave YPB Bldg - rm 133, Box 208071, New Haven, CT 06520-8071; **Phone:** 203-737-5656; **Board Cert:** Orthopaedic Surgery 1975; **Med School:** Univ Mich Med Sch 1969; **Resid:** Surgery, Michigan Med Ctr 1971; Orthopaedic Surgery, Yale-New Haven Hosp 1974; **Fellow:** Musculoskeletal Oncology, Mass Genl Hosp 1983; **Fac Appt:** Prof OrS, Yale Univ

Jokl, Peter MD (OrS) - **Spec Exp:** Knee Surgery; Sports Medicine; **Hospital:** Yale - New Haven Hosp (page 984); **Address:** Yale Sports Med, Dept Orthopaedics, 800 Howard Ave, New Haven, CT 06519-1369; **Phone:** 203-785-2579; **Board Cert:** Orthopaedic Surgery 1974; **Med School:** Yale Univ 1968; **Resid:** Orthopaedic Surgery, Yale-New Haven Hosp 1972; **Fac Appt:** Prof OrS, Yale Univ

Marsh, James S MD (OrS) - **Spec Exp:** Pediatric Orthopaedic Surgery; **Hospital:** Yale - New Haven Hosp (page 984); **Address:** 17 Woodland Rd, Madison, CT 06443; **Phone:** 203-453-1088; **Board Cert:** Orthopaedic Surgery 2000; **Med School:** Harvard Med Sch 1981; **Resid:** Orthopaedic Surgery, Stanford Univ 1986; **Fellow:** Pediatric Orthopaedic Surgery, Mass Genl Hosp 1987; **Fac Appt:** Assoc Prof OrS, Yale Univ

OTOLARYNGOLOGY

Kveton, John MD (Oto) - **Spec Exp:** Ear Disorders; Cochlear Implants; Acoustic Neuroma; **Hospital:** Yale - New Haven Hosp (page 984), Hosp of St Raphael; **Address:** 46 Prince St, Ste 601, New Haven, CT 06519-1634; **Phone:** 203-752-1726; **Board Cert:** Otolaryngology 1982; Neurotology 2004; **Med School:** St Louis Univ 1978; **Resid:** Otolaryngology, Yale-New Haven Hosp 1982; **Fellow:** Neurotology, The Otology Group 1983; **Fac Appt:** Clin Prof Oto, Yale Univ

Sasaki, Clarence T MD (Oto) - **Spec Exp:** Head & Neck Cancer; Skull Base Surgery; Voice Disorders; Swallowing Disorders; **Hospital:** Yale - New Haven Hosp (page 984), Hosp of St Raphael; **Address:** Yale Sch Med, Dept Otolaryngology, 333 Cedar St, Box 208041, New Haven, CT 06520-8041; **Phone:** 203-785-2592; **Board Cert:** Otolaryngology 1973; **Med School:** Yale Univ 1966; **Resid:** Surgery, Dartmouth-Mary Hitchcock Hosp 1968; Otolaryngology, Yale-New Haven Hosp 1973; **Fellow:** Head and Neck Surgery, Univ of Milan 1978; Skull Base Surgery, Univ Zurich 1982; **Fac Appt:** Prof Oto, Yale Univ

Vining, Eugenia MD (Oto) - **Spec Exp:** Sinus Disorders/Surgery; **Hospital:** Yale - New Haven Hosp (page 984), Hosp of St Raphael; **Address:** 46 Prince St, Ste 601, New Haven, CT 06519; **Phone:** 203-752-1726; **Board Cert:** Otolaryngology 1993; **Med School:** Yale Univ 1987; **Resid:** Otolaryngology, Yale-New Haven Hosp 1991; Otolaryngology, Yale-New Haven Hosp 1992; **Fellow:** Sinus Surgery, Univ Penn Med Ctr 1993

PEDIATRIC ENDOCRINOLOGY

Carpenter, Thomas O MD (PEn) - **Spec Exp:** Calcium Disorders; Metabolic Bone Disease; Thyroid Disorders; **Hospital:** Yale - New Haven Hosp (page 984); **Address:** Yale Sch Med, Dept Peds, 333 Cedar St, Box 208064, New Haven, CT 06520-8064; **Phone:** 203-764-9199; **Board Cert:** Pediatrics 1982; Pediatric Endocrinology 1999; **Med School:** Univ Ala 1977; **Resid:** Pediatrics, Univ Alabama Hosp 1980; **Fellow:** Pediatric Endocrinology, Children's Hosp 1983; **Fac Appt:** Prof Ped, Yale Univ

Tamborlane, William V MD (PEn) - **Spec Exp:** Diabetes; **Hospital:** Yale - New Haven Hosp (page 984); **Address:** Yale Pediatric Endocrinology, 333 Cedar St, rm 3091-LMP, New Haven, CT 06510-3289; **Phone:** 203-764-6747; **Board Cert:** Pediatrics 1978; Pediatric Endocrinology 1986; **Med School:** Georgetown Univ 1972; **Resid:** Pediatrics, Georgetown Univ Hosp 1975; **Fellow:** Pediatric Endocrinology, Yale Univ Sch Med 1977; **Fac Appt:** Prof Ped, Yale Univ

PEDIATRIC HEMATOLOGY-ONCOLOGY

Beardsley, Diana MD/PhD (PHO) - **Spec Exp:** Hemophilia; Hemangiomas; **Hospital:** Yale - New Haven Hosp (page 984); **Address:** Yale Univ, Dept Peds-Hem/Onc, 333 Cedar St, LMP 2073, Box 208064, New Haven, CT 06520-8064; **Phone:** 203-785-4640; **Board Cert:** Pediatrics 1987; Pediatric Hematology-Oncology 1987; **Med School:** Duke Univ 1976; **Resid:** Pediatrics, Chldns Hosp 1978; **Fellow:** Pediatric Hematology-Oncology, Chldns Hosp 1981; **Fac Appt:** Assoc Prof Ped, Yale Univ

PEDIATRIC INFECTIOUS DISEASE

Andiman, Warren A MD (PInf) - **Spec Exp:** AIDS/HIV; Viral Infections; **Hospital:** Yale - New Haven Hosp (page 984); **Address:** 333 Cedar St, rm 418 LSOG, Box 208064, New Haven, CT 06520-8064; **Phone:** 203-785-4730; **Board Cert:** Pediatrics 1975; **Med School:** Albert Einstein Coll Med 1969; **Resid:** Pediatrics, Babies Hosp-Columbia Presby 1971; **Fellow:** Pediatric Infectious Disease, Yale Univ Sch Med 1973; **Fac Appt:** Prof Ped, Yale Univ

Baltimore, Robert MD (PInf) - **Spec Exp:** Neonatal Infections; Hospital Acquired Infections; **Hospital:** Yale - New Haven Hosp (page 984); **Address:** Yale Univ Sch Med, Dept Pediatrics, 333 Cedar St, Box 208064, New Haven, CT 06520-8064; **Phone:** 203-785-4655; **Board Cert:** Pediatrics 1975; Pediatric Infectious Disease 2002; **Med School:** SUNY Buffalo 1968; **Resid:** Pediatrics, Univ Chicago Hosps 1971; **Fellow:** Infectious Disease, Boston City Hosp-Harvard 1976; **Fac Appt:** Prof Ped, Yale Univ

Shapiro, Eugene D MD (PInf) - **Spec Exp:** Lyme Disease; Vaccines; **Hospital:** Yale - New Haven Hosp (page 984); **Address:** Yale Univ Sch Med, Dept Peds, 333 Cedar St, Box 208064, New Haven, CT 06520-8064; **Phone:** 203-688-4518; **Board Cert:** Pediatrics 1980; Pediatric Infectious Disease 2002; **Med School:** UCSF 1976; **Resid:** Pediatrics, Chldns Hosp 1979; **Fellow:** Pediatric Infectious Disease, Chldns Hosp 1981; Research, Yale Univ 1983; **Fac Appt:** Prof Ped, Yale Univ

PEDIATRIC RHEUMATOLOGY

McCarthy, Paul L MD (PRhu) - **Spec Exp:** Lupus/SLE & Vasculitis; Juvenile Arthritis; Dermatomyositis; **Hospital:** Yale - New Haven Hosp (page 984); **Address:** Yale Schl Med, 333 Cedar St, Box 208064, New Haven, CT 06520-3289; **Phone:** 203-688-2475; **Board Cert:** Pediatrics 1974; Pediatric Rheumatology 2000; **Med School:** Georgetown Univ 1969; **Resid:** Pediatrics, Chldns Hosp 1972; **Fellow:** Pediatrics, Chldns Hosp 1974; **Fac Appt:** Prof Ped, Yale Univ

PEDIATRIC SURGERY

Moss, R Lawrence MD (PS) - **Spec Exp:** Minimally Invasive Surgery; Pelvic Surgery-Complex; **Hospital:** Yale - New Haven Hosp (page 984); **Address:** Dept Surgery-Ped Surgery, PO Box 208062, New Haven, CT 06520-8062; **Phone:** 203-785-2701; **Board Cert:** Surgery 1999; Pediatric Surgery 1996; **Med School:** UCSD 1986; **Resid:** Surgery, Virginia Mason Med Ctr 1991; Surgical Critical Care, Chldns Mem Hosp 1992; **Fellow:** Pediatric Surgery, Chldns Mem Hosp 1994; **Fac Appt:** Assoc Prof S, Yale Univ

Touloukian, Robert MD (PS) - **Spec Exp:** Neonatal Surgery; Cancer Surgery; Trauma; **Hospital:** Yale - New Haven Hosp (page 984); **Address:** Yale-New Haven Hospital, Dept Ped Surgery, 333 Cedar St, New Haven, CT 06510-3206; **Phone:** 203-785-2701; **Board Cert:** Surgery 1967; Pediatric Surgery 1993; **Med School:** Columbia P&S 1960; **Resid:** Surgery, Columbia-Presby Hosp 1964; Surgery, Bellevue Hosp 1965; **Fellow:** Pediatric Surgery, Babies Hosp 1966; **Fac Appt:** Prof S, Yale Univ

PEDIATRICS

Angoff, Ronald MD (Ped) `PCP` - **Hospital:** Hosp of St Raphael, Yale - New Haven Hosp (page 984); **Address:** 200 Orchard St, Ste 108, New Haven, CT 06511; **Phone:** 203-865-3737; **Board Cert:** Pediatrics 1978; **Med School:** Univ Cincinnati 1973; **Resid:** Pediatrics, Yale-New Haven Hosp 1975; **Fellow:** Child Development, Yale-New Haven Hosp 1977; **Fac Appt:** Assoc Prof Ped, Yale Univ

Canny, Christopher R MD (Ped) - **Spec Exp:** Behavioral Disorders; Developmental Disorders; **Hospital:** Yale - New Haven Hosp (page 984), Hosp of St Raphael; **Address:** 9 Washington Ave, Hamden, CT 06518; **Phone:** 203-287-0552; **Board Cert:** Pediatrics 2002; **Med School:** Washington Univ, St Louis 1976; **Resid:** Pediatrics, Yale-New Haven Hosp 1978; **Fellow:** Child Development, Yale Child Study Ctr 1980; **Fac Appt:** Assoc Clin Prof Ped, Yale Univ

Gruskay, Jeffrey MD (Ped) **PCP** - **Hospital:** Milford Hosp, Yale - New Haven Hosp (page 984); **Address:** 20 Commerce Park, Milford, CT 06460; **Phone:** 203-882-2066; **Board Cert:** Pediatrics 1985; Neonatal-Perinatal Medicine 1987; **Med School:** Yale Univ 1981; **Resid:** Pediatrics, Childrens Hosp 1984; **Fellow:** Neonatal-Perinatal Medicine, Childrens Hosp 1986; **Fac Appt:** Assoc Clin Prof Ped, Yale Univ

Morgan, James L MD (Ped) **PCP** - **Spec Exp:** Sports Medicine; **Hospital:** Yale - New Haven Hosp (page 984), Hosp of St Raphael; **Address:** 339 Boston Post Rd, Ste 250, Orange, CT 06477; **Phone:** 203-795-6025; **Board Cert:** Pediatrics 1983; **Med School:** Med Coll VA 1978; **Resid:** Pediatrics, Childrens Hosp 1982

Robert, Marie F MD (Ped) **PCP** - **Hospital:** Yale - New Haven Hosp (page 984), Hosp of St Raphael; **Address:** 339 Boston Post Rd, Ste 250, Orange, CT 06477; **Phone:** 203-795-6025; **Board Cert:** Pediatrics 1984; **Med School:** McGill Univ 1976; **Resid:** Pediatrics, Childrens Hosp 1978; Allergy & Immunology, Yale-New Haven Hosp 1979; **Fellow:** Infectious Disease, Yale Univ 1984

Shaywitz, Sally E MD (Ped) - **Spec Exp:** Learning Disorders; Dyslexia; **Hospital:** Yale - New Haven Hosp (page 984); **Address:** Yale Univ Sch Med, Dept Peds, 333 Cedar St, rm LMP-3089, New Haven, CT 06520; **Phone:** 203-785-4641; **Board Cert:** Pediatrics 1971; **Med School:** Albert Einstein Coll Med 1966; **Resid:** Pediatrics, Albert Einstein Coll Med 1970; **Fellow:** Pediatrics, Bronx Muni Hosp Ctr 1968; Behavioral Pediatrics, Albert Einstein Coll Med 1970; **Fac Appt:** Prof Ped, Yale Univ

Zelson, Joseph MD (Ped) **PCP** - **Spec Exp:** Adoption-International; **Hospital:** Yale - New Haven Hosp (page 984), Hosp of St Raphael; **Address:** 339 Boston Post Rd, Ste 250, Orange, CT 06477-3517; **Phone:** 203-795-6026; **Board Cert:** Pediatrics 1971; **Med School:** NYU Sch Med 1965; **Resid:** Pediatrics, Yale-New Haven Hosp 1969; **Fellow:** Pediatric Hematology-Oncology, Yale-New Haven Hosp 1971; **Fac Appt:** Clin Prof Ped, Yale Univ

PLASTIC SURGERY

Ariyan, Stephan MD (PlS) - **Spec Exp:** Melanoma; Head & Neck Surgery; Reconstructive Surgery; **Hospital:** Yale - New Haven Hosp (page 984); **Address:** 60 Temple St, Ste 7C, New Haven, CT 06510-2716; **Phone:** 203-786-3000; **Board Cert:** Plastic Surgery 1978; **Med School:** NY Med Coll 1966; **Resid:** Surgery, Yale-New Haven Hosp 1975; Plastic Surgery, Yale-New Haven Hosp 1976; **Fellow:** Surgical Oncology, Yale-New Haven Hosp 1971; **Fac Appt:** Clin Prof S, Yale Univ

Persing, John A MD (PlS) - **Spec Exp:** Craniofacial Surgery; Vascular Anomalies; Skin Cancer; Cosmetic Surgery; **Hospital:** Yale - New Haven Hosp (page 984); **Address:** Yale Plastic Surgery, 330 Cedar St Boardroom Bldg Fl 3, New Haven, CT 06519; **Phone:** 203-785-2570; **Board Cert:** Plastic Surgery 1985; Neurological Surgery 1986; **Med School:** Univ VT Coll Med 1974; **Resid:** Surgery, Univ Arizona Med Ctr 1976; Neurological Surgery, Univ Virginia Med Ctr 1982; **Fellow:** Plastic Surgery, Univ Virginia Med Ctr 1984; **Fac Appt:** Prof PlS, Yale Univ

Restifo, Richard MD (PlS) - **Spec Exp:** Skin Laser Surgery; Breast Reconstruction; Liposuction & Body Contouring; **Hospital:** St Vincent's Med Ctr - Bridgeport, Yale - New Haven Hosp (page 984); **Address:** 59 Elm St, Ste 560, New Haven, CT 06510; **Phone:** 203-772-1444; **Board Cert:** Plastic Surgery 1995; **Med School:** Harvard Med Sch 1986; **Resid:** Surgery, Georgetown Univ Hosp 1991; Plastic Surgery, Univ Pittsburgh Med Ctr 1993

Stahl, Richard S MD (PlS) - **Spec Exp:** Abdominal Wall Reconstruction; Bronchopleural Fistula Repair; **Hospital:** Yale - New Haven Hosp (page 984); **Address:** 5 Durham Rd, Guilford, CT 06437; **Phone:** 203-458-4440; **Board Cert:** Surgery 2001; Plastic Surgery 1984; **Med School:** Vanderbilt Univ 1976; **Resid:** Surgery, Yale New Haven Hosp 1981; Plastic Surgery, Emory Univ Med Ctr 1983; **Fac Appt:** Clin Prof S, Yale Univ

PSYCHIATRY

Bowers Jr, Malcolm B MD (Psyc) - **Spec Exp:** Schizophrenia; Psychopharmacology; **Hospital:** Yale - New Haven Hosp (page 984); **Address:** Yale Univ - Dept Psychiatry, 300 George St, Ste 901, New Haven, CT 06511; **Phone:** 203-785-2121; **Board Cert:** Psychiatry 1970; **Med School:** Washington Univ, St Louis 1958; **Resid:** Psychiatry, Yale-New Haven Hosp 1965; **Fellow:** Psychiatry, Yale-New Haven Hosp 1964; **Fac Appt:** Prof Psyc, Yale Univ

McGlashan, Thomas MD (Psyc) - **Spec Exp:** Schizophrenia-Early Detection/Treatment; Personality Disorders; **Hospital:** Yale - New Haven Hosp (page 984), Connecticut Mental Hlth Ctr; **Address:** Yale Univ Sch Med, Dept Psychiatry, PO Box 208068, New Haven, CT 06520-8068; **Phone:** 203-737-2077; **Board Cert:** Psychiatry 1973; **Med School:** Univ Pennsylvania 1967; **Resid:** Psychiatry, Mass Mental Hlth Ctr 1971; **Fac Appt:** Prof Psyc, Yale Univ

Riordan, Charles E MD (Psyc) - **Hospital:** Hosp of St Raphael; **Address:** 1450 Chapel St, New Haven, CT 06511; **Phone:** 203-789-4196; **Board Cert:** Psychiatry 1970; **Med School:** Harvard Med Sch 1963; **Resid:** Psychiatry, St Vincent's Hosp & Med Ctr 1967; **Fac Appt:** Clin Prof Psyc, Yale Univ

Yonkers, Kimberly A MD (Psyc) - **Spec Exp:** Anxiety & Mood Disorders; Premenstrual Dysphoric Disorder; **Hospital:** Yale - New Haven Hosp (page 984); **Address:** 142 Temple St, Ste 301, New Haven, CT 06510; **Phone:** 203-764-6621; **Board Cert:** Psychiatry 1991; **Med School:** Columbia P&S 1986; **Resid:** Psychiatry, McLean Hosp- Harvard 1990; **Fellow:** Psychiatry, McLean Hosp-Harvard 1992; **Fac Appt:** Assoc Prof Psyc, Yale Univ

PULMONARY DISEASE

Elias, Jack A MD (Pul) - **Spec Exp:** Asthma; Emphysema; Chronic Obstructive Lung Disease (COPD); **Hospital:** Yale - New Haven Hosp (page 984); **Address:** Yale Sch Med, Pulmonary Section, 300 Cedar St, S441-TAC, New Haven, CT 06520-8057; **Phone:** 203-785-4163; **Board Cert:** Internal Medicine 1979; Allergy & Immunology 1981; Pulmonary Disease 1982; **Med School:** Univ Pennsylvania 1976; **Resid:** Internal Medicine, Tufts-New England Med Ctr 1978; Internal Medicine, Hosp Univ Penn 1979; **Fellow:** Allergy & Immunology, Hosp Univ Penn 1982; Pulmonary Disease, Hosp Univ Penn 1982; **Fac Appt:** Prof Med, Yale Univ

Enelow, Richard Ian MD (Pul) - **Spec Exp:** Interstitial Lung Disease; Lung Disease; **Hospital:** VA Conn Hlthcre Sys, Yale - New Haven Hosp (page 984); **Address:** Chief Pulm Crit Care Sect-111A, VA Conn Hlth Care Syst, 950 Campbell Ave, West Haven, CT 06516; **Phone:** 203-932-5711; **Board Cert:** Internal Medicine 1986; Pulmonary Disease 2002; **Med School:** Boston Univ 1983; **Resid:** Internal Medicine, New Eng-Deaconess Med Ctr 1986; **Fellow:** Pulmonary Disease, Univ VA Hlth Scis Ctr 1992; **Fac Appt:** Asst Prof Med, Yale Univ

Friedman, Lloyd Neal MD (Pul) - **Spec Exp:** Tuberculosis; Critical Care; **Hospital:** Milford Hosp, Yale - New Haven Hosp (page 984); **Address:** Milford Hospital, 300 Seaside Ave, Milford, CT 06460; **Phone:** 203-876-4288; **Board Cert:** Internal Medicine 1983; Pulmonary Disease 1988; Critical Care Medicine 1999; **Med School:** Yale Univ 1979; **Resid:** Internal Medicine, Beth Israel Med Ctr 1980; Internal Medicine, Oregon Hlth Scis Univ 1983; **Fellow:** Pulmonary Intensive Care, Yale-New Haven Hosp 1988; **Fac Appt:** Clin Prof Med, Yale Univ

Matthay, Richard MD (Pul) - **Spec Exp:** Lung Cancer; Asthma; Lupus/SLE; Scleroderma; **Hospital:** Yale - New Haven Hosp (page 984); **Address:** 333 Cedar St, rm 105-LCI, Box 208057, New Haven, CT 06520-3206; **Phone:** 203-785-4198; **Board Cert:** Internal Medicine 1973; Pulmonary Disease 1976; Critical Care Medicine 1997; **Med School:** Tufts Univ 1970; **Resid:** Internal Medicine, Univ Colorado Med Ctr 1973; **Fellow:** Pulmonary Disease, Univ Colorado Med Ctr 1975; **Fac Appt:** Prof Med, Yale Univ

Redlich, Carrie MD (Pul) - **Spec Exp:** Occupational Lung Disease; **Hospital:** Yale - New Haven Hosp (page 984); **Address:** Yale Occupational & Environmental Med, 135 College St Fl 3 - Ste 392, New Haven, CT 06510; **Phone:** 203-785-4197; **Board Cert:** Internal Medicine 1986; Pulmonary Disease 2002; Occupational Medicine 1990; **Med School:** Yale Univ 1982; **Resid:** Internal Medicine, Yale-New Haven Hosp 1986; Occupational Medicine, Yale-New Haven Hosp 1987; **Fellow:** Pulmonary Disease, Univ Washington 1989; **Fac Appt:** Assoc Prof Med, Yale Univ

Rochester, Carolyn MD (Pul) - **Spec Exp:** Chronic Obstructive Lung Disease (COPD); **Hospital:** VA Conn Hlthcre Sys, Yale - New Haven Hosp (page 984); **Address:** Yale Univ Sch Med, Pulm & Crit Care Sect, 333 Cedar St, Box 208057, New Haven, CT 06520-8057; **Phone:** 203-785-3207; **Board Cert:** Internal Medicine 1986; Pulmonary Disease 2002; **Med School:** Columbia P&S 1983; **Resid:** Internal Medicine, Columbia Presby Med Ctr 1986; **Fellow:** Pulmonary Disease, Colombia Presby Med Ctr 1988; **Fac Appt:** Asst Prof Med, Yale Univ

Tanoue, Lynn MD (Pul) - **Spec Exp:** Lung Cancer; Sarcoidosis; **Hospital:** Yale - New Haven Hosp (page 984); **Address:** Yale Univ Sch Med, Div Pulm & Critical Care, 333 Cedar St, Box 208057, New Haven, CT 06520-8057; **Phone:** 203-785-6359; **Board Cert:** Internal Medicine 1985; Pulmonary Disease 1988; Critical Care Medicine 2002; **Med School:** Yale Univ 1982; **Resid:** Internal Medicine, Yale-New Haven Hosp 1985; **Fellow:** Pulmonary Disease, Yale-New Haven Hosp 1988; Critical Care Medicine, Yale-NEw Haven Hosp 1988; **Fac Appt:** Assoc Prof Med, Yale Univ

RADIATION ONCOLOGY

Knisely, Jonathan MD (RadRO) - **Spec Exp:** Brain Tumors; Stereotactic Radiosurgery; Gastrointestinal Cancer; **Hospital:** Yale - New Haven Hosp (page 984); **Address:** Yale Univ Sch Med, Dept Therapeutic Radiology, 15 York St Bldg Hunter - Ste HRT 1, New Haven, CT 06520-8040; **Phone:** 203-785-2960; **Board Cert:** Internal Medicine 1989; Radiation Oncology 1993; **Med School:** Univ Pennsylvania 1986; **Resid:** Internal Medicine, Michael Reese Hosp 1989; Radiation Oncology, Univ Toronto Med Ctr 1992; **Fac Appt:** Assoc Prof Rad, Yale Univ

Peschel, Richard E MD (RadRO) - **Spec Exp:** Prostate Cancer; **Hospital:** Yale - New Haven Hosp (page 984); **Address:** Yale-New Haven Hosp, Dept Radiology, 15 York St, rm HRT 142, New Haven, CT 06510; **Phone:** 203-785-2958; **Board Cert:** Therapeutic Radiology 1982; **Med School:** Yale Univ 1977; **Resid:** Radiation Oncology, Yale-New Haven Hosp 1981; **Fac Appt:** Prof RadRO, Yale Univ

Roberts, Kenneth MD (RadRO) - **Spec Exp:** Pediatric Cancers; Lymphoma; Hodgkin's Disease; **Hospital:** Yale - New Haven Hosp (page 984), Backus Hosp, Norwich; **Address:** Yale Univ School of Medicine, 333 Cedar St, HRT 138, New Haven, CT 06520; **Phone:** 203-785-2957; **Board Cert:** Internal Medicine 1987; Medical Oncology 1989; Radiation Oncology 1995; **Med School:** Duke Univ 1984; **Resid:** Internal Medicine, Ohio State Univ Hosps 1987; Radiation Oncology, Duke Univ Med Ctr 1992; **Fellow:** Hematology & Oncology, Duke Univ Med Ctr 1989; **Fac Appt:** Assoc Prof Rad, Yale Univ

Wilson, Lynn D MD (RadRO) - **Spec Exp:** Lymphoma, Cutaneous T Cell (CTCL); Lymphoma, Cutaneous B Cell (CBCL); Lung Cancer; Head & Neck Cancer; **Hospital:** Yale - New Haven Hosp (page 984); **Address:** Yale Univ Sch Med, Dept Therapeutic Rad, PO Box 208040, New Haven, CT 06520-8040; **Phone:** 203-688-1861; **Board Cert:** Radiation Oncology 2004; **Med School:** Geo Wash Univ 1990; **Resid:** Therapeutic Radiology, Yale-New Haven Hosp 1994; **Fac Appt:** Prof RadRO, Yale Univ

Reproductive Endocrinology

Arici, Aydin M MD (RE) - **Spec Exp:** Pregnancy Loss; Infertility-IVF; Endometriosis; Uterine Fibroids; **Hospital:** Yale - New Haven Hosp (page 984); **Address:** 150 Sargent Drive, New Haven, CT 06511; **Phone:** 203-785-4708; **Board Cert:** Obstetrics & Gynecology 1997; Reproductive Endocrinology 1997; **Med School:** Turkey 1979; **Resid:** Obstetrics & Gynecology, Harlem Hosp/Columbia 1986; **Fellow:** Reproductive Endocrinology, U Tex SW Med Branch 1992; **Fac Appt:** Prof ObG, Yale Univ

Patrizio, Pasquale MD (RE) - **Spec Exp:** Infertility; Infertility-IVF; Fertility Preservation in Cancer; **Hospital:** Yale - New Haven Hosp (page 984); **Address:** Yale Fertility Ctr, Dept OB/GYN, 150 Sargent Drive, New Haven, CT 06511; **Phone:** 203-785-4708; **Board Cert:** Obstetrics & Gynecology 1997; Reproductive Endocrinology 1999; **Med School:** Italy 1983; **Resid:** Obstetrics & Gynecology, Univ Naples 1987; Reproductive Endocrinology, Univ Pisa 1990; **Fellow:** Infertility, UC Irvine 1995; **Fac Appt:** Prof ObG, Yale Univ

Rheumatology

Craft, Joseph MD (Rhu) - **Spec Exp:** Lupus Nephritis; Lupus/SLE; Lyme Disease; **Hospital:** Yale - New Haven Hosp (page 984); **Address:** Yale Univ, Dept Internal Med-Rheum Sect, 300 Cedar St, rm S-541D - PO Box 208031, New Haven, CT 06520-8031; **Phone:** 203-785-2454; **Board Cert:** Internal Medicine 1980; Rheumatology 1988; **Med School:** Univ NC Sch Med 1977; **Resid:** Internal Medicine, Yale-New Haven Hosp 1978; **Fellow:** Rheumatology, Yale-New Haven Hosp 1985; **Fac Appt:** Prof Med, Yale Univ

Hutchinson, Gordon J MD (Rhu) - **Hospital:** Hosp of St Raphael; **Address:** 136 Sherman Ave, Ste 104, New Haven, CT 06516; **Phone:** 203-785-0885; **Board Cert:** Internal Medicine 1980; Rheumatology 1982; **Med School:** Switzerland 1976; **Resid:** Internal Medicine, Hosp St Raphael 1980; **Fellow:** Rheumatology, Yale Univ 1982; **Fac Appt:** Assoc Clin Prof Med, Yale Univ

Liebling, Anne MD (Rhu) - **Spec Exp:** Arthritis; Juvenile Arthritis; Fibromyalgia; **Hospital:** Yale - New Haven Hosp (page 984); **Address:** 60 Temple St, Ste 6A, New Haven, CT 06510; **Phone:** 203-789-2255; **Board Cert:** Pediatrics 1998; Pediatric Rheumatology 2002; Internal Medicine 2000; Rheumatology 2004; **Med School:** SUNY Downstate 1986; **Resid:** Internal Medicine & Pediatrics, Univ Chicago Hosps 1990; **Fellow:** Rheumatology, Univ Chicago Hosps 1993; Pediatric Rheumatology, Univ Chicago Hosps 1993

Schoen, Robert T MD (Rhu) - **Spec Exp:** Rheumatoid Arthritis; Lyme Disease; Osteoporosis; **Hospital:** Yale - New Haven Hosp (page 984), Hosp of St Raphael; **Address:** 60 Temple St, Ste 6A, New Haven, CT 06510-2716; **Phone:** 203-789-2255; **Board Cert:** Internal Medicine 1979; Rheumatology 1982; **Med School:** Columbia P&S 1976; **Resid:** Internal Medicine, Yale New Haven Hosp 1979; **Fellow:** Rheumatology, Brigham & Womens Hosp 1981; **Fac Appt:** Clin Prof Med, Yale Univ

SURGERY

Cronin II, David C MD/PhD (S) - **Spec Exp:** Transplant-Liver; Pediatric Transplant Surgery; Liver & Biliary Surgery; Pancreatic Surgery; **Hospital:** Yale - New Haven Hosp (page 984); **Address:** Yale New Haven Organ Transplant Ctr, 333 Cedar St, PO Box 208062, New Haven, CT 06520-8062; **Phone:** 203-785-2565; **Board Cert:** Surgery 2005; **Med School:** Mount Sinai Sch Med 1987; **Resid:** Surgery, Univ Chicago Hosps 1995; **Fellow:** Surgical Critical Care, Univ Chicago Hosps 1997; **Fac Appt:** Assoc Prof S, Yale Univ

Dudrick, Stanley MD (S) - **Spec Exp:** Laparoscopic Surgery; Critical Care; **Hospital:** St Mary's Hosp - Waterbury, Yale - New Haven Hosp (page 984); **Address:** St Mary's Hosp, Dept Surg, 56 Franklin St, Waterbury, CT 06706; **Phone:** 203-709-6314; **Board Cert:** Surgery 1968; **Med School:** Univ Pennsylvania 1961; **Resid:** Surgery, Hosp Univ Penn 1967; **Fellow:** Research, Hosp Univ Penn 1967; **Fac Appt:** Prof S, Yale Univ

Friedman, Amy L MD (S) - **Spec Exp:** Transplant-Living Kidney Donor; Laparoscopy; Transplant-Pancreas; **Hospital:** Yale - New Haven Hosp (page 984); **Address:** Yale-New Haven Hosp, Dept Surgery, 333 Cedar St, Box 208062, New Haven, CT 06520-8062; **Phone:** 203-785-2565; **Board Cert:** Surgery 1999; **Med School:** SUNY Downstate 1983; **Resid:** Surgery, SUNY Downstate Med Ctr 1990; **Fellow:** Transplant Surgery, Hosp Univ Penn 1992; **Fac Appt:** Assoc Prof S, Yale Univ

Salem, Ronald R MD (S) - **Spec Exp:** Cancer Surgery; Liver & Biliary Surgery; **Hospital:** Yale - New Haven Hosp (page 984); **Address:** Yale Univ Sch Med, Dept Surg, 333 Cedar St, Box 208062, New Haven, CT 06520-8062; **Phone:** 203-785-3577; **Board Cert:** Surgery 2000; **Med School:** Zimbabwe 1978; **Resid:** Surgery, Hammersmith Hosp 1985; Surgery, New Eng-Deaconess Hosp 1989; **Fac Appt:** Assoc Prof S, Yale Univ

Stein, Stephen A MD (S) - **Hospital:** Yale - New Haven Hosp (page 984), Hosp of St Raphael; **Address:** 46 Prince St, Ste 301, New Haven, CT 06519; **Phone:** 203-787-2862; **Board Cert:** Surgery 1973; **Med School:** Harvard Med Sch 1967; **Resid:** Surgery, Yale-New Haven Hosp 1972; **Fac Appt:** Assoc Clin Prof S, Yale Univ

Udelsman, Robert MD (S) - **Spec Exp:** Parathyroid Cancer; Adrenal Tumors; Thyroid Cancer; **Hospital:** Yale - New Haven Hosp (page 984); **Address:** Yale Sch Med, Rm FMB102, 330 Cedar St, Box 208062, New Haven, CT 06520-3218; **Phone:** 203-785-2697; **Board Cert:** Surgery 1999; **Med School:** Geo Wash Univ 1981; **Resid:** Surgery, Natl Inst Hlth 1986; Surgery, Johns Hopkins Hosp 1989; **Fellow:** Gastrointestinal Surgery, Johns Hopkins Hosp 1990; **Fac Appt:** Prof S, Yale Univ

THORACIC SURGERY

Detterbeck, Frank C MD (TS) - **Spec Exp:** Lung Cancer; Mediastinal Tumors; Esophageal Cancer; **Hospital:** Yale - New Haven Hosp (page 984); **Address:** Yale Sch Medicine - Thoracic Surg, 333 Cedar St, Box 208062, New Haven, CT 06520-8062; **Phone:** 203-785-4931; **Board Cert:** Thoracic Surgery 2001; **Med School:** Northwestern Univ 1983; **Resid:** Surgery, Virginia Mason Hosp 1988; **Fellow:** Cardiothoracic Surgery, Univ North Carolina Hosps 1991; **Fac Appt:** Prof S, Yale Univ

Elefteriades, John MD (TS) - **Spec Exp:** Aneurysm-Thoracic Aortic; Transplant-Heart; Ventricular Assist Device (LVAD); **Hospital:** Yale - New Haven Hosp (page 984); **Address:** Yale Sch of Med, Dept Cardiothoracic Surg, Box 208039, New Haven, CT 06520; **Phone:** 203-785-2705; **Board Cert:** Thoracic Surgery 1994; **Med School:** Yale Univ 1976; **Resid:** Surgery, Yale-New Haven Hosp 1981; Cardiothoracic Surgery, Yale-New Haven Hosp 1983; **Fellow:** Cardiothoracic Surgery, Yale-New Haven Hosp 1983; **Fac Appt:** Prof S, Yale Univ

Kopf, Gary S MD (TS) - **Spec Exp:** Cardiac Surgery; Pediatric Cardiothoracic Surgery; Congenital Heart Disease; **Hospital:** Yale - New Haven Hosp (page 984); **Address:** Surgery, 333 Cedar St, FMB-121, Box 2089039, New Haven, CT 06510; **Phone:** 203-785-2702; **Board Cert:** Thoracic Surgery 2000; **Med School:** Harvard Med Sch 1970; **Resid:** Surgery, Peter Bent Brigham Hosp 1977; Cardiothoracic Surgery, Chldns Hosp Med Ctr 1980; **Fellow:** Cardiothoracic Surgery, Harvard/Brigham Hosp 1980; **Fac Appt:** Prof S, Yale Univ

UROLOGY

Flanagan, Michael J MD (U) - **Spec Exp:** Prostate Disease; Incontinence; **Hospital:** Waterbury Hosp, St Mary's Hosp - Waterbury; **Address:** Urology specialists, PC, 160 Robbins St, Waterbury, CT 06708; **Phone:** 203-757-8361; **Board Cert:** Urology 2003; **Med School:** UMDNJ-Univ Med Dent NJ 1985; **Resid:** Surgery, Waterbury Hosp 1988; Urology, Temple Univ Hosp 1992

Weiss, Robert M MD (U) - **Spec Exp:** Pediatric Urology; **Hospital:** Yale - New Haven Hosp (page 984); **Address:** Yale Univ Sch Med, Dept Urol, 800 Howard Ave, Box 208041, New Haven, CT 06520-8041; **Phone:** 203-785-2815; **Board Cert:** Urology 1970; **Med School:** SUNY Downstate 1960; **Resid:** Surgery, Beth Israel Hosp 1962; Urology, Columbia Presby Hosp 1967; **Fellow:** Pharmacology, Columbia Presby Hosp 1965; **Fac Appt:** Prof U, Yale Univ

VASCULAR & INTERVENTIONAL RADIOLOGY

White, Robert I MD (VIR) - **Spec Exp:** Uterine Fibroid Embolization; Pelvic Congestion Syndrome; Varicocele Embolization; Vascular Malformations; **Hospital:** Yale - New Haven Hosp (page 984); **Address:** Yale Univ Sch Med, Vasc & Interventional Rad, PO Box 208042, New Haven, CT 06520-8042; **Phone:** 203-737-5395; **Board Cert:** Diagnostic Radiology 1970; Vascular & Interventional Radiology 1994; **Med School:** Baylor Coll Med 1963; **Resid:** Radiology, Johns Hopkins Hosp 1969; **Fellow:** Cardiovascular Disease, Johns Hopkins Hospital 1958; Cardiovascular Radiology, Univ Minn Medical Ctr 1971; **Fac Appt:** Prof Rad, Yale Univ

VASCULAR SURGERY

Gusberg, Richard J MD (VascS) - **Spec Exp:** Endovascular Surgery; Aneurysm-Aortic; Renovascular Disease; **Hospital:** Yale - New Haven Hosp (page 984); **Address:** Yale Univ School of Medicine-Dept Surgery, 333 Cedar St, Box 208062, New Haven, CT 06520-8062; **Phone:** 203-785-6217; **Board Cert:** Surgery 1996; Vascular Surgery 1997; **Med School:** Columbia P&S 1970; **Resid:** Surgery, Columbia-Presby Med Ctr 1975; **Fellow:** Vascular Surgery, Columbia-Presby Med Ctr 1976; **Fac Appt:** Prof S, Yale Univ

Sumpio, Bauer E MD/PhD (VascS) - **Spec Exp:** Diabetic Leg/Foot; Endovascular Surgery; **Hospital:** Yale - New Haven Hosp (page 984); **Address:** Yale Univ School Medicine, Dept Surgery, 333 Cedar St, rm FMB137, Box 208062, New Haven, CT 06520; **Phone:** 203-785-6217; **Board Cert:** Vascular Surgery 1997; Surgery 1998; **Med School:** Cornell Univ-Weill Med Coll 1980; **Resid:** Surgery, Yale-New Haven Hosp 1986; **Fellow:** Vascular Surgery, Unic NC Hosp 1987; **Fac Appt:** Prof S, Yale Univ

YALE-NEW HAVEN HOSPITAL

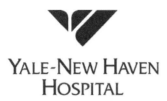

YALE-NEW HAVEN HOSPITAL

20 York Street
New Haven, CT 06510
PHONE: (203) 688-4242

www.ynhh.org

Sponsorship	Private Not-for-Profit
Beds	944 beds
Accreditation	Joint Commission on Accreditation of Healthcare Organizations (JCAHO)

Yale-New Haven Hospital is a 944-bed tertiary referral center which includes the 201-bed Yale-New Haven Children's Hospital and the 70-bed Yale-New Haven Psychiatric Hospital. Yale-New Haven Hospital offers the largest emergency center in the state which includes a Level 1 trauma service, an acute stroke program and a chest pain center staffed 24 hours a day, seven days a week.

Medical Center
Yale-New Haven's medical staff includes nearly 2,400 university-based and community physicians practicing in more than 100 medical specialties.

Yale Medical Group is one of the largest academic multi-specialty group practices in the U.S. Consisting of the full-time faculty of the Yale School of Medicine, physicians of the Yale Medical Group are leaders in their fields committed to combining a caring, individual approach to patient care with cutting edge research and advances in their respective fields.

Specialty Services
Yale-New Haven Heart Center provides a focused approach to cardiovascular disease that provides patients, their families and heart center physicians an optimal environment to deliver cardiac care. The Heart Center integrates all aspects of cardiac care including adult and pediatric cardiology and cardiac surgery.

Yale Cancer Center is one of only 39 centers in the U.S. and the only one in Southern New England designated as a comprehensive cancer center by the National Cancer Institute.

High Risk Maternity Services provides care for women whose pregnancies require special monitoring and treatment. Diagnostic tests such as chorionic villus sampling (CVS) and fetal echocardiography were developed here, bringing dramatic changes to the field of perinatal care.

Patient Health Information is available through the Yale-New Haven Health Call Center. Patients can access provider information for more than 900 participating members of the YNHH medical staff.

- **Yale-New Haven Health Call Center 1-888-700-6543**

- **Nurse Advice Line 1-877-688-1101**

- **Women's Heart Advantage 1-866-HEART-10**

- **Cancer Center Line 1-800-4-CANCER**

Sponsored Page

Section Four

Centers of Excellence

Cancer Care

CANCER CARE

Morristown Memorial Hospital • Overlook Hospital

THE PASSION TO LEAD

Goryeb Children's Hospital • Atlantic Neuroscience Institute
Carol G. Simon Cancer Center/The Cancer Center at Overlook Hospital
Gagnon Heart Hospital • Atlantic Rehabilitation Institute

P.O. Box 1905, Morristown, NJ 07962 • 1-800-247-9580 • atlantichealth.org

◢ CANCER CARE

At Atlantic Health, we do more than just treat cancer — we ease minds, educate and comfort families and renew hope. Whether you need minimally invasive surgery, robotic surgery, image-guided radiation or other treatment options, you don't have to go far for world-renowned cancer care.

We are partners with the Cancer Institute of New Jersey and affiliated with the University of Medicine and Dentistry of New Jersey. Our services are accredited by the American College of Surgeons, the American College of Radiology, and the Joint Commission on Accreditation.

◢ CAROL G. SIMON CANCER CENTER

Located at Morristown Memorial Hospital, the Carol G. Simon Cancer Center offers the most advanced methods to diagnose, treat, and manage all types of cancers. We have access to the latest clinical trials and research. We combine state-of-the-art medical technologies, such as minimally invasive surgeries, image-guided radiation, and cytogenetics, with complementary medicine, including relaxation, guided imagery, meditation, yoga, and massage. Our highly trained physicians and oncology professionals work together in a collaborative setting that promotes a coordinated multidisciplinary approach to cancer care.

◢ THE CANCER CENTER AT OVERLOOK HOSPITAL

Overlook Hospital is one of New Jersey's leading providers of superior cancer care. It was the first medical center in the Northeast U.S. to offer CyberKnife - a revolutionary radiosurgical device that uses a combination of robotics and sophisticated image-guidance technology to deliver precisely targeted doses of radiation to tumors - even tumors that are beyond the reach of other radiosurgery systems. The CyberKnife is non-invasive, highly accurate and painless.

◢ DIAGNOSTIC SERVICES

The Carol G. Simon Cancer Center and The Cancer Center at Overlook Hospital have kept pace with the latest cancer care innovations provided through weekly Tumor Boards, an essential forum to provide multidisciplinary consultative cancer care review services for patients.

Clinical Research

Our physicians are involved in regional and national research protocols for new cancer treatments. Patients may be offered to participate in clinical trials of the latest and most innovative cancer treatments.

Pain Management

Our programs provide assistance for patients with cancer or a history of cancer through medical, integrative and procedural therapies. A collaborative approach is utilized between oncologists and the team to effectively diagnose and treat syndromes of cancer pain, allowing patients to heal faster and experience less discomfort.

Continuum Cancer Centers

Beth Israel Medical Center
Roosevelt Hospital
St. Luke's Hospital
Long Island College Hospital
New York Eye and Ear Infirmary

Continuum Cancer Centers of New York

Continuum Cancer Centers of New York

Phone: (212) 844-6027

The hospitals of Continuum – Beth Israel Medical Center, St. Luke's and Roosevelt Hospitals, Long Island College Hospital and the New York Eye and Ear Infirmary – are leading providers of cancer care through Continuum Cancer Centers of New York. Our integrated system allows us to build on the clinical strengths found at each of our partner hospitals.

The goal – and result – is delivery of care in ways that are more efficient, more attractive and more convenient for patients. Specifically, it means that cancer patients at any Continuum hospital can benefit from system-wide cancer expertise, facilities and resources. Continuum Cancer Centers feature world-renowned cancer specialists, including top-rated surgeons, medical oncologists, radiation oncologists, radiologists, pathologists, and oncology nurses.

Comprehensive diagnostic and treatment services are available for breast cancer, prostate cancer, head and neck and thyroid cancers, skin cancer, lung cancer, colorectal and other gastrointestinal cancers, lymphoma/Hodgkin's Disease, gynecological cancers, and cancers of the brain and central nervous system. Delivered efficiently in a friendly and supportive environment, our services include prevention programs – such as community education, screenings and early detection – expert diagnosis, outpatient treatment, inpatient services and home care. In addition, our Research Program offers patients access to investigational protocols through a wide number of clinical trials. Our physicians are leaders in both non-invasive and minimally invasive cancer treatments that focus on maximizing both the cure rate and the quality of life.

Support services play an important role at Continuum Cancer Centers.

Nurses, social workers, psychiatrists, chaplains, pharmacists, rehabilitation therapists and nutritionists all have specialized knowledge and expertise in the field of oncology.

At the hospitals of Continuum Cancer Centers, we all work together to ensure that patients' medical, emotional and family needs are addressed appropriately and in a timely manner.

For help finding the services and care you need, please call us at (212) 844-6027.

536

Sponsored Page

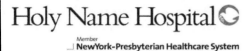

Holy Name Hospital ⟲

Member
NewYork-Presbyterian Healthcare System
Affiliate: Columbia University College of Physicians & Surgeons

718 Teaneck Road
Teaneck, NJ 07666
(201) 833-3000
www.holyname.org

THE REGIONAL CANCER CENTER AT HOLY NAME HOSPITAL

Holy Name now offers a level of cancer care unsurpassed in Bergen County—and, in some cases, the world. Housing some of the most sophisticated technology available, the center is staffed by an exceptional team of physicians, technicians, technologists and nurses dedicated to fighting cancer.

A FULL RANGE OF SERVICES

The Regional Cancer Center features a one-stop concept with a full range of services. Patients can arrange for a consultation with their medical, radiation or surgical oncologist; receive their radiation treatment or chemotherapy; and expedite imaging procedures, biopsies and other tests. They can seek the assistance of the center's dietitian or meet with one of our social workers or mental health professionals for direction on psychosocial or job issues.

TECHNOLOGY PIONEERS

The center not only offers surgery, radiation therapy and chemotherapy, it has pioneered new technologies to diagnose and treat cancer. Holy Name Hospital is part of an elite group worldwide combining PET/CT scanning, respiratory gating and IMRT to fight cancer. Using a combination PET (Positron Emission Tomography) and CT (Computerized Tomography) scan, Holy Name cancer specialists are able to view metabolic activity and pinpoint the location of abnormal lesions. The fusion of these two separate images allows for precise targeting of the disease. Discovery LS PET/CT radiation technology with "smart beam/sliding window" IMRT (intensity modulated radiation therapy) spares healthy tissue, decreases side effects and increases chances of a cure.

Respiratory gating uses a PET/CT scan to track motion within the patient's breathing cycle, significantly enhancing treatment accuracy. The radiation beam works with a patient's breathing cycle and turns on only when the tumor is in the targeted range. This synchronized treatment reduces complications, minimizes side effects and improves outcomes.

Holy Name's Cancer Center is accredited by the American College of Surgeons—Commission on Cancer and the American College of Radiology and is a member of the NewYork-Presbyterian Healthcare System.

For more information about the Regional Cancer Center, call 201-541-5900.

The Regional Cancer Center at Holy Name Hospital offers:

- High-resolution computerized tomography (CT)

- Magnetic resonance imaging (MRI)

- Positron emission tomography (PET)

- Digital mammography

- IMRT (intensity modulated radiation therapy)

- PET/CT

- Respiratory-gated PET/CT

- High dose rate (HDR) brachytherapy

- Stereotactic radiosurgery

- GliaSite®

- MammoSite®

- Participation in Clinical Research

- Radiofrequency Ablation (RFA)

- Radioimmunotherapy

- Cancer Risk Assessment Program

760

Maimonides Medical Center
MAIMONIDES CANCER CENTER

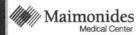
Maimonides
Medical Center

6300 Eighth Avenue • Brooklyn, New York
Phone: (718) 765-2500
www.maimonidesmed.org

Maimonides Cancer Center offers a fully integrated approach to cancer care that includes prevention, education, screening, diagnostics, treatment, palliative care and clinical research – all in one location. Staffed by a multidisciplinary team of leading oncologists, nurses, social workers and treatment specialists, the Maimonides Cancer Center provides compassionate, patient-centered, state-of-the-art care that is both accessible and comfortable. This freestanding, 50,000 square foot facility contains the following specialty centers:

Radiation Oncology Center: equipped with state-of-the art imaging and treatment delivery technologies; offers patients the most precise treatments available, yet does so in an airy, life-affirming environment.

Medical Oncology Center: provides oral drug therapies, intravenous chemotherapy infusions, transfusions, intravenous hydration, and antibiotics.

Pediatric Oncology Center: treats children with cancer in a child-friendly environment, and features special areas set aside for parent conferences.

Surgical Oncology Center: provides a convenient location for minor surgical procedures relating to cancer, including biopsies; and pre- and post-surgical care for the most complex cases.

Women's Center: provides mammography, sonography, computerized interpretation, biopsy procedures, same-day reading of results, treatment plans tailored for each patient.

Resource Center: offers access to integrative (complementary) oncology services, a library with Internet resources, social services, and dietary advice.

Research Center: conducts clinical trials that not only help advance science but also offer appropriately screened patients, who wish to volunteer, new therapies and medications.

Physicians at Maimonides are among the eight percent in the US who use computers to enter patient orders, thereby reducing the risk of errors, increasing efficiency, and speeding the healing process. Maimonides has appeared on the American Hospital Association's "Most Wired" and "Most Wireless" lists more often than any other healthcare institution in the metropolitan area. Advanced technology allows our doctors to focus more attention on caring for their patients.

Maimonides Medical Center – passionate about medicine, compassionate about people.

572

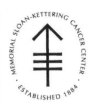

Memorial Sloan-Kettering Cancer Center

The Best Cancer Care. Anywhere.

1275 York Avenue
New York, NY 10021
Phone: (212) 639-2000
Physician Referral: (800) 525-2225
www.mskcc.org

Sponsorship: Private, Non-Profit
Beds: 432
Accreditation: Awarded Accreditation from the Joint Commission on Accreditation of Healthcare Organizations (JCAHO).

At Memorial Sloan-Kettering Cancer Center, our sole focus is cancer. Our doctors have unparalleled expertise in diagnosing and treating all types of cancer, and they use the latest technology and the most innovative, advanced therapies to increase the chances of a cure.

SUB-SPECIALIZED CLINICAL EXPERTISE

Physicians at MSKCC work within Disease Management teams that are sub-specialized by cancer type (breast, lung, etc.). The members work together to guide each patient through every aspect of their care, from diagnosis through treatment and into recovery. These teams have a depth and breadth of experience that is unsurpassed. Treatment plans reflect the combined expertise of many medical professionals, including surgeons, medical oncologists, radiologists, radiation oncologists, pathologists, psychologists and social workers. This approach ensures that patients who need several different therapies to treat their cancer will receive the best combination for them. It also provides a remarkable level of care, often resulting in better outcomes than those of patients treated at other hospitals.

RESEARCH AND EDUCATION

One of Memorial Sloan-Kettering's great strengths is the close relationship between scientists and clinicians. The constant collaboration between our doctors and research scientists means that new drugs and therapies developed in the laboratory can be moved quickly to the bedside, offering patients improved treatment options and better chances for a cure. The Center's renowned training programs prepare today's physicians, scientists, nurses and other health professionals for tomorrow's leadership roles in science and medicine, especially as it relates to cancer.

NURSING AND SUPPORTIVE CARE

Our nurses are an essential part of the healthcare team. Their support, encouragement, and deep sense of caring bring tremendous comfort to our patients and their families. Our specially trained oncology nurses care for patients before, during and after surgery, educate patients about what to expect when they go home from the hospital, and communicate with family members to address their needs and concerns. To help ensure a continuum of care, patients are typically cared for by the same nurses throughout their stay.

At Memorial Sloan-Kettering, we have long understood that cancer is not solely a physical disease. For more than 50 years, we have provided expert assistance in dealing with cancer-related distress, and have developed a range of comprehensive programs and services to help patients, families and caregivers manage the unique set of changes that often accompany serious illness. Many of our programs now serve as models for other cancer centers around the world.

A TRADITION OF EXCELLENCE

From its founding more than a century ago, Memorial Sloan-Kettering Cancer Center has been guided by a clear mission: to offer the best possible care for patients today, and to seek strategies to prevent, control and ultimately cure cancer in the future. We are proud of our designation as one of the few select National Cancer Institute Comprehensive Cancer Centers.

To see one of our specialized cancer experts, call us at (800) 525-2225.

763

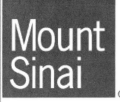

THE MOUNT SINAI MEDICAL CENTER
ONCOLOGY / CANCER CARE

One Gustave L. Levy Place (Fifth Avenue and 100th Street)
New York, NY 10029-6574
Physician Referral: 1-800-MD-SINAI (636-4624)
www.mountsinai.org

A TRADITION OF COMMITMENT AND DEDICATION
Mount Sinai has dedicated itself to one of the most widespread life-threatening diseases.

SUPERB CARE
In an atmosphere of learning, clinical excellence, and superb patient care, Mount Sinai coordinates a full-service diagnostic and treatment program for cancer patients.

A WIDE RANGE OF PROGRAMS
Programs include medical chemotherapy, radiation, surgery, bone marrow and stem cell transplants, clinical trials for adults and children, and palliative care.

ADVANCED TECHNIQUES
Mount Sinai specialists use the most recent advances in the diagnosis and treatment of all cancers and especially, breast, colorectal, liver, lung, prostate, head and neck, gynecological and genitourinary cancers, and cancers of the blood and lymph systems.

TEAMWORK
Using a multidisciplinary approach, the Medical Center's cancer specialists work with colleagues in Medical Oncology, Radiation Oncology, Radiology, Surgery, and Pathology to treat the wide spectrum of types and locations of cancer.

INNOVATION
In addition, the Medical Center takes innovative approaches to the treatment of cancer patients: minimal access, local therapy for endocrine tumors, high risk screening, genetics of breast cancer, multi-modality therapy for gastrointestinal cancer, melanoma screening, vaccine program, and minimal access surgery for cancer in the elderly. In addition, with the knowledge gained through the Human Genome Project, Mount Sinai researchers are working on a gene therapy program for colon, prostate and breast cancer.

PROSTATE HEALTH CENTER
Under the auspices of the Barbara and Maurice A. Deane Prostate Health Center, patients can access the expertise of experienced urologists, medical oncologists, and radiation oncologists, so that a patient may ultimately choose his definitive therapy with full knowledge of the risks and benefits of each treatment option. The focus of the Integrated Prostate Cancer Program is the provision of care for patients for whom standard treatments for localized disease, locally advanced disease, or metastatic disease have failed.

THE DERALD H. RUTTERBERG CANCER CENTER

The mission of the Derald H. Ruttenberg Cancer Center at The Mount Sinai Medical Center is to reduce the burden of human cancer through its outstanding interdisciplinary programs in research and patient care, including cancer prevention, treatment, early detection, and education. The Ruttenberg Treatment Center builds on this multidisciplinary model to provide state-of-the-art ambulatory cancer care.

The members of the Center—scientists and medical professionals—are working together to develop cancer therapies and prevention strategies to improve cancer care. New translational cancer research initiatives, from "bench to bedside" are being developed in a number of research laboratories with funding from the National Cancer Institute.

614

Sponsored Page

⌐ NewYork-Presbyterian
⌐ The University Hospital of Columbia and Cornell
NewYork-Presbyterian Cancer Centers

Affiliated with Columbia University College of Physicians and Surgeons and Weill Medical College of Cornell University

Herbert Irving Comprehensive Cancer Center
At NewYork-Presbyterian Hospital
Columbia University Medical Center
161 Fort Washington Avenue
New York, NY 10032

Weill Cornell Cancer Center
At NewYork-Presbyterian Hospital
Weill Cornell Medical Center
525 East 68th Street
New York, NY 10021

OVERVIEW:

NewYork-Presbyterian Cancer Centers are dedicated to reducing cancer morbidity and mortality by providing

- a full continuum of multidisciplinary, state-of-the-art screening, diagnostic, treatment and support services for all phases of the disease process;
- cutting-edge basic, clinical, and public health research;
- full range of cancer-related educational programs and resources to clinicians, scientists, patients and survivors, families, and the cancer prevention community.

The Cancer Centers, which treat over 6,000 new patients annually, draw on the innovation and excellence of the NCI- designated Herbert Irving Comprehensive Cancer Center at NewYork-Presbyterian Hospital/Columbia University Medical Center and oncology services at NewYork-Presbyterian Hospital/Weill Cornell Medical Center. Programs include:

- AIDS-related Malignancies
- Bone Marrow Transplant
- Breast Cancer
- Dermatologic/Skin Cancer
- Gastrointestinal Cancers
- Genitourinary Cancers
- Gynecologic Cancers
- Head and Neck Cancers
- Hematologic Malignancies, such as lymphoma, myeloma and leukemias
- Lung Cancer
- Neurologic Cancer
- Ophthalmic Cancer
- Pediatric Hematology/Oncology
- Urologic Cancers, including bladder, kidney and prostate cancer
- Sarcomas and Mesotheiliomas

The Centers are frequent recipients of major grants and gifts to support research programs. Recent highlights include:

- Avon Products Foundation $10 million award to NewYork-Presbyterian Hospital/Columbia University Medical Center and Columbia University for establishment of the Avon Products Breast Center to support basic, clinical and public health research in breast cancer;
- The Leukemia and Lymphoma Society five-year $7.5 million grant to NewYork-Presbyterian Hospital/Weill Cornell Medical Center to study fundamental causes of multiple myeloma

Physician Referral: For a physician referral call toll free **1-877-NYP-WELL** (1-877-697-9355) to learn more about our Cancer Centers visit our website at **www.nypcancer.org**

COMPREHENSIVE SERVICES INCLUDE:

- Access to over 400 clinical trials supported by the National Institutes of Health and many prominent pharmaceutical companies.

- Bone marrow and blood stem cell transplant, including New York State approval to perform transplants using unrelated donors for patients with hematologic malignancies

- CT screening for early lung cancer detection

- Sentinel node biopsy to assess spread of breast cancer

- Skin-sparing mastectomy and reconstruction

- Laparoscopic surgery for colon cancer

- Intraoperative brachytherapy for GI, prostate and other cancers

- Stereotactic biopsies for breast cancer and brain cancer

- Stereotactic gamma radiation for brain tumors

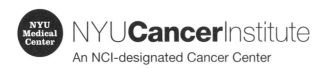

NYU**Cancer**Institute
An NCI-designated Cancer Center

Looking for information on our expert physicians?
1-212-731-5000

NYU Clinical Cancer Center
160 East 34th Street
New York, New York 10016
www.nyuci.org

NYU Medical Center
550 First Avenue (at 31st Street)
New York, New York 10016
www.nyumc.org

A Collaborative Approach
The NYU Cancer Institute, an NCI designated center, is a "matrix cancer center" without walls operating within the larger NYU Medical Center. With over 250 members and a research funding base of over $80 million, this structure strengthens our capabilities to forge collaborations across medical and scientific disciplines, which translates to comprehensive care for our patients and discoveries that will influence the future of this disease.

Renowned Expertise
Our highly skilled Magnet™ nursing team not only plays a pivotal role in coordinating direct patient care, but is also a source of invaluable patient education. Team members' compassion and expertise help patients better manage the symptoms of their disease as well as their special needs.

A Patient-Focused Setting
The NYU Clinical Cancer Center, with over 60 faculty members from various disciplines at the New York University School of Medicine, is the principal outpatient facility of the Cancer Institute and serves as home base for our patients and their caregivers. The center and its multidisciplinary team of experts provide access to the latest treatment options and clinical trials along with a variety of programs in cancer prevention, screening, diagnostics, genetic counseling, and supportive services. Our affiliation with Bellevue Hospital, the oldest public hospital in the country, affords clinically distinctive opportunities to learn and care for patients with cancer by observing its presentation and behavior in a variety of patient groups.

Sponsored Page

THE CANCER HOSPITAL OF NEW JERSEY AT ROBERT WOOD JOHNSON UNIVERSITY HOSPITAL

One Robert Wood Johnson Place • New Brunswick, NJ 08903-2601
General Information (732) 828-3000 • Physician Referral 888-44-RWJUH
www.rwjuh.edu

The Cancer Hospital of New Jersey at Robert Wood Johnson University Hospital is the flagship hospital of The Cancer Institute of New Jersey (CINJ), the state's only National Cancer Institute-designated Comprehensive Cancer Center and one of only 39 such centers nationwide.

ACADEMIC MEDICAL CENTER

The 123-bed Cancer Hospital of New Jersey and The Cancer Institute of New Jersey are physically linked and together integrate state-of-the-art care with cutting-edge translational research. Patients gain access to clinical trials, new therapies and a multi-disciplinary team of specialists including medical, surgical and radiation oncologists, Magnet Award-winning nurse specialists, pharmacists and social workers.

COMPREHENSIVE CARE

The Cancer Hospital of New Jersey provides a full spectrum of screening, diagnostic services and specialized treatments including same-day chemotherapy, medical oncology, hematology-oncology, surgical oncology, bone marrow transplantation and radiation therapy.

Led by physicians listed in *America's Top Doctors* (Castle Connolly), the **Radiation Oncology Department's** advanced capabilities include IMRT (intensity modulated radiation therapy), brachytherapy, stereotactic radiosurgery and CT simulation. The TomoTherapy Hi-Art System will be available in late 2006. A proton beam radiation center is also in development.

The Cancer Hospital of New Jersey at RWJUH is the state's **highest volume center** for lung and esophageal cancer surgery, and one of a select few centers using the **daVinci Robotic System for minimally-invasive prostate cancer surgery**.

For women, the hospital's **Women's Imaging Center** offers state-of-the-art digital mammography technology, as well as breast and gynecological ultrasound. The Center performs stereotactic breast biopsy, ultrasound-guided core breast biopsy and ultrasound-guided fine-needle biopsy, as well as needle-localization for breast biopsy and lumpectomy.

COMPASSIONATE SUPPORT

Another dimension of care is provided through an array of supportive services and oncology specialists including nutritionists, social workers, chaplains, and numerous support groups, patient education programs and complementary therapies. In addition, all patient rooms are private with room-service dining, hotel-style amenities and sleeping accommodations for family members.

Robert Wood Johnson University Hospital is the principal teaching hospital of UMDNJ-Robert Wood Johnson Medical School and the flagship hospital of the Robert Wood Johnson Health System & Network.

For Children, The Bristol-Myers Squibb Children's Hospital (www.bmsch.org) provides pediatric hematology/oncology services under the direction of nationally-renowned physicians in a child- focused environment. The hospital campus includes a Ronald McDonald House.

The Bristol-Myers Squibb Children's Hospital and The Cancer Hospital of New Jersey are part of Robert Wood Johnson University Hospital, one of the nation's leading academic medical centers. RWJUH was named in 2005 as one of the top five hospitals in the nation for patient safety by *Consumers Digest Magazine.*

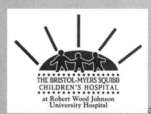

THE BRISTOL-MYERS SQUIBB
CHILDREN'S HOSPITAL
at Robert Wood Johnson
University Hospital

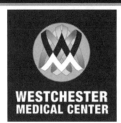

WESTCHESTER MEDICAL CENTER

Valhalla Campus
Valhalla, NY 10595
Tel. (914) 4-CANCER
http://www.worldclassmedicine.com

OVERVIEW

Groundbreaking research, state-of-the-art treatment, internationally renowned physicians and surgeons and the highest level of compassionate care make the Arlin Cancer Institute at Westchester Medical Center the choice for people from the region and beyond who are facing cancer. The Cancer Institute's team strives to partner with patients in their treatment and recovery, and fully supports patients and families in living with and fighting cancer. Through a multidisciplinary approach involving experts in the field of medical and surgical oncology and radiation medicine, every aspect of care is available in one location at Westchester Medical Center.

The Cancer Institute is home to a nationally renowned leukemia program, one of the world's oldest bone marrow transplant programs, and one of the few programs in New York State approved by the National Marrow Donor program as an unrelated bone marrow transplant and collection center.

Actively involved in a broad spectrum of research initiatives, the Cancer Institute collaborates with key national study groups and universities in dozens of cutting-edge research projects for such cancers as leukemia, lymphoma, myeloma and prostate, brain, breast, lung and an array of gynecologic cancers. Patients are able to participate in and benefit from scientific advances in oncologic medicine and technology years before they are available to the general public. The Arlin Cancer Institute continues to break ground in therapeutic anticancer approaches, including matched unrelated marrow and cord blood transplantation, stereotactic radiosurgery, high-dose-rate brachytherapy, hyperthermia and cryosurgical procedures. A gene screening and therapy program and expansion of molecular biology services are among the many innovations on the horizon at Westchester Medical Center.

As part of a large university medical center, expert diagnostic services are provided by highly skilled members of the Department of Pathology of New York Medical College, who are experienced in cancer diagnosis and have access to the most advanced technology available in cytogenetics, cytometry and immunohistology. Same day diagnoses are provided on fine needle biopsy specimens of office patients. Each year more than 25,000 radiation therapy procedures performed at Westchester Medical Center help Cancer Institute patients battle cancer. 50 years ago only one cancer patient in five survived. Today nearly half of all cancer patients win their fight against cancer. Research at Westchester Medical Center has made significant contributions to the enhanced survival of cancer patients in the U.S. and abroad.

CANCER INSTITUTE AT WESTCHESTER MEDICAL CENTER

At the forefront of medical technology, Westchester Medical Center offers Novalis® Shaped Beam Surgery —the least invasive and most precise treatment option available to patients diagnosed with cancer, brain tumors, and neurologic and vascular disorders. This revolutionary system, comprised of four state-of-the-art radiosurgery and radiotherapy applications, custom shapes the treatment beam to better target affected tissue while protecting healthy tissue.

For more information on Novalis® Shaped Beam Surgery, call 1-866-BEAMCENTER

786

Sponsored Page

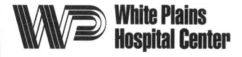

White Plains Hospital Center

The Cancer Program
White Plains Hospital Center
Davis Avenue at East Post Road
White Plains, NY 10601
(914) 681-2700
www.wphospital.org

COMPREHENSIVE CANCER CARE

The White Plains Hospital Center (WPHC) Cancer Program provides expert, comprehensive and compassionate cancer care at a level often found in more specialized hospitals and academic medical centers. Treatment and recovery success rates meet and often exceed national standards.

The Cancer Program has achieved accreditation as a Community Hospital Comprehensive Cancer Program by the American College of Surgeons, the highest designation possible for a community hospital.

DICKSTEIN CANCER TREATMENT CENTER

Opened in 1999, the Dickstein Cancer Treatment Center (DCTC) is the only freestanding outpatient cancer treatment facility in Westchester County. The modern and well-appointed DCTC building houses a linear accelerator for radiation therapy, the Lowenthal Infusion Center for chemotherapy treatment, and space for a wide variety of educational and complementary care programs. Even if a patient is diagnosed at another facility, it is possible for treatment to be provided closer to home at the Dickstein Center.

PREVENTION, DIAGNOSIS & TREATMENT

The Cancer Program at WPHC has a comprehensive range of tests and procedures available to identify cancers at their earliest stages. These resources include WPHC's **world-class Radiology Department** which employs the latest technologies, including a Positron Emission Tomography (PET) Scanner, standard and digital mammography, and breast MRI. The Hospital also offers a **Cancer Genetics Program** which measures susceptibility to various cancers based on family genetics.

In the treatment arena, the increased use of **minimally invasive surgery** shortens recovery and reduces complications. One of the best examples is the use of the da Vinci surgical robot in the removal of a cancerous prostate gland. Benefits include smaller incisions, less blood loss, fewer complications and less discomfort for the patient.

At the **Lowenthal Infusion Center,** patients can receive chemotherapy and other infusion therapies in a convenient, comfortable and clinically superior environment.

The **Breast Imaging Center** provides preventive care and screenings for women. Located within the hospital and at a satellite office in Rye Brook, NY, the services include analog and digital mammography, breast ultrasound, breast MRI, and stereotactic breast biopsy.

The Dickstein Center's **Radiation Oncology Department** is accredited by the American College of Radiology. In addition to a linear accelerator, the Department offers brachytherapy, where radioactive seeds are implanted directly into an organ or near a tumor, thereby reducing risk to adjacent body structures.

White Plains Hospital Center Comprehensive Cancer Program

- Performs more prostate, colon and breast cancer surgeries than any other hospital in Westchester County

- Minimally invasive surgery, including the da Vinci robot

- Cancer Genetics Program

- World-class radiology services, including interventional radiology, CT and PET/CT for cancer diagnosis, staging, and treatment planning

- Breast Imaging Center, including MRI and stereotactic biopsy

- Lowenthal Infusion Center

- Linear Accelerator for radiation therapy

- Complementary Care Program

- Ongoing community education programs

- Clinical research

- Screening programs

767

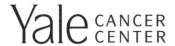

Yale CANCER CENTER

A Comprehensive Cancer Center Designated
by the National Cancer Institute

333 Cedar Street
New Haven, CT 06520
1-866-YALECANCER

Dedicated to tomorrow's cancer treatments, today.

As a National Cancer Institute designated comprehensive cancer center, **Yale Cancer Center** is a leader in developing and implementing new approaches to cancer prevention and cancer care. Beginning with the first use of chemotherapy in 1942, researchers at Yale have continued to identify innovative treatments to benefit our patients.

Yale Cancer Center currently has numerous clinical trials available to cancer patients in search of novel therapies. These trials are evaluating new methods of prevention, detection and treatment of cancer. Clinical trials give patients at **Yale Cancer Center** immediate access to the future of cancer care.

Clinical trials are currently available for patients in the following disease areas:

- Bladder Cancer
- Brain Cancer
- Breast Cancer
- Colorectal Cancer
- Cutaneous T Cell Lymphoma
- Gynecologic Malignancies
- Head and Neck Cancer
- Leukemia
- Liver Cancer
- Lung Cancer
- Lymphoma
- Melanoma
- Multiple Myeloma
- Pancreatic Cancer
- Prostate Cancer
- Thyroid Cancer

For more information on the trials currently open for accrual at Yale Cancer Center, please visit **www.yalecancercenter.org** or call **1-866-YALECANCER**

Yale Cancer Center is affiliated with:

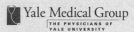

Yale Medical Group
THE PHYSICIANS OF
YALE UNIVERSITY

is one of the largest academic multispecialty group practices in the United States. Comprised of the full-time faculty of the Yale School of Medicine, YMG physicians are leaders in their fields, dedicated to combining a compassionate, individual approach to patient care with the latest clinical and technologic developments.

www.yalemedicalgroup.org

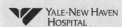

YALE-NEW HAVEN HOSPITAL

is a 944-bed tertiary referral center, the primary teaching hospital for the Yale University School of Medicine, and the only hospital in Connecticut consistently recognized as one of America's Best Hospitals by US News & World Report.

www.ynhh.org

Sponsored Page

Cardiac Imaging

ST. FRANCIS HOSPITAL
THE HEART CENTER®
100 Port Washington Blvd. • Roslyn, New York 11576
516-562-6000 • 1-888-HEARTNY
http://stfrancisheartcenter.chsli.org

NON-INVASIVE CARDIAC IMAGING

Using the latest in non-invasive cardiac imaging technology, St. Francis Hospital's physicians have immediate access to information regarding blood flow, heart muscle strength, anatomy, and coronary artery blockages that allows them to more effectively guide a patient's course of treatment.

Among the most recent introductions to St. Francis Hospital's range of services are:

• 64-Slice Computed Tomography
St. Francis Hospital is the first hospital on Long Island to offer 64-slice MultiDetector Computed Tomography (MDCT) for coronary imaging and other applications. The new technology provides previously unobtainable visualization of the coronary arteries. Faster scanning also increases patient comfort by reducing breath holds to ten seconds or less.

• Cardiac MRI
The first center on Long Island to introduce a dedicated cardiac MRI system, St. Francis Hospital has the ability to non-invasively capture images of the heart that provide a level of information not available with other technologies. Cardiac MRI allows physicians to evaluate effects of heart attack, effects of coronary artery blockages and the causes of heart failure to determine whether or not patients will benefit from heart surgery or other therapies. World-renowned cardiac MRI authority Nathaniel Reichek, M.D. leads St. Francis Hospital's clinical and research applications with cardiac MRI.

• Three-dimensional echocardiography
St. Francis Hospital was the first on Long Island to acquire a three-dimensional echocardiography system for quantifying the effects of heart disease. In creating a 3-D reconstruction of the heart, this technology can provide detail on the extent of a patient's heart disease.

• Nuclear Imaging
Nuclear imaging is being used at St. Francis Hospital to evaluate patients who are not candidates for the simple exercise stress test. Especially in cases where coronary artery disease is suspected, nuclear imaging improves the accuracy of the stress test. St. Francis Hospital offers single-photon emission computed tomography (SPECT), which involves the injection of nuclear isotopes and continuous imaging by a gamma camera that circles the patient's body. The nuclear cardiology laboratory at St. Francis Hospital is among the first facilities in the U.S. to have received accreditation from The Intersocietal Commission for the Accreditation of Nuclear Medicine Laboratories.

NON-INVASIVE IMAGING AT ST. FRANCIS HOSPITAL

Non-invasive imaging services at St. Francis Hospital include:

- 64-slice multidetector computed tomography
- cardiac MRI
- SPECT nuclear imaging
- transesophageal echocardiography
- three-dimensional echocardiography
- electron beam CT scanning (ultrafast CT scanning)
- thallium stress testing

St. Francis Hospital's highly precise non-invasive imaging technology is also being applied in its research of the cardiovascular disease process. Applying its depth of experience with various imaging modalities, the Hospital has launched a multi-disciplinary effort to improve methods for the diagnosis and treatment of cardiac disease, at its St. Francis Cardiac Research Institute. Past research efforts at the Hospital include The St. Francis Heart Study – the largest study to be conducted at any single center – which supported the use of electron beam CT scanning as a tool for cardiac risk evaluation.

766

Cardiovascular Services

GAGNON HEART HOSPITAL

Morristown Memorial Hospital • Overlook Hospital

THE PASSION TO LEAD

**Goryeb Children's Hospital • Atlantic Neuroscience Institute
Carol G. Simon Cancer Center/The Cancer Center at Overlook Hospital
Gagnon Heart Hospital • Atlantic Rehabilitation Institute**

P.O. Box 1905, Morristown, NJ 07962 • 1-800-247-9580 • atlantichealth.org

◢ National Leadership in Cardiac Care, Close To Home

Expert care and comprehensive cardiovascular services are available at Overlook Hospital and Morristown Memorial Hospital, which has the state's largest cardiac surgery program, serving patients from both facilities. We are a national leader in the research and treatment of cardiac disease and more heart surgery is performed at Morristown Memorial than at any other NJ hospital. In fact, Morristown Memorial is second in the New York Metro region in the number of heart surgeries performed. Our heart surgery survival rates rival the state benchmark. Overlook Hospital is the first hospital in New Jersey granted state approval to perform emergency angioplasty without on-site cardiac surgery as part of a clinical trial. We also offer the innovative "Cardiac Classroom" in cooperation with Liberty Science Center where students can view heart surgery live via satellite.

◢ Gagnon Heart Hospital in 2008

Morristown Memorial will soon be home to the new Gagnon Heart Hospital, a state-of-the-art facility opening in 2008 with private patient rooms, new operating and procedure rooms and convenient access to all facets of cardiac care.

◢ Newest Diagnostic and Treatment Options

64-Image Cardiac CT Angiography - The latest in non-invasive cardiac imaging technologies, 64-image Cardiac CT Angiography or Volume Computed Tomography (VCT) produces an image comparable in detail to traditional cardiac catheterization. It gives our cardiologists another powerful tool to diagnose and manage heart disease.

Robotic Surgery - This groundbreaking technology is now in use at Morristown Memorial Hospital.

◢ Interventional Cardiology

Every year, Morristown Memorial and Overlook doctors perform more than 7,500 successful cardiac catheterizations and angioplasties, saving thousands of lives.

◢ **Balloon Angioplasty**	◢ **Coronary Stenting**
◢ **Rotoblator**	◢ **Atherectomy**
◢ **Valvuloplasty**	◢ **Radiation Seed Implant Therapy or Brachytherapy**

◢ Cardiac Rhythm Management Program

The cardiac rhythm management team performs comprehensive electrophysiology studies, radiofrequency ablations for supraventricular and ventricular tachycardias, pacemaker and defibrillator implantations, and tilt table testing. The team also participates in important clinical trials to advance the standard of patient care.

◢ Enhanced External Counterpulsation

(EECP) is a non-invasive procedure that can reduce the symptoms of angina. EECP involves the use of a device to inflate and deflate a series of compressive cuffs wrapped around the patient's calves, lower thighs, and upper thighs. This program can be prescribed by your physician as a means to enhance your quality of life if you suffer from persistent angina.

Swift intervention and treatment are vital to save lives, and our medical expertise, state-of-the-art technology, clinical excellence, and compassionate care give thousands of patients each year the opportunity to live longer, more productive lives.

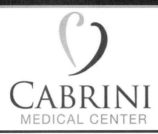

CABRINI
MEDICAL CENTER

227 East 19th Street
New York, N.Y. 10003

CABRINI CARDIOVASCULAR DIVISION

INTEGRATED CARDIOVASCULAR IMAGING
Cabrini Medical Center has one of the most advanced and comprehensive integrated cardiovascular imaging programs in the nation. Using state-of-the-art cardiac magnetic resonance imaging (MRI) and computed tomography (CAT Scan) in conjunction with nuclear medicine and ultrasound. Cabrini physicians are able to accurately diagnose and treat many cardiovascular and pulmonary diseases in the most timely and efficient manner.

CLINICAL RESEARCH
Clinical trials of several novel treatments of high blood pressure and early detection of coronary artery disease are currently underway. Cabrini is also actively involved with Chase Medical in the development of an endoventricular shaper (TRISVR) for performing surgical reshaping of the heart in patients with end stage ischemic cardiomyopathy.

TECHNOLOGY DEVELOPMENT
Advanced cardiac imaging software and protocols are currently being developed at Cabrini in collaboration with Siemens, Terarecon, and Chase Medical, Inc.

CLINICAL SERVICE
The Cardiology program at Cabrini Medical Center is actively involved in a collaborative effort with Mount Sinai School of Medicine in providing the full array of cardiology services to the Cabrini community, ranging from early and accurate diagnosis of coronary artery disease using advanced imaging methods, rapid assessment and specialized treatment of congestive heart failure, the use of drug-eluting stents, implantable pacemakers and defibrillators, and chronic infusion therapy for severe pulmonary hypertension. The ongoing collaborations include the development of clinical and research programs in advanced cardiac imaging, atherosclerosis, congestive heart failure, implantable device-therapy, and pulmonary hypertension. The Cardiologists speak fluent Cantonese, Madarin, Fuchow, Spanish and Ukranian.

Call us at 212.995.6865 to speak to a patient representative.

752

PHYSICIAN LEADERSHIP

Cabrini Medical Center is in the forefront of the New York metropolitan area for the early diagnosis and treatment of heart and vascular disease. Cabrini Medical Center physicians Michael Poon, MD, Director of Cardiology, Jurij Stecko, MD and Rose Marie Carrera, MD bring world-class cardiac diagnostic and treatment to Cabrini and the neighboring community.

Dr. Poon is a leading expert in non-invasive cardiovascular magnetic resonance MR) and computed tomography (CT) imaging and in the treatment of coronary artery disease and pulmonary hypertension.

Dr. Stecko is a recognized expert in Cardiac CT imaging. Dr. Carrera specializes in cardiovascular ultra-sound imaging. Both Dr. Stecko and Dr. Carrera are experts in nuclear cardiology imaging.

For more information, visit our website at www.cabrininy.org

Sponsored Page

Continuum Heart Institute

Beth Israel Medical Center
Roosevelt Hospital
St. Luke's Hospital
Long Island College Hospital

Phone (800) 420-4004
www.chpnyc.org

The Continuum Heart Institute combines the strengths of the cardiac programs at Beth Israel Medical Center, Roosevelt Hospital, St. Luke's Hospital and Long Island College Hospital for clinical, technological and innovative excellence. The skill and caliber of its cardiologists, cardiovascular surgeons, and other physician specialists is matched only by its state-of-the-art facilities—including the most technologically advanced cardiac care units, catheterization and electrophysiology labs, cardiac surgery suites, and open heart recovery units.

The Continuum Heart Institute offers every clinical expertise needed to prevent, diagnose, and treat heart disease, including leading-edge cardiac surgery, catheter-based diagnosis and treatment, hypertension diagnosis and treatment, heart failure diagnosis and treatment, and a hypertrophic cardiomyopathy program. Strong believers in prevention and early detection, the professionals throughout the Continuum Heart Institute also provide complete medical evaluations, echocardiography, nuclear cardiology services, coronary artery disease prevention, treatment centers for obesity and diabetes, smoking cessation programs, and complementary techniques for relaxation and stress reduction, such as massage therapy and therapeutic touch.

Some of the unique features available at the hospitals of the Continuum Heart Institute include a robotic surgical suite for closed-chest coronary artery bypass surgery; the Ross procedure—a pulmonary autograft replacement of the aortic valve; and a nationally recognized arrhythmia service.

Our cardiac surgery program is recognized by the New York State Department of Health as having one of the lowest mortality rates of any New York City hospital, and is consistently ranked among the best programs in New York State.

CONTINUUM HEART INSTITUTE

The Continuum Heart Institute was established in an effort to bridge the many cardiac care programs of our partner hospitals and provide patients with more streamlined access to our full range of services. This interdisciplinary cardiology, cardiac surgery and cardiac rehabilitation team consists of clinicians, surgeons, nurses and nurse practitioners, physician assistants, social workers, complementary care experts and rehabilitation specialists—all working together to give patients a full range of individualized treatment choices and services.

603

Holy Name Hospital ⊙

Member
NewYork-Presbyterian Healthcare System
Affiliate: Columbia University College of Physicians & Surgeons

718 Teaneck Road
Teaneck, NJ 07666
(201) 833-3000
www.holyname.org

CARDIOVASCULAR CARE AND CHEST PAIN

Holy Name Hospital received a 5-star rating from HealthGrades® two years in a row, placing it among the top 5 percent of hospitals in the nation for treatment of atrial fibrillation and heart attacks. In the Emergency Department patients with chest pain are evaluated by board-certified cardiologists, emergency medicine physicians and cardiac-certified emergency nurses. Cardiologists are on call around the clock if needed. Treatment of acute myocardial infarction (heart attack) may include emergency angioplasty and placement of a coronary stent.

CUTTING-EDGE STRESS-FREE STRESS TESTING AND MORE.

Holy Name Hospital became the first and only hospital in New Jersey to offer Cardiac PET Nuclear Stress Testing to identify coronary artery disease—providing improved accuracy in detecting coronary artery disease. Other services include pacemaker implantation, transthoracic and transesophageal echocardiography and numerous forms of stress testing.

For more information about the cardiology services at Holy Name Hospital, call 201-833-3211.

STROKE CARE CENTER

Holy Name Hospital received Primary Stroke Care Center Certification—a distinction awarded by the Joint Commission on Accreditation of Healthcare Organizations—and a 5-star rating from HealthGrades® for treatment of strokes.

Patients who are experiencing a stroke are immediately assessed in the Emergency Department. If the stroke is ischemic it may be treated within three hours with the clot-busting drug t-PA (tissue plasminogen activator). All stroke patients undergo a comprehensive evaluation by neurologists and other health specialists to help the patient toward recovery. Holy Name Hospital's designated stroke unit is staffed with board-certified neurologists and specially trained and certified nurses.

For more information about stroke care, please call 201-833-7053.

The Cardiac Services available at Holy Name Hospital include:

- Unicath cardiac catheterization system

- Pacemaker implantations

- Electrocardiography (ECG)

- Echocardiography

- Transesophageal echocardiography

- PET/CT stress testing

- Stress testing using a treadmill

- Stress echocardiography

- Thallium stress testing

- Holter monitoring

- A two-phase cardiac rehabilitation program

757

Sponsored Page

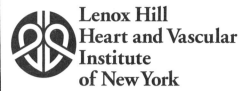

Lenox Hill Heart and Vascular Institute of New York

100 East 77th Street, New York, NY 10021
1-877-HEARTBEAT — www. lenoxheart.org

SIX SPECIALTIES UNDER ONE ROOF
The Lenox Hill Heart and Vascular Institute is among the leading cardiovascular care programs nationwide. From diagnosis to treatment and recovery, the Institute provides comprehensive care through its distinguished team of cardiologists, interventional cardiologists, electrophysiologists, cardiothoracic and vascular surgeons, and radiologists.

DEPTH OF EXPERIENCE
Lenox Hill Hospital has been a leader in cardiovascular care for decades, developing groundbreaking techniques to minimize heart damage and speed recovery:
• 1938 -- Lenox Hill Hospital cardiologists performed first angiogram in U.S.
• 1978 -- first coronary angioplasty in country performed at Lenox Hill Hospital
• 1991 -- Lenox Hill Hospital doctors implanted first coronary stent in NYC
• 1994 -- Lenox Hill Hospital surgeons introduced minimally invasive direct coronary artery bypass surgery to nation
• 2003 -- First FDA approved drug coated stent in the nation was implanted at Lenox Hill Hospital in a procedure our doctors now perform over 3,000 times each year
• 2004 -- Largest carotid stent program in U.S.
• 2005 -- Largest minimally invasive heart assist program in tri-state area; second largest nationally

A WIDE RANGE OF TREATMENTS
Physicians at the Institute constantly seek to broaden the understanding of heart and vascular disease and expand the boundaries of care through research and clinical trials. The interventional cardiology team is recognized for leadership in the use of angioplasty to clear clogged arteries. The endovascular specialists are involved in groundbreaking research involving the use of carotid stents to provide lower-risk treatment of arterial blockages without surgery and also perform minimally invasive procedures to treat complex abdominal aneurysms. The Institute's cardiothoracic surgeons are pioneers in "beating heart" surgery, and the use of robotics and minimally invasive procedures including coronary bypass, valve repair, atrial fibrillation surgery, and heart failure surgery. Surgeons specializing in vascular surgery perform surgery on the aorta, and the carotid and lower extremity arteries, including aneurysms. The Institute's electrophysiology specialists perform diagnostic, treatment and curative procedures for abnormal heart rhythms.

TIME IS MUSCLE

It's a fact. The faster a person is treated for a heart attack, the greater the chances of saving precious heart muscle and making a full recovery. That's why doctors say "time is muscle."

Today, using the most advanced technologies and sophisticated emergency communications from our ambulance directly to our cardiologists, Lenox Hill Hospital doctors have drastically reduced the time it takes for a heart attack patient to get lifesaving treatment. After all, time is muscle — and you know how important that is.

606

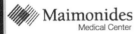

Maimonides
Medical Center

Having pioneered numerous heart care innovations through the years, The Cardiac Institute offers a rapidly growing number of diagnostic studies and therapeutic treatments, procedures and surgeries. Our patients are the beneficiaries of cutting-edge drug therapies, electrophysiology studies and therapies, interventional cardiology procedures, and cardiothoracic surgeries.

Cardiology
Among the most published and respected in the field, the Maimonides cardiology team continuously sets higher standards for patient care. Edgar Lichstein, MD, Chairman of Medicine, has been chief investigator of NIH-sponsored cardiac drug trials, and our Congestive Heart Failure (CHF) Program has been cited as the best in the Northeast.

Interventional Cardiology
New York State statistics and national independent reports have repeatedly confirmed that the Maimonides Catheterization Lab yields the best possible outcomes for patients. Led by Cardiac Institute Chairman Jacob Shani, MD, drug-eluting stents were trialed here and numerous therapeutic devices were developed and implemented. Our Electrophysiology Lab has a superb record of achievement in diagnosing and treating arrhythmias. A close collaboration with the Department of Emergency Medicine ensures that chest pain patients are evaluated immediately and that interventional procedures are used to stop heart attacks in progress whenever necessary.

Cardiothoracic Surgery
The Maimonides Cardiothoracic Surgery program has an illustrious history, setting the national standard for advances in service. Under the direction of Stephen Lahey, MD, minimally invasive and robotic heart surgeries are offered in state-of-the-art facilities. Maimonides provides one of the most prestigious cardiothoracic residency programs in the US.

Historic Moments
• The pacemaker was developed and implanted in 1961.
• In 1967, the first successful human heart transplant in the nation was performed at Maimonides.
• The intra-aortic balloon pump was developed here in 1970.
• Surgical techniques that protect the spine during cardiothoracic surgery were perfected here in 1982.
• Revolutionary cardiac catheterization devices were invented here in 1992 and 1997.
• Maimonides was the first hospital in US to implement fully automatic external cardiac defibrillators in 2001.

Physicians at Maimonides are among the eight percent in the US who use computers to enter patient orders, thereby reducing the risk of errors, increasing efficiency, and speeding the healing process. Maimonides has appeared on the American Hospital Association's "Most Wired" and "Most Wireless" lists more often than any other healthcare institution in the metropolitan area. Advanced technology allows our doctors to focus more attention on caring for their patients.

Maimonides Medical Center – passionate about medicine, compassionate about people.

72

Sponsored Page

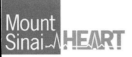

THE MOUNT SINAI MEDICAL CENTER
MOUNT SINAI HEART - CARDIOVASCULAR HEALTH

One Gustave L. Levy Place (Fifth Avenue and 100th Street)
New York, NY 10029-6574
Physician Referral: 1-800-MD-SINAI (636-4624)
www.mountsinai.org

At Mount Sinai Heart, we take a global view of cardiovascular health. Our system of integrated care combines some of the world's most accomplished physicians, research scientists, educators, and professional staff with innovative thinking, creative programs, and an unwavering commitment to the prevention and treatment of cardiovascular disease. With the rapid translation of innovative research concepts into improved preventive, diagnostic, and therapeutic care, patients receive multidisciplinary treatment of unprecedented quality.

In addition to consultative and noninvasive cardiology, cardiac catheterization, heart and lung transplantation, cardiovascular surgery, heart failure, pulmonary hypertension, lipid management, and hypertension, we also specialize in the following areas:

• *Noninvasive diagnostic imaging* - leading techniques for echocardiography, nuclear cardiology, PET, CT, and MR imaging cardiology ;
• *Coronary artery disease* - ranked as the state's safest center for patients undergoing coronary angioplasty and other catheter-based interventions;
• *Cardiac rhythm disturbances* - expert management of all aspects of heart rhythm disorders such as atrial fibrillation and tachycardia, and the insertion of implantable devices including pacemakers and defibrillators;
• *Valvular heart disease* - a wide range of medical and surgical options including a leading program for valve repair and long-term follow-up care;
• *Aortic diseases* - pioneered techniques for stent-graft repair of thoracic and abdominal aortic aneurysms, and for surgical correction of the most complex aortic pathology;
• *Congenital heart disease* - specialists in pediatric cardiology and experts in minimally invasive approaches to the correction of congenital heart defects in children and adults;
• *Cardiac failure and transplantation* - a multidisciplinary team approach to comprehensive, compassionate care for the most advanced forms of heart failure and cardiomyopathy patients;
• *Comprehensive cardiac disease prevention and rehabilitation* - a unique synergism that provides unparalleled patient care, while yielding breakthroughs in the prevention and treatment of cardiovascular disease;
• *Vascular medicine and surgery* - noninvasive diagnostic procedures and an interdisciplinary approach to disease management including medical, surgical, catheter-based, and gene therapy techniques to arterial obstruction, limb salvage, venous, and lymphatic diseases.

Mount Sinai's Cardiac Catheterization Laboratories offer leading-edge technologies of all kinds, including diagnostic angiography, angioplasty, and biopsy. We study the heart with the greatest precision available. We are pioneering new genetic techniques to help hearts with diseased arteries grow new vessels, and to help a damaged heart muscle repair itself.

MOUNT SINAI HEART

Under the creative direction of internationally renowned cardiologist Valentin Fuster, MD, PhD, Mount Sinai is recognized worldwide for its expertise in evaluating, managing and preventing cardiovascular disease through the integration of patient care, education and research. Mount Sinai Heart encompasses The Zena and Michael A. Wiener Cardiovascular Institute and the Marie-Josée and Henry R. Kravis Center for Cardiovascular Health at The Mount Sinai Medical Center, preeminent resources for the study and treatment of heart and blood vessel diseases.

Following are some of the cardiac conditions we treat at Mount Sinai Heart: arrhythmia (including atrial fibrillation, pacemakers, defibrillators and other implanted devices), coronary artery disease, heart attack and angina, heart failure and transplantation, hyperlipidemia (cholesterol), hypertension, mitral valve prolapse, myocarditis, pericardial disease, peripheral vascular disease and claudication, pulmonary hypertension, and valvular heart disease.

621

NewYork-Presbyterian
The University Hospital of Columbia and Cornell

NewYork-Presbyterian Heart

Affiliated with Columbia University College of Physicians and Surgeons and Weill Medical College of Cornell University

NewYork-Presbyterian Hospital
Columbia University Medical Center
622 West 168th Street
New York, NY 10032

NewYork-Presbyterian Hospital
Weill Cornell Medical Center
525 East 68th Street
New York, NY 10021

OVERVIEW:

The NewYork-Presbyterian Heart has a reputation for treating some of the highest risk cases in the world – healing those patients who cannot be helped anywhere else. We are committed to delivering the finest possible care to adult and pediatric patients by:

- combining the finest minds and cutting-edge technology with the most compassionate care

- helping patients make sense of the complex steps involved in treating their heart condition;

- providing them with a full set of appropriate treatment options for consideration after a complete diagnosis;

- listening, guiding and fully informing patients so that together we can confidently choose the best treatment.

The NewYork-Presbyterian Heart has:

- A well-deserved reputation for clinical excellence – the only heart center in the New York area ranked among the nation's best by *U.S. News & World Report*;

- World-renowned expertise in all areas of cardiac care, including transplantation, open-heart surgery, arrhythmia control, left ventricular assist devices (LVAD) and robotics;

- One of the country's largest and most successful pediatric cardiology, cardiology interventional and cardiac surgery programs.

- The latest heart-imaging technology, including such innovative tools as advanced digital equipment for stress echocardiography SPECT, state-of-the-art MRI, intravascular/intracoronary ultrasound, electrophysiologic studies, nuclear scanning and an outstanding cardiac catheterization laboratory;

- A state-of-the-art Interventional Cardiology Center to diagnose and treat heart disease without surgery, on an inpatient or outpatient basis, including: angioplasty, balloon valvuloplasty, stenting, and intracoronary radiation for restenosis.

Physician Referral: For a physician referral or to learn more about the NewYork-Presbyterian Heart call toll free **1-877-NYP-WELL** (1-877-697-9355) visit our website at **www.nypheart.org**

HIGHLIGHTS INCLUDE:

- Performed more heart transplants than any other hospital in the world over the last two decades.

- First Robotics-Assisted Coronary Artery Bypass Surgery in the U.S.

- One of the principal investigators (12 institutions throughout the United States) involved in ongoing FDA clinical trials to explore the use and effectiveness of robotics in cardiac surgery.

- Lead medical center in a three-year landmark study of 129 patients – REMATCH (Randomized Evaluation of Mechanical Assistance for the Treatment of Congestive Heart Failure) — which found that implanted heart pumps can extend and improve the quality of life of terminally ill heart failure patients.

- Participating in FDA-approved randomized clinical trial to evaluate use of drug-coated stents versus regular stents on incidence of reoccurrence of renarrowing inside stent.

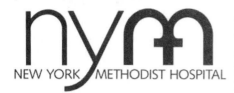

THE INSTITUTE FOR CARDIOLOGY AND CARDIAC SURGERY
New York Methodist Hospital

506 Sixth Street , Brooklyn, N.Y. 11215
Phone 866 84-HEART (866 844-3278)
http://www.nym.org

SPECIALISTS AND MEDICAL SERVICES

The Institute is the Hospital's program, for the prevention, diagnosis and treatment of all types of heart disease. The Institute brings together a panel of specialists and a range of services in all areas related to cardiac disease. These services, which range from screening and diagnostic procedures to emergency and ongoing treatment for heart attacks and chronic heart disease, are provided at the Hospital's specialized laboratories and clinical units, on both an inpatient and outpatient basis. New York Methodist houses state-of-the-art diagnostic and surgical facilities, including three cardiac catheterization laboratories and the most modern cardiac surgery suite in the area. The Institute's staff of physicians includes specialists in all areas of cardiology, electrophysiology, interventional cardiology and cardiac surgery.

PROGRAMS OFFERED

The programs and services offered by the Institute include consultative services, a chest pain emergency center (located in the Emergency Department), diagnostic evaluation and medical treatment for heart disease, interventional cardiology procedures, electrophysiology, and cardiac surgery.

***

Referrals to the specialists or to cardiac programs and services can be made through an individual's primary care physician or requested directly through the Institute's referral service. More information (and on-line physician referral) is available at the Hospital's website, http://www.nym.org.

THE NEW YORK METHODIST-CORNELL HEART CENTER

The New York Methodist-Cornell Heart Center is one of only three programs approved to perform cardiac surgery in Brooklyn. It is staffed by physicians from the prestigious Weill Cornell Medical Center of New York-Presbyterian Hospital. The Center is located in a new state-of-the-art cardiac surgery suite.

Procedures performed at the Center include coronary bypass surgery, off-pump bypass surgery, valve replacement and repair, thoracic aneurysm repair and bloodless heart surgery.

738

Sponsored Page

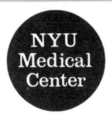

NYU Medical Center

550 First Avenue (at 31st Street)
New York, NY 10016
Physician Referral:
(888)7-NYU-MED (888-769-8633)
www.nyumc.org

ADULT CARDIOVASCULAR SERVICES

Minimally Invasive Cardiac Surgery
NYU Medical Center's cardiac surgeons are internationally recognized for pioneering minimally invasive cardiac surgery and introduced minimally invasive mitral valve repair to the U.S. in 1996. Since that time, NYU surgeons have performed more than 3000 minimally valve repair or replacement procedures, changing the standard of care for heart surgery.

Minimally invasive cardiac surgery is performed through a small incision on the side of the chest, rather than cutting the breastbone as is done with traditional open-chest surgery. Data have shown that this approach not only lowers the risk of complications, such as bleeding and infection, but also reduces postoperative pain and scarring, speeds the recovery process and helps patients resume their normal lives in record time.

The Cardiac Catheterization Laboratory
At the cutting edge of interventional cardiology, the Cardiac Catheterization Laboratory at NYU continues to set the standard of care for catheter-based diagnosis and evaluation of cardiac health. Located at Tisch Hospital, the Cath Lab provides a full range of procedures to evaluate how well the heart muscle and valves are working, detect and measure any narrowing in the coronary arteries, and recommend appropriate treatment if needed.

Electrophysiology – Heart Rhythm Center
NYU's Heart Rhythm Center treats many cardiac arrhythmias with "catheter based" procedures utilizing long, flexible wires entering the heart to apply energy that ablates the source of the arrhythmia. For atrial fibrillation, NYU is one of the few centers in the country using cutting edge, emerging technology for navigating within the heart, mapping the focus, ablating it with an energy source and, in many cases, curing this troublesome arrhythmia. We also provide the latest implantable devices for those patients who need them.

The Cardiac Rehabilitation Center
Follow-up care for cardiac patients is all about rehabilitation. What distinguishes cardiac rehab at NYU Medical Center is its quality of organization, rigorousness, and individualized patient care. At the Cardiac Rehab Center, physical rehabilitation takes place in a state-of-the-art gym, replete with spectacular views of the river and the Manhattan skyline. Patients work out to build both aerobic capacity and strength, and are fully supervised to maximize safety. Patient care at the Rehab Center is premised on the powerful idea that it takes a "village" to treat a patient. At NYU, that village is a team of cardiologists, physiatrists, nurses, physical and occupational therapists, psychologists, social workers, exercise physiologists, nutritionists, and other healthcare professionals. The goal is to return patients to their normal lives, rehabilitated and ready to meet the challenges of the world.

NYU MEDICAL CENTER

"The truly remarkable thing about minimally invasive surgery, for me, is that I've had this major heart surgery and I don't even think about it. You can't see my scar. I'm back to my normal life in much better health."

– Sandy Katz, minimally invasive MVR

"I'm a millwright welder and use everything from precision instruments to heavy machinery. I don't think I'd be ableto do my job now if I had my chest split open. I was able to get home and start moving around right away."

– Vincent Cirillo, minimally invasive CABG

686

St. Francis Hospital, The Heart Center®

100 Port Washington Blvd.
Roslyn, New York 11576
www.stfrancisheartcenter.com
(516) 562-6000
1-888-HEARTNY

A Leader in Cardiac Care

St. Francis Hospital, The Heart Center® is New York State's only specialty designated cardiac center and is the busiest heart center in the Northeast. Located in Roslyn, New York, on Long Island's North Shore, St. Francis Hospital has been ranked among the best heart centers in the United States by *U.S.News & World Report* and *Modern Maturity*, the magazine of AARP.
St. Francis:

- Performs more open heart surgeries and cardiac interventional procedures than any other hospital in New York State

- Continues to maintain the highest level of quality of care – St. Francis is the only hospital in the New York metropolitan area with risk-adjusted mortality rates significantly below the statewide average for heart valve and valve/coronary artery bypass surgery, the most challenging forms of common cardiac surgery

- Offers innovative approaches to cardiac surgery, including minimally-invasive procedures and off-pump coronary artery bypass surgery, designed to minimize trauma and reduce surgical complications

- Performed more abdominal aortic aneurysm repairs than any hospital in New York State, with risk-adjusted mortality rates significantly lower than the statewide average

- Treats more patients with congestive heart failure than any other Long Island hospital and was the only Long Island hospital with risk-adjusted mortality rates lower than the statewide average for the treatment of this condition

- Performs one of the region's highest volumes of catheter-based techniques to close atrial septal defects (ASDs) and patent foramen ovale (PFO)

- Operates a nationally recognized Arrhythmia and Pacemaker Center staffed with electrophysiologists with over a decade of experience in radiofrequency ablation, a permanent cure for certain arrhythmias, including atrial fibrillation

- Maintains a high volume center for the implantation of cardiac pacemakers and defibrillators

- Continues leadership in noninvasive imaging, including cardiac MRI, three-dimensional echocardiography, and CT scanning, and was the first Long Island hospital to offer state-of-the-art 64-slice CT scanning for coronary imaging and other applications

St. Francis Hospital has near-perfect patient satisfaction ratings, with over 99 percent of patients saying they would recommend the hospital to family and friends.

"Our large cardiac caseload and our growing research program put us in an excellent position to introduce new techniques that can benefit thousands of people in need each year." -- Alan D. Guerci, M.D. President and Chief Executive Officer, St. Francis Hospital, The Heart Center®

726

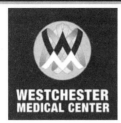

WESTCHESTER
MEDICAL CENTER

CARDIOVASCULAR SERVICES

All of Westchester Medical Center's highly regarded heart services are organized within its George E. Reed Heart Center. The Heart Center provides advanced cardiac medical diagnosis, treatment and surgery to infants, children and adults with every conceivable heart disorder. Ranked among the top 10% in the nation for cardiology services and angioplasty/stents, the Heart Center is also rated number one in the Hudson Valley region for cardiac services, heart surgery and angioplasty/stents.

Some of the world's top cardiologists and cardiac surgeons are at Westchester Medical Center, performing thousands of successful procedures each year—including heart transplant, open-heart surgery, cardiovascular surgery, angioplasty and cardiac catheterizations. The Heart Center's Cardiac Catheterization Lab is one of the busiest on the East Coast, performing more than 5,000 diagnostic cardiac catheterizations and 1,600 angioplasty and coronary stent procedures annually. The Heart Center is also home to a specialized Coronary Care Unit, a dedicated Cardiology Unit and a state-of-the-art Cardiac Diagnostic Center. In addition, Westchester Medical Center's Heart Transplant and Aortic Aneurysm Programs are life-saving resources for patients and referring physicians from throughout the Hudson Valley. The Program's renowned physicians are on-call 24/7 to treat complex aortic problems.

All physicians and surgeons at the George E. Reed Heart Center are highly skilled in latest medical and surgical technologies and techniques—from congenital heart defect surgery on babies just hours old to cardiac-assist devices, heart transplant and special treatments for congestive heart failure. As the teaching hospital for New York Medical College, patients benefit from the Heart Institute's participation in most major cardiac studies on new techniques and drug therapies.

VASCULAR SERVICES

Westchester Medical Center offers a complete range of vascular diagnostic, interventional and surgical services. Our vascular specialists are committed to the prevention of vascular disease and are known nationally and internationally for their clinical research interests. In addition to providing comprehensive diagnostic services, physicians are on the leading edge of vascular peripheral interventional and surgical procedures, including: aortic endovascular stent grafts; peripheral angiography/angioplasty/stent; carotid angiography/stent; aneurysm resection/stent; carotid endarterectomy; and limb salvage.

METABOLIC CENTER

The Metabolic Center at Westchester Medical Center offers the highest quality specialized care for adults with all types of metabolic disorders, including diabetes. From metabolic syndrome evaluation to diabetes evaluation and cardiovascular risk assessment, physicians at the Metabolic Center provide a comprehensive range of services that involve the expertise of an extensive network of related specialists that are on-call and available 24/7 as needed.

Heart Center At Westchester Medical Center

Home to some of the world's top cardiologists, cardiac surgeons and vascular surgeons, the Heart Center at Westchester Medical Center offers advanced cardiology services and the latest cardiovascular and vascular surgical techniques, including:

- Aortic Aneurysm, including arch and thoracoabdominal repairs
- Aortic and Thoracic Endovascular Stent Grafting
- AICD Implants
- Angioplasty
- Cardiac Catheterization
- Congestive Heart Failure/Specialized Treatments
- Coronary Artery Bypass Grafting
- Coronary Stents
- Endoscopic Vein Harvesting
- Off-Pump Coronary Artery Bypass
- Minimally Invasive Cardiac Surgery
- Pacemakers/Bi-Ventricular Pacemaker Insertion
- Radio Frequency Ablation
- Valve Repair
- Ventricular Assist Devices
- Heart Transplant

1-866 –WMC-HEART

Call for a physician referral or a specialty office near you.

Clinical Genetics

Clinical Genetics

One Gustave L. Levy Place (Fifth Avenue and 100th Street)
New York, NY 10029-6574
Physician Referral: 1-800-MD-SINAI (636-4624)
www.mountsinai.org

The Department of Human Genetics at The Mount Sinai Medical Center is one of the largest medical genetics units in the country, providing expert diagnostic, therapeutic, and counseling services for patients and families with genetic disorders, birth defects, and pregnancy loss. The Department performs sophisticated diagnostic tests in its state-of-the-art DNA, biochemical, and cytogenetics laboratories.

The Department has over 30 internationally recognized physician and scientist faculty members, 10 experienced genetic counselors, and a full support and research staff of over 150 people who provide expert clinical services.

Programs offered by the Department include:

• Comprehensive Genetic Diagnostic and Counseling Services

• Clinical and Laboratory Evaluation of Patients with Genetic Disorders, Birth Defects and Reproductive Loss

• Genetic Screening Program

• Prenatal Diagnostic Services

• Cancer Genetic Counseling Program

• The Center for Jewish Genetic Disease (the first such center in the world)

• Program for Inherited Metabolic Diseases

• The Comprehensive Gaucher Disease Treatment Program

• The International Center for Fabry Disease

• The International Center for Types A and B Niemann-Pick Disease

GROUNDBREAKING RESEARCH AND NEW FORMS OF TREATMENT

Almost everyone has a disease or condition that runs in their family. In fact, there are over 10,000 known genetic disorders and current research is identifying the genetic susceptibilities or predispositions for many common diseases and cancers. Moving toward this goal, the Department of Human Genetics at Mount Sinai is performing research to develop new and improved methods for the diagnosis, prevention, and treatment of these diseases and disorders. The Human Genome Project and advances in gene therapy have accelerated this research.

ADVANCES IN DIAGNOSIS AND DISEASE TREATMENT

In the past two years alone, Mount Sinai researchers have had remarkable success identifying the genes responsible for seven genetic diseases and in developing new treatments for two inherited disorders. The following are some examples and results of this important work:

• Research pioneered by Mount Sinai's Department of Human Genetics resulted in the development of a safe and effective FDA-approved treatment for Fabry Disease, an inherited metabolic disorder that results in kidney failure, heart disease, stroke, and premature death.

• Our department has made remarkable progress toward the development of treatment for Niemann-Pick Type B Disease, a hereditary disorder that results in death in childhood or early adulthood.

• We have recently identified the genes responsible for several diseases, including a debilitating juvenile arthritis syndrome. The identification of this gene may lead to greater understanding and new treatments for arthritis.

• Our researchers have identified the gene causing Noonan Syndrome, a common genetic disorder that causes congenital heart defects, so now affected families can receive early diagnosis and prevention.

610

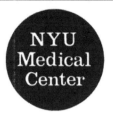

NYU Medical Center

550 First Avenue (at 31st Street)
New York, NY 10016
Physician Referral:
(888)7-NYU-MED (888-769-8633)
www.nyumc.org

CLINICAL GENETICS

The Clinical Genetics Program at NYU Medical Center offers a comprehensive program of genetic evaluation, counseling, and testing, supported by vital, ongoing research efforts and active treatment protocols. Our integrated team approach includes centralized, easy access to medical geneticists and genetic counselors. We are nationally known for groundbreaking work identifying genetic markers for breast, colorectal, ovarian, and prostate cancer, and assessing cancer risks.

BREAST AND OVARIAN CANCER - a leading participant in the New York Breast Cancer Study and the National Ovarian Cancer Early Detection Program; latest blood test can help identify early indications of ovarian cancer.

COLORECTAL CANCER - diagnostic evaluations followed by tests for identifying high-risk individuals.

PROSTATE CANCER - the latest research and ongoing protocols.

EARLY DETECTION - in the absence of a targeted test, we provide screening tests to identify high-risk patients in need of follow-up care.

COUNSELING - personalized, confidential insight into matters related to prevention, surveillance, and early diagnosis and treatment in a non-judgmental atmosphere.

Specialists at the NCI-designated NYU Cancer

Institute seek to enhance and coordinate the extensive resources of NYU Medical Center to optimize research, treatment, and the ultimate control of cancer.

Our new NYU Clinical Cancer Center is located at 160 East 34th Street. This state-of-the-art 13-level, 85,000-square-foot building serves as "home base" for patients, by providing the latest cancer prevention, screening, diagnostic treatment, genetic counseling, and support services in one central location. The NYU Clinical Cancer Center stands to dramatically improve the lives of people with cancer. As part of NYU Medical Center, patients can access a variety of other noncancer services throughout the institution.

PHYSICIAN REFERRAL
1-888-7-NYU-MED
(1-888-769-8633)
www.nyumc.org
www.nyuci.org

Sponsored Page

Clinical Research

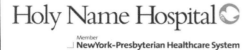

Holy Name Hospital ⟲

Member
NewYork-Presbyterian Healthcare System
Affiliate: Columbia University College of Physicians & Surgeons

718 Teaneck Road
Teaneck, NJ 07666
(201) 833-3000
www.holyname.org

THE INSTITUTE FOR CLINICAL RESEARCH

The Institute for Clinical Research at Holy Name Hospital provides exceptional investigators, facilities and services for sponsoring agencies that seek to advance patient care through superior clinical research. We're dedicated to conducting expeditious, high-quality clinical trials to test new medications, devices, diagnostic modalities and treatment protocols.

A FULL-SERVICE CENTER

Our full-service center conducts all types of clinical research (both drug and device). Because of our size and scope, we can offer sponsors high-quality data and accruals more efficiently than academic clinical research centers. There is a single point of contact for budgets, contracts, and regulatory and patient recruitment issues. We ensure efficiency through the centralized processing of all aspects of clinical trials, including identifying diligent, well-trained investigators; recruiting, enrolling and retaining study subjects; planning protocol strategies; and preparing and submitting regulatory documents. We maintain a database of active and potential investigators, and we can match your needs with an appropriate physician(s). We utilize a swift investigator selection and enrollment process. We have a large electronic patient database from which we can enroll study patients to meet your needs.

EXPERIENCED LEADERSHIP

Our research director has extensive experience in administration and clinical research. The research team includes certified clinical research coordinators, administrators and support staff and is dedicated to meeting sponsors' expectations. Our investigators have vast experience in conducting government-and industry-sponsored research.

Our research facility meets regulatory and industry standards and includes space for administrators and coordinators and storage for regulatory documents and study records. Our drug/device storage area was specially built to meet FDA requirements, industry standards, and regulatory guidelines.

To learn more about our Institute for Clinical Research call 201-541-6312.

We'll help you meet your goals by providing:

- Identification of qualified investigators

- Experienced recruiters and coordinators

- Western IRB submissions and correspondence

- Preparation and negotiation of budgets

- Agreement negotiation and execution

- Subject selection, accruals, and enrollments

- High-quality, valid data

- Clinical, laboratory, and clerical support

- On-site quality assurance program

- Performance tracking

- Comprehensive standard operating procedures (SOP)

- Study tracker software

761

Gastroenterology/ Digestive Diseases

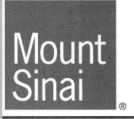

THE MOUNT SINAI MEDICAL CENTER
GASTROINTESTINAL AND SURGICAL SPECIALTIES

One Gustave L. Levy Place (Fifth Avenue and 100th Street)
New York, NY 10029-6574
Physician Referral: 1-800-MD-SINAI (636-4624)
www.mountsinai.org

Mount Sinai's *Divisions of Gastroenterology, Colon and Rectal Surgery, Liver Diseases,* and *Pediatric Gastroenterology, Nutrition,* and *Liver Diseases* are renowned for their delivery of patient care, research, and education in diseases of the gastrointestinal tract. In 2000, the National Institutes of Health (NIH) recognized the importance of Mount Sinai as a research center with a grant for GI/Liver fellowship training, making Mount Sinai the only medical school in New York City to earn this prestigious award.

Successes within the *Division of Gastroenterology* include breakthroughs in the medical and surgical management of inflammatory bowel disease (IBD) (ulcerative colitis and Crohn's disease). Mount Sinai spearheaded novel therapies for treating severe IBD, and helped establish the role of colonoscopy for preventing colon cancer by removing precancerous polyps. More recent innovations include employing a tiny camera within a swallowable capsule to capture images in the stomach and intestines. Mount Sinai's small intestine transplantation program is one of only four such programs in the country. Mount Sinai's IBD Center, Women's GI Health Center, and GI Cancer Center offer patients the latest comprehensive, interdisciplinary care, newer agents through clinical trials, and services such as psychologists and nutritionists.

Mount Sinai surgeons have a distinguished history in the surgical treatment of gastrointestinal disorders and today, surgeons in the *Division of Colon and Rectal Surgery* continue that tradition, focusing on surgical therapies for all diseases involving the colon, rectum, and anus. With special expertise in the treatment of Crohn's disease (which was first described at Mount Sinai in 1932), ulcerative colitis, colon and rectal cancer and diverticulitis, we specialize in the newer techniques of rectal surgery with special emphasis on colostomy avoidance. The newest minimally invasive techniques are offered as well as other cutting-edge technologies for the treatment of such disorders as hemorrhoids, fistulas, and rectal tumors.

Mount Sinai's *Division of Liver Diseases* has a long history of outstanding clinical care and scientific investigation with a tradition of excellence in several clinical areas, including liver transplantation; diagnosis and treatment of viral hepatitis; treatment of scarring, or fibrosis; management of primary biliary cirrhosis, an autoimmune disease of bile ducts; diagnosis and treatment of genetic liver diseases, including Wilson's disease (copper overload) and hemachromatosis (iron overload). With a steadily growing research budget, Mount Sinai carries out a diverse portfolio of research projects.

The *Division of Pediatric Gastroenterology, Nutrition,* and *Liver Diseases* provides consultative services and treatment for the full range of children's digestive and nutritional diseases. The Children's IBD Center is the only multidisciplinary center for pediatric patients with Crohn's disease and ulcerative colitis in the tri-state area and receives referrals from all over the country. The Transplant Program is one of the largest in the nation and was the first program in New York to perform liver transplants, and later small bowel transplants. The Division is active in clinical research in IBD, focusing on issues of genetic factors, psychosocial interactions, and drug trials. Several NIH grants support research in the areas of biliary atresia, bile salt absorption, and outcome analysis in children with liver failure.

Mount Sinai provides a comprehensive center, uniting the medical disciplines of gastroenterology and its related surgical specialties, as well as an array of minimally invasive surgical programs. The Center houses renowned programs for the treatment of IBD, colorectal diseases, as well as reconstructive and laparoscopic surgery programs through the *Division of Laparoscopic Surgery*, which is internationally known for pioneering a number of minimally invasive procedures for the treatment of Crohn's disease and ulcerative colitis.

608

Sponsored Page

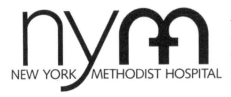

THE INSTITUTE FOR DIGESTIVE AND LIVER DISORDERS
New York Methodist Hospital
506 Sixth Street, Brooklyn, N.Y. 11215
Phone 866 DIGEST-1 (866 344-3781)
http;//www.nym.org

SPECIALISTS AND MEDICAL SERVICES

The Institute's panel of physician specialists includes gastroenterologists, hepatologists, surgeons, laparoscopic surgeons, radiologists, medical and radiation oncologists and pathologists. Nutritionists and psychologists are also members of the team. The latest advances in the diagnosis and treatment of the gastrointestinal tract and the liver are available. These include endoscopic ultrasound, pediatric and adult capsule endoscopy and advanced laparoscopic surgery. In addition, the Endoscopy Suite at New York Methodist Hospital enables physicians to perform highly advanced diagnostic and treatment procedures that can detect and describe disorders of the gastrointestinal tract and bile ducts as well as the non-surgical removal of bile duct gallstones.

PROGRAMS OFFERED

Among the programs and services offered by the Institute are a Colorectal Cancer Program, Heartburn (GERD) Program, Chronic Hepatitis B & C Program, Liver Transplantation Evaluation Program, Ulcer Program, Bowel Disorders Program and Pediatric Gastroenterology Program. Gallbladder and pancreatic conditions are also treated.

***

Referrals to the Institute's specialists, programs and services can be made through an individual's primary care physician or requested directly through the Institute's telephone referral service. More information (and on-line physician referral) is available at the Hospital's website, http://www.nym.org.

CAPSULE ENDOSCOPY

Capsule endoscopy is available at New York Methodist Hospital. A tiny camera, embedded in a capsule tiny enough to swallow, is used to examine the small intestine and diagnose possible disease. As the patient goes about his or her day, the camera travels through the small intestine, taking thousands of pictures. The patient wears a special belt that holds multiple lightweight sensors, which detect the capsule's location in the body while the capsule takes pictures.

737

Sponsored Page

⌐ NewYork-Presbyterian

⌐ The University Hospital of Columbia and Cornell

NewYork-Presbyterian Digestive Disease Services

Affiliated with Columbia University College of Physicians and Surgeons and Weill Medical College of Cornell University

NewYork-Presbyterian Hospital
Weill Cornell Medical Center
525 East 68th Street
New York, NY 10021

NewYork-Presbyterian Hospital
Columbia University Medical Center
622 West 168th Street
New York, NY 10032

OVERVIEW:

The Digestive Disease Services of NewYork-Presbyterian Hospital provide expert capabilities in research, education and clinical care of patients with gastrointestinal, liver and bile duct, pancreatic and nutritional disorders.

The Hospital offers a wide range of diagnostic tests including,
* Routine procedures, such as endoscopy, capsule endoscopy, colonoscopy and flexible sigmoidoscopy.

* Endoscopic retrograde cholangiopancreatography (ERCP) to evaluate the ducts of the gallbladder, pancreas and liver

* Endoscopic ultrasonography (EUS)to provide detailed images of the upper and lower gastrointestinal tract and for the staging of patients with esophageal, gastric and rectal cancers. The Hospital is one of the few centers using EUS for needle aspiration of pancreatic cysts and tumors.

* Laparoscopy for direct examination of the liver, gallbladder and spleen and in the diagnosis, staging and treatment of pancreatic, gastric, esophageal and colorectal cancer.

The Hospital is a leader in treating gastrointestinal (GI) conditions. For example,
* The Minimal Access Surgery Center (MASC) is at the forefront of developing and applying new technologies, such as robotics, computerized image processing and enhanced optics. It is improving the outcomes of GI surgical patients and speeding their recovery from conditions such as GERD, gallbladder disease, and benign and malignant colon and rectal disease.

* Our surgeons also perform endoscopic sewing (endocinch) and radiofrequency treatment (Stretta procedure) for GERD.

* Our surgeons are internationally renowned in the use of laparoscopic methods for cancer and other colorectal conditions. They are highly experienced with the Whipple procedure to remove a pancreas tumor, which improves the survival rates and life expectancies of patients with pancreatic cancer and other less common pancreas problems.

Additionally, our physicians are involved in numerous clinical trials, (including studies on Cox-2 inhibitors) for preventing colorectal cancer and familial polyposis (a precursor to colorectal cancer), and antiviral therapy for chronic hepatitis C.

Physician Referral: For a physician referral or to learn more about the NewYork-Presbyterian Digestive Disease Services call toll free **1-877-NYP-WELL** (1-877-697-9355) or visit our website at www.nypdigestive.org

COMPREHENSIVE CARE

Patients benefit from the collaboration of gastroenterologists, hepatologists, surgeons and diagnostic and pathology experts who develop optimal treatment plans. Areas of expertise include:

* GI Cancer, including esophageal, colorectal, liver, pancreatic and gastric tumors

* Inflammatory Bowel Diseases (Ulcerative Colitis and Crohn's Disease)

* Liver Diseases. The Hospital has a comprehensive Hepatitis C Center and the Center for Liver Disease and Transplantation

* Esophageal Disorders, including gastroesophageal reflux disease (GERD) and Barrett's esophagus

* Pancreatic and Biliary Disorders

* Celiac Disease

* Polyps of the Colon

* Peptic Ulcer Disease/Helicobacter Pylori Infections

* Gallbladder and Bile Duct Disorders

* Restorative surgery to avoid colostomies in diseases like rectal cancer, Crohn's disease, ulcerative colitis, and incontinence

* Anal diseases, such as hemorrhoids, fistulas, vascular tumors, abscesses and others

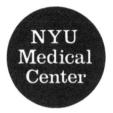

550 First Avenue (at 31st Street)
New York, NY 10016
Physician Referral:
(888)7-NYU-MED (888-769-8633)
www.nyumc.org

GASTROENTEROLOGY

The mission of the Division of Gastroenterology at NYU Medical Center is excellence in the delivery of patient care, research, and education in diseases of the gastrointestinal tract. Its physicians bring with them a rich body of knowledge in the diagnosis and management of inflammatory bowel disease, peptic ulcer disease, esophageal disorders, gastrointestinal cancer, and liver, biliary, and pancreatic diseases. Their multidisciplinary approach insures the greatest possible patient care at NYU's three acclaimed, academically integrated teaching hospitals: Tisch Hospital (New York University Hospital), Bellevue Hospitals Center, and the New York Harbor Health Care System (Manhattan Veterans Hospital).

Members of the Division of Gastroenterology are nationally recognized leaders who are involved in numerous studies in the field of gastroenterology and hepatology, including clinical research in liver diseases (especially hepatitis C), endoscopy, colon cancer screening, acute and chronic GI bleeding, and Helicobacter pylori.

Always at the forefront of new technologies, NYU's gastroenterologists work side-by-side with radiologists to perform virtual colonoscopies, a new minimally invasive technique for finding early-stage cancers in the colon.

Virtual colonoscopy is a new screening test in which a radiologist uses a CAT (Computer Assisted Tomography) scanner and sophisticated image processing computers to actually recreate and evaluate the inner surface of the colon. The CAT scanner provides the x-ray images; the image-processing computers create the 3-D display for the final interpretation by the referring gastroenterologist. The study gives a complete evaluation of the entire surface of the colon and can be performed quickly, with little discomfort and extremely accurate readings.

NYU MEDICAL CENTER

The colon and the rectum are the final sections of the large intestine. In the United States, approximately 150,000 people are diagnosed with colorectal cancer every year and of these, approximately 55,000 will die of the disease. Cancer of the colon is the second leading cause of cancer death in the United States. Most experts agree that it is preventable, and NYU is on the cutting edge of 21st century research into quicker, safer, and more accurate diagnosis and treatment, with its advanced video colonoscopy and noninvasive radiologic techniques.

**Physician Referral
(888) 7-NYU-MED
(888-769-8633)
www.nyumc.org**

696

Sponsored Page

Geriatrics

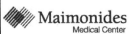

Maimonides
Medical Center

Maimonides serves one of the oldest populations in New York City, with one in ten of our patients over the age of 85. The Geriatrics Program at Maimonides is fully equipped to meet the special needs of this growing segment of the population. Directed by Barbara Paris, MD, the program encompasses inpatient and outpatient services, featuring the Acute Care for Elderly (ACE) Unit. The staff of this unit is focused on the continuity, coordination, quality and dignity of care provided.

Patient Evaluation

ACE Unit services focus on acute medical care and account for the complex needs of hospitalized elderly patients. Special attention is given to the assessment of memory loss and understanding the underlying causes of geriatric syndromes such as incontinence, falls and frailty. Psychosocial issues affecting elderly patients such as loneliness and end-of-life care are also addressed.

Wound Care

Because patients can have wounds that do not heal easily, we provide special attention through our wound care team.

Discharge and Medical Care at Home

Caregiver support groups are initiated while patients are in the hospital and are available after discharge. Once at home, if indicated, patients can receive a home visit from a member of our geriatric team, ensuring the coordination and continuity of their care.

Community & Nursing Home Liaison

The ACE Unit team serves as a bridge between hospital and community health care providers. Discharged patients are given a comprehensive plan that, if needed, includes a one-time home visit by our nurse practitioner, continued follow-up by geriatric specialists and referrals to community services. Maimonides has long established relationships with many nursing and rehabilitation facilities in Brooklyn.

Outpatient Geriatric Services

Our geriatric team offers comprehensive assessment and primary care services throughout Southern Brooklyn.

Physicians at Maimonides are among the eight percent in the US who use computers to enter patient orders, thereby reducing the risk of errors, increasing efficiency, and speeding the healing process. Maimonides has appeared on the American Hospital Association's "Most Wired" and "Most Wireless" lists more often than any other healthcare institution in the metropolitan area. Advanced technology allows our doctors to focus more attention on caring for their patients.

Maimonides Medical Center – passionate about medicine, compassionate about people.

731

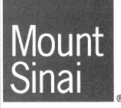

THE MOUNT SINAI MEDICAL CENTER
GERIATRICS AND ADULT DEVELOPMENT

One Gustave L. Levy Place (Fifth Avenue and 100th Street)
New York, NY 10029-6574
Physician Referral: 1-800-MD-SINAI (636-4624)
www.mountsinai.org

THE BEST IN CLINICAL CARE

In recognition of the care offered to older patients, Mount Sinai specialists are cited time and time again as the finest in the nation. In its 2006 "Best Graduate Schools" issue, *US News & World Report* ranked Mount Sinai School of Medicine at number 30 for Research and ranked its geriatrics specialty third in the nation for the second straight year.

We offer a full spectrum of patient care including a specialized care unit for the elderly (to minimize complications sometimes associated with an older person's hospital stay), a primary care geriatrics practice for older adults living in the community, a hospital-based consultation service for patients throughout Mount Sinai, a number of community-linked programs and partnerships, and a palliative care team dedicated to assuring quality care and support for patients and families facing serious illnesses.

GROUNDBREAKING RESEARCH

Mount Sinai's researchers continue to advance the understanding, prevention and treatment of age-related disorders.

The extensive research on aging conducted by the Department includes studies on health services, medical decision making and ethical dilemmas, palliative care, neurobiology of aging, and clinical interventions to promote independence in old age. The Department's expertise serves as a renowned educational resource for all Mount Sinai affiliates and other institutions in teaching geriatrics and gerontology to medical students, medical residents, geriatrics fellows, established physicians, and health professional trainees in other disciplines.

HISTORY OF EXCELLENCE

The Mount Sinai Medical Center is a pioneer in geriatric medicine. In 1909, a Mount Sinai physician coined the term "geriatrics," and in 1914, he wrote the first textbook on medical care for older adults.

Today, the Brookdale Department of Geriatrics and Adult Development continues to break new ground, offering comprehensive care, disease prevention, and the promotion of healthy and productive aging. The Department's enhanced expertise in assessing and managing patients with dementia greatly complements its established, interdisciplinary approach to patient care, in which medical staff and social workers address patients' needs as a team.

In 2007, the Martha Stewart Center for Living at Mount Sinai will open. It will be a new site for the outpatient clinical practice of geriatric medicine and will provide clinical care and education for patients, serve as a training ground for physicians-in-training, and coordinate research on healthy aging. The Coffey Geriatrics Practice will be housed within the new Center.

THE MOUNT SINAI MEDICAL CENTER

Mount Sinai's Brookdale Department of Geriatrics and Adult Development was the first freestanding department of geriatrics established by a US medical school, and it continues to be one of the very best. It offers unparalleled inpatient and outpatient care and numerous treatment programs designed to meet the unique needs of older adults. Mount Sinai is also home to world-class researchers dedicated to advancing our understanding of Alzheimer's disease and other common geriatric conditions. At the Department's heart are our patients, and the geriatricians of The Mount Sinai Medical Center work hard to improve life and longevity for New York's elderly.

609

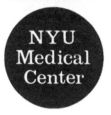

GERIATRIC MEDICINE
CARING FOR THE ELDERLY

Geriatrics, like Pediatrics, is by its nature a multidisciplinary endeavor. All geriatricians are experts in spotting and treating the unique ways that common medical problems manifest themselves in the elderly. But the elderly also have problems and issues that other groups do not face, such as loss of bone density, changes in skin health and appearance, memory disorders, incontinence, partial or complete loss of vision, and many others. Our geriatricians are also expert in these.

Some of these disorders are still incurable and the guidelines for treating patients with them are unclear. When that is the case, as it is with Alzheimer's disease, NYU Medical Center geriatricians have first-hand access to the basic laboratories where studies of the disease and its manifestations have been carried out since 1973. In fact, The William and Sylvia Silberstein Aging and Dementia Research Center at NYU Medical Center is one of the oldest and largest centers of its kind in the nation. It is a National Institute on Aging designated Center of Excellence devoted to the diagnosis and treatment of Alzheimer's disease.

The Diane and Arthur Belfer Geriatrics Center is one of the oldest and largest hospital-based clinical programs in the country. Focused on primary care and prevention, the Center treats thousands of patients at Tisch Hospital, The Hospital for Joint Diseases, Bellevue Hospital Center and the Manhattan Veterans Administration Hospital. A cooperative and integrated approach between all members of the healthcare team underscores the program's philosophy. The Geriatric Falls Prevention Program is specifically dedicated to the prevention, diagnosis and treatment of falls in the elderly. The primary goal of the Geriatric Service is to maintain a safe and independent lifestyle for older adults. A comprehensive array of specialists, such as neurologists, orthopedists, and therapists, are always available for referrals when needed.

NYU MEDICAL CENTER

The William and Sylvia Silberstein Aging and Dementia Research Center provides:

• comprehensive diagnostic evaluations to determine if memory loss is "normal" or more serious

• a memory enhancement program for age-related memory decline

• pharmaceutical clinical trials for mild memory loss and for Alzheimer's treatment

• state-of-the-art brain imaging techniques

• methods to prevent excess disability in Alzheimer's disease patients

• and comprehensive, on-going counseling and support groups for patients, caregivers and family members. Its longitudinal study of Alzheimer's patients is the most comprehensive ongoing study of its kind in the world.

697

Home Care

CALVARY HOSPITAL

CALVARY HOSPITAL

*The Model for the Relief
of Cancer Pain and Symptoms
for Over a Century*

1740 Eastchester Road
Bronx, NY 10461
Tel: (718) 518-2300
www.calvaryhospital.org

Calvary@Home
Home Care, Hospice, and Nursing Home Hospice

Calvary@Home
The umbrella for Home Care, Hospice, and Nursing Home Hospice, bringing compassionate care to patients who can be cared for at home. Our inter-disciplinary team includes physicians, nurses, aides, social workers, pastoral caregivers, volunteers, bereavement workers and other providers as needed.

The National Hospice and Palliative Care Organization and the National Island Peer Review Organization place Calvary@Home above state and national averages for relief of pain, patient/family education, and other parameters.

Calvary Certified Home Health Agency
Established in 1985, serves patients with all acute, chronic or life-limiting illnesses. Provides a full range of specialized home healthcare experts to support patients and families. We strive to ensure continuity of care by assigning a core group of caregivers to each patient. Our community health nurses work with referring physicians or a Calvary doctor to deliver appropriate care.

Areas We Serve
- Manhattan
- Queens
- Bronx
- Westchester

Hospice
Established in 1998, brings comprehensive care to people with all end-stage illnesses. Calvary assembles a core group of permanent staff to care for each patient, creating continuity of service for patients and families. Patients who require short-stay inpatient care can be admitted to Calvary in a seamless process.

In addition to physicians, nurses, and aides who address physical symptoms, we also assign visits by social workers, pastoral caregivers, and volunteers. We provide bereavement services for 13 month for families. Staffing exceeds national recommendations.

Areas We Serve
- Manhattan
- Brooklyn
- Westchester County
- Bronx
- Nassau County
- Queens
- Rockland County

Nursing Home Hospice
Brings comprehensive palliative care to nursing home residents suffering from all end-stage illnesses. Provides appropriate care to dually eligible (Medicare/Medicaid) residents, and bereavement services for loved ones.

Calvary Nursing Home Hospice has contracts with 15 nursing homes in:
- Manhattan
- Brooklyn
- Westchester County
- Bronx
- Queens
- Rockland County

For information about nursing home hospice, please call 718-518-2465.

Calvary Nursing Home Hospice

Established in 2001, nursing home hospice now serves residents of 15 homes in the NYC metro area.

Residents we care for suffer from a wide range of illnesses. We offer pain and symptom relief, pastoral care, and social work. We also consult about ethical issues that arise at the end of life. Our primary goal is to prevent complications, manage symptoms, and avert anticipated complications of illness, to promote overall quality of life and reduce frequent re-hospitalizations.

This innovative program has won major funding from the Fan Fox & Leslie R. Samuels Foundation, the Altman Foundation, New York Community Trust, the Alfred E. Smith Memorial Foundation, and the John H. and Ethel G. Noble Charitable Trust.

755

Maternal & Fetal Medicine

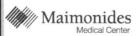
Maimonides
Medical Center

4802 Tenth Avenue • Brooklyn, New York 11219
Phone: (718) 283-7048 • Fax: (718) 283-7167
www.maimonidesmed.org

The Birthing Center at Maimonides is ranked among the best hospitals in the nation for maternity care by HealthGrades, the nation's leading source for independent healthcare quality information. More babies were delivered at Maimonides Medical Center in 2005 than at any other hospital in New York State.

The Maimonides Birthing Center features private suites with hardwood floors and a home-like environment. At the same time, physician coverage is provided 24/7 in our advanced Neonatal Intensive Care Unit. Our 36 obstetricians and 26 midwives have found that most families appreciate having the best of both worlds available to them.

Maimonides provides other unique services to its maternity patients. The largest doula program in the metropolitan area can be found at Maimonides. These fully-trained childbirth assistants are available to patients before, during and after delivery at no cost to families. And the maternity units utilize an electronic patient record that sets industry standards for patient safety and hospital efficiency.

This combination of family-centered services and advanced technology continues to have enormous appeal to the women we serve – over 6,700 of them last year alone. Our highly trained staff includes the finest nurses, physicians, midwives and specialists to ensure the safety and comfort of our patients. Several physicians specialize in high-risk pregnancy, including the Chairman of Obstetrics and Gynecology, Howard Minkoff, MD.

In recognition of its excellence in obstetrics and pediatrics, Maimonides was designated a Regional Perinatal Center by the New York State Department of Health. Women who give birth at Maimonides also have a variety of other services available to them, including:

• A Perinatal Testing Center, directed by Shoshana Haberman, MD, offering amniocentesis, 3-D ultrasound, fetal echocardiograms and other diagnostic exams.

• Neonatologists onsite around-the-clock. This vital service is always available during high-risk deliveries, working closely with the obstetrician. The Norma Sutton Center for Neonatology adjoins the Payson Birthing Center and provides the most sophisticated care in a family-friendly environment.

Physicians at Maimonides are among the eight percent in the US who use computers to enter patient orders, thereby reducing the risk of errors, increasing efficiency, and speeding the healing process.
Maimonides has appeared on the American Hospital Association's "Most Wired" and "Most Wireless" lists more often than any other healthcare institution in the metropolitan area.
Advanced technology allows our doctors to focus more attention on caring for their patients.

Maimonides Medical Center – passionate about medicine, compassionate about people.

729

Minimally Invasive Surgery

THE MOUNT SINAI MEDICAL CENTER
MINIMALLY INVASIVE SURGERY

One Gustave L. Levy Place (Fifth Avenue and 100th St)
New York, NY 10029-6574
Physician Referral: 1-800-MD-SINAI (636-4624)
www.mountsinai.org

The expert surgeons at Mount Sinai continue to be at the forefront of highly advanced minimally invasive surgery. Using the latest instrumentation, Mount Sinai surgeons have applied these techniques to a broad spectrum of general and vascular surgical procedures including aortic aneurysm repair, kidney transplantation, colon cancer resection, Crohn's disease surgery, robotic prostatectomy, and bariatric (weight loss) surgery.

Cardiac Surgeries
We perform many procedures using minimally invasive approaches, including aortic valve replacement, mitral valve replacement, mitral valve repair, and offpump coronary artery bypasses.

Weight Loss Surgeries
At Mount Sinai we use the latest minimally invasive techniques to perform laparoscopic gastric bypass, lap band placement, duodenal switch and sleeve gastrectomy. A full multidisciplinary team follows all aspects of pre and postoperative care.

Urologic Surgeries
We can perform most traditional open surgeries laparoscopically, including: nephrectomy, nephroureterectomy, radical prostatectomy, and cystectomy.

Transplant Surgeries
With laparoscopic kidney donation, we can remove kidneys from living donors using laparoscopic techniques.

Vascular Surgeries
Our vascular surgeons provide minimally invasive durable treatments for vascular diseases such as aortic aneurysms, peripheral arterial occlusions, acute and chronic venous disease, vascular trauma and long-term vascular access for medical therapy or dialysis.

Abdominal Surgeries
We offer minimally invasive approaches for the treatment of diseases of the alimentary tract (esophagus, stomach), gastrointestinal tract (small and large intestine, colon and rectum) as well as benign and malignant diseases of the hepatobiliary system.

Gynecologic Surgeries
We routinely treat endometriosis, uterine fibroids, ovarian cysts, and urinary incontinence laparoscopically. Surgeries for uterine, cervical, and ovarian cancers are also performed laparoscopically by our expert gynecologic oncologists.

ENT Surgeries
Top specialists in otolaryngologic surgery at Mount Sinai offer minimally invasive procedures and surgeries to treat many conditions involving the ear, nose and throat, including cranial based lesions, head and neck cancers, and nasal and sinus conditions.

THE MOUNT SINAI MEDICAL CENTER

In surveys of the area's top minimally invasive surgeons in a variety of specialties, Mount Sinai's physicians are consistently at the top of the lists, in areas including gynecologic oncology surgery, obstetrical surgery, colon and rectal surgery, liver and bilary surgery, thyroid surgery, hernia surgery, gastrointestinal surgery, thoracic surgery, and vascular surgery.

Compared with traditional open surgery, minimally invasive procedures result in less tissue trauma, less scarring, and faster postoperative recovery time. Although the techniques vary from procedure to procedure and among different surgical subspecialties, minimally invasive surgical procedures typically employ video cameras and lens systems to provide anatomic visualization within a region of the body.

611

NYU Medical Center

550 First Avenue (at 31st Street)
New York, NY 10016
Physician Referral:
(888)7-NYU-MED (888-769-8633)
www.nyumc.org

MINIMALLY INVASIVE SURGERY

NYU Medical Center has been at the forefront of minimally invasive surgery for two decades, treating conditions from heart disease, to prostate cancer, to obesity, to fetal anomalies in utero. Today, more patients are opting for minimally invasive procedures, a decision resulting in less pain, scarring, and surgical trauma. Post-operative recovery is also significantly reduced, allowing patients to resume their normal activities much sooner than with traditional surgery.

In 1996, surgeons at NYU Medical Center performed the world's first minimally invasive valve repair and replacement, as well as the world's first triple cardiac bypass surgery. NYU vascular surgeons and radiologists helped pioneer minimally invasive aneurysm repair. In 1997, the Center installed the city's first Gamma Knife, a neurosurgical tool that allows surgeons to remove brain tumors that were once inoperable.

The Department of Surgery at New York University School of Medicine is a highly regarded and nationally recognized academic department. The department comprises divisions of:

• Cardiothoracic Surgery
• Minimally Invasive Surgery
• Pediatric Surgery
• Plastic Surgery (reconstructive and cosmetic)
• Surgical Oncology
• Transplantation Surgery
• Vascular Surgery
• Weight-Loss Surgery

Many faculty members receive national and international recognition for their work and hold leadership positions in both regional and national surgical societies. The department's goal is to develop leaders in clinical surgery and to provide the optimal academic surgical environment for patients, residents, and staff.

NYU MEDICAL CENTER

NYU is also taking the lead in noninvasive diagnostic procedures such as colonoscopy and bronchoscopy. MRI and CT scans have in many instances replaced the traditional angiogram to diagnose aortic aneurysm and vascular disease. For more information about these and other noninvasive tests, call 212-263-8904.

Physician Referral
(888) 7-NYU-MED
(888-769-8633)
www.nyumc.org

722

Sponsored Page

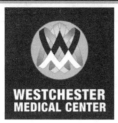

WESTCHESTER MEDICAL CENTER

Valhalla Campus
Valhalla, NY 10595
Tel. 1-877-WMC-DOCS
http://www.worldclassmedicine.com

Surgeons at Westchester Medical Center are widely recognized for their expertise in the use of minimally invasive surgical techniques to perform a wide range of advanced procedures, both in our University Hospital and Maria Fareri Children's Hospital. At the forefront of laparoscopic surgery since its introduction, Westchester Medical Center houses the region's only Surgical Skills Laboratory—a training center in which Medical Center physicians teach doctors from other hospitals the latest minimally invasive approaches.

CARDIOVASCULAR AND VASCULAR SURGERY
The Heart Center performs life-saving procedures for infants, children and adults using state-of-the-art minimally invasive techniques, including aortic valve replacement, mitral valve replacement, mitral valve repair and off-pump coronary artery bypass, ventricular assist devices, pacemakers and defibrillators, and heart transplant. We are also on the leading edge of minimally invasive vascular procedures, including aortic endovascular stent grafts and peripheral and carotid stents. Our researchers are involved in the Carotid Revascularization Endarterectomy versus Stenting Trial (CREST).

WEIGHT-LOSS SURGERY
Over 99% or 350 of the weight-loss procedures performed annually are performed laparoscopically, including gastric bypass, adjustable gastric banding, vertical banded gastroplasty, biliopancreatic diversion, sleeve gastrectomy and gastric stimulator device implants.

TRANSPLANT SURGERY
Our renowned kidney transplant surgeons are experts in laparoscopic donation, the minimally invasive removal of a kidney from a living donor. Our liver surgeons are experts in hepatobiliary surgery including the use of minimally invasive techniques. Our heart transplant surgeons are world-renowned.

NEUROSURGERY
Westchester Medical Center offers Novalis® Shaped Beam Surgery, the least invasive and most precise treatment option available to treat certain types of cancer, brain tumors and neurologic and vascular disorders. Our new Cerebrovascular Suite is available for the minimally invasive treatment of brain aneurysms and arteriovenous malformations (AVMs).

UROLOGIC SURGERY
Most surgeries for adult and childhood urologic disorders can be performed laparoscopically, including donor nephrectomy. Many urologic procedures are performed robotically-assisted or endoscopically.

GYNECOLOGIC SURGERY
Gynecologic procedures are routinely employed to treat such gynecological conditions as endometriosis, uterine fibroids, ovarian cysts and urinary incontinence. Gynecologic oncologists also perform surgeries for uterine, cervical and ovarian cancers laparoscopically.

ABDOMINAL AND THORACIC SURGERY
Minimally invasive surgical solutions are offered for all surgeries in adults and children of the abdominal cavity, including fundoplication for gastric reflux disease, colon and rectal resection, splenectomy, adrenalectomy and ventral and inguinal hernia repair. Diagnostic and therapeutic procedures are also performed for biliary and pancreatic benign and malignant diseases. Thoracic surgeons continue to advance minimally invasive access surgery of the esophagus and lung using video-assisted thoracic surgery (VATS).

EAR, NOSE AND THROAT SURGERY
Top specialists offer minimally invasive procedures to treat conditions of the ear, nose and throat, including cranial-based lesions, head and neck cancers, and nasal and sinus surgery, as well as minimally invasive dental and craniofacial dental services.

MINIMALLY INVASIVE SURGERY AT WESTCHESTER MEDICAL CENTER

Westchester Medical Center's physicians at both our University Hospital and Maria Fareri Children's Hospital are among the region's top minimally invasive surgeons in a full range of specialties, including:

- Cardiovascular and Vascular Surgery
- Weight-Loss Surgery
- Transplant Surgery
- Neurosurgery
- Urologic Surgery
- Gynecologic Surgery
- Abdominal and Thoracic Surgery
- Ear, Nose and Throat Surgery
- Dental Surgery

A pioneer in the use of minimally invasive techniques, Westchester Medical Center is home to the region's only Surgical Skills Laboratory—a training center devoted to assisting physicians from other hospitals in mastery of the latest minimally invasive tools and techniques. In addition, Westchester Medical Center recently opened a new state-of-the-art Cerebrovascular Suite for the minimally invasive treatment of brain tumors and arteriovenous malformations (AVMs).

795

Neurology/Neurosurgery

Goryeb Children's Hospital • Atlantic Neuroscience Institute
Carol G. Simon Cancer Center/The Cancer Center at Overlook Hospital
Gagnon Heart Hospital • Atlantic Rehabilitation Institute

P.O. Box 1905, Morristown, NJ 07962 • 1-800-247-9580 • atlantichealth.org

Atlantic Neuroscience Institute

The Atlantic Neuroscience Institute, a premier provider of neuroscience services in the New Jersey region, delivers quality health care that is compassionate and broadly accessible. We apply the most advanced new treatments and diagnostic tools, leading the way in the application of evidence-based medicine and technological innovation. We collaborate with other Atlantic Health professionals to provide superior, comprehensive, multidisciplinary care to all of our patients.

Based at Overlook Hospital, the Atlantic Neuroscience Institute uses the expertise of adult and pediatric neurologists and neurosurgeons, neuroradiologists, and specialists in related fields. Our Institute, including our state-of-the-art Neuroscience Inpatient Unit and Intensive Care Unit, is staffed by some of the most dedicated, highly rated neuroscience physicians and nurses. Among the many cutting edge technologies we use are neuro-imaging, image-guided neurosurgery and CyberKnife radiosurgery to provide optimal diagnostic and treatment services.

Services and programs offered at the Atlantic Neuroscience Institute include:

- Stroke Center and Regional Stroke Network
- The Atlantic Neuroscience Institute Epilepsy Center
- Brain Tumor Center of New Jersey
- CyberKnife
- Neuroradiology
- Interventional Neuroradiology
- Mild Traumatic Brain Injury Program
- Memory and Cognitive Disorders Program
- Pain Management Centers
- Spine Program
- Neuro Critical Care Transport
- Diagnostic Neurophysiology

CyberKnife

The CyberKnife is a revolutionary radiosurgical device that combines robotics and sophisticated image-guidance technology to deliver precisely targeted doses of radiation to tumors - even tumors that are beyond the reach of other radiosurgery systems. The CyberKnife is non-invasive, highly accurate and painless.

The Atlantic Neuroscience Institute was the first center in the New York City region to offer the CyberKnife for the treatment of tumors and lesions in the brain, spine, lung, liver, pancreas and prostate.

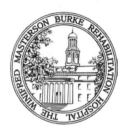

THE BURKE REHABILITATION HOSPITAL

785 Mamaroneck Avenue
White Plains, NY 10605
914-597-2500   1-888-99-BURKE
Admission Hotline 914-946-0865
www.burke.org

THE BURKE REHABILITATION HOSPITAL specializes in treating physical disabilities including stroke, brain and spinal cord injuries, Parkinson's disease and other neurological disorders, cardiac disease, pulmonary disease, arthritis, orthopedics and amputation. Patients receive intensive medical and therapeutic services carefully tailored to their individual needs.

Burke ranks among the top rehabilitation hospitals in the country. The rehabilitation care team includes board certified physicians and rehabilitation registered nurses on-site 24-hours a day. The Commission on Accreditation of Rehabilitation Facilities (CARF) accredits Burke's brain injury, spinal cord injury and medical rehabilitation programs.

BRAIN INJURY REHABILITATION PROGRAM: Led by Dr. Barry Jordan, M.D., a neurologist, the exceptional team of nurses, therapists and neuro-psychologists help patients reach their potential in a safe, structured and secure environment. Physical and occupational therapists work with patients on strengthening muscles and building endurance, on improving and strengthening visual, perception and cognitive skills, and on self-care activities. Speech-language therapists help brain injured patients with production and clarity of speech. Neuro-psychologists, who are specially trained in evaluating brain-behavior relationships, treat the behavioral and cognitive impairments that result from brain injury. Burke's team also works with patients' families to help them cope with the many changes that result from a traumatic brain injury.

SPINAL CORD INJURY REHABILITATION PROGRAM: Alan David, D.O., works with an expert team to maximize the neurological and physical recovery of each patient. The treatment team includes physical, occupational, speech and therapeutic recreational therapists, neuro-psychologists, nurses, social workers and chaplains who help patients manage their daily activities and stay healthy. The team develops a treatment plan that will help patients develop the skills and attitudes necessary to achieve a fulfilling and independent life. The rehabilitation plan includes short and long-term goals and also addresses follow-up services including referrals for less acute care and home modifications. Support for families is offered.

STROKE RECOVERY PROGRAM: Acute Inpatient Stroke Rehabilitation at Burke includes a minimum of three hours and routinely five hours of intensive therapy a day. All therapists, nurses, social workers and physicians on our stroke recovery unit are specially trained in stroke rehabilitation. Michael Reding, M.D., Stroke Recovery Program Director, works with an expert team to maximize the recovery of each patient. Therapy offered includes MIT-Manus upper limb robotic therapy, treatment for visual neglect, dysphagia retraining, custom bracing of the paretic leg, and a body weight supported treadmill training for gait recovery. Cutting-edge research protocols for neuro-pharmacologic enhancement of recovery following stroke and a wide range of follow-up care including outpatient therapy, support groups and exercise programs are available.

Burke is academically affiliated with the Weill Medical College of Cornell University and the New York-Presbyterian Healthcare System.

CONTINUUM HEALTH PARTNERS

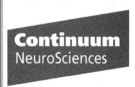

NEUROLOGY AND NEUROSURGERY EXPERTISE
Phone (800) 420-4004
www.chpnyc.org

St. Luke's and Roosevelt Hospitals, Beth Israel Medical Center and Long Island College Hospital are home to many international leaders in neurology, neurosurgery, neuro-radiology and endovascular neurosurgery.

At St. Luke's and Roosevelt Hospitals, the Center for Cranial Base Surgery and the Division of Spine and Minimally Invasive Neurosurgery offer advanced treatments for complex brain tumors, tumors of the skull base, spine and spinal cord. Our neurosurgeons are experts in surgery for chordomas, meningiomas, acoustic neuromas and treatment of trigeminal neuralgia and hemifacial spasm. The hospital also is home to The Headache Institute, which enjoys a solid reputation for its advanced treatments.

The Hyman-Newman Institute for Neurology and Neurosurgery (The INN) is dedicated to treating disorders of the brain, spinal cord, peripheral nerves and muscles. The INN has specialized programs for cerebrovascular diseases, epilepsy, movement disorders, neuro-ophthalmology and neurooncology. It is also home to the Center for Endovascular Surgery, where disorders of the brain, spine, head and neck are treated using minimally invasive endovascular techniques. It is a premier center where patients from all over the world come for the treatment of cerebrovascular and spinal vascular disorders. The Vascular Birthmarks Institute provides the most advanced treatment options for an array of medical and surgical options for birthmarks, hemangiomas, and vascular malformations in children.

Long Island College Hospital is recognized as a leader in providing treatment for acute stroke and has earned the distinguished stroke center designation by the New York State Department of Health. The Stanley S. Lamm Institute for Child Neurology and Developmental Medicine provides care for children with developmental disabilities.

Stroke prevention and treatment programs are located throughout Continuum's Manhattan and Brooklyn service area, offering 24-hour diagnosis and treatment, including the use of clot-busting thrombolytic medications.

604

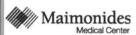

Maimonides
Medical Center

The Maimonides Stroke Center is ranked among the top 5% in the nation, and the top two in New York State. There are several other stroke centers in Brooklyn, but the services at Maimonides are far more advanced than at any other institution.

After the onset of stroke symptoms, there is a three-hour window of opportunity for the administration of a clot-busting drug. With highly specialized training, experts at certified stroke centers can administer that drug to appropriate patients. But there is a nine-hour window of opportunity for an advanced treatment, and Maimonides is one of only a handful of hospitals in the New York metropolitan area with the capability to provide that treatment – and the ONLY one in Brooklyn.

Dr. Jeffrey Farkas, Director of Interventional Neuroradiology, can insert a special instrument into a blood vessel, thread it up to the brain, and remove a stroke-causing blood clot. This procedure can greatly reduce stroke damage, and in some cases has completely reversed all symptoms. Dr. Farkas is among an elite few in the nation with significant experience utilizing this advanced technology for stroke patients.

Dr. Steven Rudolph, the neurologist Stroke Director at Maimonides, has just been selected as investigator in two clinical trials for the newest medical stroke therapies. This distinction is bestowed only on the most respected clinicians in that specialty. These therapies, too, will be able to provide treatment up to nine hours after the onset of symptoms.

In addition, Maimonides has a multidisciplinary team of stroke experts that includes physicians and nurses from the Department of Emergency Medicine, providing the vital first line of defense in combating stroke. The ER at Maimonides is equipped with telemedicine, an interactive system that allows consultation with a stroke neurologist in real time, even when the doctor is at a remote location.

In our stroke unit and interventional neuroradiology suite, nurses are certified and experienced in these specialties, and they coordinate recovery plans that include numerous technicians and therapists.

Physicians at Maimonides are among the eight percent in the US who use computers to enter patient orders, thereby reducing the risk of errors, increasing efficiency, and speeding the healing process. Maimonides has appeared on the American Hospital Association's "Most Wired" and "Most Wireless" lists more often than any other healthcare institution in the metropolitan area. Advanced technology allows our doctors to focus more attention on caring for their patients.

Maimonides Medical Center – passionate about medicine, compassionate about people.

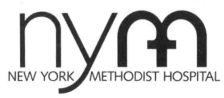

THE INSTITUTE FOR NEUROSCIENCES
New York Methodist Hospital
506 Sixth Street, Brooklyn, N.Y. 11215
Phone: 866-DO-NEURO (866-366-3876)
http://www.nym.org

SPECIALISTS AND MEDICAL SERVICES

The Institute for Neurosciences at New York Methodist Hospital brings together a unique group of specialists and medical services, offering diagnosis and treatment of a broad range of neurological conditions, ranging from frequent headaches to syncope to multiple sclerosis.

The Institute's panel of physician specialists includes neurologists, neurosurgeons, psychiatrists, endocrinologists, neuroradiologists, radiation oncologists, physiatrists, geriatricians, psychologists and physical therapists.

All diagnostic and therapeutic procedures are performed at New York Methodist Hospital or at individual physicians' offices. State-of-the-art equipment to perform computerized tomography (CT), magnetic resonance imaging (MRI), and magnetic resonance angiography (MRA) is located in the Hospital's Radiology Department. In addition, equipment and specialists trained to perform neurological diagnostic tests, such as electrocephalography (EEG), electromyography (EMG), and evoked potential examinations are available on the Hospital campus.

PROGRAMS OFFERED:

Special programs and services offered by the Institute include an Alzheimer's disease/memory center, a neuropathy program, pediatric and adult epilepsy programs that offer diagnosis via video EEG, a Parkinson's disease and other movement disorders program, a pituitary program, a balance disorders center and a stroke program. Neurosurgeons on the Institute's panel perform highly sophisticated procedures, including deep brain stimulation surgery, vascular neurosurgery, skull base surgery and spinal surgery. A stereotactic radiosurgery service is also available at the Hospital's regional radiation oncology center.

***

Referrals to the Institute, its programs and physicians can be made through an individual's primary care physician or requested directly through the Institute's telephone referral service. More information (and on-line physician referral) is available at the Hospital's website, http://www.nym.org.

741

THE STROKE PROGRAM

The Institute's Stroke Program is a New York State designated stroke center and was rated a stroke center of excellence in 2006 by Healthgrades, an independent research firm. The Program received five stars and was rated among the top ten percent in the nation for treatment of stroke.

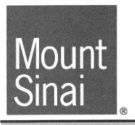

THE MOUNT SINAI MEDICAL CENTER
NEUROLOGY AND NEUROSURGERY

One Gustave L. Levy Place (Fifth Avenue and 100th Street)
New York, NY 10029-6574
Physician Referral: 1-800-MD-SINAI (636-4624)
www.mountsinai.org

The Estelle and Daniel Maggin Department of Neurology at The Mount Sinai Medical Center is the oldest neurology department in the country. From the beginning it has been an intensively productive center for research and patient care and over the past century, it has seen its reputation for excellence grow.

The Department of Neurosurgery at The Mount Sinai Medical Center was established in 1910, and has gained an international reputation for excellence. Its residency program began in 1946 and is a nationally recognized center of excellence. Areas of expertise include the skull-base, cerebrovascular, pituitary, acoustic, spinal reconstruction, epilepsy, radiosurgery, stereotactic, primary brain tumor surgery, functional, minimally invasive and neuroendoscopy. Neurosurgery research at Mount Sinai includes clinical programs, case presentations, and laboratories in the following areas: cerebrovascular, skull-base dissection, spinal cord injury, pituitary endocrinology, cerebral blood flow regulation, gene therapy and brain tumors, and movement disorders.

NEUROSURGICAL BRAIN AND SPINE TUMOR PROGRAM
Our program is world-renowned for pituitary adenomas, acoustic neuromas, meningiomas, and skull-base lesions. Using a multidisciplinary approach and state-of-the-art techniques, we provide diagnosis and comprehensive management of brain and spinal cord tumors.

STEREOTACTIC AND BRAIN TUMOR PROGRAM
As pioneers in computer assisted stereotactic techniques since 1993, we have extended the scope of operable brain tumors by using techniques such as frame-based or frameless stereotaxy, awake and asleep brain mapping, micro-neurosurgery, and endoscopic surgery. The development of a precision navigation system at Mount Sinai has resulted in substantial reductions of wound and neurosurgical morbidity, length of surgery, length of stay, and hospital costs. The addition of the Novalis Shaped Beam™ Surgery system gives our patients even more sophisticated options.

THE DIVISION OF FUNCTIONAL AND RESTORATIVE NEUROSURGERY
Equipped with the latest technology, we are focused on the development of minimally invasive neurosurgical techniques that either modulate neural function, replace lost neuronal populations, or halt the neurodegenerative process altogether. Presently, deep brain stimulation (DBS) dominates this field; but many new technologies with great potential are on the horizon. Our physicians have been honored by the Dystonia Medical Research Foundation for their pioneering work treating dystonia with DBS. They also use cutting edge techniques in the treatment of patients with Parkinson's disease, essential tremor, facial nerve disorders, epilepsy and pain.

Sponsored Page

THE NEUROSURGICAL SPINE PROGRAM
Our specially trained and highly skilled spine surgeons perform a range of spinal and peripheral nerve procedures with an emphasis on minimally invasive techniques. These include, for the spine, lumbar diskectomies, lumbar fusions, open biopsies, thoracoscopic treatments and extensive spinal reconstructions for deformities, tumors, degenerative conditions, and trauma, and for peripheral nerves, carpal tunnel releases, sympathectomies, brachial plexus decompressions and exploration, as well as exploration and grafts for various major nerve problems. Active clinical research projects include a novel experimental treatment for acute spinal cord injury.

THE CLINICAL PROGRAM FOR CEREBROVASCULAR DISORDERS
We provide expertise in the evaluation, treatment, and rehabilitation of patients with cerebrovascular diseases. Complementing the highly experienced team of medical experts are state-of-the-art facilities for surgical and endovascular treatment of cerebrovascular pathologies, a specialized Neurointensive Care Unit, and a brand new inpatient stroke unit. Video-telemedicine is utilized for the early diagnosis and treatment of stroke.

DIVISION OF NEUROMUSCULAR DISEASES
We provide unparalleled diagnosis, treatment, and compassionate care of patients with disorders in neuromuscular transmission, diseases of the muscles, or peripheral nerve problems.

THE MDA/ALS PROGRAM
This program, dedicated to Muscular Dystrophy and Amyotrophic Lateral Sclerosis, provides comprehensive, multidimensional, and seamless patient- and family-centered care for those afflicted with these disorders.

NEUROLOGICAL TUMOR PROGRAM
Mount Sinai is world-renowned for treatment of pituitary adenomas, acoustic neuromas, meningiomas, and skull-base lesions.

THE CORINNE GOLDSMITH DICKINSON CENTER FOR MULTIPLE SCLEROSIS
This program offers services in all aspects of diagnosis, disease management, rehabilitation, and support services, as well as the opportunity to participate in state-of-the-art experimental trials.

THE ROBERT AND JOHN M. BENDHEIM PARKINSON'S DISEASE CENTER
One of the world's first major centers for the study of Parkinson's Disease, we are a nucleus for multi-disciplinary translational research studies and a forum for collaboration. The Center offers state-of-the-art research programs, fostering the development of new medical and surgical therapies for the disease.

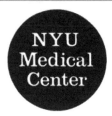

NYU Medical Center

550 First Avenue (at 31st Street)
New York, NY 10016
Physician Referral:
(888)7-NYU-MED (888-769-8633)
www.nyumc.org

NEUROLOGY

Dedicated to exceptional patient care, advanced scientific research, and high-quality graduate education, the Department of Neurology at NYU Medical Center evaluates and treats children and adults with a broad spectrum of neurological diseases. Specialty groups within the department deliver integrated care to patients with behavioral disorders and dementia, brain tumor, genetic and degenerative diseases, headache and pain sydromes, movement disorders including Parkinson's disease, multiple sclerosis, neuromuscular diseases, and diseases of children. NYU Medical Center is home to the largest multiple sclerosis program in New York.

The clinical mission especially benefits from a 30-bed neurorehabilitation unit, a state-of-the-art neurophysiology laboratory, and neurogenetics testing facility, each conducted under departmental auspices.

NYU COMPREHENSIVE EPILEPSY CENTER

Among the department's core programs is the NYU Comprehensive Epilepsy Center – the largest epilepsy program in the Eastern United States. The center offers testing, evaluation, treatment, drug trials, alternative therapies, and surgical intervention for patients with all forms of epilepsy. Beyond control of seizures, the center aims to improve quality of life by addressing problems of social isolation and helping patients achieve gratification at school, at work, at home, and in their communities.

At present, medications adequately control about 75 percent of those who suffer from recurrent epileptic seizures. But when medications fail to bring these debilitating seizures under control, a patient may be a candidate for surgery.

In the past two decades, enormous strides in understanding, technology, and surgical techniques have made surgery a safe and effective option for patients with intractable seizure disorders. Key to surgical success is functional mapping, which involves testing the brain to make sure it is safe to remove the tissues that are responsible for the seizures. Using a variety of imaging technologies, including MRI, PET, and SPECT, NYU's epileptologists are able to visualize abnormal anatomy and physiology and define a surgical target. Video-EEG recording is the most important test of all for characterizing and localizing seizures.

The most common surgical procedure for epilepsy is temporal lobe resection, often involving the removal of the deepest temporal structures. A low incidence of permanent complications makes this surgery a safe and attractive option when appropriate. At NYU, temporal lobe resection is performed without removing the patient's hair, using computer-assisted navigation and microscopic techniques. Patients are normally able to leave the hospital in 4 to 5 days. Vagus nerve stimulation (VNS), a reversible technique that was approved by the FDA in 1997, is just one of several additional surgical options for patients with particular types of seizures.

Brain diseases can cause intellectual impairments of profound complexity. The diagnosis and management of the cognitive disabilities accompanying traumatic brain injury or such diseases as stroke, Alzheimer's disease, epilepsy, and systemic illness often require an integrated approach. The Cognitive Neurology Program is an outpatient specialty clinic that serves adults with brain-based memory, perceptual, cognitive, or emotional impairments. Its specialists work closely with other branches of the Department of Neurology, and have close ties with Rusk Institute for Rehabilitation Medicine, where patients receive cognitive rehabilitation and speech therapy.

PHYSICIAN REFERRAL
1-888-7-NYU-MED
(1-888-769-8633)
WWW.NYUMC.ORG

702

Sponsored Page

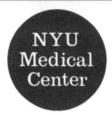

NYU Medical Center

550 First Avenue (at 31st Street)
New York, NY 10016
Physician Referral:
(888)7-NYU-MED (888-769-8633)
www.nyumc.org

NEUROSURGERY

The Department of Neurosurgery at NYU Medical Center offers the most advanced surgical procedures available anywhere in the world, along with compassionate care and supportive services for patients and their families. In an environment of leading-edge research and medical education, the department's interdisciplinary team of physicians, nurses, and allied health professionals are world-renowned for their highly specialized training and their down-to-earth approach to clinical care. The department also is home to the most sophisticated surgical instrumentation in the region.

Because of the large number of cases referred from all over the world, NYU neurosurgeons have been able to subspecialize in order to develop specific expertise and to provide the best and most up-to-date treatment in a broad range of conditions in adults and children. These include brain, skull base and spinal cord tumors, vascular disorders such as aneurysms and arteriovenous malformations, Parkinson's disease, ruptured disks, degenerative spine disease, epilepsy, peripheral nerve injuries and tumors and many other conditions. Notwithstanding the high technology focus and sophisticated surgical methodology, we firmly believe that quality of our patients' lives is the most important measure of our success.

The Center for the Study and Treatment of Movement Disorders
The Center for Study and Treatment of Movement Disorders provides surgical care for patients with Parkinson's disease and other movement disorders. Its highly focused surgeons implant neuroaugmentative devices ("brain pacemakers") and also have considerable experience in pallidotomy and thalamotomy for those with disabling tremor who may not be candidates for neuroaugmentative surgery. These procedures are performed using the latest computer localization and imaging technology in conjunction with precision electrophysiologic monitoring.

The Gamma Knife
In the recent past, patients with brain abnormalities considered too deep or too delicate to reach with a scalpel had little reason for hope. But with the Gamma Knife, neurosurgeons at NYU Medical Center can now remove deep-seated tumors, vascular malformations, and other sites of dysfunction with outstanding results. Aided by three-dimensional MRI technology that pinpoints the problem area, the neurosurgeon uses the Gamma Knife to destroy tumors with precise doses of radiation. Unlike conventional surgery, this noninvasive procedure is entirely bloodless and woundless, and achieves improved outcomes at lower cost and dramatically reduced recovery time.

Spine Surgery
NYU spinal neurosurgeons stress minimally invasive methods in treating a variety of degenerative spine conditions and in the removal of tumors of the spinal cord and spinal column. Dr. Paul Cooper, Ricciardi Professor of Neurosurgery and Dr Tony Frempong are internationally respected authorities in the management of spinal tumors, spinal reconstruction and stabilization procedures. On-line electrophysiologic monitoring has dramatically improved the neurological postoperative outcome over the past several years. Patients considered to have "inoperable" conditions at other institutions are treated here on a routine basis with excellent postoperative results and a very high level of patient satisfaction..

The Tumor Surgery Program at NYU Medical Center treats patients referred from all over the world. Dr Patrick J Kelly, Ransohoff Professor and Chairman of the Department of Neurosurgery has personally operated on over 6,600 brain tumors and is one of the most experienced brain tumor surgeons in the world. He developed computer-assisted stereotactic volumetric resection, a minimally invasive method for the precision and complete removal of brain tumors with excellent postoperative results. Methods for noninvasive brain mapping using magnetoencephalotomography (MEG), functional MRI and preoperative computer surgical simulations, allow selection of the safest surgical approach that minimizes risk and ensures the best possible clinical outcomes.

With this technology, "Inoperable tumors" become operable tumors at NYU.

689

⌐ NewYork-Presbyterian

The University Hospital of Columbia and Cornell

NewYork-Presbyterian Neuroscience Centers

Affiliated with Columbia University College of Physicians and Surgeons and Weill Medical College of Cornell University

The Neurological Institute of New York at
NewYork-Presbyterian Hospital
Columbia University Medical Center
710 West 168th Street
New York, NY 10032

Weill Cornell Neuroscience Institute at
NewYork-Presbyterian Hospital
Weill Cornell Medical Center
525 East 68th Street
New York, NY 10021

OVERVIEW:

The NewYork-Presbyterian Neuroscience Centers are consistently ranked among the top providers of neurological services in the United States, according to *U.S. News & World Report*. The Centers provide the most innovative, up-to-date treatments to combat the full range of neurological disorders, including:

- Stroke and Cerebrovascular Services – Diagnoses and treatments of Stroke (brain attack), Aneurysms, and Arteriovenous Malformations (AVMs) by leading neurologists, neurosurgeons and interventional neuroradiologists.

- Epilepsy – Comprehensive Epilepsy Centers provide round-the-clock surveillance of adults and children in monitoring unit and functional brain mapping to identify source of a seizure and the most effective treatment.

- Pediatric Neurology/Neurosurgery – Expertise and state-of-the-art care tailored to special needs of children.

- Spinal Disorders – The Spine Center integrates physicians specializing in neurology, neurosurgery, neuroradiology, orthopedics, physiatry (rehabilitative medicine) and anesthesiology/pain management, as well as physical and occupational therapy.

- Neuro-Oncology – Therapeutic interventions include the full spectrum of traditional as well as new and innovative treatments including: surgery, radiation therapy, stereotactic radiosurgery immune therapy and complementary therapies.

- Neuro-Immunology – One of the country's largest Multiple Sclerosis treatment and research programs.

- Neuro-Infectious Diseases – Rapid diagnosis and a wide range of experts.

- Neuromuscular Diseases –Diagnosis and appropriate therapies for improving pain management and quality of life.

- Movement Disorders – Largest regional program offering latest protocols and Deep Brain Stimulation Surgery to reduce/eliminate tremors.

- Memory Disorders – A premier center offering early detection/diagnosis and standard and investigational treatments to help slow or reverse progression of symptoms.

Physician Referral: For physician referral or to learn more about NewYork-Presbyterian Neuroscience Centers call toll free **1-877-NYP-WELL** (1-877-697-9355) or visit our website at **www.nypneuro.org**

HIGHLIGHTS INCLUDE:

- Leading interventional neuroradiology service providing minimally invasive endovascular surgery including carotid stenting, arterial stenosis in the brain and neck, acute stroke, cerebral aneurysms, brain tumors, arteriovenus fistulas and AVMs.

- Participating in NIH-CREST randomized clinical trial evaluating carotid artery stenting as compared to carotid endarterectomy.

- Country's largest program for Parkinson's Disease and other movement disorders; provides deep brain stimulation surgery for controlling Parkinson's.

- Only multidisciplinary academic neurointensive care units in the greater New York area.

- One of 28 specialized Alzheimer's Disease Research Centers sponsored by the National Institute on Aging.

- Intraoperative MRI

1052   Sponsored Page

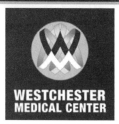

WESTCHESTER MEDICAL CENTER

Valhalla Campus
Valhalla, NY 10595
Tel. 1-877-WMC-DOCS
http://www.worldclassmedicine.com

OVERVIEW

The Neuroscience Center at Westchester Medical Center is a leader in the diagnosis and treatment of medical and surgical disorders of the nervous system. Our team of highly experienced neurologists, neurosurgeons and neuroradiologists employ the latest technologies to diagnose and treat a wide spectrum of cranial and spinal disorders. An entire floor of the Medical Center is dedicated to caring for patients with neurological and neurosurgical disorders, which includes a specialized Neurology/Neurosurgery Intensive Care Unit, Epilepsy Monitoring Unit and Stroke Unit for management of critically ill patients. Specialized operating rooms allow surgeons to perform an array of brain and spine procedures, many utilizing advanced "minimally invasive" techniques and intraoperative computer guidance. The Neuroscience Center also includes the expertise of psychiatrists from our Behavioral Health Center and the talents of a team of on-site rehabilitation specialists.

SPECIALIZED TEAM

The Neuroscience Center offers a comprehensive range of specialized programs for adult and pediatric patients, including:

• **Brain Tumor Section:** Offers aggressive multimodality treatments, including sophisticated open surgery, the latest chemotherapy protocols and minimally invasive, computer-guided radiosurgery.

• **Cerebrovascular Section**: Treats a variety of disorders, including aneurysms and strokes, with the latest in medical and surgical therapies. The University Hospital is home to a new state-of-the-art Cerebrovascular Center for the minimally invasive treatment of brain aneurysms and stroke.

• **Spine Section**: Offers advanced surgical treatment for disorders of the spinal column, including degenerative disc disease, deformities and tumors.

• **Neuromuscular Section**: Diagnoses and treats disorders such as myasthenia gravis, neuropathies, myopathies and motor neuron diseases such as ALS.

• **Epilepsy Section**: Manages patients with "simple" and complex seizure disorders through both medical and surgical treatment.

• **Movement Disorders Section:** Treats patients with a wide variety of illnesses, including Parkinson's disease, dystonias, Tourette's syndrome and tremors. The latest in both medical and surgical therapies are utilized, including deep brain stimulation.

Comprehensive outpatient and inpatient services are offered. In addition, our multidisciplinary approach to patient care involves allied specialists in such disciplines as ophthalmology, otology, urology, rehabilitation and psychiatry, as required.

NEUROSCIENCE CENTER AT WESTCHESTER MEDICAL CENTER

Specialists at the Neuroscience Center at Westchester Medical Center are leaders in the treatment of complex disorders of the central and peripheral nervous system.

Neurology:
Brij M. Singh Ahluwalia, MD, Chairman
Stephen J. Marks, MD
Venkat Ramani, MD
Tatyana Gitlevich, MD
Frances M. Dyro, MD
Jin Li, MD, PhD
Maria R. Sangiorgio, MD, MS
Baldev K. Singh, MD

Neurosurgery:
Raj Murali, MD, Chairman
Kaushik Das, MD
Prithvi Narayan, MD
John Abrahams, MD
Charles P. Garell, MD

Neuroradiology &
Neurointerventional Radiology:
Michael Tenner, MD
Kuo Chao, MD

Direct Telephone Numbers:
Neurology: (914) 345-1313
Neurosurgery: (914) 345-8111
Neuroradiology:
 (914) 493-2400, Ext. 340
Behavioral Health Center:
 (914) 493-7282

Sponsored Page

Obstetrics & Gynecology/ Birthing

WOMEN'S HEALTH

Morristown Memorial Hospital • Overlook Hospital

THE PASSION TO LEAD

Goryeb Children's Hospital • Atlantic Neuroscience Institute
Carol G. Simon Cancer Center/The Cancer Center at Overlook Hospital
Gagnon Heart Hospital • Atlantic Rehabilitation Institute

P.O. Box 1905, Morristown, NJ 07962 • 1-800-247-9580 • atlantichealth.org

Specialized Care, Just for Women

No matter what stage of life you are in, Atlantic Health offers specialized care to meet your unique needs as a woman, including preventative wellness programs and the most advanced diagnostic and treatment tools available. Whether you are making your first trip to the gynecologist, welcoming a new baby into your family, or going through menopause - Atlantic Health is here for you.

Our women's health specialists focus on:

- **Obstetrics and Gynecology**
- **Maternity**
- **High Risk Pregnancy**
- **Gynecological cancer**
- **Breast cancer**
- **Osteoporosis**
- **Depression**
- **Urogynecology**
- **Menopause**

- **Gynecology** - Our board-certified gynecologists handle a range of women's health issues. Areas of specialization include infertility programs, menopause management and osteoporosis.

- **Maternity** - At Atlantic Health, you'll deliver your baby in a supportive, family-oriented environment, staffed with caring professionals who provide the very best in medical care and the extra pampering new mothers deserve. Our maternity services include parent education classes, private and comfortable labor rooms, lactation consultants and complimentary massage.

- **High Risk Pregnancy** - Women with high-risk pregnancies are referred to Atlantic Health's Maternal-Fetal Medicine Center for evaluation and treatment. Morristown Memorial is a Regional Perinatal Referral Center and Overlook Hospital is a Level III Perinatal Hospital. Both hospitals also have Neonatal Intensive Care Units to provide advanced care to our smallest patients.

- **Women's Imaging** - The Atlantic Health hospitals offer comprehensive imaging technologies for women. Whether it's an ultrasound for pregnancy, a bone densitometry for osteoporosis or a mammography for breast cancer, we offer the diagnostic imaging procedures you need.

- **Breast Health** - Atlantic Health offers specialized services for evaluating and managing breast health and abnormalities. At the Carol W. and Julius A. Rippel Breast Center at Morristown Memorial Hospital and the Overlook Hospital Women's Imaging and Breast Center, a multidisciplinary team of physicians, nurses and technicians familiar with all aspects of breast disease participate in evaluation and treatment.

- **Women's Cancer Center** – At the Women's Cancer Center, we've created a wide range of services to help you meet the physical and emotional challenges associated with cancers unique to women including uterine, ovarian, and other gynecologic cancers. Our program offers minimally invasive surgery, participation in clinical trials, ovarian cancer genetics screening, and an early detection program for cervical cancer.

- **North Jersey Regional Arthritis Center** – For women who are affected by arthritis and osteoporosis, The North Jersey Regional Arthritis Center located at Morristown Memorial Hospital provides information and outreach, physical activity classes and self-management programs designed to increase quality of life.

Holy Name Hospital ☯

Member
NewYork-Presbyterian Healthcare System
Affiliate: Columbia University College of Physicians & Surgeons

718 Teaneck Road
Teaneck, NJ 07666
(201) 833-3000
www.holyname.org

OBSTETRICS AND GYNECOLOGY

Holy Name Hospital's maternal and child unit, The BirthPlace, received a 5-star rating from HealthGrades®, a leading information resource and provider of objective health care ratings. At Holy Name, comfort and technically superior medical care coexist. The BirthPlace was the first LDRP (Labor, Delivery, Recovery and Postpartum) design of its kind in New Jersey. Rooms are equipped with advanced monitoring and child-care equipment and furniture you'd expect to find in a luxurious hotel bedroom, complete with a private bathroom. The bed easily converts to a birthing bed, and special equipment to support the birthing process is concealed until it's needed.

LEVEL II NURSERY AND SUBSPECIALISTS

Along with having aesthetic appeal, The BirthPlace is equipped to meet emergencies and cesarean sections with 24-hour anesthesia coverage, boasts an intermediate level II special care nursery with board-certified obstetricians and pediatricians on site 24 hours a day, has a neonatologist available around the clock, and has experienced board-certified obstetrical and pediatric subspecialists on staff.

Fertility specialists and genetic counselors are also available for couples who have difficult conceiving or may be at risk for conceiving a child with a genetic or congenital disorder or who have a history of miscarriages or stillbirths. There are Parent Education services to help families prepare for the new arrival, including a Warm Line, 201-833-3124, linking new parents to a nursing consultant, and a Cord Blood Stem Cell Program, enabling parents to preserve and store the umbilical cord blood of their newborn, which could later aid treatment in the event of a life-threatening illness.

**For more information about The BirthPlace,
call 201-833-3124 or email birthplace@holyname.org.**

Holy Name Hospital's Obstetrics and Gynecology services include:

• Private LDRP suites

• Experienced labor and delivery, postpartum and neonatal care nurses

• Fully equipped cesarean section rooms

• 24-hour access to board-certified anesthesiologists, pediatricians and neonatologists

• State-of-the-art electronic alarm system

• Support programs, classes and services

• Participation in Cord Blood Stem Cell Program

• Genetic testing

• Fertility specialists

759

Sponsored Page

THE MOUNT SINAI MEDICAL CENTER
OBSTETRICS AND GYNECOLOGY

One Gustave L. Levy Place
(Fifth Avenue and 100th Street)
New York, NY 10029-6574
Physician Referral: 1-800-MD-SINAI (636-4624)
www.mountsinai.org

Building on more than a century of leadership in providing healthcare to women, the Department of Obstetrics, Gynecology, and Reproductive Science at The Mount Sinai Medical Center offers special expertise in:

• General obstetrics, including genetic counseling, prenatal care, labor and delivery management, and postpartum care. In addition to our talented physicians, other healthcare professionals are integrated into our practice, including genetic counselors, nutritionists, social workers, nurse midwives, childbirth educators, and lactation/breastfeeding specialists.

• High-risk obstetrics, including advanced techniques in prenatal diagnosis and consultations in the management of complicated pregnancies. Our ultrasound unit is recognized for its expertise in fetal anatomy ultrasound assessments. The latest technology, including 4D imaging, is utilized. Antepartum testing, including amniocentesis, chorionic villus sampling, and fetal blood sampling are all routinely performed at Mount Sinai.

• Reproductive endocrinology and infertility, including diagnosis and treatment of both female and male factor infertility. Treatment options for women include fertility medications, intrauterine insemination, in vitro fertilization, intracytoplasmic sperm injections, and ovum donation.

• General gynecology, including cancer screening, management of abnormal Pap smears, family planning, surgical management of fibroids, endometriosis, and other benign gynecologic conditions. Minimally invasive surgery is offered for many conditions.

• Gynecologic infectious diseases, including the treatment and prevention of sexually transmitted infections and consultations in obstetrical and gynecological infections.

• Gynecologic oncology, including care for women with cancers of the ovary, uterus, cervix, vulva, and vagina. Minimally invasive surgery is offered for many conditions.

• Urogynecology and reconstructive pelvic surgery, including lower urinary tract disorders.

THE MOUNT SINAI MEDICAL CENTER

Known worldwide for excellence and innovative approaches to prenatal diagnosis and fetal therapy, Mount Sinai's Department of Obstetrics, Gynecology, and Reproductive Science has a long tradition of advancing clinical practice through patient oriented research. Faculty members are pioneering work in diverse areas including first and second trimester screening for fetal chromosomal abnormalities, vaccines for the prevention of sexually transmitted infections, minimally invasive surgical techniques, and new approaches to the diagnosis and treatment of gender specific cancers.

612

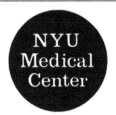

NYU Medical Center

550 First Avenue (at 31st Street)
New York, NY 10016
Physician Referral:
(888)7-NYU-MED (888-769-8633)
www.nyumc.org

WOMEN'S HEALTH

NYU Medical Center supports a comprehensive group of programs and services designed specifically for women's medical needs. Services range from primary care to the most specialized clinical care programs available in the nation. Supported by the most sophisticated research and advanced training at NYU School of Medicine, the Department of Obstetrics and Gynecology at NYU Medical Center offers a unique, abundant blend of high quality therapies and regimens, as well as leading-edge research technologies and methods.

Along with routine gynecological care, many other services are offered including: pelvic ultrasound; aspiration of breast cysts; evaluation of infertility, including the special needs of same-sex couples; colposcopy (a diagnostic evaluation of abnormal pap smears); LEEP (a loop electrosurgical procedure used to diagnose and treat cervical cancer); cryotherapy for vaginal warts; and bone density testing for osteoporosis prevention and treatment.

The Obstetrics program also offers a broad range of services. Among these are prenatal care that gives equal emphasis to the well-being of the mother and of the fetus; fetal monitoring through ultrasound and other techniques; childbirth preparedness and breastfeeding classes; and consultation for high-risk pregnancies, including treatment for women who experience recurrent pregnancy loss.

At NYU Medical Center, the backbone of patient care is the continued research into gynecologic diseases. With world-class faculty leading clinical investigations into disorders that can occur at any stage of a woman's life, doctors at NYU Medical Center are equipped with the latest findings to treat women throughout their lives.

NYU MEDICAL CENTER

Women's Health at
NYU Medical Center

• Obstetrics

• Gynecology

• Maternal-Fetal Medicine

• Gynecologic Oncology

• Reproductive Endocrinology and Infertility

• Reconstructive Pelvic Surgery and Urogynecology

• Endoscopic Pelvic Surgery and Family Planning

• Ultrasound Imaging

• Gynecological Pathology

PHYSICIAN REFERRAL
(888) 7-NYU-MED
(888-769-8633)
WWW.NYUMC.ORG

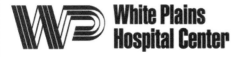

White Plains Hospital Center

**The William & Sylvia Silberstein
Neonatal & Maternity Center at
White Plains Hospital Center**

Davis Avenue at East Post Road
White Plains, New York 10601
Main Number: 914-681-0600
Physician Referral Service: 914-681-1010
www.wphospital.org

White Plains Hospital Center's (WPHC) William & Sylvia Silberstein Neonatal & Maternity Center offers a comprehensive approach to caring for mothers and newborns. More than 2,000 babies a year are born at the hospital, making it the busiest maternity program in Westchester County. The program was recently recognized with a five-star rating for clinical excellence in maternity care by HealthGrades™, the nation's leading provider of independent hospital ratings. This is the highest level of distinction possible from this rating service.

PERINATOLOGY SERVICES
Under the direction of a full-time perinatologist, WPHC's Center for Maternal-Fetal Medicine manages high-risk pregnancies. The center offers a full range of pre-conception and prenatal screening services including genetic counseling.

SPACIOUS LABOR & DELIVERY SUITES
The seven recently renovated Labor and Delivery suites are spacious and comfortably designed, with state-of-the-art technology. The private atmosphere allows family members more flexibility for visiting and provides in-room sleeping accommodations for fathers or labor support persons. Three of the rooms are private LDRP (Labor, Delivery, Recovery, Postpartum) suites, which allow the mother to remain in the same room throughout her hospital stay. Four are LDR suites which allow the mother to stay in the same room through the recovery phase, before being moved to a postpartum room in the well-appointed Mother/Baby Unit. A specialized surgical suite is available for Cesarean births.

COMFORTABLE MOTHER/BABY UNIT
The state-of-the-art Mother/Baby Unit features 14 private and six semi-private rooms. All rooms feature comfortable rocking chairs and sleeping accommodations for the baby's father or other support person to stay overnight. "Rooming in" is encouraged to promote family bonding.

LEVEL III NICU
White Plains Hospital Center's Charles A. Mastronardi Neonatal Intensive Care Unit (NICU) is designated a Level III Nursery by New York State, the highest level designation available to a community hospital. This unit offers the most technologically advanced developmental care for premature babies as young as 25 weeks, as well as newborns who are critically ill or in need of surgery. 24-hour coverage is provided by board-certified neonatologists and neonatal-trained registered nurses.

PARENT AND CHILD EDUCATION PROGRAM
Family-focused services and support groups include tours for expectant families, childbirth classes, infant care classes, and pre- and post-natal exercise. The Hospital also offers a telephone "Warm Line," where nurses are available to answer questions 24 hours a day.

The William & Sylvia Silberstein Neonatal & Maternity Center at White Plains Hospital Center

- Perinatology Program

- Management of high-risk pregnancies

- Spacious, modern renovated LDRP, LDR, and Mother/Baby Rooms

- Level III Neonatal Intensive Care Unit

- Extensive Parent & Child Education Program

- Lactation Center

- 24-hour "Warm Line"

Call (914) 681-1234 for more information or for a tour of the William & Sylvia Silberstein Neonatal & Maternity Center.

768

Sponsored Page

Occupational Medicine

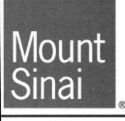

THE MOUNT SINAI MEDICAL CENTER
OCCUPATIONAL AND ENVIRONMENTAL MEDICINE

One Gustave L. Levy Place (Fifth Avenue and 100th Street)
New York, NY 10029-6574
Physician Referral: 1-800-MD-SINAI (636-4624)
www.mountsinai.org

A REPUTATION FOR EXCELLENCE

The Irving J. Selikoff Clinical Center for Occupational and Environmental Medicine is an internationally respected diagnostic and treatment center. The mission of the Center is to prevent occupational disease in the workplace and reduce morbidity and mortality associated with work. To achieve this goal, we utilize a preventive medicine model that includes three integrated components:

• *Clinical Care* – These services include the diagnosis, treatment, and management of occupational diseases and work-related musculoskeletal disorders for current and retired workers. We offer disability assessment and rehabilitation services to facilitate safe return to work and appropriate accommodations. Our social work services include counseling regarding the financial, social, and psychological aspects of occupational disease.

• *Disease Prevention Services* – These services include educating patients, health care providers, workers, unions, employers, and communities on the signs and symptoms of occupational disease. Comprehensive industrial hygiene and ergonomic services are available to evaluate exposures and recommend effective preventive measures. Technical assistance and consultation services are provided for employers, unions, and public health agencies.

• *Surveillance & Data Management* – We study the pattern and prevalence of occupational disease and identify new associations between workplace exposure and disease.

To promote disease prevention, the Center treats each newly identified case of occupational disease as a potential sentinel health event, that is, as a signal that there may be other similar cases of disease in the patient's co-workers. This approach, coupled with our efforts to reduce workplace hazards, places the Center's impact well beyond individual patient evaluations. To help achieve our goal of improving public health by preventing occupational and environmental disease, we work closely with labor unions, employers, government and service organizations, health care providers, and community organizations.

The Clinical Center has satellite sites in Westchester County and Queens, where staff physicians see patients several days a week. Some of the services available at the Irving J. Selikoff Center for Occupational and Environmental Medicine include:

• Medical evaluations for WTC workers and volunteers
• Assistance in evaluating specific workplace environments and suggesting ways of eliminating dangerous conditions
• Educational programs for unions and workers on workplace health issues
• Aid in getting worker compensation and other available legal benefits
• Social work services to help with the social, psychological, and financial problems caused by work-related health problems
• Epidemiologic services

Pediatric Environmental Health Specialty Unit

We provide consultation and medical care for children with toxic environmental exposures and with diseases of suspected environmental origin. This unit serves New York, New Jersey, Puerto Rico, and the Virgin Islands.

613

Ophthalmology

THE MOUNT SINAI MEDICAL CENTER
OPHTHALMOLOGY

One Gustave L. Levy Place (Fifth Avenue and 100th Street)
New York, NY 10029-6574
Physician Referral: 1-800-MD-SINAI (636-4624)
www.mountsinai.org

Specializing in the prevention, diagnosis, and treatment of eye disorders, The Department of Ophthalmology at Mount Sinai offers a variety of sophisticated tests for evaluating patient conditions, including electroretinography, visually evoked potentials, electro-oculography, fundus photography, fluorescein angiography, corneal topography, CT scanning, and MR imaging, as well as new techniques for assessing glaucoma. Ultrasound biomicroscopy (UBM) is a noninvasive method to achieve high-resolution imaging of the inside of the eye. In certain cases of glaucoma (those involving lesions behind the iris or behind a cloudy cornea), it is the only non-invasive way to identify the exact cause of the condition and ascertain optimal treatment. UBM is also an ideal tool to diagnose and manage certain cataract and corneal surgery complications. The pain-free procedure takes about 45 minutes.

Ophthalmology at Mount Sinai features faculty with wide experience in special eye problems and offers comprehensive eye care for the full range of eye disorders, including glaucoma, eye infections, retinal disorders (diabetic retinopathy, macular degeneration, and retinitis pigmentosa), dry eyes (Sjogren's syndrome), allergic reactions to contact lenses, neuro-ophthalmic disorders (double vision and droopy eyelids), corneal and external diseases of the eye, trauma, orbital tumors, and thyroid-related eye problems. We also offer minimally invasive procedures to treat eye disease, including non-laser refractive surgeries, small incision cataract surgery, bladeless laser procedures, and intacs for keratoconus.

Our highly skilled eye surgeons perform corneal transplants, refractive surgery, glaucoma surgery, cataract surgery, ophthalmic plastic surgery, ophthalmic reconstructive surgery, vitreous surgery for complicated retinal detachment, and corneal transplant surgery. We also specialize in the treatment of children with eye conditions.

We feature new imaging methods to assess and follow patients with OCT, HRT II, confocal for corneal problems, glaucoma, and retinal disease. These methods allow for faster, more accurate diagnosis and help determine the best treatment plan for each individual patient.

THE MOUNT SINAI MEDICAL CENTER

Mount Sinai ophthalmologists helped pioneer a new radiofrequency method of correcting farsightedness. Known as Conductive Keratoplasty (CK), the brief procedure is performed in the doctor's office with only topical anesthesia (eye drops). For most farsighted patients—especially those over age 40 whose eyes are naturally aging—the CK procedure eliminates the need for glasses.

623

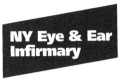

Continuum Health Partners, Inc.

THE NEW YORK EYE AND EAR INFIRMARY

310 East 14th Street
New York, New York 10003
Tel. 212.979.4000   Fax. 212.228.0664
http://www.nyee.edu

PROVIDING EXCEPTIONAL EYE CARE

The Department of Ophthalmology is the region's most comprehensive center for the delivery of primary through tertiary eye care. It is also by far the largest provider of eye care in the metropolitan area—with some 82,000 outpatient visits and 14,000 surgical cases performed each year. More than 250 board-certified ophthalmologists located throughout New York City and its tri-state area comprise the attending Medical Staff.

IN A HIGHLY SPECIALIZED SETTING

As a specialty hospital, the Infirmary is uniquely qualified to handle the most complicated cases. It serves as a nationwide referral center with a commitment to teaching, research, and high-technology based patient care. Computerized ocular imaging equipment includes the new combination of scanning laser ophthalmoscopy with optical coherence tomography, to provide highest resolution in-depth images which detect the smallest defects and assist in the earliest and most accurate diagnosis of diseases such as glaucoma and macular degeneration. Highly experienced staff using state-of-the-art instrumentation have made the Infirmary's 17 operating rooms a national benchmark in efficiency in eye surgery cases.

FOR PATIENTS OF ALL AGES

Staff at the Infirmary are sensitive to the specific needs of patients of all ages. Senior citizens are the vast majority of the Infirmary's 8,000 yearly cataract patients, as well as individuals receiving treatment for age-related macular degeneration. Young children are now 25 percent of the patient population, with conditions such as strabismus, acquired and congenital cataracts, corneal diseases and ocular trauma. For those rare cases of children who have a disease ordinarily associated with age, the Infirmary runs New York's only Pediatric Glaucoma Service. Active adults of all ages utilize the New York Eye Trauma Center and Oculoplastic and Orbital Surgery Services.

Ophthalmology Clinical Services

Ambulatory Care Services

Comprehensive Eye Care

Cornea & Refractive Surgery

Eye Trauma

Glaucoma

Low Vision

Neuro-Ophthalmology

Oculoplastic & Orbital Surgery

Ocular Tumor

Pediatric Ophthalmology & Strabismus

Retinal-Vitreal

Uveitis

Facilities

Ambulatory Surgery Center

Eye Trauma Center

Retina Center

About The New York Eye and Ear Infirmary

Founded in 1820, it is the nation's oldest, continuously operating specialty hospital. More than 10 million people have sought treatment here since its inception.

Physician Referral
1.800.449.HOPE (4673)

Sponsored Page

Orthopaedics

ORTHOPEDIC SERVICES

Morristown Memorial Hospital • Overlook Hospital

THE PASSION TO LEAD

**Goryeb Children's Hospital • Atlantic Neuroscience Institute
Carol G. Simon Cancer Center/The Cancer Center at Overlook Hospital
Gagnon Heart Hospital • Atlantic Rehabilitation Institute**

P.O. Box 1905, Morristown, NJ 07962 • 1-800-247-9580 • atlantichealth.org

Orthopedics

At Morristown Memorial Hospital, our orthopedic surgeons offer the latest in minimally invasive surgical techniques for faster recovery from both minor joint injuries and major impairments. Each year, we perform more than 1,300 joint replacements and treat more than 1,200 people with complex injuries at our Level II Trauma Center.

◢ North Jersey Regional Arthritis Center
Everything the arthritis patient needs is right here: referrals to physicians for early, accurate diagnosis, medical and surgical interventions, physical and occupational therapy, pain management, community disease management and health education.

◢ Orthopedic Trauma
Atlantic Health orthopedic surgeons at Morristown Memorial Hospital's Level II Trauma Center treat more than 1,200 people annually with complex injuries resulting from motor vehicle collisions or other incidents.

◢ Total Joint Replacement
Atlantic Health maintains superior surgical outcome rates that rival some of the nation's largest medical centers.

◢ Pediatric Orthopedics
Whether your child has a fracture or an orthopedic disorder such as scoliosis, you can be sure they will receive expert care from our pediatric orthopedists.   Our specialists provide diagnosis, treatment and rehabilitation services specifically for children.

◢ Spine Program
Atlantic Health surgeons perform surgeries and minimally invasive procedures to correct spinal disorders and alleviate back pain.

◢ Sports Medicine
Our orthopedic surgeons specializing in sports-related injuries understand your desire to get back into action as soon as possible.   Our treatment plans are designed to maximize performance, while minimizing recovery time.

◢ Rehabilitation
Our multidisciplinary team of rehabilitation professionals start you on the road to recovery following injury, illness or surgery. Additional physical rehabilitation is also available as needed at Atlantic Rehabilitation Institute.

◢ Patient Education and Resources
Atlantic Health provides patients and referring physicians with the information they need before, during and after treatment.

◢ Diagnostic Services
Our Department of Radiology provides a complete spectrum of state-of-the-art imaging services and image-guided interventional procedures for the musculoskeletal system.

Holy Name Hospital ⊙

Member
NewYork-Presbyterian Healthcare System
Affiliate: Columbia University College of Physicians & Surgeons

718 Teaneck Road
Teaneck, NJ 07666
(201) 833-3000
www.holyname.org

ORTHOPEDIC SERVICES

Holy Name's Orthopedic Services are on par with any tertiary care center. Holy Name's orthopedic surgeons are experienced in traditional hip and knee arthroscopy and in performing joint replacements using new materials including ceramics, metals and plastics to help joint replacements last longer.

INNOVATIVE NEW SURGICAL OPTIONS

Minimally invasive navigation systems for total joint replacements enable our orthopedic surgeons to perform high-precision joint replacements and view the surgical field using three-dimensional images during a procedure. A Picture Archiving Communications System, which digitally processes and stores radiologic images, enables surgeons to call up patients' X-rays, CT scans, MRI studies and other images on computers while they are performing surgery. Gender Solutions™ Innovations, an orthopedic innovation based on the distinct differences between women and men, is a system that creates gender-specific reconstructive implants resulting in improved quality of life. Minimally invasive bone grafting reduces healing and recovery time. Birmingham hip resurfacing preserves the existing bone and reduces the risk of microfractures.

Sophisticated methods of pain management—and physical therapy and satellite physical therapy units right on the surgical floor—help patients regain their independence more quickly and completely.

To learn more about the Holy Name Hospital orthopedics team or for a physician referral, call 1-888-464-7497.

The Orthopedic Services available at Holy Name Hospital include:

- Arthroscopic surgery

- Kyphoplasty

- Minimally invasive grafting

- Joint replacement

- Birmingham resurfacing

- X-LIFT

- Computer-assisted hip and knee surgery

- Extremity MRI

- Gender-specific joint replacement

758

Sponsored Page

HOSPITAL
FOR
**SPECIAL
SURGERY**

HOSPITAL FOR SPECIAL SURGERY

Orthopaedic Services

535 East 70th Street • New York, NY 10021
Physician Referral: 800-854-0071 • hss.edu

FIRST IN ITS FIELD
Founded in 1863, Hospital for Special Surgery is the nation's leading specialty hospital for orthopaedics and rheumatology.

FIRST IN JOINT REPLACEMENTS
HSS pioneered designs and surgical techniques for the first modern total knee replacement. HSS performs more joint replacements than any other hospital in the world.

PIONEERING MINIMALLY INVASIVE SURGERY
HSS surgeons developed smaller instruments and surgical techniques allowing minimally invasive total hip replacement and minimally invasive total knee replacement. HSS anesthesiologists, world leaders in regional anesthesia, developed special pain blocks required for minimally-invasive surgery. HSS surgeons are innovators in hand, elbow, shoulder, and spine surgery techniques. They are leading experts in arthroplasty. Over 75% of all knee procedures performed at HSS are minimally invasive.

WORLD'S MOST EXPERIENCED
MUSCULOSKELETAL RADIOLOGISTS
HSS Radiologists revolutionized diagnostic imaging for orthopaedics. They developed the landmark MRI pulse-sequencing techniques that reveal early degenerative changes in cartilage and other soft tissue. HSS is the only academic center with five high field MR Units dedicated exclusively to musculoskeletal imaging.

SPECIALTIES INCLUDE:

- **Arthroscopy**
- **Hip Replacements**
- **Knee Replacements**
- **Joint Replacements**
- **Back Pain**
- **Sports Medicine**
- **Physiatry**
- **Hand & Upper Extremity Problems**
- **Hip & Knee Problems**
- **Foot & Ankle Problems**
- **Shoulder Problems**
- **Ligament Injuries**
- **Spinal Problems**
- **Carpal Tunnel Syndrome**

- **Orthopaedic Trauma**
- **Musculoskeletal Nerve Damage**
- **Osteogenesis Imperfecta (OI)**
- **Osteoporosis**
- **Pediatric Orthopedics**
- **Physical Therapy**
- **Scoliosis**
- **Skeletal Dysplasia**
- **Pain Management**
- **Spina Bifida**
- **Birth defects of the bones and joints**
- **Cerebral Palsy Mobility**
- **And more, see hss.edu**

**Top Ranked in
Orthopaedics &
Rheumatology in
the Northeast by**
U.S. News & World Reports
for 16 Years in a Row

**Winner of Nursing's Highest
Honor: Magnet Status for
Nursing Excellence**

**Winner of NY's First
Patient Safety Award**

**Team Physicians for
NY Mets, NY Giants,
Association of Tennis
Professionals, St. John's
University and other
Professional and
College Teams**

**Largest Physiatry
Department Dedicated to
the Non-operative Treatment
of Musculoskeletal Disorders**

**First Women's Sports
Medicine Center, a model
across the nation**

**New at HSS: Institute for
Cartilage Research**

**Sports Medicine Institute for
Young Athletes: first in NYC**

hss.edu
**Every
Musculoskeletal
Specialty.
One Innovative
Web Site.**

ORTHOPEDIC SURGERY & SPORTS MEDICINE
Lenox Hill Hospital

100 East 77th Street, New York, NY 10021
Tel. 212-434-2710
www.lenoxhillhospital.org

Lenox Hill Hospital is recognized internationally as a leading center for orthopedic surgery and sports medicine. The Hospital's orthopedic surgeons and sports medicine specialists, pioneers in minimally invasive techniques that are widely used today, are experts in treating a broad range of musculoskeletal conditions, including disorders of the knees, hips, spine, feet, ankles, shoulders, elbows and hands.

JOINT REPLACEMENT FOR RESTORED MOBILITY
Lenox Hill Hospital's outstanding orthopedic surgeons are leaders in joint replacement surgery, offering the most advanced technologies and techniques to increase the durability of hip and knee implants. Their expertise includes surgery to lessen tissue trauma, and pain control techniques to significantly reduce post operative pain, resulting in earlier recovery of function. They perform both total and partial knee replacement surgery, as well as total replacement of the hip and shoulder joints. Surgery is followed by physical therapy to assist patients in gaining mobility and realizing the full potential of their bodies post-surgery. Lenox Hill Hospital orthopedic surgeons perform approximately 1,400 total joint replacements annually.

SPORTS MEDICINE FOR WEEKEND WARRIORS AND PROFESSIONAL ATHLETES
The Hospital's Nicholas Institute of Sports Medicine and Athletic Trauma (NISMAT), founded in 1973, is one of the largest programs of its kind and was the first hospital-based center in the U.S. dedicated to the advancement of research in sports medicine. Its expert staff of sports medicine specialists and physical therapists also provides treatment and rehabilitation to injured athletes, including players on the New York Jets and Islanders. NISMAT conducts comprehensive research, performs exercise stress tests, and educates professionals as well as the general public on the latest fitness information.

SPINE SURGERY
Lenox Hill Hospital's spine surgeons perform more than 1,000 spine procedures annually, including spinal fusion, cervical spine surgery, lumbar surgery and endoscopic scoliosis surgery, a minimally invasive procedure to correct curvature of the spine. The Hospital is one of the few spine centers in the country to perform total disc replacement, a procedure that treats severe low back pain by replacing a damaged or worn out spinal disc with an artificial one. The Hospital also offers Kyphoplasty™, a new minimally invasive procedure to treat vertebral compression fractures due to osteoporosis.

Need an orthopedic specialist?
Call the Lenox Hill Hospital
Physician Referral Service at 1-888-RIGHT MD.

AN INTERNATIONAL LEADER IN ORTHOPEDIC SURGERY AND SPORTS MEDICINE

The orthopedic surgery and sports medicine specialists at Lenox Hill Hospital treat thousands of patients each year, from recreational athletes to members of New York's professional sports teams. They provide a full range of services, including:

_ Total and partial joint replacement

_ Reconstructive knee surgery

_ Surgery of the shoulders, elbows and ankles

_ Hand surgery

_ Spine surgery, including spinal fusion and disc replacement

_ Exercise stress testing

_ Physical therapy

Sponsored Page

Mount Sinai ®

THE MOUNT SINAI MEDICAL CENTER
ORTHOPAEDICS

One Gustave L. Levy Place (Fifth Avenue and 100th Street)
New York, NY 10029-6574
Physician Referral: 1-800-MD-SINAI (636-4624)
www.mountsinai.org

In addition to offering depth and breadth of expertise, **The Leni and Peter W. May Department of Orthopaedics** is known for personalized care. The faculty and staff invest the time to get to know their patients as individuals, ensuring that they receive direct care from subspecialty-trained orthopaedists. The faculty share expertise in surgery of the foot and ankle, knee, hip, hand, elbow, shoulder, and spine; total joint replacement (knee, hip, foot and ankle, and shoulder); microvascular surgery; cancer surgery; and minimally invasive surgery. Taking a whole-patient approach to care, they work in close collaboration with specialists in geriatrics, neurology, oncology, pathology, and rehabilitation medicine.

INVESTIGATION AND INNOVATION

Recent years have seen successive refinements in the techniques of orthopaedic surgery at Mount Sinai, including the design and composition of the prostheses used in joint replacements that has lead to improved postoperative function. Faculty members have also been instrumental in the design and perfection of hip and shoulder prosthesis. Additionally, Mount Sinai has broadened the applications of arthroscopic surgery—the fiberoptic technology that first heralded the arrival of minimally invasive surgery.

Mount Sinai orthopaedic scientists are also known for their studies of "wear and tear" diseases of the skeletal system. Researchers are currently investigating bone wear at the microscopic level, rotator cuff degeneration, factors that predict hip fractures, the effects of microgravity on aging of bones and tissue, how joints of the foot degenerate, methods of determining bone strength, and how genetic alterations change the skeleton's function.

USE OF CUTTING-EDGE TECHNOLOGY

Mount Sinai uses 3-D imaging technology during many of its total knee and total hip replacement surgeries. This allows the surgeon to see multiple views of the anatomy, provides a more exact placement of implants, and lets the surgeon review the joint's range of motion with the implant installed in its final position.

THE MOUNT MEDICAL CENTER

Today at Mount Sinai, arthroscopy is used to repair not only the knee, but virtually every joint. Converting what used to be major open surgery to outpatient procedures, this has dramatically shortened rehabilitation and return-to-work times. Even more significantly, it has allowed many more patients to get help for painful, function-limiting conditions. That is the case for many elderly or frail patients who would be physically unable to undergo major surgery. The fact that such procedures are now more widely accessible is enhancing the quality of life for many patients and allowing them to lead more active lives.

624

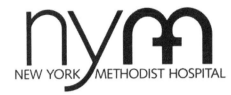

THE INSTITUTE FOR ORTHOPEDIC MEDICINE AND SURGERY
New York Methodist Hospital

506 Sixth Street, Brooklyn, N.Y. 11215
Phone: 866-ORTHO-11 (866-678-4611)
http://www.nym.org

SPECIALISTS AND MEDICAL SERVICES

The Institute for Orthopedic Medicine and Surgery at New York Methodist Hospital brings together a unique team of specialists, facilities, and medical services to provide comprehensive treatment of a broad range of orthopedic disorders.

The Institute's panel of physicians includes specialists in adult and pediatric orthopedic surgery, emergency medicine, rheumatology, podiatric medicine and surgery, endocrinology, sports medicine, pain management, orthopedic oncology, and neurosurgery. Other important health care team members include podiatrists and physical and occupational therapists. All diagnostic and therapeutic procedures are performed at New York Methodist Hospital or in the offices of the referred physicians.

PROGRAMS OFFERED

In addition to emergency orthopedic services, programs offered through the Institute include joint replacement, arthroscopic knee surgery and cartilage restoration and medical treatments for arthritis, medical and surgical treatment for hand and shoulder injuries and degenerative conditions, spine surgery, physical therapy and pain management. Podiatric physicians specialize in all foot disorders, including reconstructive foot surgery. In addition, the Institute offers complementary medicine services including chiropractic care, acupuncture, and medical massage.

***

Referrals to the Institute, its programs and physicians can be made through an individual's primary care physician or requested directly through the Institute's telephone referral service. More information (and on-line physician referral) is available at the Hospital's website, http://www.nym.org.

THE SPINE & ARTHRITIS CENTER

Focusing on conservative treatment, this unique facility is dedicated to the diagnosis and treatment of spinal and rheumatologic disorders. The Center uses a patient management program for all patients who undergo joint replacement of the hip or knee. Located on the Hospital campus, the Center provides patients with easy access to the MRI/CT, x-ray, laboratory and other resources needed to diagnose and treat all types of arthritis and back problems.

739

Sponsored Page

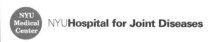

NYU**Hospital for Joint Diseases**

550 First Avenue (at 31st Street)
New York, NY 10016
Physician Referral:
(888)7-NYU-MED (888-769-8633
www.nyumc.org

301 East 17th Street (at 2nd Ave.)
New York, NY 10003
Physician Referral:
(888) HJD-D OCS (888-453-3627)
www.nyuhjd.org

ORTHOPAEDIC SERVICES

Leaders in the treatment of adult and children's bone and joint disorders.

The NYU Hospital for Joint Diseases Department of Orthopaedic Surgery offers the following services and treatments:

General Orthopaedics
The Spine Center
Pediatric Orthopaedics
Foot and Ankle Surgery
Limb Lengthening and Bone Growth
Sports Medicine
Center for Neuromuscular and Developmental Disorders
Immediate Orthopaedic Care Center

Joint Replacement Center
Arthroscopic Surgery
Bone Tumor Service
Hand Surgery
Occupational and Industrial Orthopaedic Care
Shoulder Institute
The Harkness Center for Dance Injuries

NYU Hospital for Joint Diseases provides care at NYU Tisch Hospital, NYU Hospital for Joint Diseases, Manhattan VA, Jamaica Hospital, and Bellevue Hospital Center, where more than 12,000 surgical procedures are performed each year. The orthopaedic faculty maintains offices in all five boroughs as well as in Rockland County and New Jersey.

NYUHJD Orthopaedic Programs and Services

More than 12,000 surgical procedures are performed at the NYU Hospital for Joint Diseases annually. Among our programs and services, we offer the following:

The Joint Replacement Center of NYC: Patients have access to physicians and surgeons highly specialized in treating degenerative joint conditions. Utilizing state-of-the-art techniques, the Center's surgeons are renowned for their expertise in knee, hip and shoulder replacements, complex joint revisions, as well as minimally invasive surgeries. Our center is one of the most active in the world, performing over 2,500 joint replacements annually.

The Spine Center: Provides comprehensive treatment of adult and pediatric spine disorders including lower back pain, neck pain, scoliosis, osteoporosis and the most complex spine problems. We perform minimally invasive spinal fusions that reduce incision size and lead to a speedier recovery. Our Spine Center is distinguished as one of the first in the country to successfully perform artificial disc implantation. We perform over 1,200 spinal procedures each year.

Pediatric Orthopaedic Service: Our skilled specialists provide orthopaedic care for children of all ages with the full spectrum of clinical conditions including neuromuscular diseases such as cerebral palsy, spina bifida and muscular dystrophies and congenital conditions such a clubfoot, hip dysplasia, and limb deformities. Our interdisciplinary approach teams orthopaedic surgeons with pediatric specialists to provide the most up-to-date continuity of care.

Diabetes Foot and Ankle Center: Our main goal is the prevention of foot problems and their recurrence. We offer patients an interdisciplinary team of dedicated medical professionals to provide the most advanced treatment for these complications and prevent further damage.

705

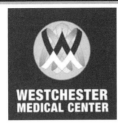

WESTCHESTER MEDICAL CENTER

Valhalla Campus
Valhalla, NY 10595
Tel. 1-866-WMC-ORTHO
http://www.worldclassmedicine.com

A LEADER IN THE DIAGNOSIS AND TREATMENT OF ADULTS AND CHILDREN WITH MUSCULOSKELETAL DISORDERS

Westchester Medical Center's Department of Orthopaedics is a model for excellence and innovation in the diagnosis and treatment of musculoskeletal disorders—performing more than 2,500 complex surgical procedures annually. Dedicated to providing comprehensive, individualized care, our board-certified physicians provide patients with a quality of care that is unsurpassed in the Hudson Valley region.

The Department of Orthopaedics employs a multidisciplinary approach to the diagnosis, treatment and rehabilitation of adults and children suffering from spinal pathology, fractures, degenerative joint diseases, rheumatologic conditions, sports-related injuries and hand and upper extremity injuries. Our board-certified surgeons, each an expert in their respective sub-specialty, work in concert with physiatrists, rheumatologists, neurologists, oncologists and other specialists as needed in order to improve patients' mobility and quality of life.

As an academic teaching hospital affiliated with New York Medical College, the faculty is recognized for its active involvement in research and education as well as for its clinical expertise in all sub-specialty areas of orthopaedic surgery—including hand and upper extremity, arthritis, joint replacement, spine and scoliosis surgery, pediatric orthopaedic surgery, arthroscopic surgery and trauma surgery.

All inpatient pediatric services are provided in Westchester Medical Center's state-of-the-art Maria Fareri Children's Hospital. This offers young patients a total healing environment in which parents can participate fully in their child's care and recovery.

As part of the Regional Trauma Center at Westchester Medical Center (Level 1), orthopaedic surgeons are available 24/7 to treat the most seriously injured adults and children who are victims of trauma.

Orthopaedic Services At Westchester Medical Center

The Department of Othopaedics at Westchester Medical Center provides comprehensive adult and pediatric Orthopaedic and Muscoloskeletal Services, including:

• Arthritis

• Arthroscopy

• Hand & Upper Extremity

• Joint Replacement

• Orthopaedic Trauma

• Pediatric Orthopaedics

• Spine and Scoliosis

• Sports Medicine

Call 1-866-WMC-ORTHO for a physician referral or a specialty office near you.

For more information, go to www.worldclassmedicine.com

784

Sponsored Page

Otolaryngology

Mount Sinai ®

THE MOUNT SINAI MEDICAL CENTER
OTOLARYNGOLOGY – EAR, NOSE, AND THROAT

One Gustave L. Levy Place (Fifth Avenue and 100th Street)
New York, NY 10029-6574
Physician Referral: 1-800-MD-SINAI (636-4624)
www.mountsinai.org

Mount Sinai's Multidisciplinary Head and Neck Cancer Team has gained national recognition for its expertise and innovation in the management of head, neck, and skull-base cancer. Mount Sinai has a nationally recognized team of experts in minimally invasive and endoscopic head and neck surgery. The team is comprised of a group of surgeons and oncologists focused on the curative treatment for head and neck malignancies. The expert team works to cure tumors of the oral cavity, jaw, and larynx and preserve each patient's quality of life. Speech and swallowing rehabilitation therapists work with patients to help them fully recover. Mount Sinai is on the cutting edge of head and neck cancer therapy, reconstruction, and rehabilitation.

Cranial Base Surgery – Surgeons at Mount Sinai have developed techniques to endoscopically remove skull-base tumors through the nose, leaving no visible sign of surgery. Interdisciplinary teams provide expertise in the diagnosis and treatment of tumors, vascular lesions, and trauma at the base of the brain.

Thyroid and Parathyroid Surgery – Minimally invasive thyroidectomy and parathyroidectomy can be performed through a one-inch incision. We believe that a team approach involving an experienced surgeon, a dedicated endocrinologist, and a team of physicians trained in nuclear medicine is of critical importance for the treatment of thyroid cancers.

Audiology – All aspects of audiology are covered at Mount Sinai, including the performance and interpretation of audiograms, brainstem evoked potentials, otoacoustic emission testing, neonatal hearing screening, and evaluations for assisted listening devices.

Facial Plastic and Cosmetic Surgery – Our reconstructive facial surgeons and specialists in facial cosmetic surgery use state-of-the-art endoscopic techniques.

Head and Neck Reconstructive Surgery – The Department has some of the most experienced reconstructive surgeons in the world, specializing in microvascular free tissue transfer.

Hearing, Facial Nerve, and Balance Disorders – Multidisciplinary teams provide treatment for a broad range of adult and pediatric neuro-otologic and otologic disorders.

Maxillofacial Prosthodontics – Complete services to restore speech and chewing abilities and minimize cosmetic defects, are offered.

Nasal and Sinus Surgery – Renowned rhinologists treat all inflammatory and infectious diseases of the nose and sinuses.

Oral and Maxillofacial Surgery – All treatment options are provided for patients with congenital, acquired, or traumatic problems of the oral cavity, jaws, and associated structures.

Additionally, The **Grabscheid Voice Center** offers the highest level of medical care for the professional voice, along with a profound understanding of the special medical, psychological, and professional needs of singers, actors, and lecturers.

THE MOUNT SINAI MEDICAL CENTER

One of the oldest and most respected departments in the nation, Mount Sinai's Department of Otolaryngology is consistently ranked among the top in the nation. In 2006, *US News & World Report* ranked Mount Sinai's Department of Otolaryngology New York City and #19 in the nation.

In a special issue of "The Best Hospitals in New York," *New York Magazine* said of otolaryngology: "... the leading hospital in this area is Mount Sinai, home to one of the oldest and busiest otolaryngology departments in the country. Sinai handles virtually every subspecialty in otolaryngology with finesse." In the Department of Otolaryngology at Mount Sinai, all physicians are board-certified specialists dedicated to healing disorders of the ear, nose, throat, head, and neck.

615

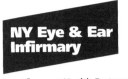

NY Eye & Ear Infirmary

Continuum Health Partners, Inc.

THE NEW YORK EYE AND EAR INFIRMARY

310 East 14th Street
New York, New York 10003
Tel. 212.979.4000   Fax. 212.228.0664
http://www.nyee.edu

PROVIDING EXCEPTIONAL CARE OF THE EAR, NOSE, THROAT, AND HEAD & NECK

Established in 1820 the Department of Otolaryngology/Head & Neck Surgery is the first training program in this specialty in the Western Hemisphere. Over nearly two centuries the department has evolved to be an international referral center for the medical and surgical treatment of diseases of the ear, nose, and throat.

OUTSTANDING SERVICES:

Facial Plastic Surgery: In-office or ambulatory procedures utilizing computer imaging, new techniques and materials produce outstanding results with minimal incisions, rapid recovery and a natural, youthful appearance.

Head & Neck Oncology: A multi-disciplinary team including board-certified surgeons, medical & radiation oncologists, nutritionists and rehabilitation specialists insure rapid recovery from complex, life-saving surgical procedures and return to daily activities.

Thyroid Center: A comprehensive program to streamline the diagnosis and treatment of thyroid diseases and cancers. A highly skilled team of surgeons, endocrinologists and radiologists manage the patient's care.

Voice & Swallowing Institute: Combining the expertise of physicians, speech pathologists and a voice physiologist to diagnose and treat voice problems – not only for performing artists but also for teachers, stockbrokers, receptionists, salespeople – anyone for whom voice is an important part of life.

Ear Institute (Otology – Neuro-otology): Specializing in the care of chronic ear disease including hearing loss, cochlear implantation, dizziness, tinnitus, intra cranial tumors and facial nerve disorders. Our advanced otologic and vestibular diagnostic labs assist physicians in treatment.

Pediatric Otolaryngology: Treating children has long been a priority at the Infirmary. Pediatric care ranges from middle ear infection, tonsil and adenoid disease, and neck masses to complex sinus and airway diseases.

Rhinology and Sinus Surgery: Internationally known specialists utilize minimally invasive techniques to treat disorders from sinusitis to intra cranial tumors

Otolaryngology Clinical Services

Facial Plastic & Reconstructive Surgery

Head & Neck Oncology

Thyroid Center

General Otolaryngology

Laryngology

Swallowing Disorders

Voice & Vocal Dynamics

Otology & Neuro-otology

Cochlear Implantation

Pediatric Otolaryngology

Rhinology & Sinus Surgery

Facilities

Ambulatory Care Services

Faculty Practice

Teaching Practice

Hearing Aid Dispensary

Vestibular Rehabilitation

About The New York Eye and Ear Infirmary

The Infirmary is the nation's oldest, continuously operating specialty hospital and one of the most experienced in terms of the number of patients it treats and complexity of its cases. Each year the otolaryngology department performs more than 6,000 surgeries and sees more than 60,000 visits from outpatients

Physician Referral
1.800.449.HOPE (4673)

NYU Medical Center

NYU Medical Center

550 First Avenue (at 31st Street)
New York, NY 10016
Physician Referral:
(888)7-NYU-MED (888-769-8633)
www.nyumc.org

OTOLARYNGOLOGY (EAR, NOSE AND THROAT)

Treating the full spectrum of ear, nose, throat, head and neck disorders, the Department of Otolaryngology at NYU Medical Center provides state-of-the-art patient care and research through the following programs:

Cochlear Implants – the first center in the U.S. to use a multichannel cochlear implant in a profoundly deaf adult, in 1984. Since then we have implanted more than 1400 adults and children from the age of 6 months to 85 years.

Sinus and Nasal Disorders – comprehensive diagnosis and minimally invasive treatment of sinus and nasal disorders

Facial Plastic Surgery – plastic and reconstructive surgery for a variety of problems, including nasal obstruction, facial trauma, defects left after removing skin and other facial cancers, facial paralysis and spasm, congenital malformations.

Head and Neck Surgery – state of the art treatment for benign and cancerous diseases of the nasopharynx, larynx, tongue, mouth, mandible, neck and face.

Sleep Apnea – repairing the collapse of soft tissue that leads to snoring and sleep apnea (a dangerous condition in which snorers stop breathing repeatedly during the night, taxing the heart and leaving the snorer unrested)

Skull Base Surgery – minimally invasive and advanced surgical approaches to the tumors of the anterior and posterior skull base such as acoustic neuroma, esthesioneuroblastoma, NF2, chordoma, chondrosarcoma, encephalocele.

Swallowing Disorders – the only center of its kind in New York City, providing comprehensive diagnosis, treatment and therapy for swallowing disorders

Voice Center – state-of-the-art biofeedback and therapy to rectify problems in speech

Advanced Otologic Medicine & Surgery – treating patients with disorders of the ear and conditions that affect hearing, balance and facial nerve function

The cochlear implant program at NYU Medical Center is one of the nation's finest. Since it set the standard in 1984 by implanting a profoundly deaf adult, the Division has been the site of numerous studies and research trials that will continue to improve the technologies available.

Adults and children travel from all over the world to get their cochlear implant at NYU Medical Center.

Physician Referral
(888) 7-NYU-MED
(888-769-8633)
www.med.nyu.edu

687

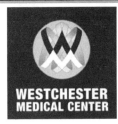

WESTCHESTER MEDICAL CENTER

Valhalla Campus
Valhalla, NY 10595
Tel. (914) 693-7636
http://www.worldclassmedicine.com

EXCELLENCE IN EAR, NOSE, THROAT AND HEAD & NECK CARE FOR ADULTS AND CHILDREN

The Department of Otolaryngology and Head & Neck Surgery at Westchester Medial Center offers state-of-the-art medical and surgical solutions for disorders that affect the ears, nose, sinuses, face, voice box, throat, head and neck.

All of the specialists within the Department of Otolaryngology are board-certified by the American Board of Otolaryngology/Head and Neck Surgery and have fellowship trained at some of the nation's top institutions in their respective sub-specialties, including Pediatric Otolaryngology, Head and Neck Surgery, Thyroid Surgery, Sinus Surgery, Facial Plastic and Reconstructive Surgery,Laryngology/Voice and Swallowing Disorders, and Otology/Neuro-otology.

Physicians within the Department also serve as full-time faculty of New York Medical College, Westchester Medical Center's academic affiliate. In addition to exploiting the most current diagnostic and treatment technologies, all physicians are devoted to excellence in teaching and research—ensuring that patients receive the most progressive and professional care available in the greater New York area.

All inpatient pediatric otolaryngology services are provided in Westchester Medical Center's state-of-the-art Maria Fareri Children's Hospital, which offers young patients a total healing environment in which parents can participate fully in their child's care and recovery.

OTOLARYNGOLOGY AND HEAD & NECK SURGERY

The Department of Otolaryngology and Head & Neck Surgery at Westchester Medical Center provides a comprehensive range of adult and pediatric clinical services, including:

- Head and Neck Surgery
- Thyroid/Parathyroid Surgery
- Head and Neck Cancer
- Skull Base Surgery
- Pediatric Otolaryngology
- Tonsillectomy and Adenoidectomy
- Ear Tube Placement
- Pediatric Airway Management
- Pediatric Sinus Surgery
- Pediatric Swallowing Disorders
- Congenital Tumors
- Endoscopic Sinus Surgery
- Sleep Apnea
- Surgery Facial Plastic and Reconstructive Surgery
- Nasal Surgery/Rhinoplasty
- Facelifts
- Eyelid/Brow Surgery
- Cosmetic Threadlift
- Scar Revision
- Facial Trauma
- Voice Disorders
- Laryngopharyngeal Reflux
- Fiberoptic Endoscopic Evaluation of Swallowing and Sensory Testing
- Video-stroboscopy
- Trans-nasal Esophagoscopy Otology and Neuro-otology
- Balance Function Center

Specialty offices conveniently located throughout Westchester and Putnam counties

For more information, go to www.worldclassmedicine.com

794

Sponsored Page

Yale Head and Neck Cancer Program

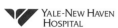 YALE-NEW HAVEN HOSPITAL

 Yale CANCER CENTER

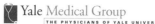 Yale Medical Group
THE PHYSICIANS OF YALE UNIVERSITY

20 York Street	333 Cedar Street	300 George Street, 6th Floor
New Haven, CT 06510	New Haven, CT 06520	New Haven, CT 06519
(203) 688-2000	1-866-YALECANCER	(203) 785-2140
www.ynhh.org	www.yalecancercenter.org	www.yalemedicalgroup.org

The Yale Head and Neck Cancer Program offers the most effective treatment options for diseases that affect the head and neck. Affiliated with Yale Cancer Center, the program is unique in Connecticut and combines the most advanced and comprehensive surgical and medical treatment approaches.

Led by **Clarence T. Sasaki, MD**, an internationally renowned head and neck cancer surgeon, the program is composed of an integrated team of specialists, including otolaryngologists, medical oncologists, plastic surgeons, neurosurgeons, dermatologists, radiation oncologists, head and neck radiologists, surgical pathologists and oral surgeons. All physicians are board-certified and fellowship-trained. The multidisciplinary nature of the program provides coordinated access to necessary physicians, streamlines the evaluation process and ensures optimal care in an efficient manner. New patients can usually be seen within 3 to 5 days.

Complementing the multi-specialty physicians and surgeons is a skilled team of rehabilitation specialists in speech, swallowing and hearing restoration, nutrition counseling, social services support and patient education.

The surgeons offer the latest advances in laser assisted endoscopic tumor resections and microvascular free tissue reconstructions. Emphasis is on organ-sparing. In select cases, the successful combination of brachytherapy, surgery and external beam radiation is available. Many clinical trials are also available for patients with special needs.

Patients benefit from specialized resources available at **Yale-New Haven Hospital**, such as the newest diagnostic imaging technologies, external beam radiation including IMRT, and gamma knife for select candidates. **The Yale-New Haven Gamma Knife Center** is the only dedicated stereotactic radiosurgical facility in Connecticut.

For more information or to make an appointment, please call **(203) 785-2593** or email **HNpatientadvocate@yale.edu.** Information is also available at www.yaleheadandneck.org.

Yale Medical Group is one of the largest academic multispecialty group practices in the United States. Comprised of the full-time faculty of the Yale School of Medicine, YMG physicians are leaders in their fields, dedicated to combining a compassionate, individual approach to patient care with the latest clinical and technologic developments.

Yale-New Haven Hospital is a 944-bed tertiary referral center, the primary teaching hospital for the Yale University School of Medicine, and the only hospital in Connecticut consistently recognized as one of America's Best Hospitals by US News & World Report.

Yale Cancer Center is one of 39 National Cancer Institute designated comprehensive cancer centers and the only one in southern New England.

Palliative Care

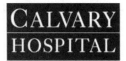

CALVARY HOSPITAL

*The Model for the Relief
of Cancer Pain and Symptoms
for Over a Century*

1740 Eastchester Road
Bronx, NY 10461
Tel: (718) 518-2300
www.calvaryhospital.org

Palliative Care Institute
Calvary's Teaching and Research Arm

Founded in 1985, to transmit, through research and education, Calvary's competence in the care of patients with advanced disease.

Each year, we train more than 800 medical students, residents and fellows in palliative care. This includes formalized palliative care observership rotations for residency and fellowship programs throughout the New York area, including Memorial Sloan-Kettering Cancer Center, Mount Sinai School of Medicine, and State University of New York Health Science Center at Brooklyn.

In 2004, the PCI established INSIDE CALVARY: COMPASSION AND COMPETENCE IN PALLIATIVE CARE, a national, three-day on-site program for health professionals.

A Model for Excellent Care
Calvary earned a reputation for skillful and compassionate control of patients' symptoms long before palliative and hospice care became popular disciplines.

In 2005, the National Cancer Institute (NCI) designated Calvary Hospital an "International Center for Training in Palliative Care." In April 2005, the NCI sponsored Robert Brescia, MD, Director of the PCI, and two Calvary nurses to visit Israel and Jordan to begin collaboration with the Middle East Cancer Consortium (MECC), with the aim of improving palliative care throughout the Middle East. In June 2005, health care professionals from Israel, Jordan, Egypt, Turkey, Cyprus, and the Palestinian Authority, sponsored by the NCI and MECC, came to Calvary for palliative care training. MECC professionals from the Middle East are scheduled to visit Calvary in fall of 2006.

Wound Care
The PCI directs Calvary Hospital's Center for Curative and Palliative Wound Care, dedicated to the treatment of complex, intractable wounds related to diabetes, cancer, peripheral vascular disease, and other disorders.

For information about our outstanding wound care, please call (718) 518-2577.

Research Initiatives
The PCI conducts research focusing on wound care, the psychological and emotional impact of terminal illness on patients and families, pain management, and ethical issues concerning end-of-life care.

INSIDE CALVARY: COMPASSION AND COMPETENCE IN PALLIATIVE CARE

A three-day on-site program offering direct patient/family observation and interaction in the actual treatment setting. INSIDE CALVARY is taught by staff from every discipline, including medicine, nursing, pastoral care, hospice/home care, wound care, family care, and bereavement.

Offers a unique teaching experience and unparalleled access to Calvary's palliative care team. In addition to didactic lectures, participants round with attending physicians, observe a patient admission work-up, and interact directly with patients/families. We believe INSIDE CALVARY is one of the nation's finest educational programs in palliative care.

**For information
and to register,
call (718) 518-2147.**

754

Parkinson's Disease

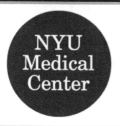

550 First Avenue (at 31st Street)
New York, NY 10016
Physician Referral: (888) 7-NYU-MED
(888-769-8633) www.nyumedicalcenter.org

PARKINSON'S DISEASE

PARKINSON'S TREATMENT AT NYU MEDICAL CENTER

To help patients and their families cope with the progressively debilitating symptoms of Parkinson's disease and essential tremor (a more common, and lesser known condition), the Rusk Institute of Rehabilitation Medicine at NYU Medical Center offers several non-drug interventions.

Physiatrists and physical and occupational therapists at Rusk Institute work intensively with patients, coaching them in techniques that can help patients manage day-to-day living. Vestibular rehabilitation is available for patients with balance disorders, and a specialized dysphagia program helps patients with swallowing disorders.

For many years, treatment options have been limited primarily to drug therapy, whose effectiveness can decrease over time and whose side effects can be significant. While there is still no cure, additional treatment options are now available. NYU Medical Center, a pioneer in the field of movement disorder surgery, has created The Center for the Study and Treatment of Movement Disorders, a multidisciplinary facility that offers patients with Parkinson's disease or essential tremor a number of state-of-the-art treatments. The core team that works collaboratively to provide these options comprises neurologists, neurosurgeons, and neurophysiologists.

Supplementing the range of traditional drug therapies, the Center offers several surgical interventions that reduce tremor and bradykinesia (slowness of movement). In addition to addressing the symptoms of Parkinson's disease, some of these surgeries can alleviate the side effects that patients experience after prolonged use of the drugs typically prescribed for the disease—side effects such as dyskinesias (uncontrollable movements), gait problems, and balance disorders.

Deep Brain Stimulation (DBS) is the preferred surgical procedure for Parkinson's disease, primarily because it is reversible and does virtually no damage to brain tissue. In addition, it can be used to treat symptoms other than tremor. In DBS, the neurosurgeon implants twin electrodes deep within the brain, aided by computer guidance and 3-D physiological mapping.

Each electrode is connected to a thin, insulated wire that is threaded under the skin from the top of the skull to the chest. That wire leads to a battery-operated pulse generator (like that used in a pacemaker), which is implanted beneath the skin in the chest. The electrodes send mild electrical pulses to stimulate the brain and block the signals that cause tremor. Using a hand-held magnet, the patient can turn the stimulator on or off.

The technology and expertise is available for other neurosurgical procedures, too (including stereotactic thalamotomy and stereotactic pallidotomy), but in most cases, DBS is the preferred procedure, for both safety reasons and the ability to make post-surgical adjustments.

NYU MEDICAL CENTER

The surgeons at the Center for the Study and Treatment of Movement Disorders are members of the Department of Neurosurgery at NYU Medical Center, a department that has long been recognized as one of the finest in the world. At the forefront of surgical technology and innovation, its surgeons are internationally renowned leaders in their specialty areas. Each is also a faculty member at the NYU School of Medicine, a leading site for groundbreaking research in neuroscience. The close, collaborative relationship between researchers and clinicians brings to patients an unsurpassed level of clinical excellence.

801

Pediatrics

THE GORYEB CHILDREN'S HOSPITAL

Morristown Memorial Hospital • Overlook Hospital

THE PASSION TO LEAD

Goryeb Children's Hospital • Atlantic Neuroscience Institute
Carol G. Simon Cancer Center/The Cancer Center at Overlook Hospital
Gagnon Heart Hospital • Atlantic Rehabilitation Institute

P.O. Box 1905, Morristown, NJ 07962 • 1-800-247-9580 • atlantichealth.org

Nationally-Recognized Pediatric Care

Your child will benefit from the expertise of nationally-recognized, board certified pediatric specialists who are actively involved in clinical research, enabling them to offer your child the newest medications, treatments and technologies. Experts at the Goryeb Children's Hospital at Morristown Memorial and the Goryeb Inpatient Pediatric Unit at Overlook Hospital partner with you and your child's physicians to manage emergencies, chronic conditions and serious illnesses. Both facilities feature a family-focused, child-friendly environment. In addition, the Morristown campus includes a pediatric intensive care unit and more.

Services available through the Goryeb Children's Hospital include:

- **Newborn nursery** – Teaching families in the care of their newly born infant is central to our mission.

- **Inpatient pediatrics** – The Inpatient Pediatric Unit provides direct care and consultative services for infants, children and adolescents who require inpatient care.

- **Family Health Center and HealthStart Clinic** – These two sites provide academic, evidence-based, primary care to children of Morris and Union counties in New Jersey who otherwise would lack access to health care services.

- **Madison Pediatrics** – Madison Pediatrics provides routine health supervision, acute and chronic illness care to infants, children and adolescents and serves as a training site for first year pediatric residents in a private practice setting.

- **Community Pediatrics** – Community Pediatrics provides medical services and educational programs for local schools, daycare centers and businesses. The program has also established close-working relationships with the local and state organizations involved in the prevention of child abuse and neglect.

- **Pediatric Critical Care** – The Pediatric Intensive Care Unit (PICU) treats children, from infants to adolescents, for post-operative management after major surgical procedures including neurosurgical, trauma, and orthopedic procedures. The PICU staff is made up of physicians who are board-certified in pediatric critical care as well as experienced caregivers from various specialties to provide your child with the best possible care.

- **Pediatric Infectious Diseases** – We provide comprehensive and specialized medical care to infants, children and adolescents with acute and chronic infectious diseases such as lyme disease, meningitis and viral infections.

- **Respiratory Center for Children** – The Respiratory Center for Children offers expertise in the evaluation of illnesses such as respiratory disorders related to neuromuscular and neurological disease, exercise limitations, lung immunology, and birth defects.

- **Pediatric Neurosurgery** – Pediatric Neurosurgery services are provided through Atlantic Neurosurgical Specialists (ANS). They offer surgical care for hydrocephalus, pediatric brain tumors, brain and spinal cord injuries and developmental and congenital anomalies in infants, children and adolescents. ANS's attending neurosurgeons provide pediatric care at the Goryeb Children's Hospital at Morristown Memorial and Overlook Hospital.

Sponsored Page

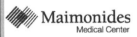

Maimonides Medical Center
MAIMONIDES INFANTS & CHILDREN'S HOSPITAL

4802 Tenth Avenue • Brooklyn, New York 11219
Phone: (718) 283-7500
www.maimonidesmed.org

The Maimonides Infants & Children's Hospital is a NACHRI-certified children's hospital-within-a-hospital. Offering over 30 sub-specialty divisions as well as primary care, the Pediatrics program is unrivaled in the region and serves one of the largest pediatric populations in the nation.

Steven Shelov, MD, head of the Children's Hospital and author of several bestselling books on childrearing, has built a family-centered pediatrics program in a state-of-the-art medical environment, where babies, children and adolescents receive the best and most appropriate care. For most children, this involves preventing illness and promoting healthy growth. For those whose problems are more complicated, Maimonides specialists can treat every manner of childhood disorder no matter how rare or complex. The level and quality of critical care provided is evidenced by the demand for the Maimonides Pediatric Transport Program, through which critically ill children from other hospitals are transferred to Maimonides.

In recognition of its excellence in obstetrics and pediatrics, Maimonides was designated a Regional Perinatal Center by the New York State Department of Health.

Pediatric Specialties include:

Allergy
Cardiology
Critical Care Medicine
Emergency Medicine
Gastroenterology
Hematology/Oncology
Infectious Disease
Nephrology
Ophthalmology
Otolaryngology
Pulmonology
Surgery

Behavioral
& Developmental Pediatrics
Dentistry and Dental Surgery
Endocrinology
Genetics
Immunology
Neonatology
Neurology
Orthopaedic Surgery
Psychiatry/Psychology
Rheumatology
Urology

Physicians at Maimonides are among the eight percent in the US who use computers to enter patient orders, thereby reducing the risk of errors, increasing efficiency, and speeding the healing process. Maimonides has appeared on the American Hospital Association's "Most Wired" and "Most Wireless" lists more often than any other healthcare institution in the metropolitan area. Advanced technology allows our doctors to focus more attention on caring for their patients.

Maimonides Medical Center – passionate about medicine, compassionate about people.

NewYork-Presbyterian
The University Hospital of Columbia and Cornell

Morgan Stanley
Children's Hospital of NewYork-Presbyterian
Columbia University Medical Center

3959 Broadway
New York, NY 10032

Phyllis and David
Komansky Center for Children's Health
NewYork-Presbyterian Hospital/Weill Cornell Medical Center

525 East 68th Street
New York, NY 10021

Sponsorship:	Voluntary Not-for-Profit
Beds:	387
Accreditation:	Joint Commission on Accreditation of Healthcare Organizations (JCAHO)

OVERVIEW:

NewYork-Presbyterian brings together the outstanding pediatric services and resources of the Morgan Stanley Children's Hospital and the Komansky Center for Children's Health to create one of the largest, most comprehensive children's hospital in the world.

With more than 1,000 pediatricians and medical and surgical subspecialists on staff, and teams of specially trained pediatric health professionals, NewYork-Presbyterian provides the highest level of care from infancy to adolescence. The Hospital's expertise in addressing simple and complex medical conditions and the psychological and emotional issues that accompany them is unparalleled. The Hospital offers:

- Adolescent Medicine
- Allergy
- Anesthesiology and Pain Management
- Cardiology
- Child Development and Behavioral Medicine
- Critical Care
- Dermatology
- Diabetes and Endocrinology
- Gastroenterology
- Genetics
- Hematology
- Infectious Disease
- Neonatal-Perinatal Medicine
- Nephrology
- Neurology
- Neurosurgery
- Oncology
- Primary Care
- Psychiatry and Mental Health
- Rheumatology
- Laboratory and Radiology Diagnostic Services
- Pediatric Emergency Care in emergency medicine, burn and trauma
- Surgical Services in cardiac, dental, oral and maxillofacial, general neurosurgery, ophthalmology, orthopedics, otolaryngology, plastic surgery, transplantation and urology

Physician Referral: For a physician referral or for information, call **1-800-245-KIDS** (1-800-245-5437) or visit our website at **www.childrensnyp.org**

CHILDREN'S HOSPITAL HIGHLIGHTS INCLUDE:

- One of the country's largest and most successful pediatric cardiology and cardiac surgery programs.

- Only provider in the region to offer three major transplant surgeries – heart, liver and kidney.

- One of three Level 1-designated Pediatric Trauma Centers in New York State and only one in New York City.

- Nationally recognized pediatric oncologists. Bone marrow transplantation program is one of the largest in the nation.

- Sophisticated neonatal intensive care that sets standards nationwide.

- Referral center and regional resource for hospitals needing expertise of our pediatric intensive care units. Seriously ill children can be transferred to NewYork-Presbyterian through the Pediatric Critical Care Transport Program.

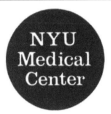

NYU Medical Center

550 First Avenue (at 31st Street)
New York, NY 10016
Physician Referral:
(888)7-NYU-MED (888-769-8633)
www.nyumc.org

NYU CHILDREN'S HEALTH

NYU Medical Center's Children's Health Team is comprised of some of the best clinical specialists in the country. Among the programs they offer are:

Apnea/SIDS Program –identifying and treating of infants with apnea and infants who are are at increased risk for SIDS

Center for Child and Adolescent Sports Medicine – developmentally sensitive and comprehensive evaluation and treatment of sports-related injuries in children

NYU- Hospital for Joint Diseases Center for Children – holistic outpatient treatment of children and adolescents with a wide range of orthopaedic and neurological conditions

Child Study Center – advancing the field of mental health for children and adolescents through evidence-based practice, science, and education

Cochlear Implant Program – restoring hearing to profoundly deaf children

Craniofacial Program – treating facial deformities discovered at birth
Epilepsy Program – state-of-the-art evaluation and multidisciplinary treatment of children with epilepsy

Familial Dysautonomia Program – the only center in the U.S. providing care to individuals affected with this genetic disorder

Hassenfeld Children's Center – comprehensive outpatient care for children with cancer and blood disorders

Headache Center – thorough diagnosis and evaluation to help pediatric patients manage frequency and severity of chronic headaches

Hemangiomas and Vascular Malformation Program – multidisciplinary care for children with hemangiomas and vascular malformations

Orthopaedic Immediate Care Center at the Hospital for Joint Diseases– evaluation and treatment of urgent pediatric and adult orthopaedic problems, such as fractures

Pediatric Rehabilitation Service – multi-disciplinary pediatric rehabilitation for a variety of congenital and acquired disabilities on an inpatient and outpatient basis

Preschool and Early Intervention Program – individualized educational and early intervention services for children under five

Stem Cell Transplant Program – Using stem cell transplant to treat brain and other solid tumors, under the auspices of the Hassenfeld Children's Center, which was the site of much of the original stem cell harvest and transplantation research.

NYU MEDICAL CENTER

Children's Services at NYU Medical Center provides comprehensive, family-centered care for children with all types of conditions. Specialized care for children are provided in the following areas:

* Adolescent Medicine
* Allergy
* Anesthesia
* Cardiology
* Cardio-Vascular Surgery
* Critical Care
* Dermatology
* Developmental Pediatrics
* Dysautonomia
* Emergency Medicine
* Endocrinology
* Epilepsy
* Gastroenterology
* Genetics
* Hematology
* Infectious Diseases
* Neonatology
* Nephrology
* Neurology
* Neurosurgery
* Oncology
* Ophthamology
* Orthopaedics
* Otolaryngology
* Pediatrics
* Plastic Surgery/Cranial Facial
* Psychiatry
* Pulmonology
* Radiology
* Rehabilitation Medicine
* Rheumatology
* Surgery
* Urology

706

Sponsored Page

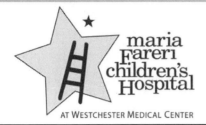

WESTCHESTER MEDICAL CENTER

Valhalla Campus
Valhalla, NY 10595
Tel. 1-866-WMC-PEDS
http://www.worldclassmedicine.com

A NEW STANDARD FOR CHILDREN'S HOSPITALS

Maria Fareri Children's Hospital at Westchester Medical Center continues to set the standard for children's hospitals in our region. The 118-bed hospital—located in a state-of-the-art child- and family-friendly building—provides the highest level of pediatric care in all medical and surgical specialties, with more than 300 professionals dedicated specifically to children's healthcare. Each year, over 25,000 infants and children benefit from the specialized staff and treatment available at Maria Fareri Children's Hospital, a member of the National Association of Children's Hospitals.

As part of a large university medical center, Maria Fareri Children's Hospital is the site for the region's only Pediatric Intensive Care and Level IV Regional Perinatal Centers, the region's only Cystic Fibrosis Center, Children's Cancer Center, Pediatric Bone Marrow Transplant Program, Fetal Medicine Program and Children's Ambulatory Surgery Center. Maria Fareri Children's Hospital also houses the only Pediatric Trauma Center in the region. The Children's Hospital has the region's largest pediatric cardiology and only pediatric cardiac surgery programs, and offers pediatric neurosurgery, pediatric orthopedics and pediatric corneal, kidney and liver transplant, among other pediatric specialty programs. Maria Fareri Children's Hospital is one of the few infant metabolic disease centers in New York State.

A model facility for family-centered care, this 250,000 square-foot facility provides a total healing environment in which parents can participate fully in their child's care and recovery. The Hospital includes dedicated pediatric operating rooms and a pediatric emergency department and trauma center. Nearly all rooms are single occupancy and designed to provide a non-threatening environment with ample room for parents to spend the night with their child. A Ronald McDonald Suite offers additional comfort for parents' extended stay. A certified Child Life program coordinates numerous support services to ease the burden of hospitalization for children and their families.

Maria Fareri Children's Hospital faculty are funded by the National Institutes of Health, the American Lung Association, the March of Dimes and other agencies to study pediatric cardiovascular disease, kidney disease, cystic fibrosis, asthma, prematurity and other life-threatening problems. Doctors also participate in the Rotarian Gift of Life heart surgery program, saving the lives of children from around the world.

A network of 11 offices in the lower Hudson Valley, Connecticut and the Bronx that are linked to the Children's Hospital allows children's specialty medical care to be provided close to home.

Maria Fareri Children's Hospital at Westchester Medical Center

Maria Fareri Children's Hospital at Westchester Medical Center provides the highest level of pediatric care in all medical and surgical specialties, including:

- Cardiology/Cardiothoracic Surgery
- Critical Care Medicine
- Developmental Pediatrics
- Emergency Medicine
- Endocrinology
- Fetal Medicine Program
- Gastroenterology
- General Pediatrics
- Hematology/Oncology
- Immunology/Infectious Diseases
- Medical Genetics/Metabolic Diseases
- Neonatology
- Nephrology
- Neurology
- Neurosurgery
- Orthopaedics
- Pediatric Gynecology
- Plastic Surgery
- Psychology
- Pulmonology/Allergy
- Rheumatology
- Sleep Center
- Sports Medicine Program
- Surgery
- Urology

Call 1-866-WMC-PEDS for a physician referral or a specialty office near you.

783

Yale Pediatric Surgery

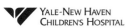

YALE-NEW HAVEN
CHILDREN'S HOSPITAL

20 York Street
New Haven, CT 06510
(203) 688-2000

www.ynhh.org

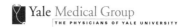

300 George Street, 6th Floor
New Haven, CT 06519
(203) 785-2140

www.yalemedicalgroup.org

Yale Pediatric Surgery is a group of world-class surgeons who treat congenital conditions, benign and malignant disease, traumatic injury, and other surgically correctable disorders in newborns, babies, children and adolescents. Surgeons use both minimally invasive and traditional approaches to treat the full range of general, abdominal, thoracic, head and neck, pelvic and soft tissue conditions. Each is nationally recognized for his or her clinical expertise and reputation for innovative and critical thinking in pediatric surgery.

All surgical procedures—whether inpatient, outpatient or diagnostic—are performed at the **Pediatric Surgery Center** of the **Yale-New Haven Children's Hospital**, which serves the region as a referral center. The facility offers dedicated pediatric operating rooms where patients are cared for by specialty-trained pediatric anesthesiologists. Preoperative tours provide parents and children with an invaluable orientation to pediatric anesthesia services, the operating suite and the post-anesthesia care unit.

The surgeons at the Children's Hospital direct the only Level 1 Pediatric Trauma Center in the state, which offers specialized care of injured children.

Appropriate referrals to Yale Pediatric Surgery include:
- Neonatal Surgery and Repair of Major Congenital Anomalies
- Tumors, Masses and Cysts of the Neck, Chest, Abdomen, Pelvis and Extremities
- ECMO – Heart Lung Bypass for Neonates and Children
- Advanced Minimally Invasive Surgery for Infants and Children
- Appendicitis and Other Common Surgical Problems of the Abdomen
- Thoracic Surgery In Children
- Hernias, Hydroceles and Undescended Testicles
- Skin and Soft Tissue Masses and Lesions

Referral from a primary care doctor is welcome but not required. Patients are seen within a week of the initial contact. To make an appointment please call **(203) 785-2701**.

For more information please visit **www.yalepediatricsurgery.org**.

Yale Medical Group is one of the largest academic multispecialty group practices in the United States. Comprised of the full-time faculty of the Yale School of Medicine, YMG physicians are leaders in their fields, dedicated to combining a compassionate, individual approach to patient care with the latest clinical and technologic developments.

Yale-New Haven Children's Hospital: With 201 beds, the Yale-New Haven Children's Hospital offers the region's largest and most comprehensive maternity and pediatric services, a 24-hour pediatric surgery center, a pediatric specialty center and a Level 1 pediatric trauma center.

Sponsored Page

Physical Medicine & Rehabilitation

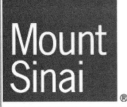

THE MOUNT SINAI MEDICAL CENTER
REHABILITATION MEDICINE

One Gustave L. Levy Place (Fifth Avenue and 100th Street)
New York, NY 10029-6574
Physician Referral: 1-800-MD-SINAI (636-4624)
www.mountsinai.org

The Department of Rehabilitation Medicine at The Mount Sinai Medical Center is a center of excellence in the delivery of complete care for people with disabilities. A wide range of comprehensive patient care services are available for individuals with spinal cord injuries, brain injuries, and a variety of neuromuscular, musculoskeletal, and chronic conditions. We are CARF-accredited for our inpatient spinal cord and brain injury programs, the only such accredited programs in New York State, as well as for our comprehensive rehabilitation medicine program.

Our Team-Oriented Approach is pivotal to successful rehabilitation. The interdisciplinary team approach at Mount Sinai takes advantage of each discipline's expertise to provide quality coordinated care. Our experienced professionals evaluate each patient and meet regularly to develop and implement individualized treatment plans in partnership with patients and their families. Our goal is to make each individual with a disability maximally self-sufficient and mobile and able to return to community life.

The Mount Sinai Rehabilitation Center team is led by Kristjan T. Ragnarsson, MD, whose leadership and innovative approach to patient care has had a major impact in the field of Rehabilitation Medicine. The Center includes physicians, primary rehab nurses, nurse practitioners, and professional staff in physical therapy, occupational therapy, speech therapy, nutrition, social work, psychology, therapeutic recreation, and vocational counseling. Special rehabilitation medicine programs include:

• **The Spinal Cord Injury (SCI) Rehabilitation Program** provides comprehensive care to individuals with spinal cord injuries. This includes a full range of innovative medical and rehabilitation services. For example, our "Do It" program is a unique outpatient program that facilitates community integration.

• **The Brain Injury (BI) Rehabilitation Program** provides comprehensive care to individuals with brain injuries. It is well recognized that the treatment of individuals with cognitive and behavioral challenges is critical to community integration. Our program contains specialists uniquely qualified to meet these challenges.

• **Sports Therapy Center** is a comprehensive outpatient physical and occupational therapy facility offering individualized treatments for individuals with a variety of musculoskeletal conditions. It is conveniently located in midtown Manhattan.

THE MOUNT SINAI MEDICAL CENTER

Mount Sinai's Department of Rehabilitation Medicine is consistently ranked among the top rehabilitation centers in the nation by *US News & World Report*; one of 16 programs designated by the National Institute on Disability and Rehabilitation Research (NIDRR) as a Model System of Care for Spinal Cord Injury; one of 16 programs designated by the NIDRR as a Model System of Care for Traumatic Brain Injury; the only Research and Training Center for Traumatic Brain Intervention; the only Model System for Spinal Cord Injury in New York State; the only Model System for Traumatic Brain Injury in New York State; and one of only a few programs in the country designated by NIDRR as Model Systems of Care in Spinal Cord Injury, Traumatic Brain Injury, and as a Research and Training Center.

618

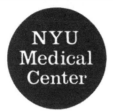

NYU Medical Center

550 First Avenue (at 31st Street)
New York, NY 10016
Physician Referral:
(888)7-NYU-MED (888-769-8633)
www.nyumc.org

Physical Medicine and Rehabilitation

Founded by Dr. Howard A. Rusk in 1948, the Rusk Institute of Rehabilitation Medicine is the world's first and one of the largest university centers for the treatment of adults and children with disabilities. Every year since 1989 when *U.S. News & World Report* initiated its hospital rankings, the Rusk Institute has ranked the number one rehabilitation center in New York and one of the top ten in the nation. It treats adults and children with neurologic, orthopaedic, and a wide variety of physical disabilities on both an inpatient and outpatient basis.

These include:

Aphasia	Amputation	Arthritis
Back Pain	Brain Injury	Brain Tumor Related Disabilities
Cardiac Dysfunction	Cerebral Palsy	Hand Disabilities
Hip and Lower Extremity Fractures	Joint Replacements	Lymphedema
	Multiple Sclerosis	Neurological Disorders
Neuromuscular Diseases	Orthopaedic Surgery	Osteoporosis
Pain (acute and chronic)	Parkinson's Disease	Pediatric Rehabilitation
Pulmonary Diseases (Asthma, Bronchitis, Emphysema)	Rhizotomy	Scoliosis
Spasticity	Spina Bifida	Spinal Cord Injury
Sports Injuries	Stroke	Swallowing Disorders
Traumatic Injuries	Urinary Incontinence	Vestibular (balance) Disorders

The Hospital for Joint Diseases Rehabilitation Services Programs provide comprehensive inpatient (72 beds) rehabilitation care for ortho-rehab and neuro-rehab patients. Both programs are CARF (Commission on the Accreditation of Rehabilitation Facilities) accredited. There are five outpatient centers to serve patients as well:

Sports Therapy & Rehabilitation Center, 614 Second Avenue -Suite 26; Orthopaedic and Sports Therapy Center, 305 Second Avenue Outpatient Physical and Occupational Center at Hospital for Joint Diseases, Fourth Floor, Occupational and Industrial Orthopaedic Center (OIOC), The Center for Pediatric Rehab and Pediatric Medicine at the Hospital for Joint Diseases.

NYU MEDICAL CENTER

The relationship between Rusk Institute and other clinical and research units within the Medical Center—including Tisch Hospital, a 726-bed acute-care facility—contributes to an environment which provides the optimal rehabilitation setting for patients. Should the need arise, patients at Rusk Institute have immediate access to Tisch Hospital's superb teritary-care faciltiites, with its full range of medical and surgical services. Physicians at Rusk also enjoy a close collaboration with the specialists from Hospital for Joint Diseases, a 72-bed facility dedicated to the treatment of orthopaedic, rheumatologic, and neurologic disorders.

717

Sponsored Page

Plastic Surgery

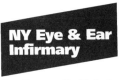

NY Eye & Ear Infirmary

Continuum Health Partners, Inc.

THE NEW YORK EYE AND EAR INFIRMARY

310 East 14th Street
New York, New York 10003
Tel. 212.979.4000   Fax. 212.228.0664
http://www.nyee.edu

PROVIDING EXCEPTIONAL CARE

The Department of Plastic & Reconstructive Surgery is one of the region's most comprehensive centers for surgery which restores the body and spirit. More than 1,500 procedures a year are performed here, and 50 of the most noted board-certified plastic surgeons located throughout New York City and tri-state area comprise the attending medical staff.

IN A HIGHLY SPECIALIZED SETTING

As a specialty hospital, the Infirmary is uniquely qualified to handle the most complicated cases. It serves as a nationwide referral center with a commitment to teaching, research, and high-technology based patient care. Highly experienced staff using state-of-the-art instrumentation have made the Infirmary's 17 operating rooms a national benchmark in efficiency. In addition, private premium patient accommodations are available to assure that the hospital experience is as comfortable and convenient as possible.

FOR PATIENTS OF ALL AGES

Clinical innovations are improving people's lives. A unique procedure to transfer tissue is performed by microvascular surgeons to repair or reattach missing digits and thumbs. Infirmary surgeons perform miracles on children born with cleft lip and palate malformation. Those seeking elective cosmetic surgery are offered an array of options including endoscopic face lifts, a refinement of the facial plastic operation that uses straw-like telescopic instrument inserted through small incisions to smooth wrinkles from "beneath" the skin; no-incision eyelid plasty; and liposuction for reshaping body contours.

Plastic Surgery Clinical Services

Facial plasty

Eyelid plastic operations

Nasal plastic operations

Breast augmentation
Breast reduction procedures
and suspension

Liposuction

Abdominoplasty

Facial resurfacing and
dermabrasion

Botox

About
The New York Eye
and Ear Infirmary

Founded in 1820, it is the nation's oldest, continuously operating specialty hospital Throughout its history, the Infirmary has led clinical advances and research in vision, hearing, speech and restoration of the physical appearance.

Physician Referral
1.800.449.HOPE (4673)

Psychiatry/Behavioral Health

Mount Sinai ®

THE MOUNT SINAI MEDICAL CENTER
PSYCHIATRY

One Gustave L. Levy Place (Fifth Avenue and 100th Street)
New York, NY 10029-6574
Physician Referral: 1-800-MD-SINAI (636-4624)
www.mountsinai.org

The Psychiatry Department at Mount Sinai serves infants, children, adolescents, adults, and seniors, offering mental health evaluation and treatment for such conditions as: autism, Attention-Deficit Hyperactivity Disorder (ADHD), behavioral disorders, care of children after trauma, schizophrenia, Alzheimer's disease, mood and anxiety disorders, Obsessive-Compulsive Disorder (OCD), substance abuse (with co-occurring disorders), Posttraumatic Stress Disorder (PTSD), eating disorders, reproductive psychiatry, impulse control disorders, and personality disorders.

CLINICAL SERVICES
We offer the full range of diagnostic and treatment services, including psychotherapy, psychopharmacology, crisis intervention and emergency services, electroconvulsive therapy (ECT), psychological and neuropsychological testing, and a new clinical initiative that focuses on the management of difficult clinical cases. The Department of Psychiatry has also been deeply engaged in Mount Sinai's World Trade Center Worker and Volunteer Screening Program, which has screened thousands of people for 9/11-related physical and mental health problems. We also offer special programs for Holocaust survivors and children of Holocaust survivors.

NEW AND EXPANDING PROGRAMS
We have recently created a new Center for Eating and Weight Disorders that serves adults and children, offering innovative, proven-effective treatment for anorexia nervosa, bulimia nervosa, binge eating disorder, and obesity. In parallel, our Mood and Anxiety Disorders Program is being expanded, applying brain imaging techniques to aid in diagnosis, and offering the latest treatment strategies for patients who suffer from panic attacks, generalized anxiety disorder, social phobia, depression, and related conditions.

MADISON EAST
Mount Sinai's Department of Psychiatry operates Madison East, a secure, eight-bed, amenities unit within the Hospital for patients seeking meaningful recovery. Under the leadership of world-renowned co-occurring disorders specialist Dr. Harris B. Stratyner, Madison East emphasizes his technique of "Carefrontation" by utilizing the latest motivational engagement skills in an environment of respect and dignity which stresses responsibility for dealing with one's addiction or mental health condition.

With experienced addiction professionals and medical management not available at other non-hospital rehabilitation programs, Madison East serves patients in need of medical and psychological stabilization before proceeding further in their continuum of care; patients who have completed rehabilitation treatment or are already in recovery, but yet remain at risk; and patients who experience chronic relapses and require further neuropsychological testing and medical consultations.

All rooms in Madison East have private baths with hotel-quality linens and accessories. The unit includes a tastefully furnished dining room, common areas that encourage scalability and allow for privacy, as well as a 24-hour concierge. Other amenity services include gourmet meals, a personal trainer, yoga instruction, and supervised exercise facilities. In addition to telephone service, television and DVD players, the unit offers business services such as Internet and fax connections.

Translating Knowledge into New Solutions

Psychiatry at Mount Sinai is at the very forefront of unlocking the interactions between biological processes and the myriad states of the human mind. At our Conte Center for the Neuroscience of Mental Disorders, for example, we are studying schizophrenia—pursuing breakthrough insights into the underlying neurobiology of the disease and applying cutting-edge technology to convert those insights into new patient solutions.

Among our other major research programs in Psychiatry include the Alzheimer's Disease Research Center, which conducts both basic science and clinical research; and the Seaver and New York Autism Center of Excellence, which is dedicated to unraveling the biological components of this developmental disorder and to developing effective new therapies.

In shedding important new light on mental illness, psychiatrists at Mount Sinai are frequently able to offer the treatments of tomorrow—therapies that will not be widely available for several years.

616

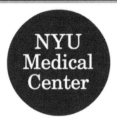

NYU Medical Center

550 First Avenue (at 31st Street)
New York, NY 10016
Physician Referral: (888) 7-NYU-MED
(888-769-8633) www.nyumedicalcenter.org

BEHAVIORAL HEALTH

TREATING MENTAL ILLNESS AND EMOTIONAL DISORDERS

The Behavioral Health Program at NYU Medical Center offers the most up-to-date, scientifically validated treatments available for a wide range of disorders, including: stress/anxiety, schizophrenia, depression, shyness, insomnia, low self-esteem, women's issues, sexual difficulties, panic attacks and phobias, manic-depression, obsessions and compulsions, and attention deficit/hyperactivity disorder.

The Program serves its patients through a variety of approaches, including career counseling, assertiveness training, marital/couples counseling, and individual, group, or family therapy.

BEHAVIORAL HEALTH AT NYU COMPRISES THREE COMPONENTS:

• A 22 bed inpatient unit services an adult population including a Young Adult Program. The service combines comprehensive diagnostic assessment and treatment including psychopharma-cology, neuropsychology, psychotherapies, and electroconvulsive therapy. A multidisciplinary team approach provides a continuum of behavioral and therapeutic modalities.

• The Outpatient Psychiatry Program provides expert yet affordable treatment to individuals and families. In conjunction with the renowned faculty of the Department of Psychiatry, residents evaluate each individual and recommend a treatment plan. Treatment options include psychotherapy, medication, or a combination of the two. Neuropsychological testing and treatment attending physicians are also available.

• The Program in Human Sexuality addresses a wide spectrum of sexual disorders, such as erectile disorder, premature ejaculation, male orgasmic disorder, female orgasmic and arousal disorders, and sexual incompatibility between partners, among other problems. In addition to patient care, Behavioral Health oversees a Clinical Research Service, dedicated to enhancing the understanding of the diagnosis, pathophysiology, and treatment of psychiatric illness. With an emphasis on mood and anxiety disorders, the Service includes phases two and three clinical trials, larger multi-center clinical studies, and small, pilot exploratory treatment trials.

PEACE OF MIND

At NYU Medical Center, scientific innovation goes hand in hand with patient care. Our physician-scientists continue to lead the way in the burgeoning field of psychopharmacology. With the rapid pace of scientific discovery at NYU, people with mood disorders and their families stand to reap the benefits of medical research sooner rather than later. A number of clinical studies are currently under way to test new treatments for depression and bipolar disorder, with potentially lifealtering results for the millions who suffer from these debilitating mental illnesses.

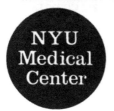

NYU Medical Center

550 First Avenue (at 31st Street)
New York, NY 10016
Physician Referral:
(888)7-NYU-MED (888-769-8633)
www.nyumc.org

PSYCHIATRY

In close collaboration with the NYU School of Medicine, which has one of thev largest and most distinguished psychiatry faculties in the United States, the NYU Medical Center Department of Psychiatry offers these special services:

Behavioral Health Program - A full complement of inpatient and outpatient psychiatric services

Silberstein Aging and Dementia Research Center - home to a 30-year longitudinal study of Alzheimer's disease with comprehensive psychosocial support for patients and caregivers

BRAIN STIMULATION SERVICES

Child Study Center - the first multi-specialty program in the New York area to offer complete child and adolescent psychiatric care fully integrated with scientific research and education. The NYU Child Study Center is home to several comprehensive programs including:

• Adolescent & Child Psychiatry Program
• Alcoholism and Drug Abuse Program
• Anxiety and Affective Disorders Service
• Attention Deficit Hyperactivity Disorder Program
• Family Studies Program
• Furman Diagnostic Service
• Human Sexuality and Sex Therapy
• Infancy and Early Childhood Development Program
• Institute for Children at Risk
• Institute for Learning and Academic Achievement
• NYU Summer Program for Kids with ADHD
• ParentCorps
• Parenting Institute
• Sex Therapy Clinic
• Young Adult Inpatient Program

The NYU Child Study Center's premiere clinicians implement the knowledge gained from research, resulting in care that incorporates the most up-to-dateinformation about the causes, symptoms, and treatments of mental disorders. They are an important part of NYU Child Study Center's enriched environment for scientific research into the risks and causes of childhood mental disorders.

The NYU Child Study Center's educational outreach programs teach thousands of parents, educators, pediatricians and other mental health professionals about normal child development and how to promptly recognize and intervene when achild needs help.

NYU MEDICAL CENTER

NYU Medical Center is a national training center for mental health professionals, offering a fully-accredited graduate program whose goal is to train and prepare the next generation of mental health professionals to meet the demands of a complex and expanding field and to translate research into advanced clinical care and effective treatments.

Committed to patient care, research, and training, the Department of Psychiatry at NYU Medical Center is home to some of the nation's most respected clinical psychiatrists and psychologists, with specialties in psychoanalysis, psychopharmacology, behavioral therapy, child psychiatry, geriatric psychiatry, neuropsychiatry, and positron emission tomography.

Physician Referral
(888) 7-NYU-MED
(888-769-8633)
www.nyumc.org

718

Behavioral Health Center
Westchester Medical Center

WESTCHESTER MEDICAL CENTER

Valhalla Campus
Valhalla, NY 10595
(914) 493-7282
http://www.worldclassmedicine.com

OVERVIEW

The Behavioral Health Center at Westchester Medical Center has been a leading provider of comprehensive Behavioral Health services since 1929. Located in a free-standing facility, the Behavioral Health Center offers a full continuum of inpatient, outpatient, community and emergency care for individuals, families, and concerned friends from toddlers to seniors. World-class medical services by Westchester Medical Center, combined with strong clinical leadership from the Department of Psychiatry at New York Medical College, keep the Behavioral Health Center at the forefront of meeting the needs of those afflicted or affected by mental illness.

Unique features of the Behavioral Health Center include the Comprehensive Psychiatric Emergency Program. This 24-hour-a-day, 365-day-a-year program consists of Mobile Crisis Teams dispatched from three service sites in Westchester County, six 72-hour observation beds, the only free-standing psychiatric emergency room between New York City and Albany, and a variety of brief treatment options for those in crisis. The Behavioral Health Center provides consultation-liason services for all patients, adult and child, who are admitted to Westchester Medical Center and its Maria Fareri Children's Hospital. The consultations are also available to families struggling to cope with the serious illness of a loved one.

The Behavioral Health Center continues its 75-year tradition of serving children and adolescents with two separate units in addition to three adult care units consisting of an acute stabilization wing and a unit for patients with combined psychiatric and medical problems. Extensive outpatient programming exists for adults, children and adolescents with expertise in treating those experiencing anxiety, or stress, difficulty coping at home or on the job, or because of medical illness such as cancer, heart disease or stroke. Specialty programming also exists for seniors, Spanish speaking individuals, gays and lesbians, families and college-age persons.

BEHAVIORAL HEALTH CENTER AT WESTCHESTER MEDICAL CENTER

For over 70 years, the Behavioral Health Center at Westchester Medical Center has been providing the highest quality care to adults, children and adolescents in times of crisis. The Behavioral Health Center offers a full array of treatment programs and services, including:

• Comprehensive Psychiatric Emergency Program (CPEP)

• Adult & Child Outpatient Treatment

• Adolescent Treatment for Emotional and Drug or Alcohol Problems

• Community Outreach & Treatment

• Inpatient Services for Adults and Children— including an Acute ICU

785

Sponsored Page

Pulmonology

THE MOUNT SINAI MEDICAL CENTER
PULMONARY MEDICINE

One Gustave L. Levy Place (Fifth Avenue and 100th Street)
New York, NY 10029-6574
Physician Referral: 1-800-MD-SINAI (636-4624)
www.mountsinai.org

Patients at Mount Sinai have access to a number of special programs and services designed by our specialists in Pulmonary Medicine, including:

- *Asthma Program*, which uses a multidisciplinary team approach, focusing on patient education and skill-building to foster self management;
- *Chronic Obstructive Pulmonary Disease (COPD) Program*, offering —for one of the nation's most underdiagnosed conditions—a coordinated approach of exercise, treatment, and education that improves quality of life and clinical outlook;
- *Critical Care Medicine Program*, featuring state-of-the-art medical intensive care and respiratory care units;
- *Interventional Pulmonary Service*, which performs diagnostic and therapeutic procedures for patients with advanced pulmonary diseases;
- *Lung Transplant Program,* for patients with advanced lung disease that has progressed despite optimal medical therapy;
- *Occupational Lung Disorders Program*, specializing in diagnosis and management of occupational lung disorders, such as occupational asthma and bronchitis, asbestosis, silicosis, and heavy metal lung injury;
- *Pulmonary Fibrosis/Interstitial Lung Disease Program*, which treats patients with chronic inflammatory and scarring disorders of the lungs, including collagen vascular associated pulmonary diseases;
- *Pulmonary Physiology Laboratory*, a service that has recently doubled in capacity and that performs the full range of physiological testing for lung disease;
- *Pulmonary Vascular Program*, offering diagnosis and management of pulmonary hypertension;
- *Pulmonary Rehabilitation Program,* which provides occupational, physical, and cardiopulmonary rehabilitation programs for patients with disabling lung disorders, as well as pre and postoperative consultation and therapy;
- *Respiratory Care Unit*, recently opened for chronic ventilator-dependent patients and those with advanced lung disease;
- *Thoracic Oncology Service*, which provides multidisciplinary medical care for lung cancer as a joint effort with the Department of Cardiothoracic Surgery.

THE MOUNT SINAI MEDICAL CENTER

Mount Sinai's Sarcoidosis Service, the largest service of its kind in the world, is an NIH Center of Excellence for research in sarcoidosis. It is the only site that performs the diagnostic Kveim-Siltzbach skin test for sarcoidosis, which eliminates the need for more invasive, uncomfortable, and expensive procedures.

Through its Pulmonary Physiology Laboratory, Mount Sinai has been instrumental in establishing normal values for various pulmonary function tests and is currently conducting clinical studies of new tests for sarcoidosis, asthma, and lung cancer. Other pulmonary specialists at Mount Sinai are performing studies of asthma and emphysema, lung cancer, sarcoidosis, collagen vascular diseases, pulmonary infections, occupational lung diseases, and critical care outcomes.

625

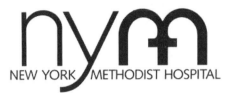

THE INSTITUTE FOR ASTHMA AND OTHER LUNG DISEASES
New York Methodist Hospital

506 Sixth Street, Brooklyn, N.Y. 11215
Phone: 866-ASK-LUNG (866-275-5864)
http://www.nym.org

SPECIALISTS AND MEDICAL SERVICES

The Institute for Lung Diseases Asthma and brings together a unique group of specialists and medical services to offer comprehensive diagnosis and treatment of a broad range of lung conditions. The Institute's panel of physician specialists includes both pediatric and adult pulmonologists and allergists. A larger constellation of physicians—medical oncologists, radiologists, radiation oncologists, and surgeons—is available, as needed. For diagnostic purposes, state-of-the-art specialty facilities—including the interventional bronchoscopy suite, the pulmonary function laboratory, and the Sleep Disorders Center—are conveniently located on the Hospital campus. These facilities are used to diagnose and treat a variety of lung disorders and are staffed by registered respiratory therapists, board-certified pulmonary function technologists, and exercise physiologists.

PROGRAMS OFFERED

In addition to the treatment of pediatric and adult asthma, physicians affiliated with the Institute diagnose and care for patients with chronic obstructive lung disease (COPD), interstitial lung disease, infectious lung disease, pulmonary hypertension and lung cancer. Highly sophisticated interventional pulmonary services as well as advanced thoracic surgery procedures are performed at the Hospital.

***

Referrals to the Institute, its programs and physicians can be made through an individual's primary care physician or requested directly through the Institute's telephone referral service. More information (and on-line physician referral) is available at the Hospital's website, http://www.nym.org.

THE INTERVENTIONAL PULMONOLOGY CENTER

New York Methodist Hospital's new Interventional Pulmonology Program is the only one of its kind in Brooklyn. This service offers state-of-the-art diagnostic and therapeutic pulmonary procedures, many of which are minimally invasive. Minimally invasive procedures are efficient and desirable because they typically cause less pain and are less time consuming than conventional investigative surgery. Furthermore, these procedures enable earlier diagnosis of certain forms of lung cancer, thereby enhancing the chances for successful treatment.

Radiology

Holy Name Hospital

Member
NewYork-Presbyterian Healthcare System
Affiliate: Columbia University College of Physicians & Surgeons

718 Teaneck Road
Teaneck, NJ 07666
(201) 833-3000
www.holyname.org

THE INTERVENTIONAL INSTITUTE

Patients facing uterine fibroids, spine fractures or even cancer can be offered innovative non-surgical treatment options. The Interventional Institute at Holy Name Hospital—under the direction of John Rundback, MD, an international leader in the field—is using revolutionary technology to shrink fibroids, deliver chemotherapy directly into cancer cells, cement spine fractures and even eliminate varicose veins. All without surgery. So there's less risk, a faster recovery and better quality of life.

REVOLUTIONARY TECHNIQUES

Interventional radiology is a medical specialty devoted to advancing patient care through minimally invasive, targeted treatments that are performed using imaging for guidance. It is a rapidly growing area of medicine. The Interventional Institute at Holy Name Hospital uses revolutionary imaging techniques to "see" inside the body while guiding narrow tubes (catheters) and other very small instruments through the blood vessels and other pathways of the body to the site of a problem. It enables patients to receive treatment for a variety of medical disorders without surgery. Shrinking uterine fibroid tumors that once meant a hysterectomy. Clearing a life-threatening blood clot in a deep leg vein. Eliminating leg pain and amputation risk due to a buildup of plaque in the peripheral arteries. Eliminating enlarged, swollen leg veins that are unsightly and restrict blood flow. Curing painful spine fractures due to osteoporosis. All of these conditions are now treatable with minimally invasive surgical techniques. Procedures at Holy Name are performed by a board-certified interventionalist and are generally less costly and involve shorter hospital stays.

To learn more or make an appointment with the Interventional Institute, call 201-833-3310.

The Radiology Institute at Holy Name Hospital can:

• Treat uterine fibroid tumors by blocking the blood supply and causing them to shrink

• Deliver cancer treatment directly to a tumor

• Eliminate varicose veins

• Insert stents into peripheral arteries to prevent plaque buildup

• Open blocked leg arteries, kidney arteries and carotid arteries using balloon angioplasty and other techniques

• Break up a blood clot in the leg due to deep vein thrombosis and restore blood flow

• Stabilize collapsed vertebrae using bone cement or an orthopedic balloon

762

Sponsored Page

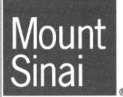

THE MOUNT SINAI MEDICAL CENTER
RADIOLOGY

One Gustave L. Levy Place (Fifth Avenue and 100th Street)
New York, NY 10029-6574
Physician Referral: 1-800-MD-SINAI (636-4624)
www.mountsinai.org

Mount Sinai offers patients one of the world's most comprehensive and sophisticated arrays of diagnostic and interventional radiology. Our imaging system is now based on filmless, digital technology that spans magnetic resonance imaging (MRI), multi-slice computed tomography (CT), positron emission tomography CT (PET-CT), single photon tomography CT (SPECT-CT), advanced ultrasound, and digital mammography. The Department of Radiology is utilizing state-of-the-art PACS technology.

COMPREHENSIVE DIAGNOSTIC SERVICES
Mount Sinai offers the entire range of diagnostic radiology services in a patient-friendly environment for the diagnosis of degenerative, infectious, vascular, neoplastic, genetic, traumatic, and toxic metabolic disorders of the brain, spine, bones and joints, heart, lungs, abdomen, pelvis, breast, and blood vessels.

EARLY DETECTION PROGRAMS
With funding from the Sharp Foundation, we are developing special screening approaches for early disease detection. Radiological screenings for colon cancer and Alzheimer's disease are joining those already in place for breast and lung cancer, and atherosclerosis. The early detection programs use a variety of imaging techniques (e.g., CT and MRI for atherosclerosis, CT for colon cancer, PET for oncology and digital mammography, MRI, and computer aided diagnosis for breast cancer).

MINIMALLY INVASIVE PROCEDURES
Radiology at Mount Sinai has moved beyond diagnosis to therapeutic intervention. Biopsies, vascular therapies, uterine artery embolization for fibroids (an alternative to hysterectomy), as well as treatments for aneurysms, atherosclerosis, and some types of cancer are all performed at Mount Sinai in the suites of Interventional Radiology.

Developing New Diagnostic Tools

Radiology at Mount Sinai is an active center of imaging research and development. Mount Sinai physicians and scientists developed a special form of MRI to non-invasively diagnose heart disease and atherosclerosis and thereby identify patients at greatest risk for stroke and heart attack.

We actively collaborate with other disciplines to develop and refine imaging tools that will make prevention, diagnosis, and prognosis increasingly effective. That is the case, for example, in neuroscience, where the work encompasses neurodegenerative conditions such as Parkinson's disease, as well as multiple sclerosis, stroke and brain tumors; and cardiovascular disease, where studies are underway for the peripheral, renal, abdominal, pulmonary, and coronary arteries; and liver disease, where radiology and the transplant team work closely together.

617

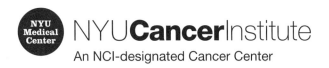

NYU**Cancer**Institute
An NCI-designated Cancer Center

Looking for information on our expert physicians?
1-212-731-5000

NYU Clinical Cancer Center
160 East 34th Street
New York, New York 10016
www.nyuci.org

NYU Medical Center
550 First Avenue (at 31st Street)
New York, New York 10016
www.nyumc.org

A Collaborative Approach
The NYU Cancer Institute, an NCI designated center, is a "matrix cancer center" without walls operating within the larger NYU Medical Center. With over 250 members and a research funding base of over $80 million, this structure strengthens our capabilities to forge collaborations across medical and scientific disciplines, which translates to comprehensive care for our patients and discoveries that will influence the future of this disease.

Renowned Expertise
Our highly skilled Magnet™ nursing team not only plays a pivotal role in coordinating direct patient care, but is also a source of invaluable patient education. Team members' compassion and expertise help patients better manage the symptoms of their disease as well as their special needs.

A Patient-Focused Setting
The NYU Clinical Cancer Center, with over 60 faculty members from various disciplines at the New York University School of Medicine, is the principal outpatient facility of the Cancer Institute and serves as home base for our patients and their caregivers. The center and its multidisciplinary team of experts provide access to the latest treatment options and clinical trials along with a variety of programs in cancer prevention, screening, diagnostics, genetic counseling, and supportive services. Our affiliation with Bellevue Hospital, the oldest public hospital in the country, affords clinically distinctive opportunities to learn and care for patients with cancer by observing its presentation and behavior in a variety of patient groups.

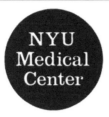

NYU Medical Center

550 First Avenue (at 31st Street)
New York, NY 10016
Physician Referral:
(888)7-NYU-MED (888-769-8633)
www.nyumc.org

RADIOLOGY:
The Diagnostic Core of Modern Medicine

LEADING EDGE TECHNOLOGY

Focusing on a broad variety of cancers including breast, colon, & lung, NYU Medical Center houses some of the most advanced radiology equipment in the world, including:

- Multi-detector 64 slice CT

- New multi-Channel MRI technology including two 3-Tesla clinical scanners and 7-Tesla research scanner

- Brand new, high resolution/high sensitivity PET/CT

- Full-field digital mammography as well as standard analog films

- Stereotactic biopsy capability

- Bone densitometry

- Advanced breast MR Imaging

- Digital fluoroscopy

- Advanced digital subtraction angiography with 3D Capabilities

- Minimally invasive techniques including radiofrequency ablation and chemoembilization

- State-of-the-art SPECT gamma cameras

- Radioimmunotherapy for Non-Hodgkin's Lymphoma

ON THE HORIZON

As part of a major academic medical center, our cancer experts collaborate in other aspects of medicine as well. The Department is the 9th largest recipient of NIH research funding in the U.S. and first in New York.

A DRIVER OF CROSS-DISCIPLINARY CLINICAL EXCELLENCE

Radiology plays an increasingly pivotal role in medical, clinical, and translational research. With an explosion of imaging technologies, researchers at NYU are making rapid strides in the understanding of complex diseases. No longer merely a supportive discipline, radiology has been transformed into a dynamic driver of medical knowledge itself. For example, the new imaging technologies allow physicians to observe minute changes in tumor activity during cancer treatment, adjust the dosage accordingly, and monitor the disease process with a depth and precision that would have previously been unimaginable.

**PHYSICIAN REFERRAL
1-888-7-NYU-MED
(1-888-769-8633)
www.nyumc.org**

Sponsored Page

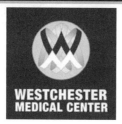

WESTCHESTER MEDICAL CENTER

Valhalla Campus
Valhalla, NY 10595
Tel. 1-877-WMC-DOCS
http://www.worldclassmedicine.com

NOVALIS® SHAPED BEAM SURGERY AT WESTCHESTER MEDICAL CENTER

At the forefront of medical technology, Westchester Medical Center was one of the first hospitals in the nation to offer Novalis® Shaped Beam Surgery, the least invasive and most precise treatment option available to patients diagnosed with a range of cancers, brain tumors, vascular malformations and neurologic disorders. A joint initiative by the Cancer Institute and Neuroscience Center at Westchester Medical Center, Novalis® Shaped Beam Surgery is widely considered the most significant advance in radiosurgery technology in the last decade.

Although it is called "surgery," there is no incision and the procedure is performed on an outpatient basis. Driven by digital diagnostic imaging, Novalis® Shaped Beam Surgery uses precise and detailed computer generated images that exactly mirror the shape and size of a patient's tumor or malformation. Each beam of radiation is shaped to conform to the tumor's precise dimensions, treating diseased tissue while leaving healthy tissue unharmed.

RADIATION MEDICINE AT WESTCHESTER MEDICAL CENTER

Accredited as "first-rate" by the American College of Radiation Oncologists, the Radiation Medicine team plays an integral role in the evaluation and treatment of patients cared for at the Cancer Institute at Westchester Medical Center. As an academic teaching hospital and the only American College of Surgeon Commission on Cancer-approved teaching hospital in the Hudson Valley region, the Cancer Institute brings together some of the nation's finest researchers, physicians, surgeons, nurses, scientists, and technicians—all dedicated to providing cutting-edge, customized cancer care and innovative therapeutic approaches to cancer management in a patient-centered, quality-driven environment.

Featuring state-of-the-art radiation facilities designed for ultimate patient comfort, physicians employ the very latest technologies and equipment with precision to achieve the best possible cure rates. The Radiation Medicine team treats patients of all ages, and offers a comprehensive range of therapeutic services, including external beam, electron beam and brachytherapy treatments with conventional low-dose rate and high-dose rate sources to treat malignancies of the breast, prostate, lung and chest, brain, stomach, pancreas, uterus and other sites.

All inpatient pediatric therapeutic radiology patients stay in Westchester Medical Center's state-of-the-art Maria Fareri Children's Hospital, which offers young patients a total healing environment in which parents can participate fully in their care and recovery.

For more information, go to www.worldclassmedicine.com

RADIOSURGERY

Targeted Novalis® Radiosurgery improves treatment for a range of body cancers, brain tumors, vascular malformations and neurologic disorders, including:

- Arteriovenous Malformations
- Brain Metastases and Gliomas
- Acoustic Neuromas
- Cavernous Angiomas
- Intractable Seizures
- Pediatric Brain Tumors
- Recurrent Brain Tumors
- Pituitary Adenomas
- Meningiomas of the Skull Base
- Carniopharyngiomas
- Spinal Tumors
- Functional Disorders

1-866-BEAM-CENTER

RADIATION MEDICINE

Among the comprehensive, state-of-the-art radiation therapy services offered are:

- Conventional External Beam Radiation
- 3-D Conformal Radiation Therapy (3-CRT)
- Intensity Modulated Radiation Therapy (IMRT)
- Image-Guided Radiation Therapy (IGRT)
- Stereotactic Radiosurgery
- Body Radiosurgery
- Total Body Irradiation
- Total Skin Electro Beam
- Brachytherapy (low- and high-dose rates)
- Hyperthermia

1-914-493-8516

Sponsored Page

Reproductive Medicine

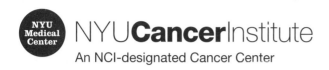

NYU**Cancer**Institute

An NCI-designated Cancer Center

Looking for information on our expert physicians?
1-212-731-5000

NYU Clinical Cancer Center
160 East 34th Street
New York, New York 10016
www.nyuci.org

NYU Medical Center
550 First Avenue (at 31st Street)
New York, New York 10016
www.nyumc.org

A Collaborative Approach

The NYU Cancer Institute, an NCI designated center, is a "matrix cancer center" without walls operating within the larger NYU Medical Center. With over 250 members and a research funding base of over $80 million, this structure strengthens our capabilities to forge collaborations across medical and scientific disciplines, which translates to comprehensive care for our patients and discoveries that will influence the future of this disease.

Renowned Expertise

Our highly skilled Magnet™ nursing team not only plays a pivotal role in coordinating direct patient care, but is also a source of invaluable patient education. Team members' compassion and expertise help patients better manage the symptoms of their disease as well as their special needs.

A Patient-Focused Setting

The NYU Clinical Cancer Center, with over 60 faculty members from various disciplines at the New York University School of Medicine, is the principal outpatient facility of the Cancer Institute and serves as home base for our patients and their caregivers. The center and its multidisciplinary team of experts provide access to the latest treatment options and clinical trials along with a variety of programs in cancer prevention, screening, diagnostics, genetic counseling, and supportive services. Our affiliation with Bellevue Hospital, the oldest public hospital in the country, affords clinically distinctive opportunities to learn and care for patients with cancer by observing its presentation and behavior in a variety of patient groups.

Rheumatology

HOSPITAL FOR
**SPECIAL
SURGERY**

HOSPITAL FOR SPECIAL SURGERY

Rheumatology

**535 East 70th Street • New York, NY 10021
Physician Referral: 800-854-0071 • hss.edu**

FIRST IN ITS FIELD
Founded in 1863, Hospital for Special Surgery is the nation's leading specialty hospital for orthopaedics and rheumatology.

AMERICA'S LARGEST GROUP OF RHEUMATOLOGISTS
HSS Rheumatologists are international authorities and pioneering researchers in every known rheumatological and autoimmune condition and treatment.

The Godsen-Robinson Early Arthritis Center provides treatment plans and education on the disease modifying importance of early intervention in osteoarthritis and rheumatoid arthritis for patients and primary care physicians.

The Barbara Volcker Center for Women and Rheumatic Diseases focuses on mobility, chronic pain, pregnancy, and osteoporosis in women with rheumatic diseases, such as rheumatoid arthritis, systemic lupus erythematosus, osteoporosis, and scleroderma. Research on these topics is conducted within the Weill Medical College of Cornell University.

Mary Kirkland Center for Lupus Research is dedicated to the advancement of knowledge about the causes, pathogenesis and genetics of systemic lupus erythematosus, to define its cure and to improve the quality of the lives of lupus patients.

Integrative Care Center affiliated with Hospital for Special Surgery providing effective, safe, evidence-based alternative and complementary medicine, including acupuncture, massage, yoga and movement classes, and mind body healing.

SPECIALTIES INCLUDE:
- Osteoarthritis
- Rheumatoid Arthritis
- Systemic Lupus Erythematosus
- Ankylosing Spondylitis
- Antiphospholipid Syndrome
- Arthritis associated with ulcerative colitis
- Bursitis
- Childhood/Teenage Arthritis
- Crohn's Disease
- Dermatomyositis
- Fibromyalgia syndrome
- Gout
- Pediatric Rheumatoid Arthritis
- Infectious arthritis
- Lyme Disease
- Myositis Paget's Disease
- Polymyositis
- Psoriatic arthritis
- Reiter's Syndrome
- Scleroderma
- Sjogren's syndrome
- Tendonitis
- Vasculitis
- And more, see all on hss.edu

Top Ranked in Orthopaedics & Rheumatology in the Northeast by *U.S. News & World Reports* **for 16 Years in a Row**

Winner of Nursing's Highest Honor: Magnet Status for Nursing Excellence

Winner of NY's First Patient Safety Award

Largest Physiatry Department Dedicated to the Non-operative Treatment of Musculoskeletal Disorders

Noted Osteoporosis Prevention Center, a model across the nation

Largest Academic Center in the World Devoted to Musculoskeletal Imaging

Renown Physical Therapy at the Virginia F. and William R. Salomon Rehabilitation Department

Innovative Education and Patient Support Programs

hss.edu
Every Musculoskeletal Specialty. One Innovative Web Site.

NYU Medical Center

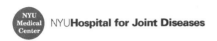

NYU**Hospital for Joint Diseases**

550 First Avenue (at 31st Street)
New York, NY 10016
Physician Referral:
(888)7-NYU-MED (888-769-8633
www.nyumc.org

301 East 17th Street (at 2nd Ave.)
New York, NY 10003
Physician Referral:
(888) HJD-D OCS (888-453-3627)
www.nyuhjd.org

RHEUMATOLOGY

The Department of Rheumatology at NYU Hospital for Joint Diseases (NYUHJD) is dedicated to the diagnosis and treatment of patients with rheumatic diseases and also focuses on autoimmune diseases. The department accomplishes its mission through a balanced combination of education, research, and clinical care. The NYUHJD Department and the Division of Rheumatology at NYU were recognized in the 2006 edition of *U.S. News and World Report* as one of the top ten rheumatology programs in the country.

Patients receive care at the following centers:

Center for Arthritis and Autoimmunity
Staffed by a select group of leading academic researchers and physicians, it provides a comprehensive program for the prevention, diagnosis, and treatment of all rheumatologic conditions. The Center integrates patient care across a variety of disciplines. Patients receive complete rheumatologic evaluations, orthopaedic and neurological consultative services, sophisticated diagnostic testing, physiotherapy, and complementary medicine.

Osteoporosis Center
The Osteoporosis Center offers comprehensive care for the prevention, evaluation and treatment of osteoporosis. The Center includes a state-of-the-art bone densitometer which affords patients all-inclusive care for this condition.

Psoriatic Arthritis Center
The Psoriatic Arthritis Center is a collaborative effort with the Department of Dermatology at NYU. Patients are seen at the NYU Skin and Cancer Center for two half-day sessions on Monday and Wednesday and in the presence of both a rheumatologist and dermatologist with particular expertise in psoriatic arthritis.

Lupus Clinic
The Lupus Clinic is devoted solely to the treatment of patients with this multifaceted disease. Patients are seen regularly by rheumatologists, and have ready access to specialists in dermatology, nephrology, orthopaedics, and neurology, all of whom have expertise in systemic lupus erythematosus. Also offers expertise in pregnancy and hormonal issues.

Clinical Research Center
Basic science and medicine converge at the Peter D. Seligman Center for Advanced Therapeutics. The Center was established to promote new initiatives in clinical and translational investigation, focusing on developing improved treatments for rheumatic diseases. Researchers conduct protocols using a wide variety of new medications for the treatment of rheumatoid arthritis, osteoarthritis, systemic lupus erythematosus, and osteoporosis.

The infusion unit at the Seligman Center for Advanced Therapeutics provides a setting to administer available agents to patients. In close collaboration with the American Behcet's Disease Association, the only North American Behcet's Center was established at Seligman for research and the evaluation and treatment of patients with Behcet's Syndrome. The Seligman Center is a satellite site of the NYU Department of Medicine NIH-funded General Clinical Research Center (GCRC).

694

Sleep Disorders

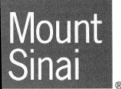

THE MOUNT SINAI MEDICAL CENTER
SLEEP MEDICINE

One Gustave L. Levy Place (Fifth Avenue and 100th Street)
New York, NY 10029-6574
Physician Referral: 1-800-MD-SINAI (636-4624)
www.mountsinai.org

Mount Sinai's recently expanded Center for Sleep Medicine is a full-service program that specializes in the comprehensive, compassionate, personalized care of adults and children with sleep disorders. This is the first truly multidisciplinary sleep center in New York City, staffed by board-certified sleep physicians who are also board-certified in pulmonary medicine, neurology and pediatrics.

We use state-of-the-art equipment to diagnose and treat all aspects of sleep pathology, including breathing-related disorders, insomnia, restless leg syndrome, periodic limb movements, and narcolepsy. An initial consultation includes a medical and surgical history, and physical examination. In some cases, the diagnosis and treatment plan can be completed in a single visit. In other cases, the evaluation requires a sleep study (typically over one or two nights) or other tests. As overnight tests are completed by 8 am, it is usually not necessary to miss a day of work. In rare instances, daytime studies are recommended, as well.

Services available at the Center for Sleep Medicine, include:

• Consultations with board-certified sleep specialists;

• Overnight sleep testing and daytime testing, provided by physicians and technicians who are experts at treating adults and children. During a sleep study, the patient is monitored by painless, noninvasive technology (PSG) that records breathing, heart rate, brain waves, oxygen levels, and eye and leg movement;

• Treatment for a sleep disorder, which may include a device to aid the patient's breathing while sleeping (called CPAP or BiPAP), medication, or light therapy as well as neuropsychiatric interventions, including biofeedback. If indicated, consultations with other specialists are available to aid in diagnosis and therapy;

• Mechanical, behavioral, surgical, dental, and pharmacological therapies, as required. Consultations can also be arranged with pulmonologists, ENT surgeons, bariatric surgeons, dentists, and psychiatrists.

THE MOUNT SINAI MEDICAL CENTER

Approximately 20 million Americans suffer from Obstructive Sleep Apnea (OSA), which occurs when muscles of the back of the mouth and the throat relax during sleep, causing a complete (apnea) or partial (hypopnea) blockage of the airway. Each time that happens, the oxygen level may fall, causing the heart to work harder. When untreated, this disorder can lead to hypertension, heart failure and stroke, as well as to bouts of daytime sleepiness that increase the risk of motor vehicle and industrial accidents. In seniors, sleepiness is often misperceived as a natural consequence of aging.

If you are concerned that you might have OSA, take the Epworth Sleepiness Test, a simple questionnaire available on the Mount Sinai Center for Sleep Medicine Web site, www.nysleep.com. If you score higher than 10 on the Epworth Sleepiness Test or if you are overweight and snore, you may have sleep apnea or another sleep disorder.

626

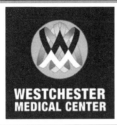

A FULL SERVICE SLEEP CENTER

Nearly 1 in 10 people will experience a sleep disorder, with the majority going undiagnosed and untreated. Advances in sleep medicine and technology have made it possible to restore the good night's sleep that is fundamental to health and well-being. The Sleep Center at Westchester Medical Center is a full service, state-of-the-art laboratory equipped to treat a wide range of sleep disorders in both adults and children.

SPECIALIZED TEAM OF PROFESSIONALS

Under the direction of Stuart G. Lehrman, M.D, Diplomate of the American Board of Sleep Medicine, the Sleep Center's experienced team of adult and pediatric physicians and sleep specialists employ state-of-the-art technology to diagnose and manage sleep apnea, insomnia, restless leg syndrome, nocturnal leg movements, narcolepsy, excessive daytime sleepiness and other less common disorders. As part of a major academic medical center, the Sleep Center works in concert with on-site specialists in such adult and pediatric disciplines as neurology, sleep medicine, cardiology, otolaryngology, pulmonology and oral and maxillofacial surgery to develop a comprehensive, individualized treatment plan.

STATE-OF-THE-ART FACILITIES

Comprehensive sleep studies are conducted in the comfort of private, well-furnished rooms for patients (and parents). Utilizing the latest digital equipment, the sleep study is a non-invasive test in which a patient's sleep patterns, breathing, oxygen level, heart rate and rhythm, and muscle tone are monitored throughout the night. The results of the study are fully evaluated and physicians work closely with the patient and family to diagnose the sleep disorder and develop an effective treatment program.

SLEEP CENTER AT WESTCHESTER MEDICAL CENTER

The Sleep Center at Westchester Medical Center is a full-service, state-of-the-art facility equipped to diagnose and treat a wide range of sleep disorders in children and adults, including:

- Sleep Apnea
- Insomnia
- Restless Leg Syndrome
- Nocturnal Leg Movements
- Narcolepsy
- Excessive Daytime Sleepiness

If you think you, your partner or your child have a sleep disorder, talk with your doctor or call the Sleep Center directly at 914.493.1105 to schedule a consultation with one of our Sleep Medicine specialists.

Sponsored Page

Thoracic Surgery

Mount Sinai ®

THE MOUNT SINAI MEDICAL CENTER
THORACIC SURGERY

One Gustave L. Levy Place (Fifth Avenue and 100th Street)
New York, NY 10029-6574
Physician Referral: 1-800-MD-SINAI (636-4624)
www.mountsinai.org

Thoracic Surgery at Mount Sinai is famed for its advancements in the application of minimally invasive techniques, its focus on state-of-the-art multidisciplinary treatment of difficult tumors, and its commitment to treating patients whose conditions others believe to be incurable.

Clinical care at Mount Sinai draws upon its expertise in behavioral medicine, genetic testing, and environmental medicine. In addition to radiation, chemotherapy, and surgical treatments to combat cancers in every stage, Mount Sinai offers:

• *Minimally invasive lung cancer surgery* – Our faculty have led national trials in VATS lobectomy, making Mount Sinai the leader in minimally invasive approaches in the New York tri-state area. Advances in this area include robotic techniques using the DaVinci system.

• *Photodynamic therapy (PDT)* – For individuals with unresectable tumors of the airway and esophagus, especially those experiencing difficulty in breathing or swallowing.

• *Laser therapy and stenting for esophageal and lung cancer* – Laser therapy can be used to burn away portions of an unresectable tumor that blocks the esophagus or airway, while stenting may be recommended either following laser therapy to make its effects more durable or when laser therapy cannot be used.

• *Access to Mount Sinai-led clinical trials.*

LUNG CANCER
Mount Sinai offers the widest possible spectrum of screening and diagnostic tests, including CT screenings for the early detection of lung cancer, advanced endoscopic techniques designed to detect early lesions and survey for early recurrence, advanced CT and PET capabilities, and innovative MRI technology with ultrasensitive resolution.

ESOPHAGEAL CANCER
Mount Sinai offers the widest possible spectrum of screening and diagnostic tests. Treatment of esophageal cancer can involve minimally invasive surgery with or without chemotherapy and radiation.

THE MOUNT SINAI MEDICAL CENTER

One of the strengths of Mount Sinai's Thoracic Oncology Program is the teamwork that its multidisciplinary experts bring to patient care. Your team may include: thoracic surgeons, medical oncologists, radiation oncologists, pathologists, radiologists, pulmonologists, gastroenterologists, plastic surgeons, oncology-dedicated nurses, respiratory therapists, physical and occupational therapists, nutritionists, social workers, and psychiatrists and psychologists.

Coordinating information among team members to ensure seamless care for the patient is one of the program's highest priorities. Our team also provides a seamless approach to the diagnosis, treatment and follow-up of patients who are affected by swallowing and reflux disorders, including expertise in the areas of gastroenterology, otolaryngology, speech and swallowing therapy, thoracic surgery, medical and radiation oncology, and radiology.

627

THE MOUNT SINAI MEDICAL CENTER
CARDIOTHORACIC SURGERY

One Gustave L. Levy Place (Fifth Avenue and 100th Street)
New York, NY 10029-6574
Physician Referral: 1-800-MD-SINAI (636-4624)
www.mountsinai.org

Mount Sinai ®

The Department of Cardiothoracic Surgery at Mount Sinai is one of the country's most prestigious programs. Cardiothoracic surgical patients benefit from an integrated and personalized care plan designed in coordination with expert cardiologists, anesthesiologists, perfusionists, and intensive care physicians. Mount Sinai is quaternary referral center, meaning we often operate on the sickest and most complicated patients. In addition to conventional coronary artery bypass and cardiac valve replacement surgery, we offer the latest technologies and procedures consistent with cutting-edge cardiothoracic surgical care.

The Mitral Valve Repair Program at Mount Sinai is one of the most advanced in the country. The superiority of mitral valve repair, instead of replacement with a mechanical or bioprosthetic valve, is now well-established. The mitral valve repair program at Mount Sinai offers patients one of the highest percentages of successful valve repair anywhere in the world. For example, in patients with mitral valve prolapse, our success rate in avoiding valve replacement approaches 100 percent. Our physicians are also experts in mitral valve repair for patients with advanced cardiomyopathy. If patients have associated atrial fibrillation, we offer the latest in concomitant arrhythmia surgery, including the MAZE procedure. We can also perform mitral valve repair with minimally invasive approaches, when appropriate.

The Thoracic Aortic Surgery Program is internationally renowned for its leadership role in surgical therapy of complex aortic disease. This program specializes in the operative management of all diseases of the ascending aorta, arch, and descending thoracic aorta. Aortic valve sparing root replacement, valve-conduit root replacement, trifurcation-graft arch replacement, acute aortic dissection repair, and preoperative aortic surgery are all commonly performed procedures at Mount Sinai. Special emphasis is placed on cerebral and spinal protection, where we also have a significant clinical and scientific research interest. Our surgeons have also been involved in the early development of minimally invasive aortic stent grafting.

The Minimally Invasive Cardiac Surgery Program offers patients the latest technologically-advanced surgery available. The minimally invasive efforts at Mount Sinai include robotic surgery using the DaVinci robot, off pump coronary artery bypass surgery, small incision valve surgery, and new frontiers including small incision atrial fibrillation surgery. We have been involved in pioneering research with a new generation of anastomotic devices which may one day replace conventional suturing in minimally invasive surgery.

The Cardiac Transplant and Assist Program is one of the largest in the United States. We have been involved in the field of mechanical cardiac assistance from its inception and we have experience with most of the currently available FDA-approved devices. We have also played an active role in multi-institutional studies exploring permanent mechanical heart support.

THE MOUNT SINAI MEDICAL CENTER

The Department of Cardiothoracic Surgery at Mount Sinai is chaired by David Adams, MD, the Marie-Josée and Henry R. Kravis Professor.

Randall Griepp, MD, Professor of Cardiothoracic Surgery, is focusing his leadership and energies toward the thoracic aortic surgery program. These leaders of cardiothoracic surgery work in concert with other members of Mount Sinai Heart, which is under the direction of world-renowned cardiologist Valentin Fuster, MD, PhD, to deliver unparalleled possibilities for patients with cardiovascular disease.

62

Sponsored Page

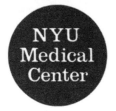

NYU Medical Center

550 First Avenue (at 31st Street)
New York, NY 10016
Physician Referral:
(888)7-NYU-MED (888-769-8633)

NYU Hospital Center Thoracic Surgery: Aggressive use of the Newest Technologies and Laboratory Discovery to Treat Thoracic Diseases

The Division of Thoracic Surgery of the NYU Hospital Center is a leader in diagnosing and treating both benign and malignant neoplasms (tissue growths), as well as providing management of other disorders of the lungs, esophagus, mediastinum and the chest wall.

The NYU Thoracic Oncology Program's multidisciplinary approach unites the disciplines of medical oncology, surgery, radiation therapy, pulmonary medicine, radiology and pathology. We use evidence-based discussion and multifaceted expert opinions to tailor care to individual patients' needs. Weekly discussions of new and existing patients are held to decide the appropriate management, and see if patients are eligible to participate in new clinical trials.

The involvement of multiple sites at the Manhattan VA, Bellevue Hospital and Tisch Hospital allows us to provide the greatest number of patients with the newest developments in treatment available through NYU Medical Center.

Our minimally invasive surgery program incorporates video-assisted and "open chest" techniques along with new methods for post-operative pain relief. Procedures include:

- video-assisted thoracoscopy for the chest
- video-assisted laparoscopy for the abdomen
- video-assisted procedures on benign lesions of the esophagus and lungs
- minimally invasive esophagectomy and pulmonary resection

We also place a unique emphasis on the treatment of pleural mesothelioma using a multimodal approach.

A key part of providing compassionate clinical care is research. That's why NYU Thoracic Surgery is committed to state-of-the-art surgical management and to developing novel treatment strategies using clinical trials. We also use the resources at the New York Thoracic Surgery Laboratory housed at Bellevue Hospital to launch investigations at the gene or protein level. Through studies like these we make clinically relevant "bench to bedside" discoveries in early detection and develop targeted therapies.

We also provide the newest in pioneering treatments, including:

- early detection of airway malignancies with fluorescence bronchoscopy
- novel diagnostic and staging modalities including endobronchial ultrasound
- novel endobronchial treatment strategies including photodynamic therapy
- investigation of non-surgical techniques selectively used for destruction of lung cancer nodules, including radiofrequency ablation and stereotactic radiation
- use of stents to relieve blockages of the windpipe and esophagus
- investigation of the use of replaceable stents in the windpipe and esophagus

685

Transplantation

THE MOUNT SINAI MEDICAL CENTER TRANSPLANTATION

Mount Sinai ®

One Gustave L. Levy Place (Fifth Avenue and 100th Street)
New York, NY 10029-6574
Physician Referral: 1-800-MD-SINAI (636-4624)
www.mountsinai.org

Technological advances, along with improved medical therapies, continue to make hopes of a normal life after organ transplantation a reality. Today, transplantation has become an accepted form of treatment for adults and children with a wide variety of diseases. Intensely committed to clinical and basic science research, members of Mount Sinai's Recanati/Miller Transplantation Institute investigate ways to improve organ preservation, reduce post-transplant complications, and the side effects of immunosuppression. They also focus on the prevention of disease after a transplant, and overall quality of life after this relatively new medical miracle.

A HISTORY OF ACHIEVEMENT
Mount Sinai surgeons were the first in New York State to perform liver transplantation, and also the first in the state to perform living donor liver transplantation.

CONTINUING THE TRADITION OF EXCELLENCE
Mount Sinai is one of the few hospitals in the country with expertise in small intestine/small bowel transplantation. Working closely with each patient's referring physician, state-of-the-art procedures are performed that profoundly affect patients' lives. Treatment at the Medical Center is not the end of the relationship. Caregivers at Mount Sinai continue to work with the referring physician to help maintain the patient's optimum health level.

A SAMPLING OF OUR INNOVATIVE PROGRAMS
The Kidney/Pancreas Transplant Program began over 30 years ago, making Mount Sinai one of the first kidney transplant programs in the region. Today, the Medical Center has performed over 1,000 kidney transplants and approximately 70 pancreas transplants or combination kidney/pancreas procedures, both for adults and children. Although pancreas transplantation has gained widespread acceptance in the United States, Mount Sinai is one of the few centers in the greater New York area that performs the operation, and is among the largest programs in the Northeast. Our Intestinal Transplant Program is one of the most established and respected in the country. We offer a comprehensive approach to intestinal failure, and have developed a team approach that includes specialists from different fields working together to achieve the best possible result for the patient.

THE MOUNT SINAI MEDICAL CENTER

The Recanati/Miller Transplantation Institute brings together clinical programs in adult and pediatric liver, kidney, pancreas, and intestine transplantation and includes major research initiatives. Meanwhile, within the Department of Cardiothoracic Surgery, heart and lung transplants are also offered.

We are one of the largest transplant centers in the United States, performing over 350 procedures annually. Patients from around the world come to Mount Sinai for transplants, including living-donor and traditional surgeries. The total volume of organ transplants at Mount Sinai places the hospital among the top academic medical centers nationally.

619

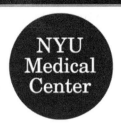

NYU Medical Center

550 First Avenue (at 31st Street)
New York, NY 10016
Physician Referral: (888) 7-NYU-MED
(888-769-8633) www.nyumedicalcenter.org

TRANSPLANT

TRANSPLANT AT NYU MEDICAL CENTER

The Mary Lea Johnson Richards Transplant Center at NYUMedical Center offers a variety of services including liver transplantation, living donor liver transplantation, kidney transplantation, living donor kidney transplantation, laparoscopic kidney transplantation, kidney-pancreas transplantation and pancreas transplantation. The transplant team follows each patient preoperatively, interoperatively, and postoperatively.

Our team consists of four transplant surgeons, two transplant fellows, six transplant coordinators/nurse practitioners, two inpatient nurse practitioners, three social workers, a designated transplant hepatologist, nephrologist, hematologist, cardiologist, pulmonologist, nutritionist, physiatrist, pharmacist, and endocrinologist, as well as radiologists and pathologists.

At NYU we pride ourselves on our ability to provide comprehensive care to patients with end stage liver and renal disease. Our approach is nondiscriminatory, regardless of patients' age, race, sex or insurance.

Patient education is designed specifically to meet the individual needs of the patient, whether the patient is fluent in English or has language barriers, or has learning disabilities or physical disabilities. There are three full-time designated social workers who follow patients both in the inpatient and outpatient settings.

In response to a decreasing organ donor pool coupled with growing liver and kidney transplant waiting lists, the Mary Lea Johnson Richards Transplant Center at NYU Medical Center has implemented a living donor liver and kidney transplant program.

Living Donor Liver Transplantation

This state-of-the-art procedure allows patients to bypass the UNOS waiting list by having a family member or close friend donate half of his/her liver. This allows surgery to be scheduled when both donor and recipient are stable and in the healthiest state possible. Because of the liver's unique ability to regenerate, both the donor and the recipient's livers grow back to full size in approximately three months following the surgery.

Living Donor Kidney Transplantation

NYU Medical Center offers living donor kidney transplantation to patients with end stage renal failure. New surgical techniques including minimally invasive kidney extraction are making it easier for family members and other donors to donate a kidney to a loved one in need.

The success rate of liver transplantation at NYU Medical Center at one and two years is 92% and 86% respectively. The one-year patient survival after kidney transplantation at NYU is over 90%, the pancreas graft survival is 85% and the kidney graft survival is 87%.

NYU MEDICAL CENTER

The Mary Lea Johnson Richards Transplant Center prides itself on its comprehensive approach to patient care. Involvement of all disciplines including: pharmacy, nutrition, physiatry, social work, hepatology, nephrology, radiology, infectious disease, cardiology, and oncology, ensure that the patient is cared for in a comprehensive manner. In addition to performing transplantation, the transplant team at NYU works very closely with our transplant physicians in providing "bridges to transplantation," such as chemoembolization, TIPS procedures, as well as innovative research and pharmacological trials.

Sponsored Page

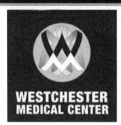

WESTCHESTER MEDICAL CENTER

Valhalla Campus
Valhalla, NY 10595
Tel. 1-877-WMC-DOCS
http://www.worldclassmedicine.com

OVERVIEW

The Transplant Center at Westchester Medical Center provides hundreds of people of all ages with a new lease on life every year. Our multidisciplinary team of physicians, nurse coordinators, social workers, nutritionists, psychiatrists and financial counselors work with patients and family members through each phase of the transplant experience. Our physicians and surgeons are able to provide the latest techniques in transplantation, and the team is committed to remaining at the forefront of this constantly evolving area of medicine.

In 1996, Westchester Medical Center performed the first-ever liver transplant in the Hudson Valley. Since then, the Liver Transplant Program has performed nearly 400 transplants. As an academic medical center, many of our patients benefit from drug studies currently underway prior to even considering liver transplantation.

Westchester Medical Center has performed more than 1,700 kidney transplants—making it one of the largest and busiest programs in all of New York State. Living-donor kidney transplants are now performed regularly, providing improved graft survival rates, a decrease in immunosupressive therapy and the ability to plan the time of transplantation. Today, kidney donors benefit from minimally invasive procedures, reducing surgery and recovery time. While awaiting transplant, patients receive leading-edge renal replacement therapy with all home and on-site modalities available. State-of-the-art dialysis access placement and access care are also available surgically and minimally invasively.

Westchester Medical Center's ophthalmologic surgeons perform hundreds of corneal transplants a year (mostly for children).

Westchester Medical Center is dedicated to all aspects of transplant and organ and tissue donation. For many years, Westchester Medical Center has been honored by the New York Organ Donor Network for our efforts in support of organ and tissue donation.

Transplant Center at Westchester Medical Center

At the Transplant Center at Westchester Medical Center, we pride ourselves on providing transplant services that rival any other major medical center. Our renowned physicians and surgeons work closely with a team of nurse coordinators, social workers, nutritionists, psychiatrists and financial counselors to guide patients and families through each phase of the transplant experience. We are committed to providing the latest techniques in transplantation and to staying at the forefront of this dynamic medical field.

Services at the Transplant Center include:

• Liver Transplant:
  (914) 493-8916

• Kidney Transplant:
  (914) 493-1990

• Renal Dialysis Services:
  (914) 493-7701

• Corneal Transplant:
  (914) 493-1599

• Bone Marrow Transplant:
  (914) 493-8374

780

Sponsored Page

The Yale-New Haven Transplantation Center

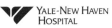 YALE-NEW HAVEN HOSPITAL

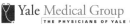 Yale Medical Group
THE PHYSICIANS OF YALE UNIVERSITY

20 York Street
New Haven, CT 06510
(203) 688-2000

www.ynhh.org

300 George Street, 6th Floor
New Haven, CT 06519
(203) 785-2140

www.yalemedicalgroup.org

The Yale-New Haven Transplantation Center provides multi-disciplinary care for patients with end-stage organ failure who might benefit from transplantation. The team includes outstanding surgeon and physician specialists, nurse coordinators, transplant social workers, financial coordinators and nutrition experts to support patient needs. Our commitment to superior clinical care and new knowledge generation and education, delivered by internationally recognized expert surgeons, physicians and staff, ensures delivery of the most advanced treatment available.

Calls from referring physicians, patients or their families are received by Center staff who provide an individualized evaluation to identify the best treatment approach. Specifically, candidates undergo a detailed medical, psychosocial and nutritional evaluation to determine if transplantation is the proper treatment. Eligible patients are also invited to consider appropriate clinical research projects ensuring continuing delivery of state-of-the-art care.

A full range of services are offered for children and adults with end-stage kidney disease, liver disease and diabetes, as well as for other forms of organ failure. A partial list of available services includes: minimally invasive living kidney donation; kidney, liver and pancreas transplantation; surgical treatment of liver and biliary disease; and hemodialysis and peritoneal dialysis surgical access. We also offer comprehensive tissue typing and immune evaluation, state-of-the-art immunosuppression treatment options, and thorough follow-up and psychosocial support.

Yale Medical Group is one of the largest academic multispecialty group practices in the United States. Comprised of the full-time faculty of the Yale School of Medicine, YMG physicians are leaders in their fields, dedicated to combining a compassionate, individual approach to patient care with the latest clinical and technologic developments.

Yale-New Haven Hospital is a 944-bed tertiary referral center, the primary teaching hospital for the Yale University School of Medicine, and the only hospital in Connecticut consistently recognized as one of America's Best Hospitals by US News & World Report.

Medical Staff:		
	Marc I. Lorber, MD, FACS	YNHTC Director, Transplant Surgery
	David C. Cronin, II, MD, PhD, FACS	Director, Liver Transplantation
	Sanjay Kulkarni, MD	Director, Kidney & Pancreas Transplant
	Amy L. Friedman, MD	Transplant Surgery
	Richard N. Formica, MD	Director, Transplant Nephrology
	Mario Strazzabosco, MD, PhD	Director, Transplant Hepatology
	Pramod K. Mistry, MD, PhD, FRCP	Director, Pediatric Gastroenterology
	Thomas L. Kennedy, MD	Pediatric Nephrology
	Margaret J. Bia, MD	Transplant Nephrology
	David Rothstein, MD	Transplant Nephrology

Please call **(203) 785-2565** for more information or you may visit: **www.ynhh.org/transplantation**.

Sponsored Page

Urology

THE MOUNT SINAI MEDICAL CENTER
UROLOGY

One Gustave L. Levy Place (Fifth Avenue and 100th Street)
New York, NY 10029-6574
Physician Referral: 1-800-MD-SINAI (636-4624)
www.mountsinai.org

The Milton and Carroll Petrie Department of Urology at The Mount Sinai Medical Center prides itself on adapting the latest technologic advancements and results of translational and clinical research to the assessment and treatment of urologic problems. Urology treatments utilized at Mount Sinai include:

• *Prostate Cancer* – Building on the successful collaboration with Radiation Oncology to pioneer the use of radioactive seeds, the Milton and Carroll Petrie Department of Urology strives to offer the full range of surgical and radiation treatments in the management of localized prostate cancer, including laparoscopic and robotic prostatectomies. For more advanced disease, treatment is integrated through the Deane Prostate Health & Research Center, exploring the use of cancer vaccines, gene therapy, new agents in chemotherapy, and hormonal therapy.

• *Bladder Cancer* – As recognized leaders in the assessment and treatment of all forms of bladder cancer, Mount Sinai's specialists employ knowledge of tumor markers and new diagnostic techniques to determine the most effective treatment approaches and exploit the latest techniques in reconstructing urinary diversions, which help preserve and maximize quality of life.

• *Kidney Cancer* – The majority of kidney tumors can be approached via minimally invasive surgical techniques, reducing pain and recovery time. Laparoscopic surgery may be applied to remove all or a portion of a kidney. Other less invasive modalities–such as freezing, or radio frequency ablation–may be recommended to treat small kidney cancers while preserving maximum function.

• *Prostatic Enlargement* – The latest technologies and treatments are applied for their effect in relieving urinary problems, including frequency, pain, burning, and retention, many in the outpatient setting, thus avoiding hospitalization.

• *Urinary Dysfunction* – For men and women, Mount Sinai provides comprehensive resources for the evaluation and treatment, both medical and surgical, of urinary incontinence, neuro-urologic problems, and pelvic pain syndrome.

• *Urologic Stone Disease* – Mount Sinai's expertise in kidney stone disease ranges from stone prevention to minimally invasive therapies with lasers, sonic energies, and extracorporeal shock wave lithotripsy.

• *Pediatric Conditions* – Mount Sinai has a strong reputation in the treatment of urologic problems in children, especially in reconstructive treatment, involving, when appropriate, minimally invasive procedures.

• *Male Infertility* – State-of-the-art approaches using medications and in vitro fertilization techniques result in a high success rate.

• *Sexuality-related Health Concerns* – For both men and women, **sexuality**-related issues are addressed through application of current medical and surgical approaches.

The Barbara and Maurice A. Deane Prostate Health & Research Center offers a new multidisciplinary facility for the assessment and treatment of all aspects of prostatic disease, including cancer, benign enlargement, and inflammation. Activities through the Center are designed to empower the patient and his family to understand the nature of his prostatic condition and decide upon the optimum treatment that may create lasting benefit and enhance quality of life.

Mount Sinai has developed an extensive **Minimally Invasive Urologic Surgery** program and is a leader in the greater New York area for complex procedures performed laparoscopically, robotically, and endoscopically. A variety of urologic cancers are treated, stone disease is managed, and reconstruction is provided for various urologic cancers, and anatomic abnormalities. These approaches provide for a rapid and virtually painless recovery and rapid return to normal activity.

620

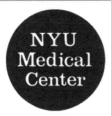

NYU Medical Center

550 First Avenue (at 31st Street)
New York, NY 10016
Physician Referral:
(888)7-NYU-MED (888-769-8633)
www.nyumc.org

UROLOGY

NYU Medical Center's urologists are internationally renowned specialists who have pioneered numerous advances in the surgical and pharmacological treatment of urological disease. They are an interdisciplinary team of physicians, nurses, and allied health professionals dedicated to providing the highest-quality state-of-the-art care. All of our doctors are also faculty at NYU School of Medicine who specialize in all aspects of urological disease. Our programs include:

Urologic Oncology – aggressively treating and curing urologic cancers while maintaining the highest quality of life. Cancers of the prostate, kidney, bladder, and testes are the most common malignancies treated in this program. Since treating cancer often requires a multidisciplinary approach, urologists work closely with NYU's medical and radiation oncologists to tailor treatment to each patient's priorities and objectives.

Minimally Invasive Surgery – committed to developing new technologies to treat even the most complex disorders more effectively and less invasively, so patients experience less pain and a quicker recovery.

Male Fertility and Sexual Health – collaborating closely with the world-renowned NYU In Vitro Fertilization Program, the fertility treatment program uses state-of-the-art technology and a multidisciplinary approach to diagnose and treat the underlying causes of both male and female sexual dysfunction.

Benign Prostatic Diseases – developing innovative medical and surgical therapies for benign prostatic diseases, such as benign prostatic hyperplasia (BPH, or enlarged prostate) and prostatitis (infection in the prostate).

Female Urology and Incontinence –expertise in the many urological problems unique to women, including recurrent urinary tract infections, pelvic pain, prolapse, and sexual dysfunction.

Pediatric Urology and Reconstructive Surgery – treating urologic diseases in children.

NYU MEDICAL CENTER

National Institutes for Health funding for NYU urological research is among the highest for a Urology department in the nation. To assure the continued cross-fertilization of research and patient care, basic scientists with primary academic appointments work closely with the NYU Medical Center urologists on research, leading to a superior understanding of clinical problems.

**Physician Referral
(888) 7-NYU-MED
(888-769-8633)
www.nyumc.org**

Sponsored Page

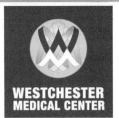

WESTCHESTER MEDICAL CENTER

Valhalla Campus
Valhalla, NY 10595
Tel. (914) 347-1900
http://www.worldclassmedicine.com

COMPREHENSIVE ADVANCED UROLOGICAL CARE FOR MEN AND WOMEN

The Urology Center at Westchester Medical Center, a tertiary level urology practice, is dedicated to providing cutting-edge advanced urological care for men and women with a wide variety of urologic conditions. The Urology Center offers the highest level of specialized care in a comfortable, patient-friendly environment.

All physicians at the Urology Center are certified by the American Board of Urology and fellowship trained in urology specialties. Physicians at the Urology Center are respected leaders in their fields and are consistently recognized by peers as being among the best urologists in the New York area.

As part of a large university hospital, the Urology Center is able to provide emergency medical care 24/7 as well as bedside care for those patients requiring hospitalization. Physicians utilize state-of-the-art diagnostic and therapeutic procedures, including the latest minimally invasive techniques, to treat such conditions as symptomatic enlargement of the prostate; cancer of the prostate, kidney, bladder and other genito-urinary organs; urinary incontinence and bladder control problems; male infertility and sexual dysfunction; kidney stones; and other urologic disorders.

As the clinical arm of New York Medical College's Department of Urology, the academic affiliate of Westchester Medical College, Urology Center of Westchester Medical Center physicians are also charged with educating and training the doctors of today and tomorrow in general urology and all urology sub-specialties.

UROLOGY CENTER AT WESTCHESTER MEDICAL CENTER

The Urology Center at Westchester Medical Center provides the highest level of specialized care in all areas of urology, including:

- General Urology
- Urologic Cancer
- Prostate Cancer
- Robotic Surgery
- Laparoscopic Surgery
- Complex Stone Disease
- Endourology
- Shock Wave Lithotripsy
- Male Infertility
- Sexual Dysfunction
- Office Vasectomy
- Vasectomy Reversal
- Microwave Office Treatment for B.P.H.
- Laser Surgery for B.P.H.
- Female Urology and Incontinence
- Bladder Reconstruction

For more information, go to www.worldclassmedicine.com

790

Vascular Surgery

Maimonides Medical Center
MAIMONIDES VASCULAR INSTITUTE

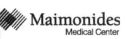
Maimonides
Medical Center

4802 Tenth Avenue • Brooklyn, New York 11219
Phone: (718) 283-7957 • Fax: (718) 283-8599
www.maimonidesmed.org

Established in 1992 by Enrico Ascher, MD, The Vascular Institute at Maimonides provides comprehensive diagnostic, clinical and vascular surgical services for patients with diseased or malfunctioning circulatory systems. It is one of only five centers in New York certified to train vascular surgeons.

One of the most successful vascular centers in the United States, providing care for more than 6,000 patients a year, The Institute has helped thousands of patients prevent the most serious of circulatory complications related to hypertension, diabetes, arteriosclerosis and other diseases. The Vascular Institute consists of the following specialty centers:

Division of Vascular Surgery
One of the busiest of its kind, the Vascular Surgery Division offers patients rapid diagnosis, personalized attention and the use of minimally invasive techniques and treatments to repair aneurysms and blocked arteries. Procedures such as balloon angioplasties and stents often eliminate the need for major surgery.

The Vein Center
The Vein Center offers several methods to remove unwanted varicose veins, including sclerotherapy, stab avulsion and laser therapy. Many of these effective and safe procedures are performed under local anesthesia on an outpatient basis.

Vascular Diagnostic Laboratory
The largest noninvasive vascular lab in New York State, it employs the most advanced technology to assess patients. Precise determinations of blood flow to vital organs and limbs are obtained here and reported rapidly, enabling physicians to make timely and informed decisions about the future course of therapy for their patients.

Wound Treatment Center
The first such center in the region, the Wound Center focuses on the needs of patients with chronic non-healing wounds of the arms and legs. The Center offers the most technologically advanced and least invasive techniques, including the use of hyperbaric chambers for the treatment of chronic wounds and infections.

Physicians at Maimonides are among the eight percent in the US who use computers to enter patient orders, thereby reducing the risk of errors, increasing efficiency, and speeding the healing process. Maimonides has appeared on the American Hospital Association's "Most Wired" and "Most Wireless" lists more often than any other healthcare institution in the metropolitan area. Advanced technology allows our doctors to focus more attention on caring for their patients.

Maimonides Medical Center – passionate about medicine, compassionate about people.

733

⌐ NewYork-Presbyterian

⌐ The University Hospital of Columbia and Cornell

NewYork-Presbyterian Vascular Center

Affiliated with Columbia University College of Physicians and Surgeons and Weill Medical College of Cornell University

NewYork-Presbyterian Hospital
Columbia University Medical Center
622 West 168th Street
New York, NY 10032

NewYork-Presbyterian Hospital
Weill Cornell Medical Center
525 East 68th Street
New York, NY 10021

OVERVIEW:

Vascular disease can affect people of all ages and requires a wide range of expertise for appropriate and effective therapies. The NewYork-Presbyterian Hospital Vascular Care Center offers a comprehensive and integrated program for the prevention, diagnosis and treatment of diverse problems relating to arteries and veins throughout the body, including the heart, abdomen, kidneys, legs, neck and brain.

The Center brings together medical and surgical experts of two internationally renowned academic medical centers – NewYork-Presbyterian Hospital/Columbia University Medical Center and NewYork-Presbyterian Hospital/Weill Cornell Medical Center – who bring a depth of experience to treating even the most unusual vascular conditions. Patients benefit from the Vascular Care Center's proven cutting edge technologies, innovative programs and groundbreaking research.

The NewYork-Presbyterian Vascular Care Center meets the needs of its patients through:
- Programs that emphasize prevention measures;

- Rigorous screenings and integrated care for patients at risk for life-threatening vascular diseases, such as strokes and abdominal aortic aneurysms;

- Innovative applications of non-invasive diagnostic technologies, including CT scans, ultrasound, MRI and MRA;

- Advances in the latest drug therapies;

- State-of-the-art surgical and minimally invasive treatments;

- New approaches in the treatment of blood clots;

- Basic and clinical research to develop more effective procedures for diagnosis and treatment.

Physician Referral: For a physician referral or to learn more about the NewYork-Presbyterian Vascular Center call toll free **1-877-NYP-WELL** (1-877-697-9355) or visit our website at **www.nypvascular.org**

COMPREHENSIVE SERVICES INCLUDE:

- Lipid Control Centers, where adults and children at risk for inherited or acquired cholesterol and lipid are evaluated and treated.

- Comprehensive Stroke Centers with an interdisciplinary Acute Stroke Team on call round the clock.

- Comprehensive Abdominal Aortic Aneurysm Program to detect and treat one of the leading causes of death, particularly in men.

- Hypertension Center for treating blocked kidney arteries, which can cause high blood pressure and kidney failure.

- Amputation Prevention Program for treating vascular blockages leading to difficulty walking or the loss of a leg.

- Gene Therapy Center includes a program to treat blocked arteries in legs.

- Wound Healing Program offers a hyperbaric oxygen chamber, growth factors and gene therapy to treat poorly healing wounds.

Sponsored Page

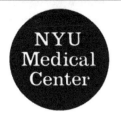

NYU Medical Center

550 First Avenue (at 31st Street)
New York, NY 10016
Physician Referral:
(888)7-NYU-MED (888-769-8633)
www.nyumc.org

VASCULAR SURGERY
A Kinder, Gentler Approach to Aneurysm Repair

When a patient has heart disease, aneurysms, or bulges in the aorta are often an unfortunate, potentially deadly symptom. Most aortic aneurysms occur in areas damaged by artherosclerosis, a condition in which the arteries become hardened from the buildup of cholesterol and other material over many years. It is estimated that one to five percent of people over the age of 65 have an aneurysm. There are usually few symptoms, although some people may feel deep back pain. Severe, excruciating pain is usually the first symptom of a rupture.

Ten years ago, a patient with an aortic aneurysm would have undergone an extensive operation to repair it. Today, NYU Medical Center is among a select group of institutions worldwide that offer minimally invasive surgical solutions to complex aortic problems.

The new, minimally invasive procedure involves making small incisions in the groin and inserting a stent graft, which the surgeon guides to the exact position in the artery needed to ease pressure and prevent rupture. Usually, patients require no blood transfusion and are able to leave the hospital just one or two days after surgery.

As the site of early FDA testing of one of the newest devices used in endovascular surgery, NYU Medical Center is leading the way in both clinical and scientific research in the burgeoning field of vascular surgery. It also is a major training center, where vascular surgeons learn and perfect the latest minimally invasive techniques. NYU's outstanding specialists continue to achieve high rates of success with the new stent graft procedure, even in patients over 75 years of age. Judging from the pace of research at NYU, it is extremely likely that the new techniques will be used to treat other types of conditions in the very near future.

NYU MEDICAL CENTER

At NYU Medical Center, we pride ourselves on delivering the highest quality care. Our emphasis on the newest surgical technologies is not an end in itself, but a way to ease pain and decrease recovery time, as well as achieve the best possible outcomes. In conventional aneurysm repair, the surgeon performs an open-chest procedure, involving blood transfusions, intensive care, and lengthy hospital stays. With the new devices and minimally invasive techniques, our patients not only get well – they return to normal activity and improved quality of life as soon as one week after surgery.

Physician Referral
(888) 7-NYU-MED
(888-769-8633)
www.mininvasive.med.nyu.edu

724

Wound Care

CALVARY HOSPITAL

1740 Eastchester Road
Bronx, NY 10461
Tel: (718) 518-2300
www.calvaryhospital.org

CENTER FOR
CURATIVE & PALLIATIVE
WOUND CARE

*Offering a continuum
of treatment options for
non-healing wounds*

Center for Curative and Palliative Wound Care

Calvary Hospital

Calvary Hospital, founded in 1899, is the nation's only acute care specialty hospital dedicated to caring for inpatients with advanced cancer, and supporting their loved ones. We serve people of all faith traditions in a restraint-free environment that offers 24/7 visiting hours and extensive bereavement support for families and friends.

In addition to inpatient care, we offer outpatient care, home care, hospice, nursing home hospice, and wound care. All Calvary care is guided by the core values of compassion, respect for the dignity of every patient, and non-abandonment of patients and families.

Calvary Wound Care: A Proud Tradition

In the course of caring for people with advanced cancer, Calvary has developed outstanding expertise in care of complex, intractable wounds. We extend this care to people in the community through our outpatient clinic. In 2004, we established the Center for Curative and Palliative Wound Care, where we treat cancer patients and people with diabetes, peripheral vascular disease, and other disorders that can cause wounds.

A Personalized Approach

Our personalized approach to wound management goes beyond established curative protocols to address the larger goals of patient care, by seeking to enhance quality of life for patients and families. We strive to relieve the suffering of patients when wounds do not respond to standard interventions, or when demands of treatment are beyond their tolerance or stamina.

The Center for Curative and Palliative Wound Care offers treatment options for wounds associated with such underlying medical conditions as:

- Venous disease
- Arterial disease
- Immobility
- Chronic inflammatory conditions
- Diabetes
- Autoimmune disease
- Blood disorders
- Neuropathy
- Arthritis
- Lymphedema

We also treat post-operative wounds and wounds caused by cancer, chemotherapy, and/or radiation therapy. Wound care personnel are available to consult with nursing homes and long-term care facilities on request. Specially trained visiting nurses and therapists provide expert wound care services for patients at home.

We are a community resource for Hispanic patients in the Bronx, who have a high incidence of diabetes.

Support for Families

Family members often serve as caregivers. Our physicians and nurses strive to build a foundation of trust and open communication with patients and families. We teach family members to clean wounds and change dressings, and we are always available to answer questions or offer guidance about wound care.

Calvary services such as pastoral care, family care, nutrition counseling, and others are available to patients and families of the Center for Curative and Palliative Wound Care.

Research is integral to the mission of the Center, which is now pursuing a number of protocols focusing on novel treatments for wounds related to diabetes and other disorders.

For information or to refer a patient, please call (718) 518-2577.

756

Section Five

Appendices

Appendix A:
Medical Boards

Intro to ABMS and Osteopathic Specialties

The following pages contain descriptions of the "official" medical specialties, approved by the American Board of Medical Specialists (for M.D.s) or by the American Osteopathic Association (for D.O.s). These are important because they are the only specialties recognized by the official governing boards. There may be physicians who call themselves one kind of specialist or another, but they may not be certified by the "official" boards. There are, in fact, over 100 such "self-designated" boards, some simply groups of physicians interested in a given area of medicine with no qualifications for membership to other groups with very specific qualifications for membership.

It is important for the medical consumer to seek out physicians certified by the ABMS or AOA to assure their doctor has had the appropriate training and passed the board certification exam.

ABMS

The ABMS is an organization of ABMS approved medical specialty boards. The mission of the ABMS is to maintain and improve the quality of medical care by assisting the Member Boards in their efforts to develop and utilize professional and educational standards for the evaluation and certification of physician specialists. The intent of certification of physicians is to provide assurance to the public that a physician specialist certified by a Member Board of the ABMS has successfully completed an approved educational program and evaluation process which includes an examination designed to assess the knowledge, skills, and experience required to provide quality patient care in that specialty. The ABMS serves to coordinate the activities of its Member Boards and to provide information to the public, the government, the profession and its Members concerning issues involving specialization and certification in medicine.

Following is a list of the addresses of the various medical specialty boards approved by the ABMS. Note that there are 24 board organizations for 25 medical specialties. Psychiatry and Neurology share the same board.

Appendix A: Medical Boards

To find out if a physician is certified, consumers can call the individual boards which may charge a fee for the information, or they can contact the ABMS at 866-275-2267 (no fee) or www.abms.org.

American Board of Allergy and Immunology
510 Walnut Street, Suite 1701
Philadelphia, PA 19106-3699
(215) 592-9466, (866) 264-5568

General Certification in Allergy and Immunology. Certifications awarded since 1989 are valid for 10 years. For those certified prior to 1989 there is no recertification requirement.

American Board of Anesthesiology
4101 Lake Boone Trail
Raleigh, NC 27607-7506
(919) 881-2570

General Certification in Anesthesiology; with Special and Added Qualifications in Critical Care Medicine and Pain Management. Certifications awarded since 2000 are valid for 10 years.

American Board of Colon and Rectal Surgery
20600 Eureka Road, Suite 600
Taylor, MI 48180
(734) 282-9400

General Certification in Colon and Rectal Surgery. Certifications awarded since 1990 are valid for 10 years.

American Board of Dermatology
Henry Ford Health System
Detriot, MI 48202-3450
(313) 874-1088

General Certification in Dermatology; with Special Qualifications in Clinical and Laboratory Dermatological Immunology, Dermatopathology, and Pediatric Dermatology. Certifications awarded since 1991 are valid for 10 years.

American Board of Emergency Medicine
3000 Coolidge Road
East Lansing, MI 48823-6319
(517) 332-4800

General Certification in Emergency Medicine; with Special and Added Qualifications in Medical Toxicology, Pediatric Emergency Medicine, Sports Medicine and Undersea and Hyperbaric Medicine. Certifications awarded since 1980 are valid for 10 years.

American Board of Family Practice
2228 Young Drive
Lexington, KY 40505-4294
(859) 269-5626, (888) 995-5700

General Certification in Family Practice; with Added Qualifications in Adolescent Medicine, Geriatric Medicine and Sports Medicine. Certifications awarded since 1970 are valid for 7 years.

American Board of Internal Medicine
510 Walnut Street, Suite 1700
Philadelphia, PA 19106-3699
(215) 446-3500, (800) 441-ABIM

General Certification in Internal Medicine; with Special Qualifications in Cardiovascular Disease, Endocrinology, Diabetes and Metabolism, Gastroenterology, Hematology, Infectious Disease, Medical Oncology, Nephrology, Pulmonary Disease, and Rheumatology; and Added Qualifications in Adolescent Medicine, Clinical Cardiac Electrophysiology, Critical Care Medicine, Geriatric Medicine, Interventional Cardiology, Sleep Medicine, Sports Medicine and Transplant Hepatology. Certifications awarded since 1990 are valid for 10 years.

American Board of Medical Genetics
9650 Rockville Pike
Bethesda, MD 20814-3998
(301) 634-7315

General Certification in Clinical Genetics (MD), PhD Medical Genetics, Clinical Biochemical Genetics, Clinical Cytogenetics and Clinical Molecular Genetics; with Added Qualifications in Molecular Genetic Pathology. Certifications awarded since 2002 are valid for 2 years.

American Board of Neurological Surgery
6550 Fannin Street, Suite 2139
Houston, TX 77030-2701
(713) 441-6015

General Certification in Neurological Surgery. Certifications awarded since 1999 are valid for 10 years.

American Board of Nuclear Medicine
4555 Forest Park Boulevard, Suite 119
St. Louis, MO 63108
(314) 367-2225

General Certification in Nuclear Medicine. Certifications awarded since 1992 are valid for 10 years.

American Board of Obstetrics and Gynecology
2915 Vine Street, Suite 300
Dallas, TX 75204
(214) 871-1619

General Certification in Obstetrics and Gynecology; with Special Qualifications in Gynecologic Oncology, Maternal and Fetal Medicine, Reproductive Endocrinology; and Added Qualifications in Critical Care Medicine. Certifications awarded since 1986 are valid for 6 years.

American Board of Ophthalmology
111 Presidential Boulevard, Suite 241
Bala Cynwyd, PA 19004-1075
(610) 664-1175

General Certification in Orthopaedic Surgery; with Added Qualifications in Hand Surgery and Orthopaedic Sports Medicine. Certifications awarded since 1986 are valid for 10 years.

American Board of Orthopaedic Surgery
400 Silver Cedar Court
Chapel Hill, NC 27514
(919) 929-7103

General Certification in Orthopaedic Surgery; with Added Qualification in Hand Surgery.

American Board of Otolaryngology
5615 Kirby Drive, Suite 600
Houston, TX 77005
(713) 850-0399

General Certification in Otolaryngology; with Added Qualifications in Neurotology, Pediatric Otolaryngology and Plastic Surgery within the Head and Neck. Certifications awarded since 2002 are valid for 10 years.

American Board of Pathology
P.O. Box 25915
Tampa, FL 33622-5915
(813) 286-2444

General Certification in Anatomic and Clinical Pathology, Anatomic Pathology and Clinical Pathology; with Special Qualifications in Blood Banking/Transfusion Medicine, Chemical Pathology, Dermatopathology, Forensic Pathology, Hematology, Medical Microbiology, Molecular Genetic Pathology, Neuropathology and Pediatric Pathology; and Added Qualifications in Cytopathology. Certifications awarded since 1997 are valid for 10 years.

American Board of Pediatrics
111 Silver Cedar Court
Chapel Hill, NC 27514-1651
(919) 929-0461

General Certification in Pediatrics; with Special Qualifications in Adolescent Medicine, Developmental-Behavioral Pediatrics, Neonatal-Perinatal Medicine, Pediatric Cardiology, Pediatric Critical Care Medicine, Pediatric Emergency Medicine, Pediatric Endocrinology, Pediatric Gastroenterology, Pediatric Hematology-Oncology, Pediatric Infectious Diseases, Pediatric Nephrology, Pediatric Pulmonology, and Pediatric Rheumatology; and Added Qualifications in Medical Toxicology, Neurodevelopmental Disabilities, Pediatric Transplant Hepatology and Sports Medicine. Certifications awarded since 1988 valid for 7 years.

American Board of Physical Medicine and Rehabilitation
3015 Allegro Park Lane, S.W.
Rochester, MN 55902-4139
(507) 282-1776

General Certification in Physical Medicine and Rehabilitation; with Special Qualifications in Pain Medicine, Pediatric Rehabilitation Medicine, and Spinal Cord Injury Medicine. Certifications awarded since 1993 are valid for 10 years.

Appendix A: Medical Boards

American Board of Plastic Surgery
  Seven Penn Center, Suite 400
  Philadelphia, PA 19103-2204
  (215) 587-9322

  General Certification in Plastic Surgery; with Added Qualifications in Hand Surgery.
  Certifications awarded since 1995 are valid for 10-years.

American Board of Preventive Medicine
  330 South Wells Street, Suite 1018
  Chicago, IL 60606-7106
  (312) 939-ABPM [2276]

  General Certification in Aerospace Medicine, Occupational Medicine and Public Health
  and General Preventive Medicine; with Added Qualifications in Undersea and
  Hyperbaric Medicine and Medical Toxicology. Certifications awarded since 1997 are
  valid for 10 years.

American Board of Psychiatry and Neurology
  500 Lake Cook Road, Suite 335
  Deerfield, IL 60015-5349
  (847) 945-7900

  General Certification in Psychiatry, Neurology and Neurology with Special Qualification
  in Child Neurology; with Special Qualifications in Child and Adolescent Psychiatry, Pain
  Medicine and Sleep Medicine; and Added Qualifications in Addiction Psychiatry,
  Clinical Neurophysiology, Forensic Psychiatry, Geriatric Psychiatry, Neurodevelopmental
  Disabilities, Psychosomatic Medicine and Vascular Neurology . Certifications awarded
  since 1994 are valid for 10 years.

American Board of Radiology
  5441 E. Williams Boulevard, Suite 200
  Tucson, AZ 85711
  (520) 790-2900

  General Certification in Diagnostic Radiology or Radiation Oncology; with Special
  Competency in Nuclear Radiology; and Added Qualifications in Neuroradiology,
  Pediatric Radiology and Vascular and Interventional Radiology. Radiological Physics is a
  non-clinical certification. Certificates are valid for 10 years.

American Board of Surgery
> 1617 John F. Kennedy Boulevard, Suite 860
> Philadelphia, PA 19103-1847
> (215) 568-4000
>
> General Certification in Surgery and Vascular Surgery; with Special Qualifications in Pediatric Surgery and Surgery of the Hand; and Added Qualifications in Surgical Critical Care. Certifications awarded since 1976 are valid for 10 years.

American Board of Thoracic Surgery
> 633 North St. Clair Street, Suite 2320
> Chicago, IL 60611
> (312) 202-5900
>
> General Certification in Thoracic Surgery. Certifications awarded since 1976 are valid for 10 years.

American Board of Urology
> 2216 Ivy Road, Suite 210
> Charlottesville, VA 22903
> (434) 979-0059
>
> General Certification in Urology. Certifications awarded as of 1985 are valid for 10 years.

Osteopathic

The American Osteopathic Association (AOA) is a member association representing more than 56,000 osteopathic physicians (D.O.s). The AOA serves as the primary certifying body for D.O.s, and is the accrediting agency for all osetopathic medical colleges and healthcare facilities. The AOA's mission is to advance the philosophy and practice of osteopathic medicine by promoting excellence in education, research, and the delivery of quality, cost-effective healthcare within a distinct, unified profession.

American Osteopathic Association
142 E Ontario Street
Chicago, IL 60611

Consumers may call the American Osteopathic Association at (800) 621-1773 or visit the website, www.osteopathic.org, for general certification information.

Appendix A: Medical Boards

American Osteopathic Board of Anesthesiology

General certification in Anesthesiology; with Added Qualifications in Addiction Medicine, Critical Care Medicine, and Pain Management. Certifications awarded since 2004 are valid for 10 years. For those certified prior to 2004 there is no recertification requirement.

American Osteopathic Board of Dermatology

General certification in Dermatology; with Added Qualifications in Dermatopathology and Mohs'-Micrographic Surgery. Certifications awarded since 2004 are valid for 10 years.

American Osteopathic Board of Emergency Medicine

General certification in Emergency Medicine; with Added Qualifications in Emergency Medical Services, Medical Toxicology, and Sports Medicine. Certifications awarded since 1994 are valid for 10 years.

American Osteopathic Board of Family Physicians

General certification in Family Practice and Osteopathic Manipulative Treatment (OMT); with Added Qualifications in Geriatric Medicine and Sports Medicine. Certifications awarded since March 1,1997 are valid for 8 years.

American Osteopathic Board of Internal Medicine

General certification in Internal Medicine; with Special Qualifications in Allergy/Immunology, Cardiology, Endocrinology, Gastroenterology, Hematology, Infectious Disease, Nephrology, Oncology, Pulmonary Disease, Rheumatology; with Added Qualifications in Addiction Medicine, Critical Care Medicine, Clinical Cardiac Electrophysiology, Geriatric Medicine, Interventional Cardiology and Sports Medicine. Certifications awarded since 1993 are valid for 10 years.

American Osteopathic Board of Neurology and Psychiatry

General certification in Neurology and Psychiatry; with Special Qualifications in Child/Adolescent Psychiatry and Child/Adolescent Neurology; with Added Qualifications in Addiction Medicine, Neurophysiology, and Sports Medicine. Certifications awarded since 1995 are valid for 10 years.

American Osteopathic Board of Neuromusculoskeletal Medicine

(Formerly American Osteopathic Board of Special Proficiency in Osteopathic Manipulative Medicine)

American Osteopathic Board of Nuclear Medicine

General certification in Nuclear Medicine. Certifications awarded since 1995 are valid for 10 years.

American Osteopathic Board of Obstetrics and Gynecology

General certification in Obstetrics and Gynecology; with Special Qualifications in Gynecologic Oncology; Maternal and Fetal Medicine and Reproductive Endocrinology. Certifications awarded since June 2002 are valid for 6 years.

American Osteopathic Board of Ophthalmology and Otolaryngology/Head and Neck Surgery

General certification in Ophthalmology, Otolaryngology, Facial Plastic Surgery and Otolaryngology/Facial Plastic Surgery; with Added Qualifications in Otolaryngic Allergy. Certifications awarded in Ophthalmology since 2000 are valid for 10 years. For those certified prior to 2000 there is no recertification requirement. Certifications awarded in Otolaryngology and/or Otolaryngology/Facial Plastic Surgery since 2002 are valid for 10 years.

American Osteopathic Board of Orthopaedic Surgery

General certification in Orthopaedic Surgery; with Added Qualifications in Hand Surgery. Certifications awarded since 1994 are valid for 10 years.

American Osteopathic Board of Pathology

General certification in Laboratory Medicine, Anatomic Pathology and Anatomic Pathology and Laboratory Medicine; with Special Qualifications in Forensic Pathology; and with Added Qualifications in Dermatopathology. Certifications awarded since 1995 are valid for 10 years.

American Osteopathic Board of Pediatrics

General certification in Pediatrics with Special Qualifications in Adolescent and Young Adult Medicine, Neonatology, Pediatric Allergy/Immunology and Pediatric Endocrinology; with Added Qualifications in Sports Medicine. Certifications awarded since 1995 are valid for 7 years.

American Osteopathic Board of Physical Medicine and Rehabilitation Medicine

General certification in Physical Medicine and Rehabilitation; with Added Qualifications in Sports Medicine. Certifications awarded since 2004 are valid for 10 years.

Appendix A: Medical Boards

American Osteopathic Board of Preventive Medicine

General certification in Preventive Medicine/Aerospace Medicine, Preventive Medicine/Occupational-Environmental Medicine and Preventive Medicine/Public Health; with Added Qualifications in Occupational Medicine and Sports Medicine. Certifications awarded since 1994 are valid for 10 years.

American Osteopathic Board of Proctology

General certification in Proctology. Certifications awarded since 2004 are valid for 10 years.

American Osteopathic Board of Radiology

General certification in Diagnostic Radiology and Radiation Oncology; with Added Qualifications in Body Imaging, Diagnostic Ultrasound, Neuroradiology, Pediatric Radiology and Vascular and Interventional Radiology. Certifications awarded since 2002 are valid for 10 years.

American Osteopathic Board of Surgery

General certification in Surgery, Neurological Surgery, Plastic and Reconstructive Surgery, Cardiothoracic Surgery, Urological Surgery and General Vascular Surgery; with Added Qualifications in Surgical Critical Care. Certifications awarded since 1997 are valid for 10 years.

Appendix B:
Self-Designated Medical Specialties

This list of self-designated medical specialty groups was obtained from the American Board of Medical Specialties. However, it is important to point out that these groups are not recognized by the ABMS, the governing board for the recognized twenty-four medical specialty boards (listed in Appendix A).

The organizations listed below range from highly organized groups that are attempting to formalize training and certification in their field to informal groups interested in a particular aspect of medicine.

If you wish to obtain information from any of these groups you will have to do some detective work. Because so many are informal, the location, phone and mailing addresses change frequently, depending upon the person who is functioning as secretary or administrator.

The best way to track down one of these groups is to consult the doctor listings to find a doctor who has expressed a special interest in that field, and call his or her office. You might also call a nearby academic health center in the area to see if they have a faculty or staff member known to be involved in that particular medical interest. If that fails, take the same approach with your community hospital.

A

Abdominal Surgeons

Acupuncture Medicine

Addiction Medicine

Addictionology

Adolescent Psychiatry

Aesthetic Plastic Surgery

Alcoholism and Other Drug
    Dependencies (AMSAODD)

Algology (Chronic Pain)

Alternative Medicine

Ambulatory Anesthesia

Ambulatory Foot Surgery

Anesthesia

Arthroscopic Surgery

Arthroscopy (Board of North America)

B

Bariatric Medicine

Bionic Psychology

Bloodless Medicine & Surgery

C

Chelation Therapy

Chemical Dependence

Clinical Chemistry

Clinical Ecology

Clinical Medicine and Surgery

Clinical Neurology

Clinical Neurophysiology

Clinical Neurosurgery

Clinical Nutrition

Clinical Orthopaedic Surgery

Clinical Pharmacology

Clinical Polysomnography

Clinical Psychiatry

Clinical Psychology

Clinical Toxicology

Cosmetic Plastic Surgery

Cosmetic Surgery

Council of Non-Board Certified Physicians

Critical Care in Medicine & Surgery

D

Disability Analysis

Disability Evaluating Physicians

E

Electrodiagnostic Medicine

Electroencephalography

Electromyography & Electrodiagnosis

Environmental Medicine

Epidemiology (College)

Eye Surgery

F

Facial Cosmetic Surgery

Facial Plastic & Reconstructive Surgery

Family Practice, Certification

Forensic Examiners

Forensic Psychiatry

Forensic Toxicology

H

Hand Surgery

Head, Facial & Neck Pain & TMJ Orthopaedics

Health Physics

Homeopathic Physicians

Homeotherapeutics

Hypnotic Anesthesiology, National Board for

I

Independent Medical Examiners

Industrial Medicine & Surgery

Insurance Medicine

International Cosmetic & Plastic
    Facial Reconstructive Standards

Interventional Radiology

L

Laser Surgery
Law in Medicine
Longevity Medicine/Surgery

M

Malpractice Physicians
Maxillofacial Surgeons
Medical Accreditation (American Federation for)
Medical Hypnosis
Medical Laboratory Immunology
Medical-Legal Analysis of Medicine & Surgery
Medical Legal & Workers
    Comp. Medicine & Surgery
Medical-Legal Consultants
Medical Management
Medical Microbiology
Medical Preventics (Academy)
Medical Psychotherapists
Medical Toxicology
Microbiology (Medical Microbiology)
Military Medicine
Mohs' Micrographic Surgery &
    Cutaneous Oncology

N

Neuroimaging
Neurologic & Orthopaedic Dental
    Medicine and Surgery
Neurological & Orthopaedic Medicine
Neurological & Orthopaedic Surgery
Neurological Microsurgery
Neurology
Neuromuscular Thermography
Neuro-Orthopaedic Dental Medicine
Neuro-Orthopaedic Electrodiagnosis
Neuro-Orthopaedic Laser Surgery
Neuro-Orthopaedic Psychiatry
Neuro-Orthopaedic Thoracic Medicine
Neurorehabilitation
Nutrition

O

Orthopaedic Medicine
Orthopaedic Microneurosurgery
Otorhinolaryngology

P

Pain Management (American Academy of)
Pain Management Specialties
Pain Medicine
Palliative Medicine
Percutaneous Diskectomy
Plastic Esthetic Surgeons
Prison Medicine
Professional Disability Consultants
Psychiatric Medicine
Psychiatry (American National Board of)
Psychoanalysis (American Examining
    Board in)
Psychological Medicine (International)

Q

Quality Assurance & Utilization Review

R

Radiology & Medical Imaging
Rheumatologic Surgery
Rheumatological & Reconstructive Medicine
Ringside Medicine & Surgery

S

Skin Specialists
Sleep Medicine (Polysomnography)
Spinal Cord Injury
Spinal Surgery
Sports Medicine
Sports Medicine/Surgery

T

Toxicology
Trauma Surgery
Traumatologic Medicine & Surgery
Tropical Medicine

U

Ultrasound Technology
Urologic Allied Health Professionals
Urological Surgery

W

Weight Reduction Medicine

APPENDIX C:
Hospital Listings

The following is an alphabetical listing of all hospitals that have at least one Castle Connolly Top Doctor in this guide. Institutions listed in **Bold** are profiled in this Guide in association with Castle Connolly's *Partnership for Excellence* program. The abbreviations as they appear in the listings are in *italics* below. Due to the many changes taking place in the hospital industry, the names on this list may have changed subsequent to publication of this guide.

Barnert Hospital (973) 977-6600
Barnert Hosp
680 Dr. Martin Luther King Jr. Way   Paterson, NJ 07514-1472   PASSAIC

Bayonne Medical Center (201) 858-5000
Bayonne Med Ctr
29 E 29th St   Bayonne, NJ 07002   HUDSON

Bayshore Community Hospital (732) 739-5900
Bayshore Community Hosp
727 North Beers Street   Holmdel, NJ 07733   MONMOUTH

Bellevue Hospital Center (212) 562-4516
Bellevue Hosp Ctr
462 First Avenue   New York, NY 10016   NEW YORK (MANHATTAN)

Beth Israel Medical Center - Kings Highway Division (718) 252-3000
Beth Israel Med Ctr- Kings Hwy Div
3201 Kings Highway   Brooklyn, NY 11234   KINGS (BROOKLYN)

Beth Israel Medical Center - Milton & Caroll Petrie Division (212) 420-2000
Beth Israel Med Ctr - Petrie Division
First Avenue @ 16th Street   New York, NY 10003   NEW YORK (MANHATTAN)

Bridgeport Hospital (203) 384-3000
Bridgeport Hosp
267 Grant St   Bridgeport, CT 06610   FAIRFIELD

Bronx Children's Psychiatric Center (718) 239-3621
Bronx Children's Psych Ctr
1000 Waters Place   Bronx, NY 10461   BRONX

Bronx Lebanon Hospital Center   (718) 590-1800
Bronx Lebanon Hosp Ctr
1650 Grand Concourse   Bronx, NY 10457   BRONX

Bronx Psychiatric Center   (718) 931-0600
Bronx Psych Ctr
1500 Waters Place   Bronx, NY 10461   BRONX

Brookdale University Hospital Medical Center   (718) 240-5000
Brookdale Univ Hosp Med Ctr
One Brookdale Plaza   Brooklyn, NY 11212   KINGS (BROOKLYN)

Brookhaven Memorial Hospital & Medical Center   (631) 654-7100
Brookhaven Meml Hosp & Med Ctr
101 Hospital Road   Patchogue, NY 11772   SUFFOLK

Brooklyn Hospital Center-Downtown   (718) 250-8000
Brooklyn Hosp Ctr-Downtown
121 DeKalb Avenue   Brooklyn, NY 11201   KINGS (BROOKLYN)

Brunswick General Hospital   (631) 789-7000
Brunswick Gen Hosp
366 Broadway   Amityville, NY 11701   SUFFOLK

Burke Rehabilitation Hospital   (914) 597-2500
Burke Rehab Hosp
785 Mamaroneck Avenue   White Plains, NY 10605   WESTCHESTER

Cabrini Medical Center   (212) 995-6000
Cabrini Med Ctr
227 East 19th Street   New York, NY 10003   NEW YORK (MANHATTAN)

Calvary Hospital   (718) 518-2000
Calvary Hosp
1740 Eastchester Road   Bronx, NY 10461   BRONX

Capital Health System - Fuld Campus   (609) 394-6000
Capital Health Sys - Fuld Campus
750 Brunswick Avenue   Trenton, NJ 08638   MERCER

Capital Health System - Mercer Campus   (609) 394-4000
Capital Hlth Sys - Mercer Campus
446 Bellevue Avenue   Trenton, NJ 08618   MERCER

CentraState Medical Center   (732) 431-2000
CentraState Med Ctr
901 West Main Street   Freehold, NJ 07728   MONMOUTH

Children's Hospital of NJ at Newark   (973) 926-4000
Chldns Hosp NJ at Newark
201 Lyons Ave N New Jersey   Newark, NJ 07112   ESSEX

Children's Specialized Hospital   (908) 233-3720
Children's Specialized Hosp
150 New Providence Rd   Mountainside, NJ 07092   UNION

Chilton Memorial Hospital   (973) 831-5000
Chilton Meml Hosp
97 West Parkway   Pompton Plains, NJ 07444   MORRIS

Christ Hospital   (201) 795-8200
Christ Hosp
176 Palisade Avenue   Jersey City, NJ 07306   HUDSON

Clara Maass Medical Center   (973) 450-2000
Clara Maass Med Ctr
One Clara Maass Drive   Belleville, NJ 07109   ESSEX

Clara Maass Medical Center - West Hudson Division   (201) 955-7000
Clara Maass Med Ctr - West Hudson Div
206 Bergen Avenue   Kearny, NJ 07032   HUDSON

Columbus Hospital   (973) 268-1400
Columbus Hosp
495 N 13th Street   Newark, NJ 07107   ESSEX

Community Hospital - Dobbs Ferry   (914) 693-0700
Comm Hosp - Dobbs Ferry
128 Ashford Ave   Dobbs Ferry, NY 10522-1924   WESTCHESTER

Coney Island Hospital   (718) 616-3000
Coney Island Hosp
2601 Ocean Parkway   Brooklyn, NY 11235   KINGS (BROOKLYN)

Danbury Hospital   (203) 797-7000
Danbury Hosp
24 Hospital Avenue   Danbury, CT 06810   FAIRFIELD

Eastern Long Island Hospital   (631) 477-1000
Eastern Long Island Hosp
201 Manor Place   Greenport, NY 11944   SUFFOLK

Elmhurst Hospital Center   (718) 334-4000
Elmhurst Hosp Ctr
79-01 Broadway   Elmhurst, NY 11373   QUEENS

Englewood Hospital & Medical Center (201) 894-3000
Englewood Hosp & Med Ctr
350 Engle Street   Englewood, NJ 07631   BERGEN

Flushing Hospital Medical Center (718) 670-5000
Flushing Hosp Med Ctr
45th Ave @ Parsons Blvd   Flushing, NY 11355   QUEENS

Four Winds Hospital (914) 763-8151
Four Winds Hosp
800 Cross River Road   Katonah, NY 10536   WESTCHESTER

Franklin Hospital Medical Center (516) 256-6000
Franklin Hosp Med Ctr
900 Franklin Avenue   Valley Stream, NY 11580   NASSAU

Good Samaritan Hospital - Suffern (845) 368-5000
Good Samaritan Hosp - Suffern
255 Lafayette Ave   Suffern, NY 10901   ROCKLAND

Good Samaritan Hospital Medical Center - West Islip (631) 376-3000
Good Samaritan Hosp Med Ctr - West Islip
1000 Montauk Highway   West Islip, NY 11795   SUFFOLK

Gracie Square Hospital (212) 988-4400
Gracie Square Hosp
420 E 76th St   New York, NY 10021   NEW YORK (MANHATTAN)

Greenville Hospital (201) 547-6100
Greenville Hosp
1825 Kennedy Boulevard   Jersey City, NJ 07305   HUDSON

Greenwich Hospital (203) 863-3000
Greenwich Hosp
Five Perryridge Road   Greenwich, CT 06830   FAIRFIELD

Hackensack University Medical Center (201) 996-2000
Hackensack Univ Med Ctr
30 Prospect Avenue   Hackensack, NJ 07601   BERGEN

Harlem Hospital Center (212) 939-1000
Harlem Hosp Ctr
506 Lenox Avenue   New York, NY 10037   NEW YORK (MANHATTAN)

Helen Hayes Hospital (845) 786-4000
Helen Hayes Hosp
Route 9 W   West Haverstraw, NY 10993   ROCKLAND

Holy Name Hospital (201) 833-3000
Holy Name Hosp
718 Teaneck Road   Teaneck, NJ 07666   BERGEN

Hospital for Joint Diseases (212) 598-6000
Hosp For Joint Diseases
301 East 17th Street   New York, NY 10003   NEW YORK (MANHATTAN)

Hospital for Special Surgery (212) 606-1000
Hosp For Special Surgery
535 East 70th Street   New York, NY 10021   NEW YORK (MANHATTAN)

Hospital of St Raphael   (203) 789-3000
Hosp of St Raphael
1450 Chapel Street   New Haven, CT 06511   NEW HAVEN

Hudson Valley Hospital Center   (914) 737-9000
Hudson Valley Hosp Ctr
1980 Crompond Road   Cortland Manor, NY 10567   WESTCHESTER

Hunterdon Medical Center   (908) 788-6100
Hunterdon Med Ctr
2100 Wescott Dr   Flemington, NJ 08822-4604   HUNTERDON

Huntington Hospital   (631) 351-2000
Huntington Hosp
270 Park Avenue   Huntington, NY 11743   SUFFOLK

Interfaith Medical Center - St John's Episcopal Hospital (718) 613-4000
Interfaith Med Ctr - St John's Episcopal Hosp
1545 Atlantic Avenue   Brooklyn, NY 11213   KINGS (BROOKLYN)

Jacobi Medical Center   (718) 918-5000
Jacobi Med Ctr
1400 Pelham Parkway South   Bronx, NY 10461   BRONX

Jamaica Hospital Medical Center   (718) 206-6000
Jamaica Hosp Med Ctr
8900 Van Wyck Expressway   Jamaica, NY 11418   QUEENS

Jersey City Medical Center   (201) 915-2000
Jersey City Med Ctr
355 Grand Street   Jersey City, NJ 07302   HUDSON

Jersey Shore University Medical Center   (732) 775-5500
Jersey Shore Univ Med Ctr
1945 Route 33   Neptune, NJ 07754   MONMOUTH

JFK Medical Center - Edison   (732) 321-7000
JFK Med Ctr - Edison
65 James Street   Edison, NJ 08818   MIDDLESEX

John T Mather Memorial Hospital of Port Jefferson   (631) 473-1320
John T Mather Meml Hosp of Port Jefferson
75 N Country Rd   Port Jefferson, NY 11777   SUFFOLK

Kessler Institute for Rehabilitation - East Orange   (973) 414-4700
Kessler Inst for Rehab - East Orange
240 Central Ave   East Orange, NJ 07018   ESSEX

Kessler Institute for Rehabilitation - West Orange   (973) 243-6800
Kessler Inst for Rehab - W Orange
1199 Pleasant Valley Way   West Orange, NJ 07052-1499   ESSEX

Kings County Hospital Center   (718) 245-3131
Kings County Hosp Ctr
451 Clarkson Avenue   Brooklyn, NY 11203   KINGS (BROOKLYN)

Kingsboro Psychiatric Center   (718) 221-7700
Kingsboro Psyc Ctr
681 Clarkson Ave   Brooklyn, NY 11203   KINGS (BROOKLYN)

Kingsbrook Jewish Medical Center   (718) 604-5000
Kingsbrook Jewish Med Ctr
585 Schenectady Avenue   Brooklyn, NY 11203   KINGS (BROOKLYN)

Lawrence Hospital Center   (914) 787-1000
Lawrence Hosp Ctr
55 Palmer Avenue   Bronxville, NY 10708   WESTCHESTER

Lenox Hill Hospital   (212) 434-2000
Lenox Hill Hosp
100 East 77th Street   New York, NY 10021   NEW YORK (MANHATTAN)

Lincoln Medical & Mental Health Center   (718) 579-5000
Lincoln Med & Mental Hlth Ctr
234 East 149th St.   Bronx, NY 10451   BRONX

Long Beach Medical Center   (516) 897-1000
Long Beach Med Ctr
455 East Bay Drive   Long Beach, NY 11561   NASSAU

Long Island College Hospital   (718) 780-1000
Long Island Coll Hosp
339 Hicks Street   Brooklyn, NY 11201   KINGS (BROOKLYN)

Long Island Jewish Medical Center   (516) 470-7000
Long Island Jewish Med Ctr
270-05 76th Avenue   New Hyde Park, NY 11040   NASSAU

Lutheran Medical Center - Brooklyn   (718) 630-7000
Lutheran Med Ctr - Brooklyn
150 55th Street   Brooklyn, NY 11220   KINGS (BROOKLYN)

Maimonides Medical Center   (718) 283-6000
Maimonides Med Ctr
4802 Tenth Avenue   Brooklyn, NY 11219   KINGS (BROOKLYN)

Manhattan Eye, Ear & Throat Hospital   (212) 838-9200
Manhattan Eye, Ear & Throat Hosp
210 East 64th Street   New York, NY 10021   NEW YORK (MANHATTAN)

Mary Immaculate Hospital   (718) 558-2000
Mary Immaculate Hosp
152-11 89th Avenue   Jamaica, NY 11432   QUEENS

Massachusetts General Hospital   (617) 726-2000
Mass Genl Hosp
55 Fruit St   Boston, MA 02114   SUFFOLK

Meadowlands Hospital Medical Center   (201) 392-3100
Meadowlands Hosp Med Ctr
55 Meadowland Parkway   Secaucus, NJ 07096   HUDSON

Memorial Sloan-Kettering Cancer Center   (212) 639-2000
Meml Sloan Kettering Cancer Ctr
1275 York Avenue   New York, NY 10021   NEW YORK (MANHATTAN)

Mercy Medical Center - Rockville Centre   (516) 705-2525
Mercy Med Ctr - Rockville Centre
1000 North Village Avenue   Rockville Centre, NY 11570   NASSAU

Metropolitan Hospital Center - NY   (212) 423-6262
Metropolitan Hosp Ctr - NY
1901 First Avenue   New York, NY 10029   NEW YORK (MANHATTAN)

Milford Hospital   (203) 876-4000
Milford Hosp
300 Seaside Ave   Milford, CT 06460   NEW HAVEN

Monmouth Medical Center   (732) 222-5200
Monmouth Med Ctr
300 Second Ave   Long Branch, NJ 07740   MONMOUTH

Montefiore Medical Center   (718) 920-4321
Montefiore Med Ctr
111 East 210 Street   Bronx, NY 10467   BRONX

Montefiore Medical Center - Weiler-Einstein Division   (718) 904-2000
Montefiore Med Ctr - Weiler-Einstein Div
1825 Eastchester Road   Bronx, NY 10461   BRONX

Morristown Memorial Hospital   (973) 971-5000
Morristown Mem Hosp
100 Madison Avenue   Morristown, NJ 07960   MORRIS

Mount Sinai Hospital of Queens   (718) 932-1000
Mount Sinai Hosp of Queens
25-10 30th Avenue   Long Island City, NY 11102   QUEENS

Mount Sinai Medical Center   (212) 241-6500
Mount Sinai Med Ctr
One Gustave L. Levy Pl   New York, NY 10029   NEW YORK (MANHATTAN)

Mount Vernon Hospital   (914) 664-8000
Mount Vernon Hosp
12 N Seventh Ave   Mount Vernon, NY 10550   WESTCHESTER

Mountainside Hospital   (973) 429-6000
Mountainside Hosp
One Bay Avenue   Montclair, NJ 07042   ESSEX

Muhlenberg Regional Medical Center   (908) 668-2000
Muhlenberg Regional Med Ctr
Park Avenue and Randolph Road   Plainfield, NJ 07061   UNION

Nassau University Medical Center   (516) 572-0123
Nassau Univ Med Ctr
2201 Hempstead Tpke   East Meadow, NY 11554   NASSAU

New Island Hospital   (516) 579-6000
New Island Hosp
4295 Hempstead Turnpike   Bethpage, NY 11714   NASSAU

New York Community Hospital   (718) 692-5300
New York Comm Hosp
2525 Kings Highway   Brooklyn, NY 11229   KINGS (BROOKLYN)

New York Downtown Hospital   (212) 312-5000
NY Downtown Hosp
170 William Street   New York, NY 10038   NEW YORK (MANHATTAN)

New York Eye & Ear Infirmary   (212) 979-4000
New York Eye & Ear Infirm
310 East 14th Street   New York, NY 10003   NEW YORK (MANHATTAN)

New York Hospital Queens   (718) 670-1231
NY Hosp Queens
56-45 Main Street   Flushing, NY 11355   QUEENS

New York Methodist Hospital   (718) 780-3000
New York Methodist Hosp
506 Sixth Street   Brooklyn, NY 11215   KINGS (BROOKLYN)

New York State Psychiatric Institute   (212) 543-5000
NY State Psychiatric Inst
1051 Riverside Dr   New York, NY 10032   NEW YORK (MANHATTAN)

New York Westchester Square Medical Center   (718) 430-7300
NY Westchester Sq Med Ctr
2475 St Raymond Ave   Bronx, NY 10461   BRONX

Newark Beth Israel Medical Center   (973) 926-7000
Newark Beth Israel Med Ctr
201 Lyons Ave   Newark, NJ 07112   ESSEX

NewYork-Presbyterian Hospital   (212) 305-2500
NY-Presby Hosp
161 Fort Washington Ave   New York, NY 10032   NEW YORK (MANHATTAN)

North General Hospital   (212) 423-4000
N Genl Hosp
1879 Madison Ave   New York, NY 10035   NEW YORK (MANHATTAN)

North Shore University Hospital at Forest Hills   (718) 830-4000
N Shore Univ Hosp at Forest Hills
102-01 66th Rd   Forest Hills, NY 11375   QUEENS

North Shore University Hospital at Glen Cove   (516) 674-7300
N Shore Univ Hosp at Glen Cove
101 St Andrew's Ln   Glen Cove, NY 11542   NASSAU

North Shore University Hospital at Manhasset   (516) 562-0100
N Shore Univ Hosp at Manhasset
300 Community Dr   Manhasset, NY 11030   NASSAU

North Shore University Hospital at Plainview   (516) 719-3000
N Shore Univ Hosp at Plainview
888 Old Country Rd   Plainview, NY 11803   NASSAU

North Shore University Hospital at Syosset		(516) 496-6400
N Shore Univ Hosp at Syosset		
221 Jericho Tpke	Syosset, NY 11791-4536	NASSAU

Northern Westchester Hospital		(914) 666-1200
Northern Westchester Hosp		
400 East Main Street	Mount Kisco, NY 10549	WESTCHESTER

Norwalk Hospital		(203) 852-2000
Norwalk Hosp		
34 Maple Street	Norwalk, CT 06856	FAIRFIELD

Nyack Hospital		(845) 348-2000
Nyack Hosp		
160 North Midland Avenue	Nyack, NY 10960	ROCKLAND

NYU Medical Center		(212) 263-7300
NYU Med Ctr		
550 First Avenue	New York, NY 10016	NEW YORK (MANHATTAN)

Ocean Medical Center		(732) 840-2200
Ocean Med Ctr		
425 Jack Martin Blvd	Brick, NJ 08724	OCEAN

Our Lady of Mercy Medical Center		(718) 920-9000
Our Lady of Mercy Med Ctr		
600 E 233rd St	Bronx, NY 10466	BRONX

Overlook Hospital		(908) 522-2000
Overlook Hosp		
99 Beauvoir Ave	Summit, NJ 07901	UNION

Palisades Medical Center		(201) 854-5000
Palisades Med Ctr		
7600 River Road	North Bergen, NJ 07047	HUDSON

Parkway Hospital		(718) 990-4100
Parkway Hosp		
70-35 113th Street	Forest Hills, NY 11375	QUEENS

Pascack Valley Hospital		(201) 358-3000
Pascack Valley Hosp		
250 Old Hook Rd	Westwood, NJ 07675	BERGEN

PBI Regional Medical Center		(973) 365-4300
PBI Regional- Passaic		
350 Boulevard	Passaic, NJ 07055	PASSAIC

Peconic Bay Medical Center   (631) 548-6000
Peconic Bay Med Ctr
1300 Roanoke Avenue   Riverhead, NY 11901   SUFFOLK

Peninsula Hospital Center   (718) 734-2000
Peninsula Hosp Ctr
51-15 Beach Channel Drive   Far Rockaway, NY 11691   QUEENS

Phelps Memorial Hospital Center   (914) 366-3000
Phelps Meml Hosp Ctr
701 N Broadway   Sleepy Hollow, NY 10591   WESTCHESTER

Queens Hospital Center - Jamaica   (718) 883-3000
Queens Hosp Ctr - Jamaica
82-68 164th Street   Jamaica, NY 11432   QUEENS

Raritan Bay Medical Center - Perth Amboy Division   (732) 442-3700
Raritan Bay Med Ctr - Perth Amboy
530 New Brunswick Avenue   Perth Amboy, NJ 08861   MIDDLESEX

Riverview Medical Center   (732) 741-2700
Riverview Med Ctr
1 Riverview Plaza   Red Bank, NJ 07701   MONMOUTH

Robert Wood Johnson University Hospital - Hamilton   (609) 586-7900
Robert Wood Johnson Univ Hosp Hamilton
1 Hamilton Health Pl   Hamilton, NJ 08690   MERCER

Robert Wood Johnson University Hospital - New Brunswick   (732) 828-3000
Robert Wood Johnson Univ Hosp - New Brunswick
1 Robert Wood Johnson Pl   New Brunswick, NJ 08901   MIDDLESEX

Robert Wood Johnson University Hospital at Rahway   (732) 381-4200
Robert Wood Johnson Univ Hosp at Rahway
865 Stone St   Rahway, NJ 07065   UNION

Rockefeller University   (212) 327-8000
Rockefeller Univ
1230 York Avenue   New York, NY 10021   NEW YORK (MANHATTAN)

Rusk Institute of Rehabilitation Medicine   (212) 263-2606
Rusk Inst of Rehab Med
400 East 34th Street   New York, NY 10016   NEW YORK (MANHATTAN)

Rye Hospital Center   (914) 967-4567
Rye Hosp Ctr
754 Boston Post Rd   Rye, NY 10580   WESTCHESTER

Saint Joseph's Medical Center - Yonkers   (914) 378-7000
Saint Joseph's Med Ctr - Yonkers
127 South Broadway   Yonkers, NY 10701   WESTCHESTER

Saint Michael's Medical Center   (973) 877-5000
Saint Michael's Med Ctr
111 Central Avenue Blvd   Newark, NJ 07102   ESSEX

Saint Vincent Catholic Medical Centers - St Vincent's Manhattan   (212) 604-7000
St Vincent Cath Med Ctrs - Manhattan
170 West 12th Street   New York, NY 10011   NEW YORK (MANHATTAN)

Saint Vincent Catholic Medical Centers - St Vincent's Staten Island   (718) 818-1234
St Vincent Cath Med Ctr - Staten Island
355 Bard Ave   Staten Island, NY 10310-1699   RICHMOND (STATEN ISLAND)

Saint Vincent Catholic Medical Centers - St. Vincent's Westchester   (914) 967-6500
St Vincent Cath Med Ctrs - Westchester
275 North Street   Harrison, NY 10528   WESTCHESTER

Schneider Children's Hospital   (718) 470-3000
Schneider Chldn's Hosp
269-01 76th Ave   New Hyde Park, NY 11040   NASSAU

Silver Hill Hospital   (203) 966-3561
Silver Hill Hosp
208 Valley Rd   New Canaan, CT 06840-3899   FAIRFIELD

Somerset Medical Center   (908) 685-2200
Somerset Med Ctr
110 Rehill Ave   Somerville, NJ 08876   SOMERSET

Sound Shore Medical Center - Westchester   (914) 632-5000
Sound Shore Med Ctr - Westchester
16 Guion Pl   New Rochelle, NY 10802   WESTCHESTER

South Nassau Communities Hospital   (516) 632-3000
South Nassau Comm Hosp
1 Healthy Way   Oceanside, NY 11572   NASSAU

South Oaks Hospital   (631) 264-4000
S Oaks Hosp
400 Sunrise Hwy   Amityville, NY 11701   SUFFOLK

Southampton Hospital   (631) 726-8200
Southampton Hosp
240 Meeting House Ln   Southampton, NY 11968   SUFFOLK

Southside Hospital	(631) 968-3000
Southside Hosp	
301 E Main St　　　　Bay Shore, NY 11706	**SUFFOLK**

St Barnabas Hospital - Bronx	(718) 960-9000
St Barnabas Hosp - Bronx	
4422 Third Avenue　　　　Bronx, NY 10457	**BRONX**

St Barnabas Medical Center	(973) 322-5000
St Barnabas Med Ctr	
94 Old Short Hills Rd　　　　Livingston, NJ 07039-5672	**ESSEX**

St Catherine's of Siena Medical Center	(631) 862-3000
St Catherine's of Siena Med Ctr	
50 Rt 25A　　　　Smithtown, NY 11787	**SUFFOLK**

St Charles Hospital	(631) 474-6000
St Charles Hosp	
200 Belle Terre Rd　　　　Port Jefferson, NY 11777	**SUFFOLK**

St Clare's Hospital - Denville	(973) 625-6000
St Clare's Hosp - Denville	
25 Pocono Road　　　　Denville, NJ 07834	**MORRIS**

St Clare's Hospital - Dover	(973) 989-3000
St Clare's Hosp - Dover	
400 W Blackwell St　　　　Dover, NJ 07801	**MORRIS**

St Francis Hospital - The Heart Center	(516) 562-6000
St Francis Hosp - The Heart Ctr	
100 Port Washington Boulevard　　　　Roslyn, NY 11576	**NASSAU**

St Francis Medical Center - Trenton	(609) 599-5000
St Francis Med Ctr - Trenton	
601 Hamilton Avenue　　　　Trenton, NJ 08629	**MERCER**

St John's Episcopal Hospital - South Shore	(718) 869-7000
St John's Epis Hosp - S Shore	
327 Beach 19th Street　　　　Far Rockaway, NY 11691	**QUEENS**

St John's Queens Hospital	(718) 558-1000
St John's Queens Hosp	
90-02 Queens Boulevard　　　　Elmhurst, NY 11373	**QUEENS**

St John's Riverside Hospital	(914) 964-4444
St John's Riverside Hosp	
967 N Broadway　　　　Yonkers, NY 10701	**WESTCHESTER**

St Joseph Wayne Hospital   (973) 942-6900
St Joseph's Wayne Hosp
224 Hamburg Tpke   Wayne, NJ 07470   PASSAIC

St Joseph's Regional Medical Center - Paterson   (973) 754-2000
St Joseph's Regl Med Ctr - Paterson
703 Main St   Paterson, NJ 07503   PASSAIC

St Lawrence Rehabilitation Center   (609) 896-9500
St Lawrence Rehab Ctr
2381 Lawrencville Rd   Lawrencville, NJ 08648   MERCER

St Luke's - Roosevelt Hospital Center - Roosevelt Division   (212) 523-4000
St Luke's - Roosevelt Hosp Ctr - Roosevelt Div
1000 Tenth Avenue   New York, NY 10019   NEW YORK (MANHATTAN)

St Luke's - Roosevelt Hospital Center - St Luke's Hospital   (212) 523-4000
St Luke's - Roosevelt Hosp Ctr - St Luke's Hosp
1111 Amsterdam Ave   New York, NY 10025   NEW YORK (MANHATTAN)

St Mary Hospital - Hoboken   (201) 418-1000
St Mary Hosp - Hoboken
308 Willow Ave   Hoboken, NJ 07030   HUDSON

St Mary's Hospital - Passaic   (973) 470-3000
St Mary's Hosp - Passaic
211 Pennington Ave   Passaic, NJ 07055   PASSAIC

St Mary's Hospital - Waterbury   (203) 709-6000
St Mary's Hosp - Waterbury
56 Franklin St   Waterbury, CT 06706-1200   New Haven

St Peter's University Hospital   (732) 745-8600
St Peter's Univ Hosp
254 Easton Ave   New Brunswick, NJ 08901-1780   MIDDLESEX

St Vincent's Medical Center - Bridgeport   (203) 576-6000
St Vincent's Med Ctr - Bridgeport
2800 Main St   Bridgeport, CT 06606   FAIRFIELD

St. Joseph's Wayne Hospital   (973) 942-6900
Wayne Hosp
224 Hamburg Turnpike   Wayne, NJ 07470   PASSAIC

St. Mary's Hospital For Children   (718) 281-8800
St Mary's Hosp for Chldn
29-01 216th St   Bayside, NY 11360-2899   QUEENS

St. Vincent's Midtown Hospital (212) 586-1500
St. Vincent's Midtown
415 W 51st St   New York, NY 10019   NEW YORK (MANHATTAN)

Stamford Hospital (203) 325-7000
Stamford Hosp
30 Shelburne Rd @ W Broad St, Box 9317 Stamford, CT 06902   FAIRFIELD

Staten Island University Hospital - North Site (718) 226-9000
Staten Island Univ Hosp-North Site
475 Seaview Avenue   Staten Island, NY 10305   RICHMOND (STATEN ISLAND)

Staten Island University Hospital - South Site (718) 226-2000
Staten Island Univ Hosp - South Site
375 Seguine Avenue   Staten Island, NY 10309   RICHMOND (STATEN ISLAND)

Stony Brook University Hospital (631) 689-8333
Stony Brook Univ Hosp
Nicolls Rd   Stony Brook, NY 11794-8410   SUFFOLK

Stony Lodge Hospital (914) 941-7400
Stony Lodge Hosp
40 Croton Dam Road   Ossining, NY 10562   WESTCHESTER

Summit Oaks Hospital (908) 522-7000
Summit Oaks Hosp
19 Prospect St   Summit, NJ 07902   UNION

SUNY Downstate Medical Center (718) 270-1000
SUNY Downstate Med Ctr
450 Clarkson Ave   Brooklyn, NY 11203   KINGS (BROOKLYN)

Trinitas Hospital (908) 994-5000
Trinitas Hosp
225 Williamson St   Elizabeth, NJ 07207   UNION

UMDNJ-University Behavioral HealthCare (732) 235-5500
UMDNJ-Univ Behavioral HealthCare
671 Hoes   Piscataway, NJ 08854-5635   MIDDLESEX

UMDNJ-University Hospital-Newark (973) 972-4300
UMDNJ-Univ Hosp-Newark
150 Bergen St   Newark, NJ 07103-2406   ESSEX

Union Hospital - New Jersey (908) 687-1900
Union Hosp - NJ
1000 Galloping Hill Rd   Union, NJ 07083   UNION

University Medical Center at Princeton   (609) 497-4000
Univ Med Ctr - Princeton
253 Witherspoon St   Princeton, NJ 08540   MERCER

VA Connecticut Healthcare System   (203) 932-5711
VA Conn Hlthcre Sys
950 Campbell Ave   West Haven, CT 06516   NEW HAVEN

VA Hudson Valley Health Care System-FDR/Montrose   (914) 737-4400
VA Hudson Valley-FDR/Montrose
622 Albany Post Rd   Montrose, NY 10548   WESTCHESTER

VA Medical Center - Bronx   (718) 584-9000
VA Med Ctr - Bronx
130 W Kingsbridge Rd   Bronx, NY 10468   BRONX

VA Medical Center - Brooklyn   (718) 836-6600
VA Med Ctr - Bklyn
800 Poly Pl   Bay Ridge, NY 11209   KINGS (BROOKLYN)

VA Medical Center - Manhattan   (212) 686-7500
VA Med Ctr - Manhattan
423 E 23rd St   New York, NY 10010   NEW YORK (MANHATTAN)

Valley Hospital   (201) 447-8000
Valley Hosp
223 N Van Dien Ave   Ridgewood, NJ 07450   BERGEN

Victory Memorial Hospital - Brooklyn   (718) 567-1234
Victory Memorial Hosp - Bklyn
699 92nd Street   Brooklyn, NY 11228   KINGS (BROOKLYN)

Waterbury Hospital   (203) 574-6000
Waterbury Hosp
56 Franklin St0   Waterbury, CT 06706-1200   NEW HAVEN

Westchester Medical Center   (914) 493-7000
Westchester Med Ctr
95 Grasslands Road   Valhalla, NY 10595   WESTCHESTER

White Plains Hospital Center   (914) 681-0600
White Plains Hosp Ctr
Davis Ave at E Post Rd   White Plains, NY 10601   WESTCHESTER

Winthrop - University Hospital   (516) 663-0333
Winthrop - Univ Hosp
259 1st St   Mineola, NY 11501   NASSAU

Woodhull Medical & Mental Health Center   (718) 963-8000
Woodhull Med & Mental Hlth Ctr
760 Broadway   Brooklyn, NY 11206   KINGS (BROOKLYN)

Wyckoff Heights Medical Center   (718) 963-7272
Wyckoff Heights Med Ctr
374 Stockholm Street   Brooklyn, NY 11237   KINGS (BROOKLYN)

Yale - New Haven Hospital   (203) 688-4242
Yale - New Haven Hosp
20 York St   New Haven, CT 06510   NEW HAVEN

Zucker Hillside Hospital   (718) 470-8000
Zucker Hillside Hosp
75-29 263rd St   Glen Oaks, NY 11004   QUEENS

Appendix D:
Selected Resources

GENERAL RESOURCES

AMERICAN AMBULANCE ASSOCIATION (AAA)
The American Ambulance Association represents emergency and non-emergency medical transportation providers, advocating high quality pre-hospital care and keeping these providers aware of legislation and news that may affect them.

8201 Greensboro Drive, Ste 300
McLean, VA 22102

800-523-4447
703-601-9018
fax 703-610-9005
www.the-aaa.org/

AMERICA'S HEALTH INSURANCE PLANS (AHIP)
America's Health Insurance Plans is a national trade association representing nearly 1,300 member companies providing health benefits to more than 200 million Americans.

601 Pennsylvania Ave, NW
South Building Suite 500
Washington, DC 20004

202-778-3200
fax: 202-331-7487
www.ahip.org/

AMERICAN BOARD OF MEDICAL SPECIALTIES (ABMS)
The ABMS is the authoritative body for the recognition of medical specialties, coordinating 24 medical specialty boards (including 25 medical specialties) and providing information on the board certification of doctors.

1007 Church Street, Suite 404
Evanston, IL 60201-5913

847-491-9091 or 866-ASK-ABMS
fax 847-328-3596
www.abms.org

AMERICAN HOSPITAL ASSOCIATION (AHA)
A national health advocacy organization, the AHA represents hospitals and healthcare networks in legislative and regulatory matters. In 1973 the AHA adopted the Patient Bill of Rights to help patients understand their rights and responsibilities.

1 North Franklin
Chicago, IL 60606

325 7th St. NW
Washington, DC 20004

800-424-4301 or 312-422-3000
fax 312-422-4796
www.aha.org/
800-424-4301 or 202-638-100
fax 202-626-3245

AMERICAN MEDICAL ASSOCIATION (AMA)
The AMA is an association that maintains information on physicians practicing throughout the nation. Healthcare consumers can use their database to check the location, licensing, education and specialty of many doctors in the United States.

515 North State Street
Chicago, IL 60610

800-621-8335
www.ama-assn.org/

CENTER FOR MEDICAL CONSUMERS

Provides volume and outcome data on certain medical procedures performed in New York state.

239 Thompson St.
New York, NY 10012

212-674-7105
fax 212-674-7100
medconsumers@earthlink.net
www.medicalconsumers.org

CENTERS FOR DISEASE CONTROL AND PREVENTION (CDC)

Part of the Department of Health and Human Services, the CDC's mission is to prevent and manage diseases and illnesses. Its website contains information on a range of illnesses and the research being pursued to manage them. It also provides free faxed reports on disease risk and prevention in various parts of the world.

Public Inquiries/MASO
Mailstop E11
1600 Clifton Road
Atlanta, GA 30333

1-800-311-3435

toll free number for international travelers 877 FYI-TRIP or 404-639-3534
fax information service for international travelers 888-232-3299
www.cdc.gov/netinfo.htm

THE CENTERWATCH CLINICAL TRIALS LISTING SERVICE

Profiles centers conducting clinical research by therapeutic area and geographic region, including more than 41,000 international industry and government-sponsored clinical trials and new FDA approved drug therapies, as well as 5,200 clinical trials that are actively recruiting patients.

22 Thomson Place, 47F1
Boston, MA 02210-1212

617-856-5900
fax 617-856-5901
www.centerwatch.com

HEALTH CARE CHOICES

Provides information on volume and outcomes of certain medical procedures performed in hospitals in various states throughout the country.

P.O. Box 21039
Columbus Circle Station
New York, NY 10023

212-724-9395
www.healthcarechoices.org

INTERNATIONAL ASSOCIATION FOR MEDICAL ASSISTANCE TO TRAVELLERS (IAMAT)

IAMAT is a non-profit organization that disseminates information on health and sanitary conditions worldwide. Membership is free but donations are appreciated. Members will receive a membership card making them eligible to access English speaking physicians all over the world. The organization also provides information on immunization requirements, malaria, and other tropical diseases, and sanitary and climactic conditions around the world. For information, send request in writing.

1623 Military Road #279
Niagra Falls, NY 14304-1745

716-754-4883
www.iamat.org

JOINT COMMISSION ON ACCREDITATION OF HEALTHCARE ORGANIZATIONS

The Joint Commission (JCAHO) is an independent, not-for-profit organization, which evaluates the quality and safety of care for nearly 17,000 health care organizations. To maintain and earn accreditation, organizations must have an extensive on-site review by a team of JCAHO health care professionals, at least once every three years. JCAHO is governed by a board that includes physicians, nurses, and consumers. JCAHO sets the standards by which health care quality is measured in America and around the world.

One Renaissance Boulevard
Oakbrook Terrace, IL 60181

630-792-5000
fax 630-792-5005
www.jcaho.org

MEDIC ALERT FOUNDATION

The Medic Alert Foundation (a non-profit organization) provides an "ID tag" engraved with personal medical facts, as well as a 24-hour emergency response center which can release additional personal medical details. Membership is $20/year (waived for the first year) and members need to purchase the "ID tag" which sells for as low as $35.

2323 Colorado Avenue
Turlock, CA 95382

888-633-4298
Fax 209-669-2450
www.medicalert.org

MEDLINE

One Medline Place
Mundelein, IL 60060

1-800-MEDLINE (800-633-5463)
fax 1-800-351-1512
www.medline.com

A medical database including millions of medical references and abstracts from thousands of scientific and medical journals.

THE NATIONAL CANCER INSTITUTE (NCI)

Part of the NIH, the NCI sponsors cancer clinical trials at more than 100 sites in the United States. Trials are carried out in major medical research centers, such as teaching hospitals, as well as in community hospitals, specialized medical clinics and even in doctors' offices.

Clinical Studies Support Center (CSSC)
6116 Executive Boulevard
Bethesda, MD 20892-8322

800-4-CANCER (800-422-6237)
www.nci.nih.gov
www/cancer.gov
cancergovstaff@mail.nih.gov

NATIONAL CENTER FOR COMPLEMENTARY AND ALTERNATIVE MEDICINE CLEARINGHOUSE (NCCAMC)

The NCCAMC facilitates the evaluation of alternative medical treatment modalities to help determine their effectiveness and bring alternative medicine into mainstream medicine. This agency does not provide referrals.

9000 Rockville Pike
Bethesda, MD 20892

888-644-6226
fax 866-464-3616
www.nccam.nih.gov
info@nccam.nih.gov

NATIONAL CONSUMERS LEAGUE (NCL)

NCL is a private, nonprofit consumer advocacy organization. NCL strives to investigate, educate, and advocate on a variety of issues including healthcare. Membership is $20 annually, but individuals can also write to the organization for a list of publications that non-members can purchase.

1701 K Street, NW, Suite 1200
Washington, DC 20006

202-835-3323
fax 202-835-0747
www.nclnet.org
info@nclnet.org

THE NATIONAL INSTITUTES OF HEALTH (NIH)

An organization operated by the U.S. government, the NIH operates its own hospital at which the care provided is usually related to clinical studies its researchers are undertaking. Information about the Warren G. Magnuson Clinical Center is also available.

Patient Recruitment Referral Center
9000 Rockville Pike
Bethesda, MD 20892

800-411-1222 or 301-496-4000
www.nih.gov
www.clinicaltrials.gov
nihinfo@od.nih.gov

NATIONAL INSURANCE INFORMATION INSTITUTE

The National Insurance Information Institute Helpline advises consumers on how to choose an insurance company or broker. It also offers an analysis of life insurance and assists in insurance complaints.

110 William Street
New York, NY 10038

800-942-4242 or 212-346-5500
www.iii.org

THE PATIENT ADVOCATE FOUNDATION

A national non-profit organization that provides consultation, referrals and case management to patients to ensure that they are not denied access to healthcare, insurance coverage, employment and public assistance programs during an illness. In particular, the organization maintains comprehensive information on cancer treatment options that are available to consumers through a separate website: www.oncology.com.

700 Thimble Shoals Boulevard, Suite 200
Newport News, VA 23606

800-532-5274
fax 757-873-8999
www.patientadvocate.org/
help@patientadvocate.org

PEOPLE'S MEDICAL SOCIETY

The People's Medical Society, a nonprofit organization, is focused on educating the healthcare consumer about healthcare issues and medical rights. Their website provides information on useful books and publications as well as the latest healthcare developments.

P.O. Box 868
Allentown, PA 18105

610-770-1670
fax 610-770-0607
www.peoplesmed.org/index.html
cbi@peoplesmed.org

PERSONS UNITED LIMITING SUBSTANDARDS AND ERRORS IN HEALTHCARE (P.U.L.S.E.)

A support group for the survivors of medical malpractice and substandard healthcare, this nonprofit group also advocates patient education and patient-doctor communication.

PO Box 353
3300 Park Avenue
Wantagh, NY 11793-0353

800-96-pulse (800-967-8573) or
516-579-4711
fax: 516-520-8105
www.PULSEamerica.org
www.PULSEofNY.com
pulse516@aol.com

Colorado Office

719-250-1286
PULSECOLO@YAHOO.COM

PUBLIC CITIZEN'S HEALTH AND RESEARCH GROUP

A non-profit organization, the Public Citizen's Group acts as a watchdog agency by advocating accountability and the open use of doctors' disciplinary backgrounds.

1600 20th Street NW
Washington, DC 20009

202-588-1000
www.citizen.org/hrg/

VERITAS MEDICINE

An organization that allows individuals to perform confidential, personalized searches of their clinical trials database and to access information on new treatment and drug options. The text is submitted by Harvard-affiliated doctors.

11 Cambridge Center
Cambridge, MA 02142

617-234-1500 or
877-5-TRIALS (877-587-4257)
fax 617-234-1555
www.veritasmedicine.com
info@veritasmedicine.com

Appendix E:
State Agencies

While there is a wealth of information available through these state agencies, much of it is not user-friendly. Complicated contractual agreements and other legal documents contain information that might prove to be valuable, providing a consumer can locate it and then review it with some understanding. Often a department will suggest that a consumer visit the office for guidance in reviewing the documents. However, some of these agencies provide useful information on doctors, hospitals, and HMOs. They may also offer statistical reports and consumer-oriented studies.

CONNECTICUT

DOCTORS

Department of Public Health State of Connecticut
Practitioner Licensing and Investigations Section
410 Capitol Avenue, MS#12MQA
P.O. Box 340308
Hartford, CT 06134-0308
(860) 509-7603
www.dph.state.ct.us
Attn: Physician renewal of verification

Department of Public Health State of Connecticut
Legal Office
410 Capitol Avenue, MS#12LEG
P.O. Box 340308
Hartford, CT 06134-0308
(860) 509-7600

HOSPITALS

Department of Public Health State of Connecticut
Facilities Licensing and Investigations Section
410 Capitol Avenue, MS#12HSR
P.O. Box 340308
Hartford, CT 06134-0308
(860) 509-7400

HMOs

Department of Insurance (Location address)
153 Market Street, 7th Floor
Hartford, CT 06103-0816
(860) 297-3800

Department of Insurance (Mailing address)
P.O. Box 816
Hartford, CT 06142-0816
(860) 297-3800

www.ct.gov/cid/site/default.asp

Office of Health Care Access
410 Capitol Avenue, MS#13HCA
P.O. Box 340308
Hartford, CT 06134-0308
800-797-9688

TDD 860-418-7058

www.ct.gov/ohca/site/default.asp

NEW JERSEY

Doctors

New Jersey State Board of Medical Examiners (Location address)
140 East Front Street, 2nd Floor
Trenton, NJ 08608
(609) 826-7100

New Jersey State Board of Medical Examiners (Mailing address)
P.O. Box 183
Trenton, NJ 08625-0183

http://www.state.nj.us/lps/ca/bme/index.html
bme@dca.lps.state.nj.us

Hospitals

Department of Health
Division of Health Facilities Evaluation and Licensing
P.O. Box 360
Trenton, NJ 08625
(609) 633-6800

http://www.nj.gov/health/

HMOs

Department of Health
Division of Health Facilities Evaluation and Licensing
P.O. Box 360
Trenton, NJ 08625
(609) 633-6800

Department of Health
Office of Managed Care
Market and Warren Streets
P.O. Box 360
Trenton, NJ 08625
(609) 292-8949

http://www.state.nj.us/dobi/managed.htm

Department of Banking & Insurance (Location address)
Division of Insurance, Life and Health Division
Managed Healthcare Bureau
20 West State Street, 11th Floor
Trenton, NJ 08625
(609) 292-8949

http://www.state.nj.us/dobi/

Department of Banking & Insurance (Mailing address)
Division of Insurance, Life and Health Division
Managed Healthcare Bureau
P.O. Box 325
Trenton, NJ 08625
(609) 292-5427

Office of Managed Care Hotline: 1-888-393-1062
Office of managed Care Fax: (609) 633-0807
Consumer Protection Services Main Line: (609) 292-5316

NEW YORK

DOCTORS

New York State Department of Health
Office of Professional Medical Conduct
433 River Street, Suite 303
Troy, NY 12180
(518) 402-0836
www.health.state.ny.us
For information about doctors prior to 1990, call (800) 663-6114 Mon.-Fri. 9-5.

opmc@health.state.ny.us

New York State Education Department
Division of Professional Licensing Services
State Education Building - 2nd floor
89 Washington Avenue
Albany, NY 12234
(518) 474-3817
http://www.op.nysed.gov/home.html

op4info@mail.nysed.gov

Hospitals

Office of Health Systems Management
Corning Tower, Room 1415
Empire State Plaza
Albany, NY 12237
(518) 474-7028

New York State Department of Health
Bureau of Biometrics
Corning Tower, Room 2348
Empire State Plaza
Albany, NY 12237
(518) 474-3189

HMOs

New York State Insurance Department
Health Bureau
1 Commerce Plaza, Suite 1909
Albany, NY 12257
(518) 474-4098

New York State Insurance Department
Life Policy Bureau
1 Commerce Plaza, Suite 1910
Albany, NY 12257
(518) 474-4552

New York State Department of Health
Office of Managed Care
Corning Tower, Room 1911
Albany, NY 12237
(518) 473-4178

New York State Department of Health
Records Access Office
Corning Tower, Room 2348
Empire State Plaza
Albany, NY 12237
(518) 474-8734

Indices

Subject Index

A

Academic Medical Center 12

Acute illness 21

Advertising 9, 13

Alternative medicine 44, 45, 51

Alternative therapy 38, 45

American Board of Medical Specialties (ABMS) 12, 15

American Board of Radiology 17, 19

American Medical Association (AMA) 9, 33, 54

American Medical News 26

B

Bachelor of Medicine 9

Baseline tests 30, 34

Board certification 8, 13, 17, 18, 19, 23, 41, 54

Board eligibility 18

C

Capitation 58, 63, 64

Chiropractors 10

Chronic condition 51

Clinical trials 40, 45, 46

Community hospitals 13, 21

Compendium of Certified Medical Specialists 15

Confidence in the healer 55, 59

Subject Index

G

General internists 10

Generic drugs 30

Group Model HMO 58

Group practice 20

H

Harvard/Beth Israel Center 44

Health Maintenance Organization (HMO) 7, 58

Hippocratic Oath xiii, 33

Hospital appointment 20, 21

Hospital referral services 7

I

Indemnity insurance 12, 30, 62, 66, 67

IPA 58, 62, 63

J

J.D. Power and Associates 66

L

LEXIS/NEXIS 54, 59

Licensed nurse practitioners 24

Licensure 12, 16, 24

Louis Harris Associates 66

Lupus 2, 6

Lyme disease 2, 6, 23

M

Malpractice insurance 21, 25

Managed care 2, 6, 7, 19, 21, 30, 33, 42, 51, 58, 59, 61-66, 68

Medical history 5, 34, 35, 53

Medical records 31, 35, 49, 52, 53

Medical school faculty appointment 22

Medical schools 15-17, 21, 22, 27

Medical societies 8, 9

MedStat Group 66

Midlevel providers 24, 25, 33

Multi-specialty group 24

N

National Practitioner Data Bank 48, 54

New England Journal of Medicine 44, 45

O

Office and practice arrangements 14, 15, 24

P

Q

R

S

Subject Index

T

Teaching hospitals 12,13, 21

Tertiary care 21

Third party payer 30

Towers Perrin 19, 21, 26

U

Usual and customary fee 63, 67

W

"Withholds" and "set-asides" 64

Special Expertise Index

This index lists the areas that the physicians listed in the Guide have identified as their "special expertise." These are not medical specialties. They are specific elements of disease, procedures, techniques and treatments for which these physicians are best known and are referred patients.

Spec	Name	St	Pg

A

Abdominal Imaging

Spec	Name	St	Pg
DR	Baer, J	NY	149
DR	Lubat, E	NJ	726
DR	McClennan, B	CT	968
DR	Megibow, A	NY	152
DR	Weinreb, J	CT	968

Abdominal Radiology

DR	Brancaccio, W	NY	615
DR	Newhouse, J	NY	152

Abdominal Surgery

S	Barone, J	NY	413
S	Corvalan, J	NY	346
S	Hornyak, S	NY	521
S	Raniolo, R	NY	706
S	Zeitlin, A	NY	502

Abdominal Surgery-Laparoscopic

S	Katz, L	NY	349
S	Pomp, A	NY	352
S	Schmidt, H	NJ	754

Abdominal Wall Reconstruction

PlS	Petro, J	NY	695
PlS	Stahl, R	CT	979
PS	Weinberg, G	NY	406

Abdominoplasty

PlS	Feinberg, J	NY	578
PlS	Godfrey, P	NY	304
PlS	Goldstein, R	NY	410
PlS	Hawrylo, R	NJ	883
PlS	Wells, S	NY	309

Abuse/Neglect

AM	Diaz, A	NY	120
AM	Johnson, R	NJ	767
Ger	Lachs, M	NY	171
Ger	Paris, B	NY	434

Acid-Base Disorders

Nep	Aronson, P	CT	973
Nep	Lowenstein, J	NY	213
Nep	Rastegar, A	CT	973

Acne

D	Almeida, L	NJ	874
D	Aprile, G	NY	536
D	Aranoff, S	NY	141
D	Berson, D	NY	141
D	Blank, E	NJ	799
D	Bruckstein, R	NY	536
D	Burke, K	NY	142
D	Davis, J	NY	142
D	Deitz, M	NY	427
D	Demar, L	NY	143
D	Dolitsky, C	NY	536
D	Eisert, J	NY	655
D	Falcon, R	NY	536
D	Feldman, P	NY	427
D	Fine, H	NJ	724
D	Fox, A	NJ	902
D	Fried, S	NJ	724
D	Goldberg, N	NY	655
D	Gordon, M	NY	143
D	Hefter, H	NY	536
D	Hisler, B	NY	536
D	Huh, J	NY	614
D	Lerman, J	NY	655
D	Lukash, B	NY	656
D	Maier, H	NJ	891
D	Notaro, A	NY	615
D	Pacernick, L	NY	537
D	Rosen, D	NY	382
D	Rozanski, R	NJ	771
D	Shalita, A	NY	427
D	Simon, S	NY	427
D	Stillman, M	NY	656
D	Sweeney, E	NJ	725
D	Tom, J	NY	615
D	Treiber, R	NY	657
D	Waldorf, D	NY	601
D	Walther, R	NY	148
D	Wexler, P	NY	149
Ped	Panzner, E	NJ	922

Acne & Rosacea

D	Baldwin, H	NY	426
D	Danziger, S	NY	427

Acoustic Neuroma

NS	Benjamin, V	NY	214
NS	Davis, R	NY	625
NS	Golfinos, J	NY	215
NS	Gutin, P	NY	216
NS	Hodosh, R	NJ	918
NS	Post, K	NY	217
NS	Sisti, M	NY	217
NS	Stieg, P	NY	218
Oto	Chandrasekhar, S	NY	269
Oto	Feghali, J	NY	403
Oto	Kohan, D	NY	271

Oto	Kveton, J	CT	976
Oto	Kwartler, J	NJ	920
Oto	Linstrom, C	NY	273
Oto	Roland, J	NY	274
Oto	Selesnick, S	NY	275
Oto	Storper, I	NY	276

Acupuncture

AdP	Smith, M	NY	378
IM	Ehrlich, M	NY	188
IM	Gazzara, P	NY	512
IM	Strauss, M	NY	196
N	Chernik, N	NY	625
N	Lazar, M	NJ	838
Onc	Boyd, D	CT	943
PM	Agin, C	NY	631
PM	Lu, G	NY	687
PM	Moqtaderi, F	NY	278
PM	Ngeow, J	NY	278
PMR	Agri, R	NJ	819
PMR	Atakent, P	NY	463
PMR	Dillard, J	NY	298
PMR	Lee, M	NY	300
PrM	Mamtani, R	NY	696
Psyc	Gurevich, M	NY	581
Rhu	Meed, S	NY	341
SM	Hamner, D	NY	343

ADD/ADHD

ChAP	Abright, A	NY	134
ChAP	Bartlett, J	NJ	770
ChAP	Bird, H	NY	134
ChAP	Burkes, L	NY	134
ChAP	Carlson, G	NY	613
ChAP	Coffey, B	NY	134
ChAP	Cohen, L	NY	652
ChAP	Greenberg, R	NJ	912
ChAP	Hajal, F	NY	652
ChAP	Hertzig, M	NY	134
ChAP	Hirsch, G	NY	134
ChAP	Holzer, B	NY	425
ChAP	Levine, A	NJ	722
ChAP	Newcorn, J	NY	135
ChAP	Shabry, F	NY	425
ChAP	Turecki, S	NY	136
ChiN	Andriola, M	NY	613
ChiN	Grossman, E	NJ	874
ChiN	Jacobson, R	NY	653
ChiN	Kutscher, M	NY	653
ChiN	Molofsky, W	NY	137
ChiN	Nass, R	NY	137
ChiN	Traeger, E	NJ	912
FMed	Gottesfeld, P	NY	660
Ped	Bases, H	NJ	745
Ped	Buchalter, M	NJ	745
Ped	Greenberg, W	NY	605
Ped	Kanter, A	NJ	746

Special Expertise Index

Special Expertise Index

Special Expertise Index

Spec	Name	St	Pg
Psyc	Rubin, K	NJ	865
Psyc	Russakoff, L	NY	699
Psyc	Sadock, B	NY	323
Psyc	Salkin, P	NY	323
Psyc	Schechter, J	CT	955
Psyc	Schein, J	NY	324
Psyc	Schleifer, S	NJ	790
Psyc	Schwartz, B	NY	411
Psyc	Seaman, C	NY	699
Psyc	Shear, M	NY	324
Psyc	Silver, B	NJ	924
Psyc	Smith, J	CT	956
Psyc	Spitz, H	NY	325
Psyc	Taylor, N	NY	326
Psyc	Turato, M	NY	700
Psyc	Villafranca, M	NJ	924
Psyc	Viswanathan, R	NY	465
Psyc	Wager, S	NY	326
Psyc	Wagle, S	NJ	749
Psyc	Zolkind, N	NY	700
Psyc	Zykorie, D	NJ	846

Aphasia

N	Mohr, J	NY	223

Appendix Cancer

S	Paty, P	NY	351

Arrhythmias

Spec	Name	St	Pg
CE	Batsford, W	CT	965
CE	Chinitz, L	NY	122
CE	Correia, J	NJ	767
CE	Costeas, C	NJ	768
CE	Evans, S	NY	122
CE	Fisher, J	NY	379
CE	Garan, H	NY	123
CE	Gomes, J	NY	123
CE	Lerman, B	NY	123
CE	Levine, J	NY	529
CE	Matos, J	NY	123
CE	Rubin, D	NY	648
CE	Slater, W	NY	123
CE	Steinberg, J	NY	123
CE	Suri, R	NY	483
CE	Turitto, G	NY	421
CE	Wilbur, S	NY	421
CE	Winters, S	NJ	873
Cv	Askanas, A	NY	124
Cv	Beauregard, L	NJ	857
Cv	Berkowitz, W	NJ	719
Cv	Besser, L	NY	507
Cv	Cramer, M	NY	530
Cv	Gelles, J	NY	422
Cv	Giardina, E	NY	126
Cv	Gliklich, J	NY	126
Cv	Greenberg, S	NY	531
Cv	Gupta, P	NY	423
Cv	Haft, J	NJ	720
Cv	Hecht, A	NY	127
Cv	Lotongkhum, V	NY	424
Cv	Matos, M	NY	650
Cv	Nacht, R	NY	424
Cv	Reiffel, J	NY	130
Cv	Sacchi, T	NY	425

Spec	Name	St	Pg
Cv	Saroff, A	NJ	769
Cv	Tartaglia, J	NY	651
Cv	Weissman, R	NY	652
IC	Schoenfeld, M	CT	971
IM	Qadir, S	NY	491
PCd	Agarwal, K	NJ	842
PCd	Hordof, A	NY	282
PCd	Kaplovitz, H	NY	457
PCd	Kurer, C	NJ	842
PCd	Rutkovsky, L	NY	496
PCd	Walsh, C	NY	404
PCd	Woolf, P	NY	688

Arrhythmias & Pacemakers

Cv	Kalischer, A	NJ	911
Cv	Shimony, R	NY	131
Cv	Varriale, P	NY	133
Cv	Vlay, S	NY	612

Art & Creativity

ChAP	Seaver, R	NY	653

Arterial Bypass Surgery

S	Vitale, G	NY	591
TS	Bercow, N	NY	591
VascS	Haimov, M	NY	370
VascS	Shin, C	NY	477
VascS	Tannenbaum, G	NY	709

Arterial Bypass Surgery-Leg

VascS	Dietzek, A	CT	960
VascS	Harrington, E	NY	370
VascS	Harrington, M	NY	370
VascS	Schanzer, H	NY	371
VascS	Wolodiger, F	NJ	758
VascS	Yatco, R	NY	503

Arterial Disease

VascS	Blumenthal, J	NY	369
VascS	Manno, J	NJ	757
VascS	Schwartz, K	NY	709
VascS	Stein, J	NY	371

Arterial Switch

PS	Quaegebeur, J	NY	292

Arteriovenous Malformations

NRad	Meyers, P	NY	228
NRad	Tenner, M	NY	677
NS	Beyerl, B	NJ	878
NS	Solomon, R	NY	217

Arthritis

FMed	Vincent, M	NY	431
HS	Beasley, R	NY	175
HS	Ende, L	NJ	876
HS	Kamler, K	NY	546
HS	Kulick, R	NY	389
HS	Lane, L	NY	546

Spec	Name	St	Pg
HS	Melone, C	NY	176
HS	Monsanto, E	NY	435
HS	Palmieri, T	NY	546
HS	Patel, M	NY	435
HS	Raskin, K	NY	176
IM	Joseph, J	NY	490
OrS	Bindelglass, D	CT	949
OrS	Buly, R	NY	256
OrS	Burak, G	NY	683
OrS	Deland, J	NY	257
OrS	Habermann, E	NY	684
OrS	Levy, R	NY	262
OrS	Stuchin, S	NY	266
OrS	Toriello, E	NY	496
OrS	Zelicof, S	NY	685
PMR	De Araujo, M	NY	409
PMR	Lanyi, V	NY	299
PMR	Levin, S	NY	409
PRhu	Lehman, T	NY	291
Rhu	Abramson, S	NY	338
Rhu	Brodman, R	NJ	924
Rhu	Cohen, D	NY	586
Rhu	Crane, R	NY	339
Rhu	Futran-Sheinberg, J	NY	703
Rhu	Liebling, A	CT	981
Rhu	Mascarenhas, B	NY	703
Rhu	McWhorter, J	NJ	906
Rhu	Panush, R	NJ	791
Rhu	Patel, J	NY	470
Rhu	Repice, M	NY	639
Rhu	Schwartzman, S	NY	342
Rhu	Solitar, B	NY	342

Arthritis Hand Surgery

HS	Ark, J	NJ	812
HS	Botwinick, N	NY	175
HS	Coyle, M	NJ	833
HS	Gurland, M	NJ	729
HS	Lenzo, S	NY	176
HS	Pruzansky, M	NY	176
HS	Rosenstein, R	NJ	730

Arthroplasty Imaging

DR	Potter, H	NY	153

Arthroscopic Surgery

HS	Miller-Breslow, A	NJ	730
OrS	Abrams, J	NJ	817
OrS	Bigliani, L	NY	255
OrS	Botwin, C	NJ	919
OrS	Brown, C	NY	683
OrS	Capozzi, J	NY	257
OrS	Carolan, P	CT	949
OrS	Costa, L	NJ	817
OrS	Esformes, I	NJ	739
OrS	Eswar, S	NY	496
OrS	Flynn, M	NY	516
OrS	Garfinkel, M	NJ	840
OrS	Garroway, R	NY	565
OrS	Giannaris, T	NY	496
OrS	Goldman, A	NY	496
OrS	Gomez, W	NJ	817
OrS	Gutowski, W	NJ	817
OrS	Harwin, S	NY	260

Special Expertise Index

Spec	Name	St	Pg
Pul	Benton, M	NJ	884
Pul	Bergman, M	NY	466
Pul	Bernardini, D	NY	637
Pul	Bernstein, C	NY	466
Pul	Bernstein, M	NY	466
Pul	Bevelaqua, F	NY	328
Pul	Binder, R	NY	700
Pul	Birns, R	NJ	749
Pul	Blair, L	NY	328
Pul	Blum, A	NY	581
Pul	Bondi, E	NY	466
Pul	Breidbart, D	NY	581
Pul	Brill, J	NY	700
Pul	Casino, J	NY	700
Pul	Castellano, M	NY	519
Pul	Cerrone, F	NJ	924
Pul	Chadha, J	NY	499
Pul	Chodosh, R	NY	700
Pul	Cohen, M	NY	581
Pul	Cooke, J	NY	329
Pul	De Matteo, R	NY	700
Pul	Delorenzo, L	NY	701
Pul	Dhar, S	NY	467
Pul	Di Pasquale, L	NJ	750
Pul	DiCosmo, B	NY	701
Pul	Donath, J	NY	499
Pul	Eden, E	NY	329
Pul	Elamir, M	NJ	804
Pul	Elias, J	CT	979
Pul	Fein, A	NY	582
Pul	Gagliardi, A	NY	329
Pul	Garay, S	NY	329
Pul	Goldberg, J	NJ	847
Pul	Goldblatt, K	NJ	821
Pul	Gordon, R	NY	582
Pul	Greenberg, M	NJ	790
Pul	Gribetz, A	NY	329
Pul	Grizzanti, J	NJ	896
Pul	Groopman, J	NY	467
Pul	Gulrajani, R	NY	467
Pul	Hammer, A	NY	467
Pul	Jacobowitz, M	NY	701
Pul	Kamelhar, D	NY	329
Pul	Karbowitz, S	NY	499
Pul	Karetzky, M	NJ	790
Pul	Karp, J	NY	582
Pul	Klapper, P	NY	412
Pul	Kolodny, E	NY	330
Pul	Krasnogor, L	CT	956
Pul	Krinsley, J	CT	956
Pul	Kurtz, C	CT	956
Pul	Kutnick, R	NY	330
Pul	Labissiere, J	NJ	790
Pul	Lee, M	NY	330
Pul	Lehrman, S	NY	701
Pul	Levine, S	NJ	750
Pul	Libby, D	NY	330
Pul	Lowy, J	NY	330
Pul	Mandel, M	NY	701
Pul	Maniatis, T	NY	519
Pul	Marino, A	CT	956
Pul	Marino, W	NY	412
Pul	Marks, C	NY	330
Pul	Martins, P	NY	519
Pul	Matthay, R	CT	980
Pul	McCalley, S	CT	956
Pul	Mehra, S	NY	500
Pul	Meixler, S	NY	701
Pul	Melillo, N	NJ	847
Pul	Menon, L	NY	412
Pul	Mensch, A	NY	583
Pul	Mermelstein, S	NY	583
Pul	Miarrostami, R	NY	467
Pul	Miller, R	NY	330
Pul	Nash, T	NY	331
Pul	Nath, S	NY	500
Pul	Newmark, I	NY	583
Pul	O'Donnell, T	NJ	896
Pul	Osei, C	NY	606
Pul	Pinsker, K	NY	412
Pul	Plottel, C	NY	331
Pul	Polkow, M	NJ	750
Pul	Posner, D	NY	331
Pul	Prager, K	NY	331
Pul	Prezant, D	NY	412
Pul	Pulle, D	NY	412
Pul	Raskin, J	NY	331
Pul	Rose, H	NJ	750
Pul	Rothman, N	NY	583
Pul	Rubenstein, R	NY	583
Pul	Sachs, P	CT	957
Pul	Safirstein, B	NJ	790
Pul	Saleh, A	NY	468
Pul	Sanders, A	NY	332
Pul	Sasso, L	NY	519
Pul	Scheuch, R	NY	637
Pul	Schiffman, P	NJ	847
Pul	Schneyer, B	NY	637
Pul	Schreiber, M	NY	702
Pul	Schulster, R	NY	583
Pul	Sender, J	NY	412
Pul	Silverman, J	NY	500
Pul	Simon, C	NJ	750
Pul	Sklarek, H	NY	638
Pul	Smith, P	NY	468
Pul	Steiger, D	NY	332
Pul	Steinberg, H	NY	584
Pul	Sukumaran, M	NY	332
Pul	Sussman, R	NJ	924
Pul	Tessler, S	NY	468
Pul	Thomashow, B	NY	332
Pul	Volcovici, G	NY	333
Pul	Weinberg, H	NY	702
Pul	Wolf, B	NJ	847
Pul	Wyner, P	NY	584
Pul	Yang, C	NY	584
Pul	Yip, C	NY	333
Pul	Zupnick, H	NY	584

Asthma & Allergy

Spec	Name	St	Pg
A&I	Caucino, J	NJ	901
A&I	Corriel, R	NY	527
A&I	Fonacier, L	NY	528
A&I	Fusillo, C	NY	647
A&I	Kadar, A	NY	121
A&I	Leibner, D	NJ	827
FMed	Gradler, T	NY	430
FMed	Leeds, G	NY	158
IM	Seicol, N	NY	669
Oto	Vecchiotti, A	NY	687
Pul	Amin, H	NY	466

Asthma & Chronic Lung Disease

Spec	Name	St	Pg
PPul	Loughlin, G	NY	291
Pul	Bakoss, I	NY	466

Asthma & Emphysema

Spec	Name	St	Pg
Pul	Demetis, S	NY	466
Pul	Maxfield, R	NY	330

Asthma & Sinusitis

Spec	Name	St	Pg
A&I	Harish, Z	NJ	719
A&I	Sher, E	NJ	857
PA&I	Hicks, P	NJ	743

Asthma in Pregnancy

Spec	Name	St	Pg
A&I	Ricketti, A	NJ	809
PA&I	Hicks, P	NJ	743

Asthma-Adult & Pediatric

Spec	Name	St	Pg
A&I	Novick, B	NY	528
PA&I	Colenda, M	NJ	742
Pul	Bohensky, P	NY	637
Pul	Marcus, P	NY	582

Asthma-Occupational

Spec	Name	St	Pg
Pul	Miller, A	NY	500

Atopic Dermatitis

Spec	Name	St	Pg
A&I	Rosenstreich, D	NY	378
D	Aprile, G	NY	536
D	Bagel, J	NJ	810
D	Schwartz, R	NJ	771
Ped	Kushner, S	NJ	746

Atrial Fibrillation

Spec	Name	St	Pg
CE	Gomes, J	NY	123
CE	Levine, J	NY	529
CE	Steinberg, J	NY	123
Cv	Friedman, H	NY	125
Cv	Halperin, J	NY	127
Cv	Hayes, J	NY	127
Cv	Kerstein, J	NY	423
Cv	Shimony, R	NY	131
Cv	Tenenbaum, J	NY	132
TS	Graver, L	NY	592
TS	La Mendola, C	NY	592

Atrial Septal Defect

Spec	Name	St	Pg
IC	Brown, D	NY	623
PCd	Levchuck, S	NY	570
PCd	Sommer, R	NY	283

Autism

Spec	Name	St	Pg
ChAP	Abright, A	NY	134
ChAP	Leckman, J	CT	966
ChAP	Pomeroy, J	NY	613
ChAP	Volkmar, F	CT	967
ChiN	De Carlo, R	NY	509

Special Expertise Index

Spec	Name	St	Pg
Hem	Billett, H	NY	389
Hem	Cohen, A	NJ	775
Hem	Coller, B	NY	178
Hem	De La Fuente, B	NY	178
Hem	Diaz, M	NY	178
Hem	Distenfeld, A	NY	178
Hem	Diuguid, D	NY	178
Hem	Goldenberg, A	NY	179
Hem	Hymes, K	NY	179
Hem	Kempin, S	NY	179
Hem	Rader, M	NY	603
Hem	Rand, J	NY	390
Hem	Saidi, P	NJ	833
IM	Etingin, O	NY	188
Onc	Bashevkin, M	NY	442
Onc	Burd, R	CT	944
Onc	Schleider, M	NJ	733
Onc	Waintraub, S	NJ	734
PHO	Bussel, J	NY	286
PHO	Flug, F	NJ	743
PHO	Karayalcin, G	NY	572
PHO	Parker, R	NY	633
PHO	Radel, E	NY	405
PHO	Truman, J	NY	288
PHO	Weinblatt, M	NY	573

Blepharoplasty

Spec	Name	St	Pg
Oph	Garber, P	NY	563
Oto	Pearlman, S	NY	274
PlS	Di Gregorio, V	NY	578
PlS	Silich, R	NY	307

Blistering Diseases

Spec	Name	St	Pg
D	Bystryn, J	NY	142

Blount's Disease

Spec	Name	St	Pg
OrS	Lehman, W	NY	262

Body Contouring

Spec	Name	St	Pg
PlS	Lipson, D	NJ	747
PlS	Rosen, A	NJ	789
PlS	Salisbury, R	NY	696
PlS	Verga, M	NY	308

Body Contouring after Weight Loss

Spec	Name	St	Pg
PlS	Dudick, S	NJ	864
PlS	Rose, M	NJ	865
PlS	Roth, M	NY	463

Bone & Joint Pathology

Spec	Name	St	Pg
Path	Schiller, A	NY	280

Bone & Soft Tissue Tumors

Spec	Name	St	Pg
HS	Athanasian, E	NY	175
OrS	Friedlaender, G	CT	975

Bone Cancer

Spec	Name	St	Pg
DR	Panicek, D	NY	153
OrS	Benevenia, J	NJ	783

Spec	Name	St	Pg
OrS	Lane, J	NY	261
PHO	Wexler, L	NY	288

Bone Densitometry

Spec	Name	St	Pg
DR	Barone, C	NY	150
DR	Berson, B	NY	150
DR	Klein, R	NY	657
EDM	Cosman, F	NY	602
ObG	Moss, R	NY	235

Bone Disorders

Spec	Name	St	Pg
DR	Brill, P	NY	150
DR	Donnelly, B	NJ	913
OrS	Rozbruch, S	NY	265

Bone Disorders-Metabolic

Spec	Name	St	Pg
EDM	Becker, C	NY	154
EDM	Bilezikian, J	NY	154
EDM	Bockman, R	NY	155
EDM	Shane, E	NY	157
EDM	Siris, E	NY	158

Bone Imaging

Spec	Name	St	Pg
DR	Lefkovitz, Z	NY	152
NuM	Scharf, S	NY	230

Bone Infections

Spec	Name	St	Pg
Inf	Klein, A	NY	620
Inf	Levine, J	NJ	731
Inf	Sensakovic, J	NJ	834

Bone Marrow Failure

Spec	Name	St	Pg
Hem	Castro-Malaspina, H	NY	178
PHO	Lipton, J	NY	573

Bone Marrow Pathology

Spec	Name	St	Pg
Path	Chadburn, A	NY	279
Path	Knowles, D	NY	280

Bone Marrow Transplant

Spec	Name	St	Pg
Hem	Bar, M	CT	939
Hem	Castro-Malaspina, H	NY	178
Hem	Cook, P	NY	178
Hem	Nimer, S	NY	180
Hem	Schuster, M	NY	180
Hem	Scigliano, E	NY	180
Hem	Strair, R	NJ	833
Onc	Ahmed, T	NY	671
PHO	Cairo, M	NY	286
PHO	Garvin, J	NY	287
PHO	Kernan, N	NY	287
PHO	Kushner, B	NY	287
PHO	Lipton, J	NY	573
PHO	O'Reilly, R	NY	287

Bone Pathology

Spec	Name	St	Pg
Path	Bullough, P	NY	279
Path	Kahn, L	NY	569
Path	Vigorita, V	NY	457

Bone Tumors

Spec	Name	St	Pg
OrS	Habermann, E	NY	684
OrS	Healey, J	NY	260
OrS	Kenan, S	NY	261
Path	Dorfman, H	NY	404
Path	Huvos, A	NY	279
Path	Schiller, A	NY	280
PHO	Aledo, A	NY	286
PHO	Harris, M	NJ	744
PHO	Meyers, P	NY	287
PHO	Miller, S	NY	459
PHO	Rausen, A	NY	287

Bone/Joint Infections

Spec	Name	St	Pg
Inf	Brause, B	NY	182
Inf	Romagnoli, M	NY	184
Inf	Smith, L	NJ	776
Inf	Weinstein, M	NJ	834

Botox for Facial Spasms/Dystonia

Spec	Name	St	Pg
N	Sadeghi, H	NJ	801

Botox Therapy

Spec	Name	St	Pg
D	Albom, M	NY	141
D	Bank, D	NY	654
D	Berry, R	NY	426
D	Downie, J	NJ	771
D	Gendler, E	NY	143
D	Gordon, M	NY	143
D	Greenberg, R	NY	144
D	Grodberg, M	NJ	724
D	Grossman, M	NY	144
D	Hochman, H	NY	144
D	Kline, M	NY	145
D	Kurtin, S	NY	145
D	Levine, L	NY	537
D	Maiocco, K	CT	936
D	Narins, R	NY	656
D	Notaro, A	NY	615
D	Polis, L	NY	146
D	Sklar, J	NY	537
D	Sobel, H	NY	148
D	Tesser, M	NY	148
D	Treiber, R	NY	657
D	Urbanek, R	NY	509
D	Vogel, L	NY	148
D	Wexler, P	NY	149
N	Friedlander, D	NJ	904
N	Salgado, M	NY	448
Oph	Forman, S	NY	680
Oph	Wagner, R	NJ	782
Oto	Blitzer, A	NY	269
Oto	Sclafani, A	NY	275
PlS	Diktaban, T	NY	303
PlS	Funt, D	NY	578

Special Expertise Index

Breast Cancer & Surgery

Breast Cancer - Young Women

Breast Cancer in Elderly

Special Expertise Index

Special Expertise Index

Special Expertise Index

Special Expertise Index

Special Expertise Index

Special Expertise Index

Special Expertise Index

Special Expertise Index

Spec	Name	St	Pg
Nep	Charytan, C	NY	395
Nep	Friedman, E	NY	444
Nep	Gorkin, J	NY	395
Nep	Kaufman, A	NY	213
Nep	Kozin, A	NY	604
Nep	Kozlowski, J	NJ	735
Nep	Laitman, R	NY	395
Nep	Mattana, J	NY	555
Nep	Parnes, E	NY	445
Nep	Ruddy, M	NJ	814
Nep	Shein, L	NY	446
Nep	Singhal, P	NY	556
Nep	Spitalewitz, S	NY	446

Diabetic Leg/Foot

Spec	Name	St	Pg
EDM	Sheehan, P	NY	157
VascS	Faust, G	NY	596
VascS	Giangola, G	NY	370
VascS	Simpson, A	NJ	851
VascS	Sumpio, B	CT	983
VascS	Tannenbaum, G	NY	709

Diabetic Leg/Foot Infections

Spec	Name	St	Pg
Inf	Farrer, W	NJ	915
NuM	Palestro, C	NY	559

Diabetic Neuropathy

Spec	Name	St	Pg
N	Weintraub, M	NY	677

Diagnostic Problems

Spec	Name	St	Pg
ChAP	Burkes, L	NY	134
FMed	Tamarin, S	NY	159
Ge	Walfish, J	NY	170
Ger	Libow, L	NY	172
IM	Fulop, R	NY	512
IM	Glowacki, J	NJ	860
Inf	Wormser, G	NY	666
Oph	Boniuk, V	NY	494
Oph	Lederman, M	NY	681
Ped	Asnes, R	NJ	745
Ped	Brown, J	NY	693
Ped	Zoltan, I	NY	409

Dialysis Access Surgery

Spec	Name	St	Pg
S	Greenstein, S	NY	414
S	Lois, W	NY	473
S	Rajdeo, H	NY	706
S	Shapiro, M	NJ	754
S	Tellis, V	NY	414
VascS	Chaudhry, S	NY	596
VascS	Schwartz, K	NY	709
VascS	Weintraub, N	NY	709
VascS	Yatco, R	NY	503

Dialysis Care

Spec	Name	St	Pg
Ger	Russell, R	NY	389
IM	Lebofsky, M	NY	668
IM	Stein, R	NY	195
IM	Walsh, F	CT	942
Nep	Ames, R	NY	211
Nep	Chan, B	CT	945

Spec	Name	St	Pg
Nep	Cheigh, J	NY	212
Nep	Chou, S	NY	444
Nep	Croll, J	NY	395
Nep	Das Gupta, M	NY	674
Nep	Dave, M	NY	395
Nep	Delano, B	NY	444
Nep	Feintzeig, I	CT	945
Nep	Fine, P	NJ	878
Nep	Fishbane, S	NY	555
Nep	Garrick, R	NY	674
Nep	Garvey, M	NY	212
Nep	Grodstein, G	NJ	735
Nep	Hines, W	CT	946
Nep	Kaufman, A	NY	213
Nep	Kostadaras, A	NY	493
Nep	Kozlowski, J	NJ	735
Nep	Levin, D	NJ	735
Nep	Lipner, H	NY	445
Nep	Louis, B	NY	445
Nep	Lyman, N	NJ	779
Nep	Lynn, R	NY	396
Nep	Mailloux, L	NY	555
Nep	Matalon, R	NY	213
Nep	Mittman, N	NY	445
Nep	Mossey, R	NY	556
Nep	Nathin, D	NJ	735
Nep	Pannone, J	NY	445
Nep	Pannone, J	NY	445
Nep	Parnes, E	NY	445
Nep	Pattner, A	NJ	735
Nep	Rigolosi, R	NJ	735
Nep	Shapiro, W	NY	445
Nep	Sherman, R	NJ	837
Nep	Tartini, A	NJ	735
Nep	Wagner, J	NY	556
Nep	Weizman, H	NJ	735
Nep	Winston, J	NY	214
Nep	Yablon, S	NY	604
PNep	Kaskel, F	NY	405
PNep	Salcedo, J	NJ	895
PNep	Schoeneman, M	NY	460

Diaphragm Dysfunction

Spec	Name	St	Pg
Pul	Yip, C	NY	333

Diaphragmatic hernia

Spec	Name	St	Pg
PS	Stolar, C	NY	293

Diarrheal Diseases

Spec	Name	St	Pg
Ge	Gerson, C	NY	163
Ge	Kornbluth, A	NY	165
Ge	Pochapin, M	NY	168
Inf	Blaser, M	NY	181
PGe	Glassman, M	CT	951

Disaster Psychiatry

Spec	Name	St	Pg
ChAP	Perlmutter, I	NY	484
Psyc	Dulit, R	NY	697

Disaster Relief Medicine

Spec	Name	St	Pg
PrM	Cahill, J	NY	309

Dissociative Disorders

Spec	Name	St	Pg
ChAP	Lewis, D	CT	966

Diving Medicine

Spec	Name	St	Pg
FMed	Maselli, F	NY	386
IM	Spero, M	NY	195
N	Katz, A	CT	974
PA&I	Torre, A	NJ	785

Divorce/Family Issues

Spec	Name	St	Pg
ChAP	Burkes, L	NY	134
Psyc	Oberfield, R	NY	320

Dizziness

Spec	Name	St	Pg
N	Bronster, D	NY	219
N	Klein, P	NJ	736
Oto	Lehrer, J	NJ	741

Down Syndrome

Spec	Name	St	Pg
CG	Marion, R	NY	381

Drug Abuse

Spec	Name	St	Pg
AdP	Galanter, M	NY	119
AdP	Kleber, H	NY	119
AdP	Schottenfeld, R	CT	965
AdP	Weiss, C	NY	119
N	Daras, M	NY	219
Psyc	McGowan, J	NY	319

Drug Development

Spec	Name	St	Pg
Onc	Fine, R	NY	201
Onc	Miller, V	NY	205
Onc	Spriggs, D	NY	208
PHO	Kamen, B	NJ	844

Drug Sensitivity

Spec	Name	St	Pg
A&I	Bosso, J	NY	601
A&I	Boxer, M	NY	527
A&I	Fine, S	NY	483
A&I	Fonacier, L	NY	528
A&I	Fusillo, C	NY	647
A&I	Goldman, N	NY	647
A&I	Krol, K	NJ	901
PA&I	Sampson, H	NY	281
PA&I	Sicherer, S	NY	281
Rhu	Gorevic, P	NY	339

Dual Diagnosis

Spec	Name	St	Pg
AdP	Levin, F	NY	119

Dupuytren's Contracture

Spec	Name	St	Pg
HS	Coyle, M	NJ	833
HS	Hurst, L	NY	620
HS	Miller, J	NJ	876

Special Expertise Index

Spec	Name	St	Pg
PMR	Atakent, P	NY	463
PMR	Diamond, M	NJ	923
PMR	Feinberg, J	NY	299
PMR	Filippone, M	NJ	803
PMR	Malanga, G	NJ	883
PMR	Mulford, G	NJ	883
PMR	Nelson, M	NY	694
PMR	Novick, E	NJ	923
PMR	Pechman, K	NY	694

Electrolyte Disorders

Spec	Name	St	Pg
Nep	Aronson, P	CT	973
Nep	Shein, L	NY	446
PNep	Trachtman, H	NY	574

Electromyography

Spec	Name	St	Pg
N	Alweiss, G	NJ	736
N	Herskovitz, S	NY	397
N	Kaplan, J	NY	398
N	Kelemen, J	NY	557
N	Knep, S	NJ	893
N	Kulick, S	NY	514
N	Maccabee, P	NY	447
N	Rapoport, S	NY	224
N	Roohi, F	NY	448
N	Sander, H	NY	225
N	Schlesinger, I	NY	558
N	Van Engel, D	NJ	737
N	Van Slooten, D	NJ	737
N	Witte, A	NJ	816
PMR	Braddom, R	NJ	864
PMR	Brown, A	NY	298
PMR	Cole, J	NJ	788
PMR	De Araujo, M	NY	409
PMR	Ma, D	NY	300
PMR	Root, B	NY	577
PMR	Vallarino, R	NY	463

Electrophysiologic Testing

Spec	Name	St	Pg
CE	Evans, S	NY	122
Cv	Lafferty, J	NY	508
Oph	Carr, R	NY	240

Emphysema

Spec	Name	St	Pg
IM	Bromberg, A	NJ	731
IM	Feuer, M	NY	189
IM	Horovitz, L	NY	190
IM	Kapoor, S	NY	668
IM	Minkowitz, S	NY	193
IM	Stein, S	NY	196
Pul	Abott, M	NY	465
Pul	Baskin, M	NY	328
Pul	Benton, M	NJ	884
Pul	Bernardini, D	NY	637
Pul	Bernstein, C	NY	466
Pul	Birns, R	NJ	749
Pul	Bohensky, P	NY	637
Pul	Castellano, M	NY	519
Pul	Chadha, J	NY	499
Pul	Cohen, M	NY	581
Pul	De Matteo, R	NY	700
Pul	Delorenzo, L	NY	701
Pul	Eden, E	NY	329

Spec	Name	St	Pg
Pul	Elias, J	CT	979
Pul	Goldblatt, K	NJ	821
Pul	Gordon, R	NY	582
Pul	Greenberg, M	NJ	790
Pul	Groopman, J	NY	467
Pul	Klapholz, A	NY	329
Pul	Klapper, P	NY	412
Pul	Kolodny, E	NY	330
Pul	Krasnogor, L	CT	956
Pul	Krinsley, J	CT	956
Pul	Kurtz, C	CT	956
Pul	Lee, M	NY	330
Pul	Marino, A	CT	956
Pul	Martins, P	NY	519
Pul	Mehra, S	NY	500
Pul	Meixler, S	NY	701
Pul	Miarrostami, R	NY	467
Pul	Nath, S	NY	500
Pul	Niederman, M	NY	583
Pul	Osei, C	NY	606
Pul	Plottel, C	NY	331
Pul	Rose, H	NJ	750
Pul	Rubenstein, R	NY	583
Pul	Scheuch, R	NY	637
Pul	Schneyer, B	NY	637
Pul	Schreiber, M	NY	702
Pul	Silverman, J	NY	500
Pul	Sklarek, H	NY	638
Pul	Steinberg, H	NY	584
Pul	Sussman, R	NJ	924
Pul	Thomashow, B	NY	332
Pul	Volcovici, G	NY	333
Pul	Wyner, P	NY	584
Pul	Yang, C	NY	584
Pul	Yip, C	NY	333
TS	Kline, G	NY	592

Encephalocele

Spec	Name	St	Pg
Oto	Linstrom, C	NY	273

Endocarditis

Spec	Name	St	Pg
IM	Matkovic, C	NY	622
Inf	Hartman, B	NY	182
Inf	Krieger, R	NJ	892
Inf	Quagliarello, V	CT	971

Endocrine Radiology

Spec	Name	St	Pg
DR	Knopp, E	NY	151

Endocrine Surgery

Spec	Name	St	Pg
S	Boyarsky, A	NJ	849
S	Brief, D	NJ	792
S	Budd, D	NJ	896
S	Fahey, T	NY	348
S	Ferzli, G	NY	520
S	Pertsemlidis, D	NY	351
S	Raina, S	NJ	793

Endocrine Tumors

Spec	Name	St	Pg
EDM	Amorosa, L	NJ	830
EDM	Kantor, A	NY	659

Endocrinology

Spec	Name	St	Pg
CG	Angulo, M	NY	535
EDM	Guzman, R	NY	385
EDM	Mann, D	NY	429
IM	Grajower, M	NY	392
IM	Liu, G	NY	192
IM	Rosa, J	CT	942

Endocrinology & Joint Disorders

Spec	Name	St	Pg
Rhu	Lahita, R	NJ	804

Endocrinology & Thyroid Disease

Spec	Name	St	Pg
IM	Rivlin, R	NY	194

Endometriosis

Spec	Name	St	Pg
ObG	Goldman, G	NY	233
ObG	Luciani, R	NJ	781
ObG	Tydings, L	NY	561
RE	Annos, T	NJ	791
RE	Arici, A	CT	981
RE	Copperman, A	NY	335
RE	Doyle, M	CT	957
RE	Fateh, M	NY	336
RE	Ginsburg, F	CT	957
RE	Kemmann, E	NJ	848
RE	Kenigsberg, D	NY	639
RE	Reyniak, J	NY	337
RE	Rosenfeld, D	NY	585
RE	Stangel, J	NY	703

Endoscopic Sinus Surgery

Spec	Name	St	Pg
Oto	Drake, W	NJ	920
Oto	Edelstein, D	NY	270
Oto	Farmer, H	NJ	818
Oto	Fleming, G	NJ	881
Oto	Fried, M	NY	403
Oto	Gold, S	NY	270
Oto	Henick, D	NJ	741
Oto	Jacobs, J	NY	271
Oto	Jay, J	NY	685
Oto	Josephson, J	NY	271
Oto	Krevitt, L	NY	272
Oto	Pincus, R	NY	274
Oto	Rosner, L	NY	568
Oto	Ryback, H	NY	686
Oto	Shapiro, B	NY	687
Oto	Snyder, G	NY	496

Endoscopic Surgery

Spec	Name	St	Pg
Oto	Anand, V	NY	268
Oto	Branovan, D	NY	269
Oto	Schaefer, S	NY	275
S	Nunez, D	NY	351

Endoscopic Ultrasound

Spec	Name	St	Pg
Ge	Dworkin, B	NY	661
Ge	Hertan, H	NY	387
Ge	Lightdale, C	NY	166
Ge	Pochapin, M	NY	168
S	Yiengpruksawan, A	NJ	755

Special Expertise Index

Special Expertise Index

Special Expertise Index

Special Expertise Index

Spec	Name	St	Pg
IM	Courtney, B	NJ	860
IM	Hoffman, P	CT	941
IM	Scaduto, P	NJ	877
IM	Sennett, M	CT	942
IM	Yamane, M	NJ	813

Giant Cell Arteritis
Rhu	Belilos, E	NY	585

Glanzmann's Thrombasthenia
Hem	Coller, B	NY	178

Glaucoma
Spec	Name	St	Pg
Oph	Ackerman, J	NY	451
Oph	Aries, P	NY	627
Oph	Bansal, R	NY	680
Oph	Barker, B	NY	239
Oph	Berke, S	NY	562
Oph	Bogaty, S	NY	627
Oph	Broderick, R	NY	562
Oph	Charles, N	NY	240
Oph	Cook, J	NY	562
Oph	D'Amico, R	NY	241
Oph	Davidson, L	NJ	782
Oph	Dieck, W	NY	680
Oph	Dinnerstein, S	NY	242
Oph	Dolan, R	NY	451
Oph	Engel, M	NJ	862
Oph	Esposito, D	NY	242
Oph	Feinstein, N	NY	452
Oph	Fong, R	NY	243
Oph	Freedman, J	NY	452
Oph	Friedman, A	NY	243
Oph	Girardi, A	NY	563
Oph	Glassman, M	NY	680
Oph	Goldberg, R	NY	495
Oph	Grasso, C	NY	495
Oph	Grayson, D	NY	244
Oph	Harmon, G	NY	245
Oph	Hayworth, R	NY	401
Oph	Jaffe, H	NY	452
Oph	Kaiden, J	NJ	738
Oph	Kasper, W	NY	563
Oph	Kazam, E	NJ	879
Oph	Klapper, D	NY	245
Oph	Klein, N	NY	245
Oph	Klein, R	NY	563
Oph	Kramer, P	NY	515
Oph	Lazzaro, E	NY	452
Oph	Lester, R	NY	246
Oph	Liebmann, J	NY	246
Oph	Liva, D	NJ	738
Oph	Lombardo, J	NY	452
Oph	Lombardo, J	NY	453
Oph	Manjoney, D	CT	948
Oph	Matossian, C	NJ	816
Oph	McDermott, J	NY	247
Oph	McKee, H	NY	681
Oph	Mignone, B	NY	681
Oph	Miller, B	NY	681
Oph	Miller, P	NY	782
Oph	Mitchell, J	NY	249
Oph	Mooney, R	NY	681
Oph	Nelson, D	NY	563

Spec	Name	St	Pg
Oph	Obstbaum, S	NY	250
Oph	Palmer, E	NY	401
Oph	Pinke, R	NJ	879
Oph	Podell,, D	NY	250
Oph	Podos, S	NY	250
Oph	Prince, A	NY	250
Oph	Prywes, A	NY	564
Oph	Ritch, R	NY	251
Oph	Romanelli, J	NY	629
Oph	Rosenbaum, P	NY	401
Oph	Rothberg, C	NY	629
Oph	Rubin, L	NY	564
Oph	Safran, S	NJ	816
Oph	Salzman, J	NY	682
Oph	Schneider, H	NY	252
Oph	Seidenberg, B	NJ	738
Oph	Serle, J	NY	252
Oph	Sherman, S	NY	252
Oph	Sherman, S	NY	453
Oph	Sidoti, P	NY	252
Oph	Solomon, I	NY	682
Oph	Soloway, B	NY	253
Oph	Stein, A	NY	454
Oph	Sturm, R	NY	564
Oph	Sussman, J	NY	682
Oph	Tchorbajian, K	NJ	919
Oph	Tiwari, R	NY	401
Oph	Tsai, J	NY	253
Oph	Wasserman, E	CT	949
Oph	Weinberg, M	NJ	739
Oph	Weiss, D	NY	402
Oph	Whitmore, W	NY	254
Oph	Wong, M	NJ	816
Oph	Zweibel, L	NY	629
Oph	Zweifach, P	NY	255

Glaucoma-Pediatric
Oph	Medow, N	NY	248
Oph	Raab, E	NY	250

Gliomas
N	Rosenfeld, S	NY	225
NS	Kelly, P	NY	216

Glomerulonephritis
Nep	Adler, S	NY	674
Nep	Appel, G	NY	211
Nep	Brown, E	CT	945
Nep	Chan, B	CT	945
Nep	Cohen, D	NY	212
Nep	Fogel, M	CT	945
Nep	Goldstein, C	NJ	917
Nep	Kabis, S	NJ	904
Nep	Lowenstein, J	NY	213
Nep	Rastegar, A	CT	973
Nep	Sherman, R	NY	213
Nep	Wasser, W	NY	214
PNep	Johnson, V	NY	289
PNep	Kaplan, M	NY	460
PNep	Lieberman, K	NJ	744
PNep	Seigle, R	NY	289

Glycogen Storage Diseases
PEn	Slonim, A	NY	571

Gout
Rhu	Crane, R	NY	339
Rhu	Faller, J	NY	339
Rhu	Fields, T	NY	339
Rhu	Meredith, G	NY	587
Rhu	Reinitz, E	NY	703

Graves' Disease
EDM	Davies, T	NY	155

Growth Disorders
Ped	Cohen, M	NJ	882
Ped	Rosenbaum, M	NY	297
Ped	Schutzengel, R	CT	953
Ped	Siegal, E	NY	605
Ped	Softness, B	NY	297
PEn	Anhalt, H	NJ	785
PEn	Avruskin, T	NY	458
PEn	Chin, D	NJ	881
PEn	Franklin, B	NY	284
PEn	Kohn, B	NY	284
PEn	Lebinger, T	NY	689
PEn	Oberfield, S	NY	284
PEn	Salas, M	NJ	843
PEn	Starkman, H	NJ	881
PEn	Torrado-Jule, C	NY	517
PEn	Wilson, T	NY	632

Growth Disorders in Childhood Cancer
PEn	Sklar, C	NY	285

Growth Hormone Therapy-Adult
EDM	Inzucchi, S	CT	969

Growth/Development Disorders
AM	Lopez, R	NY	120
NP	Brion, L	NY	394
Ped	Keller, B	CT	953
Ped	Zimmerman, S	NY	298
PEn	Aranoff, G	NY	404
PEn	Castro-Magana, M	NY	571
PEn	David, R	NY	284
PEn	Fennoy, I	NY	284
PEn	Fort, P	NY	571
PEn	Frank, G	NY	571
PEn	Kreitzer, P	NY	571
PEn	Noto, R	NY	689
PEn	Novogroder, M	NJ	743
PEn	Romano, A	NY	689
PEn	Speiser, P	NY	497

Gynecologic Cancer
DR	McCarthy, S	CT	968
GO	Brown, C	NY	173
GO	Carlson, J	NJ	832
GO	Chalas, E	NY	620
GO	Chuang, L	NY	173

Special Expertise Index

H

Special Expertise Index

Special Expertise Index

Spec	Name	St	Pg
HIV Retinitis			
Oph	El Baba, F	NY	628
Hives			
A&I	Blum, J	NJ	827
A&I	Bukosky, R	NJ	911
A&I	Lusman, P	NY	611
A&I	Pollowitz, J	NY	647
A&I	Southern, D	NJ	901
A&I	Weinstock, G	NY	528
Hodgkin's Disease			
Hem	Berliner, N	CT	970
Hem	Kolitz, J	NY	546
Onc	Coleman, M	NY	201
Onc	De Vita, V	CT	972
Onc	Portlock, C	NY	206
PHO	Karayalcin, G	NY	572
PHO	Weiner, M	NY	288
RadRO	Roberts, K	CT	981
RadRO	Yahalom, J	NY	335
Home Care			
Ger	Nichols, J	NY	172
Homocystinuria			
IM	Grieco, A	NY	190
Hormonal Disorders			
EDM	Freeman, R	NY	384
EDM	Goldenberg, A	NY	617
EDM	Wexler, C	NY	617
PEn	Aranoff, G	NY	404
Hospice-Palliative Care			
IM	Federman, H	NY	667
Onc	Forlenza, T	NY	513
Hospital Acquired Infections			
Inf	Corpuz, M	NY	390
Inf	Hammer, G	NY	182
Inf	Levine, J	NJ	731
Inf	Louie, E	NY	183
Inf	McLeod, G	CT	939
Inf	Press, R	NY	184
Inf	Rahal, J	NY	490
Inf	Slim, J	NJ	775
Inf	Turett, G	NY	185
PInf	Baltimore, R	CT	977
PInf	Litman, N	NY	405
PInf	Saiman, L	NY	289
HPV-Human Papillomavirus			
ObG	Corio, L	NY	232
ObG	Krause, C	NY	234
ObG	Levine, R	NY	234

Spec	Name	St	Pg
Huntington's Disease			
N	Marder, K	NY	223
Hydrocephalus			
NS	Cardoso, E	NY	446
NS	Lansen, T	NY	675
NS	Milhorat, T	NY	556
NS	Wisoff, J	NY	218
Hydronephrosis			
U	Hanna, M	NY	594
Hyperbaric Medicine			
FMed	Maselli, F	NY	386
S	Salzer, P	NY	591
S	Silvestri, F	NJ	754
S	Yurt, R	NY	355
Hypertension			
Cv	Akinboboye, O	NY	483
Cv	Anto, M	NY	529
Cv	Berkowitz, W	NJ	719
Cv	Bloomfield, D	NY	507
Cv	Clark, J	NY	422
Cv	Cole, W	NY	125
Cv	Cooper, J	NY	648
Cv	D'Agostino, R	NY	530
Cv	De Martino, A	NY	648
Cv	Devereux, R	NY	125
Cv	Epstein, S	NY	648
Cv	Fass, A	NY	648
Cv	Friedman, H	NY	125
Cv	Frishman, W	NY	649
Cv	Goodman, M	NY	531
Cv	Kamen, M	NY	128
Cv	Kleeman, H	NY	423
Cv	Kostis, J	NJ	828
Cv	Krakoff, L	NJ	721
Cv	Lazar, E	NY	128
Cv	Leff, S	NY	424
Cv	Lense, L	NY	612
Cv	Lucariello, R	NY	379
Cv	Matilsky, M	NY	612
Cv	Meller, J	NY	129
Cv	Mueller, R	NY	129
Cv	Ozick, H	NY	651
Cv	Pumill, R	NJ	721
Cv	Raska, K	NJ	873
Cv	Romanello, P	NY	130
Cv	Rosenfeld, I	NY	130
Cv	Siegel, S	NY	132
Cv	Siepser, S	NJ	891
Cv	Silver, M	NY	651
Cv	Sklaroff, H	NY	132
Cv	Sonnenblick, E	NY	380
Cv	Stroh, J	NJ	902
Cv	Unger, A	NY	133
Cv	Weinstock, M	NY	722
Cv	Wolk, M	NY	133
Cv	Zema, M	NY	613
EDM	Burroughs, V	NY	155
EDM	Leder, M	NY	486
FMed	Catanese, V	NJ	859

Spec	Name	St	Pg
FMed	De Blasio, M	NY	386
FMed	Eisenstat, S	NJ	914
FMed	Fisher, G	NY	487
FMed	Ibelli, V	NY	602
FMed	Johnson, M	NJ	773
FMed	Klein, S	NY	618
FMed	Krotowski, M	NY	430
FMed	Leeds, G	NY	158
FMed	Levine, M	NJ	800
FMed	Levites, K	NY	618
FMed	Levy, A	NY	158
FMed	McCampbell, E	NJ	773
FMed	Molnar, T	NY	487
FMed	Moynihan, B	NY	541
FMed	Roth, A	NY	487
Ger	Bullock, R	NJ	832
Ger	Kellogg, F	NY	171
Ger	Perskin, M	NY	172
IM	Altbaum, R	CT	940
IM	Ammazzalorso, M	NY	548
IM	Bell, N	NJ	904
IM	Blum, D	NY	490
IM	Blumberg, J	CT	940
IM	Brewer, M	NY	490
IM	Burkett, E	NJ	860
IM	Butt, A	NY	438
IM	Cardiello, G	NJ	801
IM	Case, D	NY	187
IM	Cohen, M	NY	187
IM	Cohn, S	NY	438
IM	Constantiner, A	NY	188
IM	Covey, A	NY	621
IM	Cusumano, S	NY	549
IM	Ditchek, A	NY	438
IM	Dreyer, N	CT	940
IM	Fazio, N	NY	667
IM	Federbush, R	NY	549
IM	Feldman, J	NJ	915
IM	Fields, S	NJ	732
IM	Fisch, M	NY	189
IM	Galton, B	NJ	893
IM	Gil, C	NJ	834
IM	Goldstein, M	NY	190
IM	Gribbon, J	NJ	777
IM	Haggerty, M	NJ	777
IM	Hendricks, J	NY	512
IM	Isaacs, E	NY	668
IM	Kaiser, S	NY	439
IM	Lebofsky, M	NY	668
IM	Lebowitz, A	NY	191
IM	Lerner, H	NY	622
IM	Masterson, R	NJ	860
IM	Melman, M	NY	669
IM	Minkowitz, S	NY	193
IM	Mojtabai, S	NY	392
IM	Molloy, E	CT	941
IM	Mutterperl, M	NJ	801
IM	Pecker, M	NY	193
IM	Pollak, H	NY	550
IM	Reuben, S	NY	491
IM	Rodman, J	NY	194
IM	Romanelli, J	NY	440
IM	Rosch, E	NY	669
IM	Rucker, S	NY	551
IM	Scaduto, P	NJ	877
IM	Solomon, G	NY	195
IM	Soltren, R	NY	670
IM	Tal, A	NY	441

Special Expertise Index

Spec	Name	St	Pg
IM	Teffera, F	NY	393
IM	Volpe, A	NJ	732
IM	Walsh, F	CT	942
IM	Weine, G	NJ	877
IM	Weinstein, M	NY	551
Nep	Adler, S	NY	674
Nep	Alterman, L	NJ	917
Nep	Ames, R	NY	211
Nep	August, P	NY	211
Nep	Bellucci, A	NY	555
Nep	Blumenfeld, J	NY	212
Nep	Brown, E	CT	945
Nep	Buzzeo, L	NY	674
Nep	Byrd, L	NJ	778
Nep	Charytan, C	NY	395
Nep	Chou, S	NY	444
Nep	Coco, M	NY	395
Nep	Covit, A	NJ	837
Nep	Croll, J	NY	395
Nep	Das Gupta, M	NY	674
Nep	De Fabritus, A	NY	212
Nep	Del Monte, M	NY	444
Nep	Fein, D	NJ	734
Nep	Feinfeld, D	NY	212
Nep	Feintzeig, I	CT	945
Nep	Fine, P	NJ	878
Nep	Flis, R	NJ	861
Nep	Galler, M	NY	492
Nep	Garfinkel, H	CT	945
Nep	Garrick, R	NY	674
Nep	Glabman, S	NY	213
Nep	Goldstein, C	NJ	917
Nep	Gorkin, J	NY	395
Nep	Grodstein, G	NJ	735
Nep	Hines, W	CT	946
Nep	Kabis, S	NJ	904
Nep	Kaufman, A	NY	213
Nep	Kleiner, M	NY	514
Nep	Kostadaras, A	NY	493
Nep	Kozin, A	NY	604
Nep	Kozlowski, J	NJ	735
Nep	Levin, D	NJ	735
Nep	Lief, P	NY	396
Nep	Lipner, H	NY	445
Nep	Louis, B	NY	445
Nep	Lowenstein, J	NY	213
Nep	Lynn, R	NY	396
Nep	Mailloux, L	NY	555
Nep	Manning, E	NJ	861
Nep	Mattana, J	NY	555
Nep	McAnally, J	NJ	917
Nep	Michelis, M	NY	213
Nep	Mittman, N	NY	445
Nep	Mossey, R	NY	556
Nep	Nathin, J	NY	735
Nep	Neelakantappa, K	NY	445
Nep	Pannone, J	NY	445
Nep	Parnes, E	NY	445
Nep	Pattner, A	NJ	735
Nep	Rascoff, J	NY	493
Nep	Reda, D	NY	674
Nep	Rie, J	NY	674
Nep	Rigolosi, R	NJ	735
Nep	Ruddy, M	NJ	814
Nep	Saltzman, M	NY	675
Nep	Schwarz, R	NY	625
Nep	Scott, D	NY	493
Nep	Shapiro, K	NY	604

Spec	Name	St	Pg
Nep	Shapiro, W	NY	445
Nep	Shein, L	NY	446
Nep	Sherman, R	NY	213
Nep	Singhal, P	NY	556
Nep	Somerstein, M	NJ	815
Nep	Spinowitz, B	NY	493
Nep	Spitalewitz, S	NY	446
Nep	Tartini, A	NJ	735
Nep	Thomsen, S	NJ	779
Nep	Uday, K	NY	396
Nep	Vitting, K	NJ	893
Nep	Wagner, J	NY	556
Nep	Wang, J	NY	214
Nep	Wei, F	NY	815
Nep	Weizman, H	NJ	735
Nep	Yablon, S	NY	604
Nep	Yoo, J	NY	396
NuM	Blaufox, M	NY	399
PNep	Flynn, J	NY	405
PNep	Johnson, V	NY	289
PNep	Kaplan, M	NY	460
PNep	Kennedy, T	CT	952
PNep	Lieberman, K	NJ	744
PNep	Salcedo, J	NJ	895
PNep	Satlin, L	NY	289
PNep	Schoeneman, M	NY	460
PNep	Trachtman, H	NY	574
PNep	Weiss, L	NJ	844
Pul	Pulle, D	NY	412

Hypertension in Pregnancy

Spec	Name	St	Pg
MF	Bond, A	CT	943
MF	Hsu, C	NY	670
Nep	August, P	NY	211

Hypertension-Postoperative

Spec	Name	St	Pg
CCM	Halpern, N	NY	140

Hypnosis

Spec	Name	St	Pg
Psyc	Zimberg, S	NY	327

Hypogonadism

Spec	Name	St	Pg
IM	Condon, E	NY	549

Hypohidrosis/Axillary Liposuction

Spec	Name	St	Pg
D	Vine, J	NJ	810

Hypospadias

Spec	Name	St	Pg
U	Burbige, K	CT	960
U	Giella, J	NY	607
U	Hanna, M	NY	594
U	Schlussel, R	NY	366
U	Wasnick, R	NY	643

Hysterectomy Alternatives

Spec	Name	St	Pg
GO	Khulpateea, N	NY	435
ObG	Burns, L	NJ	894
ObG	Goldman, G	NY	233
ObG	Gonzalez, O	NY	514
ObG	Nimaroff, M	NY	560

Spec	Name	St	Pg
ObG	Reilly, J	NY	515

Hysteroscopic Surgery

Spec	Name	St	Pg
ObG	Brennan, J	NY	449
ObG	Corio, L	NY	232
ObG	Haselkorn, J	NY	560
ObG	Iammatteo, M	NJ	879
ObG	Loiacono, A	NY	678
ObG	Nimaroff, M	NY	560
ObG	Rifkin, T	NY	561
ObG	Sailon, P	NY	236
ObG	Schneider, R	NY	679
ObG	Seiler, J	NY	237
RE	Grunfeld, L	NY	336
RE	Kelly, A	NY	336

I

Immune Deficiency

Spec	Name	St	Pg
A&I	Bernstein, L	NY	483
A&I	Bonagura, V	NY	527
A&I	Dattwyler, R	NY	647
A&I	Falk, T	NJ	719
A&I	Frieri, M	NY	528
A&I	Kadar, A	NY	121
A&I	Klein, N	NY	421
A&I	Litchman, M	CT	933
A&I	Michelis, M	NJ	719
A&I	Rubinstein, A	NY	378
A&I	Sicklick, M	NY	528
A&I	Siegal, F	NY	122
Inf	Berkey, P	NY	665
PHO	Kernan, N	NY	287
PInf	Munoz, J	NY	690
PRhu	Haines, K	NJ	744
Rhu	Parrish, E	NY	341

Immune Deficiency-Skin Disorders

Spec	Name	St	Pg
D	Edelson, R	CT	968

Immunodeficiency Disorders

Spec	Name	St	Pg
A&I	Cunningham-Rundles, C	NY	121
Rhu	Lahita, R	NJ	804

Immunologic Lung Disease

Spec	Name	St	Pg
Pul	Grizzanti, J	NJ	896

Immunotherapy

Spec	Name	St	Pg
A&I	Cunningham-Rundles, C	NY	121
Hem	Pecora, A	NJ	730
Onc	Chapman, P	NY	200
Onc	Hesdorffer, C	NJ	733
Onc	Houghton, A	NY	203
Onc	Livingston, P	NY	205
Onc	Scheinberg, D	NY	207
Onc	Slovin, S	NY	208

Special Expertise Index

Spec	Name	St	Pg
Infectious Mononucleosis			
Inf	Lutwick, L	NY	437
Infective Endocarditis			
Inf	Andriole, V	CT	971
Inf	Weinstein, M	NJ	834
Infertility			
ObG	Cherry, S	NY	231
ObG	Debrovner, C	NY	232
ObG	Friedman, A	NJ	816
ObG	Friedman, L	NY	232
ObG	Lemmerling, L	NJ	816
ObG	Mack, L	NY	560
ObG	Ott, A	NY	627
ObG	Panter, G	NY	235
ObG	Reiss, R	NY	236
ObG	Spector, I	NY	561
ObG	Tesauro, W	NY	627
ObG	Wallis, J	NJ	879
ObG	Young, B	NY	238
RE	David, S	NY	336
RE	Dlugi, A	NJ	906
RE	Fateh, M	NY	336
RE	Ginsburg, F	CT	957
RE	Kelly, A	NY	336
RE	Lesorgen, P	NJ	751
RE	Licciardi, F	NY	336
RE	Matera, C	NY	336
RE	Patrizio, P	CT	981
RE	Quagliarello, J	NY	337
RE	Ransom, M	NJ	896
RE	Santoro, N	NY	702
RE	Scott, R	NJ	884
RE	Seifer, D	NY	469
RE	Treiser, S	NJ	906
RE	Warren, M	NY	338
RE	Weiss, G	NJ	751
U	Litvin, Y	NJ	867
Infertility-Advanced Maternal Age			
RE	Seifer, D	NY	469
Infertility-IVF			
ObG	Melnick, H	NY	235
ObG	Sandler, B	NY	236
ObG	Scher, J	NY	236
RE	Annos, T	NJ	791
RE	Arici, A	CT	981
RE	Bergh, P	NJ	884
RE	Berkeley, A	NY	335
RE	Brenner, S	NY	585
RE	Cholst, I	NY	335
RE	Copperman, A	NY	335
RE	Davis, O	NY	336
RE	Dlugi, A	NJ	906
RE	Doyle, M	CT	957
RE	Grazi, R	NY	469
RE	Grifo, J	NY	336
RE	Grunfeld, L	NY	336
RE	Kemmann, E	NJ	848
RE	Kenigsberg, D	NY	639
RE	Kofinas, G	NY	469
RE	Lesorgen, P	NJ	751
RE	Licciardi, F	NY	336
RE	Mukherjee, T	NY	337
RE	Navot, D	NJ	751
RE	Noyes, N	NY	337
RE	Patrizio, P	CT	981
RE	Reyniak, J	NY	337
RE	Rosenfeld, D	NY	585
RE	Rosenwaks, Z	NY	337
RE	Sauer, M	NY	337
RE	Schmidt-Sarosi, C	NY	337
RE	Scott, R	NJ	884
RE	Slowey, M	NJ	751
RE	Stangel, J	NY	703
RE	Sultan, K	NY	337
RE	Treiser, S	NJ	906
RE	Witt, B	CT	958
Infertility-Male			
ObG	Melnick, H	NY	235
U	Bar-Chama, N	NY	360
U	Basralian, K	NJ	755
U	Fisch, H	NY	362
U	Goldstein, M	NY	362
U	Lifland, J	NJ	907
U	Lizza, E	NY	364
U	Mandel, E	NY	476
U	Matthews, G	NY	708
U	Mellinger, B	NY	594
U	Nagler, H	NY	365
U	Roberts, L	NY	708
U	Sadeghi-Nejad, H	NJ	756
U	Schlegel, P	NY	366
Infertility-Male & Female			
RE	Slowey, M	NJ	751
Infertility-Male in Spinal Cord Injury			
U	Linsenmeyer, T	NJ	794
Inflammatory Arthritis			
Rhu	Rackoff, P	NY	341
Inflammatory Bowel Disease			
CRS	Eisenstat, T	NJ	829
CRS	Longo, W	CT	967
CRS	McConnell, J	NJ	723
CRS	Milsom, J	NY	139
CRS	Moskowitz, R	NJ	874
CRS	Nizin, J	NJ	723
CRS	Ozuner, G	NY	601
CRS	Rothberg, R	NJ	770
CRS	Sonoda, T	NY	139
CRS	Zinkin, L	NJ	829
Ge	Abemayor, E	NY	661
Ge	Aisenberg, J	NY	159
Ge	Bank, S	NY	542
Ge	Bartolomeo, R	NY	542
Ge	Bleicher, R	NJ	892
Ge	Blumstein, M	NY	542
Ge	Bonheim, N	CT	938
Ge	Brandt, L	NY	387
Ge	Chinitz, M	NY	661
Ge	Finkelstein, W	NJ	774
Ge	Greenberg, R	NY	543
Ge	Grossman, E	CT	938
Ge	Gruss, C	CT	938
Ge	Itzkowitz, S	NY	164
Ge	Kahn, O	NY	663
Ge	Katz, S	NY	543
Ge	Kerner, M	NJ	914
Ge	Korelitz, B	NY	165
Ge	Kornbluth, A	NY	165
Ge	Kressner, M	NY	663
Ge	Landau, S	NY	663
Ge	Levinson, J	NJ	914
Ge	Liss, M	NY	663
Ge	Ludwig, S	NJ	859
Ge	Maizel, B	NY	432
Ge	Marin, G	NJ	811
Ge	Meirowitz, R	NJ	811
Ge	Milman, P	NY	544
Ge	Mogan, G	NJ	774
Ge	Nagler, J	NY	167
Ge	Nussbaum, M	NY	488
Ge	Panella, V	NJ	728
Ge	Roth, J	NJ	728
Ge	Rubin, K	NY	728
Ge	Rubin, P	NY	168
Ge	Sable, R	NY	388
Ge	Sachar, D	NY	169
Ge	Sachs, J	NJ	812
Ge	Salik, J	NY	169
Ge	Scherl, E	NY	169
Ge	Schrader, Z	NJ	774
Ge	Shapiro, N	NY	664
Ge	Sloan, W	NJ	774
Ge	Spielberg, A	NY	620
Ge	Spira, R	NJ	800
Ge	Tattet, S	NY	664
Ge	Taubin, H	CT	938
Ge	Turtel, P	NJ	859
Ge	Weissman, G	NY	544
Ge	Wolfson, D	NY	433
IM	Bains, Y	NJ	776
PGe	Daum, F	NY	572
PGe	Halata, M	NY	689
PGe	Kazlow, P	NY	285
PGe	Levine, J	NY	572
PGe	Newman, L	NY	690
PGe	Rabinowitz, S	NY	517
PGe	Rosh, J	NJ	882
PGe	Sunaryo, F	NJ	786
PGe	Treem, W	NY	458
PS	Harris, B	NY	406
S	Bauer, J	NY	344
S	Eng, K	NY	347
S	Harris, M	NY	349
S	Rolandelli, R	NJ	885
Inflammatory Bowel Disease/Chrohn's			
Ge	Lebwohl, O	NY	166
Inflammatory Bowel Disease/Crohn's			
CRS	Gingold, B	NY	139
CRS	Procaccino, J	NY	535
CRS	Steinhagen, R	NY	139

Special Expertise Index

Special Expertise Index

Special Expertise Index

Spec	Name	St	Pg
OrS	Scott, W	NY	265
OrS	Scuderi, G	NY	265
OrS	Sculco, T	NY	266
OrS	Seebacher, J	NY	685
OrS	Tischler, H	NY	455
OrS	Westrich, G	NY	267
OrS	Wilson, A	NY	403
OrS	Windsor, R	NY	268
OrS	Zuckerman, J	NY	268

Knee Replacement-Partial

Spec	Name	St	Pg
OrS	Bronson, M	NY	256

Knee Surgery

Spec	Name	St	Pg
OrS	Alpert, S	NY	630
OrS	Bauman, P	NY	255
OrS	Berman, M	NJ	739
OrS	Bleifeld, C	NY	630
OrS	Bosco, J	NY	256
OrS	Botwin, C	NJ	919
OrS	Brown, C	NY	683
OrS	Di Cesare, P	NY	258
OrS	Doidge, R	NJ	739
OrS	Fabian, D	NY	258
OrS	Figgie, M	NY	258
OrS	Garroway, R	NY	565
OrS	Glashow, J	NY	259
OrS	Grossman, R	NJ	863
OrS	Haas, S	NY	260
OrS	Hurley, J	NJ	880
OrS	Jokl, P	CT	975
OrS	Levin, H	NY	684
OrS	Levy, H	NY	262
OrS	Lubliner, J	NY	262
OrS	Menche, D	NY	263
OrS	Rokito, A	NY	264
OrS	Rozbruch, J	NY	265
OrS	Schwartz, E	NY	496
OrS	Turtel, A	NY	267
OrS	Wickiewicz, T	NY	267
SM	Altchek, D	NY	343
SM	Hershman, E	NY	343
SM	Kelly, M	NJ	752
SM	Orlin, H	NY	587
SM	Yerys, P	NY	587

Knee-Patella Problems

Spec	Name	St	Pg
OrS	Grelsamer, R	NY	260

L

Lacrimal Gland Disorders

Spec	Name	St	Pg
Oph	Dweck, M	NY	452
Oph	Garber, P	NY	563
Oph	Hornblass, A	NY	245

Langerhans Cell Histiocytoma

Spec	Name	St	Pg
PHO	Tugal, O	NY	690

Laparoscopic Abdominal Surgery

Spec	Name	St	Pg
S	Borao, F	NJ	867
S	Edye, M	NY	347
S	Fan, P	NJ	753
S	Garber, S	NY	589
S	Grieco, M	NY	589
S	Hofstetter, S	NY	349
S	Liang, H	NY	350
S	Pereira, S	NJ	754
S	Walsh, B	NY	706

Laparoscopic Cholecystectomy

Spec	Name	St	Pg
S	Bull, S	CT	958
S	Christoudias, G	NJ	753
S	Lansigan, N	NY	521
S	Pomeranz, L	NY	590
S	Rao, A	NY	473

Laparoscopic Colon Surgery

Spec	Name	St	Pg
S	Grieco, M	NY	589
S	Wegryn, R	NJ	925

Laparoscopic Hernia Repair

Spec	Name	St	Pg
S	Christoudias, G	NJ	753
S	Fan, P	NJ	753

Laparoscopic Hysterectomy

Spec	Name	St	Pg
ObG	Goldstein, S	NJ	862
ObG	Mendelowitz, L	NY	679

Laparoscopic Kidney Surgery

Spec	Name	St	Pg
U	Esposito, M	NJ	756
U	Wasserman, G	NJ	757

Laparoscopic Surgery

Spec	Name	St	Pg
CRS	Arvanitis, M	NJ	858
CRS	Brandeis, S	NY	138
CRS	Cohen, M	NY	654
CRS	Greenwald, M	NY	535
CRS	Groff, W	NJ	912
CRS	Holmes, N	NJ	770
CRS	Milsom, J	NY	139
CRS	Ozuner, G	NY	601
CRS	Sonoda, T	NY	139
CRS	Thornton, S	CT	935
CRS	Waxenbaum, S	NJ	723
CRS	Whelan, R	NY	140
GO	Barakat, R	NY	173
GO	Chuang, L	NY	173
GO	Curtin, J	NY	174
GO	Dottino, P	NY	174
GO	Herzog, T	NY	174
GO	Serur, E	NY	435
ObG	Afif, J	NY	399
ObG	Banzon, M	NJ	802
ObG	Brodman, M	NY	231
ObG	Carolan, S	NY	677
ObG	Cooperman, A	NJ	781
ObG	Florio, P	NY	677
ObG	Gallousis, S	NY	450
ObG	Goldman, M	NY	626
ObG	Goldstein, M	NY	233
ObG	Gonzalez, O	NY	514
ObG	Grano, V	NY	678
ObG	Guarnaccia, G	NY	494
ObG	Guirguis, F	NY	450
ObG	Haselkorn, J	NY	560
ObG	Hurst, W	NJ	737
ObG	Iammatteo, M	NJ	879
ObG	Lemmerling, L	NJ	816
ObG	Loiacono, A	NY	678
ObG	Luciani, R	NJ	781
ObG	Lynch, V	CT	975
ObG	Meacham, K	NY	678
ObG	Nimaroff, M	NY	560
ObG	Pascario, B	NY	235
ObG	Razmzan, S	NY	679
ObG	Reiss, R	NY	236
ObG	Rifkin, T	NY	561
ObG	Sailon, P	NY	236
ObG	Sassoon, R	NY	236
ObG	Schneider, R	NY	679
ObG	Strongin, M	NY	237
ObG	Taubman, R	NY	561
ObG	Tydings, L	NY	561
ObG	Wallis, J	NJ	879
PS	Friedman, D	NJ	745
PS	Gandhi, R	NJ	745
PS	Saad, S	NJ	864
PS	Shlasko, E	NY	461
RE	Copperman, A	NY	335
RE	Fateh, M	NY	336
RE	Grunfeld, L	NY	336
RE	Kelly, A	NY	336
RE	Kofinas, G	NJ	469
RE	Matera, C	NY	336
RE	Sultan, K	NY	337
S	Adler, H	NY	471
S	Amory, S	NY	344
S	Ballantyne, G	NJ	753
S	Bauer, J	NY	344
S	Befeler, D	NJ	925
S	Bessler, M	NY	345
S	Buch, E	NJ	907
S	Bufalini, B	NJ	753
S	Capizzi, A	NY	640
S	Cehelsky, J	NY	704
S	Chamberlain, R	NJ	792
S	Cohen, B	NY	640
S	Colaco, R	NJ	925
S	Corvalan, J	NY	346
S	Cosgrove, J	NY	588
S	Dasmahapatra, K	NJ	849
S	Davison, H	NJ	822
S	Denoto, G	NY	588
S	Dudrick, S	CT	982
S	Facelle, T	NY	607
S	Fahoum, B	NY	472
S	Ferzli, G	NY	520
S	Fleischer, L	NY	607
S	Fried, K	NJ	753
S	Friedman, S	NY	588
S	Frost, J	NJ	925
S	Gecelter, G	NY	589
S	Genato, R	NY	472

Special Expertise Index

Special Expertise Index

Special Expertise Index

M

Special Expertise Index

Special Expertise Index

Spec	Name	St	Pg
Metabolic Bone Disease			
EDM	Nydick, M	NY	157
EDM	Schwartz, E	NY	385
EDM	Wysolmerski, J	CT	969
OrS	Lane, J	NY	261
PEn	Carpenter, T	CT	976
Metabolic Disorders			
ChiN	De Vivo, D	NY	136
ChiN	Patterson, M	NY	137
Metabolic Genetic Disorders			
CG	Bialer, M	NY	535
CG	Willner, J	NY	138
Microsurgery			
HS	Pruzansky, M	NY	176
HS	Thomson, J	CT	970
NS	Camins, M	NY	215
Oph	Saffra, N	NY	453
PlS	Grant, R	NY	304
PlS	Liebling, R	NY	410
PlS	Siebert, J	NY	307
U	Bar-Chama, N	NY	360
U	Fisch, H	NY	362
U	Sadeghi-Nejad, H	NJ	756
Microvascular Surgery			
HS	Hurst, L	NY	620
HS	King, W	NY	176
PlS	Dagum, A	NY	635
Migraine			
ChiN	Chutorian, A	NY	136
ChiN	Grossman, E	NJ	874
ChiN	Maytal, J	NY	534
ChiN	Wolf, S	NY	137
N	Anselmi, G	NJ	801
N	Herman, M	NJ	862
N	Hughes, J	NY	398
N	Lepore, F	NJ	838
N	Marks, D	NJ	780
N	Nealon, N	NY	223
N	Newman, S	NY	558
N	Silbert, P	NJ	862
Oph	Friedman, A	NY	243
Minimally Invasive & Laser Surgery			
ObG	Hayworth, S	NY	678
Minimally Invasive Cardiac Surgery			
TS	Bercow, N	NY	591
TS	Colvin, S	NY	356
TS	Connolly, M	NJ	793
TS	Elmann, E	NJ	755
TS	Frymus, M	CT	959
TS	Goldenberg, B	NJ	897
TS	Grossi, E	NY	357
TS	Lafaro, R	NY	706
TS	Lang, S	NY	358

Spec	Name	St	Pg
TS	Loulmet, D	NY	358
TS	Oz, M	NY	358
TS	Robinson, N	NY	593
TS	Smith, C	NY	359
TS	Subramanian, V	NY	359
Minimally Invasive Heart Valve Surgery			
TS	Filsoufi, F	NY	356
TS	Galloway, A	NY	356
TS	Hartman, A	NY	592
TS	La Mendola, C	NY	592
Minimally Invasive Spinal Surgery			
OrS	Casden, A	NY	257
OrS	Goldstein, J	NY	259
OrS	Goodwin, C	NY	259
Minimally Invasive Surgery			
CRS	Guillem, J	NY	139
GO	Chuang, L	NY	173
GO	Rahaman, J	NY	174
NS	Snow, R	NY	217
ObG	Bernstein, R	NY	559
ObG	Burns, E	NY	677
ObG	Coady, D	NY	231
ObG	Goldstein, S	NJ	862
ObG	Sadarangani, B	NY	236
ObG	Seigel, M	NJ	862
ObG	Smilen, S	NY	237
ObG	Young, B	NY	238
OrS	Bindelglass, D	CT	949
OrS	Buly, R	NY	256
OrS	Figgie, M	NY	258
OrS	Haas, S	NY	260
OrS	Laskin, R	NY	262
OrS	Sandhu, H	NY	265
OrS	Sculco, T	NY	266
Oto	Kuriloff, D	NY	272
PS	Bethel, C	NJ	787
PS	Hong, A	NY	574
PS	Lee, T	NY	633
PS	Moss, R	CT	977
PS	Stringel, G	NY	691
PS	Zitsman, J	NY	692
RE	Slowey, M	NJ	751
S	Coppa, G	NY	520
S	Fowler, D	NY	348
S	Inabnet, W	NY	349
S	Roslin, M	NY	352
S	Rosser, J	NY	352
S	Shapiro, M	NY	641
S	Starker, P	NJ	925
S	Wilbanks, T	NY	415
S	Yiengpruksawan, A	NJ	755
TS	Connery, C	NY	356
TS	Crawford, B	NY	356
TS	Laub, G	NJ	822
TS	Lazzaro, R	NY	475
TS	Okadigwe, C	NY	475
TS	Rose, D	CT	959
TS	Saunders, C	NJ	794
TS	Swistel, D	NY	359
TS	Walker, C	CT	959
U	Davis, J	NY	361

Spec	Name	St	Pg
U	Grunberger, I	NY	475
U	Owens, G	NY	708
U	Raboy, A	NY	521
U	Sandhaus, J	NY	502
U	Schiff, H	NY	366
U	Waxberg, J	CT	960
Minimally Invasive Surgery-Pediatric			
U	Poppas, D	NY	365
U	Stock, J	NJ	795
Minimally Invasive Thoracic Surgery			
TS	Fox, S	NY	592
TS	Gorenstein, L	NY	607
TS	Krellenstein, D	NY	357
TS	Lee, P	NY	502
TS	Lettera, J	CT	959
TS	Sonett, J	NY	359
TS	Widmann, M	NJ	885
Minimally Invasive Urologic Surgery			
U	Esposito, M	NJ	756
U	Hall, S	NY	363
U	Landman, J	NY	364
U	Lanteri, V	NJ	756
U	Munver, R	NJ	756
U	Savino, M	NY	522
Minimally Invasive Vascular Surgery			
VascS	Brener, B	NJ	795
VascS	Dietzek, A	CT	960
VascS	Todd, G	NY	372
Miscarriage			
ObG	Friedman, L	NY	232
Miscarriage-Recurrent			
MF	Lockwood, C	CT	972
MF	Shiffman, R	NY	442
ObG	Antoine, C	NY	230
ObG	Baxi, L	NY	230
ObG	Ordorica, S	NY	235
ObG	Scher, J	NY	236
RE	David, S	NY	336
RE	Kelly, A	NY	336
Mitral Valve Disease			
Cv	D'Agostino, R	NY	530
Cv	Schwartz, A	NY	131
Cv	Teicholz, L	NJ	722
IM	Kennish, A	NY	191
Mitral Valve Prolapse			
Cv	Freed, L	CT	966
Cv	Gupta, P	NY	423
Cv	Kobren, S	NY	532
IC	Wasserman, H	CT	943

Special Expertise Index

Special Expertise Index

Special Expertise Index

Spec	Name	St	Pg
Oculoplastic Surgery			
Oph	Della Rocca, R	NY	242
Oph	Di Leo, F	NY	628
Oph	Grasso, C	NY	495
Oph	Kazim, M	NY	245
Oph	Langer, P	NJ	782
Oph	Lisman, R	NY	247
Oph	Milite, J	NY	248
Oph	Millman, A	NY	248
Oph	Moskowitz, B	NY	249
Oph	Musto, A	CT	948
Oph	Podell, D	NY	250
Oph	Relland, M	NY	250
Oph	Stabile, J	NJ	739
Olfactory Disorders			
Oto	Kimmelman, C	NY	271
Ophthalmic Pathology			
Path	McCormick, S	NY	280
Ophthalmic Plastic Surgery			
Oph	Chern, R	NY	241
Oph	Garber, P	NY	563
Oph	Meltzer, M	NY	248
Oph	Reich, R	NY	453
Opiate Addiction			
AdP	Kleber, H	NY	119
AdP	Paul, E	NY	119
IM	Salsitz, E	NY	194
PM	Gevirtz, C	NY	687
Psyc	Bronheim, H	NY	311
Optic Nerve Disorders			
Oph	Odel, J	NY	250
Oph	Slamovits, T	NY	401
Oph	Unterricht, S	NY	454
Orbital Diseases			
Oph	Dweck, M	NY	452
Oph	Finger, P	NY	242
Oph	Sibony, P	NY	629
Orbital Diseases & Tumors			
Oph	Kazim, M	NY	245
Orbital Inflammation/Tumors			
Oph	Hornblass, A	NY	245
Orbital Surgery			
Oph	Guillory, S	NY	244
Oph	Langer, P	NJ	782
Oph	Maher, E	NY	247
Oph	Schneck, G	NY	629

Spec	Name	St	Pg
Orbital Tumors/Cancer			
Oph	Abramson, D	NY	238
Oph	Della Rocca, R	NY	242
Oph	Turbin, R	NJ	782
Orthopaedic Imaging			
DR	Haramati, N	NY	383
Osteoarthritis			
IM	Kazdin, H	NY	439
IM	Levin, N	NY	440
PMR	Liss, D	NJ	747
Rhu	Adlersberg, J	NY	338
Rhu	Bennett, R	NY	639
Rhu	Crane, R	NY	339
Rhu	Danehower, R	CT	958
Rhu	Fields, T	NY	339
Rhu	Garner, B	NY	470
Rhu	Goldberg, M	NJ	896
Rhu	Greenwald, R	NY	586
Rhu	Hamburger, M	NY	639
Rhu	Hoffman, M	NY	586
Rhu	Honig, S	NY	340
Rhu	Lee, S	NY	340
Rhu	Lipstein-Kresch, E	NY	586
Rhu	Magid, S	NY	340
Rhu	Markenson, J	NY	341
Rhu	Radin, A	NY	341
Rhu	Reinitz, E	NY	703
Rhu	Ricciardi, D	NY	471
Rhu	Schwartzberg, M	NJ	866
Rhu	Stern, R	NY	342
Rhu	Sullivan, J	NY	587
Rhu	Tiger, L	NY	587
Osteomyelitis			
IM	Matkovic, C	NY	622
Inf	Middleton, J	NJ	834
Inf	Mullen, M	NY	184
OrS	Strauss, E	NY	266
Osteoporosis			
EDM	Aloia, J	NY	539
EDM	Balkin, M	NY	616
EDM	Becker, C	NY	154
EDM	Bergman, D	NY	154
EDM	Bilezikian, J	NY	154
EDM	Bloomgarden, D	NY	658
EDM	Blum, D	NY	658
EDM	Bockman, R	NY	155
EDM	Bucholtz, H	NJ	830
EDM	Cam, J	NJ	799
EDM	Cohen, N	NY	510
EDM	Cosman, F	NY	602
EDM	Eufemio, M	NY	658
EDM	Felig, P	NY	155
EDM	Freeman, R	NY	384
EDM	Friedman, S	NY	539
EDM	Fuhrman, R	NJ	913
EDM	Goldberg-Berman, J	CT	937
EDM	Greene, L	NY	155
EDM	Greenfield, M	NY	539
EDM	Hershon, K	NY	539

Spec	Name	St	Pg
EDM	Hochstein, M	NJ	726
EDM	Hupart, K	NY	539
EDM	Jacobs, D	NY	156
EDM	Josef, M	NY	602
EDM	Kantor, A	NY	659
EDM	Kennedy, J	NJ	810
EDM	Kukar, N	NY	486
EDM	Nydick, M	NY	157
EDM	Park, C	NY	157
EDM	Resta, C	NY	486
EDM	Rosenbaum, R	NJ	913
EDM	Rosman, L	NY	486
EDM	Ross, H	NY	659
EDM	Rothman, J	NY	510
EDM	Saxena, A	NY	429
EDM	Schmidt, P	NY	429
EDM	Shane, E	NY	157
EDM	Sherry, S	NJ	773
EDM	Silverberg, A	NY	429
EDM	Silverberg, S	NY	157
EDM	Siris, E	NY	158
EDM	Tohme, J	NJ	726
EDM	Vaswani, A	NY	540
EDM	Weinerman, S	NY	540
EDM	Wiesen, M	NJ	727
EDM	Wysolmerski, J	CT	969
EDM	Young, I	NY	158
FMed	Blyskal, S	NY	617
FMed	Eisenstat, S	NJ	914
Ger	Bloom, P	NY	171
Ger	Jacobs, L	NY	389
Ger	Solomon, R	NJ	915
IM	Alpert, B	NY	666
IM	Altbaum, R	CT	940
IM	Grajower, M	NY	392
IM	Joseph, J	NY	490
IM	Lans, D	NY	668
IM	Lebowitz, A	NY	191
IM	Seicol, N	NY	669
IM	Wozniak, D	NJ	801
IM	Zackson, D	NY	197
Nep	Tartini, A	NJ	735
NuM	Gupta, S	CT	947
NuM	Pierson, R	NY	229
ObG	Bednoff, S	NY	559
ObG	Berman, A	NY	231
ObG	Concannon, P	NY	494
ObG	Florio, P	NY	677
ObG	Lieberman, B	NY	234
ObG	Rothbaum, D	NY	561
OrS	Cataletto, M	NY	565
OrS	Toriello, E	NY	496
Rhu	Bauer, B	NY	338
Rhu	Brodman, R	NJ	924
Rhu	Cannarozzi, N	NJ	791
Rhu	Cohen, D	NY	586
Rhu	Goldberg, M	NJ	896
Rhu	Goldstein, M	NY	520
Rhu	Green, S	NY	470
Rhu	Honig, S	NY	340
Rhu	Jarrett, M	NY	520
Rhu	Kaell, A	NY	639
Rhu	Lipstein-Kresch, E	NY	586
Rhu	Marcus, R	NJ	752
Rhu	Mascarenhas, B	NY	703
Rhu	McWhorter, J	NJ	906
Rhu	Miller, K	CT	958
Rhu	Mitnick, H	NY	341

Special Expertise Index

Spec	Name	St	Pg
Pain-Back & Neck			
N	Mendelsohn, F	NY	625
N	Rapoport, S	NY	224
N	Weintraub, M	NY	677
NS	Pizzi, F	NJ	815
PM	Bram, H	NJ	863
PM	Haber, D	NJ	863
PM	Lu, G	NY	687
PM	Richman, D	NY	278
PMR	Lieberman, J	NY	300
PMR	Malanga, G	NJ	883
PMR	Novick, E	NJ	923
PMR	Ragnarsson, K	NY	300
PMR	Rosenberg, C	NY	635
Pain-Cancer			
Onc	Reed, M	NY	394
PM	Foley, K	NY	277
PM	Freedman, G	NY	277
PM	Gargiulo, J	NY	632
PM	Jain, S	NY	277
PM	Kestenbaum, A	NY	687
PM	Kloth, D	CT	951
PM	Kreitzer, J	NY	278
PM	Portenoy, R	NY	278
PM	Staats, P	NJ	864
PM	Weinberger, M	NY	279
Psyc	Breitbart, W	NY	311
Pain-Chronic			
N	Hainline, B	NY	557
N	Kanner, R	NY	557
NS	Brown, J	NY	556
PM	Gargiulo, J	NY	632
PM	Gusmorino, P	NY	277
PM	Kaplan, R	NY	278
PM	Levin, A	NJ	842
PM	Vaillancourt, P	NY	632
PMR	Lee, M	NY	300
PMR	Moldover, J	NY	300
Pain-Facial			
N	Green, M	NY	221
N	Newman, L	NY	224
Pain-Facial (TMJ)			
Psyc	McMullen, R	NY	319
Pain-Knee			
PMR	Goldberg, R	NY	299
Pain-Knee & Shoulder			
PMR	Gotlin, R	NY	299
PMR	Vad, V	NY	301
Pain-Low Back			
PM	Lefkowitz, M	NY	457
PMR	De Araujo, M	NY	409
PMR	Lutz, G	NY	300

Spec	Name	St	Pg
Pain-Mind/Body Disorder			
PM	Sarno, J	NY	278
Pain-Muscle & Nerve			
PM	Haber, D	NJ	863
Pain-Musculoskeletal			
Ped	Lazarus, H	NY	295
PM	Moqtaderi, F	NY	278
PMR	Levin, S	NY	409
Pain-Musculoskeletal-Spine & Neck			
PM	Ngeow, J	NY	278
Pain-Neuropathic			
PM	Agin, C	NY	631
PM	Ashendorf, D	NJ	921
PM	Kreitzer, J	NY	278
PM	Ngeow, J	NY	278
PM	Thomas, G	NY	279
PM	Waldman, S	NY	279
Pain-Pelvic			
ObG	Coady, D	NY	231
ObG	Lafontant, J	NY	400
PM	Jain, S	NY	277
Pain-Spine			
PM	Waldman, S	NY	279
Palliative Care			
Ge	Mehta, R	NY	387
Ger	Goldberg, R	NY	388
Ger	Meier, D	NY	172
Hem	Forte, F	NY	511
Hem	Lerner, W	NJ	860
IM	Berger, J	NY	548
IM	Bharathan, T	NY	438
IM	Cimino, J	NY	391
IM	Comfort, C	NY	392
IM	Fahey, J	NY	622
IM	Fiorentino, T	NY	667
IM	Selwyn, P	NY	392
Ped	Okun, A	NY	408
PInf	Oleske, J	NJ	786
PM	Foley, K	NY	277
PM	Gevirtz, C	NY	687
PM	Portenoy, R	NY	278
Psyc	Breitbart, W	NY	311
Psyc	Fleishman, S	NY	314
Palmar Hyperhidrosis			
S	Sekons, D	NY	353
TS	Fox, S	NY	592
TS	Gorenstein, L	NY	607
TS	Keller, S	NY	415

Spec	Name	St	Pg
Pancreatic Cancer			
Ge	Pochapin, M	NY	168
Onc	Bruckner, H	NY	442
Onc	Casper, E	NJ	877
Onc	Fine, R	NY	201
Onc	Macdonald, J	NY	205
Onc	O'Reilly, E	NY	206
Onc	Sherman, W	NY	207
RadRO	Ennis, R	NY	333
S	Blumgart, L	NY	345
S	Brennan, M	NY	345
S	Chabot, J	NY	346
S	Chamberlain, R	NJ	792
S	Coit, D	NY	346
S	Conte, C	NY	588
S	Datta, R	NY	588
S	Eng, K	NY	347
S	Fahey, T	NY	348
S	Fong, Y	NY	348
S	Gecelter, G	NY	589
S	Gouge, T	NY	348
S	Kaleya, R	NY	414
S	Kemeny, M	NY	501
S	Lieberman, M	NY	350
S	Michelassi, F	NY	350
S	Newman, E	NY	351
S	Pachter, H	NY	351
S	Shamamian, P	NY	353
Pancreatic Disease			
Ge	Bank, S	NY	542
Ge	Basuk, P	NY	160
Ge	Cohen, J	NY	161
Ge	Gendler, S	NY	662
Ge	Grendell, J	NY	543
Ge	Pitchumoni, C	NJ	832
Ge	Soterakis, J	NY	544
Ge	Stein, J	NY	170
Ge	Stevens, P	NY	170
Ge	Tempera, P	NJ	915
Pancreatic Surgery			
S	Attiyeh, F	NY	344
S	Coppa, G	NY	520
S	Cronin, D	CT	982
S	Gagner, M	NY	348
S	Gordon, M	NY	705
S	Inabnet, W	NY	349
S	Ratner, L	NY	352
S	Salky, B	NY	353
S	Savino, J	NY	706
S	Shamamian, P	NY	353
S	Zenilman, M	NY	474
Pancreatic/Biliary Endoscopy (ERCP)			
Ge	Ben-Zvi, J	NY	160
Ge	Clain, D	NY	161
Ge	Cohen, J	NY	161
Ge	Cohen, S	NY	161
Ge	Friedrich, I	NJ	727
Ge	Gendler, S	NY	662
Ge	Gutwein, I	NY	387
Ge	Heier, S	NY	662
Ge	Iswara, K	NY	432

Special Expertise Index

Special Expertise Index

Special Expertise Index

Special Expertise Index

Special Expertise Index

Special Expertise Index

Special Expertise Index

Spec	Name	St	Pg
U	Colton, M	NJ	886

Robotic Surgery-Pediatric

Spec	Name	St	Pg
U	Poppas, D	NY	365
U	Stock, J	NJ	795

Robotic Urologic Surgery

Spec	Name	St	Pg
U	Friedman, S	NY	475
U	Rosen, J	NJ	756

Rosacea

Spec	Name	St	Pg
D	Maier, H	NJ	891
D	Rozanski, R	NJ	771
D	Schwartz, R	NJ	771
D	Shalita, A	NY	427

Ross Procedure for Aortic Valve Disease

Spec	Name	St	Pg
TS	Stelzer, P	NY	359

Rotator Cuff Surgery

Spec	Name	St	Pg
HS	Monsanto, E	NY	435
OrS	Flatow, E	NY	258
OrS	Pollock, R	NJ	740
SM	Cavaliere, G	NY	704

Running Injuries

Spec	Name	St	Pg
OrS	Walsh, W	NY	685
SM	Hamner, D	NY	343
SM	Maharam, L	NY	343

S

Salivary Gland Surgery

Spec	Name	St	Pg
Oto	Myssiorek, D	NY	568
Oto	Urken, M	NY	276

Salivary Gland Tumors

Spec	Name	St	Pg
Oto	Komisar, A	NY	272
Oto	Smith, R	NY	403

Sarcoidosis

Spec	Name	St	Pg
Oph	Frohman, L	NJ	782
Pul	Adams, F	NY	328
Pul	Blair, L	NY	328
Pul	Breidbart, D	NY	581
Pul	Brill, J	NY	700
Pul	Demetis, S	NY	466
Pul	Eden, E	NY	329
Pul	Efferen, L	NY	582
Pul	Gribetz, A	NY	329
Pul	Gulrajani, R	NY	467
Pul	Kutnick, R	NY	330
Pul	Lee, M	NY	330

Spec	Name	St	Pg
Pul	Marcus, P	NY	582
Pul	Miller, A	NY	500
Pul	Padilla, M	NY	331
Pul	Paz, H	NJ	847
Pul	Pinsker, K	NY	412
Pul	Polkow, M	NJ	750
Pul	Posner, D	NY	331
Pul	Safirstein, B	NJ	790
Pul	Schiffman, P	NJ	847
Pul	Sender, J	NY	412
Pul	Tanoue, L	CT	980
Pul	Teirstein, A	NY	332
Rhu	Agus, B	NY	338
Rhu	Yee, A	NY	342

Sarcoma

Spec	Name	St	Pg
Onc	Blum, R	NY	200
Onc	Casper, E	NJ	877
Onc	Hesdorffer, C	NJ	733
Onc	Taub, R	NY	209
PHO	Meyers, P	NY	287
S	Bloom, N	NY	345
S	Brennan, M	NY	345

Sarcoma-Soft Tissue

Spec	Name	St	Pg
OrS	Benevenia, J	NJ	783
OrS	Healey, J	NY	260
PHO	Harris, M	NJ	744
PHO	Wexler, L	NY	288
S	August, D	NJ	849
S	Rosenberg, V	NY	352
S	Singer, S	NY	354

Scar Revision

Spec	Name	St	Pg
D	Rapaport, J	NJ	725

Schizophrenia

Spec	Name	St	Pg
Psyc	Benjamin, J	NY	580
Psyc	Bowers, M	CT	979
Psyc	Kahn, D	NY	316
Psyc	Kaufmann, C	NY	316
Psyc	Lee, C	NY	519
Psyc	Lindenmayer, J	NY	318
Psyc	Mendelowitz, A	NY	498
Psyc	Schwartz, B	NY	411
Psyc	Siris, S	NY	498
Psyc	Sullivan, T	NY	699
Psyc	Weiden, P	NY	465

Schizophrenia-Early Detection/Treatment

Spec	Name	St	Pg
Psyc	McGlashan, T	CT	979

Sciatica

Spec	Name	St	Pg
PM	Lefkowitz, M	NY	457
PM	Waldman, S	NY	279

Scleroderma

Spec	Name	St	Pg
D	Franks, A	NY	143
PRhu	Lehman, T	NY	291
Pul	Matthay, R	CT	980

Spec	Name	St	Pg
Rhu	Ash, J	NY	703
Rhu	Belmont, I I	NY	338
Rhu	Bernstein, L	NY	470
Rhu	Blau, S	NY	586
Rhu	Kerr, L	NY	340
Rhu	McWhorter, J	NJ	906
Rhu	Spiera, H	NY	342
Rhu	Spiera, R	NY	342
Rhu	Whitman, H	NJ	907

Scoliosis

Spec	Name	St	Pg
OrS	Bendo, J	NY	255
OrS	Boachie-Adjei, O	NY	256
OrS	Burke, S	NY	256
OrS	Cammisa, F	NY	257
OrS	Delbello, D	NY	683
OrS	Errico, T	NY	258
OrS	Lonner, B	NY	262
OrS	Merola, A	NY	455
OrS	Moskovich, R	NY	263
OrS	Neuwirth, M	NY	263
OrS	Olsewski, J	NY	402
OrS	Rieger, M	NJ	880
OrS	Roye, D	NY	265
OrS	Spivak, J	NY	266
OrS	Taddonio, R	NY	685
OrS	Tindel, N	NY	402
OrS	Ulin, R	NY	267
OrS	Widmann, R	NY	267
OrS	Wolpin, M	NY	456

Seizure Disorders

Spec	Name	St	Pg
ChiN	Kutscher, M	NY	653
ChiN	Molofsky, W	NY	137
N	Azhar, S	NY	446
N	Bronster, D	NY	219
N	Ettinger, A	NY	557
N	Jutkowitz, R	NY	514
N	Katz, A	CT	974
N	Sadeghi, H	NJ	801

Seizure Disorders in the Aging

Spec	Name	St	Pg
N	Rowan, A	NY	225

Seizure Disorders-Pediatric

Spec	Name	St	Pg
N	Moshe, S	NY	398

Sentinel Node Surgery

Spec	Name	St	Pg
S	Bernik, S	NY	345
S	Blackwood, M	NJ	792
S	Geller, P	NY	348
S	O'Hea, B	NY	641
S	Swistel, A	NY	354
S	Tartter, P	NY	354

Sepsis

Spec	Name	St	Pg
CCM	Melamed, M	NJ	723
CCM	Nierman, D	NY	140
Ped	Parker, M	NY	635
Pul	Davis, G	NJ	865
Pul	Multz, A	NY	500

Special Expertise Index

Special Expertise Index

Special Expertise Index

Spec	Name	St	Pg
Sports Medicine-Aging Athlete			
FMed	Farrell, M	CT	937
Sports Medicine-Cardiology			
Cv	Gitler, B	NY	649
Cv	Zimmerman, F	NY	652
Sports Medicine-Golf & Tennis Injuries			
PMR	Vad, V	NY	301
Sports Medicine-Hand			
HS	Rosenwasser, M	NY	177
Sports Medicine-Women			
OrS	Hannafin, J	NY	260
Sports Neurology			
N	Casson, I	NY	493
N	Jordan, B	NY	676
Stem Cell Transplant			
Hem	Fruchtman, S	NY	179
Hem	Nimer, S	NY	180
Hem	Pecora, A	NJ	730
Hem	Savage, D	NY	180
Onc	Cooper, D	CT	972
Onc	Dobbs, J	NY	623
Onc	Hesdorffer, C	NJ	733
PHO	Kernan, N	NY	287
PHO	Lipton, J	NY	573
Stereotactic Radiosurgery			
NS	Anant, A	NY	446
NS	Beyerl, B	NJ	878
NS	Golfinos, J	NY	215
NS	Lansen, T	NY	675
NS	Rosenblum, B	NJ	861
NS	Sisti, M	NY	217
NS	Spitzer, D	NY	604
NS	Torres-Gluck, J	NY	397
NS	Zampella, E	NJ	878
RadRO	Knisely, J	CT	980
RadRO	Schwartz, L	NJ	924
RadRO	Wong, J	NJ	884
Stomach Cancer			
S	Coit, D	NY	346
S	Fong, Y	NY	348
Strabismus			
Oph	Campolattaro, B	NY	240
Oph	Caputo, A	NJ	781
Oph	Cossari, A	NY	628
Oph	Deutsch, J	NY	451
Oph	Eggers, H	NY	242
Oph	Flynn, J	NY	243
Oph	Gallin, P	NY	244

Spec	Name	St	Pg
Oph	Hall, L	NY	245
Oph	Horowitz, M	NY	681
Oph	Magramm, I	NY	247
Oph	Most, R	NY	682
Oph	Muchnick, R	NY	249
Oph	Raab, E	NY	250
Oph	Rubin, S	NY	564
Oph	Steele, M	NY	253
Oph	Wagner, R	NJ	782
Oph	Wang, F	NY	254
Oph	Wisnicki, H	NY	254
Stress Echocardiography			
Cv	Golier, F	NY	649
Cv	Mercurio, P	NY	650
Stress Management			
ChAP	Bartlett, J	NJ	770
Cv	Rozanski, A	NY	130
Psyc	Aronoff, M	NY	310
Stroke			
Ger	Jacobs, L	NY	389
IM	Butt, A	NY	438
IM	Kernan, W	CT	971
N	Azhar, S	NY	446
N	Brust, J	NY	219
N	Caronna, J	NY	219
N	Charney, J	NY	219
N	Chodosh, E	NJ	893
N	Cohen, D	NY	625
N	Cohen, J	NY	397
N	Fellus, J	NJ	780
N	Foo, S	NY	220
N	Gerber, O	NY	625
N	Gropen, T	NY	447
N	Herbert, J	NY	221
N	Klein, P	NJ	736
N	Koppel, B	NY	222
N	Levine, D	NY	222
N	Levine, S	NY	222
N	Libman, R	NY	558
N	Mallin, J	NY	558
N	Marks, S	NY	676
N	Mayer, S	NY	223
N	Mohr, J	NY	223
N	Murphy, J	CT	947
N	Oh, Y	NJ	838
N	Rosenbaum, D	NY	448
N	Rudolph, S	NY	448
N	Sacco, R	NY	225
N	Schaefer, J	NY	225
N	Schanzer, B	NJ	918
N	Sena, K	CT	947
N	Singh, A	NY	677
N	Sobol, N	NY	448
N	Somasundaram, M	NY	448
N	Stacy, C	NY	226
N	Vas, G	NY	448
N	Vester, J	NJ	816
N	Weinberger, J	NY	227
N	Weiss, A	NY	227
NRad	Drayer, B	NY	227
NRad	Litt, A	NY	228

Spec	Name	St	Pg
NRad	Tenner, M	NY	677
NS	Murali, R	NY	675
VascS	De Groote, R	NJ	757
Stroke Prevention			
VascS	Simpson, A	NJ	851
Stroke Rehabilitation			
N	Feinberg, T	NY	220
PMR	Ahn, J	NY	298
PMR	Atakent, P	NY	463
PMR	Braddom, R	NJ	864
PMR	Lanyi, V	NY	299
PMR	Myers, S	NY	300
PMR	Petrillo, C	CT	954
PMR	Stein, A	NY	301
Substance Abuse			
AdP	Frances, R	NY	119
ChAP	Pincus, E	NY	652
IM	O'Connor, P	CT	971
N	Brust, J	NY	219
ObG	Allen, M	NY	230
Psyc	Nunes, E	NY	320
Psyc	Steinglass, P	NY	325
Psyc	Sussman, R	NY	700
Psyc	Tamerin, J	CT	956
Substance Abuse Effects in Newborn			
NP	Rosen, T	NY	211
Substance Abuse in ADHD Patients			
AdP	Levin, F	NY	119
Sudden Death Prevention			
CE	Levine, J	NY	529
Sudden Infant Death Syndrome (SIDS)			
NP	Perl, H	NJ	734
NP	Steele, A	NY	555
Ped	Altman, R	NY	692
Suicide			
ChAP	Pincus, E	NY	652
ChAP	Shaffer, D	NY	135
Psyc	Dulit, R	NY	697
Surgical Infections			
Inf	Press, R	NY	184
Surgical Pathology			
Path	Barnard, N	NJ	842
Path	Hoda, S	NY	279
Path	Wenig, B	NY	281

Special Expertise Index

Spec	Name	St	Pg
Nep	Cohen, D	NY	212
Nep	Friedman, E	NY	444
Nep	Markell, M	NY	445
Nep	Mulgaonkar, S	NJ	779
Nep	Pepe, J	NY	514
Nep	Shapiro, K	NY	604
Nep	Williams, G	NY	214
PNep	Kaskel, F	NY	405
PNep	Roberti, M	NJ	786
PNep	Saland, J	NY	289

Transplant Medicine-Liver

Spec	Name	St	Pg
Ge	Bodenheimer,, H	NY	160
Ge	Martin, P	NY	167
Ge	Wolf, D	NY	664
PGe	Lobritto, S	NY	285

Transplant Medicine-Lung

Spec	Name	St	Pg
Pul	Arcasoy, S	NY	328
Pul	Kamholz, S	NY	582

Transplant Surgery

Spec	Name	St	Pg
S	Shapiro, M	NJ	754

Transplant-Heart

Spec	Name	St	Pg
PS	Mosca, R	NY	292
TS	Elefteriades, J	CT	983
TS	Lansman, S	NY	706
TS	Oz, M	NY	358
TS	Rose, E	NY	358
TS	Smith, C	NY	359
TS	Spielvogel, D	NY	706

Transplant-Heart & Lung

Spec	Name	St	Pg
TS	Naka, Y	NY	358

Transplant-Kidney

Spec	Name	St	Pg
S	Bromberg, J	NY	346
S	Butt, K	NY	704
S	Chung-Loy, H	NJ	849
S	Greenstein, S	NY	414
S	Hardy, M	NY	349
S	Hong, J	NY	472
S	Ratner, L	NY	352
S	Schechner, R	NY	414
S	Tellis, V	NY	414
S	Teperman, L	NY	355
U	Fleisher, M	NJ	850
U	Frischer, Z	NY	642
VascS	Benvenisty, A	NY	369

Transplant-Liver

Spec	Name	St	Pg
S	Cronin, D	CT	982
S	Emond, J	NY	347
S	Schwartz, M	NY	353
S	Teperman, L	NY	355

Transplant-Liver-Adult & Pediatric

Spec	Name	St	Pg
S	Emre, S	NY	347

Transplant-Living Kidney Donor

Spec	Name	St	Pg
S	Edye, M	NY	347
S	Friedman, A	CT	982

Transplant-Lung

Spec	Name	St	Pg
TS	Ginsburg, M	NY	357
TS	Sonett, J	NY	359
TS	Waters, P	NY	360

Transplant-Pancreas

Spec	Name	St	Pg
S	Bromberg, J	NY	346
S	Friedman, A	CT	982
S	Ratner, L	NY	352

Trauma

Spec	Name	St	Pg
HS	Botwinick, N	NY	175
Oph	DeLuca, J	NJ	738
OrS	Arvan, G	NY	630
OrS	Butler, M	NJ	840
OrS	Cornell, C	NY	257
OrS	Helfet, D	NY	261
OrS	Hermele, H	CT	949
OrS	Kleinman, P	NY	402
OrS	Lyden, J	NY	262
OrS	Piskun, A	NJ	841
OrS	Reilly, J	NY	516
OrS	Schneider, S	NJ	905
OrS	Weiner, L	NY	267
PS	Cooper, A	NY	292
PS	Harris, B	NY	406
PS	Touloukian, R	CT	977
PS	Weinberg, G	NY	406
S	Barie, P	NY	344
S	Barone, J	NY	413
S	Benson, D	NJ	753
S	Blau, S	NY	588
S	Boyarsky, A	NJ	849
S	Deitch, E	NJ	792
S	Di Giacomo, J	NJ	804
S	Dresner, L	NY	472
S	Savino, J	NY	706
S	Walsh, B	NY	706
U	Furey, R	NY	362

Trauma Psychiatry

Spec	Name	St	Pg
ChAP	Fornari, V	NY	534
Psyc	Napoli, J	NJ	749

Trauma Radiology

Spec	Name	St	Pg
DR	Garner, S	NY	428

Trauma Reconstruction

Spec	Name	St	Pg
PlS	Cimino, E	NJ	819

Trauma-Pediatric

Spec	Name	St	Pg
OrS	Price, A	NY	264

Travel Medicine

Spec	Name	St	Pg
FMed	Clements, J	NY	158
FMed	Greenberg, M	NY	618
FMed	Strongwater, R	NY	661
Ge	Connor, B	NY	162
IM	Barry, M	CT	971
IM	Carmichael, L	NY	187
IM	Friedman, J	NY	189
IM	Haber, S	NY	190
IM	Kaminsky, D	NY	191
IM	Lewin, S	NY	192
IM	Rendel, M	NY	194
IM	Schneider, S	NY	195
Inf	Bell, E	NY	181
Inf	Berger, J	NY	390
Inf	Berkey, P	NY	665
Inf	Birch, T	NJ	730
Inf	Busillo, C	NY	182
Inf	Cervia, J	NY	547
Inf	Chapnick, E	NY	436
Inf	Farrer, W	NJ	915
Inf	Gekowski, K	NY	812
Inf	Gross, P	NJ	731
Inf	Gumprecht, J	NY	182
Inf	Helfgott, D	NY	183
Inf	Herman, D	NJ	903
Inf	Hilton, E	NY	547
Inf	Horowitz, H	NY	665
Inf	Johnson, D	NY	548
Inf	Johnson, W	NY	183
Inf	Klein, A	NY	620
Inf	Lerner, C	NY	183
Inf	Martinez, H	NJ	903
Inf	McLeod, G	CT	939
Inf	Neibart, E	NY	184
Inf	Perlman, D	NY	184
Inf	Roland, R	NJ	915
Inf	Rush, T	NY	666
Inf	Sabetta, J	CT	939
Inf	Sacks-Berg, A	NY	621
Inf	Singer, C	NY	548
Inf	Stein, A	NY	437
Inf	Weisholtz, S	NJ	731
OM	Mendelsohn, S	NY	562
PA&I	Morrison, S	NJ	784
Ped	Levitt, M	NY	693
Ped	Mayers, M	NY	408

Treatment Resistant Mental Illness

Spec	Name	St	Pg
Psyc	Hoffman, J	NY	316

Trigeminal Neuralgia

Spec	Name	St	Pg
NS	Bederson, J	NY	214
NS	Brown, J	NY	556
NS	Frank, D	NJ	779
NS	Goodman, R	NY	215
NS	Mechanic, A	NY	556
NS	Murali, R	NY	675
NS	Stern, J	NY	675

Tropical Diseases

Spec	Name	St	Pg
IM	Barry, M	CT	971
IM	Kaminsky, D	NY	191
Inf	Allegra, D	NJ	876

Special Expertise Index

Spec	Name	St	Pg
Inf	Masci, J	NY	489
Inf	Sabetta, J	CT	939
Inf	Tanowitz, H	NY	391
PrM	Cahill, J	NY	309
PrM	Imperato, P	NY	464

Tropical Medicine

FMed	Kelly, S	NY	660
PrM	Cahill, K	NY	309

Tuberculosis

Inf	Badshah, C	NY	181
Inf	Ellner, J	NJ	775
Inf	Sepkowitz, D	NY	437
Inf	Sepkowitz, K	NY	185
Inf	Telzak, E	NY	391
Ped	Mayers, M	NY	408
PInf	Rubin, L	NY	573
PInf	Saiman, L	NY	289
PInf	Sood, S	NY	573
PPul	Aguila, H	NJ	786
Pul	Adler, J	NY	328
Pul	Ankobiah, W	NY	499
Pul	Bondi, E	NY	466
Pul	Dhar, S	NY	467
Pul	Efferen, L	NY	582
Pul	Friedman, L	CT	980
Pul	Gagliardi, A	NY	329
Pul	Kamholz, S	NY	582
Pul	Reichman, L	NJ	790
Pul	Schluger, N	NY	332

Tuberous Sclerosis

ChiN	Miles, D	NY	137
N	Devinsky, O	NY	220

Tumor Banking

Path	Melamed, J	NY	280

Tumor Imaging

NuM	Brunetti, J	NJ	737

Tumor Surgery

PS	Ginsburg, H	NY	292
PS	Holgersen, L	NY	691
PS	Kessler, E	NY	575
PS	San Filippo, J	NY	691

Turner's Syndrome

PEn	Saenger, P	NY	689

Twin to Twin Transfusion Syndrome (TTTS)

ObG	Young, B	NY	238

U

Spec	Name	St	Pg

Ulcerative Colitis

CRS	Arvanitis, M	NJ	858
CRS	Levin, L	NY	535
CRS	Oliver, G	NJ	829
Ge	Abreu, M	NY	159
Ge	Auerbach, M	NY	661
Ge	Ehrlich, J	NY	662
Ge	Field, B	NY	662
Ge	Finkelstein, W	NJ	774
Ge	Gould, P	NY	543
Ge	Horowitz, L	NY	164
Ge	Korelitz, B	NY	165
Ge	Lebwohl, O	NY	166
Ge	Mayer, L	NY	167
Ge	Present, D	NY	168
Ge	Sachar, D	NY	169
Ge	Schneider, L	NY	169
Ge	Talansky, A	NY	544
Ge	Ullman, T	NY	170
IM	Klein, N	CT	941
PGe	Spivak, W	NY	286
PS	Dolgin, S	NY	574
S	Michelassi, F	NY	350

Ulcerative Colitis/Crohn's

Ge	Lustbader, I	NY	166
Ge	Magun, A	NY	167
Ge	Zucker, I	NJ	729
PGe	Bangaru, B	NY	497
PGe	Gold, D	NY	632

Ultrasound

CRS	McConnell, J	NJ	723
DR	Adler, R	NY	149
DR	Chisolm, A	NY	657
DR	Claps, R	NJ	875
DR	Cohen, S	CT	936
DR	Ford, R	NJ	810
DR	Fried, K	NY	150
DR	Geller, M	NY	602
DR	Goodman, K	NY	538
DR	Kazam, E	NY	151
DR	Koenigsberg, M	NY	383
DR	Kutcher, R	NY	657
DR	Laks, M	NY	383
DR	LoRusso, D	NY	658
DR	Mollin, J	NY	485
DR	Rambler, L	NJ	726
DR	Rifkin, M	NY	616
DR	Rosenfeld, S	NY	153
DR	Sitron, A	NY	538
DR	Whelan, C	NJ	772
DR	Yaghoobian, J	NY	428
MF	Chervenak, F	NY	198
MF	Kofinas, A	NY	441
MF	Rebarber, A	NY	199
MF	Rochelson, B	NY	552
MF	Smith, L	NJ	778
MF	Thornton, Y	NJ	835
MF	Vintzileos, A	NJ	835
NuM	Gerard, P	NY	449

Spec	Name	St	Pg
ObG	Divon, M	NY	232
ObG	Goldstein, S	NJ	862
ObG	Kirshenbaum, N	NY	678
ObG	Lederman, S	NY	450
ObG	Reilly, K	NY	679
Oph	Coleman, D	NY	241
Oph	Fisher, Y	NY	243

Undescended Testis

PS	Beck, A	NY	292
PS	Kutin, N	NY	575
PS	Schwartz, D	NY	575
PS	Winick, M	NY	633
U	Brock, W	NY	593
U	Wasnick, R	NY	643

Unknown Primary Cancer

Onc	Kelsen, D	NY	204
Onc	Stoopler, M	NY	208

Upper Extremity Surgery

OrS	Crowe, J	CT	949

Urinary Abnormalities

PNep	Nash, M	NY	289

Urinary Reconstruction-Pediatric

U	Burbige, K	CT	960

Urinary Tract Infection

PNep	Schoeneman, M	NY	460
U	Friedman, S	NY	475

Urinary Tract Infections

Inf	Andriole, V	CT	971
Inf	Glatt, A	NY	547
Inf	McCormack, W	NY	437
U	Boorjian, P	NJ	794
U	Marans, H	NY	364
U	Moldwin, R	NY	594
U	Rosenberg, S	NJ	823
U	Sperber, A	NY	367

Uro-Gynecology

ObG	Besser, G	CT	948
ObG	Blanco, J	NY	231
ObG	Maggio, J	NY	234
ObG	Pillari, V	NY	515
ObG	Ullman, J	NY	679
U	Blaivas, J	NY	361
U	Frischer, Z	NY	642
U	Staskin, D	NY	367

Urodynamics

U	Kaplan, S	NY	363
U	Nitti, V	NY	365

Special Expertise Index

Spec	Name	St	Pg
Varicocele Microsurgery			
U	Goldstein, M	NY	362
U	Nagler, H	NY	365
Varicose Veins			
D	Sadick, N	NY	147
S	Kim, Z	NY	705
S	Mansouri, H	NY	590
VascS	Arnold, T	NY	643
VascS	Blumenthal, J	NY	369
VascS	Elias, S	NJ	757
VascS	Garvey, J	NY	596
VascS	Goldman, K	NJ	823
VascS	Karanfilian, R	NY	709
VascS	Mendes, D	NY	371
VascS	Pollina, R	NY	643
VascS	Sales, C	NJ	926
VascS	Stein, J	NY	371
Vascular Access			
S	Butt, K	NY	704
S	Hong, J	NY	472
VascS	Shindelman, L	NJ	851
VIR	Siegel, R	NJ	851
Vascular Anomalies			
D	Garzon, M	NY	143
PlS	Persing, J	CT	978
Vascular Lesions of the CNS			
NRad	Litt, A	NY	228
Vascular Malformations			
Oto	Waner, M	NY	277
VIR	Haskal, Z	NY	368
VIR	Rosen, R	NY	369
VIR	Sclafani, S	NY	477
VIR	White, R	CT	983
Vascular Malformations/Birthmarks			
D	Skrokov, R	NY	615
Vascular Surgery			
S	Arbour, R	NJ	866
S	Balsano, N	NY	413
S	Butt, K	NY	704
S	D'Anna, J	NY	520
S	Daliana, M	NY	347
S	Davidson, J	NJ	822
S	Fletcher, H	NJ	792
S	Francfort, J	NY	640
S	Friedman, S	NY	588
S	Gallagher, J	NY	640
S	Glass, D	NY	472
S	Lois, W	NY	473
S	Martin, W	NY	641
S	McGovern, P	NJ	804
S	Popovich, J	NJ	804
S	Prichep, R	NY	641
S	Vitale, G	NY	591

Spec	Name	St	Pg
S	Wegryn, R	NJ	925
S	Wilbanks, T	NY	415
S	Zeitlin, A	NY	502
TS	Acinapura, A	NY	474
TS	Dranitzke, R	NY	642
TS	Forman, M	NJ	793
TS	Moideen, A	NY	502
TS	Rubenstein, R	NY	642
Vascular Ultrasound			
DR	Fried, K	NY	150
IM	Kaplan, K	NY	668
NuM	Gerard, P	NY	449
Vasculitis			
D	Soter, N	NY	148
PRhu	Kimura, Y	NJ	745
Rhu	Blume, R	NY	338
Rhu	Furie, R	NY	586
Rhu	Kaell, A	NY	639
Rhu	Kopelman, R	NJ	751
Rhu	Spiera, H	NY	342
Rhu	Spiera, R	NY	342
Vasectomy Reversal			
U	Berdini, J	NJ	755
U	Fisch, H	NY	362
U	Goldstein, M	NY	362
U	Nagler, H	NY	365
Vasectomy-Scalpelless			
U	Cruickshank, D	NY	642
U	Goldstein, M	NY	362
U	Rossman, B	NJ	823
U	Sandhaus, J	NY	502
U	Sunshine, R	NY	595
Vein Disorders			
S	Bruck, H	NJ	753
S	Buch, E	NJ	907
S	Lutchman, G	NY	473
S	Nitzberg, R	NJ	925
VascS	Adelman, M	NY	369
VascS	Chideckel, N	NY	369
VascS	Elias, S	NJ	757
VascS	Fantini, G	NY	370
VascS	Ilkhani, R	NY	477
VascS	Jacobowitz, G	NY	371
VascS	Padberg, F	NJ	795
VascS	Rivers, S	NY	416
VascS	Schanzer, H	NY	371
VascS	Schwartz, K	NY	709
VascS	Suggs, W	NY	416
Ventricular Assist Device (LVAD)			
TS	Elefteriades, J	CT	983
Cv	Smart, F	NJ	874
TS	Lansman, S	NY	706
TS	Michler, R	NY	415
TS	Naka, Y	NY	358
TS	Rose, E	NY	358

Spec	Name	St	Pg
Vertigo			
Oto	Goldofsky, E	NY	567
Oto	Shulman, A	NY	456
Video Assisted Thoracic Surgery (VATS)			
TS	Caccavale, R	NJ	907
TS	Lee, J	NJ	755
TS	Streisand, R	NY	707
TS	Swanson, S	NY	359
TS	Widmann, M	NJ	885
VascS	Shin, C	NY	477
Video-playback Therapy			
Psyc	Alger, I	NY	310
Viral Infections			
D	Hatcher, V	NY	144
Inf	Baum, S	NY	181
Inf	Gross, P	NJ	731
Inf	Polsky, B	NY	184
PInf	Andiman, W	CT	976
Vision Loss-Unexplained Loss			
Oph	Frohman, L	NJ	782
Oph	Slamovits, T	NY	401
Oph	Wolintz, A	NY	454
Vocal Cord Disorders			
Oto	Aviv, J	NY	268
Oto	Berkower, A	NY	403
Oto	Shapshay, S	NY	275
Voice Disorders			
Oto	Aviv, J	NY	268
Oto	Baredes, S	NJ	783
Oto	Blitzer, A	NY	269
Oto	Draizin, D	NY	567
Oto	Haroldson, O	NJ	818
Oto	Josephson, J	NY	271
Oto	Li, R	NJ	818
Oto	Libin, J	NY	273
Oto	Pincus, R	NY	274
Oto	Rothstein, S	NY	274
Oto	Sadowski, J	NY	605
Oto	Sasaki, C	CT	976
Oto	Schley, W	NY	275
Oto	Siglock, T	NY	687
Oto	Slavit, D	NY	276
Oto	Snyder, G	NY	496
Oto	Steckowych, J	NJ	742
Oto	Surow, J	NJ	742
Oto	Taylor, H	NJ	881
Oto	Woo, P	NY	277
Oto	Zbar, L	NJ	784
PO	Goldsmith, A	NY	497
Voice Disorders/Professional Voice Care			
Oto	Jahn, A	NJ	784
Oto	Krevitt, L	NY	272

Special Expertise Index

Spec	Name	St	Pg
Wrist & Upper Extremity Surgery			
OrS	Pianka, G	NY	264

Spec	Name	St	Pg
Wrist Surgery			
HS	Melone, C	NY	176
HS	Pruzansky, M	NY	176
HS	Wolfe, S	NY	177
OrS	Hotchkiss, R	NY	261

Spec	Name	St	Pg
Wrist/Hand Injuries			
HS	Gurland, M	NJ	729
HS	Miller-Breslow, A	NJ	730
HS	Raskin, K	NY	176
HS	Roger, I	NY	489
HS	Weiland, A	NY	177

Alphabetical Listing of Doctors

Name	Specialty	Pg	Name	Specialty	Pg
A			Adler, Albert (NY)	Ped	633
			Adler, Edward (NY)	OrS	255
Abdel-Dayem, Hussein M (NY)	NuM	228	Adler, Harry (NY)	S	471
Abelow, Arthur (NY)	Ge	386	Adler, Howard (NY)	Ge	159
Abemayor, Elie M (NY)	Ge	661	Adler, Jack (NY)	Pul	328
Abenavoli, Tancredi J (NY)	IM	666	Adler, Kenneth (NJ)	Onc	877
Abittan, Meyer H (NY)	IC	551	Adler, Mitchell (NY)	IM	186
Abott, Michael (NY)	Pul	465	Adler, Ronald S (NY)	DR	149
Abouchedid, Claude (NJ)	S	822	Adler, Stephen (NY)	Nep	674
Abrams, Jeffrey (NJ)	OrS	817	Adlersberg, Jay (NY)	Rhu	338
Abramson, Allan (NY)	Oto	567	Afif, Juan Simon (NY)	ObG	399
Abramson, David H (NY)	Oph	238	Afridi, Shariq (NJ)	Ge	811
Abramson, Sara (NY)	DR	149	Agarwal, Kishan (NJ)	PCd	842
Abramson, Steven B (NY)	Rhu	338	Agarwal, Nanakram (NY)	S	413
Abreu, Maria T (NY)	Ge	159	Agdere, Levon (NY)	PEn	458
Abright, Arthur Reese (NY)	ChAP	134	Aggarwal, Renu (NY)	NP	554
Abrol, Sunil (NY)	TS	474	Agin, Carole (NY)	PM	631
Abu-Rustum, Nadeem R (NY)	GO	173	Agri, Robyn (NJ)	PMR	819
Abud, Alfredo (NJ)	VascS	823	Agrin, Richard (NJ)	EDM	830
Abud, Ariel (NJ)	NS	815	Aguila, Helen (NJ)	PPul	786
Abularrage, Joseph J (NY)	Ped	497	Agulnek, Milton (NY)	Ped	575
Accardi, Frank E (NY)	Oph	239	Agus, Bertrand (NY)	Rhu	338
Accettola, Albert (NY)	OrS	516	Agus, Saul G (NY)	Ge	159
Accurso, Charles (NJ)	Ge	903	Aharon, Raphael (NY)	Oph	494
Acinapura, Anthony (NY)	TS	474	Ahlborn, Thomas N (NJ)	S	752
Acker, Peter J (NY)	Ped	692	Ahluwalia, Brij M Singh (NY)	N	676
Ackerman, A Bernard (NY)	D	141	Ahmad, Mahnaz (NY)	Ger	433
Ackerman, Jacob (NY)	Oph	451	Ahmed, Fakhiuddin (NY)	Onc	442
Ackert, John (NY)	Ge	159	Ahmed, Maher (NY)	VascS	369
Acosta, Rod (CT)	FMed	937	Ahmed, Tauseef (NY)	Onc	671
Acquista, Angelo (NY)	Pul	328	Ahn, Christina Y (NY)	PlS	301
Adachi, Akinori (NY)	ObG	399	Ahn, Jung Hwan (NY)	PMR	298
Adams, David H (NY)	TS	355	Ahronheim, Judith (NY)	Ger	434
Adams, Francis (NY)	Pul	328	Aiges, Harvey (NY)	PGe	571
Adams, Marc (NY)	RadRO	520	Aisenberg, James (NY)	Ge	159
Addonizio, Gerard C (NY)	Psyc	696	Aisner, Joseph (NJ)	Onc	835
Adelman, Mark (NY)	VascS	369	Ajl, Stephen (NY)	Ped	461
Adelman, Ronald (NY)	Ger	171	Akerman, Michael (NY)	Pul	465
Adelson, Richard (NJ)	Cv	857	Akinboboye, Olakunle (NY)	Cv	483
Adesman, Andrew (NY)	Ped	575	Albin, Joan (NY)	EDM	658

Alphabetical Listing of Doctors

Name	Specialty	Pg	Name	Specialty	Pg
Albom, Michael (NY)	D	141	Amiruddin, Qamar (NY)	S	471
Alderman, Elizabeth (NY)	AM	378	Amis, E Stephen (NY)	DR	382
Alderson, Philip (NY)	DR	149	Amler, David (NY)	Ped	692
Aldrich, Thomas K (NY)	Pul	411	Ammazzalorso, Michael (NY)	IM	548
Aledo, Alexander (NY)	PHO	286	Amodio, John (NY)	DR	149
Aledort, Louis (NY)	Hem	177	Amorosa, Louis (NJ)	EDM	830
Alexiades, Michael (NY)	OrS	255	Amorosi, Edward (NY)	Hem	177
Alexopoulos, George (NY)	Psyc	696	Amoruso, Robert (NJ)	Pul	895
Alfonso, Antonio (NY)	S	471	Amory, Spencer E (NY)	S	344
Alger, Ian (NY)	Psyc	310	Anand, Vijay (NY)	Oto	268
Allegra, Donald (NJ)	Inf	876	Anant, Ashok (NY)	NS	446
Allen, Carol B (NY)	EDM	384	Andiman, Warren A (CT)	PInf	976
Allen, Jeffrey (NY)	ChiN	136	Andrade, Joseph (NY)	Ped	406
Allen, Machelle (NY)	ObG	230	Andrews, Joseph (CT)	IM	940
Allen, Steven (NY)	Hem	546	Andriani, Rudy (CT)	U	959
Allendorf, Dennis (NY)	Ped	293	Andriola, Mary (NY)	ChiN	613
Almeida, Laila (NJ)	D	874	Andriole, Vincent (CT)	Inf	971
Almeyda, Elizabeth (NY)	PlS	301	Angioletti, Louis V (NY)	Oph	239
Aloia, John (NY)	EDM	539	Angoff, Ronald (CT)	Ped	977
Alper, Kenneth (NY)	Psyc	310	Angulo, Moris (NY)	CG	535
Alpert, Barbara (NY)	IM	666	Anhalt, Henry (NJ)	PEn	785
Alpert, Scott W (NY)	OrS	630	Ankobiah, William (NY)	Pul	499
Altbaum, Robert (CT)	IM	940	Annabi, Iyad N (NY)	FMed	660
Altchek, David (NY)	SM	343	Annos, Thomas (NJ)	RE	791
Altchek, Edgar (NY)	PlS	301	Anselmi, Gregory (NJ)	N	801
Alter, Sheldon (NY)	IM	666	Anto, Maliakal J (NY)	Cv	529
Alterman, Lloyd (NJ)	Nep	917	Antoine, Clarel (NY)	ObG	230
Altholz, Jeffrey (NY)	IM	666	Anton, John R (NY)	PlS	635
Altman, R Peter (NY)	PS	292	Antonacci, Anthony (NY)	S	344
Altman, Robin (NY)	Ped	692	Antonelle, Robert (NY)	Ge	661
Altman, Wayne (NJ)	OrS	739	Antony, Michael (NY)	Ge	386
Altmann, Dory B (NJ)	IC	835	Anyane-Yeboa, Kwame (NY)	CG	137
Altorki, Nasser (NY)	TS	355	Apatoff, Brian R (NY)	N	218
Altschul, Larry (NY)	Cv	611	Aponte, Alex M (NY)	FMed	617
Alweiss, Gary (NJ)	N	736	Appel, David (NY)	Pul	411
Aly, Sayed (NJ)	NP	801	Appel, Gerald (NY)	Nep	211
Alyskewycz, Roman (NY)	U	593	Applebaum, Eric (NJ)	A&I	873
Ames, John W (NY)	RadRO	584	April, Max M (NY)	PO	289
Ames, Richard (NY)	Nep	211	Aprile, Georgette (NY)	D	536
Amin, Hossam H (NY)	Pul	466	Apuzzio, Joseph (NJ)	ObG	781
Amin, Mahendra (NY)	IM	490	Apuzzo, Thomas (NY)	FMed	660
Amin, Ravindra (NY)	GerPsy	434	Aranoff, Gaya S (NY)	PEn	404

Name	Specialty	Pg	Name	Specialty	Pg
Aranoff, Shera (NY)	D	141	Askenase, Philip (CT)	A&I	965
Arbour, Robert (NJ)	S	866	Asnes, Russell (NJ)	Ped	745
Arcasoy, Selim M (NY)	Pul	328	Asnis, Deborah (NY)	Inf	436
Arcati, Anthony T (NY)	FMed	541	Asnis, Gregory (NY)	Psyc	410
Arcati, Robert J (NY)	FMed	541	Asnis, Stanley (NY)	OrS	565
Arden, Martha (NY)	AM	527	Aston, Sherrell (NY)	PlS	301
Arens, Raanan (NY)	PPul	406	Astrow, Alan (NY)	Onc	442
Argenziano, Michael (NY)	TS	355	Atakent, Pinar (NY)	PMR	463
Argyros, Thomas (NY)	Rhu	338	Athanail, Steven (NY)	FMed	430
Arici, Aydin M (CT)	RE	981	Athanasian, Edward (NY)	HS	175
Aries, Philip (NY)	Oph	627	Atkin, Suzanne (NJ)	IM	776
Ariyan, Stephan (CT)	PlS	978	Atlas, Arthur B (NJ)	PPul	882
Ark, Jon Wong Tze-Jen (NJ)	HS	812	Atlas, Ian (NJ)	U	885
Arkow, Stan D (NY)	Psyc	310	Attas, Lewis (NJ)	Onc	733
Armbruster, Robert (NY)	ObG	677	Attia, Albert (NY)	Ge	160
Armenakas, Noel (NY)	U	360	Attia, Evelyn (NY)	Psyc	310
Armento, Michael J (NJ)	PMR	922	Attiyeh, Fadi F (NY)	S	344
Arno, Louis (NJ)	Pul	906	Auchincloss, Elizabeth (NY)	Psyc	310
Arnold, Thomas E (NY)	VascS	643	Auerbach, Mitchell E (NY)	Ge	661
Arnon, Rica (NY)	PCd	281	Auerbach, Robert (NY)	D	141
Arnstein, Ellis (NY)	Ped	293	Aufiero, Patrick (NJ)	Inf	812
Aron, Alan (NY)	ChiN	136	August, David (NJ)	S	849
Aronne, Louis J (NY)	IM	186	August, Phyllis (NY)	Nep	211
Aronoff, Michael S (NY)	Psyc	310	Auguste, Louis J (NY)	S	588
Aronson, Peter S (CT)	Nep	973	Augustine, Viruppamattan M (NY)	Ped	634
Aronson, Thomas (NY)	Psyc	636	Auld, Peter (NY)	NP	210
Arpadi, Stephen (NY)	Ped	293	Austin, John H M (NY)	DR	149
Arvan, Glenn Douglas (NY)	OrS	630	Ausubel, Herbert (NY)	IM	548
Arvanitis, Michael (NJ)	CRS	858	Aviv, Jonathan (NY)	Oto	268
Arya, Yashpal (NY)	Ge	431	Avram, Marc R (NY)	D	141
Asarian, Armand (NY)	S	471	Avruskin, Theodore W (NY)	PEn	458
Asbell, Penny (NY)	Oph	239	Avvento, Louis (NY)	Hem	620
Ascheim, Robert (NY)	IM	186	Axelrod, Deborah (NY)	S	344
Ascher, Enrico (NY)	VascS	477	Axelrod, Randi (NJ)	NP	814
Ascherman, Jeffrey (NY)	PlS	301	Ayoub, Thomas (CT)	ObG	948
Ash, Julia Y (NY)	Rhu	703	Ayyanathan, K (NJ)	Ped	921
Ashamalla, Hani (NY)	RadRO	468	Azhar, Salman (NY)	N	446
Ashendorf, Douglas (NJ)	PM	921			
Ashikari, Andrew Y (NY)	S	704			
Ashinoff, Robin (NJ)	D	724			
Ashley, Richard (NY)	U	593			
Askanas, Alexander (NY)	Cv	124			

Alphabetical Listing of Doctors

Name	Specialty	Pg	Name	Specialty	Pg
B			Baram, Daniel (NY)	Pul	637
			Barandes, Martin (NY)	EDM	154
Babu, Sateesh (NY)	VascS	709	Baranetsky, Nicholas G (NJ)	EDM	772
Bacall, Charles (NY)	ObG	230	Barasch, Kenneth (NY)	Oph	239
Baccash, Emil (NY)	Ger	434	Barbaccia, Ann (NY)	ObG	559
Bach, John (NJ)	PMR	788	Barbasch, Avi (NY)	Onc	200
Bachmann, Gloria (NJ)	ObG	839	Barbuto, Joseph (NY)	Psyc	311
Bade, Harry A (NJ)	OrS	863	Bardeguez, Arlene D (NJ)	MF	777
Badikian, Arthur (NY)	Psyc	697	Baredes, Soly (NJ)	Oto	783
Badlani, Gopal (NY)	U	593	Barie, Philip (NY)	S	344
Badshah, Cyrus S (NY)	Inf	181	Barile, Gaetano (NY)	Oph	239
Baer, Jeanne (NY)	DR	149	Barker, Barbara Ann (NY)	Oph	239
Bagel, Jerry (NJ)	D	810	Barmakian, Joseph (NJ)	OrS	919
Bagg, Jennifer G (NY)	IM	666	Barnard, Nicola (NJ)	Path	842
Bahler, Alan (NJ)	Cv	768	Barone, Clement (NY)	DR	150
Bahr, Gerald (NY)	CCM	140	Barone, James (NY)	S	413
Bailey, Michele L (NY)	Ped	692	Barone, Richard P (NY)	Rhu	703
Bailine, Samuel (NY)	Psyc	579	Barrett, Leonard O (NY)	TS	591
Bains, Manjit (NY)	TS	355	Barron, O Alton (NY)	HS	175
Bains, Yatinder (NJ)	IM	776	Barry, Michele (CT)	IM	971
Baiser, Dennis (NJ)	Ped	819	Barst, Robyn J (NY)	PCd	281
Bajorin, Dean (NY)	Onc	199	Bartlett, Jacqueline (NJ)	ChAP	770
Bakal, Curtis (NJ)	VIR	795	Bartolomeo, Robert (NY)	Ge	542
Baker, Daniel (NY)	PlS	302	Barzegar, Hooshang (NY)	ObG	449
Baker, David A (NY)	ObG	626	Basch, Samuel (NY)	Psyc	311
Bakoss, Imad John (NY)	Pul	466	Bases, Hugh (NJ)	Ped	745
Baldasar, Jack L (NJ)	DR	725	Bashevkin, Michael (NY)	Onc	442
Baldwin, Hilary (NY)	D	426	Baskin, David (NY)	IM	186
Balk, Sophie (NY)	Ped	406	Baskin, Martin (NY)	Pul	328
Balkin, Michael (NY)	EDM	616	Baskind, Larry (NY)	Ped	692
Ballantyne, Garth (NJ)	S	753	Basralian, Kevin R (NJ)	U	755
Balot, Barry (NY)	IM	621	Bastawros, Mary (NY)	Ped	517
Balsano, Nicholas (NY)	S	413	Basuk, Pamela (NY)	D	614
Baltimore, Robert (CT)	PInf	977	Basuk, Paul M (NY)	Ge	160
Bangaru, Babu (NY)	PGe	497	Bateman, David (NY)	NP	210
Bank, David (NY)	D	654	Batsford, William P (CT)	CE	965
Bank, Simmy (NY)	Ge	542	Bauer, Bertha (NY)	Rhu	338
Bansal, Rajendra K (NY)	Oph	680	Bauer, Joel (NY)	S	344
Banzon, Manuel (NJ)	ObG	802	Baum, Howard B (NJ)	Ge	892
Bar, Michael (CT)	Hem	939	Baum, Stephen (NY)	Inf	181
Bar-Chama, Natan (NY)	U	360	Bauman, James S (CT)	DR	936
Barakat, Richard (NY)	GO	173	Bauman, Jonathan (NY)	Psyc	697

Name	Specialty	Pg	Name	Specialty	Pg
Bauman, Phillip (NY)	OrS	255	Bennett, Harvey S (NJ)	ChiN	874
Baumann, John (NJ)	RadRO	821	Bennett, Ronald (NY)	Rhu	639
Baxi, Laxmi Vibhakar (NY)	ObG	230	Benovitz, Harvey (NY)	IM	186
Baydin, Jeffrey (NJ)	OrS	880	Benson, Douglas (NJ)	S	753
Beardsley, Diana (CT)	PHO	976	Benson, Mitchell C (NY)	U	360
Beasley, Robert (NY)	HS	175	Benton, Marc (NJ)	Pul	884
Beauregard, Lou-Anne M (NJ)	Cv	857	Benvenisty, Alan I (NY)	VascS	369
Bebawi, Magdi (NY)	S	345	Beraka, George (NY)	PlS	302
Beccia, David (NY)	U	642	Bercow, Neil R (NY)	TS	591
Beck, A Robert (NY)	PS	292	Berdini, Jeffrey L (NJ)	U	755
Becker, Alfred (NY)	Rhu	606	Berdoff, Russell (NY)	Cv	124
Becker, Carolyn (NY)	EDM	154	Berenson, Murray J (NY)	Ge	160
Beckett, MarieAnne G (NJ)	D	799	Berenstein, Alejandro (NY)	NRad	227
Bederson, Joshua (NY)	NS	214	Berezin, Marc (NY)	SM	606
Bednarek, Karl (NY)	Ge	160	Berezin, Stuart (NY)	PGe	689
Bednoff, Stuart (NY)	ObG	559	Berger, Bernard (NY)	D	614
Befeler, David (NJ)	S	925	Berger, E Roy (NY)	Onc	623
Behm, Dutsi (NY)	IM	438	Berger, Jack (NY)	Rhu	703
Behr, Raymond (NY)	Psyc	580	Berger, Jeffrey (NY)	IM	548
Behrens, Myles (NY)	Oph	239	Berger, Judith (NY)	Inf	390
Beil, Arthur (NY)	TS	591	Berger, Marvin (NY)	Cv	124
Belilos, Elise (NY)	Rhu	585	Berger, Matthew (NY)	IM	391
Bell, Evan (NY)	Inf	181	Bergh, Paul A (NJ)	RE	884
Bell, Jonathan (CT)	A&I	933	Bergman, Donald (NY)	EDM	154
Bell, Kevin (NJ)	IM	904	Bergman, Michael I (NY)	Pul	466
Bello, Jacqueline A (NY)	NRad	399	Bergmann, Steven (NY)	Cv	124
Bello, Mary (NJ)	FMed	727	Berk, Paul D (NY)	IM	186
Bellucci, Alessandro (NY)	Nep	555	Berke, Andrew D (NY)	IC	551
Belmont, Howard Michael (NY)	Rhu	338	Berke, Stanley J (NY)	Oph	562
Belok, Lennart (NY)	N	218	Berkeley, Alan S (NY)	RE	335
Bemporad, Jules (NY)	Psyc	697	Berkey, Peter (NY)	Inf	665
Ben-Zvi, Jeffrey (NY)	Ge	160	Berkower, Alan (NY)	Oto	403
Bender-Cracco, Joan (NY)	ChiN	426	Berkowitz, Howard (NY)	Psyc	464
Bendo, John A (NY)	OrS	255	Berkowitz, Leonard B (NY)	Inf	436
Benedicto, Milagros A (NY)	ObG	493	Berkowitz, Norman (NY)	Ped	692
Benevenia, Joseph (NJ)	OrS	783	Berkowitz, Rhonda (NY)	D	654
Benisovich, Vladimir I (NY)	Onc	492	Berkowitz, Richard (NY)	MF	198
Benito, Carlos W (NJ)	MF	835	Berkowitz, Richard H (NJ)	EDM	892
Benjamin, Ernest (NY)	CCM	140	Berkowitz, Walter (NJ)	Cv	719
Benjamin, John (NY)	Psyc	580	Berkwits, Kieve (CT)	PCd	951
Benjamin, Vallo (NY)	NS	214	Berlet, Anthony C (NJ)	PlS	788
Benkov, Keith J (NY)	PGe	285	Berlin, Arnold (NY)	S	414

Alphabetical Listing of Doctors

Name	Specialty	Pg	Name	Specialty	Pg
Berliner, Nancy (CT)	Hem	970	Beyda, Bernadette (NY)	D	485
Berman, Alvin (NY)	ObG	231	Beyerl, Brian D (NJ)	NS	878
Berman, Daniel (NY)	IM	666	Bharathan, Thayyullathil (NY)	IM	438
Berman, David H (NY)	Oph	451	Bhatt, Anjani (NY)	EDM	539
Berman, Ellin (NY)	Onc	200	Bhatt, Ashok (NY)	Psyc	580
Berman, Mark (NJ)	OrS	739	Biagiotti, Wendy (NY)	FMed	385
Berman, Morton (NY)	Ped	692	Bialer, Martin G (NY)	CG	535
Berman, Richard E (NY)	Ge	619	Bialkin, Robert (NY)	ObG	559
Berman, Sandra (NY)	IM	438	Biancaniello, Thomas (NY)	PCd	632
Berman, Sheldon S (NY)	Psyc	580	Biasetti, John (NY)	IM	621
Berman, Steven (NY)	U	360	Bickers, David (NY)	D	142
Bernard, Robert (NY)	IM	621	Bielory, Leonard (NJ)	A&I	767
Bernard, Robert W (NY)	PlS	695	Bienenstock, Harry (NY)	Rhu	470
Bernardini, Dennis (NY)	Pul	637	Bierman, Fredrick (NY)	PCd	569
Bernhardt, Bernard (NY)	Onc	671	Bigajer, Charles (NY)	Ge	431
Bernik, Stephanie F (NY)	S	345	Bigliani, Louis (NY)	OrS	255
Bernstein, Brett B (NY)	Ge	160	Bilezikian, John P (NY)	EDM	154
Bernstein, Chaim (NY)	Pul	466	Bilfinger, Thomas (NY)	TS	642
Bernstein, Charles (NY)	D	509	Billett, Henny (NY)	Hem	389
Bernstein, David E (NY)	Ge	542	Bilmes, Ernest (NY)	FMed	617
Bernstein, Harvey (NY)	Ped	634	Bilsky, Mark H (NY)	NS	214
Bernstein, Larry (NY)	A&I	483	Bindelglass, David (CT)	OrS	949
Bernstein, Lawrence J (NY)	Rhu	470	Binder, Ralph E (NY)	Pul	700
Bernstein, Martin (NY)	Pul	466	Binns, Joseph (NJ)	Ge	859
Bernstein, Michael O (NY)	S	471	Birch, Thomas (NJ)	Inf	730
Bernstein, Robert M (NY)	ObG	559	Bird, Hector (NY)	ChAP	134
Bernstein, Robert M (NY)	D	141	Birkhoff, John (NY)	U	360
Bernstein, William H (NY)	Ped	605	Birnbaum, Audrey (NY)	PGe	689
Berroya, Renato (NY)	VascS	595	Birnbaum, Jay (NY)	PlS	302
Berry, Richard (NY)	D	426	Birns, Douglas (NY)	U	361
Berson, Anthony M (NY)	RadRO	333	Birns, Robert (NJ)	Pul	749
Berson, Barry (NY)	DR	150	Biro, David (NY)	D	426
Berson, Diane S (NY)	D	141	Biro, Laszlo (NY)	D	427
Besser, Gary (CT)	ObG	948	Bisaccia, Emil (NJ)	D	874
Besser, Louis (NY)	Cv	507	Bisberg, Dorothy Stein (NJ)	PPul	786
Besser, Walter (NY)	OrS	495	Bitan, Fabien D (NY)	OrS	256
Bessey, Palmer Q (NY)	S	345	Bivona, James J (CT)	IM	940
Bessler, Marc (NY)	S	345	Blackman, Edward (NJ)	Ped	845
Bethel, Colin (NJ)	PS	787	Blackwood, M Michele (NJ)	S	792
Better, Donna (NY)	PCd	569	Blady, David (NJ)	N	780
Bevelaqua, Frederick (NY)	Pul	328	Blair, Lester (NY)	Pul	328
Beyda, Allan (NY)	IM	490	Blaivas, Jerry G (NY)	U	361

Name	Specialty	Pg	Name	Specialty	Pg
Blake, James (NY)	Cv	124	Bochner, Ronnie (NJ)	ObG	839
Blanck, Richard (NY)	N	557	Bockman, Richard (NY)	EDM	155
Blanco, Jody (NY)	ObG	231	Boczko, Stanley (NY)	U	361
Blank, Ellen (NJ)	D	799	Bodenheimer, Monty (NY)	Cv	529
Blaser, Martin J (NY)	Inf	181	Bodenheimer,, Henry C (NY)	Ge	160
Blau, Sheldon P (NY)	Rhu	586	Bodis-Wollner, Ivan (NY)	N	446
Blau, Steven (NY)	S	588	Bodner, William (NY)	RadRO	413
Blaufox, M Donald (NY)	NuM	399	Bogaty, Stanley (NY)	Oph	627
Blaugrund, Stanley (NY)	Oto	268	Bogin, Marc (NY)	Cv	507
Bleiberg, Melvyn (NY)	Cv	648	Bohensky, Paul (NY)	Pul	637
Bleicher, Robert (NJ)	Ge	892	Bohrer, Stuart (NY)	PS	574
Bleifeld, Charles (NY)	OrS	630	Boim, Marilynn (NJ)	PEn	819
Bleiweiss, Ira J (NY)	Path	279	Bojko, Thomas (NJ)	PCCM	843
Blitzer, Andrew (NY)	Oto	269	Bolanowski, Paul J P (NJ)	TS	926
Block, Jerome M (NY)	N	218	Bolognia, Jean (CT)	D	967
Blood, David K (NJ)	Cv	720	Boltin, Harry (NY)	DR	601
Bloom, Norman (NY)	S	345	Bomback, Fredric (NY)	Ped	692
Bloom, Patricia A (NY)	Ger	171	Bonagura, Vincent R (NY)	A&I	527
Bloomenstein, Richard (NJ)	PlS	747	Bond, Annette L (CT)	MF	943
Bloomfield, Dennis A (NY)	Cv	507	Bondi, Elliott (NY)	Pul	466
Bloomfield, Diane (NY)	Ped	406	Bone, Stanley (NY)	Psyc	311
Bloomgarden, David K (NY)	EDM	658	Bonforte, Richard J (NJ)	Ped	803
Bloomgarden, Zachary (NY)	EDM	154	Bonheim, Nelson (CT)	Ge	938
Blum, Alan (NY)	Pul	581	Bonilla, Mary Ann (NJ)	PHO	895
Blum, Conrad (NY)	EDM	154	Boniuk, Vivien (NY)	Oph	494
Blum, Daniel N (NY)	IM	490	Boodish, Wesley (NJ)	Ped	787
Blum, David (NY)	EDM	658	Boorjian, Peter (NJ)	U	794
Blum, Jay (NJ)	A&I	827	Bopaiah, Vinod (NY)	CRS	509
Blum, Manfred (NY)	EDM	155	Borah, Gregory (NJ)	PlS	845
Blum, Mark A (NJ)	Cv	873	Borao, Frank J (NJ)	S	867
Blum, Ronald (NY)	Onc	200	Borbely, Antal (NY)	Psyc	311
Blumberg, Joel M (CT)	IM	940	Borek, Mark (NY)	Cv	611
Blume, Ralph S (NY)	Rhu	338	Borer, Jeffrey (NY)	Cv	124
Blumenfeld, Jon D (NY)	Nep	212	Borg, Morton (NY)	PCd	282
Blumenfield, Michael (NY)	Psyc	697	Borgen, Patrick I (NY)	S	345
Blumenthal, David S (NY)	Cv	124	Borkowsky, William (NY)	PInf	288
Blumenthal, Jesse (NY)	VascS	369	Borriello, Raffaele (NY)	S	471
Blumgart, Leslie H (NY)	S	345	Bortniker, David (NJ)	Oto	905
Blumstein, Meyer (NY)	Ge	542	Boscamp, Jeffrey R (NJ)	PInf	744
Blyskal, Stanley (NY)	FMed	617	Bosco, Joseph (NY)	OrS	256
Boachie-Adjei, Oheneba (NY)	OrS	256	Bosl, George (NY)	Onc	200
Bobroff, Lewis M (NY)	DR	601	Bosso, John (NY)	A&I	601

Alphabetical Listing of Doctors

Name	Specialty	Pg	Name	Specialty	Pg
Bosworth, Jay L (NY)	RadRO	584	Brenner, Steven H (NY)	RE	585
Botet, Jose (NY)	DR	657	Bressman, Susan (NY)	N	218
Botti, Anthony Charles (NJ)	Onc	778	Brewer, Marlon (NY)	IM	490
Botwin, Clifford (NJ)	OrS	919	Brickman, Alan (NY)	EDM	428
Botwinick, Nelson (NY)	HS	175	Brickner, Gary R (NJ)	ObG	816
Bourla, Steven (NY)	Nep	555	Brief, Donald (NJ)	S	792
Bowers, Malcolm B (CT)	Psyc	979	Brill, Joseph (NY)	Pul	700
Boxer, Harriet (NY)	NP	554	Brill, Paula (NY)	DR	150
Boxer, Mitchell (NY)	A&I	527	Brion, Luc (NY)	NP	394
Boyarsky, Andrew (NJ)	S	849	Brisson, Paul M (NY)	OrS	256
Boyd, D Barry (CT)	Onc	943	Brittis, Robert J (NY)	Ped	693
Boyer, Joseph (NY)	Ped	693	Britton, Carolyn B (NY)	N	218
Braddom, Randall L (NJ)	PMR	864	Brock, William A (NY)	U	593
Brademas, Mary Ellen (NY)	D	142	Broderick, Robert (NY)	Oph	562
Bradley, Thomas P (NY)	Onc	552	Brodherson, Michael (NY)	U	361
Braff, Robert (NY)	Cv	125	Brodie, Jonathan D (NY)	Psyc	311
Bram, Harris (NJ)	PM	863	Brodkin, Roger (NJ)	D	771
Brancaccio, Ronald R (NY)	D	427	Brodman, Michael (NY)	ObG	231
Brancaccio, William R (NY)	DR	615	Brodman, Richard R (NJ)	Rhu	924
Brand, Howard A (NY)	EDM	616	Brody, Samuel (NY)	Ger	489
Brandeis, Steven (NY)	CRS	138	Brodyn, Nicholas (NJ)	Cv	911
Brandt, Lawrence (NY)	Ge	387	Brolin, Robert E (NJ)	S	849
Brandt-Rauf, Paul W (NY)	OM	238	Bromberg, Assia (NJ)	IM	731
Branovan, Daniel Igor (NY)	Oto	269	Bromberg, Jonathan S (NY)	S	346
Brauner, Gary (NJ)	D	724	Bromberg, Warren (NY)	U	707
Braunstein, Richard E (NY)	Oph	239	Bromley, Gary S (NY)	PIS	302
Brauntuch, Glenn R (NJ)	Pul	749	Bronheim, Harold (NY)	Psyc	311
Brause, Barry (NY)	Inf	182	Bronin, Andrew (NY)	D	654
Braverman, Irwin (CT)	D	968	Bronson, Michael (NY)	OrS	256
Brecher, Rubin (NY)	Oph	451	Bronster, David (NY)	N	219
Breen, William (NY)	Cv	529	Brookler, Kenneth (NY)	Oto	269
Breidbart, David (NY)	Pul	581	Broumand, Stafford (NY)	PIS	302
Breitbart, Arnold (NY)	PIS	577	Brovender, Bruce J (NY)	Ped	293
Breitbart, William (NY)	Psyc	311	Brower, Mark (NY)	Onc	200
Brem, Harold (NY)	S	345	Brown, Alan (NY)	Oph	240
Brener, Bruce J (NJ)	VascS	795	Brown, Andrew (NY)	PMR	298
Brenholz, Pauline (NY)	CG	654	Brown, Arthur E (NY)	Inf	182
Brennan, George (NJ)	Ped	845	Brown, Carol (NY)	GO	173
Brennan, John P (NY)	ObG	449	Brown, Charles B (NY)	OrS	683
Brennan, Murray (NY)	S	345	Brown, David K (NJ)	A&I	911
Brenner, David A (NY)	Ge	161	Brown, David L (NY)	IC	623
Brenner, Ronald (NY)	Psyc	311	Brown, Eric (CT)	Nep	945

Name	Specialty	Pg	Name	Specialty	Pg
Brown, Jeffrey (NY)	Ped	693	Bulgarelli, Christopher (NY)	Psyc	312
Brown, Jeffrey A (NY)	NS	556	Bull, Sherman (CT)	S	958
Brown, John (NJ)	TS	885	Bullock, Richard B (NJ)	Ger	832
Brown, Karen T (NY)	VIR	368	Bullough, Peter (NY)	Path	279
Brown, Lawrence S (NY)	IM	438	Buly, Robert L (NY)	OrS	256
Brown, Lionel (CT)	HS	939	Burack, Joshua H (NY)	TS	474
Brown, Mitchell Lee (NJ)	Ger	800	Burak, George (NY)	OrS	683
Brown, Richard P (NY)	Psyc	312	Burbige, Kevin (CT)	U	960
Brown, Robert B (CT)	Pul	956	Burd, Robert (CT)	Onc	944
Bruce, Christopher J (NY)	CRS	654	Burg, Richard (NY)	CRS	654
Bruce, Jeffrey (NY)	NS	215	Burk, Peter (NY)	D	382
Bruck, Harold M (NJ)	S	753	Burke, Gary R (NY)	IM	186
Bruckner, Howard W (NY)	Onc	442	Burke, Karen (NY)	D	142
Bruckstein, Alex (NY)	Ge	510	Burke, Patricia (NJ)	Oph	738
Bruckstein, Robert (NY)	D	536	Burke, Stephen W (NY)	OrS	256
Brunckhorst, Keith (NY)	Onc	200	Burkes, Lynn (NY)	ChAP	134
Brunetti, Jacqueline (NJ)	NuM	737	Burkett, Eric N (NJ)	IM	860
Brunnquell, Stephen (NJ)	IM	731	Burns, Elisa (NY)	ObG	677
Bruno, Anthony (NY)	U	593	Burns, Godfrey (NY)	Nep	212
Bruno, Peter (NY)	IM	186	Burns, Les A (NJ)	ObG	894
Brust, John C M (NY)	N	219	Burns, Mark (NY)	Rhu	703
Brustein, Harris (NY)	Oph	680	Burns, Paul (NY)	PM	605
Brustman, Lois (NY)	ObG	231	Burroughs, Valentine (NY)	EDM	155
Buatti, Elizabeth (NY)	IM	391	Burstin, Harris E (NY)	Ped	293
Buch, Edward (NJ)	S	907	Buscaino, Giacomo J (NY)	Cv	422
Buchalter, Maury (NJ)	Ped	745	Busch-Devereaux, Erna (NY)	S	640
Buchbinder, Ellen (NY)	A&I	120	Bush, Jacqueline (NY)	MF	441
Buchbinder, Mitchell (NY)	U	593	Bush, Michael (NY)	IM	187
Buchbinder, Shalom (NY)	DR	509	Busillo, Christopher (NY)	Inf	182
Buchman, Myron (NY)	ObG	231	Bussel, James (NY)	PHO	286
Buchness, Mary Ruth (NY)	D	142	Butler, David (NJ)	ObG	737
Bucholtz, Harvey K (NJ)	EDM	830	Butler, Mark S (NJ)	OrS	840
Buckley, Michael Kevin (NJ)	S	896	Butt, Ahmar A (NY)	IM	438
Budd, Daniel (NJ)	S	896	Butt, Khalid M H (NY)	S	704
Budin, Joel A (NJ)	DR	725	Buxton, Douglas F (NY)	Oph	240
Budman, Cathy L (NY)	Psyc	580	Buyon, Jill P (NY)	Rhu	339
Budman, Daniel (NY)	Onc	552	Buzzeo, Louis (NY)	Nep	674
Budow, Jack (NY)	Cv	529	Bye, Michael R (NY)	PPul	290
Bufalini, Bruno (NJ)	S	753	Byk, Cheryl (NJ)	DR	799
Bukberg, Judith (NY)	Psyc	312	Byrd, Lawrence H (NJ)	Nep	778
Bukberg, Phillip (NY)	EDM	155	Bystryn, Jean-Claude (NY)	D	142
Bukosky, Richard (NJ)	A&I	911			

Alphabetical Listing of Doctors

Name	Specialty	Pg	Name	Specialty	Pg
C			Cardiello, Gary P (NJ)	IM	801
			Cardoso, Erico R (NY)	NS	446
Cabbad, Michael (NY)	MF	441	Carew, John F (NY)	Oto	269
Cabin, Henry S (CT)	Cv	965	Carey, Dennis (NY)	PEn	570
Caccavale, Robert J (NJ)	TS	907	Carlin, Elizabeth (NJ)	NP	734
Caccese, William (NY)	Ge	542	Carlson, Gabrielle A (NY)	ChAP	613
Cafferty, Maureen (NY)	N	219	Carlson, Harold E (NY)	EDM	616
Cahan, Anthony (NY)	S	704	Carlson, John (NJ)	GO	832
Cahill, John (NY)	FMed	385	Carlson, Michelle Gerwin (NY)	HS	175
Cahill, John (NY)	PrM	309	Carmel, Peter (NJ)	NS	779
Cahill, Kevin M (NY)	PrM	309	Carmichael, L David (NY)	IM	187
Cairo, Mitchell S (NY)	PHO	286	Carney, Alexander (NJ)	Rhu	821
Calanog, Anthony (NY)	GO	173	Carniol, Paul (NJ)	Oto	920
Calem-Grunat, Jaclyn A (NJ)	DR	725	Carolan, Patrick J (CT)	OrS	949
Call, Pamela (NY)	Psyc	312	Carolan, Stephen (NY)	ObG	677
Callahan, Lisa (NY)	SM	343	Caron, Philip C (NY)	Hem	665
Calman, Neil (NY)	FMed	158	Carone, Patrick F (NY)	Psyc	580
Cam, Jenny Rose (NJ)	EDM	799	Caronna, John J (NY)	N	219
Camacho, Fernando J (NY)	Onc	393	Carpenter, Duncan (NJ)	NS	736
Camel, Mark (CT)	NS	946	Carpenter, Thomas O (CT)	PEn	976
Camilien, Louis (NY)	ObG	449	Carr, Ronald (NY)	Oph	240
Camins, Martin B (NY)	NS	215	Carroll, William L (NY)	PHO	286
Cammarata, Angelo (NY)	S	346	Carson, Jeffrey (NJ)	IM	834
Cammisa, Frank P (NY)	OrS	257	Carsons, Steven (NY)	Rhu	586
Camp, Walter A (CT)	N	947	Caruana, Salvatore (NY)	Oto	269
Campbell, Deborah (NY)	NP	394	Caruso, Anthony (NY)	Oto	630
Campion, Robert E (NY)	Psyc	312	Caruso, Rocco (NY)	Onc	623
Campolattaro, Brian (NY)	Oph	240	Casale, Linda (CT)	Cv	933
Camunas, Jorge L (NY)	TS	356	Casden, Andrew M (NY)	OrS	257
Cancellieri, Russell (NY)	A&I	611	Case, David B (NY)	IM	187
Cangemi, Francis E (NJ)	Oph	781	Casey, Joan (NY)	Inf	390
Cannarozzi, Nicholas (NJ)	Rhu	791	Casino, Joseph (NY)	Pul	700
Canny, Christopher R (CT)	Ped	977	Casper, Daniel (NY)	Oph	240
Cantor, Michael C (NY)	Ge	161	Casper, Ephraim (NJ)	Onc	877
Capizzi, Anthony J (NY)	S	640	Casper, Theodore (NY)	Pul	412
Capobianco, Luigi (NY)	FMed	541	Cassell, Lauren (NY)	S	346
Caponegro, Robert (NY)	U	502	Cassidy, Brian (NJ)	IM	834
Capozzi, James (NY)	OrS	257	Casson, Ira (NY)	N	493
Caputo, Anthony R (NJ)	Oph	781	Castellano, Bartolomeo (NY)	Oto	516
Caputo, Thomas A (NY)	GO	173	Castellano, Michael A (NY)	Pul	519
Caracci, Giovanni (NJ)	Psyc	789	Castro-Magana, Mariano (NY)	PEn	571
Caraccio, Babette (CT)	Psyc	955	Castro-Malaspina, Hugo (NY)	Hem	178

Alphabetical Listing of Doctors

Name	Specialty	Pg	Name	Specialty	Pg
Cataletto, Mauro (NY)	OrS	565	Chaudhry, Saqib S (NY)	VascS	596
Catanese, Vincent J (NJ)	FMed	859	Chavez, Alberto (NJ)	NP	904
Caucino, Julie (NJ)	A&I	901	Cheigh, Jhoong S (NY)	Nep	212
Cavaliere, Gregg (NY)	SM	704	Chen, Jonathan M (NY)	TS	356
Cayten, C Gene (NY)	S	414	Chengot, Mathew (NY)	Cv	611
Cece, John (NJ)	Oto	894	Chern, Relly (NY)	Oph	241
Cehelsky, John Ihor (NY)	S	704	Chernack, William J (NJ)	A&I	873
Cemaletin, Nevber (NY)	Cv	125	Chernaik, Richard (NY)	IM	391
Cerny, Kenneth (NJ)	N	878	Chernaik, Robert (NY)	IM	621
Cerrone, Federico (NJ)	Pul	924	Chernik, Norman (NY)	N	625
Cerulli, Maurice A (NY)	Ge	431	Chernobilsky, Lev (NY)	Ped	634
Cervia, Joseph (NY)	Inf	547	Cherofsky, Alan (NY)	PIS	518
Chabot, John A (NY)	S	346	Cherry, Sheldon (NY)	ObG	231
Chachoua, Abraham (NY)	Onc	200	Chertoff, Harvey (NJ)	Psyc	748
Chadburn, Amy (NY)	Path	279	Chervenak, Francis A (NY)	MF	198
Chadda, Kul (NY)	Cv	529	Chesner, Michael (NY)	Cv	529
Chadha, Jang B S (NY)	Pul	499	Chess, Jeremy (NY)	Oph	400
Chaiken, Barry (NY)	Oph	240	Chessin, Robert (CT)	Ped	952
Chaikin, David C (NJ)	U	885	Chessler, Richard (NJ)	Ge	727
Chalal, Jeffrey (NJ)	DR	858	Chia, Gloria (NY)	Onc	671
Chalas, Eva (NY)	GO	620	Chianese, Maurice (NY)	Ped	575
Chamberlain, Ronald S (NJ)	S	792	Chideckel, Norman (NY)	VascS	369
Chambers, Joseph (NY)	GO	434	Chin, Daisy (NJ)	PEn	881
Chan, Brenda (CT)	Nep	945	Chin, Jean (NY)	ObG	231
Chandler, Michael (NY)	A&I	120	Chinitz, Larry (NY)	CE	122
Chandra, Pradeep (NY)	Onc	442	Chinitz, Marvin (NY)	Ge	661
Chandra, Prasanta C (NY)	ObG	449	Chiorazzi, Nicholas (NY)	Rhu	586
Chandrasekhar, Sujana (NY)	Oto	269	Chisolm, Alvin (NY)	DR	657
Chang, John (NY)	VascS	596	Chitkara, Dev (NY)	Oto	631
Chang, Patrick KS (NJ)	S	792	Chiu, David (NY)	PIS	302
Chang, Stanley (NY)	Oph	240	Chiurco, Anthony (NJ)	NS	815
Chapman, Mark (NY)	Ge	161	Cho, Hyun (NY)	Oto	269
Chapman, Paul (NY)	Onc	200	Chodosh, Eliot (NJ)	N	893
Chapnick, Edward (NY)	Inf	436	Chodosh, Ronald (NY)	Pul	700
Charap, Mitchell (NY)	IM	187	Choe, Dai-sun (NY)	S	472
Charap, Peter (NY)	IM	187	Choi, Mihye (NY)	HS	175
Charles, Norman (NY)	Oph	240	Choi, Young K (NJ)	PM	921
Charney, Jonathan (NY)	N	219	Cholst, Ina N (NY)	RE	335
Charnoff, Judah (NY)	Cv	422	Chorney, Gail (NY)	OrS	257
Charytan, Chaim (NY)	Nep	395	Chou, Shyan-yih (NY)	Nep	444
Chase, Mark (NJ)	OrS	783	Choudhury, Muhammad (NY)	U	707
Chaudhry, M Rashid (NY)	Oto	456	Chrisanderson, Donna (NJ)	IM	776

Alphabetical Listing of Doctors

Name	Specialty	Pg	Name	Specialty	Pg
Christakos, Manny (NJ)	TS	897	Cohen, Ben (NY)	Oph	241
Christoudias, George (NJ)	S	753	Cohen, Bradley (NY)	S	640
Chu, Edward (CT)	Onc	972	Cohen, Burton A (NY)	DR	150
Chu, Wing (NY)	Oph	241	Cohen, Carl (NY)	GerPsy	434
Chuang, Linus (NY)	GO	173	Cohen, Carmel (NY)	GO	173
Chung, Henry (NY)	Psyc	312	Cohen, Charmian (NY)	EDM	384
Chung-Loy, Harold (NJ)	S	849	Cohen, Daniel (NY)	N	625
Chutorian, Abraham (NY)	ChiN	136	Cohen, Daniel H (NY)	Rhu	586
Ciccarelli, Ciro (NY)	IM	549	Cohen, David J (NY)	Nep	212
Ciccone, John (NJ)	Cv	768	Cohen, Harris L (NY)	DR	616
Ciccone, Patrick (NJ)	U	794	Cohen, Herbert J (NY)	Ped	407
Cicogna, Cristina E (NJ)	Inf	731	Cohen, Howard A (NY)	Cv	125
Cimino, Ernest (NJ)	PlS	819	Cohen, Ivan S (CT)	D	935
Cimino, James E (NY)	IM	391	Cohen, Jacob L (NY)	Ge	542
Cimino, James J (NY)	IM	187	Cohen, Joel S (NY)	N	397
Cimino, Joseph (NY)	PrM	696	Cohen, Jon (NY)	VascS	596
Ciocon, Hermogenes (NJ)	TS	897	Cohen, Jonathan (NY)	Ge	161
Cioroiu, Michael (NY)	S	346	Cohen, Lawrence B (NY)	Ge	161
Cipollaro, Vincent (NY)	D	142	Cohen, Lawrence S (CT)	Cv	966
Cirello, Richard (NJ)	FMed	773	Cohen, Lee (NY)	ChAP	652
Citron, Marc L (NY)	Onc	553	Cohen, Leeber (NY)	Oph	241
Clain, David (NY)	Ge	161	Cohen, Marc (NJ)	IC	777
Claps, Richard J (NJ)	DR	875	Cohen, Martin (NJ)	Ped	882
Clark, Luther T (NY)	Cv	422	Cohen, Martin A (NY)	CRS	654
Clark, Richard (NY)	D	614	Cohen, Martin B (NY)	CE	647
Clark, Sheryl (NY)	D	142	Cohen, Michael H (NY)	IM	187
Clarke, James (NY)	S	346	Cohen, Michael L (NY)	Pul	581
Cleary, Joseph (NY)	S	346	Cohen, Michel (NY)	Ped	293
Cleman, Michael W (CT)	Cv	965	Cohen, Neil (NY)	EDM	510
Clements, Jerry (NY)	FMed	158	Cohen, Paul (NY)	Ge	431
Close, Lanny G (NY)	Oto	269	Cohen, Richard (NJ)	Ped	845
Coady, Deborah (NY)	ObG	231	Cohen, Richard P (NY)	IM	187
Cobelli, Neil (NY)	OrS	402	Cohen, Robert L (NY)	IM	187
Cobin, Rhoda (NJ)	EDM	726	Cohen, Seth A (NY)	Ge	161
Coco, Maria (NY)	Nep	395	Cohen, Seymour M (NY)	Onc	201
Coffey, Barbara J (NY)	ChAP	134	Cohen, Steven (NJ)	Oph	781
Coffey, Tom (CT)	Oto	950	Cohen, Steven M (CT)	DR	936
Cofsky, Richard (NY)	Inf	437	Cohen, Steven R (NY)	D	382
Cohen, Alice (NJ)	Hem	775	Cohn, Steven (NY)	IM	438
Cohen, Arnold R (NY)	Psyc	312	Cohn, William J (NY)	Ge	619
Cohen, Barry A (NY)	IM	438	Coit, Daniel G (NY)	S	346
Cohen, Barry H (NJ)	Nep	814	Colaco, Rodolfo (NJ)	S	925

Name	Specialty	Pg	Name	Specialty	Pg
Colangelo, Daniel (NY)	IM	667	Cooper, Arthur (NY)	PS	292
Cole, Jeffrey L (NJ)	PMR	788	Cooper, Dennis (CT)	Onc	972
Cole, William J (NY)	Cv	125	Cooper, Jay (NY)	RadRO	468
Colella, Frank (NY)	Onc	442	Cooper, Jerome (NY)	Cv	648
Coleman, D Jackson (NY)	Oph	241	Cooper, Paul (NY)	NS	215
Coleman, Morton (NY)	Onc	201	Cooper, Robert (CT)	Onc	944
Colen, Helen S (NY)	PlS	302	Cooper, Robert B (NY)	Ge	162
Colen, Stephen (NY)	PlS	302	Cooper, Rubin (NY)	PCd	282
Colenda, Maryann (NJ)	PA&I	742	Cooper, Seymour (NY)	Ped	575
Coll, Raymond (NY)	N	219	Cooperman, Alan S (NJ)	ObG	781
Collens, Richard (NY)	IM	188	Copel, Joshua (CT)	MF	972
Coller, Barry (NY)	Hem	178	Copen, David (CT)	Cv	934
Collins, Adriane (NY)	Inf	620	Coplan, Jeremy (NY)	Psyc	464
Collins, Allen H (NY)	Psyc	312	Coppa, Gene F (NY)	S	520
Coloka-Kump, Rodika (NY)	FMed	660	Copperman, Alan B (NY)	RE	335
Colon, Francisco G (NJ)	PlS	883	Coppola, John T (NY)	Cv	125
Colton, Marc D (NJ)	U	886	Corapi, Mark (NY)	IM	549
Colvin, Stephen (NY)	TS	356	Corbo, Emanuel (NJ)	Ped	921
Comfort, Christopher P (NY)	IM	392	Cordeiro, Peter G (NY)	PlS	303
Compito, Gerard (NJ)	DR	810	Cordero, Evelyn (NY)	FMed	385
Comrie, Millicent (NY)	ObG	450	Cordon, David (NY)	Psyc	312
Concannon, Patrick (NY)	ObG	494	Coren, Charles (NY)	PS	574
Condo, Dominick (NJ)	Ger	800	Corey, Timothy (NJ)	D	724
Condon, Edward M (NY)	IM	549	Corio, Laura E (NY)	ObG	232
Confino, Joel (NJ)	Oph	919	Corn, Beth E (NY)	A&I	121
Connery, Cliff (NY)	TS	356	Cornell, Charles (NY)	OrS	257
Connolly, Adrian L (NJ)	D	771	Cornell, James (NJ)	CCM	723
Connolly, Mark W (NJ)	TS	793	Corpuz, Marilou (NY)	Inf	390
Connor, Bradley A (NY)	Ge	162	Correia, Joaquim (NJ)	CE	767
Connor, Thomas M (NJ)	PCd	785	Corriel, Robert (NY)	A&I	527
Connors, Richard (CT)	D	935	Corso, Salvatore (NY)	OrS	565
Conroy, Daniel P (NJ)	Cv	720	Corson, Richard L (NJ)	FMed	902
Constad, William H (NJ)	Oph	802	Cortes, Engracio P (NY)	Onc	492
Constantiner, Arturo (NY)	IM	188	Cortes, Hiram (NY)	Inf	437
Constantinides, Minas (NY)	Oto	270	Corvalan, Jose (NY)	S	346
Conte, Charles Carmine (NY)	S	588	Cosgrove, John M (NY)	S	588
Conway, Edward E (NY)	PCCM	283	Cosman, Felicia (NY)	EDM	602
Cook, Jack (NY)	Oph	562	Cossari, Alfred (NY)	Oph	628
Cook, Perry (NY)	Hem	178	Costa, Leon N (NJ)	OrS	817
Cook, Stuart (NJ)	N	780	Costantino, Peter D (NY)	Oto	270
Cooke, Joseph T (NY)	Pul	329	Costantino, Thomas (NY)	Cv	507
Cooney, Leo M (CT)	Ger	969	Costanzo, Joseph (CT)	IM	940

Alphabetical Listing of Doctors

Name	Specialty	Pg
Costeas, Constantinos A (NJ)	CE	768
Costin, Andrew (NJ)	Cv	809
Coupey, Susan (NY)	AM	378
Cournos, Francine (NY)	Psyc	313
Courtney, Barbara (NJ)	IM	860
Coven, Barbara (NY)	Ped	693
Covey, Alexander J (NY)	IM	621
Covit, Andrew (NJ)	Nep	837
Cox, Kathryn (NY)	ObG	232
Coyle, Michael P (NJ)	HS	833
Coyle, Patricia K (NY)	N	625
Craft, Joseph (CT)	Rhu	981
Craig, Edward V (NY)	OrS	257
Craig, Nicholas (NY)	S	640
Cramer, Marvin (NY)	Cv	530
Crane, Richard (NY)	Rhu	339
Crasta, Jovita M (NY)	Psyc	580
Crawford, Bernard (NY)	TS	356
Cristofaro, Robert (NY)	OrS	683
Croen, Kenneth (NY)	IM	667
Croll, James (NY)	Nep	395
Cronin, David C (CT)	S	982
Crowe, John F (CT)	OrS	949
Cruickshank, David (NY)	U	642
Cruz, Merle Correa (NJ)	Cv	799
Crystal, Howard (NY)	N	447
Crystal, Kenneth (NY)	VIR	595
Cubelli, Ken (NJ)	OrS	880
Cullen, Mark R (CT)	OM	975
Cunha, Burke A (NY)	Inf	547
Cunningham, Joseph N (NY)	TS	475
Cunningham-Rundles, Charlotte (NY)	A&I	121
Cunningham-Rundles, Ward (NY)	IM	188
Cuomo, Frances (NY)	OrS	257
Curtin, John P (NY)	GO	174
Cusumano, Barbara (NY)	Ped	634
Cusumano, Stephen (NY)	IM	549
Cutolo, Louis Carmine (NY)	PlS	518
Cutting, Court (NY)	PlS	303
Cuttner, Janet (NY)	Hem	178
Cykiert, Robert (NY)	Oph	241
Cynamon, Jacob (NY)	VIR	416

D

Name	Specialty	Pg
D'Agostini, Robert (NJ)	OrS	905
D'Agostino, Ronald (NY)	Cv	530
D'Alton, Mary Elizabeth (NY)	MF	198
D'Amico, Richard (NJ)	PlS	747
D'Amico, Robert (NY)	Oph	241
D'Anna, John (NY)	S	520
D'Aversa, Gerard (NY)	Oph	562
D'Ayala, Marcus D (NY)	VascS	477
D'Esposito, Michael (NY)	FMed	618
Dadaian, Jack (NJ)	Pul	790
Dagum, Alexander B (NY)	PlS	635
Dalena, John M (NJ)	Ge	875
Daliana, Maurizio (NY)	S	347
Dalton, Jack F (NY)	RadRO	500
Daly, Jane (NY)	Onc	492
Damien, Miguel (NJ)	RE	866
Damus, Paul S (NY)	TS	592
Danehower, Richard L (CT)	Rhu	958
Daniels, Jeffrey (NJ)	Cv	857
Dankner, Richard (NY)	Oph	400
Danon, Moris Jak (NY)	N	219
Danziger, Stephen (NY)	D	427
Daras, Michael (NY)	N	219
Dardik, Herbert (NJ)	VascS	757
Das, Seshadri (NY)	EDM	510
Das Gupta, Manash K (NY)	Nep	674
Dasgupta, Indira (NY)	PHO	405
Dash, Greg (NY)	Oto	631
Dasmahapatra, Kumar (NJ)	S	849
Datta, Rajiv (NY)	S	588
Dattwyler, Raymond (NY)	A&I	647
Daum, Fredric (NY)	PGe	572
Dave, Mahendraray (NY)	Nep	395
Davenport, Deborah M (NY)	ObG	626
David, Raphael (NY)	PEn	284
David, Sami (NY)	RE	336
Davidson, Dennis (NY)	NP	554
Davidson, J Thomas (NJ)	S	822
Davidson, Lawrence (NJ)	Oph	782
Davidson, William D (NJ)	Oto	818

Name	Specialty	Pg	Name	Specialty	Pg
Davies, Richard (NJ)	S	753	Deitz, Marcia (NY)	D	427
Davies, Terry (NY)	EDM	155	Del Monte, Mary (NY)	Nep	444
Davis, Alan (NJ)	PCCM	785	Del Priore, Lucian (NY)	Oph	241
Davis, George (NJ)	Pul	865	Del Rowe, John (NY)	RadRO	584
Davis, Ira C (NY)	D	655	DeLacure, Mark D (NY)	Oto	270
Davis, Jessica G (NY)	CG	138	Deland, Jonathan T (NY)	OrS	257
Davis, Jonathan M (NY)	NP	555	Delaney, Brian (NY)	FMed	386
Davis, Joseph E (NY)	U	361	Delano, Barbara (NY)	Nep	444
Davis, Joyce (NY)	D	142	Delbello, Damon (NY)	OrS	683
Davis, Kenneth J (NJ)	Ped	921	Deleo, Vincent A (NY)	D	142
Davis, Owen (NY)	RE	336	Delerme, Milton (NY)	Oph	242
Davis, Raphael P (NY)	NS	625	Della Rocca, Robert (NY)	Oph	242
Davison, Edward (NY)	Cv	530	Delman, Michael (NY)	IM	621
Davison, Henry (NJ)	S	822	Delorenzo, Lawrence (NY)	Pul	701
Daya, Rami (NY)	Onc	443	DeLuca, Joseph A (NJ)	Oph	738
De Angelis, Arthur (NY)	IM	667	Demar, Leon (NY)	D	143
De Angelis, Lisa (NY)	N	219	Demento, Frank (NY)	D	536
De Antonio, Joseph (NJ)	Ge	811	Demetis, Spiro (NY)	Pul	466
De Araujo, Maria (NY)	PMR	409	Denehy, Thad (NJ)	GO	775
De Blasio, Maria-Pia (NY)	FMed	386	Dennett, Ronald (NY)	IM	667
De Carlo, Regina (NY)	ChiN	509	Denny, Donald F (NJ)	VIR	850
De Fabritus, Albert (NY)	Nep	212	Denoto, George (NY)	S	588
De France, John (CT)	TS	959	Denton, John (NY)	OrS	495
De Giacomo, Frank (NJ)	IM	892	Derespinis, Patrick (NY)	Oph	515
De Groote, Robert (NJ)	VascS	757	DeRisi, Dwight (NY)	S	588
De La Fuente, Beatriz (NY)	Hem	178	Dershaw, D David (NY)	DR	150
de Lotbiniere, Alain (NY)	NS	974	Dervan, John (NY)	Cv	612
De Martino, Anthony G. (NY)	Cv	648	Desai, Rajesh (NY)	Psyc	580
De Matteo, Robert (NY)	Pul	700	DeSilva, Derrick M (NJ)	IM	834
De Pasquale, Joseph (NJ)	Ge	773	Desnick, Robert J (NY)	CG	138
De Pietro, William (NY)	D	536	Desposito, Franklin (NJ)	CG	770
De Vita, Vincent T (CT)	Onc	972	Detterbeck, Frank C (CT)	TS	982
De Vivo, Darryl C (NY)	ChiN	136	Deutsch, Alexander (NY)	Psyc	313
DeBellis, Robert H (NY)	Onc	201	Deutsch, James A (NY)	Oph	451
Debrovner, Charles (NY)	ObG	232	Devereux, Richard B (NY)	Cv	125
Deck, Michael (NY)	NRad	227	Devinsky, Orrin (NY)	N	220
DeCosimo, Diana R (NJ)	IM	776	DeVita, Gregory (NY)	PlS	577
Decter, Edward (NJ)	OrS	783	DeVito, Bethany S (NY)	Ge	542
Decter, Julian A (NY)	Onc	201	Dhar, Santi (NY)	Pul	467
Degann, Sona (NY)	ObG	232	Dharmarajan, Thiruvinvamvalai (NY)	Ger	388
Deitch, Edwin (NJ)	S	792	Di Bella, Louis J (NJ)	U	805
Deitz, Joel (NJ)	Pul	820	Di Buono, Mark (NY)	Psyc	519

Alphabetical Listing of Doctors

Name	Specialty	Pg	Name	Specialty	Pg
Di Cesare, Paul (NY)	OrS	258	Doidge, Robert (NJ)	OrS	739
Di Giacinto, George V (NY)	NS	215	Dolan, Anna (NY)	Psyc	697
Di Giacomo, Jody C (NJ)	S	804	Dolan, Rory (NY)	Oph	451
Di Giacomo, William A (NJ)	IM	776	Dolgin, Stephen (NY)	PS	574
Di Gregorio, Vincent (NY)	PlS	578	Dolich, Barry (NY)	PlS	409
Di Leo, Frank (NY)	Oph	628	Dolitsky, Charisse (NY)	D	536
Di Maso, Gerald (NY)	IM	511	Dolitsky, Jay (NY)	PO	290
Di Pasquale, Laurene (NJ)	Pul	750	Donahue, Bernadine R (NY)	RadRO	468
Di Scala, Reno (NY)	FMed	486	Donath, Joseph (NY)	Pul	499
Diamant, Esther (NY)	Ped	605	Donnellan, Joseph (NJ)	Psyc	906
Diamond, Ezriel (NY)	RadRO	584	Donnelly, Brian (NJ)	DR	913
Diamond, Martin (NJ)	PMR	923	Donnelly, Christine (NJ)	PCd	881
Diamond, Sharon (NY)	ObG	232	Donnenfeld, Eric D (NY)	Oph	562
Diamond, Steven (NJ)	PHO	743	Dor, Nathan (NY)	ObG	450
Diaz, Angela (NY)	AM	120	Dorfman, Howard D (NY)	Path	404
Diaz, Michael (NY)	Hem	178	Dosik, David (NY)	Onc	443
DiBernardo, Barry E (NJ)	PlS	788	Dosik, Harvey (NY)	Hem	436
Dickler, Maura N (NY)	Onc	201	Dottino, Peter R (NY)	GO	174
Dickoff, David (NY)	N	676	Douglas, Carolyn (NY)	Psyc	313
DiCosmo, Bruno F (NY)	Pul	701	Douglas, Montgomery (NY)	FMed	487
Dieck, William (NY)	Oph	680	Dower, Samuel (NJ)	EDM	772
Dieterich, Douglas (NY)	Ge	162	Dowling, Sean (CT)	RadRO	957
Dietrich, Marianne (NY)	FMed	386	Dowling, Thomas (NY)	OrS	630
Dietzek, Alan M (CT)	VascS	960	Dowling, William (NJ)	OrS	880
Digioia, Julia (NJ)	S	925	Downie, Jeanine B (NJ)	D	771
Diktaban, Theodore (NY)	PlS	303	Doyle, Michael (CT)	RE	957
Dila, Carl (CT)	NS	946	Dozor, Allen J (NY)	PPul	691
Dillard, James N (NY)	PMR	298	Drachtman, Richard (NJ)	PHO	843
Dillon, Robert (NY)	U	361	Draizin, Dennis L (NY)	Oto	567
Dimaio, Mary (NY)	PPul	290	Drake, William (NJ)	Oto	920
Dines, David M (NY)	OrS	565	Dranitzke, Richard (NY)	TS	642
Dinnerstein, Stephen (NY)	Oph	242	Drascher, Gary (NJ)	S	907
Distenfeld, Ariel (NY)	Hem	178	Drayer, Burton P (NY)	NRad	227
Ditchek, Alan (NY)	IM	438	Dresdale, Robert (NY)	Cv	530
Dittmar, Klaus (NY)	Hem	546	Dresner, Lisa (NY)	S	472
Diuguid, David L (NY)	Hem	178	Drexler, Ellen (NY)	N	447
Divon, Michael Y (NY)	ObG	232	Dreyer, Neil P (CT)	IM	940
Dlugi, Alexander M (NJ)	RE	906	Dreyfuss, Patricia (NJ)	ObG	879
Do Rosario, Arnold (CT)	IM	940	Driesman, Mitchell (CT)	IC	943
Dobbs, Joan (NY)	Onc	623	Drillings, Gary (NJ)	OrS	894
Doctor, Naishad (NY)	PlS	578	Drimmer, Marc A (NJ)	PlS	820
Dodick, Jack M (NY)	Oph	242	Droller, Michael J (NY)	U	361

Alphabetical Listing of Doctors

Name	Specialty	Pg
Elmann, Elie (NJ)	TS	755
Elwyn, Katherine E (NY)	S	704
Emond, Jean C (NY)	S	347
Emre, Sukru (NY)	S	347
Emre, Umit Berk (NY)	PPul	460
Ende, Leigh (NJ)	HS	876
Enelow, Richard Ian (CT)	Pul	979
Eng, Kenneth (NY)	S	347
Engel, Harry (NY)	Oph	401
Engel, J Mark (NJ)	Oph	840
Engel, Lenore (NY)	ChAP	425
Engel, Mark (NJ)	Oph	862
Engel, Murray (CT)	N	947
Engler, Mitchell (NJ)	Pul	750
Enker, Warren (NY)	S	347
Ennis, Ronald D (NY)	RadRO	333
Epstein, Lawrence J (NY)	PM	687
Epstein, Robert (NJ)	DR	830
Epstein, Stanley (NY)	Cv	648
Erber, William (NY)	Ge	431
Ergin, M Arisan (NJ)	TS	755
Erlebacher, Jay A (NJ)	Cv	720
Ernst, Jerome (NY)	IM	392
Errico, Thomas (NY)	OrS	258
Ertl, John (CT)	PHO	951
Esformes, Ira (NJ)	OrS	739
Eshghi, A Majid (NY)	U	707
Esposito, Donna (NY)	Oph	242
Esposito, Michael P (NJ)	U	756
Estabrook, Alison (NY)	S	347
Esteban-Cruciani, Nora (NY)	Ped	407
Eswar, Sounder (NY)	OrS	496
Eth, Spencer (NY)	Psyc	313
Etingin, Orli (NY)	IM	188
Ettinger, Alan (NY)	N	557
Ettinger, Lawrence (NJ)	PHO	844
Eufemio, Michael (NY)	EDM	658
Evans, Mark I (NY)	ObG	232
Evans, Steven J (NY)	CE	122
Eviatar, Lydia (NY)	ChiN	534
Ezratty, Ari M (NY)	Cv	530

F

Name	Specialty	Pg
Faber, Mark (NJ)	Psyc	789
Fabian, Christopher (NY)	Psyc	313
Fabian, Dennis (NY)	OrS	258
Facelle, Thomas (NY)	S	607
Fagin, Bernard H (NY)	U	707
Fagin, James (NY)	PA&I	569
Fahey, Julia A (NY)	IM	622
Fahey, Thomas J (NY)	S	348
Fahn, Stanley (NY)	N	220
Fahoum, Bashar (NY)	S	472
Fakharzadeh, Frederick (NJ)	HS	729
Falco, Thomas (NY)	Cv	612
Falcon, Ronald (NY)	D	536
Falk, Theodore (NJ)	A&I	719
Faller, Jason (NY)	Rhu	339
Fan, Peter (NJ)	S	753
Fantini, Gary A (NY)	VascS	370
Farber, Bruce (NY)	Inf	547
Farber, Charles (NY)	Ge	542
Farber, Charles (NJ)	Onc	878
Farcy, Jean-Pierre (NY)	OrS	258
Farkas, Edward (NJ)	Psyc	748
Farkas, John J (NJ)	Ge	892
Farmer, Howard S (NJ)	Oto	818
Farrell, Matthew (CT)	FMed	937
Farrell, Robert (NY)	U	502
Farrer, William (NJ)	Inf	915
Farris, R Linsy (NY)	Oph	242
Fass, Arthur (NY)	Cv	648
Fass, Daniel E (CT)	RadRO	957
Fast, Avital (NY)	PMR	409
Fastenberg, David M (NY)	Oph	562
Fateh, Majid (NY)	RE	336
Faust, Glenn (NY)	VascS	596
Faust, Michael (NY)	IM	188
Faust, Michael (NJ)	ObG	737
Fawwaz, Rashib (NY)	NuM	228
Fazio, Nelson M (NY)	IM	667
Fazio, Richard (NY)	Ge	510
Federbush, Richard (NY)	IM	549

Alphabetical Listing of Doctors

Name	Specialty	Pg	Name	Specialty	Pg
Federman, Harold (NY)	IM	667	Festa, Robert S (NY)	Ped	634
Feghali, Joseph G (NY)	Oto	403	Feuer, Martin (NY)	IM	189
Feigenbaum, Howard (NJ)	S	896	Fialk, Mark A (NY)	Onc	672
Fein, Alan (NY)	Pul	582	Fidanzato, Michael (NJ)	Ge	811
Fein, Deborah A (NJ)	Nep	734	Fiedler, Robert (NY)	IM	189
Feinberg, Joseph (NY)	PlS	578	Field, Barry E (NY)	Ge	662
Feinberg, Joseph Hunt (NY)	PMR	299	Field, Steven P (NY)	Ge	162
Feinberg, Todd E (NY)	N	220	Fielding, George (NY)	S	348
Feinfeld, Donald A (NY)	Nep	212	Fieldman, Robert (NJ)	Oto	783
Feinstein, Neil (NY)	Oph	452	Fields, Sheila (NJ)	IM	732
Feintzeig, Irwin (CT)	Nep	945	Fields, Theodore (NY)	Rhu	339
Feit, Alan (NY)	Cv	422	Fiest, Thomas (NJ)	Ge	859
Feit, David (NJ)	Ge	727	Figgie, Mark (NY)	OrS	258
Feld, Michael (NY)	Cv	648	Filiberto, Cosmo (CT)	FMed	937
Felderman, Leonora (NY)	D	143	Filippone, Mark A (NJ)	PMR	803
Feldman, B Robert (NY)	A&I	121	Filsoufi, Farzan (NY)	TS	356
Feldman, David J (NJ)	OrS	880	Fine, Emily A (CT)	ObG	975
Feldman, David L (NY)	PlS	463	Fine, Eugene M (NY)	U	361
Feldman, David N (NJ)	OrS	740	Fine, Herbert (NJ)	D	724
Feldman, David S (NY)	OrS	258	Fine, Paul (NJ)	Nep	878
Feldman, Frieda (NY)	DR	150	Fine, Robert (NY)	Onc	201
Feldman, Jeffrey (NJ)	IM	915	Fine, Stanley (NY)	A&I	483
Feldman, Philip (NY)	D	427	Fineman, Sanford (NJ)	NS	917
Feldman, Sheldon M (NY)	S	348	Finger, Paul T (NY)	Oph	242
Feldman, Stuart (NY)	Onc	672	Fink, Matthew E (NY)	N	220
Feldstein, Neil A (NY)	NS	215	Finkel, Jay (NY)	Psyc	313
Feliccia, Joseph (NY)	OrS	454	Finkelstein, Jacob (NY)	S	704
Felig, Philip (NY)	EDM	155	Finkelstein, Martin S (NY)	Ger	171
Fellus, Jonathan L (NJ)	N	780	Finkelstein, Michael (NY)	IM	667
Felman, Yehudi M. (NY)	D	427	Finkelstein, Warren (NJ)	Ge	774
Felsenstein, Jerome M (NY)	D	655	Finnerty, James (CT)	IM	941
Feltheimer, Seth (NY)	IM	188	Fiore, John J (NY)	Onc	624
Fennoy, Ilene (NY)	PEn	284	Fiorentino, Thomas (NY)	IM	667
Ferges, Mitchell (NJ)	Ge	903	First, Michael B (NY)	Psyc	313
Fernandes, David R (NY)	Ped	461	Fisch, Arthur (NJ)	Cv	873
Fernandes, John (NJ)	PCd	785	Fisch, Harry (NY)	U	362
Fernbach, Barry R (NJ)	Hem	730	Fisch, Morton (NY)	IM	189
Ferran, Ernesto (NY)	Psyc	313	Fischer, Harry (NY)	Rhu	339
Ferrier, Genevieve (NY)	Ped	294	Fischer, Rita (NY)	NP	210
Ferriter, Pierce (NY)	OrS	258	Fish, Bernard (NY)	PCd	688
Ferrone, Philip J (NY)	Oph	562	Fish, Irving (NY)	ChiN	136
Ferzli, George (NY)	S	520	Fishbach, Mitchell (NY)	Cv	649

Name	Specialty	Pg	Name	Specialty	Pg
Fishbane, Steven (NY)	Nep	555	Foley, Conn J (NY)	IM	549
Fisher, George C (NY)	FMed	487	Foley, Kathleen M (NY)	PM	277
Fisher, John D (NY)	CE	379	Folman, Robert S (CT)	Onc	944
Fisher, Laura (NY)	IM	189	Fomberstein, Barry (NY)	Rhu	413
Fisher, Lawrence (CT)	Cv	934	Fonacier, Luz (NY)	A&I	528
Fisher, Martin M (NY)	AM	527	Fong, Raymond (NY)	Oph	243
Fisher, Yale (NY)	Oph	243	Fong, Yuman (NY)	S	348
Fishkin, Michael (NY)	FMed	618	Foo, Sun-Hoo (NY)	N	220
Fishman, Allen J. (NY)	Oph	495	Foong, Anthony (NY)	Ge	162
Fishman, David A (NY)	GO	174	Ford, Robert R (NJ)	DR	810
Fishman, Donald (NY)	IM	189	Forget, Bernard (CT)	Hem	970
Fishman, Miriam (NJ)	D	724	Forlenza, Thomas (NY)	Onc	513
Fiske, Steven (NJ)	Ge	774	Forley, Bryan G (NY)	PlS	303
Fitzgerald, Denis (NJ)	Onc	860	Forman, Mark (NJ)	TS	793
Flamm, Eugene (NY)	NS	396	Forman, Scott (NY)	Oph	680
Flanagan, Michael J (CT)	U	983	Formenti, Silvia C (NY)	RadRO	333
Flanagan, Steven Robert (NY)	PMR	299	Fornari, Victor (NY)	ChAP	534
Flatow, Evan (NY)	OrS	258	Forster, George (NY)	N	220
Fleischer, Adiel (NY)	ObG	560	Fort, Pavel (NY)	PEn	571
Fleischer, Lee S (NY)	S	607	Forte, Francis A (NJ)	Onc	733
Fleischer, Marian (NY)	CRS	426	Forte, Frank J (NY)	Hem	511
Fleischer, Norman (NY)	EDM	384	Fortunato, Dana (NJ)	IM	777
Fleischman, Jay (NY)	Oph	680	Fosl, Arthur (NJ)	PA&I	784
Fleischman, Jean K (NY)	Pul	499	Foster, Craig A (NY)	PlS	303
Fleisher, Michael (NJ)	U	850	Foster, Jeffrey (NY)	Psyc	314
Fleishman, Stewart (NY)	Psyc	314	Fowler, Dennis (NY)	S	348
Fleming, Gregory (NJ)	Oto	881	Fox, Alissa (NJ)	D	902
Fletcher, H Stephen (NJ)	S	792	Fox, Herbert (NY)	Psyc	314
Flis, Raymond S (NJ)	Nep	861	Fox, James (NJ)	A&I	901
Flores, Lucio (NY)	VascS	477	Fox, Joyce (NY)	CG	535
Florio, Francis (NY)	U	475	Fox, Mark (NY)	Oto	685
Florio, Philip (NY)	ObG	677	Fox, Martin L (NY)	Oph	243
Flug, Frances (NJ)	PHO	743	Fox, Sarah J (NY)	ChAP	134
Flynn, John T (NY)	Oph	243	Fox, Stewart (NY)	TS	592
Flynn, Joseph T (NY)	PNep	405	Fox, Stuart (NJ)	N	879
Flynn, Maryirene (NY)	OrS	516	Fracchia, John (NY)	U	362
Fochios, Steven (NY)	Ge	162	Frager, Joseph (NY)	Ge	387
Fogel, Joyce (NY)	Ger	171	Fram, Daniel K (NJ)	RadRO	821
Fogel, Mitchell A (CT)	Nep	945	Frances, Richard J (NY)	AdP	119
Fogler, Richard (NY)	S	472	Francfort, John (NY)	S	640
Fojas, Antonio (NY)	IM	392	Francis, Kathleen (NJ)	PMR	788
Foley, Carmel (NY)	ChAP	534	Franck, Jeanne M (NY)	D	536

Alphabetical Listing of Doctors

Name	Specialty	Pg	Name	Specialty	Pg
Franco, John (NY)	FMed	618	Friedman, Eli A (NY)	Nep	444
Frank, Donald (NJ)	NS	779	Friedman, Eugene B (NY)	Ped	576
Frank, Graeme (NY)	PEn	571	Friedman, Gerald (NY)	Ge	163
Frank, Martin (NJ)	Hem	876	Friedman, Howard S (NY)	Cv	125
Frank, Michael (NY)	Ge	162	Friedman, Jeffrey Paul (NY)	IM	189
Franklin, Bonita (NY)	PEn	284	Friedman, Lloyd Neal (CT)	Pul	980
Franks, Andrew G (NY)	D	143	Friedman, Lynn (NY)	ObG	232
Franzetti, Carl (NY)	FMed	386	Friedman, Richard Alan (NY)	Psyc	314
Freddo, Lorenza (NY)	N	397	Friedman, Ricky (NY)	ObG	232
Freed, Lisa A (CT)	Cv	966	Friedman, Robert (NY)	Oph	243
Freedman, Gordon (NY)	PM	277	Friedman, Sam (NY)	IM	603
Freedman, Jeffrey (NY)	Oph	452	Friedman, Sanford (NY)	Cv	126
Freedman, Michael L (NY)	Ger	171	Friedman, Scott L (NY)	Ge	163
Freedman, Pamela (NJ)	Ge	875	Friedman, Seth G (NY)	EDM	539
Freedman, Richard (CT)	Ped	952	Friedman, Stanley N (NY)	DR	383
Freeman, Leonard M (NY)	NuM	399	Friedman, Steven C (NY)	U	475
Freeman, Ruth (NY)	EDM	384	Friedman, Steven I (NY)	S	588
Freilich, Dennis (NY)	Oph	243	Friedman-Kien, Alvin (NY)	D	143
Freiman, Hal (NY)	Ge	162	Friedrich, Ivan (NJ)	Ge	727
Frenkel, Renata (NY)	A&I	121	Frieri, Marianne (NY)	A&I	528
Freund, Robert M (NY)	PlS	303	Frimer, Richard (NY)	Pul	701
Frey, Howard (NJ)	U	756	Frischer, Zelik (NY)	U	642
Fried, Karen O (NY)	DR	150	Friscia, Philip (NY)	Onc	513
Fried, Kenneth (NJ)	S	753	Frishman, William (NY)	Cv	649
Fried, Marvin P (NY)	Oto	403	Frisoli, Anthony (NJ)	FMed	902
Fried, Richard (NY)	IM	189	Frohman, Larry P (NJ)	Oph	782
Fried, Sharon (NJ)	D	724	Fromer, Mark D (NY)	Oph	244
Frieden, Faith (NJ)	MF	732	Frosch, William (NY)	Psyc	314
Friedlaender, Gary E (CT)	OrS	975	Frost, James H (NJ)	S	925
Friedlander, Beverly (NJ)	PlS	788	Fruchtman, Steven M (NY)	Hem	179
Friedlander, Charles (NY)	Ge	163	Frymus, Michael (CT)	TS	959
Friedlander, Devin (NJ)	N	904	Fuchs, Richard (NY)	Cv	126
Friedlander, Marvin E (NJ)	NS	917	Fuchs, Wayne (NY)	Oph	244
Friedling, Steven (NY)	IM	622	Fuhrman, Robert (NJ)	EDM	913
Friedman, Alan (NJ)	ObG	816	Fukilman, Oscar J (NY)	IM	490
Friedman, Alan H (NY)	Oph	243	Fuks, Joachim (NY)	Onc	393
Friedman, Alan J (NY)	Oph	243	Fulop, Robert (NY)	IM	512
Friedman, Amy L (CT)	S	982	Funt, David (NY)	PlS	578
Friedman, David Jay (NY)	PlS	303	Funt, Tina K (NY)	D	536
Friedman, David L (NJ)	PS	745	Furey, Robert J (NY)	U	362
Friedman, David Wayne (NY)	HS	175	Furie, Richard (NY)	Rhu	586
Friedman, Deborah (NJ)	PCd	785	Fusillo, Christine (NY)	A&I	647

Alphabetical Listing of Doctors

Name	Specialty	Pg	Name	Specialty	Pg
Fuster, Valentin (NY)	Cv	126	Garfein, Oscar (NY)	Cv	126
Futran-Sheinberg, Jacobo (NY)	Rhu	703	Garfinkel, Burton (NY)	ObG	560
Fyer, Abby J (NY)	Psyc	314	Garfinkel, Howard B (CT)	Nep	945
Fyer, Minna R (NY)	Psyc	314	Garfinkel, Matthew J (NJ)	OrS	840
			Gargano, Robert M (NY)	Oto	631
			Gargiulo, Juan (NY)	PM	632
			Garjian, Peggy Ann (NY)	Rhu	520
			Garner, Bruce (NY)	Rhu	470

G

Name	Specialty	Pg	Name	Specialty	Pg
Gabel, Richard (NY)	Psyc	697	Garner, Steven (NY)	DR	428
Gabelman, Gary (NY)	Cv	649	Garratt, Kirk N (NY)	IC	197
Gabrilove, Janice (NY)	Onc	201	Garrick, Renee (NY)	Nep	674
Gaffney, Joseph W (NJ)	PCd	842	Garrow, Eugene (NY)	PS	461
Gafori, Iraj (NJ)	GO	729	Garroway, Robert (NY)	OrS	565
Gagliardi, Anthony (NY)	Pul	329	Garvey, Julius W (NY)	VascS	596
Gagner, Michel (NY)	S	348	Garvey, Michael (NY)	Nep	212
Gajdos, Robert (NJ)	IM	893	Garvin, James (NY)	PHO	287
Galanter, Marc (NY)	AdP	119	Garzon, Maria C (NY)	D	143
Galeno, John (NY)	OrS	683	Gasalberti, Richard (NY)	PMR	498
Galinkin, Lawrence (NY)	Ped	576	Gately, Adrian (NY)	Ped	461
Gallagher, John F (NY)	S	640	Gayle, Lloyd (NY)	PlS	303
Gallagher, Pamela M (NY)	PlS	578	Gaynor, Mitchell (NY)	Onc	202
Galland, Leopold (NY)	IM	189	Gazzara, Paul (NY)	IM	512
Galler, Marilyn (NY)	Nep	492	Gecelter, Gary (NY)	S	589
Gallick, Gregory (NJ)	OrS	919	Geders, Jane (NY)	Ge	662
Gallin, Pamela F (NY)	Oph	244	Geisler, Edward (NY)	U	415
Gallousis, Spiro (NY)	ObG	450	Gejerman, Glen (NJ)	RadRO	751
Galloway, Aubrey (NY)	TS	356	Gekowski, Kathleen (NJ)	Inf	812
Galton, Barry (NJ)	IM	893	Gelato, Marie (NY)	EDM	617
Gamache, Francis (NY)	NS	215	Gelb, Bruce (NY)	PCd	282
Gammon, G Davis (CT)	ChAP	966	Gelberg, Burt (NY)	IM	549
Ganchi, Parham A (NJ)	PlS	895	Gelbfish, Joseph (NY)	Cv	422
Gandhi, Govindan (NY)	S	705	Gelfand, Janice (NY)	Psyc	411
Gandhi, Lajpat (NY)	ChAP	613	Geller, Eric B (NJ)	N	780
Gandhi, Rajinder (NJ)	PS	745	Geller, Mark E (NY)	DR	602
Ganepola, G.A.P. (NJ)	S	753	Geller, Peter (NY)	S	348
Garan, Hasan (NY)	CE	123	Gelles, Jeremiah (NY)	Cv	422
Garay, Kenneth (NJ)	Oto	741	Geltzeiler, Jules (NJ)	U	867
Garay, Stuart (NY)	Pul	329	Gemson, Donald H (NY)	PrM	310
Garber, Perry (NY)	Oph	563	Genato, Romulo (NY)	S	472
Garber, Shawn (NY)	S	589	Gendelman, Seymour (NY)	N	220
Gardenswartz, Mark (NY)	Nep	212	Gendler, Ellen C (NY)	D	143
Gardner, Peter (CT)	Ge	938	Gendler, Seth (NY)	Ge	662

Alphabetical Listing of Doctors

Name	Specialty	Pg	Name	Specialty	Pg
Genieser, Nancy B (NY)	DR	150	Gilbert, Marvin (NY)	OrS	259
Genn, David A (NY)	Ge	662	Gildengers, Jaime (NJ)	S	804
Gennace, Ronald (NJ)	OrS	740	Giliberti, Orazio (NJ)	Oph	894
Gentile, Ralph (NY)	U	415	Gilson, Noah (NJ)	N	861
Gentile, Ronald (NY)	Oph	244	Gindea, Aaron (NY)	Cv	530
Gentilesco, Michael (NY)	ObG	626	Gingold, Bruce S (NY)	CRS	139
George, Abraham (NJ)	Cv	809	Ginsberg, Gerald D (NY)	PlS	304
Georgsson, Sverrir (NY)	U	362	Ginsburg, Frances (CT)	RE	957
Geraci-Ciardullo, Kira (NY)	A&I	647	Ginsburg, Howard B (NY)	PS	292
Geraghty, Michael (NY)	Onc	443	Ginsburg, Mark (NY)	TS	357
Gerard, Perry (NY)	NuM	449	Ginzler, Ellen (NY)	Rhu	470
Gerber, Oded (NY)	N	625	Gioia, Leonard (NY)	EDM	617
Gerberg, Lynda Frances (NY)	Ped	576	Girardi, Anthony (NY)	Oph	563
Gerbino-Rosen, Ginny (NY)	Psyc	411	Girardi, Leonard N (NY)	TS	357
German, Harold (NY)	IM	622	Gitler, Bernard (NY)	Cv	649
Geronemus, Roy (NY)	D	143	Gitler, Ellen (NY)	EDM	659
Gershell, William J (NY)	Psyc	314	Giuffrida, Regina (NY)	ObG	678
Gershon, Anne (NY)	PInf	288	Giusti, Robert (NY)	PPul	460
Gerson, Charles (NY)	Ge	163	Gizzi, Martin (NJ)	N	837
Gersony, Welton Mark (NY)	PCd	282	Glabman, Sheldon (NY)	Nep	213
Gesner, Matthew (NY)	PInf	460	Gladstein, Michael (NY)	D	485
Gettenberg, Gary (NY)	Ge	431	Gladstone, James (NY)	OrS	259
Geuder, James (NJ)	VascS	757	Gladstone, Lenore (NY)	PMR	409
Gevirtz, Clifford (NY)	PM	687	Glanzman, Barry (NY)	Ge	619
Gewirtz, George (NJ)	EDM	773	Glaser, Amy (NY)	Ped	461
Gewirtz, Harold (CT)	PlS	954	Glaser, Jordan (NY)	Inf	511
Gewitz, Michael (NY)	PCd	688	Glaser, Morton (NY)	Pul	637
Gewolb, Eric B (NJ)	Psyc	803	Glasgold, Alvin (NJ)	Oto	841
Gharibo, Christopher G (NY)	PM	277	Glashow, Jonathan (NY)	OrS	259
Giaimo, Thomas (NY)	DR	509	Glass, David (NY)	S	472
Giammarino, Anthony (NY)	ObG	626	Glass, Richard (NY)	Psyc	314
Giangola, Gary (NY)	VascS	370	Glassberg, Kenneth (NY)	U	362
Giannaris, Theodore (NY)	OrS	496	Glassman, Alexander (NY)	Psyc	315
Giardina, Elsa-Grace (NY)	Cv	126	Glassman, Ben (NY)	Ped	693
Giardina, Patricia (NY)	PHO	287	Glassman, Charles F (NY)	IM	603
Gibofsky, Allan (NY)	Rhu	339	Glassman, Charles N (NY)	U	707
Gibralter, Richard P (NY)	Oph	244	Glassman, Mark (CT)	PGe	951
Giegerich, Edmund W (NY)	EDM	428	Glassman, Morris (NY)	Oph	680
Giella, John (NY)	U	607	Glatt, Aaron E (NY)	Inf	547
Gifford, Irina (NY)	PMR	463	Glatt, Herbert (NJ)	Oph	782
Gil, Constante (NJ)	IM	834	Glatt, Hershel (NY)	Ped	576
Gilbert, Fred (NY)	CG	138	Gleckel, Louis Wade (NY)	Cv	530

Alphabetical Listing of Doctors

Name	Specialty	Pg	Name	Specialty	Pg
Glick, Ronald (NJ)	OrS	817	Golden, Flavia (NY)	IM	189
Glickel, Steven (NY)	HS	176	Goldenberg, Alan (NY)	EDM	617
Glicksman, Caroline (NJ)	PlS	865	Goldenberg, Alec (NY)	Hem	179
Gliedman, Paul (NY)	RadRO	469	Goldenberg, Bruce (NJ)	TS	897
Gliklich, Jerry (NY)	Cv	126	Goldenberg, David (NJ)	Ge	914
Glowacki, Jan S (NJ)	IM	860	Goldenberg, David (CT)	PlS	954
Gluck, Ian (NJ)	ObG	879	Goldfarb, C Richard (NY)	NuM	229
Gochfeld, Michael (NJ)	OM	839	Goldfarb, Joel (NJ)	Ge	728
Godec, Circil (NY)	U	475	Goldfarb, Michael A (NJ)	S	867
Godfrey, Norman (NY)	PlS	304	Goldfarb, Steven (NY)	IM	622
Godfrey, Philip (NY)	PlS	304	Goldfischer, Jerome D (NJ)	Cv	720
Goland, Robin (NY)	EDM	155	Goldin, Howard (NY)	Ge	163
Golbe, Lawrence (NJ)	N	838	Goldman, Arnold (NY)	OrS	496
Gold, Alan (NY)	PlS	578	Goldman, Gary (NY)	ObG	233
Gold, Arnold (NY)	ChiN	136	Goldman, Ira S (NY)	Ge	543
Gold, David (NY)	PGe	632	Goldman, Jack S (NY)	IM	667
Gold, Jeffrey L (NJ)	IM	893	Goldman, Joel M (NY)	EDM	428
Gold, Joan (Ny)	PMR	299	Goldman, Kenneth Alan (NJ)	VascS	823
Gold, Scott (NY)	Oto	270	Goldman, Martin E (NY)	Cv	127
Goldberg, Arthur I (NY)	Onc	202	Goldman, Michael (NJ)	EDM	726
Goldberg, Daniel (NJ)	Oph	862	Goldman, Mitchell (NY)	ObG	626
Goldberg, Douglas (NY)	Cv	530	Goldman, Neil C (NY)	A&I	647
Goldberg, Gary L (NY)	GO	389	Goldman, Neil S (NY)	Psyc	315
Goldberg, Harvey (NY)	Cv	126	Goldofsky, Elliot (NY)	Oto	567
Goldberg, Jeffrey (NY)	Psyc	464	Goldsmith, Ari J (NY)	PO	497
Goldberg, Jory (NJ)	Pul	847	Goldsmith, Michael (NY)	Onc	202
Goldberg, Leslie (NY)	Oph	563	Goldsmith, Stanley J (NY)	NuM	229
Goldberg, Marc A (NJ)	Rhu	896	Goldstein, Carl (NJ)	Nep	917
Goldberg, Michael I (NJ)	GO	833	Goldstein, Jeffrey A (NY)	OrS	259
Goldberg, Myron D (NY)	Ge	163	Goldstein, Jonathan (NY)	S	589
Goldberg, Neil S (NY)	D	655	Goldstein, Jonathan E (NJ)	Cv	768
Goldberg, Nieca (NY)	Cv	127	Goldstein, Jonathan M (CT)	N	974
Goldberg, Robert B (NY)	PMR	299	Goldstein, Judith (NY)	Ped	294
Goldberg, Robert T (NY)	Oph	495	Goldstein, Marc (NY)	U	362
Goldberg, Roy J (NY)	Ger	388	Goldstein, Mark A (NY)	Rhu	520
Goldberg, Steven M (NY)	Cv	531	Goldstein, Martin (NY)	ObG	233
Goldberg-Berman, Judith C (CT)	EDM	937	Goldstein, Marvin (NY)	IM	190
Goldberger, Marianne (NY)	Psyc	315	Goldstein, Paul H (NY)	IM	190
Goldblatt, Kenneth (NJ)	Pul	821	Goldstein, Robert (NY)	PlS	410
Goldblatt, Robert (NY)	Ge	662	Goldstein, Stanley (NY)	A&I	528
Goldblum, Lester (NY)	Ge	543	Goldstein, Steven (NJ)	ObG	862
Golden, Brian D (NY)	Rhu	470	Goldstein, Steven I (NY)	Oto	403

Name	Specialty	Pg	Name	Specialty	Pg
Goldstein, Steven J (NY)	Ped	497	Gorenstein, Lyall (NY)	TS	607
Goldstein, Steven R (NY)	ObG	233	Gorevic, Peter D (NY)	Rhu	339
Goldstein, Susanna (NY)	Psyc	315	Gorfine, Stephen (NY)	CRS	139
Goldweit, Richard (NJ)	Cv	720	Gorkin, Janet U (NY)	Nep	395
Golfinos, John G (NY)	NS	215	Gorman, Lauren (NY)	Psyc	315
Golier, Francis (NY)	Cv	649	Gorski, Lydia E (NY)	IM	549
Golimbu, Mircea N (NY)	U	362	Gotfried, Fern (NJ)	Ped	882
Golinko, Richard J (NY)	PCd	282	Gotkin, Robert (NY)	PlS	304
Goltzman, Carey (NY)	PCCM	688	Gotlin, Robert S (NY)	PMR	299
Gomes, J Anthony (NY)	CE	123	Gottesfeld, Peter (NY)	FMed	660
Gomez, William (NJ)	OrS	817	Gottesman, Lester (NY)	CRS	139
Gomolin, Irving (NY)	Ger	545	Gottlieb, Beth (NY)	PRhu	574
Gonzalez, Orlando (NY)	ObG	514	Gottridge, Joanne (NY)	IM	550
Good, Leonard (NY)	Ped	576	Gouge, Thomas (NY)	S	348
Goodgold, Abraham (NJ)	IM	916	Goulart, Hamilton (NJ)	NS	736
Goodgold, Albert (NY)	N	220	Gould, Eric (NY)	Ped	576
Goodman, Alan (NJ)	A&I	911	Gould, Perry (NY)	Ge	543
Goodman, Berney (NY)	Psyc	315	Gould, Richard (NY)	Ge	662
Goodman, Elliot R (NY)	S	348	Goydos, James S (NJ)	S	849
Goodman, Ken J (NY)	DR	538	Grabowski, Wayne (NJ)	Oph	840
Goodman, Mark A (NY)	Cv	531	Grace, William (NY)	Onc	202
Goodman, Michael (NY)	IM	549	Grad, Joel (NY)	HS	176
Goodman, Robert L (NJ)	RadRO	791	Gradler, Thomas (NY)	FMed	430
Goodman, Robert R (NY)	NS	215	Graham, Alan M (NJ)	VascS	851
Goodman, Susan (NY)	Rhu	339	Grajower, Martin (NY)	IM	392
Goodrich, James T (NY)	NS	396	Granatir, Charles (NJ)	OrS	802
Goodstein, Carolyn E (NJ)	A&I	719	Granet, Kenneth M (NJ)	IM	860
Goodwin, Charles (NY)	OrS	259	Granick, Mark S (NJ)	PlS	789
Gopinathan, Govindan (NY)	N	221	Grano, Vanessa (NY)	ObG	678
Gordon, Bernard (NY)	Oph	628	Granstein, Richard (NY)	D	143
Gordon, Garet M (NY)	Cv	379	Grant, Alfred (NY)	OrS	259
Gordon, Jeffrey (NY)	EDM	539	Grant, Linda (CT)	PMR	954
Gordon, Lawrence A (NY)	S	589	Grant, Robert (NY)	PlS	304
Gordon, Marc L (NY)	N	557	Grasso, Cono M (NY)	Oph	495
Gordon, Mark S (NY)	S	705	Grasso, Michael (NJ)	Nep	778
Gordon, Marsha (NY)	D	143	Grasso, Michael (NY)	U	362
Gordon, Michael A (NY)	Oto	567	Graver, L Michael (NY)	TS	592
Gordon, Neil A (CT)	Oto	950	Grayson, Douglas (NY)	Oph	244
Gordon, Richard D (NJ)	Rhu	821	Grazi, Richard (NY)	RE	469
Gordon, Richard Eric (NY)	Pul	582	Greaney, Edward J (NY)	IM	190
Gordon, Stanley L (NY)	OrS	454	Grebler, Arnold (NJ)	U	867
Gorecki, Piotr J (NY)	S	472	Grecco, Michael (NY)	ObG	514

Alphabetical Listing of Doctors

Name	Specialty	Pg	Name	Specialty	Pg
Gredysa, Leslaw (NY)	VascS	643	Greig, Fenella (NY)	PEn	284
Greeley, Norman (NY)	A&I	421	Greisman, Stewart (NY)	Rhu	340
Green, Abraham (NY)	Ped	576	Grello, Ciro T (NY)	Ped	634
Green, Mark W (NY)	N	221	Grelsamer, Ronald P (NY)	OrS	260
Green, Peter (NY)	Ge	163	Grendell, James H (NY)	Ge	543
Green, Richard M (NY)	VascS	370	Grenell, Steven (NY)	N	397
Green, Robert (NY)	Oto	270	Grenis, Michael S (NJ)	OrS	817
Green, Stephen (NY)	Cv	531	Gribbin, Dorota (NJ)	PMR	819
Green, Stephen (NY)	S	640	Gribbon, John (NJ)	IM	777
Green, Steven (NY)	OrS	259	Gribetz, Allen (NY)	Pul	329
Green, Stuart (NY)	Rhu	470	Gribetz, Irwin (NY)	Ped	294
Greenbaum, Allen (NY)	Oph	680	Gribetz, Michael (NY)	U	362
Greenberg, Harly (NY)	Pul	582	Grieco, Anthony (NY)	IM	190
Greenberg, Howard (NY)	Onc	492	Grieco, Michael B (NY)	S	589
Greenberg, Judith J (NY)	ChAP	613	Grieg, Adolfo (NY)	NP	443
Greenberg, Mark (NY)	Cv	379	Griepp, Randall (NY)	TS	357
Greenberg, Martin J (NJ)	Pul	790	Grifo, James A (NY)	RE	336
Greenberg, Maury J (NY)	FMed	618	Grijnsztein, Jacob (NY)	Ped	576
Greenberg, Robert (NY)	D	144	Grizzanti, Joseph (NJ)	Pul	896
Greenberg, Ronald (NY)	Ge	543	Grodberg, Michele (NJ)	D	724
Greenberg, Rosalie (NJ)	ChAP	912	Grodman, Richard (NY)	Cv	507
Greenberg, Steven C (NY)	Oph	680	Grodstein, Gerald (NJ)	Nep	735
Greenberg, Steven M (NY)	Cv	531	Groeger, William (NY)	PlS	578
Greenberg, Susan (NJ)	Onc	861	Groff, Walter (NJ)	CRS	912
Greenberg, William (NY)	Ped	605	Groisser, Victor (NJ)	Ge	774
Greenblatt, Louis (NY)	FMed	618	Groopman, Jacob (NY)	Pul	467
Greene, Jeffrey (NY)	Inf	182	Gropen, Toby I (NY)	N	447
Greene, Loren Wissner (NY)	EDM	155	Grosman, Irwin (NY)	Ge	432
Greenfield, Martin (NY)	EDM	539	Gross, Dennis (NY)	D	144
Greengart, Alvin (NY)	Cv	422	Gross, Elliott (NY)	N	676
Greenlee, Robert (NY)	ObG	678	Gross, Gary L (NJ)	A&I	857
Greenman, James L (NJ)	Inf	731	Gross, Harvey (NJ)	FMed	727
Greenspan, Alan H (NY)	D	144	Gross, Ian (CT)	NP	973
Greenspan, Joel (NY)	Inf	547	Gross, Jeffrey (CT)	N	947
Greenstein, Bruce (NY)	PlS	410	Gross, Joshua (NY)	DR	151
Greenstein, Stuart (NY)	S	414	Gross, Michael L (NJ)	SM	752
Greenwald, Blaine (NY)	GerPsy	489	Gross, Peter A (NJ)	Inf	731
Greenwald, Bruce M (NY)	PCCM	283	Gross, Susan (NY)	CG	381
Greenwald, David A (NY)	Ge	387	Grossbard, Lionel (NY)	Onc	202
Greenwald, Marc (NY)	CRS	535	Grossbard, Michael L (NY)	Onc	202
Greenwald, Robert (NY)	Rhu	586	Grossi, Eugene A (NY)	TS	357
Greif, Richard (NY)	Cv	649	Grossi, Robert (NY)	VascS	370

Name	Specialty	Pg	Name	Specialty	Pg
Grossman, Bernard (NJ)	Onc	813	Gupta, Sanjeev (NY)	Ge	387
Grossman, Edward (CT)	Ge	938	Gupta, Shiv (CT)	NuM	947
Grossman, Elliot (NJ)	ChiN	874	Gurevich, Michael (NY)	Psyc	581
Grossman, Kenneth (NJ)	D	858	Gurland, Frances E (NJ)	Psyc	748
Grossman, Marc E (NY)	D	655	Gurland, Judith (NY)	Oph	401
Grossman, Melanie (NY)	D	144	Gurland, Mark (NJ)	HS	729
Grossman, Robert B (NJ)	OrS	863	Gusberg, Richard J (CT)	VascS	983
Grossman, Robert I (NY)	NRad	227	Gusmorino, Paul (NY)	PM	277
Grossman, Susan (NY)	Nep	513	Gusset, George (NY)	Ge	432
Grossman, Will (NY)	Cv	127	Guthrie, James (CT)	CRS	935
Grosso, John (NY)	Oto	567	Gutin, Philip (NY)	NS	216
Grubb, William R (NJ)	PM	842	Gutman, David (NY)	Ge	543
Gruber, Gabriel (NJ)	D	913	Gutowski, W Thomas (NJ)	OrS	817
Gruber, Michael L (NY)	N	221	Gutwein, Isadore Phillip (NY)	Ge	387
Grubman, Jerold (NJ)	U	850	Guzman, Rodolfo (NY)	EDM	385
Grubman, Samuel (NY)	A&I	121			
Gruenstein, Steven (NY)	Onc	202			
Gruenwald, Laurence D (NJ)	Ped	787			
Grunberger, Ivan (NY)	U	475			
Grunebaum, Amos (NY)	MF	199	**H**		
Grunfeld, Lawrence (NY)	RE	336			
Grunzweig, Milton (NY)	IM	439	Haas, Alexander (NJ)	RadRO	848
Gruskay, Jeffrey (CT)	Ped	978	Haas, Steven B (NY)	OrS	260
Gruss, Claudia (CT)	Ge	938	Haber, Daran (NJ)	PM	863
Gruss, Leslie (NY)	ObG	233	Haber, Patricia (NY)	Ped	407
Guarini, Ludovico (NY)	PHO	459	Haber, Stuart (NY)	IM	190
Guarnaccia, Gary (NY)	ObG	494	Habermann, Edward (NY)	OrS	684
Gudavalli, Madhu R (NY)	NP	444	Habib, Mohsen (NY)	Oto	456
Guida, Robert (NY)	Oto	271	Haddad, Joseph (NY)	PO	290
Guillem, Jose (NY)	CRS	139	Haffty, Bruce (NJ)	RadRO	848
Guillen, Gregorio (NJ)	IM	834	Haft, Jacob I (NJ)	Cv	720
Guillory, Samuel L (NY)	Oph	244	Hagaman, John (NJ)	Cv	809
Guirguis, Fayez (NY)	ObG	450	Hages, Harry (NJ)	Ped	746
Gulati, Subhash C (NY)	Onc	203	Haggerty, Mary A (NJ)	IM	777
Gulotta, Stephen J (NY)	Cv	531	Haher, Jane N. (NY)	PlS	304
Gulrajani, Ramesh (NY)	Pul	467	Hahn, John C (NJ)	Ge	800
Gumbs, Milton (NY)	S	414	Haight, David (NY)	Oph	244
Gumprecht, Jeffrey Paul (NY)	Inf	182	Hailoo, Wajdy (NY)	OM	627
Gundy, Edward (NY)	OrS	683	Haimov, Moshe (NY)	VascS	370
Gundy, John (CT)	Ped	952	Haimovic, Itzhak (NY)	N	557
Gupta, Jagdish (NY)	IM	439	Haines, Kathleen A (NJ)	PRhu	744
Gupta, Prem (NY)	Cv	423	Hainline, Brian (NY)	N	557
			Hait, William (NJ)	Onc	835
			Hajal, Fady (NY)	ChAP	652

Alphabetical Listing of Doctors

Name	Specialty	Pg	Name	Specialty	Pg
Hajjar, John H (NJ)	U	756	Harden, Cynthia L (NY)	N	221
Halata, Michael (NY)	PGe	689	Hardy, Howard (NJ)	CRS	809
Hall, Craig D (NJ)	PlS	747	Hardy, Mark (NY)	S	349
Hall, Lisabeth (NY)	Oph	245	Harin, Anantham (NY)	NP	513
Hall, Simon J (NY)	U	363	Harish, Ziv (NJ)	A&I	719
Hallal, Edward (NY)	IM	622	Harlam, Dean (NY)	Psyc	698
Halmi, Katherine (NY)	Psyc	697	Harlow, Paul (NJ)	Ped	746
Halperin, Alan (NY)	D	655	Harman, John (NJ)	Pul	821
Halperin, Ira (NY)	Hem	179	Harmon, Gregory K (NY)	Oph	245
Halperin, John (NJ)	N	918	Haroldson, Olaf (NJ)	Oto	818
Halperin, Jonathan L (NY)	Cv	127	Harooni, Robert (NY)	Ge	487
Halpern, Allan C (NY)	D	144	Harper, Harry (NJ)	Hem	730
Halpern, Brian (NJ)	SM	866	Harrington, Elizabeth (NY)	VascS	370
Halpern, Neil (NY)	CCM	140	Harrington, Martin (NY)	VascS	370
Halpern, Steven (NJ)	PHO	743	Harris, Burton H (NY)	PS	406
Hamburger, Max (NY)	Rhu	639	Harris, Leon (NY)	Pul	606
Hamby, Robert I (NY)	Cv	531	Harris, Matthew N (NY)	S	349
Hamet, Marc R (CT)	VIR	960	Harris, Michael (NY)	S	349
Hametz, Irwin (NJ)	D	858	Harris, Michael B (NJ)	PHO	744
Hamilton, William (NY)	OrS	260	Harris, Steven (NY)	U	594
Hammel, Jay (NY)	DR	538	Harrison, Aaron R (NY)	Ge	619
Hammer, Arthur (NY)	Pul	467	Harrison, Louis (NY)	RadRO	334
Hammer, Glenn (NY)	Inf	182	Hart, Catherine (NY)	IM	190
Hammer, Scott M (NY)	Inf	182	Hart, Sidney (CT)	Psyc	955
Hammerman, Hillel (NY)	Ge	164	Hartman, Alan (NY)	TS	592
Hammerschlag, Paul E (NY)	Oto	271	Hartman, Barry Jay (NY)	Inf	182
Hamner, Daniel (NY)	SM	343	Hartz, Cindi (NY)	Ped	693
Hand, Ivan (NY)	Ped	407	Hartzband, Mark A (NJ)	OrS	740
Handelsman, Dan (NY)	PEn	688	Harwin, Steven F (NY)	OrS	260
Handelsman, Richard E (NY)	IM	603	Haselkorn, Joan (NY)	ObG	560
Handler, Elliot (NY)	DR	602	Haskal, Ziv (NY)	VIR	368
Handler, Robert (NJ)	Ped	882	Hatcher, Virgil (NY)	D	144
Hankin, Dorie (NY)	Ped	576	Hatsis, Alexander (NY)	Oph	563
Hanley, Gerard (NY)	Cv	423	Hauptman, Allen S (NY)	IM	190
Hann, Lucy (NY)	DR	151	Hausman, Michael R (NY)	OrS	260
Hanna, Moneer (NY)	U	594	Haveson, Stephen (NY)	VascS	370
Hannafin, Jo (NY)	OrS	260	Hawrylo, Richard (NJ)	PlS	883
Har-El, Gady (NY)	Oto	271	Hayes, Joseph (NY)	Cv	127
Haramati, Linda B (NY)	DR	383	Hayes-McKenzie, Leslie (NY)	AM	421
Haramati, Nogah (NY)	DR	383	Hayworth, Robin (NY)	Oph	401
Harangozo, Andrea (NJ)	Pul	847	Hayworth, Scott (NY)	ObG	678
Harary, Albert (NY)	Ge	164	Heald, Peter (CT)	D	968

Alphabetical Listing of Doctors

Name	Specialty	Pg	Name	Specialty	Pg
Hodes, Steven (NJ)	Ge	831	Horovitz, Len (NY)	IM	190
Hodgson, W John B (NY)	S	414	Horowitz, Harold (NY)	Inf	665
Hodosh, Richard M (NJ)	NS	918	Horowitz, Lawrence (NY)	Ge	164
Hoffman, Anthony (NY)	Onc	393	Horowitz, Marc (NY)	Oph	681
Hoffman, Ira (NY)	IM	190	Horowitz, Mark D (NY)	Rhu	340
Hoffman, Janet C (NY)	DR	538	Horowitz, Steven (CT)	Cv	934
Hoffman, Joel (NY)	Psyc	316	Hotchkiss, Edward (NY)	IM	550
Hoffman, Lloyd (NY)	PlS	304	Hotchkiss, Robert (NY)	OrS	261
Hoffman, Michael L (NY)	Rhu	586	Houghton, Alan N (NY)	Onc	203
Hoffman, Pamela (CT)	IM	941	Housman, Arno (NY)	U	707
Hoffman, Richard S (NY)	EDM	510	Hricak, Hedvig (NY)	DR	151
Hoffman, Robert S (NY)	PrM	310	Hsu, Chaur Dong (NY)	MF	670
Hoffman, Ronald (NY)	Oto	271	Hsu, Daphne (NY)	PCd	282
Hoffman, Saul (NY)	PlS	305	Hsueh, John Tzu-Lang (NY)	Cv	483
Hofstetter, Steven (NY)	S	349	Hsuih, Terence CH (NY)	IM	439
Holden, Melvin (NY)	IM	550	Hubschmann, Otakar R (NJ)	NS	779
Holder, Jonathan L (NY)	OrS	684	Hudis, Clifford A (NY)	Onc	203
Holgersen, Leif (NY)	PS	691	Hughes, John T (NY)	N	398
Holland, Claudia (NY)	ObG	233	Hughes, Peter (CT)	OrS	949
Holland, Elbridge (NJ)	FMed	875	Huh, Julie (NY)	D	614
Holland, James F (NY)	Onc	203	Huh, Sun (NY)	RadRO	469
Holland, Neil R (NJ)	N	862	Hunter, John G (NY)	PlS	305
Hollander, Eric (NY)	Psyc	316	Hupart, Kenneth (NY)	EDM	539
Hollander, Gerald (NY)	Cv	423	Hurley, John A (NJ)	OrS	880
Hollis, Peter H (NY)	NS	556	Hurst, Lawrence C (NY)	HS	620
Hollister, Dickerman (CT)	Onc	944	Hurst, Wendy (NJ)	ObG	737
Holmes, Nathaniel J (NJ)	CRS	770	Huston, Jan A (NJ)	S	925
Holtzman, Robert N N (NY)	NS	216	Hutcherson, Hilda Y (NY)	ObG	233
Holzer, Barry D (NY)	ChAP	425	Hutchinson, Gordon J (CT)	Rhu	981
Holzman, Ian (NY)	NP	210	Hutson, J Milton (NY)	MF	199
Homan, William P (NY)	S	705	Huvos, Andrew G (NY)	Path	279
Homayuni, Ali (NY)	Cv	508	Hwang, Cheng-hong (NJ)	IM	916
Hong, Andrew (NY)	PS	574	Hyatt, Alexander C (NJ)	Ped	746
Hong, Joon Ho (NY)	S	472	Hyde, Phyllis (NY)	Hem	436
Honig, Stephen (NY)	Rhu	340	Hyler, Irene (NY)	ChAP	652
Hopkins, Arthur (NY)	IM	668	Hyman, David B (NY)	CG	614
Horbar, Gary (NY)	IM	190	Hyman, George (NY)	Oph	452
Hordof, Allan (NY)	PCd	282	Hymes, Kenneth (NY)	Hem	179
Hornblass, Albert (NY)	Oph	245			
Horner, Neil (NJ)	NRad	918			
Hornyak, Stephen W (NY)	S	521			
Horovitz, Joel (NY)	S	473			

Name	Specialty	Pg
I		
Iammatteo, Matthew (NJ)	ObG	879
Ibelli, Vincent (NY)	FMed	602
Ibrahim, Ibrahim M (NJ)	S	754
Idupuganti, Sudharam (NY)	Psyc	464
Igel, Gerard (NY)	Ped	407
Ilkhani, Rahman (NY)	VascS	477
Illman, Arnold (NY)	OrS	565
Ilowite, Norman T (NY)	PRhu	406
Imber, Gerald (NY)	PlS	305
Imperato, Pascal James (NY)	PrM	464
Imperato-McGinley, Julianne (NY)	EDM	156
Inabnet, William B (NY)	S	349
Inamdar, Sarla (NY)	Ped	294
Inglis, Steven R (NY)	MF	491
Ingrassia, Joseph (NY)	FMed	602
Innella, Robin (NJ)	OrS	919
Innerfield, Michael (NY)	Cv	601
Inra, Lawrence A (NY)	Cv	128
Inwald, Gary (NY)	PMR	299
Inzucchi, Sylvio (CT)	EDM	969
Iqbal, Riaz (NJ)	Ge	811
Irving, Henry C (NJ)	OrS	802
Irwin, Mark (NY)	U	475
Isaacs, Ellen (NY)	IM	668
Isaacson, Steven (NY)	RadRO	334
Isay, Richard A (NY)	Psyc	316
Isom, O Wayne (NY)	TS	357
Israel, Alan (NJ)	Hem	730
Issenberg, Henry (NY)	PCd	688
Istrico, Richard A (NY)	FMed	487
Iswara, Kadirawel (NY)	Ge	432
Itzkowitz, Steven H (NY)	Ge	164
Iyengar, Devarajan P (NJ)	Onc	801
J		
Jackson, Rosemary (NY)	Ped	461
Jacob, Jessica (NY)	ObG	560
Jacobowitz, Glenn R (NY)	VascS	371

Name	Specialty	Pg
Jacobowitz, Marilyn (NY)	Pul	701
Jacobs, Allan J (NY)	GO	489
Jacobs, David R (NY)	EDM	156
Jacobs, Elliot (NY)	PlS	305
Jacobs, Jonathan (NY)	Inf	183
Jacobs, Joseph (NY)	Oto	271
Jacobs, Laurie (NY)	Ger	389
Jacobs, Michael (NY)	D	144
Jacobs, Morton (NY)	DR	151
Jacobs, Theodore (NY)	Psyc	316
Jacobs, Thomas (NY)	EDM	156
Jacobson, Ira (NY)	Ge	164
Jacobson, Marc S (NY)	AM	527
Jacobson, Ronald (NY)	ChiN	653
Jacoby, Jacob H (NJ)	Psyc	803
Jafar, Jafar (NY)	NS	216
Jaffe, Fredrick F (NY)	OrS	261
Jaffe, Herbert (NY)	Oph	452
Jaffe, William (NY)	OrS	261
Jagannath, Sundar (NY)	Onc	204
Jahn, Anthony (NJ)	Oto	784
Jahre, Caren (NY)	NRad	228
Jaile-Marti, Jesus (NY)	NP	673
Jain, Subhash (NY)	PM	277
Jamal, Habib (NY)	Oto	685
James, David F (NY)	ObG	233
Jamil, Zafar (NJ)	VascS	795
Januzzi, James (NY)	Ge	164
Jarowski, Charles (NY)	Onc	204
Jarrett, Mark (NY)	Rhu	520
Jawetz, Harold (NJ)	IM	893
Jay, Judith (NY)	Oto	685
Jayabose, Somasundaram (NY)	PHO	690
Jayaram, Nadubeethi (NY)	OrS	516
Jeffries, James M (NJ)	PlS	923
Jelin, Abraham (NY)	PGe	458
Jelks, Glenn (NY)	PlS	305
Jelveh, Mansoor (NY)	Cv	531
Jewel, Kenneth (NJ)	DR	771
Jobanputra, Kishor (NJ)	FMed	903
Johns, William (CT)	NuM	947
Johnson, Albert (NJ)	OrS	905

Alphabetical Listing of Doctors

Name	Specialty	Pg	Name	Specialty	Pg
Johnson, Diane H (NY)	Inf	548	Kalinich, Lila J (NY)	Psyc	316
Johnson, Mark S (NJ)	FMed	773	Kalinsky, Jay (NY)	ObG	678
Johnson, Robert L (NJ)	AM	767	Kalischer, Alan (NJ)	Cv	911
Johnson, Valerie (NY)	PNep	289	Kalman, Jeffery (NY)	Ge	510
Johnson, Warren (NY)	Inf	183	Kamalakar, Peri (NJ)	PHO	786
Jokl, Peter (CT)	OrS	975	Kamelhar, David (NY)	Pul	329
Jonas, Murray (NY)	Inf	437	Kamen, Barton A (NJ)	PHO	844
Jones, Frank A (NJ)	Psyc	846	Kamen, Mazen (NY)	Cv	128
Jones, Jacqueline (NY)	PO	290	Kamholz, Stephan (NY)	Pul	582
Jones, Vann (NY)	IM	439	Kaminetsky, Jed (NY)	U	363
Jordan, Barry D (NY)	N	676	Kaminsky, Donald (NY)	IM	191
Jordan, Lawrence (NJ)	S	822	Kaminsky, Sari J (NY)	ObG	233
Josef, Minna (NY)	EDM	602	Kamler, Kenneth (NY)	HS	546
Joseph, John (NY)	IM	490	Kane, Michael J (NJ)	Onc	778
Joseph, Patricia (NJ)	S	754	Kanengiser, Steven (NJ)	PPul	744
Josephson, Jordan S (NY)	Oto	271	Kang, Harriet (NY)	ChiN	653
Josephson, Lynn (NY)	S	705	Kang, Pritpal S (NY)	Cv	423
Joshi, Anil (NY)	Nep	674	Kanner, Ronald (NY)	N	557
Joy, Mark (NY)	IM	191	Kanter, Alan (NJ)	Ped	746
Jutkowitz, Robert (NY)	N	514	Kantor, Alan (NY)	EDM	659
			Kantrowitz, Niki E (NY)	Cv	423
			Kaplan, Barry (NY)	Onc	492
			Kaplan, Gabriel (NJ)	Psyc	923
			Kaplan, Jerry (NY)	N	398
K			Kaplan, Kenneth C (NY)	IM	668
Kabakow, Bernard (NY)	Onc	204	Kaplan, Martin (NY)	Ped	634
Kabis, Suzanne (NJ)	Nep	904	Kaplan, Matthew (NY)	PNep	460
Kadar, Avraham (NY)	A&I	121	Kaplan, Ronald (NY)	PM	278
Kaell, Alan (NY)	Rhu	639	Kaplan, Sherri (NY)	D	655
Kahan, Norman (NY)	U	415	Kaplan, Steven (NY)	U	363
Kahn, David A (NY)	Psyc	316	Kaplovitz, Harry (NY)	PCd	457
Kahn, Leonard B (NY)	Path	569	Kapoor, Satish (NY)	IM	668
Kahn, Martin (NY)	Cv	128	Kappel, Bruce (NY)	Onc	553
Kahn, Max (NY)	Ped	294	Karanfilian, Richard (NY)	VascS	709
Kahn, Oren (NY)	Ge	663	Karas, Evan (NY)	OrS	684
Kahn, Steven P (NJ)	S	822	Karasu, T Byram (NY)	Psyc	316
Kaiden, Jeffrey (NJ)	Oph	738	Karatoprak, Ohan (NJ)	FMed	727
Kairam, Indira (NY)	Ge	164	Karayalcin, Gungor (NY)	PHO	572
Kaiser, Paul (NJ)	N	815	Karbowitz, Stephen (NY)	Pul	499
Kaiser, Stephen (NY)	IM	439	Karetzky, Monroe (NJ)	Pul	790
Kalafatic, Alfredo (NY)	CRS	535	Karmen, Carol (NY)	IM	668
Kalchthaler, Thomas (NY)	Ger	664	Karp, Adam (NY)	IM	191
Kaleya, Ronald (NY)	S	414			

Alphabetical Listing of Doctors

Name	Specialty	Pg	Name	Specialty	Pg
Kemeny, Nancy (NY)	Onc	204	Khulpateea, Taru (NY)	ObG	560
Kemmann, Ekkehard (NJ)	RE	848	Kierce, Roger (NJ)	ObG	894
Kempin, Sanford Jay (NY)	Hem	179	Kiernan, Howard (NY)	OrS	261
Kenan, Samuel (NY)	OrS	261	Kim, Hong (NY)	U	476
Kenefick, Timothy (CT)	Ped	953	Kim, Joyce M (NY)	ObG	234
Kenet, Barney J (NY)	D	145	Kim, Jung Yong (NY)	Onc	624
Kenigsberg, Daniel (NY)	RE	639	Kim, Zung Wan (NY)	S	705
Kennedy, Gary (NY)	GerPsy	389	Kimball, Annetta (NY)	Ge	164
Kennedy, James (NY)	IM	191	Kimmelman, Charles P (NY)	Oto	271
Kennedy, John W (NJ)	EDM	810	Kimmelstiel, Fred (NY)	S	350
Kennedy, Thomas (CT)	PNep	952	Kimura, Yukiko (NJ)	PRhu	745
Kennish, Arthur (NY)	IM	191	King, Robert A (CT)	ChAP	966
Kenny, Raymond (NJ)	Ge	774	King, William (NY)	HS	176
Kent, Joan (NY)	ObG	234	Kipen, Howard (NJ)	OM	840
Kent, K Craig (NY)	VascS	371	Kirschenbaum, Alexander M (NY)	U	363
Kernan, Nancy A (NY)	PHO	287	Kirshblum, Steven C (NJ)	PMR	788
Kernan, Walter (CT)	IM	971	Kirshenbaum, Nancy (NY)	ObG	678
Kernberg, Otto (NY)	Psyc	698	Kirtane, Sanjay (NY)	Cv	532
Kerner, Michael (NJ)	Ge	914	Kitsis, Richard N (NY)	Cv	379
Kerr, Angela (NY)	ObG	450	Kitzis, Hugo D (NJ)	ObG	802
Kerr, Leslie D (NY)	Rhu	340	Kizelshteyn, Grigory (NY)	PM	687
Kerstein, Joshua (NY)	Cv	423	Klagsbrun, Samuel C (NY)	Psyc	698
Kesarwala, Hemant (NJ)	A&I	827	Klapholz, Ari (NY)	Pul	329
Kessler, Alan (NY)	ObG	234	Klapholz, Marc (NJ)	Cv	768
Kessler, Bradley (NY)	PGe	633	Klapper, Daniel (NY)	Oph	245
Kessler, Edmund (NY)	PS	575	Klapper, Philip (NY)	Pul	412
Kessler, Jeffrey (NY)	N	558	Klar, Tobi (NY)	D	655
Kessler, Leonard (NY)	Onc	553	Klarsfeld, Jay (CT)	Oto	950
Kessler, Martin E (NY)	PlS	579	Klass, Evan (NY)	EDM	540
Kessler, William (NJ)	Hem	915	Klausner, Stanley (NY)	S	640
Kestenbaum, Alan (NY)	PM	687	Kleber, Herbert (NY)	AdP	119
Kestenbaum, Clarice J (NY)	ChAP	135	Kleeman, Harris J (NY)	Cv	423
Khafif, Rene (NY)	S	473	Klein, Arthur (NY)	Inf	620
Khalife, Michael (NY)	S	590	Klein, Donald (NY)	Psyc	317
Khan, Arfa (NY)	DR	538	Klein, George (NY)	U	363
Khan, Farida (NY)	EDM	429	Klein, Irwin (NY)	EDM	540
Khandji, Alexander G (NY)	NRad	228	Klein, Natalie (NY)	Inf	548
Khimani, Karim (NJ)	IM	916	Klein, Neil (CT)	IM	941
Khouri, Philippe J (NJ)	Psyc	820	Klein, Noah (NY)	Oph	245
Khoury, F Frederic (NY)	PlS	695	Klein, Norman (NY)	A&I	421
Khoury, Paul (NY)	DR	657	Klein, Patricia (NJ)	N	736
Khulpateea, Neekianund (NY)	GO	435	Klein, Robert (NJ)	A&I	891

Name	Specialty	Pg	Name	Specialty	Pg
Klein, Robert J (NY)	Oph	563	Kohn, Brenda (NY)	PEn	284
Klein, Robert M (NY)	DR	657	Kolitz, Jonathan E (NY)	Hem	546
Klein, Steven (NY)	FMed	618	Kolker, Adam R (NY)	PlS	305
Klein, Victor (NY)	MF	552	Kolker, Harvey A (NY)	Ped	634
Klein, Walter A (NJ)	Ge	728	Kolodny, Edwin H (NY)	N	221
Kleinbaum, Jerry (NY)	EDM	659	Kolodny, Erwin (NY)	Pul	330
Kleinberg, David (NY)	EDM	156	Kolsky, Neil (NJ)	Ped	746
Kleiner, Morton (NY)	Nep	514	Komisar, Arnold (NY)	Oto	272
Kleinman, Andrew (NY)	PlS	695	Koniaris, Soula (NJ)	PGe	843
Kleinman, Paul (NY)	OrS	402	Konigsberg, Stephen (NJ)	VascS	851
Klenk, Rosemary (CT)	Ped	953	Konka, Sudarsanam (NY)	IM	439
Klenoff, Bruce (CT)	Oto	950	Kopec, Anna V (NJ)	D	799
Kliger, Alan (CT)	Nep	973	Kopel, Samuel (NY)	Hem	436
Kligfield, Paul (NY)	Cv	128	Kopelman, Rima G (NJ)	Rhu	751
Kline, Gary (NY)	TS	592	Kopf, Gary S (CT)	TS	983
Kline, Mitchell (NY)	D	145	Koplewicz, Harold (NY)	ChAP	135
Klingenstein, Jeffrey (NY)	Ge	487	Koplin, Richard (NY)	Oph	246
Klion, Franklin (NY)	Ge	165	Koppel, Barbara (NY)	N	222
Kloss, Robert (CT)	Onc	944	Koreen, Amy R (NY)	Psyc	636
Kloth, David S (CT)	PM	951	Korelitz, Burton I (NY)	Ge	165
Klotman, Mary E (NY)	Inf	183	Kornbluth, Arthur Asher (NY)	Ge	165
Klotman, Paul E (NY)	Nep	213	Kornel, Ezriel (NY)	NS	675
Klug, Jonathan (NY)	DR	151	Kornfeld, Donald S (NY)	Psyc	317
Klugman, Susan (NY)	ObG	678	Korsten, Mark A (NY)	Ge	387
Klyde, Barry J (NY)	EDM	156	Korval, Arnold (CT)	Ped	953
Knapp, Albert B (NY)	Ge	165	Kosinski, Edward (CT)	Cv	934
Knee, Robert (NJ)	RadRO	848	Kososky, Charles (NJ)	N	815
Knep, Stanley (NJ)	N	893	Koss, Jerome (NY)	Cv	532
Knisely, Jonathan (CT)	RadRO	980	Kostadaras, Ari (NY)	Nep	493
Knopp, Edmond A. (NY)	DR	151	Kostis, John B (NJ)	Cv	828
Knowles, Daniel (NY)	Path	280	Kostroff, Karen (NY)	S	590
Ko, Wilson (NY)	TS	357	Kotin, Neal (NY)	Ped	294
Ko, Wilson (NY)	Oph	495	Kotler, Donald P (NY)	Ge	165
Kobren, Steven (NY)	Cv	532	Kottler, William (NJ)	PPul	787
Kocher, Jeffrey (NJ)	Inf	731	Koulos, John (NY)	GO	174
Kocsis, James (NY)	Psyc	317	Kowallis, George (NY)	Psyc	317
Koenig, Eli (NY)	NP	444	Kozicky, Orest (NY)	Ge	663
Koenigsberg, Mordecai (NY)	DR	383	Kozin, Arthur (NY)	Nep	604
Kofinas, Alexander (NY)	MF	441	Kozlowski, Jeffrey (NJ)	Nep	735
Kofinas, George (NY)	RE	469	Kraft, Robert L (NY)	PlS	498
Kogan, Stanley J (NY)	U	708	Krakoff, Lawrence (NJ)	Cv	721
Kohan, Darius (NY)	Oto	271	Krakovitz, Evan (NY)	S	705

Alphabetical Listing of Doctors

Name	Specialty	Pg	Name	Specialty	Pg
Kramer, Elissa (NY)	NuM	229	Kukar, Narinder (NY)	EDM	486
Kramer, Mitchell (NY)	ObG	626	Kula, Roger W (NY)	N	558
Kramer, Neil (NJ)	Rhu	791	Kulick, Roy G (NY)	HS	389
Kramer, Philip (NY)	Oph	515	Kulick, Stephen A (NY)	N	514
Kranzler, Elliot (NY)	Psyc	317	Kulpa, Jolanta (NY)	PHO	459
Kranzler, L Stephan (NY)	N	676	Kumar, Sampath (NY)	S	473
Krasinski, Keith M (NY)	PInf	288	Kummer, Bart (NY)	Ge	165
Krasnogor, Lester (CT)	Pul	956	Kuncham, Sudha (NY)	ObG	560
Kraus, Dennis (NY)	Oto	272	Kunzman, Kenneth (NJ)	Oto	905
Krause, Cynthia (NY)	ObG	234	Kupersmith, Mark (NY)	Oph	246
Kraushaar, Barry S (NY)	OrS	605	Kupfer, Yizhak (NY)	Pul	467
Krauss, Alfred N (NY)	NP	210	Kurani, Devendra (NJ)	Psyc	803
Krauthamer, Martin (CT)	Cv	934	Kurer, Cheryl C (NJ)	PCd	842
Kreitzer, Joel (NY)	PM	278	Kurfist, Lee (NY)	Ped	634
Kreitzer, Paula (NY)	PEn	571	Kuriloff, Daniel (NY)	Oto	272
Krellenstein, Daniel J (NY)	TS	357	Kurtin, Stephen (NY)	D	145
Kremberg, M Roy (NY)	Psyc	317	Kurtz, Caroline (CT)	Pul	956
Krespi, Yosef (NY)	Oto	272	Kurtz, Lewis (NY)	S	590
Kressner, Michael (NY)	Ge	663	Kurtz, Neil J (NY)	OrS	630
Krevitt, Lane (NY)	Oto	272	Kurtz, Robert C (NY)	Ge	165
Kriegel, David (NY)	D	145	Kurz, Larry (NY)	IM	439
Krieger, Ben-Zion (NY)	Ped	461	Kushner, Brian H (NY)	PHO	287
Krieger, Karl (NY)	TS	357	Kushner, Susan (NJ)	Ped	746
Krieger, Richard (NJ)	Inf	892	Kutcher, Rosalyn (NY)	DR	657
Krilov, Leonard (NY)	PInf	573	Kutin, Neil (NY)	PS	575
Krim, Eileen (NY)	ObG	560	Kutnick, Richard (NY)	Cv	128
Krinick, Ronald M (NY)	SM	343	Kutnick, Robert (NY)	Pul	330
Krinsky, Glenn (NJ)	DR	725	Kutscher, Martin (NY)	ChiN	653
Krinsley, James (CT)	Pul	956	Kuzniecky, Ruben (NY)	N	222
Kris, Mark G (NY)	Onc	204	Kveton, John (CT)	Oto	976
Kristal, Leonard (NY)	D	537	Kwartler, Jed A (NJ)	Oto	920
Krivo, James (NY)	D	537	Kwon, Tae (NY)	GO	665
Krol, Kristine (NJ)	A&I	901			
Kroll, Richard (NY)	U	607			
Kron, Leo (NY)	ChAP	135			
Kronzon, Itzhak (NY)	Cv	128	# L		
Krotowski, Mark (NY)	FMed	430	La Bagnara, James (NJ)	Oto	894
Krown, Susan (NY)	Onc	204	La Gamma, Edmund F (NY)	NP	674
Krumholz, Michael (NY)	Ge	165	La Marca, Charles (NY)	Oto	496
Krutchik, Allan (NJ)	Onc	733	La Mendola, Christopher (NY)	TS	592
Kuflik, Paul (NY)	OrS	261	La Quaglia, Michael (NY)	PS	292
Kuhel, William (NY)	Oto	272	Labar, Douglas (NY)	N	222

Alphabetical Listing of Doctors

Name	Specialty	Pg	Name	Specialty	Pg
Labissiere, Jean-Claude (NJ)	Pul	790	Lansen, Thomas A (NY)	NS	675
Lachman, Reid (NJ)	Oto	881	Lansigan, Nicholas (NY)	S	521
Lachmann, Elisabeth A (NY)	PMR	299	Lansing, Martha (NJ)	FMed	831
Lachs, Mark (NY)	Ger	171	Lansman, Steven (NY)	TS	706
Lacqua, Frank (NY)	CRS	426	Lanteri, Vincent J (NJ)	U	756
Lacy, Jill (CT)	Onc	973	Lanyi, Valery (NY)	PMR	299
Lafaro, Rocco J (NY)	TS	706	Lanzkowsky, Philip (NY)	PHO	572
Lafferty, James (NY)	Cv	508	Lara, Jonathan F (NJ)	Path	784
Lafontant, Jennifer (NY)	ObG	400	Laraque, Danielle (NY)	Ped	294
Lahita, Robert G (NJ)	Rhu	804	Larson, Signe S (NY)	Ped	295
Laifer, Steven A (CT)	MF	943	Larson, Steven M (NY)	NuM	229
Laitman, Robert (NY)	Nep	395	LaSala, Patrick (NY)	NS	397
Laks, Mitchell (NY)	DR	383	Laskey, Richard S (NJ)	Oto	803
Lalli, Corradino (NY)	IM	622	Laskin, Richard (NY)	OrS	262
Lalwani, Anil Kumar (NY)	Oto	272	Latov, Norman (NY)	N	222
Lamarque, Madeleine (NY)	ObG	450	Lau, Henry (NJ)	Cv	721
Lambert, George (NJ)	NP	836	Laub, Glenn W (NJ)	TS	822
Lambroza, Arnon (NY)	Ge	166	Laucella, Michael (NY)	DR	616
Lamm, Carin (NY)	PPul	291	Lauer, Robert (NJ)	Cv	828
Lamm, Steven (NY)	IM	191	Lauricella, Joseph (NJ)	Cv	721
Lan, Vivian E (NJ)	IM	732	Lavyne, Michael H (NY)	NS	216
Lancefield, Margaret (NJ)	IM	813	Lawrence, David (NY)	Oto	686
Landau, Leon (NY)	Hem	390	Lawson, William (NY)	Oto	273
Landau, Steven (NY)	Ge	663	Lax, James (NY)	Ge	166
Landers, David B (NJ)	Cv	721	Layne, Jeffrey (NY)	U	594
Landesman, Richard Howard (CT)	Cv	934	Lazar, Eliot J (NY)	Cv	128
Landesman, Sheldon (NY)	Inf	489	Lazar, Mark H (NJ)	N	838
Landman, Jaime (NY)	U	364	Lazar, Robert (NY)	Ge	619
Landrigan, Philip (NY)	OM	238	Lazarus, George M (NY)	Ped	295
Landzberg, Joel (NJ)	Cv	721	Lazarus, Herbert (NY)	Ped	295
Lane, Dorothy S (NY)	PrM	636	Lazzaro, E Clifford (NY)	Oph	452
Lane, Frederick M (NY)	Psyc	317	Lazzaro, Richard (NY)	TS	475
Lane, Joseph (NY)	OrS	261	Le Benger, Kerry S (NJ)	A&I	911
Lane, Lewis B (NY)	HS	546	Leach, Thomas A (NJ)	PlS	820
Lang, Paul (NY)	A&I	528	Leahy, Mary (NY)	IM	603
Lang, Samuel (NY)	TS	358	Leb, Alvin (NY)	Ge	432
Lange, Dale J (NY)	N	222	Lebinger, Martin (NY)	Psyc	411
Lange, David J (NJ)	PlS	883	Lebinger, Tessa (NY)	PEn	689
Langer, Paul (NJ)	Oph	782	Lebofsky, Martin (NY)	IM	668
Langsner, Alan (NJ)	PCd	785	Lebovics, Edward (NY)	Ge	663
Lanman, Geraldine (NY)	Ger	545	Lebovics, Robert (NY)	Oto	273
Lans, David (NY)	IM	668	Lebowicz, Joseph (NY)	Onc	443

Alphabetical Listing of Doctors

Name	Specialty	Pg	Name	Specialty	Pg
Lebowitz, Arthur (NY)	IM	191	Lehrman, David B (NY)	RadRO	702
Lebowitz, Mark (NY)	Oph	452	Lehrman, Gary R (NY)	Pul	701
Lebwohl, Mark (NY)	D	145	Lehrman, Stuart (NY)	Pul	701
Lebwohl, Oscar (NY)	Ge	166	Leib, Martin L (NY)	Oph	246
Lechner, Michael (NY)	IM	669	Leibner, Donald (NJ)	A&I	827
Leckman, James F (CT)	ChAP	966	Leiboff, Arnold (NY)	CRS	614
Leddy, Joseph (NJ)	OrS	840	Leichter, Donald (NJ)	PCd	921
Leder, Marvin (NY)	EDM	486	Leifer, Bennett (NJ)	Ger	729
Lederman, Jeffrey A (NY)	Inf	665	Leifer, Marvin W (NJ)	Psyc	820
Lederman, Josiane (NY)	D	509	Leikin, Enid (NY)	MF	670
Lederman, Martin E (NY)	Oph	681	Leipzig, Rosanne (NY)	Ger	171
Lederman, Sanford (NY)	ObG	450	Leipziger, Lyle S (NY)	PlS	579
Lee, April (NY)	AM	507	Lemmerling, L J (NJ)	ObG	816
Lee, Carol (NY)	Oph	246	Lempel, Herbert (NY)	IM	490
Lee, Chol (NY)	Psyc	519	Lenger, Ellis S (NJ)	Ge	832
Lee, Douglas S (NY)	ObG	626	Lense, Lloyd (NY)	Cv	612
Lee, Haesoon (NJ)	PPul	787	Lenzo, Salvatore (NY)	HS	176
Lee, Huey-jen (NJ)	DR	772	Leon, Martin (NY)	IC	197
Lee, Kwang Soo (NY)	Psyc	636	Leonard, John P (NY)	Hem	179
Lee, Marjorie (NY)	Pul	330	Leong, Pauline (NY)	IM	550
Lee, Mathew H M (NY)	PMR	300	Lepor, Herbert (NY)	U	364
Lee, Paul C (NY)	TS	502	Lepore, Frederick (NJ)	N	838
Lee, Roberta A (NY)	IM	192	Leppard, John (NY)	OrS	566
Lee, Ronald (CT)	DR	936	Lerman, Bruce (NY)	CE	123
Lee, Sicy H (NY)	Rhu	340	Lerman, Jay E (NY)	DR	428
Lee, Thomas Kang-Ming (NY)	PS	633	Lerman, Jay S (NY)	D	655
Lee, Youngick (NJ)	TS	755	Lerner, Chester (NY)	Inf	183
Leeds, Gary (NY)	FMed	158	Lerner, Elliot (NJ)	NRad	737
Leeds, Richard (NJ)	Cv	901	Lerner, Harvey (NY)	IM	622
Lefer, Jay (NY)	Psyc	318	Lerner, Seth E (NY)	U	708
Leff, Charles (NJ)	Onc	916	Lerner, William (NJ)	Hem	860
Leff, Sanford (NY)	Cv	424	Lescale, Keith B (NY)	MF	671
Leffell, David J (CT)	D	968	Lesesne, Carroll B (NY)	PlS	306
Lefkovitz, Zvi (NY)	DR	152	Leslie, Denise (NY)	DR	658
Lefkowitz, Harvey (NY)	DR	538	Lesniewski, Peter J (NY)	OrS	566
Lefkowitz, Mathew (NY)	PM	457	Lesorgen, Philip (NJ)	RE	751
Legato, Marianne J (NY)	IM	192	Lesser, Robert (NY)	Rhu	470
Lehach, Joan (NY)	A&I	378	Lessing, Jeffrey (NY)	U	521
Lehman, Thomas (NY)	PRhu	291	Lester, Richard (NY)	Oph	246
Lehman, Wallace B (NY)	OrS	262	Lester, Thomas J (NY)	Hem	665
Lehrer, Joel (NJ)	Oto	741	Lettera, James V (CT)	TS	959
Lehrhoff, Bernard (NJ)	U	805	Levchuck, Sean G (NY)	PCd	570

Alphabetical Listing of Doctors

Name	Specialty	Pg	Name	Specialty	Pg
Levenberg, Steven (NJ)	IM	813	Levy, Andrew S (NJ)	SM	925
Levendoglu, Hulya (NY)	Ge	432	Levy, Howard J (NY)	OrS	262
Leventhal, Arnold (NY)	U	594	Levy, I Martin (NY)	OrS	402
Leventhal, Elaine (NJ)	Ger	832	Levy, Joseph (NY)	PGe	285
Levey, Robert (NY)	IM	440	Levy, Judith (NY)	ObG	400
Levin, Aaron (NY)	PCd	688	Levy, Lauren S (NJ)	DR	725
Levin, Alexander (NJ)	PM	842	Levy, Lewis (NJ)	N	558
Levin, Andrew Paul (NY)	Psyc	698	Levy, Michael I (NY)	Psyc	606
Levin, David N (NJ)	Nep	735	Levy, Miriam (NY)	DR	152
Levin, Frances R (NY)	AdP	119	Levy, Morton (NY)	Ped	577
Levin, Howard (NY)	OrS	684	Levy, Norman B (NY)	Psyc	464
Levin, Leroy (NY)	CRS	535	Levy, Roger N (NY)	OrS	262
Levin, Nathan (NY)	IM	440	Levy, Ross (NY)	D	656
Levin, Richard (CT)	Oto	950	Lew, Arthur (NY)	Psyc	698
Levin, Sheryl (NY)	PMR	409	Lewin, Margaret (NY)	IM	192
Levin, Stephen M (NY)	OM	238	Lewin, Sharon (NY)	IM	192
Levin Carmine, Linda (NY)	AM	120	Lewis, Benjamin H (NY)	Cv	129
Levine, Allwyn (NJ)	ChAP	722	Lewis, Blair (NY)	Ge	166
Levine, David N (NY)	N	222	Lewis, Dorothy Otnow (CT)	ChAP	966
Levine, Dorothy (CT)	Ped	953	Lewis, Lawrence (NY)	Oto	686
Levine, Evan (NY)	Cv	650	Lewko, Michael (NJ)	Ger	892
Levine, Jeremiah (NY)	PGe	572	Li, Ronald (NJ)	Oto	818
Levine, Jerome F (NJ)	Inf	731	Liang, Howard (NY)	S	350
Levine, Joseph H (NY)	CE	529	Liang, Vera (NY)	Psyc	636
Levine, Laurie J (NY)	D	537	Libby, Daniel (NY)	Pul	330
Levine, Martin S (NJ)	FMed	800	Libin, Jeffrey (NY)	Oto	273
Levine, Mitchell E (NY)	NS	556	Libman, Richard (NY)	N	558
Levine, Randy (NY)	Hem	179	Libow, Leslie (NY)	Ger	172
Levine, Richard U (NY)	ObG	234	LiCalzi, Luke K (NY)	VascS	596
Levine, Selwyn (NJ)	Pul	750	Licata, Joseph J (NJ)	S	754
Levine, Seth (NJ)	U	897	Licciardi, Frederick L (NY)	RE	336
Levine, Steven B (CT)	Oto	950	Lichstein, Edgar (NY)	Cv	424
Levine, Steven R (NY)	N	222	Licht, Arnold (NY)	Psyc	464
Levine, William (NY)	SM	343	Lichtbroun, Alan (NJ)	Rhu	848
Levinson, Joel (NJ)	Ge	914	Lichter, Stephen M (NY)	Onc	443
Levitan, Stephan (NY)	Psyc	318	Lieber, Ernest (NY)	CG	381
Levites, Kenneth (NY)	FMed	618	Lieberman, Beth (NY)	ObG	234
Levitt, Miriam (NY)	Ped	693	Lieberman, David M (NY)	Oph	452
Levitz, Craig L (NY)	OrS	566	Lieberman, Elliott (NY)	U	594
Levitzky, Munro (NY)	Oph	246	Lieberman, James S (NY)	PMR	300
Levitzky, Susan (NY)	Ped	295	Lieberman, Kenneth (NJ)	PNep	744
Levy, Albert (NY)	FMed	158	Lieberman, Michael (NY)	S	350

Alphabetical Listing of Doctors

Name	Specialty	Pg	Name	Specialty	Pg
Lieberman, Theodore (NY)	Oph	246	Liu, George CK (NY)	IM	192
Liebert, Peter (NY)	PS	691	Liva, Douglas (NJ)	Oph	738
Liebeskind, Arie (NY)	NuM	229	Livingston, Lawrence (NJ)	OrS	740
Liebling, Anne (CT)	Rhu	981	Livingston, Philip (NY)	Onc	205
Liebling, Ralph (NY)	PlS	410	Lizza, Eli (NY)	U	364
Liebmann, Jeffrey (NY)	Oph	246	Lloyd, J Mervyn (NJ)	OrS	740
Lief, Philip (NY)	Nep	396	Lo, K M Steve (CT)	Onc	944
Lifland, John (NJ)	U	907	Lo Galbo, Peter (NJ)	A&I	719
Lifshitz, Benjamin (NY)	IM	440	Lobritto, Steven (NY)	PGe	285
Liftin, Alan (NJ)	D	771	Lockshin, Michael D (NY)	Rhu	340
Lightdale, Charles (NY)	Ge	166	Lockwood, Charles (CT)	MF	972
Liguori, Michael (NY)	IM	192	Lodge, Henry S (NY)	IM	192
Lindenmayer, Jean-Pierre (NY)	Psyc	318	Loeb, Laurence (NY)	Psyc	698
Lindner, Paul S (CT)	A&I	933	Logan, Bruce (NY)	IM	193
Lindsay, Gaius K (NY)	U	476	Logio, Thomas (NJ)	CRS	912
Linsenmeyer, Todd (NJ)	U	794	Loiacono, Anthony F (NY)	ObG	678
Linstrom, Christopher (NY)	Oto	273	Lois, William A (NY)	S	473
Lipkowitz, Marvin (NY)	Psyc	465	Lomasky, Steven (NY)	EDM	540
Lipner, Henry I (NY)	Nep	445	Lombardi, Joseph (NJ)	OrS	841
Lipow, Kenneth (CT)	NS	946	Lombardo, Gerard (NY)	Pul	467
Lippman, Alan (NJ)	Onc	778	Lombardo, James (NY)	Oph	452
Lippman, Jay (NY)	Oph	681	Lombardo, John (NY)	Oph	453
Lipson, David E (NJ)	PlS	747	Lombardo, Peter C (NY)	D	145
Lipstein-Kresch, Esther (NY)	Rhu	586	Lomonaco, Salvatore (NY)	Psyc	411
Lipsztein, Roberto (NY)	RadRO	500	London, Ronald (NY)	Ped	407
Lipton, Brian (NY)	Psyc	318	Longo, Walter E (CT)	CRS	967
Lipton, Jeffrey M (NY)	PHO	573	Lonner, Baron S (NY)	OrS	262
Lipton, Mark Scott (NY)	IM	192	Loo, Marcus Hsieu-Hong (NY)	U	364
Lipton, Richard J (CT)	Oto	950	Lopez, Clark (NY)	FMed	430
Liquori, Frances (NJ)	FMed	859	Lopez, Ralph (NY)	AM	120
Lisman, Richard D (NY)	Oph	247	Lopez, Robert (NY)	Oph	563
Liss, Donald (NJ)	PMR	747	Lorber, Daniel (NY)	EDM	486
Liss, Mark (NY)	Ge	663	Lorefice, Laurence (CT)	Psyc	955
Litchman, Mark (CT)	A&I	933	Loren, Gary M (NJ)	PM	818
Liteplo, Ronald (NY)	D	382	LoRusso, Diane (NY)	DR	658
Litman, Nathan (NY)	PInf	405	Lotongkhum, Vichai (NY)	Cv	424
Litman, Richard (NY)	Oto	631	Loughlin, Gerald M (NY)	PPul	291
Litman, Steven (NY)	PM	632	Louie, Eddie (NY)	Inf	183
Litt, Andrew W (NY)	NRad	228	Louis, Bertin M (NY)	Nep	445
Littlejohn, Charles E (CT)	CRS	935	Loulmet, Didier (NY)	TS	358
Lituchy, Andrew (NY)	IC	551	Lovecchio, John (NY)	GO	545
Litvin, Y Samuel (NJ)	U	867	LoVerme, Paul J (NJ)	PlS	789

Name	Specialty	Pg
Low, Ronald B (NJ)	Oto	742
Lowe, Franklin (NY)	U	364
Lowenheim, Mark Saul (NY)	PGe	633
Lowenstein, Jerome (NY)	Nep	213
Lowenthal, Dennis (NJ)	Onc	917
Lowenthal, Diana (NY)	PPul	691
Lowry, Stephen (NJ)	S	849
Lowy, Joseph (NY)	Pul	330
Lozner, Jerrold (NJ)	TS	926
Lu, Bing (NY)	IM	440
Lu, Gabriel (NY)	PM	687
Lubat, Edward (NJ)	DR	726
Lubell, Harry R (NY)	Ped	694
Lublin, Fred (NY)	N	222
Lubliner, Jerry (NY)	OrS	262
Lucak, Basil K (NY)	Ge	166
Lucariello, Richard (NY)	Cv	379
Lucente, Frank (NY)	Oto	456
Luciani, Richard L (NJ)	ObG	781
Luciano, Daniel J (NY)	N	222
Ludwig, Shelly (NJ)	Ge	859
Lukash, Barbara (NY)	D	656
Lukash, Frederick (NY)	PlS	579
Luks, Howard J (NY)	SM	704
Lundberg, Walter B (CT)	Onc	973
Luria, Martin (NJ)	EDM	858
Lusman, Paul (NY)	A&I	611
Lustbader, Ian J (NY)	Ge	166
Lustig, Ilana (NY)	ObG	234
Lutchman, Gordon (NY)	S	473
Lutwick, Larry Irwin (NY)	Inf	437
Lutz, Gregory (NY)	PMR	300
Lutzker, Letty G (NJ)	DR	772
Lux, Michael (NJ)	IC	916
Lyden, John (NY)	OrS	262
Lyman, Neil (NJ)	Nep	779
Lynch, Vincent J (CT)	ObG	975
Lynn, Robert (NY)	Nep	396
Lyon, Valerie (NY)	FMed	159

M

Name	Specialty	Pg
Ma, Dong M (NY)	PMR	300
Maccabee, Paul J (NY)	N	447
Macchia, Richard (NY)	U	476
Maccia, Clement (NJ)	A&I	911
Macdonald, John S (NY)	Onc	205
Macher, Mark (NJ)	RadRO	848
Machler, Brian (NJ)	D	771
Macina, Lucy (NY)	Ger	545
Mack, Laurence (NY)	ObG	560
MacKay, Cynthia J (NY)	Oph	247
Mackenzie, C Ronald (NY)	IM	193
Mackessy, Richard P (NJ)	OrS	919
Mackler, Karen (NY)	D	656
Mackool, Richard (NY)	Oph	495
Madajewicz, Stefan (NY)	Onc	624
Maddalo, Anthony (NY)	OrS	684
Madigan, Janet (CT)	ChAP	967
Magaro, Joseph (NY)	Oph	681
Maggio, John (NY)	ObG	234
Magid, Steven K. (NY)	Rhu	340
Maglaras, Nicholas (NJ)	IM	916
Magramm, Irene (NY)	Oph	247
Magriples, Urania (CT)	MF	972
Magun, Arthur (NY)	Ge	167
Mahal, Pradeep (NJ)	Ge	915
Maharam, Lewis G (NY)	SM	343
Maher, Elizabeth (NY)	Oph	247
Mahler, Richard J (NY)	EDM	156
Mahon, Eugene (NY)	Psyc	318
Mahoney, Maurice J (CT)	CG	967
Maidman, Jack (NY)	ObG	234
Maier, Herbert (NJ)	D	891
Mailloux, Lionel (NY)	Nep	555
Maiman, Mitchell (NY)	GO	511
Maiocco, Kenneth (CT)	D	936
Maizel, Barry (NY)	Ge	432
Maklansky, Daniel (NY)	DR	152
Malach, Barbara (NY)	IM	512
Malamud, Stephen C (NY)	Onc	205
Malanga, Gerard (NJ)	PMR	883

Alphabetical Listing of Doctors

Name	Specialty	Pg	Name	Specialty	Pg
Malik, Asim (NY)	IM	440	Margulies, Paul (NY)	EDM	540
Malik, Parvaiz (NJ)	PlS	820	Margulis, Stephen (NJ)	Ge	728
Mallin, Jeffrey (NY)	N	558	Marin, Deborah B (NY)	Psyc	318
Mallozzi, Angelo (CT)	FMed	937	Marin, Geobel (NJ)	Ge	811
Malovany, Robert (NJ)	Pul	750	Marin, Lorraine A (NY)	RadRO	585
Malpeso, James (NY)	Cv	508	Marin, Michael L (NY)	VascS	371
Maman, Arie (NJ)	EDM	831	Marinaro, Robert (NJ)	D	874
Mamtani, Ravinder (NY)	PrM	696	Marino, A Michael (CT)	Pul	956
Mandel, Edmund (NY)	U	476	Marino, John (NY)	Onc	553
Mandel, Eric R (NY)	Oph	247	Marino, Ronald (NY)	Ped	577
Mandel, Michael (NY)	Pul	701	Marino, William (NY)	Pul	412
Mandelbaum, Sid (NY)	Oph	247	Marion, Robert (NY)	CG	381
Mandeville, Edgar (NY)	ObG	494	Markell, Mariana Sari (NY)	Nep	445
Manevitz, Alan (NY)	Psyc	318	Markenson, Joseph A (NY)	Rhu	341
Manginello, Frank (NJ)	NP	734	Markovics, Sharon B (NY)	PA&I	569
Mani, John (NY)	OrS	454	Markowitz, Allan (NY)	Oph	681
Maniatis, Theodore (NY)	Pul	519	Markowitz, Arlene (NY)	Oto	273
Maniscalco, Anthony (NY)	N	447	Markowitz, Daniel (NJ)	Pul	865
Manjoney, Delia (CT)	Oph	948	Markowitz, David (NY)	Ge	167
Mankes, Seth (NY)	DR	616	Markowitz, James (NY)	PGe	572
Mann, Charles (NY)	ObG	626	Markowitz, John (NY)	Psyc	319
Mann, David (NY)	EDM	429	Marks, Alan (NY)	Oph	563
Mann, Ronald L (NY)	OrS	684	Marks, Andrea (NY)	AM	120
Manners, Richard (NY)	Ped	634	Marks, Clement E (NY)	Pul	330
Manning, Eric (NJ)	Nep	861	Marks, David A (NJ)	N	780
Manning, Frank A (NY)	MF	199	Marks, Jon O (NY)	U	364
Manno, Joseph (NJ)	VascS	757	Marks, Stephen (NY)	N	676
Manolas, Panagiotis (NY)	S	501	Marron-Corwin, Mary (NY)	NP	210
Mansour, E Hani (NJ)	S	793	Marsh, Franklin (NY)	Ge	167
Mansouri, Hormoz (NY)	S	590	Marsh, James S (CT)	OrS	975
Mansouri, Mehran (NY)	S	590	Marshall, Merville (NY)	EDM	659
Marans, Hillel (NY)	U	364	Martin, George (NY)	Ge	488
Marcus, Eric R (NY)	Psyc	318	Martin, Paul (NY)	Ge	167
Marcus, Judith R (NY)	PHO	690	Martin, Sidney A (NY)	Oph	628
Marcus, Michael (NY)	PPul	517	Martin, William (NY)	S	641
Marcus, Norman (NY)	PM	278	Martinez, Homar (NJ)	Inf	903
Marcus, Philip (NY)	Pul	582	Martins, Publius (NY)	Pul	519
Marcus, Ralph (NJ)	Rhu	752	Marush, Arthur (NY)	IM	440
Marcus, Richard (NJ)	Ped	787	Mascarenhas, Bento (NY)	Rhu	703
Marcus, Stephen (NY)	OrS	566	Masci, Joseph (NY)	Inf	489
Marder, Karen (NY)	N	223	Masciello, Michael (NY)	Cv	612
Margouleff, Donald (NY)	NuM	559	Maselli, Frank (NY)	FMed	386

Alphabetical Listing of Doctors

Name	Specialty	Pg	Name	Specialty	Pg
Masino, Frank A (CT)	RadRO	957	McCann, Peter (NY)	OrS	262
Massad, Susan (NY)	IM	440	McCarthy, Joseph G (NY)	PlS	306
Masson, Lalitha (NJ)	ObG	802	McCarthy, Paul L (CT)	PRhu	977
Masterson, Raymond M (NJ)	IM	860	McCarthy, Shirley M (CT)	DR	968
Mastrantonio, John (NY)	ObG	400	McCarton, Cecelia (NY)	Ped	295
Matalon, Martin (NY)	ObG	627	McClelland, Shearwood J (NY)	OrS	263
Matalon, Robert (NY)	Nep	213	McClennan, Bruce (CT)	DR	968
Matarasso, Alan (NY)	PlS	306	McClung, John A (NY)	Cv	650
Matera, Cristina (NY)	RE	336	McConnell, John (NJ)	CRS	723
Matilsky, Michael (NY)	Cv	612	McConnell, Robert John (NY)	EDM	156
Matkovic, Christopher (NY)	IM	622	McCormack, Barbara (NJ)	ObG	738
Matos, Jeffrey (NY)	CE	123	McCormack, Patricia (NY)	D	509
Matos, Marshall (NY)	Cv	650	McCormack, William M (NY)	Inf	437
Matossian, Cynthia (NJ)	Oph	816	McCormick, Beryl (NY)	RadRO	334
Matta, Raymond J (NY)	Cv	129	McCormick, Ellen (NY)	S	641
Mattana, Joseph (NY)	Nep	555	McCormick, Paul C (NY)	NS	216
Mattel, Stephen (NJ)	Oto	895	McCormick, Steven (NY)	Path	280
Mattes, Leonard (NY)	Cv	129	McDermott, John A (NY)	Oph	247
Matthay, Richard (CT)	Pul	980	McFarlane-Ferreira, Yvonne B (NY)	PGe	458
Matthews, Gerald J (NY)	U	708	McGill, Frances (NY)	ObG	235
Mattison, Timothy (NY)	D	656	McGinn, Joseph (NY)	TS	521
Mattoo, Nirmal (NY)	Nep	493	McGinn, Thomas (NY)	IM	193
Mattucci, Kenneth (NY)	Oto	567	McGlashan, Thomas (CT)	Psyc	979
Mauer, Kenneth (CT)	Ge	938	McGovern, Patrick Joseph (NJ)	S	804
Maulik, Dev (NY)	MF	552	McGovern, Thomas P (NY)	U	364
Mauskop, Alexander (NY)	N	223	McGowan, James M (NY)	Psyc	319
Maxfield, Roger (NY)	Pul	330	McGrath, Patrick J (NY)	Psyc	319
May, Louis (NY)	Ge	603	McHugh, Margaret T (NY)	Ped	295
Mayer, Daniel L (NY)	A&I	611	McIlveen, Stephen J (NJ)	OrS	740
Mayer, Fern (CT)	D	936	McKee, Heather (NY)	Oph	681
Mayer, Ira E (NY)	Ge	432	McKiernan, James M (NY)	U	364
Mayer, Lloyd (NY)	Ge	167	McKinley, Matthew (NY)	Ge	543
Mayer, Stephan A (NY)	N	223	McLeod, Gavin (CT)	Inf	939
Mayers, Marguerite (NY)	Ped	408	McManus, Edward (NJ)	Inf	876
Mayers, Martin (NY)	Oph	401	McManus, Susan (NJ)	S	907
Mayeux, Richard (NY)	N	223	McMeeking, Alexander (NY)	Inf	183
Maytal, Joseph (NY)	ChiN	534	McMullen, Robert (NY)	Psyc	319
Mazza, David S (NY)	A&I	121	McNutt, N Scott (NY)	Path	280
Mazzarino, Aldo (NY)	U	476	McVeigh, Anne Marie (NY)	Oph	247
McAnally, James (NJ)	Nep	917	McWhorter, John (NJ)	Rhu	906
McCalley, Stuart (CT)	Pul	956	McWhorter, Philip (CT)	S	958
McCampbell, Edwin (NJ)	FMed	773	Meacham, Kevin (NY)	ObG	678

Alphabetical Listing of Doctors

Name	Specialty	Pg	Name	Specialty	Pg
Mears, John Gregory (NY)	Hem	180	Mendes, Donna (NY)	VascS	371
Mechanic, Alan (NY)	NS	556	Mendes, John (NJ)	OrS	783
Mechanick, Jeffrey I (NY)	EDM	157	Mendoza, Francis (NY)	OrS	263
Medina, Emma (NY)	Cv	650	Mendoza, Glenn (NY)	NP	603
Medow, Norman (NY)	Oph	248	Menegus, Mark (NY)	Cv	380
Meed, Steven D (NY)	Rhu	341	Menezes, Placido (NY)	OrS	455
Meek, Allen (NY)	RadRO	638	Menon, Latha (NY)	Pul	412
Megibow, Alec J (NY)	DR	152	Mensch, Alan (NY)	Pul	583
Megna, Daniel (NY)	Ge	511	Menza, Matthew (NJ)	Psyc	846
Mehra, Sunil (NY)	Pul	500	Menzin, Andrew (NY)	GO	545
Mehta, Rajeev (NJ)	NP	837	Merav, Avraham (NY)	TS	415
Mehta, Rekha (NY)	Ge	387	Mercando, Anthony (NY)	Cv	650
Mehta, Uday (NJ)	Ped	922	Mercurio, Peter (NY)	Cv	650
Meier, Diane (NY)	Ger	172	Meredith, Gary (NY)	Rhu	587
Meirowitz, Robert (NJ)	Ge	811	Merer, David M (NY)	Oto	686
Meisenberg, Gene (NY)	U	476	Merhige, Kenneth (NY)	Oph	248
Meixler, Steven (NY)	Pul	701	Merkatz, Irwin R (NY)	MF	393
Meizlish, Jay Lewis (CT)	Cv	934	Merker, Edward (NY)	FMed	660
Melamed, Jonathan (NY)	Path	280	Mermelstein, Erwin (NJ)	Cv	828
Melamed, Marc S (NJ)	CCM	723	Mermelstein, Harold (NY)	D	656
Melillo, Nicholas (NJ)	Pul	847	Mermelstein, Steve (NY)	Pul	583
Meller, Jose (NY)	Cv	129	Merola, Andrew A (NY)	OrS	455
Mellinger, Brett (NY)	U	594	Merriam, John C (NY)	Oph	248
Mellins, Robert (NY)	PPul	291	Messana, Ida (NY)	IM	490
Mellman, Lisa (NY)	Psyc	319	Messina, John (NJ)	PCd	743
Melman, Arnold (NY)	U	416	Metzl, Jordan D (NY)	SM	343
Melman, Martin (NY)	IM	669	Meyer, Richard (NY)	IM	193
Melnick, Hugh (NY)	ObG	235	Meyers, Barnett (NY)	Psyc	698
Melone, Charles P (NY)	HS	176	Meyers, John H (NY)	D	537
Melton, R Christine (NY)	Oph	248	Meyers, Paul (NY)	PHO	287
Meltzer, Murray (NY)	Oph	248	Meyers, Philip M (NY)	NRad	228
Melville, Gordon (NJ)	DR	902	Mezey, Andrew (NY)	Ped	462
Menche, David S (NY)	OrS	263	Miarrostami, Rameen M. (NY)	Pul	467
Menchell, David (NY)	A&I	483	Mich, Robert (NJ)	IC	916
Mendelowitz, Alan (NY)	Psyc	498	Michaelson, Richard (NJ)	Onc	778
Mendelowitz, Lawrence (NY)	ObG	679	Michalos, Peter (NY)	Oph	628
Mendelsohn, Frederic (NY)	N	625	Michelassi, Fabrizio (NY)	S	350
Mendelsohn, Lois (NY)	A&I	647	Michelis, Mary Ann (NJ)	A&I	719
Mendelsohn, Michael (NY)	Oto	456	Michelis, Michael F (NY)	Nep	213
Mendelsohn, Sara L (NY)	OM	562	Michels, Robert (NY)	Psyc	319
Mendelsohn, Steven (NY)	DR	538	Michler, Robert (NY)	TS	415
Mendelson, Joel S (NJ)	A&I	911	Mickley, Diane W (CT)	IM	941

Name	Specialty	Pg	Name	Specialty	Pg
Mickley, Steven P (CT)	IM	941	Milone, Richard (NY)	Psyc	698
Miclat, Marciano (NY)	PlS	695	Milowsky, Matthew I (NY)	Onc	205
Middleton, John R (NJ)	Inf	834	Milsom, Jeffrey W (NY)	CRS	139
Mieres, Jennifer (NY)	Cv	532	Milstein, David (NY)	NuM	399
Mignone, Biagio (NY)	Oph	681	Mindel, Joel (NY)	Oph	248
Miguel, Eduardo (NJ)	IM	732	Minikes, Neil (NJ)	A&I	719
Milano, Andrew (NY)	Ge	167	Minkoff, Howard L (NY)	ObG	450
Milburn, Peter (NY)	D	427	Minkowitz, Susan (NY)	IM	193
Mildvan, Donna (NY)	Inf	183	Minsky, Bruce (NY)	RadRO	334
Miles, Daniel K (NY)	ChiN	137	Mintz, Abraham (CT)	NS	946
Miles, Richard J (CT)	Oto	951	Mirra, Suzanne S (NY)	Path	457
Milgraum, Sandy (NJ)	D	829	Miskoff, A Richard (NJ)	Onc	836
Milhorat, Thomas H (NY)	NS	556	Miskovitz, Paul (NY)	Ge	167
Milite, James (NY)	Oph	248	Misra, Sabita (NY)	PA&I	517
Miller, Aaron (NY)	N	223	Mitchell, John P (NY)	Oph	249
Miller, Albert (NY)	Pul	500	Mitnick, Hal J (NY)	Rhu	341
Miller, Andrew J (NJ)	Oto	841	Mitnick, Julie (NY)	DR	152
Miller, Ann Marie (NY)	N	398	Mitsumoto, Hiroshi (NY)	N	223
Miller, Brian (NY)	Oph	681	Mittelman, Abraham (NY)	Onc	672
Miller, Daniel (NY)	FMed	660	Mittman, Neal (NY)	Nep	445
Miller, David G (NJ)	Psyc	923	Mitty, Harold (NY)	DR	152
Miller, Dennis K (NY)	Inf	184	Mizrachy, Benjamin (NY)	S	350
Miller, Ellen G (NY)	FMed	660	Mogan, Glen (NJ)	Ge	774
Miller, Jeffrey K (NJ)	HS	876	Mohr, J P (NY)	N	223
Miller, John I (NY)	NS	446	Mohr, Robert F (NJ)	ObG	879
Miller, Karen L (NY)	DR	658	Mohrer, Jonathan (NY)	IM	490
Miller, Kenneth Alan (CT)	Rhu	958	Moideen, Ahamed S (NY)	TS	502
Miller, Kenneth Paul (NJ)	Cv	768	Moisa, Idel (NY)	Oto	567
Miller, Lawrence (NY)	Psyc	519	Mojtabai, Shaparak (NY)	IM	392
Miller, Philip (NJ)	Oph	782	Moldover, Jonathan (NY)	PMR	300
Miller, Rachel L (NY)	Pul	330	Moldwin, Robert (NY)	U	594
Miller, Richard L (NY)	D	615	Mollin, Joel (NY)	DR	485
Miller, Scott T (NY)	PHO	459	Molloy, Edward Michael (CT)	IM	941
Miller, Seth (NY)	Ge	544	Molnar, Thomas (NY)	FMed	487
Miller, Vincent A (NY)	Onc	205	Molofsky, Walter (NY)	ChiN	137
Miller-Breslow, Anne (NJ)	HS	730	Mondrow, Daniel (NJ)	Cv	828
Millman, Arthur (NY)	Oph	248	Mones, Richard (NJ)	PGe	882
Millman, Robert B (NY)	Psyc	319	Mongillo, Nicholas (CT)	Ped	953
Mills, Carl (NY)	U	642	Monheit, Alan G (NY)	MF	623
Mills, Christopher B (NY)	S	350	Monrad, E Scott (NY)	Cv	380
Mills, Nancy Ellyn (NY)	Onc	672	Monsanto, Enrique (NY)	HS	435
Milman, Perry (NY)	Ge	544	Monteferrante, Judith (NY)	Cv	651

Alphabetical Listing of Doctors

Name	Specialty	Pg	Name	Specialty	Pg
Monteleone, Bernard B (NY)	Cv	532	Moss, Richard (NY)	ObG	235
Monteleone, Frank (NY)	S	590	Mossey, Robert (NY)	Nep	556
Montero, Carlos Felix (NY)	OrS	566	Most, Richard W (NY)	Oph	682
Monti, Louis G (NY)	Ped	295	Motzer, Robert J (NY)	Onc	205
Mooney, Robert M (NY)	Oph	681	Moulton, Thomas (NY)	PHO	405
Moore, Anne (NY)	Onc	205	Moussa, Ghias (NJ)	Cv	799
Moore, Eric (NY)	S	350	Moynihan, Brian (NY)	FMed	541
Moore, Frank M (NY)	NS	216	Moynihan, Gavan D (NY)	D	615
Moore, Joanne (NY)	Psyc	319	Muchnick, Richard (NY)	Oph	249
Moorthy, Chitti (NY)	RadRO	702	Mueller, F Carl (CT)	Psyc	955
Mootabar, Hamid (NY)	MF	671	Mueller, Richard L (NY)	Cv	129
Moqtaderi, Farideh (NY)	PM	278	Muggia, Franco (NY)	Onc	205
Morabito, Carmine D (NY)	Oph	628	Muhlbauer, Helen (NY)	Psyc	320
Moraille, Pascale (NJ)	Psyc	803	Mukherjee, Tanmoy (NY)	RE	337
Moreau, Donna (NY)	ChAP	135	Muldoon, Thomas O (NY)	Oph	249
Morehouse, Helen (NY)	DR	383	Mulford, Gregory (NJ)	PMR	883
Morelli, Alan (CT)	Ped	953	Mulgaonkar, Shamkant (NJ)	Nep	779
Morello, Robert (NY)	Oph	682	Mulhall, John P (NY)	U	365
Moreta, Henry (NY)	N	625	Mullen, David (CT)	DR	936
Moretti, Michael (NY)	MF	513	Mullen, Michael (NY)	Inf	184
Morgan, Daniel J (NY)	OrS	455	Multz, Alan S (NY)	Pul	500
Morgan, James L (CT)	Ped	978	Munoz, Eric (NJ)	S	793
Morris, Robert P (NY)	Oph	628	Munoz, Jose Luis (NY)	PInf	690
Morrison, Susan (NJ)	PA&I	784	Munver, Ravi (NJ)	U	756
Morrissey, Kevin (NY)	S	350	Muraca, Glenn (NY)	FMed	541
Morrow, Robert (NY)	FMed	386	Murali, Raj (NY)	NS	675
Morrow, Todd (NJ)	Oto	784	Murphy, John (CT)	N	947
Mosca, Lori J (NY)	Cv	129	Murphy, Ramon JC (NY)	Ped	295
Mosca, Ralph S (NY)	PS	292	Murphy, Robert (NJ)	Ped	864
Moscatello, Augustine L (NY)	Oto	686	Muscillo, George (NY)	ObG	400
Moses, Brett (NJ)	Oto	818	Musiker, Seymour (NY)	Ped	635
Moses, Jeffrey W (NY)	IC	197	Muskin, Philip (NY)	Psyc	320
Moshe, Solomon L (NY)	N	398	Musto, Anthony (CT)	Oph	948
Moskovich, Ronald (NY)	OrS	263	Mutterperl, Mitchell (NJ)	IM	801
Moskovits, Norbert (NY)	Cv	424	Myers, Stanley J (NY)	PMR	300
Moskovits, Tibor (NY)	Hem	180	Myers, Wayne A (NY)	Psyc	320
Moskowitz, Bruce K (NY)	Oph	249	Myskowski, Patricia L (NY)	D	145
Moskowitz, George (NY)	FMed	430	Myssiorek, David (NY)	Oto	568
Moskowitz, Richard L (NJ)	CRS	874			
Moskowitz, Sam (NY)	Ge	488			
Moss, Charles M (NJ)	VascS	758			
Moss, R Lawrence (CT)	PS	977			

Name	Specialty	Pg	Name	Specialty	Pg
N			Neff, Richard A (NY)	VIR	369
			Neibart, Eric (NY)	Inf	184
Nachajon, Roberto (NJ)	PPul	895	Neibart, Richard (NJ)	TS	867
Nachman, Sharon (NY)	PInf	633	Nejat, Moosa (NY)	Cv	532
Nacht, Robert (NY)	Cv	424	Nelson, David B (NY)	Oph	563
Nadel, Alfred (NY)	Oph	249	Nelson, Deena (NY)	IM	193
Nadel, William (NJ)	Psyc	906	Nelson, John C (NY)	Hem	665
Nadelman, Robert (NY)	Inf	666	Nelson, John M (NY)	OrS	684
Naftolin, Frederick (NY)	ObG	235	Nelson, Mario (NY)	PMR	694
Nagel, Ronald (NY)	Hem	390	Nelson, William S (NY)	ObG	679
Nagler, Harris M (NY)	U	365	Nersessian, Edward (NY)	Psyc	320
Nagler, Jerry (NY)	Ge	167	Nerwen, Clifford (NY)	Ped	577
Nahass, Ronald (NJ)	Inf	812	Neschis, Ronald (NY)	Psyc	698
Naidich, David P (NY)	DR	152	Neuspiel, Daniel (NY)	Ped	296
Najarian, James (NJ)	IM	877	Neuwirth, Michael (NY)	OrS	263
Naka, Yoshifumi (NY)	TS	358	Nevins, Stuart (NY)	Oto	686
Namerow, David (NJ)	Ped	746	New, Maria I (NY)	PEn	284
Namm, Joel (NJ)	DR	810	Newburger, Amy (NY)	D	656
Napoli, Joseph C (NJ)	Psyc	749	Newcorn, Jeffrey H (NY)	ChAP	135
Narins, Rhoda (NY)	D	656	Newhouse, Jeffrey (NY)	DR	152
Narula, Amarjot S (NJ)	Psyc	749	Newman, Elliot (NY)	S	351
Narula, Pramod (NY)	PPul	460	Newman, Fredric A (CT)	PlS	954
Nascimento, Joao M A (CT)	Rhu	958	Newman, Lawrence C (NY)	N	224
Nash, Bernard J (NY)	Inf	621	Newman, Leonard (NY)	PGe	690
Nash, Martin (NY)	PNep	289	Newman, Scott E (NY)	PlS	695
Nash, Thomas (NY)	Pul	331	Newman, Stephen (NY)	N	558
Naso, Kristin (NY)	Ge	619	Newman-Cedar, Meryl (NY)	Ped	296
Nass, Jack (NY)	Psyc	636	Newmark, Ian H (NY)	Pul	583
Nass, Richard (NY)	Oto	273	Newton, Michael (NY)	Oph	249
Nass, Ruth (NY)	ChiN	137	Ng, John Paul Tracy (NY)	RadRO	334
Nassberg, Barton (NJ)	EDM	858	Ngeow, Jeffrey (NY)	PM	278
Natale, Benjamin (NJ)	Oph	919	Nguyen, Khanh H (NY)	TS	358
Nath, Sunil (NY)	Pul	500	Nicholas, Stephen J (NY)	OrS	263
Nathin, Donald (NJ)	Nep	735	Nicholas, Stephen W (NY)	Ped	296
Nattis, Richard (NY)	Oph	628	Nichols, Jeffrey (NY)	Ger	172
Navot, Daniel (NJ)	RE	751	Nickerson, Katherine (NY)	Rhu	341
Nayak, Asha D (NY)	Onc	443	Nicosia, Thomas A (NY)	Cv	532
Nayak, Devdutt (NY)	Psyc	465	Niederman, Michael (NY)	Pul	583
Nayak, Kumbla (NY)	Psyc	498	Nierman, David (NY)	CCM	140
Nealon, Nancy (NY)	N	223	Nightingale, Jeffrey (NY)	Oph	249
Neelakantappa, Kotresha (NY)	Nep	445	Nijensohn, Daniel (CT)	NS	946
Neeson, Francis (CT)	Cv	935	Nikias, George A (NJ)	Ge	728

Alphabetical Listing of Doctors

Name	Specialty	Pg
Nimaroff, Michael (NY)	ObG	560
Nimer, Stephen D (NY)	Hem	180
Nini, Kevin (NJ)	PlS	846
Nininger, James (NY)	Psyc	320
Nir, Yehuda (NY)	Psyc	320
Nisonson, Barton (NY)	SM	344
Nissenblatt, Michael (NJ)	Onc	836
Nitti, Victor (NY)	U	365
Nitzberg, Richard (NJ)	S	925
Nizin, Joel (NJ)	CRS	723
Noble, Kenneth (NY)	Oph	249
Nolan, William (CT)	PlS	954
Norden, Richard (NJ)	Oph	738
Nori, Dattatreyudu (NY)	RadRO	334
Norton, Karen (NJ)	DR	772
Norton, Larry (NY)	Onc	206
Nosher, John (NJ)	VIR	851
Nosko, Michael (NJ)	NS	837
Notar-Francesco, Vincent J (NY)	Ge	432
Notaro, Antoinette (NY)	D	615
Noto, Richard (NY)	PEn	689
Notterman, Daniel A (NJ)	PCCM	843
Notterman, Robyn (NJ)	D	810
Nouri, Shahin (NY)	N	447
Novich, Ira (NY)	DR	658
Novick, Brian (NY)	A&I	528
Novick, Ellen (NJ)	PMR	923
Novick, Mark D (NY)	DR	152
Novitch, Richard (NY)	Pul	702
Novogroder, Michael (NJ)	PEn	743
Nowak, Eugene (NY)	S	351
Nowygrod, Roman (NY)	VascS	371
Noyes, Nicole (NY)	RE	337
Nucci, Annamaria (NJ)	Psyc	789
Nunes, Edward (NY)	Psyc	320
Nunez, Domingo (NY)	S	351
Nussbaum, Michel E (NY)	Ge	488
Nussbaum, Moses (NY)	S	351
Nuzzo, Roy (NJ)	OrS	920
Nydick, Martin (NY)	EDM	157
Nyer, Kenneth (NY)	IM	392

O

Name	Specialty	Pg
O'Brien, Daryl H (NJ)	Ped	746
O'Connell, Joseph B (CT)	PlS	954
O'Connor, Kathleen (NY)	D	382
O'Connor, Patrick (CT)	IM	971
O'Donnell, Timothy (NJ)	Pul	896
O'Hea, Brian (NY)	S	641
O'Leary, Patrick (NY)	OrS	263
O'Malley, Grace M (NY)	Oph	629
O'Malley, Martin J (NY)	OrS	263
O'Reilly, Eileen M (NY)	Onc	206
O'Reilly, Richard (NY)	PHO	287
Oberfield, Richard (NY)	Psyc	320
Oberfield, Sharon E (NY)	PEn	284
Obstbaum, Stephen (NY)	Oph	250
Odel, Jeffrey G (NY)	Oph	250
Oeffinger, Kevin (NY)	Ped	296
Offit, Kenneth (NY)	Onc	206
Ofodile, Ferdinand (NY)	PlS	410
Oghia, Hady (NY)	Ped	462
Oh, Youn (NJ)	N	838
Ohki, Takao (NY)	VascS	416
Okadigwe, Chukuma (NY)	TS	475
Okun, Alex (NY)	Ped	408
Olanow, C Warren (NY)	N	224
Olarte, Marcelo (NY)	N	224
Olds, David (NY)	Psyc	321
Oleske, James (NJ)	PInf	786
Olichney, John (NY)	IM	193
Olin, Craig H (CT)	IM	941
Oliver, Gregory C (NJ)	CRS	829
Olsewski, John M (NY)	OrS	402
Olson, Robert (NJ)	PlS	846
Opler, Lewis (NY)	Psyc	699
Oppedisano, Carlyn (NY)	Ped	408
Oppenheim, Jeffrey (NY)	NS	604
Oppenheimer, John (NY)	IM	622
Orbuch, Philip (NY)	D	145
Ordorica, Steven A (NY)	ObG	235
Orentreich, David (NY)	D	146
Orland, Steven (NJ)	U	823

Name	Specialty	Pg	Name	Specialty	Pg
Orlin, Harvey (NY)	SM	587	Palmieri, Thomas J (NY)	HS	546
Orlow, Seth (NY)	D	146	Palsky, Glenn (NJ)	Ped	819
Orsher, Stuart (NY)	IM	193	Paltzik, Robert (NY)	D	537
Osborne, Michael P (NY)	S	351	Pane, Carmela (NJ)	NP	734
Osei, Clement (NY)	Pul	606	Panella, Vincent S (NJ)	Ge	728
Osei-Tutu, John (NY)	Psyc	411	Panetta, Thomas F (NY)	VascS	522
Osnoss, Kenneth (CT)	IM	941	Panicek, David (NY)	DR	153
Oster, Martin W (NY)	Onc	206	Pannone, John (NY)	Nep	445
Ostrer, Harry (NY)	CG	138	Panter, Gideon (NY)	ObG	235
Ostrovsky, Paul (NY)	DR	153	Panush, Richard (NJ)	Rhu	791
Ostrow, Stanley (NY)	Onc	624	Panza, Robert (NJ)	Ped	922
Ott, Allen (NY)	ObG	627	Panzner, Elizabeth (NJ)	Ped	922
Ottaviano, Lawrence (NY)	Ge	168	Papadakos, Stylianos P (NY)	IC	491
Overby, M Chris (NY)	NS	557	Papish, Steven (NJ)	Onc	878
Owens, George (NY)	U	708	Papp, Laszlo A (NY)	Psyc	321
Oxman, David (NJ)	Ped	922	Pappas, Steven (NY)	IM	669
Oz, Mehmet C (NY)	TS	358	Pappas, Thomas W (NY)	Cv	533
Ozick, Hershel (NY)	Cv	651	Pappert, Amy S (NJ)	D	830
Ozuah, Philip (NY)	Ped	408	Parekh, Aruna (NY)	NP	444
Ozuner, Gokhan (NY)	CRS	601	Paris, Barbara (NY)	Ger	434
			Parisier, Simon C (NY)	Oto	273
			Park, Constance (NY)	EDM	157
P			Park, Tae (NY)	RadRO	638
			Parker, Margaret (NY)	Ped	635
Pace, Benjamin (NY)	S	501	Parker, Robert (NY)	PHO	633
Pacernick, Lawrence (NY)	D	537	Parles, James G (NY)	Ped	635
Pachter, H Leon (NY)	S	351	Parnell, Vincent (NY)	PS	575
Pacia, Steven (NY)	N	224	Parnes, Eliezer (NY)	Nep	445
Packard, William (NY)	Psyc	636	Parness, Ira A (NY)	PCd	283
Packer, Samuel (NY)	Oph	564	Parr, Grant (NJ)	TS	885
Padberg, Frank (NJ)	VascS	795	Parrish, Edward (NY)	Rhu	341
Padilla, Alfred (CT)	EDM	937	Parry, Michael (CT)	Inf	939
Padilla, Maria L (NY)	Pul	331	Pascal, Mark (NJ)	Onc	733
Paget, Stephen (NY)	Rhu	341	Pascario, Ben (NY)	ObG	235
Pahuja, Murlidhar (NY)	S	521	Pascaru, Adina (NY)	IM	550
Paiusco, A Dino (NY)	Cv	424	Pasik, Deborah (NJ)	Rhu	885
Pak, Jayoung (NJ)	ChiN	770	Pasmantier, Mark (NY)	Onc	206
Palatt, Terry (NY)	TS	642	Pass, Harvey (NY)	TS	358
Palestro, Christopher (NY)	NuM	559	Pass, Helen (NY)	S	705
Pallotta, John (NY)	ObG	627	Passeri, Daniel J (CT)	S	958
Palmer, Edward (NY)	Oph	401	Pastore, Louis T (NY)	U	643
Palmer, Melissa (NY)	Ge	544	Pastorek, Norman (NY)	Oto	273

Alphabetical Listing of Doctors

Name	Specialty	Pg	Name	Specialty	Pg
Patel, Jitendra K (NY)	Rhu	470	Perry, Bradford (NY)	Psyc	699
Patel, Mukund (NY)	HS	435	Perry, Henry (NY)	Oph	564
Patrick, Sharon (NY)	MF	199	Perry, Kathleen (NY)	ObG	515
Patrizio, Pasquale (CT)	RE	981	Perry, Richard (NY)	ChAP	135
Patterson, Marc (NY)	ChiN	137	Perry-Bottinger, Lynne (NY)	Cv	651
Pattner, Austin (NJ)	Nep	735	Persing, John A (CT)	PlS	978
Paty, Philip B (NY)	S	351	Perskin, Michael (NY)	Ger	172
Paul, Edward (NY)	AdP	119	Persky, Mark S (NY)	Oto	274
Pavlov, Helene (NY)	DR	153	Person, Ethel (NY)	Psyc	321
Pawel, Michael A (NY)	Psyc	321	Pertsemlidis, Demetrius (NY)	S	351
Pawl, Nancy (NY)	ObG	679	Pesce, Joseph (CT)	D	936
Paz, Harold L (NJ)	Pul	847	Peschel, Richard E (CT)	RadRO	980
Pearlman, Steven J (NY)	Oto	274	Pesiri, Vincent (NY)	S	590
Pearlstein, Eric (NY)	Oph	453	Peterson, Stephen J (NY)	IM	669
Pechman, Karen M (NY)	PMR	694	Petito, Frank (NY)	N	224
Peck, Harvey (NY)	DR	602	Petrillo, Claudio R (CT)	PMR	954
Pecker, Mark S (NY)	IM	193	Petro, Jane (NY)	PlS	695
Pecora, Andrew L (NJ)	Hem	730	Petrone, Sylvia (NJ)	S	793
Pedinoff, Andrew (NJ)	A&I	901	Petrossian, George A (NY)	IC	552
Pedley, Timothy A (NY)	N	224	Petrylak, Daniel P (NY)	Onc	206
Pegler, Cynthia (NY)	AM	120	Pettei, Michael (NY)	PGe	572
Pelavin, Martin (NJ)	IM	732	Peyser, Donald (NJ)	IM	777
Pellettieri, John (NY)	ObG	494	Pfetter, Cynthia (NY)	Psyc	321
Pellicci, Paul (NY)	OrS	264	Pfister, David G (NY)	Onc	206
Peng, Benjamin (NY)	U	365	Phillips, Elizabeth (NY)	Onc	672
Pennacchi, John (NJ)	Onc	814	Phillips, Howard (NY)	Oph	682
Pepe, John (NY)	Nep	514	Phillips, Malcolm (NY)	Cv	380
Pereira, Frederick (NY)	D	485	Pianka, George (NY)	OrS	264
Pereira, Stephen (NJ)	S	754	Picciano, Anne (NJ)	AM	827
Perel, Allan (NY)	N	514	Piccione, Paul (NY)	Ge	433
Peress, Richard (NY)	OrS	684	Piccirilli, Dora (NY)	FMed	661
Perez-Soler, Roman (NY)	Onc	393	Pici, Ralph A (NY)	PMR	694
Perin, Noel I (NY)	NS	217	Picone, Frank J (NJ)	A&I	857
Perl, Harold (NJ)	NP	734	Pierson, Richard N. (NY)	NuM	229
Perla, Elliott (NY)	IM	194	Pile-Spellman, John (NY)	NRad	228
Perlman, Barry B (NY)	Psyc	699	Pili, Manuel (NY)	ObG	451
Perlman, David (NY)	Inf	184	Pillari, Vincent (NY)	ObG	515
Perlman, Donald B (NJ)	A&I	767	Pincus, Emile (NY)	ChAP	652
Perlman, Jeffrey M (NY)	NP	211	Pincus, Robert (NY)	Oto	274
Perlmutter, Ilisse (NY)	ChAP	484	Pines, Jeffrey (NY)	Psyc	321
Perron, Reed C (NJ)	N	736	Pinke, Robert S (NJ)	Oph	879
Perry, Arthur (NJ)	PlS	905			

Alphabetical Listing of Doctors

Name	Specialty	Pg	Name	Specialty	Pg
Pinsker, Kenneth (NY)	Pul	412	Porder, Michael (NY)	Psyc	321
Pinsky, Steven (NY)	PM	569	Poretsky, Leonid (NY)	EDM	157
Piskun, Andrew (NJ)	OrS	841	Porges, Andrew (NY)	Rhu	587
Pitchumoni, Capecomorin S (NJ)	Ge	832	Portenoy, Russell (NY)	PM	278
Pitem, Michael (NY)	N	448	Portlock, Carol S (NY)	Onc	206
Pitman, Gerald H (NY)	PlS	306	Porwancher, Richard (NJ)	Inf	812
Pizzarello, Louis (NY)	Oph	629	Posner, David (NY)	Pul	331
Pizzi, Francis (NJ)	NS	815	Posner, Jerome (NY)	N	224
Pizzurro, Joseph (NJ)	OrS	740	Possick, Paul (NJ)	D	725
Plancher, Kevin D (NY)	SM	344	Post, Kalmon (NY)	NS	217
Plesset, Maxwell (NY)	IM	669	Post, Martin (NY)	Cv	130
Plestis, Konstadinos (NY)	TS	358	Post, Robert (NY)	ObG	235
Plottel, Claudia (NY)	Pul	331	Postley, John E (NY)	IM	194
Plumser, Allan (NJ)	Ge	832	Potaznik, Daniel (NY)	PHO	517
Pochapin, Mark B (NY)	Ge	168	Potter, Hollis J (NY)	DR	153
Podell,, David L (NY)	Oph	250	Powell, Jeffrey S (NY)	EDM	659
Podos, Steven M (NY)	Oph	250	Prabhu, H. Sudhakar (NY)	IM	440
Podwal, Mark (NY)	D	146	Prager, Kenneth (NY)	Pul	331
Policastro, Anthony (NY)	S	705	Prakash, Anaka (NJ)	Ge	800
Polin, Richard (NY)	NP	211	Preis, Oded (NY)	Ped	462
Polis, Laurie (NY)	D	146	Present, Daniel (NY)	Ge	168
Polkow, Melvin (NJ)	Pul	750	Press, Robert (NY)	Inf	184
Pollack, Geoffrey (NY)	Oto	274	Presti, Salvatore (NY)	PCd	457
Pollack, Jed (NY)	RadRO	585	Pretto, Zorayda (NY)	EDM	659
Pollak, Harvey (NY)	IM	550	Preven, David (NY)	Psyc	321
Pollina, Robert M (NY)	VascS	643	Prezant, David (NY)	Pul	412
Pollock, Jeffrey (NJ)	N	918	Prezioso, Paula (NY)	Ped	296
Pollock, Roger G (NJ)	OrS	740	Price, Andrew (NY)	OrS	264
Pollowitz, James (NY)	A&I	647	Price, Mitchell (NJ)	PS	845
Polsky, Bruce (NY)	Inf	184	Price, Thomas J (NY)	Cv	651
Pomeranz, Lee (NY)	S	590	Prichep, Robert (NY)	S	641
Pomeroy, John C (NY)	ChAP	613	Prince, Alice (NY)	Ped	296
Pomp, Alfons (NY)	S	352	Prince, Andrew (NY)	Oph	250
Pomper, Stuart (NY)	VascS	522	Prioleau, Philip G (NY)	D	146
Ponamgi, Suri (NJ)	PlS	748	Procaccino, Angelo (NY)	S	590
Poole, Thomas (NY)	Oph	250	Procaccino, John (NY)	CRS	535
Poon, Eric Sin-Kam (NY)	Ped	296	Provenzano, Anthony (NY)	Onc	672
Poon, Michael (NY)	Cv	129	Provet, John (NY)	U	365
Popovich, Joseph F (NJ)	S	804	Pruzan, Debra L (CT)	D	936
Poppas, Dix P (NY)	U	365	Pruzansky, Mark E (NY)	HS	176
Popper, Laura (NY)	Ped	296	Prystowsky, Barry (NJ)	Ped	787
Porder, Joseph B (NY)	Cv	129	Prystowsky, Janet (NY)	D	146

Alphabetical Listing of Doctors

Name	Specialty	Pg	Name	Specialty	Pg
Prywes, Arnold (NY)	Oph	564	Rahal, James (NY)	Inf	490
Puccio, Carmelo (NY)	Onc	672	Rahaman, Jamal (NY)	GO	174
Pucillo, Anthony (NY)	Cv	651	Rahmin, Michael G (NJ)	Ge	728
Puder, Douglas (NY)	Ped	605	Rai, Kanti (NY)	Hem	547
Pujol-Morato, Fernando (NY)	Inf	437	Raina, Suresh (NJ)	S	793
Pulle, Dunstan (NY)	Pul	412	Rajagopal, Venktesalu (NY)	Ped	462
Pumill, Rick (NJ)	Cv	721	Rajdeo, Heena (NY)	S	706
Purcell, Ralph (NY)	OrS	684	Rajpal, Sanjeev (NY)	S	473
Purow, Henry (NY)	Ped	518	Raju, Raghava (NY)	PlS	518
Putignano, Joseph (NY)	U	708	Raju, Ramanathan (NY)	S	473
Putterman, Eric A (NY)	SM	587	Rakowitz, Frederic (NY)	IM	550
			Rakowski, Thomas (NJ)	Onc	733
			Ramanathan, Kumudha (NY)	DR	428
			Ramaswamy, Prema (NY)	PCd	457
Q			Rambler, Louis (NJ)	DR	726
Qadir, Shuja (NY)	IM	491	Ramgopal, Mekala (NY)	Ge	488
Quaegebeur, Jan M (NY)	PS	292	Ramirez, Mark A (NY)	Onc	394
Quagliarello, John (NY)	RE	337	Ramsay, David L (NY)	D	146
Quagliarello, Vincent (CT)	Inf	971	Ranawat, Chitranjan (NY)	OrS	264
Quartell, Anthony C (NJ)	ObG	781	Rand, Jacob H (NY)	Hem	390
Quest, Donald (NY)	NS	217	Rand, James (NY)	Ge	488
Quinn, Joseph (NY)	Ped	635	Randazzo, Jean (NJ)	IM	877
Quittell, Lynne (NY)	PPul	291	Randolph, Audrey (NY)	PMR	695
			Raniolo, Robert (NY)	S	706
			Ransom, Mark (NJ)	RE	896
			Ranta, Jeffrey A (CT)	U	960
R			Rao, Addagada (NY)	S	473
Raab, Edward L (NY)	Oph	250	Rao, Madu (NY)	PPul	461
Rabin, Aaron (NJ)	N	736	Rao, Yalamanchi K (NY)	A&I	507
Rabinowicz, Morris (NY)	Ped	577	Raoof, Suhail (NY)	Pul	468
Rabinowitz, Simon S (NY)	PGe	517	Rapaport, Jeffrey A (NJ)	D	725
Raboy, Adley (NY)	U	521	Rapaport, Robert (NY)	PEn	285
Rackoff, Paula (NY)	Rhu	341	Raphael, Bruce (NY)	Hem	180
Radel, Eva (NY)	PHO	405	Rapin, Isabelle (NY)	ChiN	381
Rader, Michael (NY)	Hem	603	Rapoport, David (NY)	Pul	331
Radin, Allen (NY)	Rhu	341	Rapoport, Samuel (NY)	N	224
Rafizadeh, Farhad (NJ)	PlS	883	Rapp, Lynn (NY)	ObG	515
Rafla, Sameer Demetrious (NY)	RadRO	469	Rappaport, Irwin (NY)	PA&I	281
Ragnarsson, Kristjan T (NY)	PMR	300	Rascoff, Joel (NY)	Nep	493
Ragno, Philip D (NY)	Cv	533	Raska, Karel (NJ)	Cv	873
Rago, Thomas (CT)	HS	939	Raskin, Jonathan (NY)	Pul	331
			Raskin, Keith (NY)	HS	176

Name	Specialty	Pg	Name	Specialty	Pg
Rastegar, Asghar (CT)	Nep	973	Reilly, Thomas (NY)	IM	491
Rathauser, Robert (NJ)	ObG	839	Rein, Joel (CT)	PlS	955
Ratner, Desiree (NY)	D	146	Reiner, Dan (NY)	S	591
Ratner, Lloyd Evan (NY)	S	352	Reiner, Mark (NY)	S	352
Ratner, Lynn (NY)	Onc	207	Reinersman, Gerald (NY)	NP	395
Raucher, Harold S (NY)	Ped	296	Reinitz, Elizabeth (NY)	Rhu	703
Rauscher, Gregory (NJ)	PlS	748	Reisberg, Barry (NY)	GerPsy	172
Rausen, Aaron (NY)	PHO	287	Reisner, Michelle (NJ)	Ger	800
Ray, Audell (NY)	Oph	682	Reison, Dennis (NY)	Cv	130
Raymond, Gerald M (NJ)	Ped	819	Reiss, Ronald J (NY)	ObG	236
Razaboni, Rosa (NY)	PlS	306	Reitman, Milton (NY)	PCd	570
Razmzan, Shahram (NY)	ObG	679	Reizis, Igal (NY)	ObG	451
Reader, Robert (NY)	S	352	Relkin, Norman (NY)	N	225
Rebarber, Andrei (NY)	MF	199	Relland, Maureen (NY)	Oph	250
Rebold, Bruce (NY)	ObG	561	Remy, Prospere (NY)	Ge	388
Rechter, Lesley (NY)	FMed	541	Ren, Christine J (NY)	S	352
Reckler, Jon M (NY)	U	365	Rendel, Michael T (NY)	IM	194
Reda, Dominick (NY)	Nep	674	Rentrop, K Peter (NY)	Cv	130
Reddy, Chatla (NY)	Cv	424	Repice, Michael (NY)	Rhu	639
Reddy, Gaddam D (NY)	Ped	497	Reppucci, Vincent (NY)	Oph	250
Reddy, Mallikarjuna (NY)	FMed	487	Resmovits, Marvin (NY)	Ped	577
Reding, Michael (NY)	N	676	Resnick, David (NY)	A&I	378
Redlich, Carrie (CT)	Pul	980	Resnick, Richard (NY)	Psyc	322
Redner, Arlene (NY)	PHO	573	Resor, Louise (CT)	N	947
Rednor, Jeffrey (NJ)	FMed	811	Respler, Don (NJ)	PO	744
Reed, Lawrence S (NY)	PlS	306	Resta, Christine (NY)	EDM	486
Reed, Mary K (NY)	Onc	394	Restifo, Richard (CT)	PlS	978
Rees, Ellen (NY)	Psyc	322	Reuben, Stephen (NY)	IM	491
Reese, Ronald (NJ)	DR	772	Reyniak, J Victor (NY)	RE	337
Rehnstrom, Jaana (NY)	ObG	235	Rezvan, Masoud (NJ)	U	823
Reich, Raymond (NY)	Oph	453	Rho, Dae-Sik (NY)	PMR	300
Reich, Steven (NJ)	OrS	841	Rhoads, Frances (NJ)	Ped	845
Reicher, Oscar (NJ)	OrS	894	Ricciardi, Daniel D (NY)	Rhu	471
Reichman, Lee B (NJ)	Pul	790	Rice, Emanuel (NY)	Psyc	322
Reichstein, Robert P (NY)	Cv	130	Rice, Stephen G (NJ)	SM	866
Reidenberg, Marcus (NY)	IM	194	Rich, Daniel (NY)	OrS	566
Reiffel, James (NY)	Cv	130	Richards, Arnold D (NY)	Psyc	322
Reiffel, Robert S (NY)	PlS	695	Richards, Renee (NY)	Oph	251
Reilly, James G (NY)	ObG	515	Richardson, William T (NJ)	Psyc	923
Reilly, John (NY)	OrS	516	Richel, Peter (NY)	Ped	694
Reilly, Kevin B (NY)	ObG	679	Richheimer, Michael (NY)	A&I	611
Reilly, Kevin D (NY)	ObG	400	Richman, Daniel (NY)	PM	278

Alphabetical Listing of Doctors

Name	Specialty	Pg	Name	Specialty	Pg
Richman, Susan M (CT)	ObG	975	Rockwell, William (CT)	A&I	933
Ricketti, Anthony J (NJ)	A&I	809	Rodke, Gae (NY)	ObG	236
Ricotta, John (NY)	VascS	643	Rodman, John (NY)	IM	194
Ridge, Gerald (NY)	IM	669	Rodriguez, Lorna (NJ)	GO	833
Rie, Jonathan (NY)	Nep	674	Rodriguez-Sains, Rene S (NY)	Oph	251
Riechers, Roger (NY)	U	708	Rogal, Gary J (NJ)	Cv	769
Rieder, Ronald F (NY)	Hem	436	Roger, Ignatius Daniel (NY)	HS	489
Rieger, Mark (NJ)	OrS	880	Rogers, Murray (NY)	IM	194
Rifkin, Arthur (NY)	Psyc	498	Rokito, Andrew (NY)	OrS	264
Rifkin, Matthew (NY)	DR	616	Roland, John Thomas (NY)	Oto	274
Rifkin, Terry (NY)	ObG	561	Roland, Robert (NJ)	Inf	915
Rifkind, Kenneth M (NY)	S	501	Rolandelli, Rolando (NJ)	S	885
Rigel, Darrell S (NY)	D	147	Romagnoli, Mario (NY)	Inf	184
Rigolosi, Robert S (NJ)	Nep	735	Romanelli, John (NY)	Oph	629
Rigtrup, Edward (NJ)	Ped	787	Romanelli, John (NY)	IM	440
Riles, Thomas (NY)	VascS	371	Romanello, Paul P (NY)	Cv	130
Riley, David (NJ)	Pul	847	Romano, Alicia (NY)	PEn	689
Ring, Kenneth S (NJ)	U	926	Romano, Angela (NY)	PCd	570
Riordan, Charles E (CT)	Psyc	979	Romano, John (NY)	D	147
Ritch, Robert (NY)	Oph	251	Romano, Rosario (NY)	IM	623
Ritter, Joseph (NJ)	U	926	Romas, Nicholas A (NY)	U	365
Rivers, Steven P (NY)	VascS	416	Romero, Carlos (NY)	S	591
Rivlin, Richard S (NY)	IM	194	Romeu, Jose (NY)	Ge	168
Rizvi, Hasan (NY)	Onc	624	Romita, Mauro C (NY)	PlS	306
Robbins, John (NY)	NS	675	Rommer, James A (NJ)	IM	777
Robbins, Kim P (CT)	Oph	948	Romo, Thomas (NY)	Oto	274
Robbins, Michael (NY)	Cv	484	Roohi, Fereydoon (NY)	N	448
Robbins, Noah (NY)	Inf	390	Roose, Steven (NY)	Psyc	322
Robert, Marie F (CT)	Ped	978	Root, Barry (NY)	PMR	577
Roberti, M Isabel (NJ)	PNep	786	Rosa, Joseph (CT)	IM	942
Roberts, Calvin (NY)	Oph	251	Rosch, Elliott (NY)	IM	669
Roberts, Kenneth (CT)	RadRO	981	Rose, Arthur L (NY)	ChiN	426
Roberts, Larry P (NY)	U	708	Rose, Daniel (CT)	TS	959
Robilotti, James (NY)	Ge	168	Rose, Donald J (NY)	OrS	264
Robins, Perry (NY)	D	147	Rose, Eric A (NY)	TS	358
Robinson, John C (NY)	S	641	Rose, Henry J (NJ)	Pul	750
Robinson, Newell B (NY)	TS	593	Rose, Howard Anthony (NY)	OrS	264
Robson, Mark Emerson (NY)	Onc	207	Rose, John (NJ)	U	868
Rochelson, Burton (NY)	MF	552	Rose, Michael I (NJ)	PlS	865
Rochester, Carolyn (CT)	Pul	980	Rosello, Lori (NY)	Ped	297
Rochford, Joseph (NJ)	Psyc	906	Rosemarin, Jack (NY)	Ge	663
Rochman, Andrew J (NY)	S	591	Rosen, Allen D (NJ)	PlS	789

Name	Specialty	Pg	Name	Specialty	Pg
Rosen, Arie (NJ)	Oto	742	Rosenstein, Roger G (NJ)	HS	730
Rosen, Arnold M (NY)	Psyc	322	Rosenstock, Arthur (CT)	PlS	955
Rosen, Bruce I (NY)	Psyc	636	Rosenstreich, David (NY)	A&I	378
Rosen, Douglas (NY)	D	382	Rosenthal, David S (NY)	EDM	540
Rosen, Evelyn (NY)	GerPsy	434	Rosenthal, Elizabeth (NY)	D	656
Rosen, Jay S (NJ)	U	756	Rosenthal, Jeanne L (NY)	Oph	251
Rosen, Norman (NY)	Onc	673	Rosenthal, Jesse (NY)	Psyc	322
Rosen, Paul P (NY)	Path	280	Rosenthal, Kenneth J (NY)	Oph	564
Rosen, Richard (NY)	Oph	251	Rosenthal, Richard N (NY)	Psyc	322
Rosen, Robert J (NY)	VIR	369	Rosenthal, Sheldon (NY)	U	476
Rosen, Tove S (NY)	NP	211	Rosenwaks, Zev (NY)	RE	337
Rosenbaum, Alfred (NY)	RadRO	334	Rosenwasser, Melvin (NY)	HS	177
Rosenbaum, Daniel (NY)	N	448	Roses, Daniel F (NY)	S	352
Rosenbaum, Jeffrey (NJ)	Oto	841	Rosh, Joel (NJ)	PGe	882
Rosenbaum, Michael (NY)	Ped	297	Roshan, Daniel (NY)	MF	199
Rosenbaum, Pearl (NY)	Oph	401	Roslin, Mitchell S (NY)	S	352
Rosenbaum, Robert (NJ)	EDM	913	Rosman, Lawrence (NY)	EDM	486
Rosenberg, Alan (NY)	IM	550	Rosman, Sidney (NY)	Ge	488
Rosenberg, Amy (NJ)	FMed	914	Rosner, Bruce (NJ)	Ge	811
Rosenberg, Craig H (NY)	PMR	635	Rosner, Louis (NY)	Oto	568
Rosenberg, Kenneth P (NY)	AdP	119	Rosner, Richard (NY)	Psyc	323
Rosenberg, Michael (NJ)	N	838	Rosner, Saran (NY)	NS	675
Rosenberg, Peter (NY)	Cv	484	Rosner, Steven (NJ)	Rhu	752
Rosenberg, Stanley (NJ)	U	823	Ross, Herbert (NY)	EDM	659
Rosenberg, Vladimiro (NY)	S	352	Ross, Marc (NY)	PMR	301
Rosenblatt, Ruth (NY)	DR	153	Rossakis, Constantine (NJ)	Cv	721
Rosenblatt, William B (NY)	PlS	306	Rosser, James C (NY)	S	352
Rosenbloom, Charles (NY)	Psyc	322	Rossi, Dennis (NY)	DR	538
Rosenblum, Bruce (NJ)	NS	861	Rossman, Barry R (NJ)	U	823
Rosenfeld, Alvin (NY)	ChAP	135	Rossoff, Leonard (NY)	Pul	583
Rosenfeld, David (NY)	RE	585	Rossos, Paul (NJ)	Oto	863
Rosenfeld, David (NJ)	DR	830	Roston, Alfred (NY)	Ge	664
Rosenfeld, David N (NJ)	Psyc	749	Roth, Alan (NY)	FMed	487
Rosenfeld, Isadore (NY)	Cv	130	Roth, Joseph (NJ)	Ge	728
Rosenfeld, Richard M (NY)	PO	460	Roth, Malcolm Z (NY)	PlS	463
Rosenfeld, Stanley (NY)	DR	153	Roth, Patrick A (NJ)	NS	736
Rosenfeld, Steven S (NY)	N	225	Roth, Philip (NY)	NP	513
Rosenfeld, Suzanne (NY)	Ped	297	Roth, Richard (NY)	Cv	601
Rosenheck, David (NJ)	Ge	832	Roth, Ronald (NY)	FMed	618
Rosenman, Stephen (CT)	ObG	948	Rothbard, Malcolm (NY)	ObG	236
Rosenstein, C Cory (CT)	NS	946	Rothbart, Stephen (NJ)	CE	768
Rosenstein, Elliot D (NJ)	Rhu	792	Rothbaum, David (NY)	ObG	561

Alphabetical Listing of Doctors

Name	Specialty	Pg	Name	Specialty	Pg
Rothberg, Charles (NY)	Oph	629	Ruddy, Michael (NJ)	Nep	814
Rothberg, Robert (NJ)	CRS	770	Ruderman, Marvin (NJ)	N	780
Rothenberg, Bennett C (NJ)	PlS	748	Rudick, A Joseph (NY)	Oph	251
Rothman, Howard (NJ)	Cv	722	Rudikoff, Donald (NY)	D	382
Rothman, Ivan (NY)	Onc	553	Rudin, Leonard (NY)	U	607
Rothman, Jeffrey (NY)	EDM	510	Rudman, Michael E (NJ)	PM	881
Rothman, Nathan (NY)	Pul	583	Rudolph, Steven (NY)	N	448
Rothstein, Stephen G (NY)	Oto	274	Ruggiero, Joseph (NY)	Onc	207
Rotman, Marvin (NY)	RadRO	469	Ruoff, Michael (NY)	Ge	168
Rotolo, James (NJ)	U	868	Rush, Stephen (NY)	RadRO	585
Roubin, Gary (NY)	IC	197	Rush, Thomas (NY)	Inf	666
Rowan, A James (NY)	N	225	Russakoff, L Mark (NY)	Psyc	699
Rowland, Lewis P (NY)	N	225	Russell, Robin (NY)	Ger	389
Roychowdhury, Sudipta (NJ)	NRad	839	Russo, John A (NJ)	IM	777
Roye, David (NY)	OrS	265	Russo, Paul (NY)	U	366
Rozanski, Alan (NY)	Cv	130	Russo, Robert (CT)	DR	936
Rozanski, Reuben (NJ)	D	771	Rutherford, Thomas (CT)	GO	970
Rozbruch, Jacob D (NY)	OrS	265	Rutkovsky, Edward (NY)	Cv	533
Rozbruch, S Robert (NY)	OrS	265	Rutkovsky, Lisa Rosner (NY)	PCd	496
Rozenblit, Alla (NY)	DR	383	Ruzicka, Petr (NJ)	NS	837
Ruben, Robert (NY)	Oto	403	Ryan, Joseph (NJ)	Ger	876
Rubenstein, Jack (NY)	IM	550	Ryback, Hyman (NY)	Oto	686
Rubenstein, Janet (NY)	ObG	451	Rydzinski, Mayer (NY)	Cv	484
Rubenstein, Richard B (NY)	TS	642			
Rubenstein, Roy (NY)	Pul	583			
Rubin, David Albert (NY)	CE	648			
Rubin, James (NY)	A&I	121			
Rubin, Kenneth (NJ)	Psyc	865	**S**		
Rubin, Kenneth (NJ)	Ge	728			
Rubin, Laurence (NY)	Oph	564	Saad, Saad A (NJ)	PS	864
Rubin, Lorry (NY)	PInf	573	Saada, Simon (NY)	U	476
Rubin, Marc R (NJ)	Ge	812	Saal, Stuart (NY)	Nep	213
Rubin, Moshe (NY)	Ge	168	Sabatino, Dominick P (NY)	PHO	573
Rubin, Peter (NY)	Ge	168	Sabetta, James (CT)	Inf	939
Rubin, Steven (NY)	Oph	564	Sable, Robert (NY)	Ge	388
Rubinoff, Mitchell (NJ)	Ge	729	Sacchi, Terrence J (NY)	Cv	425
Rubinstein, Arye (NY)	A&I	378	Sacco, Ralph L (NY)	N	225
Rubinstein, Boris (NY)	ChAP	653	Sachar, David (NY)	Ge	169
Rubinstein, Joshua (NY)	PlS	410	Sachs, Jonathan R (NJ)	Ge	812
Rubinstein, Mort (NY)	Psyc	323	Sachs, Paul (CT)	Pul	957
Rucinski, James (NY)	S	473	Sachs, R Gregory (NJ)	Cv	912
Rucker, Steve (NY)	IM	551	Sachs, Ronald (NJ)	Oph	880
			Sachs, Stephen (NJ)	N	918
			Sacker, Ira (NY)	Ped	297

Name	Specialty	Pg	Name	Specialty	Pg
Sacks, Michael (NY)	Psyc	323	Salkin, Paul (NY)	Psyc	323
Sacks, Steven (NY)	Oto	274	Salky, Barry A (NY)	S	353
Sacks-Berg, Anne (NY)	Inf	621	Salmon, Jane (NY)	Rhu	342
Sadan, Sara (NY)	Onc	673	Salsitz, Edwin A (NY)	IM	194
Sadanandan, Swayam (NY)	PHO	459	Saltstein, Elliott (NJ)	Ped	819
Sadarangani, Balvinder (NY)	ObG	236	Saltz, Leonard B (NY)	Onc	207
Sadarangani, Gurmukh J (NY)	RadRO	334	Saltzman, Martin (NY)	Nep	675
Sadeghi, Hooshang (NJ)	N	801	Saltzman, Simone (NY)	Inf	391
Sadeghi, Hossein (CT)	PPul	952	Saltzman-Gabelman, Lori (NY)	IM	669
Sadeghi-Nejad, Hossein (NJ)	U	756	Salvati, Eduardo A (NY)	OrS	265
Sadick, Neil (NY)	D	147	Salwitz, James (NJ)	Onc	836
Sadler, Daniel (NJ)	CRS	902	Salz, Alan (NJ)	Oph	904
Sadock, Benjamin (NY)	Psyc	323	Salzberg, C Andrew (NY)	PlS	696
Sadock, Virginia (NY)	Psyc	323	Salzer, Peter (NY)	S	591
Sadovsky, Richard (NY)	FMed	430	Salzer, Richard L (NJ)	OrS	741
Sadowski, John (NY)	Oto	605	Salzer, Stephen (CT)	Oto	951
Saenger, Paul (NY)	PEn	689	Salzman, Jacqueline (NY)	Oph	682
Safai, Bijan (NY)	D	147	Samach, Michael (NJ)	Ge	875
Saffra, Norman (NY)	Oph	453	Samberg, Eslee (NY)	Psyc	323
Safier, Henry L (NY)	Ge	433	Sami, Sherif (NY)	Psyc	581
Safirstein, Benjamin (NJ)	Pul	790	Sampogna, Dominick A (NY)	Oto	631
Safran, Steven (NJ)	Oph	816	Sampson, Hugh (NY)	PA&I	281
Sage, Jacob (NJ)	N	838	Samra, Said (NJ)	PlS	865
Sagorin, Charles (NJ)	Onc	778	Samuel, Steven (NJ)	Cv	809
Sagy, Mayer (NY)	PCCM	570	Samuelly, Israel (NY)	GerPsy	434
Saha, Chanchal (NY)	TS	593	Samuels, Steven (NY)	Inf	621
Saidi, Parvin (NJ)	Hem	833	Samuels, Steven (NJ)	Psyc	749
Sailon, Peter (NY)	ObG	236	San Filippo, J Anthony (NY)	PS	691
Saiman, Lisa (NY)	PInf	289	San Roman, Gerardo (NY)	ObG	627
Salama, Meir (NY)	Ge	664	Sanchez, Juan A (CT)	TS	959
Saland, Jeffrey M (NY)	PNep	289	Sanchez, Miguel A (NJ)	Path	742
Salas, Max (NJ)	PEn	843	Sanchez, Miguel R (NY)	D	147
Salcedo, Jose (NJ)	PNep	895	Sander, Howard (NY)	N	225
Saleh, Anthony (NY)	Pul	468	Sander, Norbert (NY)	IM	392
Salem, Noel (NJ)	Rhu	752	Sanders, Abraham (NY)	Pul	332
Salem, Ronald R (CT)	S	982	Sanders, Linda (NJ)	DR	772
Salerno, William (NJ)	Cv	722	Sanderson, Rhonda (NJ)	ObG	904
Sales, Clifford (NJ)	VascS	926	Sandhaus, Jeffrey (NY)	U	502
Salgado, Miran (NY)	N	448	Sandhu, Harvinder S (NY)	OrS	265
Salik, James (NY)	Ge	169	Sandler, Benjamin (NY)	ObG	236
Salimi, Mostafa (NJ)	Cv	891	Sandoval, Claudio (NY)	PHO	690
Salisbury, Roger E (NY)	PlS	696	Sands, Andrew (NY)	OrS	265

Alphabetical Listing of Doctors

Name	Specialty	Pg	Name	Specialty	Pg
Sanford, Marie (NY)	Ped	297	Schaefer, Steven D (NY)	Oto	275
Sanger, Joseph J (NY)	NuM	229	Schaeffer, Henry (NY)	Ped	462
Sanjana, Veeraf (NY)	Inf	184	Schaeffer, Janis (NY)	PPul	574
Santamaria, Jaime (NJ)	Oph	840	Schaeffer, Mark A (NJ)	IM	813
Santiamo, Joseph (NY)	IM	512	Schaffer, Dean (NY)	Oto	686
Santilli, John (CT)	A&I	933	Schanler, Richard (NY)	NP	555
Santilli, Veronica (NY)	Ped	462	Schantz, Stimson P (NY)	Oto	275
Santoro, Elissa J (NJ)	S	793	Schanzer, Bernard (NJ)	N	918
Santoro, Nanette (NY)	RE	702	Schanzer, Harry (NY)	VascS	371
Sapala, James A (NY)	S	474	Scharf, Richard (NJ)	Oto	920
Saphir, Richard L (NY)	Ped	297	Scharf, Robert D (NY)	Psyc	323
Saponara, Eduardo M (NY)	Onc	673	Scharf, Stephen (NY)	NuM	230
Sara, Gabriel (NY)	Onc	207	Scharfman, Edward L (NY)	Psyc	699
Saraiya, Narendra (NJ)	Ped	922	Schaul, Neil (NY)	N	493
Sarno, John E (NY)	PM	278	Schechner, Richard (NY)	S	414
Saroff, Alan (NJ)	Cv	769	Schechter, Justin (CT)	Psyc	955
Sarokhan, Alan (NJ)	OrS	920	Schechter, Miriam (NY)	Ped	408
Sas, Norman (NY)	S	414	Scheer, Max (NY)	Inf	548
Sasaki, Clarence T (CT)	Oto	976	Scheidt, Stephen (NY)	Cv	131
Sasso, Louis (NY)	Pul	519	Schein, Jonah (NY)	Psyc	324
Sassoon, Robert I (NY)	ObG	236	Scheinberg, David (NY)	Onc	207
Satlin, Lisa M (NY)	PNep	289	Schell, Harold S (NJ)	S	822
Satnick, Steven (NY)	A&I	611	Scher, Howard (NY)	Onc	207
Sauer, Mark (NY)	RE	337	Scher, Jonathan (NY)	ObG	236
Saul, Zane (CT)	Inf	940	Scherl, Ellen (NY)	Ge	169
Saulino, Patrick (NJ)	Cv	901	Scherl, Michael (NJ)	Oto	742
Saunders, Craig R (NJ)	TS	794	Scherl, Sharon (NJ)	D	725
Savage, David G (NY)	Hem	180	Scherr, Douglas S (NY)	U	366
Savatsky, Gary (NJ)	SM	752	Scheuch, Robert (NY)	Pul	637
Savin, Ronald (CT)	D	968	Scheuer, James (NY)	Cv	380
Savino, John (NY)	S	706	Schick, David (NY)	Cv	380
Savino, Michael (NY)	U	522	Schiff, Carl (NY)	Rhu	471
Sawczuk, Ihor S (NJ)	U	757	Schiff, Howard (NY)	U	366
Sawyer, David (NY)	Psyc	323	Schiff, Peter B (NY)	RadRO	335
Saxena, Anil (NY)	EDM	429	Schiff, Russell (NY)	PCd	570
Scaccia, Frank J (NJ)	Oto	863	Schiff, William (NY)	Oph	251
Scaduto, Philip (NJ)	IM	877	Schiffer, Mark B (NY)	Cv	131
Scardino, Peter T (NY)	U	366	Schiffman, Philip (NJ)	Pul	847
Scarpa, Nicholas P (NJ)	Rhu	804	Schiller, Alan L (NY)	Path	280
Scarpinato, Vincent M (NY)	S	353	Schiller, Myles (NY)	PCd	283
Schaebler, David (NJ)	Onc	814	Schiller, Robert (NY)	FMed	159
Schaefer, John A (NY)	N	225	Schiowitz, Emanuel (NY)	FMed	430

Name	Specialty	Pg	Name	Specialty	Pg
Schlecker, Burton A (NJ)	U	897	Schreiber, Zwi (NY)	Hem	390
Schlegel, Peter (NY)	U	366	Schroeder, Karl (NY)	Psyc	606
Schleider, Michael (NJ)	Onc	733	Schubert, Hermann (NY)	Oph	252
Schleifer, Steven (NJ)	Psyc	790	Schulder, Michael (NJ)	NS	780
Schlesinger, Irwin (NY)	N	558	Schulhafer, Edwin (NJ)	A&I	901
Schley, W Shain (NY)	Oto	275	Schulman, Ira (NY)	Cv	131
Schliftman, Alan (NY)	D	656	Schulman, Norman (NY)	PlS	307
Schluger, Neil (NY)	Pul	332	Schulman, Philip (NY)	Hem	620
Schlussel, Richard (NY)	U	366	Schulster, Rita B (NY)	Pul	583
Schmerin, Michael (NY)	Ge	169	Schultz, Neal (NY)	D	147
Schmidt, Hans J (NJ)	S	754	Schulze, Ruth (NJ)	ObG	738
Schmidt, Philip (NY)	EDM	429	Schuss, Steven A (NJ)	Ped	746
Schmidt-Sarosi, Cecilia (NY)	RE	337	Schussler, George (NY)	EDM	429
Schnabel, Freya (NY)	S	353	Schuster, Michael (NY)	Hem	180
Schneck, Gideon (NY)	Oph	629	Schuster, Stephen (NY)	ObG	494
Schneebaum, Cary (NY)	IM	195	Schuster, Victor L (NY)	Nep	396
Schneider, Arlene (NY)	A&I	421	Schutzengel, Roy (CT)	Ped	953
Schneider, George (NJ)	EDM	773	Schwartz, Allan (NY)	Cv	131
Schneider, Howard J (NY)	Oph	252	Schwartz, Bruce (NY)	Psyc	411
Schneider, Kenneth L (NY)	Oto	275	Schwartz, Charles A (NY)	Cv	508
Schneider, Lewis (NY)	Ge	169	Schwartz, David L (NY)	PS	575
Schneider, Marcie (CT)	AM	933	Schwartz, Ernest (NY)	EDM	385
Schneider, Robert (NY)	Onc	673	Schwartz, Evan (NY)	OrS	496
Schneider, Ronald (NY)	ObG	679	Schwartz, Gary (NY)	Ge	544
Schneider, Samuel (NJ)	Psyc	820	Schwartz, Joel M (NY)	DR	602
Schneider, Stephen (NJ)	OrS	905	Schwartz, Judith W (NY)	ObG	236
Schneider, Steven J (NY)	IM	195	Schwartz, Kenneth S (NY)	VascS	709
Schneyer, Barton (NY)	Pul	637	Schwartz, Louis (NJ)	RadRO	924
Schob, Clifford (NJ)	OrS	783	Schwartz, Michael (NY)	Psyc	637
Schoen, Robert T (CT)	Rhu	982	Schwartz, Michael L (NY)	VascS	607
Schoeneman, Morris J (NY)	PNep	460	Schwartz, Mitchell S (NJ)	Ge	859
Schoenfeld, Mark (CT)	IC	971	Schwartz, Myron (NY)	S	353
Schonfeld, Steven (NJ)	NRad	839	Schwartz, Paula R (NY)	Onc	553
Schore, Arthur (NY)	Psyc	324	Schwartz, Peter E (CT)	GO	970
Schorn, Karen (NY)	Rhu	639	Schwartz, Robert A (NJ)	D	771
Schottenfeld, Richard (CT)	AdP	965	Schwartz, Simeon (NY)	Onc	673
Schrader, Zalman (NJ)	Ge	774	Schwartz, William (NY)	Cv	131
Schrager, Alan (NY)	U	708	Schwartzberg, Mori (NJ)	Rhu	866
Schreiber, Carl (NY)	Cv	533	Schwartzman, Alexander (NY)	S	474
Schreiber, Klaus (NY)	ChAP	653	Schwartzman, Sergio (NY)	Rhu	342
Schreiber, Martha (NJ)	S	867	Schwarz, Michael (NJ)	Cv	891
Schreiber, Michael (NY)	Pul	702	Schwarz, Richard B (NY)	Nep	625

Alphabetical Listing of Doctors

Name	Specialty	Pg	Name	Specialty	Pg
Schwarz, Steven M (NY)	PGe	458	Selesnick, Samuel H (NY)	Oto	275
Schweitzer, Philip E (NY)	Ge	388	Self, Edward (NJ)	OrS	741
Schwinn, Hans Dieter (NY)	FMed	618	Seliger, Glenn (NY)	N	604
Sciales, John (NY)	IM	491	Selman, Jay E (NY)	N	676
Scibetta, Maria (NJ)	IM	732	Seltzer, Murray H (NJ)	S	793
Scigliano, Eileen (NY)	Hem	180	Seltzer, Terry (NY)	IM	195
Sciortino, Patrick (NY)	Oph	453	Seltzer, Vicki (NY)	GO	545
Sclafani, Anthony P (NY)	Oto	275	Selwyn, Peter (NY)	IM	392
Sclafani, Lisa (NY)	S	641	Selzer, Jeffrey A (NY)	Psyc	498
Sclafani, Michael (NJ)	SM	866	Seminara, Donna (NY)	IM	512
Sclafani, Salvatore (NY)	VIR	477	Sen, Chandranath (NY)	NS	217
Scofield, Lisa (NJ)	Ped	895	Sen, Dilip (NY)	Ped	462
Sconzo, Frank (NY)	CRS	614	Sena, Kanaga N (CT)	N	947
Scott, David (NY)	Nep	493	Sender, Joel (NY)	Pul	412
Scott, Norman (NY)	FMed	430	Sennett, Margaret A (CT)	IM	942
Scott, Richard T (NJ)	RE	884	Sensakovic, John W (NJ)	Inf	834
Scott, Susan M (NY)	PlS	307	Sepkowitz, Douglas (NY)	Inf	437
Scott, W Norman (NY)	OrS	265	Sepkowitz, Kent (NY)	Inf	185
Scuderi, Giles R (NY)	OrS	265	Seplowitz, Alan (NY)	EDM	157
Sculco, Thomas P (NY)	OrS	266	Serby, Michael J (NY)	GerPsy	172
Seaman, Cheryl (NY)	Psyc	699	Sergiou, Harry (NY)	Ped	462
Seashore, Margretta (CT)	CG	967	Serle, Janet (NY)	Oph	252
Seaver, Robert (NY)	ChAP	653	Serur, Eli (NY)	GO	435
Seebacher, J Robert (NY)	OrS	685	Setzen, Michael (NY)	Oto	568
Seedor, John A (NY)	Oph	252	Shabry, Fryderyka (NY)	ChAP	425
Seelagy, Marc (NJ)	Pul	821	Shabsigh, Ridwan (NY)	U	366
Segarra, Pedro R (NY)	ObG	237	Shabto, Uri (NY)	Oph	252
Segura-Bustamante, Alina (NY)	Psyc	465	Shaffer, David (NY)	ChAP	135
Seibt, R Stephen (NJ)	D	771	Shah, Darsit K (NJ)	Oto	863
Seicol, Noel (NY)	IM	669	Shah, Jatin P (NY)	S	353
Seidenberg, Boyd (NJ)	Oph	738	Shah, Smita (NJ)	CCM	770
Seidenfeld, Andrew (NY)	Oph	495	Shaha, Ashok (NY)	S	353
Seidenstein, Michael (NJ)	OrS	783	Shahid, Syed Javed (CT)	NS	946
Seidman, Barry (NJ)	U	794	Shahrivar, Farrokh (NY)	NP	211
Seidman, Mitchell (NY)	Oph	453	Shalit, Shimon (NY)	U	709
Seifer, David B (NY)	RE	469	Shalita, Alan (NY)	D	427
Seigel, Mark J (NJ)	ObG	862	Shamamian, Peter (NY)	S	353
Seigle, Robert (NY)	PNep	289	Shamoon, Fayez E (NJ)	Cv	769
Seiler, Jerome (NY)	ObG	237	Shamoon, Harry (NY)	EDM	385
Seinfeld, David (NY)	Cv	131	Shanahan, Andrew (NJ)	IC	813
Seiter, Karen (NY)	Onc	673	Shane, Elizabeth (NY)	EDM	157
Sekons, David (NY)	S	353	Shani, Jacob (NY)	IC	441

Alphabetical Listing of Doctors

Name	Specialty	Pg	Name	Specialty	Pg
Shapir, Yehuda (NY)	PCd	570	Sher, Ellen R (NJ)	A&I	857
Shapiro, Barry M (NY)	Oto	687	Sheridan, Bernadette (NY)	FMed	430
Shapiro, Bruce (CT)	Psyc	955	Sherling, Bruce E (NY)	Pul	702
Shapiro, Ellen (NY)	U	366	Sherman, Frederic (NY)	IM	440
Shapiro, Eugene D (CT)	PInf	977	Sherman, Fredrick T (NY)	Ger	172
Shapiro, Jonathan (NJ)	IM	732	Sherman, Howard (NY)	Ge	388
Shapiro, Kenneth (NY)	Nep	604	Sherman, John E (NY)	PlS	307
Shapiro, Lawrence (NY)	EDM	540	Sherman, Mark F (NY)	OrS	516
Shapiro, Lawrence R (NY)	CG	654	Sherman, Orrin (NY)	OrS	266
Shapiro, Marc (NY)	S	641	Sherman, Raymond (NY)	Nep	213
Shapiro, Michael E (NJ)	S	754	Sherman, Richard A (NJ)	Nep	837
Shapiro, Neil (NY)	Ge	664	Sherman, Scott J (NY)	DR	538
Shapiro, Peter (NY)	Psyc	324	Sherman, Spencer (NY)	Oph	252
Shapiro, Richard L (NY)	S	354	Sherman, Steven I (NY)	Oph	453
Shapiro, Theodore (NY)	Psyc	324	Sherman, Warren (NY)	Cv	131
Shapiro, Warren (NY)	Nep	445	Sherman, William H (NY)	Onc	207
Shaps, Jeffrey (NY)	Ge	511	Sherry, Stephen (NJ)	EDM	773
Shapshay, Stanley M (NY)	Oto	275	Sherwin, Robert (CT)	EDM	969
Sharma, Chandra (NY)	N	225	Shiffman, Rebecca L (NY)	MF	442
Sharma, Samin (NY)	IC	197	Shike, Moshe (NY)	Ge	169
Sharon, David (NJ)	Onc	861	Shikowitz, Mark (NY)	Oto	568
Shaw, Ronda R (NY)	Psyc	324	Shimony, Rony (NY)	Cv	131
Shaywitz, Bennett A (CT)	ChiN	967	Shin, Choon S (NY)	VascS	477
Shaywitz, Sally E (CT)	Ped	978	Shinbach, Kent (NY)	Psyc	324
Shear, M Katherine (NY)	Psyc	324	Shindelman, Larry (NJ)	VascS	851
Sheares, Beverley J (NY)	PPul	291	Shindler, Daniel (NJ)	Cv	828
Shebairo, Raymond (NY)	OrS	566	Shindo, Maisie L (NY)	Oto	631
Sheehan, Peter (NY)	EDM	157	Shinnar, Shlomo (NY)	ChiN	381
Sheehy, Albert (NY)	IM	670	Shinya, Hiromi (NY)	Ge	169
Sheftell, Fred (CT)	Psyc	955	Shlasko, Edward (NY)	PS	461
Sheikh, Shahid (NY)	Cv	651	Shlofmitz, Richard A (NY)	Cv	533
Shein, Leon (NY)	Nep	446	Shorofsky, Morris (NY)	IM	195
Sheinbaum, Richard (CT)	Ge	938	Short, Joan (NY)	Ped	518
Sheinfeld, Joel (NY)	U	367	Shugar, Joel (NY)	Oto	276
Shell, Roger (NJ)	Cv	828	Shulman, Abraham (NY)	Oto	456
Shelley, Gabriela (NY)	Psyc	324	Shulman, Julius (NY)	Oph	252
Shelmet, John J (NJ)	IM	813	Shulman, Yale (NJ)	U	805
Shelov, Steven (NY)	Ped	462	Shum, Kee (NY)	Onc	492
Shelton, Ronald M (NY)	D	147	Shupack, Jerome L (NY)	D	148
Shemen, Larry (NY)	Oto	276	Shypula, Gregory (NJ)	Onc	836
Shepard, Barry R (NY)	U	594	Sibony, Patrick (NY)	Oph	629
Shepherd, Gillian M (NY)	A&I	122	Sibrack, Laurence (CT)	D	936

Alphabetical Listing of Doctors

Name	Specialty	Pg	Name	Specialty	Pg
Sibulkin, David (NY)	D	148	Silverman, Marc (NY)	SM	501
Sicherer, Scott H (NY)	PA&I	281	Silverman, Mitchell (NJ)	EDM	913
Sicklick, Marc (NY)	A&I	528	Silverman, Rubin (NY)	Cv	380
Siderides, Elizabeth (CT)	Oph	948	Silvers, David (NY)	D	148
Sidoti, Paul (NY)	Oph	252	Silvestri, Fred (NJ)	S	754
Siebert, John W (NY)	PlS	307	Simberkoff, Michael S (NY)	Inf	185
Siegal, Elliot (NY)	Ped	605	Simmons, Rache M (NY)	S	354
Siegal, Frederick P (NY)	A&I	122	Simon, Clifford J (NJ)	Pul	750
Siegal, Michael S (NY)	Cv	132	Simon, John (NY)	S	641
Siegel, Beth (NY)	S	501	Simon, Jonathan (NJ)	Rhu	792
Siegel, Daniel M (NY)	D	615	Simon, Lawrence (NY)	S	607
Siegel, Jerome H (NY)	Ge	169	Simon, Lloyd (NY)	IM	623
Siegel, Judy F (NY)	U	709	Simon, Sheldon R (NY)	OrS	266
Siegel, Kenneth C (CT)	N	947	Simon, Steven (NY)	D	427
Siegel, Randall (NJ)	VIR	851	Simonson, Barry G (NY)	OrS	566
Siegel, Robert (NY)	CCM	381	Simpson, Alec (NJ)	VascS	851
Siegel, Stephen (NY)	Cv	132	Simpson, David M (NY)	N	226
Siegler, Eugenia (NY)	Ger	172	Simpson, Roger (NY)	PlS	579
Siepser, Stuart (NJ)	Cv	891	Singer, Carol (NY)	Inf	548
Sierocki, John (NJ)	Onc	814	Singer, Elliot (NY)	Psyc	699
Siever, Larry J (NY)	Psyc	325	Singer, Lewis (NY)	PCCM	404
Siglock, Timothy (NY)	Oto	687	Singer, Samuel (NY)	S	354
Silberman, Deborah (NY)	Oph	453	Singh, Anup (NJ)	PNep	844
Silberman, Mark (NY)	PlS	579	Singh, Avtar (NY)	N	677
Silbert, Glenn (NJ)	Oph	739	Singhal, Pravin C (NY)	Nep	556
Silbert, Paul (NJ)	N	862	Sinnreich, Abraham (NY)	Oto	516
Silich, Robert C (NY)	PlS	307	Sipzner, Robert (NJ)	Nep	779
Silich, Robert J (NY)	S	521	Siracuse, Jeffrey F (NY)	NP	513
Silva, Jose V (NY)	U	367	Siris, Ethel (NY)	EDM	158
Silva, Waldemar (NJ)	IM	877	Siris, Samuel G (NY)	Psyc	498
Silver, Bennett (NJ)	Psyc	924	Siskind, Steven Jay (NY)	Cv	484
Silver, David A. (NY)	U	476	Sison, Joseph (NJ)	NP	734
Silver, Jonathan M (NY)	Psyc	325	Sisti, Michael B (NY)	NS	217
Silver, Lester (NY)	PlS	307	Sitron, Alan (NY)	DR	538
Silver, Michael (NY)	Cv	651	Sivak, Mark A (NY)	N	226
Silver, Richard (NY)	Onc	208	Skinner, Kristin A (NY)	S	354
Silverberg, Arnold (NY)	EDM	429	Sklansky, B Donald (NY)	PlS	579
Silverberg, Shonni J (NY)	EDM	157	Sklar, Barrett (NY)	FMed	541
Silverman, Barney (NY)	ObG	679	Sklar, Charles A (NY)	PEn	285
Silverman, Cary (NJ)	Oph	880	Sklar, Jeffrey (NY)	D	537
Silverman, David (NY)	IM	195	Sklarek, Howard (NY)	Pul	638
Silverman, Joel (NY)	Pul	500	Sklarin, Nancy (NY)	Onc	208

Name	Specialty	Pg	Name	Specialty	Pg
Sklaroff, Herschel (NY)	Cv	132	Smith, Lawrence (NY)	IM	551
Sklower, Jay A (NJ)	FMed	800	Smith, Leon G (NJ)	Inf	776
Sklower Brooks, Susan (NJ)	CG	829	Smith, Leon G (NJ)	MF	778
Skluth, Myra (CT)	IM	942	Smith, Marilyn (CT)	Ped	953
Skolnick, Lawrence (NJ)	NP	878	Smith, Michael O (NY)	AdP	378
Skolnik, Richard A (NY)	PlS	307	Smith, Miriam (NY)	Inf	548
Skripkus, Aldona (NJ)	Ped	803	Smith, Peter R (NY)	Pul	468
Skrokov, Robert (NY)	D	615	Smith, Richard V (NY)	Oto	403
Skupski, Daniel (NY)	MF	491	Smith, Stephen M (NJ)	Inf	776
Skuza, Kathryn (NJ)	PEn	843	Smithy, William (NY)	CRS	614
Sladowski, Catherine (NJ)	ObG	781	Smotkin, David (NY)	GO	546
Slama, Robert (NJ)	Cv	912	Smotrich, Gary (NJ)	PlS	820
Slamovits, Thomas (NY)	Oph	401	Snow, Robert (NY)	NS	217
Slankard, Marjorie (NY)	A&I	122	Snyder, Barbara K (NJ)	AM	827
Slater, Gary (NY)	S	354	Snyder, David (NY)	N	226
Slater, James (NY)	IC	198	Snyder, Gary M (NY)	Oto	496
Slater, Jonathan (NY)	ChAP	653	Snyder, Jon R (NY)	ObG	237
Slater, William (NY)	CE	123	Snyder, Michael (CT)	PCd	951
Slavit, David H (NY)	Oto	276	Soave, Rosemary (NY)	Inf	185
Slim, Jihad (NJ)	Inf	775	Sobel, Howard (NY)	D	148
Sloan, Don (NY)	ObG	237	Sobol, Norman (NY)	N	448
Sloan, William (NJ)	Ge	774	Sockolow, Robbyn (NY)	PGe	285
Sloane, Lori (NY)	Rhu	704	Sofair, Jane (NJ)	Psyc	884
Slogoff, Frederick B (CT)	IM	942	Soffen, Edward (NJ)	RadRO	821
Slonim, Alfred E (NY)	PEn	571	Soffer, Jeffrey (NJ)	ObG	918
Slotwiner, Paul (NY)	N	448	Softness, Barney (NY)	Ped	297
Slovin, Alvin (NY)	TS	502	Sogani, Pramod (NY)	U	367
Slovin, Susan F (NY)	Onc	208	Soifer, Todd (NY)	OrS	455
Slowey, Michael J (NJ)	RE	751	Sokal, Myron (NY)	NP	444
Small, Steven (NY)	OrS	685	Solitar, Bruce M (NY)	Rhu	342
Smallberg, Gerald (NY)	N	226	Solomon, Edward (NJ)	Oph	739
Smart, Frank W (NJ)	Cv	874	Solomon, Gary (NY)	Rhu	342
Smilen, Scott (NY)	ObG	237	Solomon, Gregory (NY)	IM	195
Smirnov, Viktor (NY)	VascS	596	Solomon, Ira (NY)	Oph	682
Smith, Aloysius G (NY)	PlS	696	Solomon, Joel (NY)	Oph	253
Smith, Arthur D (NY)	U	595	Solomon, Michael J (NJ)	U	850
Smith, Charles R (NY)	N	398	Solomon, Robert A (NY)	NS	217
Smith, Craig R (NY)	TS	359	Solomon, Robert B (NJ)	Ger	915
Smith, David I (NY)	Ped	297	Solomon, Ronald (NY)	HS	435
Smith, Edward (NY)	Oph	454	Solomon, Sherry (NY)	Oph	682
Smith, Jo Ann (CT)	Psyc	956	Solomon, William (NY)	Onc	443
Smith, Julia A (NY)	Onc	208	Soloway, Barrie D (NY)	Oph	253

Alphabetical Listing of Doctors

Name	Specialty	Pg	Name	Specialty	Pg
Soloway, Bruce (NY)	FMed	386	Spielberg, Alan (NY)	Ge	620
Soltren, Rafael (NY)	IM	670	Spielvogel, David (NY)	TS	706
Som, Peter (NY)	DR	153	Spiera, Harry (NY)	Rhu	342
Somasundaram, Mahendra (NY)	N	448	Spiera, Robert (NY)	Rhu	342
Somerstein, Michael (NJ)	Nep	815	Spiler, Ira (NJ)	EDM	831
Sommer, Robert J (NY)	PCd	283	Spina, Christopher (NY)	A&I	421
Sommers, Gara M (NJ)	GO	801	Spindola-Franco, Hugo (NY)	DR	383
Sonett, Joshua R (NY)	TS	359	Spinelli, Henry M (NY)	PlS	307
Sonnenblick, Edmund (NY)	Cv	380	Spinowitz, Alan (NY)	D	537
Sonnenblick, Emily (NY)	DR	153	Spinowitz, Bruce (NY)	Nep	493
Sonoda, Toyooki (NY)	CRS	139	Spira, Robert S (NJ)	Ge	800
Sonpal, Girish (NY)	Rhu	501	Spitalewitz, Samuel (NY)	Nep	446
Sood, Sunil (NY)	PInf	573	Spitz, Henry (NY)	Psyc	325
Sorabella, Philip (NJ)	DR	726	Spitzer, Daniel (NY)	NS	604
Soriano, John (NJ)	Ge	875	Spivack, Barney (CT)	Ger	939
Soroko, Theresa (NJ)	Inf	776	Spivak, Jeffrey M (NY)	OrS	266
Sorra, Toomas (NY)	Ge	433	Spivak, William (NY)	PGe	286
Sosa, R Ernest (NY)	U	367	Splain, Shepard (NY)	OrS	455
Soskel, Neil (NY)	FMed	541	Spotnitz, Alan J (NJ)	TS	850
Sosulski, Richard (NY)	NP	624	Spotnitz, Henry (NY)	TS	359
Soter, Nicholas A (NY)	D	148	Sprecher, Stanley (NY)	DR	485
Soterakis, Jack (NY)	Ge	544	Spriggs, David (NY)	Onc	208
Sotsky, Gerald (NJ)	Cv	722	Squire, Anthony (NY)	Cv	132
Southern, D Loren (NJ)	A&I	901	St Louis, Yolaine (NY)	PEn	571
Souweidane, Mark (NY)	NS	217	Staats, Peter (NJ)	PM	864
Spadaro, Louise A (NY)	Cv	533	Stabile, John (NJ)	Oph	739
Spaide, Richard (NY)	Oph	253	Stabile, Richard (NJ)	RadRO	791
Spak, James I (CT)	OrS	949	Stabinsky, Susan (NY)	Psyc	699
Sparano, Joseph A (NY)	Onc	394	Stacy, Charles B (NY)	N	226
Sparr, Steven (NY)	N	398	Staffenberg, David A (NY)	PlS	410
Spector, Ira (NY)	ObG	561	Stahl, Richard S (CT)	PlS	979
Spector, Scott (CT)	Oph	949	Stahl, Theodore (NJ)	NuM	839
Speiser, Phyllis W (NY)	PEn	497	Stam, Lawrence (NY)	Nep	446
Spencer, Dennis D (CT)	NS	974	Stampfer, Morris (NY)	Cv	381
Spencer, E Kay (NY)	ChAP	136	Stanford, Paulette D (NJ)	AM	767
Spencer, Susan S (CT)	N	974	Stangel, John (NY)	RE	703
Spera, John A (CT)	RadRO	957	Starke, Charles (NY)	IM	670
Sperber, Alan B (NY)	U	367	Starker, Isaac (NJ)	PlS	883
Spergel, Gabriel (NY)	EDM	429	Starker, Paul (NJ)	S	925
Sperling, Neil M (NY)	Oto	456	Starkman, Harold (NJ)	PEn	881
Spero, Marc (NY)	IM	195	Starr, Joanne P (NJ)	TS	794
Speyer, James (NY)	Onc	208	Starr, Michael (NY)	Oph	253

Alphabetical Listing of Doctors

Name	Specialty	Pg	Name	Specialty	Pg
Staskin, David R (NY)	U	367	Stelzer, Paul (NY)	TS	359
Steckel, Joph (NY)	U	595	Stern, Harvey (NY)	DR	384
Steckowych, Jayde (NJ)	Oto	742	Stern, Jack (NY)	NS	675
Steele, Andrew M (NY)	NP	555	Stern, Richard (NY)	Rhu	342
Steele, Mark (NY)	Oph	253	Sternschein, Michael (NJ)	PlS	748
Steer, Robert (NJ)	ObG	879	Stevens, Peter D (NY)	Ge	170
Steiger, David (NY)	Pul	332	Stieg, Philip E (NY)	NS	218
Steigman, Elliott G (NJ)	U	805	Stiller, Robert J (CT)	MF	943
Stein, Adam (NY)	PMR	301	Stillman, Michael (NY)	D	656
Stein, Alan J (NY)	Inf	437	Stock, Jeffrey A (NJ)	U	795
Stein, Alvin (NY)	Onc	553	Stock, Richard (NY)	RadRO	335
Stein, Arnold (NY)	Oph	454	Stolar, Charles JH (NY)	PS	293
Stein, Barry B (NY)	Ped	297	Stoller, Gerald (NY)	Oph	629
Stein, Cy A (NY)	Onc	394	Stone, Alex (NY)	S	354
Stein, David F (NY)	Ge	388	Stone, Gregg W (NY)	IC	198
Stein, Elliott (NJ)	Cv	912	Stone, Michael H (NY)	Psyc	325
Stein, Jeffrey A (NY)	Ge	170	Stone, Peter L (NY)	U	416
Stein, Jeffrey S (NY)	VascS	371	Stone, Richard K (NY)	Ped	298
Stein, Lawrence B (NJ)	Ge	875	Stoopler, Mark (NY)	Onc	208
Stein, Mark (NY)	U	416	Storch, Kenneth J (NJ)	IM	877
Stein, Mitchell (NY)	Oph	682	Storper, Ian (NY)	Oto	276
Stein, Perry (NY)	PMR	463	Stovell, Peter (CT)	OrS	949
Stein, Richard (NY)	IM	195	Stover-Pepe, Diane E (NY)	Pul	332
Stein, Richard A (NY)	Cv	132	Strain, James (NY)	Psyc	325
Stein, Ruth E.K. (NY)	Ped	408	Strair, Roger (NJ)	Hem	833
Stein, Sidney (NY)	IM	196	Strange, Theodore (NY)	IM	512
Stein, Stefan (NY)	Psyc	325	Strashun, Arnold M (NY)	NuM	449
Stein, Stephen A (CT)	S	982	Strassberg, Barbara E (NY)	Ped	408
Steinberg, Charles (NY)	IM	196	Strauch, Robert (NY)	HS	177
Steinberg, Harry (NY)	Pul	584	Straus, David J (NY)	Onc	209
Steinberg, Jonathan S (NY)	CE	123	Strauss, Barry (NY)	Onc	624
Steinberg, L Gary (NY)	PCd	458	Strauss, Bernard (NJ)	U	795
Steinberger, Alfred A (NY)	NS	218	Strauss, Edward (CT)	DR	937
Steinbruck, Richard (NY)	S	521	Strauss, Elton (NY)	OrS	266
Steiner, Henry (NY)	S	474	Strauss, H William (NY)	NuM	230
Steinfeld, Leonard (NY)	PCd	283	Strauss, Michael (NY)	IM	196
Steingart, Richard (NY)	Cv	132	Streisand, Robert (NY)	TS	707
Steinglass, Kenneth (NY)	TS	359	Striker, Paul (NY)	PlS	308
Steinglass, Peter (NY)	Psyc	325	Stringel, Gustavo (NY)	PS	691
Steinhagen, Randolph (NY)	CRS	139	Strobeck, John E (NJ)	Cv	891
Steinherz, Laurel (NY)	PCd	283	Stroh, Jack (NJ)	Cv	902
Steinherz, Peter G (NY)	PHO	288	Strong, Leslie (NY)	S	354

Alphabetical Listing of Doctors

Name	Specialty	Pg	Name	Specialty	Pg
Strongin, Michael J (NY)	ObG	237	Swanson, Scott J (NY)	TS	359
Strongwater, Allan (NY)	OrS	266	Swee, David (NJ)	FMed	831
Strongwater, Richard F (NY)	FMed	661	Sweeney, Eugene (NJ)	D	725
Stubgen, Joerg-Patrick (NY)	N	226	Swerdlow, Michael (NY)	N	398
Stuchin, Steven (NY)	OrS	266	Swidler, Sanford (CT)	Ped	954
Sturm, Richard (NY)	Oph	564	Swiller, Hillel (NY)	Psyc	326
Sturza, Jeffrey (NY)	D	657	Swirsky, Michael (NY)	DR	384
Subramanian, Valavanur (NY)	TS	359	Swistel, Alexander (NY)	S	354
Suchy, Frederick J (NY)	PGe	286	Swistel, Daniel (NY)	TS	359
Suda, Anjuli (NJ)	Ped	882	Syracuse, Donald (NJ)	TS	794
Sudhakar, Telechery (NJ)	Nep	815	Szabo, Andrew John (NY)	EDM	158
Sugarman, Lynn B (NJ)	Ped	747			
Suggs, William D (NY)	VascS	416			
Sukumaran, Muthiah (NY)	Pul	332			
Sulkowicz, Kerry (NY)	Psyc	325	**T**		
Sullivan, Ann Marie (NY)	Psyc	499	Tabachnick, John F (NJ)	FMed	914
Sullivan, Christopher A (NY)	MF	671	Tabaddor, Kamran (NY)	NS	397
Sullivan, James (NY)	Rhu	587	Tabbal, Nicolas (NY)	PlS	308
Sullivan, Timothy B (NY)	Psyc	699	Tabershaw, Richard (NY)	OrS	630
Sullum, Stanford (NY)	ObG	237	Taddonio, Rudolph (NY)	OrS	685
Sultan, Joseph A. (NY)	Psyc	465	Taffet, Berton (NJ)	OrS	880
Sultan, Khalid (NY)	RE	337	Taffet, Sanford (NY)	Ge	664
Sultan, Mark (NY)	PlS	308	Taitsman, James (NJ)	OrS	818
Sultan, Ronald H (NJ)	S	804	Tal, Avraham (NY)	IM	441
Sumpio, Bauer E (CT)	VascS	983	Talansky, Arthur L (NY)	Ge	544
Sunaryo, Francis (NJ)	PGe	786	Talansky, Marvin (NJ)	Oph	862
Sundaram, Revathy (NY)	PHO	459	Tamarin, Steven (NY)	FMed	159
Sung, Kap-jae (NY)	S	501	Tamborlane, William V (CT)	PEn	976
Sunshine, Robert D (NY)	U	595	Tamerin, John (CT)	Psyc	956
Suri, Ranjit (NY)	CE	483	Tan, Mark (NY)	Rhu	639
Surks, Martin (NY)	EDM	385	Tanchajja, Supoj (NY)	S	474
Surow, Jason (NJ)	Oto	742	Tancredi, Laurence R (NY)	Psyc	326
Sussman, Barry (NJ)	S	754	Taneja, Samir S (NY)	U	367
Sussman, John (NY)	Oph	682	Tanenbaum, Diane (NY)	D	148
Sussman, Norman (NY)	Psyc	326	Tannenbaum, Gary (NY)	VascS	709
Sussman, Robert (NJ)	Pul	924	Tanoue, Lynn (CT)	Pul	980
Sussman, Robert B (NY)	Psyc	700	Tanowitz, Herbert B (NY)	Inf	391
Sutton, Ira (NY)	FMed	661	Tarasuk, Albert (NY)	U	503
Suvannavejh, Chaisurat (NY)	ObG	679	Tardiff, Kenneth (NY)	Psyc	326
Svitra, Paul (NY)	Oph	564	Tartaglia, Joseph J (NY)	Cv	651
Swaminathan, A P (NJ)	S	850	Tartell, Jay (NY)	DR	485
Swamy, Samala (NY)	Cv	508	Tartini, Albert (NJ)	Nep	735

Name	Specialty	Pg	Name	Specialty	Pg
Tartter, Paul (NY)	S	354	Thomsen, Stephen (NJ)	Nep	779
Taub, Peter J (NY)	PlS	308	Thomson, J Grant (CT)	HS	970
Taub, Robert (NY)	Onc	209	Thorne, Charles (NY)	PlS	308
Taubin, Howard L (CT)	Ge	938	Thornton, Scott (CT)	CRS	935
Taubman, Lowell (NY)	IM	551	Thornton, Yvonne S (NJ)	MF	835
Taubman, Richard (NY)	ObG	561	Tibaldi, Joseph (NY)	EDM	486
Tavill, Michael A (NJ)	PO	864	Tierney, Peter (NJ)	FMed	831
Tawfik, Bernard (NY)	Oto	568	Tiger, Louis (NY)	Rhu	587
Tay, Steven (NY)	IM	196	Timpone, Leonard (NY)	IM	551
Taylor, Howard (NJ)	Oto	881	Tindel, Nathaniel L (NY)	OrS	402
Taylor, Noel (NY)	Psyc	326	Tinetti, Mary E (CT)	Ger	969
Taylor, William C (NY)	IM	196	Tinger, Alfred (NY)	RadRO	702
Tchorbajian, Kirk (NJ)	Oph	802	Tischler, Henry (NY)	OrS	455
Tchorbajian, Kourkin (NJ)	Oph	919	Tiszenkel, Howard (NY)	CRS	485
Te, Alexis E (NY)	U	367	Tiwari, Ram (NY)	Oph	401
Teffera, Fassil (NY)	IM	393	Tobias, Geoffrey (NJ)	Oto	742
Teicher, Joel (NY)	OrS	455	Tobias, Hillel (NY)	Ge	170
Teichholz, Louis (NJ)	Cv	722	Todd, George (NY)	VascS	372
Teirstein, Alvin (NY)	Pul	332	Tohme, Jack (NJ)	EDM	726
Tejani, Nergesh (NY)	MF	671	Tolchin, Deborah (NY)	Ped	408
Tellis, Vivian (NY)	S	414	Tolchin, Joan G (NY)	Psyc	326
Telzak, Edward E (NY)	Inf	391	Toles, Allen (NY)	ObG	561
Tempera, Patrick (NJ)	Ge	915	Tolston, Evelyn (NY)	A&I	122
Tendler, Michael (NJ)	Ge	859	Tom, Jack (NY)	D	615
Tenenbaum, Joseph (NY)	Cv	132	Tomao, Frank (NY)	Onc	554
Tenet, William (NY)	Cv	484	Tonnesen, Marcia (NY)	D	615
Tenner, Michael (NY)	NRad	677	Toomey, Kathleen C (NJ)	Hem	903
Teperman, Lewis W (NY)	S	355	Topilow, Arthur (NJ)	Hem	860
Tepler, Jeffrey (NY)	Onc	209	Topilow, Harvey (NY)	Oph	253
Tepler, Melvin (NY)	OrS	455	Toppmeyer, Deborah (NJ)	Onc	836
Tepper, Deborah E (CT)	IM	942	Toriello, Edward (NY)	OrS	496
Tepper, Howard (NJ)	PlS	923	Torman, Julie (NY)	Ge	664
Tesauro, William (NY)	ObG	627	Tornos, Carmen (NY)	Path	632
Tesser, Mark (NY)	D	148	Torrado-Jule, Carmen (NY)	PEn	517
Tessler, Sidney (NY)	Pul	468	Torre, Arthur (NJ)	PA&I	785
Testa, N Noel (NY)	OrS	266	Torres-Gluck, Jose (NY)	NS	397
Teusink, J Paul (NY)	Psyc	326	Tortolani, Anthony J (NY)	TS	360
Tewari, Ashutosh (NY)	U	368	Touloukian, Robert (CT)	PS	977
Theofanidis, Stylianos (CT)	NP	945	Tow, Tony (NY)	Pul	638
Thomas, Bryon S (CT)	IM	942	Tozzi, Robert (NJ)	PCd	743
Thomas, Gary (NY)	PM	279	Tracer, Robert (NY)	Ge	433
Thomashow, Byron (NY)	Pul	332	Trachtman, Howard (NY)	PNep	574

Alphabetical Listing of Doctors

Name	Specialty	Pg	Name	Specialty	Pg
Traeger, Eveline (NJ)	ChiN	912	Uhm, Kyudong (NJ)	Onc	893
Trainin, Eugene (NY)	Ped	462	Ulin, Richard (NY)	OrS	267
Traister, Michael (NY)	Ped	298	Ullman, Joel (NY)	ObG	679
Tranbaugh, Robert (NY)	TS	360	Ullman, Thomas A (NY)	Ge	170
Traquina, Diana N (NJ)	PO	844	Underberg-Davis, Sharon (NJ)	DR	830
Traube, Charles (NY)	Cv	425	Unger, Allen (NY)	Cv	133
Travis, William (NY)	Path	280	Unis, George (NY)	OrS	267
Treem, William R (NY)	PGe	458	Unterricht, Sam (NY)	Oph	454
Treiber, Ruth Kaplan (NY)	D	657	Upadhyay, Yogendra (NY)	Psyc	637
Treiser, Susan L (NJ)	RE	906	Urbanek, Richard W (NY)	D	509
Trokel, Stephen (NY)	Oph	253	Urken, Mark (NY)	Oto	276
Troy, Allen (CT)	OrS	950	Ushay, H Michael (NY)	PCCM	404
Troy, Kevin (NY)	Hem	181	Uy, Rodolfo (NY)	Ped	408
Truman, John (NY)	PHO	288	Uy, Vena (NJ)	ObG	802
Tsai, James C (NY)	Oph	253			
Tsin, Daniel (NY)	ObG	494			
Tuchman, Alan (NY)	N	226			
Tugal, Oya (NY)	PHO	690			
Turato, Mariann (NY)	Psyc	700	**V**		
Turbin, Roger E (NJ)	Oph	782			
Turcios, Nelson (NJ)	PPul	844	Vad, Vijay B (NY)	PMR	301
Turecki, Stanley K (NY)	ChAP	136	Vahdat, Linda (NY)	Onc	209
Turetsky, Arthur (CT)	IM	942	Vaillancourt, Philippe D (NY)	PM	632
Turett, Glenn (NY)	Inf	185	Valda, Victor (NJ)	PS	745
Turitto, Gioia (NY)	CE	421	Vallarino, Ramon (NY)	PMR	463
Turk, Jon B (NY)	Oto	276	Vallejo, Alvaro (NY)	RadRO	335
Turner, Ira (NY)	N	558	van Dyck, Christopher H (CT)	GerPsy	969
Turner, James (NY)	S	502	Van Engel, Daniel (NJ)	N	737
Tursi, William (NY)	IM	512	Van Heertum, Ronald L (NY)	NuM	230
Turtel, Andrew (NY)	OrS	267	Van Praagh, Ian (NY)	ObG	237
Turtel, Penny (NJ)	Ge	859	Van Slooten, David (NJ)	N	737
Tutino, Jody (NY)	Ge	433	Vapnek, Jonathan M (NY)	U	368
Tyberg, Theodore (NY)	Cv	133	Vardi, Joseph R (NY)	GO	435
Tydings, Lawrence (NY)	ObG	561	Varriale, Philip (NY)	Cv	133
Tyshkov, Michael (NJ)	PGe	921	Varsos, George (NY)	RadRO	500
			Vas, George A (NY)	N	448
			Vasavada, Balendu (NY)	Cv	425
			Vastola, A Paul (NY)	Oto	456
			Vasudeva, Kusum (NY)	ObG	561
			Vaswani, Ashok N (NY)	EDM	540
U			Vaughan, Edwin D (NY)	U	368
Uday, Kalpana (NY)	Nep	396	Vazzana, Thomas (NY)	Cv	508
Udell, Ira J (NY)	Oph	564	Vecchiotti, Arthur (NY)	Oto	687
Udelsman, Robert (CT)	S	982	Velcek, Francisca (NY)	PS	293

Alphabetical Listing of Doctors

Name	Specialty	Pg
Veloso, Manuel (NY)	ObG	561
Vera, Reinaldo (NY)	ChAP	426
Verga, Michele (NY)	PlS	308
Versfelt, Mary (NY)	Ped	694
Vester, John (NJ)	N	816
Vickery, Carlin (NY)	PlS	308
Videtti, Nicholas F (NJ)	Psyc	749
Vieira, Jeffery (NY)	IM	441
Vigorita, John (NJ)	Ped	922
Vigorita, Vincent J (NY)	Path	457
Villafranca, Manuel (NJ)	Psyc	924
Villamena, Patricia (NY)	Pul	333
Vincent, Miriam (NY)	FMed	431
Vinciguerra, Vincent (NY)	Onc	554
Vine, John (NJ)	D	810
Viner, Nicholas (CT)	U	960
Vingan, Roy D (NJ)	NS	736
Vining, Eugenia (CT)	Oto	976
Vintzileos, Anthony M (NJ)	MF	835
Visco, Ferdinand (NY)	Cv	484
Visconti, Ernest (NY)	Ped	518
Viswanathan, Kusum (NY)	PHO	459
Viswanathan, Ramaswamy (NY)	Psyc	465
Vitale, Gerard (NY)	S	591
Vitenson, Jack (NJ)	U	757
Vitting, Kevin E (NJ)	Nep	893
Vivek, Seeth (NY)	Psyc	499
Vlay, Stephen C (NY)	Cv	612
Vogel, James M (NY)	Onc	209
Vogel, Louis (NY)	D	148
Vogel, Mitchell (NJ)	Oph	894
Vogelman, Arthur (NY)	Ge	488
Vogl, Steven Edward (NY)	Onc	394
Volcovici, Guido (NY)	Pul	333
Volkmar, Fred R (CT)	ChAP	967
Volpe, Anthony Peter (NJ)	IM	732
Volpi, David (NY)	Oto	276
Vukasin, Alexander P (NJ)	U	823

W

Name	Specialty	Pg
Wachtel, Alan (NY)	Psyc	326
Wachtel, Daniel (NJ)	Oph	905
Wadler, Scott (NY)	Onc	209
Wager, Marc (NY)	Ped	694
Wager, Steven (NY)	Psyc	326
Wagle, Sharad (NJ)	Psyc	749
Wagner, Ira J (NY)	CCM	141
Wagner, John (NY)	Nep	556
Wagner, Rudolph (NJ)	Oph	782
Wainstein, Sasha (NY)	U	477
Waintraub, Stanley (NJ)	Onc	734
Walczyk, John (NY)	D	537
Waldbaum, Robert (NY)	U	595
Waldman, Seth (NY)	PM	279
Waldorf, Donald (NY)	D	601
Waldstreicher, Stuart (CT)	Ge	938
Walfish, Jacob (NY)	Ge	170
Walker, Michael J (CT)	TS	959
Wallach, Frances (NY)	Inf	185
Wallach, Robert C (NY)	GO	174
Wallack, Joel J (NY)	Psyc	327
Wallack, Marc (NY)	S	355
Wallerstein, Robert (NJ)	CG	722
Wallis, Joseph J (NJ)	ObG	879
Walser, Lawrence (NY)	Pul	638
Walsh, B Timothy (NY)	Psyc	327
Walsh, Bruce (NY)	S	706
Walsh, Christina (NJ)	Onc	861
Walsh, Christine A (NY)	PCd	404
Walsh, Francis X (CT)	IM	942
Walsh, Joseph (NY)	Oph	254
Walsh, Raymond (NY)	OrS	455
Walsh, William (NY)	OrS	685
Walsky, Robert (NJ)	S	754
Walther, Robert (NY)	D	148
Waner, Milton (NY)	Oto	277
Wang, Frederick (NY)	Oph	254
Wang, Jen Chin (NY)	Hem	547
Wang, John (NY)	Nep	214
Wangenheim, Paul (NJ)	Cv	769

Alphabetical Listing of Doctors

Name	Specialty	Pg	Name	Specialty	Pg
Ward, Barbara (CT)	S	958	Weinberg, Jeffrey (NY)	PMR	518
Ward, Robert (NY)	PO	290	Weinberg, Marc (NY)	Cv	612
Wardlaw, Sharon (NY)	EDM	158	Weinberg, Martin (NJ)	Oph	739
Warner, Robert (NY)	D	149	Weinberger, George I (NJ)	D	913
Warren, Michelle (NY)	RE	338	Weinberger, Jesse (NY)	N	227
Warren, Ronald (NJ)	IM	813	Weinberger, Michael L (NY)	PM	279
Warren, Russell (NY)	OrS	267	Weinberger, Sylvain M (NY)	Ped	298
Wasnick, Robert (NY)	U	643	Weinblatt, Mark (NY)	PHO	573
Wasser, Kenneth (NJ)	Rhu	866	Weine, Gary (NJ)	IM	877
Wasser, Walter (NY)	Nep	214	Weiner, Bernard M (NY)	Nep	396
Wasserman, Eric (CT)	Oph	949	Weiner, Jay (CT)	IM	942
Wasserman, Eugene (NY)	Ped	694	Weiner, Jerome (NY)	Pul	638
Wasserman, Gary D (NJ)	U	757	Weiner, Lon S (NY)	OrS	267
Wasserman, Hal S (CT)	IC	943	Weiner, Michael (NY)	PHO	288
Wasserman, Kenneth (NJ)	IM	732	Weiner, Richard L (NY)	Ped	409
Wasserman, Patricia G (NY)	Path	569	Weinerman, Stuart (NY)	EDM	540
Wasson, Dennis (CT)	S	959	Weingarten, Jacqueline (NY)	PCCM	404
Waters, Cheryl H (NY)	N	226	Weingarten, Phyllis (NY)	Oph	604
Waters, Paul F (NY)	TS	360	Weinreb, Jeffrey C (CT)	DR	968
Watson, Rita (NJ)	Cv	858	Weinstein, Alan S (NY)	D	427
Wax, Michael (NJ)	Onc	917	Weinstein, David B (CT)	ObG	948
Waxberg, Jonathan (CT)	U	960	Weinstein, Jay (NY)	IM	196
Waxenbaum, Steven (NJ)	CRS	723	Weinstein, Joseph (NY)	Oph	565
Waxman, Samuel (NY)	Hem	181	Weinstein, Joshua (NY)	Rhu	413
Waye, Jerome (NY)	Ge	170	Weinstein, Larry (NJ)	PlS	884
Wayne, Peter (NY)	Ge	664	Weinstein, Mark (NY)	IM	551
Weber, Michael (NY)	U	503	Weinstein, Melvin P (NJ)	Inf	834
Weber, Pamela (NY)	Oph	629	Weinstein, Michael A (NY)	CRS	140
Weck, Steven (NY)	DR	538	Weinstein, Paul (CT)	Onc	944
Wedderburn, Raymond (NY)	S	355	Weinstein, Toba (NY)	PGe	572
Weg, Arnold (NY)	Ge	488	Weinstock, Gary (NY)	A&I	528
Weg, Ira (NY)	Cv	533	Weinstock, Judith (NY)	ObG	451
Wegryn, Robert (NJ)	S	925	Weinstock, Murray (NJ)	Cv	722
Wehmann, Robert (NJ)	EDM	726	Weintraub, Gerald (NY)	IM	196
Wei, Fong (NJ)	Nep	815	Weintraub, Joshua L (NY)	VIR	369
Weiden, Peter (NY)	Psyc	465	Weintraub, Michael (NY)	N	677
Weiland, Andrew J (NY)	HS	177	Weintraub, Neil (NY)	VascS	709
Weill, Terry (NY)	Psyc	327	Weisblatt, Steven (NY)	GerPsy	389
Wein, Paul (NY)	Cv	425	Weisbrot, Deborah M (NY)	ChAP	613
Weinberg, Gerard (NY)	PS	406	Weiselberg, Lora (NY)	Onc	554
Weinberg, Harlan (NY)	Pul	702	Weisenseel, Arthur Charles (NY)	Cv	133
Weinberg, Harold (NY)	N	227	Weiser, Robert (NY)	VascS	478

Alphabetical Listing of Doctors

Name	Specialty	Pg	Name	Specialty	Pg
Weisholtz, Steven (NJ)	Inf	731	Wexler, Leonard (NY)	PHO	288
Weiss, Arthur H (NY)	N	227	Wexler, Patricia (NY)	D	149
Weiss, Carol J (NY)	AdP	119	Wey, Philip D (NJ)	PlS	846
Weiss, Daniel I (NY)	Oph	402	Whelan, Charles (NJ)	DR	772
Weiss, E Michael (NJ)	Cv	891	Whelan, Richard L (NY)	CRS	140
Weiss, Gabriella A (NJ)	Inf	892	White, Dorothy (NY)	Pul	333
Weiss, Gerson (NJ)	RE	751	White, Robert I (CT)	VIR	983
Weiss, Karen (NY)	ObG	561	White, Ronald A (NJ)	CRS	723
Weiss, Louis (NY)	Inf	391	Whitley-Williams, Patricia (NJ)	PInf	844
Weiss, Lynne (NJ)	PNep	844	Whitman, Hendricks (NJ)	Rhu	907
Weiss, Melvin (NY)	Cv	652	Whitmore, Wayne (NY)	Oph	254
Weiss, Michael H (NY)	Oto	457	Wickiewicz, Thomas L (NY)	OrS	267
Weiss, Michael J (NY)	Oph	254	Wickremesinghe, Prasanna (NY)	Ge	511
Weiss, Nancy L (NY)	IM	196	Widmann, Mark D (NJ)	TS	885
Weiss, Paul R (NY)	PlS	309	Widmann, Roger F (NY)	OrS	267
Weiss, Rita (NY)	Onc	554	Wiesen, Mark (NJ)	EDM	727
Weiss, Robert A (NY)	Ge	170	Wiesenthal, Carl (NY)	Oto	517
Weiss, Robert A (NY)	PNep	690	Wilbanks, Tyr (NY)	S	415
Weiss, Robert E (NJ)	U	850	Wilbur, Sabrina L (NY)	CE	421
Weiss, Robert M (CT)	U	983	Wilchinsky, Mark (CT)	OrS	950
Weiss, Stanley H (NJ)	PrM	789	Williams, Christine (NY)	Ped	298
Weiss, Steven J (NJ)	A&I	767	Williams, Daniel T (NY)	ChAP	534
Weissman, Gary (NY)	Ge	544	Williams, Edward (NJ)	Cv	912
Weissman, Ronald (NY)	Cv	652	Williams, Gail S (NY)	Nep	214
Weisstuch, Joseph (NY)	Nep	214	Williams, John J (NY)	U	368
Weitzman, Lee (NY)	Cv	533	Williams, Riley J (NY)	OrS	268
Weizman, Howard (NJ)	Nep	735	Willner, Joseph H (NJ)	N	737
Welch, Peter (NY)	IM	670	Willner, Judith P (NY)	CG	138
Wells, Scott B (NY)	PlS	309	Wilner, Philip (NY)	Psyc	327
Welsh, Howard (NY)	Psyc	327	Wilson, Arnold B (NY)	OrS	403
Welshinger, Marie (NY)	GO	489	Wilson, Lynn D (CT)	RadRO	981
Wenig, Bruce M (NY)	Path	281	Wilson, Madeline S (CT)	IM	971
Werres, Roland (NJ)	Cv	769	Wilson, Thomas (NY)	PEn	632
Wert, Sanford (NY)	OrS	456	Winant, John (NJ)	A&I	809
Wertkin, Martin (NY)	S	706	Winawer, Sidney J (NY)	Ge	170
Weseley, Peter E (NY)	Oph	254	Winchester, Patricia (NY)	DR	153
Wesson, Michael (NJ)	RadRO	751	Windsor, Russell (NY)	OrS	268
Westfried, Morris (NY)	D	428	Winick, Martin (NY)	PS	633
Westrich, Geoffrey H (NY)	OrS	267	Winston, Arnold (NY)	Psyc	327
Wetherbee, Roger (NY)	Inf	185	Winston, Jonathan (NY)	Nep	214
Wetzler, Graciela (NY)	PGe	459	Winter, Robin Okner (NJ)	FMed	831
Wexler, Craig B (NY)	EDM	617	Winter, Stephen (CT)	Pul	957

Alphabetical Listing of Doctors

Name	Specialty	Pg	Name	Specialty	Pg
Winter, Steven (NY)	Cv	508	Wright, Albert (NY)	S	474
Winterkorn, Jacqueline (NY)	Oph	254	Wrone, David A (NJ)	D	902
Winters, Richard A (NY)	Psyc	327	Wu, Chia F (NJ)	Cv	769
Winters, Stephen Leslie (NJ)	CE	873	Wu, Ching-hui (NY)	EDM	617
Wisch, Nathaniel (NY)	Hem	181	Wu, Hen-vai (NJ)	Onc	904
Wise, Arthur (NY)	PlS	635	Wu, Jason J (NY)	Ped	463
Wise, Gilbert J (NY)	U	477	Wyner, Perry A (NY)	Pul	584
Wiseman, Paul (NY)	IM	196	Wysolmerski, John J (CT)	EDM	969
Wisnicki, H Jay (NY)	Oph	254			
Wisoff, Jeffrey H (NY)	NS	218			
Witt, Barry R (CT)	RE	958			
Witte, Arnold S (NJ)	N	816			
Wohlberg, Gary (NY)	Pul	638	**Y**		
Woldenberg, David (NY)	Cv	133	Yablon, Steven (NY)	Nep	604
Wolf, Barry (NJ)	Pul	847	Yadoo, Moshe (NY)	Ped	498
Wolf, David C (NY)	Ge	664	Yaffe, Bruce (NY)	IM	197
Wolf, David J (NY)	Onc	209	Yaghoobian, Jahangui (NY)	DR	428
Wolf, Ellen L (NY)	DR	384	Yagoda, Arnold (NY)	Oph	255
Wolf, Kenneth (NY)	Oph	402	Yahalom, Joachim (NY)	RadRO	335
Wolf, Steven M (NY)	ChiN	137	Yalamanchi, Krishan (NJ)	Ped	922
Wolf-Klein, Gisele (NY)	Ger	545	Yale, Suzanne (NY)	ObG	238
Wolfe, Mary J (NY)	IM	670	Yamane, Michael (NJ)	IM	813
Wolfe, Scott W (NY)	HS	177	Yancovitz, Stanley (NY)	Inf	185
Wolff, Steven D (NY)	DR	154	Yang, Chin-tsun (NY)	Pul	584
Wolfson, David (NY)	Ge	433	Yang, Roger (NJ)	DR	902
Wolintz, Arthur H (NY)	Oph	454	Yang, S Steven (NY)	HS	177
Wolk, Michael (NY)	Cv	133	Yankelowitz, Stanley (NY)	Oto	403
Wollack, Jan B (NJ)	ChiN	829	Yannuzzi, Lawrence (NY)	Oph	255
Wolodiger, Fred (NJ)	VascS	758	Yatco, Ruben (NY)	VascS	503
Wolpin, Martin (NY)	OrS	456	Yee, Arthur (CT)	Inf	940
Wong, James R (NJ)	RadRO	884	Yee, Arthur M F (NY)	Rhu	342
Wong, Martha Shih (NY)	Ped	409	Yellin, Joseph (NY)	N	449
Wong, Michael Y (NJ)	Oph	816	Yerys, Paul (NY)	SM	587
Wong, Raymond F (NY)	Oph	254	Yi, Peter (NJ)	Onc	814
Wong, Richard H (NJ)	Oph	817	Yiengpruksawan, Anusak (NJ)	S	755
Wong, W Douglas (NY)	CRS	140	Yip, Chun (NY)	Pul	333
Woo, Peak (NY)	Oto	277	Yonkers, Kimberly A (CT)	Psyc	979
Wood-Smith, Donald (NY)	PlS	309	Yoo, Jinil (NY)	Nep	396
Woolf, Paul (NY)	PCd	688	Youner, Craig (NY)	DR	485
Wormser, Gary (NY)	Inf	666	Young, Bruce (NY)	ObG	238
Worth, David (NJ)	Rhu	924	Young, Constance (NY)	ObG	680
Wozniak, Deborah (NJ)	IM	801	Young, George Pei Herng (NY)	U	368
			Young, Iven (NY)	EDM	158

Name	Specialty	Pg	Name	Specialty	Pg
Young, Melvin (NY)	Cv	534	Zelman, Warren H (NY)	Oto	568
Young, Stuart H. (NY)	A&I	122	Zelson, Joseph (CT)	Ped	978
Younger, Joseph (NY)	Oph	565	Zema, Michael (NY)	Cv	613
Youngerman, Jay (NY)	Oto	568	Zenilman, Michael (NY)	S	474
Younus, Bazaga (NY)	ObG	494	Zerykier, Abraham (NY)	Oph	515
Yudin, Howard (NY)	FMed	661	Zevon, Scott (NY)	PlS	309
Yung, Elizabeth (NY)	NuM	559	Zide, Barry M (NY)	PlS	309
Yurt, Roger (NY)	S	355	Ziedonis, Douglas M (NJ)	AdP	827
			Ziegelbaum, Michael M (NY)	U	595
			Ziemba, David (NY)	IM	441
			Ziering, Thomas (NJ)	FMed	903
# Z			Zimbalist, Eliot (NY)	Ge	433
			Zimberg, Sheldon (NY)	Psyc	327
Zablow, Andrew (NJ)	RadRO	791	Zimmerman, Franklin (Bud) (NY)	Cv	652
Zackson, David A (NY)	IM	197	Zimmerman, Jerald R (NJ)	PMR	747
Zager, Robert (NJ)	Hem	775	Zimmerman, Sol (NY)	Ped	298
Zahtz, Gerald (NY)	Oto	568	Zingale, Robert (NY)	S	641
Zaidman, Gerald (NY)	Oph	683	Zingler, Barry (NJ)	Ge	729
Zairis, Ignatios (NJ)	TS	755	Zinkin, Lewis (NJ)	CRS	829
Zalkowitz, Alan (NJ)	Rhu	752	Zitsman, Jeffrey (NY)	PS	692
Zaloom, Robert (NY)	Cv	425	Zolkind, Neil (NY)	Psyc	700
Zalusky, Ralph (NY)	Hem	181	Zoltan, Irving (NY)	Ped	409
Zambetti, George J (NY)	OrS	268	Zonszein, Joel (NY)	EDM	385
Zampella, Edward J (NJ)	NS	878	Zornitzer, Michael (NJ)	Psyc	790
Zanger, Norman (NJ)	Ped	922	Zubowski, Robert (NJ)	PlS	748
Zanzi, Italo (NY)	NuM	559	Zucker, Ira (NJ)	Ge	729
Zarbin, Marco (NJ)	Oph	782	Zucker, Mark Jay (NJ)	Cv	769
Zaremski, Benjamin (NY)	Cv	133	Zucker, Michael (CT)	IM	943
Zaret, Barry L (CT)	Cv	966	Zuckerman, Howard L (CT)	U	960
Zarich, Stuart (CT)	Cv	935	Zuckerman, Joseph (NY)	OrS	268
Zarowitz, William (NY)	IM	670	Zupnick, Henry (NY)	Pul	584
Zauber, N Peter (NJ)	Hem	775	Zweibel, Lawrence (NY)	Oph	629
Zbar, Lloyd (NJ)	Oto	784	Zweibel, Stuart M (NY)	D	657
Zeale, Peter (NY)	IM	197	Zweifach, Philip (NY)	Oph	255
Zeitels, Jerrold R (NJ)	PlS	923	Zykorie, David (NJ)	Psyc	846
Zeitlin, Alan (NY)	S	502			
Zeldis, Steven M (NY)	Cv	534			
Zelefsky, Melvin (NY)	DR	384			
Zelefsky, Michael J (NY)	RadRO	335			
Zelenetz, Andrew D (NY)	Onc	210			
Zelicof, Steven B (NY)	OrS	685			
Zelkowitz, Richard S (CT)	Onc	944			
Zellner, James H (NY)	Oph	454			

Acknowledgments

The publishers would like to thank the entire staff for their many hours and days of intense and precise work on this Guide in order to further its goal of assisting consumers in making the best healthcare choices.

Castle Connolly Executive Management:

Chairman	John K. Castle
President & CEO	John J. Connolly, Ed.D.
Vice President,	
Chief Medical & Research Officer	Jean Morgan, M.D.
Vice President,	
Chief Strategy & Operations Officer	William Liss-Levinson, Ph.D.

We also would like to extend our gratitude to the American Board of Medical Specialties (ABMS) for allowing us to use excerpts, especially the descriptions of medical specialties and subspecialties, from the text of their publication "Which Medical Specialist for You?"

We wish to thank our research coordinators Maryann Hynd, RN, Monica Joaquin and Lauren Davis, with additional thanks to our layout/editorial staff: Stephenie Galvan, Russell Hodgson and Matt Pretka

Other Publications from Castle Connolly Medical Ltd.:
America's Top Doctors™; Top Doctors: New York Metro Area;
America's Top Doctors for Cancer; Top Doctors: Chicago Metro Area;
America's Cosmetic Doctors and Dentists; Cancer Made Easier: New York—
Metro Area and others...

Order online at http://www.castleconnolly.com/books

Doctor-Patient Advisor

Doctor-Patient Advisor is a Castle Connolly Medical Ltd. service providing one-on-one consultations with a physician or nurse to individuals who have serious or complex medical problems or to anyone who feels he/she needs assistance finding the right physician for any purpose. Each client will receive personalized assistance in identifying the appropriate specialists for his/her condition. The Castle Connolly Medical Ltd. database of physicians and hospitals, as well as individual searches, to locate the best resources to meet the client's needs.

Fee: $275. For further information, call (212) 367-8400 x16.

Strategic Partnerships

Castle Connolly Medical Ltd. has a number of strategic partnerships that may be of interest to consumers and physicians.

Access Medical, LLC

Access Medical, LLC is a diversified healthcare company that has partnered with Castle Connolly to help expand its Top Doctors database. Through its various resources and proprietary technologies, Access and Castle Connolly hope to build upon Castle Connolly's core nomination survey, research and selection process, thereby enabling Castle Connolly to identify 2-3 times more top doctors than it currently does.

BML Medical Records Alert

A secure, private and affordable program to electronically store and retrieve your advance directives and personal healthcare information—24 hours a day, 7 days a week. MedRecords Alert members carry an ID card, wear an ID bracelet with their personal access code, or even have the option to carry their complete medical records and advance directives at all times on a secure pocket-sized USB memory key that utilizes the latest flash-disc technology. Thus, your physician or other healthcare providers can easily retrieve your information. Through Castle Connolly Medical Ltd., members receive a $5.00 discount from the $36.00 annual fee. For more information, visit www.medrecordsalert.com.

Castle Connolly Healthcare Navigation Ltd. (CCHN)
This company offers a comprehensive program for individuals and families to assist them with a range of critical healthcare issues and service needs. CCHN identifies top doctors and hospitals through the resources of Castle Connolly Medical Ltd., provides assistance in resolving problems with medical bills and insurance statements, provides a 24/7 electronic medical record, assists in identifying geriatric care managers, provides research on diseases and medical conditions, and assists in the management and care of illness when abroad through health insurance and medical transport.
For further information, visit www.cchealthcarenavigation.com
or call (203) 333-2244.

Empowered Doctor

Empowered Doctor develops practice websites for physicians, all of whom must first be screened and vetted by Castle Connolly Medical Ltd.'s physician-led Research Department. Websites are designed for new patients to easily find the physician and request an appointment, as well as to serve as a resource for existing patients. Website features include: practice brochures; appointment and prescription refill request forms; patient intake forms; a patient education library; and, a library of the latest news stories related to the physician's medical specialty. For further information, call toll-free (866) 375-4007, or visit www.empowereddoctor.net.

Trio Health, LLC

Trio Health is a healthcare services company which is an innovator in the rapidly growing executive health and wellness space. It provides a range of services—including "Physician Find" and "Access and Disease Research" provided through Castle Connolly—to its clients at specially designed centers that are created in partnership with some of the nation's most outstanding academic medical centers. The first such center, opened in 2006, is the Center for Partnership Medicine, developed and operated in conjunction with Northwestern Memorial Hospital in Chicago. Trio anticipates creating at least a dozen more centers within the next few years. For further information visit www.triohealth.com or call (312) 926-9289.

Work & Family Benefits, Inc.

Work & Family Benefits is the nation's leading provider of "work-life benefits" which are designed to help employees manage their everyday family responsibilities with less stress and effort. WFB specializes in offering highly personalized referrals for employees' dependent care needs, including their children, elders, and family members with disabilities. Employees access WFB's services by calling counselors who have expertise in listening and finding effective solutions when and where help or care is needed. Employees can also use WFB's web site for self-guided access to dependent care solutions, and best-in-class physical and behavioral health articles, videos and information. For further information, visit www.wfbenefits.com or call toll-free (800) 644-2363.

For Reference

Not to be taken from this room

60984 81800

National Physician of the Year Awards

Castle Connolly Medical Ltd. proudly hosted our first annual National Physician of the Year Awards on March 15, 2006 at the elegant Metropolitan Club in Manhattan, New York. It was a spectacular evening which allowed us to recognize both the outstanding honorees and the excellence of the many thousands of physicians throughout the nation.

The Genesis of the National Physician of the Year Award

Each year we receive thousands of nominations from physicians and the medical leadership of major medical centers, specialty hospitals, teaching hospitals and regional and community medical centers across the U.S. as an integral part of our research, screening and selection process to identify *America's Top Doctors*™. The selected physicians, while spread across all 50 states and involved in more than 70 medical specialties and subspecialties, all share one distinguishing professional attribute: an unwavering dedication to their patients and to medicine as a whole. Each and every one of these outstanding medical professionals is a symbol of the clinical excellence that characterizes American medicine. In honor of these exemplary physicians, Castle Connolly Medical Ltd. has created the National Physician of the Year Awards to recognize the thousands of excellent, dedicated physicians across the United States. Our Medical Advisory Board selected the three honorees from the hundreds nominated in a special nomination process conducted months before the event.

Our three honorees, Drs. Barlogie, Bull and Zinner, are shining examples of excellence in clinical medical practice. In addition to these awards, Castle Connolly Medical Ltd. honored Dr. Michael DeBakey for his lifetime achievement in the medical community. His career in cardiovascular surgery has spanned more than seven decades and he has contributed countless revolutionary procedures and instruments to the specialty, making him the ideal honoree for the Lifetime Achievement Award. Princess Yasmin Aga Khan, a tireless fundraiser for the Alzheimer Association, was an exemplary recipient of our first National Health Leadership Award. Her fundraising efforts have helped extend the Alzheimer Association's many programs and services, reaching millions of people devastated by this disease, providing both education and hope. Neither the medical community nor the public would ever have reaped the benefits of years of research and medical breakthroughs if not for the gallant and tireless efforts of individuals such as Dr. Michael DeBakey and Princess Yasmin Aga Khan.

Each honoree received Imagination, a beautiful and distinctive porcelain figurine from the world renowned Lladro. Portraying an angel with soaring wings, this statue represents the hope and comfort all five honorees have brought to the world through their devotion to their patients and their profession.

National Physician of the Year Awards 2006 Honorees

For Clinical Excellence

Bart Barlogie, M.D., Ph.D.
Director, Myeloma Institute for Research Therapy,
University of Arkansas for Medical Sciences

Marilyn J. Bull, M.D.
Morris Green Professor of Pediatrics,
Riley Hospital for Children

Michael J. Zinner, M.D.
Moseley Professor of Surgery,
Harvard Medical School,
Surgeon-in-Chief,
Brigham & Women's Hospital

For Lifetime Achievement

Michael E. DeBakey, M.D.
Chancellor Emeritus
Baylor College of Medicine

For National Health Leadership

Princess Yasmin Aga Khan
President, Alzheimer's Disease International